ELIZABETH R. McANARNEY, M.D.
Professor of Pediatrics and Associate Chair
(Academic Affairs)
Chief, Division of Adolescent Medicine
University of Rochester Medical Center
Rochester, New York

RICHARD E. KREIPE, M.D.
Associate Professor of Pediatrics
Director, Adolescent Services
University of Rochester Medical Center
Rochester, New York

DONALD P. ORR, M.D.
Professor of Pediatrics
Director, Section of Adolescent Medicine
Indiana University Medical Center
Indianapolis, Indiana

GEORGE D. COMERCI, M.D.
Medical Director
Pediatric and Adolescent Medicine
Desert Hills Center for Youth and Families
Tucson, Arizona

TEXTBOOK of ADOLESCENT MEDICINE

W. B. SAUNDERS COMPANY
A Division of Harcourt Brace & Company
Philadelphia London Toronto Montreal Sydney Tokyo

W.B. SAUNDERS COMPANY
A Division of
Harcourt Brace & Company

The Curtis Center
Independence Square West
Philadelphia, Pennsylvania 19106

Library of Congress Cataloging-in-Publication Data

Textbook of adolescent medicine / Elizabeth R. McAnarney . . . [et al.].

p. cm.

ISBN 0–7216–3077–4

1. Adolescent medicine.   I. McAnarney, Elizabeth R.

[DNLM: 1. Adolescent Medicine. WS 460 T355]

RJ550.T49 1992

616′.00835—dc20

DNLM/DLC   91-46868

Editor: Lisette Bralow
Developmental Editor: Kathleen McCarthy
Designer: Bill Donnelly
Cover Designer: B. J. Crim
Production Manager: Bill Preston
Manuscript Editors: Arlene Friday, Jodi von Hagen, and Louise Robinson
Illustration Specialist: Walt Verbitski
Indexer: Julie Figures

TEXTBOOK OF ADOLESCENT MEDICINE   ISBN 0–7216–3077–4

Printed in the United States of America

Last digit is the print number: 9   8   7   6   5   4   3   2

To the Young People of the World,
Who Are the Future

Consulting Editors

Contributors

STEVEN M. ADAIR, D.D.S., M.S.
Associate Professor and Chairman, Department of Pediatric Dentistry, School of Dentistry, Medical College of Georgia; Active Staff, Medical College of Georgia Hospital and Clinics; Consultant, University Hospital, Augusta, Georgia
Oral Conditions

MARK C. ADAMS, M.D.
Assistant Professor of Urology, Indiana University School of Medicine; Attending Pediatric Urologist, James Whitcomb Riley Hospital for Children, Indiana University Hospital, Wishard Memorial Hospital, Indiana University Medical Center, Indianapolis, Indiana
Urologic Conditions

HOOVER ADGER, JR., M.D., M.P.H.
Assistant Professor of Pediatrics, Johns Hopkins University School of Medicine; Johns Hopkins Hospital, Baltimore, Maryland
Prevention of Alcohol and Other Drug Use

MARGARET ALTEMUS, M.D.
Clinical Neuroendocrinology Branch, National Institute of Mental Health, Bethesda, Maryland
Neurotransmitters, Stress, and Depression

CORRIE T.M. ANDERSON, M.D.
Assistant Clinical Professor of Anesthesiology, and Assistant Clinical Professor of Pediatrics, University of California, Los Angeles; Chief, Division of Pediatric Anesthesiology, Co-Director of the UCLA Pediatric Pain Service, Los Angeles, California
Pain in Adolescence

TRINA M. ANGLIN, M.D., PH.D.
Associate Professor of Pediatrics, and Director, Center for Adolescent Health, Case Western Reserve University School of Medicine; Head, Division of Adolescent Medicine, Department of Pediatrics, MetroHealth Medical Center, Cleveland, Ohio
Nontraditional Settings

BRUNO J. ANTHONY, PH.D.
Assistant Professor, Department of Psychiatry, University of Maryland School of Medicine; Chief Psychologist, Child Psychiatry Inpatient Service, University of Maryland Medical System, Baltimore, Maryland
Attention Deficit Hyperactivity Disorder

MARTHA R. ARDEN, M.D.
Assistant Professor of Pediatrics, Albert Einstein College of Medicine, Bronx, New York; Division of Adolescent Medicine, Schneider Children's Hospital of Long Island Jewish Medical Center, New Hyde Park, New York
Nutritional Conditions: Obesity

JAMES F. BALE, JR., M.D.
Professor, Division of Pediatric Neurology, Departments of Pediatrics and Neurology, University of Iowa College of Medicine, Iowa City, Iowa
Inflammatory Conditions Affecting the Central and Peripheral Nervous Systems

ROBERTA K. BEACH, M.D., M.P.H.
Associate Professor of Pediatrics, University of Colorado School of Medicine; Director of Adolescent Ambulatory Services, Denver Department of Health and Hospitals, Denver, Colorado
Breast Disorders

DAVID C. BECK, M.D.
Assistant Clinical Professor of Psychiatry, UCLA School of Medicine; Director, Pediatric Consultation Liaison Program, UCLA Center for Health Sciences, Los Angeles, California
Liaison and Consultation

D. WOODROW BENSON, JR., M.D., PH.D.
Professor of Pediatrics, Northwestern University; Chief, Division of Cardiology, Children's Memorial Hospital, Chicago, Illinois
Disturbances of Cardiac Conduction and Rhythm

JERRY MICHAEL BERGSTEIN, M.D.
Professor and Head, Section of Nephrology, Department of Pediatrics, Indiana University School of Medicine; Director, Section of Nephrology, James Whitcomb Riley Hospital for Children, Indianapolis, Indiana
Renal Conditions

ROBERT J. BIDWELL, M.D.
Assistant Professor of Pediatrics, and Director of Adolescent Medicine, John A. Burns School of Medicine, University of Hawaii; Director of Adolescent Medicine, Kapiolani Medical Center for Women and Children, Honolulu, Hawaii
Gay and Lesbian Youth

FRANK M. BIRO, M.D.
Assistant Professor of Pediatrics and Medicine, University of Cincinnati; Associate Director, Division of Adolescent Medicine, Children's Hospital Medical Center, Cincinnati, Ohio
Disorders of Eyes, Ears, Nose, and Mouth; Reproductive Care in the Office: Screening Methods

BRUCE BLACK, M.D.
Adjunct Assistant Professor, Department of Psychiatry, Division of Child and Adolescent Psychiatry, University of Maryland School of Medicine, Baltimore, Maryland; Senior Staff Fellow and Director, Anxiety Disorders Outpatient Program, Biological Psychiatry Branch, Intramural Research Program, National Institute of Mental Health, Bethesda, Maryland
Neurotransmitters, Stress, and Depression; Obsessive-Compulsive Disorder

HEATHER MUNROE BLUM, PH.D.
Professor and Dean, Faculty of Social Work, University of Toronto, Toronto, Ontario, Canada
Schizophrenia

ROBERT WILLIAM BLUM, M.D., M.P.H., PH.D.
Professor and Director, Division of General Pediatrics and Adolescent Health, Department of Pediatrics, University of Minnesota, Minneapolis, Minnesota; University of Minnesota Hospitals, Minneapolis Children's Medical Center, Minneapolis, Minnesota; Gillette Children's Hospital, Children's Hospital, St. Paul, Minnesota
International Profile; Chronically Ill Youth

ANNE M. BOWEN, PH.D.
Assistant Professor of Psychology, Northern Arizona University, Flagstaff, Arizona
Behavior Therapy

LAURENCE A. BOXER, M.D.
Professor, and Director, Pediatric Hematology/Oncology, University of Michigan Medical School; Director, Pediatric Hematology/Oncology, C. S. Mott Children's Hospital, Ann Arbor, Michigan
Hematologic Disorders: Disorders of the Polymorphonuclear Leukocyte

CLAIRE D. BRINDIS, DR.P.H.
Assistant Adjunct Professor of Pediatrics, Division of Adolescent Medicine, Department of Pediatrics, School of Medicine, and Co-Director, Center for Reproductive Health Policy Research, Institute for Health Policy Studies, University of California, San Francisco, San Francisco, California
United States Profile

RICHARD R. BROOKMAN, M.D.
Professor of Pediatrics, Medical College of Virginia Commonwealth University; Director of Adolescent Health Services, Medical College of Virginia Hospitals, Richmond, Virginia
Appendices: Reference Data for Physical Assessment of Adolescents

MARILYN R. BROWN, M.D.
Associate Professor of Pediatrics, University of Rochester Medical Center; Pediatric Gastroenterologist, and Medical Director, Nutrition Support Service, Strong Memorial Hospital, Rochester, New York
Chronic Constipation

RICHARD C. BROWN, M.D.
Clinical Professor, Department of Pediatrics, University of California, San Francisco; Director, Children's Health Center, San Francisco General Hospital, San Francisco, California
Incarcerated Youth

DEDRA BUCHWALD, M.D.
Assistant Professor of Medicine, University of Washington School of Medicine; Director, Chronic Fatigue Clinic, Harborview Medical Center, Seattle, Washington
Viral Infections: Chronic Fatigue

NANCY J. BUNIN, M.D.
Assistant Professor of Pediatrics, University of Pennsylvania School of Medicine;

Children's Hospital of Philadelphia, Philadelphia, Pennsylvania
Oncologic Disorders: Non-Hodgkin Lymphomas

DOUGLAS W. BUNNELL, PH.D.
Assistant Professor of Pediatrics, Albert Einstein College of Medicine, Bronx, New York; Voluntary Psychologist, Lenox Hill Hospital, New York, New York; Attending Psychologist, Craig House Hospital, Beacon, New York
Nutritional Conditions: Bulimia Nervosa

THOMAS CAMPBELL, M.D.
Associate Professor of Family Medicine and Psychiatry, University of Rochester Medical Center; Staff, Highland Hospital, Rochester, New York
Family-oriented Care

DENNIS P. CANTWELL, M.D.
Joseph Campbell Professor of Child Psychiatry, UCLA School of Medicine, Los Angeles, California
Psychotropic Drug Treatment

MARY T. CASERTA, M.D.
Senior Instructor in Pediatrics and Infectious Diseases, University of Rochester Medical Center; Assistant Attending Pediatrician, Strong Memorial Hospital, Rochester, New York
Bacterial Infections: Haemophilus influenzae *Infections*

EDWARD B. CLARK, M.D.
Professor of Pediatrics, and Chief of Division of Pediatric Cardiology, University of Rochester Medical Center; Strong Memorial Hospital, Rochester, New York
Overview of Cardiovascular Evaluation; High Blood Pressure in Adolescents

C. ROBERT CLONINGER, M.D.
Professor in Psychiatry and Genetics, and Head, Department of Psychiatry, Washington University School of Medicine; Psychiatrist-in-Chief, Barnes and Allied Hospitals, St. Louis Children's Hospital; Jewish Hospital, Malcolm Bliss Mental Health Center, St. Louis, Missouri
Personality Development and Structure; Personality Disorders

PINCHAS COHEN, M.D.
Fellow in Pediatric Endocrinology, Stanford University School of Medicine; Pediatric Endocrine Fellow, Stanford University Medical Center, Stanford, California
Disorders of Growth

JAMES J. CORRIGAN, JR., M.D.
Professor of Pediatrics, Section of Pediatric Hematology/Oncology, and Vice Dean, Tulane University School of Medicine; Tulane University Medical Center Hospital and Clinics, Charity Hospital, New Orleans, Louisiana
Hematologic Disorders: Disorders of Hemostasis

MARJORIE CRAGO, PH.D.
Research Specialist, Department of Family and Community Medicine, College of Medicine, University of Arizona, Tucson, Arizona
Cigarette Smoking

LAWRENCE J. D'ANGELO, M.D., M.P.H.
Professor of Pediatrics, Medicine, and Health Care Sciences, The George Washington University School of Medicine and Health Sciences; Chairman, Department of Adolescent and Young Adult Medicine, Children's National Medical Center, Washington, D.C.
Interdisciplinary Teams

SHERMINE DARBAUGH, M.D.
Associate Professor of Pediatrics, Wayne State University School of Medicine; Department of Nephrology, Children's Hospital of Michigan, Detroit, Michigan
Hypertension

FREDRIC DAUM, M.D.
Professor of Pediatrics, Cornell University Medical College, New York, New York; Co-Chief, Division of Pediatric Gastroenterology, North Shore University Hospital, Manhasset, New York
Inflammatory Bowel Disease

ROBERT W. DEISHER, M.D.
Professor Emeritus of Pediatrics, University of Washington School of Medicine; Staff, Children's Hospital and Medical Center, University of Washington Medical Center, Seattle, Washington
Gay and Lesbian Youth

CYNTHIA A. DeLAAT, M.D.
Assistant Professor of Pediatrics, University of Cincinnati College of Medicine; Assistant Professor of Pediatrics, Children's Hospital Medical Center, Cincinnati, Ohio
Oncologic Disorders: Acute and Chronic Leukemias

EFSTRATIOS DEMETRIOU, M.D., M.P.H.
Clinical Assistant Professor of Pediatrics, Boston University School of Medicine, Boston, Massachusetts; Director of Adolescent Services, North Shore Children's Hospital, Salem, Massachusetts
Male Reproductive Conditions

G. PAUL DeROSA, M.D.
Professor and Chairman, Department of Orthopaedic Surgery, Indiana University School of Medicine, Indianapolis, Indiana
Orthopedic Conditions

REGGIE E. DUERST, M.D.
Assistant Professor of Pediatrics, Division of Pediatric Hematology/Oncology, University of Rochester Medical Center, Rochester, New York
Bone Marrow Failure and Transplantation

BURRIS DUNCAN, M.D.
Professor of Pediatrics, Department of Pediatrics, University of Arizona College of Medicine, Tucson, Arizona
Giardia lamblia *Infections*

ROBERT H. DuRANT, PH.D.
Assistant Professor of Pediatrics, Medical College of Georgia School of Medicine, Augusta, Georgia
Compliance

ANKE A. EHRHARDT, PH.D.
Professor of Clinical Psychology, Department of Psychiatry, Columbia University College of Physicians and Surgeons; Director, HIV Center for Clinical and Behavioral Studies, New York State Psychiatric Institute; Pediatric Behavioral Endocrinologist in Psychiatry Service, Presbyterian Hospital, New York, New York
Sexual Orientation

HOWARD EIGEN, M.D.
Professor of Pediatrics, Indiana University; Director of Pediatric Pulmonology and Intensive Care, James Whitcomb Riley Hospital for Children, Indianapolis, Indiana
Maturation of the Respiratory System at Puberty and Related Respiratory System Considerations

ARTHUR B. ELSTER, M.D.
Director, Adolescent Health, American Medical Association, Chicago, Illinois
Health Promotion

ABIGAIL ENGLISH, J.D.
Director, Adolescent Health Care Project, National Center for Youth Law, San Francisco, California
Legal Aspects of Care

GIUSEPPE ERBA, M.D.
Professor of Neurology and Pediatrics, University of Rochester Medical Center; Director of Comprehensive Epilepsy Program, Strong Memorial Hospital, Rochester, New York
Epilepsy and Seizure Disorders

DEBRA FANURIK, PH.D.
Assistant Professor of Research, and Psychologist, Pediatric Pain Program, Division of Neurology, Department of Pediatrics, UCLA School of Medicine, Los Angeles, California
Pain in Adolescence

MARIANNE E. FELICE, M.D.
Professor of Pediatrics, Vice Chair, Department of Pediatrics, and Director, Division of Adolescent Medicine, University of Maryland School of Medicine; University of Maryland Medical System, Baltimore, Maryland
Cross-Cultural Youth

JONATHAN L. FINLAY, M.B., CH.B.
Associate Professor of Pediatrics, Cornell University Medical College; Associate Attending and Vice Chairman, Department of Pediatrics, Memorial Sloan-Kettering Cancer Center, New York, New York
Oncologic Disorders: Brain Tumors

SAMUEL S. FLINT, PH.D.
Director, Department of Child Health Care Finance and Organization, American Academy of Pediatrics, Elk Grove, Illinois; Lecturer, Department of Pediatrics, University of Chicago, Chicago, Illinois
Financing of Adolescent Care

GILBERT B. FORBES, M.D.
Professor of Pediatrics and Biophysics, University of Rochester Medical Center; Pediatrician, Strong Memorial Hospital, Consultant, Rochester General Hospital, Genesee Hospital, Rochester, New York
Nutrition and Growth

GREGORY K. FRITZ, M.D.
Professor of Psychiatry and Human Behavior, Brown University; Director of Child and Family Psychiatry, Rhode Island Hospital, Providence, Rhode Island
Chronic Illness and Psychological Health

VINCENT A. FULGINITI, M.D.
Dean and Professor of Pediatrics, Tulane University School of Medicine, Tulane

Medical Center, Charity Hospital at New Orleans, New Orleans, Louisiana
Infectious Conditions: Developmental Overview

RICHARD GALLAGHER, Ph.D.
Assistant Professor of Psychiatry, Albert Einstein College of Medicine, Bronx, New York; Senior Staff Psychologist, Coordinator of Cognitive Behavior Therapy Program, Division of Child and Adolescent Psychiatry, Long Island Jewish Medical Center, New Hyde Park, New York
School-related Anxiety and Related Conditions

JAMES G. GARRICK, M.D.
Director, Center for Sports Medicine, Saint Francis Memorial Hospital, San Francisco, California
Sports Injuries and the Osteochondroses

GAYLE GEBER, M.P.H.
Community Health Specialist, Hennepin County Community Health Department, Minneapolis, Minnesota
Chronically Ill Youth

BRADLEY A. GEORGE, M.D.
Associate in Pediatric Hematology-Oncology, Geisinger Medical Center, Danville, Pennsylvania
Oncologic Disorders: Acute and Chronic Leukemias

BERTIL E. GLADER, Ph.D., M.D.
Professor of Pediatrics, Division of Hematology-Oncology, Stanford University School of Medicine; Chief, Hematology/Oncology Service, Lucile Packard Children's Hospital at Stanford, Stanford, California
Hematologic Disorders: Disorders of the Erythrocyte

PHILIP W. GOLD, M.D.
Clinical Neuroendocrinology Branch, National Institute of Mental Health, Bethesda, Maryland
Neurotransmitters, Stress, and Depression

MICHAEL P. GOLDEN, M.D.
Resident in Psychiatry, University of Washington, Seattle, Washington
Diabetes Mellitus

ANDREW D. GOODMAN, M.D.
Assistant Professor and Director, Neuroimmunology Unit, Department of Neurology, University of Rochester Medical Center; Attending Neurologist, Strong Memorial Hospital, Rochester, New York
Multiple Sclerosis

JOANNE GOODWIN, M.Sc.
Doctoral Student, Clinical Psychology, Dalhousie University, Halifax, Nova Scotia, Canada
Psychogenic Pain Conditions

ESTHERANN GRACE, M.D.
Assistant Clinical Professor of Pediatrics, Harvard Medical School; Associate in Medicine, Children's Hospital, Boston, Massachusetts
Normal Sexuality

DEBORAH L. GRAY, R.N., M.S.N., C.D.E.
Adjunct Clinical Instructor, Indiana University School of Nursing; Clinical Nurse Specialist, James Whitcomb Riley Hospital for Children, Indianapolis, Indiana
Diabetes Mellitus

DONALD E. GREYDANUS, M.D.
Professor of Pediatrics and Human Development, Michigan State University College of Human Medicine, East Lansing, Michigan; Pediatrics Program Director, Michigan State University/Kalamazoo Center for Medical Studies, Kalamazoo, Michigan
Contraception

ALAN B. GRUSKIN, M.D.
Professor and Chairman, Department of Pediatrics, Wayne State University School of Medicine; Pediatrician in Chief, Children's Hospital of Michigan, Detroit, Michigan
Hypertension

CAROLINE BREESE HALL, M.D.
Professor of Pediatrics and Medicine, University of Rochester Medical Center; Strong Memorial Hospital, Rochester, New York
Viral Infections: Influenza Infections

DANA S. HARDIN, M.D.
Fellow, Department of Pediatric Endocrinology, and Fellow, Department of Endocrinology and Metabolism, Indiana University School of Medicine; Indiana University Hospitals, Indianapolis, Indiana
Precocious Puberty

J. PETER HARRIS, M.D.
Associate Professor of Pediatrics, and Director, Clinical Pediatric Cardiology, University of Rochester Medical Center, Rochester, New York
Cardiovascular Aspects of Systemic Disease

FELIX P. HEALD, M.D.
Professor of Pediatrics, University of Maryland School of Medicine, Baltimore, Maryland
The History of Adolescent Medicine

KAREN HEIN, M.D.
Professor of Pediatrics, Albert Einstein College of Medicine; Director, Adolescent AIDS Program, Montefiore Medical Center, Bronx, New York
Acquired Immunodeficiency Syndrome and Human Immunodeficiency Virus–Related Syndromes

ALBERT C. HERGENROEDER, M.D.
Associate Professor of Clinical Pediatrics, Baylor College of Medicine; Chief, Adolescent Medicine, and Director, Sports Medicine Clinic, Texas Children's Hospital, Houston, Texas
Management of Common Sports Injuries

ROBERTA A. HIBBARD, M.D.
Associate Professor of Pediatrics, Indiana University School of Medicine; Attending Physician, Indiana University Hospitals, and Wishard Memorial Hospital, Indianapolis, Indiana
Sexual Abuse

ROGER HICKS, B.A.
Assistant Research Scientist, New York State Psychiatric Institute, New York, New York
Suicide and Suicidal Behaviors

J. D. HIGLEY, PH.D.
Senior Staff Fellow, Laboratory of Clinical Sciences, National Institute on Alcohol Abuse and Alcoholism, Bethesda, Maryland
Primate Models of Behavioral and Physiologic Change in Adolescence

CHRISTOPHER H. HODGMAN, M.D.
Professor of Psychiatry and Pediatrics, and Director, Division of Child and Adolescent Psychiatry, University of Rochester Medical Center, Rochester, New York
Interviewing; Approaching the Adolescent with Psychological Symptoms; Pearls from Clinical Practice

ADELE D. HOFMANN, M.D.
Professor of Pediatrics, University of California, Irvine, California College of Medicine; Director, Adolescent Medicine, Department of Pediatrics, University of California, Irvine, Medical Center, Irvine, California
Adoption

JOHN J. HUTTER, M.D.
Associate Professor of Pediatrics, University of Arizona College of Medicine; Chief, Section of Pediatric Hematology/Oncology, University of Arizona Medical Center, Tucson, Arizona
Oncologic Disorders: Overview

CRAIG L. HYSER, M.D.
St. Paul, Minnesota
Neurologic Conditions: Biochemical and Molecular Markers

WALTER K. IMAI, M.D.
Clinical Assistant Professor of Pediatrics, Texas Tech School of Medicine, Lubbock, Texas; Chief, Adolescent Medicine Service, Tripler Army Medical Center, Honolulu, Hawaii
Youth in the Military

GARY M. INGERSOLL, PH.D.
Professor of Counseling and Educational Psychology, Indiana University, Bloomington, Indiana
Psychological and Social Development

CHARLES E. IRWIN, JR., M.D.
Professor of Pediatrics, and Director, Division of Adolescent Medicine, Department of Pediatrics, School of Medicine, University of California, San Francisco, San Francisco, California
United States Profile

MARY SUE JACK, PH.D., R.N.
Assistant Professor, University of Rochester School of Nursing, Rochester, New York
Interviewing

MARC S. JACOBSON, M.D.
Associate Professor of Pediatrics, Albert Einstein College of Medicine, Bronx, New York; Director, Center for Atherosclerosis Prevention, Schneider Children's Hospital of Long Island Jewish Medical Center, New Hyde Park, New York
Nutritional Conditions: Hyperlipidemia

HILLEL K. JANAI, M.D.
Clinical Assistant Professor, Department of Pediatric Infectious Diseases, Ohio State University College of Medicine, Columbus, Ohio; Pediatrics and Pediatric Infectious Diseases, Hocking Valley Community Hospital, Logan, Ohio; and Columbus Children's Hospital, Columbus, Ohio
Bacterial Infections: Rickettsia rickettsii (Rocky Mountain Spotted Fever)

M. SUSAN JAY, M.D.
Professor, Department of Pediatrics, Loyola University, Stritch School of Medicine, Maywood, Illinois
Compliance

RENÉE R. JENKINS, M.D.
Associate Professor, Department of Pediatrics and Child Health, Howard University College of Medicine; Director of Adolescent Medicine, Howard University Hospital, Washington, D.C.
Nontraditional Settings; Cross-Cultural Youth

JAMES F. JONES, M.D.
Professor of Pediatrics, University of Colorado School of Medicine; Staff Physician, Department of Pediatrics, National Jewish Center for Immunology and Respiratory Medicine, and Children's Hospital, Denver, Colorado
Viral Infections: Epstein-Barr Virus Infections

NEIL KALTER, PH.D.
Professor, Departments of Psychology and Psychiatry, University of Michigan; Director, University of Michigan Center for the Child and the Family, Ann Arbor, Michigan
Divorce

MAUREEN A. KAYS, M.D.
Fellow, Pediatric Infectious Disease, Columbia University College of Physicians and Surgeons; Babies Hospital, New York, New York
Bacterial Infections: Bordetella pertussis Infection and Pertussis Syndromes

MICHAEL A. KEATING, M.D.
Assistant Professor of Urology, Indiana University School of Medicine; Attending Pediatric Urologist, James Whitcomb Riley Hospital for Children, Indiana University Hospital, Wishard Memorial Hospital, Indiana University Medical Center, Indianapolis, Indiana
Urologic Conditions

MICHELE D. KIPKE, PH.D.
Assistant Professor of Pediatrics, University of Southern California School of Medicine; Director, Substance Abuse Program, Division of Adolescent Medicine, Children's Hospital of Los Angeles, Los Angeles, California
Acquired Immunodeficiency Syndrome and Human Immunodeficiency Virus–Related Syndromes

HAROLD S. KOPLEWICZ, M.D.
Assistant Clinical Professor of Psychiatry, Columbia University College of Physicians and Surgeons, New York, New York; Chief, Division of Child and Adolescent Psychology, Long Island Jewish Medical Center, New Hyde Park, New York
School-related Anxiety and Related Conditions

HOWARD E. KULIN, M.D.
Professor of Pediatrics, and Chief, Division of Pediatric Endocrinology, Pennsylvania State University College of Medicine; University Hospital, M. S. Hershey Medical Center, Hershey, Pennsylvania
Neuroendocrine Regulation of Puberty; Delayed Pubertal Development

BEATRICE C. LAMPKIN, M.D.
Professor of Pediatrics, University of Cincinnati College of Medicine; Professor of Pediatrics, Children's Hospital Medical Center, Cincinnati, Ohio
Oncologic Disorders: Acute and Chronic Leukemias

JUDITH LANDAU-STANTON, M.B., CH.B.
Associate Professor of Psychiatry and Family Medicine, University of Rochester School of Medicine and Dentistry, Rochester, New York
Family Therapy

ALFRED T. LANE, M.D.
Associate Professor of Dermatology and Pediatrics, Stanford University; Lucile Salter Packard Children's Hospital at Stanford University, Stanford, California
Skin Disorders

JANE LAVELLE, M.D.
Assistant Professor of Pediatrics, University of Pennsylvania School of Medicine; Attending Physician, Emergency Department and Adolescent Clinic, Children's Hospital of Philadelphia, Philadelphia, Pennsylvania
Adolescent Emergency Conditions

RICHARD J. LAWLOR, J.D., Ph.D
Assistant Professor of Clinical Psychology, Department of Psychiatry, Indiana University School of Medicine; Indiana University Hospitals, Indianapolis, Indiana
Psychological Assessment of Adolescents

MICHAEL D. LEBOWITZ, Ph.D.
Professor of Internal Medicine, and Associate Director, Respiratory Sciences Center, University of Arizona College of Medicine, Tucson, Arizona
Environmental Conditions, Cigarette Smoking, and Occupational Conditions

RICHARD J. LEMEN, M.D.
Professor, Department of Pediatrics, University of Arizona, Steele Memorial Children's Research Center; University of Arizona Medical Center, Tucson Medical Center, Tucson, Arizona
Lung Diseases

DOROTHY OTNOW LEWIS, M.D.
Professor of Psychiatry, New York University School of Medicine, New York, New York; Clinical Professor, Yale University Child Study Center, New Haven, Connecticut; Attending Physician, NYU–Bellevue Medical Center, New York, New York
Disorders of Conduct and Delinquency

RICHARD LIVINGSTON, M.D.
Wohdan Associate Professor of Psychiatry and Pediatrics, University of Arkansas for Medical Sciences; Psychiatrist-in-Chief, Arkansas Children's Hospital; Staff Psychiatrist, University Hospital of Arkansas; Consulting Psychiatrist, Youth Home, Inc., and Rivendell of America, Little Rock, Arkansas
Somatization, Conversion, and Related Disorders

STEPHEN LUDWIG, M.D.
Professor of Pediatrics, University of Pennsylvania School of Medicine; Division Chief, General Pediatrics, Children's Hospital of Philadelphia, Philadelphia, Pennsylvania
Adolescent Emergency Conditions

RICHARD G. MacKENZIE, M.D.
Associate Professor of Pediatrics, University of Southern California School of Medicine; Director, Division of Adolescent Medicine, Children's Hospital of Los Angeles, Los Angeles, California
At-Risk Youth

M. JOAN MANSFIELD, M.D.
Instructor in Pediatrics, Harvard Medical School; Assistant in Medicine, Division of Adolescent and Young Adult Medicine, Division of Endocrinology, Children's Hospital, Boston, Massachusetts
Menstrual Conditions: Normal Female Reproductive Development and Amenorrhea

JAMES F. MARKOWITZ, M.D.
Associate Professor, Cornell University Medical College, New York, New York; Associate Chief, Division of Pediatric Gastroenterology, North Shore University Hospital, Manhasset, New York
Acid Peptic Disease; Inflammatory Bowel Disease

ANDREA MARKS, M.D.
Clinical Associate Professor of Pediatrics, Cornell University Medical College; Associate Attending Pediatrician, The New York Hospital, New York, New York
Well Adolescent Care

MELVIN I. MARKS, M.D.
Professor and Vice Chair, Department of Pediatrics, University of California, Irvine, California College of Medicine, Irvine, California; Medical Director, Memorial Miller Children's Hospital, Long Beach, California
Bacterial Infections: Rickettsia rickettsii (Rocky Moutain Spotted Fever)

SUSAN H. McDANIEL, Ph.D.
Associate Professor of Psychiatry and Family Medicine, University of Rochester Medical Center, Rochester, New York
Family-oriented Care; Family Therapy

PATRICK J. McGRATH, Ph.D.
Professor of Psychology, Pediatrics and Psychiatry, Dalhousie University, Halifax, Nova Scotia, Canada; Izaak Walton Killam Hospital for Children, Camp Hill Medical Centre, Halifax, Nova Scotia, Canada; Children's Hospital of Eastern Ontario, Ottawa, Ontario, Canada
Psychogenic Pain Conditions

WARREN A. McGUIRE, M.D.
Fellow, Department of Therapeutic Radiology/Radiation Oncology, University of Minnesota School of Medicine, Minneapolis, Minnesota
Oncologic Disorders: Lymphomas

JULIA A. McMILLAN, M.D.
Associate Professor of Pediatrics, Johns Hopkins University School of Medicine; Deputy Director, Department of Pediatrics, and Residency Program Director, Johns Hopkins Hospital, Baltimore, Maryland
Bacterial Infections: Mycoplasma pneumoniae *Infections*

BARBARA G. MELAMED, PH.D.
Professor and Dean, Ferkauf Graduate School of Psychology, Yeshiva University; Clinical Professor, Departments of Psychiatry and of Epidemiology and Social Medicine, Albert Einstein College of Medicine, Bronx, New York
Fears and Phobias

SUSAN L. MILLARD, M.D.
Pediatric Pulmonary Fellow, University of Arizona; University of Arizona Medical Center, Tucson Medical Center, Tucson, Arizona
Lung Diseases

SUSAN G. MILLSTEIN, PH.D.
Associate Adjunct Professor of Pediatrics, and Director of Research, Division of Adolescent Medicine, Department of Pediatrics, School of Medicine, University of California, San Francisco, San Francisco, California
United States Profile

JOSEPH MIRRA, M.D.
Professor of Pathology, UCLA Center for the Health Sciences; Director, Orthopedic Oncology, and Attending Pathologist, Hospital of the Good Samaritan, Los Angeles, California
Oncologic Disorders: Musculoskeletal Neoplasia

GARY MONTGOMERY, M.D.
Scottish Rite Children's Medical Center, Atlanta, Georgia
Maturation of the Respiratory System at Puberty and Related Respiratory System Considerations

KATHI NADER, D.S.W.
Director of Evaluations, Program in Trauma Violence and Sudden Bereavement, UCLA Department of Psychiatry and Biobehavioral Sciences, Neuropsychiatric Institute and Hospital, Los Angeles, California
Post-traumatic Stress Disorder

MICHAEL P. NUSSBAUM, M.D.
Clinical Associate Professor of Pediatrics, State University of New York at Stony Brook, Stony Brook, New York
Nutritional Conditions: Anorexia Nervosa

DILIP R. PATEL, M.D.
Assistant Professor of Pediatrics, Department of Pediatrics and Human Development, Michigan State University College of Human Medicine, East Lansing, Michigan; Director of Adolescent Medicine, Michigan State University/Kalamazoo Center for Medical Studies, Kalamazoo, Michigan
Contraception

ROBERT A. PENDERGRAST, JR., M.D., M.P.H.
Assistant Professor of Pediatrics, Johns Hopkins University School of Medicine; Active Staff, Johns Hopkins Hospital, Baltimore, Maryland
Sports Medicine

ORA HIRSCH PESCOVITZ, M.D.
Associate Professor of Pediatrics, Physiology and Biophysics, and Director, Pediatric Endocrinology/Diabetology, Indiana University School of Medicine; James Whitcomb Riley Hospital for Children, Indianapolis, Indiana
Precocious Puberty

ANNE C. PETERSEN, PH.D.
Vice President for Research, and Dean of the Graduate School, University of Minnesota, Minneapolis, Minnesota
Hormones and Behavior

SHERIDAN PHILLIPS, PH.D.
Associate Professor, Departments of Psychiatry and Pediatrics, University of Maryland School of Medicine; Affiliate Medical Staff, University of Maryland Medical System, Baltimore, Maryland
Attention Deficit Hyperactivity Disorder

MICHAEL E. PICHICHERO, M.D.
Clinical Professor of Pediatrics, Division of Pediatric Infectious Diseases, Elmwood Pediatric Group, University of Rochester Medical Center; Attending Physician, Strong Memorial Hospital, Rochester, New York
Bacterial Infections: Streptococcal Infections; Bacterial Infections: Haemophilus influenzae *Infections; Bacterial Infections:* Bordetella pertussis *Infection and Pertussis Syndromes*

KEITH R. POWELL, M.D.
George Washington Goler Professor and Associate Chair for Clinical Affairs, Department of Pediatrics; Chief, Division of Infectious Diseases, University of Rochester Medical Center; Strong Memorial Hospital, Rochester, New York
Selecting Antimicrobial Agents

DEBORAH PROTHROW-STITH, M.D.
Lecturer, Department of Health Policy and Management; Assistant Dean for Government and Community Programs, Harvard School of Public Health, Boston, Massachusetts
Violence

ROBERT S. PYNOOS, M.D., M.P.H.
Associate Professor, Department of Psychiatry and Biobehavioral Sciences, UCLA School of Medicine; Director, Program in Trauma Violence and Sudden Bereavement, UCLA Department of Psychiatry and Biobehavioral Sciences, Neuropsychiatric Institute and Hospital, Los Angeles, California
Post-traumatic Stress Disorder

MICHAEL RADETSKY, M.D.
Clinical Professor of Pediatrics, University of California School of Medicine, Davis, California; Director, Pediatric Critical Care and Infectious Diseases, Kaiser-Permanente Medical Care System; Department of Pediatrics, Kaiser Medical Center, Sutter Memorial Hospital, University of California Medical Center, Sacramento, California
Viral Infections: Measles, Rubella, and Other Viral Exanthems

KATHLYN L. R. RASMUSSEN, PH.D.
Senior Staff Fellow, Laboratory of Comparative Ethology, National Institute of Child Health and Human Development, Bethesda, Maryland
Primate Models of Behavioral and Physiologic Change in Adolescence

JOSEPH L. RAUH, M.D.
Professor of Pediatrics and Medicine, University of Cincinnati College of Medicine; Director, Division of Adolescent Medicine, Children's Hospital Medical Center, Cincinnati, Ohio
Mentally Retarded Youth

EDWARD O. REITER, M.D.
Professor of Pediatrics, Tufts University School of Medicine, Boston, Massachu-

setts; Chairman, Department of Pediatrics, Baystate Medical Center, Springfield, Massachusetts
Neuroendocrine Regulation of Puberty; Delayed Pubertal Development

ROBERT H. REMIEN, PH.D.
Instructor in Clinical Psychology, Department of Psychiatry, Columbia University College of Physicians and Surgeons; Research Scientist, New York State Psychiatric Institute, New York, New York
Sexual Orientation

AMY C. RICHARDSON, M.D.
Assistant Professor of Pediatrics, Case Western Reserve University School of Medicine; Child Protection Program, Rainbow Babies and Childrens Hospital, Cleveland, Ohio
Physical and Emotional Abuse

RICHARD C. RINK, M.D.
Associate Professor of Urology, Indiana University School of Medicine; Chief, Pediatric Urology, James Whitcomb Riley Hospital for Children; Attending Pediatric Urologist, Indiana University Hospital, Wishard Memorial Hospital, Indianapolis, Indiana
Urologic Conditions

ROBERT L. ROBERTS, M.D., PH.D.
Assistant Clinical Professor, Division of Immunology/Allergy, Department of Pediatrics, UCLA School of Medicine; UCLA Hospital and Clinics, Los Angeles, California
Immunologic Aspects of Adolescence

ALBERT P. ROCCHINI, M.D.
Professor of Pediatrics, and Ruben/Bentson Professor of Pediatric Cardiology, University of Minnesota; Director, Pediatric Cardiology, University of Minnesota Hospitals, Minneapolis, Minnesota
Cardiovascular Risk Factors and Prevention

PAUL C. J. ROGERS, M.B., F.R.C.P., F.R.C.P.(C)
Professor, Department of Pediatrics, University of British Columbia; Head, Division of Pediatric Hematology/Oncology, British Columbia's Children's Hospital, Vancouver, British Columbia, Canada
Oncologic Disorders: Germ Cell Tumors

GERALD ROSEN, M.D.
Associate Clinical Professor, UCLA Center for Health Sciences; Medical Director, Cedars-Sinai Cancer Center; Attending Physician, Divisions of Medical and Pediatric Oncology, Cedars-Sinai Medical Center and UCLA Center for Health Sciences, Los Angeles, California
Oncologic Disorders: Musculoskeletal Neoplasia

RON G. ROSENFELD, M.D.
Professor of Pediatrics, Stanford University School of Medicine; Professor of Pediatrics, Stanford University Medical Center, Stanford, California
Disorders of Growth

CAROLYN L. RUSSO, M.D.
Assistant Professor of Pediatrics, Division of Hematology-Oncology, Stanford University School of Medicine; Assistant Professor of Pediatrics, Lucile Packard Children's Hospital at Stanford, Stanford, California
Hematologic Disorders: Disorders of the Erythrocyte

NEAL D. RYAN, M.D.
Associate Professor of Psychiatry, University of Pittsburgh School of Medicine, Pittsburgh, Pennsylvania
Depression: Unipolar and Bipolar

OLLE JANE Z. SAHLER, M.D.
Professor of Pediatrics, Psychiatry, Medical Humanities and Medical Informatics, University of Rochester Medical Center; Strong Memorial Hospital, Rochester, New York
Grief and Bereavement

JOE M. SANDERS, JR., M.D.
Associate Executive Director, American Academy of Pediatrics, Elk Grove, Illinois; Clinical Professor of Pediatrics, University of Chicago, Chicago, Illinois
Financing of Adolescent Care

MARK SANFORD, M.D.
Assistant Professor, Department of Psychiatry, McMaster University; Chedoke Child and Family Center, Chedoke-McMaster Hospitals, Hamilton, Ontario, Canada
Schizophrenia

RICHARD SATRAN, M.D.
Professor and Associate Chair, Department of Neurology, University of Rochester Medical Center; Attending Physician, Strong Memorial Hospital, Rochester, New York
Sleep Disorders

S. KENNETH SCHONBERG, M.D.
Professor of Pediatrics, Albert Einstein College of Medicine; Director, Division of Adolescent Medicine, Montefiore Medical Center, Bronx, New York
Substance Use and Abuse

MANUEL SCHYDLOWER, M.D.
Clinical Associate Professor of Pediatrics, Uniformed Services University of the Health Sciences, Bethesda, Maryland; and Texas Tech School of Medicine, Lubbock, Texas; Consultant in Adolescent Medicine to the Army Surgeon General; Director, Adolescent Medicine Program; Chief, Department of Clinical Investigation, William Beaumont Army Medical Center, El Paso, Texas
Youth in the Military

DAVID B. SEABURN, M.S.
Associate, Departments of Psychiatry and Family Medicine, University of Rochester Medical Center, Rochester, New York
Family-oriented Care

RUTH ANDREA SEELER, M.D.
Director, Pediatric Education, University of Illinois College of Medicine; Associate Chief of Service, Humana Hospital Michael Reese, Chicago, Illinois
Developmental Overview of Hematology and Oncology

STEVEN M. SELBST, M.D.
Associate Professor of Pediatrics, University of Pennsylvania School of Medicine; Director, Emergency Department, Children's Hospital of Philadelphia, Philadelphia, Pennsylvania
Adolescent Emergency Conditions

MARY-ANN SHAFER, M.D.
Associate Professor of Pediatrics, University of California, San Francisco; Division of Adolescent Medicine, University of California, San Francisco, San Francisco, California
Sexually Transmitted Disease Syndromes

DAVID SHAFFER, M.B., F.R.C.P., F.R.C.PSYCH.
Irving Philips Professor of Child Psychiatry, Columbia University; Director, Division of Child Psychiatry, Columbia-Pres-

byterian Hospital, New York, New York
Suicide and Suicidal Behaviors

I. RONALD SHENKER, M.D.
Professor of Pediatrics, Albert Einstein
College of Medicine, Bronx, New York;
Chief, Division of Adolescent Medicine,
Schneider Children's Hospital of Long Is-
land Jewish Medical Center, New Hyde
Park, New York
Nutritional Conditions: Bulimia Nervosa

CATHERINE M. SHISSLAK, PH.D.
Associate Professor, Department of Fam-
ily and Community Medicine, College of
Medicine, University of Arizona; Allied
Health Professional Staff, Palo Verde
Hospital; Associate Medical Staff, Tucson
Medical Center; Medical Staff, University
Medical Center, Tucson, Arizona
Cigarette Smoking

DAVID M. SIEGEL, M.D., M.P.H.
Assistant Professor of Pediatrics and Med-
icine, and Co-Director, Pediatric Arthritis
Clinic, University of Rochester Medical
Center; Strong Memorial Hospital, Roch-
ester General Hospital, Rochester, New
York
Collagen Vascular Disorders

TOMAS J. SILBER, M.D., M.A.S.S.
Professor of Pediatrics and Health Care
Sciences, The George Washington Univer-
sity School of Medicine and Health Sci-
ences; Vice-Chairman, Department of Ad-
olescent and Young Adult Medicine,
Children's National Medical Center,
Washington, D.C.
Interdisciplinary Teams

LARRY B. SILVER, M.D.
Clinical Professor of Psychiatry, and Di-
rector of Training in Child and Adolescent
Psychiatry, Georgetown University School
of Medicine, Washington, D.C.
*Underachievement and Learning
Disabilities*

JAMES Q. SIMMONS, III, M.D.
Professor of Psychiatry, UCLA School of
Medicine; Chief, Clinical Services, UCLA
Neuropsychiatric Hospital, Los Angeles,
California
Liaison and Consultation

GAIL B. SLAP, M.D.
Associate Professor of Medicine and Pediatrics, Departments of Medicine and Pe-

diatrics, University of Pennsylvania School
of Medicine; Director of Adolescent Medicine, Hospital of the University of Pennsylvania, and Children's Hospital of Philadelphia, Philadelphia, Pennsylvania
Youth in Transition to Adult Health Care

MARK SCOTT SMITH, M.D.
Associate Professor of Pediatrics, Univer-
sity of Washington School of Medicine;
Chief, Adolescent Services, Children's
Hospital and Medical Center, Seattle,
Washington
Viral Infections: Chronic Fatigue

BARBARA K. SNYDER, M.D.
Chief, Division of Adolescent Medicine,
and Clinical Assistant Professor of Pediatrics, University of Medicine and Dentistry of New Jersey, Robert Wood Johnson Medical School, Piscataway, New
Jersey; Robert Wood Johnson University
Hospital, New Brunswick, New Jersey
Stress and the Immune System

ANTHONY SPIRITO, PH.D.
Associate Professor of Psychiatry and
Human Behavior, Brown University Pro-
gram in Medicine; Director of Psychology,
Rhode Island Hospital, Providence,
Rhode Island
Behavior Therapy

HOWARD R. SPIVAK, M.D.
Associate Professor in Pediatrics and
Community Health, Tufts University
School of Medicine; Chief, General Pedi-
atrics, New England Medical Center/
Floating Hospital for Infants and Children,
Boston, Massachusetts
Violence

CATHERINE STEVENS-SIMON, M.D.
Assistant Professor of Pediatrics, Univer-
sity of Colorado Health Sciences Center;
Children's Hospital, Denver, Colorado
Adolescent Pregnancy

E. RICHARD STIEHM, M.D.
Professor of Pediatrics; Head, Division of
Immunology, and Vice Chair, Department
of Pediatrics, UCLA School of Medicine;
Attending Pediatrician, UCLA Center for
Health Sciences, Los Angeles, California
Immunologic Aspects of Adolescence

MARY STORY, PH.D., R.D.
Associate Professor, Division of Human
Development and Nutrition, School of
Public Health and Nutrition, and Adoles-

cent Health Program, University of Minnesota, Minneapolis, Minnesota
Nutritional Requirements During Adolescence

VICTOR STRASBURGER, M.D.
Associate Professor of Pediatrics, Division of Adolescent Medicine, University of New Mexico, Albuquerque, New Mexico
Normal Sexuality

WILLIAM B. STRONG, M.D.
Leon Henri Charbonnier Professor of Pediatrics; Chief, Section of Pediatric Cardiology; Director, Georgia Institute for the Prevention of Human Disease and Accidents, Medical College of Georgia; Active Staff, Medical College of Georgia Hospital and Clinics, Augusta, Georgia
Sports Medicine

MARGARET L. STUBER, M.D.
Assistant Professor of Psychiatry, Division of Child Psychiatry, University of California, Los Angeles; Attending Psychiatrist, UCLA Neuropsychiatric Institute and Hospital, UCLA Center for Health Sciences, Los Angeles, California
Psychological Care of Adolescents Undergoing Transplantation

HARRIS R. STUTMAN, M.D.
Assistant Professor of Pediatrics, University of California, Irvine, California College of Medicine, Irvine, California; Director, Pediatric Infectious Diseases, Memorial Miller Children's Hospital, Long Beach, California
Bacterial Infections: Rickettsia rickettsii (Rocky Mountain Spotted Fever)

STEPHEN J. SUOMI, PH.D.
Chief, Laboratory of Comparative Ethology, National Institute of Child Health and Human Development, Bethesda, Maryland
Primate Models of Behavioral and Physiologic Change in Adolescence

ELIZABETH J. SUSMAN, PH.D.
Professor of Biobehavioral Health, The Pennsylvania State University, University Park, Pennsylvania
Hormones and Behavior

DRAGAN M. SVRAKIC, M.D., PH.D.
Instructor in Psychiatry, Washington University School of Medicine; Barnes Hospital, Jewish Hospital of St. Louis, St. Louis, Missouri
Personality Development and Structure; Personality Disorders

PETER SZATMARI, M.D.
Associate Professor, Department of Psychiatry, McMaster University; Chedoke Child and Family Center, Chedoke-McMaster Hospitals, Hamilton, Ontario, Canada
Schizophrenia

JAMES K. TODD, M.D.
Professor of Pediatrics and Microbiology and Immunology, University of Colorado School of Medicine; Director of Epidemiology, Children's Hospital, Denver, Colorado
Bacterial Infections: Staphylococcal Infection (Toxic Shock Syndrome)

JOHN N. UDALL, JR., M.D., PH.D.
Associate Professor of Pediatrics, University of Arizona College of Medicine; Chief, Pediatric Gastroenterology, University Medical Center, Tucson, Arizona
Diseases of the Liver and Pancreas During Adolescence

HAZEL J. VERNON, M.D.
Assistant Clinical Professor, Departments of Pediatrics and Dermatology, Medical College of Virginia; Attending, Medical College of Virginia Hospital, Richmond, Virginia
Skin Disorders

MARY L. VOORHESS, M.D.
Professor of Pediatrics, Department of Pediatrics, School of Medicine and Biomedical Sciences, State University of New York at Buffalo; Co-Director, Division of Endocrinology, Children's Hospital of Buffalo, Buffalo, New York
Endocrine Conditions

RUSSELL WALKER, M.D.
Associate Professor of Neurology, Cornell University Medical College; Associate Attending Neurology and Pediatrics, Memorial Sloan-Kettering Cancer Center, New York, New York
Oncologic Disorders: Brain Tumors

REGINALD L. WASHINGTON, M.D.
Associate Clinical Professor of Pediatrics, University of Colorado School of Medicine; Children's Hospital, AMI Presbyterian–St. Luke's Medical Center, Rose Medical Center, Denver, Colorado
Cardiovascular Aspects of Systemic Disease

JOHN M. WATKINS, PH.D.
Assistant Clinical Professor, Stanford Uni-

versity School of Medicine, Stanford, California
Cognitive Neuroscience and Adolescent Development

IRVING B. WEINER, PH.D.
Professor of Psychiatry and Behavioral Medicine, University of South Florida College of Medicine; Director of Psychological Services, University of South Florida Psychiatry Center, Tampa, Florida
Normality During Adolescence

LEONARD B. WEINER, M.D.
Professor of Pediatrics and Pathology, State University of New York Health Science Center at Syracuse; Attending Physician, Pediatric Infectious Disease, University Hospital, and Crouse-Irving Memorial Hospital, Syracuse, New York
Bacterial Infections: Mycoplasma pneumoniae *Infections*

JOAN B. WENNING, M.D., F.R.C.S.(C)
Assistant Professor of Obstetrics and Gynaecology, Dalhousie University; Active Staff, Izaak Walton Killam Hospital for Children, Halifax Infirmary, Grace Maternity Hospital, Halifax, Nova Scotia, Canada
Menstrual Conditions: Dysfunctional Uterine Bleeding; Menstrual Conditions: Dysmenorrhea; Menstrual Conditions: Premenstrual Syndrome; Genital Tract Cysts and Tumors; Chronic Pelvic Pain

MARIAN E. WILLIAMS, PH.D.
Staff Psychologist, Departments of Psychology and Psychiatry, University of California, Los Angeles, Los Angeles, California
Cognitive Neuroscience and Adolescent Development

MENG XIANGDONG, M.D.
Doctor-in-Charge, Child and Adolescent Health, Department of School Health, The Center of Health and Anti-Diseases of Ji-Lin Province, Chang Chun City, People's Republic of China
International Profile

W. SAM YANCY, M.D.
Clinical Professor of Pediatrics, and Associate Clinical Professor of Psychiatry, Duke University Medical Center; Attending Pediatric Staff, Durham County General Hospital; Department of Pediatrics, Duke University Hospital, Durham, North Carolina
Office Practice

KENNETH G. ZAHKA, M.D.
Associate Professor of Pediatrics, Case Western Reserve University School of Medicine; Director of Pediatric Cardiology, Rainbow Babies and Childrens Hospital, Cleveland, Ohio
Structural Cardiovascular Defects

LONNIE K. ZELTZER, M.D.
Professor of Pediatrics, and Director, Pediatric Pain Program, Division of Neurology, Department of Pediatrics, UCLA School of Medicine, Los Angeles, California
Pain in Adolescence

DEWEY K. ZIEGLER, M.D.
Professor Emeritus of Neurology, University of Kansas; University of Kansas Medical Center, Kansas City, Kansas
Headache; Syncope and Dizziness

ROBERT G. ZIEGLER, M.D.
Clinical Instructor in Psychiatry, Harvard Medical School; Assistant in Psychiatry, Children's Hospital, Boston, Massachusetts
Epilepsy and Seizure Disorders

Foreword

During the past quarter of a century, an extraordinary amount of information has emerged concerning youth, their biologic and psychological development, and their health status. Although the amassed information is extensive, its appearance in a single volume has been infrequent. This new textbook represents a welcome addition and fills a significant void. Additionally, many of these previous data were utilized to support the doctrine of a singular pattern of development, and by implication all deviations from this pervasive normal developmental track were labeled as aberrant or dysfunctional. This book represents a fresh, new look at the adolescent and the multiple paths toward normal adulthood and helps focus our attention on impressive advances in the field of adolescent medicine as we near the twenty-first century.

A number of critical themes emerge as one reads this text, but central to fully appreciating the value of this book is recognizing the absence of certainty about many facts and positions currently held regarding youth. Adolescent health is still emerging as a field of human study, and most, if not all, tenets concerning biologic, psychological, and sociologic development need to be held to gently, questioned vigorously, and challenged frequently. The many contributors to this volume subscribe to this philosophy, but it is equally critical that the reader also approach this body of knowledge with enthusiastic skepticism. It is only then that the field can and will continue to advance.

Reliable data on adolescents in all the dimensions of their lives are difficult to obtain. Adolescents are culturally diverse, crossing all economic strata, and they are biologically or, more specifically, genetically very heterogeneous. Perhaps most important, they display multiple patterns of maturation, which, although different from each other, must be considered normal—normal in the variability of their phenotypic expression and normal in the differences in temporal expression. Readers often look for a single set of reference standards, but in this field of study heterogeneity reigns, and the reader is urged to become comfortable with wide ranges of biologic and psychosocial norms. The concept of a single linear developmental curve seems to be yielding to the view that multiple normal pathways exist.

All medical texts, by their very nature, tend to describe healthy or diseased states in terms of cohorts of patients, but adolescents, like all patients, have unique and idiosyncratic lives. This individual quality is a critical feature to remember as the reader applies medical fact to a single patient management plan. This dictum is important in all clinical medicine but is especially so in adolescent medicine. It is at the heart of what special training programs offer in preparing students in this field. The exuberance or the pain of an adolescent is best appreciated in the context of the individual and not the group, and certainly from the unique vantage point of the patient as well as from the viewpoint of the health provider.

Within each adolescent, whether he or she is highly successful in negotiating this second decade of life or is markedly dysfunctional, there commonly are entire clusters of biologic, social, psychological, cultural, and even specific environmental factors that interact in rather unique ways. Interactive processes, however, do not easily lend themselves to textual presentation. The readers are thus urged to look for coexistent relationships. Identifying known clusters of successful interactive processes helps immeasurably as one plans health promotion strategies. Alternatively, identifying the covariation of dysfunctional states is extremely useful in planning interdictive strategies for more vulnerable youth. This book offers examples of both types of clusters.

A special word is necessary about our most vulnerable youth. They are frequently minority teenagers. They are termed minority not because of their racial or ethnic origins, which certainly produce intragroup differences, but because of poverty and low socioeconomic status. These most disadvantaged and vulnerable youth are overrepresented in virtually all national or regional morbidity and mortality data. They are very complex young people with what appear to be even more complex developmental pathways. They often exist at the periphery of the adolescent environment rather than within its central milieu. While you read this text, pay particular attention to the data on these socially and economically impaired minorities, since they are in urgent need of more targeted activity in both health promotion and disease prevention.

Thus, future directions in adolescent medicine appear to be delineating several clear tracks for exploration and study, and all are outlined in this volume. They include the need to adopt the concept of multiple and complex but normal developmental patterns rather than a singular pathway from childhood to adulthood; the need to learn how to translate adolescent cohort data into individual patient-specific actions; the need to vigorously pursue the covariation of healthy and unhealthy clusters of behaviors or diseases; and the need to explore the lives of our most vulnerable adolescents.

This textbook discusses all these issues in great detail and thus points the way for future initiatives. The editors and authors are not the first, nor will they be the last, to attempt to address these central health themes of young people, but they, like me, await the arrival of the very best who are yet to come—our students and trainees. It is they who will really answer the challenges outlined in this book and for whom this volume was so carefully prepared.

MICHAEL I. COHEN, M.D.
Professor and Chairman
Department of Pediatrics
Albert Einstein College of Medicine

Preface

The *Textbook of Adolescent Medicine* attempts to define and present the body of knowledge that we know as adolescent medicine, focusing on the aspects of health and illness that occur during this developmental period. Our choice of topics has been deliberate. We have attempted to be as comprehensive as possible within our self-imposed parameters. This text focuses on conditions that are affected by adolescence or have a special effect on adolescents. Discussion of other conditions can be found in traditional textbooks of pediatrics, internal medicine, and psychiatry.

We have chosen authors from many areas, representing specialists in adolescent medicine, pediatrics, nutrition, family and internal medicine, psychiatry, clinical psychology, and other pertinent fields. Their challenge has been to define and discuss, for practicing clinicians, these unique aspects of adolescent medicine. In some areas this is relatively easy. In other important areas, however, data specific to adolescence are not available. In these circumstances, data are presented relating to children and adolescents or to adolescents and adults.

The text is organized rather traditionally. The scientific background (Part 1) is meant to reflect the most recent data about adolescent development and newer areas such as the biology-behavior interface. This part is expected to change the most in future editions as our scientific and technologic competence increases. Gradually this information will be absorbed into the medical and behavioral sections of future editions. Clinical approach (Part 2) covers various aspects relating to the practice of adolescent medicine and includes a section on prevention. The astute reader will note that the prevention section is brief and does not include information about accidental injury or risk-taking behaviors. Unfortunately, this reflects the current state of the art of primary prevention. Secondary and tertiary interventions are also discussed in their respective medical (Part 3) or psychological (Part 4) sections. As knowledge about prevention increases, it will be incorporated into future editions of the textbook.

The health care of adolescents focuses on the health problems that occur in the second decade and early in the third decade of life. Although many adolescents are well, some develop health problems that first become symptomatic at this time. Others bring chronic illnesses and conditions of childhood into their adolescence. And for many, the lifestyle habits and behaviors that are developed during adolescence result in major morbidity or mortality in adulthood. As our understanding of this age group increases, so does our appreciation of the complex interactions among biologic, psychological, and social health. It is clear that many of the major problems and morbidity of adolescents are related to underlying societal problems such as poverty, lack of education, and family disorganization. These social problems have a great impact on the health and well-being of youth. However, solutions often lie beyond the scope of the practice of medicine as we know it today. Our authors discuss the social and societal problems within the context of each condition. When sufficient information of use to the clinician becomes available, appropriate sections will be added to the textbook.

The major limitations of this first edition relate to those of all multiauthored texts. Overlap among chapters has been a matter of debate for the editors on several occasions. We have left some overlap in areas where the content is important to the practice of adolescent medicine and where readers may look in one of several sections for that information.

We, as editors, would like to thank many persons for supporting us through this challenge. First, we would like to recognize our families, and our close colleagues, who often become our professional families. We would like to especially thank our section editors for the commitment, unselfish sharing of knowledge, and direction they have provided us. These individuals are Drs. Dennis P. Cantwell, Edward B. Clark, S. Jean Emans, Stephen A. Feig, Vincent A. Fulginiti, Robert J. Joynt, David Shaffer, James Q. Simmons, III, and Lynn M. Taussig. They have been most patient with us as we as editors have wrestled with the data, clarifying what is known about adolescents and what is not known. In addition, there have been a number of colleagues who have participated in the peer-review process: Drs. Robert J. Bidwell, Marilyn R. Brown, Margaret T. Colgan, Molly Coulter, Philip W. Davidson, Marianne E. Felice, Gilbert B. Forbes, Caroline B. Hall, Adele D. Hofmann, Michelle Hooper, John J. Hutter, Richard A. Insel, Kenneth V. Jackman, Julie A. Jaskiewicz, Nicholas Jospe, John S. Lambert, Gregory S. Liptak, Marvin E. Miller, Daniel B. Ornt, Keith R. Powell, Ronald Rabinowitz, Mark A. Shelly, Mary T. Story, Stephen B. Sulkes, Peter G. Szilagyi, John Udall, Élise van der Jagt, and Kathleen A. Woodin. We also wish to acknowledge the contributions of Jennifer Meyer Harris, Pharm.D., and William F. Buss, Pharm.D., of the Indiana University Medical Center, who checked the accuracy of all drug dosages in this text. We particularly want to thank our close colleague and friend over the years, Dr. Christopher Hodgman, who has reviewed a number of the chapters and whose guidance throughout the process of developing this book and throughout the years of working at the University of Rochester is highly valued.

We also want to recognize the staff in our offices for herculean efforts. Mrs. Carole Berger at the University of Rochester kept the entire process together with impeccable accuracy, remarkable energy, and indomitable spirit. We are grateful to Carole for her many contributions to the realization of this book. In addition, we want to thank Mrs. Karin Gavin in the Indiana University office and Ms. Annette Spurr in the University of Arizona office. In Rochester, Mrs. Berger was assisted by Mrs. Sandra Fedrizzi, Ms. Christine Guthrie, Mrs. Marcy Inglese, and Mrs. Debbie Shannon. We also would particularly like to thank our colleague, Dr. Molly Coulter, who reviewed a number of the chapters and gave us her suggestions as a skilled practitioner.

Both Mrs. Lisette Bralow and Ms. Kathleen McCarthy at W.B. Saunders have provided us direction, inspiration, and support. In addition to all those who worked directly on the book, we would like to thank our Rochester-based colleagues, Dr. Robert A. Hoekleman, Professor and Chair of the Department of Pediatrics, Dr. Gilbert B. Forbes, Professor Emeritus of Pediatrics, and Ms. Sydney Sutherland, whose counsel and availability are gratefully acknowledged.

ELIZABETH R. McANARNEY, M.D.
RICHARD E. KREIPE, M.D.
DONALD P. ORR, M.D.
GEORGE D. COMERCI, M.D.

Contents

Dosage Notice

Introduction

I had not been aware of the advent of this book prior to a telephone call from one of its four editors at a time when they were nearing completion of their task. I was told that the four of them found themselves in accord that the body of literature on the various aspects of adolescent medicine had grown and was accumulating at such a rate that there was a need to assemble it in a single volume. Apparently their concept from the beginning was that the book would be constructed as a Textbook of Adolescent Medicine and could function as a text for both the undergraduate and the postgraduate student as well as a source of reference for the practitioner and the investigator.

I saw no reason to disagree with their intentions, other than to warn them of the demanding and confining nature, as well as the rigid responsibilities, of the roles they had chosen. Then "the other shoe fell"—they invited me to write the introduction. There can be no gain in detailing the broad pattern and logic of my resistance. Suffice it to say, I did agree.

I was provided with the Foreword, the Preface, and the Table of Contents. Appraisal of the Table of Contents will reveal the care and thought that has gone into the planning of this text in an attempt to provide an overall perspective of the field as well as the specific topics covered in the subdivisions of each section. Initially, one is aware that there are four principal parts, each divided into chapters prepared by selected contributors. When it is realized that there are 126 chapters with some 200 authors, chosen because of acknowledged interest and concern for the specific issues assigned to them, one senses the extent of their confidence that the goals of the editors for this book were achievable.

It should be clear that the editors had set a gigantic task for themselves in their attempt to create a cohesive text of the assembled material: an entity that would create the impression of having a commonness in literary structure and in writing style. Furthermore, they must have been aware from the beginning that they would have to contend with apparent as well as real differences among the contributors in personal interpretations of like situations and comparable data. In such situations, when reconciliation between respective authors was not currently justified and it was not practical to include each position in the respective chapters, appropriate cross-references were inserted so that the reader would be aware of the currently "unsettled" state. I suspect that only one who has lived with these "necessary uncertainties" can appreciate the time and effort required for their arbitrary solutions. (Should you, the user of this book, note an occasional editorial failure in the above respect, you may be confident that the editors will be in your debt should you call it to their attention.)

The categorized arrangement of the text into four parts seems most appropriate and should enhance the repeated use of the book for reference purposes. The second part promises a sharing of the practical aspects of an organized approach to the individual patient. The third and fourth parts are more or less traditional coverages of the medical and psychological disorders, respectively, that are encountered among the youth of today. It is the first part, "Scientific Basis of Adolescent Medicine," that intrigues me most and that raises my hopes, and I look forward impatiently to receipt of my copy. My anticipation of this part promises me several evenings of quiet exploration.

Finally, the timing of publication of this book, even if not planned, seems quite pragmatic. There have been rumors that the creation of a sub-board of adolescent medicine, with its consequent examinations for certification, has been under way through the conjoined efforts of the respective parent Boards of Pediatrics and of Internal Medicine. I am now told by "Chapel Hill" that the rumor has been replaced by accomplishment.

A comrade has suggested that I am placing a blessing on this book. I am not. I have no divine right. But I shall be more than surprised if it does not come to be an accepted guide for the preparation of those whose careers are to be principally in the health care and welfare of the adolescent, as well as for those who are established in this field.

WALDO E. NELSON, M.D.
Professor of Pediatrics
Medical College of Pennsylvania and
Temple University School of Medicine
Attending Physician
St. Christopher's Hospital for Children
Philadelphia, Pennsylvania

CHAPTER 1

The History of Adolescent Medicine

FELIX P. HEALD

EARLY ORIGINS

The origins of adolescent medicine as we know them are listed in Table 1–1.

From 1790 to the present, there have been references in the literature to the medical needs of adolescents. During the mid-nineteenth century, the modern concept of adolescence, defined as a biologic phenomenon, was introduced, focusing on middle-class young people. A classic study of adolescent growth was published by Bowditch in 1877. Health services for adolescents were originally organized for boarding-school boys, and a group of physicians caring for them established the Medical Officers of School Association in 1884. In 1885, this group published their first Code of Rules in an attempt to prevent the outbreak and spread of preventable diseases.

A review of the *Index Medicus* from 1879 to the present revealed interesting historical data. From 1879 until 1904, there was no item in the *Index* under the listing of adolescence. In 1904, the classic treatise by G. Stanley Hall was published, "Adolescence: Its Psychology and Its Relationship to Physiology, Anthropology, Sociology, Sex, Crime, Religion and Education." In 1905, Jastrow published an eight-page article entitled "The Natural History of Adolescence." Subsequently articles were published by Baldwin (1913 and 1917), Fuller (1914–1915), Mapes (1917), and Bridgman (two articles in 1918). (Complete references to all these publications appear in the bibliography at the end of this chapter.)

The first description of a special clinic for adolescents was contained in an 1918 article by Amelia Gates entitled "The Work of the Adolescent Clinic of Stanford University Medical School." Because of its historical importance, the second paragraph of that particular paper is quoted:

> When we started this work we had certain medical aims in view, but we found that in this particular clinic we could hardly confine ourselves to medical work alone. The Clinic soon had to busy itself with the social and educational aspect of our problems and in proportion as we successfully dealt with these, did our work become more effective. (Gates, 1918, p 236.)

Gates and colleagues noted that adolescent care demanded attention to the whole person, not just to a particular illness. As her article stated: "For it is not only the physical ailments we have to deal with in this clinic, but also the ills that come from the various social maladjustments of our modern life" (Gates, 1918, p 236). Gates listed specific medical problems, including anemias, menstrual disturbances, conditions of the thyroid, vasomotor disturbances, nervous disorders, postural defects, and different forms of enuresis. Many of the basic principles that guide modern adolescent clinics were recognized by Gates and colleagues in 1918.

By 1927, there were 11 medical articles and six reports on adolescence. The medical papers varied from "Basal Metabolism in Puberal Obesity" to "Muscles Before and After Puberty: Influence of Endocrine Glands." The psychology articles included "A Critique of Present Day Psychology of Puberty" and "Psychopathology of Puberty: Unfitness of Girls Leaving School for Employment." By 1930, the numbers of papers had increased significantly over the previous contributions. There were 45 papers primarily focusing on medical disorders or growth disorders, and 14 papers focusing on the psychology of adolescence.

In the 1920s and the 1930s, individuals who had a common interest in adolescence collaborated to study adolescent problems. Adolescence research with a strong focus on biologic development and nutrition was carried out in the universities, whereas clinical care took place in the health clinics at boarding schools.

A series of longitudinal studies on anthropometric growth, personality development, and nutrition of normal children through adolescence was initiated during the 1920s and continued into the early 1940s. Their results have greatly shaped our current understanding of the growth and development of teenagers. These classic studies were performed at Antioch College, Harvard University, Stanford University, the University of California at Berkeley, Western Reserve University, and Yale University. During the same period, Lawrence K. Frank, a psychologist, promoted long-term longitudinal studies in child and adolescent development at Yale.

The Adolescence Study Unit of the School of Medicine and the Institute of Human Relations at Yale University was the first of its kind to be developed. The Unit incorporated several disciplines to study the normal biology and psychology of puberty, and had representatives from the Departments of Anatomy, Physiology,

TABLE 1–1. Early Origins of Adolescent Medicine: 1790s to 1904

1790 to present	Medical interest in the adolescent
1850s	Biology of adolescence
	Middle-class population
1877	Bowditch's classic study of adolescent growth
1884	Medical Officers of School Association (boarding-school boys)
1904	G. Stanley Hall's treatise

Physiological Chemistry, Pediatrics, and Psychology. The Yale studies included endocrinologic studies (measurements of estrogen, androgens, and pituitary-gonadotropic hormones) as well as studies of skeletal growth and other bodily changes.

In 1937, Dorfman and colleagues published a seminal paper on the excretion of androgenic and estrogenic substances in the urine of children. Twenty-one of the 23 subjects were either preteens or adolescents. The authors noted the wide variation in developmental status of adolescents of the same age:

> In view of the marked variation in the developmental status of children of the same chronological age, it seems desirable to attempt to relate the sex hormone excretion more directly to the degree of physical maturity. (Dorfman et al, 1937, p 743.)

It was from this observation that William Greulich developed the sexual maturation staging in boys and girls so widely used today and discussed later in this chapter. About the same time, Priesel and Wagner in Vienna reported the order of appearance of the extra-genital sexual characteristics in girls (quoted in Pryor, 1936, p 53), and this was confirmed by Pryor in the United States. The stages for breast development were first described by Stratz in 1909 (quoted in Reynolds and Wines, 1948, p 332) and later modified by Pryor and Greulich in the United States.

In 1942, Greulich and colleagues published a major document entitled "Somatic and Endocrine Studies of Puberal and Adolescent Boys." This document is notable for the numerous subjects and the correlation of sex hormone excretion with secondary sexual development and skeletal growth. Of particular importance is their publication of the first staging system for puberty assessment. These original maturational ratings were known as Greulich stages of sexual development. This method for maturational ratings was later refined and used by Tanner in the 1950s and 1960s.

Greulich and colleagues also reported on the sequence of the physical changes in boys associated with sexual maturation. Their proposed method classified pubertal and adolescent boys into five maturity groups. They also published data on gonadotropin excretion plotted against chronologic age and against developmental status. They showed, as is now known, that the variance around developmental status was reduced when compared with chronologic age (Figs. 1–1 and 1–2).

In the 1930s, in addition to studies of puberty, there was also considerable interest in nutrition. The first study of juvenile atherosclerosis was reported by Zeek and soon forgotten. In 1932, Wait and Roberts published their classic paper on the energy and protein requirements of adolescents. The methodology and design of this research have not been surpassed. In the 1930s, Johnston (a pediatrician at the Henry Ford Hospital) initiated a series of investigations into the nutritional status of teenage girls who were hospitalized because of recent conversion to a positive tuberculin test or because of active tuberculosis. His studies focused on the correlations between nitrogen balance and physiologic events such as menarche. Johnston initially published data on the increased energy and protein needs of

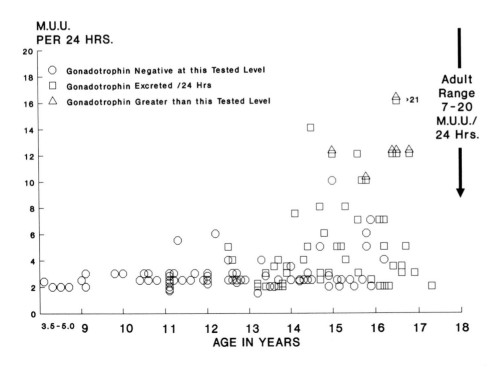

Figure 1–1. Gonadotropin excretion plotted against chronologic age. M.U.U., mouse uterine units. (With permission from Greulich WW, Dorfman RI, Catchpole HR, et al: Somatic and endocrine studies of puberal and adolescent boys. Monogr Soc Res Child Dev 7(3):54, 1942.)

Figure 1–2. By plotting gonadotropin excretion against developmental status, variance is reduced when compared to age. M.U.U., mouse uterine units. (With permission from Greulich WW, Dorfman RI, Catchpole HR, et al: Somatic and endocrine studies of puberal and adolescent boys. Monogr Soc Res Child Dev 7(3):55, 1942.)

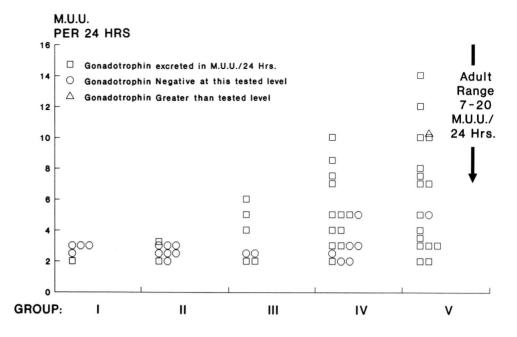

GROWTH OF THE DISCIPLINE OF ADOLESCENT MEDICINE

In the early 1940s, the subject of adolescence first attracted the attention of the American Academy of Pediatrics. In 1941, Region 1 in New Haven, Connecticut, and Region 3 in Chicago, Illinois, independently developed programs for half-day symposia on adolescent medicine. The *Journal of Pediatrics* published the proceedings of these two meetings in a single volume, issued in September 1941. There were a total of 10 presentations, five papers presented in New Haven and five papers delivered in Chicago; an additional paper on metabolism was added (see bibliography).

A. Graeme Mitchell presided over the program in Chicago 2 weeks before his death on June 1, 1941. His remarks are of some historical interest:

> As you see by the program, we are going to discuss . . . only certain phases of adolescence. In the Academy there have been . . . discussions on the subject of adolescence and our discussions have not been completed as yet, and I doubt if they will be for some time to come. To me it is rather significant that we are carrying on a discussion on adolescence. The pediatrician is manifesting not only an increasing interest but an increasing activity in the problems of the adolescent. I see no reason myself why he should not. The pediatrician has a background of interest in the subject. He is the fellow who perhaps more than anyone else is and should be interested in growth and development, and furthermore, often in the individual instance he has the background of the individual child whom he has seen through the early part of childhood, and hence I know of no one better able than he to carry on the studies and the direction of adolescence. (Mitchell, 1941, pp 290–291.)

After World War II, there were minimal developments in adolescent medicine because of reduced research activity during the war. By the late 1940s and the early 1950s, focus on the adolescent resumed in a significant way. The modern clinical care of adolescents began with the development of the Adolescent Unit at the Children's Medical Center in Boston, Massachusetts, in 1951. Sidney Farber foresaw the development of an adolescent unit as a new program for the Children's Hospital and appointed J. Roswell Gallagher as director of this new unit.

The Boston unit set the tone in adolescent care for the 1950s and 1960s. Its primary focus was on the uniqueness, individuality, and difference of adolescents from younger children. The Boston program was the first formal clinical training program in an academic medical center.

By the end of the 1950s, programs for adolescent medicine were expanding across the country at the same time as other pediatric specialties were also developing. Cardiology, neurology, nephrology, and hematology all began as clinical programs that had their intellectual bases in either biochemistry or physiology. Of all the subspecialties in pediatrics, adolescent medicine and ambulatory pediatrics were primarily clinical and did not develop their base in one of the basic sciences. Adolescent medicine focused primarily on clinical research; the more basic research in adolescent-related issues was accomplished in the pediatric specialties, such as endocrinology and cardiology. James Tanner, using the Harpenden Growth Study material, dominated research in growth during adolescence, and Melvin Grumbach performed the pioneering work in the endocrinology of puberty.

In 1965, the first issue of the *Society for Adolescent Medicine Newsletter* was published. The first paragraph summarized the then current state of adolescent medicine:

> The growth and development of clinics for the medical care of adolescents has been most rapid in the last 5 years. Well over 30 clinics are now in existence and 35 inpatient services have been established. Interest is extremely high

pubertal girls in 1936; his publications continued through the 1940s and into the 1950s.

among pediatricians, internists, and generalists to develop additional programs in the future. Adolescent medical care is being taught in many medical schools throughout the country. It has become part of the regular rotation in the training of residents and has offered postgraduate courses to physicians in the community interested in improving their skills in dealing with the adolescent-age patient. Research activities have increased in clinical investigation as well as basic research. (Soc Adolescent Med Newsletter, 1965, Vol 1, p 20.)

This newsletter was the forerunner of the *Journal of Adolescent Health Care.*

Arthur Lesser, then acting head of the Children's Bureau in Washington, D.C., was responsible for funding of the first training program in adolescent health care at the Boston Children's Hospital and two months later at the Division of Adolescent Medicine at the Children's Hospital in the District of Columbia. Lesser's own early commitment to adolescent health care gradually grew into a major emphasis on this subspecialty and eventually to greater funding by this government agency of several adolescent medicine training programs.

Increasingly, there was a perceived need for special educational seminars for the leaders of adolescent medicine. The first seminar, led by Felix P. Heald, focused on adolescent gynecology and was held in Washington, D.C., on March 16 and 17, 1965. The seminar was also funded by the Children's Bureau. This was the first of the yearly in-service programs that lasted until 1974 and provided an opportunity for professionals interested in adolescent medicine to meet yearly.

The second seminar, in 1966, focused on nutrition. At that gathering there was a perceived need for a meeting of colleagues to discuss the challenges of running adolescent medicine programs. A small group of physicians committed to working full-time in adolescent medicine were the major participants. A separate meeting focused on the teaching of adolescent medicine. The second such meeting, held 1 year later, focused on experimental design in adolescent medicine research. These two meetings were the forerunners of the Society for Adolescent Medicine. At the seminar in 1967, a committee was appointed to develop a plan and a constitution for the Society for Adolescent Medicine.

At the Washington, D.C., meeting in 1968, the plan was approved, and the Society for Adolescent Medicine was formally established on April 28, 1968. The stated goals were

To improve the quality of health care for adolescents, to encourage the investigation of normal growth and development during adolescence, and of those diseases that affect adolescents, to stimulate the creation of health services for adolescents, to increase communication among health professionals who care for adolescents, to foster and improve the quality of training of those individuals providing health care to adolescents.

The Society for Adolescent Medicine's first business meeting was held on March 2, 1969, as a part of the fifth annual adolescent medicine seminar in Washington. In 1979, its goals were later modified to place greater emphasis on research and the dissemination of scientific information.

In 1969, the Society for Adolescent Medicine developed a program separate from the Washington, D.C., seminars. The first meeting was held in conjunction with the American Academy of Pediatrics on October 16, 1970, in San Francisco, California. Despite the clinical orientation within the Society for Adolescent Medicine, some members were developing the scientific basis of adolescent medicine. Largely through the efforts of Michael I. Cohen and Stanford B. Friedman, the first 12 clinical and experimental research papers of the Society for Adolescent Medicine were presented at the Chicago, Illinois, meeting on October 20, 1973. In 1976, again through the efforts of Cohen, the American Pediatric Society and The Society for Pediatric Research created a session for research papers on adolescent medicine.

In 1977, the American Board of Pediatrics developed a 3-year core curriculum in pediatrics that included adolescent medicine. In 1979, the American Academy of Pediatrics created a Section on Adolescent Health. In 1979, the Maternal and Child Health section of the Department of Health and Human Services funded eight training centers for interdisciplinary adolescent health care.

In 1980, the *Journal of Adolescent Health Care* became the official publication of the Society. The 1980s were characterized by increased funding for the delivery of adolescent medicine at a national level. The Robert Wood Johnson Foundation funded an initiative in adolescent health care, linking health services in academic centers and local health agencies in 1982. In 1986, the Robert Wood Johnson Foundation funded a program to establish school-based clinics for adolescents. These clinics created considerable controversy because of the concern of community leaders and parents about the distribution of contraceptive knowledge or devices in public schools. Another area of concern was the possible disruption of already existing primary care services to adolescents, with the potential for minimal communication between school-based clinic providers and primary care physicians (see Chapter 18).

National debate during the 1980s over controversial teenage issues (adolescent consent for sexuality-related services, including abortion, financing of adolescent health care, and access to services) resulted in several national reviews of adolescent development and adolescent health. The American Medical Association's House of Delegates issued a report on adolescent health and passed a resolution about adolescent health care, establishing an initiative focused on research and education in adolescent health care. In June 1988, this initiative was formalized with the development of a Department of Adolescent Health.

In 1987, the Carnegie Foundation established a Council on Adolescent Development. The Council's initiatives resulted in the publication of three books about adolescent issues. In addition, a number of position papers have been published. The Congress of the United States directed the Office of Technology Assessment to study the health status of adolescents, which published a report in April 1991.

By 1990, adolescent medicine had become well established on the American medical scene. Certification of adolescent medicine as a subspecialty has now been approved, and development of sub-boards is proceeding. The increasing body of research knowledge, the presence of adolescent training programs in most major medical centers, the influence of the leaders in adolescent medicine on national policy, the federal government's involvement in adolescent health care at many levels, and the interest on the part of primary care practitioners in caring for adolescents all testify to the maturation of a movement that now has become part of the nation's medical and societal agenda.

Acknowledgments: The author wishes to thank Dr. Joseph Rauh for supplying historical material about the seminars and the Society for Adolescent Medicine. Dr. Michael I. Cohen supplied additional information and many of the key dates used to identify significant events in the more recent history of adolescent medicine. This chapter would not have been possible without their cooperation and help. Heather Prescott's scholarly work on the history of adolescent health care is gratefully appreciated.

BIBLIOGRAPHY

Dorfman RI, Greulich WW, Solomon CI: The excretion of androgenic and estrogenic substances in the urine of children. Endocrinology 21:741, 1937.

Gallagher JR: The origins, development and goals of adolescent medicine. J Adolesc Health Care 3:57, 1982.

Greulich WW, Dorfman RI, Catchpole HR, et al: Somatic and endocrine studies of puberal and adolescent boys. Monogr Soc Child Dev 7(3):1, 1942.

Johnston JA: Nutritional Studies in Adolescent Girls and Their Relation to Tuberculosis. Springfield, IL, Charles C Thomas, 1953.

Kett JF: Rites of Passage: Adolescence in America 1790 to the Present. New York, Basic Books, Inc, 1977.

Mitchell AG: Symposium on adolescence. J Pediatr 19:289, 1941.

Prescott HM: Medicine tackles the problems of growing up: The emergence of adolescent medicine as a clinical sub-field, 1950–70. Unpublished paper presented at the American Association for the History of Medicine Annual Meeting, Baltimore, MD, May 12, 1990.

Pryor HB: Certain physical and physiologic aspects of adolescent development in girls. J Pediatr 8:52, 1936.

Reynolds EL, Wines JV: Individual differences in physical changes associated with adolescence in girls. Am J Dis Child 75:329, 1948.

Society for Adolescent Medicine Newsletter. Garell DC (ed). Vol 1, February 1965.

Society for Adolescent Medicine Newsletter. Garell DC (ed). Vol 3, December 1967.

Tanner JM: Growth at Adolescence, 2nd ed. Oxford, Blackwell Scientific Publications, 1962.

US Congress, Office of Technology Assessment: Adolescent Health, Vol 1: Summary and Policy Options, OTA-H-468. Washington, DC, Government Printing Office, 1991.

Wait B, Roberts LJ: Studies in the food requirement of adolescent girls. III. The protein intake of well-nourished girl 10 to 16 years of age. J Am Diet Assoc 8:403, 1932.

Zeek P: Juvenile atherosclerosis. Arch Pathol 10:417, 1930.

Publications on Adolescence, 1904–1918

Hall GS: Adolescence: Its Psychology and Its Relationship to Physiology, Anthropology, Sociology, Sex, Crime, Religion and Education. 2 vols. New York, D. Appleton & Co, 1904.

Jastrow J: The natural history of adolescence. Popular Science Monthly 66:457–465, 1904–5.

Baldwin BT: Adolescence. Psychol Bull 10:197–419, 1913.

Fuller FM: Adolescence, its relation to primary and secondary disease. J Iowa State M Soc 4:369–374, 1914–15.

Mapes CC: The ethics of adolescence. Urology and Cutaneous Review 21:130–132, 1917.

Baldwin BT: Adolescence. Psychol Bull 14:336–340, 1917.

Gates AE: The work of the adolescent clinic of Stanford University Medical School. Arch Pediatr 35:236–243, 1918.

Bridgman OL: Some special problems in abnormal adolescent psychology. Med Press 106:118–122, 1918.

Bridgman OL: Some special problems in abnormal adolescent psychology. Arch Pediatr 35:172–181, 1918.

1941 American Academy of Pediatrics' Presentations in New Haven, Connecticut, and Chicago, Illinois

General Considerations. Certain Problems of Puberty and Adolescence. Lawrence K. Frank, New York, NY, Vice-President, Josiah Macy, Jr., Foundation.

Some Observations on the Growth and Development of Adolescent Children. William W. Greulich, Ph.D., Cleveland, OH, Director of the Brush Foundation, Western Reserve University.

Examination of the Adolescent Female. Joseph L. Baer, M.D., Chicago, IL, Professor of Obstetrics and Gynecology, Rush Medical School.

Menstrual Abnormalities of Adolescence. E.L. Sevringhaus, M.D., Madison, WI, Professor of Medicine, University of Wisconsin.

Endocrine Problems in Adolescence. Ephraim Shorr, M.D., New York, NY, Assistant Professor of Medicine, Cornell University Medical College.

The Standard Metabolism of Adolescence. Bruce Webster, M.D., Helen Harrington, and L.M. Wright, New York, NY, Department of Medicine, New York Hospital, and Cornell University Medical College.

Obesity in Relation to Puberty. Hilde Bruch, M.D., New York, NY, Department of Pediatrics, College of Physicians and Surgeons, Columbia University.

What to Do About the Fat Child at Puberty. Fred W. Schultz, M.D., Chicago, IL, Professor of Pediatrics, University of Chicago.

Athletic Activity at Puberty, with Special Reference to the Cardiac and Tuberculous Patient. Stanley Gibson, M.D., Chicago, IL, Professor of Pediatrics, Northwestern University.

Sexual Education of the Adolescent. George Mohr, M.D., Chicago, IL, Associate Professor, Department of Criminology, University of Illinois.

Psychologic Aspects of Adolescence. Douglas A. Thom, M.D., Boston, MA, Director of the Habit Clinic for Child Guidance.

SCIENTIFIC BASIS OF

ADOLESCENT MEDICINE

Introduction

Adolescence is usually defined as the period of rapid physical and psychological growth and development occurring during the second decade of life. Adolescent medicine focuses on the medical, psychological, and social care of adolescents.

The growth of modern adolescent medicine has resulted from several occurrences. They include early observations about the biologic and psychological differences of adolescents as compared with children and adults; fascination with the process of adolescent growth and development, including the profound changes resulting from puberty; and most recently, the remarkable changes in modern society, including technologic breakthroughs in science and medicine and profound changes in the family, the economy, and the world, all of which have had a major impact on adolescents and on the science of and practice of adolescent medicine.

The first part of this text provides the scientific background of adolescent medicine. The scope of the content is broad, as it moves from a section on the demography of adolescence to chapters containing the most sophisticated modern science of adolescent medicine.

The first two chapters in Section I provide data on the demography of adolescence, both nationally and internationally. The national data portray a somber picture. Despite what is perceived as the relatively "healthy" status of adolescents as a group, violence has resulted in untoward morbidity and mortality among our youngest most vital citizens, who have potentially many productive years ahead. Steps to prevent morbidity and mortality from violence must be taken by the family, the schools, and the community. Early and unprotected sexual activity perpetuates the dilemmas of adolescent pregnancy and sexually transmitted diseases, including acquired immunodeficiency syndrome (AIDS). Adolescent pregnancy has consequences for the vulnerable, often uneducated adolescent parents, their offspring, and society. Sexually transmitted diseases account for morbidity in adolescents such as subsequent infertility and ectopic pregnancies, and pain and suffering for the infected. The specter of AIDS is one of the gravest facing modern society. Of those who become infected during adolescence with the human immunodeficiency virus (HIV), many become symptomatic and die in their 20s.

Many adolescents who experience violent behaviors are the same young people who initiate early sexual activity. Substance use is also a part of the culture of these young people, with all its attendant morbidity for those using the substances and for society, against which crimes are perpetrated to support the use of expensive, dangerous drugs.

The international data are perhaps somewhat less graphic than the national data, as they are not always as readily available as data are in the United States. The problems of high-risk youth, however, are becoming international in scope, defying geographic borders and cultural traditions. As developing countries move toward development, their youth become increasingly vulnerable to the influences of modern society.

The chapters in the Sections II and III address what is known about the biology of and behavioral issues of adolescent development. We have learned a great deal recently about the neuroendocrine regulation of puberty. Despite the vast knowledge we now have about the complexities of the neuroendocrine control of puberty, we still are challenged to understand exactly why puberty begins when it does for individual adolescents. We do know, however, vastly more than previously about the relationship between the central nervous system and the endocrine end-organs. Understanding of the somatic development of adolescents has gradually increased over the years, with in-depth observations of and study of the growth of many adolescents: the secular trend of adolescent growth, the sequence of appearance of secondary sexual changes, and the definition of sexual maturity ratings (SMR). The topics covered in the chapters on nutrition and growth and nutritional requirements are central to our appreciation of the importance of and our understanding of growth and nutrition during adolescence. As noted, the rate of adolescent growth is a sensitive indicator of adolescent nutritional status.

Behavioral issues and the psychological development of adolescence have filled volumes. The question of whether adolescents are by nature distressed psychologically is addressed in the chapter on normality during adolescence. The overall conclusion is that, indeed, most adolescents are not psychologically distressed; that is, the implication should not be that adolescence and distress are synonymous, as recent studies do not support that historical notion. The complexities of psychological and social development are discussed in detail in the next chapter. The complexities result from the ongoing processes of independence, identity formation, sexual identity, social skills, and cognitive development. Cognitive development that transforms the early adolescent's abilities from concrete operational, present-oriented capacities to the late adolescent's formal operational, insightful, future-oriented capacities is among the most dramatic transformations in human development. Often the most creative and the highest levels of cognitive capabilities are developed during adolescence. The chapter on cognitive neuroscience illustrates the application of modern technology to our understanding of this most fascinating portion of human development.

Section IV provides the reader with an overview of some of the most exciting scientific areas in adolescent medicine. The topics were chosen because they combine data from the biologic sciences and the behavioral sciences in a way that is uniquely the challenge of adolescent medicine—the interface between adolescent biology and behavior. Using the most sophisticated scientific techniques in biology and in the social sciences, topics such as neurotransmitters, stress, and depression; hormones and behavior; stress and the immune system; primate models and adolescence; and pain in adolescents are explored. These topics provide a glimpse of what the future science of adolescent medicine holds.

In future volumes, we expect that not only will there be more known about these most important areas, but also there will be more known in areas such as the etiology and prevention of violent behaviors; the etiology and prevention of addiction to substances such as alcohol, marijuana, and cocaine; the etiology and prevention of cardiovascular diseases, including congenital heart disease; and the etiology and prevention of genetic diseases such as cystic fibrosis and the degenerative neurologic conditions that adversely affect the lives of adolescents and young adults on the verge of productive adult lives. We also expect that we shall know more about the etiology of mental disorders such as the affective disorders that have a genetic basis and that become manifest during the second decade of life.

The world of adolescent medicine, like all areas in medicine, is exploding with new challenges, new hope, and new directions. In this background section, we hope to set the stage for what follows in the subsequent sections of the book: the clinical approach to adolescents, medical conditions, and psychological issues.

SECTION I

Demographic Profile

CHAPTER 2

United States Profile

CLAIRE D. BRINDIS, CHARLES E. IRWIN JR., and SUSAN G. MILLSTEIN

INTRODUCTION

Adolescence is often perceived as one of the healthiest periods in the life cycle. An increasing body of knowledge raises concerns about this perception. Profiles of adolescents and their health status have undergone dramatic changes during the past 3 decades, and these shifts have major implications for health care providers. In the past, the absence of adequate data sources and the failure of documentation to differentiate the chronologic adolescent years (defined as ranging from ages 10 to 19 to reflect the earlier physical maturation of young people and its extension until the years of early adulthood) from children in other age groups or from young adults have often masked the health conditions of youth. More recent research, however, has begun to document the distinct and unique mortality and morbidity patterns of adolescents.

Several limitations remain in the available data. The first is that currently available population-based surveys generally utilize secondary informants to document the health status of adolescents. For example, the National Health Interview Survey, which provides much helpful information on the health status of the adolescent population, is restricted because it uses interviews with parents, usually the adolescent's mother, to ascertain the adolescent's health status and health utilization patterns. While parents may be a source of information, they may not be aware of a number of health problems that adolescents may experience or of the self-perception of health status, and furthermore they may not know that their children may have sought confidential health services. The National Ambulatory Care Survey is also used to describe the health care utilization patterns of adolescents, relying primarily on survey data based on the experiences of physicians working in private practice ambulatory settings. Thus, the health status of adolescents seeking care in hospital-based or community-based clinic settings is excluded from this profile (see Chapter 18). In addition, the health status of institutionalized (incarcerated [see Chapter 34] and residential-based)

adolescents represents another gap in the documentation of adolescent health.

A second problem relates to the limited number of adolescent populations that are included for studies. Data are often collected on accessible populations, for example, adolescents attending school, whereas out-of-school youth or those absent who may be experiencing higher rates of morbidity may be overlooked. For example, national surveys documenting the use of substances and other risk behaviors are often conducted in school settings and do not reach other populations at risk.

A third problem occurs because there has been little consensus regarding what ages constitute adolescence, and as a result, data may be reported regarding different age cohorts (e.g., 5 to 14, 10 to 19, and 12 to 17). Furthermore, many data bases aggregate adolescents with young adults, for example, 15 to 24 years. Finally, minimal data exist that consider differences inherent within the developmental phases of adolescence. For example, few studies use comparisons between early (ages 10 to 14), middle (ages 15 to 17), and late (ages 18 to 21) adolescence (see Chapter 9).

Although many adolescents avoid the health problems of older people, their generally healthy state is compromised by the health consequences of risk behaviors, including the combination of alcohol and substance use (see Chapter 111) with unsafe driving, interpersonal violence (see Chapter 117) and access to weapons, and early initiation of sexual activity (see Chapter 68). For adolescents, health problems are frequently medical manifestations of problems that have social, economic, or behavioral causes. For example, injuries, suicides, and homicides account for 80% of all deaths among adolescents.

This chapter presents a demographic profile of adolescents, including future population projections and a population overview; descriptive data on their mortality and morbidity patterns; a profile of their health care utilization patterns; patterns of substance use and abuse; a profile of their sexual and contraceptive behavior, adolescent pregnancy, and sexually transmitted diseases; and the interrelationship of risk behavior profiles. For the purposes of this chapter, chronologic age (ages 10 to 19) is used as the definition of the adolescent years. When possible, we have reported the data by ages 10 to 14 and 15 to 19, reflecting the important differences between early and late adolescence. Whenever data analyzed have not been aggregated in these age groups,

---

Because persons of Hispanic origin have been classified into any one of the three racial groups and because they are most frequently classified as white, Hispanics have often been hidden as a distinct minority population. With special adjustments to Bureau of the Census data, Hispanics can be disaggregated from the estimates of the white population so that the size of their population can be more carefully documented.

these data will be reported as close to this adolescent age breakdown as possible. Racial and ethnic data, focusing primarily on the three most prevalent populations living in the United States (whites, blacks, and Hispanics), have also been reported whenever available.

CURRENT AND FUTURE POPULATIONS

Population Overview

The size, age, and racial and ethnic composition of the adolescent population will undergo major changes during the 1990s. In 1990, the number of adolescents ages 10 to 19 decreased to 33.8 million from a total of 35.7 million in 1985. This trend will reverse during the 1990s, and the adolescent population will reach a peak of 38.3 million in the year 2000 (US Bureau of the Census, 1984, 1986a). In spite of the increase in absolute numbers, adolescents will constitute a lower proportion of the overall population by 2000. The adolescent population as a relative percentage of the total population fell from 14.8% in 1985 to 13.5% in 1990 and will rise to 14.3% by 2000. This trend reflects the increasing numbers of aging post–World War II baby boomers in the population (Fig. 2–1).

In addition, the age composition of the adolescent population will change in important ways between 1980 and 2000, with decreases among older adolescents (ages 15 to 19) and increases among younger adolescents (ages

10 to 14). The older adolescent population is expected to decline by 11.0%, compared with a 7.0% increase among younger adolescents. As a result, the adolescent population in the year 2000 will be a younger one than it is today (US Bureau of the Census, 1984) (Table 2–1).

The racial and ethnic composition of the adolescent population is changing. Demographers expect that by the year 2000, 31.2% of the adolescent population will be composed of individuals of a racial or ethnic minority group, as compared with 25.6% of the total population. In 1985, minorities constituted 26.9% of the adolescent population, as compared with 21.8% of the total population. Overall, minority groups will grow at a faster rate than other population segments, reaching 20% to 25% of the total population in 1990, as compared with 17% in 1980.

Population pattern shifts will occur for blacks, whites, and Hispanics. Between 1985 and the year 2000, there will be an increase of 16% in the total number of black adolescents, with the greatest increase occurring in the younger age group (ages 10 to 14). Although the absolute numbers of black adolescents will increase, their rates of growth will be smaller than those for Hispanic and Asian youth. Thus, although blacks will continue to be the largest group among the adolescent minority population, their overall proportion will decrease from 55% in 1985 to 52% in 2000. Projections also indicate that the white adolescent population will increase in size by 1%. There will be a 42% increase in the overall number of Hispanic adolescents, and as a result, they will represent approximately 11.9% of the adolescent population (Table 2–2, Fig. 2–2). The growth among Hispanics reflects both an increased number of new immigrants and improvements in the manner in which Hispanics are accounted for in the population (US Bureau of the Census, 1986).

In addition, as a result of Asian migration, demographers also estimate that, in the year 2000, 11% of all school-age children will be of Asian or Pacific Island descent (Millstein, Irwin, and Brindis, 1991).

These ethnic and racial shifts reflect a significant demographic change in the number of new immigrants. Since 1970, nearly 400,000 legal immigrants have entered the country each year. In addition, an estimated 250,000 to 400,000 enter the country each year as undocumented immigrants. The sum of these numbers is almost as large as the numbers entering during the great waves of immigration at the turn of the century. Compounding the effect of the wave of new immigration is the younger age of immigrant groups as the result of high fertility rates (McCarthy, 1983). In contrast to the low birth and death rates for the overall population, the Hispanic population is increasing dramatically. Because of large influxes of Spanish-speaking immigrant populations and their high fertility rates, demographers predict that Hispanics will increase from 4.5 million in 1980 to 13.6 million by 2030. Hispanics are a young population with a median age of 23.1, as compared with 34.4 for non-Hispanic whites in 1980 (McCarthy, 1983).

Thus, a variety of factors will have a dramatic effect on the evolving profile of American adolescents. Increasing our understanding of cultural differences that

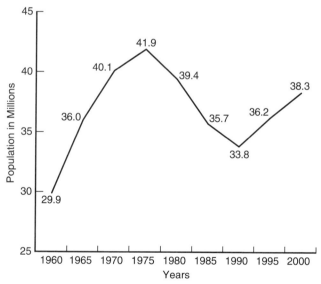

Figure 2–1. Actual and projected adolescent population, ages 10–19 years; 1960–2000 (in millions). Data from 1960–1985 are enumerated; data after 1985 are estimated. (Sources: Millstein SG, Irwin CE, Jr, Brindis CD: Sociodemographic trends and projections in the adolescent population. In Hendee WR (ed): The Health of Adolescents. San Francisco, Jossey-Bass, 1991; US Bureau of the Census. Current Population Reports, Series P-25, No. 985, Estimates of the Population of the United States, by Age, Sex, and Race: 1980–1985. Washington, DC, US Government Printing Office, 1986; US Bureau of the Census. Current Population Reports, Series P-25, No. 952, Projections of the Population of the United States, by Age, Sex, and Race: 1983 to 2080. Washington, DC, US Government Printing Office, 1984.)

TABLE 2–1. Number* of Adolescents in Thousands (Ages 10–14, 15–19, and 10–19) by Sex in 5-Year Intervals, 1980–2000

YEAR	AGE 10–14		AGE 15–19		AGE 10–19 (TOTAL)	
	Female	Male	Female	Male	Female	Male
1980	8923	9314	10,382	10,776	19,305	20,090
1985	8340	8762	9110	9477	17,450	18,239
1990	8207	8586	8299	8670	16,506	17,256
1995	9170	9602	8300	9170	17,470	18,772
2000	9532	9986	9262	9532	18,794	19,518

*Numbers for 1980 and 1985 are estimates; after 1985, the numbers represent projections.
Sources: US Bureau of the Census: Estimates of the Population of the United States, by Age, Sex, and Race: 1980 to 1985. Current Population Reports, Series P-25, No. 985. Washington, DC, US Government Printing Office, 1986; US Bureau of the Census: Projections of the Population of the United States, by Age, Sex, and Race: 1983 to 2080. Current Population Reports, Series P-25, No. 952. Washington, DC, US Government Printing Office, 1984.

affect health, health seeking, and health utilizing behaviors will be an important component of the way the health system responds to these demographic changes (see Chapter 28).

Location of Future Adolescent Population

While the rate of the population growth has slowed, migration within the United States has become increasingly significant for adolescents and their families. For economic, social, and climatic reasons, there has been a significant shifting from the North and Midwest to the South and West. As of 1990, 19% of Americans live in the West, and the South has over 30% of the United States population. The states expected to grow most dramatically by the year 2000 are Florida, California, Texas, Arizona, Colorado, Washington, Oregon, Utah, New Mexico, Hawaii, Idaho, and Nevada. Population changes in different racial and ethnic groups will also affect growth in particular parts of the country. Among Hispanics, approximately two thirds of youth will reside in three states: California, New York, and Texas. Within

the Hispanic population, there will be variations in residence among immigrants from different Latin American countries. For example, California and Texas will continue to be the home for Mexican-Americans and Central Americans, and New York will have larger numbers of adolescents who are Puerto Rican and Dominican Republican (US Immigration and Naturalization Service, 1987).

As of 1980, the majority of adolescents resided in metropolitan areas, reflecting areas that included either a city of at least 50,000 or a Census Bureau–defined urbanized area of at least 50,000 with a total population area of at least 100,000. Twenty-eight percent of teenagers were living in large central cities (Millstein, Irwin, and Brindis, 1991). Urban cities are the ones most likely to be populated by adolescents reflecting different racial and ethnic minority groups. In 1980, 56% of black youth (ages 15 to 24) lived in central cities, as compared with 23% of white youth. Because of economic factors and decreasing opportunities to work in more rural areas, these trends are expected to continue into the twenty-first century, especially among minority youth who have recently migrated to the United States.

Economic Status

Although the proportion of adolescents in the total population will somewhat diminish, it is probable that their health care needs will actually increase, primarily as a result of the changing economic conditions of adolescents and the increasing number of adolescents who reside in single-parent families. The percentages of families headed by one parent increased from 19.5% in 1980 to 26.1% in 1985, reflecting high rates of divorce and separation as well as a higher incidence of out-of-wedlock births. Single-parent families are likely to have low incomes, partly as a result of pay inequities faced by women and lack of paternal financial support. On average, single-parent households have about 40% less income than two-parent families. Fewer than one half of all children living with their mothers received child support from their fathers (Glick, 1984).

In 1988, the percentage of children younger than 6 years of age living in poverty grew to 23%, with the highest rates among black and Hispanic children (Bane and Ellwood, 1989). In 1987, among adolescents and young adults ages 14 to 21, 15.9% lived below the

TABLE 2–2. Racial and Hispanic Ethnicity Distribution of Total Population and Adolescents (Ages 10–19): 1985 and 2000

RACE/ETHNICITY	% OF TOTAL POPULATION		% OF ADOLESCENTS 10–19	
	1985	2000	1985	2000
Black	11.8	12.9	14.8	16.0
Hispanic	7.2	9.4	9.0	11.9
White	78.2	74.4	73.1	68.8
Other	2.8	3.3	3.1	3.3
	100.0	100.0	100.0	100.0

For blacks, whites, and others, percentages are based on estimates for 1985 and projections for 2000. For Hispanics, percentages are based on projections for both 1985 and 2000. Middle-series projections were used for all calculations.
Sources: US Bureau of the Census: Projections of the Population of the United States, by Age, Sex, and Race: 1983 to 2080. Current Population Reports, Series P-25, No. 952. Washington, DC, US Government Printing Office, 1984; US Bureau of the Census: Estimates of the Population of the United States, by Age, Sex, and Race: 1980 to 1985. Current Population Reports, Series P-25, No. 985. Washington, DC, US Government Printing Office, 1986; US Bureau of the Census: Projections of the Hispanic Population: 1983 to 2080. Current Population Reports, Series P-25, No. 995. Washington, DC, US Government Printing Office, 1986.

Figure 2–2. Racial and ethnic distribution of Adolescents, 1985–2000. (Sources: US Bureau of the Census, Current Population Reports, Series P-25, Nos. 952, 985, and 995. US Government Printing Office, Washington, DC, 1984–86; Millstein SG, Irwin CE, Jr, Brindis CD: Sociodemographic trends and projections in the adolescent population. In Hendee WR (ed): The Health of Adolescents. San Francisco, Jossey-Bass, 1991.)

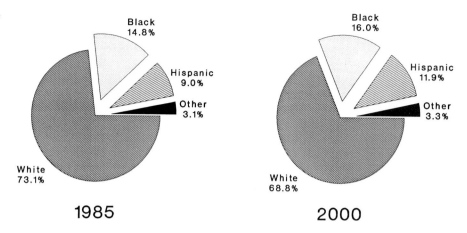

1985

2000

poverty line, compared with 13.9% in 1980 (Bureau of the Census, 1987, cited by Rosen et al, 1990). It is estimated that there will be more than 20 million children (18 years of age or younger) living in poverty by the year 2020, representing an increase of about 37% since 1985. These trends are already becoming apparent in the last decades of the twentieth century. In 1987, 37.6% of black youth and 30.2% of Hispanic youth ages 14 to 21 were impoverished by federal standards, compared with 11.8% among white youth (Bureau of the Census, 1987, cited by Rosen et al, 1990).

The picture for young families is also bleak, as a result of the poor economic outlook for many young adults. Less than one half of males aged 20 to 24 earn above the three-person poverty level (reflecting a male, female partner, and one child), with minority youth earning the lowest wages. The proportion of young families (head of household younger than 25 years of age) whose income was below the poverty level rose to 32.6% in 1986, an increase of more than one third over 1979 (William T. Grant Commission, 1988). This profile often reflects the high levels of unemployment among adolescents, which has risen dramatically over the past 35 years. Between 1950 and 1980, the unemployment rate for 16- to 19-year-olds increased from 12.2% to 17.8%, compared with rates among adults of 4.4% to 5.1%. Black adolescents experienced even higher rates of unemployment, with 40% of black youth unemployed in 1984.

As a result of labor force participation and greater levels of economic dependence when children are younger, adolescents constitute slightly more than one third of the 7 million children whose families receive benefits from the largest social service program, Aid to Families with Dependent Children (AFDC). The increasing numbers of poor children reflect, in part, an increase in the proportion of Hispanic children who are living in poverty, which rose to 40% in 1985. In addition, there is a significant contrast between Hispanic populations that reflects their national origin, with 42% of Hispanics from Puerto Rico living in poverty in 1985, compared with 24% of Mexicans and Central and South Americans and 13% of Cubans living in poverty. This increase in poverty is taking place among the fastest growing population group and will therefore be associated with greater overall levels of poverty among youth in the future (Millstein, Irwin, and Brindis, 1991).

There is a strong relationship between poverty and health status. As shown in the 1983 and 1984 National Health Interview Surveys, adolescents living in families with incomes below the poverty level are three times as likely to be reported in only fair or poor health (see Chapter 18), and are 47% more likely to suffer from disabling chronic illnesses (see Chapter 30) than adolescents living in families with incomes above the poverty level. Use of inpatient hospital services was similar in adolescents from poor and nonpoor families when health status was controlled. However, adolescents from poor families were 35% more likely than those from nonpoor families to have waited 2 or more years between physician contacts. In addition, poor adolescents made 13% fewer physician contacts on an annual basis when compared with nonpoor adolescents (Newacheck, 1989b).

Family Structure and Living Conditions

In the United States, the family is undergoing major changes in its composition, and children and adolescents often experience the consequences of these changes. Increases in the numbers of divorces and separations and the incidence of children born to unmarried women have resulted in larger numbers of youth being raised in nontraditional families. For example, using census data one author projects that 59% of the children born in 1983 will live with only one parent before reaching age 18, creating important changes in the life experiences of the majority of children and adolescents (Hodgkinson, 1985). Decreases in the proportion of families classified as intact (those comprising two parents raising children in the same home) have occurred across all racial and ethnic groups, although their proportions differ significantly. In 1985, 80% of white children (18 years and younger) were living with both parents, compared with 67.8% of Hispanic children and 39.5% of black children. As previously stated, an important consequence of living in a single-parent household is the economic impact. Of children from single-parent, female-headed households, the percentage (age 18 and younger) being raised in poverty was 53.6%, more than twice the overall rate (US Bureau of the Census, 1986b). The economic consequences are most damaging among minorities who raise their children in single-parent homes. Among children being raised in single-parent families headed by a Hispanic female, 72.5% were living in poverty; among children from families with black female heads of household the percentage was 66.9%; and among non-Hispanic whites the proportion was 37.0%. Minorities living in nonmetropolitan areas fare even worse. Seventy-five percent of black single-parent families residing in nonmetropolitan areas live below the poverty line, as do 67.3% of Hispanics (US Bureau of the Census, 1986c).

The "traditional" United States family consisting of a working father, a housewife mother, and two or more school-age children is becoming an anomaly, reflecting the profile of only 7% of American homes in 1985. As a result of job opportunities, the economic necessity of employment, particularly for single heads of household, and changes in the labor market for women, more than 70% of mothers with children between the ages of 6 and 17 were in the job market by the end of the 1980s. Limited and often expensive child care available to these families creates an at-risk situation for early adolescents, with over three quarters of the 13- to 14-year-old adolescents in the United States left in self-care with a younger sibling for more than 10 hours a week. This trend seems certain to continue.

Alternative Living Conditions

Although the majority of adolescents live in related family units, a significant minority of youth live in nonfamily situations. In 1985, more than 6% of adolescents lived in alternative living situations, including 3.2% of adolescents between the ages of 15 and 19 who were married and living with their spouse, 2.8% who were living with unrelated individuals, and 0.7% who were living alone (US Bureau of the Census, 1989).

In addition, approximately 500,000 youth younger than 22 years of age are placed in correctional institutions each year (see Chapter 34). On any given day, almost 50,000 youth are in detention. Almost 13,500 nonoffenders are held in juvenile custody facilities. A profile of juveniles held in custody indicates that the majority are males (87%), white (57%), and between the ages of 14 and 17 years (81%). Racial and ethnic minorities are overrepresented in correctional institutions, with black youth between the ages of 15 and 19 years being four times more likely than white youth to be placed there.

The proportion of juveniles placed in custody has been rising, from a rate of 167 per 100,000 in 1979, to a rate of 185 per 100,000 in 1985. It is likely that these rates will continue to increase, given the large numbers of adolescents who will live in poor, metropolitan areas and who have limited educational and employment opportunities (Wetzel, 1987).

Youth in military service also reflects a primarily male profile: 90% of the youth serving in the armed forces are male (see Chapter 29). The military attracts an adolescent and young adult population; 55% of recruits and soldiers are between the ages of 16 and 24 years. Black youth are more likely to serve than are white youth; among 16- to 24-year-old males, 6.8% of blacks and 4.9% of whites are in the military service. No comparable data are available on Hispanics.

An additional group of adolescents living in nontraditional settings includes the estimated 1 million adolescents who are runaways or homeless (see Chapter 33). While data documenting this number are inadequate, their numbers appear to be increasing (Rosen et al, 1990). A 1983 study by the Office of the Inspector General of the Department of Health and Human Services estimated that 558,000 runaway and homeless teenagers made contact mostly with nongovernmental agencies in the preceding year (US Department of Health and Human Services, 1983). This finding clearly indicates a fraction of the total number of adolescents, since many are never reported as missing and many others have no contact with agencies.

EDUCATION

As cited in the William T. Grant Foundation's report of 1987, nearly 86% of 25- to 29-year-olds are high school graduates, compared with only 38% in 1940. The breakdown by race is 86.5% of whites, 82.5% of blacks, and about 70% of Hispanics (US Bureau of the Census, 1987a).

Across the country, almost 3 out of 10 students who enter high school will not graduate, however, resulting in approximately 700,000 students dropping out of school each year. Without even a basic high school diploma, adolescents severely restrict their future opportunities, often resulting in higher rates of unemployment, lower yearly and lifelong earnings, and ultimately dependence on public assistance. School dropouts also experience poorer health outcomes than do individuals who complete at least high school. The highest rate of dropouts occurs among those who are from minority groups, are poor, live in inner cities, and live in the western and southern states.

Data from the High School and Beyond Survey document a dropout rate of 29% in Native Americans, 18% in blacks, 17% in Hispanics, 12% in whites, and 3% in Asians. Other analyses that consider wider time spans than "high school and beyond" show the dropout rate to be 35% in Hispanic youth, 24% in blacks, and 18% in whites. Differences also exist within subgroups of the Hispanic population; higher dropout rates exist in the Cuban and Mexican-American subgroups. Poverty is a more significant predictor of school dropout rates than is either ethnicity or race. A 1985 comparison of dropout rates among poor 18- to 21-year-olds showed that 56% of the poor black youth, compared with 53% of the poor white youth, failed to graduate from high school (Millstein, Irwin, and Brindis, 1991).

Youth at risk for school dropout often begin their pattern of truancy and disengagement from the educational system long before they actually leave or are "pushed" out of school. Poor children often enter school with academic backgrounds poorer than those of their economically advantaged peers. Children whose academic performance is poor have a much greater chance of dropping out of school. The gap widens as students progress through school; there are an estimated 1.4 million students who are enrolled 2 or more years below their expected grade level. As a result of language barriers, migration and immigration patterns, and other factors, such as poverty, Hispanic youth experience the highest incidence of school delay, with 10% of Hispanic children between the ages of 8 and 13 years and 25% of those between 14 and 20 being held back a grade in school.

HEALTH CARE UTILIZATION

Acute and Chronic Medical Care

Adolescents are in relatively good physical health compared with adults, who have greater numbers of chronic conditions. For the most part, adolescents experience fewer short-term hospital stays, have fewer days when they stay home sick in bed, and are more likely to be assessed in excellent or very good health than are children and adults (Adams and Hardy, 1989). Among adolescents, acute nonfatal injuries account for the largest number of hospital days for both males and females, excluding pregnancy, and for approximately 16% of ambulatory visits.

Office-based visits are frequent (245 visits per 100 children) for children younger than 11 years of age, whereas the frequency for early adolescents ages 11 to 14 decreases to 140 per 100 (see Chapters 17 and 18). The number of visits gradually increases throughout the life span to a rate of 438 visits per 100 persons for the elderly (65 years and older). Nonwhite children and adolescents on average have fewer office visits than do white children and adolescents. The mean number of medical care visits for white children and youth from birth to 18 years of age was 3.7 in 1980, compared with 2.1 for blacks and 2.4 for Hispanics. The pattern of physician visit utilization by gender changes after age 15, with females visiting physician's offices more frequently than do males, primarily related to reproductive health issues (see Section XVII). Pediatricians and family practitioners care for the largest numbers of early adolescents in their practices; family physicians, obstetricians/gynecologists, dermatologists, and pediatricians see the largest numbers of patients during the late adolescent age period (see Chapter 17).

There is a strong relationship between poverty and access to health care. The highest number of visits (3.6) was for those children and youth (18 years old and younger) who live in families above 200% of poverty. The lowest number (2.6) was for children and youth in families between 100% to 150% of poverty, who are least likely to have either private or public insurance. Children (18 years and younger) whose family's income is under $10,000 are nearly seven times more likely to be in fair or poor health than are children in families with incomes over $35,000. Children in poverty are 2.5 times more likely to be limited in a daily activity, such as going to school, because of a chronic condition (Adams and Hardy, 1989).

The percentage of uninsured children and early adolescents (ages 5 to 14) has increased from 11.7% in 1980 to 15.3% in 1986. Lack of insurance is higher among late adolescents (ages 15 to 18) than early adolescents (ages 10 to 14) (17.1% vs. 13.8%), owing to a lack of both public and private coverage (Adams and Hardy, 1989) (see Chapters 21 and 35). On average, adolescents aged 10 to 18 years accumulated annual medical care charges of $525 in 1988 dollars. Families paid an average of $151 (29%) of total charges out-of-pocket for each adolescent, and the remaining expenses were paid by insurance or other payment resources (Newacheck and McManus, 1990). Mean charges per year for medical care are twice as high for older adolescents (ages 15 to 18) as for younger adolescents (ages 10 to 14) ($720 vs. $349 per year). On average, white adolescents had medical expenses twice those of nonwhites ($573 for whites, as compared with $289 for nonwhites).

Adolescents living in families with incomes below the poverty level experienced substantially higher charges for medical services than those in families with incomes above the poverty line ($768 for those living below the poverty line, as compared with $491 for those living above the poverty line) (Newacheck and McManus, 1990). Payment for health care varies substantially according to the setting in which health care is delivered; traditional health insurance coverage is more generous in paying for inpatient hospital bills as compared with ambulatory services or nonphysician services (e.g., counseling services). Thus, the average share of medical care bills paid out-of-pocket ranged from only 15% for inpatient hospital services to 74% for other medical items, such as medical equipment and supplies (Newacheck and McManus, 1990).

Nearly 2 million adolescents ages 10 to 18 (6%) have a serious chronic condition (Newacheck, 1989a). The leading source of chronic disability for adolescents is some form of mental disorder, which affects 634,000 adolescents. The majority of these adolescents are either learning disabled or mentally retarded, with a small proportion experiencing a severe emotional or psychological disorder (Newacheck, 1989a) (see Chapters 30 and 31).

White children younger than 18 years of age were more likely than black children to have more days of limited activities due to poor health, spend more days in bed because of health reasons, and miss more days of school for health reasons (Adams and Hardy, 1989; Newacheck, 1989a). However, rates of activity limitation are very similar for black and white children younger than 18 years of age. Children and adolescents in poverty have twice as many short-term hospital stays and 1.6 times more disability days in which they miss school, compared with youth in families with incomes over $35,000 per year (Adams and Hardy, 1989). Among 12- to 14-year-olds, whites were slightly more likely than blacks to be hospitalized (2.3% and 1.7%, respectively), but 3.5% of both black and white adolescents 15 to 17 years of age had a hospital visit, excluding giving birth.

In the future a greater proportion of adolescents are likely to be disabled, because advances in medical technology have extended life expectancy among the disabled (see Chapters 30 and 35). An important factor that will affect these adolescents' access to health care services will be whether their families have adequate health insurance coverage (see Chapters 21, 30, and 35).

Psychiatric Care

Adolescents are more likely to be hospitalized for psychiatric conditions than are any other age group. Rates of hospitalization for adolescents have increased over the past decade, with admission rates to psychiatric hospitals rising dramatically for young people between 1970 and 1986 (Burns and Taube, 1991). For children 17 years of age or younger, the number of inpatient admissions increased by 34.6% between 1975 and 1986 (from 83,368 to 112,215). Most of this growth has occurred in general hospitals and private psychiatric hospitals. Because of changes in insurance coverage, the growth in the numbers of psychiatric admissions in private hospitals may reflect the influence of payer source (Burns and Taube, 1991).

The proportion of nonwhite adolescents in all types of psychiatric hospitals has decreased from 20% in 1975 to 13% in 1986. There has also been a decrease in the length of stays in hospital admissions, decreasing from 48.6 days to 42.3 days for adolescents (NAPPH, 1988). Overall, there has been a dramatic shift by hospital type in the proportion of relatively short stays (less than 8 days). These brief evaluations or crisis interventions constituted 30% of all admissions in 1986, as compared with 14% in 1975 (Burns and Taube, 1991). The 15- to 17-year-old group is more likely to be admitted to a psychiatric hospital than is the younger 10- to 14-year-old group, with older adolescents admitted almost 3.5 times as often in 1975. This trend decreased in 1986 when the ratio for admissions for older and younger adolescents was 2.6:1. Although psychiatric admission rates to state, county, and nonfederal general hospitals have been decreasing for young adults, they continue to have high rates of admission as compared with the general population. For example, in 1980, males aged 18 to 24 were admitted to state and county hospitals at a rate of 388 per 10,000, compared with rates of 26 per 10,000 for persons younger than 18, and 164 per 10,000 for the total population (Burns and Taube, 1991).

Two important factors have influenced the patterns of hospital admissions and causes for the admission. With the introduction of the Diagnostic and Statistical Manual (DSM) III in 1980, psychiatrists and psychologists can provide more accurate diagnoses, and thus the causes of admissions have been primarily the affective and behavior disorders (see Chapters 100–113), diminishing the number of youth with a diagnosis of schizophrenia. Second, the shift toward the diagnosis of affective disorders may be influenced by the growth of private psychiatric hospitals and general hospital psychiatry units, which provide most of the care for these conditions (Burns and Taube, 1991; Witkin, Atay, and Fell, 1987.)

MORTALITY
Trends in Mortality Data

This section highlights the details of the mortality statistics of adolescents in the United States. Over the past 50 years the leading causes of death have changed from natural causes (e.g., illness and birth defects) to injury and violence. For example, in 1933, 75% of deaths among teenagers ages 15 to 19 were due to natural causes, but by 1987, 21% of deaths in this age group were due to natural causes.

Age-specific mortality rates were as follows in 1987: for early adolescents, 26.9 per 100,000; for late adolescents, 84.6 per 100,000; for young adults (20 to 24 years old), 113.2 per 100,000. Since 1970, this represents the following decreases: 34% for early adolescents, 23% for late adolescents, and 24% for young adults. Since 1985, mortality rates for late adolescents and young adults have reversed direction for the first time since 1970. The mortality rates for late adolescents and young adults increased by 4.2% and 3.9%, respectively (see Fig. 2–3).

Comparing data from early and late adolescence, there is a 300% increase in overall mortality, the largest increase of mortality in any two consecutive age cohorts. There are dramatic differences in mortality rates between early adolescents and late adolescents for the seven leading causes of death. Violent causes of death are responsible for this major increase, with motor vehicle accidents increasing by 400%, non–motor vehicle accidents increasing by 85%, and homicide and suicide rates increasing by over 500% (NCHS, 1990b). Violence and injury account for three of every four adolescent deaths. As shown in Table 2–3, the major causes of mortality due to violence and injury peak among young adults and remain relatively high into early adulthood; they then decrease throughout the remainder of the life cycle (NCHS, 1990b).

Many of the deaths during adolescence are preventable. The National Adolescent Student Health Survey reports that more than 50% of students did not wear a seatbelt the last time they rode in a motor vehicle, 92% never wear a helmet when riding a bike, and 72% never use a light at night when riding a bike (NASHS, 1989).

Adolescents of all ages and young adults experience the highest rates of mortality from motor vehicle accidents, suicide, and homicide. Accidents and injuries are the leading cause of death in this age group and account for 60% of all deaths; motor vehicle injuries account for 80% of these deaths. The motor vehicle accident death rate for young people ages 15 to 24 is nearly double that of any other age group except those over 75 years (NCHS, 1990b).

Suicide is the second leading cause of death for youth (Chapter 101). In 1987, 2152 young people ages 10 to 19 took their own lives, and an additional 3022 suicide deaths occurred among those ages 20 to 24. Overall, adolescent suicides account for fewer than 20% of suicides for all age groups, although this loss during adolescence is a particular tragedy. There have been dramatic increases in the incidence of deaths by suicide over time. The death rate for suicide in early adolescence has increased by 200% since 1960, from 0.5 per 100,000 in 1960 to 1.5 per 100,000 in 1987; for late adolescents the rate has increased by almost 200% since 1960, from 3.6 per 100,000 in 1960 to 10.3 per 100,000 in 1987. For young adults the rates of suicide have also sharply increased by over 100% since 1960, from 7.1

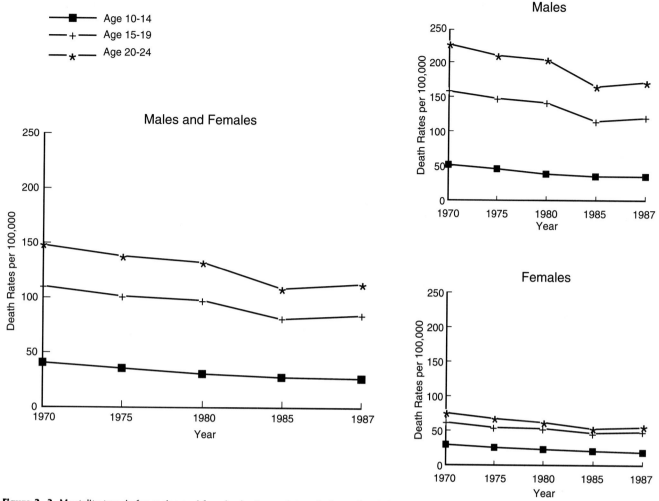

Figure 2–3. Mortality trends for males and females by 5-year intervals, by early adolescents 10–14, late adolescents 15–19, and young adults 20–24; 1970–1987. (Source: National Center for Health Statistics. Vital Statistics of the United States, Volume II, Mortality, Part A, Individual Years, Public Health Service. Washington, DC, US Government Printing Office, 1989.)

Mortality Graph for Males and Females (death rates per 100,000)				**Mortality Graph for Males** (death rates per 100,000)				**Mortality Graph for Females** (death rates per 100,000)		
		Ages				Ages				Ages
Year	10–14	15–19	20–24	Year	10–14	15–19	20–24	Year	10–14	15–19	20–24
1970	40.6	110.3	148.0	1970	51.3	157.8	225.7	1970	29.5	61.7	75.3
1975	35.7	101.5	138.2	1975	45.5	147.4	209.6	1975	25.6	54.4	67.2
1980	30.8	97.9	132.7	1980	38.3	141.4	203.5	1980	22.9	53.1	61.9
1985	27.9	81.2	108.9	1985	34.9	114.7	164.8	1985	20.5	46.5	52.8
1987	26.9	84.6	113.2	1987	34.8	119.6	171.2	1987	18.7	48.2	55.0

per 100,000 in 1960 to 15.3 per 100,000 in 1987 (NCHS, 1990b). Although females attempt suicide far more frequently than do males, the rising suicide rate is largely the result of the increasing rate among males, particularly white males.

Homicide is the third leading cause of death for adolescents and has also shown a dramatic increase over time. In 1987, 1744 adolescents were murdered. The death rate from homicides has increased from 0.4 per 100,000 in 1960 to 1.6 deaths per 100,000 for early adolescents in 1987 and from 0.5 per 100,000 in 1960 to 10.0 deaths per 100,000 for late adolescents in 1987. For young adults, the rate has increased from 4.0 to 17.8

per 100,000 during the same time period (NCHS, 1990b). Most homicide victims aged 10 to 19 are killed by guns. In 1987, firearms accounted for 68% of the 1744 adolescents murdered. Another 18% of adolescent homicide victims were murdered with knives and other cutting or stabbing instruments. Fourteen percent were killed with a club or other blunt instrument or with personal weapons (hands, fists, and so forth) or were strangled or murdered by some other means (Federal Bureau of Investigation 1987, cited in Gans, Blyth, and Elster, 1990).

Gender is an important demographic factor that influences the cause of death (Table 2–3). Male adolescents

TABLE 2–3. Death Rates per 100,000 Due to Seven Leading Causes of Death for Adolescents and Young Adults (Ages 10–14, 15–19, and 20–24) by Sex: 1987

CAUSE	MALES			FEMALES		
	10–14	15–19	20–24	10–14	15–19	20–24
Motor vehicle accident	10.3	51.0	59.7	4.8	22.2	17.4
Other accidents	8.2	15.6	21.5	2.2	2.9	4.0
Suicide	2.3	16.2	26.1	0.6	4.2	4.4
Homicide	2.0	15.3	26.0	1.2	4.4	7.4
Malignant neoplasms	3.4	5.1	6.9	2.7	3.7	4.5
Cardiovascular disease	1.4	3.2	1.3	1.3	2.1	3.6
Congenital anomalies	1.3	1.6	1.0	1.0	1.0	1.1

Source: National Center for Health Statistics: Vital Statistics of the United States, 1987, Vol II, Mortality, Part A. DHHS Publication No. (PHS)90-1101. Public Health Service, Washington, DC, US Government Printing Office, 1990.

die at twice the rate of adolescent females. Adolescent males of all ages have considerably higher death rates from motor vehicle accidents, other accidents, homicides, and suicides (particularly the 15- to 19-year-olds) than do females.

Race and ethnicity are also important demographic factors that influence mortality (Table 2–4). In 1987, the rate of homicide for black adolescents of all age groups was six times higher than it was for white adolescents (Figure 2–4). The homicide rates for black males 15 to 24 years old have increased markedly between 1978 and 1988. In contrast, whites experienced suicide rates nearly 2.5 times as high as those for black adolescents. Rates for motor vehicle accidents also show differences, with white adolescents ages 15 to 19 experiencing nearly 2.7 times as many motor vehicle deaths as do blacks or adolescents from other ethnic groups (including Asian/Pacific Islanders and Native Americans) of the same age. These patterns continue into the early adult years of 20 to 24, with increasing differences among racial groups, depending upon the cause of death.

Trends indicate that all racial groups across all ages will experience a decrease in their mortality rates between the years 1979 and 2000. By ethnicity and racial groups, white youth and youth of racial groups other than black will experience the most dramatic decreases. For example, white youth ages 15 to 19 will experience a 17% decrease in mortality rates, and youth in other racial groups (not including blacks) will experience nearly a 27% decrease (Irwin et al, 1991). The increases from 1985 to 1987 in the mortality rates in late adoles-

cents and young adults raise questions, however, about the long-term projections.

Combining gender and race reveals the following data. The rate of suicide among white males is nearly four times as high as it is for white females ages 10 to 14 (2.4 per 100,000 for males and 0.7 for females), but white females experience nearly twice the rate of suicide as do black and other females (0.7 per 100,000 for white females and 0.4 for black females). Death rates from motor vehicle accidents and homicides among females of all racial groups in early adolescence are more similar. For females ages 15 to 19, the rate of suicide is twice as high for white females as for black females, and the trends remain stable (4.1 for white females and 2.1 for black females). The death rate from motor vehicle accidents for white females ages 15 to 19 (24.8 per 100,000) is three times as high as the death rate experienced by black females (8.0 per 100,000) (Irwin et al, 1991).

RATES AND CAUSES OF MORBIDITY

Morbidity is generally defined as the incidence of negative health outcomes. In earlier sections of this chapter, the health care utilization patterns of adolescents with acute and chronic conditions have been documented. In this section, risk behaviors that emerge during adolescence and are associated with morbidity in adolescence and adulthood are emphasized.

TABLE 2–4. Death Rates per 100,000 Due to Seven Leading Causes of Death for Adolescents and Young Adults (Ages 10–14, 15–19, and 20–24) by Race:* 1987

CAUSE	BLACK			WHITE			OTHER		
	10–14	15–19	20–24	10–14	15–19	20–24	10–14	15–19	20–24
Motor vehicle accident	5.6	17.7	27.7	8.0	40.9	40.5	5.9	19.5	29.5
Other accidents	8.9	11.0	14.8	4.6	9.1	12.4	8.2	10.4	14.2
Suicide	1.0	5.8	9.5	1.6	11.2	16.2	1.0	6.5	10.9
Homicide	4.6	36.2	66.4	1.0	5.2	9.8	4.1	30.7	55.8
Malignant neoplasms	2.7	5.2	6.6	3.1	4.2	5.6	2.7	5.0	6.2
Cardiovascular disease	2.2	4.8	9.5	1.2	2.3	3.8	2.0	4.1	8.5
Congenital anomalies	1.7	1.3	1.8	1.0	1.4	1.2	1.5	1.2	1.6

*Hispanics may be of any race.
Source: National Center for Health Statistics: Vital Statistics of the United States, 1987. Vol II, Mortality, Part A. DHHS Pub. No. (PHS) 90-1101. Public Health Service, Washington, DC, U.S. Government Printing Office, 1990.

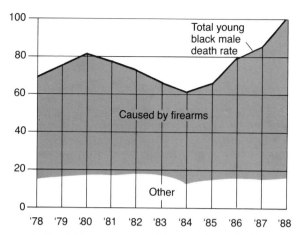

Figure 2–4. Homicide rates per 100,000 population, for black males ages 15–24. (From The New York Times, National Edition, Friday, December 7, 1990. Source: Centers for Disease Control. Copyright © 1990 by the New York Times Company. Reprinted by permission.)

Increasingly, the associations between adolescent high-risk behaviors and the major morbidities are being identified (see Chapter 3). Adolescents engage most frequently in three risk behaviors: substance use and abuse, sexual behavior, and motor or recreational vehicle use (see Chapters 3, 68, and 111). Many of these behaviors are initiated during early adolescence, with a marked increase in frequency from early to late adolescence. They are prevalent in all socioeconomic and racial and ethnic groups, differ by gender and racial and ethnic groups, and account for the majority of morbidity during adolescence (Blum, 1987; Irwin, 1990; Irwin and Ryan, 1989). The prevalence of these three risk behaviors has remained high over the past decade, and together they account for 24% of hospital discharges for early adolescents, 51% for late adolescents, and 65% for young adults (McManus et al, in press).

Substance Use and Abuse

High rates of substance use during adolescence have been reported in national surveys since 1975. The 1989

adolescent lifetime prevalence rates of marijuana and cocaine use are 43.7% and 8.5%, respectively. These rates have declined markedly since the peak of marijuana use in 1979 and of cocaine use in 1985. The reported rates of "crack" cocaine and cocaine use probably underestimate the actual frequency of use because surveys were conducted among high school and college students, and adolescents who do not attend school probably have higher rates of use. The rates of cigarette and alcohol use in 1989 continue to remain high at 65.7% and 90.7%, respectively (Johnston, O'Malley, and Bachman, 1989) (Table 2–5).

In 1989, the daily use of cigarettes by high school seniors was reported at 18.9%, with 11.2% reporting smoking more than one-half pack per day (see Chapters 38 and 49). Females have consistently reported greater daily use than have males since 1978. Twelve years of age is the mean self-reported age of onset (age at which cigarette use began). In addition to the high prevalence of daily smoking among high school seniors, there is evidence to suggest that boys are using smokeless tobacco as an alternative to cigarettes (Johnston, O'Malley, and Bachman, 1989) (see Chapter 38 and 41).

Alcohol remains the most commonly used substance. Reported daily use of alcohol in 1989 remained high at 4.2%, with 33% of high school seniors stating that they had had five or more drinks in a row in the previous 2 weeks. Alcohol consumption also begins early in adolescence, with a mean age of onset of 12.6 years. Males consistently reported more frequent and heavier use by a factor of 2:1 as compared with females. The use of alcohol often contributes to adolescents' deaths; close to one fifth of all deaths of 15- to 20-year-olds are due to an alcohol-related car accident, and more than 21 adolescents are killed each day in alcohol-related fatalities (National Commission Against Drunk Driving, 1988, cited in Gans, Blyth, and Elster, 1990).

Apart from alcohol, cigarettes and marijuana are reported to be the most commonly abused substances among adolescents. In 1989, reported daily use of marijuana by high school seniors was 2.9%, and the mean age of onset was 14.4 years. Forty-four percent of high school seniors in 1989 had reported having tried marijuana at least once, and one fifth of the sample reported

TABLE 2–5. Trends in Lifetime Prevalence (Percentage Ever Used) of Substance Use Among High School Seniors for Selected Substances: 1980–1989

SCHOOL YEAR	SUBSTANCE								
	Alcohol	Cigarettes	Cocaine	Crack Cocaine	Hallucinogens*	Heroin	Inhalants	Marijuana/ Hashish	Stimulants*
1980	93.2	71.0	15.7	NA	15.6	1.1	17.3	60.3	NA
1981	92.6	71.0	16.5	NA	15.3	1.1	17.2	59.5	NA
1982	92.8	70.1	16.0	NA	14.3	1.2	17.7	58.7	27.9
1983	92.6	70.6	16.2	NA	13.6	1.2	18.2	57.0	26.9
1984	92.6	69.7	16.1	NA	12.3	1.3	18.0*	54.9	27.9
1985	92.2	68.8	17.3	NA	12.1	1.2	18.1*	54.2	26.2
1986	91.3	67.6	16.9	NA	11.9	1.1	20.1*	50.9	23.4
1987	92.2	67.2	15.2	5.6	10.6	1.2	18.6*	50.2	21.6
1988	92.0	66.4	12.1	4.8	9.2	1.1	17.5*	47.2	19.8
1989	90.7	65.7	8.5	4.7	9.9	1.3	18.6	43.7	19.1

*Adjusted data.

Sources: Johnston LD, O'Malley PM, Bachman JG: Drug use, drinking, and smoking: National survey results from high school, college and young adult population, 1975–1988. National Institute on Drug Abuse. US Department of Health and Human Services. Public Health Service. Alcohol, Drug Abuse, and Mental Health Administration. DHHS Publication No. (ADM)89-1638. Washington, DC, US Government Printing Office, unpublished data from Johnston et al, 1989.

having used it during the past month. Besides its documented effect on cognitive functioning, marijuana is recognized as a "gateway" drug among adolescents, associated with the use of harder drugs (Johnston, O'Malley, and Bachman, 1989). Cocaine, particularly in its formulation as crack, has also been a major threat to adolescent health. Over one-half million 12- to 17-year-olds reported having used cocaine in 1988, and close to 250,000 of these adolescents reported having used the drug within the past month (National Institute on Drug Abuse, 1989). Among high school seniors, 10% reported having tried cocaine, and 3% reported using it within the past month (Johnston, O'Malley, and Bachman, 1989).

Adolescents also report using other drugs, including diet pills, steroids, MMDA ("ecstasy"), and crystal methamphetamine ("ice"). One in six adolescents reported using diet pills to help control their weight (Gans, Blyth, and Elster, 1990) (see Chapter 60). The 1989 high school senior survey found that nearly 5% of high school males reported having used anabolic/androgenic steroids to enhance either their athletic performance or appearance (Johnston, O'Malley, and Bachman, 1989) (see Chapter 81). A large number of adolescents have also reported using inhalants; 19% of 12- to 17-year-olds have reported sniffing glue. The use of tranquilizers among this age group is reported as less common; 7.6% of high school seniors in 1989 reported having tried tranquilizers, and 1.3% reported having used them in the past month. A somewhat larger proportion (9.9%) of high school seniors in 1989 indicated that they had tried hallucinogens (e.g., lysergic acid diethylamide [LSD] or phencyclidine [PCP]), and 2.9% reported having used them in the past month (Johnston, O'Malley, and Bachman, 1989).

The overall decrease in drug use among this population may reflect a shift in the level of disapproval expressed by high school students regarding the use of illicit drugs. The vast majority of students do not condone regular use of any of the illicit drugs, including marijuana; 89% of students indicated a disapproval of regular marijuana use. For other illicit drugs (cocaine, barbiturates, etc.), their regular use was disapproved of by 94% to 97% of students. Although occasional drug use is perceived as of less risk, trends indicate a change in social norms since the late 1970s regarding the use of illicit drugs (Johnston, O'Malley, and Bachman, 1989).

Lifetime prevalence (percentage ever used) also varies by gender and race or ethnicity. More males tend to use substances, with the exception of marijuana and hallucinogens, than do females. For adolescents ages 12 to 17, more males reported using alcohol (53.4% for males and 46.8% for females), cigarettes (45.3% for males and 39.2% for females), and smokeless tobacco (25.8% for males and 3.6% for females). Cocaine use is similar for both genders (National Institute on Drug Abuse, 1989).

Lifetime prevalence rates among racial and ethnic groups document that white adolescents have overall higher rates of substance use than do black or Hispanic adolescents. For adolescents ages 12 to 17, 53.7% of whites reported ever having used alcohol, as compared to 36.6% among black and 47.1% among Hispanic youth. Similar patterns are found in the reported use of

marijuana; 18.2% of white youth ages 12 to 17 indicated that they have used the drug, and 16.9% of Hispanic and 13.5% of black youth reported using it. Patterns of cocaine use vary, with higher reported use among Hispanic youth (4.6%) as compared with white (3.6%) and black youth (2.1%). The reported use of both cigarettes and smokeless tobacco is higher among white adolescents (46.7% and 18.6%, respectively), as compared with black (27.4% and 4.7%) and Hispanic youth (35.9% and 6.1%).

Sexual Behavior: Sexual Intercourse and Contraceptive Use

SEXUAL INTERCOURSE (see Chapter 68)

The incidence of sexual activity has increased dramatically from 1971 to the late 1980s in both younger and older age cohorts of adolescents. By age 15, 24% of black females, 26% of white females and males, and 69% of black males have experienced coitus at least once. By age 19, 83% of black females, 76% of white females, 86% of white males, and 98% of black males have had coitus at least once. White adolescent females report more frequent intercourse with more partners than their age-related black peers (Pratt, unpublished data from NSFG, Cycle IV, 1990; Sonenstein, Pleck, and Ku, 1989). Little is known about sexual behaviors other than coitus in adolescents (Brooks-Gunn and Furstenberg, 1989). Although specific data on Hispanic adolescents were not reported in the 1988 survey, previous research in 1982 documented that patterns of sexual activity among Hispanic youth fell between that of black and white youth. For example, among females ages 15 to 19, 59% of black females had initiated sexual activity, as compared with 50% of Hispanics and 44% of whites.

USE OF CONTRACEPTION (see Chapter 73)

Age and race or ethnicity are significant factors in the adoption of contraception among sexually active adolescents. For female adolescents as a whole, the percentage of sexually active adolescents who reported ever having used contraceptives increased from 58% to 83% between the ages of 15 and 16 years and reached 91% by age 19 years. Sexually active black female adolescents are the most likely to report ever having used contraception at the youngest ages. At age 15 years, 71% of black females have ever used contraception, as compared with 58% of white females and only 10% of Hispanic females. By age 19 years, however, 83% of black females, 94% of white females, and 81% of Hispanic females have initiated contraception.

While patterns of contraceptive choice change during adolescence, a key factor in the adoption and use of contraceptives appears to be related to their use at the point of sexual debut. In a recent survey, only about one half of whites and one third of blacks used a method of contraception at first intercourse. Only a small proportion of adolescents (19% of whites and 13% of blacks) subsequently became contraceptive users during the next 2 months. The slow rate of subsequent adoption of a contraceptive method leaves a large group of adolescents at continued high risk for an unintended pregnancy (Kahn, Rindfuss, and Guilkey, 1990).

The reported percentages of adolescents who currently use contraception are dramatically lower than the percentages of adolescents who have ever used contraception. In 1982, 65% used ineffective or no contraception at first intercourse; by 1988, that proportion had dropped to 41%. Younger adolescents continue to be less likely to use effective contraception, so their exposure to risk is high, resulting in high pregnancy and birth rates among those who are sexually active (Pratt, unpublished data from NSFG, Cycle IV, 1990).

Whereas about one half of 17-year-old black and white adolescents report current use of contraception, only 12% of Hispanics reported routine contraception use. Differences in use of contraception may reflect marriage patterns as well as cultural and religious differences regarding the acceptability of the use of contraception and of premarital sexual activity (Irwin et al, 1991).

Outcomes of Sexual Behavior: Pregnancies and Births (see Chapter 74)

PREGNANCIES

Approximately 1 million adolescents become pregnant each year in the United States, which is a pregnancy rate of approximately 110 per 100,000. Dramatic differences exist between racial and ethnic groups in the percentages of 10- to 19-year-olds who have experienced a pregnancy. More than twice as many blacks as whites in every age group have been pregnant. Hispanics have the highest and whites have the lowest "ever been pregnant" percentages in all age groups except age 17, for which Hispanics are lowest (6%) and blacks are highest (24%) (Irwin et al, 1991).

BIRTHS

In 1987, there were a total of 472,623 births among mothers ages 10 to 19, reflecting a 16% decline since 1980 (562,330 births in 1980). Overall, the birthrates have declined during the past 4 decades.

In 1987, 24% of all births were among unmarried women; 64% of births among women younger than 20 years of age were out-of-wedlock. This figure has changed dramatically since 1980, when 18% of all births were among unmarried women, and 48% of all births among adolescents were out-of-wedlock. The younger the adolescent mother, the greater the likelihood that she is unmarried. In 1984, 91% of all births among adolescents younger than 15 occurred among unmarried adolescents, contrasted with 54% of births among unmarried 18-year-olds. The birthrate for black unmarried adolescents has generally decreased by 4% between 1970 and 1987, from 96.9 per 1000 in 1970 to 92.6 per 1000 in 1985, whereas for white unmarried adolescents,

the rate has increased by 109%, from 10.9 per 1000 in 1970 to 22.8 per 1000 in 1987.

Birthrates for early adolescents (10 to 14 years) remain low; however, since 1960 they have increased by 225%, from 0.4 per 1000 to 1.3 per 1000 births in 1987. Within the 15- to 19-year-old category there are some interesting trends since 1966: the birthrate in the 15- to 17-year-old age group has decreased from 35.7 per 1000 in 1966 to 31.8 per 1000 in 1987; the rate in the 17- to 19-year-old age group has decreased from 120.3 per 1000 in 1966 to 80.2 per 1000 in 1987.

Comparing the birthrates of black and white adolescents during a 20-year period (1966–1987), there has been a 27% decrease among 15- to 17-year-old black adolescents (from 99.5 to 72.9 per 1000) and a 6% decrease (from 25.7 to 24.1 per 1000) among white adolescents in this age group. Similar trends also are seen for 18- to 19-year-olds. The birthrates for adolescents have decreased by 43% between 1960 and 1987 among all races (89.6 per 1000 and 51.1 per 1000 in 1987). During the same time period, the rate among blacks decreased by 36% (156.1 per 1000 to 100.3 per 1000) and among whites by 47% (79.4 per 1000 to 41.9 per 1000). During the same years, the percentage of total births among unmarried adolescents increased significantly. In 1980, 85% of births among black adolescents and 33% of births among white adolescents occurred among unmarried females.

ABORTION

Approximately 300,000 to 400,000 abortions are performed on adolescents annually. Since the legalization of abortion in 1973, both the number of estimated abortions and the abortion rates (percentage of pregnancies terminated by abortion) for all females up to age 24 have risen. The percentages of females ages 15 to 19 who have ever had an abortion increase with age from 3% for 15-year-olds to 15% for 19-year-olds with all races combined. Among 15-year-olds, the percentages are 3% for blacks, 2% for whites, and 14% for Hispanics. At age 19, 12% of black females, 14% of whites, and 36% of Hispanics have had an abortion (Irwin et al, 1991). It should be noted that the lack of a national reporting system for abortions provided in both the private and the public sectors may well contribute to an overall underestimation of the total number of abortions that are performed on a yearly basis. Data are not based on a national representative sample of adolescents receiving abortion care. Differences in the use of publicly subsidized clinics and private practice physicians and clinics where abortion services are delivered may also affect the ethnic profile of adolescents having had an abortion.

Outcomes of Sexual Behavior: Sexually Transmitted Diseases

GONORRHEA (see Chapter 75)

There were approximately 195,312 cases of gonorrhea reported in young people 15 to 19 years old in 1988.

There has been a 325% increase in the incidence of gonorrhea among 10- to 14-year-olds and a 170% increase among 15- to 19-year-olds between 1960 and 1988, whereas for young adults ages 20 to 24 there was a 43% increase. These rates have contributed to the overall doubling in the incidence of gonorrhea among the general population (Centers for Disease Control, unpublished data, cited in Irwin et al, 1991). Among adolescents ages 15 to 19 years, males have experienced nearly a twofold increase in the incidence of gonorrhea and females nearly a fourfold increase between 1960 and 1985. Younger adolescents ages 10 to 14 experienced nearly a fourfold increase among males and a threefold increase among females in the incidence of gonorrhea (Irwin et al, 1991).

Differences in the incidence of gonorrhea also vary by race and ethnicity. Incidence rates per 100,000 in 1988 were as follows: white males ages 15 to 19, 151.0; black males, 5469.6; Hispanic males, 389.1; and males from other ethnic groups, 111.5. For females, comparable numbers were 359.2 for whites, 5645.5 for black females, 389.1 for Hispanic females, and 133.7 for females of other ethnic groups. The incidence of gonorrhea increases among young adults ages 20 to 24. Among males, for example, the incidence is 262.2 for whites, 8563.7 for blacks, 819.9 for Hispanics, and 234.3 for other ethnic groups. Among white females ages 20 to 24, the incidence is 297.4 for whites, 5375.7 for blacks, 430.1 for Hispanic females, and 274.0 for females of other ethnic groups (Centers for Disease Control, 1989, cited in Irwin et al, 1991).

SYPHILIS

There were approximately 3969 cases of syphilis reported in young people 15 to 19 years old in 1988. Although the rates of syphilis in the 10- to 14-year-old and 15- to 19-year-old age groups remained relatively stable between 1960 and 1988, there have been some significant changes in the incidence of syphilis among adolescents between 1980 and 1988. Among males ages 15 to 19, there has been a 16% decrease in the incidence of syphilis between 1980 and 1988, from 19.2 to 16.2 per 100,000. However, among females, there has been an 83% increase over the same time period, with the incidence rising from 15.1 to 27.7 per 100,000 for this age group. Incidence rates of syphilis vary by race and ethnicity. In 1988, the incidence of syphilis among males was 1.4 for whites, 80.8 for blacks, 30.4 for Hispanics, and 1.1 for other ethnic groups. For females, the incidence was 4.2 for whites, 146.1 for blacks, 21.7 for Hispanics, and 2.4 for other females. Rates for both males and females increase among young adults ages 20 to 24. For males, the incidence is 7.5 for whites, 323.9 for blacks, 85.4 for Hispanics, and 6.2 for other racial groups. For females, the incidence is 6.1 for whites, 276.2 for blacks, 37.3 for Hispanics, and 6.8 for other ethnic groups (Centers for Disease Control, 1989, cited in Irwin et al, 1991).

HUMAN IMMUNODEFICIENCY VIRUS (HIV) AND ACQUIRED IMMUNODEFICIENCY SYNDROME (AIDS)

The demographic background for HIV-related conditions is found in Chapter 76. While the numbers of AIDS cases among adolescents have been relatively low, this population is particularly vulnerable to HIV infection and the AIDS disease, which may not manifest itself until after an extensive incubation period of up to 10 years. Although adolescent AIDS cases account for only 1% of the nation's total, the number of cases doubles every 14 months. Adolescents place themselves at risk for AIDS by engaging in a variety of behaviors, including intravenous drug use (see Chapter 111) and having a relatively large number of sexual partners. Recent data from the departments of education in 30 states, 10 cities, and two territories in the winter and spring of 1989 report the following median behaviors: 3% of students reported using intravenous drugs, 0.9% reported sharing needles, 56% reported having had coitus, 21% reported having had four or more sexual partners. Throughout all the sites, more males reported having had sexual intercourse and having had four or more sex partners. Another study documenting the seroprevalence rate of HIV among adolescent applicants (below the age of 20 years) for the United States military service also demonstrates that infections with the virus are not rare among teenagers (see Chapter 29). Serum specimens from more than 1 million adolescents were tested for antibodies to HIV. Overall, 393 teenagers were found to be seropositive (incidence of 0.39 per 1000). The incidence of seropositivity varied according to geographic locations, with a rate of less than 0.1 per 1000 found among applicants from the north and central states, compared with more than 2 per 1000 in urban counties in Maryland, Texas, New York, and the District of Columbia. In addition, the incidence among black teenage applicants (1.06 per 1000) was greater than that among white (0.18 per 1000) or Hispanic (0.31 per 1000) teenage applicants. However, overall rates for males and females were comparable (0.35 incidence for males and 0.32 for females) (Burke et al, 1990). Health providers will need to consider ways in which they can play a major role in educating their clients regarding their risks of getting sexually transmitted diseases, especially the risk of acquiring HIV.

Interrelationships of Behavior and Covariation of Risk Behaviors

(see Chapter 3)

Increasingly there is a recognition of the covariation of the risk-taking behaviors and outcomes, as well as the mechanisms by which specific behaviors are interrelated among adolescents, with some investigators postulating a developmental trajectory of behaviors (Irwin, 1987; Irwin, 1990; Irwin and Millstein, 1986). Adolescents ages 12 to 17 who smoke cigarettes are more likely than nonsmokers to use other drugs, and adolescents who consume alcohol or use marijuana are also more likely to use other substances (National Institute on Drug Abuse, 1989). For example, adolescents who drank alcohol in the past month were six times more likely than nondrinkers to have smoked cigarettes. They were also 10 times more likely than nondrinkers to have used marijuana and 11 times more likely to have recently used cocaine. Adolescents who used marijuana in the past month were more than 20 times more likely to have tried cocaine, compared with adolescents who had not tried marijuana (National Institute on Drug Abuse, 1989).

In addition, substance use has been shown to have a relationship to other risk-taking behaviors. For example, substance use is positively correlated with early initiation of sexual behavior. Jessor used drinking status as a marker for at-risk youth and found that 80% of adolescent drinkers had initiated marijuana use and more than 50% had initiated sexual intercourse (Jessor, 1984). Other investigators have documented the association of early sexual activity and ineffective contraceptive use with the use of cigarettes and alcohol.

The association of alcohol use and unintentional injury has been well established. Alcohol-related motor vehicle injuries remain the leading cause of mortality in late adolescence. Alcohol is also associated with a large number of injuries involving nonmotorized vehicles (bicycles and skateboards), drownings, falls, and fires. The role of other substances in unintentional injuries remains to be established.

Within the area of substance use, substances are associated in predictable ways. Alcohol and tobacco use predict the use of illicit substances. Kandel and colleagues have documented the progression in a cohort of adolescents followed through young adulthood (Kandel, Kessler, and Margulies, 1978). The sequence of progression is as follows: cigarettes, alcohol, and marijuana precede other illicit substances (including psychedelics, cocaine, heroin, and other nonprescribed stimulants, sedatives, and tranquilizers), and the use of prescribed psychoactive drugs follows all other illicit substances. Cigarettes appear to be the drug of initiation for females. Recently a 5-year longitudinal study in Los Angeles County has monitored the initiation of cocaine use and its association with other substances. Alcohol use in the preceding year was an important predictor of marijuana use. Marijuana use in the preceding year was an important predictor of cocaine use in the following year (Newcomb and Bentler, 1986).

CONCLUSION

During the next decade, the size, ethnic composition, geographic distribution, environmental conditions, educational patterns, economics, and health status of the adolescent population will change. These changes will have a profound effect upon the ways in which the health care system provides for this population during the second decade of life.

The absolute numbers of adolescents in the United States will increase; however, the relative proportion of adolescents in the population in general will decrease. With the population becoming more aged, there is some question about the amount of resources that will be allocated to adolescents. Adolescents of the future will be more likely to come from minority backgrounds, speak languages other than English, and come from impoverished, single-parent (usually the mother) living conditions in metropolitan areas. There will continue to

be a major shift in where adolescents will reside in the United States; increasingly adolescents will live in the South, Southwest, and West, with the Midwest and Northeast experiencing significant declines in the number of adolescents.

Acknowledgments: During the preparation of this chapter the authors were supported in part by a grant from the Bureau of Maternal and Child Health, Department of Health and Human Services (MCJ000978A). The authors thank Mr. Roy Rodriguez, Assistant Administrator, Division of Adolescent Medicine for his editorial and data analyses in the chapter.

BIBLIOGRAPHY

Adams PF, Hardy AM: Current estimates from the National Health Interview Survey, 1988. Vital and Health Statistics, Series 10, No. 173, DHHS Publication No. (PHS)89-1501. National Center for Health Statistics. Washington, DC, US Government Printing Office, 1989.

Baker SP, O'Neill B, Karpf RS: The Injury Fact Book. Lexington, MA, Lexington Books, 1984.

Bane MJ, Ellwood DT: One-fifth of the nation's children: Why are they poor? Science 245:1047, 1989.

Blum R: Contemporary threats to adolescent health in the United States. JAMA 257:3390, 1987.

Brooks-Gunn J, Furstenberg F, Jr: Adolescent sexual behavior. Am Psychol 44:249, 1989.

Burke DS, Brundage JF, Goldenbaum M, et al: Human immunodeficiency virus infections in teenagers: Seroprevalence among applicants for US military services. JAMA 263:2074, 1990.

Burns BJ, Taube CA: Mental health services for adolescents: Office of Technology Assessment background paper for U.S. Congress, Office of Technology Assessment. In Adolescent Health, Vol I: Summary and Policy Options, OTA-H-468. Washington, DC, US Government Printing Office, 1991.

Centers for Disease Control: HIV AIDS Surveillance Report. Atlanta, Division of HIV/AIDS, October 1990a.

Centers for Disease Control: HIV-related knowledge and behaviors among high school students, selected U.S. sites. MMWR 39:385, 1990b.

Fingerhut LA, Kleinman JC: Trends and current status in childhood mortality, United States 1900–1985. Vital and Health Statistics, Series 3, No. 26. DHHS Publication No. (PHS)89-1410. National Center for Health Statistics. Washington, DC, US Government Printing Office, 1989.

Gallagher SS, Finison K, Guyer R, et al: The incidence of injuries among 87,000 Massachusetts children and adolescents: Results of the 1980–1981 Statewide Childhood Injury Prevention Program Surveillance System. Am J Public Health 74:1340, 1984.

Gans JE, Blyth DA, Elster AB: America's adolescents: How healthy are they? Profiles of Adolescent Health Series, Vol I. Chicago, American Medical Association, 1990.

Glick PC: How American families are changing. Am Demographics 6:20, 1984.

Hill JP: Research on adolescents and their families: Past and prospect. In Irwin CE, Jr (ed): Adolescent Social Behavior and Health: New Directions for Child Development. No. 37. San Francisco, Jossey-Bass, 1987, pp 13–31.

Hodgkinson HL: All One System: Demographics of Education, Kindergarten through Graduate School. Washington, DC, Institute for Educational Leadership, 1985.

Irwin CE, Jr (ed): Adolescent Social Behavior and Health: New Directions for Child Development. No. 37. San Francisco, Jossey-Bass, 1987.

Irwin CE, Jr: The theoretical concept of at-risk adolescents. Adolescent Medicine: State of the Art Reviews 1:1, 1990.

Irwin CE, Jr, Brindis C, Brodt S, et al: The Health of America's Youth—A Prelude to Action. Washington, DC, DHHS, Bureau of Maternal and Child Health, 1991.

Irwin CE, Jr, Millstein SG: Biopsychosocial correlates of risk-taking behaviors during adolescence. J Adolesc Health Care 7:82S, 1986.

Irwin CE, Jr, Ryan SA: Problem behaviors of adolescents. Pediatr Rev 10:235, 1989.

Irwin CE, Jr, Vaughan E: Psychosocial content of adolescent development: Study group report. J Adolesc Health Care 9(Suppl):115, 1988.

Jessor R: Adolescent development and behavioral health. In Matarazzo JD, Weiss SM, Herd JA, et al (eds): Behavioral Health: A Handbook of Health Enhancement and Disease Prevention. New York, John Wiley & Sons, 1984, pp 69–90.

Johnston LD, O'Malley PM, Bachman JG: Drug use, drinking and smoking: National survey results from high school, college and young adult population, 1975–1988. DHHS Publication No. (ADM)89-1638. Washington, DC, US Government Printing Office, 1989.

Kahn JR, Rindfuss RR, Guilkey DK: Adolescent contraceptive method choices. Demography 27:323, 1990.

Kandel DB, Kessler RC, Margulies RZ: Antecedents of adolescent initiation into stages of drug use: A developmental analysis. In Kandel DB (ed): Longitudinal Research on Drug Use: Empirical Findings and Methodological Issues. Washington, DC, Hemisphere, 1978.

McCarthy KF: Immigration and California: Issues for the 1980's. Rand Paper Series P-6846. Santa Monica, CA, Rand Corporation, 1983.

McManus P, McCarty E, Kozak L, Newacheck P: Hospital use by adolescents and young adults. J Adolesc Health Care, in press.

Millstein S, Irwin C, Brindis C: Sociodemographic trends and projections in the adolescent population. In Hendee WR (ed): The Health of Adolescents. San Francisco, Jossey-Bass, 1991, pp 1–15.

National Adolescent Student Health Survey: A Report on the Health of America's Youth. Oakland, CA, Third Party Publishing, 1989.

National Association of Private Psychiatric Hospitals: 1988 NAPPH Annual Survey. Washington, DC, National Association for Private Psychiatric Hospitals, 1988.

National Center for Health Statistics: Health USA, 1988. DHHS Publication No. (DHS)89-1232. Washington, DC, US Government Printing Office, 1989a.

National Center for Health Statistics: Vital Statistics for the United States, 1985, Vol I. DHHS Publication No. (DHS)88-1113. Public Health Service, Washington, DC, US Government Printing Office, 1989b.

National Center for Health Statistics: Vital Statistics of the United States, 1985, Vol II, Mortality, Part A, Individual Years. Public Health Service, Washington, DC, US Government Printing Office, 1989c.

National Center for Health Statistics: Vital Statistics of the United States, 1987, Vol II, Mortality, Part B. DHHS Publication No. (DHS)89-1102. Washington, DC, US Government Printing Office, 1989d.

National Center for Health Statistics: Vital Statistics of the United States, 1987, Vol I, Natality. Public Health Service, Washington, DC, US Government Printing Office, 1990a.

National Center for Health Statistics: Vital Statistics of the United States, 1987, Vol II, Mortality, Part A. DHHS Publication No. (PHS)90-1101. Public Health Service, Washington, DC, US Government Printing Office, 1990b.

National Commission Against Drunk Driving: Youth driving without impairment: A community challenge. Report on the Youth Impaired Driving Public Hearings. Washington, DC, National Highways Traffic Safety Administration, 1987.

National Institute on Drug Abuse, National Household Survey on Drug Abuse: Population Estimates, 1988. DHHS Publication No. (ADM)89-1636. Washington, DC, US Government Printing Office, 1989.

National Vital Statistics Division: Vital statistics of the United States, 1960, Vol II, Mortality, Part A. Washington, DC, US Department of Health, Education, and Welfare, 1963a.

National Vital Statistics Division: Vital statistics of the United States, 1960, Vol II, Mortality, Part B. Washington, DC, US Department of Health, Education, and Welfare, 1963b.

Newacheck PW: Adolescents with special health needs: Prevalence, severity, and access to health services. Pediatrics 84:872, 1989a.

Newacheck PW: Improving access to health services for adolescents from economically disadvantaged families. Pediatrics 84:1056, 1989b.

Newacheck PW, McManus MA: Health care expenditure patterns for adolescents. J Adolesc Health Care 11:133, 1990.

Newcomb MD, Bentler PM: Cocaine use among adolescents: Longitudinal associates with social context, psychopathology and use of other substances. Addict Behav 11:263, 1986.

Paulson J: Injuries: The leading cause of morbidity and mortality in adolescents. Adolescent Medicine: State of the Art Reviews 1:97, 1990.

Pratt W: National Survey of Family Growth, Cycles III and IV for 1988. Unpublished Tabulations, Ohio State University, Columbus, OH, 1990.

Preston SH: Children and the elderly in the U.S. Sci Am 251:6, 1984.

Rosen DS, Xiangdong M, Blum RW: Adolescent health: Current trends and critical issues. Adolescent Medicine: State of the Art Reviews 1:15, 1990.

Sonenstein FL, Pleck JH, Ku LC: Sexual activity, condom use and AIDS awareness among adolescent males. Fam Plann Perspect 21:152, 1989.

Spencer G: Projections of the Hispanic Population: 1983–2080. US Bureau of the Census, Current Population Reports, Series P-25, No. 995. Washington, DC, US Government Printing Office, 1986.

US Bureau of the Census: Persons below the poverty level by family status, sex of head, race and Spanish origin, 1966, 1967, 1971, 1973, and 1975. Money Income and Poverty Status of Families and Persons in the United States: 1975 and 1974 Revisions, Series P-60, No. 103, Table 17, September, 1976. Washington, DC, US Government Printing Office, 1977a.

US Bureau of the Census: Persons in families—Persons by total family income in 1975, by relationship to family head, age, race, Spanish origin and sex. Money Income in 1975 of Families and Persons in the United States, Series P-60, No. 105, June, 1977. Washington, DC, US Government Printing Office, 1977b.

US Bureau of the Census: Projections of the population of the United States, by age, sex, and race: 1983 to 2080. Current Population Reports, Series P-25, No. 952. Washington, DC, US Government Printing Office, 1984.

US Bureau of the Census: Estimates of the population of the United States, by age, sex, and race: 1980–1985. Current Population Reports, Series P-25, No. 985. Washington, DC, US Government Printing Office, 1986a.

US Bureau of the Census: Metropolitan and non-metropolitan residence and region—Poverty status in 1985 of persons, by family status, type of family and race. Current Population Reports—Consumer Income, Series P-60, No. 158, Table 6. Poverty in the United States, 1985. US Department of Commerce, Washington, DC, US Government Printing Office, 1986b.

US Bureau of the Census: Persons below the poverty level, by family status, type of family, race, and Spanish origin, 1959, 1960, 1965, 1968 to 1984. Characteristics of the Population Below the Poverty Level: 1984. Current Population Reports, Series P-60, No. 152. Washington, DC, US Government Printing Office, 1986c.

US Bureau of the Census: Age and sex—Poverty status in 1985 of persons, by family relationship, type of family, race, and Hispanic origin, Table 7. Current Population Reports, Series P-60, No. 158. Washington, DC, US Government Printing Office, 1987a.

US Bureau of the Census: Current Population Reports, Series P-20, Nos. 303 and 429. Washington, DC, US Government Printing Office, 1987b.

US Bureau of the Census: Metropolitan and non-metropolitan and poverty area residence by region—Persons by poverty status in 1975, by family status, sex of head, and race. Characteristics of the Population Below the Poverty Level, 1975. Series P-60, No. 106, Population Reports, Consumer Income. Washington, DC, US Government Printing Office, 1987c.

US Bureau of the Census: Rates of income of poverty level in 1985, persons by family status, sex of household and race, Table 4. Poverty in the United States, 1985, Series P-60, No. 158. Washington, DC, US Government Printing Office, 1987d

US Bureau of the Census: Age, type of residence, region and work experience—Poverty status in 1985 of persons by race and Spanish origin. Current Population Reports, Series P-60, Money Income 1986, Table 18. Washington, DC, US Government Printing Office, 1988.

US Bureau of the Census: Marital status and living arrangements, March 1982, 1985, 1987 and 1988. Current Population Reports, Series P-20, Nos. 380, 410, 423, and 433. Washington, DC, US Government Printing Office, 1989.

US Department of Health and Human Services, Office of the Inspector General, Region X: Report on Runaway and Homeless Youth. Washington, DC, 1983.

US Department of Health and Human Services: Sexually Transmitted Disease Statistics: 1985. Issue No. 135. Atlanta, Centers for Disease Control, 1987.

US Department of Health and Human Services: Health USA 1988. DHHS Publication 89-1232. Hyattsville, MD, US Government Printing Office, 1989.

US Department of Health and Human Services: Sexually Transmitted Disease Statistics, Unpublished data. Atlanta, Centers for Disease Control, 1990.

US Federal Bureau of Investigation: Uniform crime reports for the United States. Washington, DC, US Government Printing Office, 1987.

US Government: Reauthorization of the Juvenile Justice and Delinquency Prevention Act: Runaway and Homeless Youth. Hearing before the Subcommittee on Human Resources, Committee on Education and Labor, House of Representatives. Publication 100-72. Washington, DC, US Government Printing Office, 1988.

US Immigration and Naturalization Service: Statistical Yearbook. Washington, DC, US Government Printing Office, 1987.

US Preventive Services Task Force: Guide to clinical preventive services: An assessment of the effectiveness of 169 interventions. Report of the US Preventive Services Task Force. Baltimore, Williams & Wilkins, 1989.

Wetzel JR: American Youth: A Statistical Snapshot. The William T. Grant Commission on Work, Family, and Citizenship. Washington, DC, The William T. Grant Foundation, 1987.

William T. Grant Commission on Work, Family, and Citizenship: The Forgotten Half: Pathways to Success for America's Youth and Young Families. Youth and America's Future. Washington, DC, The William T. Grant Foundation, 1988.

Williams AF, Carsten O: Driver age and crash involvement. Am J Public Health 79:326, 1989.

Witkin MJ, Atay JE, Fell AS: Specialty mental health system characteristics. In Maderscheid RW, Barrett SA (eds): Mental Health, United States, 1987. Rockville, MD, US Department of Health and Human Services, NIMH, 1987.

CHAPTER 3

International Profile

ROBERT W. BLUM and MENG XIANGDONG

INTRODUCTION

Dramatic reductions in infant mortality in many developing nations over the last 20 years along with major population shifts within and between countries have resulted in a rising international awareness of the health and social concerns of adolescents and young adults.

In the 2 decades between 1960 and 1980 the rate of growth in the number of young people 10 to 24 years of age increased at a pace nearly 50% above that of the general global population growth—a staggering 66%! Today, 30% of the world's population is between 10 and 24 years of age; and increasingly these young people are residing in developing countries.

There has been a dramatic increase in infant survival without a concomitant reduction in birthrates in many developing countries, and there have been important population shifts as well, which have resulted in an increasing focus on education; rural to urban migration; international migration, including the rise in the number of refugees and the influx of youths, especially women, into the city; unemployment; and the changing role of women in many societies.

These changes have had and will continue to have a dramatic impact on the national profiles of countries throughout the world. Within an agrarian society of early marriage and low educational aspirations, early childbearing is beneficial. But, as the age of marriage is delayed and education, including the education of women, is a national priority, early childbearing conflicts with that priority, and for the first time, nations are faced with significant numbers of out-of-wedlock births. Additionally, abortion, even where illegal, is still used. Within a rural farm community, unemployment was not a significant problem. In fact, larger numbers of children ensured assistance with planting, harvesting, and herding, but with a shift to an urban, industrialized structure, there is an increasing inability for national economies to employ and to support large numbers of young people. As a consequence, many countries are faced with greatly exacerbated problems of urban violence, alcohol and substance abuse, and social unrest that result from urban migration and unemployment.

This chapter will review some of the major causes of mortality and morbidity among young people throughout the world. Where data are available, it is critical to remember that they are at best rough approximations. Many industrialized nations have only the most rudimentary data on health outcomes such as sexually trans-mitted diseases, abortions, and suicide and even less on health behaviors. Few developing nations have the capability to maintain health statistics beyond gross mortality data and census, and even then those data may be uncertain.

EDUCATIONAL TRENDS

Despite widely divergent values placed on education in countries throughout the world, there is a clear trend toward increasing school enrollment; and although the gender gap in education in many countries remains wide, it is beginning to narrow. For example, in developing countries between 1960 and 1985, the percentage of male enrollment in school increased from 28% to 52%; during the same period, female enrollment increased nearly three times (from 15% to 41% of the eligible population). Although one cannot directly extrapolate from enrollment to literacy data, here too the trends are extremely encouraging (Fig. 3–1). Today, in many developing nations male literacy exceeds 75% and female literacy is also improving.

MORTALITY IN THE SECOND DECADE

There has been a dramatic change since World War II in the causes of mortality during the teenage years in both industrialized and developing nations. In the second decade of life, deaths caused by infection have decreased markedly and have been replaced by deaths from injuries, suicide, homicide, and war (see Chapter 2). In developing nations, maternal mortality is still a primary cause of death in the teenage years.

Unintentional Injuries

There is little doubt that unintentional injuries are the major cause of death in many countries of the world, accounting for between 46% and 51% of all deaths for males 10 to 24 years of age. Especially in developing nations, the absolute numbers of injury-related fatalities among young people increased since 1960, as did the relative rank of injuries as a cause of death. For example, in the 20 years between 1955 and 1975, automotive

Figure 3–1. Percentage literate by sex for select countries, 1980–1981. (Source: US Bureau of the Census, World Population Profile, 1985.)

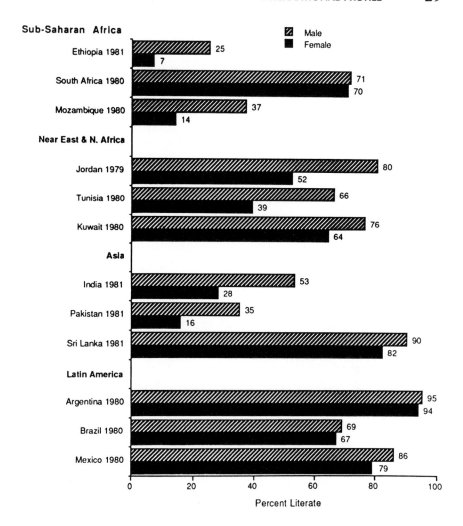

fatalities rose 600% in Mexico, 450% in Thailand, 250% in Venezuela, and 210% in Chile. Today, unintentional injuries are the leading cause of death for males 15 to 19 years of age in 48 of 58 countries for which good national mortality data exist and in 31 of those countries for females the same age (Taket, 1986).

In nearly every country males are at greater risk for death from unintentional injuries than are females (see Chapter 2). In addition, although fatalities from motor vehicles are an increasing cause of concern in many countries, other causes of unintended injury include drowning, falls, burns, poisonings, and bicycle accidents. Finally, there is cause for optimism since in the decade from 1970 to 1980 there was a reduction in deaths from unintentional injuries in 18 countries of Europe as well as in several developing countries. When analysis of unintentional injuries in the United States has been undertaken, it has been noted that many are preventable (Selbst et al, 1987) (see Chapter 2).

Suicide

Suicide is the second leading cause of death in many developed nations; data suggest rates are rising for those 15 to 24 years of age in many countries. Tables 3–1 and 3–2 provide comparison data for a number of countries.

During the decade from 1970 to 1980, youth 15 to 24 years of age in Norway experienced the largest increase in juvenile suicide (+224%),* followed by youth in Spain (+93%), in Switzerland (+80%), and in Thailand (+74%). During the same period, countries that have shown a decline in juvenile suicide rates include Guatemala (−51%), Chile (−32%), Venezuela (−28%), and Sweden (−13%) (Lester, 1988).

Historical trends associated with rising suicide rates within countries have been evaluated, and the following important correlates have been found: unemployment, divorce, homicide, alcohol use, declining church affiliation, and rising employment of women outside of the home (Diekstra, 1989a). These correlates of suicide suggest that those societies experiencing the greatest social disruption are also at greatest risk for rising suicide rates. Diekstra (1989b) suggests four strategies for suicide prevention:

1. Accurate data on causes of suicide as well as evaluation of intervention and prevention programs in a variety of cultural settings;
2. Improvement of services for those who are suicidal;
3. Effective community education;
4. Provision of special services to high-risk youth, including incarcerated youth (see Chapter 34), those

---

*Despite the significant increase in suicides among youth in Norway, Denmark has had consistently the highest rates of suicide in Scandinavia, while Iceland and Norway have had the lowest.

TABLE 3–1. Suicide Rates (per 100,000)* of Males 15 to 24 Years Old: 1973–1985

0–2.49	2.50–4.99	5.00–7.49	7.50–9.99	10.00–12.49	12.50–14.99	15.00–17.49	17.50–19.99	20.00–24.99	25.00 +
Bahamas	Barbados	England/	Argentina	Belgium	Cuba	Australia	Iceland	Czechos-	Austria
Belize	Brazil	Wales	Cape Verde	Bulgaria	France	Denmark	Japan	lovakia	Canada
Egypt	Dominican	Hong Kong	Islands	Chile	Trinidad	Luxembourg	Poland	German	El Salvador
Guatemala	Republic	Ireland	Colombia	Puerto Rico	Uruguay	New Zealand	United States	Democratic	Finland
Jordan	Fiji	Israel	Costa Rica	Thailand		Norway		Republic	Hungary
Kuwait	Greece	Martinique	Ecuador	Venezuela		Sweden		German	Sri Lanka
Malta	Italy	Netherlands	Mauritania	Yugoslavia				Federal	Switzerland
Philippines	Mexico	Northern	Scotland					Republic	
St. Lucia	Nicaragua	Ireland	Singapore					Surinam	
Syria	Panama	Portugal							
	Paraguay								
	Peru								
	Spain								

*Rates per million have been converted to rates per 100,000.
Adapted from Barraclough B: International variation in the suicide rate of 15–24 year olds. Soc Psychiatry Psychiatr Epidemiol 23:75–84, 1988.

with chronic illnesses (see Chapter 30), alcohol and substance abusers (see Chapter 111), and relatives of those who have committed suicide (see Chapter 101).

Maternal Mortality

Although not a major cause of death in industrialized nations or in those countries where abortion is legally accessible, maternal mortality remains one of the leading causes of death for young women in many developing countries (Fig. 3–2). In Ethiopia, for example, where the maternal mortality rate for women of all ages is 436 per 100,000, it is almost three times higher (1270 per 100,000) for teens 15 to 19 years old.

One major contributing factor to maternal mortality is lack of access to prenatal services. Where these services are unavailable, the World Health Organization (WHO) estimates that a young woman has a 5% to 7% chance of dying from a complication of pregnancy.

Not all maternal deaths internationally are the result of childbirth; complications from illegal abortion may account for nearly one half of all maternal deaths. In those countries where it is legal, abortion mortality is less than the mortality from childbirth; where abortion is illegal, the World Health Organization estimates that it accounts for between 150,000 and 200,000 maternal deaths annually of women of all ages. In Addis Ababa, Ethiopia, for example, 54% of all pregnancy-related deaths were the result of abortion complications; in Lagos, Nigeria, 51% of all pregnancy-related deaths also resulted from abortion. Yet for young women who are unmarried and who become pregnant, the choice is often one between risking death through abortion and risking personal ruin or expulsion from home and school through childbearing.

In most countries where abortion is legal, during the last 20 years there has been a general rise in the rate of abortion among teenage women, followed by a plateau and then a more recent decline (Fig. 3–3). For countries

TABLE 3–2. Suicide Rates (per 100,000)* of Females 15 to 24 Years Old: 1973–1985

0–2.49	2.50–4.99	5.00–7.49	7.50–9.99	10.00–12.49	12.50–14.99	15.00–17.49	17.50–19.99	20.00–24.99	25.00 +
Bahamas	Australia	Argentina	Equador	German	El Salvador	Thailand	Surinam	—	Cuba
Barbados	Belgium	Austria	Hungary	Democratic					Sri Lanka
Belize	Brazil	Bulgaria	Japan	Republic					
Egypt	Cape Verde	Canada	Mauritania	Singapore					
Fiji	Islands	Colombia	Sweden	Trinidad					
Greece	Chile	Czecho-	Switzerland						
Guatemala	Costa Rica	slovakia							
Ireland	Dominican	Denmark							
Italy	Republic	German							
Jordan	England/	Federal							
Kuwait	Wales	Republic							
Malta	Israel	Hong Kong							
Mexico	Netherlands	Luxembourg							
Nicaragua	New Zealand	Martinique							
Northern	Norway	Paraguay							
Ireland	Peru	Uruguay							
Panama	Poland	Yugoslavia							
Philippines	Portugal								
Puerto Rico	Scotland								
St. Lucia	United States								
Spain	Venezuela								
Syria									

*Rates per million have been converted to rates per 100,000.
Adapted from Barraclough B: International variation in the suicide rate of 15–24 year olds. Soc Psychiatry Epidemiol 23:75–84, 1988.

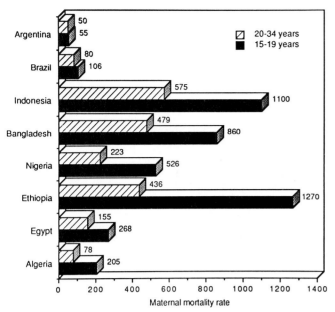

Figure 3–2. Maternal mortality rate per 100,000 live births: a comparison of adolescents with women aged 20–34 years. (For Brazil, data are for older women aged 20–29 years.) (Source: WHO, 1989.)

where abortion is illegal, it is far more difficult to quantify its incidence; however, in a study of 60 developing countries in the late 1970s, the International Planned Parenthood Federation estimated there were

207 induced abortions per 1000 live births. In South America, where abortion is uniformly illegal, 20% to 25% of pregnancies are estimated to end in abortion. Although there are no adolescent-specific data, it would be reasonable to believe that adolescent abortion rates would *at least* roughly parallel national rates.

MORBIDITY IN THE SECOND DECADE

Substance Use

TOBACCO

There is a growing awareness in both developing and industrialized countries that tobacco represents a major cause of morbidity. As Kandel and Logan (1984) have shown, in the United States cigarettes are the only substance of abuse whose use continues to increase after the age of 22. Its potency has been highlighted by showing that if a teenager is able to smoke and inhale two cigarettes nonconsecutively at any time, then there is a high likelihood that he or she will progress to being a regular smoker (Perry et al, in press).

Although data on smoking have many flaws, there are two general trends. In many industrialized nations, the incidence of juvenile smoking declined in the decade from 1970 to 1980; however, in Eastern Europe and developing nations of Africa, South America, and Asia,

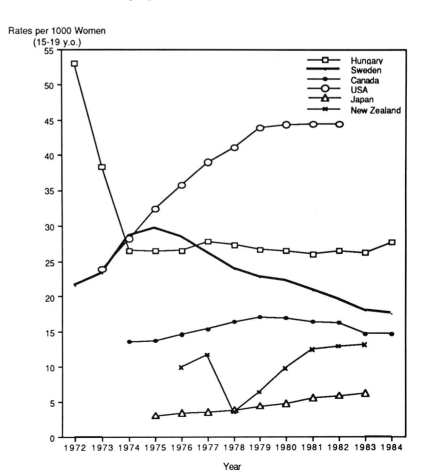

Figure 3–3. Trends in abortion rates for adolescent women 15–19 years old for selected countries, 1972–1984. (Source: Henshaw S, Tietze C: Induced Abortion: A World Review. New York, Alan Guttmacher Institute, 1986.)

**TABLE 3–3. Smoking Prevalence* Among
Young People in Selected Developing Nations:
1980–1985**

| COUNTRY | PERCENTAGE | |
	Male	Female
Brazil	10	16
Chile	52	69
Uruguay	66	72
Nepal	25	14
Papua New Guinea	66	72
Ethiopia	16	3
Nigeria	71	18
Senegal	71	52

*Based upon best approximations derived from local surveys. Ages of those
surveyed range from 14 to 25 years of age. Sample size and methodologies vary
considerably.
Source: WHO, unpublished data.

evidence suggests that rates continue to increase. In October 1990, the Soviet Union's Minister of Health commented on the heavy marketing that the tobacco industry was undertaking in that country: "There are those who suggest that we change the name of our country to Marlboro Country because of the billions of cigarettes Philip Morris recently sent." Because markets are restricted in Western Europe and North America, the tobacco industry is looking elsewhere. Table 3–3 lists the prevalence of cigarette smoking among young people in selected developing countries.

In industrialized nations, reductions in cigarette smoking are especially notable among males; however, this is misleading, for when smoking incidence takes into account switching to pipes and cigars and chewing smokeless tobacco, the gender differences almost totally disappear.

There have been substantial reductions in juvenile smoking in countries where there have been concerted smoking prevention programs combining public education through the media, restrictions on tobacco advertising, school education programs, and restrictions on public smoking. In the United States, prevalence in daily smoking among juveniles fell from 29% in 1976 to 18% in 1982 (there has been no reduction since that time). Likewise, in Norway and Sweden, where there have been intensive antismoking programs, there also have been substantial reductions in smoking (Fig. 3–4).

As industrialized nations limit advertising of tobacco and restrict public smoking, the tobacco industry is changing its marketing focus to the developing nations of Africa (especially West Africa), Southeast Asia, and Latin America. China is already the largest consumer of tobacco in the world, and the increasing incidence of tobacco use among juveniles in much of the developing world suggests that tobacco companies (in the short run, at least) may find receptive markets there.

ALCOHOL AND OTHER SUBSTANCES OF ABUSE

Adolescence is an age of experimentation in many societies; one aspect of experimentation relates to the use of distilled beverages and other mind-altering substances. As youth move from rural to urban communities, as unemployment and social ennui increase, as

access to alcohol and other substances increases, so too does the likelihood of substance abuse by young people. While a general trend toward increased substance use through the adolescent years has been shown, the specific substances and the extent of abuse are heavily influenced by cultural factors and availability (see also Chapter 111).

Reproductive Health

NONMARITAL SEXUAL BEHAVIOR
(see Chapters 2 and 68)

There is very good reason to believe that in many countries—industrialized and developing alike—large numbers of young people are engaged in early sexual intercourse. In the United States, approximately 70% have had their sexual debut prior to age 18; in Sweden this figure is 94%, and it is 50% in France, Great Britain, and the Netherlands (Jones et al, 1986). These data are consistent with findings of the Demographic and Health Survey, which reported that one half of all 20- to 24-year-old females in Colombia had had intercourse, and three fourths of them had done so prior to marriage. In Botswana, 45% of 15- to 17-year-olds report having had intercourse, a percentage comparable to that in much of southern and eastern Africa. The cultural norms more than the economic status of a nation appear to influence the age at first intercourse. In Japan, fewer than 17% of unmarried 20-year-old females had reported experiencing intercourse. Likewise, in countries of Central America rates are below 20% (Morris, 1983).

OTHER TRENDS IN REPRODUCTIVE HEALTH

Two other trends in adolescent reproductive health are worth mentioning. Evidence from the Contraceptive Prevalence Survey indicates that there is growing awareness of contraceptive options for young people around the world. In many developing countries more than 90% of young women are able to name at least one form of contraception.

This increase in contraceptive knowledge is paralleled by a desire to limit family size. In those developing countries where it has been studied, the "ideal" family size has decreased by nearly one third in the years between 1970 and 1985. In Colombia, for example, 15- to 19-year-old women considered 3.6 children to be the ideal number in 1969; in 1986, the ideal was 2.4 children.

PREGNANCY AND CHILDBEARING (see Chapters 2 and 74)

Throughout much of the past 30 years there has been a dramatic rise in adolescent fertility in most countries of Europe and North America. Concomitantly, throughout many industrialized countries there has been an equally dramatic rise in out-of-wedlock births among adolescents. This is in contrast with much of the developing world, in which—at least until recently—most childbearing occurred within marriage.

What distinguishes the industrialized from the devel-

Figure 3—4. Change in smoking incidence among adolescents between 1970 and 1980 in selected countries. (Source: WHO, unpublished data.)

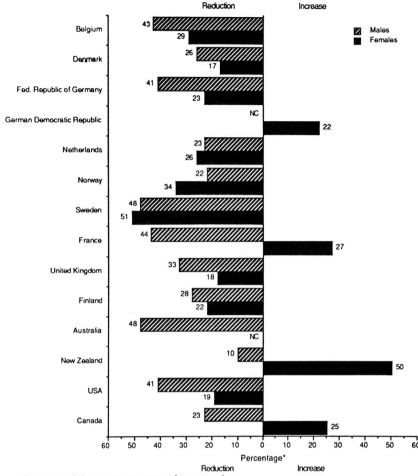

* Percentage of change, not percentages of current smokers

oping world is not so much the age at onset of intercourse, but rather the age at marriage. In Bangladesh, for example, the mean age at marriage was 11.6 years for girls in 1976. In most of sub-Saharan Africa, two thirds of girls 15 to 19 years of age live in consensual unions or marriages.

As developing countries move to limit population growth, one strategy that has been used is to delay the age at marriage. This has proved to be an effective strategy in reducing adolescent fertility. Tunisia, where the mean age at first marriage was 24 in 1981, had an adolescent fertility rate of 35 per 1000 (one half that of its neighbors). This same strategy, however, raises the likelihood for nonmarital sexual activity and out-of-wedlock pregnancies.

In conclusion, there are economic and social trends in many developing nations that parallel those that industrialized countries experienced a generation or more ago. In addition, death and morbidity from infectious causes are becoming increasingly controlled in developing countries (see Chapter 2). As a consequence, the major causes of morbidity and mortality during the second decade of life among the industrialized countries are becoming more prevalent among the developing

countries: unintentional injuries, self-inflicted trauma, violence toward others, substance abuse, and precocious childbearing.

BIBLIOGRAPHY

Blum R: Global trends in adolescent health. JAMA 265:2711, 1991.
Diekstra R: Suicidal behavior in adolescents and young adults: The international picture. Crisis 10(1):15, 1989a.
Diekstra R: Toward a comprehensive strategy for the prevention of suicidal behavior. Acta Paediatr Scand 80(Suppl 354):19, 1989b.
Jones E, Forrest J, Goldman N, et al: Teenage Pregnancy in Industrialized Countries. New Haven, CT, Yale University Press, 1986.
Kandel D, Logan J: Patterns of drug use for adolescents to young adulthood: Periods of risk for initiation, continued use and discontinuation. Am J Public Health 74:660, 1984.
Lester D: Youth suicide: A cross-cultural perspective. Adolescence 23(92):955, 1988.
Morris L: Teenage fertility data in Latin America. Paper presented at the Regional Adolescent Reproductive Health Workshop, Bahia, Brazil, November 1983 (unpublished).
Perry C, Grant M, Ernberg G, et al: W.H.O. collaborative study on alcohol education and young people: Outcomes of a four-country pilot study. Int J Addict, in press.
Selbst S, Alexander D, Ruddy R: Bicycle-related injuries. Am J Dis Child 144:140, 1987.
Taket A: Accident mortality in children, adolescents and young adults. WHO Quarterly 39(3):232, 1986.

Biologic Issues

CHAPTER 4

Neuroendocrine Regulation of Puberty

EDWARD O. REITER and HOWARD E. KULIN

Puberty is a transitional period between childhood and adulthood, during which a growth spurt occurs, secondary sexual characteristics appear, fertility is achieved, and profound psychological changes take place. The events of pubertal maturation, however, are only one part of a developmental continuum extending from initial sexual differentiation to senescence.

MATURE NEUROENDOCRINE AXIS
(Figs. 4–1 and 4–2)

The regulatory systems that control human reproduction include

1. Suprahypothalamic sites, including the limbic system, along with higher cortical centers, that influence production and release by the hypothalamus of the gonadotropin-releasing hormone (GnRH). Diverse clinical examples, such as the altered pubertal development often associated with psychiatric syndromes (e.g., anorexia nervosa), confirm the importance of higher brain neurochemical regulation.
2. The arcuate nucleus of the medial basal hypothalamus and its transducer neurosecretory neurons, whose signals are mediated by the periodic, oscillatory release of gonadotropin-releasing hormone (GnRH). GnRH is a decapeptide released from the median eminence into the primary plexus of the hypothalamic-hypophyseal portal circulation, the conduit to the anterior pituitary gland. Although direct measurements of GnRH secretion in humans are limited, studies in primates have shown that intermittent abrupt increases in pubertal blood GnRH concentrations do occur.
3. The pituitary gonadotropes, which respond to the GnRH rhythmic signal and release luteinizing hormone (LH) and follicle-stimulating hormone (FSH) in a pulsatile manner into the general circulation. The gonadotropins act to stimulate synthesis and secretion of a variety of gonadal steroids and peptides.

This neuroendocrine axis, with its three principal components, is common to all mammalian species. At each of the loci, modulating factors exert significant effects. Further, at each level within the neuroendocrine unit, target cells contain hormone-specific receptors (membrane-bound in the case of peptide hormones, and

intracellular for steroids), thereby allowing mediation of the varied input signals.

NATURE OF GONADOTROPIN SECRETION

Assay Methodologies

Techniques employed to quantify LH and FSH have included bioassay systems as well as sophisticated competitive binding assays, such as radioimmunoassays (RIA), immunoradiometric assays (IRMA), and immunofluorometric assays (IFMA). Biologic activity of the gonadotropins has been determined through *in vivo* systems such as the ventral prostate and ovarian augmentation assays, which quantitate LH and FSH on the

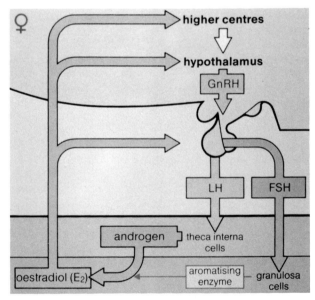

Figure 4–1. Diagrammatic representation of the hypothalamic-pituitary-ovarian axis. The interaction of gonadotropins and the components of the ovarian follicles are shown. Sex steroid feedback effects upon the brain, hypothalamus, and pituitary can also be seen. LH, luteinizing hormone; FSH, follicle-stimulating hormone; GnRH, gonadotropin-releasing hormone. (From Reiter EO: Normal and abnormal sexual development. In Besser GM, Cudworth AE [eds]: Slide Atlas of Endocrinology. London, Gower Medical Publishing, 1986, slide no. 16.14.)

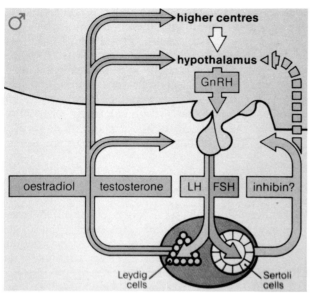

Figure 4–2. Diagram of the hypothalamic-pituitary-testicular axis. The testes differentiate into steroid-producing tissue (Leydig cells) and germinal epithelium (seminiferous tubules). The effects of gonadotropins upon the two gonadal components as well as feedback of steroids and inhibin upon the brain, hypothalamus, and pituitary are indicated. (From Reiter EO: Normal and abnormal sexual development. In Besser GM, Cudworth AE [eds]: Slide Atlas of Endocrinology. London, Gower Medical Publishing, 1986, slide no. 16.15.)

basis of change in organ weight, or *in vitro* bioassays, such as the rat interstitial cell testosterone production assay for LH or the Sertoli cell aromatase activity assay for FSH. The latter two *in vitro* assays are highly sensitive and specific in their measurements.

The competitive binding assays for gonadotropins utilize competition between purified labeled LH or FSH standard and unknown amounts of hormone in serum or urine for binding sites on highly specific antibodies. Most of the currently published studies measuring LH and FSH employed double antibody radioimmunoassays (RIA). However, these data are now being superseded by investigations using even more sensitive immunoradiometric assay ("Sandwich," IRMA) or immunofluorometric assay (IFMA) techniques because of their ability to detect extremely low serum LH and FSH concentrations, perhaps obviating the need to use urinary gonadotropin assays in prepubertal adolescents. Assays of urine extracts, however, do allow an easy means of integrating pulsatile LH and FSH secretion (see later).

Since there is considerable molecular heterogeneity of circulating LH and FSH, qualitative as well as quantitative changes in concentrations of circulating gonadotropins are important in determining gonadal steroidogenesis and maturation of germinal tissue. Post-translational synthetic modifications of gonadotropins, primarily in carbohydrate content, lead to rather striking alterations in biopotency, receptor binding activity, and plasma half-life. The very sensitive *in vitro* bioassays measure the important biologically active gonadotropins and do not quantitate the molecular subspecies, which have only immunologic potency. IFMA systems appear to measure molecular forms that more accurately reflect circulating bioactive gonadotropins than do RIA determinations.

Patterns of Gonadotropin Release

PULSATILE AND CIRCADIAN

FSH and LH are always secreted in a pulsatile or episodic (circhoral) manner with discrete bursts of hormone release from the gonadotroph separated by periods of little or no secretory activity. The frequency and amplitude of these bursts are modulated by the interaction of GnRH and sex steroids at the pituitary level to produce the various gonadotropin concentration profiles present in the peripheral circulation. In the biologically mature male, pulsatile release of LH has a periodicity of about 90 minutes; the periodicity of the LH secretory episodes is similar in adult females, except during the mid- and late-luteal phases of the menstrual cycle when the LH pulses are diminished to every 3 to 4 hours. FSH periodicity is less prominent than that for LH.

The GnRH input to the pituitary gonadotropes is also frequency coded. This intermittent nature of the GnRH signal appears to be critical in maintaining normal LH and FSH release, since inhibition of gonadotropin secretion by continuous infusion of GnRH occurs via desensitization, or down-regulation, of gonadotrope GnRH receptors.

Circadian rhythmicity is an additional characteristic of gonadotropin release in children and adolescents. A diurnal pattern with nocturnal, sleep-enhanced increments of LH and FSH release occurs until adulthood, when the nocturnal amplification diminishes and the pattern of gonadotropin release becomes relatively constant throughout the day.

TONIC AND CYCLIC

The terms *tonic* and *cyclic* are used to describe the patterns of gonadotropin concentration present in the peripheral circulation. Tonic or mean basal levels of gonadotropins result from regulation by inhibitory mechanisms whereby fluctuations in the concentration of circulating sex steroids or nonsteroidal regulators of FSH secretion produced by germinal tissue inhibins produce reciprocal changes in the episodic secretion of LH or FSH. Several blood samples for measurement of gonadotropins are required to characterize in a general way the mean circulating levels of these hormones. These gonadally mediated inhibitory processes, along with central neuroregulation, maintain gonadotropin levels for periods of days.

Cyclic secretion involves a positive (stimulatory) feedback mechanism, usually an increment in circulating estrogens to a critical level for a sufficient time. A synchronous, pulsatile burst of LH and FSH follows such a stimulus, which is characteristic of the ovulatory midcycle surge.

CONTROL OF GONADOTROPIN SECRETION
Putative Hypothalamic Regulators

Many different neurotransmitters have some regulatory input to the arcuate nucleus release of GnRH.

Catecholaminergic, noradrenergic, dopaminergic, and opioidergic neurons have been shown to modulate GnRH synthesis, secretion, and feedback regulation by sex steroids. Neuroactive amino acids (e.g., aspartate or glutamate) may also regulate GnRH secretion. N-Methyl-D-aspartate (NMDA) injections into rodents and monkeys have triggered the pubertal process and have focused investigative interest on these agents. Melatonin does not appear to play a significant role in GnRH control in primates, although it does in lower animals.

Gonadal Function

Although the testis increases significantly in size during the several years before the onset of puberty, testosterone levels appear to remain constant at less than 10 ng/dl (in boys and girls) throughout childhood. During puberty in boys, circulating testosterone levels increase more than 20-fold. Once testosterone levels begin to rise in boys, they do so relatively rapidly, usually associated with the pubertal growth spurt. A testicular length of more than 2.5 cm is consistent with early pubertal development, the change being primarily due to the tubular constituents of the gonad. Studies of the onset of spermatogenesis in boys are few, but this process may occur at a relatively early stage of sexual maturation. By age 13 or 14, sperm may be found in the urine of most boys who are appropriately studied.

Although the prepubertal ovary exhibits dramatic changes in terms of histologic development (presumably gonadotropin-induced), measurable differences in circulating 17β-estradiol (E_2) between boys and girls are not detectable before 7 or 8 years of age; blood levels of this most active gonadal estrogen are less than 10 pg/ml before the onset of puberty. Uterine size increases at about age 7, clearly before the onset of breast development. By age 10 years, levels of E_2 in girls are twofold greater than those in boys. Then there is a steady rise in estradiol concentration throughout female puberty, with wide individual fluctuations manifested by the time of menarche.

A family of gonadally produced glycoproteins, the inhibins, also regulate gonadotropin secretion through an FSH-inhibitory action. Both LH and FSH are needed for normal inhibin production by male Sertoli and female granulosa cells. Concentrations of immunoreactive inhibin rise throughout puberty, with levels in males twice those of females. In biologically mature males, inhibin and testosterone are secreted in concordant pulses. The maturational importance of gonadal inhibin production and subsequent interaction with the GnRH pulse secretion is not yet known.

Negative Feedback

The diminution of hypothalamic GnRH release and the subsequent lowering of pituitary gonadotropin secretion because of the effects of gonadally produced sex steroids or peptide products of the germinal epithelium are referred to as negative feedback. Other examples of negative feedback influencing the reproductive endocrine system include direct effects of gonadotropins upon the production and release of GnRH (short loop feedback) and the direct inhibiting effect of GnRH upon its further synthesis and secretion by the same or neighboring arcuate nucleus neurons (ultra-short loop feedback). In mature adults, negative feedback systems maintain the homeostasis of gonadotropin production; in puberty, they participate in the maturational process of altering the regulation of gonadotropin secretion.

Positive Feedback

When gonadotropin secretion is enhanced by rising levels of sex steroids, presumably estrogens, the process of positive feedback occurs. This is a developmentally sensitive system, which characterizes ovulatory menstrual cycles in mature women.

MATURATION OF THE HYPOTHALAMIC-GONADOTROPE AXIS (see Chapter 70)

In humans, the hypothalamic-pituitary-gonadal system differentiates and functions during fetal life and early infancy, is then suppressed to a low level of activity for almost a decade during childhood, and is reactivated during puberty. Therefore, puberty does not represent the initiation of pulsatile secretion of GnRH and gonadotropins, but rather the reactivation of the appropriate GnRH neurosecretory neurons in the arcuate nucleus. Experimental and clinical studies support the hypothesis that as yet undefined central nervous system (CNS) input (not the arcuate nucleus, the pituitary gonadotropes, or the gonads) restrains the activation of the hypothalamic-pituitary-gonadotropin-gonadal system in prepubertal children.

Changes in FSH and LH Secretion with Age

The human fetal pituitary gland can synthesize and store FSH and LH by 10 weeks of gestation and can secrete these hormones by 11 and 12 weeks. The pattern of changes in FSH and LH concentrations in pituitary glands and serum of fetuses reveals peak concentrations that reach adult castrate levels, followed by a decline after midgestation that persists to term.

After the decrease in sex steroid levels (especially estrogens) during the first days after birth, the concentrations of FSH and LH increase and exhibit wide perturbations during the first months of life. Intermittent high gonadotropin concentrations are associated with notably increased testosterone values in male infants and, to a lesser extent, with estradiol levels in females. By about 6 months in the male and 1 to 2 years of age in the female, concentrations of gonadotropins decrease to low levels, which persist during childhood until the onset of puberty.

Using conventional RIA techniques, basal gonadotropin concentrations increase in the peripubertal period. In girls, FSH levels rise during the early stages of puberty and then reach a plateau, whereas LH levels tend to rise during later stages. In boys, FSH concentrations rise progressively during puberty; LH levels increase sharply during early pubertal development and then gradually rise throughout the remainder of pubertal maturation.

In addition to these changes in immunoreactive gonadotropins, serum concentrations of biologically active LH (measured by sensitive, *in vitro* rodent interstitial cell testosterone generation assays) have been quantitated throughout fetal life and at all stages of extrauterine life. In human studies, bioactive LH concentrations are usually undetectable during prepubertal years, then rise dramatically during pubertal maturation. The increment in mean LH levels between prepubertal and pubertal states has generally been greater when determined using bioassays as compared with standard RIA techniques, perhaps because of assay sensitivity, but possibly related to qualitative changes in the LH molecule.

Studies utilizing measurements of urinary gonadotropin excretion as well as serum determinations with IFMA have shown as much as a 100-fold elevation of basal LH levels between prepuberty and adulthood, with an approximate sevenfold rise in FSH levels. IFMA measurements of LH appear to eliminate much of the bio/immuno-dissociation, stressing the importance of utilizing highly specific and sensitive measuring systems when assessing the very low gonadotropin levels of early prepubertal children.

Maturational Changes in Episodic and Circadian Release of Gonadotropins with Age (Fig. 4–3)

In prepubertal children, LH is secreted in a pulsatile manner, with a frequency and an amplitude lower than those in pubertal children or adults. The increase in the mean plasma concentration of LH during puberty correlates with the increase in both the magnitude of the LH pulses and the frequency of secretory episodes. Additionally, pulsatile release of FSH occurs in pubertal individuals, though the spikes are smaller than those of LH.

In addition to episodic fluctuations of gonadotropin release, a circadian rhythm exists that becomes augmented during late childhood and the adolescent years. In prepubertal boys, most studies have reported significant nocturnal augmentation of LH release. In prepubertal children, nocturnal urinary LH excretion is greater than that during the daytime, although absolute differences are small. Less striking nocturnal increments have been described in serum FSH levels in prepubertal children. During puberty, there is further maturation of sleep-enhanced LH secretion. In early pubertal subjects, pulsatile LH release with rising frequency and amplitude occurs largely during sleep. In late puberty, LH release is stable throughout a 24-hour period and simulates the adult pattern.

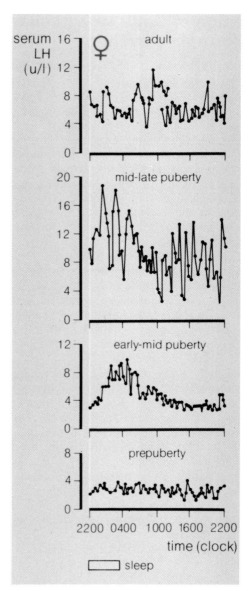

Figure 4–3. Patterns of LH secretion during pubertal development. Episodic pulses and circadian rhythms of secretion can be seen. (From Reiter EO: Normal and abnormal sexual development. In Besser GM, Cudworth AE [eds]: Slide Atlas of Endocrinology. London, Gower Medical Publishing, 1986, slide no. 16.20.)

The factors that lead to the initiation and development of this circadian rhythm remain unclear. Patients with early or premature sexual maturation, as in idiopathic precocious puberty (see Chapter 58), or glucocorticoid-treated patients with congenital virilizing adrenal hyperplasia (see Chapter 55) who have advanced bone age and early onset of true puberty exhibit the same pattern of LH secretion as do normal pubertal children. The pattern of enhanced sleep-associated LH secretion occurring in agonadal patients during the pubertal period suggests that this pattern does not depend upon gonadal function. These data, taken in aggregate, show that the increased levels of LH during the pubertal years are amplifications of preexisting modes of episodic and circadian gonadotropin release.

Interaction of GnRH with Pituitary Gonadotropin Secretion

If increased secretion of gonadotropins during the late prepubertal period is the consequence of a change in neural and hormonal restraints on synthesis and pulsatile secretion of GnRH, the disinhibition of the arcuate GnRH oscillator should lead to increased GnRH pulses (frequency and amplitude) initially, followed by increased gonadotropin secretion by the pituitary, and finally to augmented output of sex steroids by the gonad. Direct measurements of levels of GnRH in median eminence effluent have confirmed the presence of pulsatile release in prepubertal and pubertal monkeys, with an increase in pulse frequency and amplitude in the more mature animals.

With the availability of synthetic GnRH, the pituitary sensitivity to GnRH and the dynamic reserve or readily releasable pool of pituitary gonadotropins have been examined during different stages of pubertal maturation and in many disorders involving the hypothalamic-pituitary-gonadal system. The results support the concept that the prepubertal state is characterized by relative functional GnRH insufficiency.

The heightened LH response of the pituitary gonadotropes to exogenous GnRH in peripubertal children who do not yet exhibit physical signs of sexual maturation but who already have increasing levels of nocturnal gonadotrope secretion provides evidence that a self-priming effect of endogenous GnRH augments pituitary responsiveness to exogenous GnRH. The degree of previous exposure of gonadotropes to endogenous GnRH appears to affect both the magnitude and the quality of LH responses to a single dose of GnRH. As a result, the prepubertal pituitary gland has a small pool of releasable LH and thus has decreased responsiveness to acute administration of synthetic GnRH. With the approach of puberty, increased release of endogenous GnRH increases the number of LH receptors on the gonadotrope, augments pituitary sensitivity to exogenous GnRH, and enlarges the reserve of LH in the gonadotrope. The release of LH following the administration of GnRH is low in prepubertal children beyond infancy, increases strikingly during the peripubertal and pubertal periods, and is still greater in adult males and females. The change in the maturity-related patterns of FSH release after administration of GnRH is quite different from that of LH and results in a striking reversal of the FSH to LH ratio. Prepubertal and pubertal females release much more FSH than do males at all stages of sexual maturation. Prepubertal girls, in fact, have a larger readily releasable pool of pituitary FSH than do pubertal girls (Fig. 4–4).

The explanation for the discordance of FSH and LH release during maturation is not clear, but studies in the monkey with differing modes of administration of GnRH suggest that frequency of secretion of endogenous GnRH is a major factor. Altering intervals of GnRH pulse markedly affects the ratio of FSH to LH. Pulsatile GnRH can fully reestablish gonadotropin secretion in animals with lesions of the hypothalamus; similar administration of GnRH to prepubertal monkeys generates menstrual cyclicity.

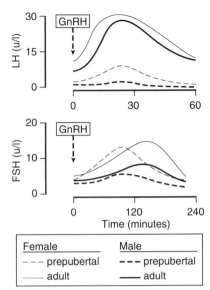

Figure 4–4. The maturity-related increment of LH is seen from prepubertal to pubertal levels. The sex differences in GnRH-induced FSH release are also demonstrated. (Redrawn from Reiter EO: Normal and abnormal sexual development. In Besser GM, Cudworth AE [eds]: Slide Atlas of Endocrinology. London, Gower Medical Publishing, 1986, slide no. 16.25.)

Administration of large doses of GnRH intravenously to patients with hypogonadotropic hypogonadism for approximately 1 week leads to normalization of previously immature responses to standard GnRH tests. In general, basal levels of FSH rise earlier than those of LH, but within several weeks, LH release in response to discrete doses of GnRH generally exceeds that of FSH, as in normal pubertal maturation.

PREPUBERTAL RESTRAINT IN GONADOTROPIN SECRETION
(Fig. 4–5)

In human and subhuman primates, the increased LH and FSH secretion in the fetus and neonate is followed by a long period during which the reproductive endocrine system is suppressed. The factors involved in this restraint of the onset of puberty are not well understood. Two mechanisms have been invoked to explain the changes in gonadotropin secretion. One is a sex steroid–dependent mechanism, a highly sensitive hypothalamic-pituitary-gonadal negative feedback system. The other is an apparently sex steroid–independent mechanism that modulates steroid or other inhibitory influences upon the arcuate nucleus or higher centers.

Negative Feedback

The inhibition of hypothalamic-GnRH release and the decrease in pituitary gonadotropin secretion after the first several years of life are hypothesized to be associated with progressively increased sensitivity of the hypothalamus, and perhaps the pituitary gland, to the inhibitory effects of sex steroids. This hypothalamic regulatory mechanism, which probably involves matu-

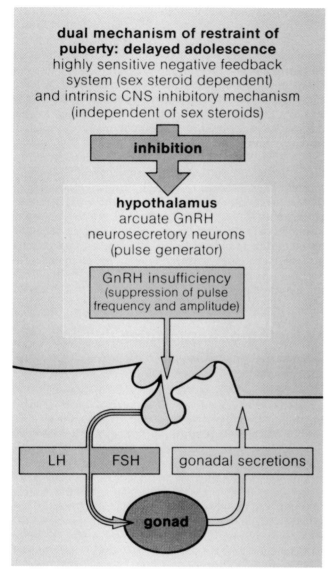

**dual mechanism of restraint of
puberty: delayed adolescence**
highly sensitive negative feedback
system (sex steroid dependent)
and intrinsic CNS inhibitory mechanism
(independent of sex steroids)

inhibition

hypothalamus
arcuate GnRH
neurosecretory neurons
(pulse generator)

GnRH insufficiency
(suppression of pulse
frequency and amplitude)

LH FSH   gonadal secretions

gonad

Figure 4–5. Diagram of the dual mechanism of restraint in puberty during midchildhood. Inhibition is great and the amount of GnRH production is small; a relative state of GnRH insufficiency is therefore present. (From Reiter EO: Normal and abnormal sexual development. In Besser GM, Cudworth AE [eds]: Slide Atlas of Endocrinology. London, Gower Medical Publishing, 1986, slide no. 16.51.)

steroids upon GnRH release, resulting in increased pulsatile GnRH release and enhanced secretion of gonadotropins.

The sensing mechanism for the set-point regulation of feedback control has been referred to as the gonadostat. It seems unlikely that a gonadostat change is the sole initiator of the fall in gonadotropin levels during middle childhood. Nonetheless, in females, acquisition of an appropriate set-point for negative feedback may be a prerequisite for appropriate gonadotropin fluctuations during the early follicular phase of the menstrual cycle to allow ripening of a mature ovum.

Direct experiments have sought to identify the site of sex steroid negative feedback upon the hypothalamic-pituitary system. Investigators using such diverse techniques as portal blood sampling, destructive lesioning of discrete hypothalamic nuclei, and microinfusion systems to administer estrogens or androgens to either hypothalamus or pituitary have accumulated data to suggest that sex steroid–induced gonadotropin suppression may occur at both hypothalamic and pituitary levels. The major inhibitory action in primates, however, appears to be at the pituitary level.

Intrinsic Central Nervous System Control (see Fig. 4–5)

The diphasic pattern of basal and GnRH-induced FSH and LH secretion from infancy to adulthood (i.e., it is higher in the first 2 to 3 years of life than in the next 8 to 10 years) is qualitatively similar in normal individuals and in patients with gonadal dysgenesis (see Chapter 55). In the agonadal individual, gonadotropin levels are strikingly higher except during the midchildhood nadir (Fig. 4–6). The striking fall in gonadotropin secretion and reserve in children with gonadal dysgenesis during middle childhood suggests the presence of CNS inhibitory influences, independent of gonadal sex steroid secretion, that may restrain gonadotropin production and delay the onset of puberty. The nature of this postulated intrinsic CNS inhibitory system during infancy and childhood and its possible interaction with gonadal steroids or peptides remain uncertain. Suppression of such a neural inhibitory mechanism would lead to reactivation of gonadotropin secretion at puberty. In some patients who develop true central precocious puberty due to a gonadotropin-dependent mechanism, the intrinsic CNS inhibitory system may be impaired, resulting in the premature appearance of the augmented, pulsatile gonadotropin secretion characteristic of puberty.

Neither the gonads nor the pituitary gland represents a rate-limiting step in the maturational process. Early findings focused attention upon the hypothalamic arcuate nucleus with its GnRH pulse generator as the site of regulation of pubertal onset. Measurements of median eminence effluent in monkeys demonstrated an increment of GnRH release from low levels in prepuberty to high amplitude frequent pulses with maturity. In contrast, substantial amounts of GnRH mRNA measured in hypothalami of immature monkeys were similar

ration of sex steroid receptors on GnRH neurons, is not fully developed at birth. During childhood, this tonic control mechanism is exquisitely and quickly sensitive to the suppressive effect of small amounts of circulating sex steroids. In contrast, considerably higher levels of estrogen are required to suppress gonadotropin secretion in adolescents and adults. Furthermore, the elevated gonadotropin concentrations during the first 2 to 3 years in patients with gonadal dysgenesis are indirect evidence that hormones secreted by the normal prepubertal gonad, despite their low level, are capable of inhibiting the highly sensitive gonadotropin secretion.

With the onset of puberty, the hypothalamic arcuate nucleus and the pituitary gonadotropes become progressively less sensitive to the inhibitory effects of sex

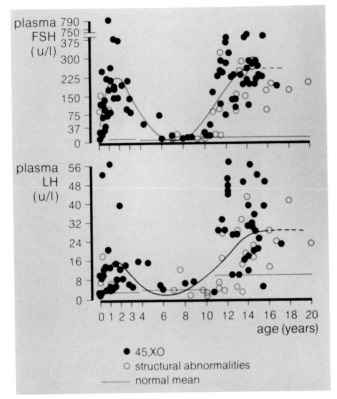

Figure 4–6. Graph demonstrating the diphasic pattern of LH and FSH levels in patients with gonadal dysgenesis. The curve is a polynomial regression plot of the data. The qualitative data shown in the normal subjects are similar to those in patients with agonadism. (From Reiter EO: Normal and abnormal sexual development. In Besser GM, Cudworth AE [eds]: Slide Atlas of Endocrinology. London, 1986, Gower Medical Publishing, slide no. 16.27.)

to quantities in pubertal animals, indicating adequate synthetic capacity for GnRH. Abundant GnRH and gonadotropin release is also evoked by administration of NMDA, an excitatory neuroamine, to juvenile monkeys. These data confirm the early potential for GnRH production, as does the ongoing release of GnRH by pulsatile administration of NMDA. Such findings suggest the hypothesis that there are suprahypothalamic neuroregulatory factors that have primary importance in the timing of puberty and eliminate arcuate nucleus secretion as the rate-limiting step in the pubertal process.

Positive Feedback and Consequent Ovulation

In normal women, the midcycle surge in LH and FSH secretion is attributed to the positive feedback effect of an increased, critical concentration of estradiol for a sufficient length of time during the latter part of the follicular phase. This stimulatory effect of estradiol upon gonadotropin secretion has not been demonstrated in prepubertal or early pubertal girls. It is a later maturational event and does not occur before midpuberty.

The development of positive feedback action of estradiol requires (1) ovarian follicles primed by FSH to secrete sufficient estradiol and maintain a critical level

in the circulation, (2) a pituitary gland that is sensitized by estrogen to amplify and augment the effect of GnRH and that contains a large enough pool of releasable LH to provide an LH surge, (3) adequate GnRH stores for the GnRH neurosecretory neurons to respond to estradiol stimulation with an acute increase in GnRH release, and (4) a sufficiently insensitive negative feedback system to allow estradiol levels to rise high enough to elicit the LH surge without shutting off GnRH and gonadotropin secretion.

Estrogen-induced positive feedback occurs directly at the pituitary level if the gonadotropes are being or have recently been exposed to GnRH. An increase in neither the frequency nor the amplitude of the GnRH pulse is required to induce a midcycle LH surge. However, available data do not exclude the possibility that, in the normal adult female, estrogen also induces an increase in GnRH release. Thus, estrogen probably exerts a positive feedback effect on both the pituitary gland and the hypothalamic GnRH neurons.

Evolution of Reproductive Capability (see Chapter 70)

Even though gonadotropin cyclicity and estrogen-induced positive feedback have been demonstrated by midpuberty, the positive feedback loop does not appear to be completely mature at that time. Indeed, the modulating action of estradiol production by the mid-pubertal ovary on the hypothalamic-pituitary-gonadotropin unit is insufficient to induce an ovulatory LH surge even in the presence of adequate pituitary stores of readily releasable LH and FSH. The ovary, from either lack of sufficient gonadotropin stimulation or decreased responsivity, does not secrete estradiol in sufficient amount or duration to induce the ovulatory LH surge. Thus, during the first 2 years postmenarche as many as 50% to 90% of cycles are anovulatory, decreasing to fewer than 20% of cycles by 5 years after menarche.

The onset of reproductive capacity in boys is not marked by an easily detectable event, such as menarche in girls. The appearance of sperm in urine (spermaturia), however, does allow an approximation of the time of spermarche, the first release of spermatozoa. The median age of spermarche is approximately 14 years, a time when mid- to late-pubertal levels of gonadotropins are being produced.

CONTROL OF THE TIME OF ONSET OF PUBERTY

The specific mechanisms involved in the timing of puberty are complex and poorly understood. The average age at menarche has shown a secular trend over the past century toward earlier occurrence (see Chapter 5). This progressive decline in the age at puberty is thought to be due to improvements in socioeconomic conditions, nutrition, and general health. In developed nations such a trend appears to have slowed or ceased over the last 20 years.

Influences other than socioeconomic ones also affect the age at puberty. An effect of nutritional factors and body composition upon the time of onset of puberty is supported by the earlier age of menarche in moderately obese girls, by delayed maturation of the reproductive endocrine system in states of malnutrition and chronic illness, and by the relationship of amenorrhea to such states of diminished body fat as anorexia nervosa and voluntary weight loss. Very vigorous physical conditioning, perhaps relating to energy expenditure, may independently affect pubertal onset and progression.

Recent studies have speculated upon potential metabolic signals during pubertal maturation. Earlier utilization of alternative energy stores (i.e., amino acids and fatty acids) by the fasting juvenile primate than by the adult primate, perhaps related to increased rates of energy consumption or diminished availability of energy substrate, suggests a linkage between metabolic alterations during maturation and the timing of pubertal onset. In contrast with their central role in nonprimate reproductive physiology, the pineal gland and melatonin do not have an important inhibitory influence on this control system in humans and other primates. Inhibitory opioidergic effects upon GnRH release have been well characterized in adults; this system, however, appears less important in the pubertal process. The more recent evidence that excitatory neuroamines may fully activate the hypothalamic-pituitary-gonadal axis in monkeys provides further support for suprahypothalamic regulation. The neurophysiologic systems that effect temporal influences on the maturing reproductive endocrine system remain undefined.

BIBLIOGRAPHY

Beitins IZ, Padmanabhan V, Kasa-Vuba J, et al: The role of biological activity of gonadotropin in puberty. In Sizonenko PC, Aubert ML (eds): Developmental Endocrinology. New York, Raven Press, 1990, pp 117–126.

Grumbach MM, Kaplan SL: The neuroendocrinology of human puberty: An ontogenetic approach. In Grumbach MM, Sizonenko PC, Aubert ML (eds): Control of the Onset of Puberty. Baltimore, Williams & Wilkins, 1990, pp 1–68.

Kulin HE: Normal pubertal development. In Rudolph AM, Hoffman JLE (eds): Pediatrics, 19th ed. Norwalk, CT, Appleton & Lange, 1991, pp 1665–1671.

Plant TM: Gonadal regulation of hypothalamic gonadotropin-releasing hormone in primates. Endocr Rev 7:75, 1986.

Plant TM: Puberty in primates. In Knobil E, Neill JD (eds): The Physiology of Reproduction. New York, Raven Press, 1988, pp 1763–1788.

Plant TM, Gay VL, Marshall GR, Arslan M: Puberty in monkeys is triggered by chemical stimulation of the hypothalamus. Proc Natl Acad Sci USA 86:2506, 1989.

Reiter EO: Neuroendocrine control process: Pubertal onset and progression. J Adolesc Health Care 8:479, 1987.

Rosenfield RL: The ovary and female sexual maturation. In Kaplan SA (ed): Clinical Pediatric Endocrinology, 2nd ed. Philadelphia, WB Saunders, 1990, pp 259–324.

Terasawa E, Claypool LE, Gore AC, et al: The timing of the onset of puberty in the female rhesus monkey. In Delemarre-van de Waal HA, Plant TM, van Rees GP (eds): Control of the Onset of Puberty III. New York, Elsevier Science Publishers, 1990, pp 123–136.

CHAPTER 5

Normal Somatic Adolescent Growth and Development

RICHARD E. KREIPE

INTRODUCTION

Several features characterize adolescent somatic growth and development. First, change is the most constant trait of the biologic process of puberty. Hormonal regulatory systems in the hypothalamus, pituitary, gonads, and adrenal glands undergo major qualitative and quantitative changes between the prepubertal and the adult states. These bring about rapid growth in height and weight, changes in body composition and tissues, and the acquisition of primary and secondary sex characteristics that result in the development of a "boy into a man" and a "girl into a woman."

Second, somatic changes vary widely in timing of onset and completion, in velocity, and in magnitude. Tanner notes that "the one generalization about puberty that one can make without fear of contradiction is that it is variable in every possible manner between individuals" (Tanner, 1987, p. 476). Defining the limits of normal is difficult in some circumstances, and the ages of occurrence for various events are best interpreted as approximations rather than precise values.

Third, even though the timing of various events of puberty is highly variable, an individual adolescent follows an orderly sequence of events in somatic growth and development (Figs. 5–1 and 5–2). For example, in normal male puberty, androgens from the enlarging testes cause elongation and then widening of the penis, sexual hair development, and rapid growth in height. Thus, testicular enlargement should precede these events. If a male undergoes secondary sex changes and growth spurt *before* enlargement of the testes, an extratesticular source of androgen, such as the adrenal gland or exogenous anabolic steroids, should be sought (see Chapters 55 and 81).

Fourth, the emergence of the secondary sex characteristics represents a somatic manifestation of gonadal activity that can be divided into a series of stages. The five stages of physical development from prepubertal (sexual maturity rating [SMR] 1) to adult (SMR 5) have been termed the *Tanner stages* (Figs. 5–3 and 5–4). Pubic hair is included as a rating criterion but is less valid than genital criteria in assessing sexual maturation, since its appearance (termed *adrenarche* or *pubarche*) is related to adrenal, rather than gonadal, development. Hence, the appearance of adrenal androgens (dehydro-

epiandrosterone and dehydroepiandrosterone sulfate) occurs around age 8, usually without any visible somatic changes, but may result in isolated pubic hair development. Nevertheless, genital activation and adrenarche do frequently coincide.

Sexual maturity ratings based on biologic variables correlate more closely with physical maturity as measured by bone age than by chronologic age. Sexual maturity ratings also relate to the appearance of medical conditions such as acne, gynecomastia, scoliosis, and slipped capital femoral epiphysis, as well as elevation of serum alkaline phosphatase levels in both sexes and hemoglobin levels in males (Table 5–1). Thus, the SMR is frequently more relevant to the clinician than is chronologic age.

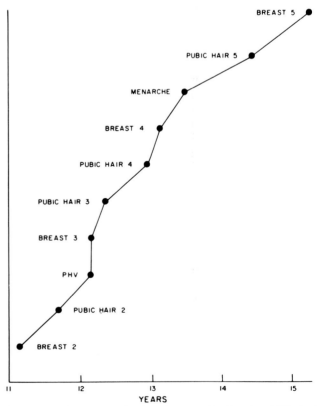

Figure 5–1. Sequence of pubertal events for females. PHV, Peak height velocity. (With permission from Root AW: Endocrinology of puberty, I: Normal sexual maturation. J Pediatr 83:1–19, 1973.)

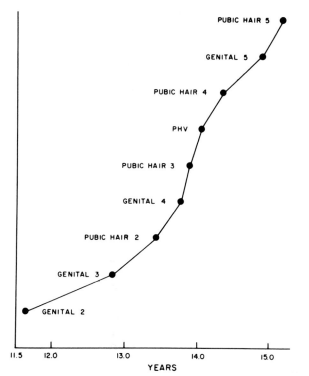

Figure 5–2. Sequence of pubertal events for males. PHV, Peak height velocity. (With permission from Root AW: Endocrinology of puberty, I: Normal sexual maturation. J Pediatr 83:1–19, 1973.)

A fifth feature of adolescent somatic growth and development is the change that has occurred over the last century in the size and age of individuals undergoing puberty. Generally attributed to improved nutrition and public health measures, this "secular" trend toward greater and earlier growth has occurred worldwide in industrialized countries and is occurring in some developing countries as well. Over the last 3 decades this trend has reached a plateau in most of North America and Europe. In addition, there are both ethnic and environmental influences on the age at onset of puberty. Compared with American whites, blacks develop slightly earlier and Mexican-Americans develop slightly later (Tables 5–2 and 5–3). Furthermore, adolescents living in rural areas tend to develop slightly later than those from urban settings.

There are certain features of somatic growth and development during puberty (such as increase in the skeletal, muscle, and fat mass; gain in weight; and biochemical alterations) that occur in both females and males, although the pattern may be different between females and males. Others, such as breast development or growth of facial hair, are relatively sex-specific.

Throughout this book, *puberty* is the term applied to the biologic processes ultimately leading to reproductive capacity. *Adolescence* refers to the psychosocial transition from childhood to adulthood. This chapter will focus on the various somatic changes that occur during puberty, including the adolescent growth spurt, the development of the gonads, the development of the secondary sex characteristics, and the changes in body composition. The normal pubertal physical changes are

presented in the context of early, middle, and late stages of development. Although such distinction is arbitrary, it does assist the clinician in determining advancing physical maturity by grouping events that commonly occur together. In addition, by breaking down pubertal development into three sequential stages, it is possible to link the biologic, psychological, and social phenomena experienced by adolescents into a comprehensive model of development as proposed recently by Vaughan and Litt (1990). The discussion will begin, however, with a summary of the central control mechanisms involved in somatic growth and development.

CENTRAL CONTROL MECHANISMS

The hypothalamus is the regulatory center for pubertal activation. Puberty is initiated as the hypothalamus becomes decreasingly sensitive to the negative feedback of sex steroids, leading to an increased output of gonadotropin releasing hormone (GnRH), as described in Chapter 4. The inhibition of tonic secretion of GnRH,

TABLE 5–1. Relationships between Clinical Conditions and Sexual Maturity Ratings (SMR)

CLINICAL CONDITION	SMR
Hematocrit rise (male)	2–5
Alkaline phosphatase peak (male)	3
Alkaline phosphatase peak (female)	2
Adolescent hormonal levels (rise in estrogen for females, testosterone for males)	2–5
Peak height velocity (male)	3–4
Peak height velocity (female)	2–3
Short male with growth potential	2
Short male with limited growth potential	4–5
Usual timing of menarche	Late 3 or early 4
Appearance of menarche	1 to 3.6 years post–stage 2
Slipped capital femoral epiphysis	(obese) 2 or 3
Acute worsening of idiopathic adolescent scoliosis (time for close monitoring)	2–4
Osgood-Schlatter disease	3
Oral contraceptive prescription	4
Diaphragm prescription	4–5
Observe for worsening of straight-back syndrome	2–4
Appearance of "normal" gynecomastia	2 or 3
Usual appearance of acne vulgaris	2 or 3
Gonococcal vaginitis	1
Gonococcal cervicitis (with or without pelvic inflammatory disease)	2+
Timing of orchiopexy	1
Decreased incidence in serous otitis media	2 or 3
Mild regression of virginal hypertrophy	5
Timing of breast reduction	5
Timing of rhinoplasty	5
Counseling for further breast growth	2
Increase levels of serum uric acid in males	2–5

With permission from Daniel WA: Growth at adolescence: Clinical correlates. Semin Adolesc Med 1:15–24, 1985.

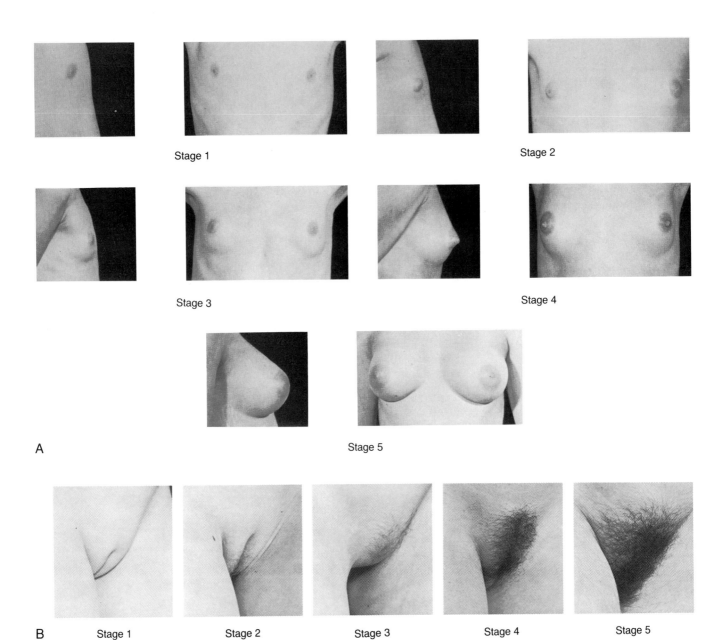

Figure 5–3. Sexual maturity ratings for females. *A,* Pubertal development in size of female breasts. Stage 1: The breasts are preadolescent. There is elevation of the papilla only. Stage 2: Breast bud stage. A small mound is formed by the elevation of the breast and papilla. The areolar diameter enlarges. Stage 3: There is further enlargement of breast and areola with no separation of their contours. Stage 4: There is a projection of the areola and papilla to form a secondary mound above the level of the breast. Stage 5: The breasts resemble those of a mature female, as the areola has recessed to the general contour of the breast.

B, Pubertal development of female pubic hair. Stage 1: There is no pubic hair. Stage 2: There is sparse growth of long, slightly pigmented, downy hair, straight or only slightly curled, primarily along the labia. Stage 3: The hair is considerably darker, coarser, and more curled. The hair spreads sparsely over the junction of the pubes. Stage 4: The hair, now adult in type, covers a smaller area than in the adult and does not extend onto the thighs. Stage 5: The hair is adult in quantity and type, with extension onto the thighs.

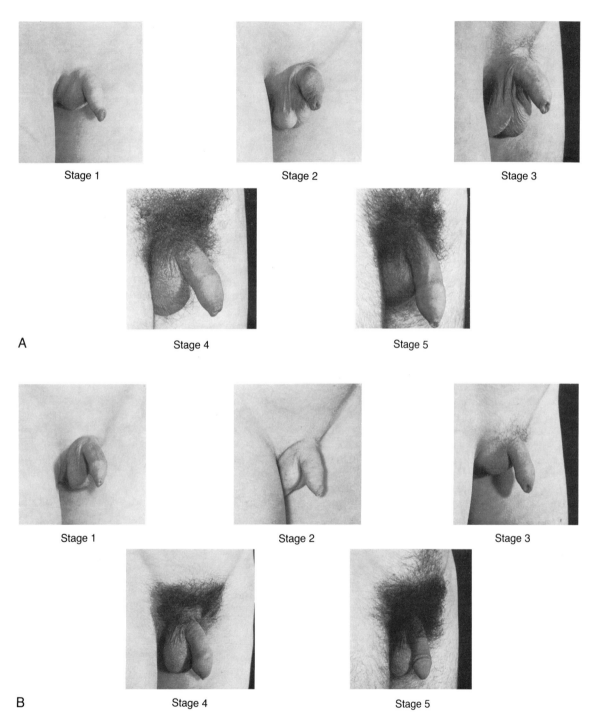

Figure 5–4. Sexual maturity ratings for males. *A,* Pubertal development in size of male genitalia. Stage 1: The penis, testes, and scrotum are of childhood size. Stage 2: There is enlargement of the scrotum and testes, but the penis usually does not enlarge. The scrotal skin reddens. Stage 3: There is further growth of the testes and scrotum, with enlargement of the penis, mainly in length. Stage 4: There is still further growth of the testes and scrotum with increased size of the penis, especially in breadth. Stage 5: The genitalia are adult in size and shape.

B, Pubertal development of male pubic hair. Stage 1: There is no pubic hair. Stage 2: There is sparse growth of long, slightly pigmented, downy hair, straight or only slightly curled, primarily at the base of the penis. Stage 3: The hair is considerably darker, coarser, and more curled. The hair spreads sparsely over the junction of the pubes. Stage 4: The hair, now adult in type, covers a smaller area than in the adult and does not extend onto the thighs. Stage 5: The hair is adult in quantity and type, with extension onto the thighs.

(*A,* With permission from van Wieringen JC, et al: Growth Diagrams. Groningen, Netherlands, Woplter-Noorhoff Publishing, 1971.)

TABLE 5–2. Maturation of White, Black, and Mexican-American Females Expressed as Percentage at SMR Stage by Age

| | PUBIC HAIR STAGES IN FEMALES (%) | | | | | | | | | | | | | | |
| | 1 | | | 2 | | | 3 | | | 4 | | | 5 | | |
AGE	W	B	M-A	W	B	M-A	W	B	M-A	W	B	M-A	W	B	M-A
12	10.2	4.5	11.0	16.5	10.3	34.0	29.5	26.9	35.0	34.9	29.8	13.0	9.2	28.2	6.5
13	2.0	0.0	1.2	9.0	2.2	19.8	22.1	17.5	39.5	44.2	42.5	22.2	21.5	37.2	17.3
14	0.4	0.0	0.0	1.0	3.0	6.3	10.8	11.0	36.3	48.4	27.0	32.5	38.9	60.0	25.0
16	0.0	0.0	0.0	0.1	0.0	1.3	2.2	1.4	10.3	30.4	20.3	20.5	67.8	78.4	68.3

| | BREAST STAGES IN FEMALES (%) | | | | | | | | | | | | | | |
| | 1 | | | 2 | | | 3 | | | 4 | | | 5 | | |
AGE	W	B	M-A	W	B	M-A	W	B	M-A	W	B	M-A	W	B	M-A
12	5.3	5.7	7.4	20.4	6.8	32.4	32.8	23.5	37.0	27.4	33.2	13.0	14.2	30.5	10.2
13	0.8	0.0	4.9	9.2	4.4	17.3	23.4	19.7	33.3	35.3	34.3	25.9	30.0	41.0	18.5
14	0.4	0.0	0.0	1.4	3.0	2.5	13.8	8.0	35.0	41.0	38.0	25.0	42.9	52.0	37.5
16	0.0	0.0	0.0	0.3	0.0	2.6	5.1	3.7	10.6	33.1	23.2	15.6	62.2	73.2	72.8

W, white; B, black; M-A, Mexican-American.
With permission from Vaughan VC, Litt IF: Child and Adolescent Development: Clinical Implications. Philadelphia, WB Saunders, 1990, p 230; as modified from Harlan WR, Harlan EA, Grillo GP: Secondary sex characteristics of girls 12 to 17 years of age: The US Health Examination Survey. J Pediatr 96:1074–1078, 1980, and Villarreal S, Martorell R, Mendoza F: Sexual maturation in Mexican-American adolescents. Am J Hum Biol 1:87–95, 1989.

the pulsatile release of GnRH, and for females, the menstrual cycle–related positive feedback of GnRH secretion all must be orchestrated for maturation of the gonads to occur. The consequent secretion of follicle-stimulating hormone (FSH) and luteinizing hormone (LH) from the anterior pituitary results in the release of sex steroids from the gonads that effect numerous biologic changes in target organs, including muscles, bones, skin, and hair follicles.

The patterns of FSH and LH secretion and resultant sex steroid release exhibit sexual dimorphism as well as diurnal variation (Figs. 5–5 and 5–6). In general, FSH levels exceed LH levels in both girls and boys in early puberty. In girls there is a later leveling off of FSH, compared with its steady rise in boys throughout puberty. There is also a lag in elevation of LH concentra-

tions relative to FSH that is more marked in girls than in boys. Although daytime estradiol concentrations in girls roughly parallel LH levels, testosterone production rises steeply in boys later in puberty, resulting in at least a 20-fold increase in testosterone during puberty. Testosterone levels in boys increase dramatically after SMR 3, even though the mean concentration of LH increases only slightly. The effect of LH is weak in early puberty because in both girls and boys there are few LH receptors.

Somatic growth during puberty occurs in response to sex steroids but also is regulated directly by two hypothalamic peptides that affect growth hormone (GH) release from the anterior pituitary: growth hormone releasing hormone (GH-RH) and somatostatin (an inhibitor of GH-RH–induced GH release). GH-RH ef-

TABLE 5–3. Maturation of White and Mexican-American Males Expressed as Percentage at SMR Stage by Age

| | PUBIC HAIR STAGES IN MALES (%) | | | | | | | | | |
| | 1 | | 2 | | 3 | | 4 | | 5 | |
AGE	W	M-A	W	M-A	W	M-A	W	M-A	W	M-A
12	26.5	57.9	41.3	28.1	21.8	11.4	8.7	2.6	1.7	0
13	9.3	22.9	26.8	32.3	28.6	20.8	23.1	13.5	12.3	10.4
14	2.7	5.9	10.5	9.9	12.4	41.6	34.9	28.7	39.6	13.9
15	0.4	0	2.5	5.4	5.1	20.3	26.8	45.9	65.1	28.4
16	0.4	0	0.8	2.9	1.8	4.3	15.5	40.0	81.4	52.9
17	0	0	0	1.6	0.4	0	5.5	7.9	94.0	90.5

| | GENITALIA STAGE IN MALES (%) | | | | | | | | | |
| | 1 | | 2 | | 3 | | 4 | | 5 | |
AGE	W	M-A	W	M-A	W	M-A	W	M-A	W	M-A
12	32.2	50.9	41.9	31.6	19.3	13.2	6.0	4.4	0.6	0
13	12.5	15.6	31.4	35.4	24.6	24.0	24.9	13.5	6.7	11.5
14	4.4	5.9	9.8	9.9	18.6	39.6	37.0	29.7	30.3	14.9
15	0.8	0	2.5	2.7	6.9	25.7	36.5	48.6	53.2	23.0
16	0	0	0.6	1.4	2.0	7.1	19.8	48.6	77.5	42.9
17	0	0	0	0	0	4.5	8.4	0	91.3	95.5

W, white; M-A, Mexican-American.
With permission from Vaughan VC, Litt IF: Child and Adolescent Development: Clinical Implications. Philadelphia, WB Saunders, 1990, p 231, as modified from Harlan WR, Grillo GP, Coroni-Huntlay J, et al: Secondary sex characteristics of boys 12 to 17 years of age: The US Health Examination Survey. J Pediatr 95:293–297, 1979, and Villarreal S, Martorell R, Mendoza F: Sexual maturation in Mexican-American adolescents. Am J Hum Biol 1:87–95, 1989.

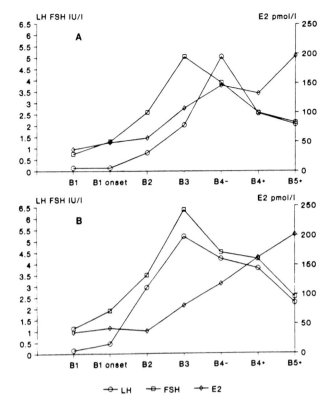

Figure 5–5. Mean plasma follicle-stimulating hormone (FSH), luteinizing hormone (LH), and estradiol (E₂) concentrations in females by sexual maturity rating, time of day, and menarcheal status. Mean plasma levels were recorded in a 6-hour sampling period during the day (A) and night (B) in girls throughout puberty. B, Sexual maturity rating of breast development; −, before menarche; +, after menarche. (With permission from Delemarre-van de Waal HA, Wennink JMB, Roelof JH: Gonadotropin secretion during puberty in man. In Delemarre-van de Waal HA, Plant TM, van Rees GP, Schoemaker J [eds]: Control of the Onset of Puberty. III. Amsterdam, Excerpta Medica, 1989, pp 151–167.)

PRIMARY AND SECONDARY SEX CHARACTERISTICS DURING PUBERTY

Ovaries

The primary female sex characteristic is the development and release of eggs from ovarian follicles approximately every 28 days. Although the full complement of ova is present at birth, it is not until early puberty (SMR 2) that FSH induces granulosa cells in numerous follicles to produce estrogen. However, the resultant estradiol concentration and the FSH-induced development of LH receptors on progesterone-producing theca cells are not yet sufficient to result in ovulation.

By the time the adolescent female reaches SMR 3 or 4, estrogens generally are produced in sufficient amounts to result in endometrial proliferation and menstruation, as described in Chapter 70. The onset of menstruation is termed *menarche*. At menarche, ova still do not generally mature to the point of being released because adequate concentrations of estrogens and progesterone cannot be sustained.

fects the release of GH, whereas somatostatin has a transient inhibitory effect on the pituitary that is followed by rebound release of GH.

Growth hormone, like GnRH, is released in pulses during sleep stages 3 and 4 in early puberty. The bursts of GH secretion are irregular and do not show the predictable periodicity of LH secretion, but they do exhibit an increased overall amplitude as puberty progresses, reaching a maximum during the height spurt (SMR 2–3). GH causes hepatocytes to secrete insulin-like growth factor I (IGF-I, also known as somatomedin C), a substance that promotes the cell multiplication required for growth in the skeleton, connective tissue, muscles, and viscera. GH is controlled by a self-regulatory, negative-feedback system that acts on the hypothalamus by stimulating somatostatin secretion and on the pituitary by inhibiting GH-RH–stimulated GH secretion. Kappy (1987) reviewed the potential value of somatomedin C therapy, not yet available, for numerous adolescents with chronic diseases associated with growth retardation (see Chapter 30).

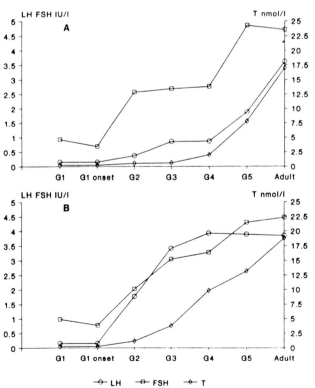

Figure 5–6. Mean plasma follicle-stimulating hormone (FSH), luteinizing hormone (LH), and testosterone concentrations in males by sexual maturity rating and time of day. Mean plasma levels were recorded in a 6-hour sampling period during the day (A) and night (B) in boys throughout puberty. G, Sexual maturity rating of genital development. (With permission from Delemarre-van de Waal HA, Wennink JMB, Roelof JH: Gonadotropin secretion during puberty in man. In Delemarre-van de Waal HA, Plant TM, van Rees GP, Schoemaker J [eds]: Control of the Onset of Puberty. III. Amsterdam, Excerpta Medica, 1989, pp 151–167.)

As puberty progresses to SMR 4 and 5, one follicle becomes dominant during each cycle and produces increasing amounts of estradiol during the follicular phase of the menstrual cycle. After ovulation, the follicle involutes into a corpus luteum that involutes after about 14 days in the absence of conception. As sex steroid concentrations subsequently fall, negative feedback on gonadotropin release declines and the concentration of FSH again begins to rise in preparation for the next ovulatory cycle.

By direct action, estrogenic compounds cause growth and development of the vagina, uterus, and fallopian tubes as well as nonsexual changes (Table 5–4). The vaginal epithelium becomes keratinized and thicker, the clitoris is slightly enlarged, and the hymenal opening almost doubles in size in response to estrogen. The skin of the labia majora, as well as that of the areola and nipple, grows and darkens under the influence of estrogen. Progesterone, too, appears to have an effect on areolar development. Breast enlargement occurs because of ductal growth and stromal development (see Chapter 77). At low levels, estrogens tend to stimulate skeletal growth, but at higher levels they inhibit growth and cause closure of the epiphyses. Estrogen also promotes growth of pubic and axillary hair, pigmentation of genital skin, and widening of the pelvic inlet and the hips.

Testes

The primary male sex characteristic is the development of viable sperm. Although the number of sperm precursors increases throughout childhood, prior to puberty the indistinct lumina of the seminiferous tubules contain undifferentiated Sertoli cells and no viable sperm, while the loose interstitium contains undifferentiated Leydig cells. During puberty, the seminiferous tubules become patent, enlarged, tortuous, and lined with Sertoli cells that have been stimulated by FSH to promote the development of viable sperm. The testicular interstitium also enlarges owing to the differentiation and growth of Leydig cells in response to LH, resulting in the production of testicular secretions including testosterone. Thus, the first visible evidence of puberty in males is the enlargement of the testes due to the growth of these cells and tissues.

In this process, males do not experience a discrete event analogous to menstruation or ovulation. However, just as the production of mature ova tends to follow the first menstrual period after an interval of more than a year, the production of viable sperm tends to follow the first ejaculation. The capacity to ejaculate appears approximately one year after initiation of SMR 2. From a clinical standpoint, however, an adolescent should be considered to be potentially fertile with her first menstrual period or his first ejaculation.

In addition to not being readily identifiable clinically, spermatogenesis also lacks the periodicity of the ovulatory cycle; the release of spermatozoa occurs without a recognizable pattern. The development of sperm within the seminiferous tubules is initiated by FSH, which has two additional actions. First, FSH stimulates the aromatization of testosterone into estradiol in the Sertoli cells of the testes. Second, it causes the development of LH receptors on the interstitial cells of Leydig. These,

TABLE 5–4. Primary Action of Major Hormones of Puberty

HORMONE	SEX	ACTION
FSH (follicle-stimulating hormone)	Male	Stimulates gametogenesis.
	Female	Stimulates development of primary ovarian follicles.
		Stimulates activation of enzymes in ovarian granulosa cells to increase estrogen production.
LH (luteinizing hormone)	Male	Stimulates testicular Leydig cells to produce testosterone.
	Female	Stimulates ovarian theca cells to produce androgens and the corpus luteum to synthesize progesterone.
		Midcycle surge induces ovulation.
Estradiol (E_2)	Male	Increases rate of epiphyseal fusion.
	Female	Stimulates breast development.
		Low level enhances linear growth, while a high level increases the rate of epiphyseal fusion.
		Triggers midcycle surge of LH.
		Stimulates development of labia, vagina, uterus, and ducts of the breasts.
		Stimulates development of a proliferative endometrium in the uterus.
		Increases fat mass of the body.
Testosterone	Male	Accelerates linear growth.
		Increases rate of epiphyseal fusion.
		Stimulates development of the penis, scrotum, prostate, and the seminal vesicles.
		Stimulates growth of pubic, facial, and axillary hair.
		Increases larynx size and thus deepens the voice.
		Stimulates sebaceous gland secretion of oil.
		Increases libido.
		Increases muscle mass.
		Increases red blood cell mass.
	Female	Accelerates linear growth.
		Stimulates growth of pubic and axillary hair.
Progesterone	Female	Converts a proliferative uterine endometrium to a secretory endometrium.
		Stimulates lobuloalveolar breast development.
Adrenal androgens	Male and female	Stimulates pubic hair and linear growth.

With permission from Neinstein LS: Adolescent Health Care: A Practical Guide, 2nd ed. Baltimore, Urban & Schwarzenberg, 1991, p 6.

in turn, mediate the production of androgens, most notably, testosterone.

Androgenic activity is also shared by different compounds; as a group these substances produce masculinization (see Table 5–4). They produce growth of the penis, scrotum, prostate, and seminal vesicles. Their tremendous growth-promoting properties also result in rapid increases in muscle mass, skeletal growth, and bone age and density. The bones of the shoulders and vertebral column, the cartilage in the larynx, and the red blood cell precursors are especially sensitive to androgenic growth promotion. In both sexes, the skin becomes thicker (and subcutaneous fat is lost in males), and hair follicles produce more sebum under androgenic stimulation. Pubic, axillary, and eventually facial and body hair develops. Clinically, increased androgenic activity is associated with such varied pubertal conditions as acne, body odor, deepening of the voice, and for males, broadening of the shoulders, the height spurt, and elevation of hemoglobin levels.

PHYSICAL GROWTH DURING PUBERTY

Growth Tempo

Because adolescents grow at varying tempos, they exhibit a variation of size and shape not seen during childhood (see Chapter 6). The average early developer (whose tempo tends to be more rapid) and the average late developer (whose tempo tends to be slower) both arrive at the same average adult height. An adolescent's growth tempo determines only *when* he or she completes growth, without an independent influence on ultimate adult size. Genetic endowment is clearly the strongest predictor of stature, accounting for more than half of the variability seen in final height. But all else being equal, early developers who grow at a slow rate tend to reach adulthood being quite short, whereas late developers who grow at a fast rate can become tall.

Similarly, the timing of the onset of breast development in girls has no relationship to breast size at the completion of puberty. Interestingly, adolescents with large breasts experience menarche about 1 year later than those who develop small breasts.

Another generalization that can be made about growth tempo is that most of the events of puberty have a gaussian distribution in the population and a standard deviation (SD) of approximately 1 year. This means that about 95% of the members of a normal population will experience a given event within 2 years (2 SD) of the mean. With respect to menarche, for which the average age is approximately 12.5 years, this means that 2.5% of normal early developing females begin to menstruate at least 2 years before that age and 2.5% of normal late maturers do not begin to menstruate until at least 2 years after that. Tanner points out that 3 in 1000 normal females do not have their first menstrual period until age 15.5 (emphasizing the importance of using clinical judgment in defining a girl as abnormal), and the same number of males do not have their peak height velocity until age 16.5 years.

All estimates of growth tempo are indirect. Bone age (BA) is the measure that best assesses the tempo of growth. Standard BA tables (Greulich and Pyle, or Bayley and Pinneau) are based on the appearance and closure of the epiphyses of bones in the hand and the wrist on radiographs; BA can then be compared to chronologic age. Individuals with a BA in advance of their chronologic age are considered early developers, whereas those with a BA less than their chronologic age are considered late developers. The velocity of attainment of SMR stages is the best clinical (and least expensive) estimate of tempo, because the physical changes occurring in both males and females, like BA, are the result of sex steroid activity.

Skeletal Growth

"Growing up" is one of the outstanding features of puberty. Immediately prior to puberty, linear growth (height velocity) is declining; during puberty it accelerates in a burst called the height spurt. When linear growth is occurring at maximal speed, adolescents are said to be experiencing their peak height velocity (PHV). Plotting an adolescent's yearly increase in height against age reveals a slightly skewed curve with an ascending limb of about 2 years' duration and a descending limb of 3 or more years' duration (Figs. 5–7 and 5–8).

Tall children tend to grow into tall adults, and short children tend to grow into short adults. The correlation between height before the height spurt and final adult height is about 0.8. Only about 30% of the variability in adult height can be accounted for on the basis of pubertal growth patterns, and less than 20% of final adult height is acquired during the growth spurt. However, adolescents who mature 2 SDs earlier than average reach a PHV that is about 1 cm/year greater and occurs 2 years before the mean. In contrast, adolescents who mature 2 SDs later than average have a PHV that is about 1 cm/year less and occurs 2 years after the mean. Wilson and colleagues (1987) developed curves to predict more accurately final adult height for early and late maturers that use sexual maturity ratings rather than radiographs, as required in other techniques of height estimation.

Close inspection of the height curves published by Tanner and Davies points out a subtle clinical feature of adolescent growth. A normal adolescent undergoing puberty does not follow normal population height curves, since these "smooth out" the effect of accelerated growth during the phase of PHV by combining early, average, and late developers. An adolescent who develops early may cross from below the 75th percentile to above the 95th percentile, with an early plateau, whereas a late developer may fall from above the 25th percentile to below the 5th percentile, followed by a late spurt. These effects are more dramatic for boys than for girls. Such an occurrence is of great concern during childhood, since moving out of one's growth "channel" at that time is often associated with a pathologic condition. However, this is merely another example of how adolescents are different from either children or adults.

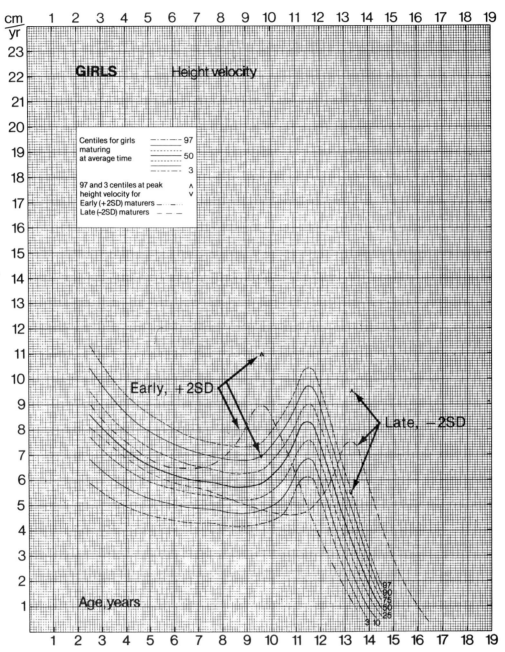

Figure 5–7. Height velocity for adolescent females. (Modified with permission from Tanner JM, Davies PW: Clinical longitudinal standards for height and height velocity for North American children. J Pediatr 107:317–329, 1985.)

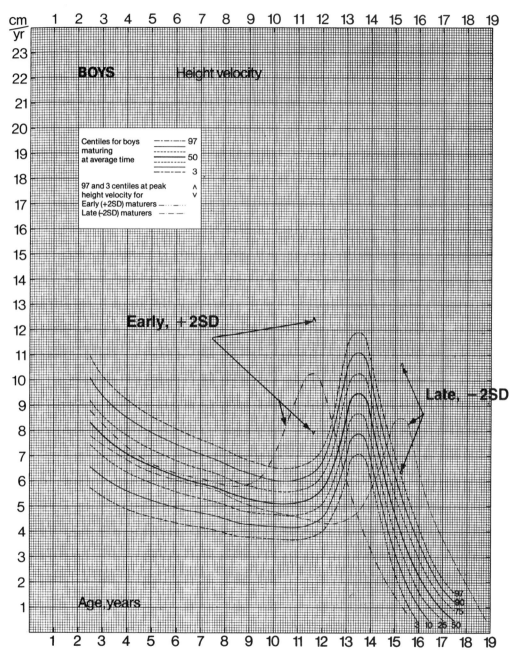

Figure 5–8. Height velocity for adolescent males. (Modified with permission from Tanner JM, Davies PW: Clinical longitudinal standards for height and height velocity for North American children. J Pediatr 107:317–329, 1985.)

The pubertal increase in linear growth follows a caudorostral progression. Thus, adolescents in early puberty tend to outgrow their shoes first, then their pants, and finally their coats. The peak velocity of lower extremity growth precedes growth of the trunk by about 6 to 9 months and that of the shoulders and chest by about 1 year. Even though boys have longer legs than girls, the increase in height during puberty in both sexes is related more to increased trunk length than to leg length. This is often not appreciated because the increase in leg length occurs first and more rapidly, whereas truncal growth comes later and is more gradual. It is interesting to note that the secular trend toward greater stature mentioned in the introduction of this chapter is due almost entirely to changes that have occurred over time in leg length and not sitting height.

Even though that portion of skeletal growth (long bones and trunk) that contributes to stature receives the most attention in analyses of puberty, it is important to recognize that all bones undergo qualitative and quantitative changes during this time. The density of the skeleton increases (more so for males than for females and more for blacks than for whites). The bones of the face undergo marked transformation; differential growth rates result most notably in a greater prominence of the nose and the jaw. The dentition also undergoes predictable development during puberty. For the secondary teeth, only the incisors and first molars are completely calcified and erupted prior to puberty. The third molars ("wisdom teeth") may not erupt until adulthood and may not become fully calcified until 25 years of age (see Appendix).

GROWTH IN FEMALES

Prior to the onset of the growth spurt, girls grow at a rate slightly more than 5.5 cm/year (range approximately 4 to 7.5). About 2 years after the initiation of the growth spurt, girls reach their PHV of slightly more than 8 cm/year (range 6 to 10.5). This maximal growth rate is reached about 6 to 12 months prior to menarche and is maintained for only a few months. Girls then begin to decelerate in linear growth over the next 2 years, reflected in a leveling off of the height curve as adult stature is approached in SMR 4 (Fig. 5–9).

One of the most outstanding and earliest features of female skeletal growth is the large spurt that occurs in hip width during puberty. The growth of the pelvis and hips (measured as the bi-iliac diameter) is quantitatively as great as that for boys. However, because girls grow less in other dimensions, their hip width appears disproportionately large in comparison with boys.

GROWTH IN MALES

Prior to the onset of their growth spurt, boys are growing at a rate of about 5 cm/year (range approximately 3.5 to 6.5). They continue to increase in height at this velocity for about 2 years, while girls are experiencing their growth spurt. Then, as the growth of their female age-mates is decelerating, boys begin to accelerate in growth, reaching a PHV of more than 9 cm/year (range 7 to 12). The mean peak height velocity for early maturing boys is more than 10 cm/year (range 8 to 12.5), compared with about 8.5 cm/year (range 6.5 to 10.5) for late maturers. Thus, during their respective growth spurts, some early maturing boys may grow at a rate of only 8 cm/year, whereas some late maturing boys may grow at more than 10 cm/year. Individuals do not grow at their peak height velocity for more than a few months. Interestingly, both boys and girls grow more in the spring and summer than in the fall and winter months. On average, boys grow about 7 cm in the first year of their spurt, 9 cm in the second year, 7 cm in the third year, 3 cm in the fourth year, and about 2 cm for each year thereafter that they continue to grow.

Broader shoulders, narrower hips, longer legs, and relatively still longer arms (particularly forearms) characterize the sexual dimorphism of male compared with female skeletal growth. The cartilage of those bones that demonstrate disproportionately greater growth (such as those in the shoulder) appears to have a heightened responsiveness to androgens. The final height differential between males (Fig. 5–10) and females of about 13 cm occurs for two reasons. First, because of a later growth spurt, boys have approximately 2 more years of prepubertal growth than girls, making them almost 10 cm taller at the initiation of the growth spurt. Second, during their growth spurt, boys have a greater PHV than that of girls.

Growth of the Heart, Lungs, and Viscera

Longitudinal studies of chest radiographs in adolescents have shown the transverse diameter of the heart to increase in parallel to overall body growth. The magnitude of the spurt in cardiac size is equal in boys and girls. The peak velocity of cardiac growth coincides with PHV. Changes in blood pressure, pulse, and electrocardiogram all are seen in relation to sexual maturation. The heart and lungs become larger not only in absolute terms but also in relation to total body size (see Chapters 42 and 45).

The lungs increase in both diameter and length during puberty (see Chapter 42). The peak velocity in diameter coincides with PHV, but the increase in length occurs approximately 6 months later. Boys and girls have an equal magnitude of growth in the lungs. Growth in the pharynx results in the hyoid bone's moving well below the level of the mandible in both sexes. The larynx exhibits significant sexual dimorphism during puberty. Under the influence of androgen, boys develop an acute 90-degree angle in their anterior thyroid cartilage (Adam's apple), in comparison with 120 degrees in girls, and vocal cords that are three times the length of those in girls.

The abdominal viscera, including the liver and kidneys, go through a growth spurt that parallels general somatic growth. Lymphatic tissue, however, such as that found in the spleen, regresses during puberty.

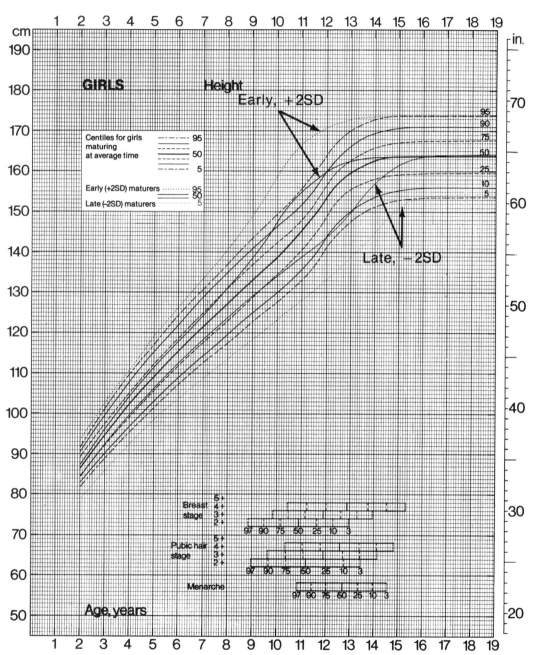

Figure 5–9. Height attained for adolescent females. (Modified with permission from Tanner JM, Davies PW: Clinical longitudinal standards for height and height velocity for North American children. J Pediatr 107:317–329, 1985.)

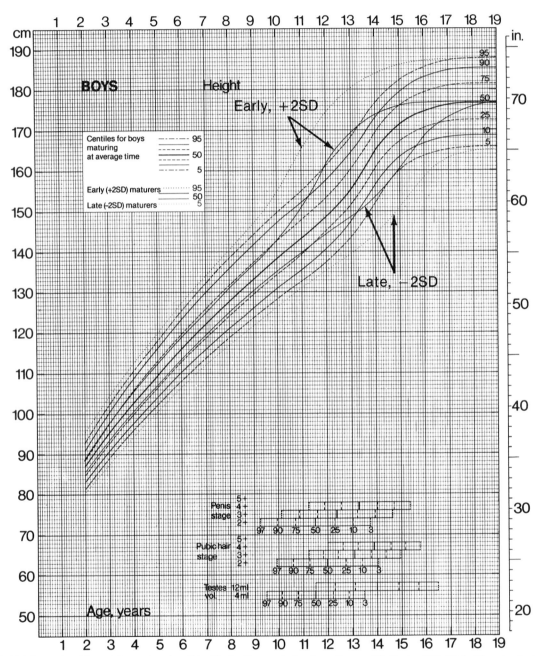

Figure 5–10. Height attained for adolescent males. (Modified with permission from Tanner JM, Davies PW: Clinical longitudinal standards for height and height velocity for North American children. J Pediatr 107:317–329, 1985.)

Growth of Muscle

All muscles grow during puberty. However, skeletal muscles receive the most attention because of their role in shaping external physical appearance, especially in males. Androgens are potent stimulators of skeletal muscle hypertrophy, as evidenced by the large increase in bulk realized by athletes taking anabolic steroids. Thus, the peak velocity for muscle growth is much greater for males than for females.

The spurt in muscle strength lags behind the spurt in muscle mass by about 1 year. Muscles first grow in size, increasing the volume of each fiber; later, increase in strength occurs owing to the effects of androgens on protein structure and enzymatic activity. Muscular strength, measured as hand grip by dynamometer, arm pull by pull-ups, or arm thrust by pushups, does not increase appreciably after menarche for females. Although the spurt in strength begins late in puberty, muscular strength continues to increase in males, especially with training, reaching a maximum by 25 years of age.

Because androgens play such an important role in determining strength, increases in strength are closely related to the SMR of an adolescent. It has been demonstrated that grip strength greater than 55 lb/in.[2] predicted an SMR higher than 3 with a high degree of accuracy in boys undergoing routine physical examinations for participation in sports.

Growth of Fat (see Chapter 6)

Data regarding changes in fat during puberty are difficult to interpret. In addition to sexual dimorphism, there is also differential deposition or loss of fat in various body locations. Furthermore, some authors describe the composite body fat changes in terms of percentage of body weight, while others describe it in absolute terms. Since change is the focus of this chapter, accumulation and loss will be described (Fig. 5–11). Subcutaneous appendicular fat (measured as triceps, biceps, and calf skinfold thickness) continues to accumulate but at a decreased velocity in both boys and girls in the year immediately prior to the peak height velocity. The accumulation of subcutaneous truncal fat (measured as subscapular, suprailiac, or abdominal skinfold thickness) is relatively constant during that period. Thus, although the velocity at which fat is accumulating is decreasing, the absolute amount of total body fat increases during early puberty for both boys and girls (see Chapter 6).

Boys actually lose fat, especially in the limbs, during their height spurt at SMR 3–4. Fat in the trunk, however, decreases little, if at all, during the male height spurt and is relatively quickly reaccumulated to prepubertal levels. Fat that is lost in the limbs of boys is much slower to reaccumulate and may never increase to prepubertal levels. Overall truncal fat increases in boys after the height spurt, adding to the weight gain that occurs relatively late in puberty. Fat normally accounts for about 12% of body weight in males by late puberty.

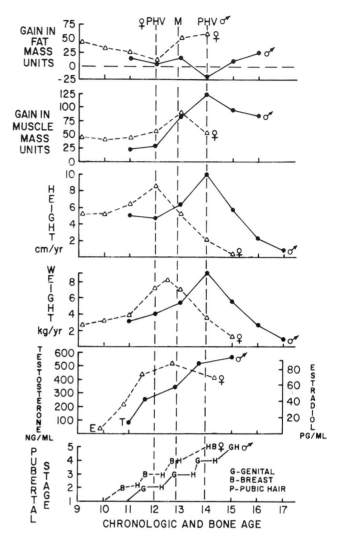

Figure 5–11. Relationships between spurt in height, weight, muscle, and fat; sex steroid levels; sexual maturity rating; and chronologic age. (Adapted with permission from Barnes HV: Adolescent medicine. In Harvey AM, Johns RJ, Owens AH, Ross RS [eds]: Principles and Practice of Medicine, 19th ed. New York, Appleton-Century-Crofts, 1976, p. 1752.)

In contrast with boys, girls have a continuous increase in body fat during puberty, interrupted only by a short-lived slowing of fat accumulation prior to their height spurt. At no time during puberty do girls normally lose fat. After their height spurt, girls lay down fat more rapidly and extensively (larger and more numerous fat cells) than do boys, resulting in more than a quarter of their weight being fat. Girls accumulate fat in both the arms and the trunk, with a predominance in the lower trunk and posterior thighs, in contrast with boys.

Frisch (1983) has noted that pubertal females experience a 44% increase in lean body mass and a 120% increase in body fat. More to the point, the lean body mass to fat ratio changes from 5:1 at the initiation of the growth spurt to 3:1 at menarche. Frisch suggests that body fat is an important mediator in the initiation of menstruation and regular ovulatory cycles because it is proportionally one of the most important components of the weight spurt for females. Although Scott and Johnston (1982) have summarized the arguments against this theory, fat cell metabolism is known to affect the levels of sex steroids. Furthermore, significant loss of body fat (as in anorexia nervosa or even "normal" dieting) to below 17% of total body weight is regularly associated with loss of menstrual periods. Using calipers, one can estimate body fat, as described in Chapter 6.

Weight Spurt

Tanner (1987) points out that because weight is easy to measure, it has an undeserved importance as a measure of growth. Weight represents the sum of many different tissue masses, and any given weight is therefore

very difficult to interpret clinically. Thus, changes in height or SMR are much more likely than weight to reflect substantive changes in growth, except in instances of acute illness or starvation. In addition, the modern emphasis on thinness, especially for females, often leads to a restriction in normal weight gain. Figures 5–12 to 5–15 show the weight and weight velocity standards for each sex.

FEMALE WEIGHT SPURT

On entering puberty, girls have attained about 60% of adult weight. For the first 3 to 6 months of the height spurt, girls continue to gain weight at prepubertal levels, approximately 2 kg/year, but then accelerate into a

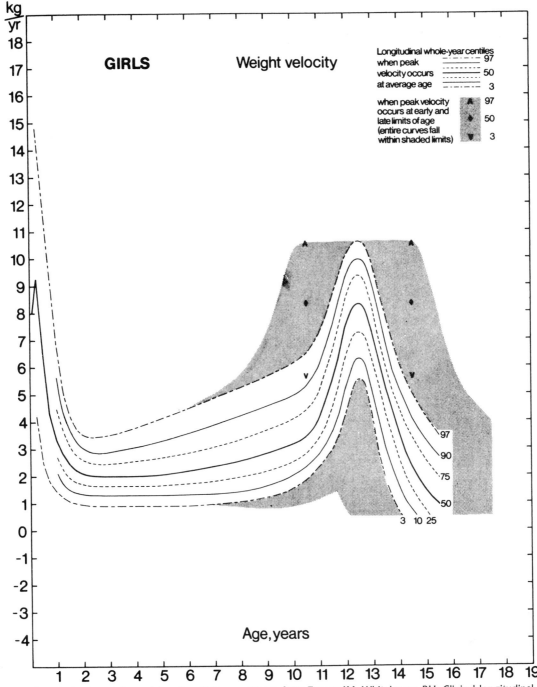

Figure 5–12. Weight velocity for adolescent females. (With permission from Tanner JM, Whitehouse RH: Clinical longitudinal standards for height, weight, height velocity, weight velocity, and stages of puberty. Arch Dis Child 51:170–179, 1976.)

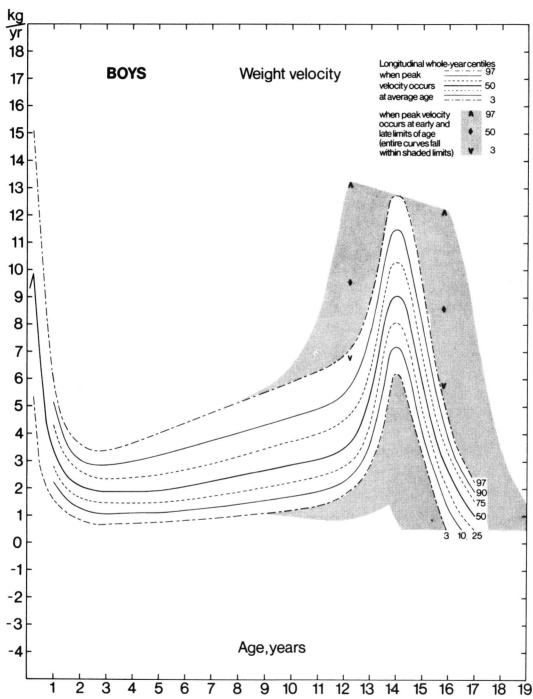

Figure 5–13. Weight velocity for adolescent males. (With permission from Tanner JM, Whitehouse RH: Clinical longitudinal standards for height, weight, height velocity, weight velocity, and stages of puberty. Arch Dis Child 51:170–179, 1976.)

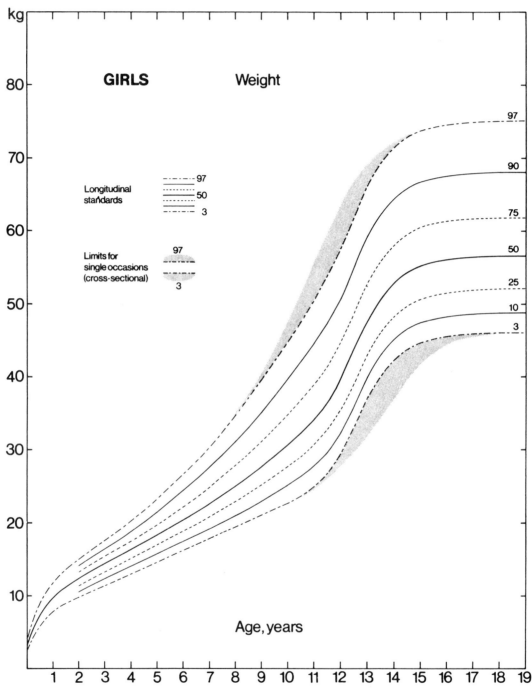

Figure 5–14. Weight attained for adolescent females. (With permission from Tanner JM, Whitehouse RH: Clinical longitudinal standards for height, weight, height velocity, weight velocity, and stages of puberty. Arch Dis Child 51:170–179, 1976.)

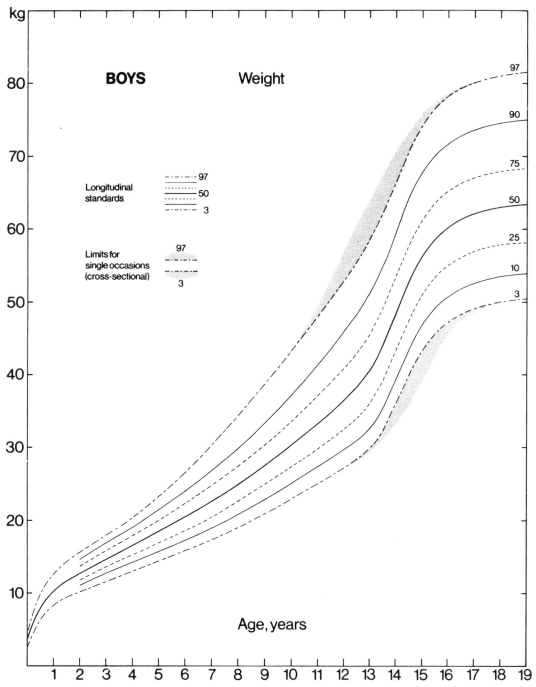

Figure 5–15. Weight attained for adolescent males. (With permission from Tanner JM, Whitehouse RH: Clinical longitudinal standards for height, weight, height velocity, weight velocity, and stages of puberty. Arch Dis Child 51:170–179, 1976.)

weight spurt, eventually attaining a weight velocity at peak growth of about 8 kg/year, with 95% of normal girls gaining weight at a rate between 5.5 and 10.5 kg/year. Interestingly, there is no difference in the rate at which early or late maturing girls put on weight. This is distinctly different from height—early maturers grow at a rate about 20% greater than late maturers. The female muscle spurt lags behind the weight spurt by another 3 to 6 months (see Fig. 5–11).

MALE WEIGHT SPURT

The male weight spurt coincides with both the height and the muscle spurts. Thus, whereas girls experience a sequence of peak height followed by peak weight followed by peak muscle velocity, boys experience these peaks simultaneously. The average weight velocity at peak growth is about 9 kg/year, with 95% of average maturing normal boys gaining between 6 and 12.5 kg/year. In contrast with girls, early maturing boys do differ from late maturing boys in the rate at which they gain weight. Boys who develop early gain an average of 9.5 kg/year at peak, with a range of 7 to 13 kg/year; late developing boys gain only about 8.5 kg/year, with a range of 6 to 12 kg/year.

Physiologic Changes of Puberty

The secondary sex characteristics of puberty that have been discussed are anatomic changes that occur in response to variations in hormonal, receptor, and enzymatic activity. During the height spurt, for example, the level of alkaline phosphatase produced by osteoblasts during bone formation is elevated. Likewise, hemoglobin levels in boys rise about 12% from the initiation to the completion of puberty as a result of testosterone stimulation of erythrocyte production.

Endocrine measures are also closely related to sexual maturation. However, for a given stage of puberty or even for a given individual, blood levels of endocrine hormones tend to have a wide range of normal values and frequently show either diurnal or pulsatile patterns. Because of fluctuations in secretion and complex neuroendocrine interactions, timed urine collections, serial blood samples, or responses to stimulation tests tend to provide more useful clinical information than a single serum determination of an endocrine substance. The Appendix lists normal values for various substances in females and males with respect to sexual maturity rating.

THE SEQUENCE OF FEMALE PUBERTAL MATURATION (Fig. 5–16)

Early Puberty (SMR 2–3)

BREAST DEVELOPMENT

The onset of breast development (thelarche) is one of the earliest manifestations of puberty and the first readily identifiable change of puberty in 85% of females. The glandular tissue under the areola enlarges in re-

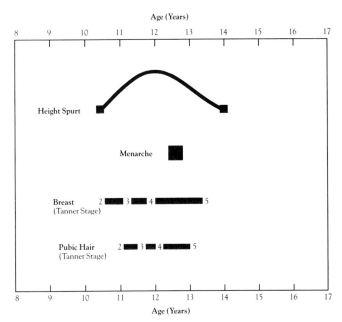

Figure 5–16. Pubertal events in females. (With permission from Copeland KC, Brookman RR, Rauh JL: Assessment of Pubertal Development. Ross Laboratories PREP Series. Columbus, OH, Ross Laboratories, August 1986, p. 6.)

sponse to estrogen produced in the ovaries, marking entry into SMR 2 (breast budding). Thelarche occurs at 11 years of age on average, with 95% of normal girls initiating breast development between ages 9 and 13 years (SD ≈ 1 year). The rate of progression to more advanced stages varies widely, but the interval between SMR 2 and 3 of breast development averages approximately 1 year (see Chapter 77).

Breast development prior to age 8 years is considered premature; if it is associated with pubic hair, a height spurt, and menstruation, it is considered the first sign of precocious puberty (see Chapter 58). There have been reports recently of premature thelarche in a large number of girls in Puerto Rico, suggesting that environmental influences can affect the onset of breast development.

SEXUAL HAIR

The first sexual hair denoting SMR 2 grows along the edges of the labia majora and is fine, long, silky, dark, sparse, and generally straight. Although its appearance at approximately 11.5 years of age is due to adrenal androgens and therefore not causally related to thelarche, it generally coincides with or closely follows thelarche temporally. Fewer than 10% of normal girls do not develop pubic hair until reaching SMR 4 breast development, and no more than 30% of girls experience adrenarche before thelarche.

GENITALIA

Prior to puberty, the cervix is about twice the size of the body of the uterus. During very early puberty, the body of the uterus enlarges to a greater degree than does the cervix, so that the two structures approximate each other in size as puberty progresses. The ovaries and other internal genital structures also grow in size. Changes attributable to increased estrogen production are direct evidence that ovarian maturation is occurring. One important sign of such maturation is cornification of the vaginal epithelium, identifiable on microscopic examination as the presence of pyknotic squamous cells in acidic vaginal secretions.

As the mucus-secreting cells lining the uterus develop, many adolescent females have a scant amount of vaginal discharge in the months preceding menarche. This is typically thin, acidic, clear or milky, and without odor. However, some girls or their mothers may be concerned about infection. They can be reassured that this normal discharge, called "physiologic leukorrhea," is a sign that the uterus is preparing for menstruation.

SOMATIC GROWTH

The height spurt is a relatively early occurrence in the female pubertal sequence, generally beginning soon after thelarche and reaching its peak about a year later. Although the majority of girls experience PHV while in SMR 3, Marshall and Tanner (1969) found that 30% to 40% of girls attain their PHV during SMR 2, and fewer than 10% do not do so until SMR 4 breast development. Later studies, such as those by Zacharias and Rand (1983), indicate that girls are not developing any earlier now than they were a generation ago. Prior to the height spurt, there is widening of the hips that is often not recognized except by the adolescent herself. Peak height velocity is typically reached between ages 11 and 12 and completed by age 13. Early developers may experience their height spurt between ages 9 and 10, whereas late developers may not experience their height spurt until between 13 and 14 years of age. During the height spurt, girls grow an average of 25 cm.

Some girls who have an early growth spurt are concerned because they are taller than boys their age and believe that they will continue to grow at their peak velocity, becoming unusually tall women. Using growth curves that take into account the SMR, such as those published by Tanner and Davies or Wilson and colleagues (1987), one can predict the approximate final height of the individual and reassure her about such concerns. This obviates the use of radiographs to determine bone age.

Bone mineral density also goes through a slight pubertal growth spurt but does not increase appreciably beyond late puberty. More than 45% of the adult complement of body calcium is acquired during the teenage years.

Middle Puberty (SMR 3–4)

BREAST DEVELOPMENT

Whereas the change from SMR 2 to 3 is mainly quantitative (breast "buds" to "mounds"), the change between SMR 3 and 4 is qualitative as well as quantitative and is marked primarily by changes in the areolae. In SMR 4 breast development, the areolae are noticeably darker and larger and elevated above the contour of the surrounding breast tissue, the so-called "double-mound" effect. The progression from SMR 3 to 4 occurs on average in slightly less than 1 year, between 12 and 13 years of age.

Growth of the breasts may not be symmetric in girls, either in size or in SMR stage. Although breast asymmetry is normal, it can be quite marked and disturbing to the individual. Most girls can be reassured that their breasts will become approximately the same size within 2 years (see Chapter 77).

Investigators have attempted to rate breast development based on areolar diameter enlargement. Although a relationship exists between areolar size and sexual maturation, genetic factors appear to have an even stronger influence. Rohn (1982) has attempted to define breast development more precisely by measuring breast papilla (nipple) diameter growth. Although not particularly useful for the earlier stages of development, this method clearly distinguishes breast SMR 4 and 5 from each other and from earlier stages.

SEXUAL HAIR

Although pubic hair generally appears soon after thelarche, its progression proceeds more rapidly. Among girls at SMR 3 breast development, 25% have no pubic hair (SMR 1) and 10% have completely adult (SMR 5) pubic hair. The time for progression from SMR 2 to 4 in pubic hair averages approximately 18 months, between ages 11.5 and 13 years.

Pubic hair in SMR 3 is thicker, coarser, and less straight than in the previous stage and spreads up onto the pubis. As is true of breast staging, the pubic hair changes between SMR 3 and 4 are qualitative as well as quantitative and are marked by the appearance of dense, curled, adult-type hair covering the outer surface of the labia and mons veneris in the characteristic triangular female escutcheon.

Axillary, facial, and adult-type body hair appears relatively late in the pubertal sequence, usually not before SMR 4 pubic hair has been established, but in a few normal girls there may be axillary hair before any breast development. There is considerable variability in sexual hair characteristics that is determined largely by the genetic background of the individual.

GENITALIA

The uterine corpus continues to enlarge, equaling the height of the cervix by menarche, and the genital organs come to lie relatively lower in the pelvis. Cells lining the uterus and cervix also begin to develop. The vagina begins to elongate to about 8 cm, and its pooled secretions become acidic. The fallopian tubes increase in diameter, and complex folds appear in the ciliated mucosa. In addition to these internal changes, the labia majora become thin, more heavily pigmented, and redundant to provide complete coverage of the introitus.

The outstanding feature of middle to late puberty is menstruation, occurring for the first time at an average age of 12.5 years, with more than 95% of girls having menarche between 10.5 and 14.5 years of age. In one study, 0.5% of girls had apparently normal menarche before thelarche. Marshall and Tanner (1969) followed a population of normal adolescents longitudinally with frequent assessment of sexual maturation and found that only 26% had experienced menarche by the time they reached SMR 3, but that 62% of girls were menstruating by the time they reached SMR 4 breast development. Almost 10% did not menstruate until late puberty at SMR 5. The mean age of menarche is highly variable, depending on the ethnic, socioeconomic, and possibly athletic background of the individual.

For girls with a normal tempo of pubertal progression, menarche occurs 1.5 to 2.5 years after thelarche and 9 to 12 months after peak height velocity. For most girls, their height velocity is decelerating rapidly when they have their first menstrual period. Peak weight velocity occurs only 3 months prior to menarche. Most notable, however, is the simultaneous occurrence of menarche, peak muscle velocity, and peak fat velocity.

As previously noted, this has led to Frisch's hypothesizing a direct link between body composition, especially related to fat, and menarche. Although this theory has not been substantiated, it is known that girls with increased amounts of fat experience earlier puberty, while vigorous athletic training or excessive dieting associated with decreased fat can delay puberty (see Chapter 60). An average of 17% of body fat seems to be needed for menarche, while about 22% is needed to initiate and maintain regular ovulatory cycles.

Measuring pregnanediol excretion in 209 adolescent females, Metcalf and colleagues (1983) found that 25% of cycles were ovulatory during the first 2 years after menarche and 45% were ovulatory 2 to 4 years after menarche. It was not until 7 years after menarche that more than 80% of cycles were ovulatory. Furthermore, in a classic longitudinal study of 298 girls, Billewicz and colleagues (1980) determined that menstrual periods gradually became more regular, most notably owing to a decrease in the proportion of long (>57 days) menstrual cycles from 27% to 1% over the 3 years after menarche. On average it takes 18 months to experience the first 12 menstrual periods. Although such anovulatory menstrual irregularity is considered physiologic at this stage of development, many adolescents and their parents are concerned about the possibility of a pathologic condition.

SOMATIC GROWTH

The growth velocity decelerates after SMR 3 breast development is attained at slightly older than 12 years of age. Because both breast development and the growth spurt occur in response to estrogen, it is extremely unusual for a normal girl to have PHV prior to thelarche. While growth in height slows down after the peak height velocity, the growth of fat and muscle accelerates. By menarche, more than 95% of a girl's final height has been achieved.

Late Puberty (SMR 4–5)

BREAST DEVELOPMENT

Girls enter SMR 5 breast development when the contour of the areola recedes to the level of the sur-

rounding breast tissue. The central papilla is generally elevated above the contour of the surrounding areola, although it may be retracted or inverted. The enlargement of and changes in the areola in SMR 4 are attributed to the effect of progesterone, so most adolescents at this stage are menstruating or very near menarche.

A few normal females never progress in their breast development beyond SMR 4 or may advance to SMR 5 only during pregnancy; some appear to pass directly from SMR 3 to 5. There is often a long lag between SMR 4 and 5 breast development. The average interval between these two stages is almost 2 years, but the interval may be as short as 1.5 or as long as 9 years. For this reason, many clinicians consider SMR 4 to be an "adult" level of development.

SEXUAL HAIR

SMR 5 occurs when adult-type pubic hair extends down the medial aspect of the thighs. As is true of breast development, there is often a lag between SMR 4 and 5 pubic hair development. This lag is generally about 18 months but can extend from only 6 to as long as 28 months. This is the same interval as that between the appearance of SMR 2 and 4 pubic hair.

GENITALIA

With the completion of sexual maturation, the body of the uterus becomes three times the height of the cervix, and the vagina lengthens to 15 cm. Prior to this, development of the external genitalia including the vestibular (Bartholin) glands is completed.

SOMATIC GROWTH

Growth in height slows dramatically after menarche. The magnitude of postmenarcheal growth averages approximately 7.5 cm but depends on the height of the individual at menarche; taller girls have proportionately greater growth. All other compartments of the body also show a decreased velocity in growth except for fat, which continues to be added, though at a much slower rate than that prior to the initiation of menstruation.

THE SEQUENCE OF MALE PUBERTAL MATURATION (Fig. 5–17)

Early Puberty (SMR 2–3)

TESTICULAR DEVELOPMENT

Each prepubertal testis is generally less than 4 ml in volume and less than 2.5 cm in greatest diameter. Testicular enlargement heralds recognizable changes in sexual development and SMR 2 stage. A testis at SMR 3 is generally 8 to 10 ml in volume. Most of this increase is caused by proliferation of the seminiferous tubules. The mean age for the initiation of male puberty is 11.5 years, only slightly later than that for the female. Normal boys may enter SMR 2 as early as 9.5 or as late as 13.5 years of age. The subsequent transition from SMR 2 to SMR 3 testicular development requires about 1 year.

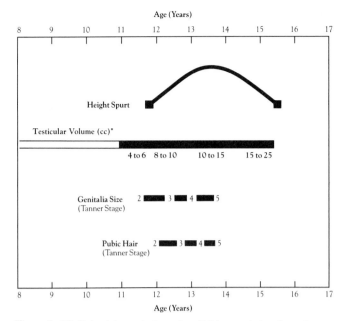

Figure 5–17. Pubertal events in males. (With permission from Copeland KC, Brookman RR, Rauh JL: Assessment of Pubertal Development. Ross Laboratories PREP Series. Columbus, OH, Ross Laboratories, August 1986, p. 4.)

Gonadal growth in males can be directly assessed by palpation of the testes in the scrotum and comparing their size to a standardized orchiometer or set of drawings. Adolescents have demonstrated that they are able to determine their own level of development if they are given standards against which to compare themselves. Self-assessment is, therefore, a generally reliable method of determining sexual maturation. Enlargement of the epididymis, seminal vesicles, and prostate occurs concurrently with testicular growth but is not appreciable externally.

The size of the testicles may be difficult to appreciate by mere visual inspection, since testosterone causes wrinkling, thinning, and increased pigmentation of the scrotal skin. The testes do not fill the scrotum fully, as in childhood. Likewise, in adolescents with a varicocele or a hydrocele (see Chapter 78), the scrotum may be enlarged without concomitant testicular enlargement, giving the false impression of sexual maturity. The left testis generally hangs lower than the right testis once puberty begins.

PENIS

The penis does not usually begin to enlarge until the testes have reached SMR 3 size, at about age 12.5 years. Growth of the penis can begin normally as early as 10.5 or as late as 14.5 years of age. When it does begin to grow, the response to testosterone is initially an increase in length from its 6 cm (stretched) prepubertal size and deepened pigmentation.

SEXUAL HAIR

Pubic hair in boys most often appears between 12 and 12.5 years of age, after puberty has begun, but before significant penile enlargement has occurred. Some re-

ports suggest an age closer to 13.5 for SMR 2 pubic hair development, but this is probably due to experimental method bias. As in girls, pubic hair is initially long, silky, dark, lightly pigmented, and straight. It is sparsely distributed, primarily at the base of the penis in early puberty. As puberty progresses and SMR 3 pubic hair is attained between 13 and 14 years of age, hair that is thicker and slightly curled extends across the pubis in a more dense patch. In addition, hair can be found on the scrotum.

SOMATIC GROWTH

During early puberty, boys continue to grow at their prepubertal rate. At the same chronologic age, girls are in their growth spurt. Therefore, in the 5th and 6th grades in school, boys are often shorter than girls. It is this 2-year discrepancy in growth spurt timing that accounts for the popular idea that boys lag 2 years behind girls in puberty. Skeletal and total body growth, including fat, occurs during early puberty in males, but not at an accelerated pace.

Middle Puberty (SMR 3–4)

TESTICULAR DEVELOPMENT

The size of each testis shows a steady enlargement during midpuberty, reaching a volume of 10 to 15 ml at SMR 4. Seminal fluid is produced in small amounts. The scrotal skin becomes thinner and the sac still larger so that the testes hang some distance from the body. Normal spermatogenesis requires a relatively constant temperature, so the ability to raise or lower the testes is an important factor in fertility. The first release of mature spermatozoa (spermarche) generally first occurs in midpuberty during masturbation or in nocturnal emissions at a mean age of 13.5 to 14.5 years but may occur at any stage of development from SMR 2 to 5.

PENIS

During midpuberty the penis continues to grow in length but also shows the first signs of increasing in width, as the result of development of the corpora cavernosa in response to testosterone. Erections occur more frequently and are especially prominent on awakening. Growth of the penis tends to occur relatively rapidly and is essentially complete (11 to 17 cm in length) before either full testicular or full pubic hair development has occurred.

SEXUAL HAIR

As in girls, there is both a qualitative and quantitative difference between pubic hair at SMR 3 and 4. The latter is defined by adult-type hair that covers the entire pubic area but does not extend down the medial thigh or up the midline. The timing of the midpubertal changes is highly variable, but they generally occur between 12.5 and 14.5 years of age. However, in the Harpenden Growth Study as many as 15% of normal males at SMR 4 testicular development had SMR 1 pubic hair. Rarely is the converse true.

Also as in girls, axillary hair in males generally does not appear before SMR 4 pubic hair. Facial hair appears only after SMR 4 pubic hair and does so in an ordered sequence: the outer corners of the upper lip first, followed by the whole upper lip, then the upper cheeks and middle of the lower lip, followed finally by hair along the sides and lower border of the chin. Body hair develops gradually after facial hair. The extent of body hair in males is determined to a large degree by genetic factors.

SOMATIC GROWTH

Although the velocity of skeletal growth begins to increase noticeably when the penis starts to enlarge (at about 12.5 years), the PHV tends to occur late in middle puberty or early in late puberty (at about 13.5 years). Simultaneously with the height spurt, boys experience a peak in muscle mass and in weight, despite actually losing total body fat. Boys can begin their growth spurt as early as 10.5 or as late as 16 years of age, but they generally lag behind girls by about 2 years. The larynx also undergoes a growth spurt, associated with a "cracking" and deepening of the voice characteristic of growing boys, that coincides with the PHV.

In addition to a cracking voice, another source of embarrassment is the development of breast tissue (gynecomastia) (see Chapter 77), occurring in as many as one third of adolescents around the time of penile lengthening. Although the areolae normally widen from 12.5 mm in boys to more than 25 mm in men, gynecomastia refers to the actual growth of breast tissue in response to estrogen in the male and should be differentiated from fatty tissue associated with obesity.

The enlargement is immediately subareolar and generally 20 to 30 mm in diameter and has been attributed to endogenous estrogen sensitivity. It may be associated with tenderness (possibly due to manipulation or heightened sensitivity) but should show no other signs of inflammation. About 60% of cases are bilateral; when unilateral, it is more likely to be left-sided. The amount of breast tissue usually regresses in 1 to 2 years, but its presence during that time can cause a great deal of concern for affected boys.

Boys who develop later than their peers may have concerns about short stature, frequently because they are teased or feel self-conscious. Although height curves that include SMR can be used in this situation, simple reassurance may not be sufficient, since there is frequently lack of evidence of sexual maturation. In such cases, bone age determination may be indicated, since it will provide the adolescent with concrete evidence about growth potential.

Late Puberty (SMR 4–5)

TESTICULAR DEVELOPMENT

The growth of the testes is considered complete (adult, SMR 5) when they attain a volume of approxi-

mately 20 to 25 ml each. From initiation to completion, pubertal growth of the testes occurs over a period of about 4 years, with most adolescents attaining SMR 5 testicular development between 13.5 and 17 years of age. However, the timing of the onset has little relationship to the velocity of change. Thus, a class of 7th grade boys could be expected to have representatives from every SMR, from prepuberty to adulthood.

PENIS

Despite continued growth of the testes, the penis grows only slightly beyond SMR 4. From initiation to completion, penile growth takes less than 3 years. The normal ages for beginning and completing penile growth are about 12.5 and 14.5 years of age, respectively. The lower and upper ranges for initiation are 10.5 and 14.5 years of age, respectively; the lower and upper ranges for completion are 12.5 and 16.5 years of age, respectively.

SEXUAL HAIR

SMR 5 pubic hair is attained when adult-type pubic hair extends onto the medial thigh. Some clinicians have suggested that hair extending up the midline of the abdomen, in the typical diamond-shaped male escutcheon, be designated SMR 6, but there is no evidence that this pattern represents a more mature stage of development than SMR 5. Pubic hair at this stage tends to blend in with body hair over the lower abdomen and legs. Although a mustache may be present at SMR 4, a beard indicates the SMR 5 level of maturation.

SOMATIC GROWTH

Although the growth spurt tends to be a relatively late event for males, they tend to continue to grow for a prolonged period of time after their peak height velocity. One fifth of normal adolescent males do not reach their PHV until SMR 5. Males can continue to grow, albeit minimally, well beyond their teenage years.

The most outstanding feature of physical development at this stage of puberty is continued increasing strength and the ability to endure hard physical labor over a longer period of time. This is due, in part, to the cardiorespiratory changes mentioned earlier.

BIBLIOGRAPHY

Billewicz WZ, Fellowes HM, Thomson AM: Post-menarchal menstrual cycles in British (Newcastle-upon-Tyne) girls. Ann Hum Biol 7:177, 1980.
Delemarre-van de Waal HA, Wennink JMB, Roelof JH: Gonadotropin secretion during puberty in man. In Delemarre-van de Waal HA, Plant TM, van Rees GP, Schoemaker J (eds): Control of the Onset of Puberty III. Amsterdam, Excerpta Medica, 1989, pp 151–167.
Frisch RE: Fatness, puberty, and fertility: The effects of nutrition and physical training on menarche and ovulation. In Brooks-Gunn J, Petersen AC (eds): Girls at Puberty: Biological and Psychosocial Perspectives. New York, Plenum Press, 1983, pp 29–49.
Kappy MS: Regulation of growth in children with chronic illness: Therapeutic implications for the year 2000. Am J Dis Child 141:489, 1987.

Kreipe RE, Sahler OJZ: Physical growth and development in normal adolescents. In WR Hendee (ed): The Health of Adolescents. Chicago, AMA, 1991.

Marshall WA, Tanner JM: Variation in the pattern of pubertal changes in girls. Arch Dis Child 44:291, 1969.

Marshall WA, Tanner JM: Variation in the pattern of pubertal changes in boys. Arch Dis Child 45:13, 1970.

Metcalf MG, Skidmore DS, Lowry GF, Mackenzie JA: Incidence of ovulation in the years after the menarche. J Endocrinol 97:213, 1983.

Odell WD: Physiology of sexual maturation and primary amenorrhea. West J Med 131:401, 1979.

Reiter EO: Neuroendocrine control processes: Pubertal onset and progression. J Adolesc Health Care 8:479, 1987.

Rohn RD: Papilla (nipple) development during female puberty. J Adolesc Health Care 2:217, 1982.

Scott EC, Johnston FE: Critical fat, menarche, and the maintenance of menstrual cycles: A critical review. J Adolesc Health Care 2:249, 1982.

Tanner JM: Issues and advances in adolescent growth and development. J Adolesc Health Care 8:470, 1987.

Tanner JM: Foetus into Man: Physical Growth from Conception to Maturity (revised and enlarged edition). Cambridge, Harvard University Press, 1990.

Tanner JM, Falkner F: Human Growth: A Comprehensive Treatise, 2nd ed. New York, Plenum Press, 1986.

Vaughan VC, Litt IF: Child and Adolescent Development: Clinical Implications. Philadelphia, WB Saunders, 1990.

Wilson DM, Kraemer HC, Ritter PL, Hammer LD: Growth curves and adult height estimation for adolescents. Am J Dis Child 141:565, 1987.

Zacharias L, Rand WM: Adolescent growth in height and its relation to menarche in contemporary American girls. Ann Hum Biol 10:209, 1983.

CHAPTER 6

Nutrition and Growth

GILBERT B. FORBES

OVERVIEW

Normal growth requires proper nutrition. The growth rate is actually a very sensitive indicator of nutritional status; therefore, growth velocity can serve as a bioassay for dietary adequacy. Investigators have long used the growth rate of rats and other animals as a means of determining the adequacy and efficiency of various diets. Indeed, it was the use of this technique that led to the discovery of some vitamins: The observation that highly purified diets did not sustain growth led to the search for missing essential ingredients. In like manner, the relative biologic value of various dietary proteins has been established.

Growth requires energy and an adequate supply of *all* essential nutrients; indeed, essentiality is often defined on the basis of growth performance. Hence there is no single dietary "growth factor." In developing areas of the world, growth is known to falter when individuals ingest diets low in vitamin A, zinc, or protein, as well as energy. In the United States, we have in recent years been rudely reminded that chloride is also a growth factor. However, in Western society diets are usually not deficient in essential nutrients because of the variety of foods available and the fact that some foods are fortified with vitamins and minerals. The one exception is iron; it is known that some adolescents are deficient in this element. Hence it is the energy content of the diet that is most frequently at fault.

The great sensitivity of the growth rate to a reduction in energy intake means that growth *per se* is an integral, inescapable part of adolescent life. Although the young infant uses about one third of its total energy intake for growth, this is not true in subsequent years. Consider for a moment the growth rate at the peak of the adolescent growth spurt: in this case the average velocity is 16 g/day for girls and 19 g/day for boys; assuming an energy cost of 8 kcal/g weight gain, the growth demand is only 130 to 150 kcal/day in excess of maintenance, or 5% to 6% of total intake. Nevertheless, the entire adolescent functional unit suffers from insufficient food—the metabolic rate, activity level, physical performance, and sexual maturation, as well as growth velocity. Growth demands its fair share of energy intake, and if this is inadequate, growth will suffer along with other bodily functions.

The growing body also responds to energy surfeit. Deliberate overfeeding of adults and adolescents results in weight gain. About two thirds of this gain is fat, and about one third is lean. Of interest is the finding that the weight increment/unit of excess food consumed is the same for women as it is for men (Forbes, 1987). It is known that obese children, who can achieve such a state only via a positive energy balance, are apt to be taller and to have a larger lean weight and larger bones than their thin peers. Longitudinal studies of children who became obese during childhood show that most of them had an increase in their height percentile status once they became obese and that this change in height status occurred either coincident with the increase in weight or sometime thereafter, but never before (Forbes, 1977).

The fact that obese children and adolescents tend to be tall and to have a larger lean body mass is proof that the food eaten is nutritious. Although some of their favorite foods may not be ideal from the nutritional standpoint, the sum total of their intake must perforce be adequate in all respects. (A clear exception is the Prader-Willi syndrome, for these children and adolescents have reduced lean weight in the face of a marked increase in body fat; in this respect they mimic the body composition changes seen in animals with experimental hypothalamic obesity [Schoeller et al, 1988]). Human beings thus behave as other mammals: Energy surfeit accelerates growth, just as energy deficit impairs growth.

The plane of nutrition also has an effect on sexual maturation. Girls who have an early menarche tend to be heavier and taller at menarche than their premenarcheal age peers, and those with a late menarche tend to be lighter than their postmenarcheal age peers, though they are of comparable stature. Thus early maturers have an elevated body mass index (BMI) (weight/height^2), and late maturers have a smaller BMI than their age peers. A plot of the data provided by Zacharias and associates (1976) shows a progressive fall in BMI with age at menarche, in distinct contrast to the progressive increase in BMI that occurs normally at this time of life (see Fig. 6–2). However, it should be noted that the preceding data are based on averages, for there is wide variation in menarcheal weight, the range being about twofold.

Underfed animals have delayed puberty. Young female rats who are underfed have reduced levels of pituitary gonadotropin-releasing hormone (GnRH), as well as fewer GnRH receptors, so gonadotropin production, release, or both is subnormal, and vaginal opening does not occur. This situation is promptly reversed by adequate food—normal hormonal function is restored, and sexual maturation takes place (Dele-marre-van de Waal et al, 1989). Of interest is the recent demonstration of compromised ovarian function in young women undergoing rather modest degrees of weight reduction (Lager and Ellison, 1990).

It has now been demonstrated that undernutrition diminishes the production of somatomedin, an important facilitator of growth produced in the liver by the action of growth hormone. Reduced plasma levels of somatomedin have been recorded in infants with kwashiorkor, and it turns out that even brief periods of undernutrition in adult subjects result in a striking reduction in plasma somatomedin levels, which are promptly restored by adequate food (Clemmons et al, 1981). Thus it is clear that hormonal factors are the prime movers in sexual maturation and that nutrition can influence hormones as well as somatic growth.

Note should be taken of the changes that have occurred in the growth of children and adolescents during the past 100 years (see Chapter 5). Such secular increases in height and weight have been noted in all industrialized societies for which reliable data exist. Male adolescents are 6 to 15 cm taller and 9 to 14 kg heavier than their age peers of a century ago, the larger values being associated with the time of the adolescent growth spurt. In addition, puberty (as judged by menarcheal age) is occurring at an earlier age (Tanner, 1962). This period of secular change witnessed the rise of modern nutritional science, and most observers favor the hypothesis that improved nutrition is responsible. However, there are two additional factors that may have played a role: the decline in chronic infection, and the phenomenon of hybrid vigor.

ASSESSMENT OF GROWTH IN HEIGHT AND WEIGHT

The most commonly used growth charts are those based on data collected by the National Center on Health Statistics from thousands of white children in the United States (see Chapter 56). Percentile plots are preferred over means and standard deviations, because the frequency distributions are often skewed. Although black children and adolescents tend to be somewhat taller and Hispanics and Asians somewhat shorter than their white counterparts, these charts have proved most satisfactory.* Every effort should be made to make an accurate measurement of height and weight and to record age to the nearest month. The best instrument for measuring height is the Holtain stadiometer,† which consists of a fixed vertical member attached to the wall, upon which rides a movable headboard maintained in a horizontal position, a direct reading dial, and a footboard with a heel plate (see Chapter 56). Unfortunately this instrument is not cheap. A satisfactory substitute is a meter stick attached to the wall next to a bare floor

and a movable headboard positioned perpendicular to the wall. The sliding stick devices attached to platform scales are not accurate and should not be used.

The subject must remove shoes and stand erect next to the measuring device in the nonlordotic position, with eyes and ears forming a horizontal plane. Some observers prefer to give a gentle upward tug on the chin. It is well to remember that individuals are often 1 to 2 cm shorter in the late afternoon than in the early morning. Weight should be taken with the subject dressed in light indoor clothing and shoes off.

In assessing the stature of a given individual, the role of heredity must be kept in mind. At all ages past infancy, there is a reasonable correlation between the heights of children and the heights of their parents. In addition, the timing of sexual maturation also follows this correlation, with daughters tending to mimic the menarcheal age of their mothers.

Older children and adolescents may want to know how tall they will be when fully grown; this is especially true of undergrown boys and tall girls. There are two techniques for making such estimates. The simplest is to average the parents' heights and then add 6.5 cm for boys and subtract 6.5 cm for girls. Another method is to obtain a roentgenogram of the wrist and to enter bone age and present stature into the tables provided by Bayley and Pinneau (1952) (see Chapter 5).

CHANGES IN BODY COMPOSITION DURING GROWTH

Body weight comprises a number of organ systems. Modern technology has made it possible to estimate several components of the body in a relatively nontraumatic manner. It will be seen that the growth of these components during adolescence differs somewhat from the growth of the body as a whole.

Methods for Estimating Body Composition

Body fluid spaces (plasma volume, total red cell mass, extracellular fluid volume, total body water) are estimated by the principle of isotopic dilution.

Lean body mass (LBM), or as some prefer fat-free mass, can be estimated in several ways, based on the facts that neither electrolytes nor water is bound by neutral fat and that LBM has a different density than that of fat. Hence a measurement of total body water or total body potassium can yield an estimate of LBM; body fat is weight minus LBM. Measurement of body density yields an estimate of the percentage of body fat and body lean. Urine creatinine excretion is used as an index of muscle mass.

Estimates of skeletal mass have been made from the size and density of various bones, using the degree of attenuation of monoenergetic gamma rays; this is referred to as single- or dual-photon absorptiometry. The cross-sectional area of the second metacarpal cortex

---

*Tanner and Davies (1985) have devised some charts that portray *height velocity* as a function of age for average adolescents and for early and late maturers. These charts are available from Serono Laboratories, Inc., 280 Pond St., Randolph, MA 02368.

†Holtain Limited, Crosswell, Crymmych, Pembrokeshire, U.K.

read from a plain roentgenogram has also been used for this purpose.

Two new techniques are now under study. Total body conductivity and bioimpedance are used to estimate lean weight. The former measures the perturbation of an electromagnetic field produced by the presence of the subject; the latter measures the resistance to a weak alternating current passed between the hand and foot.

Computed tomography (CT) and magnetic resonance imaging (MRI) can define the size and shape of various organs, as well as muscle mass and body fat.

Most of these techniques are more suitable for the research laboratory; some require expensive instrumentation and some involve radiation exposure. Details can be found in Forbes (1987) and Lukaski (1987).

Although it cannot claim a high degree of precision, anthropometry provides an inexpensive and easily used technique for estimating body fat. The two most commonly used techniques are the measurement of skinfold (really fat-fold) thickness and of various body circumferences (see Chapter 5).

Since human skin is only 0.5 to 2 mm thick, the subcutaneous fat layer contributes the bulk of the skinfold thickness. The measurement is made by grasping the skin plus subcutaneous tissue between the thumb and forefinger, shaking it gently to (hopefully) exclude underlying muscle, and stretching it just far enough to permit the jaws of a spring-actuated caliper to impinge on the tissue. Since the jaws of the caliper compress the tissue, the caliper reading diminishes for a few seconds and the dial is then read.

The most frequent measurement site is over the triceps muscle at a point halfway between the shoulder and elbow; other sites are over the biceps, at the inferior tip of the scapula, and at the iliac crest. Subjects with moderately firm subcutaneous tissue and those with very firm tissue that is not easily deformable present somewhat of a problem. In individuals who have recently lost weight, the subcutaneous tissue is often flabby; in very obese individuals, the tissue thickness may exceed the maximum jaw width (40 mm) of the caliper.

The ratio of abdomen to hip circumference can be used as an index of body fat distribution. There is some evidence to suggest that adults with high ratios have large accumulations of intraabdominal fat and are somewhat more prone to cardiovascular disease and stroke. A recent publication (Forbes, 1990) describes the changes in this ratio during the adolescent and adult years in normal individuals. It is noteworthy that sex differences first appear during adolescence, with girls having a lower ratio than boys.

One can calculate the cross-sectional area of arm muscle plus bone and fat from measurements of arm circumference and skinfold thickness.

arm muscle + bone area is $(C - \pi SF)^2/4\pi$,
and arm fat area is $SF/4\ (2C - \pi SF)$,
in which C is arm circumference and SF is skinfold thickness

Many authors use the term *arm muscle area*, which is incorrect. Although this technique yields reliable results in thin individuals, it may overestimate arm muscle plus

bone area and so underestimate arm fat area in obese individuals.

Finally, it should not be forgotten that the use of relative weight—either percentage weight for height, or BMI (weight/height[2])—though far from perfect can be useful in evaluating large numbers of individuals. Those persons with high values almost always have increased body fat, especially girls and women. Male athletes are a clear exception to this rule, since their increased weight for height often represents a larger muscle mass. A nomogram for determining BMI from weight and height is shown in Figure 6–1.

Body Mass Index

The BMI is age dependent, as shown in Figure 6–2, which depicts the 50th percentile for white children and adolescents who participated in the 1971–1974 National Health and Nutrition Examination Survey (Cronk and Roche, 1982). Values for black male adolescents tend

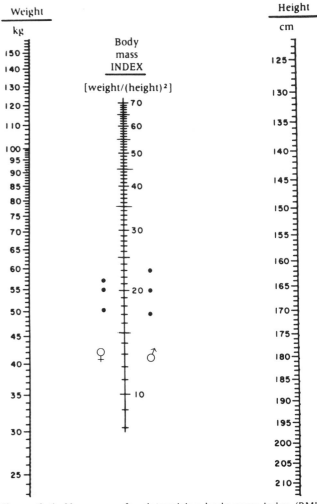

Figure 6–1. Nomogram for determining body mass index (BMI) from height and weight. A straight edge connecting weight and height allows one to read BMI (weight in kg ÷ [height in m]²). The three dots on the left side of the BMI line represent 50th percentile values for females aged 20 years *(top),* 15 years *(middle),* and 10 years *(bottom).* The dots on the right side are for similar-aged males.

Figure 6–2. Body mass index as a function of age. (Data from Cronk CE, Roche AF: Race- and sex-specific reference data for triceps and subscapular skinfolds and weight/stature[2]. Am J Clin Nutr 35:351, 1982.)

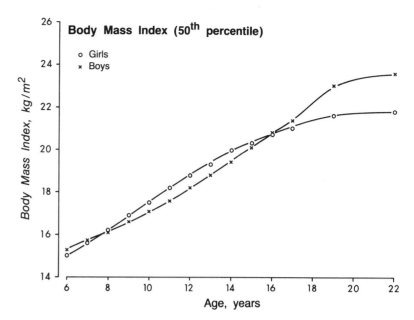

to be a little lower, and those for black female adolescents are a little higher (each by 1% to 4%) than those for whites. Values for Dutch children and for French children are comparable to those shown in Figure 6–2.

Table 6–1 lists the various percentile values for males and females. It is evident that the distributions at all ages shown are strongly skewed to the right.

Although the 50th percentile values for girls are higher than those for boys during the late childhood and early adolescent years, in keeping with the sex difference in body fat content, the situation is reversed later on. By age 18 years, males have a larger BMI despite the fact that they have less body fat. The problem is that body weight is the sum of lean and fat and that lean weight is a major contributor to body weight in boys.

SUBCUTANEOUS FAT

The region over the triceps muscle is the most commonly used site for measuring the thickness of skin plus subcutaneous tissue (really a double layer squeezed between the jaws of a caliper). Measurements at other sites usually yield different values, so the subcutaneous

fat mantle is far from uniform thickness; indeed, CT scan and MRI studies show a large fraction of total subcutaneous fat in women to be located in hips and thighs. The triceps site has the advantage of easy accessibility, and it can be said that the triceps skinfold does bear a relationship to total body fat content.

Figures 6–3 and 6–4 show the changes in triceps skinfold thickness during adolescence in white females and males who participated in the 1971–1974 National Health and Nutrition Examination Survey. The sex difference is readily apparent; it is also evident that the frequency distributions in both sexes are strongly skewed toward higher values. Of interest is what seems to be a mild fat "spurt" in boys aged 9 to 13 years. The cause of this is not known (see Chapter 5).

LEAN BODY MASS AND BODY FAT

Figure 6–5 shows the time course for body weight, LBM, and body fat (average values) for males and females. The developing sex difference in LBM during adolescence is clearly evident; by the end of the second decade of life, the male LBM is roughly equal to female

TABLE 6–1. Percentile Values for Body Mass Index (kg/m^2)

AGE (yr)	MALES							FEMALES						
	5th	10th	25th	50th	75th	90th	95th	5th	10th	25th	50th	75th	90th	95th
6	13.0	13.6	14.4	15.3	16.0	17.7	18.7	12.8	13.5	14.0	15.0	16.0	16.9	17.3
7	13.3	13.9	14.7	15.7	16.7	18.5	19.9	13.1	13.8	14.5	15.6	16.8	18.4	19.2
8	13.6	14.2	15.1	16.1	17.4	19.4	21.1	13.5	14.2	15.1	16.2	17.7	19.9	21.1
9	14.0	14.5	15.5	16.6	18.1	20.4	22.3	13.9	14.6	15.6	16.9	18.7	21.3	23.0
10	14.5	14.9	15.9	17.1	18.9	21.3	23.4	14.4	15.1	16.2	17.5	19.6	22.7	24.8
11	15.0	15.3	16.4	17.6	19.7	22.2	24.5	14.9	15.5	16.7	18.2	20.4	23.8	26.3
12	15.5	15.8	16.9	18.2	20.4	23.1	25.5	15.3	16.0	17.3	18.8	21.2	24.8	27.7
13	16.0	16.3	17.4	18.8	21.1	24.0	26.5	15.8	16.4	17.8	19.3	21.9	25.6	28.8
14	16.5	16.9	18.0	19.4	21.9	24.8	27.3	16.2	16.8	18.2	19.9	22.5	26.1	29.6
15	17.0	17.5	18.7	20.1	22.5	25.6	28.0	16.6	17.2	18.6	20.3	23.0	26.5	30.2
16	17.4	18.0	19.2	20.8	23.2	26.3	28.6	16.9	17.5	18.9	20.7	23.5	26.7	30.6
17	17.8	18.5	19.8	21.4	23.8	26.9	29.2	17.1	17.8	19.2	21.0	23.8	26.9	30.9
18–20	18.6	19.7	21.0	23.0	25.3	28.4	30.5	17.6	18.4	19.7	21.6	24.3	27.2	31.2
21–23	19.0	20.0	21.4	23.6	26.0	29.0	31.2	17.7	18.5	19.8	21.8	24.4	27.7	31.5

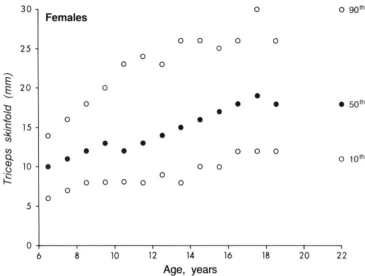

Figure 6–3. Triceps skinfold thickness for females: 90th, 50th, and 10th percentiles. (Data from Cronk CE, Roche AF: Race- and sex-specific reference data for triceps and subscapular skinfolds and weight/stature[2]. Am J Clin Nutr 35:351, 1982.)

body weight; the sex ratio for LBM is about 1.44:1, in contrast with 1.25:1 for body weight. This is one reason why boys are stronger than girls and why their energy requirement is greater.

LBM (fat-free mass) has physiologic and nutritional importance. It comprises the active metabolic mass of the body, for body fat is relatively inert. For example, there is little or no sex difference in basal metabolic rate when LBM is used as a reference point; total energy expenditure, blood volume, and maximum oxygen consumption all are functions of LBM. Accretion rates of various body constituents are more closely related to LBM than to weight with its variable component of fat.

It should be noted that LBM is a function of stature at all ages, and the same is true for total body calcium in adults; hence tall children should have an athletic advantage over those who are shorter. The variability in LBM for subjects of a given age and sex is less than that for weight, so body fat variability accounts for a large proportion of the variation in body weight.

Table 6–2 lists average values of a number of body measurements and body constituents for 10-year-old and 20-year-old individuals, together with estimates of daily accretion rates for nitrogen, calcium, and iron over the entire decade. At the peak of the adolescent growth spurt, these accretion values are two to three times greater. Although at the beginning of the decade there is little, if any, sex difference for any of these values, it is to be seen that the accretion rates, that is, the amounts added to the body as a result of growth, are considerably greater in boys. By age 20 years, the male-to-female ratios for the various measurements are in the range of 1.3:1 to 1.7:1, in contrast with a weight ratio of only 1.25:1 and a height ratio of 1.08:1. On average, the boys acquire about twice as much nitrogen, calcium, and iron and much more muscle mass, as reflected by arm muscle plus bone cross-sectional area and the daily excretion of creatinine. These are accretion rates, not dietary requirements, that must take into consideration gastrointestinal absorption and urinary, fecal, and cutaneous losses. The adolescent boy lays down muscle and bone, and the adolescent girl lays down fat.

COMPOSITION OF WEIGHT GAINS AND WEIGHT LOSSES

Generally speaking, a significant loss of weight (the result of nutritional deficit) involves both LBM and fat.

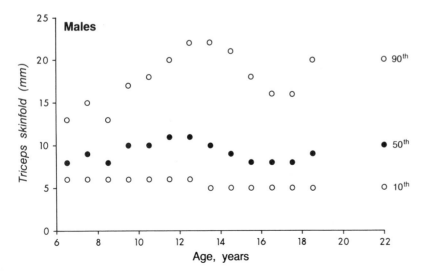

Figure 6–4. Triceps skinfold thickness for males: 90th, 50th, and 10th percentiles. (Data from Cronk CE, Roche AF: Race-and sex-specific reference data for triceps and subscapular skinfolds and weight/stature[2]. Am J Clin Nutr 35:351, 1982.)

Figure 6–5. Time course of body weight and lean body mass for males and females. Body fat is the difference between weight and LBM. Author's data based on 559 white males and 554 females by potassium-40 counting.

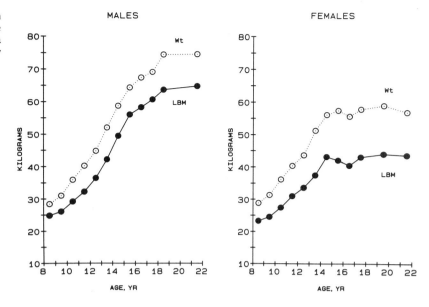

The relative contribution of these two body components to the total weight loss depends on the initial body fat content and on the magnitude of the energy deficit; thin individuals tend to lose relatively more lean tissue, and obese persons lose relatively more fat (Forbes, 1987). Very low energy diets result in considerable erosion of the LBM, even in the face of adequate protein intake, whereas diets providing more than 1000 kcal/day are less hazardous in this respect. Exercise tends to mitigate the effect of low energy intakes, but only to a degree; a weight loss of more than a few kilograms will still be accompanied by some loss of LBM. Careful studies have shown that an energy deficit that results from exercise produces about the same degree of weight loss and negative nitrogen balance as a comparable deficit from

eating less food. Athletes should be told to eat properly; the practice among high school wrestlers of trying to "make weight," that is, the next lower weight category, should be condemned.

Weight gain that is the result of nutritional surfeit also involves both LBM and fat; the fact that obese individuals usually have a somewhat larger LBM than thin individuals speaks in favor of the hypothesis that obesity is indeed a nutritional disease, the result of a positive energy balance. Indeed, obese individuals need to eat more than do thin individuals to stay in energy balance; data on free-living adults and adolescents at light physical activity show that an extra 16 to 20 kcal/day are needed for each additional kilogram of body weight (Forbes, 1987; Bandini et al, 1990). Data from dietary histories that purport to show otherwise must be regarded with great skepticism. Also of note is that obese individuals are more sedentary than their non-obese peers.

There are two exceptions to the general rule that LBM and fat rise and fall together. The first relates to the effect of anabolic agents. Androgenic-anabolic steroids given in significant amounts and for long enough periods cause an increase in LBM (including muscle) and a decrease in body fat, and the same is true of human growth hormone (see Chapter 81). This is why athletes take them and will run the risk of undesirable side effects in an effort to augment athletic performance. The second exception is the Prader-Willi syndrome (see Chapter 31), in which LBM is decreased in the face of an excess of body fat.

TABLE 6–2. Body Measurements and Constituents at Selected Ages

	AGE 10 YEARS (M/F)	AGE 20 YEARS (M/F)	DAILY ACCRETION AVERAGE ENTIRE DECADE (M/F)
Body weight (kg)*	33/34	71/57	
Lean body mass (kg)*	27/26	62/43	
Total body nitrogen (g)†	840/780	1980/1290	0.31/0.14
Total body calcium (g)‡	330/290	1100/710§	0.21/0.12
Total body iron (mg)‖	1480/1430	3560/2270	0.57/0.23
Blood volume (ml)‖	2450/2400	5350/3950	
Arm muscle + bone area (cm²)¶	24.4/22.6	59/34	
Urine creatinine (mg/24 hr)	730/700	1990/1300	
Metacarpal cortex (cm²)**	0.27/0.26	0.56/0.42	

*Author's data.

†To convert to grams of protein, multiply by 6.25.

‡Data from Christiansen et al (1975) (as cited in Forbes, 1987), extrapolated from photon density measurements of forearm bones.

§Values obtained by neutron activation (S. Cohn et al 1971, 1980, as cited in Forbes, 1987) are 1100 g for males and 830 g for females.

‖Data from Hawkins (1964) (as cited in Forbes, 1987).

¶Midarm cross-sectional area, calculated from skinfold thickness and arm circumference. Data from Frisancho (1981) (as cited in Forbes, 1987).

**Midshaft cross-sectional area, second metacarpal. Data from Garn et al (1976) (as cited in Forbes, 1987).

Exercise

A regular program of exercise over a period of several weeks can produce a modest increase (1 to 3 kg) in LBM and a fall in body fat. However, as already noted, a weight loss of more than a few kilograms will usually cause some loss of LBM even with adequate exercise. Excessive exercise can lead to fatigue and even some loss of appetite; the latter will of course lead to weight loss.

The fact that the dominant arm of professional tennis players has a larger muscle and bone mass testifies to the phenomenon of local muscle hypertrophy in response to vigorous use over prolonged periods. The large, and sometimes grotesque, muscle bulk of some bodybuilders is sometimes hailed as a result of exercise and muscle training, but without special tests (such as serum testosterone and gonadotropin levels) it is most difficult (in view of their widespread use) to exclude the effects of unreported use of anabolic-androgenic steroids. Certainly the generous deltoid muscles of some runners provides circumstantial evidence of steroid use (see Chapter 81).

Many athletes, boys and girls alike, have a larger LBM and less body fat than do nonathletes. The question is whether this is the result of training or is principally hereditary in nature. As already noted, a generous intake of food can augment the LBM.

In summary, nutrition is a most important determinant of growth. Suboptimal nutrition slows the growth processes and the rate of sexual maturation, and excess calories speed up both processes. It has now been established that significant changes in body weight incident to nutritional factors affect both the lean and the fat components of the body—both fall with undernutrition, and both rise with overnutrition.

There are several situations in adolescence for which nutritional surveillance and advice are particularly important: in adolescent pregnancy (see Chapter 74), especially in girls who are undergrown; in athletes, whose energy expenditure is high (see Chapters 80 and 81); in individuals who partake of fad diets that may be deficient in one or more essential nutrients (see Chapter 7); and in chronic illnesses, especially cystic fibrosis (see Chapter 43) and inflammatory bowel disease (see Chapter 63). Faltering growth can occur on diets low in cholesterol and saturated fat if attention is not given to energy intake.

A word should be said for the nutritional benefits of exercise for adolescents. Exercise demands more food but not necessarily more essential nutrients: Assuming a well-balanced diet, the result will be a higher intake of such nutrients and thus less likelihood of a specific deficiency.

BIBLIOGRAPHY

Bandini LG, Schoeller DA, Dietz WH: Energy expenditure in obese and nonobese adolescents. Pediatr Res 27:198, 1990.

Bayley N, Pinneau SR: Tables for predicting adult height from skeletal age: Revised for use with the Gruelich-Pyle hand standards. J Pediatr 40:432, 1952.

Clemmons DR, Klibanski A, Underwood LE, et al: Reduction of plasma immunoactive somatomedin-C during fasting in humans. J Clin Endocrinol Metab 53:1247, 1981.

Cronk CE, Roche AF: Race- and sex-specific reference data for triceps and subscapular skinfolds and weight/stature^2. Am J Clin Nutr 35:351, 1982.

Delemarre-van de Waal HA, Plant TM, vanRees GP, et al (eds): Control of the Onset of Puberty III. Amsterdam, Excerpta Medica, 1989.

Forbes GB: Nutrition and growth. J Pediatr 91:40, 1977.

Forbes GB: Human Body Composition: Growth, Aging, Nutrition, and Activity. New York, Springer-Verlag, 1987.

Forbes GB: The abdomen:hip ratio. Normative data and observations on selected patients. Int J Obes 14:149, 1990.

Frisancho AR: Anthropometric Standards for the Assessment of Growth and Nutritional Status. Ann Arbor, MI, University of Michigan Press, 1989.

Lager C, Ellison PT: Effect of moderate weight loss on ovarian function assessed by salivary progesterone measurements. Am J Hum Biol 2:303, 1990.

Lukaski HC: Methods for the assessment of human body composition: traditional and new. Am J Clin Nutr 46:537, 1987.

Schoeller DA, Levitsky LL, Bandini LG, et al: Energy expenditure and body composition in Prader-Willi syndrome. Metabolism 37:115, 1988.

Tanner JM: Growth at Adolescence, 2nd ed. Oxford, Blackwell Scientific, 1962.

Tanner JM, Davies PSW: Clinical longitudinal standards for height and height velocity for North American children. J Pediatr 107:317, 1985.

Zacharias L, Rand WM, Wurtman RJ: A prospective study of sexual development and growth in American girls: the statistics of menarche. Obstet Gynecol Surv 31:325, 1976.

CHAPTER 7

Nutritional Requirements During Adolescence

MARY STORY

The phenomenal growth in tissue deposition that occurs in adolescence, which is second only to that in the first year of life, creates increased demands for energy and nutrients. Total nutrient needs are higher during adolescence than at any other time in the life cycle. Nutrition and physical growth are integrally related; optimal nutrition is a requisite for achieving full growth potential. Failure to consume an adequate diet at this time can result in delayed sexual maturation and can slow or arrest linear growth.

NUTRIENT REQUIREMENTS

Nutrient needs parallel the rate of growth, with the greatest nutrient demands occurring during the peak velocity of growth. Because of the wide individual variability in the onset of puberty, as well as the magnitude and duration of growth, nutritional requirements should be correlated with physiologic development and the current rate of growth rather than with chronologic age (see Chapter 5). A 13-year-old boy who is prepubescent has very different nutrient needs than those of a 13-year-old boy who is in his growth spurt. The nutrient needs of adolescents are best understood in the context of changes in body composition. Prior to puberty, nutrient needs are similar between boys and girls; however, distinct sex differences in body composition, which affects nutrient needs, emerge during adolescence (see Chapter 6). Boys deposit proportionately more lean body tissue and skeletal mass, whereas girls deposit proportionately more fat, so by the time physical maturation is complete, girls have about twice the percentage of body fat as do boys but only about two thirds as much lean tissue. The relatively greater amounts of skeletal and lean body mass in boys require increased deposition of nutrients, which help account for the greater nutritional needs of boys compared with girls (Forbes, 1981). An additional reason for the larger requirements of nutrients in boys is their greater rate of growth.

Nonetheless, nutrient needs for both boys and girls increase sharply during adolescence. The rapid rate of skeletal growth increases requirements for calcium, magnesium, phosphorus, zinc, and vitamins A and D. The higher rate of tissue synthesis increases the demand for nitrogen, folacin, vitamin B_{12}, zinc, and iron. Vitamins A, C, and E are required in greater amounts for the preservation and integrity of new cells. The greater energy demands during adolescence require increased amounts of thiamine, riboflavin, and niacin for the release of energy from carbohydrates, protein, and fats. At the peak of the adolescent growth spurt, the nutritional requirements may be twice as high as those of the remaining period of adolescence. Based on changes in lean body mass, Forbes estimated the daily increments of selected nutrients during adolescent growth. Table 7–1 illustrates the deposition of nutrients during the adolescent growth spurt compared with the rest of adolescence.

Recommended Dietary Allowances

Unfortunately, data regarding specific nutrient requirements of adolescents are extremely limited. For the most part, estimates of requirements and recommendations have been interpolated from studies of adults and young children or are estimated intakes associated with good health and growth and therefore must be regarded as educated guesses. The Recom-

TABLE 7–1. Daily Increments in Body Content Due to Growth

		AVERAGE FOR PERIOD 10–20 YR (mg)	AT PEAK OF GROWTH SPURT (mg)
Calcium	M	210	400
	F	110	240
Iron	M	0.57	1.1
	F	0.23	0.9
Nitrogen*	M	320	610 (3.8 g protein)
	F	160	360 (2.2 g protein)
Zinc	M	0.27	0.50
	F	0.18	0.31
Magnesium	M	4.4	8.4
	F	2.3	5.0

*Maintenance needs (2 mg/basal calorie) at age 18 years are 3500 mg and 2700 mg for males and females, respectively.

From Forbes GB: Nutritional requirements in adolescence. In Suskind RM (ed): Textbook of Pediatric Nutrition. New York, Raven Press, 1981.

mended Dietary Allowances (RDAs) established by the Food and Nutrition Board of the National Research Council for Adolescents are based on the best scientific knowledge available and are given in terms of age, gender, and median weights and heights (Table 7–2). With the exception of the RDA for energy, the RDAs provide a safety factor specific for each nutrient, so the needs of "practically all healthy" individuals are met. Thus, the RDAs (except for energy) are designed to exceed the actual requirements of most individuals. Although best applied to groups, RDAs can be used as standards against which to compare individual nutrient intakes, averaged over a sufficient length of time, to estimate risk of deficiencies (FNB, NRC, 1989).

Survey Findings

National surveys such as the First Health and Nutrition Examination Survey (NHANES I, 1971–1974) and more recently the second Health and Nutrition Examination Survey (NHANES II, 1976–1980), as well as the Nationwide Food Consumption Survey (NFCS, 1977–1978), have provided relevant dietary (1-day intake), nutritional, and health status data on adolescents (Life Sciences Research Office, 1989). These surveys have found that although the nutritional status of adolescents as a group is good, there is evidence of inadequate individual dietary intakes of vitamins and minerals, impaired nutritional status, or both, in some subgroups of adolescents. Those at highest risk include adolescents of low socioeconomic status and girls. The minerals that teenagers most often consume in inadequate amounts are iron, calcium, and zinc. Vitamins that are often consumed at less than the recommended intake include vitamin A, riboflavin, folacin, and vitamin B_6 (Life Sciences Research Office, 1989; Greenwood and Richardson, 1979). Inadequate protein has not been found to be problematic among adolescents in the United States.

Energy

Sufficient energy is needed to support growth and development, metabolic functions, and muscle activity and to repair damage caused by illness or injury. Food energy is provided by fat, carbohydrates, protein, and alcohol, the pure forms of which provide approximately 9, 4, 4, and 7 kcal/g, respectively. The energy requirements of adolescents are determined by individual-based basal metabolic rates (BMRs), rates of growth, and activity patterns (Surgeon General's Report on Nutrition and Health, 1988). Unless levels of physical activity are high, the BMR constitutes the largest component of total energy expenditure. The BMR is closely correlated with measures of lean body mass (Forbes, 1981). Consequently, boys who have a greater percentage of lean body tissue have a higher metabolic rate than do girls. Although there is a high requirement for energy during adolescence, the energy actually required for tissue deposition and growth does not exceed 3% of the total

TABLE 7–2. Recommended Dietary Allowances of Nutrients for Adolescent and Young Adult Males, Females, and Pregnant Adolescents

	MALES			FEMALES			PREGNANT FEMALES
	11–14 Yr	15–18 Yr	19–24 Yr	11–14 Yr	15–18 Yr	19–24 Yr	
Weight (kg)*	45	66	72	46	55	58	—
Height (cm)*	157	176	177	157	163	164	—
Energy (total kcal)	2500	3000	2900	2200	2200	2200	+300
Energy (kcal/kg)	55	45	40	47	40	38	—
Protein (g)	45	59	58	46	44	46	60
Vitamin A (μg RE)	1000	1000	1000	800	800	800	800
Vitamin D (μg)	10	10	10	10	10	10	10
Vitamin E (mg α-TE)	10	10	10	8	8	8	10
Vitamin K (μg)	45	65	70	45	55	60	65
Vitamin C (mg)	50	60	60	50	60	60	70
Thiamine (mg)	1.3	1.5	1.5	1.1	1.1	1.1	1.5
Riboflavin (mg)	1.5	1.8	1.7	1.3	1.3	1.3	1.6
Niacin (mg NE)	17	20	19	15	15	15	17
Vitamin B_6 (mg)	1.7	2.0	2.0	1.4	1.5	1.6	2.2
Folate (μg)	150	200	200	150	180	180	400
Vitamin B_{12} (μg)	2.0	2.0	2.0	2.0	2.0	2.0	2.2
Calcium (mg)	1200	1200	1200	1200	1200	1200	1200
Phosphorus (mg)	1200	1200	1200	1200	1200	1200	1200
Magnesium (mg)	270	400	350	280	300	280	320
Iron (mg)	12	12	10	15	15	15	30
Zinc (mg)	15	15	15	12	12	12	5
Iodine (μg)	150	150	150	150	150	150	175
Selenium (μg)	40	50	70	45	50	55	65

*Weights and heights represent actual median weights and heights for adolescents derived from national data collected by the National Center for Health Statistics.
RE, Retinol equivalents; α-TE, α-tocopherol equivalents; NE, niacin equivalents.
Adapted from Food and Nutrition Board, National Research Council: Recommended Dietary Allowances, 10th ed. © 1989 by the National Academy of Sciences, National Academy Press, Washington, DC.

energy requirement, even during the growth spurt. Thus, the high energy requirement for teenagers reflects maintenance needs and physical activity rather than actual growth. The RDA for energy (shown in Table 7–2) represents average approximate needs and was developed by estimating resting energy expenditure and then multiplying the results by an activity factor representing light to moderate activity (FNB, NRC, 1989). Actual energy needs vary with physical activity. Inactive adolescents may become overweight even though their energy intake is less than the recommendation, whereas very active teenagers have greater needs than those recommended. In both the NHANES II and the NFCS, the mean caloric intakes for adolescent girls 12 to 15 years of age were substantially less than the RDA. In NHANES II, the mean caloric intake for girls of this age was 1821 kcal/day and 1687 kcal/day for 16- to 19-year-olds. Mean energy intakes for boys coincided with the RDAs (Life Sciences Research Office, 1989).

The adolescent growth spurt is extremely sensitive to energy and nutrient deprivation. Low energy intake may lead to growth retardation. Insufficient calorie consumption may occur because of insufficient resources to purchase food or intentional dieting, or secondary to other factors such as substance abuse or chronic illness. Energy is the primary dietary requirement. If energy needs are not met, dietary protein, vitamins, and minerals cannot be used effectively for various metabolic functions.

Protein

Protein is required for growth, development, and maintenance of body tissues and is involved in almost all metabolic processes. Protein supplies about 12% to 14% of the energy intake throughout childhood and adolescence. The peak in protein intake coincides with the peak in energy intake; thus, protein needs correlate more closely with growth patterns than with chronologic age. The RDA requirement for protein in adolescents is interpolated from results of nitrogen balance studies on young children and young adult males as well as on theoretical needs for adequate growth (FNB, NRC, 1989). The RDA for daily protein intake for teenagers ranges from 44 to 59 g, depending on gender and age. Expressed in terms of body weight, boys and girls 11 to 14 years old require 1 g/kg body weight, decreasing to 0.9 g/kg for males and 0.8 g/kg for females aged 15 to 18 years. There is little evidence of insufficient protein intake in the United States, as mean intakes are much greater than the RDAs. In NHANES II, the mean daily protein intake was 107 g/day for males and 65 g/day for females (Life Sciences Research Office, 1989). Adolescents at risk for inadequate protein intakes include those who are from low-income families and those who are strict vegetarians (vegans) or chronic dieters. When energy is limited, dietary protein is used to meet energy needs and is unavailable for new tissue synthesis. Therefore either inadequate energy or protein intake may impair growth. Growth is a sensitive indicator of protein nutrition status.

Lipids

Other than the general recommendation that 3% of total energy be obtained from essential fatty acids, there are no RDAs for fat or cholesterol (Life Sciences Research Office, 1989). Recently, several authoritative groups and agencies (American Heart Association, National Cholesterol Education Program, Year 2000 Health Objectives for the Nation) have recommended that healthy children older than 2 years of age adopt a diet that reduces dietary fat to no more than 30% of calories, saturated fat to less than 10% of calories, and daily cholesterol intake to 300 mg or less in the hope of preventing the onset of cardiovascular disease. In contrast, the American Academy of Pediatrics has advised against specific recommendations because of insufficient evidence of the safety and efficacy of such diets in children and adolescents. Whether a diet consisting of no more than 30% of calories from fat should be advised for children and teenagers remains controversial; however, a total fat intake of more than 40% of calories is excessive (LaRosa and Finberg, 1988). According to the NHANES II data, almost one third (32%) of children and teenagers had diets consisting of 40% or more of calories from fat. At present, dietary fat accounts for about 37% of the total energy intake of adolescents, both boys and girls (Life Sciences Research Office, 1989). To help reduce excessive consumption of total fat, food choices should emphasize the intake of fruits, vegetables, and whole grain products and cereals. Low-fat dairy products and lean cuts of meat should also be encouraged.

Carbohydrates

Carbohydrates, a major source of energy for the body, serve as constituents of various cellular structures and substances and are primary components of dietary fiber. Although there are no specific dietary recommendations for carbohydrates, the Food and Nutrition Board Subcommittee on the Tenth Edition of the RDAs recommends that more than half the energy requirement beyond infancy be provided by carbohydrates (FNB, NRC, 1989). At present, more than one fourth of total carbohydrates in adolescents is provided by added sweeteners, mostly sucrose and high fructose corn syrup. The current United States Department of Agriculture/Department of Health and Human Services (USDA-DHHS) Dietary Guidelines for Americans recommend limiting consumption of sugar and increasing consumption of complex carbohydrates such as whole grain foods and cereal products, vegetables, and fruits.

Minerals

During the adolescent growth spurt, the need for all minerals increases. Although minerals play a vital role in health, calcium, iron, and zinc have particular significance for growth and development.

IRON

Iron deficiency is the most prevalent nutritional deficiency in the United States. Adolescents are one group considered at great risk for iron deficiency. Although iron deficiency occurs in all socioeconomic groups, it is most common among low-income youth (Life Sciences Research Office, 1989). The best recent estimates of impaired iron status for adolescents are derived from NHANES II, as calculated by averaging the results of serum ferritin, transferrin saturation, and erythrocyte protoporphyrin determinations. Using these methods, the prevalence of iron deficiency was 2.8% in females 11 to 14 years old, 7.2% in females 15 to 19 years old, 4.1% in males 11 to 14 years old, and 0.6% in males 15 to 19 years old (Surgeon General's Report on Nutrition and Health, 1988). The major causes of iron deficiency include insufficient assimilation of iron from the diet, dilution of body iron stores by rapid growth, and blood loss.

For both boys and girls, the need for iron increases with rapid growth and the expansion of blood volume and muscle mass. Since boys gain lean body mass at a faster rate than girls do, they require more iron/kg weight gain than do girls. For example, boys in the 50th percentile require 42 mg of iron/kg weight gain compared with 31 mg/kg for girls in the 50th percentile (Greenwood and Richardson, 1979). Body composition is more important in determining iron requirements than is weight. The onset of menstruation imposes additional iron needs for girls. Another factor that must be considered in assessing the iron needs of adolescents is biologic variation of growth. For example, the requirement for iron of a boy growing at the 97th percentile for body weight may be double that of a boy growing at the 3rd percentile (Greenwood and Richardson, 1979).

The 1989 RDAs for iron were calculated to attain a target iron storage level of 300 mg for both sexes. For prepubertal children, an allowance of 10 mg/day is recommended. An additional 2 mg/day is recommended for boys during the pubertal growth spurt, and an additional 5 mg is advised for girls starting with the pubertal growth spurt and menstruation. Survey data show that few adolescent girls consume the RDA, with the mean intake being 10 mg/day (Life Sciences Research Office, 1989). The adolescent diet for both boys and girls contains about 6 mg iron/1000 kcal (Bailey and Cerda, 1988). Therefore girls, who generally have lower caloric intakes than do boys, have more difficulty in meeting their iron needs.

The availability of dietary iron for absorption is as important a factor as is the total amount of dietary iron in determining nutritional adequacy. There are two types of iron in food—heme iron (found primarily in meat) and nonheme iron (found in plant sources). Most of the iron in the diet, usually more than 80%, is present as nonheme iron, which has a much lower bioavailability than does heme iron. Nonheme iron absorption is greatly enhanced by relatively small amounts of meats

or foods containing ascorbic acid and is inhibited by tea, bran, and fiber. Adolescents who eat little or no animal protein or whose diets are low in vitamin C may require higher amounts of iron or vitamin C from food. To improve their iron status, adolescents should be encouraged to consume iron-rich foods and to consume a vitamin C source along with cereals and grains.

CALCIUM

Calcium needs during adolescence are greater than they are in either childhood or adulthood because of the dramatic increase in skeletal growth and lean body mass. During adolescence, approximately 20% of adult height is attained, and 45% of adult skeletal mass is formed. Because approximately 99% of total body calcium is found in the skeleton and teeth, the requirement for calcium closely parallels skeletal growth. During peak adolescent growth, calcium retention is on average about 200 mg/day in girls and 300 to 400 mg/day in boys (Forbes, 1981; Greenwood and Richardson, 1979). Calcium needs vary by gender, physiologic age, and body size. The peak daily increment of calcium is greater and the spurt lasts longer in boys than in girls (Forbes, 1981). The RDA for calcium increases from 800 mg/day during childhood to 1200 mg/day for both sexes from age 11 to 19 years.

Adequate calcium during adolescence is important not only for ensuring bone growth but also for achieving peak bone mass. Although the precise relationship of dietary calcium to osteoporosis has not been elucidated, it appears that higher intakes of dietary calcium could increase peak bone mass during adolescence and delay the onset of bone fractures occurring later in life (FNB, NRC, 1989). There is concern that chronically low calcium intakes, especially during adolescence, may compromise development of peak bone mass (FNB, NRC, 1989; Surgeon General's Report on Nutrition and Health, 1988).

It is of concern that many adolescents, especially girls, have calcium intakes that are much less than the RDA. More than 50% of adolescent girls are reported to consume diets containing less than 70% of the RDA for calcium, compared with 24% to 35% of boys. Adolescents' low calcium intake may be explained, in part, by the substitution of soft drinks for milk. According to NHANES II data, the mean intake of calcium for females aged 12 to 19 years was only 780 mg/day. The mean intake for males aged 12 to 19 years was 1270 mg/day (Life Sciences Research Office, 1989).

The interrelationship between calcium and other dietary components is of significance because it can affect calcium bioavailability, utilization, or both. The most important factor affecting calcium metabolism is a sufficient supply of vitamin D, either from diet or sunlight. In the past, it was believed that a high intake of phosphorus adversely affected calcium status. However, more recent studies have found no evidence to suggest that excess dietary phosphorus adversely affects calcium balance at adequate levels of calcium intake (FNB, NRC, 1989).

ZINC

Zinc is a component of 40 metalloenzymes and is involved in most major metabolic processes, including protein synthesis, wound healing, immune function, and growth and maintenance of tissues. Zinc is especially important in adolescents because of its role in growth and sexual maturation. With the onset of puberty, there is a striking increase in the retention of zinc in both sexes that is closely related to the increase in lean body mass (Greenwood and Richardson, 1979). It is estimated that for each kilogram of lean body mass gained, 20 mg of zinc is required. In boys between the ages of 11 and 17 years, the average retention exceeds 400 mg/day (FNB, NRC, 1989).

Zinc deficiency related to diet was first characterized in the early 1960s among adolescent boys living in Egypt and Iran who had growth failure and delayed sexual maturation. After treatment with zinc, the boys matured sexually and had accelerated growth. Since then, similar responses to zinc in growth failure have been reported in both adolescent boys and girls in other countries in the Middle East. A major factor in the pathogenesis of the syndrome is low dietary intake or low bioavailability of zinc from diets high in phytates. In addition, causes of conditioned zinc deficiency include parasitic infections, geophagia, malabsorption syndromes, and inflammatory diseases of the bowel (see Chapter 63).

Marginal states of zinc nutriture may exist in segments of the population in the United States. Hambidge and colleagues (1972) reported suboptimal growth, poor appetite, and impaired taste acuity among middle-income children in Denver who had low concentrations of zinc in their hair. Increasing the daily zinc intake from 0.4 to 0.8 mg/kg brought about marked improvement. Data on zinc nutriture and requirements for teenagers are limited; however, there is some evidence that dietary intakes may be low, especially among girls (Life Sciences Research Office, 1989).

The composition of the diet has an important effect on the bioavailability of zinc. Zinc from animal proteins is more available for absorption, whereas whole grain products contain the element in a less available form. Dietary fibers such as phytates, hemicellulose, and lignin may inhibit zinc absorption, and if these fibers are present in large amounts, the availability of zinc may be significantly impaired. It is estimated that the zinc content of typical mixed diets in the United States is between 10 and 15 mg/day (Greenwood and Richardson, 1979). The current RDA for adolescent boys is 15 mg/day and 12 mg/day for girls.

OTHER MINERALS

Although in recent years there has been more research on minerals and trace elements, very little is known about the requirements in adolescents for magnesium, phosphorus, iodine, copper, chromium, and selenium as well as others. Iodine nutriture was assessed in the Ten-State Nutrition Survey (1968–1970), and there was no evidence of iodine deficiency in the adolescent population surveyed. No clinical or biochemical indicators of the status of trace elements are available from national surveys for adolescents or other age groups (in most cases there are no good biochemical or clinical measurements available). Until future research and better methods of assessment of status are available for these elements and vitamins such as vitamins E and K, biotin, and pantothenic acid, the best ensurance of an adequate and safe intake is consumption of a varied diet.

Vitamins

VITAMIN A

Vitamin A is a fat-soluble nutrient that is essential for vision, bone growth, cellular differentiation, reproduction, and the integrity of the immune system. Although acute vitamin A deficiency is extremely rare in the United States, it is a major nutritional problem in developing countries, causing an estimated 250,000 cases of blindness annually in children. Dietary surveys in the United States have frequently found low dietary vitamin A intakes among adolescents, generally because of low consumption of beta-carotene–rich fruits and vegetables. Low plasma levels of vitamin A, the clinical implications of which are unknown, were found in 40% of Hispanic teenagers and 10% of white and black teenagers studied in the Ten State Nutrition Survey. More recent national data from NHANES I and II do not indicate a significant incidence of low serum vitamin A values among adolescents (Life Sciences Research Office, 1989).

VITAMIN C

Vitamin C functions in the formation of collagen; the maintenance of capillaries, bones, and teeth; the promotion of nonheme iron absorption; and the protection of other vitamins and minerals from oxidation. Based on national studies, vitamin C intakes appear to be adequate for most teenagers in the United States. For example, in NHANES II, the mean vitamin C intake for adolescent boys was 121 mg/day, and for adolescent girls, it was 80 mg/day. These intakes are much greater than the RDAs, which are 50 mg/day for teenagers 11 to 14 years of age and 60 mg/day for 15- to 18-year-olds (Life Sciences Research Office, 1989). Food preference studies have consistently shown that fresh fruits such as oranges and strawberries, and juice, which are excellent sources of vitamin C, are highly preferred foods among teens. Because fresh fruits and juice tend to be relatively expensive, low-income youth or those in geographically isolated areas may be at risk for low dietary intakes of vitamin C.

Adequate vitamin C intake is also of concern among adolescent smokers. Cigarette smokers have lower concentrations of ascorbic acid in serum and leukocytes and a markedly reduced mean half-life of vitamin C compared with nonsmokers with the same dietary intakes (FNB, NRC, 1989). One study found that the metabolic turnover of males who smoked 20 or more cigarettes daily was increased to a level 40% greater than that of nonsmokers (Kallner et al, 1981). The vitamin C requirement of smokers has been estimated to be as much as twice that of nonsmokers. The Food and Nutrition Board Subcommittee on the Tenth Edition of the RDAs recommends that regular smokers consume at least 100 mg/day of vitamin C (FNB, NRC, 1989).

FOLATE

Increased DNA synthesis associated with the rapid cellular division of adolescent growth results in increased folate needs. The RDA for folate is approximately 3 μg/kg body weight for adolescents. Inadequate folate status is relatively common among adolescents. Bailey and Cerda (1988) evaluated folate status in 400 adolescent boys and girls. Approximately 40% of the adolescents had low (<140 ng/ml) red blood cell folate concentrates. Serum folate levels were also found to decrease in both sexes with increasing sexual maturity. The high incidence of folate inadequacy in this study, as well as in others, was associated with insufficient dietary intake of folate. The most concentrated food sources of folate include green leafy vegetables and liver, which are among the teenager's least liked foods.

NIACIN, RIBOFLAVIN, AND THIAMINE

The greater energy demands during adolescence require increased supplies of niacin, riboflavin, and thiamine, which all are involved in energy metabolism. Therefore, recommendations for these nutrients are based on energy intake. Although clinically overt deficiencies are extremely rare in the United States, marginal nutritional status for some of these vitamins has been reported in adolescents (Greenwood and Richardson, 1979). For example, subclinical riboflavin deficiency, as measured by erythrocyte glutathione reductase activity, has been reported in 7% to 27% of low-income adolescents. Low consumption of dairy products, which are concentrated sources of riboflavin, is often related to poor dietary intakes. At this time, low biochemical values reported for riboflavin as well as thiamine do not have clinical correlates, and therefore their significance is unclear.

VITAMIN B₆

Vitamin B_6 is involved in protein synthesis, and therefore the requirement for vitamin B_6 increases as the intake of protein increases. The RDA for adolescents is based on 0.02 mg vitamin B_6/g protein. Evidence of impaired status and low intakes of vitamin B_6 has been reported among adolescent girls. In one study, almost half of adolescent girls had coenzyme stimulation values indicative of marginal or deficient status. The mean dietary intake was 1.25 mg/day (Driskel et al, 1987).

FACTORS INFLUENCING NUTRIENT REQUIREMENTS

Physical Activity and Performance
(see Chapter 81)

In general, the nutritional needs of adolescent athletes are similar to those of nonathletic adolescents with the exception of energy. Energy intake is the principal dietary determinant of athletic performance. Energy demands are based on individual-based basal metabolic rates plus the intensity, duration, frequency, and type of activity involved. Adolescents engaged in vigorous exercise training programs may have energy needs ranging from 3000 to 6000 kcal/day or more. Most adolescents participating in sports require an additional 600 to 1200 kcal/day, depending on the nature of the activity (AAP, 1985). Adolescents can increase their total energy intake by eating more food from the basic food groups, particularly complex carbohydrates. An optimal distribution of calories in the diet of an adolescent athlete consists of protein, 15%; fat, 30%; and carbohydrate, 55% (AAP, 1985).

An increase in muscle mass is a function of growth and physical training. A daily intake of 1 to 1.5 g/kg of high-quality animal protein, which is more than adequately met by the typical diet in the United States, should be sufficient to meet the needs of a young adolescent boy or girl in physical training. Provided that a balanced, varied diet is consumed, the additional energy intake of 600 to 1200 calories adds 22 to 45 g of protein daily. This raises the daily protein to more than adequate levels (AAP, 1985).

Physical activity increases the need for some vitamins and minerals—such as thiamine, riboflavin, and sodium—which the adolescent can easily meet by consuming a balanced diet. Vitamin and mineral supplements are unnecessary, with the possible exception of iron supplements for some athletes. Female adolescent athletes have been shown to be at a greater risk for iron deficiency and iron deficiency anemia than their nonathletic peers (AAP, 1985). It is recommended that the iron status of adolescent athletes be monitored regularly. If iron supplements are to be used, it is recommended they be in the amount of the RDA, which is 15 mg/day.

Pregnancy (see Chapter 74)

The pregnant adolescent has greater nutrient needs than does the nonpregnant adolescent. Extra energy and nutrients are needed to support growth of maternal tissues, such as the breast and uterus, and the increased metabolic demands of pregnancy, as well as the growth of the fetus and placenta. Data regarding nutrient requirements of pregnant adolescents are extremely limited. In general, the greater the amount of uncompleted growth at conception, the greater the nutritional needs of the pregnant adolescent. Although individual variability is great, the majority of growth occurs prior to menarche. Almost all residual growth occurs in the first 2 years after menarche. Therefore, an adolescent who becomes pregnant within 2 years after menarche may have increased nutrient requirements compared with adolescents who have finished their growth. A majority of older pregnant adolescents (16 years and older) or teenagers who mature early finish their growth prior to conception and will not have increased nutrient needs for growth. Their energy and nutrient needs are similar to those of an adult pregnant woman; however, these needs are still substantially increased over the nonpregnant state. The RDAs for pregnancy are shown in Table 7–2. Since the RDAs for women during pregnancy are tabulated as absolute figures rather than as additions to the basic allowance, they may underestimate pregnancy needs for the very young adolescent. An adolescent's nutritional status and lifestyle habits at conception and during gestation profoundly influence the pregnancy outcome. To improve the pregnancy outcome, emphasis should be placed on optimal energy and nutrient intakes to promote adequate weight gain and fetal development.

Oral Contraceptives

Much attention has been paid in recent years to the nutritional status of oral contraceptive users (see Chapter 73). Although early reports in the mid-1960s and 1970s indicated some adverse nutritional consequences related to oral contraceptive use, the lower doses of estrogen and progesterone used today have reduced the number of biochemical and physiologic side effects. Still, oral contraceptives cause many different metabolic alterations, including changes in carbohydrate, lipid, protein, vitamin, and mineral metabolism. Limited research has been conducted with adolescent oral contraceptive users. In young adult women, lipid levels have been found to fluctuate primarily during the first 6 months of oral contraceptive use, with an increase in plasma triglycerides and beta-lipoproteins (very low-density lipoproteins [VLDL] and [LDL]) and a decrease in plasma lipoproteins (high-density lipoproteins [HDL]). No consistent change in plasma cholesterol levels has been observed; however, girls with familial hypercholesterolemia show marked increases in plasma cholesterol levels (see Chapter 60). Vitamin and mineral changes include elevations of plasma levels of vitamin A and serum levels of iron and copper, with decreases in circulating levels or function of carotene, folacin, vitamins B_{12} and B_6, zinc, calcium, phosphorus, and magnesium. Reports on circulating levels of vitamins C and E have been variable. Mild to moderate weight gains of 1.3 to 2.7 kg have also been observed in some adolescents. The metabolic alterations in nutrients found in young adult oral contraceptive users have not been associated with any undesirable health consequences or any measurable problems in future pregnancies. Consequently, there is little evidence to suggest that increased intakes of these nutrients are required for users of oral contraceptives. However, there is still some concern for adolescents who use oral contraceptives for many months and have a diet of poor nutritional quality.

The potential exists over the long term for development of suboptimal folate or vitamin B_6 status, or both.

Chronic Illnesses and Disabling Conditions

The nutritional requirements for adolescents with disabilities or chronic illnesses may be significantly altered by either the medical condition or the therapy necessary to control the disorder (see Chapters 30, 43, 59, 60, 62, 63, and 65). These teenagers face a greater than average risk for nutritional problems, resulting from their condition, and, indeed, nutrition-related problems occur frequently. Malnutrition has been implicated as a major factor contributing to poor growth and short stature in adolescents with a variety of diseases (e.g., chronic inflammatory bowel disease, cystic fibrosis). Inadequate intake, excessive nutrient losses, malabsorption, and increased nutrient requirements all are factors leading to the chronic malnourished state. Studies have shown that the energy requirements for adolescents with cystic fibrosis or inflammatory bowel disease may be as high as 30% to 50% more than the RDA for adequate growth. In addition to the increased energy needs caused by malabsorption (or in the case of adolescents with cystic fibrosis, the increased work of breathing), fever, infection, and inflammation also increase energy requirements. For example, an increase of 1°C greater than the normal temperature requires an average increase in basal metabolism of about 13%. Whereas undernourishment is frequently seen in adolescents with chronic illnesses, obesity is common among youth with gross motor limitations or immobility (see Chapter 60). Because of limited activity, caloric requirements are lower, and the balance between intake and expenditure is often difficult, resulting in obesity. Early assessment of nutritional status followed by nutritional intervention and monitoring will substantially help ensure the health and well-being of youth with chronic and disabling conditions.

RECOMMENDED FOOD GUIDE FOR ADOLESCENTS

There are about 50 known essential nutrients required by humans. Based on current scientific knowledge, the Food and Nutrition Board of the National Research Council has established dietary allowances or estimated safe and adequate ranges for only 24 of these 50 nutrients. Obviously, a great deal of research remains to be done on nutrient requirements in general, and in adolescents more specifically. The best way to ensure that adolescents meet the nutrient needs for all 50 essential nutrients is for them to consume a variety of foods from diverse food groups that contain adequate energy. Table 7–3 provides a summary of major nutrients and includes dietary sources of these nutrients.

TABLE 7–3. Summary of Major Nutrients

Food Component	Function in Body	Good Sources in Diet	Consequences of Inadequate Intake	Consequences of Excessive Intake
Food energy	Metabolic functions: maintenance of body temperature, growth and repair of bones and tissue, and movement of muscles; body fat storage	Protein—4 kcal/g Carbohydrate—4 kcal/g Fat—9 kcal/g	Underweight, semistarvation, growth retardation	Overweight, obesity
Protein	Involved in most metabolic processes; essential for growth, development, and maintenance of body tissues; amino acids are structural elements of muscle, connective tissue, bone, enzymes, hormones, and antibodies	Meat, poultry, fish, eggs, milk, cheese	Protein-energy malnutrition	Excess protein intake converted to body fat
Fat, fatty acids, cholesterol	Concentrated source of energy; carrier for the fat-soluble vitamins; structural and functional components of cell membranes; precursors of compounds involved in many aspects of metabolism	Saturated fatty acids: butter, lard Monounsaturated fatty acids; olive oil Polyunsaturated fatty acids and soybean oils Cholesterol: liver, kidney, brains, egg yolk, meat, poultry, fish, cheese	Clinical deficiencies of essential fatty acids and fat-soluble nutrients have occurred, poor growth	Overweight, obesity; may increase risk for cardiovascular disease later in life
Carbohydrate	Energy source; stored as glycogen or converted to body fat	Simple carbohydrates: fruits, vegetables, milk, sugar, other caloric sweeteners Complex carbohydrates: grain products and vegetables	Ketosis	Contribution to excess calorie intake
Fiber	Bulk in diet; promotes normal elimination	Whole-grain products, many fruits and vegetables, dry beans, nuts	Constipation	Possible decrease in mineral absorption
Alcohol	Source of calories; depressant	Beer, wine, and other alcoholic beverages	—	Inadequate nutrient intake; possible overweight; social and public safety problems
Vitamin A (retinol)	Formation and maintenance of skin, hair, and mucous membranes; essential for vision, bone, growth, tooth development, and reproduction	Preformed retinol: liver and vitamin A–fortified foods, milk Carotene: dark green leafy vegetables, yellow and orange vegetables and fruits	Changes in eyes (keratomalacia) and skin, vision problems (xerophthalmia)	Teratogenicity; toxicity symptoms including effects on skin and bone
Vitamin E (tocopherol)	Antioxidant functions	Vegetable fats and oils, some cereal products, nuts, some seafood	Enhanced fragility of red blood cells	—
Thiamine	Component of enzymes involved in energy metabolism; required for cell reproduction, fatty acid metabolism, and nervous system functions	Pork, beef and pork liver, whole-grain and enriched grain products, milk	Loss of appetite, decreased muscle tone, depression, neurologic changes (beriberi)	—
Riboflavin	Component of enzymes involved in protein and energy metabolism	Milk, cheeses, meat, liver, enriched and fortified cereals, and grains	Cracks at corner of mouth; soreness and inflammation of mouth, lips, and tongue	—
Niacin	Involved in energy metabolism and synthesis of protein and fat	Liver, peanuts, poultry, red meat, fish (also dairy produts and eggs as sources of tryptophan)	Dermatitis, diarrhea, depression (pellagra)	Vascular dilation
Vitamin B_6 (pyridoxal)	Functions in metabolism of protein; nervous system function	Poultry, fish, bananas, red meat, milk	Depression, confusion, convulsions	Possible damage to peripheral nervous system

TABLE 7–3. Summary of Major Nutrients *Continued*

Food Component	Function in Body	Good Sources in Diet	Consequences of Inadequate Intake	Consequences of Excessive Intake
Vitamin B$_{12}$ (cobalamins)	Required for formation of red blood cells, building genetic material, function of nervous system, and metabolism of protein and fat	Liver, red meat, fish, eggs, milk	Pernicious anemia; neurologic damage	—
Vitamin C (ascorbic acid)	Formation of collagen; maintenance of capillaries, bones, and teeth; iron absorption; antioxidant	Citrus fruits, other fruits, tomatoes, potatoes, dark green vegetables	Hemorrhages in skin and gums, weakness, defects in bone development (scurvy)	Gastrointestinal symptoms
Folacin (folate)	Formation of hemoglobin and genetic material	Liver, dark green leafy vegetables, dry beans, wheat germ	Pallor, weakness, neurologic changes, anemia	—
Iron	Carrier of oxygen in body; red blood cell formation	Liver, beef, dry beans, spinach, fortified and enriched grains and cereals	Iron deficiency, iron deficiency anemia	Iron overload (persons with genetic predisposition)
Calcium	Formation and maintenance of bone and teeth; muscle contraction; blood clotting; integrity of cell membranes	Dairy products, broccoli, spinach, turnip greens, canned fish	Decreased peak bone mass (may increase risk for osteoporosis later in life)	Renal calculi; possible soft tissue calcification; constipation
Phosphorus	Structural element of bones and teeth; participates in a variety of chemical reactions	Dairy products, meat, poultry, fish (protein sources)	None of practical concern	—
Magnesium	Component of bone; protein synthesis; release of energy from glycogen; regulation of body temperature and blood pressure	Whole grain products, some dry beans, some dark beans, some dark green vegetables, nuts	Rarely—muscle spasms, tremor, nausea, apathy, convulsions, coma	—
Sodium	Regulation of body fluid volume and acid-base balance of blood; transmission of nerve impulses; principal extracellular cation	Salt (sodium chloride), sodium-containing additives and condiments, many processed foods, canned foods, salty snacks	—	Edema, hypertension
Potassium	Regulation with sodium of body fluid volume and acid-base balance; principal intracellular cation	Red meat, milk, many fruits and vegetables, seafood	—	—
Copper	Component of several proteins and enzymes; iron utilization	Shellfish, nuts, liver, kidney, corn oil, margarine, lentils	Anemia, bone disease	—
Zinc	Formation of protein; component of many enzymes; wound healing, blood formation, general growth and maintenance of all tissues	Shellfish, red meat, poultry, ricotta cheese, whole grain cereals, dry beans, eggs	Growth retardation, poor appetite, mental lethargy, skin changes, retarded sexual development	Emesis (acute intoxication)
Fluoride	Component of bones and tooth enamel	Fluoridated water, certain fish, tea (also from fluoridated toothpastes and rinses)	Impaired dental health	Mottled teeth
Selenium	Constituent of red blood cell, glutathione peroxidase	Seafoods, kidney, liver	Cardiomyopathy in children (Keshan disease)	—

Adapted from Nutrition Monitoring in the United States. US Depts HHS, and USDA, DHHS Publ. No. (PHS) 89-1255, 1989.

BIBLIOGRAPHY

American Academy of Pediatrics: Adolescent nutrition. In Forbes GB (ed): Pediatric Nutrition Handbook, 2nd ed. Elk Grove Village, IL, American Academy of Pediatrics, 1985.

Bailey L, Cerda JJ: Iron and folate nutriture during life cycle. World Rev Nutr Diet 56:56, 1988.

Driskel JA, Clark A, Mock SW: Longitudinal assessment of vitamin B_6 status in southern adolescent girls. J Am Diet Assoc 87:307, 1987.

Food and Nutrition Board, National Research Council: Recommended Dietary Allowances, 10th ed. Washington, DC, National Academy of Sciences, 1989.

Forbes GB: Nutritional requirements in adolescence. In Suskind RM (ed): Textbook of Pediatric Nutrition. New York, Raven Press, 1981.

Greenwood CT, Richardson DP: Nutrition during adolescence. World Rev Nutr Diet 31:1, 1979.

Hambidge KM, Hambidge C, Jacobs M, Baum JP: Low levels of zinc in hair, anorexia, poor growth, and hypogeusia in children. Pediatr Res 6:868, 1972.

Kallner AB, Hartmann D, Hornig DH: On the requirements of ascorbic acid in man: Steady-state turnover and body pool in smokers. Am J Clin Nutr 34:1347, 1981.

LaRosa J, Finberg L: Preliminary report from a conference entitled "Prevention of Adult Atherosclerosis During Childhood." J Pediatr 112:317, 1988.

Life Sciences Research Office, FASEB: Nutrition Monitoring in the United States. An Update Report on Nutrition Monitoring. US Depts HHS, USDA, DHHS Publ. No. (PHS) 89 1255, Hyattsville, MD, Sept 1989.

Surgeon General's Report on Nutrition and Health: Maternal and Child Nutrition. US Depts HHS, DHHS (PHS) Publ. No. 88 50210, Washington, DC, 1988.

Ten-State Nutrition Survey (1968–1970). US Dept HEW, DHEW Publ. No. (HSM) 72-8130. Washington, DC, US Government Printing Office, 1972.

Behavior Issues

CHAPTER 8

Normality During Adolescence

IRVING B. WEINER

Normal psychological development during adolescence, as at other times of life, consists of age-appropriate and adaptive patterns of behavior. Young people who are growing up normally cope reasonably effectively with the developmental tasks of their age group and think, feel, and act in much the same manner as the majority of their peers. Abnormal psychological development, in contrast, is likely to be identified by ineffective coping efforts that are not characteristic of a young person's age group.

This does not mean that uncommon behaviors are abnormal behaviors. Adolescents who are uncommonly bright, talented, energetic, self-confident, or socially adept are not clinically abnormal, except in the unlikely event that these usually desirable characteristics lead to ineffective coping.

When the current coping effectiveness of atypical behavior patterns is difficult to determine, their normality can best be judged from their future implications. Unusual or problematic behaviors that can be expected to lead to subsequent psychopathologic conditions are more likely to reflect abnormal development than are atypical behaviors. These behaviors usually disappear of their own accord, without resulting in later disturbance.

Distinguishing normal and abnormal adolescent development lays the foundation for accurate diagnosis of psychological disturbance in young people. The more that adolescents deviate from normative and effective ways of coping with their experience, the more likely they are to be suffering from diagnosable or emerging psychopathologic conditions for which treatment is indicated. Early identification of and timely intervention for the development of psychological disturbance are especially critical during the adolescent years. Adolescents are more likely than children to have matured to a point at which psychological difficulties are becoming less transient and are more likely to crystallize into adult psychopathologic conditions. When compared with adults, however, adolescents are less likely to have settled into a psychopathologic lifestyle and are more likely to change in response to therapy.

To recognize a developmental psychopathologic condition, clinicians need to be familiar with how young people ordinarily grow up and conduct themselves and how an emerging disorder is typically manifested in children and adolescents. In addition, the assessment of adolescents can be guided by clinical and research findings documenting (1) that normative adolescence is adaptive, (2) that adolescent turmoil reflects deviant adjustment, and (3) that significant symptom formation in adolescents is pathologic.

NORMATIVE ADOLESCENCE IS ADAPTIVE

Contrary to the popular belief that adolescents normally pass through a period of psychological upheaval and alienation, empirical evidence demonstrates that adolescence is typically an adaptive phase of growth characterized by developmental continuity rather than disruption, emotional stability rather than disorder, gradual identity formation rather than disabling crisis, and generational harmony rather than conflict.

Personality Development Is Continuous (see Chapter 11)

Considerable longitudinal data indicate that personality development is in many respects continuous and transitional. In well-known studies begun many years ago at the Fels Research Institute and the Institute of Human Development at the University of California at Berkeley, many adult characteristics were found to be predictable from related behaviors exhibited during childhood (including dependency, passivity, proneness to anger, and anxiety level) and from personality traits apparent during adolescence (such as introspectiveness, assertiveness, likableness, overcontrol, talkativeness, and self-satisfaction) (Kagan and Moss, 1962; Eichorn et al, 1981).

In a more recent research project that provided impressive evidence of continuity in personality development, Bachman and colleagues (1979) studied a representative national sample of 1628 boys from their entry into tenth grade until they reached the age of 23 years. Their data painted a picture primarily of stability, not change: "Contrary to what might have been expected by those who view adolescence as a period of great turbulence and stress, we found a good deal of consistency along dimensions of attitudes, aspirations, and self-concept" (Bachman et al, 1979, p 220).

These findings do not mean that personality becomes fixed and immutable early in life. What is consistent over time is not any specific set of behaviors but rather dimensions of personality along which individuals tend to maintain the same relative position. For example, people tend to become increasingly capable of self-control as they mature, and most adults manifest more self-control than they did as adolescents. However, because this is a fairly consistent dimension of personality, individuals who have relatively poor self-control as teenagers are likely as adults to show less self-control than other adults. Recent reports in this vein demonstrate that boys and girls who at age 4 and 5 years are less able than other children to delay receiving gratification show less stress tolerance than their peers at adolescence, and that 8- to 10-year-old children of both sexes who are prone to temper tantrums become relatively ill-tempered adults 30 years later (Caspi et al, 1987; Mischel et al, 1988).

Adolescents Are Emotionally Stable

Research of various kinds demonstrates that adolescence is normally a period of emotional stability rather than upset. In the first major study addressing this issue, Douvan and Adelson (1966) collected interview data from more than 3000 boys and girls representative of junior and senior high school students in the United States. Very few of these young people described their lives in terms of turmoil, conflict, and instability. Instead, the comments that Douvan and Adelson's interviewers most commonly heard from these subjects convinced them that it is only the adolescent at the extremes, not the typical young person, "who responds to the instinctual and psychosocial upheaval of puberty by disorder" (Douvan and Adelson, 1966, p 351).

In another seminal research project, using an in-depth clinical approach rather than the survey method of Douvan and Adelson, Offer and Offer (1975) conducted an 8-year study in which 73 typical middle-class American midwestern boys were assessed in interviews, on psychological tests, and from parents' reports on several occasions from their freshman to senior years of high school. Sixty-one of these young men were subsequently evaluated in the same way during four years of college. The majority of these subjects showed a pattern of calm and adaptive progress from adolescence into young adulthood, and just one fifth of the group gave evidence of noteworthy inner unrest or overt behavior problems from 14 to 22 years of age.

Offer and other researchers have obtained similar results over the last 20 years from extensive surveys using a self-report instrument called the Offer Self-Image Questionnaire (Offer et al, 1981). This 130-item questionnaire has been administered to many thousands of adolescents in many different samples of nonpatient male and female subjects living in diverse environments. Their responses strongly suggest that the vast majority of teenagers are happy, self-confident, optimistic, and socially well-adjusted individuals free from any throes of adolescent turmoil:

As far as we know, almost every researcher who has studied a representative sample of normal teenagers has come to the conclusion that by and large good coping and a smooth transition into adulthood are much more typical than the opposite. Among middle-class high school students 80 percent can, in general, be described as normal, free of symptoms, and without turmoil (Offer and Sabshin, 1984, pp 100–101).

Many other recent studies have documented that turmoil is the exception rather than the rule among representative samples of nonpatient adolescents. Reviews of this evidence leave little doubt that adolescent personality development is for the most part a relatively smooth process in which maturation occurs gradually and without tumult (Petersen, 1988; Powers et al, 1989).

Two other seminal research projects investigated the frequency with which adolescents become psychologically disturbed. Masterson (1967), in the Symptomatic Adolescent Research Project, assessed symptom patterns in 101 nonpatient 12- to 18-year-olds selected as a comparison group for a sample of adolescent patients being evaluated at the Payne Whitney Clinic. He found that 20% of these nonpatient subjects had psychological symptoms that moderately or severely impaired their ability to function in school or in social relationships; 63% had occasional symptoms—mainly anxiety and depression—that from time to time caused mild impairments of their ability to function; and the remaining 17% were completely free of symptoms.

In another clinical study of nonpatients, Rutter and colleagues (1976) examined the education, health, and behavior of all children and adolescents on the Isle of Wight, a small island of 100,000 people just off the southern coast of England and similar to it in social composition. Included in this study were detailed clinical evaluations conducted with 200 randomly selected 14- to 15-year-olds. About one half of these adolescents reported feelings of anxiety or depression, but only 16.3% were considered to have a significant psychological disorder (Rutter et al, 1976).

Numerous subsequent studies have consistently confirmed that a diagnosable psychological disorder is present in approximately 20% of the adolescent population (Kashani et al, 1987; Offer et al, 1987). Interestingly, Costello and associates (1988), in a study of several hundred 7- to 11-year-old children visiting their primary care pediatricians, found that 22% demonstrated psychological disorders, as defined in the *Diagnostic and Statistical Manual of Mental Disorders,* 3rd edition. These are about the same as the percentages that have been found in large-scale normative studies of adult adjustment. At any point in time, between 16% and 25% of American adults have suffered within the previous 6 months from moderate to severe psychological problems that constitute a clinically diagnosable disorder; 51% to 58% have, or have recently had, mild or fleeting problems; and 18% to 19% have had few or no symptoms (Myers et al, 1984). Thus, among younger and older people alike, about 60% demonstrate mild forms of symptom formation, and the remaining 40% are about evenly divided between symptom-free and moderately or severely impaired groups.

Identity Formation Is Gradual

As a reflection of the normal process of identity formation during the adolescent years, young people typically spend several years "trying on" alternative roles and ideologies. They consider various job and career possibilities; they enter into friendship and dating relationships with different kinds of people; and they weigh the merits of divergent social, political, economic, and religious points of view. Because adolescents are actively examining alternatives before choosing among them, they often vacillate in what they like to do, with whom they want to be, and what they prefer to believe. This means that young people tend to be somewhat more changeable and unpredictable, at least by adult standards, and that they typically struggle with some uncertainty while they are deciding on their future commitments (Kimmel and Weiner, 1985, Chap. 8).

However, for the most part adolescents do not experience any maladaptive distress while they are working to achieve a sense of identity, nor does their vacillation ordinarily involve any pronounced emotional disequilibrium or disturbing concerns about who or what they are at present. Empirical studies have consistently found that disruptive crises accompanying the process of identity formation are the exception, not the rule (Larson et al, 1980; Waterman, 1982).

Moreover, the process of working on identity formation is associated with increasingly stable self-concepts rather than any disruption of an adolescent's self-image. Young people are vulnerable to an unstable self-image mainly during puberty, when they are coping with major changes in the size and appearance of their bodies. Following the pubescent growth spurt, however, teenagers' views of themselves are found to change only gradually and in the direction of progressively greater stability (Dusek and Flaherty, 1981).

Generational Relationships Are Harmonious

Abundant research on relationships between the adolescent and adult generations indicates that very few young people are in rebellion against either their families or society. To the contrary, most adolescents share their parents' sense of values and get along well with them. In the previously mentioned studies by Douvan and Adelson (1966) and Offer and colleagues (1981), for example, the majority of the thousands of adolescents surveyed reported that they respected their parents, wanted to be like them, and enjoyed harmonious relationships with them and other adults as well. Most of these teenagers expressed satisfaction with their homes and described their parents as knowledgeable, reliable, understanding, and sympathetic people. Although they reported disagreeing with their parents on matters such as curfews, use of the family car, and styles of dress and grooming, arguments over such relatively trivial issues seldom threatened the basic bonds of affection within their families: "Contrary to prevailing mythology, the normal adolescents we studied do not perceive any major problems between themselves and their parents" (Offer and Sabshin, 1984, p 94).

Subsequent work involving large and socioculturally diverse groups of subjects has consistently yielded similar evidence of predominantly positive relationships between adolescents and their parents (Hill, 1987; Montemayor, 1983; Powers et al, 1989; Steinberg, 1987). Conducted at different times and in different settings, these studies confirm that the typical pattern for relationships between the adolescent and adult generations involves harmony rather than strife, affection rather than alienation, and commitment to, rather than rejection of, family life.

ADOLESCENT TURMOIL REFLECTS DEVIANT ADJUSTMENT

In those infrequent instances in which adolescent turmoil emerges, it is typically accompanied by signs and symptoms of psychological disturbance that reliably distinguish between normally and abnormally developing young people. Contrary to expectations in some quarters that adolescence is typically characterized by discontinuous personality development, emotional instability, identity crises, and disruptive family conflict, these features of a tumultuous adolescence are consistently found to reflect deviant, not normative, adjustment.

With respect to emotional instability, for example, Offer and associates (1981, Chap. 8) compared the Offer Self-Image Questionnaire responses of normative adolescent samples with responses given by three diagnostically diverse groups of 13- to 18-year-olds receiving treatment in a psychiatric facility. These patients were much more likely than the nonpatient adolescents to describe themselves as being emotionally upset, and they also reported lower self-esteem than did normative adolescents, a poorer image of their bodies, and more difficulty in getting along with their peers. Numerous other studies have demonstrated relationships between these manifestations of emotional upset and other evidence of developing psychological disorder (Kashani et al, 1987; Offer et al, 1986; Tolan et al, 1988).

Regarding identity crises, empirical findings indicate that the more adolescents perceive themselves as changing and the more uncertain they are about their sex role identity, the more likely they are to have adjustment difficulties. The relatively few adolescents who do experience an identity crisis are usually found to be sufficiently troubled to need professional help (Handel, 1980; Marcia, 1980).

As for relationships within the family, there is good evidence that adolescents who experience or report marked conflict with or alienation from their families are likely to be psychologically maladjusted. In the study by Offer and colleagues (1981), the subjects receiving treatment were markedly more likely than normative adolescents to endorse negative attitudes toward their families and markedly less likely to endorse positive attitudes. In the Isle of Wight research, Rutter and co-workers (1976) found that a group of 156 14-year-olds with diagnosable psychological disorders were substantially more likely than a comparison group of 123 14-year-olds without disorders to display communication difficulty, altercations, and physical withdrawal in their relationships with their parents.

The work of many other investigators has confirmed that conflict, dissatisfaction, and poor communication among family members occur much more frequently in the homes of disturbed adolescents than in the homes of normative adolescents (Doane, 1978; Petersen, 1988). Family strife and generational conflict are associated with disturbed adolescent development, and dramatic rebellion against closeness within the family constitutes deviant behavior. Families that are seriously at odds with each other tend to have disturbed children in their midst, and disturbed young people are much more likely than their well-adjusted peers to come from families that are not functioning comfortably as a unit.

In addition to documenting that features of adolescent turmoil differentiate maladjusted from normal adolescents, clinical studies, beginning with Masterson's Symptomatic Adolescent Research Project (1967), have identified some specific dimensions of symptom formation that help sharpen this differentiation. Compared with the approximately 60% of adolescents who are developing normally but nevertheless show some symptom formation, disturbed adolescents who need professional care display a greater number of symptoms that last longer and are more likely to include cognitive and behavioral as well as emotional components (Hudgens, 1974; Weiner, 1982). These findings provide three guidelines for differentiating normal from abnormal development in the symptomatic adolescent: (1) The more symptoms the young person displays, (2) the longer symptoms of any kind persist, and (3) the more the symptom picture is marked not only by feelings of anxiety and depression but also by disturbed thinking or antisocial behavior, the more likely it is that the young person has a diagnosable psychopathologic condition.

With further respect to the types of difficulties adolescents may present, several specific cognitive and behavioral problems are particularly likely to indicate an emerging psychopathologic condition. In the cognitive sphere, clinicians should be especially concerned about adolescents who are beginning to reason in illogical ways, to harbor unrealistic and far-fetched ideas, to communicate poorly because of peculiar and idiosyncratic ways of using language, and to perform uncharacteristically poorly in their school work. In the behavioral sphere, a psychological disorder should be suspected in adolescents who are abusing alcohol or drugs, engaging in promiscuous sexuality, committing repetitive delinquent acts independent of involvement with a subculturally delinquent peer group, or withdrawing from social interactions or recreational activities that were previously enjoyed (see Chapters 68 and 111).

SYMPTOM FORMATION IN ADOLESCENTS IS PATHOLOGIC

As just noted, the likelihood and severity of a diagnosable disorder in a young person vary with the number, kind, and persistence of symptoms he or she is manifesting. To ensure that adolescents are helped as much as possible to mature into psychologically healthy adults, however, any symptom formation they show should be regarded as at least potentially psychopathologic. This conclusion is derived from evidence in longitudinal studies of both nonpatient and disturbed individuals indicating that a person's level of adjustment relative to that of his or her peers tends to remain fairly stable during adolescence and from adolescence to adulthood, for better or worse.

Among nonpatient populations, for example, Rutter and colleagues (1976) in the Isle of Wight research found considerable continuity of poor adjustment from early to middle adolescence. Children in this survey who showed emotional problems at age 10 and 11 years were more than twice as likely as their age mates to have such problems at 14 and 15 years of age. In the previously mentioned California studies, good psychological health at age 40 years was found to be predictable from good adjustment in adolescence, for both males and females (Livson and Peskin, 1981).

Vaillant (1978) reported similar results from a 35-year study of 268 college sophomore men, 94 of whom were available to be interviewed at age 54 years. The adequacy of the high school adjustment of these men, as rated from information they gave as college students, was significantly related to the adequacy of their psychological adjustment as adults. Good social adjustment in adolescence predicted good social adjustment at midlife for these men, and poor adjustment at midlife was typically predicted by poor adjustment in adolescence.

In another prospective study, Vaillant and Vaillant (1981) followed 456 inner-city males from 14 to 47 years of age. The effectiveness with which these subjects coped as adolescents with work-related activities at home, in school, and in part-time jobs significantly predicted their mental health and capacity for interpersonal relationships as adults. Other more recent studies of normative groups, both male and female, have confirmed the stability of individual differences in coping effectiveness from childhood through adolescence and into adulthood (Caspi et al, 1987; Lerner et al, 1988; Raphael, 1988).

Follow-up evaluations of disturbed adolescents have similarly identified consistency over time in a young person's level of adjustment relative to that of his or her peers. These studies indicate that for the most part adolescents who manifest obvious symptoms of a diagnosable disorder do not outgrow them. Those who appear disturbed are likely to be disturbed and to remain disturbed unless they receive adequate treatment. In the Symptomatic Adolescent Research Project, for example, a 5-year follow-up revealed that almost two thirds of the patients continued to have moderate or severe functioning impairments.

Weiner and Del Gaudio (1976) reported comparable findings in a long-term community study of 1334 12- to 18-year-olds who had visited a mental health facility or practitioner during a 2-year period. Over the next 10 years, 52.4% of these patients returned on one or more occasions for further professional care. This rate of persistent or recurring psychological difficulty far exceeds what would be expected if the initial disturbances had been maturational phenomena destined to pass in time.

As final testimony to the psychopathologic significance of symptom formation, reports from numerous psychiatric hospitals indicate that adolescents who require inpatient treatment are at relatively high risk for poor adjustment in adulthood. Follow-up evaluations up to 10 years after hospital discharge have revealed that though these disturbed youngsters improve in the majority of cases, they are subsequently much more likely than the general adult population to experience psychological difficulties that interfere with their lives. Consistent with other data on the temporal stability of relative adjustment level, the severity of the psychopathologic conditions exhibited by the disturbed adolescents in these studies is found to predict the degree of disturbance they show as adults (Gossett et al, 1983; Welner et al, 1979).

BIBLIOGRAPHY

Bachman JG, O'Malley RM, Johnston J: Adolescent to Adulthood: Change and Stability in the Lives of Young Men. Ann Arbor, MI, Institute for Social Research, 1979.

Caspi A, Elder GH, Bem DJ: Moving against the world: Life-course patterns of explosive children. Dev Psychol 23:308, 1987.

Costello EJ, Costello AJ, Edelbrock C, et al: Psychiatric disorders in pediatric primary care. Arch Gen Psychiatry 45:1107, 1988.

Doane JA: Family interaction and communication deviance in disturbed and normal families: A review of research. Fam Proc 17:357, 1978.

Douvan E, Adelson J: The Adolescent Experience. New York, John Wiley & Sons, 1966.

Dusek JB, Flaherty JF: The development of the self-concept during the adolescent years. Mongr Soc Res Child Dev 46(4):1, 1981.

Eichorn DH, Mussen PH, Clausen JA, et al: Overview. In Eichorn DH, Clausen JA, Haan N, et al (eds): Present and Past in Midlife. New York, Academic Press, 1981.

Gossett JT, Lewis JM, Barnhart FD: To Find A Way: The Outcome of Hospital Treatment of Disturbed Adolescents. New York, Brunner/Mazel, 1983.

Handel A: Perceived change of self among adolescents. J Youth Adolesc 9:507, 1980.

Hill JP: Research on adolescents and their families: Past and prospect. In Irwin CE (ed): Adolescent Development, Social Behavior, and Health. San Francisco, Jossey-Bass, 1987.

Hudgens RW: Psychiatric Disorders in Adolescents. Baltimore, Williams & Wilkins, 1974.

Kagan J, Moss HA: Birth to Maturity: A Study in Psychological Development. New York, John Wiley & Sons, 1962.

Kashani JH, Beck NC, Hoeper EW, et al: Psychiatric disorders in a community sample of adolescents. Am J Psychiatry 144:584, 1987.

Kimmel DC, Weiner IB: Adolescence: A Developmental Transition. New York, John Wiley & Sons, 1985.

Larson R, Czikszentmihalyi M, Graef R: Mood variability and the psychosocial adjustment of adolescents. J Youth Adolesc 9:469, 1980.

Lerner JV, Hertzog C, Hooker KA, et al: A longitudinal study of negative emotional states and adjustment from early childhood through adolescence. Child Dev 59:356, 1988.

Livson N, Peskin H: Psychological health at age 40. In Eichorn DH, Clausen JA, Haan N, et al (eds): Present and Past in Midlife. New York, Academic Press, 1981.

Marcia JE: Identity in adolescence. In Adelson J (ed): Handbook of Adolescent Psychology. New York, John Wiley & Sons, 1980.

Masterson JF: The Psychiatric Dilemma of Adolescence. Boston, Little, Brown, 1967.

Mischel W, Shoda Y, Peake PK: The nature of adolescent competencies predicted by preschool delay of gratification. J Pers Soc Psychol 54:687, 1988.

Montemayor R: Parents and adolescents in conflict: All families some of the time and some families most of the time. J Early Adolesc 3:83, 1983.

Myers JK, Weissman MM, Tischler GL, et al: Six-month prevalence of psychiatric disorders in three communities. Arch Gen Psychiatry 41:959, 1984.

Offer D, Offer JB: From Teenage to Young Manhood: A Psychological Study. New York, Basic Books, 1975.

Offer D, Sabshin M: Adolescence: Empirical perspectives. In Offer D, Sabshin M (eds): Normality and the Life Cycle. New York, Basic Books, 1984.

Offer D, Ostrov E, Howard KI: The Adolescent: A Psychological Self-Portrait. New York, Basic Books, 1981.

Offer D, Ostrov E, Howard KI: Self-image, delinquency, and help-seeking behavior among normal adolescents. In Feinstein SC: Adolescent Psychiatry, Vol 13. Chicago, University of Chicago Press, 1986.

Offer D, Ostrov E, Howard KI: The epidemiology of mental health and mental illness among urban adolescents. In Call J: Significant Advances in Child Psychiatry. New York, Basic Books, 1987.

Petersen AC: Adolescent development. Annu Rev Psychol 39:583, 1988.

Powers SI, Hauser ST, Kilner LA: Adolescent mental health. Am Psychol 44:200, 1989.

Raphael D: High school conceptual level as an indicator of young adult adjustment. J Pers Assess 52:679, 1988.

Rutter M, Graham P, Chadwick OFD, et al: Adolescent turmoil: Fact or fiction? J Child Psychol Psychiatry 17:35, 1976.

Steinberg LD: Family processes at adolescence: A developmental perspective. Fam Ther 14:78, 1987.

Tolan P, Miller L, Thomas P: Perception and experience of types of social stress and self-image among adolescents. J Youth Adolesc 17:147, 1988.

Vaillant GE: Natural history of male psychological health. VI. Correlates of successful marriage and fatherhood. Am J Psychiatry 135:653, 1978.

Vaillant GE, Vaillant CO: Natural history of male psychological health. X. Work as a predictor of positive mental health. Am J Psychiatry 138:1433, 1981.

Waterman AS: Identity development from adolescence to adulthood: An extension of theory and a review of research. Dev Psychol 18:341, 1982.

Weiner IB: Child and Adolescent Psychopathology. New York, John Wiley & Sons, 1982.

Weiner IB, Del Gaudio AC: Psychopathology in adolescence: An epidemiological study. Arch Gen Psychiatry 33:187, 1976.

Welner A, Welner Z, Fishman R: Psychiatric adolescent inpatients: Eight to ten-year follow-up. Arch Gen Psychiatry 36:687, 1979.

CHAPTER 9

Psychological and Social Development

GARY M. INGERSOLL

BACKGROUND

As young people experience the biologic changes from childhood to adulthood, they also experience profound changes in their psychological and social worlds. Parents and professionals frequently view adolescents and the period of adolescence with ambivalence. On the one hand, adults admire the exuberance, enthusiasm, and idealism of youth. On the other hand, adults fear that adolescents' impulsive behaviors and egocentric demeanor will result in long-term negative health and social consequences.

Health professionals who care for adolescents can play important roles in fostering a positive transition to adulthood. To be effective in caring for adolescents, however, it must be recognized that the adolescent presents both physical and psychosocial concerns. Further, immediate psychosocial concerns may be much more salient to adolescents than warnings of potential long-term risks of negative health behaviors or lack of adherence to a medical regimen (see Chapter 26). Therapeutic interventions that do not incorporate normal cognitive, social, and affective needs of adolescents are likely to be ineffective. The purpose of this chapter is to introduce practitioners to normal developmental and psychosocial aspects of adolescence.

Definitions

Before describing the psychosocial aspects of adolescence, it is important first to define adolescence. At one level, there is an intuitive sense that adolescents are "teenagers" or that somehow adolescence is a physical phenomenon related to puberty (see Chapters 4 and 5). Adolescence, however, encompasses more than a simple age range or a stage of physical maturation. The transition from childhood to adulthood that is considered adolescence is a composite of several transitions. Thus, composing a definition of adolescence, and by inference "adolescents," is not easy.

First, limiting adolescence to the teenaged years ignores the fact that many developmental tasks of adolescence have their initiation well before the child turns 13 years of age, with other tasks continuing well into young adulthood. Second, though puberty marks one of the primary aspects of the developing adolescent, the physical transition is by no means the only major aspect of the adolescent transition (see Chapters 4 and 5). Adolescence consists of several developmental transitions in which the individual relinquishes the role of child in favor of the role of adult. Third, any definition risks masking the wide range of individual differences among young people.

With these cautions in mind, adolescence is defined as "a period of personal development during which a young person must establish a personal sense of individual identity and feelings of self-worth which include an alteration of his or her body image, adaptation to more mature intellectual abilities, adjustment to society's demands for behavioral maturity, internalizing a personal value system, and preparing for adult roles" (Ingersoll, 1989, p 2). These disparate elements of the adolescent's self-image coalesce into a general cognitive, social, and physical self-image with which the young person enters adulthood. The degree to which the process results in a positive sense of self is directly antecedent to the adequacy with which the young person enters and moves through the young adult years.

Such a global definition of adolescence is not without its problems. It fails, for example, to distinguish among early, middle, and late adolescence (Table 9–1) (see Chapter 2). Early adolescence is marked by rapid acceleration in physical growth and maturation. Not surprisingly, much of the early adolescent's intellectual and emotional energies are targeted at a reassessment and restructuring of body image. At the same time, acceptance by peers is paramount; getting along and not being viewed as different are motives that dominate much of the early adolescent's social behavior. Middle adolescence is marked by nearly completed pubertal growth, the emergence of new thinking skills, an increased recognition of impending adulthood, and a desire to establish emotional and psychological distance from parents. Late adolescence is marked by preparation for adult roles, including the clarification of vocational goals and internalizing a personal value system. The role of the practitioner caring for adolescents varies with the developmental status of the adolescent patient.

The focus of this chapter is on psychological and social aspects of the normal adolescent transition. Although the physical aspects of puberty are important to an understanding of the adolescent transition, they are discussed elsewhere in this volume (see Chapters 4 and

TABLE 9–1. Psychosocial Processes and the Substages of Adolescent Development

Substage	Emotionally Related	Cognitively Related	Socially Related
Early adolescence	Adjustment to a new body image; adaptation to emerging sexuality	Concrete thinking; early moral concepts	Strong peer effect
Middle adolescence	Establishment of emotional separation from parents	Emergence of abstract thinking; expansion of verbal abilities; conventional morality; adjustment to increased school demands	Increased health risk behavior; heterosexual peer interests; early vocational plans
Late adolescence	Establishment of a personal sense of identity; further separation from parents	Development of abstract, complex thinking; emergence of postconventional morality	Increased impulse control; emerging social autonomy; establishment of vocational capability

5). Likewise, though psychosocial maladaptation during adolescence is an issue of great concern, it too is addressed elsewhere and will be omitted from this chapter. The focus is instead on normal psychological and social developmental processes of adolescence.

Historical Background

The concept of adolescence as a separate period of psychosocial maturation is a relatively recent development. Prior to the twentieth century, few writers wrote of a distinct period of life that could be labeled *adolescence,* though lamentations about the sad state of "youth" were found even in Aristotle's writings. The systematic study of adolescence, however, is traced to the writings of G. Stanley Hall (see Chapter 1). Hall pictured adolescence as a period of transition paralleling the evolutionary transition from primate (childhood) to civilized human (adulthood). Reflective of this transition, Hall believed that adolescence was thus inherently tumultuous and anxiety-ridden.

It is from Hall that we receive the concept of adolescence as a period of "storm and stress." Although the image of adolescence as intrinsically stormy and filled with stress was, and remains, common, direct evidence in support of that image has not been strong. (Chapter 8 reviews the data in support of normality during adolescence.) Studies of adolescents confirm the impression drawn from a study conducted by Offer and Offer (1975) (see Chapter 8). Evidence of generalized anxiety during adolescence is not found. Some adolescents do experience significant tumult, and their health is potentially jeopardized. However, an image of adolescents as generally stressed, tumultuous, and anxiety-ridden is misleading and potentially harmful; it impedes a vision of adolescents as capable of maintaining a positive health orientation.

Theoretical Orientations

The psychological and social study of adolescence has been dominated by three major theoretical orientations. The psychoanalytic view of adolescence is built upon Sigmund Freud's general theory of psychosexual development. Freud gave the adolescent transition little attention, perhaps because of his focus on infantile sex-

uality. It was Anna Freud who focused attention on the psychosexual character of ego development during the adolescent years. In the psychoanalytic tradition, puberty acts as the trigger for a sudden surge of strong erotic and aggressive impulses. The emergence of these impulses and unbridled erotic thoughts often cause the young adolescent to alternate between periods of unsocialized aggression and overwhelming feelings of guilt. As such, the traditional psychoanalytic conception of adolescence is one of stress and tumult in which psychological turmoil is the norm. From the view of many psychoanalytically oriented writers, the failure of adolescents to display turmoil is seen as an indicator of concern. The adolescent's response to conflicting social and emotional stresses is a dependence upon immature defense mechanisms, including regression and rigid denial. As adolescents mature toward adult functioning, and abstract reasoning develops, ego functioning and adaptation improve.

The second dominant theoretical orientation has been provided by the cognitive developmental theorists. In their view, adolescence is marked by a set of qualitative shifts in the ways in which a young person thinks about the world. Although the primary theorist associated with this theoretical orientation is Piaget, comparable qualitative shifts in thinking are documented in a broad array of domains including morality, social interactions, vocational development, and general personality development. In each domain, cognitions progress from global, undifferentiated, and largely egocentric views, to concrete, rigid, authority-oriented views, to complex, highly differentiated, abstract views. As adolescents progress toward complex conceptual systems, they display improved adaptability to a changing and uncertain environment. (Cognitive development will be considered in greater depth in a subsequent section.)

The third orientation emerges from the behaviorist tradition of Skinner and Pavlov. The social learning theorist assumes that behavior is primarily a result of learning. The primary principle underlying the behaviorist tradition is that people behave in ways that lead to reinforcement (or rewards). In drawing upon a behavioral approach, the health care professional identifies those elements of the adolescent's world that are valued by the adolescent and attempts to make those elements (reinforcers) contingent upon desired behaviors. Since much of the adolescent's behavior is tied to the social setting, it is reasonable to focus on the social reinforcers built into each setting. More recently, social learning theorists have begun to incorporate more cognitive and affective variables into their descriptions of adolescent behavior. Of particular importance is the concept of self-efficacy—that is, adolescents will work for rewards only insofar as they feel they have the potential of achieving them. If an adolescent is convinced that regardless of how much effort is put forth no reward is forthcoming, the likelihood of continuing with a behavior is greatly reduced.

COGNITIVE DEVELOPMENT

The most visible aspect of the adolescent transition is the sudden spurt in physical and genital maturation. In addition to being a period of rapid physical development (see Chapters 4 and 5), adolescence is also a period of accelerated development in intellectual and cognitive abilities. Adolescents must adjust not only to their new body image but also to their increased cognitive powers. Since adults may expect adolescents to think more like adults, school curricula increasingly contain abstract concepts regardless of the adolescents' actual abilities to understand the information. In the same fashion, the medical community may presume that adolescents are capable of understanding concepts that are, in reality, beyond an individual adolescent's comprehension.

The writer who has had the most pervasive influence on our current understanding of children's and adolescents' thinking is Piaget (Inhelder and Piaget, 1958). He proposed that thinking in children and adolescents progresses through a series of stagewise shifts that start in infancy and continue through adolescence. He described children and adolescents as interacting with their environment in an adaptive fashion. Of central relevance to this discussion is Piaget's distinction between *concrete operational thinking* and *formal operational thinking,* which he described as the central cognitive transition of adolescence. Thinking, in Piaget's view, is an adaptive process in much the same fashion as biologic processes are adaptive. When individuals are faced with problems or tasks, they draw on existing intellectual structures, which Piaget describes as schema. To the degree that these schema are effective in aiding the individual in generating a response, little adaptation is needed. However, when there is a mismatch between the environment and the schema, a state of imbalance, or in Piaget's terms, disequilibrium, exists. To reconcile the imbalance, the individual either adapts the schema to the new information, a process called accommodation, or modifies the information to meet the demands of the schema, a process called assimilation. In reality, adaptation is often a combination of the two processes in which the person interacts with the environment in a purposeful manner.

Critical to Piaget's model, however, is a recognition of qualitative shifts in the kinds of thought processes individuals are capable of as they mature. The infant's thinking is restricted to schema that are composed of sensory and kinesthetic images. During the preschool years, children's thinking expands, but their adaptation is restricted by their inability to recognize the stability of "operations" over different conditions. However, as children enter the school-aged years, they develop an ability to maintain stability of, or conserve, schema across conditions. Cognitions are still limited because schema are possible only for events or phenomena that have a concrete referent. The ability to understand abstract concepts, or to consider what might happen if reality were to be altered, is outside the realm of possibility for the concrete operational thinker.

Beginning in middle adolescence, many young people begin to expand their range of concepts to include abstract and hypothetico-deductive, formal operational thinking. When caring for adolescents at this stage, it is common to hear them talk about abstractions as if the ideas were new discoveries. The power of their expanded thinking ability is like a new toy. They are attracted to new, and idealistic, abstractions. The ability to handle formal thought is not, however, fully developed. Although young people may operate well in one area of thought, they may still operate as concrete operational thinkers in other areas of thought. For example, time is a concept of great importance to adults. Early adolescents, in contrast, have a very limited concept of time as an abstraction. Telling young people that today's behavior may affect their health 5, 10, or 20 years from now has little meaning to them. Even as young people start to develop formal thought, the functional operation of their abstract concepts may have only limited utility.

Several misconceptions exist about adolescence and formal operational thinking. The first, and perhaps most problematic, misconception is that *all* adolescents achieve formal operational thought. It is not uncommon to read that "adolescence is a period of formal operational thought" as if the two are equal. Cognitive stages are not uniformly linked to any age group, nor does an individual always respond on one cognitive level. A stage model implies that one stage is qualitatively different and dependent upon completing the previous stage. A stage model does not, however, imply that an individual will not show attributes of multiple stages, depending on the context. Neither is formal thinking linked to some magical age or level of physical maturity. Many adolescents (and adults) never achieve formal thought. It is a safe assumption that few middle or early adolescents are routinely operating on a formal operational level. One should even be cautious about inferring formal thought among college-aged students, especially in the context of health care.

Irrespective of the generality and validity of the specific stages proposed by Piaget, the general progression in thinking from simple to complex, from concrete to abstract, and from egocentric to decentered is generally accepted. Further, the adolescent's level of cognitive maturity affects the ways in which the individual understands one's world and makes decisions. In the context of health-related behaviors, the adolescent's general cognitive social maturity and specific health-related concepts moderate the willingness and ability to respond to normal health demands. Both chronically ill and normal adolescents will ultimately understand their health status and the demands placed on them by health care professionals in light of their level of cognitive maturity (see Chapter 30).

Early researchers found that children's initial concepts of illness and health were magical and simplistic. Bibace and Walsh (1979) describe a progression in children's concepts of illness paralleling Piaget's stages of cognitive growth. Early health concepts are based on simple, sometimes magical, causation: "People get sick because they are bad"; "When you get well, 'sickness' goes someplace else." During childhood, concepts of health and illness are dominated by notions of contagion: "People get sick because they 'catch' the illness from someone else or from something." Other causes of illness are harder to conceive. During early adolescence, young people are increasingly able to understand the role of environmental causes and the concept of bacterial or viral infections. Because of this more complex understanding, they are increasingly able to understand the role of avoidance behaviors in preserving health. This understanding is, however, rigid and categorical. As adolescents approach later adolescence and young adulthood, they are increasingly able to conceive of multiple causes for illness and wellness and the role that personal behavior has in promotion of or endangerment of health. A strong relationship exists between the level of cognitive social development and the tendency to engage in behaviors that risk health. Young people at more advanced levels of cognitive maturity, regardless of age, are less likely to engage in behaviors that endanger health (Ingersoll and Orr, 1989).

Although there is little disagreement that there is a qualitative change in the thinking patterns of adolescents as they shift from childhood to adulthood, there is not yet consensus regarding the precise character of the transition or transitions. Clearly, Piaget's concept of formal operational thinking has played a central role in furthering our understanding of adolescent thinking. In caring for adolescents, however, one should keep in mind that many of the concepts underlying a health care model are intrinsically abstract.

At the same time that adolescents are adapting to their newly found cognitive powers, they must also develop a verbal repertoire to manage these new intellectual powers. Hence, the ability to relate their concerns to, and to understand the messages offered by, the physician are impeded by their lack of an adequate vocabulary. Practitioners must be willing to adapt health care messages to the cognitive characteristics of the individual adolescent. Efforts should be made to probe the level of understanding, since there is a high likelihood of initial miscommunication.

AFFECTIVE DEVELOPMENT

Of the neo-Freudian writers, few have had as profound an influence on contemporary psychology of adolescence as Erik Erikson. Erikson (1968) proposed that the fundamental psychosexual struggle defined by Freud was instead a series of psychosocial struggles. Adolescence is marked by a consolidation of an individual's identity. The social and psychological dynamics of the adolescent transition are dominated by the individual's attempts to establish a new sense of self. The hallmark of adolescent transition is a period of *identity formation.*

During middle to late adolescence, a young person may become disaffected and have an inadequate sense of personal identity. Identity formation occurs as the adolescent consolidates elements of one's childhood identity with the emerging values and goals that form the basis of one's adult identity.

A new ego identity is established when the individual has experienced a consolidation of values and vocational goals with which to enter the adult years. It is composed partly of elements of the adolescent's childhood identity, largely defined by the parents' identity, and partly of new elements that differentiate the adolescent from the parents. It represents the adolescent's personal answer to the questions "Who am I?" and "What does it mean to be me?" The actual process of establishing a personal identity may be accompanied by a period of intense emotional upheaval that Erikson defines as the *identity crisis.*

Ego identity occurs concurrently with *identity diffusion,* in which either no effort has been made to consolidate a personal identity or the effort has been disrupted and the individual has an inadequate personal identity with which to enter the adult years. Erikson's model presumes that the identity formation process of adolescence is contained within a context of a broader lifelong pattern of reconciling psychosocial developmental conflicts. The adequacy with which adolescents reconcile the identity conflict is a function of the adequacy with which they reconciled earlier psychosocial conflicts. Likewise, the adequacy with which they reconcile the psychosocial conflicts of adulthood is directly related to the adequacy of their resolution of the identity conflict of adolescence.

Attempts to document the existence of ego identity and identity diffusion have indicated that the process of identity formation may be facilitated or disrupted by internal traits or social contexts that augment or impede the normal developmental process (Marcia, 1980). Parents or authorities who disallow freedom to explore alternative roles and alternative value systems risk closing off the exploratory process. In some instances, the adolescent is presented an implied or explicit expectation of an adult role. When adolescents accept an intact identity defined by parents, they experience *identity foreclosure.* The result may be an externally defined and not well-internalized identity. Adolescents may elect to postpone temporarily the identity formation process and enter a period of *identity moratorium;* they put the process of identity formation "on hold" while exploring identity options. In caring for adolescents at this stage, the professional's role becomes one of helping the adolescent explore and recognize role and value choices.

The development of a new sense of self—a new identity—may be the central developmental task of adolescence. The self-concept is the composite of an individual's perceptions about his or her physical, social, intellectual, educational, and psychological characteristics. Like other elements of the adolescent's cognitive-social network, self-concept becomes increasingly complex and differentiated as one matures. Self-esteem is distinguished from self-concept as the valuation applied to the self-concept; the self-concept is an objective statement of personal traits, whereas self-esteem is the personal value attributed to those traits. Such a distinction may, however, be artificial, since the choices of labels for one's self-attribution are value-laden.

As central as the constructs of self-concept and self-esteem are to the adolescent transition, at the same time they are elusive targets of study. Current psychometric measures of the adolescent self-image are composites of multiple self-views. The self-image contains elements of a physical, social, sexual, and familial self, along with a sense of adequacy in coping with stress and mastery of one's external world. Rosenberg (1965) provides an important and useful distinction between one's *extant self* and one's *desired self.* The extant self is an adolescent's current view of himself or herself; it is an objective and subjective statement of how the individual describes himself or herself. The desired self, conversely, is a subjective statement of how the individual would like to be seen. There is a sense that as the discrepancy between the two increases, self-esteem, the net value attributed to one's self-concept, would be lowered. However, perfect correspondence between the two might equally reflect low self-esteem, since it would reflect limited goals for personal growth, an indicator of positive self-esteem. Beyond the images an adolescent holds defining the desired self, there are also a set of images of self the adolescent possesses that define what one does not want to become.

Despite the intrinsic appeal of the constructs of self-concept and self-esteem, their stability in predicting health outcomes has been less forthcoming. At best, statistical relationships, when controlled for intelligence or depression, are seemingly marginal. In part, the lack of stable statistical results may be a function of the lack of psychometric stability of earlier measures or the frequent dependence on global measures of self-esteem. Alternatively, the choice of physiologic outcomes as dependent measures may present problems. Self-esteem may be related more to quality of life issues. Hence, if adolescents perceive a medical regimen as causing them to be isolated from their peers, their personal sense of self-worth may be jeopardized. When self-esteem suffers, adolescents may be more likely to conform to peer demands for behaviors that present a health risk. Self-esteem and these risky behaviors are related. In an earlier study, we documented an association between early coital status and self-esteem that was mediated by the adolescent's gender. Virgin or nonvirgin status among young adolescents was not related to self-esteem among boys, but nonvirgin girls had diminished self-esteem. The relationship of self-esteem to health-related behavior may be a function of the specific behavior and the social-psychological value it holds for individuals and groups of individuals.

Practitioners may be in a position to nurture adolescents' feelings of self-acceptance, particularly, but not exclusively, as it relates to the physical self-image and its acceptability. At a time of maximum divergence in physical growth and development, adolescents desire uniformity; they do not want to be seen as different. As much as anything, listening to adolescents express their fears and concerns and helping them accept their individuality may be as important as providing a "cure" for their current complaint.

SOCIAL DEVELOPMENT

As adolescents move from their secure, dependent roles as children to less secure, but independent roles as adults, they are likewise expected to develop social maturity. Social maturity includes increased autonomy from parents and adult authority, altered interpersonal and heterosexual relations, and behavioral maturity. The need to develop behavioral maturity is reflected by the observation that the label *adolescent,* when applied to behavior, implies a degree of social immaturity and impulsiveness. Adult independence carries with it social expectations for behavioral maturity.

Social maturity in adolescents develops in patterns akin to their cognitive and emotional maturity. Their concepts of the nature and roles of interpersonal relationships are themselves linked to levels of cognitive development. Linked to their emerging cognitive maturity, however, is something of an intellectual trap. During early cognitive development, children presume that everyone sees objects the same as they do; their perceptions are egocentric. As children mature, they are increasingly capable of decentering their view, that is, they are able to conceive of a view of an object from another perspective. This decentering, however, is limited to concrete objects.

Adolescents are prone to another form of egocentricity. As they develop abstract thought, they recognize that not only do they think but also others think. The problem is that adolescents are likely to presume that since they hold a given thought, everyone else shares the same point of view. They are unable to distinguish their thoughts from those of others (Elkind, 1967). Hence, if an adolescent sees herself or himself as clumsy, she or he will presume everybody is watching every move to confirm that view. This presumption that everyone else is inordinately concerned with the adolescent's personal well-being gives rise to the "invisible audience" that is constantly attentive to the adolescent's actions. At the same time, the adolescent is likely to view himself or herself as unique. As a result, a "personal fable" evolves in which adolescents see themselves as invulnerable to harm. This sense of invulnerability contributes to adolescents' willingness to engage in high-risk activities, including failure to use contraceptives, experimenting with drugs, and reckless automobile driving (see Chapters 26, 73, and 111).

Family Issues (see Chapter 23)

A primary developmental task of the adolescent transition is the establishment of emotional and psychological independence from one's parents. As a child, one is completely dependent upon adults to provide basic necessities and to make decisions for one's personal welfare. As adolescents move toward adulthood, they are expected to assume increased personal responsibility for their well-being. It is particularly in the adolescent's struggle to assert independence that tensions may arise between the adolescent and the family. However, the degree to which the adolescent's progress toward adult autonomy is seriously stressful and stormy versus only temporarily discomforting is a function of the family dynamics that precede and continue through adolescence.

Some writers have suggested that adolescents' values are inherently discontinuous with those of their parents, and the result is a "generation gap." Research evidence suggests that the "gap" has been seriously overstated. Instead, conflict between parents and adolescents, which is usually normal, seems to be related to routine, daily activities in which the adolescent challenges the authority of the parent. Conflicts over basic value structures are less common. Conversely, continuous and excessive family conflict and disruption should not be dismissed lightly. Such conflict may be reflective of more general family dysfunction.

Routine challenges to parental authority are part of the adolescent's struggle to assert individuality and independence. Although the adolescent's challenges to parental authority are often a source of frustration to beleaguered parents, the move toward emotional and psychological autonomy is routinely presumed to be prerequisite to healthy progress toward independent adult functioning and psychological maturity. There are, however, reasons to caution against accelerated demands for autonomy: Advanced social demands made upon an adolescent who is not psychologically mature enough to handle the task may result in damaged self-esteem, depression, and "acting out." Early entry into the job market, often seen as indicative of emerging adult independence, has not been shown to be a necessarily positive process. Those who work full-time, or nearly full-time, while still attending high school have been shown to have higher rates of cigarette smoking, alcohol use, and drug use than do those who do not work or work less than 20 hours/week.

The family environment has clear and pervasive effects on adolescent self-esteem and psychosocial adjustment. Parental warmth and support in the context of clearly defined family expectations is linked with positive self-esteem and positive social adjustment, whereas harsh, rejecting parenting is associated with the converse. For example, adolescents with insulin-dependent diabetes mellitus who have cohesive, supportive, flexible families are more likely to comply with a self-care regimen than are adolescents from disruptive, nonsupportive families. Further, the degree to which the family has positive or negative perceptions of the health care system will affect the level of compliance by the adolescent.

Contemporary professionals are increasingly likely to care for young people living in a variety of alternative family settings (see Chapter 2). In the period from 1960 to 1985 there was a decline in the percent of children living in two-parent families from 87% to 75%. In the same time period, the percent of children living in single female households increased from 8% to 20%. Children and adolescents are increasingly apt to experience at least one family dissolution during their growing years. It is estimated that a child born this year will have a 50% chance of experiencing a family divorce by age 16 years and a 60% chance of living at least one year in a single parent home.

The degree to which disruption of the traditional family structure results in disruption of the adolescent's psychosocial development is unclear. In some studies, divorce is associated with impaired self-concept, increased depression, and an increase in behaviors that are a risk to health (see Chapter 115). In other studies, the relationship is less firm; divorce appears most disruptive when the family environment before the divorce was marked by hostility and conflict. Marital hostility, either in intact or separated families, is a pervasively negative factor in adolescent psychosocial development. Clearly, however, divorce may constitute a major disturbance in normal psychosocial development of adolescents, requiring referral for counseling.

Peer Influences

During early and middle adolescence, in particular, the need to be accepted by one's peer group dominates social interactions. The worst fear of young adolescents is to be excluded from the crowd. Research evidence indicates the need to conform to peers increases dramatically in early adolescence and starts to decrease by late adolescence. It is because of the powerful influence of peers on adolescent behavior that peer influence is routinely described as a causal contributor to substance abuse, early sexual experimentation, discontinuance of schooling, and engaging in delinquent behavior. As a result, adults may assume peer influences are unilaterally negative.

Research studies demonstrate that the focus of peer influence on adolescents is not uniform across all groups, and the influences on adolescent misconduct may be more unclear than previously thought. In reality, peer influence can produce a positive, socializing effect. In their attempts to establish autonomy from parents, adolescents turn to their peers for support. Peer groups offer a context within which the young person can experiment with alternative concepts of one's self, learn social skills, and clarify value systems. Just as peers can exert pressure to engage in health-jeopardizing behaviors, peers can similarly exert pressures that promote positive health behaviors.

The development of social competence during adolescence is a strong indicator of adequacy of adult psychosocial adjustment. Social competence is dependent on the individual's ability to adequately interpret environmental cues and to respond appropriately. Socially adept children and adolescents are able accurately to interpret critical cues in a social setting and are not distracted by misleading or irrelevant cues. Barring their own ability to recognize critical cues, they are likely to identify someone else who is apt to be socially adept and to follow that person's lead. Adolescents lacking in social competence are unable to make such distinctions. They are either unable to identify critical cues or are unable to respond in behaviorally appropriate fashion.

Moral Development

As young people approach their adult years, they need to develop a personal value system. This value system includes not only a template of rights and wrongs but also decision-making strategies on how one responds to ambiguous settings.

Social learning theorists' approach to the development of moral behavior during the adolescent years is to focus on the reward structures that dictate which behaviors are socially approved and which are socially disapproved. Moral development, in this view, follows the same course as other behavior development. Moral values are defined by moral behavior: One behaves in ways that are expected to lead to positive outcomes or to avoid or escape negative outcomes.

Beyond the direct use of reward structures to shape moral behavior, social learning theorists presume that considerable shaping of moral behavior occurs through modeling. Adolescents learn socially approved behaviors by observing and imitating others whom they presume to be socially competent. If the observed model is seen as socially competent and receives social reinforcement for a given behavior, the observer is likely to copy and repeat that behavior. When positive models are lacking and the primary source of information about socially acceptable behavior is the peer group or media, there is a heightened risk of negative behavior being modeled.

The primary alternative view of moral development was derived from the cognitive developmental model of Piaget. Piaget's initial formulation of a cognitive theory of moral development presumed that moral thinking progressed from other-oriented moral judgments (heteronomous morality) to self-oriented moral judgments (autonomous morality). Heteronomous moral judgments were presumed to correspond to concrete operational thinking. Heteronomous moral schema are defined by those in authority and are rigid. As adolescents develop formal reasoning and the ability to consider abstractions and multiple perspectives, autonomous, internally defined moral structures follow. Moral concepts become more general and adaptive.

Although Piaget's model recognizes the progressive character of moral thinking, it fails to discriminate adequately among the qualitative changes in moral thinking that are observed as adolescents mature. Piaget's theory of moral development has been supplanted by the work of Kohlberg (1981). Kohlberg presented moral dilemmas to children and adolescents in a clinical interview. Once a subject responded to the moral dilemma, Kohlberg probed the limits of the moral decision. Kohlberg concluded that the kinds of moral decisions made by children and adolescents follow a natural progression through three broad stages and within the broad stages, substages.

Early moral thinking, described as *preconventional morality,* results in self-centered, fundamentally hedonic moral decisions. At first, moral decisions are based on the individual's desire to avoid punishment (Level 1). In this type of moral thinking, one does not skip school—not because of any moral commitment to schooling but because "getting caught" will result in unpleasant results. Note, however, if there is little or no chance of getting caught, the reason for not engaging in an undesirable behavior is eliminated. Further, if the positive rewards (fun, peer approval) outweigh the neg-

ative sanctions, the constraints of this morality are limited. (Since they have little in the way of time perspective, warning that noncompliance to a medical regimen will result in unpleasant effects 15 years later has little meaning.) Subsequently, moral decisions are based on gaining some material outcome (Level 2); morality is defined by the highest bidder. Level 2 moral thinking can be thought of as "What's in it for me?" morality. The Level 2 adolescent's motivation for behaving morally is the satisfaction of personal, social, or physical needs. Reciprocity and "fairness" dominate decisions. "Fairness" in this sense implies that everyone is treated equally; one acts morally insofar as the recipient acts morally in return.

During early adolescence, there is a change in moral thinking to *conventional morality.* Conventional morality is tied to basic moral standards of society. Initially, motivation to act in a moral fashion is dominated by the adolescent's desire to be seen as a good or nice person (Level 3). Moral values are arbitrary and rigid; behavior (and individuals) are either good or bad, right or wrong. Authority for the Level 3 thinker is, however, a fickle master. The authority of parents and adults may be in conflict with the authority of peers. The closer the authority, the more the influence. In the later conventional morality (Level 4), the adolescent recognizes the role of rules and values in the preservation of social order. Moral decisions are made not solely because one wants to be seen as a good person but because the person has begun to identify with and internalize the values of the society within which he or she lives.

During later adolescence and young adulthood, moral thinking may progress to *postconventional morality.* As adolescents mature in their levels of cognitive thought, they are more capable of recognizing ambiguities and complex interrelationships. In the same fashion, their moral concepts become increasingly complex. At Level 5, moral decisions are based on the individuals' understanding of the standards of society as well as on their understanding of the rights of the individual. The concept of extenuating circumstances, alien to adolescents at earlier levels, now becomes important. As formal thinking progresses, adolescents are very often intrigued by issues of moral relativity. In early formulations of his theory of moral development, Kohlberg suggested that the highest level of moral development (Level 6) was seen only in a few who recognized universal ethical standards that sometimes transcended standard morality. Such a transcendent morality may, however, be achieved in later adulthood.

In Kohlberg's later research, it became clear that the distinctiveness of the higher stages of moral thought was not as clear as originally thought. As a result, he began to speculate about transitional substages and a "soft" high level of moral cognition.

Kohlberg's model of moral development has not been without its critics, however. In particular, the model has been criticized as being biased against females. Gilligan (1982) argues that males are more likely to be socialized to be independent (separated), whereas females are socialized to be interdependent (connected). Kohlberg's scales for rating moral judgments are slanted toward the male dimension. As an overall result, females score lower on measures of moral development.

Although future research is likely to refine Kohlberg's model with clearer definitions of stages of moral cognition and its assessment, the key concepts will persist—that is, the course of moral cognitive development progresses from a state of relatively simple, hedonic moral structures to concrete, rigid moral structures to complex, highly integrated and differentiated moral structures. As practitioners working with adolescents who look like adults, it is tempting to presume that they hold moral structures akin to those of adults. In fact, their moral structures may be incompatible with the value messages that adults present. Value-laden messages laced with statements about the "greater good of the family" presented to an adolescent operating at a preconventional level of morality are unlikely to be effective.

Vocational Development

If the establishment of psychological independence from parents represents a primary developmental task of adolescence, a primary reflection of that independence is the adolescent's entry into the job market. Career choice is thus a central element in the adolescent's development of a sense of identity.

Like other aspects of the adolescent's cognitive social development, the structure of vocational choice and vocational self-image change as the adolescent matures. Early vocational choices are often based in fantasy and linked to glamorous and highly visible occupations. Early choices are often made with no regard to sociocultural realities that might limit entry into those roles; ability and opportunity are irrelevant. During the adolescent years, tentative vocational choices are made and modified with some regularity. These shifts in vocational goals are frequently accompanied by indecision and uncertainty. Although some element of vocational uncertainty is normal and is expected, excessive anxieties about vocational roles may be reflective of a broader range of problems in psychological adjustment.

BIBLIOGRAPHY

Bibace R, Walsh ME: Developmental stages in children's conceptions of illness. In Stone GC, Cohen F, Adler NE (eds): Health Psychology. San Francisco, Jossey-Bass, 1979, pp 285–301.

Elkind D: Egocentrism in adolescence. Child Dev 38:1025, 1967.

Erikson EH: Identity, Youth and Crisis. New York, WW Norton, 1968.

Gilligan C: In a Different Voice: Psychological Theory and Women's Development. Cambrige, MA, Harvard University Press, 1982.

Ingersoll GM: Adolescence, 2nd ed. Englewood Cliffs, NJ, Prentice-Hall, 1989, p 2.

Ingersoll GM, Orr DP: Behavioral and emotional risk in early adolescents. J Early Adolesc 9:396, 1989.

Inhelder B, Piaget J: The Growth of Logical Thinking from Childhood to Adolescence. New York, Basic Books, 1958.

Kohlberg L: Essays on Moral Development: The Philosophy of Moral Development. New York, Harper & Row, 1981.

Marcia J: Identity in adolescence. In Adelson J (ed): Handbook of Adolescent Psychology. New York, John Wiley & Sons, 1980, pp 159–187.

Offer D, Offer J: From Teenage to Young Manhood. New York, Basic Books, 1975.

Rosenberg M: Society and the Adolescent Self-Image. Princeton, NJ, Princeton University Press, 1965.

CHAPTER 10

Cognitive Neuroscience and Adolescent Development

JOHN M. WATKINS and MARIAN E. WILLIAMS

The linking of cognitive psychology and developmental neuroscience has produced something of a revolution in our thinking about behavioral development. Theoretical and methodologic advances in the two disciplines have now made possible the discovery of meaningful links between brain development and changes in cognition. The increasing understanding of developmental neurobiology has placed important constraints on cognitive developmental theories, leading to more sophisticated and sometimes surprising new formulations. Similarly, theories of the mechanisms of cognitive development have provided a more meaningful framework for understanding environmental and developmental influences on brain organization. Although it was always assumed that brain development must somehow be related to cognitive development, early theorists focused on very general shifts in cognition, such as improvements in intelligence test performance, as they related to very general maturational processes in the brain, such as progressive myelination. It is only recently that we have been able to address the more profound issue of which particular developmental changes in the brain relate to which specific emerging cognitive capacities in children and adolescents.

CORTICAL CIRCUITRY AND COGNITIVE DEVELOPMENT DURING ADOLESCENCE

Shortly after birth, the growth of neurons and axons in the brain stops. By about 3 months of age, selective cell death and axonal elimination also appear to be complete. Thus, large neuroanatomic variations appear to be determined very early in life and are unlikely to be modified by later experience. However, despite the relatively invariant structure provided by neuronal and axonal anatomy, changes in the number and density of synapses, the structures across which nerve cells communicate, extend through adolescence and into adulthood. Greenough and colleagues (1987) have noted that in the much smaller brain of the rat, as many as a quarter of a million of these connections between nerve cells are formed each second during the first postnatal month. In addition, dendritic branching and segregation of neural input extend throughout the period of infancy, and myelination progresses gradually in the tertiary frontal, parietal, and temporal cortices well into adolescence (Yakovlev and Lecours, 1967). Finally, levels of regional cerebral glucose metabolism vary dramatically throughout childhood and into adolescence, possibly in association with changes in synaptic density (Chugani et al, 1987).

The number and density of synapses in various regions of the brain follow a developmental course that can be understood broadly as involving early overproduction during infancy, followed by selective pruning of synaptic terminals during later childhood and adolescence. In one small area of the frontal lobes—the third layer of the middle frontal gyrus—the average number of synapses grows from approximately 10,000 at birth to 100,000 by 1 year of age. Increases in synaptic density in humans begin at 8 months of age, peak at about 2 years of age, then level off and fall until adult levels are approximated at about age 7 years (Huttenlocker, 1979). Further, less dramatic modifications in synaptic architecture through elimination of excess synapses proceed throughout adolescence and into young adulthood.

Rakic and colleagues (1986) have provided evidence that developmental changes in synaptic density occur concurrently across all areas of the cortex in the infant rhesus monkey, rather than differing by anatomic location, until a final constant adult density of 15 to 20/100 μ^2 is achieved. However, adult synaptic density is reached in subcortical structures well before it is attained in the cortex. These findings indicate that different neural systems at the level of the cortex (e.g., visual, motor) develop concurrently, but that hierarchic development occurs within discrete neural systems.

The processes of synaptogenesis and synaptic pruning offer new perspectives on classic issues in cognitive development and provide a basis for translating experience during development into stable changes in cortical circuitry. Two major theories have been offered to account for the influence of synaptogenesis on cognitive development: (1) the brain growth hypothesis and (2) the theory of experience-expectant versus experience-dependent processes.

The Brain Growth Hypothesis

Goldman-Rakic (1987) has hypothesized that the cardinal cognitive functions of each cortical area emerge in some elementary form simultaneously early in ontogeny, coinciding with shifts in levels of synaptic density. This view emphasizes the integrated nature of behavior and the fact that cognitive functions are not carried out by one part of the brain in isolation. The brain growth hypothesis (Epstein, 1974; Fischer, 1987), building partly on the work of Goldman-Rakic (1987), postulates that spurts in brain growth occur concurrently with the emergence of each developmental level. Evidence for this hypothesis comes from the observation that changes in the brain, including synaptogenesis, electroencephalographic patterns, and metabolic function, appear to follow patterns of peaks and valleys during early development. These spurts in brain growth closely match the emergence of major discontinuities in behavior. Fischer describes four periods of rapid cognitive change after infancy: at approximately 4 years, 6 to 7 years, 10 to 12 years, and 14 to 16 years of age. Fischer hypothesizes that unlike the pattern in infancy, cognitive changes at later ages may emerge from formation of isolated groups of new synapses in limited cortical regions, coupled with regional pruning.

Experience-Expectant and Experience-Dependent Processes

Greenough and colleagues (1987) have proposed that experience influences the developing brain through two major mechanisms, experience-expectant and experience-dependent processes, each based upon the type of information stored in the brain and the neural mechanisms mediating storage. Experience-expectant processes are based on overproduction and pruning of synapses, as in Goldman-Rakic's theory, but Greenough suggests that which synapses are pruned during development depends upon experience. Experience-expectant processes are confined to early development and refer to storage of information that is ubiquitous in the environment and commonly experienced by all species members, such as the elements of pattern perception. Early sensory experience therefore determines which synaptic connections between nerve cells are selectively eliminated. The information stored in experience-expectant processes is consolidated early in life and remains relatively invariant across individuals. From an evolutionary viewpoint, experience-expectant processes allow rapid acquisition of information in normal environments but also offer some flexibility in adverse environments.

Experience-dependent processes, in contrast, occur throughout life and provide the neural substrate for learning. Experience-dependent processes refer to storage of environmental information that is unique to the individual, such as vocabulary in a particular language or mathematics. Greenough has provided evidence that experience-dependent processes involve formation of new synapses in specific areas of the brain in response to specific environmental events. Synapse formation in experience-dependent processes can occur as early as 10 to 15 minutes after a new experience and appears to be correlated with long-term potentiation in associated neurons and the presence of polyribosomal aggregates in the synaptic spines (Greenough et al, 1987).

The separation of experience-expectant and experience-dependent processes provides a basis for examining some fundamental differences between cognitive development during infancy and early childhood and development during adolescence and young adulthood. Experience-expectant processes occurring during early development appear to emerge from genetically regulated overproduction of synapses, followed by selective elimination of unused synapses until a functional subset remains. Experience-dependent synapse formation in later development, including adolescence, differs from early development in that it is triggered by experience and is localized to specific brain regions involved in specific information processes. Experience-expectant and experience-dependent processes are similar in that synapses may be initially formed on a relatively unpatterned basis, with neural activity arising from a specific experience, determining which subset of synapses is preserved.

Studies of synaptic density have implications for the understanding of developmental disorders of cognition. Abnormally high or low levels of synaptic density have been associated with several forms of mental retardation. About 10 to 20 synapses/100 μ^2 is considered to be biologically optimal for information processing. Higher values have been found histologically in patients with Down syndrome (see Chapter 31), and lower values have been found in other forms of mental retardation.

Positron Emission Tomography Studies

Studies using positron emission tomography (PET) have shown that rates of cortical glucose metabolism closely parallel the changes in levels of synapse formation and elimination previously described. PET employs tracer kinetic measures of metabolites labeled with positron-emitting isotopes and provides an index of regional brain energy utilization. Developmental changes in brain metabolism have been examined in two ways by researchers: (1) comparison of patterns of relative metabolic rates across brain regions at different ages and (2) examination of overall absolute values of glucose metabolism at different ages. Shifts in regional patterns of metabolism have been examined by comparing rates across specified regions of interest. Chugani and colleagues (1987) have found that there are dramatic shifts in regional metabolic rates from the period just after birth through the first year of life. These regional shifts are illustrated in Figure 10–1. In the neonate, relatively high metabolic rates are found in the sensorimotor cortex, thalamus, cerebellar vermis, and brainstem. Metabolic rates increase in the primary sensory cortex, basal ganglia, and cerebellar cortex during the second and third months of life. This shift is followed by increases in lateral prefrontal regions of the cortex at 6 months and in the medial frontal cortex and the dorsilateral occipital cortex after 8 months of age. After 1 year of age, the regional pattern appears to stabilize and remains constant through adolescence and into adulthood. In contrast with these early shifts in regional

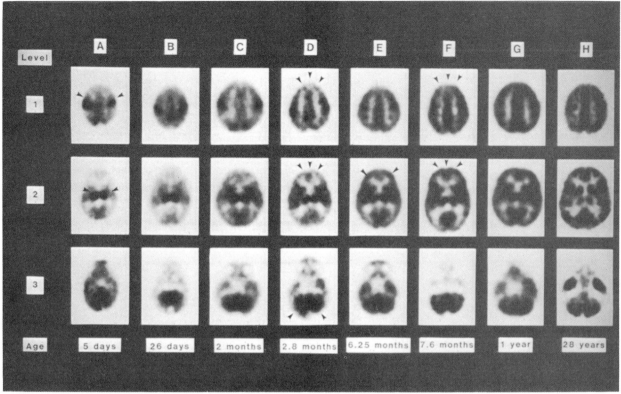

Figure 10–1. 2-Deoxy-2(^{18}F)-fluoro-D-glucose (FDG)-positron emission tomography (PET) images illustrating developmental changes in local cerebral metabolic rates for glucose (lCMRGlc) in the normal human infant with increasing age, as compared to lCMRGlc of the adult (image sizes not on same scale). Level 1 is a superior section, at the level of the cingulate gyrus. Level 2 is more inferior, at the level of caudate, putamen, and thalamus. Level 3 is an inferior section of the brain, at the level of cerebellum and inferior portion of the temporal lobes. Gray scale is proportional to lCMRGlc, with black being highest. Images from all subjects are not shown on the same absolute gray scale of lCMRGlc; instead, images of each subject are shown with the full gray scale to maximize gray scale display of lCMRGlc at each age. In each image, the anterior portion of the brain is at the top of the image and the left side of the brain is at the left of the image. *A,* In the 5-day-old, lCMRGlc is highest in sensorimotor cortex, thalamus, cerebellar vermis *(arrows),* and brainstem *(not shown). B to D,* lCMRGlc gradually increases in parietal, temporal, and calcarine cortices; basal ganglia; and cerebellar cortex *(arrows),* particularly during the second and third months. *E,* In the frontal cortex, lCMRGlc increases first in the lateral prefrontal regions by approximately 6 months. *F,* By approximately 8 months, lCMRGlc also increases in the medial aspects of the frontal cortex *(arrows),* as well as the dorsolateral occipital cortex. *G,* By 1 year, the lCMRGlc pattern resembles that of adults *(H).* (From Chugani HT, Phelps ME, Mazziotta JC: Positron emission tomography study of human brain functional development. Ann Neurol 22[4]:487–497, 1987.)

metabolic patterns during infancy, overall absolute values of brain glucose metabolism remain high and continue to change well into adolescence. Figure 10–2 shows absolute values of local cerebral metabolic rates for glucose in 29 infants and children compared with 7 adult subjects for several areas of the cortex. Similar curves were found for other cortical and subcortical structures.

Chugani and co-workers (1987) theorize that the high density of synapses and dendritic processes found by Rakic and others in the developing brain accounts for the relatively higher overall energy requirements they found in child and adolescent brains. As synaptic and dendritic density decreases steadily from age 7 years through adolescence, the corresponding energy requirements decrease. Consistent with the animal model data from Rakic and Goldman-Rakic, developmental shifts in absolute values of metabolism appear to covary across discrete brain regions, even though some regional differences may be observed early in life.

Chugani and colleagues propose several correlations between metabolic shifts within neuroanatomic structures and the emergence of behavioral functions associated with those structures. In newborns, behavior

appears to be dominated by subcortical brain structures, with the presence of intrinsic brainstem reflexes (such as Moro, root, and grasp reflexes) coinciding with high levels of subcortical metabolic activity. Cortical metabolism during this period appears to be highest in primary sensory and motor areas. As infants develop visuospatial and visuosensorimotor integration at 3 to 6 months of age, increases in parietal, primary visual, and cerebellar cortices can be observed. Later, as the older infant engages in more complex interactions, and as the ability to inhibit response on tasks such as the delayed response task emerges, increasing energy requirements begin to emerge in the prefrontal cortex. Using animal models, Chugani and colleagues found a "second" metabolic peak during adolescence, which corresponds to acquisition of complex mating and sexual behaviors. In general, these studies provide evidence that a developmental increase in metabolic rate for a particular neuroanatomic structure corresponds to the time at which that structure begins to contribute to the emerging behavioral repertoire of the individual.

Although the theories outlined earlier provide new ways of linking cognitive development and neural sub-

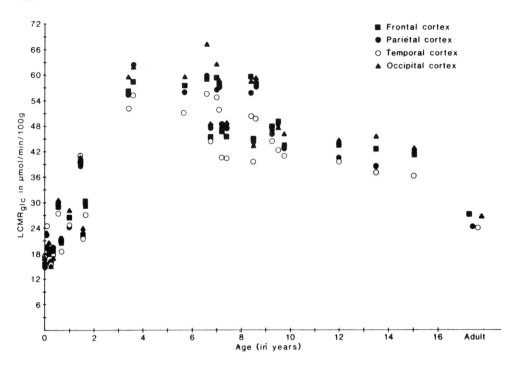

Figure 10–2. Absolute values of local cerebral metabolic rates for glucose (lCMRGlc) for selected brain regions plotted as a function of age for 29 infants and children and corresponding adult values. In infants and children, points represent individual values of lCMRGlc; in adults, points are mean values from seven subjects. (From Chugani HT, Phelps ME, Mazziotta JC: Positron emission tomography study of human brain functional development. Ann Neurol 22[4]487–497, 1987.)

strates, they focus primarily on the types of sensory and motor skills that emerge during early development (Bertenthal and Campos, 1987). Tasks that are unique to adolescence, particularly tasks pertaining to psychosexual development and conceptual thinking (see Chapter 9), cannot be fully understood by reference to synaptogenesis and pruning or even alterations in overall rates of metabolism. The mechanisms underlying much of adolescent cognitive development must necessarily include additional layers of complexity involving both the neurobiologic (e.g., neuroendocrine; see Chapter 4) and cognitive (e.g., formal operational thinking; see Chapter 9).

Neuroendocrine Influences

Studies of neuroendocrine influences on adolescent cognitive development have only begun to emerge within the past decade and have generally taken one of two approaches: (1) studies of the effect of pubertal timing on cognitive development and (2) studies of adolescents with specific endocrine disorders. Longitudinal studies of normal adolescents that correlate hormonal assays with psychological measures have generally focused on behavioral and affective variables and have not been as concerned with measures of information processing (see Chapter 13).

Several studies by Waber and colleagues have reported a divergence in verbal and spatial abilities as a function of pubertal timing, with boys and girls who mature early scoring better on verbal than on spatial tasks and late maturers scoring better on spatial than on verbal tasks (Waber et al, 1985). Waber has argued that the rate of maturation may affect patterns of hemispheric specialization for language and spatial skills. These studies remain controversial, particularly because of the confounding influences of maturational rate with

maturational status, and it is important to note that cognitive effects of pubertal timing have not been found to hold up when subjects were later examined as adults.

An illustration of the complex interaction of hormones, brain, and adolescent development is seen in growth hormone deficiency (see Chapter 56). Children with growth hormone deficiency have long been observed to be at risk for poor social adjustment during adolescence. This has been attributed to a variety of factors, including the delayed onset of puberty associated with some types of growth delay. Recent research, however, has shown this social morbidity to reflect a complex interaction of cognitive and social factors. There is increasing evidence of an association between growth hormone deficiency and information processing deficits (McCauley et al, 1987). These information-processing deficits have, in turn, become related to difficulty in evaluating nonverbal gestures and other subtle social cues. Thus, inhibited social behavior in growth hormone–deficient adolescents may result from a deficit in processing subtle social cues, as well as from societal responses to short stature.

COGNITIVE DEVELOPMENT IN ADOLESCENCE

Piaget

Any exploration of cognitive development must first recognize the work of Piaget in carefully observing and describing the cognitive growth occurring in children from infancy through adulthood. Although other approaches to cognitive development (in particular, the information-processing model explored further on) have recently emerged as alternatives or supplements to Piaget's formulation, some familiarity with Piagetian stages is essential to understanding the foundation upon which later theorists build or remodel. (A discussion of Piagetian theory is found in Chapter 9).

The Information-Processing Approach

The information-processing approach has emerged as an important alternative to Piagetian theory, although many recent studies build on Piagetian hypotheses. The information-processing approach views the human mind as a system that gathers, processes, manipulates, and stores incoming information from the environment. Although not incompatible with Piagetian theory, this approach does lead to different emphases and experiments. Piaget observed and described the behavior of small numbers of children (usually his own), posing questions and observing their approaches to problems; the information-processing approach seeks to explicate a detailed model that makes predictions about ongoing cognitive processes. Such a model focuses on, for example, determining the attentional and memory capacity of the brain, identifying strategies that people use to encode, retain, and use incoming information, or studying executive processes that monitor and direct cognitive activities as they occur.

Developmental Trends During Adolescence

FORMAL OPERATIONS

Piaget viewed adolescent and adult cognition as being characterized by formal thought (see Chapter 9), including the use of rules, deductions, hypotheses, and logic to solve problems. Although current studies support the idea that adolescents *can* think in logical ways, these studies and others also suggest that most adults do *not* habitually use their abilities as formal thinkers. In fact, some estimates indicate that only 25% of college students could be classified as using formal operations to solve Piagetian-type problems, whereas fully 50% use concrete operations. It appears, then, that although most older adolescents are capable of reasoning deductively, the odds are that any particular adolescent going about daily life will not be applying these logical rules in any consistent way. Acknowledging that adolescents do not progress stage-like through one type of thinking, researchers have recently sought to examine how adolescents select strategies for problem solving.

STRATEGIC THINKING

What distinguishes the cognition of adolescents from that of children? A major contribution of information-processing approaches is the recognition of humans' ability to use strategies to plan, learn, remember, and think about their own planning, learning, and remembering. These "metacognitive" skills are evident, for example, in the adolescent who recognizes that his or her mind is wandering during a lecture on conflict resolution and develops strategies for bringing the attention back (taking notes), avoiding drowsiness in the future (going to sleep earlier), or thinking about the relevance of the material to everyday life (e.g., remembering a recent conflict with his or her mother over the lyrics on a favorite compact disc).

Most theorists identify metacognitive strategies as developing in late childhood or early adolescence (e.g., Flavell, 1985). In earlier childhood, reasoning abilities do serve a self-regulatory function, as when children use their memory of past bedtime routines to remind themselves to brush their teeth, put on their pajamas, and ask their parent for a bedtime story. It is in adolescence, however, that reasoning abilities are applied to organize in a meaningful way not only concrete tasks such as self-care routines but also *cognition*. The metacognitive processes that develop at this time influence every other aspect of cognition. For example, the use of strategies for remembering effectively expands the short-term memory capacity of the adolescent beyond any increases in structural capacity that may occur. Just as adolescents apply metacognitive skills to increase their memory capacity, other cognitive abilities acquired during adolescence enable a dramatic expansion of knowledge and learning in a similar way. For example, the adolescent who learns to read and write well finds a wealth of new perspectives, adventures, and discoveries in innumerable libraries and bookstores. New information begins to be linked with previously learned material, and the adolescent actively seeks out new, contradictory findings in a way that is often unparalleled in either adulthood or earlier childhood.

MATHEMATICAL THINKING

The formal, logical, symbolic thinking identified by Piaget is precisely the type of approach needed to grasp the complex concepts that adolescents confront in their high school mathematics classes. Without formal thought, adolescents could not carry out operations on mathematical symbols, the ultimate in abstraction.

However, just as many adolescents and even adults do *not* think logically, so mathematical abstractions are not grasped by everyone. Wood (1988) describes a large-scale study investigating the mathematical competencies of 10,000 11- to 15-year-olds. The following striking deficiencies were among their findings: Only 2% of 13-year-olds and 30% of 15-year-olds understood that between any pair of numbers, there are theoretically an infinite number of numbers. Many adolescents do not recognize which operations they should perform on a word problem; for example, when told that they are standing 29 miles from Grange and 58 miles from Barton, two towns lying in opposite directions, many of them were unable to recognize that they needed to add the two numbers to determine the distance between the towns. Conversely, Bruner and Kenney (1965) demonstrated that a classroom of 8-year-olds could be taught to use abstract algebraic mathematical procedures.

Perhaps in mathematics more than in any other area, the method of teaching and the context of knowledge play an important role. The Russian psychologist Vygotsky emphasized focusing on what children can learn with help rather than what they know in a static sense. As Wood (1988) suggests, although we learn to use language from the very beginning of life and are strongly motivated to communicate effectively, mathematics is dependent on school learning that begins later in life and is too often unaccompanied by adequate motivation. In fact, Wood notes that mathematics is quite difficult for most children to learn, and thus many high school students prefer to avoid looking "stupid" so they put forth little effort.

DOMAIN-SPECIFIC KNOWLEDGE

A critical aspect of understanding cognitive abilities lies in identifying, in Sternberg's words, "not how much intelligence the individual has but, rather, how that intelligence is directed or exploited" (Sternberg, 1988, p 276). One of the most important tasks of adolescence is that of identifying those domains in which one wishes to apply one's intellectual skills. In school, adolescents begin to choose which courses they will take in preparation for which career. Their skills in some areas develop at a much faster rate than do skills in other areas. For example, one person directs energy at learning to play football and analyze literature and another focuses on becoming a computer whiz or an expert in chess. Success depends as much on selecting domains in which one can become proficient as on one's general level of intelligence or ability to engage in formal thought. The process of matching abilities and preferences with particular domains is, then, a central task of adolescence.

COMPONENTS OF INTELLIGENCE AND THE INFLUENCE OF CULTURE

Recent developments in the field of cognitive psychology have broadened our conception of "intelligence" to include separable components of intelligence and the ability to accomplish practical goals such as fixing a bicycle or convincing another person to help cook dinner. Further, the goals accomplished must be important to the society or culture within which the person resides (Ford, 1986). Thus, definitions of "practical intelligence" seek to encompass cultural variability, expanding our traditional Western view of intelligence as a set of skills that predict one's ability to perform in a Western school setting.

Gardner (1983) has spelled out a theory of multiple intelligences that gives concrete meaning to the term *practical intelligence*. The intelligences he has identified thus far include the following: musical, bodily-kinesthetic, logical-mathematical, linguistic, spatial, interpersonal, and intrapersonal. Thus, the South Seas navigator who can accurately chart a course without instruments possesses a high degree of spatial intelligence, which is valued by his or her culture. According to Gardner, these intelligences are independent from one another; a person may be a skilled musician while being unable to solve logical-mathematical problems.

Because expanding definitions of intelligence are relatively new, little empirical work has been done as yet to identify the developmental trajectories of different types of intelligence. It is clear, however, that a more varied conception of intelligence is accompanied by more variation in developmental paths. In Gardner's description of the development of musical intelligence, for example, the basic musical skills are usually present prior to adolescence. The shift occurring in adolescence is then twofold: First, the adolescent must formally learn aspects of musical analysis that were known intuitively as a child. Second, the gifted adolescent is said to go through a kind of "midlife crisis" in which a decision must be made as to whether to devote his or her life to music (Bamberger, 1982). Contrast this path to that of the linguistic intelligence of a writer. Technical skill with writing, memory for experiences, and a kind of self-restraint that avoids self-conscious word play or overstatement of emotion are necessary attributes of good writers that develop over time and are unlikely to be completed by the end of adolescence. The complicated task lies ahead of documenting not a single path of cognitive development in adolescence but rather multiple paths that are likely to vary across cultures as well.

The separable components of intelligence outlined by Gardner and Sternberg and others can operate in all cultures, although their specific form may differ across cultures (Sternberg, 1988). In particular, the culture may influence which components and which strategies are valued over others. Similarly, components that are essential to success in one culture may be less important in another.

Social Cognition

One of the most important areas of practical intelligence is the investigation of social cognition. How do children and adolescents reason about their friendships? How does development of formal, logical thinking interact with social development? Selman (1981) used extensive interviews to explore children's philosophies regarding friendship. He identified the following stages of friendship concepts.

At Stage 0 (approximately ages 3 to 7 years), friends are seen as momentary playmates; there is little sense of interpersonal affection or ability to recognize the other's point of view. At Stage 1 (approximately ages 4 to 9 years), friendship is seen as a one-way offer of assistance: A friend is someone who does what you want. With middle childhood comes Stage 2 friendship (approximately 6 to 12 years of age). Selman calls this stage "fair-weather cooperation": "The friends are aware of reciprocal perspectives, but the relationship is discontinuous, with specific arguments seen as severing the relationship" (Selman, 1981, p 259).

During adolescence, Selman suggests that most people reach Stage 3, in which friendships are intimate and mutually shared, and value is placed on sharing personal problems rather than simple relief from boredom or loneliness. A common pitfall of this stage is overemphasis of the two-person clique. Finally, Stage 4 friendships, achieved between age 12 years and adulthood, allow for a balance of independence and dependence.

In a recent longitudinal study, Keller and Wood (1989) explored the development of friendship reasoning and influential factors. They found that development across the stages moves in a slow and gradual manner, with most 9-year-olds reasoning between Stages 1 and 2, 12-year-olds reasoning at about Stage 2, and 15-year-olds reasoning between Stages 2 and 3. Interestingly, Keller and Wood found that cognitive ability (measured at age 7 years) exerted a stable influence on friendship reasoning over time; children who were more cognitively advanced on Piagetian tasks administered at age 7 years reached higher levels of friendship reasoning in adolescence. In addition, gender and social class were shown to influence social cognition, with girls and members of higher social classes reasoning at a higher level. These social class effects were strongest in boys and in the group with lower cognitive ability.

THEMES IN ADOLESCENT COGNITIVE DEVELOPMENT

As children enter adolescence, cognitive and brain development is far from over. Even though final brain size and the overall number of available neurons and axons are largely fixed early in infancy, continued plasticity is mediated by synaptogenesis and pruning, dendritic proliferation and elimination, progressive myelination, variations in absolute metabolic rate, and the influence of hormones. In general, brain development during adolescence involves widespread and highly generalized changes that appear to be concurrent across the entire cerebral cortex, rather than restricted to specific cortical regions. Studies of both synaptic architecture and metabolic activity converge in demonstrating that levels of synaptic density and glucose metabolism during adolescence exceed those of adults (and may peak in animals at greater than childhood levels) but then gradually decline to adult levels. These changes appear to covary across the cortex and to show little regional variation after 1 year of age.

In association with these generalized shifts in brain development, adolescent cognition undergoes profound changes in organization and application. First and chief among these changes is the development of higher level "executive" skills. These changes allow the adolescent to gain a measure of self-regulation over cognitive activities—the ability to organize and deploy components of information processing in a planned, adaptive way. This contrasts sharply with the younger child, who "knows" a variety of cognitive strategies but has not developed the skills necessary to integrate and apply these skills flexibly in uncertain environments. This contrast is captured eloquently by Vygotsky, who commented that whereas the "young child thinks by remembering, an adolescent remembers by thinking" (Luria, 1976, p 11).

A second change in adolescence involves an increasingly active and self-conscious attempt to match cognitive abilities and components to specific adaptive domains in the real world. The "match" between the adolescent's profile of cognitive abilities and the environment thus becomes a central issue in successful adaptation. Part of what makes adolescence a time of great flexibility, in which people have the time to use introspection and the intellectual ability to engage in self-reflection, is this developing ability to engage in personal experiments in testing various "fits" between self and situation.

Third, as adolescents learn new cognitive strategies, new possibilities open up in relation to cognitive self-management. Through acquisition of new skills (such as the ability to read and write well), broad new areas of knowledge become available to the adolescent. The adolescent develops universal, abstract cognitive processes and at the same time acquires specific kinds of knowledge.

These three themes have in common an emphasis on emerging cognitive self-regulation. The preoccupation of infant cognitive development is to some extent the self-regulation of perception, motor function, and social attachment, whereas self-regulation during adolescence involves gaining self-control of cognitive activity itself. These shifts in adolescent cognitive development were not explicitly recognized by Piaget, who instead focused upon the emergence of formal operations and the adolescent's shift in perspective from egocentrism to decentering. According to Piaget, the adolescent is unique among children in the ability to use formal logic to make sense of the world. Although children in middle childhood are no longer at the mercy of direct sensation, as the infant is, they still do not possess that sense of the possible—the hypothetical—that enables the adolescent to grasp abstraction, make logical deductions, and be an idealist. For Piaget, a "decentering process . . . later makes it possible for the adolescent to get beyond the early relative lack of differentiation and to cure himself of his idealistic crisis—in other words, the return to reality which is the path from adolescence to the true beginnings of adulthood" (Piaget, 1977, p 441). Piaget saw this decentering process as being triggered by social relationships, beginning with dialogues with peers but becoming most pronounced with the entrance to the professional world: "It is then that he is transformed from an idealistic reformer into an achiever" (Piaget, 1977, p 441). In fact, adolescence can be seen as representing the peak in abstract thought, so much so that although many dreams are formed, little in the way of practical, lasting work is accomplished during this time of life.

Unlike many changes in early cognitive development, in which highly general affordances in the environment may allow the normal development of what Greenough has termed experience-expectant processes, cognitive development in adolescence depends more profoundly on specific influences, particularly in the peer and school environments. Unfortunately, in many schools, a mismatch may exist between the academic environment and changes in the adolescent's approach to information processing (Eccles and Midgley, 1989). For the adolescent, self-regulation of cognition and the need to self-identify different domains for applying cognitive strengths may be prerequisites for academic or any other form of success.

BIBLIOGRAPHY

Bamberger J: Growing up prodigies: The mid-life crisis. New Dir Child Dev 17:61, 1982.

Bertenthal BI, Campos JJ: New directions in the study of early experience. Child Dev 58:560, 1987.

Bruner JS, Kenney HJ: Representation and mathematics learning. Monogr Soc Res Child Dev 30(1):50, 1965.

Chugani HT, Phelps ME, Mazziotta JC: Positron emission tomography study of human brain functional development. Ann Neurol 22:487, 1987.

Eccles JS, Midgley C: Stage/environment fit: Developmentally appropriate classrooms for early adolescents. In Ames C, Ames RE (eds): Research on Motivation in Education, Vol 3. New York, Academic Press, 1989.

Epstein HT: Phrenoblysis: Special brain and mind growth periods. Dev Psychobiol 7:207, 1974.

Fischer KW: Relations between brain and cognitive development. Child Dev 58:623, 1987.

Flavell JH: Cognitive Development, 2nd ed. Englewood Cliffs, NJ, Prentice Hall, 1985.

Ford ME: For all practical purposes: Criteria for defining and evaluating practical intelligence. In Sternberg RJ, Wagner RK (eds): Practical Intelligence. Cambridge, Cambridge University Press, 1986, pp 183–202.

Gardner H: Frames of Mind. Cambridge, MA: MIT Bradford Press, 1983.

Goldman-Rakic PS: Development of cortical circuitry and cognitive function. Child Dev 58:601, 1987.

Greenough WT, Black JE, Wallace CS: Experience and brain development. Child Dev 58:539, 1987.

Huttenlocker P: Synaptic density in human frontal cortex-developmental changes and effects of aging. Brain Res 163:195, 1979.

Keller M, Wood P: Development of friendship reasoning: A study of interindividual differences in intraindividual change. Dev Psychol 25:820, 1989.

Luria AR: Cognitive Development. Cambridge, MA, Harvard University Press, 1976.

McCauley E, Kay T, Ito J, Treder R: The Turner syndrome: Cognitive deficits, affective discrimination, and behavior problems. Child Dev 58:464, 1987.

Piaget J: The Essential Piaget (Gruber HE, Voneche JJ [eds]). New York, Basic Books, 1977.

Rakic P, Bourgeois J-P, Zecevic N, et al: Concurrent overproduction of synapses in diverse regions of the primate cerebral cortex. Science 232:232, 1986.

Selman RL: The child as a friendship philosopher. In Asher SR, Gottman JM (eds): The Development of Children's Friendships. Cambridge, MA, Cambridge University Press, 1981, pp 242–272.

Sternberg RJ: The Triarchic Mind: A New Theory of Human Intelligence. New York, Penguin Books, 1988.

Waber DP, Mann MB, Merola J, Moylan PM: Physical maturation rate and cognitive performance in early adolescence: A longitudinal examination. Dev Psychol 21:666, 1985.

Wood D: How Children Think and Learn. Cambridge, MA, Basil Blackwell, 1988.

Yakovlev PI, Lecours AR: The myelogenetic cycles of regional maturation of the brain. In Minknosky A (ed): Regional Development of the Brain in Early Life. Oxford, Blackwell Scientific, 1967, pp 3–70.

CHAPTER 11

Personality Development and Structure

DRAGAN M. SVRAKIC and C. ROBERT CLONINGER

From the standpoint of this chapter, adolescence is best defined as the final phase in the process of personality development, because there is rarely much change in personality style after 21 years of age.

PERSONALITY STRUCTURE

Temperament, character, emotionality, and personality are closely related phenomena that can be difficult to distinguish. Temperament denotes individual differences in genetically determined emotional dispositions, such as fear, anger, and love. The practical distinction between temperament and personality is questionable because there is no observable component of personality that is unchanging. Basic temperamental features are fairly stable over time, but as development proceeds, the expression of temperament becomes more influenced by experience and context.

In psychodynamic theories, character and character traits are conceived as residues of previous defense mechanisms that have become dissociated from the original conflicts that elicited their use and emerge in a person's everyday life. Individuals are often described as "characters" if they are predictably unusual in their interpersonal style; what they say and do would be unusual for more flexible people but is typical of their fixed and limited range of adaptive responses. As extensions of previous defensive responses to conflict, character traits serve to prevent a person from being involved in such situations again. Being the "code" of direct behavior, character also includes fixed patterns of behavioral adjustment as well as idiosyncratic ethical attitudes. Thus, character refers to the direct outward manifestation of personality, particularly its social and ethical aspects.

Motivation originates in the primary emotional dispositions of fear, anger, and love, which are hypothe-

sized to derive directly from the biologic goals of survival and reproduction. Under normal circumstances, after survival needs are met, the goals of normally developing individuals change to include the integrity of not only the physical but also the psychic self. An individual's behavior may also be influenced by various social goals, which are usually called secondary motives. Deviant and inflexible motivated behavior usually derives from two or three monopolistic elementary psychological needs. In contrast, normal and flexible motivation develops after basic needs are met and the person is free to experience numerous secondary motives.

At one time it was diagnostically practical to divide personality into its temperamental and character aspects. Contemporary personality theories encompass both motivational and behavioral aspects of personality. This is possible because personality is viewed in developmental terms. Biogenetic factors influence how an individual adapts to experience; in turn, prior experience modifies future adaptive tendencies. Consequently, personality traits are not expected to be fixed regardless of prior experience or the current situation.

The vast majority of modern theories of personality structure are tridimensional (e.g., those of Eysenck, Cloninger, Tellegen, Gray). Three independent, stable, and heritable personality dimensions, in addition to intelligence, have been consistently identified when observations about population are factor-analyzed, regardless of the demographics of the population or the method of measurement. According to Cloninger (1987), the underlying genetic predisposition to personality is reflected in three dimensions called novelty seeking (NS), harm avoidance (HA), and reward dependence (RD) (Table 11–1).

These basic personality dimensions can be systematically related to the three primary emotions, or basic temperamental dispositions, mentioned earlier. For example, NS and HA in Cloninger's model derive from predispositions to anger and fear, respectively. The third dimension is associated with emotional attachment (e.g., RD). The close correspondence between personality and emotionality is presented in Table 11–2.

The major difficulty in mapping variation in personality, emotions, and cognition to their underlying biologic processes arises from the following two facts: First,

Supported in part by Grant MH31302 from the National Institute of Mental Health, Grants AA07982 and AA08028 from the National Institute of Alcoholism, and a pilot research grant from the MacArthur Foundation Mental Health Research Network I (Psychobiology of Depression).

TABLE 11–1. Personality Characteristics of High and Low Scorers on Novelty-Seeking, Harm Avoidance, and Reward Dependence

PERSONALITY DIMENSION	PERSONALITY CHARACTERISTICS (Contrasting Set of Personality Traits)	
	High Scorer	Low Scorer
Novelty-seeking	Curious, exploratory, fickle, easily bored, impressionistic, impulsive, extravagant, enthusiastic, disorderly, unconventional, quick-tempered, excitable, evasive, deceptive	Content, quiet, rigid, patient, methodical, reflective, frugal, reserved, orderly, regimented, slow-tempered, stoic forthright, honest
Harm avoidance	Cautious, worrying, pessimistic, restrained, fearful, shy, fatigable, asthenic	Confident, carefree, optimistic, risk-taking, bold, outgoing, energetic, vigorous
Reward dependence	Sentimental, socially sensitive, persistent, "tender-hearted," dedicated	Practical, insensitive, irresolute, "cold-blooded", detached

factor analysis can determine only the minimal number of distinguishing personality traits, not their underlying causative factors; and second, the observed phenotypic personality structure may differ from the biogenetic structure because learning and environmental factors also influence phenotypic variation.

One of the authors (C.R.C.) has recently formulated a unified biosocial model of personality based on a synthesis of data from longitudinal studies of development, family and adoption studies, psychometric studies of personality structure, and a growing body of neuropharmacologic and neuroanatomic data on behavior and learning in humans and other animals. The biosocial model recognizes the personality dimensions of HA, NS, and RD, mentioned earlier, or, more precisely, recognizes genetic predispositions to adaptive personality traits that comprehensively define one's personality and motivation.

Each of these personality dimensions follows a normal gaussian distribution in the general population, with most people having intermediate values. The term *dimension* is intended to emphasize quantitative variation in the understanding of both normal and deviant personality structures. HA, NS, and RD represent bipolar scales between two extremes in the same dimension of behavior, and each of them is defined by contrasting sets of personality traits, shown in Tables 11–1 and 11–2. (For a more detailed description of personality dimensions postulated in the unified biosocial model, see Cloninger [1987].)

The unified biosocial model of personality postulates a functional association between three basic dimensions and three major brain systems for the activation, maintenance, and inhibition of behaviors. (For the neuroanatomic and biochemical networks that underlie the personality dimensions of HA, NS, and RD and regulate emotional and learning processes, see Cloninger [1987].)

The three major brain systems, their principal neuromodulators, and corresponding learning and personality characteristics are summarized in Table 11–3.

With the exclusion of psychotic disorders and related phenomena like schizotypal personality disorder (PD), which are likely to be qualitative defects rather than extreme variants of normal variation, factor analyses repeatedly show that deviant personality traits have a tridimensional structure that corresponds to that observed with normal traits. In contrast with intermediate values of HA, NS, and RD in general population samples, personality disorders are characterized by high or low scores on one or more of the basic personality dimensions. Various combinations of over- and under-pronounced personality dimensions and their relation to traditional categories of PDs are summarized in Figure 11–1.

The close correspondence between traditional categories of PDs and those predicted as extreme variants of normal personality traits suggests that "normal" and "deviant" personalities share the same biogenetic structure. An important implication is that individuals who can adapt flexibly to the full range of environmental situations (an ability usually called normality) are those who are nearly average on all three personality dimensions. This is also in accord with the genetic principle of balanced selection against extreme high or low deviations, which leads to an intermediate phenotype being optimal from the standpoint of reproductive fitness.

Continuity of Personality from Childhood to Adulthood

Empirical data regarding fundamental questions about the development and change of personality over one's life span are rather limited. Several longitudinal studies of children and adolescents have demonstrated the stability of certain behaviors (e.g., aggressiveness) or personality traits (e.g., shyness, timidity, passivity). Other studies have followed the effects of certain environmental (e.g., social status) or biologic (e.g., parental illness) variables on individual personality and adjustment across time.

TABLE 11–2. Correspondence Between Personality and Emotionality

PERSONALITY DIMENSION	CHARACTERISTIC EMOTIONALITY TRAITS	
	High Scorer	Low Scorer
Novelty-seeking	Quick-tempered, excitable, curious, enthusiastic, exuberant, easily bored	Slow-tempered, stoic, uninquiring, inexuberant, tolerant, unenthusiastic
Harm avoidance	Fearful, doubtful, timid, dismayed, disgusted, fatigable	Relaxed, self-assured, bold, daring, dauntless, vigorous
Reward dependence	Loving, sensitive, warm, dedicated, sad if separated	Unfriendly, insensitive, cool, indifferent if alone

TABLE 11–3. Three Major Brain Systems, Their Neuromodulators, and Their Associated Learning and Personality Characteristics

BRAIN SYSTEM (RELATED PERSONALITY DIMENSION)	PRINCIPAL MONOAMINE NEUROMODULATOR	LEARNING CHARACTERISTICS		PERSONALITY CHARACTERISTICS	
		Relevant Stimuli	Behavioral or Learned Response	High Scorer	Low Scorer
ACTIVATION (Novelty-seeking)	Dopamine	Novelty (potential reward)	Exploratory pursuit	Curious, exploratory	Content, quiet
		Monotony	Active avoidance	Fickle, easily bored	Rigid, patient
		Complexity	Collative approach	Impressionable, impulsive	Methodical, reflective
		Cues to reward	Appetitive approach	Extravagant, enthusiastic	Frugal, reserved
		Conditioned signals of punishment or nonreward	Active avoidance	Disorderly, unconventional	Orderly, regimented
		Punishment or frustrative nonreward	"Fight or flight"	Quick-tempered, excitable, evasive, deceptive	Slow-tempered, stoic, forthright, honest
INHIBITION (Harm avoidance)	Serotonin	Conditioned signals of punishment	Passive avoidance	Cautious, worrying	Confident, carefree
		Conditioned signals of frustrative nonreward	Extinction	Pessimistic, restrained	Optimistic, risk-taking
		Novelty (potential danger)	Slow habituation, passive avoidance	Fearful, shy	Bold, outgoing
		Inescapable or unpredictable punishment	Sensitization, helpless inactivity	Fatigable, asthenic	Energetic, vigorous
MAINTENANCE (Reward dependence)	Norepinephrine	Pairing of collative (novel) stimuli with rewards or relief from punishment	Classic appetitive conditioning	Sentimental, socially sensitive	Practical, insensitive
		Frustrative nonreward or punishment of previously rewarded behavior	Resistance to extinction, "fight or flight"	Persistent, "tender-hearted," dedicated	Irresolute, "cold-blooded," detached

Many short-term and a few long-term follow-up studies have shown considerable stability of temperamental dispositions during the first few years of life. However, they do not permit reliable predictions on the relationship between childhood and adult personality.

Wolf and Chick (1980) showed that schizoid personality characteristics, such as solitariness, emotional detachment, hypersensitivity, mental rigidity, and eccentricity, tend to be fairly stable over a period of 15 years (from 5 to 14 years to 17 to 28 years of age).

Studies of personality development and changes in twins indicate that the stable components of personality are genetically determined and that personality changes are attributable largely to transient environmental influences. Sigvardsson and co-workers (1987) studied the stability of personality dimensions postulated by Cloninger in 431 children from 10 to 27 years of age. The structure of personality in childhood observed by Sigvardsson and associates was remarkably similar to that in adults described by Cloninger (1987). Most personality traits derived by factor analysis were found to involve the interaction of two or more of the dimensions of HA, NS, and RD at all ages studied. The cardinal finding was that the predictive ability of childhood ratings did not appear to decrease as children grew older, suggesting that the personality dimensions are stable adaptive tendencies rather than fixed traits or acquired habit patterns.

Further, personality ratings at age 10 to 11 years were predictive of most personality traits at ages 15, 18, and 27 years. For example, individual differences in NS at age 11 years were predictive of later differences in maturity, activity, and aggression at age 15 years, logical reasoning and leadership at age 18 years, and risk of antisocial behavior in adulthood. Differences in HA were predictive of differences in maturity, sociability, and aggression (age 15 years), leadership and obesity (age 18 years), and violent crime (age 27 years). Finally, differences in RD at age 11 years were predictive of maturity and academic achievement (age 15 years), social skills (age 18 years), and risk of violent crime in adulthood (Sigvardsson et al, 1987). However, childhood personality does not explain more than half of the observed variation in later behavior, so the important influence of environmental factors on personality development needs careful consideration.

PERSONALITY DEVELOPMENT

Today it is widely accepted that personality develops through a process of genetic and environmental inter-

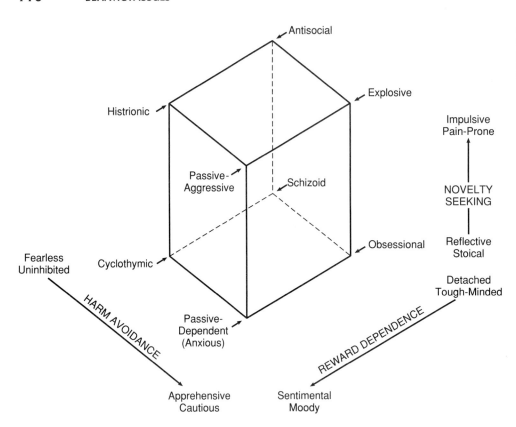

Figure 11–1. Traditional personality disorders related to the three personality dimensions of novelty seeking, harm avoidance, and reward dependence.

action. According to twin, adoption, and family studies, genetic differences among individuals account for about one half of the variance in most normally distributed personality traits, and the rest is explained mostly by nonfamilial environmental effects. Contrary to the common belief about the importance of family environment in personality formation, environmental influences shared by members of the same family have little or no role in influencing the style of personality characteristics.

Nonshared environment denotes individually unique experiences in the same family, such as birth order, gender differences, illnesses, or differential parental treatment. Nonshared environmental effects and heritable differences in personality explain the existence of "resilient" adolescents who, despite numerous negative circumstances, become well adjusted and healthy individuals.

The contemporary concept of normal psychic development has been derived from the pioneering works of Freud, Klein, Mahler, Kohut, Spitz, Kernberg, Winicott, Hartmann, and Erikson. Basically eclectic, the concept reconciles classic instinctual theory, direct observations of childrens' development, ego psychology, and object-relations theory in an attempt to understand normal personality development (see Chapter 9).

The process of personality development begins with the symbiotic phase (from 3 to 18 months of age), which is characterized by the complete mental fusion between a newborn and his or her caregiver. During this phase, the child's feelings, thoughts, and actions are almost entirely dependent on the caregiver. The immature personality and views of others are composed of "all good" self-images (determined by positive affects) that

are separated from "all bad" self-images (determined by negative affects). Children often have a self-centered view of the world in which they assume that whatever they need or want is the same as that of others. They do not realize that their desires may be in conflict with those of others. Figure 11–2 summarizes the contemporary psychodynamic concept of the normal childhood development of mental representations of one's self and other objects.

During the separation-individuation phase (from 18 to 36 months of age), which coincides with the development of perception, memory, and the capacity to walk, contradictory self- and object-images are integrated into more realistic concepts. Children begin to be able to feel guilt, and they develop an increased capacity to be alone or to tolerate frustration and loss.

Between 3 and 6 years of age, children begin to show an increased capacity for maintaining interests and emotional bonds despite temporary frustration or dissatisfaction. This increased persistence in relations with other people and things is sometimes called *object constancy*.

After 6 years of age, there is little maturation of personality until puberty, that is, personality is highly stable during the primary school years (ages 7 to 12 years) except in response to unusual social pressures.

Adolescence is frequently referred to as the second separation-individuation phase, during which several major steps in personality development occur. The most important of these changes are physical and sexual maturation (see Chapter 5), cognitive maturation (see Chapters 9 and 10), progression from dependence to independence, and the establishment of personal identity and interpersonal intimacy.

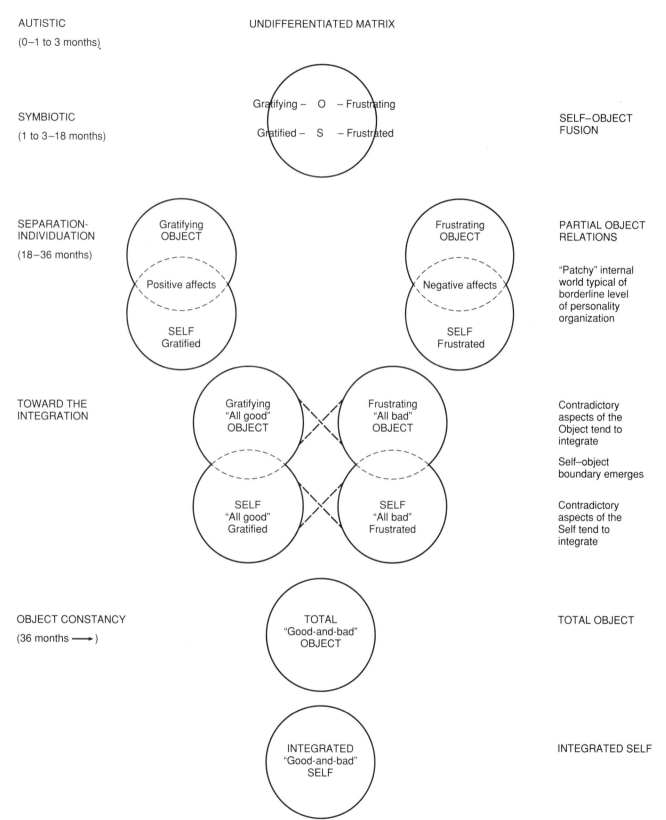

Figure 11–2. Normal development of self- and object representations.

BIBLIOGRAPHY

American Psychiatric Association: Diagnostic and Statistical Manual of Mental Disorders, 3rd ed revised. Washington, DC, American Psychiatric Association, 1987.

Cloninger CR: A systematic method for clinical description and classification of personality variables: A proposal. Arch Gen Psychiatry, 44:573, 1987.

Feinstein S: Identity and adjustment disorder of adolescence. In Kaplan H, Sadock B (eds): Comprehensive Textbook of Psychiatry, 4th ed. Baltimore, Williams & Wilkins, 1985, pp 1760–1765.

Gunderson J: Personality disorders. In Nicholi A (ed): The New Harvard Guide to Psychiatry. Cambridge, MA, Belknap Press, 1988, pp 337–357.

Kernberg O: Borderline Conditions and Pathological Narcissism. New York, Jason Aronson, 1975.

Klar H, Siever L: The psychopharmacologic treatment of personality disorders. Psychiatr Clin North Am 7(4):791, 1984.

Masterson J: From Borderline Adolescent to Functioning Adult: The Test of Time. New York, Brunner/Mazel, 1980.

Sigafoos A, Feinstein C, Diamond M, Reiss D: The measurement of behavioral autonomy in adolescence: The autonomous functioning checklist. In Feinstein S (ed): Adolescent Psychiatry Vol 15. Chicago, University of Chicago Press, 1988, pp 432–462.

Sigvardsson S, Bohman M, Cloninger CR: Structure and stability of childhood personality: Prediction of later social adjustment. J Child Psychol Psychiatry 28(6):929, 1987.

Wolf S, Chick J: Schizoid personality in childhood: A controlled follow up study. Psychol Med 10:85, 1980.

Biology and Behavior: Interface

CHAPTER 12

Neurotransmitters, Stress, and Depression

MARGARET ALTEMUS, BRUCE BLACK, and PHILIP W. GOLD

A fundamental biologic concept introduced by Empedocles in 500 B.C. is that organisms must maintain harmony or homeostasis in order to survive. Empedocles wrote that counterbalancing (adaptive) forces were essential to neutralize the harmful impact of disturbing forces. Building on a foundation spanning more than 2000 years, Selye in 1938 introduced the modern concept of the general adaptation response, corresponding to what Empedocles and Hippocrates called the counterbalancing forces and what Galen referred to as the *vis medicatrix naturae,* the healing forces of nature. Selye's major contribution was the description of a generalized syndrome that followed a wide variety of physical stresses and included secretion of glucocorticoids and catecholamines. Later it became clear that psychological stresses alone could stimulate the general adaptational response.

In this chapter we first describe the central biologic components of the generalized stress response and then argue that dysregulated stress responses predispose individuals to depression and other psychiatric illnesses. Our interest is in the connection between neurotransmitters, stress, and depression, particularly during adolescence. Unfortunately, there have been very few useful studies of the biology of adolescent stress responses or depression. Although the incidence of depression increases dramatically following puberty, we actually know less about adolescent depression than we do about prepubertal depression, and far less than we do about depression in adulthood. Therefore, we must rely heavily on studies of the neurobiology of depression in adults and in prepubertal children and extrapolate from there, taking into account the few studies that have been completed in adolescents. Such a course is not without its perils, for it is clear that dramatic changes occur from puberty to adolescence to adulthood in neuroendocrine status, in the development of neurotransmitter systems, and in the complex interactions between the various neuroendocrine and neurotransmitter systems (see Chapter 4). Therefore, much of what we will discuss can be applied only very cautiously to depression in adolescents.

PRINCIPAL CENTRAL COMPONENTS OF THE STRESS RESPONSE

The two principal central effectors of the generalized stress response are the locus ceruleus–norepinephrine (LC-NE) system and the hypothalamic-pituitary-adrenal (HPA) axis (Fig. 12–1). These two systems perform many overlapping functions and seem to participate in a mutually reinforcing, positive feedback loop.

Locus Ceruleus–Norepinephrine System

The LC-NE system was the first of the central stress responsive systems to be described in detail. The locus ceruleus (LC) is a nucleus of noradrenergic neurons located in the midpons with terminal fields in the hypothalamus, hippocampus, and amygdala and throughout the cerebral cortex. The LC provides 90% of the brain's supply of norepinephrine (NE). In addition, the LC is a central nucleus of the peripheral sympathetic nervous system and sympathomedullary system, both of which release catecholamines to mediate the fight-or-flight response. Numerous findings have demonstrated the importance of the LC in mediating arousal. Electrical stimulation of the LC in unanesthetized primates produces intense anxiety, hypervigilance, and inhibition of exploratory behavior. Spontaneous firing of the LC increases during threatening situations and diminishes during sleep, grooming, and feeding. Finally, acute stress in animals causes increased release of NE in several brain areas, including the hypothalamus and LC, and chronic stress increases the activity of tyrosine hydroxylase, the rate-limiting enzyme for NE synthesis.

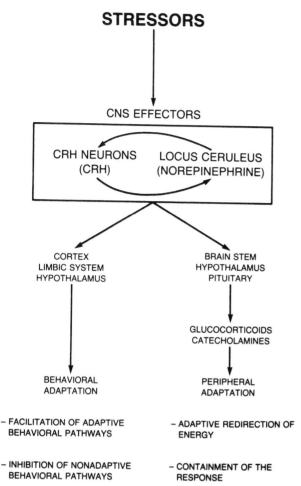

STRESSORS

CNS EFFECTORS

CRH NEURONS (CRH) ⟷ LOCUS CERULEUS (NOREPINEPHRINE)

CORTEX LIMBIC SYSTEM HYPOTHALAMUS

BRAIN STEM HYPOTHALAMUS PITUITARY

GLUCOCORTICOIDS CATECHOLAMINES

BEHAVIORAL ADAPTATION

PERIPHERAL ADAPTATION

- FACILITATION OF ADAPTIVE BEHAVIORAL PATHWAYS

- ADAPTIVE REDIRECTION OF ENERGY

- INHIBITION OF NONADAPTIVE BEHAVIORAL PATHWAYS

- CONTAINMENT OF THE RESPONSE

Figure 12–1. Schematic diagram of stress-mediated central effectors. Arrows show the function of central effectors in facilitating a characteristic behavioral and peripheral response to stress. CNS, Central nervous system; CRH, corticotropin-releasing hormone. (With permission from Gold PW, Goodwin FK, Chrousos GP: Clinical and biochemical manifestations of depression. Relation to the neurobiology of stress [two parts]. N Engl J Med 319:348–353, 413–420, 1988.)

Hypothalamic-Pituitary-Adrenal Axis

The other major central component of the generalized stress response is corticotropin-releasing hormone (CRH), a 41–amino acid peptide located primarily in the paraventricular nucleus of the hypothalamus. The well-documented rise in plasma cortisol in response to stress is initiated by release of hypothalamic CRH, which is transported from the median eminence through the portal system to cause adrenocorticotropic hormone (ACTH) release from the pituitary. ACTH then acts at the adrenals to stimulate release of glucocorticoids. The HPA axis, like all neuroendocrine axes, has feedback loops that maintain a homeostatic set point. Both glucocorticoids and ACTH act via hypothalamic and pituitary feedback loops to limit activation of the system.

CRH is released not only at the median eminence into the portal blood, but also into the cerebrospinal fluid (CSF) through hypothalamic projections to numerous brain areas, including the floor of the third ventricle.

Extrahypothalamic CRH cell bodies and terminal fields are located in disparate regions of the central nervous system (CNS), particularly in close association with the central autonomic system and the LC and in many periventricular locations. The anatomic distribution of CRH within and beyond the boundaries of the hypothalamus correlates with the observation that CRH can simultaneously activate and coordinate a series of metabolic, cardiovascular, and behavioral responses that are adaptive during threatening or stressful situations. For example, intracerebroventricular administration of CRH in rats leads to activation of the pituitary-adrenal axis, producing energy mobilization to meet acute metabolic demands, and also to several other adaptive behavioral changes characteristic of the stress response. These include decreased feeding and sexual behavior and increased context-dependent changes in motor activity. In larger doses, CRH produces anxiety-like behavioral effects, including hyperresponsiveness to acoustic startle and decreased exploration in an open field.

Several lines of evidence indicate that the LC-NE and CRH systems influence each other through a positive feedback loop. Direct application of CRH onto LC neurons in awake free-ranging rats markedly increases the LC firing rate. Conversely, NE is a potent stimulus to the *in vitro* release of hypothalamic CRH. Propranolol, a β-adrenergic receptor blocker, has been shown to attenuate the arousal producing-effects of centrally administered CRH.

Other Stress-Responsive Neurotransmitter Systems

The LC-NE and CRH-glucocorticoid systems do not constitute the only neuroendocrine and neurotransmitter responses to stress. Vasopressin, growth hormone (GH), and thyroid hormone are also released in response to acute stress, and luteinizing hormone release may be inhibited. These stress-responsive systems are intimately interrelated, and all contribute to the maintenance of homeostasis in the course of responding to environmental stresses. In the present discussion, we shall focus our attention on the CRH and LC-NE systems and their perturbations, but we shall also explore the potential role of other elements.

Recently, it has become evident that, like CRH, other stress-responsive hypothalamic releasing hormones and peptides are synthesized in cell bodies lying outside the hypothalamus, are widely distributed throughout the brain, and act in the CNS to exert specific receptor-mediated biologic actions and to coordinate complex behavioral and physiologic processes. Dissociation between the location of neuropeptides and their receptors is the rule rather than the exception in the CNS. This suggests that parasynaptic, hormonally mediated events constitute a significant mode of information processing in the brain. Moreover, recent work has shown that both neuropeptides and their receptors are particularly enriched in the areas of the brain known as the limbic system.

Pathophysiologic Mechanisms and Clinical Implications

To be successful, the generalized stress response not only must be poised to respond quickly and appropriately to a variety of stresses but also must have the capacity to respond quickly with counterregulatory elements in order not to hyperrespond or overshoot. The principal counterregulating elements of the generalized stress response are the adrenal glucocorticoids, which serve to restrain the CRH neuron, the LC-NE system, and the immunologic or inflammatory responses associated with injury incurred during a fight-or-flight situation.

Illnesses may arise from either deficient or excessive counterregulation of the stress response, with behavioral, endocrinologic, and immunologic consequences. Whereas a failure to counterregulate adequately the stress response has been described as an etiologic factor in melancholic depression (see later), recent data also suggest that excessive counterregulation of the stress response can result in certain behavioral syndromes, as well as alter susceptibility and resistance to inflammatory and infectious disease. For example, a rat strain that has excessive restraint of the CRH neuron during exposure to inflammatory stimuli has enhanced susceptibility to illnesses such as inflammatory arthritis, compatible with the hyperresponsive immune reaction expected in the absence of adequate glucocorticoid responses.

The hypothesis that adrenal cortical activity can reflect an individual's degree of emotional arousal or distress has been extensively studied during the past 3 decades. Over time, a consensus has developed that novelty and unpredictability, particularly if they overwhelm coping resources, are potent inducers of adrenal cortical activation. This model accounts for observations of normalization of HPA activity during chronic, stable stress situations. In addition, if an individual has an available behavioral or intrapsychic coping response, the glucocorticoid activation is reduced.

Although an individual's coping response is partly determined by social milieu, experience, and cognitive maturity, there appears to be a significant genetic component contributing to individual variability in stress responsiveness. Inhibited or fearful reactivity to novel stimuli in childhood is a trait that appears to show significant stability from infancy into childhood and adolescence. Twin studies have shown that this trait is inherited, and that the degree of physiologic reactivity to stress is also inherited and closely correlated to behavioral measures.

Recent studies in humans and animals have examined the neurobiologic mechanisms underlying these differences. Consistently inhibited children may have lower thresholds of excitability in the limbic system, particularly the amygdala and hypothalamus, leading to activation of the HPA axis and sympathetic nervous system. In support of this model, peripheral indications of increased sympathetic nervous system and HPA reactivity in cohorts of inhibited children have been demonstrated. In macaque monkeys, as in children, timid behavior and

exaggerated physiologic stress responses are stable and heritable traits. A similar stable trait has been identified in cats. In inhibited cats, electrical stimulation of the amygdala leads to greater propagation of activity from the amygdala to the hypothalamus than in noninhibited cats. When inhibited cats are presented with threatening stimuli, they have more prolonged increases in neural activity in the amygdala and hypothalamus than noninhibited cats. A role for the amygdala in the stress response is supported by evidence of abundant projections from the amygdala to the hypothalamic nuclei involved in neuroendocrine stress responses and the finding that electrical stimulation of the amygdala in a number of species leads to release of glucocorticoids.

A developmental phase of exaggerated behavioral responses to novelty appears to be a normal part of development for most mammalian species. In humans this occurs at approximately 7 months (manifested by stranger anxiety), in monkeys at 2 months, and in kittens at about 27 days of age. This period corresponds to the phase in cat brain development when the amygdala begins to modulate activity of hypothalamic nuclei involved in the stress response.

Despite the evidence of inherited sensitivity of limbic systems underlying inhibited behavior, animal work also suggests that hyperresponsiveness to stress may be created by repeated stimulation of central stress systems. Rats subjected to maternal deprivation during the neonatal period or situations of inescapable stress (the "learned helplessness" paradigm) show long-lasting hyperactivity of the HPA axis in response to stress. Perinatal handling of rats, which reliably alters adult levels of fearfulness, is also associated with altered binding of glucocorticoids in the prefrontal cortex and hippocampus.

These findings are intriguing in light of clinical evidence in humans that repeated trauma predisposes an individual to depression and anxiety disorders. It raises the possibility that a "kindling mechanism" could be involved in altering an individual's vulnerability to depression or other maladaptive neuroendocrine and behavioral responses to stress. *Kindling* refers to the process whereby the repeated application of electrical stimulation to the brain that is originally insufficient to produce seizures eventually leads to a permanent alteration in seizure threshold, so that the previously subthreshold stimuli produce major motor seizures. Continued application of these stimuli leads to the development of spontaneous seizure activity. Kindling can also be produced through the repeated administration of small doses of epileptogenic drugs. Although narrowly defined, kindling is a process resulting in the production of major motor seizures; the model may also be applicable to long-term alterations in neuronal excitability unrelated to seizure activity. Thus, repeated stress could increase the sensitivity of stress-responsive neuronal systems in the limbic system. For example, lasting inhibited behavior can be produced in noninhibited cats by repeated electrical stimulation of the ventromedial hypothalamic-hippocampal system. Of note, CRH is one of the few endogenous agents that, when given to rats via repeated intracerebroventricular injection, can induce seizures in the limbic system.

DEPRESSION (see Chapter 100)

Exaggerated physiologic reactivity may be a trait that places individuals at risk for development of depression and other psychiatric disorders (Table 12–1). For example, heightened reactivity to novel stimuli could impair development of social skills, self-esteem, and a sense of self-regulation. On a biologic level, dysregulation of stress-responsive systems may produce CNS changes manifested as psychiatric disturbance. A few long-term follow-up studies have shown correlations between childhood hyperresponsivity to novel stimuli and later psychiatric pathology.

Depression as a Syndromal Illness

Nonpsychiatric medical illnesses are most commonly discrete disease syndromes, with a characteristic constellation of symptoms, predictable course and response to treatment, and, most important, known etiology in the form of a demonstrable morphologic lesion or infectious agent. Illness categories, such as pneumococcal pneumonia or rheumatoid arthritis, are established in order that individuals may be grouped together and regarded as suffering from the same underlying disorder. The *diagnostic validity* of an illness generally refers to the extent to which the individuals so categorized do in fact represent a meaningful grouping and the extent to which the category is distinct from other similar disease

categories. *Diagnostic reliability,* on the other hand, refers to the extent to which different clinicians can agree in assigning a diagnosis to individuals. The issues of diagnostic validity and reliability are seldom given much consideration in those areas of medicine where the etiologic agent or lesion is demonstrable. However, few psychiatric illnesses are associated with known lesions. Therefore, diagnostic validity and reliability are of great importance in psychiatric research aimed at uncovering pathophysiologic mechanisms or demonstrating the efficacy of a treatment.

In adults, major depressive disorder is a syndromal diagnosis with well-established diagnostic validity, supported by a highly characteristic and cohesive constellation of clinical manifestations, a fairly predictable natural history and response to treatment, and evidence of familial inheritance and demonstrable biologic derangements (albeit no single, identifiable lesion). Diagnostic reliability, using modern diagnostic criteria, is excellent in research settings and fairly good in community clinical practice.

In adolescents, the syndrome of major depressive disorder can also be reliably identified in research settings with the use of standardized, structured diagnostic interviews. The essential clinical features are similar in children, adolescents, and adults. The diagnostic validity of child and adolescent depressive disorders and their continuity with adult depressive disorders is supported by familial aggregation studies and follow-up studies assessing outcome of depressed adolescents. The greatest familial morbidity for affective illness occurs in families of patients with onset of depression in childhood and adolescence. Outcome studies have demonstrated

TABLE 12–1. Parallels Between the General Adaptational Response to Stress and the Syndrome of Depression

TYPE OF CHANGE	STRESS	DEPRESSION
Redirection of behavior by the central nervous system	Acute facilitation of adaptive neural pathways	Chronic maladaptive facilitation of neural pathways
	Arousal, alertness	Dysphoric hyperarousal and anxiety
	Increased vigilance, focused attention	Hypervigilance, constricted focus, obsessiveness
	Aggressiveness when appropriate	Assertiveness inappropriately restrained by anxiety
	Acute inhibition of nonadaptive pathways	Maladaptive inhibition of neural pathways
	Decreased eating	Decreased eating
	Decreased libido and sexual behavior	Decreased libido and sexual behavior
	Appropriate caution or restraint	Excessive caution, regardless of context
Redirection of energy in the periphery	Oxygen and nutrients to the stressed body site	Oxygen and nutrients to the central nervous system
	Increased blood pressure, heart, and respiratory rates	Increased blood pressure, heart, and respiratory rates
	Increased gluconeogenesis	Increased gluconeogenesis
	Increased lipolysis	Increased lipolysis
	Inhibition of programs for growth and reproduction	Inhibition of programs for growth and reproduction
	Acute glucocorticoid-mediated counterregulatory responses (containment)	Chronic inadequate or maladaptive counterregulatory responses (containment)
	Restraint of the corticotropin-releasing hormone system and the pituitary-adrenal axis	Inadequate restraint of the corticotropin-releasing hormone system and the pituitary-adrenal axis
	Restraint of the norepinephrine–locus ceruleus system	Inadequate restraint of the norepinephrine–locus ceruleus system
	Restraint of the expected immunologic or inflammatory response	Chronic immunosuppression

With permission from Gold PW, Goodwin FK, Chrousos GP: Clinical and biochemical manifestations of depression. Relation to the neurobiology of stress [two parts]. N Engl J Med 319:348–353, 413–420, 1988.

recurrence of prepubertal and adolescent affective disorders in later life.

However, there are also reasons to question the validity of this diagnostic category in adolescents and to question the continuity between adolescent-onset and adult-onset depression. First, empirical studies using multivariate statistical techniques to analyze symptom reports of psychiatrically disturbed children and adolescents have suggested that misery and unhappiness are common and continuously distributed symptoms in behaviorally and emotionally disturbed children and adolescents, but they have provided only partial validation for the concept of major depression as a distinct diagnostic category in these age groups. Second, some of the neuroendocrine studies that have been completed in both adults and adolescents (discussed later) have yielded conflicting results in the two age groups (e.g., decreased nocturnal GH secretion in depressed adults, increased nocturnal growth hormone secretion in depressed adolescents). Finally, tricyclic antidepressant drugs that are effective in treating depression in adults have not been shown to be effective in the treatment of depression in adolescents.

More questionable syndromal diagnostic validity in adolescence compared with adulthood means that in studying depressed adolescents as a group and in comparing them with depressed adults we may be lumping together individuals with similar symptomatic presentations who in fact are suffering from different disease processes with different pathophysiologies. This would certainly obscure the results of research studies and must be kept in mind in assessing the meaning of negative findings.

Despite the evidence of differences between adolescent-onset and adult-onset depression, we feel that the weight of evidence, particularly family studies and follow-up studies, demonstrates that the two are closely linked, and that findings in adults are relevant to an understanding of adolescent depression. Therefore, we will review what is known with regard to the biology of depression in both adults and adolescents (and, to a lesser extent, in prepubertal children), keeping in mind that the disparate findings in similarly affected individuals of different ages may have as much to tell us as do the common findings. (See Table 12–2 for a summary of biologic findings in depression.)

Hypothalamic-Pituitary-Adrenal Axis

The clinical phenomenology of depressive illness points to several aspects of hypothalamic dysfunction. Depressed patients can demonstrate anorexia or hyperphagia, insomnia or hypersomnia, decreased libido, hypothalamic amenorrhea, and an apparent phase advance of rapid eye movement sleep and body temperature rhythms. These striking physiologic symptoms have made neuroendocrine investigations a principal focus of research efforts in depression. Furthermore, depression is associated with alterations in the synthesis and release of hypothalamic hormones into hypophyseal portal blood and the systemic circulation.

Pathologic activation of the HPA axis in depression is the most consistent and widely investigated biologic abnormality in psychiatry. Melancholic depression, the prototype of severe depressive illness, is characterized by an intensely painful, dysphoric hyperarousal, excessive guilt, and obsessional preoccupation with personal inadequacy and the inevitability of loss. Patients with this syndrome display early morning awakening, loss of appetite, and worsening of mood in the morning. The melancholic depressive syndrome may be conceptualized as a pathologic activation of the principal effectors of the generalized adaptational response, which have escaped their usual glucocorticoid-mediated counterregulation. This pathologic hyperarousal seems analogous to the behavioral changes noted in rats following central CRH administration.

ACTIVATION OF THE HPA AXIS IN MELANCHOLIC DEPRESSION

Several types of measures have been used to demonstrate activation of the HPA axis in melancholic depression. Twenty-four-hour blood sampling studies have shown elevation of the plasma cortisol level in patients with melancholic depression, with preservation of a circadian rhythm. Measurements of urinary free cortisol are also elevated. The dexamethasone suppression test (DST) has been intensively studied in depression. Patients tend not to show the normal suppression of cortisol secretion in response to a dose of the long-acting synthetic glucocorticoid dexamethasone. These measures of cortisol hypersecretion generally normalize with recovery from a depressive episode. HPA activation is less consistent in studies of depressed patients who are not selected for melancholic symptoms.

Three lines of evidence suggest that hypercortisolism in major melancholic depression reflects a defect at or above the hypothalamus, resulting in the hypersecretion of CRH. First, plasma ACTH responses to synthetic ovine CRH are attenuated in major depression, indicating that the pituitary corticotroph cell is appropriately restrained by the negative feedback effects of elevated glucocorticoids. Second, normal control subjects given a continuous infusion of CRH have a pattern and magnitude of hypercortisolism consistent with that seen in depression. Third, CRH in the CSF of depressed patients correlates positively with indices of pituitary-adrenal activation. In addition, elevated levels of CRH have been found in the CSF of patients with major depression.

HPA AXIS IN DEPRESSED CHILDREN AND ADOLESCENTS

HPA activity is less consistently elevated in studies of children and adolescents with major depression, consistent with the observation that the melancholic syndrome is less common in younger age groups. In studies using the DST, abnormal results have been found in several

TABLE 12–2. Biologic Findings in Depression

	DEPRESSED PREPUBERTAL CHILDREN	DEPRESSED ADOLESCENTS	DEPRESSED ADULTS
Hypothalamic-pituitary-adrenal axis			
Serum cortisol	NS	NS	↑
Urinary free cortisol	NS	NS	↑
DST nonsuppression	+/−	+/−	+
CRH levels in cerebrospinal fluid	−	−	↑
Hypothalamic-pituitary-thyroid axis			
TSH response to TRH	NS	NS	↓
TRH concentrations in CSF	−	−	↑
Locus ceruleus–norepinephrine system			
NE concentrations in plasma	−	−	↑
NE concentrations in CSF	−	−	↑
MHPG concentrations in urine	−	−	↑
MHPG concentrations in CSF	−	−	↑
GH response to clonidine	↓	NS	↓
GH response to GH-RH	−	−	↓
GH response to hypoglycemia	↓	−	↓
GH response to desipramine	NS	↓	↓
GH secretion during wakefulness	NS	↑	↑
GH secretion during sleep	↑	↑	↓
Serotonin system			
5-HIAA concentrations in CSF	−	−	↓
Uptake of serotonin by platelets	−	−	↓
Platelet serotonin receptor binding	−	−	↓

CRH, corticotropin-releasing hormone; CSF, cerebrospinal fluid; DST, dexamethasone suppression test; GH, growth hormone; GH-RH, growth hormone releasing hormone; 5-HIAA, 5-hydroxyindoleacetic acid; MHPG, 3-methoxy-4-hydroxyphenylglycol; NE, norepinephrine; TRH, thyrotropin-releasing hormone; TSH, thyroid-stimulating hormone.

↑, increased; ↓, decreased; −, indicates has not been studied; +, indicates abnormal findings in patient group; +/−, indicates conflicting or unclear findings; NS, no significant difference between patients and control subjects.

studies in prepubertal and adolescent depressed inpatients, but rates of abnormality are generally lower than those in adult depressed patients, and the specificity of the DST for major depression versus anxiety disorders and minor depressive disturbances is poor. In 24-hour blood sampling studies, prepubertal children and adolescents suffering from major depression do not hypersecrete cortisol. In addition, urinary free cortisol measures are not reliably elevated in adolescents with major depression.

This relative lack of HPA axis activation in depressed children and adolescents may be explained by the positive correlation of cortisol secretion and age in both normal and depressed adults. An age effect on DST nonsuppression has also been demonstrated. Related evidence comes from animal studies reporting an age influence on stress responses. For example, compared with adult rats, prepubertal rats show less HPA axis response to prolonged stress paradigms and attenuated cortisol responses to acute immobilization stress.

The kindling model of stress-responsive systems described earlier may be applicable to clinical observations regarding the course of depressive illness in humans. For example, the frequency and intensity of episodes of recurrent affective illness tend to increase as a function of the number of prior episodes. At the same time, the relationship between external environmental stressors and the onset of affective episodes becomes weaker and eventually disappears altogether so that the illness develops its own rhythm and spontaneity, independent of life events. Furthermore, anticonvulsant medications such as carbamazepine and valproic acid are effective in controlling recurrent affective illness.

Neurotransmitter Systems

The predisposition to developing depressive illness may also be associated with particular constellations of neurotransmitter abnormalities, which in turn contribute to the dysregulation of the general adaptation syndrome. In adults, research efforts have focused on the locus ceruleus–norepinephrine (or adrenergic) system, the serotonergic system, and the cholinergic system. These three neurotransmitter systems all modulate activity of the hypothalamic CRH neuron, show functional changes in depressed adults, and are the target of pharmacologic agents known to be effective in treatment of adult depression.

LOCUS CERULEUS–NOREPINEPHRINE SYSTEM

A number of studies in recent years indicate activation of the LC-NE system in melancholic depression. In highly aroused melancholic patients, using direct assay of NE and mass-spectroscopic assay of the NE metabolite 3-methoxy-4-hydroxyphenylglycol (MHPG), these studies report normal or increased levels of NE in CSF, increased plasma levels of NE, and increased CSF and urinary levels of MHPG. In addition, positive responses to antidepressant medications, even those that do not act principally on the NE system, are consistently associated with decreases in cerebrospinal fluid and plasma MHPG. These clinical data are consistent with preclinical data indicating that monoamine oxidase inhibitors and tricyclic antidepressants decrease the firing rate of the LC, reduce tyrosine hydroxylase messenger RNA (mRNA) levels in the LC, and reduce the level of NE metabolites in the brain. Tricyclic antidepressants and electroconvulsive treatment down-regulate the cortical β-adrenergic receptors that are thought to mediate the arousal-producing effects of NE. Tricyclic antidepressants also increase the density of glucocorticoid receptors and hippocampal mineralocorticoid receptor mRNA, as well as the expression of glucocorticoid receptor mRNA, all of which turn off the CRH and LC systems.

SEROTONIN SYSTEM

There also appears to be a subgroup of depressed adults who show a functional serotonin deficiency, evidenced by low CSF levels of the serotonin metabolite 5-hydroxyindoleacetic acid (5-HIAA), decreased uptake of serotonin into platelets, and reduced binding of ligands to the serotonin reuptake site on platelets. This subgroup of depressed patients is characterized by histories of violent suicidal acts and positive family histories for affective and bipolar illness. A major serotonin pathway begins in the midbrain raphe nuclei and projects axons into the hippocampus, amygdala, and other limbic structures. The mechanism of action of antidepressants in this population may be related to their ability to cause desensitization of postsynaptic serotonin receptors as well as adrenergic receptors.

Accumulating evidence suggests decreased central serotonin activity as a biologic marker of suicidal behavior. In adults, postmortem studies of suicide victims show a decrease in the brain content of serotonin and 5-HIAA. Also, serotonin receptor density, which is a measure more reflective of chronic serotonergic activity levels, shows changes consistent with a reduction in serotonergic functioning. In adults who attempt suicide, CSF concentrations of 5-HIAA are reduced relative to those of normal subjects. This finding has been consistent across diagnostic groups, including those with personality disorders, alcoholism, and schizophrenia. In addition, studies of a variety of patient populations, criminal offenders, and normal subjects have found an association between low CSF levels of 5-HIAA and history of aggressive behavior as well as impulsiveness and sensation-seeking behavior. As yet, there have been no studies of central serotonergic activity in adolescents who attempt suicide. However, low CSF levels of 5-HIAA have been associated with aggression in children and adolescents. Studies of platelet imipramine binding, a potential marker of central serotonergic function, have shown reductions of imipramine binding sites in children with conduct disorder. In primate and human studies, decreased CSF levels of 5-HIAA have been associated with social nondominance; in human studies, decreased CSF levels of 5-HIAA have been associated with decreased social competence and increased social stress.

CHOLINERGIC SYSTEM

Cholinergic supersensitivity leading to an imbalance of adrenergic and cholinergic influences has also been proposed to play a pathophysiologic role in depressive illness. Although much of the supporting evidence for this hypothesis comes from animal models of depression and stress responsivity, there is also some evidence from human studies. For example, administration of cholinomimetic agents or withdrawal from anticholinergic agents may worsen depressive symptoms in both depressed patients and normal individuals. These agents also can provoke positive DST responses in normal subjects. Furthermore, depressed patients show greater increases in ACTH secretion in response to cholinomimetics than do control subjects.

Differences in the pathophysiology of depression in children, adolescents, and adults may reflect maturational changes in these individual neurotransmitter systems and in the balances and interactions between them. In rats, catecholamine systems are not anatomically and functionally mature until the beginning of adulthood, whereas cholinergic and serotonergic systems become fully developed much earlier during the postnatal period. In humans, evidence for changes in these systems with development includes higher CSF concentrations of 5-HIAA and homovanillic acid, a dopamine metabolite, in children.

Hypothalamic-Pituitary-Thyroid Axis

Hypothyroidism is associated with an increased incidence of major depression. A consistent finding regarding perturbation of the thyroid axis in depression is the observation that the thyroid-stimulating hormone (TSH) response to thyrotropin-releasing hormone (TRH) administration is blunted in roughly 30% of depressed patients, despite the fact that most of these patients are apparently euthyroid.

The etiology and functional significance of the blunted TSH responses to TRH in major depression have not been elucidated. Because weight loss and hypercortisolism can influence the TSH response to TRH, these factors may have a role in the pathophysiology of this abnormality. It has also been argued that blunted TSH responses reflect a primary CNS disturbance that results in the hypersecretion of TRH and consequent down-regulation of TRH receptors at the pituitary. In two of three studies, CSF TRH levels have been reported to be elevated in depressed patients, consistent with down-regulation in response to elevated TRH. It should be noted that hypersecretion of TRH, like CRH, may have central behavioral effects contributing to the depressive syndrome. In animals, TRH reverses hibernation and barbiturate-induced sedation, stimulates locomotor activity, and inhibits food and water intake.

There is some evidence that this marker is age-dependent. Consistent with these observations, the TSH response to TRH in depressed prepubertal or adolescent samples is not different from that in normal subjects.

Growth Hormone

The growth hormone (GH) axis, like the HPA axis, is sensitive to stressful stimuli. During acutely threatening situations GH levels rise quickly and significantly. The only known function of acute GH secretion during stress is to increase metabolic fuel availability. It is possible that the acute secretion of growth hormone releasing hormone (GH-RH) during stress may also have behavioral implications. In contrast with the arousal-producing effects of CRH and TRH, GH-RH promotes sedation and food consumption, which may be construed as counterregulatory to the activating and anorexigenic effects of CRH.

GH function has been intensively studied in depressed children, adolescents, and adults. GH secretion during wakefulness is increased in depressed adults but has not been studied in depressed children or adolescents. Nocturnal GH secretion, on the other hand, is decreased in depressed adults but is increased in depressed children and adolescents. In both adults and children, the abnormal patterns of nocturnal GH secretion have been shown to persist after recovery from the depressive episode, suggesting that they are trait rather than state markers of depression. Nocturnal GH secretion after recovery has not been studied in adolescents. Developmental changes in the neural control of GH secretion may contribute to the observed differences between children, adolescents, and adults.

In addition, in depressed adults GH responses to several GH releasing challenges (insulin-induced hypoglycemia, desipramine, amphetamine, and clonidine) are blunted compared with those of control subjects. Reduced GH response to insulin-induced hypoglycemia has been demonstrated in depressed prepubertal children. In depressed adolescents, the GH response to desmethylimipramine is decreased compared with that of normal control subjects. As with nocturnal GH hypersecretion, the blunted GH response to hypoglycemia in depressed prepubertal children persists after recovery.

Noradrenergic, serotonergic, and cholinergic systems, all implicated in the pathophysiology of major depression, contribute to regulation of GH secretion. Changes in these neurotransmitter systems could affect GH release at the pituitary level or by affecting release of GH-RH from the hypothalamus.

The finding that GH responses to GH-RH infusion are attenuated in depression suggests that hypersecretion of GH-RH may down-regulate the pituitary secretory cell receptors and contribute to the blunted GH responses. The hypothesis of chronic GH-RH hypersecretion is also supported by evidence of elevated peripheral somatomedin C levels that restrain the pituitary GH releasing cell in response to a variety of stimuli, including GH-RH.

Another possible central mechanism underlying GH hypersecretion in depression is impairment of the usual GH inhibitory effect of somatostatin at the pituitary. CSF levels of somatostatin are reduced in depressed adults. A negative correlation between postdexamethasone cortisol levels and CSF somatostatin levels in depressed patients and prednisone-induced decreases in CSF levels of somatostatin suggests that the reduction in CSF somatostatin may be a reflection of the hypercortisolism of depression.

Hypothalamic-Pituitary-Gonadal Axis

Major depression is frequently associated with loss of libido, and in some women, with menstrual disturbances, including secondary amenorrhea. These disturbances may stem from a reduction in the release of the hypothalamic hormone luteinizing hormone releasing hormone (LH-RH). Evidence points to a role for LH-RH in the coordination of sexual behavior and menstrual cycling. For example, in animals, intracerebroventricular administration of LH-RH can stimulate performance of mating behavior patterns.

Inhibition of sexual functioning is adaptive in situations of stress, when metabolic and behavioral resources need to be conserved for coping activities. In adults, glucocorticoid administration is associated with lower levels of LH in men and women and lower levels of testosterone in men. Glucocorticoids have been shown to inhibit reproductive function at the hypothalamic, pituitary, and gonadal levels. Hence, the pituitary-adrenal activation associated with depression could potentially act at multiple levels to inhibit both behavioral and physiologic aspects of reproductive function. The implication of this interaction for adolescents is that chronic adrenal activation in response to ongoing stress may suppress the gonadal axis, leading to delayed physical maturation and reproductive function.

Gonadal steroid levels have been shown to have striking influences on the neurotransmitter systems involved in the pathophysiology of depression and on the neurochemical substrates of psychotropic drug effects. Levels of gonadal hormones change dramatically with puberty. In nonpsychiatrically disturbed early adolescent girls, increases in depressed mood and decreases in impulse control correlate significantly with the rapid changes in hormonal status in midpuberty. Changes in androgen levels during puberty correlate with changes in self-perceptions of cognitive, social, and physical competence. Although both boys and girls show these correlations between hormone levels and changes in mood, behavior, and self-image, there are significant differences between the sexes in the characteristic patterns of changes that take place (see Chapter 13).

More information is needed about the normal patterns of development of neurotransmitter and neuroendocrine function and interaction from childhood, through puberty and adolescence, and into adulthood. Animal studies will be particularly vital in increasing our understanding of these developmental changes.

OTHER STRESS-RELATED PSYCHIATRIC ILLNESSES

Atypical Depression

The pathologic hyperarousal of melancholic depression represents the classic and best described major depressive syndrome. In contrast with this state of intense arousal, however, is the pathologic inactivation of another major depressive syndrome, commonly referred to as atypical depression. In many respects, this syndrome seems to be the antithesis of melancholic depression. Patients with atypical depression suffer from hyperphagia and hypersomnia rather than the anorexia and insomnia characteristic of melancholic depression. In contrast with the intense anxiety about self and the ruminative preoccupation with the inevitability of loss characteristic of melancholia, patients with atypical depression seem passive, anergic, and apathetic, and their sensitivity to loss is more reactive in nature.

These marked differences in the clinical manifestations of the melancholic and atypical depressive syndromes are associated with differences in associated biochemical features. For example, whereas hypercortisolism is the cardinal neuroendocrine manifestation of melancholic depression, this finding is generally absent in patients with atypical depression. Several preliminary lines of evidence suggest that there is a pathologic inactivation of the CRH or LC-NE system, or both, in atypical depression.

It is difficult to demonstrate a decrease in the functional activity of the HPA axis from the plasma cortisol level alone. Several illnesses associated with atypical depression features seem to produce an inactivation of the CRH system due to a variety of disparate pathophysiologic mechanisms. For example, the atypical depression that almost invariably accompanies Cushing disease is associated with a marked decrease in the levels of CSF CRH (see Chapter 55). Patients with the chronic fatigue syndrome show a marked reduction in plasma free cortisol concentrations associated with diminished plasma ACTH responses to exogenous CRH, indicative of possible insufficiency in the priming of the pituitary corticotroph cell by endogenous CRH (see Chapter 93). Recent data also suggest a similar central CRH deficiency in hypothyroidism, indicated by both the basal cortisol levels and their responses to CRH in patients with hypothyroidism, as well as the demonstration that hypothyroid rats show increased expression of glucocorticoid receptor number in the hippocampus. Finally, the lack of HPA activation in depressed adolescents compared with depressed adults is consistent with findings of an increased incidence of atypical symptoms in depressed adolescents.

Eating Disorders (see Chapter 60)

Anorexia nervosa is another syndrome with psychiatric manifestations with significant dysregulation in hypothalamic function, manifested by hypercortisolism, hypothalamic hypogonadism, abnormalities of plasma and CSF vasopressin secretion, and hypersecretion of GH. Women with anorexia nervosa achieve a low body weight by restricting their food intake and increasing their activity; they are obsessively preoccupied with fears of gaining weight. A related condition, bulimia nervosa (see Chapter 60), is characterized by episodic binge eating accompanied by a desire to purge by vomiting,

diuretics, laxatives, exercise, or fasting. Bulimia may be found in conjunction with anorexia nervosa or independently. Normal-weight bulimics do not show the profound hypercortisolism associated with anorexia and other starvation states. However, as a consequence of food restriction between binges, they show other metabolic signs of malnourishment. Anorexia nervosa and bulimia nervosa occur predominantly in young women, and there is an increased incidence of affective illness in the personal and family histories of women with anorexia and bulimia.

In contrast with melancholic depression, in anorexia nervosa and bulimia nervosa, indices of LC-NE system function are generally diminished. Clearly, down-regulation of the sympathetic nervous system is necessary for survival during periods of food restriction or excessive exercise, since sympathetic tone is a major determinant of thermogenesis and metabolic rate. Since it appears from human and animal data that central noradrenergic tone is down-regulated in parallel with peripheral noradrenergic activity during caloric restriction, anorectic behavior may serve to reduce anxiety by limiting activation of the LC.

Anxiety Disorders
(see Chapters 102 and 103)

A substantial body of evidence has accumulated demonstrating important relationships among depression and anxiety disorders, especially panic disorder in adolescents and adults, and separation anxiety disorder of childhood. Panic disorder is a common psychiatric disorder characterized by recurrent panic attacks—discrete periods of intense fear or discomfort accompanied by a variety of characteristic psychic and somatic symptoms that occur unexpectedly and last for minutes to hours. Depression, panic disorder, and separation anxiety disorder of childhood commonly occur together in the same individual. They also tend to occur within families, so the family members of individuals with one of these disorders are also at increased risk for the other disorders. All three disorders respond to treatment with antidepressant medications.

It has been suggested that these different clinical presentations may be the manifestations of a common underlying disorder and that the common pathophysiologic deficit is in the regulation of the affective response to the stress of separation experiences. In fact, a number of empirical studies have found an increased incidence of stressful separation experiences preceding the onset of depressive illness, panic disorder, or separation anxiety disorder. Recent work following the course of young children identified as behaviorally inhibited in novel, stressful circumstances suggests that it is even possible to identify individuals with this pathophysiologic deficit prior to the onset of psychiatric disorder, that is, to identify vulnerable individuals. As we have previously discussed, the trait appears to be heritable. Analogous behavioral response styles have been identified in a number of animal models, appear to be stable across the life span of individual animals, and also predict vulnerability to maladaptive, anxiety-like, or depression-like responses to stressful circumstances, especially separation from mother or from other familiar conspecifics (see Chapter 15). Similar neurobiologic and pharmacologic response patterns have been demonstrated in these animal models. For example, the characteristic behavioral responses to separation from peers seen in young rhesus monkeys, distress vocalization in puppies precipitated by separation from littermates, and isolation calls in adult squirrel monkeys all are blocked by imipramine. In rhesus monkeys, intra-individual differences in reactions to social separations show correlations not only with the separation responses of genetic relatives but also with environmental variables, such as the mothering style of natural or foster mothers, as well as with variations in early rearing experiences.

In light of the pathophysiologic or genetic link between panic disorder and depression, it is interesting that CRH, which seems to have a role in the pathophysiology of depression, may have an integrative role in this severe anxiety syndrome as well. The central anxiogenic effects of CRH dovetail with the clinical impression of central sympathetic nervous system activation during panic attacks because, as noted earlier, the LC-NE and CRH systems seem to participate in a mutually reinforcing feedback loop.

Studies of adult patients with panic disorder, which were conducted during the basal state between panic attacks, have demonstrated some differences from normal adults. Patients with panic disorder have greater anxiety and enhanced release of the NE metabolite MHPG in response to the alpha$_2$-adrenergic antagonist yohimbine. They also have blunted growth hormone responses to a variety of pharmacologic and physiologic stimulants of growth hormone release. Studies of HPA axis function in patients with panic disorder have produced conflicting results. Most studies of patients with panic disorder who are not depressed have failed to demonstrate increased rates of dexamethasone nonsuppression or increased levels of urinary free cortisols. Two studies have shown a blunted ACTH response to CRH infusion, suggesting hypersecretion of CRH, and these same two studies also reported lower ACTH-to-cortisol ratios, suggesting adrenal hyperresponsiveness. This pattern of response to CRH infusion parallels that seen in depression. Both studies report that blunting of the ACTH response did not correspond to the severity of depressive symptoms, suggesting hypersecretion of CRH independent of coexisting depression.

CONCLUSION

The prominent role played by stress-responsive neurotransmitters in the pathophysiology of major depression and related illnesses is consistent with clinical observations that the appearance and natural history of these illnesses are influenced by the burdens of intense conflict, counterproductive psychological defenses, and external stresses. Although the proximal cause of these illnesses has not been definitively identified, the weight of available data suggests that they may, in part, be determined by a dysregulation of the apparatus ordinarily called into play to counterregulate appropriately elements of the generalized stress response. Abnormalities in the CRH system in each of these disorders suggest a final common pathway conferring some pathophysiologic similarity among the disorders.

We have attempted to elucidate both the similarities and the dissimilarities among biologic findings in depressed adolescents and depressed adults. We have also pointed out that, given the incomplete development of neurobiologic systems and the dramatic shifts in hormonal status that occur from prepuberty to adolescence to adulthood, dissimilarities in the neuroendocrine and neurotransmitter controls over physiologic reactivity to stress and disturbances in those controls (as manifested by depressive illness) are to be expected, even among individuals who are afflicted with the same illness. In other words, these dissimilarities do not necessarily invalidate the continuity of adolescent-onset and adult-onset depression. By analogy, varicella in a toddler and varicella in a young adult are the same illness, despite the different clinical manifestations and pathophysiologic derangements that ensue following infection. In fact, many biologic findings in depressed children and adolescents are in general similar to findings in depressed adults. The markers that do differ are those that tend to show significant changes with age in normal individuals.

There are likely to be a number of pathophysiologic abnormalities that independently can contribute to dysregulation of the stress response. One or more pathophysiologic abnormalities in an individual are likely to modulate or increase vulnerability to psychiatric illness.

Similarly, environmental influences such as personal losses or adaptive role models may set in motion responses that interact with the unique physiologic strengths and vulnerabilities of an individual. We have focused exclusively on neurophysiologic processes, on the brain rather than the mind. But just as physiologic responsiveness to stress may change during the course of development, the experience of this physiologic responsiveness also changes. As young people learn to label their emotional states, put stress in context, and develop a stable sense of self and their capacity for mastery, they develop cognitive and affective capacities to modulate stress (see Chapter 9). Conversely, repetitive traumatic life experiences may induce a sense of helplessness and incompetence in the face of arousal or stress and exacerbate maladaptive physiologic responses. Because they are more susceptible to stress, physiologically vulnerable children may hamper their development by avoiding stressful circumstances, further limiting their opportunities to acquire more adaptive coping strategies. Thus, physiologic differences and environmental influences should not be regarded as independent. They interact in determining any given individual's unique responses to the vicissitudes of life.

BIBLIOGRAPHY

Altemus M, Gold PW: Neuroendocrinology and psychiatric illness. Frontiers in Neuroendocrinology 11:238, 1990.

Gold PW, Goodwin FK, Chrousos GP: Clinical and biochemical manifestations of depression. Relation to the neurobiology of stress (two parts). N Engl J Med 319:348, 413, 1988.

Kagan J, Snidman N, Reznick JS: The constructs of inhibition and lack of inhibition to unfamiliarity in children. In Palermo DS (ed): Coping with Uncertainty. Hillsdale, NJ, Laurence Erlbaum Assoc., 1989, pp 131–149.

Kreusi MJP, Rapopórt JL, Hamburger S, et al: Cerebrospinal fluid monoamine metabolites, aggression and impulsivity in disruptive behavior disorders of children and adolescents. Arch Gen Psychiatry 47:419, 1990.

Levine S: A definition of stress? In Mosberg GP (ed): Animal Stress. Bethesda, MD, American Physiological Society, 1985, pp 51–69.

Post RM, Ballenger JC: Conditioning, sensitization, and kindling: implications for the course of affective illness. In Post R (ed): Neurobiology of Mood Disorders. Baltimore, Williams & Wilkins, 1984, pp 432–465.

Puig-Antich J: Affective disorders in children and adolescents: Diagnostic validity and psychobiology. In Meltzer HY (ed): Psychopharmacology: The Third Generation of Progress. New York, Raven Press, 1987, pp 843–859.

Suomi SJ: Genetic and maternal contributions to individual differences in rhesus monkey biobehavioral development. In Krasnegor NA, Blass EM, Hofer MA, Smotherman WP (eds): Perinatal Development: A Psychobiological Perspective. Orlando, FL, Academic Press, 1987, pp 397–419.

Warren MP, Brooks-Gunn J: Mood and behavior at adolescence: Evidence for hormonal factors. J Clin Endocrinol Metab 69:77, 1989.

CHAPTER 13

Hormones and Behavior

ELIZABETH J. SUSMAN and ANNE C. PETERSEN

INTRODUCTION

Within the last few decades, associations have been demonstrated among the levels of various circulating hormones and behavior in many species, including human adolescents. These findings tend to support century-old speculations regarding the role of hormones as modulators of human behavior. This chapter presents contemporary information about the relationship of hormones and behavior during adolescence.

A brief explanation about the theoretical limitations of conducting and interpreting newer research in this area is necessary. To date, all studies have been nonexperimental. Ethically, it is not possible to manipulate hormone levels of normal humans merely in order to test specific hypotheses. Investigators must rely on either mistakes of nature (i.e., endocrine abnormalities causing states of hormone deficiency, excess, or insensitivity) or careful documentation of naturally occurring covariation of hormone levels and specific behaviors in normal subjects. Although sensitive, highly reliable methods of measuring hormones and neuropeptides are now available, interpretation of these values is sometimes difficult, because they are attempts to describe a very dynamic, biologic system in static terms. This is particularly problematic during the peripubertal period, when the previously established diurnal variations in secretion of hypothalamic, pituitary, adrenal, and gonadal hormones undergo dramatic changes. (See Chapter 4 for a discussion of secretory patterns of follicle-stimulating hormone and luteinizing hormone and Chapters 12 and 100 for hormonal changes in depression.) Moreover, it is becoming clearer that many, if not all, of the hypothalamic neuropeptides are secreted in a pulsatile fashion, with changes in amplitude and frequency over developmental periods. It is not yet clear how one best samples biologic fluids in order to describe adequately hormone secretory patterns, especially during certain developmental periods. In addition, it is well known that there is considerable transformation of one hormone to another at the cellular level. (See adrenal steroid discussion in Chapter 58.) The biologically or behaviorally active hormone may not be the one that is measured in the blood. In this instance the characteristic rate-limiting enzymes may be more important than peripheral blood hormone levels.

Parallel advances in analytic techniques for both social and behavioral science data permit investigators statistically to control for known confounding variables (fac-

tors) in order to compensate for the inability to manipulate experimentally subjects and sample selection. Unknown confounding factors become increasingly important in their ability to introduce bias when the observed relationships among variables are weak—the situation with most of the current findings in this area. These newer multivariate statistical techniques (broadly referred to as causal modeling) are powerful tools when combined with theoretically sound investigations driven by hypotheses. They permit the careful investigator to infer the direction of associations using cross-sectional and longitudinal study designs. Especially in longitudinal studies, the investigator often uses causal effects to describe these antecedent factors. The reader should keep in mind how the term *causal* is used in this chapter. It refers to a relationship between independent and dependent variables that remains statistically significant when theoretically possible alternative hypotheses have been explored. In those situations in which investigators inappropriately use biologic or social science methods, the results may simply be a meaningless array of statistically significant associations. The reader must critically evaluate all research.

HISTORICAL PERSPECTIVE

The activating effects of hormones on adolescent behavior constitute a central premise in virtually all contemporary theories of adolescent psychological development. Specifically, theories of psychosocial development (see Chapter 9) hypothesize the effects of hormones on emotions and libidinal urges. In spite of their hypothesized importance, until the last decade, the evidence of the activating influences of hormones on behavior remained anecdotal. During the 1980s, empirical findings on the concurrent associations among circulating levels of adrenal and gonadal hormones and behavior in adolescents were presented. The current interest in the activating influences of hormones stems from observations of neuroendocrine relationships in certain mental health disorders (anxiety, anorexia nervosa, depression, schizophrenia) (see Chapters 12, 100, 103, and 110) and other findings suggesting a relationship to the subtle, yet pervasive behavior changes and lability of adolescents.

Explorations of the interaction between hormone levels and behavior in adolescents were not possible until relatively recently. The animal research model previously used in behavioral-endocrine research consisted of ablation of the source of the hormone, observation of behavior, restoration of the hormone by exogenous administration, and repeated observations of behavior. An alternative approach was adopted by Beach (1975), who suggested that causal relationships could be inferred from the covariation of behavioral and hormonal events. Guided by the findings from research with small mammals and primates, hypotheses then were formulated regarding covariations between hormones and behavior in humans.

Technologic advances in endocrinology, paralleling the shifts in the hormone behavior research model, made descriptive studies of human adolescents possible. These advances included the measurement of minute amounts of circulating hormones in both prepubertal and pubertal adolescents (see Chapter 4 for related advances in the neuroendocrinology of puberty); the development of behavioral endocrinology as a new field devoted to the study of effects of hormones on animal and human behaviors and the effects of social experiences on hormone levels; and demonstration of systematic associations of endocrine abnormalities with variations in behavior that led to hypotheses about normal hormonal processes and behavior (e.g., androgen exposure and masculinized behavior) (see Chapter 120).

BEHAVIORS RELATED TO HORMONES

Many psychological characteristics have been examined to date, including aggression, moods and emotionality, and cognition.

Aggression

Aggression is behavior aimed at causing physical and psychological harm to others and includes both emotional and behavioral components. Aggression is the behavior most commonly linked to androgenic hormones. The long-standing hypothesis that androgenic hormones are related to aggression is derived from observations that males are more likely to fight and have higher levels of androgens than are females. Therefore, the two are hypothesized to be causally related.

Moods and Emotionality

In the context of this chapter we use *moods* to refer to those emotions that tend to be precipitated by specific events; they may be relatively short-lived (see Chapter 100 for discussion of moods in the context of psychological behavior). Emotionality includes a broader array of moods and emotions and is the concept now used in the study of hormones and behaviors. The hypothesis that hormone levels and degree of emotions covary is derived from the observation that hormones change rapidly and dramatically during specific developmental periods, including puberty, pregnancy, and menopause, and during the menstrual cycle. Emotions are thought to vary in intensity and lability during these periods.

In laboratory and field studies, the interactions among stress-related emotionality and the levels of adrenal and gonadal hormones are well documented. (See Chapter 12 for a discussion of the influence of emotions, including clinical depression, on the hypothalamic-pituitary-adrenal [HPA] axis.)

Cognition

Many studies have examined hormonal hypotheses to explain the gender differences in spatial ability, one of the few reliable differences in cognition between the sexes. Hormonal hypotheses have been both organizational (i.e., prenatal) and activating (i.e., pubertal). Although Waber's initial report suggesting the possibility of activating effects contained promising results (Waber et al, 1985), the preponderance of evidence suggests that prenatal hormones more probably exert influences on cognition (an organizational effect of hormones), because the gender differences in spatial ability are demonstrated well before puberty.

Hormonal effects on other aspects of cognition have been investigated through studies of variations during the menstrual cycle. Although most studies of cognitive performance find no differences, when actual responses rather than self-reports are assessed, decrements in visual acuity during ovulation have been observed. Hampson and Kimura (1988) reported that women in the midluteal phase (when estrogen and progesterone are high) showed improved performance on speeded motor coordination and on perceptual-spatial tests as compared with performance during menses. No studies to date have examined performance on cognitive tasks and concurrent levels of hormones. Despite the indirect lines of evidence suggesting the possible effects of pubertal hormones on cognition during adolescence, data are not yet available to support this hypothesis.

MECHANISMS OF HORMONE-BEHAVIOR INTERACTIONS

The major hypothesized mechanisms of hormone-behavior interactions include the effects of hormones on the central nervous system (CNS), the organizing and the activating influences of hormones on behavior, and the reciprocal interactions of hormones and behavior.

Regulation of the CNS by hormones is now well known from animal studies. Hormone-related CNS alterations, in turn, affect a diverse array of behaviors. Specifically, it is widely accepted that gonadal steroids are neuroregulators of the CNS, primarily in the thalamic and hypothalamic areas. The exact mechanisms involved in CNS regulation by gonadal and other hormones, either directly or indirectly, are not completely understood (see Chapters 4 and 12).

The original approach to explaining hormone actions on behavior was conceptualized in terms of the organizing and activating influences of hormones. Organizing influences stem from prenatal and perinatal hormone exposure that affects the structure or functioning of the CNS such that development is altered. Activating influences of hormones stem from contemporaneous effects of hormone levels on behavior. Thus, pubertal-related hormone changes are hypothesized to have primarily activating influences on behavior. An example is the increase in aggressive behavior during the pubertal period, which is attributed to hormonal influences. Current research is focused on elucidating the molecular basis of hormone action at the cellular level.

One interactive model recognized that hormones both influence and are influenced by behavior. Leshner (1977) has proposed mechanisms that involve activation of neurotransmitters in disparate brain regions. Changes in the endocrine milieu are thought to alter the responsiveness of the organism to stimulation. Under this influence of emotion-eliciting stimuli, the organism's level of reactivity or arousability is a function of the interaction of hormonal and neural baseline conditions.

The CNS also mediates hormone secretion. Stimulation of the areas of the brain known to be involved in emotionality (the amygdala, anterior medial hypothalamus, hippocampus, and septal areas) affects hormone levels. Thus, emotionality may affect stress hormones, their secretory patterns, the limbic system, and other neural structures. The fight-or-flight response is one example of the effects of behavior on the CNS.

Hormones and Adolescent Psychological Development

Two models have been used to investigate the relationship of hormones and adolescent psychological development (Petersen and Taylor, 1980). The direct-effects model specifies that the hormonal changes associated with puberty directly influence psychological development. The organizing and activating influence of puberty-related hormones on behavior is consistent with a direct-effects model. The indirect-effects model is an inclusive model that takes into account the multiple influences on adolescent psychological development. In this model, the hormone-induced physical maturational changes of puberty serve as a social stimulus to others that adolescents should begin to behave like adults. Adolescents then change their behavior to fit the demands of their environmental contexts.

SEXUAL DIFFERENTIATION AND GENDER DIFFERENCES

At conception, the brain is inherently female. Sex differences in CNS function are due, to a large degree, to the hormonally induced sexual differentiation of the brain after embryonic differentiation of the testis or ovary early in prenatal development. In male animals, sexual differentiation results from exposure of the brain to testicular hormones. In female animals, in the absence of testicular secretions during the critical period, a neural substrate develops that is responsible for the cyclical pattern of hormones necessary for reproduction.

The extent to which sexual differentiation during early gestation influences later gender differences in behavior remains controversial. At the heart of the controversy on gender differences in behavior is the issue of the relative importance of early organizing influences of hormones compared with postnatal socialization influences. One speculation is that the organizing influence of sex steroids, for instance, may sensitize individuals in such a way that males and females differ with regard to readiness for certain types of emotional responses. Prenatally, males are exposed to higher levels of testosterone and therefore may be more sensitive than females to subsequent androgen exposure. Hines (Hines and Shipley, 1984) has speculated that high exposure to either exogenous or endogenous androgens during fetal development shifts later behavior in a male-typical direction. Studies of individuals with endocrine disorders that cause abnormally high levels of hormones during the prenatal period, primarily androgens, or of offspring of women who received exogenous androgens or progestins during pregnancy have supported the belief that prenatal hormones have an organizing effect on gender-specific behavior.

Endogenous Androgen Exposure

Congenital adrenal hyperplasia (CAH) (see Chapter 55) has been of particular interest in studies examining the relationship between abnormal prenatal hormone levels and later behavioral development, since the adrenal cortex releases an excess of adrenal androgens from early fetal life. Ehrhardt and colleagues (see Chapter 120) have shown that CAH (prenatally androgenized) females, treated early to correct hormone secretory patterns and surgically corrected, exhibited significantly more tomboy behavior, identified themselves as tomboys, and showed less interest in parenting behavior (low interest in doll care) than did a sibling or a matched control.

Turner syndrome (see Chapter 55), characterized by gonadal dysgenesis resulting in defective endogenous production of estrogens, has been associated with deficits in cognition. Nyborg and Nielsen (1982) showed that long-term estrogen-treated and untreated women with Turner syndrome were more deficient in spatial skills than were their nonaffected siblings. The findings were interpreted as suggesting that estrogen deficits may influence CNS structures and thereby adversely affect the development of spatial skills.

Exogenous Hormones

The effects of administration of estrogens on cognitive abilities and cerebral lateralization were reported by Hines and Shipley (1984) as further evidence of the organizing effects of prenatal hormone exposure on behavior. Women who were exposed to diethylstilbestrol (DES), a synthetic estrogen, were compared with their nonexposed siblings on measures of cognitive abilities and cerebral lateralization. Estrogen is believed to act at the cellular level to masculinize aspects of brain and behavioral development. The DES-exposed women showed a more masculine pattern of cerebral lateralization and performance on a listening task than did their nonexposed siblings. In a parallel study of high prenatal exposure to progestins, Reinisch (1981) reported that exposed children exhibited aggressive response tendencies and masculine personality characteristics. The findings were interpreted as suggesting that the altered prenatal endocrine milieu—high prenatal estrogen exposure—propels development in the direction of masculine functioning.

Together, the findings might be interpreted as suggesting that early prenatal organizing influences have a pervasive impact on behavioral development. The caveats to this conclusion are that the observed differences in cognitive performance and personality are neither consistent nor large, the studies reporting the findings are few, and the degree of masculine or otherwise atypical appearance was not assessed. Finally, although behavior may be oriented in a masculine direction, high prenatal estrogen exposure did not result in extreme social or intellectual impairment.

RESEARCH ON HORMONES AND BEHAVIOR IN ADOLESCENTS

Money and Ehrhardt (1968) were the first to examine the role of gonadal hormones in childhood aggression by examining girls with hermaphroditism. Hermaphroditic girls were characterized by more tomboyish behavior than their nonaffected peers. The more male-like behavior cannot necessarily be attributed to the effects of hormones, since hermaphroditic girls' more male-like appearance may encourage participation in masculine behavior as compared with normal females. Circulating hormone levels were not examined in these early studies.

Scandinavian Study

A Scandinavian longitudinal study examined testosterone (T) levels and aggressive behavior in 15- to 17-year-old males (Olweus et al, 1980). The boys were rated primarily in Tanner sexual maturity stage five, with fewer than 25% in stages three and four (see Chapter 5). The adolescents completed personality inventories including self-reports of provoked and unprovoked aggression.

The mean T level was lower at the first time of testing than 1 month later. T levels were related to reports of physical and verbal aggression resulting from provocation. These data also suggested that acute states of anxiety (e.g., during venipuncture) may briefly suppress T secretion.

In a recently published report from the same study (Olweus et al, 1988), the causal role of T in provoked and unprovoked aggression was examined. Consistent with causal data analytic strategies, the variables thought to be antecedent were first controlled: mother's negativ-

ism, boy's temperament, mother's and father's power assertiveness, provoked aggressive behavior, and low frustration tolerance. Based on path analysis, the findings suggest that, at grade 9, there is a direct causal relationship between T and provoked aggressive behavior. The findings also suggest that T may lower a younger boy's frustration tolerance. The authors conclude that a higher level of T leads to an increased readiness to respond with vigor and assertion to provocation and threat.

For unprovoked aggressive behavior (starting fights and saying nasty things), the findings were somewhat different. Testosterone had no direct effect on unprovoked aggressive behavior; there was an indirect effect of T, with low frustration tolerance as the mediating variable. The authors conclude that higher levels of aggression in puberty made the boys more impatient and irritable, which, in turn, increased readiness to engage in unprovoked aggressive behavior. Overall, the findings indicate that T had effects on provoked and unprovoked aggressive behavior when selected variables were controlled.

Adolescent Study Program

The Adolescent Study Program (Brooks-Gunn and Warren, 1989) has examined puberty-related psychological and biologic processes. The study focused on emotionality (primarily depression and aggressive tendencies), life events, and hormones of gonadal and adrenal origin among white, 10- to 14-year-old, middle- to upper-middle-class girls.

Measures included self-reports of emotional states, depressed-withdrawal and aggressive affect; life events; sexual maturity rating of pubertal development; and hormonal assessment (luteinizing hormone [LH], follicle-stimulating hormone [FSH], estradiol [E_2], T, and dehydroepiandrosterone sulfate [DHEAS]).

Girls were divided into four estrogen groupings: 2–25 pg/ml; 26–50 pg/ml; 51–74 pg/ml; and greater than 75 pg/ml. Depressive affect increased between the first and third categories and decreased between the third and fourth categories. Aggressive affect was linearly and negatively associated with DHEAS; that is, the higher the aggressive affect, the lower the DHEAS. The authors concluded that although hormone effects were found, they should be considered along with other developmental processes. Age was not related to the increase in negative affect. Negative life events, however, were associated with negative affect, suggesting that social factors may overshadow hormonal factors to a great extent.

A second aspect of the study examined hormonal levels, pubertal development, self-reported psychological functioning (psychopathology, behavior problems, mastery and competence, relations with others, and body image), interest in sports, and depressive mood as perceived by mothers. The girls were again grouped according to the E_2 levels described earlier. The relationships between hormones and psychological measures were curvilinear. Removal of the effects of age enhanced the hormonal effects. The researchers concluded that certain behaviors change at midpuberty and the changes may be biologically mediated. Adolescent girls may be more vulnerable to depressive affect at certain stages of puberty, primarily at the time when there are the most rapid changes in hormone levels. For depression and psychopathology there was an increase in the middle two hormonal stages (26–50 and 51–75 pg/ml), followed by a decline. Impulse control showed a curvilinear decline from the first (2–25 pg/ml) to the second stage (26–50 pg/ml) and an increase from the second to the third and fourth stages. Interest in sports was higher in stage one than in stage three. It was also negatively correlated with serum DHEAS and T.

NIMH-NICHHD Study

A collaborative study between the National Institute of Mental Health (NIMH) and the National Institute of Child Health and Human Development (NICHHD) examined multiple aspects of social and emotional behavioral development and hormone and pubertal processes in 108 adolescent boys (ages 10 to 14 years) and girls (ages 9 to 14 years). Subjects were assessed on three occasions, at 6-month intervals. One hypothesis was that higher levels of androgens (primarily T, and to a lesser extent the adrenal androgens) were related to higher levels of aggressive behavior (Susman et al, 1987). Negative emotions were assumed to be involved in the pathway between hormone levels and aggressive behavior.

For boys only, higher levels of emotional tone (sad and anxious affect) were related to lower T-to-E_2 ratio, testosterone-estradiol–binding globulin (TeBG), and higher levels of Δ^4-androstenedione. Higher scores on delinquent behavior problems were related to lower levels of E_2 and higher levels of Δ^4-androstenedione. Higher scores on rebellious attitude were related to higher levels of LH, lower levels of FSH, and higher levels of DHEA. When emotional dispositions and aggressive attributes were considered together with hormones, the following pattern of findings emerged: Higher scores on delinquent behavior problems were related to lower T-to-E_2 ratios, lower levels of TeBG, and lower levels of DHEAS. Anxiety also was related to delinquent behavior problems.

From the same sample of adolescents, Nottelmann and colleagues (1987) reported that adjustment problems were associated with a hormone profile similar to that previously described for aggressive attributes: higher Δ^4-androstenedione and lower T levels or a lower T-to-E_2 ratio. When age and pubertal stage were controlled, the associations between hormone levels and adjustment problems remained relatively the same.

The hormone and chronologic age profile associated with adjustment problems was characterized by relatively lower sex steroid levels, lower pubertal stage, and higher Δ^4-androstenedione levels, sometimes in conjunction with higher chronologic age. The investigation suggested that during the pubertal period there may be heightened sensitivity of the gonadal axis to stress-related changes in the adrenal axis, resulting in suppression of the gonadal axis. A second interpretation was

that in some individuals higher adrenal and lower gonadal hormone levels may be a reflection of a predisposition to heightened biologic reactivity to environmental challenges.

Observations of aggressive behavior of young adolescents interacting with their parents were the focus of another aspect of the same study (Inoff-Germain et al, 1988). Relations among adolescents' hormone levels and their use of anger and power while interacting with their parents were examined. Levels of certain gonadal and adrenal steroids that increase at puberty were associated with the behavioral expressions of anger and power when the adolescents interacted with their parents. Young adolescent girls may be very sensitive to changes in E_2 level; similar suggestions have been made concerning the menopausal period. The relationships with Δ^4-androstenedione, a major androgen in girls, indicate that androgens may play a role in aggressive behavior. Since the findings involved mainly E_2 and adrenal androgens, the underlying mechanisms responsible for hormone-behavior relations for hormones of gonadal and adrenal origin may be similar.

North Carolina Study

The North Carolina program of research focused on the relations among levels of androgenic hormones and sexuality and personality in young adolescents. Boys and girls in the eighth, ninth, and tenth grades described their pubertal development, sexual motivation, and details of their sexual behavior. Sera were collected for adrenal and gonadal steroid measurements and progesterone among girls. Total circulating androgenicity was estimated by the free T index (FTI). Among boys, there was a linear relation between T and the odds of ever having had intercourse. There also was a relationship between FTI and a total sexual outlet score (number of times of masturbation, wet dreams, and coitus). Among those with the lowest FTI, only 8.7% reported having had a sexual outlet in the last month, compared with 76.2% of boys with the highest FTI. There was no relationship between stage of pubertal development and sexual outlet scores. Udry and colleagues (1985) suggest that involvement in socially determined patterns of sexual behavior is heavily influenced by serum androgenic hormones.

No variables predicted sexual intercourse among girls (Udry, Talbert, and Morris, 1986). FTI was the best predictor of masturbation and the frequency of sexual outlet. Follicular phase progesterone was inversely related to ever having masturbated; the higher the level of follicular phase progesterone, the less likely that the girls had masturbated. The authors concluded that there was some support for both the biologic (direct hormone effect) and the sociologic (indirect effect) components of the model in relation to whether the girls had ever masturbated. The anticipation for future sexual activity was predicted by the biologic component, that is, the androgenic hormones, DHEA and Δ^4-androstenedione, and LH.

In summary, the authors concluded that girls show significant hormone effects (androgen related) on certain aspects of their sexual behavior (excluding intercourse). Sexual motivation was associated with androgens, primarily of adrenal origin. In both boys and girls, the effects of hormones appear to be direct rather than indirect, operating throughout pubertal development, with the exception of masturbation, which shows age-graded and pubertal effects.

Pubertal hormones also were hypothesized to have a more general effect on personality, which in turn would predispose adolescents to sexual behavior (Udry and Talbert, 1988). Cross-sectional relations were examined between T and personality, as assessed on the Adjective Check List (ACL). The correlations between T and the ACL were factor-analyzed. A T factor emerged for both boys and girls (ACL-T). The factor contained a mixture of positive and negative attributes (e.g., dominant, robust, spontaneous, and stingy for the boy factor; discreet, showing initiative, cynical, and charming for the girl factor). There was some evidence that girls may be more sensitive to T levels than are boys. A one-unit increase in T produced a fivefold greater increase in the female ACL-T scores (the sum of the adjectives on the ACL-T common factor versus the factor score) as compared with the male scores. These findings were interpreted as suggesting that although female T levels were lower and exhibited less variability, the increase in T during the pubertal years may have an effect on female personality comparable to that in males during the same period.

CONCLUSIONS

The findings reviewed here suggest that puberty-related hormones of gonadal and adrenal origins may have activating influences on behavior. Testosterone, its binding globulin, and adrenal androgens were related to negative emotionality and aggressive behavior. Similarly, lower levels of DHEA and higher levels of Δ^4-androstenedione were related to problem behaviors and negative emotionality. These findings could not be accounted for by physical developmental changes. In the studies reported here, the effects of hormones appear to support a direct-effects model of psychological development.

An alternative interpretation of the findings reviewed here also seems justifiable. We have focused on the pubertal period of development to examine hormone-behavior associations, but individual differences in hormone levels and behavior at any stage of development might also explain the findings. Studies following adolescents from the prepubertal to the postpubertal period are needed to disentangle developmental-activating hormone influences and individual differences in psychological development.

In spite of some convergence of findings across studies, there are several qualifications to the findings. First, the associations among pubertal hormones and behavior may be mediated by the timing of the changes. For example, Nottelmann and co-workers (1987) observed lower-for-age gonadal steroid levels to be associated with problems of adjustment. Second, there are gender differences in the findings suggesting different physiologic and behavioral processes for boys and girls. Third, life events alter the relation between hormones and behavior in undefined ways. Fourth, the research methods may determine the nature of the findings. For instance, observations of girls interacting with their parents showed covariations among aggressive tendencies and gonadal steroids and adrenal androgens. However, self- or parent-report questionnaires of aggressive tendencies in girls were not related to hormone levels.

BIBLIOGRAPHY

Beach FA: Behavioral endocrinology: An emerging discipline. Am Sci 63:178, 1975.
Brooks-Gunn J, Warren MP: Biological contributions to affective expression in young adolescent girls. Child Dev 60:40, 1989.
Hampson E, Kimura D: Reciprocal effects of hormonal fluctuations on human motor and perceptual-spatial skills. Behav Neurosci 102:456, 1988.
Hines M, Shipley C: Prenatal exposure to diethylstilbestrol (DES) and the development of sexually dimorphic cognitive abilities and cerebral lateralization. Dev Psychol 20:81, 1984.
Inoff-Germain GE, Arnold GS, Nottelmann ED, et al: Relations between hormone levels and observational measures of aggressive behavior of early adolescents in family interactions. Dev Psychol 24:120, 1988.
Leshner AI: Hormones and emotions. In Candland DK, Fell JP, Keen E, et al (eds): Emotion. Pacific Grove, CA, Brooks/Cole Publishing, 1977, pp 85–145.
Money J, Ehrhardt AA: Prenatal hormone exposure: Possible effects on behaviour in man. In Michael RP (ed): Endocrinology and Human Behaviour. London, Oxford University Press, 1968, pp 32–48.
Nottelmann ED, Susman EJ, Inoff-Germain GE, et al: Developmental processes in early adolescence: Relations between adolescent adjustment problems and chronologic age, pubertal stage, and puberty-related hormone levels. J Pediatr 110:473, 1987.
Nyborg H, Nielsen J: Sex hormone treatment and spatial ability in women with Turner's syndrome. In Schmid W, Nielsen J (eds): Human Behaviour and Genetics. New York, Elsevier, 1981, pp 167–182.
Olweus D, Mattsson A, Schalling D, Löw H: Testosterone, aggression, physical, and personality dimensions in normal adolescent males. Psychosom Med 42:253, 1980.
Olweus D, Mattsson A, Schalling D, Löw H: Circulating testosterone levels and aggression in adolescent males: A causal analysis. Psychosom Med 50:261, 1988.
Petersen AC, Taylor B: The biological approach to adolescence: Biological change and psychosocial adaptation. In Adelson J (ed): Handbook of the Psychology of Adolescence. New York, John Wiley & Sons, 1980, pp 117–155.
Reinisch JM: Prenatal exposure to synthetic progestins increases potential for aggression in humans. Science 211:1171, 1981.
Susman EJ, Inoff-Germain G, Nottelmann ED, et al: Hormones, emotional dispositions, and aggressive attributes in early adolescents. Child Dev 58:1114, 1987.
Udry LM, Talbert LM: Sex hormone effects on personality at puberty. J Pers Soc Psychol 54:291, 1988.
Udry R, Billy JOG, Morris NM, et al: Serum androgenic hormones motivate sexual behavior in adolescent boys. Fertil Steril 43:90, 1985.
Udry JR, Talbert LM, Morris NM: Biosocial foundations for adolescent female sexuality. Demography 23:217, 1986.
Waber DP, Mann MB, Merola J, Moylan PM: Physical maturation rate and cognitive performance in early adolescence: A longitudinal examination. Dev Psychol 21:666, 1985.
Warren M, Brooks-Gunn J: Mood and behavior at adolescence: Evidence for hormonal factors. J Clin Endocrinol Metab 69:77, 1989.

CHAPTER 14

Stress and the Immune System

BARBARA K. SNYDER

INTRODUCTION

It has long been common wisdom that life stress can adversely affect health, but only recently have the mechanisms underlying this relationship been explored. Psychoneuroimmunology is the study of the relationships among psychosocial factors (such as life stress, affective state, coping) and resultant changes in neuroendocrine and immune function, and it offers new strategies for the study of altered susceptibility to disease. Evidence that the central nervous and immune systems interact bidirectionally includes both experimental and naturally occurring stress associated with changes in *in vivo* and *in vitro* immune function; conditioned immunologic responses in animals; and experimental manipulations of the brain and endocrine system, leading to reproducible changes in immune function, and vice versa. Many questions remain unanswered. It is clear, however, that there is not an all-or-nothing relationship between stress and disease susceptibility; rather stress is just one of many coexisting risk factors that can affect health.

Most of the psychoneuroimmunology research has focused on animal models and adults, though university students have been the subjects in a number of studies. This chapter therefore covers major concepts in psychoneuroimmunology and theories about pathophysiology and suggests implications specific for adolescence.

There is no single or best measure of immune competence, and the various components of the immune system are highly interactive. The components of immune function most widely studied in psychoneuroimmunology have been cell-mediated (or T lymphocyte) immunity and natural killer cell activity (NKCA); humoral (or B lymphocyte) immunity and phagocytic function have less often been studied as outcomes.

Measuring Stress

There is much literature discussing the semantic and methodologic problems in stress research. The term *stress* is used here to mean external stimuli or events, in contrast with the response to stress—often referred to as *distress* or *strain*. It is obvious that non-events, such as not getting a hoped for acceptance to college, can also be extremely stressful. Research has focused on three main categories of stressful events: major life events; more minor, day-to-day "hassles"; and catastrophic events, such as bereavement. The first two of

these are typically measured using one of the many available self-report checklists. These checklists are easy to administer and have common sense appeal, but there is debate about whether they really capture the nature and degree of life stress experienced by subjects. The third type of stress is the criterion by which subjects are selected, and further details are often obtained by interview.

Other methodologic issues that have been raised about stress research include infrequent use of control groups; recall bias; stress assessed at only one time; and potential confounding of events and illness outcomes. Results are often analyzed as correlations, thus making it difficult to prove temporal relationships. It is now clear that certain qualities of stressful events help determine the ultimate impact on the individual, including duration, intensity, desirability, predictability, and controllability of the stress.

Other Influences on the Stress-Illness Relationship

Stressful events always take place within the context of the individual and his or her environment. Human stress research is increasingly examining these factors to understand better the great variability (psychologically, behaviorally, and physiologically) in individual responses to stress. Table 14–1 lists some of the variables that can affect the stress-illness relationship. The nature and degree of the effects vary with the type of stress and the outcome studied. They include independent effects (e.g., biologic factors), mediating effects (e.g., personality traits), and buffering effects (e.g., social support). A variety of scales have been developed to evaluate these factors.

OVERVIEW OF PSYCHONEUROIMMUNOLOGY RESEARCH

Studies in Animals

Research with animal models has shown that stress can cause changes in immune function as well as increased susceptibility to or severity of disease (Table 14–2). However, changes have been seen following some

TABLE 14–1. Potential Influences on the Stress-Illness Relationship

Individual factors
  Personal characteristics (personality, coping style, mood, intelligence, values, attitudes, beliefs)
  Past history (prior stresses and response to them, psychiatric history)
  Sociodemographics (age, sex, race, socioeconomic status)
  Biologic variables (genetic predispositions, past medical history, current physical state, medications, health habits—diet, exercise, etc.)

Process factors
  Cognitive appraisal (meaning of an event, desirability and controllability of an event)
  Coping skills (repertoire, flexibility)

Environmental factors
  Social network (quality and quantity of available support)
  Social setting (geography, size and structure of institutions, culture, prejudice, resources)

Modified from Cohen F, Horowitz MJ, Lazarus RS, et al: Panel report on psychosocial assets and modifiers of stress. In Elliott GR, Eisdorfer C (eds): Stress and Human Health. Analysis and Implications of Research. Copyright 1982 by Springer Publishing Co., Inc., New York 10012; used with permission.

stressful stimuli but not others, or in one sex only, or in some immunologic parameters and not in others. Further, some studies have demonstrated increased resistance of the subjects to disease following experimental stress. Animal models offer unique advantages in this kind of research: the total environment can be controlled; the specific stress is known and can be manipulated; and the animals can be genetically identical or otherwise homogeneous. Generalizing from animal studies to human beings is limited by the fact that the human immune system is better developed at birth than is that of nonprimates and that human emotional and cognitive responses to stress have no obvious counterpart in animals.

A number of studies found greater immunosuppression or morbidity and mortality when animals were exposed to the antigen (e.g., infectious agent, foreign protein) before or simultaneously with the stressful stimuli; in contrast, there was less effect if the antigen was introduced following stress. This suggests that stress may interfere acutely with mounting an immune response. In addition, animals seem to be more vulnerable to the immunologic effects of stress at certain ages than at others.

Studies in Humans

The relationship between human stress and illness was first studied using an epidemiologic approach. Infections were the most common outcomes evaluated (Table 14–3), but other immune-related diseases (cancer, autoimmune disease) have also been studied. Much of this work found an association between stress and other psychosocial factors and the onset and course of illness. Unfortunately, immunologic function was not measured in any of these studies.

Unanswered questions about how psychosocial factors might influence health include the following: Do they directly affect immune function? Do they influence an individual's behavior and thus exposure to infectious and other agents? Do they mainly affect the susceptibility to or the clinical course of the disease? Do they affect outcome by influencing the individual's health behavior (e.g., seeking health care, compliance)?

More recent research has focused on altered immune function as the path by which stress can affect health. In most of this work, one or more assessments of cellular immune function have been studied in relation to stressful events or other psychosocial factors, or both. In general, immune function is diminished in stressed subjects, as compared with those less stressed or with the same subjects at a time prior to the stress.

A number of these studies have used healthy university students as subjects, asking them about past stressful events or studying them at the time of known stress—such as final examinations. Results include decreased NKCA, percentage of helper T cells, or interferon production on the first day of examination as compared with baseline; increased antibody titer to Epstein-Barr virus (a latent virus) on the day of examination; decreased NKCA in students with higher stress scores and more psychological symptoms (defined as "poor copers"); increased reporting of (mostly viral) infections around examination time; and increased ratio of helper to suppressor T cells in students practicing self-relaxation techniques.

Even more than stress alone, interaction between stressful events and other psychosocial factors (e.g., depression, loneliness, personality traits, or social support) has been associated with altered immune function. It is likely that stress in combination with these psychosocial factors impairs coping abilities, with resultant greater impact on immune function.

The relationship between stress and humoral immunity has been studied much less often than has cellular immunity, and the results have been more varied. Several studies involved giving live virus (influenza) vaccine to healthy young adults and measuring postimmunization immune responses. The results showed no consistent relationship to stress. Salivary immunoglobulin A, another measure of humoral immunity, was found to be

TABLE 14–2. Findings from Animal Studies

Nature of Stressful Stimuli	Results
Repeated noise stress (mice)	Initial ↓ then ↑ in LP
Conditioned illness-induced taste aversion (pairing cyclophosphamide with saccharin) (rats)	Conditioned animals: very suppressed Ab response to injected SRBCs
	Placebo: high Ab titer to injected SRBCs
Premature weaning, separation (rats)	↓ LP
Handling in early life (rats)	↑ Ab response to injected foreign protein
Crowding (mice): brief	↓ Ab response to injected foreign protein
long-term	↑ LP response to injected foreign protein
Chronic avoidance learning (mice)	↓ Skin homograft rejection
Preweaning handling (mice)	↓ Resistance to leukemia virus infection

LP, lymphocyte proliferation; Ab, antibody; SRBCs, sheep red blood cells.

TABLE 14–3. Findings From Studies of Stress and Infection

↑ Number of streptococcal infections in family members when family had recent acute stress (prospective)

↑ Incidence of clinical mononucleosis in previously seronegative West Point cadets who wanted military careers but had poor academic performance, or whose fathers were overachievers (prospective)

↑ Number of upper respiratory infections in college students who were socially isolated or experiencing failure (retrospective)

More severe, protracted upper respiratory infections in children whose families experienced more stress (prospective)

↑ Number of Herpes simplex recurrences in known seropositive nursing students who reported being unhappy (prospective)

Peak in undesirable events and trough in desirable events several days before illness episodes (prospective)

lower in students experiencing examination stress. A recent study focused on the relationship between stress and other psychosocial factors and immune response to a novel protein antigen. Subject-defined positive stresses were correlated with higher peak postimmunization responses, whereas negative stresses had the opposite effect. In this study, stressful events seemed to have an indirect influence on immune response, acting through the psychological state.

Several critical questions remain: Do the observed changes in immune function represent immune compromise, or are they merely *in vitro* phenomena of no clinical relevance? If there is compromise, does it increase susceptibility to disease?

PATHOPHYSIOLOGIC MECHANISMS

Although the study samples, designs, and outcomes vary a great deal, the evidence is overwhelming that there is a relationship between psychosocial factors and immune-mediated diseases. Our understanding of underlying mechanisms, still largely speculative, is based on a growing body of data of neuroendocrine–immune system interactions.

Hormones, neurotransmitters, antibodies, and lymphokines all have been named as probable messengers of these interactions. It is known that all organs of the immune system, including the bone marrow, thymus, lymph nodes, and spleen, have sympathetic and parasympathetic innervation. Further, surface receptors have been found on lymphocytes for neurotransmitters, opiates, and several hormones, including corticosteroids. Thus, through both direct innervation and a variety of biochemical mediators, there are many ways in which the central nervous system (especially the hypothalamus) can interact bidirectionally with the immune system. It is likely that the pathways involved in a given response depend on the nature of the stress and physiologic predispositions of the individual, among other factors.

The hypothalamic-pituitary-adrenal axis has been widely studied in psychoneuroimmunology. High doses of exogenous steroids have depressant effects on many immune parameters, especially cell-mediated immunity

and phagocytosis. Acute stress has frequently (but not invariably) been associated with transient high levels of corticosteroids, and it was long thought that this was the mechanism for stress-induced immune suppression. It is now clear, however, that stress is associated with increased levels of many hormones (Fig. 14–1) and that virtually all hormones can influence immunologic activity. Stress-induced changes in hormonal levels may produce immunologic effects by altering cyclic nucleotide levels in immune cells.

The role of neurotransmitters is being actively investigated. Stress tends to raise catecholamine levels, perhaps modulated by the organism's ability to cope with or control the stress. Dopamine and β-endorphins tend to have immune-enhancing effects, whereas serotonin has a net inhibitory effect on immune function.

IMPLICATIONS FOR ADOLESCENCE

University students, a typically cooperative and "captive" group, have constituted the study sample in many of the human psychoneuroimmunology studies. No studies, however, have examined children or younger adolescents for stress-related changes in immune function or health. This raises the question of how applicable the data from existing studies may be to adolescents. Little is known about interactions among behavior, the brain, and the immune system early in life. Might psychosocial factors (including life stress) influence later development of either the neuroendocrine or the immune system? Data from animal studies suggest that early life stress has greater impact on immune function than when the same stress is experienced later in life.

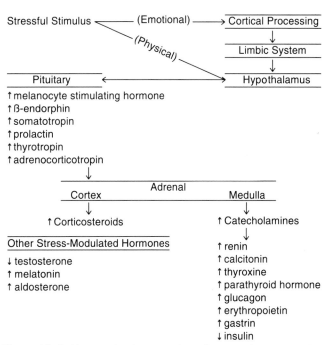

Figure 14–1. Neuroendocrine sequelae of stress; the stereotypic response to stimuli arousing the need for "fight-or-flight." (Reprinted by permission of the publisher from Stress, behavior, and immunity: Animal models and mediating mechanisms, by Borysenko M, and Borysenko J, Gen Hosp Psychiatry 4:59–67. Copyright 1982 by Elsevier Science Publishing Co., Inc.)

For a number of reasons, adolescence may be a period of increased vulnerability to the effects of stress. Little is specifically known about immune function in adolescence, but there are theoretical reasons why immune function might be different during this period. Many aspects of immune function peak with sexual maturity. Thymic involution begins in puberty, perhaps contributing to the decline in T cell activity that begins during this time. The hormonal changes of puberty, especially in growth hormone, gonadotropins, and sex steroids, may well contribute to changes in immune function.

With all the concurrent physical, psychosocial, and cognitive changes, adolescence is normally seen as stressful. An adolescent's stage of psychosocial maturity and cognitive development clearly influences how that adolescent copes with stress, and, theoretically, the capacity to cope with stress could modulate immunologic reactivity. Adolescence might therefore be a critical time for learning effective coping strategies.

CONCLUSIONS AND UNANSWERED QUESTIONS

Life stress is one of many potential risk factors for immune-related diseases. Longitudinal studies are needed to show whether stress-associated changes in immune function actually alter an individual's susceptibility to disease. It is clear that all stress is not delete-rious, and we need to better understand under what circumstances stress can enhance immunity and resistance to disease.

"Whether stress, through its effect upon various hormonal systems, can alter immunologic function in an age-specific manner is an open question" (Ader, 1981, p 213). Adolescence, a time of great physiologic and psychosocial change, may be a period of increased vulnerability to the health effects of stress. Perhaps, though, these adverse health consequences can be lessened by enhancing coping skills and other psychosocial modifiers of stress.

BIBLIOGRAPHY

Ader R (ed): Psychoneuroimmunology. New York, Academic Press, 1981.

Borysenko M, Borysenko J: Stress, behavior and immunity: Animal models and mediating mechanisms. Gen Hosp Psychiatry 4:59, 1982.

Elliott GR, Eisdorfer C (eds): Stress and Human Health. Analysis and Implications of Research. New York, Springer Publishing, 1982.

Goetzl, EJ (ed): Proceedings of a conference on neuromodulation of immunity and hypersensitivity. J Immunol 135 (2nd Suppl):739s, 1985.

Jemott JB, Locke SE: Psychosocial factors, immunologic mediation, and human susceptibility to infectious diseases. How much do we know? Psychol Bull 95:78, 1984.

Schleifer SJ, Scott B, Stein M, Keller SE: Behavioral and developmental aspects of immunity. J Am Acad Child Psychiatry 6:751, 1986.

Solomon GF: Psychoneuroimmunology: Interactions between central nervous system and immune system. J Neurosci Res 18:1, 1987.

CHAPTER 15

Primate Models of Behavioral and Physiologic Change in Adolescence

STEPHEN J. SUOMI, KATHLYN L. R. RASMUSSEN, and J. D. HIGLEY

Researchers who study developmental changes in physiology and behavior during adolescence clearly face a variety of formidable methodological challenges. On the one hand, there is a relative paucity of normative data documenting the extent and timing of change in physiologic processes and in patterns of behavior that are associated with the passage through puberty (see Chapter 13). As a consequence, it is often difficult to tell whether a dramatic change observed in any one individual's hormonal levels or particular patterns of behavior is abnormal or merely represents an appropriate, normative aspect of developmental change. On the other hand, there is an emerging body of data suggesting that physiologic and behavioral changes are far from independent and, indeed, are capable of influencing each other. In addition, certain patterns of behavior during adolescence, such as aggressive or risk-taking behavior, as well as some physiologic processes are also subject to influence by a wide range of other factors associated with pubertal change, including those intrinsic to the organism (e.g., cognitive or neurochemical processes) and those that are basically extrinsic (e.g., family, school, or societal expectations). Thus, even when pubertal changes in physiology and behavior are well documented, the actual basis for such changes may not be well understood.

In many other fields of biomedical inquiry, researchers who face comparable methodological obstacles to the direct study of human physiology or behavior often turn to animal models in order to advance knowledge of the human phenomena under scrutiny. The use of animal subjects often enables investigators to manipulate specific aspects of physiology or behavior in precise fashion under more tightly controlled conditions than is generally feasible with human subjects or patients in order to establish causal relationships. Moreover, although animal subjects obviously cannot fill out questionnaires or be interviewed about their symptoms or memories of events, it is usually possible to collect more extensive sets of physiologic and behavioral data systematically than what most human protocols would permit. Finally, most animal species mature much more rapidly than do *Homo sapiens,* so an investigator can readily follow an individual animal subject over a portion of its lifetime greater than that of a human in a longitudinal study of comparable duration. This third point is especially relevant for evaluating the effects of early experience on later functioning during adolescence or adulthood, for determining long-term consequences of pubertal events, and for investigating cross-generational phenomena.

Of course, animal models of human physiology and behavior are useful only to the extent to which the animal phenomena under study generalize to the human case. For this reason, among the most informative animal models of human pubertal phenomena are those that have utilized advanced nonhuman primates, that is, Old World monkeys and apes, as subjects. These species of nonhuman primates are our closest biologic relatives, sharing the large majority of our genes. For example, it has been estimated that more than 90% of human unreplicated DNA is present in all Old World monkeys, and for chimpanzees the degree of genetic overlap with humans is between 98% and 99% (Lovejoy, 1981). One consequence of such enormous genetic overlap is that most physiologic systems in these nonhuman primate species are highly similar, if not identical, to those in humans with respect to their component parts, patterns of development, modes of functioning, and susceptibility to the same general influences.

In addition, most species of advanced nonhuman primates living in nature reside in complex social groups characterized by long-term relationships between individuals, well-established multigenerational kinship lines, and dynamic dominance hierarchies that reflect both cooperation and competition. Although such complex social groups clearly cannot match the levels of sophistication inherent in even the most primitive human cultures, there are many obvious parallels, particularly in terms of social roles that change as a function of developmental status. For example, in virtually all Old World monkey and ape species, both males and females typically undergo major social changes during adolescence, making it feasible to study the relationship between pubertal hormonal changes and social role changes under controlled experimental conditions. Even though the actual patterns of pubertal social change in many of these species may in fact differ from those characteristic of most cultures of *Homo sapiens,* some general principles regarding these hormonal and behavioral influences and interactions may well provide useful insights into the human phenomena.

In this chapter, data from a recently developed primate model examining pubertal change in behavior and physiology as it relates to depressive phenomena will be presented to illustrate these points. The model is based on studies of rhesus monkeys *(Macaca mulatta),* a highly successful species of Old World monkey indigenous to the Indian subcontinent. These studies focus on individual differences in response to stress and risk of developing depressive reactions. The utility of the model derives in no small part from a thorough knowledge of normative biobehavioral development in this species.

SPECIES-NORMATIVE SOCIAL ORGANIZATION AND SOCIAL DEVELOPMENT IN RHESUS MONKEYS

A large body of normative developmental data has been collected on rhesus monkeys growing up both in the wild and in a variety of captive settings. Rhesus monkeys typically live in large social groups (termed *troops*) containing between several dozen and several hundred individuals. Despite differences in size, these troops all have the same basic social structure, with each troop containing several multigenerational matrilines (i.e., old females surrounded by three or more generations of adult female offspring), along with unrelated males who have entered the troop as adults (Lindburg, 1973). This species-normative social troop structure results from the fact that females stay for their entire lives in the troop in which they were born, whereas males stay in their natal troop only until puberty, at which point they leave to join all-male gangs (Sade, 1967). After spending several months or more in the all-male gangs, the young adult males emigrate to different troops, in which they typically take up long-term residence.

Rhesus monkey infants spend their first weeks of life on or in close physical proximity to their biologic mothers. Starting in the second month of life, however, the infants begin to leave their mothers for brief exploratory forays, during which time they encounter other monkeys in the troop. In succeeding months these young monkeys spend increasing amounts of time away from their mothers, and during much of this time away they become engaged in extensive interactions with peers. In fact, play with peers emerges as their predominant social activity until puberty (Suomi and Harlow, 1978), which for rhesus monkey females begins near the end of their third year of life, when menarche occurs and the females begin to have regular menstrual cycles (usually averaging 28 days in length). Puberty for males is marked by the descent of the testes into the scrotum and the production of viable sperm, usually at the beginning of their fourth year of life.

The onset of puberty is clearly associated with major life transitions for both male and female rhesus monkeys. Although females almost always remain in the troop in which they were born, after puberty their interactions with peers decline dramatically, and they redirect much of their social activities toward other members of their own matriline. In contrast, either adolescent males leave their natal troop voluntarily, or if they remain too long, they are physically expelled. In either case, these young males typically join all-male gangs for varying periods before they attempt to enter a new troop, and they also employ a variety of different strategies to get into that troop. It should be noted that the period of adolescence and young adulthood is clearly the most dangerous time in these males' lives—in the wild, the mortality rate for males from the time they leave their natal troop until the time they are successfully integrated into a new troop approaches 50% (Dittus, 1979).

This pattern of rhesus monkey social development has been observed not only in wild troops but also in groups of rhesus monkeys maintained in captivity (Suomi and Harlow, 1978). The consistency of these observations makes it clear that the onset of puberty signals the beginning of very different expected life courses for male and female rhesus monkeys. Not only do males and females undergo dramatic, sexually dimorphic changes in their physical growth and hormonal profiles, but they also take on very different social roles. At the same time, the manner in which adolescent males and females are treated by their fellow monkeys also undergoes dramatic, sexually dimorphic change from that of earlier years. The impact of such changes in external social patterns and pressures should not be underestimated. Indeed, there exist compelling data from several species of nonhuman primates indicating that the actual onset and duration of pubertal change can be significantly influenced by external social pressures and stress (Savage, Ziegler, and Snowdon, 1988).

INDIVIDUAL DIFFERENCES IN BIOBEHAVIORAL RESPONSE TO STRESS IN ADOLESCENT RHESUS MONKEYS (see Chapters 12 and 100)

Over the past decade a major research effort has been directed toward the study of individual differences in how rhesus monkeys react behaviorally and physiologically to new or stressful physical stimuli and social situations. It is now well established that some rhesus monkeys—approximately 20% of the population—consistently respond to such situations with unusual behavioral disruption and prolonged physiologic arousal as compared with their fellow troop members. Stimuli that characteristically elicit interest and physical exploration from most monkeys instead reliably produce fearful, anxious behavioral withdrawal in these individuals, along with profound and prolonged activation of the hypothalamic-pituitary-adrenal axis (as indexed by elevated levels of plasma cortisol and adrenocorticotropic hormone [ACTH]), of the sympathetic nervous system (as indexed by high, stable heart rates), and of monoamine turnover (as indexed by high cerebrospinal fluid [CSF] levels of dopamine, norepinephrine, and serotonin metabolites—homovanillic acid [HVA], methoxy-hydroxyphenylglycol [MHPG], and 5-hydroxyindole-acetic acid [5-HIAA], respectively). Moreover, these individual differences can be detected in the first few weeks of life and, in the absence of major environmental change, seem to be remarkably stable throughout childhood and adolescence and even into adulthood (Higley and Suomi, 1989). An increasing body of circumstantial data indicates that such differences in biobehavioral reactions to environmental novelty and stress are highly heritable, although other studies have demonstrated that certain early rearing experiences—especially those involving early social attachments—can significantly alter both behavioral and physiologic patterns of response (Suomi, 1991a).

As mentioned previously, these individual differences in reaction to environmental challenges tend to be quite stable through major developmental transitions. Individual rhesus monkeys who as infants were reluctant to leave their mothers and explore their immediate surroundings are also typically shy and withdrawn as juveniles in their interactions with peers. In contrast, individuals who as infants were eager to explore novel objects and new situations are likely to be especially outgoing in later interactions with peers. With the coming of adolescence, such distinctive patterns of response style carry different long-term consequences and risks for males and females.

We now know that female monkeys who were shy and withdrawn as infants and juveniles carry a relatively high risk of providing inadequate maternal care to their first-born offspring in the absence of a stable, supportive social environment. In contrast, females who were outgoing as infants and juveniles seldom, if ever, demonstrate inadequate care toward their first-born offspring, even in socially unstable and stressful social settings (Suomi and Ripp, 1983). Such knowledge has proved to be useful in developing programs for early identification of at-risk rhesus monkey mothers-to-be and for provision of stable social support systems, effectively eliminating the incidence of offspring neglect and abuse among these vulnerable adolescent females.

Individual differences in prototypic response to novelty and stress also have ramifications for adolescent male rhesus monkeys, especially as they go through the process of emigration from their natal troop. Longitudinal studies of adolescent males who live in wild troops and who were followed as they emigrated have reported that both the timing of emigration and the "strategy" that individual males utilize in trying to join a new troop appear to be related to their respective biobehavioral response styles. Males who are highly reactive in the face of stress (i.e., those who consistently respond to stress with behavioral disturbance; high, stable heart rates; and high levels of plasma cortisol) tend to leave their natal troops significantly later chronologically than do males whose prototypic stress response is more mild. Moreover, highly reactive males tend to follow much more "conservative" strategies for joining new troops than do their less reactive cohorts. They often bypass entirely the all-male gangs that most emigrating adolescents join for short periods, and they are much more likely to spend considerable time on the periphery of a new troop rather than trying to enter the troop's central core directly.

Thus, individual differences in prototypic response to stress exhibited during infancy and the juvenile years tend to carry over into adolescence and beyond. Moreover, the consequences of such differences in response style appear to be quite different for adolescent male and female rhesus monkeys.

MONKEY MODEL OF ADOLESCENT DEPRESSION

Knowledge of profound individual differences in the ways in which rhesus monkeys typically react to environmental novelty and stress has provided important insights regarding the development of a new primate model of depression. Over the last 25 years numerous investigators working with several different nonhuman primate species have reported that some (but clearly not all) individuals react to brief social separations from familiar conspecific individuals with reactions that appear to be depressive in nature. Most of these studies have focused on mother–infant separations, although disruption of other social relationships via separation has been studied in subjects of all ages. Although virtually all monkeys respond to maternal separations with initial behavioral agitation and activation of the hypothalamic-pituitary-adrenal axis and various sympathetic pathways, most appear to adjust and adapt to the separation within a few hours. In contrast, a few subjects fall into behavioral "despair" (much as Bowlby has described for human infants and children following separation), in which they become withdrawn and inactive, seem unresponsive to social or nonsocial stimulation, and exhibit gross disruption of normal sleeping and eating patterns. These individuals typically have highly elevated levels of plasma cortisol and ACTH, low CSF levels of norepinephrine (and high levels of the norepinephrine metabolite MHPG, suggesting high turnover rates), and compromised immune systems. Most, if not all, of these behavioral symptoms and physiologic patterns are reversed upon reunion or following treatment with antidepressant medication (Suomi, 1991b).

Detailed study of these different patterns of response to social separation has shown that an individual monkey's characteristic response tends to be quite stable across repeated separations and over major periods of development. Thus, an infant who exhibits a depressive reaction to brief separation from its mother at 6 months of age is likely to exhibit a depressive reaction again if the separation is repeated a week, a month, or even a year later. Moreover, monkeys who exhibit extreme reactions to maternal separations as infants are prone to displaying depressive reactions to separations from peers as juveniles or to separation from their own infants as young adults. In contrast, monkeys who exhibit relatively mild and transient biobehavioral responses to maternal separations as infants are highly unlikely to display depressive reactions to separations experienced later in life.

Who are the individuals who appear to be at risk for displaying depressive symptomatology following social separation? We now know that these are the same individuals who in other novel or mildly stressful circumstances exhibit extreme behavioral reactions and physiologic arousal. In our rhesus monkey colony, these at-risk monkeys are the same 20% of the colony that we have classified as "highly reactive," who show anxious responses in the face of novelty or challenge. Thus, as was the case for high reactivity in general, the risk of depressive responses to separation appears to be highly heritable, readily modified by certain early attachment experiences, and relatively consistent over major periods of development (Higley and Suomi, 1989; Suomi, 1991a).

The ability to identify specific rhesus monkeys early in life who are at risk for developing depressive episodes throughout their lives and to follow such individuals longitudinally has provided valuable insights regarding adolescent depressive phenomena, at least in these individuals. As suggested above, we have consistently found that those monkeys who displayed the most extreme reactions to social separations as adolescents were also those individuals who as infants or juveniles also exhibited extreme separation reactions or, in the absence of any separation experiences, displayed anxious behavior when confronted with novel or mildly stressful situations. Moreover, those adolescents who exhibit extreme reactions to separation are the same individuals who are at greatest risk for displaying depressive reactions to separation as adults. Thus, the risk of displaying extreme reactions to separation represents a developmental continuity that appears to transcend the period of adolescence (Suomi, 1991b).

However, the nature of extreme response to separation during adolescence is somewhat different for these at-risk monkeys from the response during infancy, childhood, or even adulthood. The greatest discrepancy is in the prototypic behavioral response: rather than becoming extremely passive, withdrawn, and generally unresponsive to physical or social stimulation following separation, at-risk adolescent monkeys tend to become exceedingly agitated and to engage in active stereotypies and may be unusually aggressive in their response to social stimulation (Higley and Suomi, 1989). In contrast, with two possible exceptions, the general physiologic profile of adolescent monkeys following separation is virtually identical to that of infants, juveniles, and adults: significant increases in hypothalamic-pituitary-adrenal activity, in sympathetic nervous system activity, in norepinephrine turnover, and in immunosuppression (Suomi, 1991b). One exception involves serotonergic functioning: CSF levels of 5-HIAA, the primary serotonin metabolite, appear to be elevated to a greater degree and for a longer period (especially in males) than what is typically the case for younger or older monkeys following separation. The second exception involves an apparent partial suppression of cortisol secretion in male, but not female, adolescents following separation. These latter findings seem especially interesting in light of the human depression literature, in which a major difference in the incidence of depression has consistently been reported during adolescence and adulthood but not prior to puberty.

What are the implications of findings from studies of rhesus monkeys and other nonhuman primates regarding human adolescent depressive phenomena—and what insights might they provide? Because rhesus monkeys are not furry little humans with tails but instead are members of a different (albeit closely related) species, one must be cautious in drawing direct links. Nevertheless, some general principles emerge from the primate data that do, in fact, address basic issues regarding human adolescent depression.

First, it is clear that depressive-like responses to separation in rhesus monkeys present behavioral and physiologic profiles in adolescent subjects that are somewhat different from those in infant, juvenile, and adult monkeys. There are, to be sure, some common features displayed at all ages (e.g., increases in norepinephrine turnover), but there are also "symptoms" that are unique to adolescent subjects. Second, there is striking continuity in apparent risk of depressive-like reactions to separation before, during, and following adolescence. The same individuals who display the most extreme reactions as adolescents are also likely to have exhibited extreme reactions as infants and juveniles and are likely to be at risk as adults, too. Moreover, individuals at risk for severe separation reactions also appear to be unusually sensitive to other novel or challenging circumstances, even though their reactions to those other circumstances might not be depressive in nature. Finally, it appears that both genetic and environmental factors contribute to these differences in response to challenge.

Researchers who work with animal models cannot expect to answer all the relevant questions posed by the human phenomena. At best they can provide certain insights as well as present hypotheses that might be tested at the human level. However, careful studies of rhesus monkeys and other nonhuman primates can ensure that such insights have a well-grounded empirical basis and that such hypotheses derive at least in part from our own evolutionary history. These are the real contributions that primate models can provide for our knowledge of behavioral and physiologic change in adolescence.

BIBLIOGRAPHY

Dittus WPJ: The evaluation of behaviours regulating density and age-specific sex ratios in a primate population. Behaviour 69:365, 1979.

Higley JD, Suomi SJ: Temperament in nonhuman primates. In Kohnstamm GA, Bates JE, Rothbard MK (eds): Handbook of Temperament in Children. New York, Wiley, 1989.

Lindburg DG: The rhesus monkey in North India: An ecological and behavioral study. In Rosenblum LA (ed): Primate Behavior, Vol 2. New York, Academic Press, 1973.

Lovejoy CO: The origin of man. Science 211:341, 1981.

Sade D: Determinants of dominance in a group of free-ranging rhesus monkeys. In Altman SA (ed): Social Communication Among Primates. Chicago, University of Chicago Press, 1967.

Savage A, Ziegler TE, Snowdon CT: Sociosexual development, pair bond formation, and mechanisms of fertility suppression in female cottontop tamarins (Saguinus oedipus oedipus). Am J Primatol 14:345, 1988.

Suomi SJ: Early stress and adult emotional reactivity in rhesus monkeys. In The Childhood Environment and Adult Disease (Ciba Foundation Symposium 156). Chichester, England, Wiley, 1991a.

Suomi SJ: Primate separation models of affective disorders. In Madden J (ed): Neurobiology of Learning, Emotion, and Affect. New York, Raven Press, 1991b.

Suomi SJ, Harlow HF: Early experience and social development in rhesus monkeys. In Lamb ME (ed): Social and Personality Development. New York, Holt, Rinehart & Winston, 1978.

Suomi SJ, Ripp C: A history of motherless mother monkey mothering at the University of Wisconsin Primate Laboratory. In Reite M, Caine N (eds): Child Abuse: The Nonhuman Primate Data. New York, Alan R. Liss, 1983.

CHAPTER 16

Pain in Adolescence

CORRIE T. M. ANDERSON, DEBRA FANURIK, and LONNIE K. ZELTZER

The evaluation and treatment of pain are often neglected aspects of adolescent medicine. The experience of pain associated with injury, disease, or repeated invasive diagnostic and treatment procedures can threaten the adolescent's physical, emotional, and psychological adjustment during an already vulnerable period. Untreated or undertreated pain not only may have a significant emotional impact but also may result in poor medical outcome and maladaptive behavior.

Pain may be viewed as a complex interaction of biologic, cognitive-developmental, situational, and affective factors. The adequate evaluation and management of pain in adolescents require an understanding of how these variables interact for an individual adolescent. Additionally, age, context, and cultural factors mediate the relationship between the sensory and emotional aspects of the pain experience and the adolescent's outward expression of pain. Other individuals provide feedback to the adolescent in response to the adolescent's pain behaviors, and this feedback further modifies the adolescent's future expressions of pain.

Adolescents differ in their reactivity to pain and in their natural coping styles and abilities. For example, some adolescents appear to be highly reactive and exhibit extreme distress following even minor injuries, whereas others seem to be impervious to pain. Similarly, some adolescents cope with pain by focusing on the site and the sensory aspects of the pain (attenders), whereas others cope by thinking about something else (distractors). Understanding how a particular adolescent usually copes with pain can be important in helping him or her to more effectively manage pain.

To integrate an understanding of pain in adolescents with psychological and pharmacologic pain management, this chapter reviews pain transmission and inhibition mechanisms and describes the processes that occur during adolescence that can modify pain experience and expression. Strategies for evaluating pain are proposed, and psychological and pharmacologic pain management strategies are reviewed.

PAIN TRANSMISSION AND INHIBITION

Pain, as defined by the International Association for the Study of Pain (IASP), is "an unpleasant sensory and emotional experience associated with actual or potential tissue damage, or described in terms of such damage." Integral to this definition is the emotional, cultural, behavioral, and neurophysiologic aspects of pain. Critical in the treatment of an adolescent in pain is an understanding of the basic neurophysiologic elements of pain at the sensory level. Implicit in the perception of pain is the process of transmission of signals from the periphery to the central nervous system (CNS). Afferent nerves of classes A, B, and C are the principal types of nerve fibers that carry signals from the periphery to the CNS. Noxious perturbations such as those from thermal, mechanical, or chemical stimuli that produce or can potentially produce tissue damage if prolonged typically activate specialized nerve fibers that carry signals to the CNS. This process is termed *nociception*. The receptors on the ends of these specialized nerves that are activated by noxious stimuli are termed *nociceptors*. These nociceptors generate signals that are transmitted along afferent nerve fibers to the spinal cord through the dorsal root ganglia where their cell bodies reside. Release of compounds such as substance P, histamine, certain protanoids, acetylcholine, potassium, bradykinin, and serotonin from damaged tissue increases nociceptor sensitivity and thus enhances the amount of pain experienced.

Utilizing histologic and neurophysiologic techniques, investigators have identified several specialized populations of nerve fibers that are involved primarily with nociception. When stimulated, small, thinly myelinated A-δ fibers produce sharp, rapid, well-localized pain of short duration. Other specialized fibers are the slow-conducting, unmyelinated C fibers. Activation of C fibers produces a dull, aching, poorly localized pain.

In the spinal cord, afferent A-δ and C pain fibers synapse upon a variety of neurons, including nociceptive-specific (NS) neurons, wide dynamic range (WDR) neurons, movement detection neurons, thermoreceptive neurons, low-threshold neurons, somatic motor neurons, and preganglionic autonomic neurons. The NS neurons are activated only by heavy pressure, pinch, painful stimuli, and heat greater than 45°C, whereas the WDR neurons respond to thermal, mechanical, and chemical stimuli of varying intensities. It is in the spinal cord at these first synaptic junctions that modulation of painful signals occurs. Incoming nociceptive signals are amplified or suppressed by other afferent signals and by descending signals from higher brain centers.

Immunohistochemical, radioimmune, and electrophysiologic investigations have demonstrated that the communications between the primary afferent nerve fibers and the neurons in the spinal cord on which they synapse are carried out by the calcium-dependent release of excitatory neurotransmitters. Many of these neuroactive substances have been identified during the past decade (Table 16–1). Current research is aimed at modulating the expression of the substances.

Continuing on with the course a nociceptive signal must travel after reaching the dorsal horn, nociceptive signals are carried to higher centers in the brain, such as the thalamus, reticular formation, the limbic system, and the cerebral cortex, through a number of different tracts. The nociceptive tracts that have been identified include the spinothalamic, spinoreticular, spinomesencephalic, spinocervical, trigeminal thalamic, and postsynaptic dorsal tracts. Additional pathways may have some involvement in nociceptive transmission, so surgical interventions for pain may not be curative. Besides carrying signals alerting one to the presence of potential danger, the ascending tracts also are involved with the localization of pain, activation of the autonomic and motor systems, triggering of the motivation-affective centers of the cortex, and recruiting of components of the descending analgesic system.

Multiple areas in the brain appear to be involved in modifying or modulating afferent input. Evidence of this theory includes examples of trauma resulting in severe tissue injury of which the sufferer is unaware and individuals lying on beds of nails without any sign of discomfort. Inhibition of afferent activity originating in the cortex and passing through descending neuronal tracts was postulated several decades ago and has been under considerable investigation. Researchers in the late 1960s and early 1970s demonstrated that electrical stimulation of discrete areas of the brain produced analgesia to noxious stimuli. The discovery of the binding of morphine in the periaqueductal-periventricular gray areas of the midbrain stimulated the search for endogenous opioid molecules. The first of these opioid peptides to be identified were the pentapeptides, leu-enkephalin and met-enkephalin. Several additional endogenous opioids have been characterized, including dynorphin and β-endorphin. It is now known that these peptides also exist in neurons that reside in the dorsal horn and that their release produces analgesia.

Such a dynamic, highly integrated system must be considered from a developmental perspective to understand how pain is perceived, expressed, and managed.

PAIN EXPERIENCE AND EXPRESSION: DEVELOPMENTAL CONSIDERATIONS

The stage of an adolescent's psychological development influences how pain is perceived in the cortex and how it is expressed and managed. The adolescent's maturing cognitive abilities, including the capacity for abstract thinking (see Chapters 9 and 10), contribute to an increasing understanding of and ability to cope with pain. However, increased understanding of the meaning of a particular pain (e.g., its association with disease)

TABLE 16–1. Neuropeptides Localized to Primary Afferent Neurons

Angiotensin II	Galanin
Arg-vasopressin	Gastrin-releasing peptide
Calcitonin gene-related peptide	Oxytocin
Cholecystokinin	Somatostatin
Corticotropin-releasing factor	Substance K
Dynorphin	Substance P
Enkephalin	Vasoactive intestinal polypeptide

and the likelihood of future traumatic pain experiences may serve to increase the adolescent's pain experience. This may also heighten his or her anxiety (e.g., compared with a younger child with less environmental and causal awareness in a similar situation). With higher cognitive function and more life experiences with age, the adolescent develops an increasing repertoire of cognitive and behavioral strategies to cope with pain. The adolescent also learns how to exert more self-control than does a younger child. Thus, rather than displaying overt pain behaviors such as screaming, crying, or resisting, the adolescent is likely to use controlled, subtle behaviors indicative of pain, such as muscular rigidity, flinching, or grimacing. The adolescent also has increased capacity for cognitive coping strategies, and consequently with age there is the potential for an increasing disparity between the adolescent's private suffering and the outward manifestations of pain. Therefore, asking adolescents about their pain, allowing them to individualize their experience and play a role in the control of their pain, becomes an increasingly important aspect of pain assessment during this developmental period.

The experience of pain is also related to the type of pain or pain situation. *Acute* pain is usually characterized by a sudden onset, a short duration and predictable course, and an association with a specific noxious or tissue-damaging stimulus. Acute pain includes pain that is produced by injuries or accidents, pain following surgical procedures, and pain associated with diagnostic or treatment procedures. *Chronic* or *recurring* pain has a longer duration and may or may not be associated with a definable pathologic disease process. Once pain is a persistent or recurring phenomenon, regardless of the identifiable pathophysiologic processes that may be causing the pain, other factors can contribute to its persistence and associated disability.

Acute pain, such as that associated with medical procedures, requires the adolescent to appraise the situation (especially in the case of a planned, expected procedure), plan a strategy, and then actively cope with the pain and anxiety during the painful event. However, the anticipation of a painful event (a higher function modulating event), brings a substantial amount of anxiety that the adolescent must manage. For example, past successes or failures contribute to the adolescent's perceived self-effectiveness in coping with the expected pain and to real or exaggerated memories of the pain itself. For some adolescents, the anxiety related to an anticipated pain event may become so overwhelming that he or she attempts to avoid the experience. Arguments with parents about pain may become a serious problem for adolescents with chronic illness (see Chapters 30 and 121). As parents who better understand the long-term implications of the particular illness attempt to exert control for required diagnostic and treatment procedures, the adolescent may become either more recalcitrant or more infantile. Adolescents who believe that they are unable to tolerate the procedure and who refuse to go to the clinic or to the doctor's office require intervention aimed at helping them to manage their anticipatory anxiety.

Chronic pain requires the adolescent to manage persistent or recurring distress and to learn how to accomplish the tasks of daily living while experiencing discomfort. Persistent pain may diminish the adolescent's energy and deprive him or her of the opportunities for social and emotional growth offered by physical activities and peer involvement. An adolescent in pain may become more sensitive to other somatic sensations, such as nausea or pruritus and may have sleep deprivation, rendering him or her even more vulnerable to pain-related distress. The adolescent's pain behaviors produce responses from significant people in the adolescent's environment, and these responses may serve to prolong, aggravate, or reduce the pain. Family interaction patterns, parental stress and anxiety, and family models of coping with challenges, especially with pain, can enhance or interfere with the adolescent's pain control effectiveness. Secondary gain (e.g., attention, comfort, or sympathy) for the symptoms in the family system can prolong pain long after the inciting event is past. Additionally, the parents' own stress may heighten their and their adolescent's anxiety and interfere with the parent's ability to assist their adolescent in coping with painful situations.

In addition to the clinical interview (see Chapter 22), there are a number of assessment instruments that are valuable in measuring an adolescent's pain. Behavior rating scales, often used during acute medical procedures or postoperative periods, involve an observer's assessment of the occurrence and intensity of specific pain behaviors. Visual analogue scales consist of a line with endpoints (no numerical anchors) on which a mark is made to indicate the amount of pain. Numerical scales, often pictorially presented as a thermometer or ladder with numerical anchors, are common measurement instruments, where the level of pain is conveyed by selecting shading in the thermometer or selecting a rung number. Many adolescents are able to use descriptive scales that involve endorsing pain words presented in a checklist format. Descriptive scales are useful in their inclusion of affective as well as the sensory components of pain. Pain diaries involve the recording of pain and associated influences, such as the situation and emotional state at the time. Repeated use of these assessment tools with an individual adolescent can be valuable in monitoring treatment effectiveness and providing concrete feedback to the adolescent.

PAIN MANAGEMENT

The most effective approach to adolescent pain management often is a combination of pharmacologic agents and psychological intervention. However, the approach taken depends on the type of pain and the adolescent's needs. Treatment selection should be based upon several factors: the type of pain and situation (e.g., acute or chronic, tissue damage or no identifiable underlying injury); the previous experience of the adolescent with similar or other pain situations; the environmental resources available to the adolescent, including the parents' abilities to help their adolescent; and individual characteristics (e.g., age, cognitive level, coping abilities). In general, pain management methods should be implemented within the framework of the adolescent and his or her family, assessing individual needs, capitalizing on personal resources, establishing predictability and control as appropriate, and fostering feelings of self-control and self-efficacy.

When difficulty with painful medical procedures is anticipated, a helpful general guideline for choosing an intervention (or combinations of interventions) is to maximize the intervention for the initial procedures so that anticipatory anxiety does not develop. Whether to combine pharmacologic and psychological interventions for acute medical procedures should be determined by the level of the adolescent's anxiety and the extent to which the adolescent would benefit from a sense of control over the situation. For some adolescents, pharmacologic treatment may diminish their sense of control, and psychological intervention alone may be sufficient for pain control and enhancement of mastery and self-esteem. However, if an adolescent's anxiety level is so high that he or she is unable to control his or her behavior, sedation (with or without analgesia) is effective in reducing anxiety sufficiently so that the adolescent can respond to behavioral interventions.

Psychological Interventions

There are a number of effective behavioral and cognitive-behavioral techniques for pain management. The provision of information is a widely used method of preparing adolescents for medical procedures. Although it does not provide specific coping techniques, its aim is to reduce fear, anxiety, and pain by providing procedural (what will be done) and sensory (what it may feel like) information to ensure realistic expectations. Information is usually supplemented by exposure to medical equipment and provision of coping strategies.

Interventions such as positive reinforcement, positive self-statements, and modeling may be particularly beneficial for the young or developmentally delayed adolescent. However, they can also be quite helpful to older adolescents when used with other methods. Positive reinforcement involves encouragement with verbal praise, tangible rewards, or rewards of attention immediately following cooperative and adaptive coping behavior. The use of positive self-statements involves teaching a number of simple statements that can be repeated during times of anxiety, fear, or pain. The basic premise is to modify any negative statements related to the appraisal of the situation and self-efficacy. Modeling involves a demonstration (e.g., live models, videotape) of effective coping behavior.

TABLE 16-2. Nonsteroidal Anti-Inflammatory Agents

DRUG	INDICATION	DOSE
Acetaminophen*	Mild pain; fevers	PO: 10–15 mg/kg q4h
		PR: 10–15 mg/kg q4h
Acetylsalicylic acid*	Mild to moderate pain	PO: 10–15 mg/kg q4h
Ibuprofen (Motrin)*	Acute and chronic pain; fever	PO: 5–10 mg/kg tid or qid
Naproxen (Naprosyn)*	Acute and chronic pain	PO: 2–5 mg/kg bid or tid
Tolmetin (Tolectin)*	Acute and chronic pain	PO: 6–8 mg/kg tid or qid
Choline magnesium trisalicylate (Trilisate)	Mild pain	PO: 15–20 mg/kg bid or tid

*FDA approved for use in children.

Distraction techniques aim at focusing attention on something other than the pain or the painful procedure. This can often be accomplished effectively by engaging the adolescent in a cognitive activity, for example, counting, telling a story or jokes, or playing video games. Adolescents must be encouraged to use their own adaptive coping styles. Recent attention has been directed toward understanding the relationship between children's natural coping dispositions and their response to specific interventions. There are findings that children who spontaneously employ distraction techniques for pain demonstrate greater pain tolerance when taught to use imagery than do children whose natural tendency is to focus on some aspect of the pain being experienced (Fanurik et al, 1991).

Hypnosis as a pain intervention involves a combination of distraction, reframing (putting the pain experience in a different perspective), and alterations in sensory experiences. It accomplishes these goals by helping the adolescent to become as intensely involved as possible in a fantasy experience, based upon past experiences, future hopes, the re-creation of a favorite story, or simply an imaginative creation. Involvement in this hypnotic fantasy can be enhanced by asking questions that require thought and imaginative visualization. Developmental level and individual interests can guide the choice of imagery content. Learning self-hypnosis for pain control is particularly appealing for adolescents.

Biofeedback has also been used successfully with adolescents. Biofeedback training teaches adolescents to monitor and control their physiologic responses or concomitants to pain or stress (e.g., increases in muscle tension, heart rate, or blood pressure) by providing them with a feedback signal (auditory or visual). Training in relaxation techniques may also be accomplished through biofeedback.

Pharmacologic Strategies

The pharmacologic management of the adolescent in pain, to augment psychological interventions, can be very challenging, since pain is a highly individualized phenomenon that is subject to the influences of time, cognition, extent of tissue damage or threat of damage, culture, and individual coping styles. However, an un-

derstanding of the various endogenous opioids, adrenergic, serotonergic, and gamma-aminobutyric acid (GABA) systems can help to integrate successful pharmacologic management strategies. The degree of pain, treatment goals, adolescent's clinical status, and the environment in which the adolescent is being cared for dictate the agents and the routes of drug administration. The aim of treatment should be the relief of pain, achievement of metabolic homeostasis, avoidance of toxic side effects, normalization of activity, and prevention of a chronic pain state.

NONSTEROIDAL ANTI-INFLAMMATORY DRUGS

Mild pain can be treated with a variety of nonsteroidal anti-inflammatory drugs (NSAIDs) (Table 16–2). These agents inhibit the enzymatic conversion of arachidonic acid to prostaglandins and leukotrienes, both of which act at peripheral nociceptors to produce hyperalgesia. The use of aspirin, a salicylate representative of this class of drugs, in the adolescent population has been substantially reduced in the past decade as the result of its association with Reye syndrome. Acetaminophen has gained wide acceptance as an alternative to aspirin. Several useful NSAIDs are now available. Ketorolac tromethamine (Toradol), a parenteral NSAID, is now available for clinical use. Since the NSAIDs act to block synthesis, they are best utilized prior to initiation of a painful event. Patients must be carefully monitored for side effects if long-term use is planned. Liver toxicity, hyperkalemia, hypertension, renal dysfunction, and gastrointestinal hemorrhage all are infrequently associated with long-term NSAID use.

OPIOIDS

Opioids are the next most potent class of drugs that produce analgesia (Table 16–3). They act at multiple sites in the brain and spinal cord. There is some evidence that there are peripheral opioid receptors that mediate the analgesic action of the opioids. Multiple receptors mediate the action of these agents; they include μ, κ, σ, and δ. These receptors have been identified by biochemical binding studies and the ability of synthetic and nonsynthetic compounds to produce analgesia, respiratory depression, miosis, euphoria, or physical de-

TABLE 16–3. Opioid Analgesia for Older Children and Adolescents

DRUG	ROUTE	DOSAGE*	IV:PO RATIO	COMMENTS
Codeine phosphate	PO, IM, IV, SC	PO: 0.5–1.0 mg/kg/dose q4h	1:(1.5–2)	Mild pain, more potent in combination with acetaminophen or aspirin
Oxycodone	PO, IM, IV, SC	IV: 0.05–0.15 mg/kg/dose to 10 mg/dose maximum q4–5h	1:2	Mild pain, used in Darvocet and Tylox
Morphine sulfate	PO, IM, IV	PO: 0.2–0.3 mg/kg q2–4h IV bolus: 0.1–1.0 mg/kg/dose q2–4h IV continuous infusion: 0.05–0.4 mg/kg/h (range 0.025–2.6 mg/kg/h)† SC continuous infusion: 0.06–0.1 mg/kg/h (range: 0.03–1.8 mg/kg/h)†	1:3 1:6 (with initial dose but with increasing doses decrease to 1:2–3)	Moderate to severe pain, smoother pain control with IV bolus followed by continuous infusion; SC continuous infusion provides good home care method; $T_{1/2}$ 3–4 h
Meperidine hydrochloride	PO, IM, IV	IV bolus: 1–1.5 mg/kg/dose q3–4h IV continuous infusion: 0.5–0.7 mg/kg/h	1:4	Moderate to severe pain, smoother pain control with IV bolus followed by continuous infusion
Hydromorphone hydrochloride	PO, IM, IV, SC, rectal suppository	IV: 0.05–0.1 mg/kg/dose to 5 mg/dose q6h (not recommended for young children)	1:5	Moderate to severe pain, useful as oral agent; $t_{1/2}$ 2–3 h
Methadone hydrochloride	PO, IM, IV, SC	IV: 0.2 mg/kg/dose q6h (1–5-year-old children: 0.1 mg/kg/dose to maximum of 0.7 mg/kg/24 h)	1:2	Moderate to severe pain expected for prolonged time period; oral analgesia sought ultimately; $t_{1/2}$ 15–24 h; steady state after 4–5 days with oral administration: risk of inadequate early pain relief, should be used with IV morphine initially or alone as IV boluses q2–4h until adequate pain relief; calculate oral dose from these data; amitriptyline reduces methadone clearance while phenytoin enhances it

*All dosages are only suggestions and should be verified with a pharmacist. Additionally, the patient's clinical status and drug sensitivity should be taken into account when administering these drugs.

†The range for some patients may be higher.

Adapted with permission from Zeltzer LK, Zeltzer PM: Clinical assessment and pharmacologic treatment of pain in children: Cancer as a model for the management of chronic persistent pain. Pediatrician 16:64, 1989.

pendence. All opioids depress respiration in a dose-dependent manner; however, this respiratory depression is counteracted by pain. Thus, an adolescent in pain tolerates more drug than the same adolescent without pain. Other side effects depend on the specific opiate administered, the dose, and the rate of delivery. Imperative to proper management is titration to individual analgesic levels and the concomitant use of stimulants, NSAIDs, laxatives, and antipruritics to effectively eliminate side effects.

Morphine remains the gold standard for opioids. It produces sedation and analgesia. Morphine can be administered through a number of different routes: intravenous (IV), epidural, intrathecal, enteral, intramuscular (IM), rectal, transdermal, and transmucosal. It reaches its peak after intravenous administration within 15 minutes and is most effective in antagonizing dull, intermittent pain. Patient-controlled administration of morphine via small mechanized pumps has been used increasingly. Use of these pumping devices has allowed tailoring of better individualized analgesic regimens.

Methadone is much like morphine, except that it has a much longer half-life—12 to 30 hours. This is an ideal agent for patients with chronic pain, when IV administration of opiates is not approved, when there is limited IV access, or when patient-controlled devices are not available.

Numerous synthetic opioids possessing a variety of biophysical properties are available. Fentanyl, a highly

lipid soluble agent, has a very short onset and duration of action. It suppresses the stress response associated with pain and acute injury and is approximately 300 times more potent than morphine. Sufentanil, another synthetic agent, is 7 to 10 times more potent than fentanyl, thus limiting its use to only special circumstances outside of the operating room.

OTHER ANALGESICS AND ANESTHETICS

Other agents such as meperidine (Demerol), hydromorphone (Dilaudid), and alfentanil (Alfenta) each have different biochemical characteristics that are appropriate to various clinical settings. Demerol has been a popular drug; however, the association of one of its metabolites with seizures has led to its decreased use.

Several other classes of agents can be beneficial adjuncts to a drug regimen. Benzodiazepines are anxiolytics that produce antegrade amnesia, muscle relaxation, sedation, and anticonvulsant activity. They have a wide therapeutic index and produce limited hemodynamic alterations. Midazolam is the newest of this class of agent to gain acceptance for use in the adolescent population. It is ideal for use in conjunction with medical procedures because it is water soluble and very short acting.

Ketamine, a dissociative anesthetic agent that is structurally related to phencyclidine, produces analgesia, anesthesia, and antegrade amnesia. Ketamine, 0.25 mg/

kg body weight given intravenously, is also ideal for short procedures. Administration of a benzodiazepine with ketamine reduces the incidence of unpleasant dreams associated with ketamine use.

Stimulants such as dextroamphetamine increase the analgesic effects of opioids. They reduce the nausea, respiratory depression, and sedation associated with opioid administration. The anticonvulsants carbamazepine, phenytoin, and clonidine are especially useful in treating neuropathic pain. Suppression of peripheral nerve excitability is thought to be their mode of action. Antidepressants such as fluoxetine, desipramine, doxepin, and imipramine have a direct analgesic action mediated by the inhibition of re-uptake of serotonin and norepinephrine by neurons. These drugs potentiate the actions of opioids at low nonantidepressive doses.

Regional anesthetic techniques are simple and can be safely performed. The techniques can eliminate the need for the aforementioned agents, thus reducing exposure of the patient to some drug side effects. A myriad of nerve blocks can be performed with local anesthetics to reduce nociceptive nerve transmission and to reduce the stress hormone response to pain. Epidural, intrathecal nerve blocks and sympathetic nerve blocks are being used to treat acute postoperative pain and chronic pain, such as that which may result from cancer and reflex sympathetic dystrophy.

Newer, more innovative techniques of pain control must be discovered in the future. The techniques should be cost effective and time efficient and have limited side effects. Devices such as the transdermal fentanyl patch and the transdermal local anesthetic patch will help to eliminate barriers to effective pain management, such as the use of IM injections. A working knowledge of the pharmacology of the several classes of drugs used in pain treatment, a wider acknowledgment of the variability in pain tolerance and coping styles, and a recognition that the pharmacologic and psychological management of pain are not mutually exclusive help to ensure that better treatment strategies are applied to patients in pain.

In summary, multiple interventional strategies exist for the treatment of an adolescent's pain. Future investigation must focus on finding rapid, inexpensive techniques of identifying coping styles, developing quick pain assessment tools, and creating safe, simple methods of pharmacologic intervention. Additionally, the role of pubertal development and its influence on pain perception should be studied.

BIBLIOGRAPHY

Fanurik D, Zeltzer LK, Roberts MC, Blount RL: The relationship between children's coping styles and psychological interventions for cold pressor pain. Unpublished manuscript, 1991.

McGrath PA: Pain in Children: Nature, Assessment, and Treatment. New York, Guilford Press, 1990.

Ross DM, Ross SA: Childhood Pain: Current Issues, Research, and Management. Baltimore, Urban & Schwarzenberg, 1988.

Siegel LJ, Smith KE: Children's strategies for coping with pain. Pediatrician 16:110, 1989.

Smith K, Ackerson JD, Blotcky AD: Reducing stress during invasive medical procedures. Relating behavioral interventions to preferred coping style in pediatric cancer patients. J Pediatr Psychol 14:405, 1989.

Zeltzer LK, Anderson CTM, Schecter N: Pediatric pain: Current status and new directions. Curr Prob Pediatr 20(8):411, 1990.

Zeltzer LK, Jay SM, Fisher DM: The management of pain associated with medical procedures. Pediatr Clin North Am 36:1, 1989.

CLINICAL APPROACH TO

ADOLESCENTS

Introduction

The clinical approach to adolescents is in large part determined by their unique biologic and psychological characteristics and by a need for flexibility in the delivery of their health care. Thus, information on practice settings, practice principles, and practice applications is critical to the practitioner of adolescent medicine.

Practice settings for adolescent medicine encompass a number of sites. Many adolescents are cared for by primary care physicians, in adolescent clinics, and in inpatient units; others receive care in nontraditional settings. The office practice of adolescent medicine includes consideration of the facility, the office staff, the time, and the scheduling of appointments; the practitioner who cares for adolescents; and patient and parent considerations, not the least of which are socioeconomic considerations. Most adolescents being cared for in private practices are seen within a larger practice, whether it is a pediatrician's office, an internist's office, a family physician's office, or an obstetrician-gynecologist's office. Emphasis should be placed on adequate privacy, confidentiality, comfort, and convenience. Well-trained staff enjoy adolescents and treat young people and their families with respect and dignity. Time is always at a premium for practitioners and for adolescents and their families. Flexibility in scheduling and provision of adequate time for the diagnosis and treatment of complex problems are practice challenges.

There are a number of models of nontraditional settings of practice of adolescent medicine. These include school-based health centers, community-based centers and free clinics, vocationally based services such as the Job Corps, and specific programs within given states. The strength of these sites is that they offer adolescents the ability to receive health care that might be unavailable otherwise.

Practice principles include legal aspects of providing personal, confidential adolescent health care and the financing of adolescent health care. It is imperative that practitioners of adolescent medicine know the laws governing adolescent medicine in their states and the policies in institutional settings such as hospitals where they practice. In most states, the legal age of majority is 18 years, but there are exceptions to when adolescent medical care can be rendered if the person is younger than 18 years of age. A firm understanding of the legal aspects of delivering adolescent medicine is critical for the protection of the adolescent, the adolescent's parents, and the practitioner. Financing of adolescent health care is a constant challenge in the office and at the national level. Many new strategies are being suggested to ensure adequate funding of adolescent health services.

Practice applications of adolescent medicine are challenging. Successful interviewing of adolescents combines knowledge of adolescent development, human nature, and enjoyment of talking with and helping young people. As is true of any skill, the more the practitioner interviews adolescents, the easier interviewing becomes.

A focus on family issues is at the heart of the optimum practice of adolescent medicine. Definition of the presenting symptom and differentiation of the actual symptomatic member of the family are critical to a thorough evaluation. Referral of adolescents to psychiatric care when appropriate is extremely important. Primary care practitioners should develop the skills to recognize psychological problems and should seek early consultation to optimize the adolescent's health outcome.

Guidelines to well adolescent care (health maintenance visits) are critical, but they are less well defined than those for infants and children. There is new information on immunizations, cardiovascular health, and reproductive concerns.

Compliance is a particular challenge in the practice of adolescent medicine, because adolescents, as a result of their relative immaturity and their inability to conceptualize, abstract, and think ahead, may not realize the importance of taking medication. It is important that practitioners of adolescent medicine understand the relationship between compliance and adolescent development and develop strategies to work with adolescents to help them to follow medical regimens.

As the health care issues of adolescents become increasingly complex over time, interdisciplinary teams have been found to be effective in providing services for some adolescents. Interdisciplinary teams are found in university hospital and other teaching programs, health maintenance organizations, specialty clinics for adolescents with chronic illnesses, adolescent inpatient units, and community health care clinics.

The special needs of subgroups of adolescents should be considered as practitioners provide their care. Cross-cultural youth, military youth, chronically ill and emotionally disturbed youth, mentally retarded youth, gay youth, at-risk youth, and incarcerated youth are the groups addressed in this text. Suggestions are made by the authors of these chapters as to how each of us can become sensitized to the special needs of vulnerable young people. Preparing adolescents and young adults, especially chronically ill young people, to make the transition to adult health care is a particular challenge to clinicians.

New strategies to prevent adolescent morbidity and mortality are evolving. Adolescence is an ideal time to empower young people to take care of themselves and to prevent morbidity in the future. Focuses on adolescent health promotion, prevention of alcohol and other drug use, and prevention of the initiation of cigarette smoking during the adolescent years all are critically important new areas about which information is becoming available. The strategies that are now experimental will be incorporated into the clinical practice of adolescent medicine in the future.

Practice Settings

CHAPTER 17

Office Practice

W. SAM YANCY

Adolescents constitute approximately 16% of all ambulatory visits to physicians. On the average, they visit physicians less frequently than do all other age groups, and the duration of each visit is less than 10 minutes, despite the complex nature of their health problems.

Both physicians and adolescents may perceive several barriers to the optimal delivery of adolescent health care in the office. Physicians may be concerned about reimbursement (see Chapter 21), time constraints, and a lack of skill in caring for adolescents. Adolescents may believe they are not in need of services. They may be concerned about access to and cost of services, confidentiality and privacy (see Chapter 20), and whether the physician and staff are really interested in their concerns. All these potential barriers to care are surmountable. The following provides suggestions for the physician who offers health care services to adolescents in the primary care office.

FACILITY CONSIDERATIONS

There are increasing numbers of physicians who limit their practices to adolescents only; at least one medical group has been successful in caring for adolescents by providing a separate office facility for their adolescent patients. This group provides care for their younger patients in their primary pediatric office. At age 12 or 13 years, or at the age at which they are comfortable, the patients "graduate" to the nearby adolescent center. This center is dedicated to comprehensive adolescent care and is staffed by physicians with whom the patients are already familiar. However, in most practices, adolescents share a pediatrician's office with younger patients, an internist's or gynecologist's office with adults, or a family physician's office with adults and children. If the office provides adequate privacy, comfort, and convenience, there may be no need for modification; a separate waiting room is desirable, however. Rock music and strobe lights are not necessary, but appropriate posters and a bulletin board with local school items and relevant health education materials are helpful. Reading material, for both education and entertainment, should reflect adolescent tastes. There should be additional materials for parents as well. "No smoking" signs and the lack of ashtrays provide a good example and an important message about not smoking.

Examination rooms should be large enough to accommodate the adolescent, the physician, and a parent or a chaperone when indicated. Adult-sized examination tables fitted with stirrups for pelvic examinations are necessary. Soundproofing is advisable to ensure privacy when sensitive topics are being discussed.

Other office features are similar to those for adults and young children, with a few exceptions. The laboratory should be equipped for Papanicolaou smears and sexually transmitted disease testing (see Chapter 69). There should be appropriate gowns for the adolescent age group. Small- and medium-sized specula should be available for pelvic examinations.

STAFF CONSIDERATIONS

More important than the physical arrangement of the primary care office is the attitude of the practitioner and staff. First impressions are lasting impressions, and the adolescent patient's first contact with the office may be by telephone or at the office's front desk. If the receptionist or nurse is cold or uninterested, the adolescent may expect to receive the same treatment from the physician. All staff should be comfortable talking to teenagers and should respect their need for privacy and confidentiality. If a parent calls asking for patient information, the call should be referred to the physician.

An interested and well-trained nurse may provide valuable patient education on relevant topics such as menstruation, nutrition, and contraception. This may be done on a one-to-one basis or with groups. Some offices offer monthly evening discussion groups. There may be a charge for this service or there may be no charge if it is used as a means of attracting new patients.

TIME AND SCHEDULING CONSIDERATIONS

The duration of office encounters for acute illness is similar for all ages, but health maintenance examinations, sports physicals, and especially pelvic examinations may take longer for the adolescent patient (see Chapters 25, 69, and 81). The appointment secretary needs to request the reason for a visit in order to determine how much time to allocate. If the adolescent or parent is unwilling to discuss a sensitive matter with the receptionist, the physician should be available to determine what type of appointment is needed. Another strategy may be to schedule a short visit to determine the nature of the problem for those adolescents and families who do not want to or who cannot discuss the reason for the visit on the telephone.

Although adolescents do not often require urgent visits, some walk-in or same-day appointments should be available. Even visits for a sports participation examination (see Chapter 81) may be considered urgent if the patient will not be allowed to play or practice until the examination is completed. Occasionally the complexity of unanticipated problems may require additional time that is not available. The adolescent will appreciate and have respect for the practitioner who arranges another appointment to allow sufficient time to evaluate the problem. Any attempt to dismiss the problem because of a lack of time or a hurried, cursory response will be poorly received and weaken the practitioner-adolescent relationship.

Obviously the practitioner's office time is valuable, but the adolescent patient's time should also be respected. Late afternoon appointments and evening clinics once or twice a week help adolescents avoid missing school and being absent from afterschool activities.

Adolescents should be encouraged to make their own appointments, but parents should be informed of this arrangement. If the adolescent does make the appointment, it is appropriate to see the patient alone first. This will assist in the development of rapport and a sense of trust. Subsequent visits may be with the adolescent alone or with the parent or parents present. Meeting together provides valuable information regarding family dynamics (see Chapter 25).

History forms and questionnaires can save time and provide records for future reference. They should be used not to take the place of the interview but to allow more time for important or relevant matters. Parent questionnaires may be helpful if the parent is unable to be present at the time of the initial appointment. Some questionnaires facilitate discussion or raise issues of concern to the adolescent that one otherwise might not mention.

PHYSICIAN CONSIDERATIONS
(see Chapter 22)

All physicians should be honest, fair, and sincere in interacting with their patients—the adolescent patient expects no less. It is important to be warm, friendly, and understanding, but it is not necessary to be a "buddy" or a "pal." The physician can be an advocate for adolescents and remain an authority, but he or she should not act in an authoritarian manner. The adolescent is still struggling with ambivalence about the authority status of parents and the independence he or she is seeking. It is not necessary for the practitioner to act, dress, or speak like an adolescent in order to communicate successfully. Rather, the adolescent recognizes this effort as dishonest, and it interferes with the development of a trusting relationship. The physician should not hesitate to ask the meaning of slang words or phrases, thinking that it would make him or her appear uninformed. More often the adolescent patient is impressed with the fact that the physician is trying to

understand and is interested in what he or she has to say. For parents who complain that they do not know what their adolescent thinks because he or she never talks to them, there is also an adolescent who says, "No one listens to me, so what is the use of saying anything?" Careful, concerned listening goes a long way toward successful communication with adolescents, and good communication is of prime importance.

Interviewing is more than just taking a history (see Chapter 22). It provides the information that the practitioner needs to understand and treat the patient; it also enables the patient to understand the physician's assessment and recommendations. It is the medium of communication through which the patient and the practitioner evaluate each other, negotiate their respective roles and obligations, and develop a working relationship. A good interview can be therapeutic in itself, because making another person feel truly understood provides that person with comfort and helps the individual to feel better regardless of the problem.

Many subjects that adolescents want to discuss are complex and controversial. The practitioner needs to become comfortable with questions regarding sexual matters and drug use (see Chapters 25, 75, and 111). This requires a thorough knowledge of such matters, as well as insightful thinking in order not to be encumbered by one's own unresolved adolescent and sexual problems. In brief, the practitioner must be honest and open-minded, knowledgeable, and sensitive and should encourage responsible behavior without being judgmental.

PATIENT AND PARENT CONSIDERATIONS

A general definition of adolescence is that it begins with the youth's initial psychological reaction to pubescent physical changes and extends to a reasonable resolution of personal identity (see Chapters 5 and 9). Just as the adolescent's practitioner should be familiar with the stages of physical growth and development during puberty and the normal age ranges over which they occur, so should he or she be knowledgeable about the behavioral and developmental tasks the adolescent is striving to accomplish.

The adolescent patient comes to the physician seeking confidentiality and professional advice (see Chapter 20). The pediatrician and family physician have an advantage in caring for adolescents since they often have had the opportunity to develop a background of knowledge and rapport during previous visits. The adolescent can appreciate an existing, trusting relationship and thus avoid exposing his or her body and intimate problems to a stranger.

The physician, however, must strike a balance between preserving the teenager's right to confidential medical care and respecting the parents' responsibility for their child. The goal of the physician should be to facilitate communication and understanding between the parent and the adolescent and not to interfere with that relationship.

Parents can provide the practitioner with important

information that may be unknown to the adolescent patient or that the patient is unwilling to share. Parents are valuable not only in the diagnostic evaluation but also in the treatment process and should be kept thoroughly informed within the bounds of patient confidentiality (see Chapter 22). The laws protecting the right of adolescents to seek care without parental consent usually refer to reproductive health and substance abuse, but they vary from state to state (see Chapter 20).

The issue of using a chaperone when examining the adolescent relates to both privacy and confidentiality. A survey of physicians who treat adolescents has revealed that one third use no chaperone during pelvic examinations. Younger patients may prefer to have a parent present; others may request that no one but the physician be present. The decision to use a chaperone should consider the adolescent's preference as well as the physician's. In addition to personal and medicolegal considerations, as an assistant the chaperone can improve comfort and efficiency and may allow for an optimum educational experience for the adolescent patient. Other indications for using a chaperone include a first pelvic examination, a patient with emotional problems, a history of rape or sexual abuse, and a seductive patient (see Chapters 69, 118, and 119).

FINANCIAL CONSIDERATIONS

Just as the chronologic age of the adolescent patient falls between that of the child and the adult, the fees charged for adolescent health care usually fall between those of the pediatrician and the internist. As stated earlier, there are increasing numbers of private practices limited to adolescent patients, but most adolescents continue to be seen by pediatricians and family physicians who also see younger or older patients, or both. Health maintenance organizations, independent practice associations, and preferred provider organizations will have an increasing impact on the health care delivery to all patients, and in the future, resource-based relative-value scales will allow more equitable setting of fees (see Chapter 21). Currently, the physician who serves adolescents must accept the fact that one should charge for professional time spent. Long suggests a formula for setting fees that considers professional expenses, the collection percentage, and the time spent with the patient. A simpler approach is to establish the charge for a standard office visit as the basic fee unit. Since these visits average 15 minutes in most offices, a visit or conference that lasts 30 minutes will carry a fee of twice the basic unit. Once the basic fee unit is established, the physician need only use the codes in the *Current Procedural Terminology* that are appropriate (established patient–adolescent = 90761, counseling and conference services for 30 minutes = 90843, and so on). It is advisable to discuss possible expense with adolescents and parents if longer term counseling is indicated.

At the adolescent's request it is appropriate to bill parents, who must be informed of appointments and findings. The physician must decide whether to accept the risks, both legal and financial, for seeing an adolescent without parental consent (see Chapter 20). A

TABLE 17–1. Community Resources for Adolescents

ORGANIZATION	SERVICES PROVIDED
ACLD (Association for Children with Learning Disabilities)	Advocates optimal services for the learning-disabled
Alateen	Assists adolescents to deal with their alcohol problems through meetings and group discussions
Al-Anon Family Groups	Provides fellowship with other families facing the problem of alcoholism in a relative
ARC (Association for Retarded Citizens)	Advocates optimal services for individuals with mental retardation; provides support for families
Big Brothers and Big Sisters	Provides, under professional supervision, a volunteer older "sibling" for youth who are from single-parent families and may benefit from adult guidance and companionship
Boy Scouts of America and Girl Scouts of America	Promotes group interaction, responsibility, and leadership skills, with emphasis on outdoor activities
Child Watch	Supports families who have a missing youth and assists in searching for the adolescent
Family Counseling Services	Provides family therapy and group work to individuals and families
4-H Clubs	Promotes group interaction and responsibility with emphasis on homemaking and agricultural activities
Health Department	Family planning clinics; sexually transmitted diseases clinics; prenatal clinics
Legal Aid Society	Provides legal advice and representation for civil cases to persons unable to afford a lawyer
Mental Health Department	Assesses mental health needs of the community and plans, organizes, and provides direct services to meet these needs
Planned Parenthood	Provides contraceptive assistance and abortion referral or services
Public Defender System	Provides free legal representation in criminal and juvenile proceedings
American Red Cross	Provides health education classes
SADD (Students Against Drunk Driving)	Provides peer group education and assistance
Social Service Department	Provides foster care, adoption, and protection services
Telephone Hotlines	Respond to crisis needs, including rape, suicide, runaways, and drug abuse—National Clearinghouse for Mental Health Information: (301) 433-4515
Vocational Rehabilitation	Assists the physically, mentally, or emotionally disabled in their efforts to obtain suitable employment; provides vocational assessments
Weight Reduction Centers (e.g., Shape-Down, etc.)	Provide structured, nutritional peer group approach to weight reduction
Young Men's Christian Association (YMCA) and Young Women's Christian Association (YWCA)	Provide planned programs for physical and social development, educational classes, interest groups, and self-help workshops

Adapted by permission of Elsevier Science Publishing Co., Inc. from Community resources for adolescents, by WS Yancy. Journal of Adolescent Health Care, Vol. 8, p. 221. Copyright 1987 by The Society for Adolescent Medicine.

separate account can be set up for the adolescent without sending statements to the parents. One survey has shown that some adolescents are willing to pay for confidential care, but the practitioner may wish to reduce the fees, since most adolescents are not wage earners. Laboratory studies that are sent to an outside laboratory present a more complicated problem. The physician may need to absorb these expenses to avoid statements being delivered to the parents and trust that the adolescent will reimburse the physician.

COMMUNITY RESOURCES CONSIDERATIONS

The optimal approach to adolescent problems often requires interaction with community support systems to develop a multidisciplinary diagnostic and therapeutic team (see Chapter 27). Merely providing the adolescent or the parents with a phone number does not ensure entry into a resource system. Prior communication with the agency by the physician to establish a relationship with a particular person within an agency and a call to alert that individual about the specifics of the adolescent's problem allow the practitioner to ease the entry process. It is always important to call and make sure

that parents and adolescents have followed through with the contact. Table 17–1 provides a partial list of frequently available resources. Similar programs may operate under different names in different communities. The practitioner can compile his or her own list if a local directory is unavailable, and new services can be added as they become available.

BIBLIOGRAPHY

Compendium of Resource Materials on Adolescent Health: Department of Health and Human Resources. Publication Number (HSA) 81–5245, Rockville, MD, 1981.
Felice ME, Friedman SB: Behavioral considerations in the health care of adolescents. Pediatr Clin North Am 29:399, 1982.
Friedman IM, Goldberg E: Reference materials for the practice of adolescent medicine. Pediatr Clin North Am 27:193, 1980.
Gleason CH: Our practice grew—The second time around. Med Econ 65:63, 1988.
Irwin CE (ed.): Health care of the emerging adult: Implications for the practitioner. J Adolesc Health Care 7(Suppl):1S, 1986.
Long WA: The role of the private practitioner II. Financial considerations. Adolesc Med: State of the Art Rev 1:152, 1990.
Marks A, Fisher M: Health assessment and screening during adolescence. Pediatrics 80(Suppl):135, 1987.
Neinstein LS: Consolidation of psychosocial scales. J Adolesc Health Care 9:507, 1988.
Thornburg HD: Development in Adolescence. Monterey, CA, Brooks/Cole, 1982.
Yancy WS: Considerations for the physician who treats adolescents in the office. Semin Adolesc Med 3:93, 1987.

CHAPTER 18

Nontraditional Settings

RENÉE R. JENKINS and TRINA M. ANGLIN

When compared with all other age groups, adolescents (aged 11 to 20 years) have the lowest rate of ambulatory visits per year to physicians practicing in office settings (see Chapters 2 and 17). Although this observation supports the concept that adolescents use traditional health care services less frequently than do either adults or children, it fails to consider the number of adolescents who receive health care from agencies and institutions that are considered "nontraditional." School-based health centers, vocational training centers, and juvenile detention centers are among the age-specific settings in which young people, especially those from families with a lower socioeconomic status, receive health services. Community-based public health clinics and free clinics that have special services for adolescents also function as alternative health care settings for this population. This chapter presents the rationale for the use of nontraditional settings by adolescents, describes several models of nontraditional practice, and reviews the service issues related to providing care in these unique settings.

RATIONALE FOR NONTRADITIONAL SETTINGS

Adolescents preferentially rank cost, access, and confidentiality as important factors that affect their use of health care. Recent studies on health insurance coverage of adolescents and young adults confirm that cost is a major issue (see Chapters 2 and 21).

Access issues include general concerns about the geographic location of health care facilities and their hours of operation as well as age-related concerns, such as the minor's right to consent to his or her own health care. The management of confidentiality within a health setting is the most identifiable feature of the appropriateness of a service for adolescent patients (see Chapter 20). Other subtle characteristics, as discussed in the previous chapter, include the ambience and receptiveness of the setting for providing care to adolescents, the recognition that adolescents are progressing through a rapidly changing stage of development, and an open communication style about sensitive issues relevant to the lives and health of adolescents (see Chapter 17).

Few research studies have empirically documented the demographic and morbidity profiles of adolescents who use nontraditional settings for their health and medical care. However, available research data as well as the impressions of experienced staff members who work in these settings indicate that these adolescents frequently have multiple and complex biobehavioral problems. In addition, many adolescents have confirmed that they are not able (because of financial constraints) or willing (because of concern about confidentiality or judgmental attitudes) to seek care from traditional medical settings, such as the physician's office (see Chapter 17).

Many nontraditional settings for adolescent health care were designed to address health care delivery issues: that is, the adolescents freely sought health care in that setting. Others have achieved high use through structured programs in which adolescents take part and receive health care as part of the program, such as in juvenile detention settings (see Chapter 34) or vocational training settings. The successful structured models have developed health services screening and content elements that are highly relevant to the adolescents whom they serve (see Chapters 28–35).

MODELS OF NONTRADITIONAL PRACTICE

School-based Clinics

School-based clinics are primary care health centers located on the campuses of junior and senior high schools. This controversial model for providing health care and psychosocial counseling to adolescents is becoming increasingly popular, as witnessed by its rapid growth over the past decade. The first comprehensive high school clinic opened in West Dallas in 1970. The pioneering and widely publicized St. Paul High School Clinic opened in 1973. Since then, the number of school-based clinics has grown steadily; growth has been especially rapid since 1984. In 1989, approximately 150 sites were operating across 91 communities in 32 states.

School-based clinics offer a variety of services to enhance student health. In addition to providing comprehensive primary medical care and mental health care, clinic staff members commonly mobilize existing community resources to create referral networks for students, address adolescent sexuality and reproductive health issues, and provide health and nutrition education. Most clinics also offer substance abuse programs.

The services provided by school-based clinics during 1988 are listed in Table 18–1.

The majority of school-based clinics maintain organizational and administrative independence from the school system, though 20% of current programs are actually administered by community school districts. School-based clinics were originally organized to function autonomously from the schools that housed them, as a strategy to enhance students' trust in their staff members. However, an increasing proportion of clinics are currently sponsored by school districts. These sites report that this administrative arrangement works well in practice, because it facilitates integration of school health services and decreases bureaucratic complexity. Other sponsoring agencies include hospitals and medical schools (26%), departments of public health (23%), and nonprofit organizations (19%). An additional 12% of school-based clinics function as satellites of community health centers.

The staffing of school-based clinics usually relies upon nurse practitioners and physicians to provide the majority of general health and medical care, as well as counselors or social workers to address mental health, substance use, and family issues. The most frequent reason for students to visit school-based clinics is for acute problems, including illness and injury (25%). Mental health and psychosocial problems (18%) are the second most frequent reason for visits. In contrast, relatively few students have been seen primarily for substance abuse problems (see Chapter 111). Reproductive health care visits have recently accounted for only 12% of all visits. The majority of newer school-based clinics provide a narrower range of reproductive health care services compared with older clinic sites, and they are less likely to prescribe or dispense contraceptives. An in-depth evaluation of six independent school-based clinic sites confirmed that even at sites that formally dispense contraceptive products, the large majority of visits (about 75%) are for health needs unrelated to contraception.

School-based clinics are thought to enhance adolescents' access to health care, including mental health care. More than one half (55%) of the students enrolled in school-based clinics had no other source of primary health care during 1988. In addition, about one third of enrolled students (34%) had no health insurance coverage. This figure is significantly higher than a 1984 national estimate that 14% of adolescents had no health insurance coverage. The remainder of students had either private or public (Medicaid) health insurance (see Chapter 21).

Community-based Centers and Free Clinics

The histories of community health centers and the free clinic movement parallel one another regarding both their inception and the motivation for their existence. Both health models emerged during the late 1960s during a climate of social reform. They represented a delivery model that encouraged health consumers to participate in the design and operation of new organizations trying to improve the health status of their local communities. Free clinics and community-based centers represented a grassroots response to two major issues: drug-related problems among youth and the failure of the traditional health care system to provide care for poor individuals without health insurance. The free clinic movement was the forerunner of many community-based services that are currently in existence for teenagers.

Some organizations developed services from a fixed site, whereas others used a mobile unit that interacted with a fixed site. Two examples of the fixed-site model, in which health services are delivered to patients of all ages including adolescents, are the Los Angeles Free

TABLE 18–1. Services Provided by School-based Clinics in 1988

TYPE OF SERVICE	PERCENTAGE OF SITES PROVIDING SERVICE
General Health Services	
Primary health care	98
Assessment and referral to a community health care system	98
Physical assessment for sports	95
General physical examinations	95
Laboratory tests	95
Diagnosis and treatment of minor trauma	95
Assessment and referral to a community physician	94
Prescription of medication for treatment	92
Pregnancy diagnosis and referral for antenatal care	89
Diagnosis and treatment of sexually transmitted diseases	87
Gynecologic examinations	85
Immunizations	81
Follow-up examination for users of contraceptive methods	77
Chronic illness management	75
Medications dispensed	72
Examination for selected methods of contraception	62
Referral for contraceptive method and examination	61
Early and periodic screening, diagnosis, and treatment	51
Health care for infants of adolescents	47
Prescription of contraceptive methods	46
Antenatal care	41
Dental services	41
Day care	17
Methods of contraception dispensed	15
Counseling and Educational Services	
Health education	100
Nutrition education	99
Mental health and psychosocial counseling	96
Sexuality counseling	95
Weight reduction programs	95
Pregnancy counseling	89
Contraceptive method counseling	86
Substance abuse programs	77
Sexuality education in classroom setting	73
Parenting education	67
Job counseling	27

Adapted from Lovick SR, Stern RF: School-based Clinics, 1988 Update. Washington, DC, Center for Population Options, 1988.

Clinic in California and The Free Medical Clinic of Greater Cleveland in Ohio. They were started during the original free clinic movement and were established in 1968 and 1970 respectively. Another fixed-site model is one that serves adolescents exclusively. Examples include The Door in New York City, another product of the free clinic movement, and more recent replications of that model, such as The Center for Youth Services in Washington, DC, and Threshold Center for Youth Alternative Services, Inc. in Rochester, New York. These models provide comprehensive services for adolescents. They offer health and medical services concurrently with mental health, substance abuse, educational, and employment services. This model requires young persons to work with individual primary counselors, who use a baseline assessment to guide adolescents to the services they request or that are seen as appropriate to resolve their problems. Another important component of this model is the concept of an interdisciplinary team that meets regularly to coordinate the efforts of its individual providers (see Chapter 27). The model is committed to case management, and a single, unified record is maintained for each adolescent.

The Door is a large-scale example of the fixed-site service model, with approximately 70 full-time paid positions and more than 75 volunteers. Staff members include physicians, nurse practitioners, nurses, nutritionists, pharmacists, laboratory technicians, medical assistants, psychologists, social workers, lawyers, teachers and health educators, vocational rehabilitation counselors, artists, and dancers. These staff members provide broad services for the adolescent patients of The Door. However, The Door still interacts with numerous community agencies for two purposes: referral networks for outreach to new adolescent patients and delivery of specialized services to adolescents already enrolled with The Door. The Door's annual budget is supported by more than 80 funding sources, which include federal, state, and local public agencies, as well as private foundations, corporations, and individuals. About 75% of the youth who use The Door do not have health insurance coverage, either public or private. An estimated 22% of The Door's adolescent patients are covered by Medicaid, and an estimated 3% have private third-party insurance. Although a sliding scale payment system is operational, out of pocket payments by The Door's clients are negligible.

The Bridge Over Troubled Waters Program in Boston, Massachusetts illustrates the model of a mobile unit that has relationships with fixed sites. The Bridge was established in 1970 to provide a wide range of free services to runaways, homeless street youth, and other alienated adolescents (see Chapter 33). The full program has nine parts, of which the mobile van is the oldest. The other mobile component is an outreach service in which street worker staff members contact individual young street persons who need help. The other components are fixed in buildings and include counseling services, a free dental clinic, a program for pregnant and parenting adolescents, a runaway program, educational services, and both long-term and short-term residential programs that help youth make the transition from the streets to stable and economically productive lifestyles. The hallmark of The Bridge is its strategy of taking services into the street rather than expecting homeless and street youth to go to a fixed site for initial contact with helping services. The mobile contact and medical treatment services fit the evening and nocturnal schedules of street youth (see Chapter 33).

A significant constraint of using a mobile van to provide medical care, however, is its inability to address more than a finite number of acute health problems. The two most frequent problems encountered by the mobile van's staff members are infections and trauma; together they compose 60% of the presenting problems. It is not clear why youth who have chronic medical conditions represent a relatively low proportion of adolescent visits for care by the staff members of the mobile van, but it cannot be concluded that this population has no need for or will not use medical care for other than acute problems.

Vocationally Based Services

The Job Corps program is one of the largest national vocational training programs in the United States. It was established in 1964 by the Economic Opportunity Act and is administered by the US Department of Labor. Approximately 107 Job Corps centers currently exist, and 75% of them are operated by private companies through competitive bidding. The Job Corps program was designed to address the severe employment problems faced by seriously disadvantaged youth. Young persons are eligible to enroll in Job Corps if they are between the ages of 16 and 21 years and are impoverished and unemployed and come from debilitating environments. Many Job Corps enrollees are relocated to residential centers in order to receive intensive services in a new, salutary environment. The young persons volunteer for the program and receive basic (remedial) education, vocational skills training, work experience counseling, health care (medical and dental), and related support services. They learn the responsibilities of citizenship through self-government and community volunteer work. Statistics reveal that during the 1988 program year most Corps members were male (67%), belonged to minority groups (70%), had ceased going to school (83%), and had an average reading ability that was equivalent to a sixth grade level. The mean annual family income of Corps members was $6,032 in 1988, and 38% of the families of the Corps members received public financial assistance. More than one half of Corps members were younger than 19 years, and approximately one half had prior arrest records.

The health services component requires new Corps members to complete a physical examination that includes screening for anemia, dental and visual abnormalities, and substance abuse. Residential students are also screened for the human immunodeficiency virus (HIV). Substance abuse counseling and preventive education are standard features of a Job Corps program. Because private industrial corporations subcontract the operation of Job Corps centers from the Department of Labor, health services other than those already listed may not be delivered similarly at all centers. Reproductive health services are provided on or off campus, depending on the skills of individual health center staff members. The range of dental procedures available also varies by center. Generally, however, many Corps members are exposed to preventive care at a level not experienced since early childhood.

Although the Job Corps program does not maintain statistics on health problems that are treated at its individual centers, it does have data on the health and medical problems that prompted temporary or permanent dismissal of enrollees. Almost one half of dismissals are for mental health problems (48%), and more than one quarter of the dismissals are for pregnancy (27%). A Corps member with a normal pregnancy is retained in the program until the early third trimester.

Corps members who require secondary and tertiary level medical care or who have urgent medical problems are referred to nearby hospitals and medical centers. Such referral is not financially problematic as long as the Corps member is covered by public or private health insurance. Although data are not available on the number of insured Corps members, those 18 years and older are often too old to be included in family coverage and present financing problems for centers as they seek care for these young individuals.

Statewide Programs

The models described previously provide health services for only a small proportion of young individuals living in a circumscribed geographic area, making it difficult to observe changes in health status using standard health statistics measures. These models of comprehensive care are generally considered too expensive and the staffing needs too intense to replicate on a population-based scale using a public health framework. The State of New Jersey, however, has undertaken this task and has created what it believes is a cost-effective method of providing community-based, comprehensive health care for its adolescents. The New Jersey School-based Youth Services Program, developed by the New Jersey Department of Human Services with the strong support of the governor's office, created 29 multiservice sites, which are distributed throughout the state's 21 counties. Sixteen sites are in schools, and 13 sites are located close to companion schools. The school sites include high schools, junior high schools, and vocational schools. Adolescents who are not enrolled in school are also eligible to receive services. The administrative responsibility for project sites is decentralized; a community-based managing agency is often a mental health agency or a private industry council. Each host community is required to contribute 25% toward the cost of the program, either through direct financial participation or "in-kind" services, facilities, or materials. The state has budgeted a total of $6 million annually for these projects, with each project site receiving approximately $200,000 a year in state monies. New Jersey has made a long-term commitment to the continued funding of this statewide program.

Each center provides mental health and family counseling, health and substance abuse services, employment counseling and training services, information and referral services, and recreation. Many of the centers also provide family planning (65%), transportation (62%), day care (44%), and crisis intervention hotlines (44%). State program rules require parental consent to receive direct services, but center staff members are allowed to talk with a young person at any time to determine a service need or to defuse a crisis. The services are offered during afternoon and evening hours so that conflicts with school and with parents' work schedules are reduced. Most programs initiated their operation in 1988. It is, therefore, too early for data from formal evaluation. However, the experiential anecdotes describing young persons who have been helped by this program are providing sufficient encouragement for New Jersey to continue its support.

Service Issues: Lessons Learned from Models

The primary lesson of nontraditional health care programs for adolescents is that young people *do* use special services designed especially for them, even if they have not recently sought care from traditional settings. For example, school-based centers enroll a mean of approximately 50% of students in the school per year, and well-established programs may enroll as many as 80% to 90% of students. In addition, close to 80% of enrolled students actually use their school-based health centers for care.

Single large-scale programs like The Door report 60,000 visits per year, whereas smaller programs such as The Bridge aid about 4,000 young persons annually. Job Corps enrolled approximately 68,000 youths in program year 1988. When the value of nontraditional health care programs for adolescents is considered, the type of young person enrolled for care should be counted as a second important reason for the existence of these programs. The young persons most likely to use these programs come from lower income and minority backgrounds and are unlikely to seek services from traditional health care settings. Poverty and minority status are often intertwined and are associated with both a high health risk status and poor health outcomes (see Chapter 28).

The atmosphere in health care settings is important for adolescents. Many of the process issues identified by Schorr for child health intervention programs are applicable to adolescent programs. Successful programs offer a broad range of intensive services. They do not practice "creaming," or setting barrier preconditions to screen out those who are most in need and therefore difficult to serve. The programs are flexible; they cross traditional professional and bureaucratic boundaries in order to meet the needs of individual patients. Professional discretion is encouraged in making decisions about patients. The staff is highly skilled and committed. The staff members see the youthful patients in the context of their families and their families in the context of their surroundings. The adolescents perceive the providers in the program as people who care about them, respect them, and value their trust. The services are coherent and easy to use. The programs ensure continuity of providers.

Schorr's maxims are particularly relevant for staff members who work in adolescent-oriented programs. Individuals working in nontraditional settings are interested in and trained specifically to provide health services for teenagers. Staff members who are successful working with adolescents have the following characteristics: commitment to and enjoyment in helping young people, flexible personal styles, and a good knowledge of adolescent development and behavior (see Chapter 17). In addition, a sense of humor often is helpful for health practitioners who work with adolescents. Staff members are often called upon to act as advocates and case managers and are committed to helping adolescents from becoming "lost" if referrals are needed for specialized care. These characteristics are most important for the "front-line" staff, including the receptionists and outreach workers who often represent the adolescent's first contact with a program. All staff members are challenged to communicate well and to interact constructively and effectively with young persons from differing cultural, economic, and lifestyle backgrounds (see Chapter 17 and 28–35).

Overall, noninstitutional settings located in areas with good public transportation routes have been more successful than geographically isolated programs. The best hours of operation for noninstitutional programs providing care for adolescents are late afternoon and evening, thus removing the need for teenagers to miss school as well as facilitating the involvement of working parents for programs with strong family counseling components.

EFFECTIVENESS OF NONTRADITIONAL SETTINGS: ISSUES OF PROGRAM EVALUATION

A message learned from nontraditional programs is that their effectiveness is very difficult to evaluate. Many of the problems that nontraditional programs help young people address are related to poverty, educational disadvantage, and stressed family functioning. It is usually unrealistic to expect long-term effects from short-term programmatic services, especially if the problems are complex and chronic. Complexity, costs, time constraints, and limited staff are but a few of the obstacles that limit most nontraditional programs in their attempts to provide rigorous evaluative data. Evaluation standards imposed by funding agencies have been a strain for many nontraditional health care programs, and new innovative strategies are needed to demonstrate the effectiveness of these varied and intensive programs.

BIBLIOGRAPHY

Earls F, Robins LN, Stiffman AR, et al: Comprehensive health care for high-risk adolescents: An evaluation study. Am J Publ Health 79:999, 1989.

Giblin PT, Poland ML: Primary care of adolescents: Issues in program development and implementation. J Adolesc Health Care 6:387, 1985.

Kean TH: The life you save may be your own. New Jersey addresses prevention of adolescent problems. Am Psychol 44(5):828, 1989.

Kirby D, Waszak CS, Ziegler J: An Assessment of Six School-based Clinics: Services, Impact and Potential. Washington, DC, Center for Population Options, 1989.

Lovick SR, Stern RF: School-based Clinics, 1988 Update. A Closer Look at the Numbers. Washington, DC, Center for Population Options, 1988.

Newacheck PW: Improving access to health services for adolescents from economically disadvantaged families. Pediatrics 84:1056, 1989.

Schorr LB: Within Our Reach. Breaking the Cycle of Disadvantage. New York, Anchor Press (Doubleday), 1988.

Stiffman AR, Earls F, Robins LN, et al: Problems and help seeking in high-risk adolescent patients of health clinics. J Adolesc Health Care 9:305, 1988.

Vernon MEL, Seymore C: Communicating with adolescents in alternative health care sites. Semin Adolesc Med 3:115, 1987.

US Department of Labor, Employment and Training Administration, Job Corps: Jobs Corps in Brief, Program Year 1988, Washington, DC, 1989.

Weatherly RA, Perlman SB, Levine MH, et al: Comprehensive programs for pregnant teenagers and teenage parents: how successful have they been? Fam Plann Perspect 18:73, 1986.

CHAPTER 19

Adolescent General Inpatient Unit

ELIZABETH R. McANARNEY

BACKGROUND

Inpatient adolescent services are optimally provided on a unit that is dedicated to the specialized care of adolescents who have medical, surgical, or behavioral problems. There are precedents for segregation of patients on inpatient units: Pediatric services are separated from adult services, medical services are separated from nonmedical services, including surgical services, obstetrics-gynecology services, and psychiatric services. Thus, the separation of pediatric services into age-appropriate units allows specialized interdisciplinary services for adolescents who require hospitalization.

It could be questioned why a separate unit is ideal for adolescent inpatient care. There are several reasons. First, it is developmentally appropriate; second, the adolescent is at the center of care whatever the specific diagnosis; and third, as more children with chronic illnesses survive into adolescence and young adulthood, their needs for special services are increasing (see Chapter 35).

Adolescent inpatient units provide developmentally appropriate services. Adolescents report feeling more comfortable with their peers, who provide much needed social support to adolescents who are ill. Adolescent patients can be helpful to each other, and on units in which there are flexible visiting hours, friends from outside the hospital can also visit. Most adolescents want to be treated as normally as possible during hospitalization.

Adolescent inpatient units provide the benefit of age-appropriate education and supportive services. Many units use both the tutoring services of individual school districts and inpatient unit tutors to ensure that adolescents who are well enough are able to keep up with their education. In addition, specially trained social workers and other developmentally knowledgeable professionals can support young persons as they experience the trauma of illness or surgery. Staff members who are trained to care for adolescents need to have an intimate knowledge of normal physical and psychological growth and development in order to optimally care for the adolescent who has the burden of an added acute or chronic condition.

Chronically ill young persons require special interdisciplinary services (see Chapter 30). They often undergo recurrent hospitalizations; they are struggling to maintain independence and control at a time when their health may be deteriorating; and they may be experiencing normal adolescent stresses similar to those of other young persons (see Chapters 5 and 9). Chronically ill adolescents are optimally cared for on units that are age-appropriate.

Many adolescent programs have integrated inpatient-ambulatory services. The staff from the adolescent inpatient unit relate directly to their colleagues in the ambulatory setting and facilitate the admission and discharge of adolescents between the ambulatory and inpatient settings. The same staff members who care for young persons in the ambulatory setting may provide continuity of care in the inpatient setting and facilitate admissions and discharges as well as plans for admission and plans for discharge and follow-up. These liaisons work particularly well for chronically ill adolescents who are cared for by interdisciplinary teams in hematology-oncology, for pulmonary diseases, and for eating disorders (see Chapters 42–44, 51–54, and 60).

BASIC PRINCIPLES

Basic principles guide the philosophy of adolescent inpatient units. The basic principles of privacy, confidentiality, and respecting young persons and their families are included in a number of chapters in this section. In addition, adolescents who are hospitalized need to maintain as much control over their lives as possible. Thus, if they are well enough, they should be allowed to dress in regular clothes, discuss their treatment regimens with medical and nursing staff members, and be allowed to negotiate, within limits, certain decisions—for example, when their tutors come and other issues that are appropriate.

Clear written guidelines as to what constitutes proper deportment on the unit are important, including guidelines for visitors, for noise, for going to bed at night, and for going off the unit. Flexibility is key in the development of guidelines; often the input of adolescents themselves can be helpful to staff members who are trying to develop them for the first time. Guidelines for behavior need to be clear; however, providers must know when they need to set limits, as well as when negotiation is possible. Middle adolescents often have the need to exert their independence; their need for control may be great. Providers should allow adolescents, particularly middle adolescents, as much independence and control as possible but must also know when independence and control are not possible. Most adolescents are cooperative if they understand the rationale behind staff decisions.

BASIC REQUIREMENTS

A basic requirement for an excellent unit is a well-trained, mature, professional staff. The core of this staff is a floor-based team that consists of senior nursing personnel, senior physicians trained in adolescent medicine, senior social workers, and senior psychiatric liaison colleagues (see Chapter 24). These senior staff members should meet regularly to review policies and discuss patient care issues and administrative challenges. The staff members should have frequent educational sessions that focus on the principles of adolescent medicine, discussion of individual adolescent patients and development of their care plans, and opportunities to meet with the interdisciplinary team, the adolescents, and their families.

Physical facilities should be secure and bright and should provide ample opportunity for privacy (for interviews of adolescents and their families, and for studying). A recreation room with age-appropriate activities and supervision by an adolescent life specialist is important. No procedure should be performed within this area; it should be a safe haven for the young people. Some units have a family style dining area within the recreational facility to encourage adolescents to eat together as an appropriate peer activity. The recreation room may be used on off hours as a setting for convening groups of adolescents, parents, or staff.

Special issues include safety and ownership. The unit must be reviewed for safety and security. Some providers admit young persons who have experienced suicidal behavior, but who are not actively suicidal, to a general adolescent inpatient unit. If that decision is made, it must be done with the understanding that the unit is safe: The windows should be secure and not easily opened, the staff should be able to supervise the suicidal young person, and any entrances or exits are secured. If there are exits on the back of the unit or in areas that staff members cannot monitor, alarms can be installed that are tripped if someone goes out the door and that can only be turned off with a key. The hospital administration can be involved in reviewing the security of the unit and can make suggestions.

It is also helpful for the staff members and the adolescents to feel some degree of ownership of the unit so the physical appearance of the unit is maintained. This sense of ownership is nurtured by the senior floor-based staff members who make ownership an explicit issue. This sense of ownership is nurtured by communicating its importance through printed material such as brochures and regular newsletters that the teenagers publish and through use of the artistic and creative work of the teenagers. It is a great tribute to a unit when a young person leaves art work or a message to the staff to be displayed on the unit. Visits from previously hospitalized adolescents are also a welcome experience for floor-based staff members.

SECTION VI

Practice Principles

CHAPTER 20

Legal Aspects of Care

ABIGAIL ENGLISH

Practitioners of adolescent medicine encounter numerous legal issues in caring for their young patients. An ability to differentiate those issues that are of sufficient complexity or sensitivity to require consultation with an attorney from those that may be resolved by a familiarity with basic legal principles is an important skill for clinicians.

Most legal issues of concern to practitioners of adolescent medicine fall into one of three categories: (1) consent, (2) confidentiality, and (3) payment for care. In each category, some basic questions are relevant:

1. Who has *authority* to give *consent* for care? Whose consent is *required?*

2. To what extent are the *communications* and *records* involved in the care protected as *confidential?* Who has the *authority* to *release* confidential information? Whose authorization is *required?*

3. Who is responsible for *payment* for the care—the *adolescent?* the *parent?* a *public* or *private insurer?* an *alternative* source of public or private funding?

The laws governing these issues are derived from multiple sources in state and federal law. These sources include statutes enacted by Congress and the state legislatures, decisions issued by federal and state courts, regulations promulgated by federal and state administrative agencies, and provisions of the United States Constitution and state constitutions. The state laws pertaining to adolescent health care vary significantly from state to state. Therefore, practitioners must become familiar with the relevant laws in whichever state they are working.*

Basic principles of medical ethics are also highly relevant to many of the issues of consent, confidentiality, and payment that arise in treating adolescents. The professional codes of ethics of most of the health care professions involved in adolescent care contain provisions that are specific to this age group.

Adolescents have a unique legal status different from that of both adults and younger children. Their developmental characteristics also vary from those of adults and younger children. The unique legal and developmental status of adolescents has a direct bearing on the laws that govern the provision of health care services to them. It also informs the ethical principles applicable to their care. Although many of the restrictions on liberty that apply to children generally remain applicable until they reach the age of majority, adolescents have been accorded a greater degree of autonomy in health care decisions than have younger children.

CONSENT

As with patients of all ages, the provision of health care to adolescents requires the consent of someone who is legally authorized to provide it. The failure to obtain consent may result in legal liability. Practitioners treating or performing any procedure on a patient without consent may be liable for battery (the unauthorized touching of another person), negligence, or malpractice.

Informed Consent

In most circumstances, practitioners providing medical care have an obligation to obtain the informed consent of the patient (or, when parental consent is required, of the parent). Informed consent is theoretically required for all care, but the obligation has the greatest practical relevance with respect to complex treatments or procedures and those involving significant risk. Practitioners are required to obtain informed consent in order to ensure that the patient has understood the proposed course of treatment and has agreed to go forward voluntarily.

The requirement of informed consent applies equally to the care of minors and adults. The critical question in treating adolescents is whether the informed consent must be obtained from the adolescent or from the parent or another adult. From an ethical perspective, even in situations in which there is no legal obligation to do so, it may be appropriate and desirable nevertheless for the practitioner to obtain the adolescent's informed consent before proceeding with care.

Supported by the Carnegie Corporation of New York, which is not responsible for the views expressed herein.

*Possible sources of information concerning the laws in specific states include state or local medical societies, local bar associations, children's advocacy organizations, and legal aid offices. The National Center for Youth Law in San Francisco, CA, may also be able to provide some information.

The doctrine of informed consent requires the disclosure of at least the following information:

The diagnosis

The benefits and risks of the proposed procedure or treatment

Alternative procedures or treatments with their benefits and risks

The consequences of not proceeding with the proposed procedure or treatment

There are no uniform rules establishing exactly which risks must be disclosed, but a useful guiding principle is that the more serious the risk, the stronger the obligation to disclose it. In most states, the standard for disclosure is an "objective" one, determined by the prevailing practice in the medical community; in a growing number of states, a "subjective" standard has been established, requiring disclosure of whatever would be relevant to the patient's decision.

Parental Consent

The law has traditionally required the consent of a parent for any medical care provided to a minor child. Minors include all children and adolescents younger than 18 years of age (or 19 years in Alabama, Nebraska, and Wyoming). The rationale for the requirement is at least twofold. First, the relationship between physician and patient is a contractual one, and minors ordinarily do not have the legal capacity to enter into binding contracts. Second, minors have been presumed—for developmental reasons—to lack the requisite competence or capacity for decision-making.

The requirement of parental consent often poses no barrier to the delivery of appropriate health care services to minors. In many cases, the involvement of parents occurs naturally, provides significant benefits, and furthers the adolescent's health interests. However, there are some situations—for example, those involving minors who are not living in their parents' custody or who are seeking sensitive services that they are unable or unwilling to discuss with their parents—in which the necessity for obtaining parental consent poses a serious obstacle to care. In many, though not all, of these situations, the courts and the legislatures have created exceptions and alternatives to the parental consent requirement, enabling minors to consent to their own care or allowing other adults or courts to provide the necessary authorization.

Alternatives to Parental Consent

The law has provided for alternatives to the consent of a biologic parent in numerous circumstances. Adults other than biologic parents who may be authorized by state law to provide consent for the medical care of a minor child or adolescent include legal guardians, adoptive parents, and foster parents, although foster parents are rarely authorized to consent to other than routine care. Parents may also authorize other individuals caring for a child to provide consent for medical care.

Every state has enacted laws enabling the juvenile or family court to authorize care for children and youth under its jurisdiction. These young people include delinquent minors, status offenders (runaways, truants, children beyond parental control), and abused and neglected children. In some states, this authority may be delegated to a probation officer or a social worker. It is usually also retained by the parents unless their parental rights have been permanently terminated by a court. In most states, the juvenile or family court may also provide consent for treatment of minors who are victims of medical neglect, even if they are not under the jurisdiction of the court for other reasons.

Consent of the Minor

Recognizing that there are a variety of circumstances in which a requirement of parental consent would impede an adolescent's access to necessary health care services, courts and legislatures have developed an array of exceptions to the requirement that permit minors to consent to their own care. The situations providing the impetus for these exceptions include circumstances in which adolescents are living independent of their families, as runaways or homeless youth, for example; cases in which they have been physically, sexually, or emotionally abused by their families; and situations in which they desire privacy for normal developmental reasons, because the services they seek are sensitive in nature, or both.

Minor Consent Based on Status

Courts have issued decisions and legislatures have enacted statutes permitting minors who have achieved a particular *status* to consent to their own health care (Table 20–1). Some of these laws include age limits or contain provisions pertaining to parental notification or financial responsibility. Few states' laws include all the categories listed in Table 20–1, but every state's laws include one or more of the groups. Although specific criteria and definitions vary from one state to another, certain general principles apply.

Mature minors are those who can understand the risks and benefits of proposed treatment or those who can give informed consent. Studies have found that, beginning at approximately age 14 years, the medical decision-making capacity of adolescents does not vary significantly from that of adults.

Experts agree that there is very little risk of liability in providing care to an older adolescent who is a mature minor if the care is for the adolescent's benefit or is necessary according to conservative medical opinion, and there is a good reason (including the minor's refusal to request it) for not obtaining parental consent.

Emancipated minors may attain their emancipated status by formal court declaration in many states. They may sometimes also be recognized as such by a court after the fact when a dispute has arisen (e.g., over a parent's financial responsibility). The traditional criteria for emancipation are marriage, service in the armed forces, *or* living separate from parents while managing one's own financial affairs. These criteria have been incorporated into many of the statutes providing for judicial declarations of emancipation. Emancipation generally relieves the parents of legal liability for support and enables emancipated minors to establish their own residences and to enter into binding contracts. Some, but not all, of the emancipation statutes explicitly authorize emancipated minors to consent to medical care. *Legal emancipation* should not be confused with *medical emancipation,* a term used to refer specifically to laws authorizing minors to consent to medical care.

Other categories of status include minors living independently, pregnant minors, minor parents, minors older than a specific age, and high-school graduates.

Minor Consent for Specific Services

In addition to minor consent based on status, every state has laws, contained either in court decisions or in state statutes, authorizing minors to consent to one or more *specific health services* (see Table 20–1). These laws are based on a recognition of the importance, from a public health perspective, of encouraging adolescents to seek services for certain conditions and of the overwhelming reluctance of some adolescents to involve their parents in their health care.

Some of these laws contain age limits or provisions pertaining to parental notification or financial responsibility. A few explicitly relieve the physician of liability for failure to obtain consent.

In emergency situations, the prior consent of a parent is not required, although parents should generally be notified as soon as possible of any emergency care provided. This principle is recognized for children of all ages, including adolescents. In addition, some state laws explicitly authorize minors to consent to their own care in an emergency. The definition of emergency varies, but leading authorities have suggested that a child requiring care to alleviate pain or to prevent deterioration of a physical condition should never be forced to wait for a prolonged period so that parental permission can be obtained.

The laws relating to reproductive health care, in particular, are derived from a series of decisions of state and federal courts, including the United States Supreme Court, delineating the scope of minors' constitutional rights to privacy (Table 20–2). With respect to abortion, these decisions have established that although states may require parental consent or parental notification for minors seeking abortions, they must provide the alternative of a "judicial bypass," allowing minors to go to court without notifying their parents and ensuring that courts will permit mature minors to make their own decisions and will determine whether it is in the best interest of immature minors to have an abortion without parental involvement. In two states (California and Florida), courts have ruled, at least on a preliminary basis, under privacy provisions of the state constitutions that parental consent may not be required, even with a judicial bypass provision.

With respect to contraception, the Supreme Court has decided that the right to privacy protects minors' access to contraceptives and that states may not ban the sale of nonprescription contraceptives to minors. In addition, based on federal statutes and regulations and federal court decisions, it is clear that parental consent or notification may not be required for family planning services in federally funded programs, although these programs are mandated to encourage parental involvement. Many state laws specifically authorize minors to give their own consent for contraceptive services. Most states also authorize minors to consent to pregnancy-related care, including prenatal, delivery, and postnatal care.

Every state authorizes minors to consent to the diagnosis and treatment of sexually transmitted or venereal diseases, and some states include other contagious diseases. A growing number or states allow minors to consent to human immunodeficiency virus (HIV) testing or treatment of HIV disease including acquired immunodeficiency syndrome (AIDS). Some of these laws specifically require informed consent—for HIV testing, for example. However, in view of the substantial social and psychological risks associated with HIV testing, as well as the medical risks involved in many of the

TABLE 20–1. State Minor Consent Laws*

MINORS WHO MAY CONSENT BASED ON THEIR STATUS†	SERVICES FOR WHICH MINORS MAY GIVE THEIR OWN CONSENT‡
Mature minors	Emergency care
Emancipated minors	Abortion-contraception services
Minors living independently§	Pregnancy-related care**
Pregnant minors	Diagnosis and treatment of sexually transmitted and venereal diseases††
Minor parents ‖	
Minors older than a specified age	Diagnosis and treatment of contagious diseases
High school graduates	HIV-AIDS–related care‡‡
	Substance abuse treatment§§
	Mental health services ‖‖
	Services for rape or sexual assault

*These laws may contain age limits, parental notification provisions, or other specific criteria that vary from state to state.

†Every state has laws enabling one or more categories of minors to consent to medical care.

‡Every state has laws authorizing minors to consent to one or more categories of services.

§May include minors such as runaways and homeless youth who are living apart from their parents with or without permission.

‖ May authorize minor parents to consent to care for themselves *or* for their children, *or* both.

**May include prenatal and postnatal care, childbirth delivery services, and other pregnancy-related care; may exclude sterilization.

††Every state provides for minors to consent to care for sexually transmitted and venereal diseases.

‡‡May be limited to HIV testing *or* may include other diagnostic and treatment services.

§§May include treatment of drug *or* alcohol problems, *or* both.

‖‖ May include inpatient *or* outpatient services, *or* both.

**TABLE 20–2. Minors' Right to Privacy and
Reproductive Health Care: United States
Supreme Court Decisions**

Griswold v. Connecticut, 381 US 479 (1965)
Constitutional right of privacy protected by the United States
Constitution protects decision whether to bear or beget a child
Eisenstadt v. Baird, 405 US 438 (1972)
Constitutional right of privacy protects contraceptive decisions of
both married and unmarried persons
Planned Parenthood of Central Missouri v. Danforth, 428 US 52
(1976)
Constitutional right of privacy protects minors as well as adults,
and states may not grant parents a veto over the abortion
decisions of their minor daughters
Carey v. Population Services International, 431 US 678 (1977)
Constitutional right of privacy protects minors as well as adults,
and states may not ban the sale of nonprescription
contraceptives to minors
Bellotti v. Baird, 443 US 622 (1979) (Bellotti II)
States may not require parental consent for minors' abortions
unless they provide a judicial bypass alternative that allows
minors to go to court in an anonymous and speedy proceeding
without first notifying their parents and that requires courts to
permit a mature minor to make her own decision and to
determine whether it is in the best interest of an immature
minor to have an abortion without parental involvement
H.L. v. Matheson, 450 US 398 (1981)
States may require prior parental notification for immature minors
seeking abortions
Akron Center for Reproductive Health v. City of Akron, 462 US 416
(1983)
Local government may not require parental consent or judicial
approval for all minors less than 15 years of age without
providing an opportunity for a case-by-case determination of
whether a minor is mature or an abortion is in her best interests
*Planned Parenthood Association of Kansas City, Missouri, v.
Ashcroft,* 462 US 476 (1983)
State may require minors seeking abortions to obtain the consent
of a parent or a juvenile court if a mature minor is allowed to
make her own decision and the juvenile court authorizes an
abortion for an immature minor for whom it is determined to be
in her best interests
Hodgson v. Minnesota, 58 USLW 4957 (June 25, 1990)
States may require prior parental notification of both parents of
minors seeking abortions provided judicial bypass procedure is
in place
Ohio v. Akron Center for Reproductive Health, 58 USLW 4979
(June 25, 1990)
States may require prior consent or notification of one parent for
minors seeking abortions, provided that judicial bypass
procedure is in place, and states may require proof of minors'
maturity by clear and convincing evidence in addition to
imposing other procedural requirements in judicial bypass
proceeding

treatments for HIV infection and AIDS, ethical principles would require a practitioner to obtain informed consent from any adolescent seeking HIV-related care (see Chapter 76). In addition, counseling that is developmentally and culturally appropriate should be provided to any adolescent seeking an HIV test both before and after testing.

Almost every state authorizes minors to consent to services for the treatment of substance abuse problems—including drug- or alcohol-related problems, or both. One of the most sensitive problems that arises in this context is the request by a parent or other adult for a urine drug test to be performed on an adolescent without the adolescent's knowledge or consent. The law provides only limited guidance on this issue, and, in any case,

ethical considerations are paramount. The American Academy of Pediatrics, for example, has recommended that pediatricians should not do police work and that with rare exceptions the informed consent of an older adolescent should be obtained for a drug test.

Almost one half of the states have enacted laws enabling minors to consent to outpatient mental health services. One half of the states permit older minors to apply for admission to inpatient mental health facilities, although most states also allow parents to commit their children to inpatient facilities regardless of the wishes of the child, and pursuant to a decision of the United States Supreme Court, only limited due process protections are required for these "voluntary" commitments.

Services for rape or sexual assault can be provided with the minor's consent alone in many states. These situations sometimes trigger the necessity for a child abuse report.

CONFIDENTIALITY

Adolescents desire confidentiality and privacy in their relationships with health care providers for varied reasons. For some, it is part of the natural developmental process of burgeoning autonomy; others fear adverse reactions from abusive parents in dysfunctional families. Practitioners find that assurances of confidentiality encourage adolescents to be more candid and to provide complete information about their health histories, thereby promoting the adolescents' health interests.

The legal obligation of health care professionals to maintain the confidentiality of both communications with patients and contents of medical records is derived from a wide variety of sources in the law. In addition, most of the professions involved in treating adolescents have adopted professional codes of ethics or organizational policies that address issues of confidentiality (Table 20–3). The legal sources include the constitutional right of privacy, the physician-patient and psychotherapist-patient privileges, and federal and state statutes explicitly requiring confidentiality to be maintained. For example, some states have enacted medical records legislation, and many federal funding statutes include guarantees of confidentiality (Table 20–4).

In general, communications between a practitioner and an adolescent patient and the content of medical records pertaining to the care are considered confidential and may not be disclosed without an appropriate authorization. Although a parent customarily has the right to have access to information pertaining to the health care of a minor child and to authorize release of that information, in some situations the authorization of the adolescent may be required. Under some states' laws and in some federally funded programs (e.g., family planning and substance abuse treatment), the authorization of the adolescent to release confidential information is legally required. However, some state laws enabling minors to consent to their own care permit the treating professional to notify the parents. In the case of abortion, some laws explicitly require parental notification, although they must provide a judicial bypass

TABLE 20–3. Professional Codes of Ethics and Policies of Professional Organizations*†

American Academy of Child Psychiatry: Code of Ethics. Washington, DC, 1980:

Specific confidences of the patient and the parents or guardians and others involved should be protected unless this course would involve untenable risks or betrayal of care-taking responsibility.

The release of any information regarding a minor unemancipated child or adolescent to persons outside the family (including the non-custodial parent) requires the agreement of parents or guardians. Regardless of the locus of decision, the child psychiatrist will attempt to inform the child or adolescent of the need and intent to release information and will seek his/her concurrence even though such agreement is not required.

It is necessary that the child or adolescent, within his/her capacity for understanding, be clearly apprised of confidentiality in regard both to his/her own communication and those of parents or guardians. He/she should also be informed of the limits to the general principle of confidentiality that the sharing of caretaking responsibility requires.

American Academy of Pediatrics: Policy Statement—Screening for drugs of abuse in children and adolescents. AAP News, March 1989:

[B]ecause of the potential for serious psychosocial effects of drug screening, it is a minimal requirement that there be candid discussion with the person screened regarding confidentiality and the need for informed, competent consent. In practice, therefore, a competent adolescent might be able to consent to such screening and counseling without parental knowledge. However, the pediatrician should be cautious about initiating such programs in a school setting where results might be used for punitive purposes and the maintenance of confidentiality may be difficult.

American Academy of Pediatrics, Committee on Adolescence: Role of the Pediatrician in Management of Sexually Transmitted Diseases in Children and Adolescents. Pediatrics 79:454, 1987:

The screening medical history should be performed in a setting where privacy and confidentiality can be assured. Information regarding sexuality obtained from an adolescent whose parent is not present is more likely to be accurate.

American Association for Counseling and Development: Ethical Standards. Alexandria, VA, 1988:

The counseling relationship and information resulting therefrom must be kept confidential, consistent with the obligations of the member as a professional person.

When the client's condition indicates that there is clear and imminent danger to the client or others, the member must take reasonable personal action or inform responsible authorities.

Revelation to others of counseling material must occur only upon the express consent of the client.

American College of Obstetricians and Gynecologists: ACOG Statement of Policy—Confidentiality in Adolescent Health Care. Washington, DC, 1988.‡

At the time providers establish an independent relationship with adolescents as patients, the providers should make this new relationship clear to parents and adolescents.

The same confidentiality will be preserved between the adolescent patient and the provider as between the parent/adult and the provider.

The adolescent must understand under what circumstances (e.g., life-threatening emergency) the provider will abrogate this confidentiality.

Ultimately, the health risks to the adolescent are so impelling that legal barriers and deference to parental involvement should not stand in the way of needed health care.

American Medical Association: Current Opinions of the Council on Ethical and Judicial Affairs of the American Medical Association. Chicago, IL, 1989:

The physician should not reveal confidential communications or information without the express consent of the patient, unless required to do so by law.

[Exceptions include situations] where a patient threatens to inflict serious bodily harm to another person and there is a reasonable probability that the patient may carry out the threat, . . . communicable diseases, gun shot and knife wounds.

The utmost effort and care must be taken to protect the confidentiality of all medical records.

American Nurses' Association: Code for Nurses with Interpretive Statements. Kansas City, MO, 1985:

The nurse safeguards the client's right to privacy by judiciously protecting information of a confidential nature.

The right to privacy is an inalienable human right. The client trusts the nurse to hold all information in confidence . . . The duty of confidentiality, however, is not absolute when innocent parties are in direct jeopardy.

American Psychiatric Association: The Principles of Medical Ethics, with Annotations Especially Applicable to Psychiatry. Washington, DC, 1989:

Psychiatric records, including even the identification of a person as a patient, must be protected with extreme care. Confidentiality is essential to psychiatric treatment.

A psychiatrist may release confidential information only with the authorization of the patient or under proper legal compulsion. . . . Information gained in confidence about patients seen in student health services should not be released without the student's explicit permission.

Careful judgment must be exercised by the psychiatrist in order to include, when appropriate, the parents or guardian in the treatment of the minor. At the same time the psychiatrist must assure the minor proper confidentiality.

Psychiatrists at times may find it necessary, in order to protect the patient or the community from imminent danger, to reveal confidential information disclosed by the patient.

TABLE 20–3. Professional Codes of Ethics and Policies of Professional Organizations*† *Continued*

American Psychological Association: Ethical Principles of Psychologists. Washington, DC, 1989:
Psychologists have a primary obligation to respect the confidentiality of information obtained from persons in the course of their work as psychologists. They reveal such information to others only with the consent of the person or the person's legal representative, except in those unusual circumstances in which not to do so would result in clear danger to the person or to others. Where appropriate, psychologists inform their clients of the legal limits of confidentiality.

American Psychological Association: General Guidelines for Providers of Psychological Services. Washington, DC, 1987:
Psychologists do not release confidential information, except with the written consent of the user involved, or of his or her legal representative, guardian . . . and only after being assured . . . that the user has been assisted in understanding the implications of the release.

Users are informed in advance of any limits in the setting for maintaining the confidentiality of psychological information. . . . [L]imitations on confidentiality of psychological information may be present in certain school . . . settings. . . .

In school settings, parents have the legal right to examine such psychological records, preferably in the presence of a psychologist.

National Association of Social Workers: Code of Ethics—Professional Standards. Silver Spring, MD, 1990:
The social worker should respect the privacy of clients and hold in confidence all information obtained in the course of professional service.

The social worker should inform clients fully about the limits of confidentiality in a given situation, the purposes for which information is obtained, and how it may be used.

*Statements are excerpts from complete ethical codes and policies.
†See also Moore RS, Hofmann AD (eds): American Academy of Pediatrics—Conference on Consent and Confidentiality in Adolescent Health Care. Elk Grove Village, IL, American Academy of Pediatrics, 1982.
‡The ACOG policy has been endorsed by the American Academy of Pediatrics, the American Academy of Family Physicians, and the National Medical Association.

option when they do so (see Table 20–2). In any case, it is almost always appropriate, from an ethical perspective, to request the permission of the adolescent to disclose confidential information and to explain to adolescent patients the limits of confidentiality.

In certain situations, disclosure is explicitly required by law even if the adolescent or the parent does not authorize it. For example, mandatory disclosures in some states include reports to child welfare authorities under state child abuse reporting laws, reports of gunshot and stab wounds to law enforcement, and warnings by a psychotherapist to a reasonably identifiable victim of a patient's threats of violence. In addition, health care professionals may be required to exercise judgment to determine the appropriateness or necessity for breaching confidentiality in circumstances involving danger to the patient (including suicidal ideation) or to others. Specific legal provisions in this regard vary from state to state.

PAYMENT

Parents are generally financially responsible for medical care provided to their children until they reach the age of majority or are legally emancipated. However, some of the statutes authorizing minors to consent to their own care specify that parents are not financially responsible. Other statutes that protect confidentiality sometimes specify that parents may not be notified for billing purposes. If parents are not financially responsible, that responsibility may fall upon the adolescents themselves.

As a practical matter, however, few adolescents are able to pay even for routine care. Thus their access to necessary care may depend upon the availability of payment from some other source. It is ordinarily diffi-

cult, if not impossible, for minors to depend upon their families' private insurance to cover the costs of confidential care because of the necessity for parents to be involved in the claims process. Some health maintenance organizations providing direct care have begun to make provision for confidentiality in the treatment of adolescents.

When adolescents seek confidential care or cannot rely on their families for support (e.g., runaway and homeless youth), they are usually dependent on publicly funded care. There are numerous sources of public funding for adolescent health services at the federal and state level. Many federal programs provide some funding for adolescent health services or provide direct health services to some adolescents (see Table 20–4). The level of funding in these programs is not adequate to meet the need, however, and many adolescents lack coverage for necessary health services. Only two of the federal programs operate as insurance or entitlement programs—Medicaid and the Early Periodic Screening, Diagnosis, and Treatment (EPSDT) program. The remainder provide limited funding for services, and when funds are exhausted, adolescents go unserved. Adolescents who seek funding in private physicians' offices must generally rely either on private insurance or Medicaid and EPSDT. Public and private clinics and other programs providing comprehensive health care for adolescents are unable to depend on a single source of funding and must use a combination of different sources (see Chapter 21).

CONCLUSION

Practitioners who provide health care services to adolescents need to develop a familiarity with a broad range of basic legal and ethical principles related to

TABLE 20–4. Federal Sources of Funding for Adolescent Health Services

Medicaid, Social Security Act, Title XIX (42. U.S.C. §§ 1396 *et seq.,* 42 C.F.R. §§ 430 *et seq.*)*
   Medicaid is a federal-state program providing coverage of a broad range of health care services for low-income individuals, especially those who are recipients of cash assistance to dependent, blind, or disabled children (Aid to Families with Dependent Children or Supplemental Security Income benefits). Individuals who meet federal and state eligibility requirements are *entitled* to covered services that include a minimum package of federally mandated services and additional services included by state option. As of 1990, adolescents living below the federal poverty line are covered in some, but not all, states.
Early and Periodic Screening, Diagnosis, and Treatment (EPSDT), Social Security Act, Title XIX (42 U.S.C. §§ 1396d and 1396s)*
   Created as a special component of the Medicaid program in 1967, and substantially extended by Congress in 1989, the EPSDT program provides funding for preventive and treatment services. EPSDT requires states to provide, for all Medicaid-eligible children and adolescents, periodic comprehensive health assessments (including dental, hearing, and vision screenings), further diagnostic procedures, and medically necessary treatment to address problems identified during an EPSDT screening.
Maternal and Child Health (MCH) Block Grant, Social Security Act, Title V (42 U.S.C. §§ 701 *et seq.,* 45 C.F.R. Part 96; 42 C.F.R. Parts 51d and 51f)*
   Under the MCH Block Grant, funds are provided to the states for the purpose of ensuring access to health services for low-income women and children, reducing infant mortality and preventable disease, providing rehabilitation services for blind and disabled children and youth, and providing services for children with special medical needs. Low-income women and children must be served without charge in MCH-funded programs. The federal Department of Health and Human Services is required to allocate a specific percentage of funds for special projects to promote access to primary health services for children and to promote coordinated services for children with special medical needs. Federal MCH funds have supported training for specialists in adolescent medicine and health care.
Family Planning Programs, Public Health Service Act, Title X (42 U.S.C. §§ 300 *et seq.,* 42 C.F.R. §§ 59 *et seq.*)*
   Title X authorizes funding for family planning clinics and services. Services must be made available to adolescents. Priority must be given to persons from low-income families, and persons living below the federal poverty level are entitled to receive free services.
Alcohol, Drug Abuse, and Mental Health Block Grant, Public Health Service Act, Title XIX (42 U.S.C. §§ 300x *et seq.,* 45 C.F.R. Part 96) (cf. 42 U.S.C. §§ 290aa *et seq.*)*
   Created by Congress in 1981 and administered by the Alcohol, Drug Abuse, and Mental Health Administration (ADAMHA), the block grant provides federal funds to states for prevention, treatment, and rehabilitation activities in the area of substance abuse and for community mental health services, including the identification and assessment of children and adolescents with severe mental disturbance and the provision of appropriate services to them. Funds are divided equally between substance abuse and mental health services.
Adolescent Family Life Act, Public Health Service Act, Title XX (42 U.S.C. §§ 300z *et seq.*)
   Enacted by Congress in 1981, the Adolescent Family Life Act (AFLA) provides federal funds for programs to prevent adolescent pregnancy and to provide services to pregnant adolescents and adolescent parents. AFLA grantees may offer pregnancy testing and maternity counseling, adoption counseling and referral, primary and preventive health services, nutrition counseling, referrals for treatment of sexually transmitted diseases and pediatric care, mental health services, and family planning services; abortion-related services cannot be provided. With limited exceptions, parental consent and notification are required for unemancipated adolescents.
Community Health Centers, Public Health Service Act, Title III (42 U.S.C. § 254c; 42 C.F.R. Part 51c)*
   Community Health Centers (CHCs) provide health services in low-income urban and rural communities or neighborhoods designated as medically underserved areas. CHCs must provide a range of primary health services and may provide supplemental services (including home health, vision and dental care, and mental health services). Public or private nonprofit entities may receive grants to establish and operate CHCs.
Migrant Health Centers, Public Health Service Act, Title III (42 U.S.C. § 254b; 42 C.F.R. Part 56)
   Administered by the Public Health Service, the Migrant Health Program supports primary and supplemental health services for seasonal and migratory agricultural workers and their families. State and local public agencies may apply for grants. Those with incomes less than the federal poverty level must be served free; others may be charged on a sliding fee scale.
Indian Health Programs, Indian Health Care Improvement Act (25 U.S.C. §§ 1621 *et seq.;* 42 C.F.R. Part 36; cf. 45 C.F.R. §§ 96.40 *et seq.*)
   The Indian Health Service (IHS) operates programs to provide health services to Indians living on or near reservations and to urban Indians. Services include a range of primary care services, including prenatal and postnatal care, family planning, and health education. Services are provided both in IHS facilities and under contract with other public or private facilities. Services are provided without charge to persons of Indian descent.
Preventive Health and Health Services Block Grant, Public Health Service Act, Title XIX (42 U.S.C. §§ 300w *et seq.;* 45 C.F.R. Part 96)
   Created by Congress in 1981, the block grant authorizes grants to states for preventive health and health services programs including, among others, health education services designed to prevent smoking and alcohol use among children and adolescents, home health services, and rape crisis and prevention services.
Hill-Burton, Hospital Survey and Construction Act of 1946 (42 U.S.C. §§ 291 *et seq.*); Public Health Service Act, Title XVI (42 U.S.C. §§ 300r *et seq.;* 42 C.F.R. Part 53; 42 C.F.R. Part 124)
   The Hill-Burton program has provided grants, loans, and loan guarantees for the construction and modernization of health care facilities. In exchange, facilities undertake an uncompensated care obligation (to provide services for persons unable to pay) and a community service obligation (to make services available to all persons residing in the geographic area).

*Explicit confidentiality provisions are contained in program statute or regulations.
   Data from Select Committee on Children, Youth, and Families, House of Representatives, US Congress, 100th Congress, First Session, Federal Programs Affecting Children, 1987. Washington, DC, US Government Printing Office, 1987.

consent, confidentiality, and payment. Specific laws vary from state to state, and it is important to learn local requirements. Many issues are not addressed by specific statutes, regulations, or court decisions. In these circumstances, clear policies (for physician's offices, clinics, hospitals) that are grounded in basic legal and ethical principles can facilitate the delivery of appropriate and comprehensive health care to adolescents.

BIBLIOGRAPHY

Blum RW: Adolescent health care. In Wallace HM, Ryan G Jr, Oglesby AC (eds): Maternal and Child Health Practices, 3d ed. Oakland, Third Party Publishing, 1988.

Capron AM: The competence of children as self-deciders in biomedical interventions. In Gaylin W, Macklin R (eds): Who Speaks for the Child: The Problems of Proxy Consent. New York, Plenum Press, 1982.

English A: Runaway and street youth at risk for HIV infection: Legal and ethical issues in access to care. J Adolesc Health Care, in press.

English A: Treating adolescents: Legal and ethical considerations. Pediatr Clin North Am 74:1097, 1990.

English A, Tereszkiewicz L: Adolescent Health Care: A Manual of State and Federal Law. San Francisco, CA, National Center for Youth Law, in press.

Gittler J, Quigley-Rick M, Saks MJ: Adolescent Health Care Decision Making: The Law and Public Policy. Washington, DC, Carnegie Council on Adolescent Development, 1990.

Holder AR: Legal Issues in Pediatrics and Adolescent Medicine, 2d ed. New Haven, CT, Yale University Press, 1985.

Holder AR: Disclosure and consent problems in pediatrics. Law Med Health Care 16:219, 1988.

Morrissey JM, Hofmann AD, Thrope JC: Consent and Confidentiality in the Health Care of Children and Adolescents: A Legal Guide. New York, The Free Press, 1986.

Newachek P: Improving access to health services for adolescents from economically disadvantaged families. Pediatrics 84:1056, 1989.

North RL: Legal authority for HIV testing of adolescents. J Adolesc Health Care 11:176, 1990.

CHAPTER 21

Financing of Adolescent Care

JOE M. SANDERS, JR. and SAMUEL S. FLINT

Assuming responsibility for one's own health and well-being is complicated by the ambiguity of laws regulating the health care rights of minors. In our society, an adult has a fundamental right to consent to his or her own health care and to develop a confidential relationship with the provider (see Chapter 20). Parents traditionally exercise these basic ethical and legal rights on behalf of their children. Complications develop during the transition to the legal age of majority because of a variety of circumstances that preclude the involvement of parents in certain decisions relative to the health needs of adolescents. Fortunately, the *mature minor doctrine,* a growing body of legal support that allows minors who are deemed capable to give informed consent for their own medical treatment, has effectively eliminated the requirement to notify parents when said minor requests health services. Thus, it has become the standard of practice in adolescent medicine for the health care provider to enter into a contract of confidentiality with an adolescent who is judged cognitively mature.

The dilemma that commonly occurs in these expanded opportunities for adolescents to receive health services centers around the payment for such services. Parents are generally held liable for such payment, as the majority of adolescents lack the financial capability to assume this responsibility. A potential barrier is created because the adolescent may view contact with the parent for payment as a breach of confidentiality. Specific strategies to assist the practitioner in addressing the issue of financing health care for adolescents are discussed later in this chapter.

Most 10- to 18-year-olds in the United States are covered by some form of health insurance; however, the majority of these third-party insurers require the signature of the policy holder prior to processing a claim and inevitably notify the policy holder of the claim outcome. Only in rare circumstances is the adolescent identified as a policy holder (e.g., when he or she works for a company that offers health insurance as part of an employment benefit package). In order to gain a better understanding of this complex issue, however, it is important to explore in depth the current health insurance status of adolescents in the United States.

HEALTH INSURANCE STATUS OF ADOLESCENTS IN THE UNITED STATES

There is abundant evidence that health insurance increases the use of medical services and improves the health status of covered populations. For adolescents (and children), insurance coverage exerts a particularly strong influence on the use of ambulatory services, the care most needed by the vast majority of adolescents.

This chapter focuses first on broad issues of financial coverage of adolescent health care at a national level and then addresses strategies for the individual practitioner. Information about financial considerations in office practice is also found in Chapter 17.

Despite the importance of health insurance to adolescents' health, until recently little information was known about the extent of this coverage in the 10- to 18-year-old population in the United States. Unfortunately, standard data bases grouped adolescents with children or adults (e.g., 0 to 17 years, to 0 to 14 years, 15 to 25 years). Analogous to the situation with other institutions that ignored the uniqueness of adolescence, there was little interest in collecting or analyzing health insurance data to determine whether there were any special characteristics of the adolescent age group. However, as the salience of the health risks that adolescents faced increased, comprehensive studies emerged that drew a consistent picture of the health insurance status of adolescents in the United States (see Chapter 2).

Adolescents are similar to all other age groups younger than 65 years in two respects. First, approximately 85% of adolescents have some form of health insurance coverage, and most are covered by private, employment-related plans. Second, the likelihood of having coverage is determined primarily by sociodemographic factors (e.g., family income, parental educational level), rather than need for medical care. The proportion of uninsured adolescents with disabilities (14%) is nearly identical to the proportion of uninsured and underinsured adolescents in the entire population. Specific problems faced by this group of 270,000 adolescents are discussed later.

SOURCES OF INSURANCE

In the late 1980s, approximately 72% of 10- to 18-year-olds were covered by some form of private health insurance, that is, commercial insurance, Blue Cross–Blue Shield or a health maintenance organization (HMO), preferred provider organization (PPO), or some other nongovernment-financed managed care plan. Ten percent of these individuals were insured by the federal- and state-funded Medicaid program, and approximately 3% were covered by either another public insurance plan (e.g., Civilian Health and Medical Program of the Uniformed Services [CHAMPUS], Medicare) or a combination of public and private insurance. Estimates of the uninsured adolescent population put that proportion at roughly 15%—more than 4.5 million adolescents.

SOCIODEMOGRAPHIC CHARACTERISTICS OF UNINSURED ADOLESCENTS

The majority of uninsured adolescents reside in two-parent, white families in which there is at least one full-time employed parent earning an income greater than the federal poverty line. However, the likelihood of being uninsured is significantly greater for adolescents who reside in families with incomes less than 150% of the poverty line that are either black or Hispanic or are headed by a single parent who did not complete high school. The adolescents at greatest risk of being uninsured also reside in central cities of metropolitan areas and rural areas and in the southern and western parts of the United States.

Of all the sociodemographic characteristics associated with a greater likelihood of being uninsured, family income is the best predictor of adolescent health insurance status. According to the 1984 National Health Interview Survey, approximately 70% of parents with uninsured adolescents cited the high costs of health insurance as the primary reason. Another 11% cited job layoff or job loss. Thus, more than 80% of uninsured adolescents were uninsured because of economic reasons.

When the influence of family income is controlled, the negative correlations between health insurance coverage and membership in a black or single-parent family virtually disappear. However, Hispanic adolescents are more likely to be uninsured than are non-Hispanic adolescents of equal family income. This is because of the disproportionately larger number of Hispanic household heads employed in agriculture and domestic service, in which health insurance coverage for employees and their dependents is substantially less likely than in other industries. This is also a consequence of some state Medicaid programs choosing not to cover "undocumented aliens" despite eligibility for federal Medicaid matching funds, which cover between 50% and 80% of the costs.

Another factor increasing the risk of lack of insurance that remains after the influence of family income is eliminated is the level of parental education. Adolescents in families in which the parents have had less than 9 years of education are more than ten times as likely to be uninsured as adolescents residing in homes in which the parents have had some education after college. At all income levels, adolescents whose parents have had more education are more likely to be insured than adolescents residing with parents of equal income and less formal education.

Another variable that predicts the greater likelihood of being uninsured is region of residence. Nearly one fifth of adolescents in the southern and western parts of the United States are uninsured, whereas less than one tenth of adolescents in the northeastern and midwestern portions of the United States are without coverage. A small portion of the disparity is attributable to less liberal Medicaid eligibility standards in the southern and western United States, but the greatest part of the difference is due to less private insurance coverage in these regions. The northeastern and midwestern parts of the United States have a higher percentage of the labor force in industrial manufacturing, and a larger proportion of workers in these regions are unionized. Both factors contribute to higher rates of employment-related health insurance benefits.

RECENT TRENDS IN ADOLESCENT HEALTH INSURANCE COVERAGE

A sharp 25% increase in the number of uninsured adolescents occurred between 1979 and 1984, but since that time the proportion of uninsured adolescents has been stable (see Chapter 2). The causes of the increase are threefold. First, during the early 1980s, the United States experienced the most severe economic slump since the 1930s, and many parents of adolescents lost their jobs and consequently health insurance for themselves and their dependents. This recession hit the manufacturing sector hardest, and it is these jobs that traditionally offer relatively extensive health insurance benefits to employees' dependents. By the time the business cycle improved in the mid-1980s and unemployment declined, employee health insurance costs had risen to the point that employers began insisting on a larger employee share of health insurance premiums for workers and their dependents. Many workers who earned lower wages simply could not afford their share of the health insurance premium, so they dropped family coverage.

New restrictions in eligibility for Medicaid also occurred in the 1980s, simultaneous with a steep increase in the number of adolescents residing in poor families. Between 1979 and 1983, the proportion of poor adolescents grew from less than 15% to 21%, but because of new eligibility rules, only 37% of adolescents in families with incomes less than the federal poverty line were insured by Medicaid in 1984. Particularly hard hit were adolescents in poor families whose incomes were too high for them to receive Medicaid. By the mid-1980s, a greater proportion of uninsured adolescents were in families whose incomes were between 50% and 100% of the poverty threshold than in families with income less than 50% of the poverty line.

Since the Medicaid eligibility reductions of the early 1980s, a series of eligibility expansions have been enacted. The liberalization of rules and accompanying federal funding were targeted almost exclusively at pregnant women and young children, until 1990 when new eligibility rules were enacted requiring a phase-in of older children and adolescents. Beginning July 1, 1991, all states must offer Medicaid eligibility to children born after September 30, 1983 who reside in families with incomes less than the federal poverty line. Although it is progressive, it will take 11 years before all poor adolescents through age 18 years are eligible for Medicaid. Thus, a combination of macroeconomic conditions, increasing health insurance costs, and a more conservative federal government led to a pullback by both private sector and public sector insurers in the 1980s, which harmed adolescents disproportionately with respect to health insurance coverage. Some remediation will occur in the 1990s for uninsured adolescents living in poor families.

INSURANCE PROBLEMS FACED BY ADOLESCENTS WITH SPECIAL HEALTH NEEDS

According to data from the 1984 National Health Interview Survey, 25% of adolescents whose health status was described as "fair" or "poor" were uninsured, whereas only 11% of adolescents with "excellent" health did not have coverage (see Chapter 2). Private insurers can deny coverage to individuals who have "preexisting conditions," such as epilepsy or diabetes. In addition to formal restrictions, private insurers also use other administrative approaches to limit their exposure to adolescents and individuals of other ages in poor health, for example, increased premiums for adolescents with fairly common problems, such as allergies.

The discrepancy between coverage rates for adolescents in poor health and those in excellent health is primarily due to private insurers avoiding insuring adolescents in poor health whenever they can. Medicaid and other public programs insure a little more than 10% of the entire adolescent population, but they insure 28% of adolescents in fair or poor health and only 9% of adolescents in excellent health. Private insurers, who insure between 70% and 75% of adolescents, cover only 50% of adolescents in fair or poor health, in contrast with 82% of adolescents described to be in excellent health.

In addition to insuring a disproportionately small number of adolescents in poor health, private insurance companies frequently do not provide benefits that are broad enough or deep enough to cover the special needs of adolescents with the most difficult problems. Waiting periods and exclusion waivers exist for a number of conditions, and there are annual or lifetime coverage limits, or both. In addition, restrictions on the scope of benefits frequently leave mental health and substance abuse services inadequately covered. Other health services that are not strictly medical (e.g., occupational therapy, physical therapy, payments for special diets) are typically uninsurable under private insurance plans.

Limitations on the scope of benefits also exist in most state Medicaid plans. In addition to mandatory services (e.g., inpatient hospital care, physician services), states can offer up to 32 optional services—for example, prescription drugs, dental care, inpatient psychiatric care for individuals 21 years and younger. There is a great deal of variability among states, with Wyoming offering only eight optional services and Massachusetts offering 31 of these services. In addition to the choice of services offered, mandatory Medicaid benefits can be limited in their "amount, duration, and scope," and many states impose such limits. For example, 21 states place annual limits on the number of reimbursable physician visits.

Part of the underinsurance problem for Medicaid-eligible adolescents should be remedied by federal legislation enacted in 1989. Under the provisions of the new law, liberalized benefits for health problems detected during an Early and Periodic Screening, Diagnosis, and Treatment (EPSDT) program visit must be provided by the states. However, in most states, these preventive care visits are scheduled only once every 2 or 3 years for Medicaid beneficiaries in the adolescent age range. Patients with problems diagnosed at other times still face the limitations of the standard Medicaid benefit package.

An additional problem for Medicaid-insured adolescents in poor health is the increasing difficulty of finding physicians who accept Medicaid-insured patients. Low reimbursement levels, complex claims forms, slow payment, and retroactive claim denials have discouraged many physicians from participating in the program. A marked decline in pediatrician availability to Medicaid beneficiaries has occurred throughout the last decade. Thus, private insurers restrict access to adolescents in poor health by using preexisting conditions exclusions and placing limits on covered benefits, and Medicaid, which cannot refuse eligibility based on preexisting health conditions, limits access by restricting benefits and discouraging physicians from participating in the program.

Partially filling the gap are services provided by the states from the Maternal and Child Health (MCH) Block Grant, also known as Programs for Children with Special Health Care Needs, formerly Crippled Childrens' Services. The majority of services from these programs are targeted at low-income families with specific conditions (e.g., cystic fibrosis, sickle cell anemia; see Chapters 43 and 52). Thus, some coverage is extended to low-income adolescents who have conditions identified by the state's program.

LOSS OF COVERAGE AT AGE OF MAJORITY

A problem unique to older adolescents is the loss of health insurance at the age of 18 years (or later if attending college). Since 1986, federal law requires that dependents attaining the age of majority who would be dropped from their parents' employers' insurance plan must be allowed to continue coverage for a premium no greater than 2% more than group rates, regardless of health status. However, because of high cost and other factors, most older adolescents do not purchase extended health insurance. More than one fourth of 19- to 24-year-olds have no health insurance, although many of them were eligible to continue coverage with their parent's plan at one time. Many of these young adults are employed in entry-level positions. They also tend to stay at their first jobs for short periods; thus, the likelihood of employer-sponsored insurance is low, and the income generated from entry-level positions is frequently insufficient to afford either purchasing an individual plan or paying for an extension of the parent's employer's insurance coverage.

UNDERINSURANCE

Being insured does not guarantee full financial access to needed health care for adolescents (or any other age group) because of limitations in coverage. Many services particularly important to adolescents either are not covered by private or public plans or are severely restricted. Preventive care, mental health services, substance abuse treatment, dental care, prescription drugs, physical therapy, and gynecologic care are examples of health services that are frequently paid "out-of-pocket" by the parents or the adolescents themselves, are forgone, or are delivered through direct grant-funded programs—for example, community health centers or school-based clinics (see Chapter 18).

In addition to benefit limitations, patient cost-sharing continues to grow in popularity with corporate benefits managers as a cost-containment strategy. Cost-sharing comes in three forms: (1) deductibles, (2) copayments, and (3) coinsurance. A deductible is an annual, fixed-dollar amount that an individual or family must exceed before insurance coverage begins. Only services covered by the insurance plan are accepted as payments toward the financial obligation. Thus, if an adolescent's insurance plan does not include coverage for preventive care or other ambulatory services, the patient or family not only has to be responsible for the charges but also is no closer to meeting the deductible and having the insurance begin to pay for care covered by the plan.

Coinsurance is a fixed percentage of the bill (e.g., 20%) that the insured must pay after the deductible has been reached. Copayments are fixed-dollar fees that are charged for specific coverage services (e.g., $10 for an emergency room visit).

Cost-sharing reduces payor costs in two ways. First, there is the actual expenditure made by the patient instead of the insuring entity. In addition, there is unambiguous evidence that cost-sharing reduces use of services. However, the necessity of this forgone care is not known.

It has been estimated that between limitations on benefits and cost-sharing, nearly 30% of adolescents' medical care is paid for out-of-pocket. This expense is in addition to dental care and the cost of health insurance premiums, which average about $50 per month for employee-dependent care. In 1988, 10% of adolescents had out-of-pocket expenditures greater than $300/year. This group accounted for 65% of aggregate adolescent out-of-pocket expenditures. More than 93% of this top decile live in families with incomes greater than the poverty line. Since the health status of poor individuals on average is not as good as the that of individuals who are not poor, the relatively low out-of-pocket expenditures by poor persons suggest that their access to care is compromised. To mitigate the impact on use of health care that results from high cost-sharing, there are max-

imum out-of-pocket expenditure limits for covered services in most private insurance plans. These annual "catastrophic" or "stop-loss" limits average about $1,000/family.

One other aspect of the underinsurance issue is the relatively low compensation for evaluation and management or "cognitive" services. Even if an adolescent has optimal coverage, compensation for managing a patient through means such as prescribing medication or exercise programs or providing health education is historically less than reimbursement for performing medical procedures. Thus, the time-consuming health supervision and counseling services so crucial to adolescent medicine generally are not compensated commensurate to the effort, skill, and time required of the physician providing care.

This long-held suspicion was verified in a landmark study commissioned by the Congress for the Medicare program. Hsiao and colleagues (1988) determined that relative to the cost of the resources it takes to provide medical services, invasive procedures are compensated at more than twice the rate of cognitive services. With this research as a basis, the Medicare program restructured its fee schedule. Beginning in 1992, Medicare will reimburse physicians for their services based on a "resource-based relative value scale" (RBRVS), which will result in increased compensation for primary care physicians. If Medicaid and private insurers emulate this shift, as they did to some extent when Medicare adopted prospective payments for hospital reimbursement, compensation for caring for the adolescent patient would be substantially improved.

POLICY OPTIONS TO EXPAND HEALTH INSURANCE TO ADOLESCENTS

Proposed solutions to the problem of lack of insurance and underinsurance for adolescents and others have been widely discussed in recent years. Some proposals, such as the one developed by the Physicians for a National Health Program, recommend universal coverage by a single publicly funded plan, similar to the Canadian system, which includes global hospital budgets and government controls over the number and size of residency programs. The American College of Physicians (ACP) also supports a universal system. However, they stop short of endorsing an exclusive government payor system, allowing for private insurance if universal coverage and equality of benefits can be achieved.

Other serious proposals, such as legislation introduced by Senator Edward Kennedy, would force greater private sector contributions for the financing of health care by requiring all employers to provide a minimum health benefit to employees and their dependents. If enacted, an employer mandate would extend insurance coverage to approximately two thirds of the 34 million uninsured individuals in the United States. This plan is not exceedingly costly when compared with other federal labor requirements. The cost for the proposed benefit package is estimated to be fifty-five cents/hour, which is only ten cents/hour more than federal minimum wage increases that took effect in 1990 and 1991. However, resistance from the business community, particularly small businesses, is quite strong. Also, some government policy makers believe an employer mandate will result in substantial numbers of lost jobs because of the increase in the cost for labor.

Other proposals target selected uninsured groups. Nearly 20 states have some form of risk pool through which individuals considered uninsurable because of preexisting conditions can purchase private health insurance at higher premiums. Even with state subsidies, the cost of insurance is excessive for many families; waiting periods for preexisting conditions are common, as are annual or lifetime dollar limits, or both, and the benefit packages are not expanded to include services needed by individuals with disabilities.

Expansions of the Medicaid program have been recommended by those who want to target low-income uninsured individuals, many of whom are employed or all dependents of employees. The Health Policy Agenda for the American People, which was convened by the American Medical Association (AMA) and included consumer, government, labor, and business groups, along with physicians and hospital representatives, recommends a $21 billion expansion of Medicaid. The proposal recommends expanding Medicaid eligibility to the 11 million individuals who make up the uninsured poor population, upgrading benefits, and increasing the rates of reimbursement to physicians and hospitals to improve provider participation and accessibility to services.

Combined Medicaid–employer mandate strategies have also been designed. The second-generation Kennedy proposal includes phased-in Medicaid expansions to cover the one third of the uninsured population who would remain uninsured after employers cover all workers and their dependents. Cosponsored by Congressman Henry Waxman, this legislation is entitled the Basic Health for All Americans Act.

Access proposals by the AMA, American Society of Internal Medicine (ASIM), and the American Association of Family Physicians (AAFP) also endorse Medicaid expansions coupled with an employer mandate as the basis for universal health coverage.

Two other noteworthy proposals call for an employer mandate combined with a new public sector plan that would replace Medicaid and cover the remaining uninsured population. The American Academy of Pediatrics (AAP) has proposed a plan, the Children First proposal, that would create a statutory entitlement to health insurance for pregnant women of any age and children and adolescents through age 21 years. Financing would be derived from four sources: (1) employers required to provide approved employee dependent insurance or pay a 3.2% payroll tax; (2) Medicaid funds now being spent for this population, which would be used to purchase approved private insurance plans; (3) contributions toward insurance premiums and cost-sharing for services by families with incomes greater than 133% of the federal poverty line; and (4) a federal contribution to subsidize employer payroll taxes for low-income workers. All beneficiaries would be eligible for identical private insurance plans with a comprehensive benefits package designed to reduce the underinsurance problems children and adolescents now face.

The plan's appeal is its potential for substantial social benefits at a relatively modest cost. For a 2% increase in health care spending in the United States ($12 billion in 1991), 38% of the uninsured population would gain coverage and millions more young people would have improved, age-appropriate benefits. The payoff for this social investment is the healthier, more capable work force U.S. corporations need to keep the United States competitive in world markets.

Similar in many ways to the AAP proposal, the US Bipartisan Commission on Comprehensive Health Care, more generally known as the "Pepper Commission," issued a set of recommendations in March 1990, which were adapted for legislation sponsored by Senator John D. Rockefeller IV in 1991. The Commission was composed of 3 presidential appointees and 12 senators and congressmen, including both Senator Kennedy and Congressman Waxman. This proposal recommends replacing Medicaid with a new public plan. Employers would be required to insure workers and their dependents or to contribute to the public plan to meet their costs. Small employers (i.e., firms with fewer than 100 employees) would be granted tax credits, and there would be a 7-year phase-in for employers to accommodate

TABLE 21–1. Key Features of Comprehensive Access Proposals

	EMPLOYER MANDATE	MEDICAID EXPANSION	REPLACE MEDICAID	BEGIN WITH PREGNANT WOMEN, CHILDREN, AND ADOLESCENTS	COST-SHARING (EXCEPT FOR LOW-INCOME FAMILIES)	ELIMINATE PREEXISTING CONDITION EXCLUSIONS	USE OF PRACTICE GUIDELINES
Pepper Commission	X		X	X	X	X	X
Basic Health Benefit Act	X	X			X		
AMA	X	X			X	X	X
ASIM	X	X			X	X	X
ACP	X*	X*			X		X
AAP	X		X	X	X	X	

*Acceptable only as an interim step.

AMA, American Medical Association; ASIM, American Society of Internal Medicine; ACP, American College of Physicians; AAP, American Academy of Pediatrics.

these new costs. The proposal also calls for private insurance reform that would ease the purchase of insurance by small employers and eliminate preexisting condition exclusions. The plan allows for an employee share for health insurance premiums and cost-sharing through deductibles and coinsurance. There are catastrophic limits, and low-income families would have additional out-of-pocket spending caps.

The plan recommends phasing-in coverage beginning in year one with pregnant women and children through age 6 years. Older children and adolescents would gain coverage during the second year of the proposed 7-year implementation schedule.

One other component of the Pepper Commission proposal that is shared by many of the physician association proposals is development of practice guidelines derived from medical outcomes research. Several empirical studies have demonstrated large variations in treatments for the same diagnoses with little difference in medical outcome. It is believed by many observers that expanded access to care can be financed, at least in part, through savings achieved by efficient delivery of necessary, effective, and appropriate care (Table 21–1).

STRATEGIES FOR THE INDIVIDUAL PRACTITIONER

There are some options for providing health care to adolescents without risk of violating a contract of confidentiality. Although there is a paucity of data in the literature regarding self-payment by adolescents, there are mounting anecdotal reports to support this as one option. Many adolescents have some financial resources of their own, albeit limited in most cases. Providers who accept and encourage such reimbursement methods often find it necessary to develop special arrangements for payment over a more extended period. A general observation is that these young people are very conscientious about meeting these financial obligations and are particularly appreciative of being offered these special considerations. Some physicians provide free services for selected patients, including adolescents. Although this may be laudable in certain circumstances, one must remain cognizant of the fact that in our society, a value is assigned to all products and services. Thus, a service for which no monetary fee is attached may have a similarly perceived value (see Chapter 17).

Another option that appears to be increasingly acceptable is a voluntary arrangement between parents and providers. This method of payment is not limited only to affluent families. Most parents desire the best for their children and recognize the issues involved in the emancipation process. This includes access to quality health care that is delivered in a confidential manner. Similarly, health care providers recognize the importance of parental involvement in these issues and advocate this approach whenever possible. When an environment of mutual trust is established, parents may agree to pay unitemized medical bills for services rendered to their teenagers. A variation on this theme is a plan whereby both the parent and the adolescent agree to pay a specified proportion of such bills.

In situations in which the adolescent is unable, and the parents are unwilling, to pay for services delivered, the provider may be left with no alternative but to refer the patient to other health care resources (see Chapter 18). Most communities have clinics or programs in which medical care is available free or at low cost. This is particularly true for reproductive health services, which are often subsidized by state or federal funding (see Chapter 20). The same applies for mental health services but generally to a lesser extent. The new and somewhat controversial concept of school-based clinics is gaining increased acceptance and provides another option in those communities that have established such programs. Physicians should be knowledgeable about the alternative health care resources available to their adolescent patients and can play a major role in the establishment of such programs when none currently exist.

The delivery of health care to adolescents is generally a more time-consuming process than are similar services offered to younger or older patients. Adolescents tend to be seen less frequently, so more needs to be accomplished at each visit (see Chapter 25). The anticipatory guidance is, of necessity, a critical component of each interaction, since the adolescent relies heavily on the physician for guidance and support on some very sensitive issues ranging from self-esteem to sexuality. The time required for visits will vary from 15 minutes to 1 hour, depending on the agenda; routine follow-up may take only 15 minutes, a complete examination usually requires 30 minutes, and a counseling session may take up to 1 hour (see Chapter 17). Therefore, the traditional billing procedures used by primary care physicians may be inadequate, and a more reasonable approach is the development of a fee-for-time schedule.

Formulas exist that permit calculation of unit fees based on office overhead (see Chapter 17). Such fees must be negotiated with insurers. These third-party payers are well aware of fee-for-time compensation and tend to accept the fact that this is a reasonable approach to adolescent health care. The provider must, however, be prepared to verify that he or she has the knowledge and skills to deal with the problems unique to this patient population. Board certification or some similar certification of competence in adolescent medicine will obviously enhance this process of establishing credentials (see Chapter 1).

In summary, it is clear that major reforms are needed in the United States with respect to health care financing. The number of citizens who are uninsured or underinsured is, in a word, unacceptable. The establishment of some form of universal health care coverage seems inevitable, and it would appear most likely that funding for such a plan will include a combination of public and private resources. Public funding may be the more acceptable option for adolescents, since Medicaid currently is essentially the only third-party payment source that does not require notification of the head of a household regarding a claim. Publicly financed care may also be more acceptable to physicians if fees for cognitive services are increased based upon established resource-based relative value scales. These relative costs will also likely be applicable to payments from private insurers, but the issue of claim notification will still have to be addressed. Creative mechanisms must be developed that permit third-party reimbursement while still maintaining confidentiality with respect to health care rendered to adolescents.

BIBLIOGRAPHY

Congressional Research Service: Health Insurance and the Uninsured: Background Data and Analysis. Washington, DC, US Government Printing Office, May 1988.

Gabel J, DiCarlo S, Fink S, deLissovoy G: Employer-sponsored health insurance in America. Health Aff 8:116, 1989.

Hofmann AD: Legal issues in adolescent medicine. In Hofmann AD, Greydanus, DE (eds): Adolescent Medicine. Norwalk, CT, Appleton & Lange, 1989, pp 519–530.

Hsiao WC, Braun P, Dunn D, et al: Results and policy implications of the resource-based relative-value study. N Engl J Med 319:881, 1988.

Neinstein LS: Consent and confidentiality laws for minors in the western United States. West J Med 147:218, 1987.

Newacheck PW: Adolescents with special health needs: Prevalence, severity and access to health services. Pediatrics 84:872, 1989.

Newacheck PW, McManus MA: Health insurance status of adolescents in the United States. Pediatrics 84:699, 1989.

Newacheck PW, McManus MA: Health care expenditure patterns for adolescents. J Adoles Health Care 11:133, 1990.

US Congress Office of Technology Assessment: Adolescent Health Insurance Status: Analyses of Trends in Coverage and Preliminary Estimates of the Effects of an Employer Mandate and Medicaid Expansion on the Uninsured. Washington, DC, US Congress, Office of Technology Assessment, July 1989.

Yudkowsky BK, Cartland JDC, Flint SS: Pediatrician participation in Medicaid: 1978–1989. Pediatrics 85:567, 1990.

Practice Applications

CHAPTER 22

Interviewing

CHRISTOPHER H. HODGMAN and MARY SUE JACK

Interviewing adolescents can be a challenging and yet rewarding experience. In this chapter, we present general issues to be considered by interviewers of adolescents, followed by some characteristics specific to interviews of early, middle, and late adolescents. This will be followed by special approaches that facilitate communication with adolescents, such as family interviews and group interviews (see Chapter 17).

The majority of adolescents enjoy talking about themselves and feel a sense of self-efficacy when communicating with health care providers who positively reinforce their comments and listen to them attentively. Most adolescents give honest information when provided the opportunity. Some adolescents, however, are difficult to interview no matter what approach is used. Monosyllabic responses are frustrating in any circumstance.

Why is the interview of the adolescent special, distinct from the pediatric interview on the one hand or the standard adult interview on the other hand? Interviewing adolescents emphasizes their developmental distinctions from children and adults. Too often the traditional pediatric model is followed, and the parent and the adolescent are seen together. An adult model of talking only with the patient may be equally problematic. The unique developmental needs of adolescents must be considered in order for an effective interview to transpire.

THE INTERVIEW

The interview is the health care provider's single most important tool in assessing adolescents. Its main purpose is to obtain information. The background for the interview includes the adolescent's and provider's previous contacts, if any, and the reason for the visit to the health provider. Through effective use of verbal and nonverbal communication skills, the health care provider usually can establish a trusting relationship with a young person. When trust is established early in the adolescent–health care provider encounter, the chances for a long-term relationship are good, enabling the health care provider to assist the young person with health concerns into early adulthood.

Initial Interview

An interview of an adolescent is likely to take place, at least initially, in the presence of a parent or parents (especially with younger adolescents, less so with older adolescents). Such a joint interview is just that: It is not an interview of the parents about their adolescent in front of him or her, but an opportunity to speak to both generations together, setting limits, defining confidentiality, and describing the "contract" the professional expects to fulfill. It is important that the interviewer not permit parents to deprecate the adolescent in front of him or her; correspondingly, it is important that the adolescent observe that the parents are treated respectfully and supportively by the interviewer. As described in Chapters 20 and 25, other elements of the contract include confidentiality (what the adolescent tells the interviewer is kept between them unless both agree it should be shared or unless physical risk is entailed in continued silence), readiness to reveal outside information (so that the teenager understands what the interviewer knows), and a discussion of the limits of the contract (when interviews are for consultation only or when interviews are "official," requiring that the information from the interview be shared with another agency).

Financial realities may also need to be discussed during the initial interview; to do so in front of the adolescent indicates a readiness to address important issues in his or her presence (see Chapter 21). If the primary nature of the problem leading to the interview is embarrassing or shameful, it is probably best to discuss that reality early in the interview. To do so lessens everyone's anxiety, while affording the interviewer an opportunity to demonstrate care for the feelings of the adolescent and the parents alike. Usually, the joint interview is not the time for a lengthy discussion of a teenager's difficulties, because of potential risks to the adolescent's self-esteem.

Whether to continue the initial interview jointly or to see the adolescent alone should be decided in favor of the approach that will be most productive. In family conflict, for example, joint interviews are often most worthwhile. A symptomatic teenager may prefer parental assistance in describing the problem or, in contrast, may resent parental presence as "interference." Disorders of character—that is, delinquency or sexual deviations (see Chapter 108)—require that the interviewer know facts that the parents can supply but the adolescent may be unwilling to divulge.

Weiner has described a sequence that should be followed in the initial adolescent interview: comfort, engagement, and commitment.

Comfort. The setting in which the interview occurs and the style of interviewing (individual contact versus family contact) are very much related to the adolescent's comfort. If the adolescent is not relatively comfortable during the interview, the process will suffer. Circumstances that may be acceptable to adults can be disconcerting to the adolescent. Attractive but not imposing surroundings are helpful, but of even more importance is an interviewer with a welcoming manner (see Chapter 17). The youngster needs a sense that this will be a positive process rather than an alienating or disconcerting one. Having the adolescent talk about *something,* such as biographic details, is far more important than introducing the primary problem and having a resounding silence follow. Some adolescents expect to be looked at; others find it most awkward. Unlined paper and a pencil, a lump of clay, or an inviting hand-sized object nearby may increase comfort by giving the adolescent something to do while difficult matters are discussed. Acknowledgment of the adolescent's discomfort can help, as well as an indication of a readiness to change the subject if a given topic proves too difficult. The fact that awkward things will need discussion should be acknowledged, even if the initial interview is not the ideal time.

Engagement. It is highly desirable to demonstrate the usefulness of the interview to the adolescent. A variety of ways are available to "set the hook." Encouraged to expound on a variety of biographic details, the patient demonstrates that he or she is competent. By openly discussing the patient's discomforts and responding sensitively, the interviewer indicates a sensitivity to the teenager's needs. Of most value in engaging the patient—in "setting the hook"—is the proposal of a new way of viewing a certain matter, a new angle on a familiar topic, evidence of insight and the ability of the interviewer to enlighten the adolescent patient. If such responses can occur, the interviewer demonstrates usefulness to a frequently dubious young person.

Commitment. Too often novices err by seeking commitment from the adolescent to a therapeutic regimen too early. Remembering that the adolescent is risking independence and self-definition at a vulnerable age, the interviewer should initially avoid suggesting the desirability of ongoing treatment. It is usually better to suggest to the adolescent that the interviews are being conducted on a trial basis to see if they can be useful. Only after several sessions should the issue of ongoing meetings be introduced.

Typical Features of the Successful Adolescent Interview

Certain aspects of successful interviews with adolescents may or may not distinguish them from similar interviews with adults; nonetheless, the developmental status of the adolescent is likely to impose certain distinct qualities on a successful interview.

Content. As the adolescent matures, content changes substantially. Thus, among younger adolescents it is often helpful to indicate that the adolescent is not expected to discuss matters too painful to handle. This is different from the typical expectation that an adolescent must say whatever is necessary and will be completely open with the interviewer. Some adolescents feel too guilty to continue discussing their problems with the practitioner if they are ashamed because of omissions on the one hand or embarrassing honesty on the other hand. Adults are usually more able to handle both frankness and omission, recognizing the need for one or the other under differing circumstances.

Style. Style can be important to a successful adolescent interview. A "light touch" is often helpful, as distinguished from jocularity (which may seem belittling to the patient) or teasing (which has an aggressive undercurrent difficult for the teenager to manage gracefully). A willingness to "shift gears" from serious matters to a lighter, more trivial content is helpful, especially if done openly with an acknowledgment that the adolescent can be expected to handle only a certain amount of discomfort during a given interview.

Pacing. This is another way of expressing the ability to vary tempo, to increase or decrease pressure on the adolescent, or to lighten mood as necessary.

Activity. Activity is likely to be considerably greater in a typical adolescent interview than in an interview with an adult. Such an interview often sounds more like "conversation" than a classic adult interchange. The more a natural rhythm is achieved, the easier it is for the average teenager to participate. Silence can be destructive in an interview if the adolescent feels inadequate, is expected to reveal uncomfortable material, or is too self-conscious. Experienced interviewers of adolescents vary their activity to diminish the young person's anxiety; however, anxiety can, on occasion, drive the adolescent to useful self-revelation. Sometimes the willingness of the interviewer to listen sympathetically and at length is a new experience for the adolescent.

Honesty and Genuineness. These are important attributes for the interviewer to manifest. Holmes has described the requirement for "abnormal candor" from the interviewer as important to success. Youngsters often expect adult authority figures to dissimulate, to rely on appearances, or to assert authority to cover their own discomforts. To be direct and honest under such circumstances—"abnormally candid"—marks the interviewer as different and the interview as the first such experience for many adolescent patients.

Language. Language introduces many problems for interviewers. On the one hand, it is essential to avoid stilted "professional" terminology, and on the other hand, the use of teenage jargon is often experienced as patronizing or manipulative (see Chapter 17). It can be said that as soon as an adult interviewer uses teenage jargon, that jargon is no longer age-unique or distinctive—by definition, it is obsolete for the adolescent.

Positive Issues. Every interview should touch upon positive issues. Too often adolescents feel that they are only a collection of failures to the caretaker—just diabetic, just obese, just academically incompetent. The fact that positive issues are discussed should not imply a trivializing, "cheerful" quality to the interview. Rather, it indicates to the patient that the interviewer has respect for the adolescent, whatever his or her difficulties.

Negative Issues. These should usually be discussed early in the interview so that, unspoken, they do not hang over the entire session and so that they can be dealt with and left behind if necessary.

Duration. The typical adolescent interview is often briefer than that with an adult, though there are many exceptions. It is desirable to emphasize that flexibility—permitting the interview to end early if it has been too painful or too uncomfortable—is sometimes worthwhile. Conversely, the adolescent who "arranges" to have only short exchanges with the care provider is likely to be avoiding important matters and may need to be confronted with this possibility.

THE INTERVIEWER

Just as a successful adolescent interview is more likely if the interviewer attends to developmental features and the changeability of this age group, so self-examination can materially improve the interviewer's technique. Certain issues need to be considered by the interviewer.

Authority. The interviewer may feel threatened if the adolescent appears to question his or her competence. If the interviewer defensively maintains a given position, the adolescent patient may become more resistant. If, however, the interviewer is comfortably authoritative and competent, these qualities need not be emphasized, and youthful rebelliousness may diminish (see Chapter 17).

Medical Model. The fact that a problem is brought to a practitioner does not make it medical. "Medicalizing" often means "pathologizing"; this may lead to the assumption that if something is wrong, a solution must be available to correct it.

Age. Younger interviewers often overidentify with the adolescent, assuming a mutuality of interest because of youth. It is well to remember that as young as the professional may feel within a professional field, the teenager views him or her as an adult. Older interviewers sometimes overidentify with parents, an even more dangerous trap because of the likelihood of ensuing alienation of the adolescent patient.

Conservatism. Many care providers are conservative by nature or training or are assumed to be so by the adolescent. Problems also may arise if the interviewer feels it necessary to demonstrate that this is not so.

Competence. The variety of effects on the interview imposed by the interviewer's personality and background is very broad. It is rare for most practitioners to have had much directly monitored or observed training in interviewing. The importance of direct supervision, one-way mirrors, video taping, or audio taping as a means of improving one's interviewing cannot be overemphasized. Much of the value of such observation is the opportunity it gives to the interviewer to review the assumptions and thought processes that may have dictated certain responses or outcomes in interviewing. Groups of practitioners have found it helpful to review one another's interviewing because of the difficulty of accurate self-monitoring.

THE ADOLESCENT AND THE INTERVIEW

Throughout this text, developmental aspects of adolescence are emphasized, with the reminder that the period itself is part of the continuum of the life cycle, preceded by childhood and followed by adulthood (see Chapter 9). As a group, adolescents share certain common characteristics, which should be recognized during the interview. There are also the substages of preadolescence, adolescence (early, middle, and late), and postadolescence, each having its separate characteristics. We shall first examine common characteristics of adolescents and then consider the substages and how each has an impact on the interviewing process.

Common Characteristics

Lability or Changeability. Unlike most adults, adolescents may change from day to day. The interviewer who expects the pleasant, open youngster of yesterday may be disconcerted to find an irritable and resistant adolescent today; the interviewer who girds for another difficult session may be surprised to find an eager, cooperative adolescent patient ready to make real progress.

Energy, Exhaustion, and Reenergization. Adolescents sometimes take refuge in fatigued withdrawal after emotionally draining experiences. Unlike many adults, they may not be prepared to sustain the effort required for successful interaction with a medical care provider. In addition, depression may present as boredom or apathy, both accompanied by exhaustion (see Chapter 100). If these dysphoric states are acknowledged and waited out, the adolescent often rebounds to levels of previous energy. If the adolescent does not respond that way, it may be reasonable to investigate possible underlying causes (see Chapters 98–105).

Curiosity, Skepticism, and Defensiveness. A youth's curiosity may support a positive relationship with the physician and a productive interview. Questions about the interviewer suggest identification with the practitioner or the adolescent's need to test the interviewer's reliability. Young persons deserve a courteous, direct response limited by the interviewer's sense of propriety and comfort. Correspondingly, adolescent skepticism and defensiveness may occur as a defense against positive feelings for the interviewer. They may not represent rejection of the interviewer as much as misgivings about the adult as a potential model.

Future Orientation. This is another useful index of adolescent health. The youngster who appears vague and uninterested about the future may be manifesting depression or pessimism. The "personal fable" is a less positive variant of future orientation—that is, the youth's sense of invulnerability, a belief that "the rules do not apply," that he or she cannot have an automobile accident when driving too rapidly, or that she cannot become pregnant when experiencing sexual activity.

Substages

PREADOLESCENCE

Preadolescence especially is a time during which the health care provider can prepare the child and his or her family for the future. Performing part of the interview with a preadolescent separately from the parents can teach the young person about participation in the health care interview as well as establish the expectation of increasingly independent responsibility for health care activities. By paying special attention to simple, direct vocabulary (short but open-ended questions) and appropriate concrete information the patient can readily supply, the interviewer helps the preadolescent develop confidence in participating in the health history. However, it is unrealistic to expect clear historical data from all preadolescents; in this case, the parent may supply information, with the interviewer turning to the preadolescent for corroboration from time to time.

EARLY ADOLESCENCE

The early adolescent is experiencing significant changes in the body as a result of puberty (see Chapters 4 and 5). Increased height and the appearance of secondary sexual characteristics produce heightened self-consciousness. The sense of an imaginary audience often leads early adolescents to believe that everyone is watching them and knows what they are thinking.

Approach. Health care providers must be sensitive to the early adolescent's self-consciousness. Starting with neutral, nonthreatening topics such as routine identifying data is an approach that allows trust to develop before sensitive topics are raised. Continued concrete operational thinking in the early adolescent dictates that the health care provider avoid the use of abstract concepts. Conducting the interview separately from parents is appropriate with early adolescents, since they may have questions and concerns that they are not comfortable discussing in front of parents.

Content. School activities and school performance are content areas that must be assessed in early adolescents. Junior high school is a time of increased stress, which may lead to a lowering of grades and of enjoyment of school or to social difficulties, often expressed in "acting-out" behavior. Discussion of potential pressures by the peer group to participate in exploratory behaviors helps prepare the early adolescent for future experiences.

Skills. It is helpful to focus initially on the adolescent's concerns rather than those of the parents; young patients appreciate being seen as separate individuals.

The early adolescent may respond to the health care provider's questions with "I don't know." This response may mean that the adolescent really does not know. However, it may also mean that the adolescent is not quite ready to share the information. One skill useful for eliciting information from an early adolescent is having him or her keep a diary of thoughts between visits. The health care provider and the adolescent can review the diary together at subsequent visits.

Although silence can be used effectively in therapeutic communication, it is usually best to avoid silence with early adolescents. Their feelings of self-consciousness add to the uneasiness with which silence is usually greeted by individuals in this age group.

MIDDLE ADOLESCENCE

Middle adolescence is traditionally the period when separation from parents is increasingly sanctioned (e.g., by acquisition of a driver's license). Argumentativeness and negativism are common, but more actual competence and self-confidence can make relations with adults less strident than before.

Approach. Cognitively, middle adolescents should be thinking at the formal operational level, at least in most domains. Thus they can think abstractly and can comprehend complex but clear explanations and instruction. Most middle adolescents still live with parents or other adult caregivers. Relationships with such adults need to be addressed; however, interviewing a middle adolescent alone often produces a maximum amount of information.

Content. Starting the interview with nonthreatening topics such as biographic information sets the middle adolescent at ease by providing an opportunity to demonstrate self-efficacy. Topics important to discuss with the middle adolescent include, but are not limited to, school and peer activities, responsibility, sexuality, and exposure to drug use and abuse. The power of the peer group cannot be underestimated with middle adolescents. Discussion of the influence of friends on activities such as drug experimentation and other risk-taking behaviors often is valuable to the adolescent who is exposed increasingly to this pressure in the absence of parental structure and support.

Skills. It should be established early in the interview that the health care provider is an ally to the middle adolescent. This assures the adolescent that his or her concerns and health are to be the major focus of the visit. If at all possible, power struggles should be avoided, particularly around issues of openness. In any case, complete openness is difficult for the middle adolescent because of a need for independence and autonomy. As a result, such patients often limit the amount of information they are willing to divulge about their private thoughts. Momentary regression may be followed by renewed maturation in the middle adolescent; accordingly, the interviewer may need to wait to discuss sensitive material until a propitious moment.

LATE ADOLESCENCE

Late adolescence finds identity resolution in social, sexual, moral, and occupational terms becoming increasingly pressing. Separation from parents may now become a reality. Undercurrents of dependency on adults remain, unacknowledged by the adolescent and often concealed from the interviewer.

Approach. By late adolescence, an interview with a health care provider can be accomplished completely independently from parents. Now the adolescent is more mobile, spends many hours out of the home, and seeks health care autonomously.

Content. Usually the late adolescent has an agenda for the health care provider, though it is not always immediately apparent. Among content areas to be included in the interview are future goals and responsibility. By this time, normal adolescents have begun to address the future in terms of careers, jobs, and potential mates. These topics may be discussed with the health care provider for assistance in decision-making.

Skills. It is best to avoid overestimating the maturity of the late adolescent. Occasional regression occurs and usually passes. Some intemperate or risk-taking behavior typical of younger ages can still be anticipated. For the late adolescent to take responsibility for health care is an important goal to be conveyed by the health care provider through example and teaching. Nonverbal communication may be particularly significant in late adolescents. They have been socialized to say what they believe health care providers want to hear, which may be far from the truth. Attending to nonverbal messages transmitted by late adolescents helps health care providers obtain more comprehensive views of their patients.

POSTADOLESCENCE

Adolescent features remain well into adulthood, particularly for those individuals sheltered from adult expectations by educational status or continued dependency upon parents. Many aspects of late adolescence apply to postadolescence as well. Health care providers accustomed to working with the postadolescent as an adult often overlook ongoing, unresolved developmental issues that may render compliance less than complete and that make continued adolescent care techniques appropriate.

FAMILY INTERVIEWING
(see Chapter 23)

In a sense, every interview is a family interview. Whether or not members of the family other than the identified adolescent patient are present, their salient importance to the adolescent is evident. Many adolescent interviews begin with the adolescent patient and whoever else has come along to the appointment, since presence suggests relevance to the interview. Sometimes such a joint interview proceeds for only a few minutes; at other times, it is apparent that the joint or family approach is working so well that it should continue throughout the session. Under such circumstances, the very immediacy of the process capitalizes on spontaneity and mutual supportiveness. As mentioned previously, family interviews also enable the care provider to prevent mutual abuse or recrimination, and in so doing promote positive family interchange.

In most instances, however, family interviews are scheduled by prior arrangement, permitting all participants to think about the reasons for their presence beforehand. Presence at the meeting assumes a willingness to help; with assistance, all family members can learn to generalize the problem beyond the identified adolescent patient. This permits support of the adolescent and the sharing of responsibility for recounting painful circumstances when the adolescent may be unable or unwilling to do so alone. For example, family interviews can serve to ease the problem of a teenager's silence in individual interviews; most adolescents wish to participate in any discussion regarding themselves rather than abdicate to other family members the sole responsibility for discussing their problems. Therefore, it is sometimes useful to move from a difficult interview with an unproductive, resistant, or silent adolescent to a family interview in the next session. It is especially desirable under such circumstances to make the move appear warranted and natural: "It's hard for us to discuss these things alone; let's see if the family can help us."

Family interviews permit modeling of constructive family relationships when the skilled interviewer prevents destructive attacks on the adolescent by family members or on the family by the adolescent, while acknowledging everyone's responsibility for the situation. Family interviewing can exploit natural alliances in the family or create new ones; sometimes a teenager discovers, to his or her surprise, that other family members see things the same way he or she does but have never said so.

The disadvantages of family interviewing include possible diffusion of responsibility—for example, an adolescent may feel it is unnecessary to acknowledge a problem because the family will assume it. Family interviewing may make discussion of certain topics more difficult rather than easier. Conversely, if deviant or unacceptable behavior is too shameful for an adolescent patient to discuss, hearing the unmentionable mentioned by a sympathetic family member may be helpful.

It is helpful to set the ground rules for family interviews. These rules include the fact that "scapegoating" is unacceptable and that a problem occurring in a family is everyone's problem. The presence of all members of a family may or may not be necessary for successful family interviewing. A good rule to follow is to postpone discussion about any potentially available family member not present at a given interview: "How can we get Dad in to discuss his side of the problem? May I call him?" (It is often best for the practitioner to recruit unavailable family members rather than to have others do so judgmentally or punitively.) Alternatively, assembling the whole family may be given to those present as a positive task: "How can you get everybody else in and have them feel good about coming?" Even multigenerational family sessions can be useful; at the same time it is well to remember that smaller units (e.g., siblings alone, one parent, and so on) are sometimes efficient and expeditious aids to supporting an adolescent in distress.

Family interviewing in medical illnesses is useful at many levels: Mutual concern and support are mobilized; a wider family history is made available; and opportunities to allay guilt or imagined responsibility for unavoidable illness are offered. Family members often are grateful for an opportunity to be helpful; such gratitude can be poignant when expressed by a young sibling or a grandparent of a seriously ill youngster. Family interviews are of particular importance after a family member's death. Such sessions are desirable not only immediately after the loss but also at subsequent anniversaries (see Chapter 116). A health care provider is particularly able to offer support at such times.

GROUP INTERVIEWING

Group interviews are especially useful for adolescents because of their tendency to identify with peers. In the medical or pediatric setting, the use of "network" therapy relies on the existing group of friends to support a troubled or ill adolescent. Here the opportunity for friends to ask the health care provider the questions that everyone secretly has makes an unmentionable or difficult situation comprehensible and even more bearable for the adolescent and friends alike. The fact that the health care provider, with the adolescent's permission, can answer difficult questions honestly offers other group members an opportunity to work through their anxieties and fears in order to support the adolescent more fully.

Another form of group support that is of great value to chronically or seriously ill adolescents involves groups of patients with similar diagnoses (see Chapter 30). The value of such groups for substance abuse, eating disorders, and weight control is well established. Camps for adolescents with diabetes mellitus use group therapy routinely, as do programs for youngsters with asthma, cystic fibrosis, and hematologic and oncologic illnesses. In such programs, as in all other group sessions, groups may be open (adding or losing members weekly) or closed (usually after a period of recruitment). In the latter instance, the duration may be fixed or open for negotiation. In some conditions (e.g., cystic fibrosis), group membership may be terminated by death, with subsequent groups serving to support survivors. In every instance, however, a properly conducted group can be a remarkably supportable endeavor, particularly if group members have problems or illnesses in common for which they can offer mutual support. Similarly, groups of parents or siblings of such patients can provide family members with needed support (see Chapters 43 and 45–54).

Experienced providers learn that the interview is the most productive single portion of the medical examination. It brings to bear all the wisdom, experience, and skill of the interviewer and all the concerns of the adolescent patient. In the end, good interviewing is a personal matter. For success, one must develop a personal approach, permitting the most direct and expedient access to information coupled with ongoing support of the concerned and troubled adolescent. The health care interview should change and improve as the professional matures and gains greater experience. Good interviewing is much more than the "art of medicine"—it is the science of medicine at its fullest.

BIBLIOGRAPHY

Elkind D: Egocentrism in adolescence. Child Dev 38:1025, 1967.
Holmes DJ: The Adolescent in Psychotherapy. Boston, Little, Brown, 1964.
Meeks JE, Bernet W: Fragile Alliance: An Orientation to the Outpatient Psychotherapy of the Adolescent, 4th ed. Melbourne, FL, Krieger, 1990.
Weiner IB: Psychotherapy. In Weiner IB (ed): Psychological Disturbance in Adolescence. New York, John Wiley & Sons, 1970.

CHAPTER 23

Family-oriented Care

SUSAN H. McDANIEL, DAVID SEABURN, and THOMAS CAMPBELL

Adolescents face unique developmental challenges as they struggle to make the transition from childhood to adulthood (see Chapters 5, 8, and 9). Many physicians recognize the need to support the adolescent's strivings toward autonomy in order to facilitate the tasks of adolescence. However, this support should take place with recognition of the pivotal role of the family in facilitating the adolescent's move toward autonomy. Even with the well-recognized importance of the adolescent's peer group, studies document the central role the family continues to have in the development of the adolescent's values and self-esteem. For these reasons, we believe the family is the most important resource for understanding and treating adolescents. Comprehensive adolescent health care must respect both the adolescent's growing autonomy and the parents' vital role in the adolescent's overall health and development. Psychosocial problems, in particular, require the physician to attend to the context of the adolescent's difficulties and to include family members and other relevant parties in the assessment and treatment of these problems.

A family-oriented, or systems, approach to health care is one way of treating the individual adolescent patient and that patient's symptoms in context. This approach operationalizes the biopsychosocial model and may be brought to any patient encounter, whether the visit occurs with only the individual adolescent or involves family or friends (see Chapters 22 and 24). It includes gathering information about current family relationships; patterns of health, illness, and relationships across generations; and, particularly, the history of the family's approach to adolescence and separation in previous generations. This information helps the physician to understand the adolescent's difficulties and develop a treatment plan that can draw on the strengths of both the adolescent and the persons who care for and about him or her.

There are many levels of physician involvement with families. They range from the minimal inclusion of the family (only for medical or legal necessity) to communicating with them regularly about medical issues, addressing family stress and feelings, conducting a family assessment and providing family counseling, and finally, addressing more deeply rooted family problems with family therapy. In this chapter we discuss several levels of family-oriented care, beginning with the day-to-day family-oriented medical care of adolescents, including issues such as the importance of maintaining a positive relationship with both the adolescent and the parents.

Next we describe techniques and strategies for family assessment and family counseling for the psychosocial problems of adolescence. (See Chapter 123 for a discussion of family therapy, including a review of adolescent problems that are best treated with family therapy, a description of the current state of the art, and the issues involved in adolescent specialists' collaboration with, and referral to, family therapists.)

FAMILY RESOURCES AND DAY-TO-DAY MEDICAL CARE OF ADOLESCENTS

Adolescent development does not take place in a vacuum but is part of multiple developmental transitions involving the family as a whole. Adolescent individuation is a family process. All members work together to negotiate and renegotiate issues of closeness and distance and dependence and independence; this process transforms all family members, including the adolescent. Just as the adolescent is struggling with identity issues, important changes are also occurring in the parents and the grandparents. Parents may be facing midlife identity issues about career and marriage as well as the issue of the health of their own parents. Grandparents may be reviewing their lives as they approach retirement or face the declining capacities that are associated with normal aging or illness. In addition to issues related to adolescent development, teenagers are sometimes faced with the stress of a parent's or other family member's illness or death, parents' separation and divorce, or living in a single-parent household. None of these circumstances occurs in isolation, but they are interwoven and form the fabric of this phase of family life. It is with these multiple family transitions in mind that the primary care of adolescents should occur.

Adolescent health care should be focused on the adolescent, with a family orientation. Adolescents do not fit into the pattern of younger well-child care, in which parents clearly have the primary responsibility, and yet they are not adults either. They are an in-between generation that is still attached to and dependent on family, while at the same time they seek independence and function with many adult rights regarding health care. The physician must find a balance between the emerging independence of the adolescent and the ongoing importance and responsibility of parents. This is best achieved by establishing and maintaining supportive relationships with both the adolescent and his or her parents.

It may be helpful to have both the adolescent and the parents available at an office visit so that the physician can have a complete view of the adolescent within the larger context of his or her family (see Chapter 98). This makes it easier to maintain alliances with both parents and adolescents. The adolescent should be given the option to be seen alone for most of the office visit, unless he or she specifically requests that the parent stay. The concerns of the parents should be addressed at the beginning and end of the interview. The physician needs to be sensitive to what information he or she shares with parents. When there is a disagreement between the physician and the adolescent about information to be divulged, the adolescent's wishes should be acknowledged (see Chapter 20). The physician can encourage or coach the adolescent gently on how to share the difficult information with parents on his or her own. In high-risk situations, such as when a patient is suicidal or homicidal, the adolescent should know that his or her request for confidentiality cannot be honored and that the parents will be apprised immediately of the situation (see Chapters 20 and 22).

When considering an adolescent's or parent's request for confidentiality, the physician must also assess the role that family dynamics may play in such a request. Family members may try to enlist the physician's collusion in keeping secrets about emotional or interpersonal issues in the family. A common example is a parent wanting a physician to discuss a sensitive issue with an adolescent (sex or drugs) without revealing the origin of the concern. Alternatively, an adolescent may share a concern only if the physician promises beforehand not to tell anyone. It is important for the adolescent to believe his or her confidentiality is protected, barring dangerous circumstances. However, the physician should also avoid destructive bonds of secrecy and should make every effort to help adolescents and parents talk directly to each other.

It is often tempting to side with an adolescent's efforts to pull away from parental authority; however, in most cases the physician should avoid taking sides with either the adolescent or the parents. Siding with the parent against the adolescent or the adolescent against the parent runs the risk of eventually losing the trust of both. By maintaining alliances with both the adolescent and the parents, the physician is best able to help the adolescent when there is a problem, as illustrated in the following example:

JW, aged 15 years, was sent by his pediatrician to an adolescent specialist, Dr. A, because J's parents were concerned that he had "changed" and had become very moody.

At the initial visit, Dr. A met with both Mrs. W and J and had Mrs. W explain her concerns. J said nothing. Dr. A suggested he meet with J several times alone, in addition to having a family meeting with him and his parents. In the second session, Dr. A took the opportunity to discuss some of the developmental issues of adolescence with J, who did not respond. Dr. A said J did not have to talk but should feel free to listen while Dr. A talked in a general way about some of the changes adolescents face. At the end of the session, J

finally began to talk when Dr. A turned the conversation to athletics. In the third session, J hinted at some confusion regarding relationships with his friends. Dr. A used this discussion to talk about sexuality. J listened intently but did not want to discuss it. He did say he was starting to feel better. In the last session, both Mr. and Mrs. W said J seemed brighter and that he had made the transition to a new school and seemed to be attracted to a different group of friends. Both J and his parents believed he was doing well.

Two years later, Mr. W called and said J's grades had dropped and he was again acting moody. With his parents' encouragement, J came in and hesitantly told Dr. A he had "odd feelings" toward a boy who was his best friend. J was feeling very confused. Dr. A asked if J's parents were aware of his concern. J said that they were not and he wanted to keep it that way. Dr. A offered to have several more sessions with J to address these concerns. J accepted the offer. Dr. A saw J three times over the next several weeks as J gradually began to recognize and accept his homosexuality. In addition, they discussed health concerns, such as AIDS, and Dr. A referred J to a support group. Dr. A continued to encourage J to talk with his parents, but he refused, saying they would be furious. Dr. A assured J that he had worked with other adolescents with similar concerns and that with support the love of parents usually overcomes the shock of hearing about any issue. He explained to J that his parents would always be important to him, whereas the therapy relationship was only temporary.

During this time, Dr. A saw Mr. and Mrs. W to hear about their impressions and concerns. Mr. W said J was again doing well in school, but they were concerned that J was growing up so fast and soon would leave for college. Dr. A encouraged Mr. and Mrs. W to share this with J, telling them that adolescents often need their parents' support most when they are becoming more and more independent. Dr. A convened a family conference in which Mr. and Mrs. W shared their concerns with their son, but J said little in response.

Soon after this session, J told Dr. A he had decided to tell his parents. Dr. A offered to see J and his parents together, but J wanted to tell his parents himself. Dr. A helped J clarify what he wanted to say to his parents. J's disclosure to his mother and father led initially to a great deal of conflict. Mr. W called Dr. A, and Dr. A suggested a family meeting. At the meeting it was clear that Mr. W, in particular, had difficulty accepting his son's sexual orientation. The family met twice with Dr. A, and by the end of the second session Mr. W was still upset, but with Mrs. W's support, he was willing to work on communicating with their son. They said that though they could not understand this part of J, they also recognized his many other accomplishments and did not want to "lose" him. J, for his part, was able to accept the fact that his parents did not understand entirely, but he felt good that they were openly discussing issues together.

In our culture, issues involving sexuality or sexual orientation can often tempt the physician to side with one party or another. In this case, Dr. A balanced his support of each member of the W family. He maintained J's confidentiality but, by encouraging communication among all family members, avoided creating an atmosphere of secrecy or taking over the parents' responsibility for J. Dr. A developed a relationship of trust with the whole family, which enabled them to come together and talk in a time of crisis, thereby strengthening the family bonds instead of stressing them further. Situations like this often require considerable patience and effort from the physician, but they can result in substantial change for both the adolescent and the family.

The key to comprehensive, effective care of adolescents lies in balancing the needs of the adolescent's growing autonomy and the important role of parents and family in launching the adolescent into adulthood. A physician can play a vital role in helping adolescents and their families navigate this significant life cycle transition. The alliances that a physician builds with the adolescent and family provide the foundation for assessing and treating the psychosocial problems of adolescence.

TECHNIQUES AND STRATEGY: ASSESSMENT AND COUNSELING OF ADOLESCENTS AND THEIR FAMILIES

Contrary to popular myth, research has shown that adolescence is not a time of serious turmoil for most families (see Chapters 8 and 9). Smetana found that adolescents and their parents are in frequent conflict. (They average 12 conflicts per week, even though they spend little time together.) However, the conflict was rated by both parties as mild—2 on a scale of 1 to 5, with 5 being serious conflict. Offer and Offer found that only 20% to 30% of all adolescents experience severe difficulties at any point during this developmental stage. For adolescents who do have significant problems, the physicians caring for them may wish to convene the family to conduct an assessment and consider family counseling or family therapy if needed.

To assess and treat any serious adolescent psychosocial problem, it is essential to involve both parents of the adolescent as well as other relevant family members, friends, and professionals. All adolescent psychosocial problems influence and are influenced by the family system and are often related to other family problems. The first step in the family treatment of any problem is to convene the family and conduct a comprehensive family assessment, as was done in the previous example with J's family. Conducting an initial family interview has been shown to reduce the number of problem visits and may reduce both the number of emergency room visits and the number of after-hours phone calls about young children. No such study has yet been done with adolescents.

As was discussed earlier, the most important principle in working with the families of adolescents is to maintain a strong positive alliance with the parents as well as the adolescent and to avoid siding with one party against the other. Establishing a positive collaborative relationship with the adolescent's family begins when the clinician invites them to participate in a family meeting or conference. When convening a family conference, the clinician should be clear and direct about his or her need to meet with the entire household and other relevant family members, friends, or other professionals to adequately assess the adolescent's problem. Both parents should attend the conference, as should siblings and any other member of the household. Meeting with only one parent gives a distorted view of the adolescent's

problem and the functioning of the family and may exacerbate underlying family dynamics. Including the siblings in the family conference leads to a more accurate assessment of the family; it takes some of the "heat" off the adolescent as the identified patient and communicates to the family that each member has an important role in treating the problem. When an adolescent's parents are divorced, they and any stepparents should attend the family conference together, if they can cooperate and agree to work together to help their child. If the parents cannot cooperate, it is usually necessary to meet separately with each parent and the stepfamily. It is always useful to include grandparents whenever possible, but in the case of stepfamilies it is especially important.

When convening a family conference, the focus of the meeting should be what the family identifies as the problem, not the clinician's assessment of the problem. The clinician should communicate to the parents the importance of obtaining their help in assessing and treating the adolescent's problem. It is important not to imply that there is a family problem or that the family needs counseling. Most parents already feel guilt or blame for their adolescent's difficulties and are very sensitive to any suggestion that they are at fault. Parents or other family members may resist attending a family conference if there are serious marital conflicts or family secrets, if the family has felt blame for the problem in the past, or if they believe that the clinician has sided with the adolescent against them. This resistance can be diminished by reassuring the parents that they are the adolescent's best resource and are essential to the solution. This approach mitigates against feelings of blame and guilt.

Prior to a family conference, it is helpful to review what is known about the adolescent and his or her family, to generate tentative hypotheses about the presenting problem, and to develop a strategy for conducting the meeting. The family genogram is a useful tool for gathering and recording information about the family in a pictorial form (Fig. 23–1.) Information on the genogram should include names, ages, marital status, children, household, significant illnesses, dates of traumatic events (such as deaths), and occupations. It can also include emotional closeness, distance, or conflict among members, significant relationships with other professionals, and any other information important to the case. Information gathered during the family conference can be added to the genogram. Constructing a genogram may reveal repeating problematic emotional patterns, common medical problems, and other considerations that are important in the process of evaluation and treatment planning. McGoldrick and Gerson provide a comprehensive review of how to use family genograms in family assessment and treatment.

From reviewing the family genogram, the clinician can usually understand what individual and family developmental issues are being faced by the family. Many adolescents' problems involving sexuality, substance abuse, and school failure are a reflection of parallel difficulties in one or both parents (e.g., extramarital affairs, alcohol abuse, work problems). Reviewing the family genogram in the context of the family life cycle

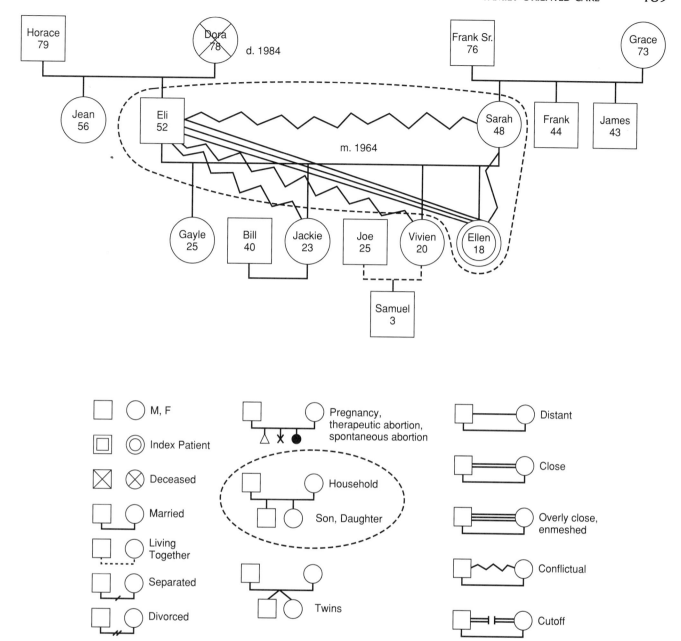

Figure 23–1. The family genogram. Eli, 52, and Sarah, 48, have been married 26 years. They have four daughters: Gayle, 25, Jackie, 23, Vivien, 20, and Ellen, 18. The family entered therapy because of Ellen's multiple suicide attempts. Each of Ellen's sisters had a difficult relationship with their father around "leaving home" issues. Ellen had a very close relationship with her father and a conflictual relationship with her mother. Eli and Sarah have a history of conflict about parenting their daughters.

assists the clinician in developing hypotheses about presenting problems prior to the family conference.

An interview with multiple participants must be structured and directed by the clinician. When first meeting with the family of an adolescent, it is usually best not to delve immediately into the presenting problem but instead to spend a few minutes socializing with the family, welcoming them, getting to know them better, and helping them to feel comfortable. Talking with each family member and finding something interesting about them (work or school activity, hobby, and so on) helps put them at ease, gains their cooperation, and gives the interviewer additional information—a process called joining. Extra time may have to be spent joining with an important family member who is quiet, resistant,

suspicious, or openly hostile to the clinician. When grandparents are present, an effort should be made to join with them early, since they are senior members of the family. It is always useful to first join with the top of the hierarchy (either the grandparents or the parents) rather than to challenge it.

The phases of a family conference and the goals of each phase are outlined in Table 23–1. The agenda for the meeting is best established by eliciting what different family members would like to accomplish during the conference. These ideas from the family can then be translated into clear, concise, and realistic goals (e.g., "Today we will focus on Donna's recent school problems and how we can all help her"). It is useful to solicit each person's view of the problem, encouraging them

TABLE 23–1. Phases of a Family Conference

PHASE 1: JOINING WITH THE FAMILY
Develop a collaborative relationship with the family by briefly
greeting and talking with each family member and helping him or
her feel more comfortable in the setting of the conference.

PHASE 2: SETTING GOALS
Establish the family's goals for the conference by soliciting ideas
from each person and helping him or her prioritize them.

PHASE 3: DISCUSSING THE PROBLEM
Exchange information about the problem with the family by
inquiring about each participant's viewpoint.

PHASE 4: IDENTIFYING RESOURCES
Recognize and highlight family strengths and internal and external
resources that can be used to help resolve the current problem.

PHASE 5: ESTABLISHING A PLAN
Develop a mutually agreeable treatment plan with the family that
includes specific tasks for each family member and appropriate
follow-up.

Adapted from McDaniel SH, Campbell TL, Seaburn D: Family-oriented
Primary Care: A Manual for Medical Providers. New York, Springer-Verlag,
1990.

to be as specific as possible and to provide examples.
The clinician should track (follow along and affirm the
importance of) each family member's contribution without taking sides. Part of tracking involves not allowing
people to speak over, answer for, or interrupt each
other, once the clinican has observed how the family
typically interacts or disagrees. For the balance of the
meeting, the clinician should avoid giving any advice or
interpretations. After obtaining a complete description
of the problem from all those present and inquiring
about recent changes and stresses on the family, the
clinician can help the family identify strengths and
resources that could be used to help solve the problem.
Many families resist this phase because of embarrassment and have to be encouraged (e.g., "What do you think
this family does really well?"). Eliciting family strengths
helps to support the family and build the self-esteem
and confidence that is necessary to deal with the presenting problem.

The final task of a family conference is to develop a
specific treatment plan that is agreeable to the adolescent and the family and to clarify each person's role in
carrying out the plan. These plans may range from
developing a simple behavioral contract to hospitalizing
the adolescent and referring the family for family therapy. During the initial family conference, the family
may agree to meet again with the adolescent's physician
to continue family counseling, or they may be referred
to a family therapist. Treatment by a professional with
advanced family therapy training is essential when the
presenting problem is life-threatening, such as suicidal-

ideation (see Chapter 101), or severe, such as psychosis,
anorexia nervosa, physical or sexual abuse, or substance
abuse (see Chapters 60, 111, 118, and 119). Chronic
psychosocial problems that have been unresponsive to
treatment or that involve serious marital conflict also
usually require treatment by a family therapist. In any
of these cases, it is most effective for the physician to
work collaboratively with a family therapist in treating
these severe problems.

This description of a family conference offers an initial
blueprint for ongoing family counseling. The amount
and type of family counseling done by the physician
caring for adolescents depend upon his or her level of
interest, training, and available time and energy. In any
case, the following principles are important: Family
counseling is most effective when it is goal-oriented and
time-limited. The clinician can contract with the family
for a specific number of sessions (usually four to six
sessions) over a specified period, with clear goals established in order to assess progress easily. If significant
progress is not made during this period, or more serious
problems emerge, the family should be referred for
family therapy. Family counseling should be problem-
focused with a clear and comprehensive treatment plan
and specific homework tasks for family members to do
between counseling visits. On occasion, a family that
has a serious problem such as substance abuse may
refuse referral. In such cases, a goal of family counseling
is to help the family recognize and accept the problem,
confront the substance abuser, and enter a family-
oriented treatment program. In this situation, as with
many referrals, the physician may be most helpful by
working closely with the family therapist, perhaps even
seeing the family together with the therapist initially, to
facilitate the referral and ensure a well-functioning collaborative relationship.

BIBLIOGRAPHY

Carter E, McGoldrick M (eds): The Changing Family Life Cycle.
New York, Gardner Press, 1988.
Doherty WJ, Baird M: Family-Centered Medical Care: A Clinical
Casebook. New York, Guilford Press, 1987.
Haley J: Leaving Home. New York, McGraw-Hill, 1980.
McDaniel SH, Campbell TL, Seaburn D: Family-oriented Primary
Care: A Manual for Medical Providers. New York, Springer-Verlag,
1990.
McGoldrick M, Gerson R: Genograms in Family Assessment. New
York, WW Norton, 1985.
Minuchin S, Rosman BL, Baker L: Psychosomatic Families. Cam-
bridge, Harvard University Press, 1978.
Offer D, Offer J: From Teenage to Young Manhood. New York,
Basic Books, 1975.
Smetana J: Adolescents' and parents' conceptions of parental author-
ity. Child Dev 50:321, 1988.

CHAPTER 24

Liaison and Consultation

JAMES Q. SIMMONS III and DAVID C. BECK

Physicians who treat adolescents know that the psychosocial problems of their patients profoundly influence and complicate their medical practices. Most clinicians have experienced the routine office visit that is rapidly transformed into a disruptive and frustrating marathon event when a serious and unsuspected problem—such as suicidal depression, drug abuse, or an eating disorder—is uncovered (see Chapters 60, 101, and 111). They also know that the probability of uncovering significant school, family, or emotional problems is quite high if a generally previously healthy teenager develops chronic complaints of headache, abdominal pain, or chest pain. Clarifying these issues is not easy when the doctor must also ensure that the teenager does not have a significant medical problem. Moreover, when an adolescent does have a serious medical problem, the physician is well aware of how psychosocial problems can rapidly complicate clinical management.

Practitioners may be sensitive to their patient's individual and family problems but may be unprepared to treat them and unable to identify other treatment. Most physicians are unable to obtain effective, practical help with adolescent psychosocial problems that complicate their practices. Requests for help from psychiatric colleagues may result in frustration or disappointment. Many studies have shown the general lack of satisfaction with psychiatric consultations resulting from the fact that the recommendations may be obscure or impractical. Patients also may fail to follow through with psychiatric recommendations or referrals. This is frustrating for both the adolescent and the health care professional.

This lack of practical, readily available psychiatric consultation has had an impact on the practice of medicine. With limited evidence for the effectiveness of many psychiatric interventions and with little formal mental health training, many primary care providers practice without benefit of contemporary psychiatric expertise. Systematic survey and interview strategies have led to significant improvement in the routine identification and diagnosis of psychiatric disorders and family dysfunction (see Chapters 98 and 99); population and genetic studies have enhanced our understanding of the genetic and biologic causes of many psychiatric disorders (see Chapter 12); more is known about the behavioral, emotional, and family contributions to somatization (see Chapter 112); a greater number of effective psychopharmacologic treatments are available (see Chapter 125); and innovative individual and family therapy techniques are increasing (see Chapter 123).

Current psychiatry is very relevant to the practice of adolescent medicine.

Close collaboration between primary care physicians and mental health specialists would seem intuitive. For complicated, important reasons, transfer of information between psychiatry and other areas of medicine has been slow. Physicians often do not practice and patients do not receive "the state of the art" treatment in this crucial domain of clinical practice.

The primary task of this chapter is to describe a working model to integrate contemporary mental health concepts into the practice of adolescent medicine. First, the problems that maintain the separation between child psychiatry and pediatrics are reviewed for illustrative purposes; the concepts can be generalized for psychiatry and general medicine. Second, clinical case studies illustrate how the current model of psychiatric consultation and referral fails to address the needs of both the adolescent and the practicing clinician. Finally, we propose a new model of collaborative care that emphasizes ways in which psychiatrists and other mental health workers can become integral to the practice of adolescent medicine.

RELATIONSHIP OF PEDIATRICS TO CHILD PSYCHIATRY

In its early years, child psychiatry was often synonymous with pediatric psychiatry and was a part of pediatrics. In the 1930s, a number of child psychiatrists, such as Leo Kanner at Johns Hopkins, worked in close relationship with pediatricians. The report of the 1932 White Conference on Child Health stated that children could not be given adequate medical care without attention to intellectual and emotional problems occurring in the course of physical disease and general growth and development. These conclusions remain valid today, especially in adolescent medicine.

From the 1940s to the 1960s, child psychiatric programs in academic centers and children's hospitals remained closely related to pediatrics, whereas those in mental hygiene clinics were closely allied to psychiatry. In the 1950s, the decision was made that child psychiatry was a subspecialty of psychiatry rather than of pediatrics and a subspecialty board was established in 1959.

Over several decades, psychoanalytic theory prepared

the psychiatrist to function more as a consultant to other physicians than as a colleague with a shared body of scientific knowledge. In this role, psychiatrists generally focused on consultation regarding primary psychiatric disorders in the pediatric population, conversion disorders (see Chapter 112), and on the so-called vegetative neuroses (a function of adaptation to recurring emotional states).

Over the last 20 years, psychiatry has developed into a sophisticated understanding of human behavior, particularly of physical symptoms and illness. Important advances in psychiatric knowledge include Engel's description of the biopsychosocial model, the role of stressful life events in physical disease, psychopharmacologic mechanisms in central nervous system function, operant and respondent learning in symptom formation, and neural imaging techniques aiding in diagnosis (see Chapter 10).

There have been parallel developments in pediatrics. The life expectancy of individuals with chronic conditions has been considerably lengthened (see Chapters 30, 53, and 121). Physical disease may place significant limitations on an adolescent's growth, strength, and expectations for vocation, marriage, and child-rearing. The physician is increasingly faced with ongoing problems in psychosocial development and long-term adherence to complicated medical treatment routines (see Chapter 26).

LIMITATIONS OF THE TRADITIONAL MODEL OF CONSULTATION LIAISON PSYCHIATRY

The following case studies illustrate challenges in the traditional model of providing care for adolescents who have psychological symptoms and who are identified in the primary care office.

The "Routine" Office Visit

During a routine office visit for a school sports physical examination, Dr. B notes that his 14-year-old patient, H, is withdrawn and depressed. Dr. B has followed her for a number of years but has seen her only for minor ailments. His inquiries about school are met with silence, but H nods her head affirmatively when Dr. B asks if there are problems at home. With some coaxing, she tearfully reveals a few details about ongoing family conflicts and admits that she took "a handful" of Tylenol 1 month ago when she was particularly despondent following a fight with her father. After some discussion, she agrees to a "no suicide" contract while Dr. B tries to help her with her problems. Dr. B gently tells her that she and her family need some help, and that he wants to refer them to a psychiatrist. The patient angrily responds, "I'm not crazy" and then refuses further discussion. He tells H that he must talk with her mother because of the seriousness of her having taken the Tylenol. He also tells her she can be with him when he speaks to her mother, or he will tell her mother alone. She chooses to have the doctor

talk to her mother alone. Dr. B speaks with the adolescent's mother and reviews his concerns. When he recommends psychiatric help, Dr. B receives a blank stare from the mother. Eventually she acknowledges Dr. B's concerns but states, "I'm not sure that my husband will agree to a psychiatrist." Frustrated, and with his schedule now in shambles, Dr. B schedules a follow-up appointment within the week.

Dr. B's next patient is a teenaged boy whose chief complaint is an earache. As the boy enters the examination room, the patient's father hurriedly mentions that he is also concerned about his son's "attitude." During the examination, the physician notes that, like his previous patient, the boy seems strikingly withdrawn and sullen. Privately thinking "not again," Dr. B asks about school and receives a very terse response. Asking a few more questions, he completes his examination, prescribes an antibiotic for otitis media, and moves on to the next patient.

Subsequently, the first patient cancels her follow-up appointment with no explanation. Three weeks later the physician learns that the second patient has taken a very serious overdose of drugs and alcohol and has been hospitalized. Upset by both situations, Dr. B questions what more could have been done for each of these adolescents in the primary care setting.

These cases are certainly familiar to the primary care practitioner. After uncovering a significant psychiatric problem, he or she invests considerable time and effort in the process and then is unable to effect a necessary referral. At other times the physician does not pursue an occult psychiatric problem, with resulting serious repercussions. Obviously, neither situation has been resolved satisfactorily. These examples highlight a significant problem in psychiatry and primary care medicine, which may be an unrealistic expectation about the role of the primary care practitioner. He or she is expected to screen patients for significant mental health problems and to refer those in need of assistance to an appropriate mental health practitioner. On the surface, this expectation seems quite logical and appropriate. In this model of practice, mental health problems are viewed as essentially no different from any other medical problem. When faced with a cardiac problem that exceeds the physician's ability to manage alone, the patient is referred to a cardiologist; a similar assumption is made for mental health problems. This process works adequately for some patients and physicians but not for many others. There are two main reasons.

First, it may be unreasonable to expect the average primary care practitioner to have the time or the expertise to identify all patients with significant mental health problems. According to recent epidemiologic data approximately 10% of the general population of children and adolescents has a recognizable psychiatric disorder in need of assessment and treatment. Also, many adolescents first seek help for mental health problems from primary practitioners rather than from mental health practitioners. The time required to perform a preliminary assessment of these problems, however, is usually far greater than the usual 15-minute office visit. Thus it becomes apparent that few primary care physicians could really screen a total patient population for significant mental health problems, particularly if it "opens up a can of worms." Unless the physician alters his or her practice, there will be a penalty for these efforts because of the excessive drain on time.

Second, the primary care physician who attempts to make a psychiatric referral frequently cannot address many of the often hidden resistances to this recommendation. After cost, the initial resistance is usually stated as the social stigma associated with mental health intervention. This was true of the adolescent who took the Tylenol. Other, equally powerful, resistances may also occur. One example is a teenager who makes a surprisingly intense emotional connection to a physician who has recognized that she is in psychological pain, who is able to draw her out, and who then tells her she has to go elsewhere to discuss these concerns. Carefully worded explanations about the need for a referral often do little to dampen the feelings of rejection that may ensue. Another example is the strong emotional reaction in a teenager's parents to the physician's referral to a mental health site, which also decreases the likelihood of a successful referral. Many parents view referral to a mental health practitioner as a judgment by the primary care physician that they have failed as parents. Shame and embarrassment may amplify their natural anxiety about having the adolescent see a psychiatrist and result in the comment "We can handle our own problems." Also, these recommendations are often conveyed directly only to the parent who usually accompanies the teenager to his or her appointment. Thus this parent acts as the "bearer of bad news" when telling the spouse that "the doctor thinks we should see a psychiatrist." It is very easy to add a tone of judgment or accusation to the communication, which can sabotage the recommendation.

If primary care practitioners are to make progress in addressing behavioral problems that arise during "routine" office visits, the problems of screening and referral must be solved. One solution, discussed later, lies in a collaborative model of care in which the screening and referral is shared by a mental health colleague who works actively with the primary care physician.

The Adolescent with Functional Somatic Complaints

A 13-year-old adolescent girl is seen for reevaluation of abdominal pain of 3 months' duration. The physician originally saw her 2½ months previously when she presented with fever, severe abdominal pain, and vomiting of 1 week's duration. Two of her siblings had similar symptoms but recovered in approximately 3 days. Finding nothing of significance on the physical examination, the physician diagnosed a probable viral gastroenteritis and reassured the mother and daughter that she was otherwise healthy and that the symptoms should disappear soon. A week later she returned with continuing symptoms of abdominal pain and nausea. She had returned to school for 1 day but had left after 2 hours and had remained at home since that time. Again, finding nothing of note on physical examination, the physician inquired about the girl's school history. He learned that she had always loved school, was an excellent student, and had many friends. There had been no prior history of recurrent abdominal pain. He ordered a complete blood count; erythrocyte sedimentation rate, serum glutamic-pyruvic transaminase, and amylase determinations; and urinalysis and urine culture and scheduled

---

a return appointment in 1 week. All studies showed normal results, but her symptoms continued. Impressed by the severity and chronicity of the symptoms, the physician ordered an upper and lower gastrointestinal series; results of both were normal. He then referred the girl to a gastroenterologist who performed a gastroscopy, which was normal. Throughout these studies she did not return to school, and her mother arranged for her to start home tutoring.

At this point, 3 months later, the physician believed that he had scrupulously eliminated any biologic problem and was now convinced that the adolescent had a functional problem. He met with the adolescent and her mother and explained that he could find nothing physically wrong with her and that he would like the consultation of a psychiatrist. The mother reacted strongly to this suggestion and stated "She's not faking!" The mother stated that she would "think about" the referral. Two weeks later, the physician receives a request for the records from another general physician who had been consulted for the same problem.

This case demonstrates another common clinical problem in the working relationship between primary care physicians and psychiatrists—the prevailing assumptions about how a functional somatic complaint should be "worked-up." Primary care physicians are constantly called upon to distinguish functional from biologic symptoms. It has been estimated that as many as 25% of children have somatoform symptoms at some time (see Chapter 112). Adolescents are particularly likely to experience somatic complaints. The majority of these minor stress responses are readily handled by physicians with a thorough examination and reassurance. A number of patients, however, demand considerable time and attention.

The general approach taken by both primary care physicians and psychiatrists is that the physician should carefully investigate and rule out any possible biologic cause for the symptoms before turning attention to any "emotional possibilities." After the "plate is swept clean" of any biologic possibilities, the physician can then confidently address the emotional issues and dynamics. At this juncture, and usually not before, the expertise of a psychiatrist may be requested. For example, primary care physicians may handle the diagnosis and care of school withdrawal or school phobia in a young child. The older the child, however, the more complex psychologically the condition usually is. Unless it is quite obvious why the adolescent did not return to school, referral to a psychiatrist is important because the cause and treatment of this condition may be complex.

Superficially, this appears to be logical and appropriate. Obviously, primary care physicians must be certain that no potentially treatable biologic condition is missed for which a specific treatment is warranted. Unfortunately, the approach described for the work-up of likely somatoform symptoms has two serious drawbacks.

First, in most cases of persistent somatic complaints involving an otherwise healthy adolescent with normal results on physical examination, a functional diagnosis is often high on the differential diagnosis list. Using the approach of "first rule out every biologic possibility," the most likely diagnosis is worked up last. In this light, the approach is really quite illogical. By postponing an investigation of the functional aspects of suspected somatoform symptoms, the adolescent patient is often subjected to many unnecessary, costly, and invasive tests and procedures. With the availability of innumerable diagnostic tests, a well-intentioned attempt to be thorough can easily escalate into a major clinical investigation unless the probability of uncovering a genuinely meaningful finding is kept clearly in mind. The primary care physician can unwittingly become an agent in the perpetuation of the patient's symptoms because of the attention that the symptoms receive via the physical work-up.

Second, another major reason for the "better to be safe than sorry" approach is that many primary care physicians assume that a careful psychiatric diagnostic assessment will not yield reliable positive or negative findings. It is as though the behavioral, emotional, and family forces that can produce or maintain somatoform symptoms are simply too intangible to be systematically assessed and produce "real" findings. Stated differently, one can generally trust a negative upper gastrointestinal series, but can one really trust a psychiatric assessment that uncovers "clinically significant separation anxiety"? The answer is "no," if the psychiatrist who uses this jargon does not actively work with a medical colleague to make the understanding of the diagnosis clear. Unfortunately, many psychiatrists tacitly accept the assumption that their assessment skills are too subjective to be relied upon and insist that a complete physical work-up be done before they see an adolescent with a suspected somatoform symptom. Obviously, a careful screening for physical illnesses is central to the assessment of suspected somatoform symptoms, but it is unreasonable for the psychiatrist to delay making a contribution until every possible biologic illness has been investigated and ruled out.

The combined (biopsychosocial approach) effect of this diagnostic approach to a somatoform symptom is profound. The most important history and clinical findings often are not assessed during the diagnostic evaluation. One searches for unknown physical disease processes with a relatively low probability of occurrence, but systematic assessment of the predisposing, precipitating, and perpetuating psychosocial factors known to be associated with somatization phenomena is often ignored. Symptoms are routinely declared to be "functional" on the basis of negative physical findings and laboratory studies. The usefulness of such conclusions is generally low, since most adolescents and families with somatoform symptoms often cannot understand how family or emotional problems can become manifested as physical symptoms. Because these matters have not been systematically explored during the patient's physical evaluation, the primary care physician does not have the information necessary to give the patient and family an adequate explanation. When the symptoms are labeled "functional," the physician generally does not know what "functions" are served by the symptom for the patient or the family, and thus cannot discuss these matters in a meaningful way. Not surprisingly, many adolescents and families view the physician's conclusions as more accusatory than helpful. Feeling anxious or misunderstood, they may come to very different conclu-sions about the negative diagnostic evaluation. Rather than being reassured, they become more fearful that the physician may have "missed something" or "given up," and they seek another opinion.

To improve the diagnostic approach to somatoform symptoms, a fundamental change must occur in the working relationship between psychiatrists and primary care physicians. Most importantly, the "linear" approach in which physical symptoms are exhaustively investigated before psychosocial variables receive any systematic attention must change. Specifically, psychiatrists must actively bring their expertise into the evaluation phase in a practical and efficient manner.

Noncompliance

For the third time in 6 months, a 14-year-old boy is admitted to the hospital for diabetic ketoacidosis. Diagnosed at 6 years of age, the boy's diabetes mellitus had been in relatively good control until the past year, when his glycosylated hemoglobin level increased markedly. His physician had multiple conferences with the adolescent and his parents about the need for better adherence to the recommended diet and insulin administration. His parents have repeatedly threatened and cajoled him; his mother is frantic about the danger to his health. Still, the noncompliance has continued. At a loss, the primary care physician once again explains to the adolescent the various complications that could occur if he does not change his behavior. The adolescent responds with stony silence. Frustrated, the primary care physician requests a psychiatric consultation. The next day he learns that the psychiatrist met only with the boy, as opposed to also meeting with the health care team and especially with the parents. The patient was generally uncooperative and upset that a psychiatrist had been called. The psychiatrist speculates that the boy has an "adjustment disorder" and is having trouble reconciling the demands of his illness with his adolescent need to be independent. He recommends individual therapy and a family assessment. Having learned nothing he did not already know, the primary care physician is frustrated, and the recurrent ketoacidosis is likely to continue (see Chapters 26 and 59).

This case is another example of the failure of both the psychiatrist and the primary care physician to integrate mental health care into another critical area—that of the chronically ill adolescent. Despite the fact that noncompliance is recognized to be an extremely serious, ubiquitous problem in health care, the exact cause is rarely addressed in a systematic manner (see Chapters 26 and 30).

It is unfortunate when the first contact between a patient or family and a psychiatrist occurs in the context of a crisis. By this time, maladaptive patterns may be deeply ingrained and difficult to change easily. This is analogous to allowing all the signs and symptoms of end-stage renal disease to develop before measuring the level of serum creatinine. Just as early medical intervention may alter the course of renal disease, so may early psychiatric care. Certainly, delay makes the physician's job more difficult, and it is even harder for the mental health professional because he or she is an "outsider." Although the psychiatrist's recommendations for a family assessment and individual therapy in the last case study presented seem absurd, they are needed (see Chapters 23 and 98). The physician's frustration is the result not of a consultation that is conceptually "unsound" but of a consultation made "unhelpful" by the physician's failure to involve the psychiatrist earlier in the problem and the psychiatrist's making recommendations without having included direct consultation with the health care team and the family before drawing conclusions. The psychiatrist, after having made his recommendations, leaves the staff to carry out the program. Thus, the psychiatrist is not a member of the team, and the patient is not considered as a "shared" patient. The physician needed practical ongoing help.

A NEW MODEL OF COLLABORATIVE CARE

Common themes run through each of the case studies presented. In each, mental health problems complicate or confound the practice of adolescent medicine. The traditional means for the primary care physician to obtain help—psychiatric referral or consultation—are inadequate or ineffective; only a small percentage of adolescent patients actively follow through with a referral once it is made. In many situations, a consultation is not helpful because the primary care physician who requests the consultation actually needs collaboration from mental health professionals, not consultation.

The idea of collaboration is not new. Collaborative team work is standard in adolescent medicine (see Chapter 27). It is accepted that primary care physicians need the coordinated help of a wide variety of health care professionals to care for certain adolescents. We will briefly examine some of the organizational and group dynamics that provide the foundation for effective collaboration. This will make it possible to identify the key changes that must take place to optimize collaboration between physicians and mental health practitioners.

Collaboration means "to work jointly or in partnership with another, especially in an intellectual endeavor." A partner is "one who shares with another in some activity, especially in a business firm in which he shares risks and profits." To work together effectively, all the involved professionals must believe that they are working on a common task, which is to maximize the patient's health status. As elementary as this sounds, it is a crucial concept in understanding the impediments to collaboration between primary care physicians and mental health professionals. This sense of sharing a common task is at the heart of the team concept and is generally taken for granted in medical care. It is also the key group dynamic that enables input from different health professionals to be readily integrated into patient care.

By sharing a common task, each participating professional psychologically "shares" the adolescent patient. Each feels that the patient is "his or hers," and that the job of each professional is to share expertise. The process also creates a sense of psychological identification with the physician who is in charge of directing the adolescent's care and who is dependent on the help of other professionals. This psychological concept of a "collaborative work group" makes it possible for advances in different disciplines to be integrated into the team's thinking and incorporated into patient care. For example, it usually is quite easy for a respiratory therapist, aware of an advance in equipment, to suggest a device. Because this expert and the primary care physician share the same goal, the primary physician accepts this advice. Despite being independent practitioners, the consultants share the same goal with regard to the adolescent patient and are strongly identified with the referring physician's problems in providing optimal care. Disagreements or differences of opinion about the adolescent patient's management do not undermine the overall integrity of the system because the sense of common purpose among participants remains constant.

The same underlying group dynamics do not appear to extend to mental health practitioners. They are rarely seen as core members of a medical team. The prevailing assumptions of the medical team reveal part of the reason. Simply put, psychiatrists may be expected to work with psychiatric problems, not medical problems. Their "mission" is thus seen as very different from that of other physicians. Consequently, the group dynamics that psychologically bond different members of the medical team and allow for automatic collaborative work-ups may not apply. In particular, many physicians do not expect that their adolescent patients will receive the same level of attention from mental health professionals as they receive from other health care professionals. They do not expect mental health professionals to identify with their problems and to join with them in the effort to provide optimal adolescent patient care.

Unfortunately, these assumptions are often quite accurate. Mental health professionals usually see their primary task as maximizing the behavioral, emotional, or family functioning of their patients. This is very different from seeing their primary task as applying their mental health expertise to maximize the adolescent's medical care or to assist a physician with mental health problems that complicate a physician's practice. Without psychological identification with the primary physician, the natural collaboration between disciplines does not occur. If an adolescent does not follow through with a referral, or if a medical team does not implement the recommendations of a consultation, the psychiatrist often does little more, because he or she feels estranged from the broader system. The disciplines remain isolated from one another, and primary care physicians do not learn about contemporary mental health practices. More importantly, adolescent patients are denied the benefits of modern mental health knowledge and interventions.

To collaborate, the mental health profession in general, and psychiatrists in particular, must join the health care team psychologically. Physicians and mental health specialists must agree that they share a common task—to deliver the highest quality health care. Both medical and mental health knowledge and expertise are necessary to accomplish this. Simply put, collaboration means that primary care physicians need a mental health "partner" with whom they work on the problems that are present in "their" practices. This emphasis on "partnership" does not refer to a legal or financial arrangement.

The idea of having a psychiatrist affiliated with a medical team is hardly new. In fact, the "liaison" aspect of consultation liaison psychiatry refers to the nonpatient-centered activities of a psychiatrist working on a medical team. Our emphasis, however, is on a model of "collaboration" as opposed to "liaison." Collaborative care means that a primary care physician and a mental health specialist actively and regularly anticipate and plan for myriad mental health problems that affect the physician's practice. It is a significant departure from a model in which the primary care physician asks for help only when it is needed. It is a recognition that the mental health problems in certain medical practices may be so ubiquitous and problemmatic that physicians cannot realistically be expected to manage all of them alone.

Practical Application of a Model of Collaborative Care

Two steps are necessary for a psychiatrist to collaborate effectively with another physician:

1. The psychiatrist must meet regularly with the other physician and his or her medical team and review with them any cases of concern and plans for their management.

2. The psychiatrist must attend the other physician's clinic on a regular basis and see adolescent patients there at specific scheduled times.

Both steps are logical extensions of the issues discussed earlier.

THE TREATMENT PLANNING MEETING

To address the issues raised in the discussion of the case studies presented earlier, one needs a treatment planning meeting. If it is accepted that many of the mental health problems encountered in medical practice are ubiquitous, complex, and at times serious and that many physicians cannot handle them alone, it follows that a standard mechanism is needed to address these problems collaboratively and thoughtfully plan for their assessment and management. An ongoing, regularly scheduled treatment planning meeting is essential.

The meeting should be held at a set time in the physician's office; all staff who are familiar with the adolescent and his or her family should be present. In general, 1 hour/week should be scheduled to allow for adequate discussion and planning. One possible format could be that the physician first presents information about the adolescent about whom there is concern. The other medical staff members contribute additional information. The main goal of this portion of the meeting is for the medical team to apprise the psychiatrist of the full dimensions of the adolescent's problems. Often the collective information known about an adolescent patient is surprisingly large, but it needs to be "harvested," or organized, and interpreted from a psychiatric perspective. The psychiatrist then outlines a plan of action

for the assessment and the kinds of support that he or she needs from the team. Assuming that the psychiatrist has established standard hours for attending the primary care setting, he or she defines the amount of time each adolescent patient requires and who should attend the initial meeting.

Next, a family contact is arranged. The team decides who should contact the family. This is a very important part of the collaborative process because it directly involves the medical team in arranging the adolescent patient's first contact with the psychiatrist. As already discussed, many adolescents do not follow through with this step in the traditional referral process. The primary care physician may need to contact the adolescent's parents directly and to use his or her authority with them to establish a firm commitment regarding the initial visit with the psychiatrist. Certain points need to be made when discussing these recommendations. Among them are the reason for referral; its value to the adolescent, the family, and the physician; the time of the appointment; and the need to follow through with the appointment or to notify the office of a cancellation. The adolescent should also be contacted and a discussion similar to that with the parents should ensue.

COLLABORATION IN THE OFFICE OR HEALTH CARE SITE

Recalling the case studies, the rationale for the psychiatrist working out of the physician's office is clear. Not only are there many psychological impediments to following through with a psychiatric referral, in many cases it really is not logical to seek psychiatric input outside the context of the medical practice.

The psychiatrist who truly collaborates with other physicians demonstrates commitment to their common task by working on the physician's "turf." This is a major departure from the traditional model of psychiatric practice, however, and the physician must demonstrate his or her support of this effort in equally tangible ways. Specifically, the primary care physician must make it possible for the psychiatrist to work effectively during scheduled appointments. The psychiatrist requires a reasonable space when he or she attends the office setting. This may range from an examination room to a conference room that permits uninterrupted privacy and is large enough to accommodate a family. The staff must recognize that the psychiatrist's time in the office is quite limited, and they must not schedule conflicting procedures or tests during these appointments. In short, the physician and staff must provide an environment that makes it possible for the psychiatrist to give adolescent patients the help they seek.

BIBLIOGRAPHY

Blum RW: Compliance with therapeutic regimens among children and youths. In Blum RW (ed): Chronic Illness and Disabilities in Childhood and Adolescence. New York, Grune & Stratton, 1984, pp 143–158.

Engel G: The need for a new medical model: A challenge for biomedicine. Science 196:129, 1977.

Fritz GK: Consultation liaison in child psychiatry and the evolution of pediatric psychiatry. Psychosomatics 31:85, 1990.

Fritz GK, Bergman AS: Child psychiatrists seen through the pediatricians eyes: Results of a national survey. J Child Psychiatry 24:81, 1985.

Jellinek MS: The present status of child psychiatry in pediatrics. N Engl J Med 306:1227, 1982.

Lipowski ZJ: Psychosomatic medicine and liaison psychiatry. New York, Plenum Medical, 1985.

Proceedings of the National Conference on Behavioral Pediatrics: J Dev Behav Pediatr 6:179, 1985.

Russo DC, Varni JW: Behavioral Pediatrics: Research and Practice. New York, Plenum Press, 1982.

Shapiro EG, Rosenfeld AA: The Somatizing Child, Diagnosis and Treatment of Conversion and Somatization Disorders. New York, Springer-Verlag, 1987.

The Future of Pediatric Education: A report by the Task Force on Pediatric Education. Elk Grove, IL, American Academy of Pediatrics, 1978.

CHAPTER 25

Well Adolescent Care

ANDREA MARKS

THE WELL ADOLESCENT VISIT

The term *well adolescent* refers to a young person who is healthy and coping reasonably well with the tasks of adolescence (see Chapter 9). The stage of adolescence has been perceived as the healthiest time of life, when the individual is unlikely to become seriously ill. It is well appreciated, however, that adolescence is also a time of physical and psychological vulnerability to significant health concerns. The well adolescent's medical visit should not be considered a trivial event but should be approached rather as a significant component of preventive health care. Indeed, visits are regularly requested by school personnel, camp administrators, sports team officials, employers, parents, and even teenagers themselves. The visit provides an opportunity to screen for a wide range of subtle diseases or dysfunctions and to establish a uniquely important relationship between the adolescent and the health care provider. Conversely, a cursory health encounter is unlikely to be productive. The ultimate goal is for the adolescent to emerge as a competent and independent health consumer.

Why Is It Important?

Although most adolescents are healthy, recent advances in medical research and changes within society have improved our understanding of adolescence as biologically and psychosocially challenging. Teenagers acquire a wide range of acute and chronic illnesses; they may have genetic disorders; and they may have physical sequelae from risk-taking behaviors (see Chapters 2, 30, 31, and 33). Numerous behavioral difficulties may be identified during adolescence. The presentations of some problems are dramatic, whereas others are subtle.

What Are the Goals?

The goals of a well adolescent visit are both immediate and long term. The first or immediate goal is to screen for disease either that is asymptomatic, and therefore unrecognized, or that may be "known" to the adolescent or the parents but is not presented directly to the health provider. Even when substantial time is allotted for such a health encounter, it is justifiable to screen only for those conditions that are potentially serious, relatively prevalent in the population, and treatable if detected early, when there are reliable and valid methods of screening.

A second or long-term goal of the visit is to establish a relationship with the adolescent that will result in the most effective health care for the future (see Chapters 17 and 22). Adolescence is an impressionable time. If the provider is friendly, direct, and interested in what the adolescent has to say; is respectful of the limits the adolescent sets; and by the questions asked indicates an understanding of the adolescent's world, chances are enhanced that the adolescent will initiate contacts in the future (see Chapters 17 and 22). A third and long-term goal of the visit, especially when caring for a younger adolescent, is to assist the adolescent in becoming an independent health consumer.

HOW SHOULD THE VISIT BE PERFORMED?

In practice, the three goals of detecting disease or dysfunction, establishing a relationship, and fostering independence are pursued simultaneously, and all three can be accomplished or, at least, initiated within a reasonable amount of time. If health problems or other patient concerns are encountered that require additional time to delineate, a return visit should be scheduled to devote to that purpose.

If the adolescent is new to the provider and younger than 18 years of age, it is advisable to interview briefly the parents and the adolescent together to review their collective concerns and the patient's past medical history, the family history, and social history (see Chapters 17 and 22).

Guidelines for confidentiality are established while the adolescent and parents are together (see Chapters 20 and 22). Both parents and adolescents should understand that there are limits to patient confidentiality (see Chapter 20). If the adolescent tells the provider something extremely serious, parents should generally be informed about the matter and should become involved in the decisions about the diagnosis and treatment of the adolescent's condition. Such issues might include, for example, suicidal thoughts or drug abuse. If this were to occur, the adolescent should have the choice of being with the health care provider when he or she meets with the parents, or the adolescent could talk with the parents alone. The adolescent should be assured that if such a situation were to arise, the provider would serve as the adolescent's advocate and not divulge information to the parents without the adolescent's knowledge. Such a candid exchange generally puts the adolescent at ease and tends to encourage openness and trust. Likewise, if the parents disclose a "family secret," such as an impending divorce that may be affecting their adolescent's health, the parents should be counseled that the adolescent needs to know, and the parents should be given options that are similar to those given the adolescent regarding whether the parents want to be with the provider when there is disclosure or have the provider present the information alone.

An initial visit may be accomplished effectively in approximately 45 to 60 minutes. In some settings—for example, a private practice office—the fee for such a visit should be higher than for visits that require substantially less time (see Chapter 17).

Some providers may consider using "waiting room" questionnaires to elicit the patient's current concerns or details of the past medical or family history. This time-saving technique is preferred by some adolescents who are reluctant to discuss certain matters directly; other adolescent patients and providers prefer a personal face-to-face approach. After the history is elicited, a complete physical examination is performed.

WHICH ISSUES SHOULD BE ADDRESSED?

The content of the well adolescent visit depends on several factors. If it is a first visit, the health care provider spends considerable time reviewing the patient's past medical history, the family history, and the social history. If the patient is known to the provider, more time can be devoted to interval and current issues.

It is important to consider the patient's age and maturity (see Chapters 5 and 9). These factors influence not only the nature of the communication but also the items to be stressed in the history and physical examination. (For discussion of interviewing and substages, see Chapter 22.)

Even if the concerns brought to the encounter by the adolescent do not appear serious to the health care provider or worthy of much time, it is crucial to address the adolescent's agenda thoroughly before proceeding on to the details of health screening. The health care provider must at all times be respectful of the adolescent's most immediate needs and address them sensitively.

HOW OFTEN SHOULD AN ADOLESCENT HAVE A VISIT?

Most health care providers introduce the idea of children spending some time alone with their health care provider at approximately 9 to 11 years of age for girls and 10 to 12 years of age for boys (see Chapter 22). Some parents may be reluctant at first to relinquish

control, whereas others may encourage a reluctant child to speak for himself or herself prematurely. The health care provider, of course, must be sensitive to these issues and must be willing to be flexible, especially with younger adolescents.

There are dramatic physical, psychological, and social changes during all stages of adolescence (see Chapters 5 and 8–11). It is therefore advisable to recommend that an adolescent have a visit no less frequently than once a year. For some patients, the health care provider may feel that more frequent visits should be scheduled, for example, at 3- or 6-month intervals, to ensure ongoing communication for evaluation of concerns the provider may have. The guidelines of the American Academy of Pediatrics for comprehensive health supervision of adolescents recommend screening every 2 years. Such infrequent visits may miss the onset or the progression of a serious pathologic condition during this time of rapid growth and would be unlikely to foster the development of a sound relationship between the adolescent and the provider.

WHO SHOULD PERFORM THESE VISITS AND WHERE SHOULD THEY BE PERFORMED?

Most adolescents go for a visit to the office of their pediatrician, family doctor, or internist (see Chapter 17). In some communities, specialists in adolescent medicine care for adolescents in private office settings, but this option is unusual. Most specialists in adolescent medicine are based in hospitals, and they see adolescent patients in clinics or in a private practice. In recent years, many adolescents have begun to receive comprehensive health care at school-based clinics located in junior and senior high schools. The care is generally provided by nurse practitioners who have expertise in adolescent medicine, and the physician serves as a consultant (see Chapter 18).

GETTING THE "BIG PICTURE"

Within a relatively brief period, the health care provider must attempt to assess the physical and emotional health of the young person. If, in fact, a year has gone by since the previous visit or the provider has never met the adolescent, the visit will focus primarily on getting the "big picture," that is, establishing that this adolescent is indeed *well* in all respects or that he or she requires additional care or intervention. Achieving this goal requires the provider to move swiftly but carefully through various components of the medical history and physical examination and to consider laboratory tests.

History

There are various components to the health history. A discussion of them follows (Table 25–1).

TABLE 25–1. Health Screening During Adolescence

PAST MEDICAL HISTORY
Perinatal period, early development
Illness, hospitalization, surgery, injury, allergies, medications
Immunizations
  Diphtheria-tetanus
  Polio
  Measles, mumps, rubella
  Tuberculosis status (BCG)

FAMILY HISTORY
Parents and siblings: health, ages, education, work, activities
Pertinent family illnesses (heart-cholesterol, blood, tuberculosis, hepatitis, asthma-allergies, neurologic illness, mental illness, addictions)

PSYCHOSOCIAL (DEVELOPMENTAL) HISTORY
Family relationships (independence)
Peer relationships (sexual identity)
School performance; career plans (societal role)
Special interests and skills

HEALTH RISK BEHAVIORS (MEDICAL-SOCIAL) HISTORY
Sexual experiences
  Dating history
  Age at first intercourse, frequency, partners
  Contraception, pregnancy, sexually transmitted disease
Cigarette smoking
Drug and alcohol use-abuse
Serious accidents/injuries
Violence/homicide
Mood swings
Suicide
Physical or sexual abuse, or both
Eating disorders

REVIEW OF SYSTEMS
Weight and dietary habits
Physical activity
Sleep patterns
Menstrual history
Dental and eye care

PHYSICAL EXAMINATION
Height and weight with percentiles
Blood pressure
Pubertal development
Breast examination (teach)
Pelvic examination (if indicated)
Testicular examination (teach)
Skin
Head and neck
Heart, lungs, abdomen, spine

LABORATORY SCREENING
Hemoglobin-hematocrit determination
Sickle cell screening
Tuberculin skin test (?BCG status)
Screening for pregnancy and sexually transmitted disease in sexually active adolescents
? Cholesterol screening

OTHER
Immunizations
  Measles, mumps, rubella
  Diphtheria, tetanus

PAST MEDICAL HISTORY

The pertinent aspects of an adolescent's past medical history include items similar to the ones generally reviewed with a child or an adult patient. The perinatal period may be reviewed quickly, with attention focused on the patient's birth weight and any significant problems during the pregnancy, labor, delivery, or newborn period. Patients born after 1971 are not at risk for having been exposed to diethylstilbestrol (DES) *in utero*. The "pediatric" developmental milestone history may be condensed into a single inquiry of whether the patient "walked and talked at a normal age." The most important aspects of *adolescent* development (relationships with parents and peers and performance at school) are generally part of the psychosocial history (discussed further on).

The most important aspects of an adolescent's past medical history include the existence of serious acute illnesses; chronic disorders; hospitalizations for illness, surgery, or injury; current allergies; current and past medications; and exact dates of immunizations.

FAMILY HISTORY

The family medical history should review the health status of the adolescent's parents and siblings and any significant illnesses in other relatives, including aunts, uncles, grandparents, and first cousins. It is also of interest to inquire about the parents' and siblings' ages, education, work, and current activities. A thorough family history alerts the provider to any potential genetic or familial disorders (e.g., hypercholesterolemia, sickle cell anemia, or polycystic kidneys) or contagious infections (e.g., tuberculosis, hepatitis A or B) that would warrant special scrutiny, screening, or treatment. The family medical history also provides insight into the "health environment" in which the adolescent is growing up and of any family health crisis the adolescent has experienced.

PSYCHOSOCIAL (DEVELOPMENTAL) HISTORY

The goal of the psychosocial history is to assess whether the adolescent is progressing appropriately for age on each of the tasks of adolescence (independence, sexual identity, and societal role) (see Chapters 9 and 22). Many adolescents have greater ease with one or two of these tasks and difficulty with another; this pattern may be perfectly normal.

Each of the developmental tasks of adolescence is focused in a specific sphere of the adolescent's world. Independence is negotiated at home with family, especially with parents; sexual identity is a peer group–centered matter; and societal role evolves primarily at school. Assessing the psychosocial development of an adolescent may be accomplished by briefly discussing each of these tasks with the adolescent and, when appropriate, with the parents as well.

Asking the adolescent simple and direct questions such as, Tell me about your parents, or What are your friends' names and ages? or How are you doing in school? may elicit meaningful responses from most adolescents. A reserved adolescent or a young adolescent may need more focused questions to achieve the same degree of assessment. Questions such as, Are your parents well? How old are they? What kind of work do they do? What school do you attend? What courses are you taking? What activities do you like? What are your grades? may structure the interview and facilitate listening and talking (see Chapter 22).

The psychosocial history is important for at least two reasons. First, adolescence may be the time when serious psychiatric disorders, such as affective disorder, schizophrenia, borderline personality, and character disorders, are first recognized (see Chapters 98–113). Second, and more frequent, adolescents may experience adjustment disorders related to the developmental tasks of adolescence. Depression related to problems at home, with peers, or at school may be mild, moderate, or severe (see Chapter 101). Adolescents may contemplate, attempt, or even complete a suicide (see Chapter 100) or become involved in an activity that is life-threatening, such as abusing drugs (see Chapter 111) or driving while intoxicated. If the health care provider is concerned about the adolescent's suicidal potential, it is best to ask directly whether the young person has thought of hurting himself or herself. If the response is affirmative, exploration of the degree of suicidal risk is critical. Screening for these possibilities, therefore, must be considered a crucial part of well adolescent care.

HEALTH RISK BEHAVIORS (MEDICAL-SOCIAL) HISTORY

Although it may be difficult for the provider to ask adolescents about "personal" matters, this part of the medical history is perhaps the *most* important when caring for an adolescent. If health screening is intended to discover common and relatively serious problems for which intervention is helpful, screening for health risk behaviors is likely to have the highest yield of any part of the well adolescent's examination. Health risk behaviors that are common during adolescence include sexual experience, cigarette smoking, use and abuse of alcohol and drugs, serious accidents, violence, mood swings, physical abuse or sexual abuse, or both, and eating disorders (see Chapters 17 and 22).

Inquiring about risk-taking behaviors or forms of victimization should be direct, nonjudgmental, and relaxed. Questions regarding dating and sexual activity (heterosexual and homosexual behavior) and use of cigarettes, drugs, and alcohol are most logically asked during the discussion of peer group activities. Inquiry about suicide, physical or sexual abuse, or nutrition (eating disorders) must also be made directly and supportively. It may be helpful to tell the adolescent that you are planning to ask about several matters that are relatively common problems for young people today, that you ask about these matters "routinely," and that you hope the adolescent will feel free to discuss with you any concerns he or she may have.

REVIEW OF SYSTEMS

In addition to the standard review of systems that inquires about all systems in sequence, the review of systems for the adolescent should take into account several other aspects of their health, including the following: (1) *weight and dietary habits*—whether the patient's weight has been stable, increasing, or decreasing and whether the adolescent eats at least three meals a day consisting of foods from all four nutrient groups (intake of iron and calcium are of particular concern, since intake is often less than the required daily allowance among adolescents (see Chapter 7); (2) *physical activity*—whether the adolescent participates regularly, sporadically, or not at all in exercise (see Chapters 49 and 81); (3) *sleep patterns*—the adolescent's usual bedtime and morning awakening times and whether the adolescent has significant difficulty in falling asleep or staying asleep throughout the night or experiences early morning insomnia (suggestive of depression) (see Chapter 86); (4) *menstrual history*—whether a female adolescent has begun to menstruate and, if so, how often and for how many days each cycle, whether she has painful menstrual periods, and the date of the last period (see Chapter 70); and (5) *dental and eye care*—whether the adolescent has regular dental evaluations (see Chapter 41) and whether he or she has ever had a formal eye examination by an ophthalmologist or optometrist (see Chapter 40).

Physical Examination

The general physical examination is similar to that of older children and adults. The reader is referred to the standard textbooks of physical diagnosis. This section highlights those portions of the physical examination that are important to the adolescent examination.

HEIGHT AND WEIGHT

Just as sequential measurements of height and weight are important components of the physical assessment of very young children (especially during the first 2 years of life when they are growing most rapidly), likewise, these parameters in the adolescent reflect the physical well-being of a rapidly growing person. Increases in height and especially weight are important hallmarks of successful puberty and relate in a specific pattern to the development of secondary sexual characteristics (see Chapter 5). If changes in height and weight proceed as expected, these measurements alone lend confidence that the adolescent is physically healthy. Many chronic illnesses that have their onset at the time of puberty, or that began prior to puberty, affect growth and development at this time (see Chapter 30).

Body composition in males and females is similar until early adolescence when girls "naturally" become fatter and boys become more muscular (see Chapters 5 and 6). A chubby 12-year-old girl will tend naturally to become fatter, whereas a chubby 12-year-old boy is likely to become leaner, even without dieting. The girl of normal weight, of course, must also be prepared to gain a considerable amount of weight, fat, and new contours. These inevitable changes are important to discuss with the adolescent as the examination proceeds, especially if he or she reacts with unhappiness at what the scale or stadiometer shows (see Chapters 5 and 6).

BLOOD PRESSURE

The blood pressure should be measured with the patient in the sitting position, with a cuff of appropriate width (covering two thirds of the upper arm). At least three readings should be taken, with the last two being averaged for the final blood pressure reading (see Chapters 48 and 67).

PUBERTAL DEVELOPMENT

Even before a child experiences an accelerated rate of growth in height and weight, the earliest signs of puberty emerge. A discussion of the actual pubertal changes is contained in Chapter 5. The assessment of individual adolescents should take into account the *interrelationship* of the pubertal events. In order to engage adolescents and interest them in their growth, some health care providers have them stage their pubertal development using the Tanner growth charts. This self-staging by adolescents is remarkably accurate. In addition, sharing the actual growth data on the growth percentiles with individual adolescents can also teach them about their growth and provide an opportunity to discuss it.

Teaching self-examination of the breasts is an important component of well adolescent care (see Chapter 77). The female adolescent should be instructed to examine her breasts after each menstrual period (see Chapter 77). A pelvic examination need not be performed on all adolescents. If an adolescent has regular periods, is not complaining of significant vaginal discharge, does not have lower abdominal pain, and has never been sexually active, the pelvic examination is best done in late adolescence or early adulthood when the patient is well prepared (see Chapter 69). If, however, the adolescent is symptomatic, a pelvic examination should be performed. If, for another reason, a pelvic examination cannot be done in a symptomatic female, a rectal examination may reveal the diagnosis.

Boys generally enter puberty a full year or more later than girls. A discussion of the actual pubertal changes are contained in Chapter 5. When the adolescent boy has become fully developed, it is a good time to review the importance of self-examination of the testicles and then to teach him to do it himself (see Chapter 78). Unlike breast cancer in females, testicular cancer is a disease of adolescents and young adult men. Approximately 70% of adolescent males develop gynecomastia during early to middle puberty. If breast development is noted during the physical examination of the adolescent male, it is helpful to mention this finding to him and provide reassurance that in nearly all cases the breast tissue will disappear within 6 to 24 months. If the breast development is large or begins before puberty or late in puberty or in a male whose genitalia are not developing normally, further evaluation is needed (see Chapter 77).

SPECIFIC ISSUES

The skin should be thoroughly examined for problems such as acne, warts, and other common lesions (see Chapter 39). Examination of the head and neck should include evaluation of visual acuity and hearing. Myopia is a particular problem during adolescence, and hearing impairment (conductive or sensorineural) may have been missed prior to adolescence (see Chapter 40). The use of a Snellen eye chart or Titmus tester is suggested for evaluation of sight; audiometric testing (pure-tone method) is suggested for adolescents with possible hearing loss. Dental caries and malocclusions should be detected (see Chapter 41). Thyroid enlargement should be detected; it possibly indicates thyroiditis, Graves' disease, and thyroid tumors (see Chapter 55). Cardiac examination seeks murmurs, clicks, and arrhythmias (see Chapters 45 to 50). Examination of the spine should include screening for idiopathic scoliosis (see Chapter 79). Screening for sexually related problems is discussed in Chapters 69 and 75.

Laboratory Screening

If a detailed medical history and physical examination do not raise any specific concerns regarding the adolescent's health, laboratory screening need not be extensive. Its purpose is to lend support to the assumption that the adolescent is, in fact, well and to screen for asymptomatic conditions that are relatively common, potentially serious, and amenable to treatment or counseling but that are "hidden" from view. Such testing would include (1) a hemoglobin or hematocrit determination, (2) a sickle cell screen in black or Hispanic patients (unless it is performed at birth as in some states), (3) tuberculin skin testing, and (4) screening for pregnancy and sexually transmitted disease.

Hemoglobin and hematocrit determinations provide a relatively inexpensive laboratory assay of the adolescent's nutritional and physical well-being. The interpretation of this screening test must consider the patient's age, sex, race, and stage of physical maturation (see Chapter 51). Black adolescents who are unaware of their sickle cell trait status should be screened for the purpose of genetic counseling. Individuals who have sickle cell trait should not have hemoglobin or hematocrits values lower than those of black individuals without the sickle cell trait.

The recommended frequency of skin testing for exposure to tuberculosis depends upon age, sex, geographic location, and other personal risk factors. Early adolescent girls are at increased risk for reactivation tuberculosis. Most adolescents' lifestyle tends to place them in contact with more potentially infected individuals than is true during childhood. Therefore, it would be pragmatic to skin-test all adolescents at least once during early adolescence, and every 1 to 2 years thereafter if the local prevalence rate of positive results on skin testing exceeds 1%. A discussion of laboratory screening for pregnancy and sexually transmitted diseases is contained in Chapters 69, 74, 75, and 76. A discussion of cholesterol screening is contained later in this chapter and in Chapters 49 and 60.

FILLING IN THE DETAILS
Immunizations
PREVIOUSLY IMMUNIZED ADOLESCENTS

Most young adolescents were last immunized at approximately 5 years of age when they received the final diphtheria, pertussis, tetanus (DPT) and oral polio vaccine (OPV) immunizations of their primary series. Adolescents born after 1976 were most likely immunized against measles, mumps, and rubella (MMR) with an MMR preparation given at 15 months rather than at 12 months of age as had previously been recommended by the Committee on Infectious Diseases of the American Academy of Pediatrics and the Immunization Practices Advisory Committee of the Centers for Disease Control. The change from 12 to 15 months came when it was recognized that long-lasting immunity for measles was optimized by later immunization. In recent years, outbreaks of measles in young children, adolescents, and college-aged young adults have necessitated a review of old practices and revised recommendations from all these groups. The new recommendations call for a second MMR immunization to be given either at entry into kindergarten or at 12 years of age or, in the case of adolescents and young adults, at the next annual visit. Colleges are beginning to require a second measles immunization or proof of immunity for entering students who have not had their second measles immunization. The second immunization may be with either measles alone or MMR, but MMR is generally recommended because of a recent increase in the number of cases of mumps and rubella in teenagers and young adults. Most adolescents at age 14 or 15 years are due for their 10-year booster of tetanus and diphtheria toxoids, Td (pertussis vaccine is not recommended for children older than age 6 years), and, if previously immunized only once with MMR, for a second dose of these live virus vaccines. Earlier immunization in female patients has the advantage of taking place prior to the onset of sexual activity. Because of the theoretical risk, live virus vaccine should not be administered to a pregnant adolescent. Trivalent live OPV boosters are not indicated beyond age 5 years in those who have had their complete primary series, except in individuals exposed to polio or traveling to an endemic region.

PREVIOUSLY UNIMMUNIZED ADOLESCENTS

Adolescents who were never immunized or those in whom the immunization was questionable or those who lack documentation of their immunization status, which is required for entry into school, should receive a three-dose primary series of Td and OPV and a two-dose primary series of MMR. At an initial visit, Td, OPV, and MMR all should be given. Two months later, the second Td and OPV should be given, with the third doses given at 6 to 12 months after the first dose. The second MMR is given at least 1 month after the first. OPV is not recommended for young people older than age 18 years who have never been immunized; the new enhanced formalin-inactivated polio vaccine (IPV) given subcutaneously should be used instead. Because of a theoretical risk, administration of OPV or IPV should be avoided during pregnancy.

Cardiovascular Risk Reduction

Detection of possible risk factors for cardiovascular disease and efforts directed at reducing cardiovascular risk are important components of well adolescent care (see Chapter 49). A thorough search for risk factors is directed toward the medical history, physical examination, and laboratory screening.

FAMILY HISTORY

An individual is at high risk for the development of cardiovascular disease if that person had a parent or sibling who had a myocardial infarction or hyperlipidemia at approximately 55 years of age (men, younger than 50 years; women, younger than 60 years). The parents and siblings of most adolescents are usually younger than age 60 years, and such a risk may not yet be apparent. Having a grandparent, aunt, or uncle with known ischemic heart disease at a relatively young age may also provide an important clue with respect to the adolescent's potential risk. Both genetic and environmental factors (such as diet, activity level, psychosocial stress, and cigarette smoking) may be important in the familial clustering of cardiovascular disease. If a positive family history exists, special vigilance should be applied to detecting associated risk factors in the adolescent.

HYPERTENSION

If the blood pressure reading is elevated above the 90th percentile for age and sex on standard blood pressure curves developed by the Second Task Force on Blood Pressure Control in Children (see Chapters 48, 49 and 67), it should be repeated at three consecutive visits in the office or in school (performed by a school nurse) during a 6- to 12-month period. An average of three systolic or diastolic readings greater than 95th percentile defines the adolescent as hypertensive (see Chapters 48, 49, and 67). Most adolescents with mild elevations in blood pressure are found to have a familial history of primary or essential hypertension rather than disorders of renal, endocrine, or vascular origin (see Chapters 48, 49, and 67). Many adolescents continue to be hypertensive into adulthood. It is well established that sustained hypertension in adults contributes to the development of cardiovascular disease, as well as central nervous system and renal disorders.

HYPERCHOLESTEROLEMIA

Elevated total cholesterol in the serum is an established risk factor for cardiovascular disease (see Chapters 49 and 60). It is not well established, however, at what age and which children or adolescents should be screened for hypercholesterolemia. Through the 1980s, the most widely held view was that only children and adolescents with a family history of early-onset cardiovascular disease or hypercholesterolemia, or both, or those adolescents who themselves had other risk factors for cardiovascular disease (such as hypertension, obesity, or diabetes mellitus) should be screened. Recent studies, however, have indicated that approximately one half of all children and adolescents found to have hypercholesterolemia on routine testing lacked any such family or personal risk factors, and their elevated cholesterol levels would have been missed if only these indicators for screening had been employed. There is

TABLE 25–2. Anticipatory Guidance Regarding Health Risk Behaviors

HISTORY	DISCUSSION-EVALUATION	INTERVENTION
DATING	Responsibility as lifelong principle Adolescent's partner (heterosexual, homosexual) Knowledge of sexual activity and consequences Partner pressure to initiate activity	Delay of premature sexual activity (discussion with partner about sexual activity) Preparation: if sexually active, to prevent adolescent pregnancy (contraception) and sexually transmitted disease (condom use)
SEXUAL ACTIVITY Heterosexual	Responsibility as lifelong principle Knowledge of risk of pregnancy, sexually transmitted diseases (particularly HIV and AIDS)	Contraception (see Chapter 73) Sexually transmitted disease prevention (see Chapters 75 and 76)
Homosexual (see Chapter 32)	Responsibility as lifelong principle Knowledge of risk of sexually transmitted diseases	Difficulties being gay Specific morbidities
CIGARETTE SMOKING	Responsibility as lifelong principle Family history of cigarette smoking Specific medical morbidities of cigarette smoking (cardiovascular, pulmonary) Specific medical morbidities from passive smoking, especially if adolescent is a parent Expense	If not started, encouragement not to start If started, discontinuation (see Chapters 38, 44, and 49)
DRUG OR ALCOHOL USE-ABUSE	Responsibility as lifelong principle Family history of use of specific substances If using, possibility of depression (decreased school grades and concentration difficulties, early morning awakening, uncontrolled anger, crying, and use of drugs as self-medication) Marijuana and cocaine—illegal drugs and legal consequences Medical and psychosocial morbidities (see Chapter 111) Driving vehicles while using substances	If not started, encouragement not to start Discussion of moderate use of alcohol Discussion of drug use and impairment of function—school, work, driving If started, discontinue individually or through participation in Alcoholics Anonymous or specific drug program Avoidance of driving while under influence of drugs
SERIOUS ACCIDENTS/INJURIES	Responsibility as lifelong principle Risk behaviors (driving too fast, use of motorcycles, other dangerous vehicles, use of cigarettes, drugs, alcohol) Possibility of depression Impulsiveness, hyperactivity Number of accidents and exact circumstances of accident Use of seat belts and helmets when driving or riding motorcycles	Discussion of thinking out consequences of behavior before doing it Discussion of peer pressure and means of handling other than joining the crowd Discussion of specific intervention if depressed (see Chapter 101)
VIOLENCE/HOMICIDE	Experience with violence: setting and circumstance Friends injured or killed through violence Carrying guns, knives, other potentially harmful instruments Peer pressures	Protection of adolescent and others by avoiding settings where violent behaviors occur (arguments, gang fights, drug trafficking) and circumstances in which violent behaviors are likely
SUICIDE	Exact nature of thoughts (general versus specific plan) History of gesture or attempt, or both Family history of depression or suicidal behavior Depression Family knowledge of distress	Discussion with provider, knowing adolescent is distressed Further evaluation, depending on immediacy and risk to adolescent Discussion with family Decision about hospitalization versus ambulatory care (see Chapter 101)
PHYSICAL OR SEXUAL ABUSE	Exact nature of abuse Perpetrator Duration What has been done Appropriate physical evaluation and documentation of injury (observation, photographs, x-ray studies) Abusive behavior on the adolescent's part	Protection of adolescent Immediate care of injuries Report to proper authorities If still at risk, consider out of home placement with Department of Social Services Psychological intervention, if adolescent is abusive
EATING DISORDERS Undereating or loss of weight (see Chapter 60)	Determination of whether purposeful Documentation of intake, perception of food, eating, perception of whether losing weight, menstrual function Constitutional symptoms: fever, rash, joint pain, vomiting, diarrhea, cough, fatigue Family history Physical examination: plot of height and weight over time; evaluation of orthostatic pulse and blood pressure; neurologic examination including visual fields; examination for lymphadenopathy, hepatosplenomegaly, evidence of malnutrition (see Chapter 60) Exercise	Demonstration of weight, height percentiles; discussion of ideal weight for height Discussion of potential effects of starvation on growth and fertility If <10% loss, ambulatory program with at least weekly follow-up; if continues to lose weight, hospitalization, set specific goals If >10% loss, consideration of hospitalization Limitation of exercise
Overeating (see Chapters 49 and 60)	Documentation of intake, perception of food, eating, perception whether gaining weight, menstrual function Family history Physical examination: plot of height and weight over time, thyromegaly, striae, buffalo hump, hypertension, distribution of adipose tissue (see Chapter 55) Exercise	Demonstration of weight percentiles Discussion of morbidity of chronic obesity (cardiovascular, pulmonary, and so on) Weight reduction plan *only* if adolescent is motivated and family will follow up (see Chapters 49 and 60) Initiation of exercise

considerable debate about the efficacy of screening all adolescents. With respect to adolescents who have never been screened, some believe it is reasonable to recommend checking total and high-density lipoprotein cholesterol levels at the completion of puberty, even though this practice is not universally accepted. By this time, secretion of testosterone and estrogen, which influence cholesterol metabolism, has stabilized, and efforts to act upon results worthy of concern may be undertaken by a fully developed and mature adolescent. Others believe it is better to delay screening until adulthood.

OBESITY

Obesity is associated with several well-established cardiovascular risk factors (hypertension, elevated cholesterol, diabetes mellitus), although its unique relationship to cardiovascular risk is less clear (see Chapter 49). Approximately 11% to 19% of adolescents in the United States are obese, which is defined as 20% greater than ideal weight for age, height, and sex (see Chapter 60). Well adolescent care should not overlook the existence of obesity, and although its treatment is often difficult, the health care provider should at least offer to play a role in helping the motivated adolescent to control his or her weight. Obese adolescents should always be carefully screened for other cardiovascular risk factors and the psychosocial sequelae of obesity.

CIGARETTE SMOKING

Most adult cigarette smokers started to smoke during adolescence, and most adolescent smokers do not worry about the serious medical risks associated with this habit that may strike them as adults (see Chapters 38, 44, and 49). Although fewer teenagers smoke now than 15 to 20 years ago, large numbers of adolescents, more commonly females, are initiating this harmful behavior (see Chapter 2). Teenagers who smoke probably will not have cancer or heart disease until many years later, but it is important to point out to them the more immediate side effects of their smoking habit, which include chronic cough and phlegm production, wheezing and shortness of breath, decreased stamina and athletic ability, and increased susceptibility to colds and other respiratory infections.

EXERCISE

Adolescence is an ideal time to initiate exercise programs, whether as a team sport (track, volleyball, baseball) or a sport one does alone. Exercise not only has therapeutic benefits of maintaining general physical and emotional health but also has specific benefits of reducing cardiovascular risk (see Chapter 49). Evaluation for competitive sports is contained in Chapter 81.

ANTICIPATORY GUIDANCE

Having thoroughly evaluated the adolescent and having identified health risk behaviors, the practitioner may be baffled by how to respond to them and what interventions are possible in the primary care office.

Table 25–2 lists the specific health risk behaviors enumerated both in Table 25–1 and in this chapter and provides suggestions for topics for discussion regarding each group of behaviors and specific interventions. The practitioner is most helpful to the adolescent by being nonjudgmental, stating his or her views clearly about the health implications of health risk behavior, and suggesting interventions. General principles, such as responsibility as a lifelong principle, knowledge of the consequences of the behavior, and possible interventions are stressed. Some adolescents may be only considering one behavior, whereas others may be engaged in one or more health risk behaviors. Further discussion of screening for high-risk behaviors is found in Chapter 33.

Well adolescent care is a challenging and gratifying aspect of medical practice. In our society, adolescents are vulnerable to a wide range of medical, psychological, and social disorders. The health care provider who establishes a meaningful and ongoing relationship with an adolescent, and who commits himself or herself to a comprehensive approach to care, is in the best position to detect problems and treat them effectively and sensitively.

BIBLIOGRAPHY

American Academy of Pediatrics, Committee on the Psychosocial Aspects of Child and Family Health: Guidelines for Health Supervision. Elk Grove Village, IL, American Academy of Pediatrics, 1988.

Cross AW: Health screening in schools. J Pediatr 107:487; 653, 1985.

Daniel WA: Hematocrit: Maturity relationship in adolescence. Pediatrics 52:388, 1973.

Denaison BA, Kikuchi DA, Srinivasan SR, et al: Parental history of cardiovascular disease as an indication for screening for lipoprotein abnormalities in children. J Pediatr 115:186, 1989.

Frankenburg WK: Selection of diseases and tests in pediatric screening. Pediatrics 54:612, 1974.

Marks A, Fisher M: Health assessment and screening during adolescence. Pediatrics 80(Suppl):135, 1987.

Marks A, Lasker S, Fisher M: Adolescent medicine in pediatric practice. J Adolesc Health Care 11:149, 1990.

Marks A, Malizio J, Hoch J, et al: Assessment of the health needs and willingness to utilize health care resources of adolescents in a suburban population. J Pediatr 102:456, 1983.

Neinstein LS: Adolescent Health Care, A Practical Guide. Baltimore, Urban and Schwarzenberg, 1984.

Newman TB, Brownes WS, Hulley SB: The case against childhood cholesterol screening. JAMA 264:3039, 1990.

Steiner NJ, Neinstein LS, Pennbridge J: Hypercholesterolemia in adolescents: Effectiveness of screening strategies based on selected risk factors. Pediatrics 88:269, 1991.

Task Force on Blood Pressure Control in Children: Report of the Second Task Force on Blood Pressure Control in Children—1987. Pediatrics 79:1, 1987.

CHAPTER 26

Compliance

M. SUSAN JAY and ROBERT H. DURANT

Compliance is an important issue in the clinical practice of adolescent medicine (see also Chapter 24). Compliance failures are costly from both a therapeutic and an economic perspective. Noncompliant adolescents do not receive the full benefit of therapy and as a result, they may not get well. Moreover, health care providers may conclude that a specific treatment is not effective when, in fact, the adolescent may have taken only a few doses of medication.

Adolescents may be perceived as nonusers of prescribed medications and abusers of nonprescribed drugs. Compliance with medical regimens and positive health practices during adolescence is complicated by developmental issues that can have an impact on adolescent health behavior (see Chapters 5 and 9). Some of the same developmental factors that are associated with risk-taking behavior, such as feelings of invulnerability, failure to connect appropriate consequences with specific behaviors, and a lack of a future time perspective, are also associated with noncompliance with care and treatment.

DEFINITION OF COMPLIANCE

Compliance has traditionally been defined as the extent to which patients are obedient and follow instructions relating to taking medications, changing lifestyle, and following diets. *Adherence* has been used recently to suggest active collaboration between patient and physicians working together to achieve therapeutic success. *Compliance* and *adherence* are used interchangeably throughout this chapter when describing the adolescent's ability and willingness to follow recommended health practices or preventive health care regimens. Because the major causes of morbidity and mortality among adolescents have changed from traditional childhood illness to substance use and abuse, sexually transmitted diseases, accidents, suicide, and homicide (see Chapters 75, 97, 101, 111, and 117), the definition of compliance should be broadened to include adherence to preventive health practices, as well as compliance with treatment regimens.

ASSESSING COMPLIANCE

A number of different measures have been used to assess compliance with taking medication, each with varying degrees of accuracy and clinical applicability. These techniques include drug assays, observational methods, patient estimates or physician estimates, pill counts, and treatment outcome. Table 26–1 presents the benefits and limitations of each method.

The most accurate measure of compliance with taking medication is drug assays. This is a direct measure that determines the presence or lack of actual levels of a prescribed medicine or its metabolite in body fluid. Serum analysis necessitates a venipuncture, which can be anxiety-provoking. Alternatively, techniques such as salivary assays for theophylline, digoxin, and anticonvulsant levels are noninvasive. Qualitative assessments using techniques such as bioassays of antibiotics in urine specimens or inactive markers such as riboflavin, which produce fluorescence in urine, have also been used successfully to assess medication compliance. Given the constraints of cost and time in medical practice, however, these direct measures are best implemented in specific situations: (1) to confirm a clinical suspicion of noncompliance, (2) to illustrate the effects of noncompliance to a teenager, or (3) to monitor compliance as one part of a therapeutic intervention.

It is important to remember that with the exception of analysis of body fluids, all other assessment methods serve only as indicators of compliance. However, the use of several methods in combination can provide useful information. Family members can provide relatively reliable observations. Patient estimates (e.g., asking the adolescent directly) are easily obtained although sometimes difficult to evaluate. Although teenaged patients may overestimate their compliance, information obtained directly from the adolescent can be reliable and accurate. It is best to be nonthreatening and nonjudgmental when asking adolescents about taking medication. Teenagers who are initiating a regimen can also be asked to estimate their compliance with past medications. The answer to this question has been shown to be positively associated with adolescent's adherence to future medical regimens. Physician estimates of compliance, although easily obtained, are also limited, since they may overestimate compliance. Pill counts of unused medication and tallies of refills have also been used to assess compliance. Treatment outcome may also be used to indicate compliance, but its validity and reliability are low. When an adolescent fails to demonstrate clinical recovery, noncompliance is suspected, whereas clinical status quo is assumed to indicate compliance. Although

TABLE 26–1. Measures of Compliance

METHOD	BENEFITS	LIMITATIONS
Drug assays	Direct	Measurement of compliance over limited time
	Quantifiable	Pharmokinetic variability
	Objective	Costliness; feasibility in private practice setting limited
Observational methods	Objective	Observer-dependent
	Done by family member and eliminates physician or patient estimates	"Nagging"
Patient estimates	Easily obtained information	Reliability and validity lacking
Physician estimates	Most common method that can be easily done in practice	Accuracy found with pill counts, observation, or assays lacking with this method
		Accuracy unrelated to physician's familiarity with patient or years of practice experience
Pill counts	Inexpensive and easily obtained	Return of medication containers; missed pills discarded prior to visit
		Overestimation of compliance
Treatment outcome	Easily obtained	Treatment outcome affected by variables other than compliance
		Relationship to compliance tenuous, often used by physicians when adolescent fails to improve

noncompliance may be a reasonable explanation for the lack of a clinical effect from a medication, the lack of clinical response may also be due to genetic, pharmacologic, or disease factors rather than to noncompliance.

Early identification of adolescents who are likely to be noncompliant is important. Information collected through a combination of measures can be used to identify the at-risk adolescent. This allows modification of subsequent clinical interactions to promote adherence.

PATTERNS OF NONCOMPLIANCE

If frustrated by a system they believe is not responsive to their needs, adolescents may become noncompliant with treatment (Table 26–2).

Ambulatory Attendance

The attendance of adolescents in ambulatory clinic settings may be inconsistent. They may delay or fail to seek care until their symptoms are severe or incapacitating. Their pattern of use of the health care system may be episodic and fragmented; the failed appointment rate in this age group can be as high as 60%. When seeking care, some adolescents may fail to attend follow-up appointments, may use emergency room services when ill, and may terminate treatment prematurely.

Behavioral Aspects

Adolescents may fail to take preventive measures for symptoms of their chronic diseases (e.g., the diabetic teenager who ignores the effects of poor metabolic control and overindulges in alcohol use or the seizure patient who takes the prescribed medication only when he or she remembers or immediately before a visit to the physician) (see Chapter 30). Another form of nonadherence is demonstrated by the teenager who sabotages the treatment regimen or fails to participate in a prescribed health protocol. This type of behavior is often observed in adolescents who have eating disorders

and alter their dietary intake or increase their exercise to avoid what they perceive to be excessive weight gain (Chapter 60). Adolescents have also been known to improvise or substitute one medication for another.

Medication Alterations

Adolescents may fail to fill their prescriptions or may take only a portion of a prescribed regimen. With antibiotics, for example, an adolescent may question why it is necessary to take a full 10-day regimen when he or she feels better after a few days of treatment. Adolescents may also borrow someone else's medication, causing improper use of medications or dangerous drug interactions. Adolescents may ignore dosage instructions, for example, failing to follow a three times a day dosage, believing that tripling the dosage and taking it once a day will suffice.

If adolescents believe that their problem has not been appropriately treated, they may adopt a nonadherent posture, manifested by failing to fill the prescription, taking only part of a prescribed regimen, or altering the dose or frequency of a medication.

TABLE 26–2. Patterns of Noncompliance
with Treatment

AMBULATORY ATTENDANCE
Delaying or failing to seek care
Failing to keep scheduled appointments
Terminating treatment prematurely

BEHAVIORAL ASPECTS
Not taking recommended preventive measures
Incompletely following with a prescribed regimen
Sabotaging treatment regimens or not participating in prescribed health programs
Improvising, creating, or substituting ready made treatment regimen

MEDICATION ALTERATIONS
Failing to fill the prescription
Taking only a portion of a prescribed regimen or none at all despite filling the prescription
Taking a medication that has not been prescribed (i.e., borrowing a friend's or relative's medications)
Altering the prescription (i.e., changing the dose or frequency of the regimen)

Adapted from Meichenbaum D, Turk DC: Facilitating Treatment Adherence: A Practitioner's Guidebook. New York, Plenum Press, 1987.

MODIFIERS OF COMPLIANCE

Adolescent Development

When the stress of physical illness is added to the stress of adolescence, an adolescent's compliance is often affected negatively. Changes in cognitive abilities and style throughout adolescence require an awareness of the relationship of the adolescent's developmental stage and compliance. With early adolescents, it is best to use concrete reasoning and to avoid intellectual or conceptually based arguments when discussing treatment regimens. When possible, it is best to simplify discussions and *avoid* the usual didactic lecture employed in adolescent-physician exchanges. Asking the patient to repeat the prescriptive instructions allows the practitioner to assess the success of the interchange. Follow-up calls made by the office nurse 24 to 48 hours after a visit allow an additional opportunity to modify a treatment plan prior to the follow-up visit, as well as emphasizing that the adolescent is an active participant in his or her medical care.

Identity, self-esteem, and autonomy are formalized during adolescence and may affect adolescent compliance. The development of adolescent identity is related to being similar to other adolescents; thus, a diabetic teenager who believes taking insulin makes him or her different from peers may fail to maintain a daily intake of take insulin. Self-esteem is related to feeling good about oneself; the cosmetic effects of certain medications such as steroids, which may cause obesity and acne, may undermine an adolescent's self-esteem. An adolescent with renal disease may stop taking his or her steroids in an effort to decrease the unsightly side effects. Adolescents seek autonomy, particularly through decision-making. This may or may not be possible regarding behavior toward medication. Whenever possible, autonomy should be encouraged. If the adolescent is mature and the parents are supportive, discussions about medication regimens can be negotiated between the adolescent and the practitioner.

Nature of the Disease and Complexity of the Regimen

The nature of the disease may also affect compliance. The duration of disease, the length of treatment, and the necessity of changing personal behavior all are inversely correlated with compliance.

The complexity of a regimen, such as taking multiple drugs several times each day, may not be readily acceptable to many adolescents. Whenever possible, the regimen should be simplified and a drug that can be taken once daily should be considered, even if it is slightly more costly. Even greater success can be achieved if the clinician can motivate the adolescent to "invest" in the regimen. For example, allowing adolescents to choose between medication that can be taken once daily rather than four times a day involves the adolescent in the development of the regimen so that successful resolution of the health problem is a result of

their behavior. Weight control is an example of a clinical situation in which the teenager can be an active participant in setting weight loss goals, scheduling appointments for weekly weigh-ins, and working with the team regarding dietary modification and exercise programs.

Confidentiality of Care

The adolescent's perception of the extent of physician confidentiality can affect compliance. The adolescent who believes care is not confidential, including arbitrary revelations of confidential information to parents, may be unwilling to follow through with prescriptive regimens as well as subsequent appointments. (see Chapter 20).

Cost of Health Care

Finally the cost of medical visits and medication remains a major burden to adolescents. To address this issue, a nominal fee-structured reimbursement schedule may allow more adolescents to avail themselves of services (see Chapter 17); medication samples can be dispensed when cost is a concern.

ADAPTIVE NONCOMPLIANCE

Control of Life

For the healthy adolescent, a component of the normal developmental process is the achievement of mastery or control of one's own life. For the teenager with chronic illness, compliance or noncompliance with therapeutic regimens offers an avenue for controlling one's own destiny (see Chapter 30). Rather than tolerate severe side effects from medication, some adolescents may alter their regimens to a point that reduces the side effects. Clinicians must weigh the possibility of noncompliance as a positive response in some cases in which adolescents do not follow their prescribed regimen.

Cultural Factors

Cultural factors must be considered when compliance is assessed (see Chapter 28). Folk medicine is often used in conjunction with traditional medical care. Such parallel use of the health care system is not uncommon among ethnic groups. It is important to remember that formal medical therapy may be just one of a number of competing coping strategies in adolescent health behavior.

FACILITATION OF COMPLIANCE

A number of interventions can increase adolescent compliance. First, the adolescent should be encouraged

TABLE 26–3. Guidelines for Adolescent Health Education Messages

1. Whenever possible, provide adolescents with instructions at the start of the encounter.
2. Stress the importance of the regimen and attempt to be selective, limiting the length of the message.
3. Verbalize the message more than once and have the adolescent repeat it to you.
4. Make your advice as specific, detailed, and concrete as possible.
5. Delineate your expectations; cue compliance to daily activity.
6. When appropriate (without infringing on the adolescent's confidentiality), enlist the support of significant others to reinforce the health education message after the adolescent leaves the office. For adolescents with chronic diseases, the use of support groups can be helpful.

to assume as much responsibility as possible for the successful treatment of any medical condition. Second, the regimen should be tailored for minimal intrusion on the adolescent's daily schedule. These interventions obviously work best for brief rather than lengthy regimens, and multiple interventions probably are more helpful than one in isolation.

Patient health education messages (Table 26–3) are frequently combined with other interventions to increase effectiveness. Adolescents with chronic illnesses, particularly if they have little experience with long-term and complex medical regimens, may benefit greatly from health education. These adolescents also require frequent reeducation, particularly if they were first diagnosed during the preadolescent years. If compliance is to be continued, the adolescent must remember medication instructions. Understanding and recall can be best enhanced by an efficient verbal presentation of information that is reinforced with a printed version of the same material for the adolescent to take home. Written handouts should describe the treatment in simple language. Studies have found that compliance with short-term oral antibiotics is significantly improved by providing supplementary written instructions.

An additional tool can be self-monitoring or asking the adolescent to record his or her own behavior. For example, adolescents with specific problems, such as eating disorders or dysmenorrhea, record their dietary practices and menstrual patterns sufficiently well to allow modification of treatment (see Chapters 60 and 70).

FOLLOW-UP

Since compliance decreases over the course of therapy, it is important to use reminders or "cues" via telephone calls, written notes, labels, or stickers to support the adolescent's resolve. Reminders have traditionally been most useful for short-term regimens. Other reminder methods can be designed to forge a link between a daily activity such as combing one's hair (cue) and applying a topical antibiotic for acne (behavior). From the start, the regimen should be tailored to the adolescent's schedule. If an adolescent needs two medications for acne, one should be introduced initially, if possible, and a cue identified. At a follow-up visit, if the initial part of the prescriptive package is going well, the second medication, such as an oral antibiotic, can be added.

Follow-up visits may also be used to monitor the progress of an adolescent who may require additional help. Greater supervision may provide reinforcement and has the additional benefit of serving as a cue to action. Studies of adolescents with epilepsy and juvenile rheumatoid arthritis (see Chapters 83 and 90) found better compliance when they were seen frequently, such as once a month as opposed to once every 3 to 6 months. Although it is not necessary that these visits be lengthy, it is best if the interaction during the follow-up monitoring is informative and nonconfrontational. This supportive approach by the health care provider is especially important when parents are asked to assist in monitoring the teenager's compliance. When the teenager and the family are not able to communicate freely, it may be better to enlist the help of a peer or a nonparental adult who can support the adolescent.

Negotiating with the adolescent to set reasonable goals is another tool used to increase compliance. This technique of developing a contract clearly defines the expected behavior; objective measures of outcome are then used for feedback. Although studies on the efficacy of this technique during adolescence are limited, it has been used successfully to enhance metabolic control in teenagers who have diabetes mellitus (see Chapter 59). When both contract setting and reinforcement are incorporated into goal setting they should be clear, positive when possible, and succinct, with defined and measurable outcomes. For example, an adolescent who has epilepsy (see Chapter 83) should be informed that a person cannot receive medical approval to get a driver's license until one is free of seizures for 1 year. If structured interventions are unsuccessful, more intense individual counseling may be a necessary adjunct to continuing medical care.

In conclusion, adolescent behavior is frequently viewed by health care providers as either wholly noncompliant or totally compliant. Although it is tempting to generalize about adolescent compliance, it is important to consider each aspect of care individually. The health care provider should entertain noncompliance as a possibility and promote adherence and positive health practices at every opportunity.

BIBLIOGRAPHY

Blum, RW (ed): Chronic Illness and Disabilities in Childhood and Adolescence. Orlando, FL, Grune & Stratton, 1984.

DuRant RH, Jay MS (eds): Communication and compliance issues in adolescent medicine. Semin Adolesc Med 3(2), 1987.

DuRant RH, Seymore C, Jay MS: Adolescents' compliance with therapeutic regimens. In Hendee WR, (ed): The Health of Adolescents. San Francisco, Jossey-Bass, 1991, pp 468–494.

Friedman IM, Litt IF: Promoting adolescents' compliance with therapeutic regimens. Pediatr Clin North Am 33:955, 1986.

Friedman IM, Litt IF: Adolescents' compliance with therapeutic regimens. J Adolesc Health Care 8:52, 1987.

Haynes RB, Taylor DW, Sackett D (eds): Compliance in Health Care. Baltimore, Johns Hopkins University Press, 1979.

Jay S, Litt IF, DuRant RH: Compliance with therapeutic regimens. J Adolesc Health Care 5:124, 1984.

Meichenbaum D, Turk DC: Facilitating Treatment Adherence: A Practitioner's Guidebook. New York, Plenum Press, 1987.

Rickert V, Jay MS, Gottlieb AA: Adolescent wellness: Facilitating compliance in the social morbidities. Med Clin North Am, 74(5):1135, 1990.

CHAPTER 27

Interdisciplinary Teams

LAWRENCE J. D'ANGELO and TOMAS J. SILBER

Interdisciplinary teams facilitate the provision of optimal health care to adolescents, whose problems are frequently complex. Delivery of adolescent health care by an interdisciplinary team can be important to the well-being of young people who become ill or who have traumatic experiences at the same time that they are trying to develop autonomy from the family. The resultant complexity of these challenges, as well as the adolescent's task of learning how to interact with the adult world, can be markedly enriched by the team approach to care. A team perspective can promote clinical views that are broader and more creative than the traditional approaches. Additional benefits of the team approach include the following:

1. *Backup for routine medical care.* Team care allows additional resources to be available and easily accessible to the adolescent who requires more than simple health care maintenance services (see Chapter 25). The adolescent rapidly identifies with the *group* of doctors, nurses, and other professionals caring for him or her and with the place in which the care is provided.

2. *Legitimization of the need for mental health services.* When mental health services are a routine part of the team approach, there is less stigma attached to the use of these services by adolescents than if they are offered separately (see Chapter 24). Since adolescent medical complaints are often accompanied by psychosomatic complaints (fatigue, pain, fainting, hyperventilation) and mental health problems (depression, suicide attempts, substance abuse), the adolescent often has need of such services but might otherwise avoid them if it would mean seeing a separate professional not associated with the health care team (see Chapters 100, 101, and 111).

3. *Avoidance of "splitting" between and among health professionals.* When separate professionals are involved in a patient's care, the adolescent may "play one off against another." This manipulation can frustrate efforts to solve a patient's problem. A team approach with joint discussions and decision-making decreases this behavior and facilitates making the necessary difficult therapeutic decisions and interventions. Team members can support one another in these decisions and interventions.

4. *Promotion of patient entry into a comprehensive health care system.* Although simple problems might prompt initial contact with a health care provider, the team approach can make it easier to provide a broad range of services.

5. *Improved problem-solving documentation and comprehensive record keeping.* A team approach to care results in improved problem solving and documentation.

TYPES OF TEAMS

A *multidisciplinary team* is a loose association of members of various disciplines who provide services to a shared population, with each member working independently. Although there is frequent interaction among team members, this is not a necessary condition for their work, which is often done in different locations and usually with an exclusive focus on a particular discipline. The *interdisciplinary team* (Table 27–1) provides joint services concentrating on a particular problem. A regular, systematized exchange of information and integration of team members constitute the hallmark of the interdisciplinary team.

GENERAL AND SPECIALIZED ADOLESCENT HEALTH CARE TEAMS

An interdisciplinary team for the care of adolescents can be (1) a general team that provides routine health care or (2) a problem-oriented specialty team. Both types of teams can be deployed in a variety of settings: health maintenance organizations, specialty clinics for adolescents with chronic illnesses, tertiary care or adolescent inpatient units, and community health care clinics.

TABLE 27–1. Interdisciplinary Team Participants

PRIMARY MEMBERS	ADDITIONAL MEMBERS
Primary practitioners (pediatrician, internist, family physician, nurse practitioner, physician's assistant)	Chaplains
	Adolescent life specialists
	Vocational rehabilitation counselors
Social workers	Recreational therapists
Mental health practitioners (psychiatrist, counselor, psychologist, educational specialist)	Physical therapists
	Occupational therapists
Professional nurses	
Nutritionists	

TABLE 27–2. Specialty Adolescent Health Care Teams

Crisis intervention
Sexual and physical abuse
Nutrition and eating disorders
Psychosomatic illness
Chronic illness and rehabilitation
Substance abuse
Grief and suicide counseling

General Teams

General teams have the advantage of providing comprehensive services to adolescents in a primary care setting. These teams can accomplish many aspects of care, for example, providing back-up, legitimizing mental health services, and facilitating easy entry into a comprehensive setting. Teams are sometimes limited, however, by their lack of sufficient expertise to cope with complicated problems. These limitations can be overcome by judicious use of consultative assistance.

Specialty Teams

A list of specialty teams is provided in Table 27–2.

Crisis Intervention Teams. These teams are usually affiliated with emergency rooms or ambulatory group practices. They provide care for adolescents in a variety of emergency situations, including trauma, rape, and suicide attempts (see Chapters 101, 117, and 119).

Sexual and Physical Abuse Teams. These teams work with the police and the judiciary system to provide optimal support for victims (see Chapters 118 and 119). They provide both medical and psychosocial follow-up and may extend their services to perpetrators as well as victims.

Nutrition and Eating Disorders Teams. These usually focus attention on adolescents who have significant nutritional problems (morbid obesity, anorexia nervosa, and bulimia) (see Chapter 60). The team helps adolescents modify their pathologic eating patterns through behavior modification, individual and family therapy,

and nutritional counseling. Often closely related to this group are the psychosomatic illness teams that follow adolescents with somatization disorders, school phobias, conversion reactions, psychogenic pain, and cyclic vomiting (see Chapters 103, 112, and 113). Chronic illness and rehabilitative teams usually care only for the impaired adolescent (see Chapters 30 and 121).

Substance Abuse Teams. These are some of the oldest subspecialty teams. Medical services for detoxification are often combined with counseling for patient and family. Although this team may operate on an ambulatory or inpatient basis, most of its successes take place in its inpatient program (see Chapter 111).

Grief and Suicide Teams. These teams become involved after major adolescent losses or adolescent suicidal behavior (see Chapters 101 and 116). They can operate in a variety of settings but usually are involved in assisting school programs in counseling adolescents following tragedies.

BIBLIOGRAPHY

Blum RW (ed): Chronic Illness and Disabilities in Childhood and Adolescence. Orlando, FL, Grune & Stratton, 1984.

Brown TM: A historical view of health care teams. In Agich G (ed): Responsibility in Health Care. Dordrecht, Reidel, 1982.

Centers for Disease Control: CDC recommendations for a community plan for the prevention and containment of suicide clusters. MMWR 375(6):1, 1988.

Dunger DB, Pritchard J, Hensman S, et al: The investigation of atypical psychosomatic illness. A team approach to diagnosis. Clin Pediatr 25:341, 1968.

Earls F, Robins LN, Stiffman AR, Powell J: Comprehensive health care for high risk adolescents. An evaluation study. Am J Publ Health 79:999, 1989.

Gallagher JR: The origins, development and goals of adolescent medicine. J Adolesc Health Care 3:57, 1982.

Irwin CE Jr: Adolescent Social Behavior and Health. New Directions for Child Development, No. 37. San Francisco, Jossey-Bass, 1982.

Noble J: Primary Care and the Practice of Medicine. Boston, Little, Brown, 1976.

Silber TJ: Adolescent medicine: Origins, segmenting, synthesis. J Adolesc Health Care 4:135, 1983.

Silber TJ, Ragsdale R, Addelstone I: A birth control clinic within an adolescent medicine program. J Sex Educ Ther 8:29, 1982.

Strasburger VC, Greydanus DE (eds): The "At-Risk" Adolescent. State of the Art Reviews. Philadelphia, Hanley and Belfus, 1990.

SECTION VIII

Youth with Special Needs

There are certain subgroups of youth who have special needs as a result of their backgrounds or their conditions. This section includes chapters focusing on specific groups of adolescents. Common themes emerge in these chapters: the need for understanding and respecting all young people, the need for access to cost-efficient services, the need for privacy and confidentiality, and often the need for interdisciplinary care because their problems are so multifaceted. As our society becomes more complex, we can expect greater diversity among the young people for whom we care.

CHAPTER 28

Cross-Cultural Youth

MARIANNE E. FELICE and RENÉE JENKINS

DEMOGRAPHICS

In the not too distant future, when today's babies are in their 60s, it is estimated that the average United States resident will trace his or her ancestors to Africa, Asia, Latin America, southern Europe, or the Pacific Islands, and very few to northern Europe. These figures clearly indicate that physicians must be prepared to care for adolescents of diverse racial and ethnic groups (see Chapter 2).

This is particularly important for clinicians in adolescent medicine, because many adolescent health problems have a behavioral context (e.g., sexuality [see Chapter 68], depression [see Chapter 100], suicide [see Chapter 101], violence [see Chapter 117]) and are heavily influenced by culture and the norms of specific groups. Problem assessments, intervention, and prevention strategies must consider cultural issues if they are to be relevant to adolescents and useful to those who design programs.

RACE, ETHNICITY, AND CULTURE

The terms *race* and *ethnicity* are not interchangeable, whereas the terms *ethnicity* and *culture* are somewhat related. There are several different races of people, based on physical characteristics, blood types, genetically transmitted diseases, geographic origin, and migration. Each race encompasses many different ethnic or cultural groups. Ethnicity refers to membership in a group of people who share a specific social heritage that is passed down from one generation to another. Culture is a set of guidelines that an individual inherits as a member of an ethnic group, which determines how he or she views the world and behaves in relation to other people, to supernatural forces or gods, and to the natural environment. Virtually all societies have more than one culture.

In this country, blacks constitute the largest minority group, but not all blacks in this country are African-American; some are Caribbean or West Indian, with different cultural mores. Latin Americans, or Hispanics, are the second largest minority. The term *Hispanic* does not refer to race, but rather to people of Spanish or Portuguese linguistic and cultural heritage, and includes Mexicans, Cubans, Puerto Ricans, Central Americans, and South Americans. Despite similar heritage, attitudes and languages vary. There are white, brown, and black Hispanics, depending on their racial origin.

Native Americans are the oldest minority, and Asian Americans are probably the newest. These populations are not homogeneous. Native Americans represent over 25 different tribal groups, each with distinctive languages, customs, and beliefs. Asian-Americans include at least 23 ethnic groups from a wide range of geographic origins who speak very different languages and represent civilizations that range from old to modern. Understanding these differences is important for appropriate adolescent care.

CULTURAL INFLUENCES ON HEALTH BEHAVIOR

Culture influences health behavior in many ways. The adolescent's support systems, health care experiences and beliefs, and social phenomena influence his or her behavior. A thorough cultural assessment is probably not necessary for every adolescent at every visit, but many clinical situations demand such assessments. Situations in which cultural assessments are most relevant are ones in which (1) the problem has a significant behavioral component, (2) the intervention proposed for a specific health problem is behaviorally based, and (3) compliance with the proposed nonbehavioral intervention is poor and compliance issues are being evaluated (see Chapter 26).

Support Systems

FAMILY

In many cultures (e.g., Hispanic, Asian), the family takes on a collective responsibility for the health problems of all members of the family, including the adolescent. This responsibility is viewed as sharing the burden of the family and is considered a very important form of family member support. Furthermore, elders in such families are treated with great respect; their opinions are sought and obeyed. Hence, parents in such families naturally expect that they will be informed of all matters related to the care of their daughter or son, including psychosexual history. The modern adolescent medicine practitioner, however, may view such familial involvement as invasive and possibly as undermining the adolescent's independence and responsibility. Failure to recognize this dilemma may have ethical ramifications for the physician and may cause confusion in the adolescent and anger in the parents.

Blacks typically value family ties and tend to maintain contact with a large network of relatives and fictive kin, a pattern especially functional for low-income families, who exchange resources, services, and emotional support. This network may confuse some clinicians who do not recognize the value of such a support system.

Future adolescent care must take into consideration the fact that all adolescents come from a familial system, and although adolescent independence is extremely important and should be encouraged, the physician should not lose sight of the fact that the adolescent is part of a family system (see Chapter 23).

RELIGION

In many cultural groups, particularly in black communities, the church is the central focus of social and civic activity. Even if blacks are not currently involved in a particular church, their religious heritage shapes their beliefs and values; their views on marital relationships, divorce, abortion, and adoption; and their child-rearing practices. Other groups may also believe strongly in their religion; whenever possible the clinician should involve the family's spiritual leader as a resource when appropriate.

Health Care Experiences and Beliefs

ACCESS

Some ethnic groups, particularly those who are recent immigrants to the United States, may not be familiar with the United States medical system and may not have knowledge of access routes to even the most routine medical care. Some families may view formalized care as an extremely rare event to be used only when the family member is near death. In many countries, good health care is available only to the elite. Other families may not be able to afford medical care, particularly the working poor, who are disproportionately represented in minority groups. Some groups, such as illegal aliens, may be afraid to seek medical advice for fear that the physician will expose them to the authorities. Hence, when a patient delays seeking care for a major problem, the clinician should explore whether the delay was based on cultural factors.

HOME REMEDIES

Nearly all cultures have a folklore of home remedies that have been handed down from generation to generation. Some of these may actually be beneficial (e.g., chamomile tea for abdominal pain, as used by Mexican families). Others are pure myths; in rare cases they may be harmful. Physicians should always inquire whether home remedies have been tried prior to coming for care.

Physicians should not scoff at such remedies but try to understand the reasons for using them.

CULTURAL BELIEFS CONCERNING ILLNESS

In many families, illness has special meaning. Being assigned a sick role in a family may have special importance to the patient, or the family may believe that the illness has a nonbiologic cause (e.g., spiritual, supernatural, or mystic). The practitioner who takes the time to explore the cultural beliefs of a family concerning illness is able to understand better what action should be taken to treat the illness and why that action should be taken.

NONTRADITIONAL HEALTH SYSTEMS

Many families have only limited experience with Western medical care. In the past, they may have relied solely on nontraditional systems, including healers or Eastern medicine practices. If in the practitioner's view non-Western healing practices will not hurt the patient, the physician is wise to encourage the dual usage of traditional and Western interventions in order to improve compliance by the adolescent. In fact, utilizing both systems may actually help the adolescent to gradually adapt to Western medicine more fully in future years.

Social Phenomena

Providers should be aware that there are special social phenomena that may influence an adolescent's behavior and, hence, his or her medical behavior. Such issues include immigration status, acculturation, and economic issues.

RECENT IMMIGRATION

Recent adolescent immigrants may view their parents as old-fashioned and rigid. More than other adolescents, these young people may experience parental constraints and pressures that they perceive as unfair and unrealistic. Migrant youth are specifically vulnerable to a particular kind of intrapsychic conflict. They do not wish to bring dishonor to their families by acting against parental expectations, but at the same time they want to adapt to the customs of their new country. Migrant youth may have experienced trauma in the process of arriving in the United States. For example, they may have witnessed the killing of family members or have heard stories of family members who were lost. They might have traveled great distances or resided in inhumane refugee camps. Their parents may have made many sacrifices to bring them to the United States, even leaving some family members behind.

ACCULTURATION

Based on information concerning European immigration in the early part of the twentieth century, it is theorized that by the third generation, immigrant families are completely integrated into the mainstream of American life. But those young people who are in the first or second generation may have a special struggle. These adolescents try to respect their own culture while adapting to a new one. They may be confused by their acculturation and the normal developmental crises of adolescence. As a result, their struggle for socialization and identity formation may be heightened. It behooves the practitioner to gather specific biographical data related to the pre- and postmigration experience. It is important to understand the expectations of the adolescent's parents and to see whether these expectations are providing undue stress upon their adolescent. These principles also apply to adolescents whose families have left established cultural communities to move into mainstream America, for example, Native Americans who relocate from the reservation to urban centers.

ECONOMIC STATUS

Many families take a decided downturn in economic status as a result of immigration to this country. This may be the result of the loss of the breadwinner, the inability to be licensed in one's trade, language difficulties, inability to find work, or lack of familiarity with the work industry. It is particularly difficult for families from farming backgrounds who migrate to urban areas. Loss of socioeconomic status may be a source of shame and confusion for the family as well as the adolescent who may not understand this situation. The family also may not be accustomed to being treated as being impoverished if they had more financial resources in their country of origin. They may feel ashamed because of their need for welfare programs.

Even for families who are not recent immigrants, socioeconomic issues are important. For example, black families historically have valued hard work, education, and social mobility. The impetus for higher education has slowed down in recent years for several reasons, including the social isolation of poor, inner-city blacks, who lack middle-class role models, the changing nature of the economy, and the government's declining commitment to affirmative action. These social changes have created a widening gap between middle-class blacks, who are able to take advantage of educational opportunities, and poor blacks, who are not even aware of these opportunities.

ISSUES RELATED TO CLINICAL CARE

Cultural Biases of Providers

ASSESSMENT VERSUS ASSUMPTIONS

Practitioners of one ethnic group who care for adolescents from another ethnic or racial group must be prepared to face their own biases and prejudices as they assess those adolescents and their families. There are times when providers make unfounded assumptions concerning other cultural groups. These assumptions may be based on their perceptions from the media or on limited previous experiences. The practitioner must recognize the difference between making an assessment of an adolescent and making assumptions about the adolescent and his or her family.

VALUES AND BIASES

Frequently, practitioners have value systems that are different from those of the adolescents for whom they care. Sometimes the differences are based on racial or ethnic backgrounds; other times the differences may be based on the different socioeconomic statuses of providers and the adolescent patient. What is important to the practitioner may not always be important to the adolescent and his or her family. Differences in values may exist between professionals and adolescents in the areas of punctuality, cleanliness, response to pain, sexual conduct, drug use, and family involvement. The practitioner must be capable of acknowledging varying world views and must develop sensitivity to different guidelines of adolescent deportment. This does not mean that the practitioner must compromise his or her own standards of care or value system, but he or she must be capable of acknowledging the adolescent's right to a value system different from the practitioner's.

Cultural Biases of Patients or Parents

Just as practitioners may have biases about adolescent patients, adolescents and their parents may have biases about the provider, particularly if that individual is from an ethnic or racial group different from that of the adolescent and his or her family. In clinical situations, adolescents or their parents may refuse to accept care from a minority practitioner or may presume that a practitioner from a different racial or ethnic group is incompetent or does not know or understand English. The provider should address these issues with the adolescent and the family gently and educate them. Responding with anger or disrespect will not solve the problem, but responding with professionalism and the best medical care may provide the optimum experience for that adolescent and his or her family.

The Use of Interpreters

Everyone is more comfortable if the provider and the adolescent both speak the same language. Unfortunately many practitioners may find themselves limited in their ability to communicate with an adolescent because they do not know the adolescent's language. This means that interpreters must be utilized. The following guidelines are offered when utilizing interpreters in a health care facility.

First, determine whether an adolescent really requires a translator. In other words, would communication, though limited, be more effective without the presence of a third person in the room? Practitioners may be tempted to use a family member as a translator, not realizing that in that situation confidential information might not be obtained successfully. Second, the provider must determine whether the gender of an interpreter will actually encumber the adolescent-practitioner interaction. For example, in Indochinese communities, a young girl may be very reluctant or in fact refuse to share information concerning her personal life (e.g., menstruation) with a male translator. Third, the practitioner should always sit directly across from the adolescent, with the translator seated at an angle, and talk directly to the adolescent or parent, not through the translator. These simple techniques ensure that the adolescent recognizes the desire of the physician to speak directly with him or her.

Medical and Psychosocial Problems of Specific Groups

Those practitioners who are caring for groups of adolescents for whom they have never provided care previously would be wise to familiarize themselves with the mores, health traditions, and the specific medical problems prevalent in that group. For example, practitioners who care for African-American youth should be familiar with the complications of sickle cell anemia and essential hypertension (see Chapters 52 and 67); clinicians who care for Indochinese youth should be aware of hemoglobin E conditions (See Chapter 52).

The influence of social class, education, and poverty on minority groups places them under adverse living conditions that affect their health behavior and outcomes. The depressed economics of the inner-city dwellings, reservations, or migrant camps with substandard housing conditions, overcrowding, and, most recently, the addition of the drug subculture places such individuals at increased risk for poverty-related health conditions.

BIBLIOGRAPHY

Felice ME, Schragg GP, James M, Hollingsworth DR: Clinical observations of Mexican-American, Caucasian, and black pregnant teenagers. J Adolesc Health Care 7:305, 1986.

Fitzpatrick SB, Fujii C, Shragg GP, et al: Do health care needs of indigent Mexican-American, black, and white adolescents differ? J Adolesc Health Care 11:128, 1990.

Gibbs JT, Huang LN: Children of Color: Psychological Interventions with Minority Youth. San Francisco, Jossey-Bass, 1989.

Harlan WR, Harlan EA, Grillo GP: Secondary sex characteristics of girls 12–17 years of age: The U.S. Health Examination Survey. J Pediatr 96:1074, 1980.

Harlan WR, Grillo GP, Cornoni-Huntley J, Leaverton PE: Secondary sex characteristics of boys 12–17 years of age: The U.S. Health Examination Survey. J Pediatr 95:293, 1979.

Johnson J, Fitzpatrick SB, Felice ME: Medical & mental health needs of adolescent Indo-Chinese refugees. Migration World 14:29, 1987.

Martorell R, Mendoza FS, Castillo RO: Genetics & environmental determinants of growth in Mexican-Americans. Pediatrics 84:864, 1989.

Nguyen NA, Williams HL: Transition from East to West: Vietnamese adolescents and their parents. J Am Acad Child Adolesc Psychiatry 28:505, 1989.

Nidorf JF, Morgan ME: Cross-cultural issues in adolescent medicine. Prim Care 14:69, 1987.

Powell GJ (ed): The Psychosocial Development of Minority Group Children. New York, Brunner-Mazel, 1983.

Rotheram-Borus MJ: Ethnic differences in adolescents' identity status and associated behavior problems. J Adolesc 12:361, 1989.

Schutte J: Growth difference between lower and middle income black male adolescents. Hum Biol 52:193, 1980.

Velez CN, Ungemack JA: Drug use among Puerto Rican youth: An exploration of generational status differences. Soc Sci Med 29:779, 1989.

CHAPTER 29

Youth in the Military

MANUEL SCHYDLOWER and WALTER K. IMAI

POPULATION AND DEMOGRAPHICS

Youth in the military represent a microcosm of youth in the United States, with the same socioeconomic, ethnic, cultural, and health backgrounds. However, they are additionally subject to the cultural influences and health risks encountered in areas of the world where they reside. From high school halls and shopping malls of US civilian communities one day, to barracks or foreign territories the following day, youth in the military share more similarities than differences with their civilian counterparts. This chapter focuses mainly on these differences and special features of this population in order to define the best approach to their comprehensive health care.

Adolescents in the military can be categorized into two distinct groups: the 223,000 active duty servicemen and women who are 17 to 19 years old and the dependents of active duty, retired, or deceased military parents. In the latter group, of the more than 1.6 million dependent children eligible for health care in the military, approximately 200,000 are adolescents. Dependents of active duty military personnel are members of Army (45%), Air Force (30%), Navy (20%), and Marine Corps (5%) families. The majority of these dependents (87%) are located in the continental United States, Alaska, Hawaii, and the US territories; those overseas reside with their families, assigned to more than 15 countries, mainly Germany (52%), Japan (10%), United Kingdom (7%), Panama (6%), Philippines (4%), Italy (4%), and Spain (3%). Other hosting countries include South Korea, Belgium, Turkey, Netherlands, Cuba, Greece, Portugal, and Iceland. The distribution of this group varies with US defense requirements related to political changes occurring overseas.

ADOLESCENTS IN UNIFORM

Common Health Problems

The most common health problems encountered in 17- to 19-year-old adolescents on active duty involve

musculoskeletal injuries, occurring mainly during their initial 8 weeks of basic training. The incidence of these injuries is between 25 and 27% for males and 46 and 51% for females. Ninety percent of these injuries occur in the lower extremity, and most represent musculoskeletal overuse conditions, strains, sprains, tendinitis, and stress fractures (see Chapters 79 and 80). The incidence of these injuries in females is twice that in males, with the incidence of stress fractures in females as much as three times higher than that in males. In effect, the overall incidence of injury in trainee populations is slightly higher than that for high school track and cross-country teams and lower than that for contact sports like football and wrestling. The major risk factor for injury in this population appears to be the low physical fitness level on entry to the military (primarily endurance fitness) and not training intensity and may reflect the overall low level of physical fitness among adolescents in the United States.

Asthma is an important disease existing prior to service that is not always identifiable at the military entrance processing station. It is the most common chronic medical problem in youth younger than 20 years of age and results in numerous discharges from the armed services (see Chapter 43).

Immunizations and Infectious Diseases

Youth in the military are among the best immunized adolescent populations in the world owing to free and readily available vaccinations and periodic reviews of their health records to meet travel requirements. Upon entry to active duty, adolescents are vaccinated against measles, rubella, tetanus, diphtheria, meningococcus (groups A, C, Y, and W-135), smallpox, influenza, and adenovirus (types 4 and 7) and later may receive hepatitis B, yellow fever, and typhoid vaccines if they are assigned to locations of high risk for these conditions. In particular, the occurrences of meningococcal disease and upper respiratory infections have significantly decreased in barracks, largely as a result of specific preventive vaccinations.

Human Immunodeficiency Virus Infection

Over a 42-month period from 1985 to 1989, 1,141,164 adolescents (17 to 19 years old) applied for entry to

The opinions or assertions contained herein are the private views of the authors and are not to be construed as official or as reflecting the views of the Department of the Army or the Department of Defense.

military service, and on mandatory testing they showed an overall incidence of human immunodeficiency virus (HIV) infection of 0.34 per 1000. Incidence was greater than 2 per 1000 in urban counties in Maryland, Texas, New York, and the District of Columbia and less than 0.1 in north-central states. They were also higher in blacks (1.00) than in Hispanics (0.29) or whites (0.17). The male-to-female ratio of HIV-infected adolescents (1:1) was lower than those reported among AIDS cases in adolescents (4:1) and adults (9:1) but still reflected the striking proportional excess risk for female adolescents, most likely due to less suspicion of the disease and underdiagnosis, more sexual contact with older infected individuals, and high-risk lifestyles (see Chapter 76).

Substance Abuse

The decrease in incidence of positive drug screens (marijuana and cocaine) from 10% in 1983 to 3% in 1988 and the decrease in incidence of substance abuse in the previous 30 days by service members (including adolescents in uniform) from 27% in 1980 to 4.8% in 1988 could be attributed to the deterrent effect of mandatory drug screening.

The percentage of positive urine specimens also decreased among applicants to the armed services (mostly among 17- to 20-year-old adolescents) from a pilot study high of 7.3% for marijuana and 1.8% for cocaine to 2.4% and 0.9%, respectively, in a subsequent systematic screening program that included advance knowledge that testing would be part of the induction physical examination. Notifying applicants of the drug testing program may deter continued use; however, it may also prompt users to withdraw from the application process or discourage application for military service (see Chapter 111).

Suicide

Reported national ratios of attempted to actual suicides of 100:1 in the 15- to 24-year-old age group are considerably higher than the 3:1 to 23:1 reported in the military. Full employment; preset medical, educational, and mental standards; and the turnover of one fourth to one third of servicemen each year may account for this difference. Age-specific suicide rates in Army populations are generally lower than those for the general US population; however, the rate of 12.8 in 100,000 soldiers 17 to 19 years of age is slightly higher than the national rate of 10.0 for the 15- to 19-year-old age group. The most common stressful problems prior to suicide were difficulties with a loved one (pending divorce, separation, break-up, marital problems, altercation, infidelity); difficulty with job, work, or Army; trouble with the law other than absence without official leave; and financial problems (see Chapter 101).

MILITARY DEPENDENT ADOLESCENTS

Military dependent youth also show excellent vaccination records and high immunity. This group is not subject to mandatory HIV and drug screening, and the incidence of these problems in this group is not known but may be similar to that of adolescents entering active duty. As with adolescents in uniform, they may live in areas of the world where there is a higher risk for conditions such as penicillinase-resistant gonorrhea, AIDS, and hepatitis B. Additionally, if exposed, they may transmit these conditions to adolescent contacts upon their return to the United States, or acquire them when dating affected active duty adolescents returning from high-risk overseas areas. They are also vulnerable abroad to the availability of alcohol without age limitations and to various illicit drugs (amphetamines, sedatives, analgesics) in local drugstores without prescription.

Myth of the Military "Brat"

Previous stereotype labeling of children and adolescents in service-connected families as military "brats" (impudent, unruly) is unfounded. The stressful circumstances of life involving frequent moves and parental absences due to duty requirements are not unique to the military and can cause behavioral and emotional reactions in all adolescents. Reported higher incidences of child abuse and alcoholism in military families, with an expected higher occurrence of adolescent reactive behaviors, are based on more frequent reporting of these situations by the military and readily available access to treatment. Reported lower rates of juvenile delinquency and illicit drug use among adolescents living on military posts may reflect the more restrictive life and environment of the military community. Also, adolescents may feel their freedom of self-expression and experimentation curtailed by a sense of obligation to stay out of trouble and avoid a negative impact on the parent's military status and career. While sensitive to this parental concern, adolescents may react to expected codes of family conduct by either complying with them or angrily defying them, as a normal manifestation of adolescent psychosocial development, whether in a military or a civilian setting.

Transiency

Frequent moves can result in emotional stress, loneliness, and feelings of alienation. In the military setting, reassignment necessitates reestablishing homes and households and to the family is a major economic stress that is not fully offset by salary and allowances. Other significant effects are interruption of education and academic programs and disruption of the spouse's career progression and plans. The military family members are also faced with culture shock stresses when moving overseas or to unfamiliar settings within the United

States. The few studies done in this area are inconclusive, but they suggest that transiency may interfere with developmental progression and may precipitate symptoms without being causative. Comparisons between military dependent youth with and without psychological problems reveal no difference in degree of mobility; however, families with well-adapted children showed positive maternal attitudes to moves and stronger parental identification with the military community. Recent studies suggest that there are no lasting negative effects of relocations on military youth, and that they in fact may provide more growth opportunities and increase coping capacities for most military families. The advantages of increased opportunity for travel and cultural experiences, increased family unity, and development of increased adaptability and interpersonal skills may offset the disadvantages for most military youth. In any case, the differences between civilian and military families may not be as great as once thought. The great mobility of families in the United States in general and the economic and political impetus to stabilize and decrease military overseas assignments combine to make both groups similar. From 1976 to 1982, military mobility went from 60% per year to 33% per year, which approaches the overall population mobility rate of about 25%. In general, there is little evidence of a significant relationship between emotional and behavioral problems and geographic mobility. Mobility appears to be less important than parental attitudes and parents' adaptability to relocation. Nevertheless, adolescents can experience significant stresses if moves occur during developmental stages when continuity of peer group relationships and growing autonomous functioning away from the family are important.

Parental Absence

Absence of the parent has been considered to interfere with the healthy development of the child's personality. Studies link reactions such as anger, denial, guilt, anxiety, fear, and depression to parental absence, most often in sons with an absent father. Stress reactions may occur with both separation and reunion and may be mediated by preexisting father-family relationships; the age, sex, and birth order of siblings; the meaning of the absence to the family; and how the mother copes with the separation. Military service may require frequent absence of a parent. The past 2 decades have seen a shift in the military from primarily an unmarried personnel force to one composed of married service members, working spouses, and single parents, reflecting the changes already taking place in the larger society. Parental absences and separation in military families may be aggravated by combat duty assignments, difficulty in communication accessibility, and having both parents as active duty members. These stresses may be mitigated, however, by support services and programs for families in all branches. Military families tend to be more traditional than their civilian counterparts and are less likely to have a working spouse or a single or divorced parent. Although military fathers may be absent frequently, civilian children are much more likely to be separated

from both parents. Most military family members deal well with the stress of separation, especially if they are well adjusted and prepared, and have available support services. With our present volunteer military, most families continue in this lifestyle by choice.

MISCELLANEOUS ISSUES

Access to Care

One of the benefits of military service is the provision of full medical care at no additional cost to all active duty service members. This care is provided by one of the largest health care systems in the world in terms of number of patients and geographic area covered. The Army, Air Force, and Navy operate interrelated but separate medical systems, ranging from large teaching medical centers to small clinics and medical corpsmen at the troop level. Dependents of active duty service members are also provided care in this system on a space available basis, and utilization is usually heavy for what is perceived as a major benefit of military service. Dependents of retired military personnel, which may include as many as 50% of adolescent patients, have a still lower priority, but access to care for children and adolescents is generally good. Medical care is generally through hospital-based clinics and may be provided by pediatricians, family practitioners, internists, general medical officers, or emergency room physicians in different settings. All services have adolescent medicine specialists, who are usually stationed at the larger medical centers and community hospitals. The Army and Navy operate adolescent medicine fellowship training programs within their graduate medical education system. Care specific to developmental stage is generally much more readily available at the medical centers as compared with the smaller community facilities. Recent developments in dependent health care include general convenience clinics run by civilian contractors. Health care in either setting, including medications and diagnostic procedures, is free of additional cost to the patient. There are minimal economic barriers to health care for teenagers as no fees are charged when they are seen, nor is a bill generated.

Consent and Confidentiality

Doctor-patient confidentiality is protected for all patients in the military health care system. Medical records of dependent adolescents are maintained as confidential by regulation in matters of reproductive care, sexually transmitted disease, and drug abuse, in accordance with civil law and precedent. Where adolescent medicine clinics are operated, teenage patients can uniformly make their own appointments, keep their records confidential, and be seen without a parent present. Lesser degrees of confidential access may exist in general medical settings. In other matters of consent and confidential medical care, the standards of legal and medical practice of the local community generally prevail (see Chapter 20).

Special Areas of Research

Studies are currently under way to identify the best diagnostic measures and preventive strategies to reduce the occurrence of musculoskeletal injuries incurred during basic training. Planned research in this young population also aims at determining the best method for diagnosing hyperactive airways and thus reducing the number of discharges due to asthma existing prior to service. All individuals on active duty, including adolescents, are subject to unannounced mandatory drug testing. There is a need to determine the possible role of compulsory drug testing, separately and together with preventive educational programs, in deterring substance use and abuse among adolescents applying for entry to the military and among those already on active duty. Access to health care is a right for youth in the military, generally available without charge and provided with usually good assurance of privacy and confidentiality. Effectiveness and cost-savings studies of this model of health care delivery may help identify better approaches to ensure this right for all youth in the United States.

BIBLIOGRAPHY

Brundage J, Scott R, Lednar W, et al: Building-associated risk of febrile acute respiratory diseases in Army trainees. JAMA 259:2108, 1988.

Burke DS, Brundage JF, Goldenbaum M, et al: Human immunodeficiency virus infection in teenagers. Seroprevalence among applicants for US military service. Walter Reed Retrovirus Research Group. JAMA 263:2074, 1990.

Centers for Disease Control: Prevalence of drug use among applicants for military service. MMWR 38:580, 1989.

Department of the Army, Headquarters: AR 40-66 Update. Washington, DC, January 31, 1985.

Department of the Army, Headquarters: AR 40-3 Update. Washington, DC, February 15, 1985.

Harrell A, Rayhawk M: Today's military families: A status report. Washington, DC, American Red Cross, 1985.

Jensen P, Lewis R, Xenakis S: The military family in review: Context, risk and prevention. J Am Acad Child Psychiatry 25:225, 1986.

Jones B, Manikowski R, Harris J, et al: Incidence of and risk factors for injury and illness among male and female Army basic trainees. Report No T19-88. Natick, MA, US Army Research Institute of Environmental Medicine, June 1988.

Rodriguez A: Special treatment needs of children of military families. In Kaslow F, Ridenour R (eds): The Military Family: Dynamics and Treatment. New York, The Guilford Press, 1984.

Rothberg J, Jones F: Suicide in the U.S. Army: Epidemiological and periodic aspects. Suicide Life Threat Behav 17:119, 1987.

Sanders J: Health needs of adolescents in the military services. Pediatr Clin North Am 27:183, 1980.

Srabstein J: Geographic distribution of military dependent children: Mental health resources needed. Milit Med 148:127, 1983.

CHAPTER 30

Chronically Ill Youth

ROBERT W. BLUM and GAYLE GEBER

POPULATION AND DEMOGRAPHICS

Estimates from the National Health Interview Survey suggest that more than 2,000,000 children aged 10 to 18 years have some degree of limitation in their school or recreational activities because of chronic health conditions (see Chapter 2). Analyses of these data indicate an increase in prevalence of activity-limiting chronic conditions among children from 1.8% in 1960 to 3.8% in 1981. Since 1970, the increase in prevalence has been due to increases in the less severe forms of limitations. Although the survival of very low birth weight infants has increased over the last 20 years, this has resulted in only modest increases in moderate or severe disabilities in children and youth.

The majority (60%) of adolescents who have disabilities have moderate limitation, 33% have mild limitation, and approximately 7% experience severe disability. Those adolescents most likely to be disabled are younger (10 to 14 years), male, and from low-income families and have parents who have little formal education.

Eighty-four percent of children who have disabilities now survive into adulthood; improvements in technology increase the likelihood that children requiring complex life support systems will live well into their adolescent and adult years (see Chapter 35). Between 1960 and 1988, disease-specific survival rates have improved dramatically. For example, survival rates for cystic fibrosis increased 700%; for congenital heart disease, rates increased 400%; for spina bifida, rates increased 200%; and for leukemia, rates increased 200%.

When viewed from another perspective, the estimated proportion of children with chronic illnesses who survive until age 20 is even more remarkable (Table 30–1).

Reliable prevalence data on the chronic illnesses of youth are difficult to acquire because the conditions have such a low incidence. National Health Interview Survey data, however, provide the following picture of chronic illness in youth ages 10 to 24 years (Table 30–2).

The health services utilization rates for adolescents (10 to 18 years) who have disabilities vary from those of adolescents without disabilities. Those who have disabilities make more visits to physicians annually (8 versus 3) and have more hospital episodes (18 per 100 persons per year vs 4 per 100 persons per year). Further, an estimated 270,000 adolescents who have disabilities (14%) have no health insurance coverage at all (see Chapter 21). The primary reason for lack of insurance is reported to be the high cost of coverage. The resulting financial burden falls either on parents or on the health system in uncompensated care. The economic worries of parents have more than financial consequences. One study of technology-dependent children living at home found that parents receiving Medicaid waiver services (with adequate coverage) experienced less psychiatric impairment than those who had private coverage (with less comprehensive coverage).

There exist other problems with health services utilization for youth who have disabilities. Several studies report a disturbing lack of primary care. Studies in Great Britain found that utilization rates dropped in young adulthood as mandated services ended. Although the British service system differs markedly from that in the United States, it seems likely that the situation here would be no better owing to our lack of transition planning (see Chapter 35).

SPECIAL ISSUES

Physiologic Maturation

The processes of puberty herald a cascade of events associated with adolescence. For healthy adolescents, the process usually occurs between 8 and 16 years of age (see Chapters 4 and 5). For the adolescent with either a chronic condition or a disability, the tempo of puberty is often different from that of peers. Pubertal timing can be influenced by the condition's impact on hypothalamic-pituitary-gonadal functioning, as is seen, for example, in spina bifida; or the impact may be mediated through the condition's impact on nutritional status, such as occurs with Crohn disease (see Chapter 63). With few exceptions, such as virilizing tumors, the process and pattern of physical development remain relatively constant and independent of condition.

Many chronic illnesses are associated with pubertal delay, which is primarily the consequence of gonadotropin deficiency. The list of chronic illnesses associated

The research for this chapter was supported in part by grant #MCJ-2736 (National Center for Youth with Disabilities), Bureau of Maternal and Child Health and Resources Development, Department of Health and Human Services, and grant #H133B90012 (The Center for Children with Chronic Illness and Disability), National Institute on Disability and Rehabilitation Research, Department of Education.

TABLE 30–1. Prevalence Estimates for Selected Chronic Conditions (Birth to 20 Years, United States)*

CONDITIONS	ESTIMATED PROPORTION SURVIVING (%)
Asthma (moderate and severe)	98
Congenital heart disease	71†
Diabetes mellitus	95
Cleft lip/palate	92
Spina bifida	50
Sickle cell anemia	90
Cystic fibrosis	60
Hemophilia	90
Acute lymphocytic leukemia	71‡
End-stage renal disease	90§
Muscular dystrophy	25

*Data from Gortmaker SL, Sappenfield W: Chronic childhood disorders: Prevalence and impact. Pediatr Clin North Am 31(1):3, 1984, with revisions as noted.

†Moller J, Anderson R: 1000 consecutive children with a cardiac malformation: 26–37 year follow-up. Unpublished data, 1991.

‡Birth through 14 years of age. Cancer Statistical Review, NIH Pub. No. 89-2789. National Cancer Institute, May 1989.

§Actuarial 2 year survival data for patients ages 10–19 with end stage renal disease begun on treatment (transplant or dialysis). US Renal Data System, USRDS 1989 Annual Report. Bethesda, MD, NIH, National Institute of Diabetes and Digestive and Kidney Diseases, 1989.

with pubertal delay is extensive; cystic fibrosis, inflammatory bowel disease, and chronic renal disease are several examples (see Chapters 43, 63, and 65). Complicating the condition's impact on pubertal maturation are the effects of certain medications such as corticosteroids, certain cancer chemotherapies, and medications for attentional deficits that may delay pubertal development. Central nervous system tumors, such as craniopharyngiomas (which have their peak incidence between 6 and 15 years of age), and other extrasellar masses encroaching on the hypothalamus can result in pubertal delay, as can germinomas, hypothalamic and optic

TABLE 30–2. Number of Cases and Prevalence of Selected Chronic Conditions for Persons 10 to 24 Years of Age (United States, 1986–1988)

CHRONIC CONDITIONS	CASES*	PREVALENCE (PER 1000 PERSONS)
Deformities or orthopedic impairments	4,874,000	90.8
Asthma	2,696,000	50.2
Hearing impairments	1,425,000	26.6
Visual impairments	1,003,000	18.7
Mental retardation	698,000	13.0
Arthritis	633,000	11.8
Speech impairments	561,000	10.5
Epilepsy	273,000	5.1
Diabetes mellitus	218,000	4.1
Paralysis of extremities (complete or partial)	97,000	1.8
Cerebral palsy	65,000†	1.2†
Cleft palate	46,000†	0.9†
Malignancies—all sites	21,000†	0.4†
Spina bifida	11,000†	0.2†
Multiple sclerosis	9,000†	0.2†

*Based on total population of 10- to 24-year-olds of 53,654,000.

†Does not meet standards of statistical reliability.

Source: National Center for Health Statistics: National Health Interview Survey. Unpublished data.

gliomas, astrocytomas, and occasionally chromophilic adenomas.

In addition, a wide range of conditions is associated with precocious puberty (see Chapter 58). Conditions such as polyostotic fibrous dysplasia, neurofibromatosis, neural tube defects such as spina bifida, and hypothalamic and pituitary tumors all may be associated with physical precocity.

Whether delayed or precocious, pubertal changes have profound social and emotional consequences for all youth (see Chapters 57 and 58). Girls who have precocious development face substantial stigma, which frequently predisposes them to name-calling, social isolation, depression, and withdrawal. Males who have delayed maturation may face similar consequences. Both adolescent females and males who have chronic illnesses have greater somatic preoccupation than do their peers. This concern translates into more questions and worries about height, weight, body changes, and appearance. For those whose development is delayed, a persistent question is "Am I normal?" For those whose development is later than that of their peers, a persistent lament is "Treat me according to my age, not my appearance."

The interrelations among pubertal maturation, body-image, and self-esteem have been well described through both research and anecdotal reports. Although it is critical for the health professional to separate the adolescent from his or her illness (e.g., the person is not a leukemic but rather an adolescent who has leukemia), it is also important to remember that for adolescents who have chronic conditions, identity is intricately related to those specific conditions.

Social messages that bombard adolescents daily serve only to further reinforce differences between healthy and chronically ill adolescents. One need only look briefly at television or magazines to see our social images of beauty. One way of diminishing such conflict is to limit contact with peers with comparable conditions or to suppress those distinguishing aspects of the condition that are controllable. It is common to see the adolescent who has cystic fibrosis who suppresses his or her cough or the adolescent who has diabetes mellitus who violates his or her diet so as not to be conspicuously different from peers. Although the health costs of these behaviors may be significant, the social costs of nonconforming to youth are great (see Chapter 26).

Likewise, it is not surprising that the social values and norms of beauty and acceptability for those who have chronic illnesses tend to parallel those of their nondisabled peers. Original research in this area has suggested a near uniformity of perspective regarding a "hierarchy of acceptability" between those with and without disabilities. However, such findings recently have been challenged, since in the "real world" it is questionable whether a hierarchy of preference of one type of disability over another has much meaning. It has been suggested that social preferences of children (both disabled and nondisabled) are related in part to the functional capability of the individual coupled with the social environment within which the disability is viewed. For the individual who has the condition, one key factor in moderating the negative body-image and diminished self-esteem is social support from parents and friends.

Research on burn-injured adolescents has indicated that the social environment can moderate a negative sense of self.

Body-Image

An adolescent's sense of self does not develop within a social vacuum. How the adolescent views himself or herself is profoundly influenced by environment, medical condition, age, and gender. Studies of chronically ill youngsters who have cystic fibrosis and sickle cell disease have found that chronically ill young people have poorer body-image and self-image than do well adolescents. Poorer body-image is not synonymous with psychopathology. In comparing teenagers who have asthma, cancer, and cystic fibrosis with non-ill peers, one study found few differences between chronically ill females and their well female counterparts. There is little evidence of greater psychopathology in most groups of chronically ill adolescents.

One study suggested that for every condition studied, the adolescent male has more somatic disturbance than does his female counterpart. Perhaps the impact of the condition on pubertal development rather than the direct impact of the condition itself predisposes those with certain conditions to have disturbance of body-image. If this is the case, adolescent boys rather than girls would have body-image distortion for those conditions that result in pubertal delay, since such delay appears to be more threatening to male self-esteem. This hypothesis has yet to be tested.

Social and Emotional Development (see Chapter 121)

One of the most psychologically devastating realities experienced by youth who have chronic illness is social isolation. While all indicate that they have a "best" friend, many such friendships are limited to a kind word in the school corridor or a smile in class. Most have fewer, more superficial friends and have less contact with friends than do their nondisabled peers.

With few friends, loneliness is the norm; and loneliness is often associated with depression. The high rates of depression associated with a variety of chronic conditions have been well documented. Contrary to conventional wisdom and still not confirmed by all studies, adolescents who have the greatest medical morbidity may not experience the greatest degree of emotional distress. Rather, at greatest risk may be those who have less visible or more minimal sequelae of the condition who risk healthy psychological development as they try to pass for being healthy. Perhaps this occurs in part because such adolescents are always striving "to pass" as healthy and feel that they are living a lie. Perhaps those who have severe involvement have been forced earlier in life to "look into the mirror" and come to terms with their limitations.

This lack of any peer or social group reference is very distressing. One 18-year-old young woman who had spina bifida with only a slight gait disturbance said it eloquently:

You don't understand what it's like—it's like living in no man's land. For kids with spina bifida, I'm able-bodied and I'm not one of them. For kids without spina bifida, I'm handicapped and I'm not one of them. I've got no group to turn to. I'm all alone.

Although loneliness and depression are common for adolescents who have chronic conditions, they are not universal phenomena. In addition, not all lonely youth who have chronic illnesses are maladapted. Most display independence comparable to that of non-ill peers. Most appear to cope quite well despite greater life uncertainties and more loss of personal control than their peers. Most are psychologically normal, and some even speak of the unique perspectives that are the results of living with illness:

Before I got sick I would do everything my friends did without even stopping to think. Now I don't have the energy any more and I have to pick and choose. You know—there are a lot of things they do which are pretty dumb.

Factors associated with resilience (successful coping) among chronically ill adolescents, particularly regarding their social and emotional development, include
Family and peer support,
Self-perception as not handicapped,
Involvement with household chores,
Having a network of friends,
Having friends who are not disabled or ill as well as some who are, and
Parental support without parental overprotectiveness.

Sexual Development

While the timing of puberty may vary significantly among youth who have chronic illnesses and disabilities, their social and sexual drives parallel those of nondisabled adolescents. In a recent study of adolescents who have spina bifida and adolescents who have cystic fibrosis, although it was rare for adolescents to date (6.9% of the entire sample), three of four hoped to marry, and more than two of three anticipated having children.

As the aspirations of chronically ill youth parallel those of able-bodied adolescents, so too are their needs comparable. Turner has identified seven core sexual health issues important to adolescents who have disabilities:

1. Personal hygiene
2. Menstruation
3. Sexually transmitted diseases
4. Birth control
5. Marriage
6. Masturbation
7. Premarital sex (sexual activity)

In addition, sexual orientation should be added to the list, for although it is known that 1 in 10 nondisabled adolescents express ambiguity on this issue (see Chapter 32), there is no literature on homosexuality or sexual orientation in teenagers who have chronic illnesses. Clearly, homosexuality does exist among these young people, but for many, social isolation, constant parental supervision, and lack of peer contact make sexual exploration more complicated than it is for their able-bodied peers.

There is usually very little communication between parents and chronically ill adolescents on sexual issues. Although this is often the case for nondisabled youth as well, data suggest that it is even more extreme for youth who have disabilities. In one study of youth who have spina bifida and cerebral palsy, only one third of adolescents who have spina bifida and fewer than one half of adolescents who have cerebral palsy had discussed puberty with a parent. For girls, a little more than one half had ever discussed menstruation. Most recalled the discussion to be brief, embarrassing, and uninformative.

Several studies have shown that youth who have chronic and disabling conditions have a markedly diminished knowledge of sexual health issues when compared with their peers. Likewise, parents believe they are ill-equipped to be the sex educators of their adolescents who have chronic illnesses and disabilities.

For adolescents, unanswered questions persist, with their needs falling into five general categories:

1. General sexual information: the anatomy and physiology of reproduction.
2. Emotional aspects of sexuality: how to know when you're "ready"; the social aspects of courtship.
3. Sexual techniques: the "how to's" of sexual relationships and safe sex techniques.
4. Genetics: the risks to offspring.
5. Contraception, if the youngster is heterosexual.

For those with limitations due to chronic illness or disability, sex education should include the following:

1. Information that is developmentally and cognitively appropriate and specific for the chronic condition—including reproductive physiology, menstruation, sexually transmitted diseases, safe sex techniques, contraception, and prevention of sexual assault.
2. Education that teaches the role that touch plays in discriminating appropriate from inappropriate behavior.
3. Education that teaches the social skills that enhance same gender and heterosexual friendships.

FAMILY ISSUES

Families of adolescents who have disabilities face ever-changing challenges. Chronicity does not in any sense imply predictability. Nor, however, does the presence of a chronic illness or disability imply inevitable dysfunction due to family disorganization. As youth with disabilities move through adolescence, they and their families experience both normative and illness-related stressors that tap family strengths. When unsettling illness-related events (e.g., relapse, marked disintegration in functional status, or lack of needed services) occur, families may appear to experience profound disruption, when in fact they simply may be working through a complex series of shifts in roles, boundaries,

and communication styles that will lead to a fully functional adaptation. The cost of care in terms of both direct and indirect lost opportunities and the burden of care on all family members can be major challenges. Families may become socially isolated.

Concerns that naturally accompany disabilities are integrated into the family's organizational structure and process and may be a source of conflict with typical adolescent and family developmental needs. Fear of death with a life-threatening illness may complicate family cohesion; time-intensive treatments (e.g., cystic fibrosis treatments) may constrain the adolescent's sense of independence; and family communications may be impaired at a critical developmental stage (e.g., if family members of a deaf adolescent have not mastered sign language).

For optimal development to occur, every adolescent who has a chronic illness or disability needs an individualized independence plan—a plan developed with adolescents and parents that begins in childhood and is focused on self-care and social mastery skills as well as the adolescent's progressive independence from the family and the family's independence from the adolescent. If the plan is developed in childhood and carried out through the adolescent years, chronically ill youth are more likely to be socially competent by adolescence than if such planning does not occur.

Families are at risk for dysfunction during transition periods as their usual patterns of functioning are disrupted and a new sense of balance is sought. During this transition, situational demands often exceed the family's capacity to respond. During times such as these, professional support and access to social services are even more critical than usual to help the family adjust to the new situation. For optimal family functioning to result, a balance must be reached between the ever-changing situation and the psychological need for stability. Support can be provided by acknowledging the family's central role and by linking family members with appropriate support services. It should never be forgotten that the family is the structure within which development occurs and that no one knows the adolescent better than his or her parents.

EDUCATION

Youth who have chronic illnesses miss more school than do their peers. Even chronically ill youth without functional impairments miss significantly more school than those without chronic illnesses. Some youth who have chronic illnesses or disabilities, however, may have conditions that do not directly affect school achievement.

Psychosocial problems are associated with missed school days, particularly when accentuated by chronic illness or disability. In addition, some chronically ill youth have other problems, such as transfers between classes, reduced cognitive function due to medications, and increased risks of exacerbation of the condition from avoiding treatments (see Chapter 26). This situation is exacerbated at times by teachers' lack of understanding of chronic illnesses and the adjustments chron-

TABLE 30–3. Secondary School Completion Status of Special Education Students 2 Years after Leaving School

DISABILITY CATEGORY	GRADUATED (%)	DROPPED OUT (%)	AGED OUT* (%)	SAMPLE SIZE
Speech impaired	62.7	32.5	4.8	222
Visually impaired	69.5	16.8	13.7	279
Deaf	71.8	11.8	16.4	354
Hearing deficit	72.3	15.5	12.2	249
Orthopedically impaired	76.5	15.6	7.9	246
Other health impaired	65.4	25.9	8.7	142
Multiply handicapped	32.2	17.6	50.2	182
Deaf and blind	43.1	7.8	49.2	45

*Past the mandatory age for school attendance.

Adapted from Wagner M, Shaver DM: Educational Programs and Achievements of Secondary Special Education Students: Findings from the National Longitudinal Transition Study. Menlo Park, CA, SRI International, 1989, p 187.

ically ill students must make, even given many teachers' extensive experience with students who have these very conditions.

Not all students who have chronic illnesses require or receive special educational services. Those who are eligible include students who have speech, hearing, or visual impairments; mental retardation (see Chapter 31); serious emotional disturbances; orthopedic impairments; multiple handicaps; learning disabilities; autism; and limitations in health, strength, vitality, or alertness. Those students who have a specific learning disability are also eligible for special education or related services as a result of their impairments. Determining which students with chronic illnesses need these special educational services is difficult. Thus, medical advocacy is often crucial for a child to receive the services he or she needs.

An array of educational and health-related services are legislated by Public Law 94-142, the 1975 Education for All Handicapped Children Act, which mandated a free, appropriate education in the least restrictive environment. This education is to be facilitated by Individualized Education Plans (IEPs) written for each student with consultation from professionals, parents, and the students themselves. Among others, this law helped to establish the special needs of individuals who have disabilities as civil rights issues. A 1981 government report on disparities in access to special education identified secondary school students and 18- to 21-year-olds as underserved groups (see Chapter 35). In 1983, an amendment to the original law was passed (PL 98-199) to establish and fund services to assist in the transition of students from school to work and the community. Further, the vocational education of young adults was aided by the Carl Perkins Vocational Technical Education Act of 1984 (PL 98-524), which mandated the development or expansion of high-quality vocational educational programs with a 10% "set aside" for individuals who have disabilities. Together, these laws establish the legally mandated services within which education takes place. If the goal of education in general is to help students achieve their potential and live successfully in the community, educating students who have disabilities or chronic illnesses can best be accomplished in a varied and flexible environment supported by individualized educational and vocational transition planning.

Public Law 94-142 established a wide array of services available to children and youth within schools to ensure that every child has access to the least restrictive educational environment. Such services include speech or language therapy; personal counseling or therapy; occupational therapy or life skills training; help from a tutor, reader, or interpreter; physical therapy or mobility therapy; hearing-loss therapy; and help in getting or using transportation.

For youth who have chronic illnesses, the problem with PL 94-142 lies in the vagueness in the legislation regarding which conditions are covered under the legislation and which are excluded. Additional debate has focused on which services are legislatively mandated. Schools are reluctant to provide and fund certain health services (e.g., intermittent catheterization), believing that these services are in the health, rather than the educational, domain. On the other hand, the health sector will not fund services that they believe the educational system should be providing. What is evident, though, is that of all special education students, youth who have chronic illnesses or speech impairments are least likely to receive additional services.

Compounding the standoff between the health and educational sectors regarding service provision responsibilities is a general lack of communication among physicians, nurses, and teachers in the student's individual educational planning. There may be a lack of communication between parents and teachers about the adolescent's participation in school. There is little agreement between parents and teachers on the need for special education services, and it diminishes proportionately with decreased parental education and income.

Although the percentage of college freshmen with disabilities rose from 2.6% in 1978 to 7.4% in 1985, this participation rate is slightly lower than what would be expected given barrier-free access. Many students who have disabilities drop out of school before ever reaching postsecondary educational institutions. These dropout rates vary markedly by disability, with multiply handicapped students showing the lowest graduation rates (Table 30–3).

There is also substantial variability in postsecondary education participation by students who have disabilities, yet this is indicative of admirable perseverance on the part of many highly challenged students (Table 30–4).

TABLE 30–4. Post-secondary Education Participation of Special Education Students (1985–1986)*

DISABILITY CATEGORY	ANY POST-SECONDARY INSTITUTION	VOCATIONAL OR TRADE SCHOOL	2-YEAR COLLEGE	4-YEAR COLLEGE	SAMPLE SIZE
Speech impaired	29.3	7.0	19.3	8.3	83
Visually impaired	42.1	2.9	15.2	27.5	110
Deaf	38.5	7.0	19.0	15.2	154
Hearing deficit	30.1	11.6	12.7	7.0	101
Orthopedically impaired	28.0	9.0	10.4	9.5	108
Other health impaired	30.7	13.2	12.1	7.6	65
Multiply handicapped	3.8	.9	4.0	.2	77
Deaf and blind	8.3	8.8	0.0	0.0	27

*Source: Parent reports.

Adapted from Wagner M: The Transition Experiences of Youth with Disabilities: A Report from the National Longitudinal Transition Study. Menlo Park, CA, SRI International, 1989, p 188.

Not surprisingly, the reasons for dropping out of school also vary by disability. When parents of adolescents who have disabilities were asked why their children dropped out of high school, one third of those with orthopedic impairments and one half of those with other health impairments cited illness-related concerns (Table 30–5). Far fewer parents of children who have other disabilities gave this reason, which is evidence apparently that although educational issues may be adequately addressed in school, health issues are not, and the consequences for the affected students are substantial.

Perception of disability is another important factor in dropout rates. Students who consider themselves handicapped over the course of their high school years have higher dropout rates than students who consider themselves handicapped for a short period of time or who do not identify themselves as handicapped at all. Although self-perception is important, disability status appears not to predict whether students pursue any type of postsecondary education within 2 years of high school.

EMPLOYMENT

When compared with their peers, youth who have chronic illnesses are found to have fewer or less definite career plans. A small but significant proportion of youth experience major problems resulting from career choices that accentuate the disabling condition. According to 1988 self-report data, 3.8% of the population ages 16 to 24 years had a work disability (4.1% for males, 3.6% for females). The US Department of Commerce defines people having a work disability as those people with a condition resulting from a physical or mental illness that affects the kind or amount of work they can do, or

TABLE 30–5. Reasons for Dropping out of School among Youth with Disabilities (as Cited by Parents)*

REASON FOR DROPPING OUT	SPEECH IMPAIRED	VISUALLY IMPAIRED	HEARING DEFICIT	DEAF	DEAF AND BLIND	ORTHOPEDICALLY IMPAIRED	OTHER HEALTH IMPAIRED	MULTIPLY HANDICAPPED
Percentage of youth reported by parents to have dropped out of secondary school because of:								
Pregnancy/ childbearing	0.0	24.0	34.2	15.4	a/	0.0	2.0	0.0
Poor grades, not doing well in school	30.0	15.7	12.6	11.3	a/	15.6	8.9	0.0
Wanting/needing a job	0.0	0.0	7.0	.0	a/	0.0	0.0	0.0
Moving	10.0	0.0	1.5	2.6	a/	4.2	4.2	0.0
Didn't like school	41.7	29.9	25.6	38.6	a/	21.5	19.6	17.9
Illness/disability	4.2	16.4	13.3	3.5	a/	32.7	49.1	39.6
Behavioral problems	12.1	0.0	3.3	2.6	a/	0.0	4.9	4.4
Didn't get in desired program	0.0	5.3	3.8	2.6	a/	0.0	0.0	10.3
Other	40.6	17.2	29.1	40.9	a/	34.4	18.5	50.3
(Number of respondents)	(19)	(14)	(24)	(20)	(2)	(21)	(16)	23

*Some parents cited more than one reason, so percentages do not total 100.

a/ Numbers too small to report.

Adapted from Butler-Nalin P, Padilla C: Dropouts: The Relationship of Student Characteristics, Behaviors, and Performance for Special Education Students. Menlo Park, CA, SRI International, 1989.

people younger than 65 years who are covered by Medicare or receive Supplemental Security Income.

In the Department of Commerce study, both the general labor force participation rates and the specific rates of those working full-time year-round were found to be lower for youth who have disabilities than for nondisabled youth. Work disabilities also affect earnings. For all 16- to 24-year-old workers in 1987, the mean earnings were $6,463 for males who have a work disability and $7,851 for those without; the comparable earnings for females were $4,910 for those with a work disability and $6,403 for those without. (Caution should be used in interpreting these data, however, because of the small numbers reported.)

While the United States Department of Commerce data are not distinguished by type of disability or educational services received, other studies demonstrate which disabilities affect hourly wages and the ability to work full-time.

Some rather disturbing trends are noted for special education youth who have disabilities, based on the length of time that they have been out of school. For some disabilities, students are more likely to be working full-time within 1 year of leaving school than they are when more time has elapsed. The average rate of pay per hour for employed youth in a few disability categories follows the same trend. Overall, wages are low and occupations have relatively low status.

Although not the original mission of the Department of Vocational Rehabilitation (DVR) throughout the United States, there is need now for the DVR to work closely with schools so as to facilitate the transition of students with disabilities into employment. To achieve this goal, a reorientation in DVR philosophy will be needed at the national and state levels, for vocational services currently tend to be provided later than is optimal. For example, of those students who do receive DVR services and successfully complete the program,

only 40% were referred from elementary or secondary schools. Clearly, there is need for closer collaboration between special education and vocational rehabilitation services to ease students with disabilities into employment settings. In addition to better interagency coordination, improved services for youth are needed, for only three of five successfully complete the vocational rehabilitation program.

BIBLIOGRAPHY

Anderson EM, Clark L: Disability in Adolescence. New York, Methuen, 1982.

Blum R (ed): Chronic Illness and Disability in Childhood and Adolescence. New York, Grune & Stratton, 1984.

Blum R, Resnick M, Nelson R, St. Germaine A: Family and peer issues among adolescents with spina bifida and cerebral palsy. Pediatrics 88:280, 1991.

Gliedman J, Roth W: The Unexpected Minority: Handicapped Children in America. New York, Harcourt, Brace, Jovanovich, 1980.

Hobbs H, Perrin JM, Ireys HT: Chronically Ill Children and Their Families. San Francisco, Jossey-Bass, 1985.

Offer D, Ostrov E, Howard K: Body image, self-perception, and chronic illness in adolescence. In Blum RW (ed): Chronic Illness and Disabilities in Childhood and Adolescence. New York, Grune and Stratton, 1984, pp 59–73.

Owings J, Stocking C: High School and Beyond: A National Longitudinal Study for the 1980's: Characteristics of High School Students Who Identify Themselves as Handicapped. Washington, DC, US Department of Education, Office of Educational Research & Improvement, 1985.

Phaneuf J: Considerations on deafness and homosexuality. Am Ann Deaf 132:52, 1987.

Turner E: Attitudes of parents of deficient children toward their child's sexual behavior. J School Health 40:548, 1970.

Wagner M, Shaver DM: Educational Programs and Achievements of Secondary Special Education Students: Findings from the National Longitudinal Transition Study. Menlo Park, CA, SRI International, 1989.

Wallace HM, Biehl RF, Oglesby AC, et al (eds): Handicapped Children and Youth. A Comprehensive Community and Clinical Approach. New York, Human Sciences Press, 1987.

CHAPTER 31

Mentally Retarded Youth

JOSEPH L. RAUH

POPULATION AND DEMOGRAPHICS

The teenager who has a developmental disability presents a multitude of challenges to the adolescent health care provider. *Developmental disability* currently is defined as a severe, chronic disability that

1. is explained by a mental and/or physical impairment,
2. is present before age 22 and is likely to continue indefinitely,
3. results in substantial functional limitations in three or more of these areas of major life activity: (a) self-care; (b) receptive and expressive language; (c) learning; (d) mobility; (e) self-direction; (f) capacity for independent living; and (g) economic self-sufficiency, and
4. reflects a need for individually planned and coordinated interdisciplinary care and treatment.

This chapter will focus on disorders and problems associated with mental retardation and will reflect the author's experience with a special interdisciplinary diagnostic and management program in adolescent medicine and developmental disabilities in Cincinnati, Ohio.

Mental retardation is characterized by significantly subaverage cognitive functioning, that is, full-scale intelligence quotient (IQ) of 70 or below on an individually administered IQ test *and* concurrent deficits or impairments in adaptive behavior for age. Mental retardation may be mild, moderate, severe, or profound. Almost 90% of adolescents with mental retardation have a mild degree of retardation (IQ between 50 and 70); they constitute 1% to 3% of the population, or approximately one-half million youth in the United States.

Generally, the diagnosis of mental retardation has been well established in early school life, and parents realize long before puberty that their child is cognitively delayed. Often there is a quiescent period during the elementary school years when the child seems to make modest progress in a special education program and can be easily managed at home. As puberty begins, the teenager becomes adult in size, and the family often becomes concerned about his or her behavior, socialization, and vocational future. Also, adolescence is a time when issues of guilt, despair, grief, and fear of the future, repressed for many years, suddenly are reawakened in the parent.

SPECIAL ISSUES

For most adolescents, the etiology of mental retardation cannot be established. For those conditions that are understood, some information is known about the onset of puberty and the medical and psychosocial characteristics at adolescence. Table 31–1 presents information for conditions that have been associated with mental retardation in some adolescents.

Parents and nonmedical professionals are most likely to approach the physician with the following questions:

1. How can we address specific medical problems such as seizures or irregular menses?
2. Why isn't he starting or progressing in pubertal development?
3. How can we control behaviors at home and school and in the community?
4. Why is she not progressing in school?
5. How independent can he be? Is she employable? How should we plan for her long-term care?
6. Can she marry and have children? Can she be protected from sexual abuse and unwanted pregnancy? Can he, or should he, have any kind of sexual life?

It cannot be overemphasized that the adaptive level and social skills of the teenager are the best indicators of future functioning, especially in late adolescence and adulthood. Many mildly retarded teenagers may be able to function close to the normal range once they are out of the school and into a vocational or task-oriented setting. The following case illustrates this point:

Vickie, now 35, was first seen at age 13 because her mother believed she was not retarded and puberty had not begun. She had always attended a classroom for developmentally handicapped children. She had several distinguishing physical findings—short stature, multiple flat congenital hemangiomas, a right sensorineural hearing loss, mild scoliosis, and lymphedema of her lower extremities. Vickie's findings were not indicative of any dysmorphic or genetic syndrome. Her adaptive skills were excellent; her parents had encouraged independence and self-help skills and had taught her sewing and cooking at an early age. Her cognitive abilities were delayed.

Vickie menstruated at 17 years of age. She married at 18 years, was divorced at 20, and started full-time employment as an office cleaner at 21 years. She remarried at 26 years of age, after requesting and receiving a tubal ligation. Both Vickie's husbands had developmental delays. The second marriage has prevailed, and Vickie continues to support herself and enjoy many family and social activities.

Vickie had strong family support during childhood and adolescence, and as a result, her adaptive skills were considerably higher than was her cognitive level. Marriage was possible, but it was challenging. Her choice of contraception is not used frequently today, but tubal ligation can be an option if appropriate legal review, medical review, and implementation process are followed.

Adolescents with mental retardation often have serious difficulty in finding competent, caring health care providers. Few primary care residency training programs for physicians provide adequate attention to adolescent patients with developmental disabilities. The physician caring for adolescents with mental retardation does need to learn and utilize the basic knowledge and skills of the allied disciplines (Table 31–2) and to know how to interpret and communicate this information to patients and their families. Physicians need to provide adequate time for these patients and their families. Sometimes the primary care physician must coordinate complicated medical and behavioral problems that involve other medical specialists in fields such as neurology, orthopedics, psychiatry, dentistry, nutrition, physiatrics, occupational therapy, and physical therapy. Close communication with an interdisciplinary team is vital to optimal care of mentally retarded adolescents (see Table 31–2).

Special health needs include dental problems, the use of psychotropic medications, and sexuality issues. Dental problems may be secondary to the underlying medical condition or due to use of seizure medications such as Dilantin (phenytoin), injury to the teeth from trauma or falls, or lack of dental care (see Chapter 41).

Parents may inquire about the use of psychotropic medications, especially for teenagers with moderate and severe retardation. Although they can be helpful in certain situations, such drugs must be used cautiously and for limited time periods with specific objectives. For example, Mellaril (thioridazine), in initial doses of 50 to 100 mg/day, and Haldol (haloperidol), in initial doses of 0.5 to 3 mg/day, have been used to help young people with volatile mood swings, severe temper outbursts, and

TABLE 31–1. Conditions Associated with Mental Retardation in Adolescents

AUTISM/PERVASIVE DEVELOPMENTAL DISORDER
Etiology: Unknown; may occur in association with other syndromes
Onset of Puberty: Normal, or depends on syndrome
Psychosocial Consequences and Behavior: The main area of difficulty is with language and interpersonal relationship abnormalities; adolescents may become withdrawn
Clinical Problems: Self-care difficulties and self-mutilation; outwardly destructive tendencies; seizures; problems related to associated syndromes
Intelligence Quotient (IQ): 80% mentally retarded, but wide variability
Incidence: 4:10,000 to 5:10,000

CEREBRAL PALSY
Etiology: Central nervous system insult in the pre- or perinatal period, or unknown
Onset of Puberty: May be early or normal
Psychosocial Consequences and Behavior: Social discrimination depending on level of involvement, especially if speech is affected
Clinical Problems: Worsening orthopedic difficulties such as progressive scoliosis; seizures; drooling; self-care difficulties
IQ: Varies from profound retardation to superior range
Incidence: 2:1000

DOWN SYNDROME
Etiology: Trisomy of chromosome 21; 3% have translocation of chromosome 21
Onset of Puberty: Normal; hypogonadism and infertility usually in males; final adult height reached around 15 years
Psychosocial Consequences and Behavior: Obvious physical features of Down syndrome may cause social discrimination; at risk for depression; poor coordination
Clinical Problems: Residual congenital heart disease with pulmonary hypertension; thyroid abnormalities; atlantoaxial instability; hearing and vision problems; increased frequency of mitral valve prolapse and aortic regurgitation; periodontal problems; infections, especially skin and respiratory. Increased risk of earlier onset of Alzheimer's disease
IQ: Moderate mental retardation, but usually IQ of 50 to 60, with social performance beyond that expected
Incidence: 1:660 to 1:1000

FRAGILE X SYNDROME
Etiology: Break point on X chromosome at Xq27.3
Onset of Puberty: Normal; macro-orchidism in some prepubertal and most postpubertal males
Psychosocial Consequences and Behavior: Occasional autistic-like features; behavior problems; hyperactivity; language deficits
Clinical Problems: Mitral valve prolapse; dilatation of the ascending aorta
IQ: Usually 30 to 55, but may be higher or lower; possible decline in IQ over time
Incidence: Unclear. >1:1000 males; 1:1000 females are carriers, and 1:3000 females are affected

MENINGOMYELOCELE
Etiology: Neural tube defect during early fetal development
Onset of Puberty: May be as early as 7 years or normal
Psychosocial Consequences and Behavior: Spectrum of disability (minimal or obvious if in brace or wheelchair, with subsequent social discrimination); social concerns if incontinent of urine or bowel; sexual function concerns; increased dependency issues if more disabled; learning disabilities; perceptual problems
Clinical Problems: Weight gain; loss of previous function such as ambulation with tethered cord; worsening renal disease; shunt dysfunction; arthritic changes; chronic restrictive lung disease; constipation; urinary tract infection
IQ: 25% mental retardation, average IQ estimated to be 80 to 90
Incidence: 4.3:10,000

NEUROFIBROMATOSIS
Etiology: Mutation of NF locus on chromosome 17 (type 1 NF)
Onset of Puberty: Early or normal
Psychosocial Consequences and Behavior: Possible visible deformities and cosmetic disfigurement, with resultant social discrimination; increased incidence of learning disabilities, perceptual problems, attention deficit disorders, and speech impediments
Clinical Problems: Tumors, especially involving the central nervous system (CNS); long bone and spine abnormalities; hypertension; headaches; seizures; constipation; pruritus
IQ: 2% to 5% in the mentally retarded range; average IQ is 88
Incidence: 1:3000

PRADER-WILLI SYNDROME
Etiology: In many patients, deletion of chromosome 15
Onset of Puberty: Usually delayed; small penis and cryptorchidism in males; diminished secondary sexual development in females who may be amenorrheic; frequent hypogonadism
Psychosocial Consequences and Behavior: Poor coordination; may have increased behavior problems during adolescence; bizarre eating patterns and foraging for food, with social consequences of morbid obesity
Clinical Problems: Obesity that can cause sleep apnea and can be life-threatening; consider need for testosterone replacement in males
IQ: Range 20 to 80, but usually 40 to 60
Incidence: 1:10,000

WILLIAMS SYNDROME
Etiology: Unknown
Onset of Puberty: May be early
Psychosocial Consequences and Behavior: Short stature may result in social discrimination; loquacious personality and may have inappropriate friendliness; immature; poor perceptual-motor skills; social problems if enuretic
Clinical Problems: Cardiac, vascular, and renal abnormalities; hypertension; musculoskeletal difficulties with joint limitation; thyroid abnormalities; hypercalcemia
IQ: Range 40 to 80
Incidence: 1:20,000

**TABLE 31–2. Discipline-Specific Focus for Multidisciplinary Evaluation
of Mentally Retarded Adolescents**

DISCIPLINE	AREA OF ASSESSMENT	SUGGESTED INSTRUMENTS	OBJECTIVES
Medicine	Physical development Medical status Etiology	History and neurodevelopmental screening, physical examination, laboratory studies	Understand physical growth and medical status
Social work	Family strengths and weaknesses	Individual and family interview	Assist adolescent and family with social, independent living skills
Psychology	Cognition	Kaufman Assessment Battery for Children Wechsler Intelligence Scale for Children (Revised) Stanford-Binet Intelligence Scale (Fourth Edition) Differential ability scale	Obtain information regarding cognitive potential
	Adaptive behavior	Vineland Adaptive Behavior Scales Child behavior checklist AAMD Adaptive Behavior Scale	Determine skills related to independent living and societal expectations
	Emotional status	Thematic apperception test, tasks of emotional development Children's apperception test The house, tree, person drawings	Perceptions of emotional outlook
Communication (speech and hearing)	Communication skills	Peabody Picture Vocabulary Test (Revised) Clinical evaluation of language fundamentals Expressive one-word vocabulary test Test of adolescent language	Receptive and expressive language skills, pragmatics, communication, competency for daily living experiences
Special education	General knowledge School-related	Woodcock-Johnson Psycho-Educational Battery (Revised) Test of Written Language–2 Kaufman Test of Educational Achievement	Skills correlating with academic expectations, general knowledge, and ability to function independently

outward or self-destructive behavior. Cogentin (benztropine), in doses of 1 to 2 mg/day, or Benadryl (diphenhydramine), in doses of 25 to 50 mg/day, probably should be added initially to the phenothiazines to prevent dystonic reactions. Careful consideration and possibly consultation should be used before prescribing psychotropic medications, since they have been overused in the past for chemical restraint and carry the risk of potentially irreversible tardive dyskinesia. Ritalin (methylphenidate) or other psychostimulants may be helpful for borderline or retarded adolescents who demonstrate evidence of attention deficit hyperactivity disorder based on the *Diagnostic and Statistical Manual III-Revised* (DSM-IIIR) criteria. Other medications that have been beneficial to adolescents with mental retardation and severe behavior problems include lithium carbonate or lithium citrate, Tegretol (carbamazepine), Inderal (propranolol), clonidine, Ativan (lorazepam), and antidepressants such as Tofranil (imipramine).

Sexuality concerns are frequent. Additional information about sexuality is contained in Chapter 30. Anxiety or fear about sexual abuse and pregnancy of mentally retarded youth is almost universal among the caretakers of these adolescents. One half of the young women with mild retardation attending our program in 1982 were sexually active; 32% of those who were moderately retarded and 9% of those who had severe retardation had had intercourse. One third of the adolescents who were mildly retarded and one fourth of the adolescents who were moderately retarded had been victims of rape or incest (see Chapter 119).

Oral contraception can be used by adolescents who are mildly retarded and who have excellent social and adaptive skills. Those with severe retardation cannot comply, and few will be able to use the barrier methods. Intrauterine devices, although successful in selected adolescents in our program a decade ago, have no place among any adolescents now because of medical complications when sexually transmitted infections occur. Injectable medroxyprogesterone acetate (MPA) (Depo-Provera) can be very effective as a contraceptive and menstrual suppressant when given in an intramuscular dosage of 150 mg every 3 months. Parents of our MPA users reported above average satisfaction. Breakthrough bleeding is the chief side effect and reason for discontinuance (see Chapter 73). Levonorgestrel implants (Norplant) may prove even more useful as experience is gained with this form of contraception in adolescents.

Attitudes about sterilization for adolescents with mental retardation vary widely among health providers, yet a high percentage of parents in our program favor a state statute that would enable sterilization under certain conditions and limitations. Caretakers frequently ask about sterilization, and care providers should be knowledgeable about their state statutes, court decisions, and the presence of a defined judicial process in their state.

Teenagers with developmental delays, like their normally developing peers, need to learn appropriate sexual behavior. It is possible to teach most adolescents with mild and moderate retardation about parts of the body, physical development, peer and family relationships, vulnerability to community risks, stranger avoidance, and appropriate peer communication skills. This individualized instruction can be done by any interested adult who is comfortable with the sexual needs of youth with developmental disabilities. This instruction should start as soon as possible, preferably before adolescence, and continue through the adolescent years.

Appropriate visual aids, including three-dimensional models, are helpful educational adjuncts. Role-playing social situations that might occur in real life, including being approached by strangers and being touched inappropriately, is very useful. It should be emphasized that we provide this instruction only if the parent or caretaker is willing to participate in each session and will repeat and reinforce the instruction at home.

MISCELLANEOUS ISSUES

Developmentally delayed adolescents have one advantage in the United States that teenagers with normal intelligence do not enjoy—political power. Parents and professionals responsible for children with special needs have made remarkable legislative progress in the past 3 decades; Congress has enacted more than 20 statutes related to disability issues. By far the most important law, the Education for All Handicapped Children Act, also known as Public Law 94-142, was passed in 1975. Please see Chapter 30 for details.

Adolescents with developmental disabilities and their families need many educational, social, recreational, vocational, financial, and legal services. Physicians are frequently asked to assist with the transition to adult employment and medical services. Referenced below are several national directories with listings by geographic or service area. Care providers obviously need to keep up with local organizations and the network they compose in their own communities. Parent support groups are a source of support in many communities.

Acknowledgments: The author is grateful to Drs. Lucia Horstein, William Klykylo, Celia Neavel, Sonya Oppenheimer, Bonnie Patterson, and Jack Rubinstein, and Vicki Jahns, M.Ed., for their contributions to this chapter.

RESOURCES AND DIRECTORIES

General

A Guide to Selected National Genetic Voluntary Organizations. January 1989, The National Center for Education in Maternal and Child Health (NCEMCH), 38th and R Streets, NW, Washington, DC 20057. (202) 625-8400.

Children with Special Health Care Needs, A Resource Guide. February 1990, The National Center for Education in Maternal and Child Health (NCEMCH), 38th and R Streets, NW, Washington, DC 20057. (202) 625-8410. Single copies available at no cost.

Clinical Programs for Mentally Retarded Children. December 1985, DHHS Publication # (HRSA) HRS-D-MC-85-1. (202) 625-8400.

Directory of National Information Sources on Handicapping Conditions and Related Services. June 1986, US Department of Education, Office of Special Education and Rehabilitative Services, National Institute of Handicapped Research, 400 Maryland Avenue, SW, Washington, DC 20202. (202) 732-1134. For sale by the Superintendent of Documents, US Government Printing Office, Washington, DC 20402. (202) 275-3648.

Exceptional Parent. Published eight times a year by Psy-Ed. Corporation, 30 Broad Street, Denville, NJ 07834. (800) 247-8080. $18.00/year.

Education for All Handicapped Children Act (P.L. 94-142): Preserving Both Children's and Teacher's Rights. American Federation of Teachers, AFL-CIO, 555 New Jersey Avenue, NW, Washington, DC 20001. (202) 879-4400. Ask for Item No. 436. Single copy free; $5.00 for 100 copies.

Parent Resource Directory for Parents and Professionals Caring for Children with Chronic Illness or Disabilities, 3rd Edition. February 1989, Association for the Care of Children's Health, 3615 Wisconsin Avenue, NW, Washington, DC 20016. (202) 244-1801 or (202) 244-8922.

Reaching Out: A Directory of National Organizations Related to Maternal and Child Health. March 1989, National Center for Education in Maternal and Child Health (NCEMCH), 38th and R Streets, NW, Washington, DC 20057 (202) 625-8400.

Resource Guide (1989) to Organizations Concerned with Developmental Handicaps. American Association of University Affiliated Programs, 8630 Fenton Street, Suite 410, Silver Spring, MD 20910. (301) 588-8252.

Sexuality

National Association for Retarded Citizens, 2509 Avenue J, P.O. Box 6109, Arlington, TX 76006. (817) 640-0204.

SIECUS (Sex Information and Education Council of the US), 1855 Broadway, New York, NY 10023. (212) 673-3850.

Stanfield House, 900 Euclid Avenue, Santa Monica, CA 90403. Write for a list of films available. (800) 421-6534. In CA call collect (213) 395-7466.

BIBLIOGRAPHY

American Academy of Pediatrics, Committee on Bioethics: Sterilization of women who are mentally handicapped. Pediatrics 85:868, 1990.

Baroff GS: Mental Retardation: Nature, Cause, and Management, 2nd ed. Washington, DC, Hemisphere Publishing Corporation, 1986.

Blum RW: Developing with disabilities: The early adolescent experience. In Levine MD, McAnarney ER (eds): Early Adolescent Transitions. Lexington, MA/Toronto, Lexington Books, 1988, pp 177–192.

Chamberlain A, Rauh J, Passer A, et al: Issues in fertility control for mentally retarded female adolescents: I. Sexual activity, sexual abuse, and contraception. Pediatrics 73:445, 1984.

Ehlers WH, Prothero JC, Langone J: Mental Retardation and Other Developmental Disabilities, A Programmed Introduction, 3rd ed. Columbus, OH, Charles E. Merrill Publishing Company, 1982.

Jones KL: Smith's Recognizable Patterns of Human Malformation, 4th ed. Philadelphia, WB Saunders, 1988.

Levine MD, Zallen BG: The learning disorders of adolescence: Organic and nonorganic failure to strive. Pediatr Clin North Am 31:345, 1984.

Levine MS, Rauh JL, Levine CW, et al: Adolescents with developmental disabilities: A survey of their problems and their management. Clin Pediatr 14:25, 1975.

Magrab PR: A primer for interpreting psychological test results. Pediatr Ann 11:470, 1982.

Passer A, Rauh J, Chamberlain A, et al: Issues in fertility control for mentally retarded female adolescents: II. Parental attitudes toward sterilization. Pediatrics 73:451, 1984.

Rauh JL, Dine MS, Biro FM, et al: Sterilization for the mentally retarded adolescent: Balancing the equities/The Cincinnati experience. J Adolesc Health Care 10:467, 1989.

CHAPTER 32

Gay and Lesbian Youth

ROBERT J. BIDWELL and ROBERT W. DEISHER

POPULATION AND DEMOGRAPHICS

Most lesbian and gay youth, like their heterosexual peers, are ordinary teenagers from ordinary families living ordinary lives. For the most part, their struggles around sexual orientation are invisible, even to their own families. Yet, there is something unique in the experience of growing up gay or lesbian in our society. This is reflected, in part, in a recent report on youth suicide by the US Department of Health and Human Services, which found that gay youth are two to three times more likely to attempt suicide than are their heterosexual peers and estimated that perhaps 30% of all teen suicides may be related to conflicts over sexual orientation (see Chapter 101).

Sexual identity, in its simplest terms, can be defined as having three aspects. The first, core morphologic identity, is an individual's basic sense of being male or female. The second, gender role behavior, refers to the congruence between an individual's behaviors and society's behavioral expectations for each gender. The third, sexual partner orientation, refers to a persistent pattern of sexual attraction to persons of the same or opposite gender. The foundations of all three aspects are generally believed to be well established before adolescence. It is only in sexual partner orientation that gay and lesbian teenagers differ from heterosexual teenagers. Another sexual minority, transsexual adolescents, may be even more confused and isolated than are gay and lesbian teenagers, as they feel that they are males or females trapped in the body of the opposite gender. Finally, whereas most adults engaging in transvestitism are heterosexual and cross-dress for erotic rather than identity reasons, a minority of gay and lesbian teenagers may adopt cross-dressing as a means of expressing their sexual orientation.

It is now generally accepted that a homosexual orientation neither is chosen by the individual nor seems to be due primarily to parental influences on the child or adolescent (as has been expressed in the early "dominant mother–passive uninvolved father" theories). Biologic and prenatal influences have recently been given more consideration, although no conclusive evidence is available. The discredited yet still widely held belief that gay and lesbian adolescents are somehow responsible for their sexual orientation often creates feelings of guilt and reinforces the rejection they face from parents,

peers, and society. Likewise, the increasingly disputed theories of parental influence on adolescent homosexuality have led to much self-recrimination and guilt among parents of gay and lesbian teenagers.

The dangers of identifying oneself or being identified by others as gay or lesbian are real and immediate. These teenagers risk rejection by family, friends, school, church, and society at large. Many have been subjected to verbal, physical, and sexual violence. Some have been forced to leave their homes or have run away from home and school to a life on the streets, where involvement in prostitution and substance use is commonplace (see Chapter 33). This in turn leads to the risks of pregnancy, sexually transmitted diseases, violence and abuse, and entrance into the juvenile justice and foster care systems (see Chapters 34, 74, 75, 118, and 119).

Most gay and lesbian adolescents, however, are "invisible," neither fitting the stereotypic notions of what it means to be gay or lesbian nor choosing to reveal their sexual feelings to others. They, too, face very real dangers. School dropout, family conflict, withdrawal from peers, substance abuse, and other acting-out behaviors are the common responses of any teenager faced with fear, isolation, anger, and guilt. More frequently, a large number of adolescents simply decide not to deal with homosexual feelings and concentrate instead on schoolwork, athletics, or other pursuits, thereby experiencing a developmental moratorium around a fundamental part of their identity. Some turn to heterosexual relationships in an attempt to deny underlying homosexual feelings or in order to "pass" among peers and family. Many gay and lesbian adolescents see their futures, in terms of relationships, parenthood, and career, as predetermined or limited by their sexual orientation. A significant number of gay and lesbian teenagers view suicide as their only alternative (see Chapter 101).

The prevalence of homosexual behaviors among adolescents is uncertain. Kinsey, Pomeroy, and Martin, in their classic studies of human sexuality, found that 8% of men and 4% of women were exclusively homosexual for at least 3 years between the ages of 16 and 55. More recently, Sorenson reported that 17% of males and 6% of females had had one or more homosexual experiences by 19 years of age. It is currently estimated that approximately 10% of the population of the United States is gay or lesbian.

Sexual behaviors, however, may or may not reflect underlying sexual orientation. Adolescence is a time of experimentation and self-discovery. Some adolescents who engage in homosexual behaviors may be predominantly heterosexual as adults. At the same time, it is clear that a homosexual orientation is the natural developmental outcome for some teenagers. It may well be that a sizable proportion of teenagers who are coming to terms with a gay or lesbian identity have never been homosexually active or, perhaps, have only been heterosexually active.

SPECIAL ISSUES

Most gay and lesbian youth have the same general medical needs and problems as do their heterosexual peers. They are at special risk for several medical problems, however, because of the dangers of growing up gay or lesbian and because of the nature of various homosexual behaviors. It should be remembered that few adolescents will identify their sexual behaviors and sexual feelings, even on direct questioning. Often they will not even acknowledge existing signs and symptoms of sexually transmitted diseases (STDs) (see Chapter 75) for fear of revealing their sexual orientation. This failure to disclose sexual behaviors may be due to personal denial, fear of physician disapproval, or simply a lack of the vocabulary or insight necessary to discuss their sexual orientation.

Sexual behaviors do not necessarily reflect sexual orientation. For example, some gay and lesbian teenagers may be heterosexually active, and others, although they are deeply aware of their homosexual orientation, may never have had sex with a person of either gender. Practitioners **must** be aware of their own discomfort in talking about sexual activity, and especially sexual orientation, with their adolescent patients. Probably the greatest barrier to the provision of care to gay and lesbian adolescents is the practitioner's reluctance to discuss sexual orientation with his or her adolescent patients.

History and Physical Examination

The history obtained at any one visit may depend on the patient and on the context of the visit. The history should include information on reasons for concerns about sexual identity, external concerns, internal concerns, and sexual experience, as shown in Table 32–1. The discussion that follows considers the sexual history specifically.

The physician should take sufficient time to establish rapport before pursuing sensitive questions related to sexual orientation. However, questions about sexual orientation and sexual behaviors should be asked of all teenagers and at regular intervals throughout their adolescent years. A nonjudgmental, accepting demeanor on the part of the practitioner maximizes patient openness. Terms about sexuality and sexual behavior should be mutually comfortable and understandable. One should not presume the gender of dating or sexual partners during questioning. Asking the question "Do you have a girlfriend?" of a gay male adolescent, for example, may give the unintended message that the

TABLE 32–1. Elements of a Sexual History

Reasons for concerns about sexual identity
    Feelings and fantasies
    Experiences
External concerns
    Family
    Peers
    School
    Support systems
Internal concerns
    Comfort with perceived identity
    Degree of isolation
    Evidence of depression: social withdrawal, declining school
        performance, substance abuse, runaway behavior, suicidal
        ideation, health (e.g., AIDS)
Sexual experience
    Sexual practices and frequency of sexual contacts
    Nature and numbers of sexual partners
    Location of sexual encounters
    History of prostitution or sexual assault
    History of sexually transmitted disease and previous treatment
    Symptoms of sexually transmitted disease or trauma from
        present sexual practices
    Use of condoms and lubricants
    Use of alcohol or other substances before or during sexual
        activity
    Other medical conditions associated with homosexual behavior
        (see Table 32–2)

Adapted from Bidwell R: The gay and lesbian teen: A case of denied adolescence. J Pediatr Health Care 2:3–8, 1988.

practitioner is not open to discussing the teenager's boyfriends. Finally, it is important to remember that because most gay and lesbian teenagers will not acknowledge their sexual orientation, the history alone may not be a reliable guide in conducting the physical examination or in providing anticipatory guidance.

A comprehensive sexual history is essential to the medical evaluation of gay and lesbian adolescents. Questioning should take place within the context of a complete medical history and move from less threatening to more sensitive areas, as shown in Table 32–1.

One might begin questioning a teenager, for example, by asking "Have you ever dated anyone?" This could be followed by "Have you ever had sex with another person?" If either question is answered affirmatively, one should inquire further, "Are the persons you date/have sex with male, female, or both?" Practitioners often fail to ask this question of teenagers because of their own discomfort, or because they fear an adolescent will react negatively. Teenagers sometimes may express disapproval of the idea of homosexual behavior, but rarely do they withdraw from the interview when the subject is addressed. One way of softening the impact of this line of questioning is to preface the question as follows: "Among my teenage patients, there are some who have sex with girls, some with boys, and some who have sex with both. Can you tell me with whom you've had sex?" Whether or not they are able to acknowledge their homosexual behaviors or attractions, these patients now know they are not alone and that the practitioner is someone to whom they can talk, when they are ready to do so.

Once gay or lesbian teenagers acknowledge homosexual behaviors, it is important to define the nature of their sexual experience (see Table 32–1). Among areas to explore are the sexual practices and frequency of sexual contacts; the nature of the sexual partners (anonymous, casual, long-term, substance-using, prostituting); numbers of sexual partners; location of sexual encounters (at home, parks, baths); a history of prostitution or sexual assault; sexually transmitted diseases (STDs) and previous treatment; types of behaviors engaged in (e.g., anal intercourse, oral-genital sex); the use of condoms and lubricants; use of alcohol or other substances before or during sexual activity; and medical conditions (Table 32–2).

Table 32–2 outlines clinical conditions related to homosexual activity. The signs and symptoms of STDs and trauma secondary to sexual practices in both male and female adolescents should be explored (see Chapter 75). All homosexually active male adolescents should have regular screenings for gonococcal (urethral, rectal, and oral) and chlamydial (urethral, rectal) infection (Table 32–2). Screening frequency depends on the kinds and the degree of sexual activity. A serologic test for syphilis, such as the Venereal Disease Research Laboratory (VDRL) test, should be performed (see Chapter 75). Evidence of immunity to hepatitis B should be sought, and if not present, hepatitis B vaccine should be administered to all homosexually active males and non–sexually active males who acknowledge being gay. Human immunodeficiency virus (HIV) antibody testing should be seriously considered for all homosexually active males, since treatment of some asymptomatic HIV carriers with zidovudine is now recommended (see Chapter 76). Such testing should be confidential and accompanied by education and counseling appropriate to the developmental and experiential background of the in-

TABLE 32–2. Clinical Conditions Related to Homosexual Behaviors

Male
Urethritis and epididymitis (*Neisseria gonorrhoeae, Chlamydia trachomatis, Mycoplasma hominis,* herpes)
Hepatitis B
HIV infection
Dermatologic disorders
    Ulcerative (syphilis, chancroid, herpes)
    Papular (venereal warts)
    Diffuse (tinea cruris, scabies, pubic lice, molluscum contagiosum)
Oropharyngeal disease (*N. gonorrhoeae, C. trachomatis,* herpes)
Gastrointestinal disorders
    Proctitis (*N. gonorrhoeae, C. trachomatis,* herpes, syphilis)
    Proctocolitis (*Shigella* spp., *C. trachomatis, Entamoeba histolytica, Campylobacter* spp.)
    Enteric syndromes (*Salmonella* spp., *Giardia lamblia, E. histolytica, Cryptosporidium* spp., *Isospora* spp., cytomegalovirus)
Traumatic
    Anal fissures
    Rectosigmoid tears
    Hemorrhoids
    Allergic proctitis
    Penile edema
    Inhaled nitrite burns

Female
Vaginitis (especially nonspecific vaginitis)

Adapted from Zenilman J: Sexually transmitted diseases in homosexual adolescents. J Adolesc Health Care 9:129–138, 1988.

TABLE 32–3. Principles of Counseling Gay and Lesbian Youth

Assure confidentiality
Be supportive and nonjudgmental
Avoid labeling
Provide role models
Address myths and stereotypes
Discuss "safer sex" guidelines
Provide supportive resources: books, films, support groups
Allow time for self-definition and acceptance by self and others
Validate both homosexual and heterosexual identities as healthy and natural

Adapted from Bidwell R: The gay and lesbian teen: A case of denied adolescence. J Pediatr Health Care 2:3–8, 1988.

dividual adolescent. The practitioner is cautioned to understand the legal implications of HIV testing in one's state, especially among minors. Treatment of STDs is discussed in Chapter 75.

Lesbian adolescents, if they and their sexual partners have not been heterosexually active, are unlikely to encounter STDs. However, both *Trichomonas* and *Gardnerella* vaginitis have been reported in lesbians with a history of only homosexual contact, although whether or not they are sexually transmitted is uncertain. It should be remembered that some young lesbians may have been heterosexually active, and appropriate STD evaluations and contraceptive counseling should be done. Lesbians, like other women, are susceptible to both breast cancer and cervical cancer. Therefore, they should be taught breast self-examination and have annual pelvic examinations with Papanicolaou smears.

MISCELLANEOUS ISSUES

The major goal in counseling adolescents coping with sexual identity issues is to help them mature into a healthy adulthood by anticipating and developing strategies to cope with society's general disapproval of homosexuality. General guidelines for counseling are outlined in Table 32–3.

Counseling can usually be accomplished through the provision of information and support by a caring and accepting health practitioner. The purpose of counseling is not to make a "diagnosis" or to change the young person's orientation. It is, rather, to convey the message to each teenager that whatever one's sexual orientation, one can lead a healthy and fulfilling life.

In counseling, it is important, first of all, to determine whether a gay or lesbian identity is seen as a problem or as an asset by the teenager. Gay and lesbian teenagers may have experienced harassment, abuse, or rejection by family, peers, teachers, and others. Also, many find their newly recognized sexual attractions in direct conflict with deeply held religious or moral values. Others are relatively comfortable with their gay or lesbian identity but may be troubled by relationship problems, career indecision, or sexual dysfunction. Adolescents belonging to ethnic minority groups may be especially isolated and doubly stigmatized (see Chapter 28).

Much of the confusion and distress gay and lesbian adolescents experience is due to lack of information about homosexuality. The practitioner should determine what being gay or lesbian means to the teenager and correct any misconceptions, myths, or stereotypes. Gay and lesbian teenagers should understand that their feelings are natural and not a matter of "something gone wrong." They should be informed that they are not alone in their feelings and that gay and lesbian people are a part of their everyday life. Positive role models in history and in the community should be identified and recognized. One should avoid easy and inappropriate reassurances such as "It's just a phase," which will alienate any teenager who is struggling with deep feelings. It may be helpful to remind the adolescent who may fear the implications of stereotypes that he or she defines what it means to be gay or lesbian rather than the converse.

Anticipatory guidance is essential for the teenager who is beginning to cope with a gay or lesbian identity. Medical counseling should include the nature of homosexual behaviors and any attendant risks. Both gay and lesbian teenagers should be aware of "safer sex" principles, which include avoiding anal intercourse, using condoms during intercourse to avoid the exchange of body fluids, and decreasing the number of sexual partners. It should be remembered that almost none of the information on AIDS presented in school curricula addresses the special needs and concerns of homosexual youth. Teenagers should be aware of the alternative forms of sexual expression such as intimate touch and masturbation. Most important, teenagers must be given an opportunity to discuss and practice skills in negotiation and decision-making related to sex and other high-risk behaviors.

Psychosocial issues should also be addressed. Gay and lesbian teenagers need guidance on how to handle harassment and discrimination, how to "come out" to parents and friends, and how to meet other gay and lesbian teenagers and explore dating relationships. Most important, however, the practitioner should help teenagers see their futures as being open to all possibilities and not limited in any significant way by their sexual orientation.

Finally, gay and lesbian teenagers should be introduced to supportive community resources. Larger cities may have gay and lesbian teen discussion groups, which provide teenagers with opportunities to socialize in a safe environment with other teenagers. Several books have been written for gay and lesbian teenagers and their parents. Practitioners might keep a small library of these in their offices. (See resource list at end of chapter.) Some physicians do not feel comfortable caring for gay youth. They might consider referral of those patients to colleagues who are more comfortable than they are.

Parents who discover that their teenager is gay or lesbian are filled with conflicting emotions, including guilt, shame, anger, fear, and grief. Their needs are similar to those of their adolescent. They should understand that their adolescent's sexual orientation is not a choice, nor is it a result of deficient parenting. The interpretation and meaning of homosexuality and a gay or lesbian identity must be explored with the teenager's parents; misconceptions about homosexuality should be corrected. Many parents will ask the practitioner to help change their adolescent's sexual orientation. The lack of proven effectiveness, the questionable ethics, and the dangers of such therapies should be discussed. Parents, like their teenage sons or daughters, need time to develop acceptance and understanding of homosexuality. Some parents never reach this point. However, all parents should be encouraged to allow their teenagers the space they need for self-discovery by providing a home environment of love and support. They should be made aware of the very real dangers to life and health for teenagers who are rejected by their families. Supportive resources such as books, pamphlets, and information about parent support organizations should also be provided. The Federation of Parents and Friends of Lesbians and Gays (ParentsFLAG), P.O. Box 27605, Washington, DC 20038, has chapters in many communities.

RESOURCES FOR ADOLESCENTS, PARENTS, AND PROVIDERS

Fairchild B, Hayward N: Now That You Know: What Every Parent Should Know About Homosexuality. San Diego, CA, Harcourt Brace Jovanovich, 1979.

Hanckel F, Cunningham J: A Way of Love, A Way of Life: A Young Person's Introduction to What It Means To Be Gay. New York, Lathrop, Lee and Shephard, 1979.

Hunt M: Gay: What Teenagers Should Know About Homosexuality and the AIDS Crisis. New York, Farrar, Straus, Giroux, 1987.

BIBLIOGRAPHY

Green R: Sexual Identity Conflict in Children and Adults. New York, Basic Books, 1974.

Johnson SR, Guenther SM, Laube DW, et al: Factors influencing lesbian gynecologic care: A preliminary study. Am J Obstet Gynecol 140:20, 1981.

Kinsey AC, Pomeroy WB, Martin CD: Sexual Behavior in the Human Male. Philadelphia, WB Saunders, 1948.

Kinsey AC, Pomeroy WB, Martin CD: Sexual Behavior in the Human Female. Philadelphia, WB Saunders, 1953.

LeVay S: A difference in hypothalamic structure between heterosexual and homosexual men. Science 253:1034, 1991.

Remafedi G: Adolescent homosexuality: Psychosocial and medical implications. Pediatrics 79:331, 1987.

Remafedi G: Homosexual youth: A challenge to contemporary society. JAMA 258:222, 1987.

Remafedi G: Sexually transmitted diseases in homosexual youth. Adol Med: State of the Art Reviews 1:3, 1990.

Robertson P, Schachter J: Failure to identify venereal disease in a lesbian population. Sex Transm Dis 8:75, 1981.

Sorenson RC: Adolescent Sexuality in Contemporary America. New York, World Publishing, 1973.

US Department of Health and Human Services: Report of the Secretary's Task Force on Youth Suicide. Washington, DC, US DHHS, 1989.

CHAPTER 33

At-Risk Youth

RICHARD G. MacKENZIE

POPULATION AND DEMOGRAPHICS

At-risk youth in this context refers to young people who participate in a number of high-risk behaviors (i.e., running away, living on the streets, dropping out of school, early sexual activity, substance use, and antisocial behavior) that compromise their physical and mental health. The risk status of homeless and runaway youth generally increases the longer they are on the streets. Delivery of clinical health services to this unique group of young people demands an approach that appreciates their vulnerability and recognizes that their distrust of authority and institutions will lead to avoidance and delays in seeking service.

The United States Department of Health and Human Services estimates the number of runaway youth (12- to 21-year-olds) to be between 730,000 to 1.3 million nationally. Although many return home within 30 days, approximately 25% will become permanently homeless (see Chapter 2). For more than one half of those who run away from home, physical or sexual abuse, or both, in the home or by family members is the precipitating cause (see Chapters 118 and 119). Others are encouraged to leave, are forced to vacate, or are abandoned because of family stress, marital discord, or the adolescent's disruptive behavior. Most who leave home are not seeking adventure but are looking for a resolution of an intolerable situation, usually as the result of a highly dysfunctional family. Many who are unable or choose not to return home gravitate to "magnet" cities, where a migrating subculture supports their new-found independence through marginal activities and high-risk lifestyles. Others remain within a 30-mile radius of home and blend into the runaway and street subculture of the nearest town or city.

A period of adaptation lasting days to weeks occurs, during which the young person develops ways of satisfying his or her basic needs—food, shelter, clothes, and so forth. The need for acceptance, security, trust, support, and sense of control governs much of the young person's decisions. Assimilation occurs as the ways of the street are learned. Many runaways are minors who are educationally impoverished, school dropouts, and without work experience; they turn to illegal activities for survival. Recent estimates suggest that 75% of street-committed youth engage in illicit activity, and approximately 50% are involved in prostitution (survival sex).

Increasing commitment to this lifestyle, negotiation of relationships that are mutually beneficial, and manipulation of social institutions for survival are the hallmarks of ultimate acculturation, that is, that point at which rescue becomes increasingly difficult.

Approximately 50% of these youth have significant alcohol problems. Eighty percent use or have used illicit drugs, 30% to 40% intravenously. Limited shelter space forces these youth to sleep in vacated buildings ("squats," "galleries," "houses"), in parks, on the streets, under freeway overpasses, or wherever else they can find some degree of comfort, safety, and security. Exposure to the weather, environment, and their fellow homeless compounds an already desperate situation. To continue to survive and to satisfy their basic physical needs, approximately two thirds participate in illegal activities such as drug dealing or drug running, survival sex, pornography, petty theft, and burglary or armed robbery. Some, particularly females, will exchange sex for drugs to sustain a habit or desired state of consciousness. The risks of unprotected sex are apparent in increased rates of sexually transmitted diseases (STDs), including human immunodeficiency virus (HIV) infection and syphilis, and pregnancy (see Chapters 74, 75 and 76). Contraceptive use is the exception rather than the rule in this population (see Chapter 73).

SPECIAL ISSUES

Trapped by life circumstances and limited resources, runaway and homeless youth enter into a number of health-compromising but developmentally directed behaviors. These survival behaviors escalate the risk of disease. Paradoxically, access to health care services is often limited by availability, expense, and sensitivity on the part of providers to the special needs of this population. Delayed medical care and lifestyle factors tend to amplify existing health problems. Homeless youth have multiple health problems that originate from the interplay of biologic, psychoemotional, and social factors. These may be grouped into seven areas: nutrition, substance abuse, mental health problems, dental problems, medical complaints (especially those related to exposure and hygiene), sexuality-related medical concerns, and problems related to victimization and abuse. Table 33–1 lists these common problems of runaway and homeless youth.

A noncategorical, integrated approach to health care

TABLE 33–1. Common Problems of Runaway and Homeless Youth

NUTRITION
  Poor intake
    Unaffordable
    Secondary to emotional problems (e.g., depression)
    Secondary to drug use (e.g., cocaine, methamphetamine)
    Chronic illness
    Vitamin deficiencies
    Anemia
  Excess loss
    Diarrhea
    Infections
SUBSTANCE ABUSE
  Detoxification/intoxication
  Habituation and dependence
  Medical problems related to
    Alcohol use
    Cocaine/crack
    Methamphetamine
    Nicotine/marijuana inhalation
  HIV risk
  Intravenous drug use
  Violence
MENTAL HEALTH PROBLEMS
  Depression
  Suicidal ideation and attempt
  Psychoses (especially schizophrenia, manic depressive disorder)
  Personality disorders (especially borderline and psychopathic
    deviance)
  Psychoneuroses (anxiety, depression)
  Sexual identity crisis
  Acting out
DENTAL PROBLEMS
  Gingivitis
  Caries
  Absent teeth
MEDICAL COMPLAINTS
  Skin problems (acne, impetigo, dermatophytosis, insect bites and
    infection, pediculosis, scabies)
  Upper/lower respiratory infections
  Asthma, tuberculosis
  Gastrointestinal complaints
  Hepatitis
  Exposure
  Poor hygiene
  Musculoskeletal complaints
  Immunizations (status unknown)
  Psychosomatic disorders
SEXUALITY-RELATED MEDICAL CONCERNS
  Sexually transmitted diseases (most common: infections with
    Neisseria gonorrhoeae, Chlamydia trachomatis, human
    papillomavirus, and herpes simplex virus, and syphilis)
  Pelvic inflammatory disease
  HIV infection and AIDS
  Pregnancy
  Menstrual disorders
  Sexual dysfunction
  Need for contraception
VICTIMIZATION AND ABUSE
  Physical and psychological trauma
  Rape
  HIV risk
  Sexual exploitation
  Risk of violent behavior

thus developed that recognizes these forces and the role they play. A hierarchical approach to identification has been proposed (Fig. 33–1). This model has several advantages. The entry symptom is the first to be addressed, and the provider appropriately focuses on the concerns of the young person. Rapport is established between the young person and the provider in an area of expertise of the health care provider and the concern of the teen. Attention is then focused on the underlying circumstances and forces that may contribute to or are the source of the presenting complaint. Questions are asked in the context of the presenting complaint. Key principles in interviewing and providing health care to the homeless or runaway teen include

1. A nonjudgmental attitude
2. Assurance of confidentiality, except for state-mandated limitations (i.e., sexual abuse, suicide, homicide)
3. Psychosocial evaluation at each visit
4. Recognition and focus on survival needs (food, shelter, security) at each visit
5. Inclusion of other team members early in problem identification
6. Maximal intervention with each visit, rather than reliance on a follow-up appointment

A logical approach to risk assessment has been proposed that utilizes the acronym HEADS (Fig. 33–2). This method has the advantage of not only providing consistency and relevancy but also exploring issues systematically, from the usually less sensitive to the more heavily charged. Documentation in the records follows the format of the physical examination findings, permitting easy retrieval and updating.

Many homeless and runaway adolescents have been forced into lifestyles and activities for survival (e.g., pornography, prostitution, drug dealing) that they find denigrating and embarrassing. Shame or guilt is unlikely to effect behavioral change. Many have come to distrust

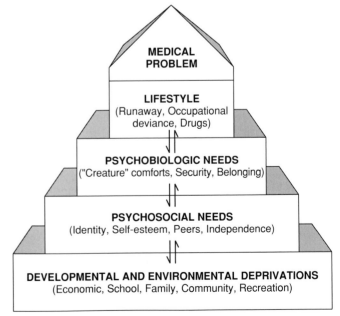

Figure 33–1. Model of integrated health care for high-risk youth.

has been shown to optimize each clinical contact with this population. The medical complaint usually serves as the entry point into the system of care. Those factors that expose, contribute to, or perpetuate the complaint are simultaneously identified. A management plan is

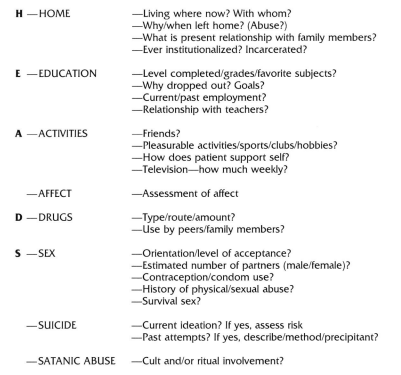

H — HOME	— Living where now? With whom?
	— Why/when left home? (Abuse?)
	— What is present relationship with family members?
	— Ever institutionalized? Incarcerated?
E — EDUCATION	— Level completed/grades/favorite subjects?
	— Why dropped out? Goals?
	— Current/past employment?
	— Relationship with teachers?
A — ACTIVITIES	— Friends?
	— Pleasurable activities/sports/clubs/hobbies?
	— How does patient support self?
	— Television — how much weekly?
— AFFECT	— Assessment of affect
D — DRUGS	— Type/route/amount?
	— Use by peers/family members?
S — SEX	— Orientation/level of acceptance?
	— Estimated number of partners (male/female)?
	— Contraception/condom use?
	— History of physical/sexual abuse?
	— Survival sex?
— SUICIDE	— Current ideation? If yes, assess risk
	— Past attempts? If yes, describe/method/precipitant?
— SATANIC ABUSE	— Cult and/or ritual involvement?

Figure 33–2. Adolescent risk profile (HEADS). (Courtesy of Childrens Hospital of Los Angeles.)

adults and authority figures. Limited formal education often lessens their personal knowledge base for decision-making and behavioral change.

Questions that are misunderstood by high risk youth often incite a negative response that promotes closure of communication. Streetwise youth know that positive responses result in more questions. Creative, empathetic approaches are more likely to be effective than perfunctory, rigid, and judgmental methods. In-depth questions asked by adults often raise suspicion on the adolescent's part. Explaining the relevance of such questions may be necessary.

Most runaway and homeless youth have decreased access to medical care, despite the complexity and severity of their medical problems. Factors contributing to diminished access include inability to pay, naiveté about the health care system and how it works, distrust of authority, fear of reprimand or being reported to authorities, shame about lifestyle, anxiety about institutions, or fear of rejection due to being misunderstood (Chapter 18). Changes in sleep patterns, which are necessary for survival, often prevent clinic attendance during the usual daytime hours. Denial plays an important role in delaying health care and usually acts to further compound the seriousness of their complaints. Misunderstanding by adolescents of their right to self-consent and to establishment of a confidential relationship with a health care provider may lead to avoidance of any care.

These factors unique to street youth are in addition to the reasons adolescents in general may avoid medical care—fear of painful procedures (e.g., phlebotomy), loss of control (e.g., pelvic examination), low priority of health complaints, anxiety about self-disclosure, and fear of not being taken seriously.

Some of the common risk behaviors are noted in Table 33–2, and the resultant problems of runaway and homeless youth are listed in Table 33–1. Many of these problems are interdependent and share a common etiology. Homeless and runaway youth usually have multiple problems, although only one may precipitate the clinical visit.

Optimum care in this population requires the physician to understand the mechanism of disease. Not only is the usual medical history important, but attention to the context in which the complaint and symptom occurred is mandatory. Homeless or street youth are exposed to many adverse environments and physical and psychological deprivations and participate in activities and behaviors that place them at risk. The street is not a homogeneous environment. Each young person has a unique risk profile. This awareness and knowledge must be integrated into the usual principles of well adolescent care (see Chapter 25).

At each contact the practitioner should emphasize the complete health assessment, review the risk profile through updating the HEADS examination or similar evaluation, assess physical and psychological growth, document, if possible, the immunization history, and correct deficiencies with attention to special needs (e.g., hepatitis B, influenza, and pneumococcal vaccines). The young person's risk profile for human immunodeficiency virus (HIV) infection should be noted, and safe sex practices that minimize the risk for infection and transmission should be reviewed (see Chapter 76).

Every visit needs to be maximized, as follow-up and compliance are not guaranteed. Team members should be available from nursing, social work, health education, patient advocacy, psychology or psychiatry, and the appropriate subspecialties (see Chapter 27). Adolescents

**TABLE 33–2. Common Risk Behaviors
in Teenagers**

Alcohol and substance abuse (including tobacco)
Driving while intoxicated
Delinquent and violent behaviors
School failure/dropout
Physical and sexual abuse in childhood/adolescence
Runaway/homelessness
Unprotected sexual intercourse
Pregnancy
Serially monogamous sexual relationships
Survival sex
Poor personal hygiene
Homosexual orientation
Decreased exercise
Poor dietary habits

who are in crisis are usually fearful and anxious. Alarming and uncoordinated actions by health workers can often exacerbate these fears and cause them to lose trust and run back to the streets. There they will receive services through drug dealers, friends, or pimps.

Laboratory evaluation should include general screening tests (i.e., hemoglobin, hematocrit, urinalysis) and, in the sexually active young persons, the serologic test for syphilis (STS), chlamydial and gonococcal cultures, and other appropriate screening tests (see Chapter 69). Other tests should be determined based on risk profile, specific complaint, and differential diagnosis. For those at risk, HIV testing is encouraged but only after appropriate counseling, consent, and assurance of confidentiality (see Chapter 76). As much as possible, assessment, examination, and treatments should be carried out at one clinical site. A single site provides a stable environment and a staff with whom the adolescents can develop trust and who understand them. The health care setting may take on added importance as a safe and supportive haven for an adolescent whose lifestyle is characterized by transience and insecurity.

Significant mental health problems occur in this population as a result of childhood and family experience, indigent lifestyle, and abusive relationships. All runaway and homeless youth could benefit from traditional psychotherapeutic interventions, but attempts at these approaches usually only frustrate the provider. Resources, especially inpatient or day care programs, are extremely limited. Successful models have included using shelters as therapeutic milieus, brief 4- to 6-week therapeutic contacts, overnight programs, trained outreach indigenous workers utilizing a crisis model of intervention, psychological emergency teams (PET), hotlines, psychotherapeutic milieu of vocational training programs, ambulatory detoxification programs, and modified inpatient programs for the severely compromised. Much mental health intervention can be accomplished in association with the medical visit by an appropriately trained clinician. This often proves to be cost effective and less confusing to the teenager. If a referral is made to another member of the team, the young person should be appropriately prepared and if possible directly introduced to the other team member. Psychotherapeutic medications must be used with extreme caution because of the unpredictable lifestyles of this population and the already high propensity for drug abuse.

BIBLIOGRAPHY

Council on Scientific Affairs: Health care needs of homeless and runaway youths. JAMA 262(10):1358, 1989.
Jessor R: Adolescent development and behavioral health. In Matarazzo JD, Weiss SM, Herd JA, et al (eds): Behavioral Health: A Handbook of Health Enhancement and Disease Prevention. New York, John Wiley & Sons, 1984, pp 69–90.
Jessor R, Jessor SL: Problem Behavior and Psychosocial Development: A Longitudinal Study of Youth. New York, Academic Press, 1977.
Patterson GR, DeBaryshe BD, Ramsey E: A developmental perspective on antisocial behavior. Am Psychol 44(2):329, 1989.
Perry CL, Jessor R: The concept of health promotion and the prevention of adolescent drug abuse. Health Educ Q 12(2):169, 1985.
Yates GL, MacKenzie RG, Pennbridge JN, Cohen EH: A risk profile comparison of runaway and non-runaway youth. Am J Public Health 78(37):820, 1988.
Yates GL, Pennbridge JN, MacKenzie RG, et al: Multiagency system of care for runaway/homeless youth. In Forst ML (ed): Missing Children—The Law Enforcement Response. Springfield, IL, Charles C Thomas, 1990, pp 219–233.

CHAPTER 34

Incarcerated Youth

RICHARD C. BROWN

POPULATION AND DEMOGRAPHICS

Youth are incarcerated for reasons such as need for protection and guardianship, status offenses, and an array of illegal activities and crimes. Incarcerated adolescents come from intact families in crisis, fragmented and disorganized families, destructive families, foster and group homes, other institutions, no family, and the streets. They include young people who are runaways, throwaways, neglected, disturbed, and substance dependent (see Chapters 33, 111, 118, and 119).

An ever-increasing number of children and adolescents are incarcerated in juvenile correctional facilities each year in the United States. Jails, detention centers, camps, ranches, and juvenile training schools form an integral part of each state's criminal justice system. More than 590,000 children are incarcerated each year in public juvenile facilities. In addition, about 90,000 children and youth are confined to adult jails each year. This is an unfortunate and tragic trend because it brings youth in contact with other criminals and increases their risk of abuse. Meeting the developmental and special needs of youth is jeopardized by such placement. Even with a declining adolescent population in the United States, the number of juveniles confined to public facilities has increased by 10% between 1983 and 1987; the volume of juvenile admissions and discharges reached its highest in 1987.

Juvenile arrest rates have actually decreased over the past decade, and the number of juveniles held for the most serious violent offenses continues to decline, down 8% from 1985 and 11% from 1983. However, in 1987, the number of juveniles held for alcohol and drug offenses increased by more than 50% since 1985. In addition to the large number of juveniles incarcerated in the United States, youth are also confined for long periods of time. The overall average length of stay in juvenile facilities is approximately 41 days. Those discharged from long-term facilities have average stays lasting 8 months. Besides the increase in rates and length of stay within institutions, juvenile institutions are also faced with rising costs. These new stresses result in severe crowding and understaffing in many institutions throughout the country.

SPECIAL ISSUES
The Health Care Provider

In the face of ever-increasing challenges within the juvenile court system, the health care provider can be pivotal in developing policy, in leading systems toward better health care, in improving evaluations and research, and in maintaining needed links with the community for both support and clinical services.

The health care provider supplies clinical services and supervises clinical care, and it is hoped that he or she is also part of an interprofessional team serving youth. A close working relationship needs to be established with the judge, the probation staff, and the counseling and administrative staff.

An institutional health council can serve as a forum for health care planning, quality assurance, and problem solving. Council members should include the superintendent of the facility, a physician, a mental health worker, the head nurse, the chief probation officer, and the judge, when possible. Other members might include a dentist, an educator, a dietitian, and a vocational counselor.

Health Services

Every institution in which juveniles are confined must have a health program designed to protect and promote the physical and mental well-being of each young person, to determine who is in need of short-term and long-term medical and dental treatment, and to contribute to each young person's rehabilitation by appropriate diagnosis, treatment, and provision of continuity of care following release. New health standards have been established in some states and for the nation to ensure that these basic health requirements are fulfilled.

The establishment of health care standards within a specific institution is an essential part of good structure and good team collaboration, and is necessary for ensuring adequate health care to the adolescent. The basic outline for such standards is available from the American Academy of Pediatrics and the American Medical Association. Standards are included for isolation policy, medical records, pharmacy services, quality assurance, dental care, physical environment, and medical protocols and procedures.

To best serve incarcerated youth, a multiprofessional team approach is ideal (see Chapter 27). Health care provision must be designed for the specific setting and for the duration of the incarceration. A detention facility may require a triage assessment and basic physical and psychological assessment, whereas long-term facilities require ongoing care from a variety of professional services.

Relationship Between Adolescents and Health Care Providers

All detained and incarcerated youth have the right to basic health care. This care must be given with the informed consent of the young person in a confidential manner as designated by state and local laws (see Chapter 20). Of particular concern are adolescents engaged in high-risk behaviors who do not want their parents or probation officer informed of their problems because of fear of consequences, such as punishment, devaluation, and physical harm. Every effort should be made to gain the confidence of the young person in order to diagnose and treat potentially harmful medical and emotional problems. These include suicidal ideation and behavior, substance abuse, sexually transmitted disease, pregnancy, and homicidal ideation (see Chapters 74, 75, 101, and 111).

In a setting where youth are often fearful of being punished or disciplined, it is especially challenging and crucial for the health care provider to make the clinic a safe haven for health care. There should be no surprises; full explanations of all procedures and tests must be provided before obtaining an informed consent from the young person. Without this general policy, adolescents will not reveal important health information vital to their future health and well-being (see Chapter 20). When court-ordered examinations are undertaken, the results of these tests should be given in confidence only to the professional who requested the tests or to the judge.

Health Screening Tests

At the time of an adolescent's admission to an institution, a nurse usually performs the health screening tests by following protocol procedures and the written standing orders for care of the adolescent's problems. Assessment should include state of consciousness, temperature, gross motor function, evidence of physical trauma, and general psychological and physical state.

A physical examination should be performed as part of the health assessment of all incarcerated youth within 24 hours of admission to the institution. The examination should be performed in a private clinical area by staff who are trained to provide basic adolescent health care and should include a complete health history and psychosocial history, a physical examination including pelvic examination when indicated, and other necessary procedures (see Chapters 25 and 69).

Clinical services must include daily sick call; acute care services; family planning counseling; and health education on prevention of sexually transmitted diseases and human immunodeficiency virus (HIV) infection, alcohol and substance abuse, dental health, contraception, and nutrition. Emergency ambulatory and hospital services and radiologic, laboratory, minor surgery, and family planning services must be available. Nurses, nurse practitioners, and physician assistants can perform many of the health care tasks under the supervision of a physician and under specific protocol direction.

The Institutional Environment

Certain health problems may be initiated or exacerbated during the time of incarceration. A significant body of literature has been accumulated on the adverse relationship of crowding to health. Not only does crowding promote transmission of infectious diseases, but it also results in significant psychological stress. There is definite evidence that spatial and social crowding has a negative impact on overall health. Associated with overcrowding are the adverse effects of excessive noise, poor ventilation, and lack of personal privacy. Each of these, singly or in combination, has adverse effects on the health of incarcerated youth.

Some juvenile correctional facilities use solitary confinement, restraints, and "experimental therapies" as a means of control and discipline. Such procedures are in direct opposition to the mental, physical, and social development and health of young people. Every effort must be taken to eliminate these destructive procedures.

A nutritionally balanced diet is necessary for normal adolescent growth and development during incarceration (see Chapter 7). During the past decade there has been considerable discussion about the potential association of dietary intake and juvenile delinquency. Data in the lay literature have suggested that reactive hypoglycemia, food additives, food allergies, nutritional deficiencies, and nutritional excesses play a role in delinquency and criminal behavior. Although the majority of criminal justice systems have not embraced these nutritional theories of criminal behavior, proponents of these theories have had a considerable impact on the juvenile justice systems. Although the controversy is not yet settled, the scientific evidence does not support these theories.

Adequate daily physical exercise is important to the overall social, psychological, and physical health of young people. Disciplinary measures resulting in solitary confinement and a lack of physical exercise can increase adolescents' anxiety and depression. Opportunities for family contact are especially important for young people who are incarcerated. Unfortunately many facilities are a great distance from the adolescent's home, which makes it very difficult, if not impossible, for families to visit. Efforts should be made to improve transportation opportunities for these families.

Pharmacy service standards should include a medication formulary and instructions for drug storage, labeling, and drug dispensing procedures. Maintaining regular pharmacist consultation should be part of the basic standards of the pharmacy. Prolonged isolation and lack of contact with the medical service must not occur. Pharmacologic control and shackling of adolescents have no place in controlling adolescent behavior and must be prevented. Valid standing orders for care of common adolescent medical conditions should be written and reviewed yearly. Medical protocols and procedures must be written and approved by the medical administration. Quality assurance must be maintained through regular evaluation of policies and procedures and inspection of the institution. All services must be reviewed in the context of caring for adolescents who are less than voluntary recipients of the medical efforts.

The guidelines for health screening were summarized by the American Academy of Pediatrics Committee on Adolescence in 1981. These guidelines include admission inspection, general health inspection, care during illness and emergencies, health protection, and health education.

Special Medical Problems

Clinical studies reveal that approximately 50% of incarcerated youth have significant health problems. Adolescents confined to correctional facilities suffer many medical and psychological disorders. In a study conducted by the American Medical Association, incarcerated adolescents were found to have a higher than average prevalence of various medical problems. The disorders include dental problems, 26.6%; skin problems (excluding acne), 25.5%; respiratory problems (including asthma), 8%; obesity and other nutritional disorders, 5.1%; orthopedic problems, 4.1%; and seizure disorders, 2.9%.

Eliciting sensitive history from a depressed, hostile, or frightened young person requires patience and skill. An initial hostile response should not be construed as the young person's final reaction or feelings. Openness and patience on the part of the health care provider are vital. However, once trust is established, the young person may become demanding and express feelings and needs openly. This transition must be viewed as a part of the normal process of establishing a relationship for disturbed youth. Adolescents are often very inexperienced in confidential and caring relationships.

The history may reveal preadmission trauma, physical abuse, and sexual abuse (see Chapters 118 and 119). Any evidence must be collected, recorded, and reported. Further investigation and counseling must be done by either a trained professional in the program or a child abuse professional. Suspected abuse by the police or by the institutional staff must be reported and investigated.

Alcoholism and addiction to other substances are frequent findings and require assessment and referral for treatment (see Chapter 111). Many communities have teen alcohol programs that offer support to the institution. In assessing youth with a history of intravenous drug use, screening must include tests for HIV, hepatitis, and sexually transmitted diseases.

The sexually active adolescent requires special attention (see Chapters 32 and 75). The incidence of sexually transmitted disease is significant in the incarcerated adolescent population. Infections include those caused by *Neisseria gonorrhoeae* and *Chlamydia trachomatis*, syphilis, hepatitis B, papillomavirus infection, and now HIV infection. Within an institution it is often difficult to find a quiet, private, trusting environment in which to obtain the sexual history and perform an appropriate physical examination. The history should include information on sexual relationships, sexual practices, gender identity, and condom and contraceptive use. Counseling and physical evaluation are dependent on knowing this important information (see Chapter 75).

The clinic must have equipment for pelvic and rectal examinations. Laboratory services should include cultures, Venereal Disease Research Laboratory (VDRL) testing, and treatment for venereal warts (see Chapter 69). Of special concern today is the possibility of HIV infection in youth involved in high-risk situations; they may be carrying the virus when they are incarcerated or may acquire the virus within the institution. HIV prevention, counseling, testing, and follow-up require staff training and careful policy development. The stress of institutionalization can potentiate the stress of determining the status of HIV infection. Every effort must be made to assess the mental status of these adolescents and to give them support through the counseling process. Some youth are too disturbed and anxious to be tested during incarceration (see Chapter 76).

Pregnancy assessment, testing, and counseling is a common and complex clinical process. State and institutional regulations guide the confidentiality and the process in counseling. Sexual abuse and incest should be considered during the initial interview (see Chapters 69, 74, 118, and 119).

Providing health care to youth with a history of mental health problems and who have mental stress as a result of incarceration requires awareness and skills in assessment, crisis intervention, and referral support. Depression is ubiquitous and must be individually assessed for degree and potential suicidal ideation (see Chapter 101). Mental health staff must be consulted for all youth who are at risk for suicidal behavior.

The crisis of institutionalization can contribute to already disturbed feelings and ideation. Psychotic and serious mental illness can become obvious during the initial health evaluation. The health care provider should be aware of impending and blatant mental disorder during this stressful time. Suicidal ideations, flight of ideas, delusions, hallucinations, and disorientation require mental health consultation.

Panic and anxiety reactions can occur throughout the institutionalized period (see Chapter 102). Hyperventilation syndrome is one example. Such an attack necessitates a careful history to elucidate the cause, which can include one or more of the following: court disposition, conflict with other youth or with staff, reaction to parents, and identity crisis. If simple and consistent support does not result in remission, consultation is necessary.

Physical injuries as a result of violence may come to the attention of the health care provider (see Chapter 117). A careful history is required to determine the cause. Gang violence has increased in many settings; victimization must be considered. Arrangements must be made for proper evaluation of injuries, including radiologic and orthopedic assessment when indicated. When head injury is considered, a conservative approach is necessary since close clinical follow-up is often not possible in the institution.

Institutionalized youth who have chronic disorders can be a particular challenge if the disorder is used to manipulate the staff and to bring needed but negative attention to the young person (see Chapters 30 and 121). Staff training helps develop skills and a consistent approach to youth with chronic disorders. Double messages, excessive control, and fighting over decisions accentuate the conflict. Seizure disorders, asthma, and diabetes mellitus are disorders requiring training and clinical protocols (see Chapters 43, 59, and 83).

Emergency kits and procedures must be part of the medical protocols. Emergency practice and planning are a part of quality assurance.

MISCELLANEOUS ISSUES

Institutional health care accreditation is a new means of evaluating and providing technical assistance to institutional programs. The process allows for assessment, correction of services, and recognition after completion of the accreditation process.

Several states have begun statewide juvenile court health conferences to convene health care providers, judges, juvenile probation personnel, and facility administrators and counseling staff. Within an efficient institution, all professionals are involved in health care policy and delivery. A medical advisory group within the institution can oversee care, address problems and incidents, and develop policy and team support.

On a local level, a community advisory committee and juvenile delinquency prevention commission can support and advocate for the health care delivery team. The advisory group should include community physicians, hospital staff, health department representatives, and other professional groups linked to the health program.

BIBLIOGRAPHY

American Academy of Pediatrics, Committee on Adolescence: Health care for children and adolescents in detention centers, jails, lockups and other court-sponsored residential facilities. Juvenile & Family Court Journal May:11, 1981.

American Medical Association: Common Health Problems of Juveniles in Correctional Facilities. Chicago, National Commission on Correctional Health Care, 1979.

American Medical Association: Standards for Health Services in Juvenile Correctional Facilities. Chicago, American Medical Association, 1979.

Bell TA, Farrow JA, Stamm WE, et al: Sexually transmitted diseases in females in a juvenile detention center. Sex Transm Dis 12:140, 1985.

National Commission on Correctional Health Care: Standards for Health Services in Juvenile Confinement Facilities. Chicago, National Commission on Correctional Health Care, 1984.

National Council on Crime and Delinquency and Hubert H. Humphrey Institute of Public Affairs: Rethinking Juvenile Justice: National Statistical Trends. Minneapolis, Hubert H. Humphrey Institute, November 1984.

State of California Department of Youth Authority: Overcrowding in Juvenile Detention Facilities and Methods to Relieve its Adverse Effects. Sacramento, CA, Department of Youth Authority, 1983.

United States Department of Justice: Bureau of Justice Statistics, Jail Inmates, 1986. Washington, DC, US Government Printing Office, 1986.

United States Department of Justice: Children in Custody: Public Juvenile Facilities, 1987. Washington, DC, US Government Printing Office, October 1988.

CHAPTER 35

Youth in Transition to Adult Health Care

GAIL B. SLAP

Adolescence marks the transition between childhood and adulthood. All older adolescents, whether well or ill, face the task of independent management of their health and well-being. The complexity of this transition has far-reaching effects for youth, their parents, health care professionals, and society (see Chapter 9). An overview of the background, issues of transitional care, knowledge and training gaps, barriers, and potential solutions for adolescents in transition to adult health care is provided in this chapter.

BACKGROUND

Adolescents are commonly perceived as being basically healthy. Twentieth-century adolescents, however, are neither uniformly healthy nor homogeneous in their risk-taking behavior and the sequelae of their risk-taking behavior. Many adolescents have survived chronic childhood disorders and seek care as adults (see Chapters 30 and 121). Furthermore, the diseases afflicting American youth do not fit the traditional disease-oriented model that typically is applied to adults. The transition from child health care to adult health care requires an interdisciplinary approach that considers medical problems, cognitive development, environment, and behavior (see Chapter 27).

The shifting demography of youth has had a major impact on the visibility of the health problems of adolescents and young adults. The proportion of American youth living in poverty has been increasing steadily. Youth in transition to adult health care are twice as likely as 10- to 14-year-olds or 25- to 44-year-olds to have no form of private or public health care insurance (see Chapter 21).

Many adolescents in transition receive no health screening tests or preventive counseling to avoid the conditions of highest morbidity and mortality, such as premature pregnancies, sexually transmitted diseases, substance abuse, and death from violence (accidents, suicide, homicide).

Health care providers for adults must manage an increasing number of adolescents who have survived previously fatal childhood diseases. Advances in medical science now allow 84% of children with chronic illness and disability to survive to adulthood (see Chapter 30). It is estimated that nearly 10% of adolescents have chronic problems and that their resultant office visits have increased threefold in the past 25 years.

Thus the nature of adolescent and young adult medicine is changing. There are discrepancies among health care utilization, patient need, service delivery, and disease complexity. Older adolescents are seeking service from health care providers who treat adults and who may be unfamiliar with developmental issues, childhood diseases, and anticipatory guidance, which are central to good pediatric care. The health care system as well as the adolescent population faces a transition to an updated, appropriate, and flexible service model.

ISSUES OF TRANSITIONAL CARE

The transition to adult medical care requires readiness and preparation on the part of the adolescent, parent(s), pediatrician, and provider of adult care. A transition failure risks the forfeit of all health care to the young adult. A successful transition prepares the adolescent and young adult to negotiate the health care system independently and to maximize personal well-being throughout adult life. As they move into adulthood, some adolescents will continue to receive health care from family medicine practitioners.

Although most adolescents begin to expect increasing involvement in the decisions pertaining to their health care, many are not ready to find their way from one site of care to another. Adolescents use services most effectively when they are comprehensive and multidimensional and located at one site (see Chapters 17 and 18). School-based health clinics, for example, offer an accessible, affordable site for primary and preventive care for many adolescents. Such programs focus on education, the management of common illnesses, and health screening tests. They allow adolescents to seek and receive primary care with little or no parental involvement yet guide them when care outside the site is indicated (see Chapter 18).

The health care professional who practices outside an adolescent program should recognize the complexities that challenge the newly independent adolescent patient. The young person must recognize the need for care, choose an appropriate site for care, meet the requirements for eligibility at that site (e.g., health insurance), articulate a health history, and comply with treatment (see Chapters 17, 21, 25, and 26). The adolescent or young adult who has difficulty assuming responsibility will require time and patience on the part of the clinician (see Chapter 17). Instructions should be explicit and written. Follow-up phone calls or letters may be required to ensure compliance (see Chapter 26).

Discussions with the adolescent patient about the level of parental involvement must also occur. Although confidentiality should be maintained whenever possible, the adolescent must understand the physician's own limits for protecting this confidentiality (see Chapter 20). When the health care provider believes that the adolescent is unable to comply and that behavior has become life threatening, it is appropriate to inform the parents with the adolescent's knowledge. Most adolescents, however, when given professional time and concern, will agree to inform and involve their parents. The clinician then becomes an important liaison between adolescent and parent, promoting objectivity and communication.

The content of care during the transitional years includes (1) anticipatory guidance to prevent the new morbidities of youth; (2) screening tests to promote health during adulthood; (3) assessment of the stage and tempo of puberty; (4) identification of the adolescent's health concerns; and (5) management of disease and disability (see Chapters 25 and 30).

When evaluating an adolescent in transition to adult health care, it is important to shift from the population perspective of morbidity and mortality to the individual perspective of health concern and disease detection. Surveys of adolescents' concerns indicate that stress, anxiety, nervousness, and worries about health are recurrent themes for youth. However, adolescents are far more likely to present with a somatic complaint such as abdominal pain, headache, or cough than with an explicit psychosocial problem. Nearly one half of the adolescents in one survey described concerns such as weight control, contraception, depression, fatigue, and drug abuse for which they never sought or received care.

The transition from childhood to adult medical care provides an important opportunity to take a new, unbiased history and to explore issues that may not have been identified previously. More important, health care professionals must recognize the adult tendency to underestimate adolescents' health concerns. This is the first step toward meeting the health needs and wishes of youth in transition.

Adolescents with chronic illness or disability present with special concerns and needs as they move from pediatric to adult care (see Chapter 30). Variation in the tempo of pubertal maturation and cognitive development is common among youth with chronic conditions. The health care provider who assumes responsibility for a 19-year-old with Crohn disease, cystic fibrosis, or Turner syndrome may discover that puberty is far from completed. Although youth with pubertal delay appear young, they deserve and often demand an adult approach to their health care (see Chapter 30).

Chronically ill adolescents often have formed very strong ties with their health care providers during childhood. Although these adolescents may request transfer to adult care, they may be unprepared for the sense of loss that follows the transfer. In addition to the emotional support that evolved over the patient's lifetime, the pediatrician's comfort in managing the patient's medical complications grows with time. The first medical crisis in the adult setting, therefore, may be met with uncertainty on the part of a clinician who cares for adults and who is less familiar with pediatric disease and has not spent years caring for the adolescent.

The alternative to transfer of care, however, is a poor one. Pediatricians usually are unprepared to meet the health care needs of adults. Adult patients who remain within the pediatric setting usually feel out of place and may cause discomfort for younger children and their families. Most importantly, the pediatrician who maintains the care of chronically ill youth inadvertently may imply that the likelihood of responsible adult function or prolonged survival is low. All chronically ill adolescents, regardless of prognosis, should be given the opportunity to move into an adult care setting. The ease of this transition depends on preparation of the adolescent and parents and communication between pediatricians and providers of adult health care.

KNOWLEDGE AND TRAINING GAPS

The decision about who should care for adolescent and young adult patients depends more on physician knowledge and comfort than on subspecialty training. Unfortunately, surveys of physician skill in adolescent medicine indicate deficiencies across most subspecialties. A 1987 survey of 351 family practitioners, pediatricians, and internists revealed that 25% of all the physicians and 75% of the internists considered themselves inadequately trained in all categories of adolescent care.

A 1989 position paper by the American College of Physicians states that adolescents need more comprehensive care and that internists must be better trained and more involved in their care. In addition to more exposure to adolescent medicine during medical school and residency, the American College of Physicians recommends that practicing physicians attend continuing medical education programs pertaining to adolescent health. The National Coalition on Adolescent Health developed by the American Medical Association brings together health care professional groups such as the American College of Physicians, the American Academy of Pediatrics, and the American Academy of Family Physicians in an attempt to address adolescent health issues in an innovative, interdisciplinary way.

In 1986, the Bureau of Maternal and Child Health, U.S. Department of Health and Human Services, convened a national conference entitled the Health Futures of Youth. One of the eight study groups explored the training of health care professionals in adolescent care. The following conclusions were outlined in the final report: (1) professional school training does not prepare graduates to meet the health needs of youth; (2) most clinicians do not seek such training once in practice; (3) training should be multidisciplinary and should emphasize normal growth and development as well as risk-taking behavior; and (4) curricula must be developed by subspecialties to ensure that professionals in training complete minimal requirements for competence in adolescent care.

Although the guidelines for education in adolescent care are improving, internists and family physicians continue to express discomfort with their skills. It will be difficult to promote a smooth transition to adult care until the professionals who assume that care are adequately trained and confident in the management of adolescents.

BARRIERS TO TRANSITION OF CARE

Adolescents in transition from child health care to adult medical care face a number of barriers. The most pressing problem is payment. Impoverished, uninsured adolescents are 35% more likely to see no physician for 2 years (see Chapter 21). When they do enter adult care, there is a consequent gap in their primary and preventive care.

Most care sites expect proof of insurance or ability to pay before enrolling a patient in the clinic or practice. Older adolescents who are trying to enter the system for the first time may be unable to either provide the proof or complete the insurance registration process. Many become overwhelmed by the requirements and forgo care.

Adolescents with chronic disabilities or special health care needs face additional financing problems. Even when these adolescents are insured, health care professionals and hospitals may find that the reimbursement does not cover the time or effort required. These young patients, therefore, may have difficulty finding a site to assume their care. Even more important, coverage under their parents' policies usually terminates at age 22 or on leaving home or school. Disabled youth may have difficulty finding work because employers are unwilling to assume the health insurance risk. Although they may be underemployed and underinsured, once employed these youth become ineligible for public health insurance. The result is a young population in need of complex service yet unable to secure either the employment or public support to pay for the service.

Another barrier to transitional health care is concern by both adolescents and health care providers about confidentiality (see Chapter 20). Adult patients and their health care providers assume confidentiality even when it is not discussed. Adolescent patients may question the new provider's guidelines about confidentiality. Clinicians may avoid discussing confidentiality if they are in conflict about withholding information from parents or uncertain about the legality of providing care to minors without parental consent (see Chapter 20).

Parents may pose a barrier to transitional care, especially when their child has had a chronic disease. They may be reluctant to leave the nurturing, informative environment of the pediatric caregivers. If their child's disease is uncommon in adulthood, they may fear suboptimal care in the adult setting. They may miss the personal ties and family support that developed over the course of their child's illness. They may feel superfluous or intrusive in the adult care setting. More important, they may believe that their child is not yet ready to manage his or her health care decisions independently. Both the adolescent and parent must be willing to separate, make mistakes, recognize limitations, and begin again.

Health care professionals may add another set of barriers to a smooth transition. Pediatricians, similar to parents, may have trouble deciding when the youth can function independently. They may worry about whether providers of adult health care have the needed expertise or whether psychosocial support will be available in the adult health care setting. Providers of adult health care may be reluctant to request pediatric consultation when challenged by the conditions of adult patients who have chronic disease of childhood. They may view adolescents as immature or their families as overinvolved. The disease-oriented model that is common in internal medicine may be unable to meet the multidisciplinary needs of youth and their families (see Chapter 27). Providers of adult health care may have less experience than providers of pediatric health care in coordinating the health care with educational services. Conversely, pediatric caregivers may be unable to counsel youth about the vocational or independent living options that are available for adults.

The barriers to a smooth transition of care are not insurmountable.

REMOVAL OF THE BARRIERS

Potential solutions for easing the transition from child-oriented to adult medical care may begin with the patient, the health care site, the health care professional, or the community. Regardless of the focus for change, successful intervention requires coordination and communication among all levels.

Methods for easing the transition at the patient level have focused on youth with chronic illness or disability (see Chapter 30). Most of the transition programs supported by the Bureau of Maternal and Child Health since the mid 1980s have explored the psychosocial needs of disabled adolescents and have developed support systems that allow adolescents and young adults to manage their own care. Proposals include training in small groups in social skills, individual training in personal case management, prevocational education to improve job readiness, support programs for genetically affected youth and their families, clarification of the transition needs of adolescents with specific diseases such as cystic fibrosis or sickle cell disease, and family support to promote adolescent empowerment and independent function (see Chapters 30 and 31).

The design of effective health care sites depends on adolescents' perceptions of attractiveness, accessibility, affordability, and need. Successful sites share several common elements. Their locations are often accessible yet offer privacy to adolescents and staff. The staff enjoy caring for adolescents and promote a relaxed, flexible, nonthreatening environment (see Chapters 17 and 18). Education and counseling begin in the waiting room and serve the dual purpose of information dissemination and peer interaction. Once the adolescent has reached the health care site, the clinician assumes primary responsibility for keeping the adolescent in ongoing care. Networking, coordination, and communication become the key concepts for clinicians involved in transitional care for youth.

Most adolescents see generalists rather than specialists. Therefore, education for all health care professionals in the issues of adolescent care must be improved. Each discipline should establish a basic curriculum that provides a minimum expected exposure for all its trainees at the school level. Postgraduate training programs, especially for those in the primary care fields, should expand on this base, with formal instruction and exposure to adolescent patients.

A critical barrier to comprehensive care for youth in the United States is the lack of adequate health insurance (see Chapter 21). Both the public and the private sectors must respond with adjustments in eligibility, grace periods, and premiums. Within the private sector, recommendations have included mandated employer coverage for dependents, private group health insurance through schools, and the creation of high-risk pools. Small businesses argue that mandated coverage would force reductions in wages or increases in the price of goods. School-based coverage would provide affordable premiums but would not reach the dropout and graduate population (see Chapter 18). In the risk-pool strategy, states would organize all insurance carriers to share the risk associated with covering individuals who have been deemed ineligible because of preexisting conditions. An extension of the risk-pool concept to the public sector involves the purchase of Medicaid by families with incomes above the eligibility cutoff. Adjustment of premiums according to risk would then create varying public pools for public insurance coverage.

Young adults pose an even more difficult insurance problem than do adolescents. They are twice as likely to be uninsured, are unconvinced about the need for insurance, are often ineligible for both employment insurance and Medicaid, and have outgrown coverage through their parents' plans. This group desperately needs bridge policies that will cover services during the transitional years. Educational and incentive strategies also are needed to encourage young adults to use such policies. Only then will youth reach adulthood with continuous, comprehensive health care services.

BIBLIOGRAPHY

American College of Physicians: Position Paper: Health care needs of the adolescent. Ann Intern Med 110:930, 1989.

Blum R (ed): Chronic Illness and Disabilities in Childhood and Adolescence. New York, Grune & Stratton, 1984.

Blum R: Physician's assessment of deficiencies and desire for training in adolescent care. J Med Ed 62:401, 1987.

Blum R, Smith M: Training of health professionals in adolescent health care: Study group report. J Adolesc Health Care 9:46S, 1988.

Cypress BK: Health care of adolescents by office-based physicians: National Ambulatory Medical Care Survey, 1980–81. Department of Health and Human Services Publication No. (PHS) 84-1250. Hyattsville, MD, National Center for Health Statistics, Public Health Service, 1984.

Hein K: Issues in Adolescent Health: An Overview. Washington, DC, Carnegie Council on Adolescent Development, Carnegie Corporation of New York, 1988.

McManus MA, Greaney AM, Newacheck PW: Health insurance status of young adults in the United States. Pediatrics 84:709, 1989.

Newacheck PW: Adolescents with special health needs: Prevalence, severity, and access to health services. Pediatrics 84:872, 1989.

Newacheck PW: Improving access to health services for adolescents from economically disadvantaged families. Pediatrics 84:1056, 1989.

Newacheck PW, McManus MA: Health insurance status of adolescents in the United States. Pediatrics 84:699, 1989.

Prevention Issues

CHAPTER 36

Health Promotion

ARTHUR B. ELSTER

Health promotion strategies for adolescents are evolving because of two major sociomedical forces. The first is a concern for the costs of human suffering and financial expenditures resulting from the immediate danger posed by addictive disorders, early pregnancy and parenthood, human immunodeficiency virus infection, motor vehicle fatalities, suicide and homicide, firearms and other accidents, and delinquency (see Chapters 74, 76, 101, and 111). Growing recognition of these costs has created a sense of urgency for finding and implementing effective preventive interventions for contemporary adolescents. The second major driving force is the realization that preventing unhealthful adult behaviors is easier than altering behaviors once they have begun. Recent studies have documented that many health-compromising behaviors that lead to adult morbidity and premature death, such as the use of tobacco and alcohol, irresponsible sexual behavior, and poor dietary and exercise habits, begin during adolescence. The strategy of trying to improve the health status of adults by focusing preventive services on children and youth is supported by consensus agreement on the relationships of lung cancer and cigarette smoking, cervical cancer and human papillomavirus infection, and heart disease and an elevated cholesterol level and a sedentary lifestyle (see Chapters 38 and 49).

Current strategies with varying conceptual orientations toward prevention are used by specialists from diverse disciplines such as adolescent medicine, public health, health education, mental health, health psychology, and preventive medicine. As stated by Coates, one of the impediments toward developing health promotion strategies for adolescents is "not the lack of knowledge about adolescents and their activities," but "the differing assumptions, professional perspectives, research paradigms, and treatment programs used with the intention of promoting adolescent health" (Coates et al, 1982).

The purpose of this chapter is to advance adolescent health promotion by synthesizing information from varied sources into a discussion of the definition and dimensions of health promotion, the focus of health promotion strategies and examples of such strategies, the theoretical framework for adolescent health promotion and its special challenges, and recommendations for action.

DEFINITION AND DIMENSIONS OF HEALTH PROMOTION

The goals of health promotion are to reduce the number of persons who have a particular disease, disorder, or condition *and* to promote an optimal state of physical and emotional well-being (wellness). These goals are met through preventive interventions directed at both assisting individuals in changing their personal health behaviors and lifestyles and altering environmental factors harmful to health (referred to at times as "health protection"). A distinction is often made between the concepts of "disease prevention" and "health promotion." The former usually refers to the prevention of classic medical disorders caused by a biologic agent, whereas the latter refers to enhancing healthy behaviors and lifestyles. For example, although disease prevention efforts attempt to reduce the transmission of sexually transmitted disease through early treatment of infected individuals and identification and treatment of case contacts, health promotion efforts attempt to both reduce the rate of sexually transmitted disease *and* promote healthy psychosexual adjustment by enhancing responsible sexual behavior (see Chapters 68 and 75). The distinction between the two approaches, however, has little practical relevance when addressing disorders that lack a single causative agent, such as the health risk behaviors of adolescents.

Major impetus to develop preventive interventions was provided by the 1979 report, *Healthy People: The Surgeon General's Report on Health Promotion and Disease Prevention.* This report was intended to initiate the second public health revolution in the United States. The first revolution, from the late nineteenth century through the first half of the twentieth century, involved the battle against infectious disease. According to Joseph Califano, former Secretary of the Department of Health and Human Services, a second public health revolution was needed because, "We are killing ourselves by our own careless habits. We are killing ourselves by carelessly polluting the environment. We are killing ourselves by permitting harmful social conditions to persist—conditions like poverty, hunger, and ignorance—which destroy health, especially for infants and children" (US Public Health Service, 1979). The Surgeon General's report galvanized efforts directed at personal behavioral change as a way of improving health status.

Comments in this paper do not necessarily reflect the views of the American Medical Association.

Basic to the strategy of individual responsibility for health is the assumption that people with the appropriate cognitive and interpersonal skills have the ability and the opportunity to alter their behaviors. Although theoretically persuasive, this assumption fails when there are excessive developmental "obstacles" and environmental impediments that either preclude or prevent behavioral change (see Chapter 37). The former occurs when the health promotion strategy is not geared to the appropriate developmental level of the adolescent. Examples of environmental impediments include peer influence, poverty, poor nutrition, parental dysfunction because of psychiatric disease or drug abuse, family discord, living in an area of high unemployment and crime, and strong media and social influences that promote unhealthful behaviors (see Chapter 37). Because these obstacles are not usually within an individual's control, the focus of health promotion is now generally perceived in broader terms. This concept is clearly described by the World Health Organization's (WHO) orientation to prevention.

WHO perceives health promotion as a "mediating strategy between people and their environments, synthesizing personal choice and social responsibility in health" (WHO, 1986). This socioecologic concept implies three types of action that extend beyond basic health education efforts: (1) action directed at the determinants of health, (2) action directed at the elicitation of a high degree of individual involvement and participation, and (3) action directed at the promotion of environmental change through legislative, organizational, and community efforts. Although increasing health education and altering personal health behaviors remain important components of health promotion, according to WHO, they are secondary to the socioeconomic factors—access to health care, development of a healthy environment, and strengthened social networks—that enable behavioral change to occur.

FOCUS OF HEALTH PROMOTION STRATEGIES

The standard public health classification of prevention distinguishes among primary, secondary, and tertiary preventive interventions. Basic to this model is the concept that the prevalence of a condition or disorder, defined as the total number of cases that exists at any one time, reflects the incidence of the condition, which can be defined as the number of new cases occurring each year, the chronicity of the condition, and the length of the condition.

The purpose of primary preventive interventions is to reduce the incidence of new cases of dysfunctional behavior, disease, or conditions in currently nonaffected populations. When applied in a traditional manner to biologic disease, primary prevention is directed at reducing the risk from disease prior to the onset of the disease process (which is usually a discrete event). When applied to personal behavior, primary prevention attempts to reduce risk from a dysfunctional developmental process that, in turn, leads to a problem behavior.

Primary prevention efforts are directed at large populations and include much of what is considered health promotion. Essential to developing primary prevention activities is the knowledge of causative factors leading to health disorders *and* the ability to alter one or more of these factors through general activities directed at the whole population. Examples of primary prevention efforts include educational messages to promote strategies directed toward the individual, such as altering one's diet, and strategies directed toward populations, including the use of bicycle helmets and health protection legislation to raise the age at which it is legal to purchase alcohol.

Secondary prevention efforts are directed at interrupting the expected pathogenic process, thus shortening the time a person has a chronic disorder or condition. Implied here is the notion that the intervention occurs early enough in the process so that disability has not yet occurred. Secondary prevention requires knowledge of the early manifestations of a disorder, a systematic risk assessment to accurately identify the target group that will receive the intervention, and the ability to alter the evolution of the disorder. Prevention of repeat adolescent pregnancies, screening for cholesterol and for anemia, and early detection and treatment of disorders such as sexually transmitted diseases and alcohol abuse are examples of secondary prevention strategies.

Tertiary prevention includes efforts to prevent recurrent episodes of a chronic condition as well as the sequelae that can result from the condition or disorder. Rehabilitation and medical interventions are involved in these efforts. Examples of tertiary prevention include reducing the cardiovascular consequences of juvenile diabetes mellitus, promoting the successful transition of a youth with a physical disability into stable employment, and preventing automobile accidents in which adolescent alcohol abusers are involved.

In general, the distinction among primary, secondary, and tertiary strategies works best with linear models of disease in which current conditions directly reflect previous health status. Prevention efforts directed at infectious disease (see Chapters 91–96), hypertension (see Chapter 67), diabetes mellitus (see Chapter 59), and attention deficit disorder (see Chapter 106) fit this model nicely. The classification does not fit particularly well, however, with the prevention of adolescent problem behavior. The differentiation between primary and secondary prevention requires the ability to identify when a disease process begins. Most problem behaviors, however, lack a singular antecedent factor whose onset is clearly delineated but result rather from a set of conditions and circumstances that interact and develop over time. Programs to prevent or reduce health-compromising behaviors, therefore, are best considered as a combination of primary and secondary prevention. This level of intervention, in turn, can be differentiated from tertiary prevention efforts directed at adolescents already heavily involved in problem behaviors.

A functional classification of preventive interventions has been developed by Gordon in which he proposes a differentiation of three strategies—universal, selective, and targeted—related to the recipient of the intervention. Gordon's approach to classification differs from the traditional approach by emphasizing the recipient of the services rather than the intended outcome and by including the possibility of untoward effects of the intervention. Health promotion activities could be directed at any of these three recipient groups.

Universal interventions are directed at an entire population or a group not necessarily at risk for the development of a health disorder. Because activities are general and broad, the chance of an unexpected negative consequence from the intervention is small. Examples of this approach include advocating seat belt use, proper diet, and immunizations. Selective interventions are directed at individuals who are at risk for one or more disorders or conditions but do not actually demonstrate signs or symptoms of the disorder or do not engage in health-threatening behavior. Examples include efforts to identify and provide preventive interventions for adolescents who live in dysfunctional families, who have a past history of central nervous system trauma, who are having academic difficulties, or whose parents have a familial medical condition. Targeted interventions are directed at adolescents who manifest a known risk factor for a disorder or condition. Because interventions provided to this group of adolescents are more intense and focused than are preventive measures provided universally or to selected populations, the risk of an adverse response is increased. Adolescents are usually identified for indicated preventive interventions through a medical history, physical examination, psychosocial history, or laboratory test.

Irrespective of the focus or the recipient of adolescent health promotion, effective strategies for changing health and well-being are best derived from sound theoretical concepts. Although many theories have been developed to explain adolescent problem behavior, health professionals have only recently begun to translate these theories into useful preventive interventions. What follows is a discussion of three theories of risk behavior that can be used to develop health promotion strategies for adolescents.

THEORETICAL FRAMEWORK FOR ADOLESCENT HEALTH PROMOTION

Although many theoretical constructs explaining health behaviors have been proposed during the past several decades, three models that represent current thought regarding adolescent risk behavior and health outcomes will be described. They are (1) the transactional model developed by Sameroff and Fiese, (2) the problem behavior model developed by Jessor and Jessor, and adapted by Perry and Jessor, and (3) the biopsychosocial model elaborated by Irwin and Millstein (see Chapters 2, 24, and 37). Central to each of these models is the fact that environmental factors (family, peer, and societal influences) interact with internal factors (constitutional, psychological, physical, and cognitive influences) to determine an adolescent's vulnerability for participating in health risk behaviors (see Chapter 37).

In the transactional model, development is viewed as a product of continuous dynamic interactions between children and their environment. Because the external and internal influences on behavior are bidirectional and progressively changing, developmental outcomes can rarely be explained by a single, identifiable cause. Conversely, single causes by themselves rarely result in a problematic outcome. Using this model, prevention can be directed at changing internal factors, external factors, or the interactive process between and among factors with the intent of disrupting the anticipated progression toward an undesirable outcome. Although developed for understanding the behavior of young children, preventive interventions directed at altering the preceding factors should also be useful with adolescents.

The preventive model used by Perry and Jessor is based on problem behavior theory (see Chapter 37) that focuses on the interactions among behavioral factors such as social skills and health-enhancing behaviors, environmental factors such as social norms and social support, and personality factors such as knowledge and values. This paradigm assumes an overlap between what Jessor calls a "problem behavior" and what experts in prevention refer to as a "health-compromising behavior." Predisposing factors are predominantly psychosocial. Prevention efforts based on this model are directed at altering social influences and promoting prosocial behaviors. This model has been applied successfully to efforts to reduce alcohol and tobacco use among adolescents (see Chapter 38).

Irwin and Millstein use a developmental model to describe adolescent risk-taking behavior (see Chapter 2). They propose that biologic maturation affects a person's cognitive scope (the degree of self-centeredness and the ability to assume future perspective), self-perceptions (self-esteem, body image, and so on), perceptions of the social environment (parental and peer influences), and personal values (achievement-orientation, independence, and so on), which, in turn, leads to the decision about engaging in health risk behaviors. This model, as distinct from the models of Sameroff and Perry, addresses the influence of the biologic and psychosocial effects of puberty on behavior (see Chapter 13). Awareness of the connection between puberty and psychosocial development provides practitioners the opportunity to offer health information and counseling directed at promoting personal adjustment to normal developmental processes.

Once the focus and theoretical framework for adolescent health promotion is understood, concrete strategies for action can be developed. Complementary strategies include promoting both personal and environmental change.

STRATEGIES FOR PROMOTING PERSONAL CHANGE

Health promotion efforts directed at personal change attempt to either strengthen health-enhancing behaviors or eliminate health-compromising behaviors (see Chapter 37). The former strategy is directed at promoting changes in general lifestyle and includes providing instruction on proper diet, encouraging regular exercise, and providing social skills training to foster the assertiveness and decision-making abilities necessary to resist peer pressure (see Chapter 37). The alternative personal change strategy, eliminating health-compromising behaviors, involves highly targeted efforts directed at reducing specific behaviors, such as the use of drugs, tobacco (see Chapter 38), and alcohol (see Chapter 37); attempted suicide; delinquent activities; teenage pregnancies; and sexually transmitted diseases. Both approaches have their strengths and their weaknesses.

Programmatic efforts to affect adolescents' general lifestyle reflect that behavioral change is more likely to persist if it occurs within a broad context of improved physical, social, psychological, and personal health. This approach, however, may become too diffuse and can fail to teach the skills necessary for producing the desired change. Efforts to reduce a specific behavior may have popular appeal because they usually target contemporary issues perceived by society as national concerns. The limitation of a targeted approach to prevention, however, is the lack of attention often given to its co-occurrence with other health problems (see Chapters 2 and 37). The categorical nature of public and private program funding often provides support for only a specified problem, thus inhibiting efforts to address multiple, related health behaviors in the clinical setting.

Although activities directed at personal change occur predominantly within schools, programs have also been developed using a broad community approach (see Chapters 37 and 38). Examples of the activities directed at personal change in this setting include comprehensive community health education, youth recreational activities, adult mentoring programs, peer counseling programs, and the use of the electronic and print media to deliver health promotion messages (see Chapter 37). Many national youth-serving organizations, corporations, and religious institutions have also developed major health promotion initiatives for adolescents.

STRATEGIES FOR PROMOTING ENVIRONMENTAL CHANGE

Until relatively recently, the focus of health promotion in the United States had been on individual change. This orientation is changing, however, and there are a growing number of efforts consistent with the broader WHO view of health promotion. These efforts include strategies to increase financial access to health care, the creation of community interventions to provide alternative programming for inner-city youth, and efforts to transform schools into healthier environments. Action taken by some cities to make their community a "kids' place" that is more nurturing to children and youth is an acknowledgment that personal health reflects the environment in which people live. In addition, strong community advocacy has led to debate regarding the labeling of rock music lyrics, community curfews, and alcohol and tobacco advertisement directed at youth.

Advocates for these regulations argue that behavior is more difficult to alter when individuals are exposed to environmental influences that are counter to health.

SPECIAL CHALLENGES OF ADOLESCENT HEALTH PROMOTION

The creation and implementation of preventive services for youth present special challenges, which are discussed in the following paragraphs.

The Lack of National Consensus on Desired Outcomes

Since problem behaviors present not only physical and emotional threats for adolescents but also ethical dilemmas for society, the goals of prevention are often debated and as a result lack clarity. Although almost all concerned groups would accept without much controversy the goal of preventing the use of tobacco products among adolescents, there is less agreement on the goals related to alcohol use and sexual behavior. Although some individuals advocate promoting total abstinence from these behaviors, others work to prevent the consequences of irresponsible use, such as driving while intoxicated and having unintended pregnancies. The result of this open debate is that adolescents receive mixed messages from society regarding proper and expected behavior.

The Symbolic Meaning of Health-threatening Behaviors

Behaviors targeted for prevention—such as drinking, irresponsible sexual behavior, and cigarette smoking—have a symbolic significance regarding advanced maturity and therefore assume strong social favor within the adolescent subculture. Other behaviors, such as use of anabolic steroids and self-induced emesis (see Chapters 60 and 81), also have assumed a certain level of prominence because of the social benefits they provide (e.g., enhanced athletic ability and thinness). The "rites of passage" of contemporary youth emanate from behaviors that are based on peer group values, such as having one's first drink, tobacco cigarette, marijuana cigarette, or sexual experience, rather than on events based in traditional family values, such as assuming family responsibilities and participating in religious ceremonies, for example. The challenge for society is to help adolescents replace health-threatening activities, many of which have symbolic meaning, with positive behaviors that have personal significance.

Developmentally Appropriate Preventive Interventions

Health promotion efforts should be age-specific. For example, young adolescents lack a future orientation for life, so they do not comprehend long-term consequences of health-compromising behaviors (see Chapter 9). Whether preventive interventions are conducted through individual counseling or large, universal health promotion activities, the emphasis on prevention for these young teenagers should be directed at concrete issues that are germane to their everyday lives. Conversely, preventive interventions with older adolescents can focus to a greater extent on cognitive approaches involving abstract concepts. Another reason health promotion should be age-specific is that the strength of peer group influence is a U-shaped curve, with less influence noted during early and late adolescence and relatively greater influence occurring during middle adolescence (i.e., 13 to 15 years of age). It should not be expected, therefore, that strategies to help youth counter peer group influences will be equally effective at all ages.

Countering the Societal Exploitation of Youth

Although a distinct "youth culture" has been present in America since the 1960s, there is a dramatic increase in the inappropriate exploitation of youth for marketing purposes. Tobacco companies, breweries, some high school and college athletic programs, and organizers of prostitution and pornography are examples of "industries" that have focused on adolescents as a means to increase revenue. Directing marketing efforts toward adolescents is not new or inherently wrong. What is different is that these industries are beginning to market products to adolescents or to use adolescents in ways that do not promote health. Because of deep economic entrenchment, countering the efforts of these industries will be difficult and will probably require regulations or health protection strategies.

CONCLUSION AND RECOMMENDATIONS FOR ACTION

Prevention of adolescent problem behaviors will not result from simple, "quick-fix" activities. Concern and fear of the current social morbidities, unlike morbidities of past decades, have led many individuals to think that something must be done and done expediently to ensure the health of America's youth. This mandate for action, however, must be managed carefully to ensure the development of thoughtful, scientifically sound initiatives and not merely programs that are costly, ineffective, and possibly associated with unexpected negative consequences.

Several recommendations for action can be made regarding the role of practitioners and other health professionals in the development and implementation of health promotion strategies for adolescents.

1. Primary care settings and hospitals should be transformed into health-promoting environments (see Chapters 17 and 18). The environments of these settings provide subtle health messages to adolescents and their parents. They should be smoke-free, display magazines that do not contain alcohol or cigarette advertisements, and provide visible health education material.

2. Primary care–based health promotion interventions that are specifically for adolescents should be identified. These interventions could include both personal health education counseling and the provision of computer-assisted health education programs to be used by adolescents either before or after their visit with the physician. Although the former method provides a personal approach, the latter method may provide an alternative to busy practice schedules and adolescents' concern with confidentiality.

Specific recommendations for office-based preventive interventions, including screening, counseling, and immunizations, can be found in the report of the US Preventive Services Task Force, *Guide to Clinical Preventive Services: An Assessment of the Effectiveness of 169 Interventions.* The recommendations contained in this guide have some degree of proven effectiveness. They are presented in a clear, easy-to-read manner and are categorized by age group. Since the effectiveness of only 169 selected interventions was reviewed, the guide should not be viewed as addressing all adolescent health issues completely.

3. Health promotion activities developed by schools and community agencies (e.g., clubs, settlement houses) should provide mutually reinforcing, consistent messages. One mechanism to implement this goal would be to develop community coordinating committees involving medical, school, and youth-serving organizations as well as adolescents, to identify and implement a comprehensive, coordinated strategy of adolescent health promotion for each specific locale.

4. Health professionals should encourage parents to actively monitor and supervise the behavior of their children. As difficult as this is for single-parent families and families in which both parents work outside the home, greater involvement by parents in the lives of their children is essential in moderating the effects of a changing social environment.

5. Health professionals, either individually or through their professional organizations, should assume an advocacy role by monitoring the influences that shape adolescents' lives. Physicians may offer their services to review school health promotion policies, use the media to promote public awareness and debate by providing expert comment on topical matters of concern, or sponsor alternative health-promoting activities for youth.

6. Health professionals should take a leadership role in critically reviewing the accessibility, availability, and appropriateness of local health services for adolescents. If barriers to quality health care are found, strategies to improve access should be identified and implemented. Because of the complexity of the health problems facing adolescents, prevention services should be coordinated within a community and should be comprehensive in nature.

BIBLIOGRAPHY

Coates TJ, Petersen AC, Perry CL: Crossing the barriers. In Coates TJ, Petersen AC, Perry CL (eds): Promoting Adolescent Health:

A Dialogue on Research and Practice. New York, Academic Press, 1982, pp 1–21.

Durlak JA: Primary prevention of school maladjustment. J Consult Clin Psychol 5:623, 1985.

Gordon RS: An operational classification of disease prevention. Public Health Rep 98:107, 1983.

Irwin CE, Millstein SG: Biopsychosocial correlates of risk-taking behaviors during adolescence: Can the physician intervene? J Adolesc Health Care 7(Suppl):82, 1986.

Lorion RP, Price RH, Eaton WW: The prevention of child and adolescent disorders: From theory to research. In Schaffer D, Philips U, Enzer NB (eds): Office of Substance Abuse Prevention Prevention Monograph-2: Prevention of Mental Disorders, Alcohol and Other Drug Use in Children and Adolescents. Washington, DC, Alcohol, Drug Abuse, and Mental Health Administration, DHHS Publication No. (ADM) 89-1646, 1989, pp 56–96.

Minkler M: Health education, health promotion and the open society: An historical perspective. Health Educ Q 16:17, 1989.

Offord DR: Prevention of behavioral and emotional disorders in children. J Child Psychol Psychiatry 28:9, 1987.

Perry CL, Jessor R: The concept of health promotion and the prevention of adolescent drug abuse. Health Educ Q 12:169, 1985.

Sameroff AJ, Fiese BH: Conceptual issues in prevention. In Schaffer D, Philips U, Enzer NB (eds): Office of Substance Abuse Prevention Prevention Monograph-2: Prevention of Mental Disorders, Alcohol and Other Drug Use in Children and Adolescents. Washington, DC, Alcohol, Drug Abuse, and Mental Health Administration, DHHS Publication No. (ADM) 89-1646, 1989, pp 23–53.

US Preventive Services Task Force: Guide to Clinical Preventive Services: An Assessment of the Effectiveness of 169 Interventions. Baltimore, Williams & Wilkins, 1989.

US Public Health Service: Healthy People: The Surgeon General's Report on Health Promotion and Disease Prevention. Washington, DC, US DHEW, PHS Publication No. 79-55071, 1979.

World Health Organization: Report of the working group on concept and principles of health promotion. Health Promotion 1:73, 1986.

CHAPTER 37

Prevention of Alcohol and Other Drug Use

HOOVER ADGER, JR.

Public concern about alcohol and other drug use among children and adolescents has stimulated a major national effort to identify effective ways of deterring or delaying the onset of this behavior. Two decades ago, when a new crisis in the abuse of alcohol and other drugs became evident, the top priority, outside of law enforcement, was treatment of heroin addiction. Subsequently, the initial and narrowly defined concern with heroin has broadened to include a wide variety of nonopiate drugs ranging from marijuana to phencyclidine piperdine (PCP) and lysergic acid diethylamide (LSD) and more recently, concern about the use of cocaine. Although reduction in supply remains an important focus in preventing the use of alcohol and other drugs, it is now widely recognized that supply reduction alone will never be sufficient to make a substantial impact because of strong mitigating forces. The importance of both reducing the demand for illicit drugs and deterring the onset of alcohol and other drug use in young people has become increasingly clear (see Chapter 111).

During the past 20 years, there has been increasing awareness of and concern about the level of drug involvement among our youth. Recognition of the epidemic nature of alcohol and other drug use and its emergence as a major adolescent health problem stimulated the implementation of large-scale epidemiologic studies, as well as the development of knowledge about the nature, trends, and consequences of such use (see Chapter 2).

At the end of the 1960s, the use of illicit drugs among adolescents and young adults was recognized as a major epidemic. Large segments of the nation's youth had begun to experiment with marijuana, PCP, and other psychoactive drugs. Moreover, misuse and abuse of prescription drugs (e.g., tranquilizers and stimulants) was on the increase. By the mid-1970s, illicit drug experimentation seemed to have become synonymous with other "rites of passage" into adulthood.

Although the rate of drug use for most psychoactive substances declined during the late 1970s and early 1980s, drug use among adolescents and young adults continues to be a significant problem (see Chapter 2). One disturbing observation is that although there has been a decrease in the reported prevalence of the use of most illicit drugs, there has been little change in the reported use of alcohol, which is the major drug of abuse. The use of alcohol and other drugs is a major factor in the deterioration of the health status of adolescents and young adults. It is a major contributor to disability and death for individuals in this age group (see Chapter 2). Of equal concern is the impact of alcohol and other drugs on the cognitive and psychosocial development of young people. These facts underscore the need for effective prevention approaches.

The physician or other health care provider should be familiar with the background, rationale, and general aspects of prevention approaches. Parents and patients, alike, look to their physician for advice. Increasingly, physicians are being asked to play a major role in assisting in the development and implementation of prevention-related activities.

HISTORICAL OVERVIEW

Historically, drug abuse prevention programs were founded on the theoretical assumption that children and adolescents used drugs because they were ignorant of the consequences of such use. It was assumed that the provision of adequate information about alcohol and other drugs would lead to changes in behavior. Hence, the primary emphasis in prevention was on providing information about the dangers of alcohol and other drugs to adolescents and young adults. Prevention campaigns involving the dissemination of information alone, however, were quickly shown to be inadequate and spurred new approaches.

In the 1970s, social scientists began to address interpersonal and intrapersonal factors that influenced drug abuse behaviors among children and adolescents. These studies, which found correlations between substance use and attitudes, beliefs, values, and personality factors such as self-esteem, self-reliance, and alienation, gave way to new enthusiasm for prevention programs that use clarification of values and affective education. The assumption behind these programs was that young people use alcohol and other drugs because they do not think through their values or do not learn how to express their feelings adequately. When these approaches failed to deter the use of alcohol and other drugs, there was a brief period of pessimism about achieving this goal.

Although traditional health education approaches have proved largely unsuccessful in reducing the rate of alcohol and other drug use, new and innovative approaches have been sought to address this problem. More recently, there has been a renewed sense of optimism about prevention, primarily sparked by a new generation of prevention programs that make use of life skills training and peer refusal techniques. New approaches incorporating the impact of the environment and a better understanding of the multiple causes of drug abuse have been adapted and have built upon some of the successes of the information and affective programs. In addition, new community-wide approaches emphasizing the role and responsibility of the family and the importance of clear guidelines for youthful behavior have become increasingly more influential and promising. Many of these new approaches have been strengthened by a better understanding of risk factors (see Chapter 36).

YOUTH AT HIGH RISK

Risk factors for the use of alcohol and other drugs fall into five broad categories: (1) genetic and family factors, (2) peer-related factors, (3) psychological factors, (4) biologic factors, and (5) environmental factors. In addition to these broad categories, there are several demographic variables that have been used to characterize youth at risk.

Genetic and Family Factors

A number of genetic and family factors put youth in high-risk categories, for example, the increasing evidence for the genetic susceptibility of sons of fathers who had an early onset of drinking problems. Twin studies especially suggest the importance of genetic factors, particularly with regard to males. Individuals with a positive family history of alcoholism have a four- to sixfold increased risk for the same disorder when compared with others in the general population. A family history of antisocial behavior is another risk factor. Children with parents or siblings who show antisocial behavior are at higher risk for the development of problems with alcohol and other drugs than are other youngsters. Additionally, there is evidence that families with poor parenting skills have a disproportionately higher risk of having children who use alcohol and other drugs. The use of alcohol and other drugs by parents, as well as attitudes favorable to such use, are other familial factors associated with a greater risk of teenage alcohol and other drug use.

Peer-related Factors

One of the most powerful predictors of alcohol or other drug use by an adolescent is the drug use behavior of the youth's best friend (see Chapter 2). Adolescents whose friends use drugs are much more likely to use them than are those whose peers do not. Having friends who are drug users is one of the strongest predictors of

use, and there is good evidence that initiation into drug use takes place more often through friends than through strangers. Additionally, youngsters with older siblings who are involved with alcohol or other drugs are more likely to become involved themselves.

Psychological Factors

A wide variety of psychological factors are known to be associated with the use of alcohol and other drugs, including school failure, a low interest in school and achievement, rebelliousness and alienation, low self-esteem, and early antisocial behavior (see Chapter 2). Although the psychological factors are less well understood, a constellation of character traits has been identified that is associated with a high risk of alcohol and other drug problems among teenagers. These characteristics include a lack of empathy for the feelings of others, easy and frequent lying, favoring immediate over delayed gratification, and insensitivity to punishment. Youths with these character traits are especially vulnerable to problems with alcohol and other drugs, as well as to other problem behaviors.

Biologic Factors

One of the most important developments in alcohol and other drug research during the past 2 decades has been the exploration of the biologic aspects of dependence on alcohol and other drugs. Although much remains unclear, it appears that once a person has been dependent on alcohol or other drugs, that individual remains biologically different from others who have never used drugs; this difference is one factor that makes relapse common.

Environmental Factors

Environmental characteristics have long been known to play a major role in the etiology of delinquency (see Chapter 108) and, by extension, in the development of alcohol and other drug use. It appears that persistent drug use and delinquent activity, as opposed to infrequent or occasional use of alcohol and other drugs, are associated with the adolescent's growing into adulthood under a condition of extraordinary deprivation and an altered sense of reality.

Demographic Factors

Demographic variables such as age, ethnicity, race, and socioeconomic status have been examined with regard to their impact on the use of alcohol and other drugs by adolescents. Each of these variables has been postulated to be associated with exposure to alcohol and other drugs and may have independent effects on use characteristics.

Age. Age is the demographic variable most consistently associated with problem drug use. Kandel and others have shown that initiation of alcohol use at a young age influences the risk of using marijuana, and that use of marijuana at an early age increases the risk of involvement with other illicit drugs (see Chapters 2 and 3). In particular, using drugs before age 15 years greatly increases the risk of later drug use. Current research on age effects suggests that delaying the onset of experimentation with alcohol and other drugs may be beneficial in preventing later and more serious drug involvement.

Gender. Gender as a single variable is not a good predictor of adolescent drug use. Differences between male and female patterns of reported drug use have declined over the past 2 decades. These differences are relatively small and vary with the type of drug, the level of drug involvement, and age. In general, although differences between male and female use patterns for cigarettes are minimal, males are more likely to report higher levels of illicit drug use when compared with females and are more likely to report episodes of binge drinking and heavy use of illicit drugs (see Chapters 2 and 3). Although there are observed differences in male and female drug use, these differences do not appear to be sufficiently large to merit gender-specific prevention programs. There are specific populations of adolescents, however, such as pregnant teenagers, in whom the needs of the target group are sufficiently different to merit an approach tailored to the special needs of the group (see Chapter 74).

Ethnic and Racial Differences. Ethnic and racial differences in the abuse of alcohol and other drugs are difficult to determine because these variables are often confounded by socioeconomic status and living conditions. Although white youth, compared with nonwhite youth, have reported consistently higher levels of use of alcohol, marijuana, cocaine, and other illicit drugs, differences between these groups are now very small. In general, however, white and Native American youth, especially those in urban areas, report the highest rates of use, Hispanic and black youth report intermediate rates of use, and Asian American youth report the lowest rates of use (see Chapter 2). Among ethnic groups, use rates vary by age and gender. Hence, in order to be effective, prevention programs need to be sensitive to cultural, environmental, economic, historical, and demographic distinctions that affect alcohol- and other drug-related behaviors within racial and ethnic groups.

Socioeconomic Status. Socioeconomic status alone is not strongly associated with substance abuse. There is little evidence that socioeconomic status *per se* influences the use of alcohol or other drugs. Substance abuse and dependency cross all income and socioeconomic categories. Although socioeconomic status itself is not related to drug use, a factor that is closely related, education, does show a correlation with the use of alcohol and other drugs. Students who are doing well in school report lower rates of use than do those who are doing poorly. In addition, students who have plans to attend college are less likely to engage in illicit drug use than are those without college expectations.

Although many of the preceding considerations point to the importance of understanding various risk factors, it is important to realize that risk factors are simply characteristics that refer only to the higher probability of a problem's occurring. Recent studies suggest the importance of multiple factors, including individual, family, and sociocultural characteristics. Although the presence of risk factors may help identify those who are most vulnerable, their presence does not predict the absolute development of problems. Many children growing up under highly adverse conditions still manage to become healthy, well-functioning adults.

A major goal in the effort to identify youth at high risk is to intervene sufficiently early to permit the interruption of behaviors that would otherwise lead to the use of alcohol and other drugs or to other dysfunctional behaviors, and to do so in a manner that identifies youths without inappropriate negative labeling. In the earliest school grades, youngsters at risk may be distinguishable from others by aggressive antisocial behavior. In particular, the combination of shyness and aggression, as well as evidence of school adjustment problems and truancy, have been shown to place this population at increased risk. By the late elementary grades, youngsters at highest risk are made still more visible by evidence of school failure. By adolescence, a low commitment to school and associated academic failure may be evident, in addition to delinquency, association with friends who use drugs, alienation from the larger society, and associated rebelliousness. Early identification of those at high risk, meaningful intervention, and avoidance of these negative consequences are issues of major concern.

THEORETICAL BASIS OF PREVENTION

The research literature identifies a number of theories on drug use. A review of some of these theories is offered here. An understanding of the basic concepts of these theories is important because they serve as a foundation for many of the past and current prevention efforts.

Problem Behavior Theory

The problem behavior theory suggests that drug use is interrelated with other problem behaviors, with which it shares common antecedents (see Chapter 36). Jessor and Jessor originally hypothesized that many problems, including abuse of alcohol and other drugs, could be explained by variations in individual personality characteristics, perceived environmental structures, socialization patterns, and demographic status. Subsequent empirical research supports the Jessors' arguments. In general, teenage drug use is associated with a low value on education or low expectations for academic achievement, a high tolerance of deviance, and a high value on personal independence. In addition, the adolescent's perceptions of parental and peer modeling of drug use, as well as perceptions that peers or parents approve or tolerate drug use, are likewise associated with the use of drugs. One of the strengths of this model is its specification of the adolescent's perception of peer values and behaviors as the antecedent variable for problem behavior.

Several others have examined the relationships among adolescent problem behaviors and have identified characteristics that commonly precede these problem behaviors. Common antecedents of drug use include early antisocial behavior, parental and sibling modeling of drug use and delinquency, poor family management, family conflict, a low value attached to education, alienation from dominant social values, community disorganization, and geographic mobility.

Social Learning Theory

Social learning theory expands problem behavior theory by suggesting that behavioral patterns will be more or less problematic, depending on the opportunities and social influences to which one is exposed, the skillfulness with which one performs, and the balance of rewards one receives from participation in these activities. According to Bandura, learning is acquired and shaped by the observation of the behavior of other individuals and the consequences of that behavior. Bandura also notes that the ability to anticipate both the consequences of one's behavior and the attitudes of others toward such behavior develops as an individual matures. This ability allows individuals to self-regulate and internalize rewards and punishments and serve as agents of their own behavioral change. Accordingly, the rewards one receives for behavior will directly affect the likelihood that one will continue that behavior. The risk of problem behavior thus is reduced when young people have an opportunity to perform skillfully in conventional settings.

McGuire has outlined "pretreatment" procedures for maintaining attitudes, values, and beliefs that favor nonuse of alcohol or other drugs. These pretreatment procedures are applied before drug use behavior is initiated and are not designed for youth who already use drugs. "Cognitive inoculation" is one pretreatment method, which, through discussion of conflicting attitudes and beliefs that one will likely encounter, attempts to prepare students for, and thereby protect them from, pressure to adopt beliefs and attitudes that are unhealthy.

Another pretreatment approach requires that a "behavioral commitment" be made on the part of the individual. This commitment can take the form of a private decision, a public announcement of one's decision, active participation on the basis of the belief, or commitment based on someone else's commitment to the belief (external commitment). The potential power of peer, parental, community, media, and societal support for nonuse behavior among youth is illustrated by the finding that external commitment is stronger than private commitment in most cases.

Addressing "cognitive dissonance" or the incompatibility of attitudes and beliefs with one's behaviors is another procedure. For example, if an adolescent strongly values his or her athletic ability, to successfully attach the belief that smoking marijuana diminishes this ability would create dissonance. Resolution of this dissonance would require that the individual either abstain from smoking marijuana or place a lower value on athletic ability.

Evans' social inoculation theory extends McGuire's theory to address the many social influences, beliefs, and attitudes that create pressure on a young person to use alcohol and other drugs. Many programs based on the social inoculation theory use modeling, as suggested by Bandura and others, to teach peer resistance skills. Other programs encourage public commitment from students as an added incentive to resist negative peer pressure and as positive social reinforcement for the group as a whole.

Stage Theory

Stage theory proposes that within normal adolescent populations, drug use tends to follow several stages, each of which is necessary but not sufficient for progressing to the next stage. Kandel and co-workers empirically tested the hypothesis that drug involvement progresses through a series of stages that begin with experimentation, progress to regular use, and then to abuse and dependence (see Chapter 2 and earlier discussion). The stage model of drug use for primary prevention would seem to suggest that avoiding or delaying the initiation of experimentation with alcohol and tobacco could be effective in reducing later and more serious involvement, as was discussed earlier.

Multiple Risk Factor Theory

Opponents of the stage theory argue that no one path leads to drug use or abuse. The multiple risk factor theory suggests that drug use is caused by a combination of factors, none of which alone causes drug use (see Chapter 2). Bry, McKeon, and Pandina developed a multiple risk factor model that examined the effects of six etiologic variables on drug use. The variables included grades, affiliation with religion, age of first use of alcohol, psychological distress, self-esteem, and perception of parental love. Although this work, as well as that of others, found that the number of risk factors was linearly associated with the use, frequency of use, and heavy use of a substance, the amount of explained variation in drug use was low and varied for different drugs. Multiple risk factor analyses imply that drug abuse prevention should seek to reduce youthful experience with risk behaviors and should seek to modify factors that already exist in the adolescent's lifestyle.

Biopsychosocial Model

The biopsychosocial model, emerging from the field of behavioral medicine and from recent interest in competence and coping, is based on two central premises (see Chapters 24 and 36). The first premise is that substances may be used as a coping mechanism to reduce or enhance desirable or undesirable feelings or emotions. The second premise is that skills used to cope with the stress of daily life situations are different from those used to cope with temptation to experiment with or experience the effects of a mood altering substance. The model suggests that substance abuse results from a deficiency in coping skills that are relevant to a variety of stressors. Hence, when faced with personal or social pressure to use substances, youth with deficits in social skills will be more likely to engage in drug use behaviors.

Social Stress Model

The social stress model proposed by Rhodes and Jason integrates the traditional emphasis on individual and family variables with recent research on competence and coping. Additionally, the social stress model attempts to address the broader social variables that influence adolescent behavior more directly. Drug use is viewed as a long-term outcome of multiple experiences with significant others and social systems from birth to adolescence. Experiences involving the family, school, and community are seen as influencing the identification with parents, peers, and role models and the development of effective coping strategies. Accordingly, adolescents who (1) make positive attachments with family, teachers, and peers; (2) develop good coping skills; (3) have school and community role models; and (4) have resources in the community that provide opportunities for success are more likely to deal with stress effectively and are less likely to engage in problem behaviors, including the use of alcohol or other drugs. The social stress model suggests that in addition to focusing on individual, family, and peer variables, it is important to examine the large-scale social, political, and economic issues that may have an impact on substance use. The model suggests that it is important to examine the broader social context in an attempt to minimize the social and institutional obstacles to adjustment for youth, such as improving the quality of school systems. Additionally, the model emphasizes the importance of examining broader variables, such as socioeconomic status, race, school environment, and community resources, which are oftentimes not considered but can be important variables in determining risk.

MODEL PROGRAMS AND APPROACHES

Effective prevention strategies begin with an understanding of the many reasons why young people begin to use alcohol and other drugs. Although many prevention programs continue to concentrate on changing the individual, research has shown that this limited approach seldom results in long-term change (see also Chapter 38). As a result, many programs are adopting a "systems" approach in an attempt to encourage the development of long-term prevention strategies and targeting multiple elements of the environment known to be associated with the use of alcohol and other drugs. Although there is no single best approach for all groups, comprehensive programs have attempted to address strategies that focus on the individual, peer group, family, community and school environment, and the larger social environment, including the mass media and prevention through regulatory and legal action.

Strategies That Focus on the Individual

Programs designed to influence the individual generally have been designed to (1) provide factual information, (2) modify perceptions of invulnerability, (3) address beliefs about alcohol and other drugs, (4) teach stress reduction and coping skills, (5) meet the social or psychological needs of young persons, (6) improve decision-making and communication skills, and (7) address early antisocial behavior.

Strategies That Focus on the Peer Group

Providing opportunities for students to observe peer role models who do not use alcohol and other drugs is a popular method for influencing norms. The process of having same-age or slightly older students conduct programs is commonly referred to as "peer or near-peer education" or "peer leadership." Programs are often a combination of both components. The peer education component provides factual information, whereas the peer leadership component addresses modeling appropriate behavior, teaching social skills, and other activities such as leading role rehearsals. There are also many programs that teach social and peer resistance skills. At present, this type of program appears to be especially popular as a method of delaying the use of tobacco, alcohol, and other drugs, though it appears to be much more effective when there is a clear nonuse norm. Schools try to influence peer norms in regard to use of alcohol and other drugs by encouraging clubs that support abstinence from these substances. In this way students learn that not everyone is using drugs and that nonuse has benefits and is socially acceptable.

Family-Focused Prevention

Increasingly, prevention experts have recognized the importance of parents and families as a valuable resource. Strategies that target parents are an important part of an effective prevention program. These strategies include parents (1) becoming informed about and aware of situations in which alcohol and other drug use can occur; (2) developing skills that help to build strong family bonds, including effective listening, building self-esteem, and clarification of values; (3) establishing clear family policies and consequences concerning alcohol and other drug use; and (4) joining with other parents and families in promoting a drug-free environment in the school, neighborhood, and extended community.

Community and School-based Strategies

The community and school, when working together, send a unified message to young people that alcohol and other drug use is unacceptable. One example of a partnership between community health agencies and the schools is the student assistance program. Modeled after the employee assistance programs found in industry, the student assistance program is a promising approach for intervention with and prevention of alcohol and other drug problems among school-aged youth. These programs offer school staff and others a mechanism for helping youth with a wide range of problems that may contribute to alcohol and other drug use. In addition, these programs also assist students who are experiencing adverse effects from parental abuse of alcohol or other drugs. It is estimated that there are 7 million children less than 18 years of age in the United States who have a parent or parents who are alcoholics. There have been positive results documented for those who participate in groups that focus on the unique problems of children who grow up with a parent who is dependent on alcohol or other drugs.

The number of student assistance programs is growing. Although the mix of alcohol and other drug-specific services may vary, most school student assistance programs include early identification of student problems, referrals to designated assessment-evaluation specialists, in-school services (e.g., support groups and individual counseling), referral to outside agencies, and follow-up services.

A number of exemplary programs were recently cited in the Office of Substance Abuse Prevention document, Communities Creating Change. A unique program in Madison, WI, Families and Schools Together, provides another innovative example of a community- and school-based strategy. This program involves schools, mental health agencies, alcohol and other drug agencies, and hard-to-reach families as collaborative partners in an effort to empower families to become primary prevention agents for their own children. The program's mission is to educate children about their right to have a life that is alcohol- and drug-free. It simultaneously provides parents the opportunity to deal with their own dependence and codependence issues so that they may ultimately become the primary prevention agents for their children.

Mass Media Approaches to Prevention

The media provide important messages to shape and reinforce societal norms, including those associated with the use of alcohol and other drugs. Mass media approaches typically include a combination of television and radio public service announcements, advertise- ments, billboards, booklets, posters, and special planned events and health education activities.

Although the ultimate goal of prevention efforts is to reduce the use of alcohol and other drugs by affecting behavior, research on the effects of media campaigns has determined that mass media efforts at best only increase awareness of the target population. It may be unrealistic to expect to accomplish changes in behavior through the use of a media campaign alone; however, increasing awareness about a problem is one of the first steps toward achieving the ultimate goal.

Mass media campaigns are most successful when the media messages are followed with and linked to efforts on a local or personal level. Parents or other role models, neighborhood institutions, public service agencies, health care professionals, or school personnel can be spokespersons who reinforce media messages. Likewise, media efforts can be used to supplement school-based or community-based prevention programs by reinforcing the information and skills being taught in these programs.

A particularly promising approach is the "cooperative consultation" technique that consists of working with media personnel so that a less glamorous, more accurate portrayal of drinking in television programs is presented. Through cooperative consultation, health professionals work closely with television producers and program developers in a variety of ways to assist them in creating programs and messages that are likely to have a more positive public health impact.

Prevention Through Regulatory and Legal Action

Many laws and regulations are aimed at limiting the availability, use, and abuse of alcohol, tobacco, and illicit drugs. Drug policy regarding illicit drugs has focused on controlling the market through enforcement of laws against the production, sale, and distribution of these substances. Although law enforcement has made some progress in reducing the availability of drugs, past increases in enforcement efforts have produced disappointing results. Strategies that address regulatory and legal actions against alcohol have been more promising. Investigators have found that simply raising the price of alcoholic beverages reduces overall consumption. Increasing the minimum drinking age from 18 to 21 years

TABLE 37–1. Components of Successful Programs

A broad spectrum of services is offered to cover multiple needs of participants

Program structures and staff are flexible and attempt to meet the individual needs of participants

An ecologic approach is used for helping youth at high risk, which recognizes the influences of the family and surrounding socioeconomic and physical environments

Services provided are coherent, accessible, and easy to use

Barriers to cost, culture, language, and inadequate transportation are eliminated

Staff members demonstrate genuine concern about clients, have time to provide intensive help, and are able to win the trust of participants has proved to significantly decrease alcohol consumption by youth and to reduce the number of alcohol-related traffic accidents in which youth are involved.

Communities can influence regulatory and legal action pertaining to alcohol use by young people by increasing public awareness of alcohol beverage policies, challenging policies that compromise efforts to prevent alcohol use, and persuading public officials and law enforcement agencies to create and enforce laws that are sensitive to prevention issues. Community advocacy groups such as Mothers Against Drunk Driving (MADD) and Students Against Drunk Driving (SADD) have been very active and instrumental in this regard.

COMPONENTS OF EFFECTIVE PROGRAMS

One conclusion that can be reached regarding alcohol and drug prevention programs is that there is no single strategy with long-term impact. More recently, a consensus has begun to emerge favoring a much broader view of prevention than had characterized past approaches, focusing on social, cultural, and legislative aspects of prevention as much as on individual responsibility. Although there appears to be no one strategy that is a guarantee for a positive outcome, successful programs are characterized by several key components (Table 37–1).

ROLE OF THE HEALTH CARE PROVIDER

The health care provider is in an ideal position to take an active role in the prevention of alcohol and drug use. As mentioned previously, parents and patients often look to the health care provider for advice and direction regarding health and lifestyle issues. In this regard, the health care provider can have a potentially important impact by presenting alcohol and other drug prevention messages as a routine component of anticipatory guidance, providing accurate information regarding the health hazards and consequences of alcohol and other drug use, and thereby becoming an important resource for parents, children, and adolescents. Moreover, practitioners can be supportive of youth who adopt nonuse behaviors and should discuss alternative strategies to alcohol and drug use.

The early identification of individuals who are at high risk for use or those who have already begun using alcohol and drugs is a critical role for the health care provider. Subsequently, appropriate intervention, management, and referral should become a part of adolescent patient service delivery.

Additionally, the health care provider can play an active role by serving as an advocate within the community. Health care professionals should take an active role in supporting community efforts and can make a valuable contribution by participating in the planning or implementation of prevention activities or by serving as content experts.

Lastly, health care providers can serve as exemplary role models. Because many young persons look to members of the medical profession as role models in the community, it is important that in their involvement with youth, practitioners model nonuse of tobacco and other drugs and either abstinence or moderate and responsible use of alcohol. In addition, physicians need to be sensitive to the possible negative consequences of overprescribing medications to youth, who may infer from their experience with prescription medications that all pain or discomfort can be cured with drugs.

BIBLIOGRAPHY

Bachman JG, Johnston LD, O'Malley PM, et al: Explaining the recent decline in marijuana use: Differentiating the effect of perceived risks, disapproval, and general lifestyle factors. J Health Soc Behav 29:92, 1988.

Bandura A: Social Learning Theory. Englewood Cliffs, NJ, Prentice-Hall, 1977.

Botvin GJ, Baker E, Renick N, et al: A cognitive behavioral approach to substance abuse prevention. Addict Behav 9:137, 1984.

Bry BH, McKeon P, Pandina RJ: Extent of drug use as a function of number of risk factors. J Abnorm Psychol 92:273, 1982.

Comerci GD, MacDonald DI: Prevention of substance abuse in children and adolescents. Adolesc Med State Art Rev 1:127, 1990.

Communities Creating Change: Exemplary Alcohol and Other Drug Prevention Programs for 1990. Office for Substance Abuse Prevention, RPO-768, 1990.

Evans RI, Rozelle RM, Mittlemark MB, et al: Deterring the onset of smoking in children: Knowledge of immediate physiological effects and coping with peer resolve, media pressure, and parent modeling. J Appl Soc Psychol 8:126, 1978.

Hawkins JD, Lishner DM, Catalano RF: Childhood predictors and the prevention of adolescent substance abuse. In Etiology of Drug Abuse: Implications for Prevention. DHHS Publication No. (ADM) 85–1335. Washington, DC, U.S. Government Printing Office, 1985.

Jessor R, Jessor SL: Problem Behavior and Psychosocial Development—A Longitudinal Study of Youth. New York, Academic Press, 1977.

Johnston LD, O'Malley PM, Bachman JG: Drug Use, Drinking, and Smoking: National Survey Results from High School, College, and Young Adult Populations, 1975–1988. Rockville, MD, National Institute on Drug Abuse, 1989.

Kandel DB, Logan JA: Patterns of drug use from adolescence to young adulthood: I. Periods of risk for initiation, continued use, and discontinuation. Am J Public Health 74:660, 1984.

McGuire WJ: Introducing resistance to persuasion. In Berkowitz L (ed): Advances in Experimental Social Psychology, Vol 1. New York, Academic Press, 1964.

Moskowitz JM: The primary prevention of alcohol problems: A critical review of the research literature. J Stud Alcohol 50(1):54, 1989.

National Institute on Drug Abuse: Biological Vulnerability to Drug Abuse. Research Monograph 89, DHHS(ADM) 88–1590. Washington, DC, U.S. Government Printing Office, 1988.

Rhodes JE, Jason LA: Preventing Substance Abuse Among Children and Adolescents. New York, Pergamon Books, 1988.

Yamaguchi K, Kandel DB: Patterns of drug use from adolescence to young adulthood: II. Sequences of progression. Am J Public Health 74:668, 1984.

CHAPTER 38

Cigarette Smoking

CATHERINE M. SHISSLAK and MARJORIE CRAGO

Recent reports by the Surgeon General of the United States indicate that cigarette smokers have a 70% greater rate of death from all causes than do nonsmokers. The earlier the onset of smoking, the greater the mortality and morbidity rates (see also Chapter 37). Individuals who have smoked since age 15 years have substantially higher mortality rates than do those who did not begin smoking until they were in their 20s. Significantly higher levels of cardiovascular risk factor levels have been found in adolescents who smoke than in adolescents who are nonsmokers (see Chapter 49). Smoking may also be associated with poor pregnancy outcome in teenaged mothers (see Chapter 74).

RISK FACTORS

One of the most important risk factors for cigarette smoking in adolescents is the social influence of parents, siblings, and friends who smoke (see Chapter 37). Media influences also play an important role in the initiation and maintenance of regular cigarette smoking by adolescents. In addition, certain personal characteristics may be important in determining which adolescents are more likely to become cigarette smokers and which adolescents will abstain. Some of the personal characteristics associated with cigarette smoking and other forms of substance use in adolescents are low self-esteem, poor interpersonal relations, and lack of adequate coping skills to cope with stress (see Chapter 37). Certain groups of adolescents are much more likely than others to become cigarette smokers. For example, cigarette smoking rates among adolescents who are school dropouts, ethnic minorities, or from a lower socioeconomic background are often as high as 75%. Recent data indicate that children who reported buying candy cigarettes more than once were more likely to have reported smoking cigarettes (see also Chapters 2 and 49).

CIGARETTE SMOKING PREVENTION PROGRAMS

Since the late 1960s, a number of cigarette smoking prevention programs have been implemented at both the grade school and high school levels (see also Chapter 37). The need for such programs is emphasized by research findings indicating that (1) cigarette smoking is associated with increased morbidity and mortality rates, especially among those who begin smoking at an early age; (2) cigarette smoking is a difficult habit to break once it is established; (3) adolescents who smoke cigarettes are more likely to use other substances such as alcohol and drugs than are nonsmokers; and (4) the age of onset of cigarette smoking is decreasing.

The first school-based anti–cigarette smoking programs were focused primarily on providing information about the health hazards of cigarette smoking. These programs were based on the assumption that if young persons knew why cigarette smoking was unhealthy, they would choose not to become smokers. Subsequent evaluations of these programs indicated that they were effective in increasing knowledge about the negative consequences of cigarette smoking and sometimes were effective in changing attitudes toward cigarette smoking, but they had very little impact on actual cigarette smoking behavior. Prevention programs that emphasize long-term health risks associated with cigarette smoking are more effective with adults than with children and adolescents, who are much more inclined to be oriented in the present than in the future (see Chapter 9).

A number of changes have taken place in school-based prevention programs since the first programs were implemented. Currently, most cigarette smoking prevention programs are based on one of two general psychosocial approaches: the social influences approach and the life skills training approach (see Chapter 37).

The social influences approach is based on the assumption that modeling is the primary factor in the initiation of smoking behavior and that children and adolescents need to be taught ways to resist the social pressures to smoke cigarettes. Most social pressures to smoke cigarettes come from parents, siblings, friends, and the media. Programs based on this approach focus on (1) helping the individual become aware of the social influences promoting the use of tobacco and (2) teaching specific skills to resist these influences. Some of the techniques used with this approach are role playing, behavior rehearsal, the use of peer leaders to deliver all or part of the program, and a public commitment not to smoke cigarettes in the future.

In contrast, the life skills training approach is based on the assumption that the cause of cigarette smoking and other forms of substance use is the lack of certain personal and social skills. Some of the personal deficits that may make an individual more susceptible to substance use include low self-esteem, lack of social and communication skills, lack of achievement motivation, and lack of coping strategies for dealing with stress. Programs based on this approach usually provide skills training in the following areas: self-esteem enhancement, assertiveness, communication, social interactions, relaxation and stress management, problem solving, and decision-making. This approach is broader than the social influences approach, and the skills that are taught can be applied not only to substance use but also to other areas of the individual's life.

EFFECTIVENESS OF CURRENT PROGRAMS

Most of the recent cigarette smoking prevention programs focus on the transition period from elementary school to junior high school, since it is during this time that there is a more than threefold increase in cigarette smoking. In a recent review of a number of school-based cigarette smoking prevention programs, the effectiveness of programs based on the social influences approach were compared with those based on the life skills training approach. Although both approaches were successful in reducing cigarette smoking in the treatment versus control groups, the effects of the life skills training approach were somewhat greater than those of the social influences approach.

Follow-up studies on both types of programs indicate that program effects last for approximately 2 years but tend to diminish over time. There are three large-scale, state-of-the-art cigarette smoking prevention programs that are currently ongoing and are designed to include longer term follow-ups. All three programs are based on the social influences approach. The first program involves more than 1600 sixth and seventh graders in eight Kansas City schools. At the 2-year follow-up, there were 30% fewer monthly smokers in program schools compared with control schools. The students will continue to be evaluated yearly for 6 years. The second program includes more than 600 sixth graders in 22 schools in Waterloo, Canada. Six years after the program was implemented, there were no significant differences in the cigarette smoking behavior of students from program versus control schools, even though there had been significant program effects at the 1- and 2-year follow-up evaluations.

Similar nonsignificant results were obtained in a 6-year follow-up of the third program, which includes more than 7000 seventh grade students in four schools in Minnesota. This is the only program, thus far, in which a follow-up evaluation has been conducted beyond high school. No long-term follow-up study (more than 2 years) of a prevention program based on the life skills training approach has been reported, so it is not known whether the effects of this approach will last longer than the effects of the social influences approach.

The results of the few long-term follow-up studies that have been reported indicate that school-based cigarette smoking prevention programs have been successful primarily in delaying the onset of cigarette smoking. Delayed onset in itself, however, has various beneficial effects such as a lower incidence of morbidity and mortality in adulthood (see also Chapter 49) and a better prognosis for stopping cigarette smoking. All in all, the short-term effects of cigarette smoking prevention programs are encouraging, but strategies need to be developed to maintain these effects over time.

FUTURE DIRECTIONS IN CIGARETTE SMOKING PREVENTION

Although school-based smoking prevention programs have yielded encouraging results, future programs in this area need to be strengthened in various ways. First, the prevention program should be of sufficient duration to produce beneficial effects. Many programs in the past consisted of only a few sessions over a few weeks' time. The ideal program would include five to ten sessions each year throughout grades 6 through 9, which is an important transition period during which substance use often begins. If the program is to be implemented for only 1 year, as many programs in the past have been, it is recommended that booster sessions be provided for the next several years.

The use of peer leaders in delivering all or part of the program has been emphasized by the positive results obtained in peer-led programs (see Chapter 37). Also, with regard to program delivery, it is important that the leaders of the program receive specialized training and that quality checks be conducted periodically to ascertain that the program is being delivered properly.

Future programs should include longer follow-up periods, since it has been found that program effects last for up to 2 years but then begin to drop off dramatically. Also, it is important to track individuals after graduation from high school whenever possible to determine whether exposure to a prevention program in grade school or junior high has a differential effect on stopping cigarette smoking during adulthood. It is also important to ascertain which students are most likely to benefit from a cigarette smoking prevention program. In this regard, future prevention programs may need to be modified in order to be effective with certain high-risk groups such as minorities, school dropouts, and those from lower socioeconomic backgrounds. More research is also needed to determine which of the program components are most effective. The differential effectiveness of different types of program providers also needs to be investigated further. There are some indications, for example, that girls may be more influenced by peer-led programs than are boys.

Future prevention programs will need to become more comprehensive and include in their approach to prevention not only the individual but also the family, school, community (clubs, settlement houses), and the media as well. The health care setting is another important site for cigarette smoking prevention. Individual teaching and intervention groups led by physicians, nurses, social workers, and peers in the health care setting or in a community setting with a liaison to the health care setting are challenges for the future. School-based clinics are ideal settings to perform such programs (see Chapter

18). Increasingly, legislative means of preventing the sale of cigarettes to minors may be implemented. States are enacting laws prohibiting the sale of tobacco to minors (persons younger than 18 years of age). Reinforcement of this legislation is now the greatest challenge.

Killen and others have emphasized the need to package effective interventions in such a way that they can be administered in different localities by individuals with different educational backgrounds and training experiences. Since remarkable progress has been made in school-based cigarette smoking prevention programs over the past 15 years, and since school-based programs are extremely cost-effective, it is likely that these programs will continue to be implemented and strengthened in the future.

BIBLIOGRAPHY

Botvin, GJ, Schinke SP, Orlandi MA: Psychosocial approaches to substance abuse prevention: Theoretical foundations and empirical findings. Crisis 10:62, 1989.

Comerci GD, MacDonald DI: Prevention of substance abuse in children and adolescents. Adolesc Med State Art Rev 1:127, 1990.

Davis RL, Tollestrup K, Milham S: Trends in teenage smoking during pregnancy, Washington State: 1984 through 1988. Am J Dis Child 144:1297, 1990.

Flay BR: Psychosocial approaches to smoking prevention: A review of findings. Health Psychol 4:449, 1985.

Flay BR, Koepke D, Thomson SJ, et al: Six-year follow-up of the first Waterloo school smoking prevention trial. Am J Public Health 79:1371, 1989.

Killen JD: Prevention of adolescent tobacco smoking: The social pressure resistance training approach. J Child Psychol Psychiatry 26:7, 1985.

Ravesloot L, Young WF, Walkington DA: Cigarette sales to minors—Colorado, 1989. MMWR 39:794, 1990.

Murray DM, Pirie P, Leupker RV, et al: Five- and six-year follow-up results from four seventh-grade smoking prevention strategies. J Behav Med 12:207, 1989.

Pentz MA, MacKinnon DP, Dwyer JH, et al: Longitudinal effects of the Midwestern Prevention Project on regular and experimental smoking in adolescents. Prev Med 18:304, 1989.

Reimers TW, Pomrehn PR, Becker SL, Lauer RM: Risk factors for adolescent cigarette smoking. Am J Dis Child 144:1265, 1990.

MEDICAL CONDITIONS

Introduction

Medical conditions affecting adolescents can represent the residua of childhood illness or the initiation of disease processes most commonly manifested in adulthood. There are also a small number of medical conditions that are relatively specific to adolescents or that have different manifestations, treatments, or prognoses from those in either childhood or adulthood. This part of the textbook addresses the various conditions considered important in adolescent medicine from an organ system point of view. Since the development of the reproductive system and the initiation of reproductive medical conditions during and following puberty represent such a large portion of adolescent medicine, we have devoted a separate section to reproductive conditions.

The first chapter of this part deals with skin disorders in adolescents. Acne, the most common skin problem of adolescents, is discussed in detail, since it represents a major medical condition bringing adolescents to health care providers. Disorders of the hair and sweat glands affecting adolescents are also described. Systemic dermatologic conditions, although not common in adolescents, are addressed because of the devastating effect they can have when present. Finally, disorders associated with exposure to ultraviolet light radiation, of special concern for light-skinned adolescents, are addressed.

Disorders of the eyes, ears, and mouth, so common during childhood, become less frequent in adolescence. The presentation, etiology, and management of conditions affecting these sites are described in the chapter by Dr. Frank Biro. Since dental conditions are an especially important aspect of oral health in adolescents, a separate chapter is devoted to periodontal disease, dental caries, malocclusion, trauma, and temporomandibular joint dysfunction in adolescents.

The respiratory tract becomes a site of major concern for clinicians treating adolescents with asthma or cystic fibrosis, immunocompromised adolescents with lung disease, and adolescents with pulmonary manifestations of systemc conditions. Each of these problems is discussed in the section on pulmonary conditions. First, however, there is a discussion of the biologic maturation of the respiratory system. Appreciating these normal developmental changes allows the clinician to place in context the conditions that are discussed. Such a developmental framework is especially important when considering the environmental, occupational, and accidental conditions affecting the pulmonary system. Environmental and occupational pulmonary medicine is a rapidly growing field, and Dr. Michael Lebowitz presents the state of the art of this subspecialty as it applies to adolescents. As adolescents enter the workplace, where they may be placed at risk at an early age, it is important for clinicians to be aware of potential problems.

Exciting new information is available regarding cardiovascular conditions; Dr. Edward Clark is the consulting editor for that section. He has brought the world's experts together regarding disturbances in cardiac conduction and rhythm, structural cardiovascular defects, cardiovascular risk factors and prevention of adult cardiovascular disease, and the cardiovascular aspects of systemic disease. As children with congenital heart defects survive into adulthood after surgical repair or correction, it is important for clinicians caring for them to have an understanding of their medical as well as psychosocial problems. In addition, new technologies, most commonly used in cardiac conduction and rhythm problems in adults, are being applied to adolescents, especially to those who have had an intracardiac repair of a congenital heart lesion. Data regarding coronary artery disease clearly indicate that it is a condition that begins before adulthood. Therefore, health care providers for adolescents must be aware of the approaches to identifying high-risk adolescents and to initiating appropriate preventive management strategies as outlined by Dr. Albert Rocchini.

Dr. Stephen Feig, the consulting editor on hematologic and oncologic conditions, has assembled leaders in the fields of hematology and oncology who also have extensive experience in working with adolescents. His guiding hand brings a comprehensive and cohesive discussion to the reader. As is true of the other organ systems, a developmental biologic framework is useful in understanding disorders of the erythrocyte, disorders of the polymorphonuclear leukocyte, and disorders of hemostasis.

The oncologic conditions most commonly seen in adolescents include acute and chronic leukemias, bone tumors, lymphomas (Hodgkin as well as non-Hodgkin), brain tumors, and germinal cell tumors. Each of these conditions can have a devastating effect on the psychosocial development of adolescents, so an overview of psychosocial issues is presented by Dr. John Hutter. One of the newest treatment modalities, which holds great hope for many adolescents affected with life-threatening illness, is bone marrow transplantation. Dr. Reggie Duerst presents the state of the art regarding this treatment modality in adolescents.

No organ system undergoes as many changes during adolescence as does the endocrine system. Dr. Mary Voorhess shares her extensive experience with adolescents affected by disorders of the thyroid, adrenal, parathyroid, and pituitary glands. Disorders of growth, presenting to the clinician as short stature or tall stature, are discussed, in addition to disorders of puberty, which present to the clinician as delayed or precocious sexual development. Diabetes mellitus, a common, lifelong, and potentially life-threatening condition that frequently is frustrating to treat because of adolescent developmental issues resulting in noncompliance or "brittle" diabetes, is discussed in a separate chapter.

Adolescents with nutritional problems are also frequently difficult to treat. Although anorexia nervosa and bulimia nervosa are generally classified as psychiatric disorders, they are included in this textbook in the chapter on nutritional disorders to emphasize the important role that medical care providers have in treating these conditions. The extensive experience of Drs. Michael Nussbaum, I. Ronald Shenker, and Douglas Bunnell in treating adolescents with eating disorders is evident in their subchapters. Obesity, statistically the most common eating disorder, is no more easy to treat during adolescence than it is during childhood or adulthood. However, by maintaining a consistent and pragmatic approach as suggested by Dr. Martha Arden, the health care provider may be able to have a positive influence on this important public health problem. Recent data regarding the importance of control of hyperlipidemia in the prevention of adult coronary artery disease necessitate a separate subchapter on hyperlipidemia. This is an area in which the knowledge base is constantly changing. Dr. Marc Jacobson presents the state of the art at the time of publication of this textbook.

Gastrointestinal conditions in adolescents frequently receive little attention, except for the problem of chronic abdominal pain. Dr. James Markowitz presents exciting new data regarding acid peptic disease as it relates specifically to adolescents. Drs. Markowitz and Daum also present new information that relates specifically to inflammatory bowel disease in adolescents. Liver and pancreatic diseases are discussed, as is the common clinical problem of chronic constipation.

Renal and urologic conditions that affect adolescents have two different presentations. First, there may be congenital or early childhood disorders that persist into adolescence. Second, some conditions arise during adolescence. Disorders of the upper and the lower urinary tracts are addressed in separate chapters. Genitourinary conditions related to sexual maturation are covered in the section on reproductive conditions, whose consulting editor is Dr. S. Jean Emans. As noted earlier, this section is one of the most important because of the frequency of these conditions and the potential for morbidity of pathologic conditions that go undetected and untreated.

The musculoskeletal conditions affecting adolescents fall into two major categories, sports-related and non–sports-related. Each of these is addressed in a separate chapter. Because athletics are such an important aspect of adolescent activity and because sports preparticipation evaluations or injuries are frequently the reason for an adolescent's seeing a clinician, an overview of sports medicine and of the medical conditions related to sports medicine is presented, as is the management of some common sports injuries.

Dr. Robert Joynt is the consulting editor for the section on neurologic conditions. Seizure disorders, headache, syncope, vertigo, and dizziness all are addressed from a symptom-based point of view. New data regarding sleep disorders in adolescents, as well as inflammatory conditions and demyelinating disease, also are presented. Biochemical and molecular markers of neurologic conditions, state-of-the-art technologic aids in assisting in the diagnosis and management of neurologic conditions, are also addressed.

Rheumatologic conditions affecting adolescents are described by Dr. David Siegel. The overlap among rheumatologic conditions, infectious conditions, and immunologic conditions can be great. The readers of this textbook are fortunate in having Dr. Vincent Fulginiti serve as the consulting editor for the section on infectious conditions. The editors made no attempt to present an exhaustive discussion of infectious conditions affecting adolescents. Rather, selected conditions were chosen, either because they were common in adolescents or because the presentation or management in adolescents is somewhat different from that in children or adults. An overview of the process of selecting an appropriate antimicrobial agent for an adolescent is described by Dr. Keith Powell.

Conditions that are likely to cause an adolescent to be brought to a hospital emergency room are addressed by Drs. Stephen Ludwig, Steven Selbst, and Jane Lavelle. Trauma is the most common reason for hospital emergency room visits in the adolescent age group. The resuscitation of an adolescent with trauma or a serious medical problem is discussed in detail. In addition, the approaches to gynecologic, neurologic, and metabolic emergencies are addressed. The evaluation and management of drug overdosage, an increasingly common problem among adolescents, especially in urban areas, are also presented.

No section of this text should be considered all-inclusive with respect to any condition possibly affecting an adolescent. The focus of this text, which is to define the body of knowledge that is relatively specific to adolescents, will necessarily leave out conditions that some readers may consider important. We hope that as the knowledge base of adolescent medicine becomes more clearly defined in the future that these areas can be addressed.

Disorders of the Skin, Eyes, Ears, Nose, and Mouth

CHAPTER 39

Skin Disorders

HAZEL J. VERNON and ALFRED T. LANE

ACNE

Incidence and Pathophysiology

Common acne occurs in 85% of adolescents. It is a disorder of the pilosebaceous glands and is characterized by follicular occlusion and inflammation. The lining of the follicle is abnormally thickened and occludes the lumen. The plugged follicle is called a microcomedo and is the primary abnormality in all acne lesions.

Sebaceous glands secrete a mixture of lipid and cellular contents that contribute to follicular occlusion and cause inflammation. These glands are stimulated by androgens and are inhibited by estrogens. Although most adolescents with acne have normal testosterone levels, increased conversion of testosterone to dihydrotestosterone appears to occur in the skin of adolescent patients with acne. Other androgenic hormones may also play a role in acne production. For example, female adolescents with partial 11- or 21-hydroxylase deficiency may develop severe acne despite having normal testosterone levels (see Chapter 55). In addition, most female adolescents relate flares of activity immediately prior to their menstrual period when estrogen levels are relatively low.

During puberty, the concentration of the microaerophilic diphtheroid *Propionibacterium acnes* in the follicles is increased. This organism produces chemotactic factors and lipases that hydrolyze triglycerides to free fatty acids, which may contribute to inflammation.

Once a microcomedo is formed, the follicular wall thins as the lumen continues to expand under pressure of epithelial cells, sebum, and bacteria. If this enlarging plug causes dilation of the follicular ostium, the resulting noninflammatory lesion is an open comedo (blackhead). If the ostium does not dilate, the resulting noninflammatory clinical lesion is a closed comedo (whitehead). Closed comedones and microcomedones may develop into inflammatory lesions, whereas open comedones usually do not. Chemotactic factors secreted by *P. acnes* attract leukocytes whose enzymes disrupt the follicular wall, releasing luminal contents into the dermis. If the resulting inflammatory process is in the upper dermis and localized, the clinical lesion will be a superficial papule or pustule. If the inflammatory process is more severe and deeper, a nodule or cyst may develop.

Clinical Manifestations

Acne commonly presents as comedones on the forehead and the nose of preadolescents. As puberty progresses, acne gradually worsens in both severity and the extent of skin surface involvement. Rarely, an adolescent may present with the explosive onset of scarring cystic acne without a prior history of other types of lesions. The severity of the disease tends to be similar to that of the adolescent's parents and siblings.

Most acne lesions are asymptomatic. However, the larger, deeper lesions may be markedly tender and can be accompanied by soft tissue edema. Superficial papules and some deeper lesions may "point," and the adolescent may express the contents, leaving only a crust (scab) at presentation. The deeper nodules and cysts usually do not "point," and squeezing increases their size and tenderness owing to rupture into the dermis rather than onto the surface of the skin.

Superficial acne lesions resolve without scarring but may leave hyperpigmented macules that fade with time. Cystic lesions, however, frequently heal with a depressed permanent scar. A cyst may occasionally result in a sinus tract.

Diagnosis

History should focus on identifying diseases associated with acne (e.g., adrenal or ovarian hyperfunction), factors causing flare-ups, prior treatments, and current skin care regimen. Physical examination must include the face and trunk and determination of sexual maturation. The types of lesions present, the number of each type, the intensity of inflammation, and the extent and severity of hyperpigmentation and scarring should be noted. No laboratory studies are indicated unless the history and physical examination suggest androgen excess or Cushing syndrome (see Chapter 55).

Differential Diagnosis and Flare Factors

Oral contraceptive therapy may improve or may exacerbate acne. The effect is usually unpredictable, depending on the adolescent and on the medication used (see Chapter 73). Corticosteroids, phenytoin, isoniazid, and lithium can cause papular or pustular acne-like

TABLE 39–1. Guidelines for Treatment of Acne Based on Severity and Extent of Disease

Comedonal Acne—no inflammatory lesions
Topical tretinoin* 0.025% cream every other night for 1 week and then every night

or

Topical benzoyl peroxide* twice daily

Mild to Moderate Inflammatory Acne—no cysts, few to no nodules
Topical tretinoin every night

and

Topical antibiotic and/or topical benzoyl peroxide every morning

If disease is resistant to above therapy:
add

Oral antibiotic

Moderate to Severe Inflammatory Acne—occasional cysts, few to many nodules
Topical tretinoin every night

and

Topical antibiotic or benzoyl peroxide every morning
and

Oral antibiotic

Severe Nodulocystic Acne
Topical tretinoin every night

and

Topical antibiotic or benzoyl peroxide every morning
and

Oral antibiotic
and

Consider isotretinoin

*Both tretinoin and benzoyl peroxide can result in skin photosensitivity in susceptible adolescents. Therefore, a noncomedogenic sunscreen with SPF >15 should be used on prolonged sun exposure.

eruptions. Anabolic steroids may cause a severe, deep inflammatory acne.

Acne may be caused or exacerbated by skin care products (acne cosmetica). Adolescents should be encouraged to use makeup bases, moisturizers, and hair care items that are labeled "oil free," "nonacnegenic," or "noncomedogenic."

Hair oil or grease frequently causes numerous closed comedones around the hair line and on the forehead (pomade acne). Patients can avoid this condition by using small amounts of a less oily gel or lotion on the ends of the hair only.

Adolescents who are employed in occupations that result in exposure to oils or greases, such as working in a fast food restaurant or automobile repair shop, may develop an acne-like eruption or flare of preexisting acne. Both comedones and inflammatory lesions occur. Treatment is similar to that of other forms of acne, with thorough skin cleansing and minimum exposure to oils or greases.

Patients who are active in sports and who wear tight or occlusive garments, such as football pads or lycra/spandex leotards, may develop acne where these items come into contact with their skin. The lesions result from the maceration, friction, and irritation from sweat and occlusive clothing (acne mechanica). This problem can be minimized by wearing a cotton T-shirt or other absorbent material under the occlusive garment and showering and changing clothing immediately after exercise.

Gram-negative folliculitis is a rare problem that pre-sents as a sudden flare of numerous pustules clustered in the nasolabial region or of numerous cysts over the face of adolescents who are taking antibiotics. Usually *Klebsiella, Enterobacter,* or *Proteus species* are found. Treatment with appropriate antibiotics based on culture results may clear the eruption. Isotretinoin has also been used successfully.

Acne fulminans is a very rare disease of male adolescents and young adults. It is characterized by the explosive onset of tender nodules and cysts, that frequently ulcerate and heal with scarring. Lesions are most common on the trunk, but there may be facial involvement. Associated systemic signs and symptoms include fever, malaise, myalgias, arthralgias, and leukocytosis. Radiographs may show osteolysis and periosteal reaction in areas of bone tenderness. Treatment requires combination therapy with topical agents, systemic antibiotics, antiinflammatory agents including systemic corticosteroids, and sometimes isotretinoin.

A pruritic or tender acneiform eruption can occur on the trunk caused by the yeast *Malassezia furfur (Pityrosporum orbiculare)*. Characteristically, the onset is sudden, and all lesions are clinically in the same stage of development. The lesions respond to topical or systemic antifungal therapy.

Acne conglobata is a severe form of nodulocystic acne with sinus tract formation. Similar lesions may be seen in the scalp, axillae, and groin. This type of acne is less common in adolescents than in adults.

Treatment

Acne can be a psychologically debilitating disease for adolescents who are particularly sensitive about their appearance. Treatment can increase self-esteem and can prevent permanent scars that might have developed without treatment. Successful acne therapy depends on the physician understanding the adolescent's goals for treatment and the patient understanding what causes his or her acne (Table 39–1).

The following points should be emphasized when counseling adolescents about acne:

1. The adolescent patient must not pick or squeeze at the lesions, especially the deeper ones, which may result in inflammation and scarring.

2. Improvement in the lesions is gradual and usually occurs in 4 to 6 weeks.

3. Acne is not caused by dirt or oil on the surface of the skin. The skin is washed gently with a mild soap. Antibacterial soaps are not necessary. Frequent or vigorous washing will traumatize the skin and result in further inflammation.

4. Astringents and rubbing alcohol make the skin surface less oily but have minimal beneficial effect on the acne; such treatment may actually irritate the skin.

5. Mechanical abrasives, such as scrubs and "buffers," traumatize the skin, can exacerbate inflammatory acne lesions, and fail to remove follicular plugs.

6. Fatty foods or chocolate do not cause an exacerbation of the acne.

7. Use of nonacnegenic skin care products is essential.

Medical treatment of acne is determined by the extent and severity of disease, prior treatments, and therapeutic goals. Each regimen must be followed for a minimum of 4 to 6 weeks before determining efficacy.

Topical treatments are used to prevent new lesions as well as to treat preexisting ones. Treatment must be used over the entire affected area, not merely on existing lesions. Adolescents with dry skin will prefer less drying medications and can use nonacnegenic moisturizers during therapy. Patients with extremely oily skin will prefer the drying products.

Tretinoin is the treatment of choice for comedonal acne. This derivative of vitamin A normalizes the abnormal epithelial lining of the follicle and loosens the compacted debris within the lumen. The result is clearing of clinical comedones as well as the microcomedones. Tretinoin has a propensity to severely irritate the skin if it is used incorrectly. To avoid irritation, therapy is begun with the low-strength 0.025% cream, which is applied every other night for 1 week and then every night. Treated skin is more sensitive to sun exposure, and sunscreen use is required. Because the amount of topical retinoic acid absorbed is small, the drug is unlikely to be teratogenic. Tretinoin may be used alone for young patients with only comedonal acne. It has no effect in clearing existing inflammatory lesions, but it should be considered as preventive therapy. In inflammatory acne, tretinoin is used in conjunction with other agents.

Benzoyl peroxide is the most widely used topical agent for acne. It decreases the number of *P. acnes* organisms on the skin, and it is also mildly comedolytic. There may be only a small increase in efficacy among the 2.5%, 5%, or 10% strengths of benzoyl peroxide. As is true of tretinoin, cream preparations are less irritating than gel forms; the liquid formulations are the most drying and irritating. Once having chosen a preparation, the adolescent should be instructed to apply the benzoyl peroxide to the skin once or twice daily. Side effects include irritation and the potential to bleach clothing; contact dermatitis may rarely occur. Benzoyl peroxide may be used alone in adolescents with mild acne, but it is more effective when used in conjunction with other agents.

Topical antibiotics decrease the quantity of *P. acnes* organisms in hair follicles. Topical erythromycin (usually 2% in solution or gel) and clindamycin (1% phosphate salt in solution, gel, or lotion) are similar in efficacy; each can be used once or twice a day. Topical antibiotics are frequently used in combination therapy with tretinoin or benzoyl peroxide. A cream containing both erythromycin and benzoyl peroxide is available. An erythromycin-zinc topical product has shown promise in the treatment of both inflammatory and noninflammatory lesions. Only small amounts of the antibiotics are absorbed systemically.

The systemic antibiotics most commonly used for acne are tetracycline and erythromycin. In addition to decreasing the quantity of *P. acnes* organisms, the efficacy of these antibiotics may also be due to their inhibition of chemotaxis and the consequent decrease in inflammation. Treatment of moderate to severe inflammatory acne is usually begun at a dose of 500 mg to 1 g daily of tetracycline or erythromycin in two or three divided doses. In the absence of an adequate clinical response, 1.5 g daily may be used. Minocycline, 100 to 200 mg daily, is very effective for many adolescents who have used tetracycline without success. Its cost, however, limits its use to those patients with severe or recalcitrant disease.

Once clinical improvement is seen, an attempt should be made to taper the patient's systemic treatment to once daily or every other day treatment over several months and then to continue with only topical therapy. However, many adolescents must remain on antibiotic therapy for several years. When tetracycline is used by a female adolescent, her pregnancy status must be monitored.

There is the potential for the broad-spectrum antibiotics used in acne therapy to alter the absorption of oral contraceptives by changing gut flora. Several isolated cases in the literature suggest this, although these reports must be considered rare in light of the number of patients who receive treatment with both antibiotics and oral contraceptives. It may be prudent for adolescents to avoid simultaneous treatment or to use an alternate method of birth control when possible (see Chapter 73).

Isotretinoin (13-*cis*-retinoic acid) can dramatically improve the cosmetic and emotional state of adolescents with severe, recalcitrant nodulocystic acne. In appropriate regimens, isotretinoin has resulted in long-term remission of acne in approximately 60% of patients treated. Because of the severity of side effects and its teratogenicity, it should be prescribed only by physicians familiar with its use.

Standard therapy begins with a dose of 0.5 to 1 mg/kg/day for 16 to 20 weeks. The dosage may be increased or decreased depending on therapeutic response or tolerance to side effects. Shorter treatment courses and lower doses produce higher recurrence rates and are not recommended.

Mucocutaneous dryness, skin fragility, and photosensitivity are expected. Less common side effects include arthralgias, myalgias, mood disturbances, and hair loss. There are reports of pseudotumor cerebri occurring with the use of isotretinoin, especially when this agent is used concurrently with tetracyclines.

An elevation in triglyceride levels occurs in 25% of adolescents and can usually be corrected with dietary changes. Less commonly, an elevation in serum liver enzyme concentration or a decrease in white blood cell count occurs. Intermittent determination of these values should continue throughout the treatment period.

Because of isotretinoin's severe teratogenicity, an intensive education program for potential female candidates is indicated. Adolescents of childbearing potential must not become pregnant during isotretinoin treatment. Current recommendations are to obtain informed consent, to perform pregnancy tests throughout treatment, to postpone initiating therapy until the menstrual period begins, and to use two effective birth control methods from the month before treatment until 1 month after discontinuing treatment.

Course and Prognosis

Most adolescents "outgrow" acne. However, 5% to 10% of young adults still complain of significant acne, and young adults who had minimal problems during their teens may develop significant inflammatory disease in their 20s.

DISORDERS OF HAIR

The hair follicle growth cycle consists of a growing phase (anagen) followed by a resting phase (telogen) and loss of the hair. Approximately 100 scalp hairs are lost daily, and approximately 85% of hairs are in anagen and 15% are in telogen at any one time. Scalp hair grows approximately 1 cm a month for 1 to 3 years before entering the resting phase. Patients with thick hair may lose up to one third to one half of their hair before a physician is able to detect the loss. Soft, usually unpigmented (vellous) hairs in the pubic and axillary region are transformed into coarser, pigmented (terminal) hairs by androgens during puberty.

Hair Loss (Table 39–2)

Hair breakage can result from trauma from various cosmetic treatments, including hair permanents, bleaching, relaxers, pressing, weaving, or hot-styling appliances. Hair stubs of variable length are seen; the scalp itself is normal. The differential diagnosis includes congenital or acquired hair shaft abnormalities and fungal infection. If further trauma is avoided, the replacement hairs are normal.

Alopecia areata is a common cause of hair loss in adolescents. The differential diagnosis includes trichotillomania, secondary syphilis, tinea capitis, and traction alopecia. Medical treatment is the same as for alopecia areata in other age groups, but in adolescents particular care must be taken to address the social and psychological consequences of hair loss.

Complete regrowth of the hair occurs in 95% of patients within 1 year. Thirty percent will have a future episode of alopecia areata. Patients who present with disease prior to puberty, with extensive disease, or with disease lasting more than 1 year have a worse prognosis for total remission.

Trichotillomania is alopecia caused by repetitive manipulation of the hair. It is most common in schoolaged children and younger adolescents. The scalp hair is most often involved. The patient either twists the hair until it is removed from the scalp or frankly plucks the hair. Trichotillomania is frequently a "nervous" habit, but in older patients or in patients with a persistent condition it is classified as an impulse disorder, closely associated with obsessive-compulsive disorder. Usually there is only one linear or angular area of partial hair loss in the frontal or temporal region. Hairs are very short and of varying lengths. The scalp is usually normal.

Therapy includes reassurance, close follow-up, and treatment of any underlying emotional problem. Clomipramine and fluoxetine may be effective in longstanding cases. Prognosis for regrowth of the hair depends on the extent of emotional disease. Regrowth usually occurs after removal of the hair ceases; scarring of the scalp may occur if the condition is chronic.

The use of hair styles and styling methods that pull on the hair can cause traction alopecia in the area of the scalp affected by the stress—the frontal scalp for ponytails, the borders of parts with cornrows or hair rollers, and the hair line circumferentially with all techniques. Hair loss is never total. Scarring is seen if damage is chronic. Similarly, the use of hot combs during the hot pressing method of hair straightening can

TABLE 39–2. Causes of Hair Loss

STRUCTURAL ABNORMALITIES OF THE HAIR SHAFT
Primary
   Menkes syndrome
   Trichothiodystrophy
Secondary
   Damage due to styling methods
NONSCARRING ALOPECIA
Infection
   Fungal
Traumatic
   Traction alopecia
   Hot comb alopecia
   Trichotillomania
Alopecia areata
Androgenetic alopecia
Alopecia associated with systemic disease
   Telogen effluvium
   Endocrine disease (thyroid, adrenal, gonadal)
   Syphilis
   Nutritional, including anorexia
Drug-associated alopecia
   Cytotoxic agents
   Retinoids
   Propylthiouracil
   Carbamazepine
   Lithium
   Haloperidol
   Clofibrate
   Anticoagulants
   Propranolol
   Bromocriptine
   Valproate
   Amitriptyline
   Ethambutol
SCARRING ALOPECIA
Lupus erythematosus
Scleroderma/morphea
Sarcoidosis
Lichen planus
Folliculitis keloidalis
Perifolliculitis associated with hidradenitis suppurativa
   Traumatic—scarring if of long standing
   Traction alopecia
   Hot comb alopecia
   Trichotillomania
   Chemical burns
Infection
   Superficial fungal (when associated with severe inflammation)
   Deep fungal, bacterial, viral less commonly
Neoplasms/hamartomas
   Nevus sebaceous
   Epidermal nevus
   Tumors of epidermal appendages
   Lymphoma
   Metastases
   Basal cell carcinoma

cause alopecia by both traumatic removal and thermal burn; scarring can result. Treatment is to change to another hair style or styling method. Prognosis depends on the degree of scarring.

Androgenetic alopecia (male-pattern baldness) affects both males and females and is either autosomal dominant with variable penetration or of multifactorial inheritance. In females, the hair loss is usually seen as diffuse thinning of the frontoparietal scalp and rarely becomes total loss. It usually has a later onset than that occurring in men. In 5% of white males, hair loss begins before the age of 20.

The entire frontal hairline recedes normally in most adolescents and does not indicate alopecia. The first sign of androgenetic alopecia is usually bilateral recession of the frontotemporal scalp with sparing of the midfrontal area. The progression is typically gradual, although patients may relate periods of relatively rapid hair loss or recession followed by fairly stable periods.

The diagnosis is usually made clinically. All female adolescents with male-pattern baldness should be screened for adrenal or ovarian hyperfunction (see Chapter 55 and 70).

During a period of emotional or physical stress, including severe dieting in anorexia nervosa (see Chapter 60), many anagen hairs abruptly enter telogen. After the stress subsides, the follicles enter anagen simultaneously. The individual presents with diffuse thinning 2 to 6 months later as a result of loss of the old telogen hairs (telogen effluvium). Adolescents need only to be reassured that the hair loss is really indicative of hair regrowth. The differential diagnosis includes the diffuse form of alopecia areata and a rapid phase of androgenetic alopecia.

Folliculitis Keloidalis and Pseudofolliculitis Barbae

Folliculitis keloidalis is a chronic inflammatory condition of the nuchal region of the scalp that frequently begins during puberty. It is seen most commonly in young black men who have closely clipped or shaved hair styles and is due to inflammation and infection with subsequent scarring associated with "ingrowing" hairs. Friction from tight clothing exacerbates the condition. Physical examination demonstrates papules and pustules or mildly pruritic 2- to 3-mm, firm, flesh-colored hypertrophic scars around hair follicles. Rarely, the entire occipital scalp area will be covered by this scarring. For mild disease, changing hair styles and avoiding occlusive, heavy hair oils may be adequate. Topical antibiotic solutions or systemic antibiotics are frequently necessary. Small scars can be treated with intralesional corticosteroids. Larger ones may require surgical excision to arrest the chronic inflammatory process.

Pseudofolliculitis barbae is a similar condition in the beard area of young men who shave and is also most common in blacks. Discontinuation of a close shave is the usual treatment. An electric razor may give acceptable results, but sometimes hair must be clipped. For very mild cases, benzoyl peroxide and intermittent use of a low-potency topical corticosteroid may allow a young man to shave. Other treatment is similar to that for folliculitis keloidalis. The differential diagnosis includes staphylococcal folliculitis; a culture of the lesions may be indicated.

DISORDERS OF SWEAT GLANDS

Eccrine sweat glands are found over the entire body surface and function in thermoregulation. Apocrine glands occur in the axillary and perineal regions and do not become functional until puberty. Apocrine glands have no role in thermoregulation but are closely related to the scent glands in other species and are stimulated in stressful or emotional situations.

Axillary Odor

The secretions from eccrine and apocrine glands have no odor until they are metabolized by skin surface bacteria. Antiodor treatment is designed to diminish both surface secretions and surface bacterial growth. The aluminum salts in antiperspirants inhibit bacterial flora and temporarily occlude the duct openings, thus preventing secretions from reaching the skin surface. A roll-on or stick antiperspirant product may be more effective than a spray. If these products are not effective, a 6.25% (e.g., Xerac AC) or 12% (e.g., Certan-Dri) aluminum chloride solution can be applied daily to weekly as needed. In addition, adolescents should use an antibacterial soap and make certain that clothes are laundered regularly.

Fox-Fordyce Disease

Fox-Fordyce disease is characterized by itchy, flesh-colored papules in the axillae and occasionally other apocrine gland areas of adolescents and young adults, especially young women. These lesions are caused by the plugging and subsequent rupture of the intraepidermal portion of apocrine ducts. Itching can be quite intense. Hair growth and apocrine odor are decreased, but eccrine sweating is unaffected. A mild corticosteroid cream or low-strength tretinoin cream may decrease symptoms, but the disease is usually chronic.

Hidradenitis Suppurativa

A chronic disease of apocrine glands, hidradenitis suppurativa begins during puberty and is characterized by the development of painful, malodorous cysts and sinus tracts in the axillae, perineum, or both. Occasionally it is associated with cystic acne and a scarring folliculitis on the scalp, known as the "follicular occlusion triad." Obesity, residence in a hot humid climate, and a family history of severe acne are associated factors.

The apocrine duct becomes plugged and dilated by

epithelial cells and entrapped bacteria. The duct and gland walls then rupture, resulting in painful abscesses that can ulcerate onto the skin surface or spread to neighboring glands. Lesions heal with scarring and sinus tract formation. An associated seronegative spondyloarthropathy has been reported. Cultures may demonstrate a solitary organism or mixed infection with gram-positive and gram-negative organisms. Anaerobes are less commonly found. The differential diagnosis includes an inflamed or infected epidermal inclusion cyst, recurrent staphylococcal furunculosis, acid-fast bacilli infections, cat-scratch disease, actinomycosis, lymphogranuloma venereum, granuloma inguinale, and inflammatory bowel disease.

Tight clothing and clothing made of nonporous synthetic material should be avoided. Shaving and antiperspirants may exacerbate the condition. Depilatories or electric shavers may be better tolerated. Antibacterial soaps, topical 6.25% aluminum chloride in anhydrous alcohol, and acne therapies such as benzoyl peroxide, topical erythromycin, or clindamycin in a drying base can be used prophylactically. A solitary lesion may respond to intralesional corticosteroids with involution within 2 to 3 days. This procedure is less likely to cause sinus tract formation than incision and drainage. Systemic antibiotics are indicated for any acute exacerbation and should be continued until the acute lesions resolve. Adolescents with mild disease can be treated with intermittent systemic therapy; however, some individuals may require chronic antibiotic therapy with tetracycline or erythromycin. Isotretinoin has been used with mixed results.

Sinus tracts require surgical excision. Occasionally, total excision of the axillae and the apocrine areas of the perineum with grafting is necessary.

If treated aggressively and early, hidradinitis suppurativa can frequently be limited to an occasional isolated lesion. In the absence of sinus tracts, many patients notice resolution of the disease after a few years. Others have progressive disease with scarring and fistula formation despite maximum therapy.

Foot Odor

Foot odor is caused by interactions between eccrine sweat, the stratum corneum of the epidermis, and cutaneous microflora. Treatment consists of keeping the feet dry, wearing absorbent socks, wearing shoes of porous materials, rotating pairs of shoes, and using antiperspirant sprays or 6.25% to 20% aluminum chloride (Drysol). Topical antibacterial agents can be helpful.

ECZEMA

Atopic Dermatitis

Fewer than half of children with classic flexural atopic dermatitis experience total remission. However, the adolescent may develop hand or foot eczema in addition to, or instead of, body eczema. Treatment of hand and foot dermatitis in the adolescent is similar to that for body involvement in the younger child, except that it typically requires more potent topical corticosteroids.

Lichen Simplex Chronicus

Constant rubbing of one particular area of the skin can result in an intensely pruritic rash lasting weeks to months. Symptoms are most severe during periods of stress. One or two elevated, lichenified 2- to 5-cm plaques are seen on the extremities, the occiput, or occasionally the buttocks. Lichen simplex chronicus is treated with higher-strength topical corticosteroids. If the patient is scratching as a way to relieve tension, therapy may be only temporarily effective.

Keratosis Pilaris

Keratosis pilaris is a disorder of hair follicle keratinization that results in plugs of follicular ostia. It may be an isolated phenomenon or may occur in association with atopy or ichthyosis vulgaris. The peak incidence (up to 50%) of keratosis pilaris occurs during adolescence. Adolescents present with concerns about the appearance of the lesions, which are numerous red, white, or flesh-colored, firm, 1- to 2-mm follicular papules on the lateral upper arms and/or the anterior thighs. Moisturizers containing lactic acid, topical keratolytics such as propylene glycol, and tretinoin decrease the roughness. Although topical corticosteroids decrease erythema, they are not indicated for this chronic disorder.

Contact Dermatitis

Dermatitis from contact with poison ivy, oak, or sumac is caused by a delayed-type hypersensitivity reaction to the oil found within any part of the plant. Before washing skin and clothing, the person may spread the oil from exposed areas to unexposed areas. For limited disease, topical antipruritics, such as lotions with camphor and menthol, and a potent topical corticosteroid are indicated. For vesicular or extensive reactions, as well as those involving the eyes and genital area, systemic prednisone at 0.5 to 2 mg/kg/day for at least 2 weeks can give dramatic relief. If corticosteroids are discontinued prematurely or if the dose is tapered too rapidly, the rash may recur. Other plants, such as those in the chrysanthemum family, can also cause hypersensitivity reactions.

Allergic contact dermatitis to the nickel found in jewelry, bra strap hooks, and jean fasteners is quite common in adolescents. For mild sensitivity the offending metal can be coated with plastic or a plastic spray. Surgical stainless steel, sterling silver, or 14-karat gold jewelry is generally well tolerated.

In comparison to dermatophyte infection or eczema, the rash of allergic contact dermatitis to shoe materials frequently occurs on the dorsal foot as well as, or instead of, the sole. Patch testing is required to determine the precise cause.

Frequent causes of contact dermatitis include fingernail polish (may cause eyelid dermatitis), acrylic nails, and lipstick. Preservatives and perfumes may also be offending agents.

PAPULOSQUAMOUS DISORDERS

Psoriasis

Psoriasis occurs in approximately 1% of the general population. The peak age at onset is the second decade for females and slightly later for males. Familial associations are more common when onset occurs in adolescence. Psoriasis is characterized by accelerated epidermal proliferation and turnover and dermal inflammation.

Adolescents may present with the common plaque psoriasis, guttate psoriasis, or scalp disease only. In plaque psoriasis, the lesions are bilaterally symmetric, well-circumscribed, red, thick, scaly plaques on the elbows, knees, sacrum, and scalp. Guttate psoriasis is characterized by the sudden onset of teardrop-shaped small plaques over the trunk and extremities. This form is frequently associated with streptococcal infections. Nail involvement may resemble dermatophyte infection. Psoriatic arthritis can mimic various forms of arthritis (see Chapter 90).

The differential diagnosis for guttate psoriasis includes pityriasis rosea and secondary syphilis. Scalp disease may resemble seborrheic dermatitis and tinea capitis. In adolescents with psoriasis most marked in the sun-exposed areas, subacute lupus erythematosus associated with Ro/SSA antibodies should be considered. In patients with psoriasis and arthritis, Reiter syndrome should be considered (see Chapter 90).

Moisturizers alone may give marked improvement. Higher-strength topical corticosteroids give good results for short periods of time, but the disease may eventually become unresponsive to these agents. Systemic corticosteroids may result in a pustular flare. Although time consuming and more difficult to use, topical tar products and anthralin provide longer remission times. Guttate psoriasis frequently responds to antistreptococcal antibiotics. Ultraviolet B phototherapy is quite effective and is considered safe in adolescents. Hospitalization and systemic therapies, such as treatment with psoralens and ultraviolet A (PUVA), methotrexate, and retinoids, are less commonly used in adolescents but are indicated for patients with debilitating disease.

Psoriasis is usually a chronic problem. In as many as 50% of patients, remissions do occur but are rarely permanent.

Pityriasis Rosea

Pityriasis rosea occurs in 1% of all patients seen in a dermatology practice. Seventy-five percent of patients are between 10 and 35 years of age. The cause is unknown, but the disorder may be caused by a viral infection. The adolescent presents with the sudden eruption of small red papules or oval plaques on the trunk and upper arms that follow the skin lines, forming the suggestion of a "fir tree" distribution. Papules may be clustered to form an oval plaque with a "collar" of scale just inside the margins. Lesions may be few or numerous. A herald patch, which is one large plaque that appears 2 weeks prior to the generalized eruption, may or may not be found. Pruritus occurs in 75% of patients and can be severe. The rash resolves spontaneously in 6 to 8 weeks, after which residual hypopigmentation or hyperpigmentation fades.

The rash of secondary syphilis can be identical to pityriasis rosea. A serologic test for syphilis should be obtained in all sexually active adolescent patients with pityriasis rosea. The differential diagnosis includes pityriasis lichenoides and guttate psoriasis.

In asymptomatic patients, no treatment is required. Mild itching can be relieved with lotions containing 0.5% menthol and 0.5% camphor. For severe disease or intense itching, relief has been achieved with a single treatment of ultraviolet B.

Pityriasis Lichenoides

Pityriasis lichenoides is characterized by crops of discrete papules, vesicles, pustules, small ulcerations, or scaly plaques over the trunk and extremities. Although uncommon, pityriasis lichenoides tends to occur in adolescents and is frequently confused with more common disorders such as varicella, leukocytoclastic vasculitis, and pityriasis rosea. The differential diagnosis also includes syphilis and guttate psoriasis. Histologic confirmation is indicated. Treatment can be difficult; tetracycline or erythromycin administered for several months and ultraviolet B therapy have been successful. The disease may resolve after several months or persist for several years.

DISORDERS CAUSED BY EXPOSURE TO ULTRAVIOLET RADIATION

The ultraviolet B (UVB) range of solar radiation primarily affects the epidermis and upper dermis. It is the major culprit in sunburn and induces tanning. UVB is carcinogenic through direct DNA damage in the form of pyrimidine dimers. Melanin appears to be photoprotective to DNA and other cellular elements by absorbing radiation and the free radicals formed by that radiation. UVB causes cutaneous immunosuppression by decreasing the number of Langerhans cells (bone marrow–derived antigen presenter cells). The amount of UVB reaching the earth's surface varies by the time of day. Ultraviolet A (UVA) radiation penetrates into the deeper portions of the epidermis and into the dermis. Evidence suggests that UVA is photoadditive with UVB in producing skin cancers. UVA is proposed to be the major cause of photoaging, the visible result of damage to collagen and blood vessels. In addition, UVA is a major cause of cataracts. The amount of UVA in sunlight, in contrast to UVB, is relatively constant throughout the day.

Skin Cancer and Cancer Prevention

There is a strong association between the cumulative exposure to ultraviolet radiation over one's lifetime and the incidence of squamous cell and basal cell carcinomas. Most ultraviolet radiation exposure occurs during childhood and adolescence. Evidence suggests that 70% to 80% of all nonmelanomatous skin cancers could be prevented with appropriate use of sunscreens from infancy to age 18. Other studies support an association between the number of sunburn episodes in childhood and adolescence and the incidence of melanoma years later. Both melanoma and nonmelanomatous skin cancers are increasing and are appearing in a younger population. The lifetime risk for melanoma in white Americans is expected to be at least 1 in 100 by the year 2000. The gradual ozone depletion may also result in an increased incidence of skin cancer.

Simple preventive measures will minimize photodamage. Noonday sun exposure should be avoided. Sand and snow reflect ultraviolet radiation; clothing provides only partial protection. UVA-blocking sunglasses should be used as well as sunscreens with a sun protective factor of 15 or greater. Occlusive sunblocks such as zinc oxide paste provide total protection. Most currently available sunscreens are excellent absorbers of UVB but are less effective absorbers of UVA. Fair-skinned adolescents are at particular risk of the adverse effects of sun exposure.

The dose of UVB needed to induce a tan is similar to the dose causing a burn. However, the dose of UVA needed to induce a tan is less than that which causes burning. Tanning booths take advantage of this property of UVA and promote "safe tanning." However, all tanning is a sign of skin injury.

Sunburn

Cutaneous symptoms of sunburn can be relieved by a cool bath followed by application of a lotion containing pramoxine. Aspirin or nonsteroidal anti-inflammatory agents ease both cutaneous and systemic symptoms.

Disorders Associated with Increased Sensitivity to Light

Many medications, including tetracycline, thiazides, tretinoin, griseofulvin, and nonsteroidal anti-inflammatory agents can cause an exaggerated sunburn in sun-exposed skin (phototoxic reaction). Other medications, such as sulfonamides and sulfonylureas, can cause a dermatitis in sun-exposed skin (photoallergic reaction).

Polymorphous Light Eruption

Polymorphous light eruption is an idiopathic syndrome characterized by pruritus, burning, or rash on sun-exposed skin occurring 2 hours to several days after sun exposure. The rash may be papular, vesicular, urticarial, or eczematous. This disorder usually begins in adolescence or early adult years. It is more common in females and may be familial in Native Americans. Patients are usually asymptomatic in the winter but develop symptoms or rash after the first significant sun exposure each spring. Two thirds of patients continue with symptoms or rash all summer long; one third become more tolerant after sequential exposures.

Treatment is difficult. Some patients find relief with routine sun avoidance and use of sunscreens. In particular, a sunscreen with butyl methoxydibenzoylmethane (e.g., Photoplex, Filteray), which blocks more UVA than other sunscreens, may be beneficial. Use of light therapy, beta carotene, or antimalarials has shown variable degrees of success. Cutaneous or systemic lupus erythematosus must be ruled out (see Chapter 90).

SKIN TUMORS AND PROLIFERATIVE DISORDERS

Acanthosis nigricans is velvety and hyperpigmented skin on the nape and sides of the neck and in the axillae. It is usually found during a routine physical examination in otherwise healthy obese adolescents. However, it can also be associated with endocrinopathies, especially insulin resistance.

Keloids are firm, shiny, elevated scars that extend outside the borders of previous trauma. They commonly occur after earpiercing and occasionally after severe acne. Currently available therapy is unsatisfactory. A series of intralesional corticosteroids may result in some flattening, but permanent hypopigmentation can occur. Surgical excision may result in recurrence.

Nevus sebaceus is a common birthmark that appears as a yellow, pebbly, hairless plaque, usually on the scalp and face. During puberty, a nevus sebaceus becomes larger and more yellow as the sebaceous glands within the lesion become active. A basal cell carcinoma develops in 5% to 10% of these lesions in adults. Other benign and malignant skin tumors can occur within these nevi as well. For these reasons, prophylactic surgical excision of these lesions at puberty is advised.

Becker nevus appears as unilateral flat hyperpigmentation on the anterior or posterior shoulder and chest. It begins in late childhood and early adolescence, usually in males. Over time the area may become slightly elevated and develop hypertrichosis.

Melanocytic Tumors

Melanocytic nevi are hamartomas of melanocytes that may be congenital or may first appear during childhood or puberty. In adolescents, flat, hyperpigmented nevi may become elevated and may or may not lose their pigment. With normal elevation, however, the entire lesion should become uniformly elevated with a smooth, slightly pebbly surface. Any nevus in which only part of the lesion is elevated is distinctly unusual.

Less than 2% of malignant melanomas occur in adolescents. However, melanoma should be considered in any nevus that is larger than 6 mm, is not uniformly pigmented, has irregular borders, is asymmetric, or has areas of depigmentation or inflammation. Acral-lentiginous melanomas, occurring more commonly in blacks and Asians, are melanomas of the palms, soles, nail beds, and mucous membranes. They are much more aggressive than the more common superficial spreading melanomas. Melanomas that are removed while still less than 0.76 mm in thickness have a 99% cure rate. Early recognition and treatment are critical.

In recent years, an autosomal dominantly inherited disease has been described in which affected members have an almost 100% lifetime risk of developing melanomas. The clinical marker for this disease is the occurrence of dysplastic nevi. Clinically these nevi are larger than usual, have only a portion that is elevated, and frequently are pink to reddish-brown. In affected family members, these nevi first appear in late childhood, then become more numerous during adolescence and continue to develop throughout life. The histology is characteristic.

Adolescents with dysplastic nevi must be followed closely, and a biopsy should be done on any lesion that changes. In contrast, other adolescents may have such a nevus and have no increased risk for melanoma above that of the general population. Unfortunately at present there are no good criteria to determine which adolescents with only one or two of these unusual nevi and no family history of melanoma will have an increased risk of malignancy and which adolescents will not. Therefore, all adolescents with one or two of these nevi are encouraged to have biopsy confirmation and frequent skin examinations until such time as dysplastic nevi are better understood.

Halo nevi are melanocytic nevi in which an immunologic response against the melanocytes results in the development of a depigmented white ring around the pigmented portion of the nevus. Rarely, only the round area of depigmentation is seen. Halo nevi commonly occur during adolescence. Halos are usually associated with normal nevi but can occur around a malignant melanoma, around a dysplastic nevus, or around normal nevi in response to a distant melanoma. For this reason, all adolescents with these nevi must have a thorough physical examination, including the genital area and scalp. Any halo nevus in which the pigmented portion appears abnormal or any other abnormal-appearing nevus should be removed.

Spitz nevus, or epithelioid and spindle cell nevus, is an unusual form of nevocellular nevus that occurs most often in children and adolescents. Classically, the lesion appears suddenly as a firm red papule that grows rapidly, reaching a size of 5 to 10 mm. A biopsy is necessary to confirm the diagnosis and to exclude other skin tumors. There are rare reports of malignancy occurring within Spitz nevi.

PRIMARY CUTANEOUS INFECTIONS

Viral Infections

Verrucae, or warts, are due to infection with human papillomaviruses. Infection is acquired during close personal contact or by contact with desquamated skin cells. Breaks in the skin and skin maceration are predisposing factors. The inoculum size and the potential host's immunity to the particular virus affect the degree of contagion. The virus stimulates epidermal proliferation. Clinical lesions usually occur 2 to 6 months after infection.

Treatment can be difficult. The extent of clinical involvement, the concerns of the adolescent about the appearance of the skin, and the potential for spontaneous resolution must be weighed against the side effects of the treatment. Most treatments require destruction of infected epidermis. The effects of salicylic acid (17%) products are improved if the wart is first pared and then soaked; the product is then applied, and the area is covered with plastic adhesive tape. Treatment takes 2 to 12 weeks of daily therapy and can cause skin irritation. Alternatively, cryotherapy with liquid nitrogen is done biweekly or triweekly for one to four treatments. Potential side effects include permanent hypopigmentation, nail dystrophy, and damage to an underlying digital nerve. With encouragement and time, plantar warts can be successfully treated with stronger salicylic acid products, such as 27% salicylic acid gel or 40% salicylic acid plasters. Adequate freezing of plantar warts is exquisitely painful. Surgery should be avoided if possible.

Molluscum contagiosum is a common cutaneous infection with a poxvirus. In adolescents, it is frequently transmitted during sexual contact. Lesions occur as discrete, shiny, flesh-colored to red papules 2 to 6 mm in diameter and may be isolated or grouped. They are common on the trunk and in genital areas. They usually respond easily to treatment. The central viral bodies can be expressed with a comedo extractor or, more commonly, the lesions are treated with topical wart therapies, cantharone, curettage, or liquid nitrogen.

Herpes labialis is a recurrent skin eruption caused by herpes simplex virus that frequently occurs during emotional stress, exposure to sunlight, menses, or fever. It appears as painful grouped vesicles or crusts on an erythematous base, usually on the lips or perioral area. In an immunocompetent patient, it is rare for herpes simplex virus to cause ulcerations of the oral mucosa except during the primary infection. No treatment is necessary for an acute recurrence. Oral acyclovir, 200 mg three times a day or 400 mg twice daily for several months, may prevent frequent recurrences while the patient is on therapy. Once therapy is stopped, the adolescent may suffer recurrences.

Fungal Infections

Dermatophyte infections of the foot (tinea pedis) increase in frequency during adolescence and may become chronic. Clinically the adolescent may have asymptomatic diffuse scaling over the entire sole, maceration in the fourth and fifth web spaces, or bullae. "Athlete's foot" is not always caused by a dermatophyte infection. The differential diagnosis includes foot eczema, superficial bacterial infection, and contact dermatitis.

Tinea cruris, dermatophyte infection of the groin, also becomes more common in adolescence. The differential diagnosis includes erythrasma, psoriasis, irritant dermatitis, and candidiasis.

Diagnosis is confirmed with a potassium hydroxide (KOH) examination under the microscope or fungal culture. Excessive moisture in the affected area should be avoided. Topical imidazole or allylamine antifungal creams are used once or twice daily. To decrease the frequency of recurrences, the cream should be used for at least 2 weeks after the rash subsides and sometimes for 6 to 8 weeks or longer. Antifungal sprays and powders are not as effective as creams or lotions. Griseofulvin may be required for severe cases. Ketoconazole is also effective. Secondary bacterial infections require treatment with appropriate antibiotics.

Tinea capitis occurs in all ages but becomes less common after puberty.

Tinea versicolor (pityriasis versicolor) is one of the most common dermatologic reasons for an adolescent to see a physician. The incidence of this disorder approaches 50% in tropical climates. It is caused by an abundance of the lipophilic yeast *Malassezia furfur (Pityrosporum ovale)*, part of the normal flora. Predisposing factors include warmth, humidity, genetics, or immune suppression. The adolescent will complain about a color change on the skin or of mild pruritus. On the upper back, and less commonly the anterior chest, shoulders, and neck, the adolescent will have hypopigmented, hyperpigmented, or erythematous macules. On scratching the skin, scaling will be marked. KOH examination under the microscope shows numerous yeast forms with short hyphae ("broken spaghetti and meat balls").

For large areas of involvement, it is most economical to use 2.5% selenium sulfide lotion applied liberally to all areas of rash and surrounding normal skin for 10 to 20 minutes each night for 1 week. Scaliness quickly resolves, but the color change takes several weeks to fade. For smaller areas of rash, any topical antifungal cream used daily or twice daily as recommended for 2 weeks usually is effective. Recurrences are common, signaled by the reappearance of scaling or color change. Application of selenium sulfide lotion once a week may prevent recurrences.

Cutaneous Infestations

SCABIES

Scabies is caused by cutaneous infestation with the mite *Sarcoptes scabiei*. During adolescence, the mite is frequently transmitted during sexual contact. The pregnant female mite burrows into the epidermis and lays eggs, which, on hatching, continue the life cycle. After 2 to 6 weeks the adolescent's immune response becomes intense and a rash occurs. Unfortunately, during those first several weeks there may be no rash, yet the patient is infectious.

Adolescent patients may present with intensely pruritic 1- to 3-mm flesh-colored or red papules, which have frequently been excoriated. Occasionally in a linear array, the papules are located on the wrists, finger webs, axillae, groin areas, nipples, waist band area, and intergluteal fold. Examination of skin scrapings demonstrates the mite, eggs, or mite feces; false-negative results are frequent.

Permethrin 5% cream (Elimite), the treatment of choice, is safe and effective. Lindane 1% lotion (Kwell), if used correctly, has minimal risk for neurotoxicity. Both agents are applied to dry skin from the neckline down, with specific attention to intertriginous areas and under the fingernails and toenails. Permethrin cream is rinsed off in 8 to 12 hours, lindane in 6 hours. Sheets, towels, and clothing should be laundered immediately after treatment. Family members and sexual partners should also be treated. Itching may continue for up to 2 weeks after treatment.

LICE

Although often acquired during sexual contact, pubic lice can be transmitted by fomites such as towels and sheets. Once infected, patients experience itching and present with red papules in the pubic hair region. The louse as well as the nits may be seen. Maculae caeruleae (bluish-gray, 5-mm macules caused by the insect bites) are uncommon but specific for pubic lice. Infection of the eyelashes may occur. Head lice are less common in adolescents than in younger children.

Pubic lice and head lice are treated similarly. Permethrin 1% cream rinse is applied after shampooing and rinsed off after 10 minutes. In most cases, retreatment is not necessary. Pyrethrins with piperonyl butoxide shampoos are applied to the affected area for 10 minutes and then rinsed. Therapy is repeated in 1 week. Lindane 1% shampoo is applied to the affected area for 4 minutes; a lather is produced and then rinsed off. Malathion 0.5% is approved for head lice and may be more effective than any of the other agents. It is applied to dry hair and shampooed out after 8 to 12 hours; re-treatment is not needed. Nit casings can be removed with a fine-toothed "nit comb." For eyelash disease, white petrolatum is applied three to five times a day for 10 days. People with whom the adolescent has close bodily contact should be treated for pubic lice. All household members must be treated for head lice. Clothing and linens must be washed and dried or put through a complete cycle in a clothes dryer. The itching and rash take a few days to subside.

BIBLIOGRAPHY

Abramowicz M: Permethrin for scabies. Med Lett 32:21, 1990.
Drake LA, et al: Guidelines of care for acne vulgaris. J Am Acad Dermatol 22:676, 1990.
Lowy DR, Androphy EJ: Warts. In Fitzpatrick TB, et al (eds): Dermatology in General Medicine. New York, McGraw-Hill, 1987, pp 2355–2364.
Orme ML, Back DJ: Interactions between oral contraceptive steroids and broad-spectrum antibiotics. Clin Exp Dermatol 11:327, 1986.

Rothman KF, Pochi PE: Use of oral and topical agents for acne in pregnancy. J Am Acad Dermatol 6:431, 1988.

Shapiro SC, Strasburger VC, Greydanus DE (eds): Adolescent Medicine: State of the Art Reviews 1(2), 1990.

Stern RS, Weinstock MC, Baker SG: Risk reduction for nonmelanoma skin cancer with childhood sunscreen use. Arch Dermatol 122:537, 1986.

Weinstock MA, Colditz GA, Willett WC, et al: Nonfamilial cutaneous melanoma incidence in women associated with sun exposure before 20 years of age. Pediatrics 84:199, 1989.

Weston WL: The use and abuse of topical steroids. Contemp Pediatr 5:57, 1988.

CHAPTER 40

Disorders of Eyes, Ears, Nose, and Mouth

FRANK M. BIRO

DISORDERS OF VISION AND THE EYES

Newly acquired myopia and eye injuries are most common in adolescence. Sports and motor vehicle accidents place teenagers at risk for hyphema. Sexual activity of adolescents increases the risk for conjunctivitis from *Neisseria gonorrhoeae* and *Chlamydia trachomatis* (see Chapter 75). Additionally, the eye can be involved in several different systemic diseases that have their onset during the teenage years (e.g., Usher syndrome and chorioretinitis).

Refractive Disorders

The highest incidence of newly acquired myopia occurs between the ages of 11 and 13. The later the onset of myopia, the smaller is the amount of final refractive error. Myopia can be divided into two varieties: simple (physiologic) and pathologic. In simple myopia there is an increased axial length of the eye or increased curvature of the cornea, or both, leading to the myopia; a major factor for simple myopia appears to be heredity. In pathologic myopia there is an abnormal axial length of the globe with thinning of the sclera and the retina. Pathologic myopia may be associated with high degrees of refractive errors.

Clinically significant hyperopia is less common than myopia. Not all subjects who have hyperopia require corrective lenses. Those whose hyperopia is +4 to +5 diopters may require a corrective prescription, especially if they have symptoms of accommodative fatigue such as eye strain, blurring after near-vision tasks, or decreased acuity for distant objects.

Refractive errors can be corrected by eyeglasses, contact lenses, or keratorefractive surgery. There are currently three types of contact lenses that are in popular use: soft (hydrogel) lenses, semi-rigid gas-permeable lenses, and hard lenses. The complications of contact lens use include an allergic reaction to lens cleaning solution and corneal epithelial degeneration secondary to the lack of oxygen, which may lead to punctate erosions. A red painful eye in a contact lens user should be considered an infectious keratitis until otherwise proved. Complications are more likely with extended use (more than 24 hours).

Strabismus and Amblyopia

Strabismus is unlikely to develop during adolescence. A tropia is diagnosed when there is failure of the fusion of an image, leading to manifest malalignment and diplopia. Phoria is a latent deviation not evident during use of the eye, only at rest, and is treated only if symptomatic.

Amblyopia is suggested if there is more than one line disparity of visual acuity between the two eyes. There are two major groups of amblyopia: organic and functional. In organic amblyopia there is disruption of the retina or visual pathways by a disease process. Functional amblyopia can be subdivided into three additional areas: deprivation, strabismic, and refractive. In deprivation amblyopia there is disuse of visual pathways; this form of amblyopia is often not responsive to therapy. In strabismic amblyopia there is decreased vision secondary to the deviation of the eye. In refractive amblyopia there is decreased vision secondary to a blurred retinal image; for example, if there is a correction of a high refractive error, there may be a difference in the image size between the two eyes, leading to the refractive amblyopia.

Eye Injury

Adolescents are one of the leading age groups for eye injuries. The majority of adolescents with eye injuries are male; over one third of injuries occur between the months of April and June. Most are ocular injuries with nonperforation; hyphema is the leading diagnosis. Sports activities are the most common cause of injury; the three sports most associated with eye injuries, in order of frequency of injury, are baseball, tennis, and soccer. Injuries from a BB gun are an especially devastating form of trauma; the majority of adolescents with penetrating injuries from pellets require enucleation of the eye.

Because of the association between eye injuries and baseball, all adolescent baseball batters should wear helmets with face protectors. An adolescent who has one eye should wear safety lenses at all times and not be allowed to participate in contact sports or those involving high-velocity missiles.

Hyphema is blood in the anterior chamber that accumulates as a result of blunt trauma; this is to be distinguished from subconjunctival hemorrhage, which is a clinically harmless although cosmetically disturbing finding in which the blood collects under the limbic conjunctiva. Hyphema has a predilection for male adolescents. Hyphemas can be graded from microscopic to grade 4, and the degree of hyphema establishes a prognosis for the disorder. When an adolescent presents with a hyphema, an examination must be performed to establish a baseline visual acuity, to rule out extraocular injuries such as a lid laceration or blowout fracture, and to evaluate the pupillary response. Evaluation of an afferent pupillary defect is done to see if the pupil reacts consensually but not directly to light, suggesting retinal or optic nerve damage.

The risk of complications for hyphema is increased with higher grades or in those individuals with sickle cell anemia or sickle trait (see Chapter 52). The complications include secondary hemorrhage, increased intraocular pressure, anterior synechiae, and corneal staining with blood. Secondary hemorrhage, also called recurrent hyphema, usually occurs 2 to 5 days after trauma. The presence of a secondary hemorrhage leads to a worse prognosis for the patient with a hyphema. Increased intraocular pressure is often associated with nausea and vomiting and may lead to subsequent optic nerve atrophy. Anterior synechiae are more likely if the hyphema has been present for more than a week and they may lead to chronic glaucoma.

Treatment of hyphema includes allowing the adolescent to ambulate with quiet indoor activities. He or she should be discouraged from near-viewing activities and should have the head of his or her bed raised 35 degrees. One month after the injury, gonioscopy should be performed.

Red Eye

There are many evaluations that have been recommended for the "red eye." Baseline data should include an inquiry regarding a history of ocular disorders as well as the onset and progression of the pain. Examination must include assessment of visual acuity, the appearance of the cornea, and the size of the pupil and its reactivity to light. Some red eye conditions require referral to an ophthalmologist, and others can be managed by a primary care physician. Conditions that should be referred include acute glaucoma, acute iritis, acute corneal tear or inflammation, and acute scleritis. Those that usually can be managed by a primary care physician include bacterial and viral conjunctivitis, allergic conjunctivitis, and foreign body.

Bacterial conjunctivitis can present as hyperacute, acute, or chronic. In hyperacute conjunctivitis, there is a copious discharge. The Gram stain usually reveals gram-negative diplococci representing *Neisseria gonorrhoeae* or *N. meningitidis*. This condition represents a medical emergency and, without prompt therapy, can result in severe rapid ulcerative keratitis. In acute bacterial conjunctivitis there is eye irritation (burning somewhat more likely than itching) with watering. On awakening, the eyelids are usually stuck together. Because of autoinoculation, the other eye is often infected after 1 or 2 days. If hemorrhagic conjunctivitis is present, the cause is usually pneumococcus or adenovirus. Although viral conjunctivitis usually requires symptomatic treatment only, because of bacterial superinfection from rubbing the eyes, viral conjunctivitis that has been present for more than 1 or 2 days requires treatment as for acute bacterial conjunctivitis. In chronic bacterial conjunctivitis, there is a foreign body sensation, with redness, itching, and the lids sticking after sleep. There is often a history of recurrent styes and a loss of eyelashes. The management of chronic bacterial conjunctivitis includes chemical scrubbing of the eyelid margins with an isotonic shampoo as well as an antibiotic and corticosteroid ointment massaged into the hair follicles.

Two other infections involved in the external eye that deserve special mention are herpes simplex virus infection and *Chlamydia trachomatis* infection. The initial infection of herpes simplex virus is usually a follicular conjunctivitis. Recurrent herpes ocular infection causes corneal scarring, often with pathognomonic dendritic keratitis. Herpes simplex keratitis is the most common cause of corneal blindness in the United States. Conjunctivitis from *C. trachomatis* occurs in approximately 1% of those who have a chlamydial-associated sexually transmitted disease (see Chapter 75). In these adolescents, there is chronic follicular conjunctivitis with a foreign body sensation, tearing, and redness. There is often unilateral involvement with mucopurulent discharge.

In allergic (vernal) conjunctivitis, the conjunctivae have a cobblestone appearance, associated with chemosis, itching, tearing, and often allergic rhinitis. The discharge may be thick and yellow, and the adolescent may pull a ropy strand from the lids. The condition is usually worse in the spring and summer. Treatment includes elimination of the allergen and use of cold compresses, systemic antihistamines, topical vasoconstrictors, cromolyn sodium, or, in advanced cases, topical corticosteroids.

The adolescent with a foreign body in the eye presents with the sudden onset of unilateral eye pain. Fluorescein staining often demonstrates the particle, which can then be removed. A topical antibiotic is administered, and the eye is covered with a patch for 24 hours. If the foreign body contains iron and had been deposited for a time, some secondary corneal staining may occur.

In distinguishing the various causes of the red eye, aspects of the history or physical examination may be very helpful. In acute conjunctivitis there is minimal pain with generally a small amount of discharge. The vision is normal, and the pupil size is normal as is the pupillary reaction to light. There is no visual halo, and the adolescent may or may not complain of mild photophobia. In acute iritis there is moderate pain with tearing but no discharge. There is normal to slightly blurred vision. The pupil is small with a poor response to light. There is no halo, and the adolescent may have moderate photophobia. In acute glaucoma the pain is mild to severe. There is tearing without discharge, vision is blurred, and the cornea is cloudy. The pupil is dilated with a poor response to light. A halo and mild photophobia are reported. On examination there will be increased intraocular pressure. In acute scleritis there is mild to moderate pain without discharge. The vision is normal, and the pupil is normal in size and reacts to light normally. There is no photophobia. An underlying condition may be present that predisposes to an ocular disorder.

Uveitis

Uveitis broadly defines any intraocular inflammatory disease and includes anterior uveitis (iritis, iridocyclitis), intermediate uveitis (involving the vitreous), and posterior uveitis (chorioretinitis). It may be infectious or autoimmune, and there is an association with some HLA antigens. Anterior uveitis can be characterized as granulomatous ("mutton-fat," as in sarcoidosis) or nongranulomatous (the "flare" seen with many connective tissue diseases) (see Chapter 90). The presentation and course of uveitis may help identify an associated connective tissue disease. Additionally, uveitis may develop not only in the ipsilateral eye after trauma but also in the contralateral eye after several weeks.

The most common cause of chorioretinitis in the United States is *Toxoplasma gondii.* Onset is typically during adolescence, and chorioretinitis may be recurrent in many cases.

Disorders of the Eyelids

There are three major conditions involving the eyelids: chalazion, hordeolum, and blepharitis. A chalazion is an obstruction of the meibomian gland. It is generally not painful except if a secondary infection occurs. A hordeolum is an infection of the gland of Zeis. There is erythema and pain and subsequent nodular swelling. A hordeolum generally responds to topical heat and antibiotics. In blepharitis there is chronic inflammation of the eyelid margin. This may result in recurrent chalazion, conjunctivitis, loss of lashes, and a thickening of the lid margin. Treatment includes the chemical scrubbing of the lid margins with an isotonic shampoo as well as an antibiotic corticosteroid ointment massaged into the eyelash follicles.

DISORDERS OF HEARING, THE EARS, AND THE SINUSES

Hearing impairment is one of the most prevalent chronic disorders, involving 16 in every 1000 adolescents. Additionally, nearly 250,000 teenagers are affected by a severe to profound hearing loss.

Audiometric hearing problems can be conductive, sensorineural, and mixed. A conductive hearing loss is caused by the interruption of sound transmission to the inner ear; these adolescents generally have good speech discrimination if the speech is loud enough. In sensorineural hearing loss, the inner ear or eighth cranial nerve is affected. These adolescents cannot monitor their own voice and therefore often speak loudly. In mixed hearing loss, there are features of both.

The practical assessment of hearing includes basic audiology and speech discrimination, which allows the health care provider to assign functional degrees of impairment. Those with thresholds of 0 to 15 dB have normal hearing. If the threshold is 16 to 25 dB, there is a slight hearing loss. When the threshold is 26 to 40 dB, there is a mild hearing loss, leading to difficulty hearing faint or distant sounds. A 41- to 65-dB threshold, or moderate hearing loss, means that most speech is being missed at a normal conversational level. At a 66- to 90-dB threshold, there is severe hearing loss with no speech sounds audible at normal levels; the adolescent cannot distinguish consonants. At a threshold of 91 dB or greater, there is a profound hearing loss, with no response to speech and sound.

In addition to basic audiometry and speech discrimination, the third area of assessment is impedance audiometry. Auditory impedance evaluates the functional status of the middle ear and the neural pathways of the stapedius muscle. The impedance battery includes tympanometry and the acoustic reflex. There are three patterns of tympanograms: (1) normal conduction, (2) flattening of the curve (e.g., from ossicle fixation or middle ear effusion), and (3) increase in negative middle ear pressure (e.g., from eustachian tube dysfunction). The acoustic reflex test measures ipsilateral and contralateral stapedius muscle contractions in response to an auditory stimulus.

The most common cause of sensorineural hearing loss in adolescents is meningitis; this hearing loss can progress for several years after meningitis, with further deterioration during the teenage years. Sensorineural hearing loss may also result from acoustic trauma; common exposure in adolescents occurs at rock concerts and discos and from high-powered stereo headphones. Recovery may occur if there is sufficient time (i.e., a week or more) between exposures. Adolescents can protect themselves against hearing loss caused by acoustic trauma by limiting the time exposure (e.g., use stereo headphones less than 20 to 30 minutes per day) or using sound protectors so that the amplitude of the sound is less than 80 dB.

Of special note, since it requires an immediate audiologic examination, is the sudden hearing loss syndrome. This is a sudden onset of loss, a fluctuation in the degree of hearing, or a deterioration in existing hearing loss. One possible cause of sudden hearing loss syndrome is a perilymphatic fistula, which is also present in as many as 6% of the "normal" hearing impaired population.

Otitis Media

Otitis media is less common in adolescents than in children because of the increased length and angulation of the eustachian tube and the decreased amount of lymphoid tissue, both of which are part of normal maturation. Otitis media can be divided into acute otitis media, otitis media with effusion (middle ear filled with fluid), and chronic otitis media (recurrent otorrhea through a perforation or a tympanostomy tube).

Audiology is of limited value in evaluation for acute otitis media, whereas typanograms are very helpful. The health care provider should evaluate the tympanic membrane concavity, mobility, and color, although erythema of the tympanic membrane is an inconsistent finding. Localized erythema and white scarring may indicate active infection; a white or yellow tympanic membrane suggests that purulent material may be behind the tympanic membrane; an amber or blue tympanic membrane suggests a chronic middle ear effusion. In acute otitis media, the two leading organisms are *Streptococcus pneumoniae* and *Haemophilus influenzae* (see Chapter 94). A third organism that is being found with increasing prevalence is *Branhamella catarrhalis*. Thus, there are two organisms that are potentially beta-lactamase producers.

The treatment of acute otitis media is a 10-day course of amoxicillin. Amoxicillin is preferred over ampicillin because of the improved compliance in a three times per day administration over a four times per day administration, particularly in adolescents (see Chapter 26). An erythromycin-sulfisoxazole combination should be used if the adolescent is allergic to penicillin. Trimethoprim-sulfamethoxazole is not effective against *Streptococcus pyogenes,* and an alternative should be considered in an adolescent with otitis and pharyngitis. Administration of antihistamines or decongestants is not effective in the treatment of otitis media, nor is self-inflation of the middle ear or the Valsalva maneuver. Clinical improvement occurs within 48 to 72 hours in 85% to 90% of patients.

When tympanocentesis is performed in nonresponders, approximately 20% of the organisms are found to be resistant to the prescribed antibiotics, and 60% have sterile fluid. The indications for tympanocentesis are otitis with severe otalgia or with an underlying serious illness such as in the immunocompromised patient, an unsatisfactory response to antibiotics, or otitis media with a suppurative complication. Of note, 40% to 50% of those patients receiving appropriate antibiotic treatment have effusion 30 days after diagnosis and treatment. Beta-lactamase–producing organisms are associated with recurrence of acute otitis media within 1 to 2 weeks after completion of treatment with amoxicillin. If the recurrence occurs 4 or more weeks after the initial episode, the organisms and their sensitivities to antibiotics are the same as in those adolescents with an initial acute otitis media.

In otitis with effusion (i.e., middle ear filled with fluid), there is a retracted or concave tympanic membrane with decreased mobility. Approximately one half of affected adolescents have pathogenic bacteria on culture (e.g., *H. influenzae, B. catarrhalis, S. pneumoniae*); thus, initial management should be with a 10-day course of antibiotics. Amoxicillin should be prescribed if the adolescent has not had antibiotics recently. If the adolescent has been taking antibiotics recently or is unresponsive to amoxicillin, an antibiotic should be instituted that is effective against ampicillin-resistant organisms. These include amoxicillin–clavulinic acid, erythromycin-sulfisoxazole, or trimethoprim-sulfamethoxazole.

If the effusion persists for more than 2 months despite therapy, the health care provider must decide whether to place the adolescent under general anesthesia. Without general anesthesia, the management would be myringotomy with aspiration; with general anesthesia, one would insert tympanostomy tubes (ventilating tubes). Other indications for tympanostomy tubes are recurrent otitis media (i.e., four or more episodes per year despite appropriate prophylactic antibiotic therapy); persistent high negative middle ear pressure with hearing loss, or with otalgia, vertigo, or retraction pockets; or suppurative complications of otitis media.

The diagnosis of cholesteatoma may be difficult to establish secondary to a paucity of symptoms. One must consider a cholesteatoma with the clinical triad of otorrhea, hearing loss, and an abnormal otoscopy. Of note, only 7% of patients have a mass behind an intact tympanic membrane. Cholesteatomas tend to be more aggressive, tend to undergo faster growth in adolescents, and often involve the ossicles. Cholesteatoma always requires an evaluation by an otolaryngologist.

Sinusitis

Acute sinusitis usually presents as a history of a recent upper respiratory tract infection (see Chapter 94); other common presentations include maxillary dental infections or atopy. In adolescents with upper respiratory tract infections or with an atopic history, inflammation and edema lead to obstruction of the sinus ostia with subsequent development of clinical signs and symptoms of sinusitis. Signs and symptoms include a low-grade temperature, nasal obstruction, a metallic taste, and cough at night. There is often pain over the involved sinus. Maxillary sinusitis (the most frequent sinus infection in adolescents) may present as pain on percussion of the cuspid or bicuspid tooth. In ethmoid sinusitis there is tenderness of the lateral wall of the nose medial to the inner canthus. If frontal sinusitis is present, there is pain with palpation on the undersurface of the medial supraorbital rim. The finding of greatest diagnostic use is a purulent discharge from the sinus ostia. In up to one half of cases there is an associated bronchitis or otitis. Sinus transillumination may be helpful in frontal and maxillary sinusitis but not in ethmoid or sphenoid sinusitis. Radiography is indicated if the diagnosis remains unclear or if there is suspected frontal sinusitis because of a higher rate of potential complications. Sinus ultrasound may also be of some diagnostic assistance. Involvement of sphenoid and ethmoid sinuses is more commonly part of a pansinusitis. Therefore, if there is isolated involvement of one of these sinuses, the health care provider should consider an investigation for an obstructing neoplasm or mucocele.

The pathogens in acute sinusitis are *Streptococcus pneumoniae, Haemophilus influenzae,* and *Branhamella catarrhalis*, in order of frequency. The culture results of the nasal or nasopharyngeal secretions have a poor correlation with bacterial isolates obtained through sinus aspiration. In chronic sinusitis there is predominance of anaerobic organisms, the majority of which are sensitive to penicillin. The treatment for acute sinusitis is amoxicillin, with an initial cure rate of 80%. If the initial course of amoxicillin fails, beta-lactamase coverage should be instituted, with the antimicrobials listed previously for otitis with effusion. Other treatment modalities include topical decongestants for 3 to 5 days, systemic decongestants, and normal saline nose drops. Antihistamines should be avoided in the management of acute sinusitis because of an increased viscosity of sinus secretions and an increase in ciliary dysfunction with use of antihistamines. Several authors recommend inpatient treatment of frontal sinusitis, secondary to a higher rate of potentially devastating complications.

The indications for sinus aspiration are failure to respond to appropriate antibiotic treatment, a compromised immune system (see Chapter 76), and a suppurative complication of sinusitis. The most common complication of sinusitis is orbital inflammation (i.e., preseptal or orbital cellulitis); likewise, the most common cause of orbital inflammation is sinusitis. The potential complications of sinusitis include cavernous sinus thrombosis; meningitis; epidural, subdural, or brain abscess; osteomyelitis; and mucoceles.

DISORDERS OF THE OROPHARYNX

Pharyngitis

Pharyngitis remains one of the more common presenting complaints in the adolescent patient (see Chapter 94). For the diagnosis of pharyngitis there must be objective evidence of inflammation, such as erythema, exudate, or ulceration. Pharyngitis can be grouped into two categories: nasopharyngitis (nearly always viral) and pharyngitis (virus predominates over bacteria). The most common cause of nasal pharyngitis is adenovirus. In adenovirus and influenza, pharyngeal findings are more prominent in the clinical presentations. Of the other respiratory tract viral infections, coryza is more notable.

More than 90% of pharyngeal infections are caused by streptococci, adenoviruses, influenza viruses, parainfluenza viruses, Epstein-Barr virus, enteroviruses, or *Mycoplasma pneumoniae*. Although cytomegalovirus causes an infectious mononucleosis–like syndrome, pharyngitis is uncommon. Features in both the history and examination are helpful in differentiating viral from streptococcal pharyngitis. Streptococcal pharyngitis typically has an acute onset and is associated with dysphagia and headache (see Chapter 94). If more than one family member has a streptococcal infection, then the adolescent patient has an increased chance of having a streptococcal pharyngitis. Outbreaks of streptococcal pharyngitis occur more often in the winter and the spring. On physical examination, those adolescents with streptococcal infection have an elevated temperature, but a temperature of more than 40°C usually indicates a viral cause (such as coxsackievirus or herpes simplex virus). A tonsillar exudate is characteristic but not diagnostic of streptococcal infections; exudates are also evident in patients with Epstein-Barr virus, adenovirus, and diphtheria. If the adolescent also has rhinitis or conjunctivitis, streptococcal infection is less likely. A follicular pharyngitis suggests adenovirus; an ulcerative pharyngitis suggests enterovirus. On examination, one should also look for swelling of the pharynx or asymmetry of the uvula, which suggests a peritonsillar or retropharyngeal abscess.

Because of the risk of rheumatic fever, it is important to identify group A beta-hemolytic *Streptococcus*. Therapy should not be started until confirmation of the causative organism through either a rapid strep test or culture, except in a toxic-appearing adolescent who presents during an outbreak of streptococcal disease or has classic findings of scarlet fever. In both these cases, however, cultures should still be obtained to confirm the diagnosis. If an adolescent presents with a clinical picture compatible with streptococcal pharyngitis, and a rapid diagnostic test is positive, appropriate treatment can be instituted. However, because rapid diagnostic tests have a sensitivity of only 70% to 95%, a negative rapid strep test must be followed by a culture for confirmation.

There are special points to be made about the adolescent who presents with pharyngitis. If rapid tests for infectious mononucleosis are positive, the patient should still receive streptococcal diagnostic tests because of the association with infectious mononucleosis and streptococcal pharyngitis. In adolescents with *N. gonorrhoeae* infection, the pharynx is the sole site of infection in only 1% to 4% of cases. Additionally, over 90% of pharyngeal infections will be asymptomatic. *C. trachomatis* also appears to be an uncommon cause of pharyngitis. Only 2% of adolescents presenting with pharyngitis had *C. trachomatis* on pharyngeal culture, with none identified in the asymptomatic group. However, previous studies have shown elevated IgG or IgM titers for *C. trachomatis* in 20% of adults seeking care for sore throats. Several studies have documented positive *C. trachomatis* cultures in less than 6% of adults with pharyngitis. *C. pneumoniae* may account for the disparity in these findings; it is known that *C. pneumoniae* can cause a bronchitis or pneumonia that often has a coincident and severe pharyngitis. The most common cause of pharyngitis in adolescents seen at sexually transmitted disease clinics is herpes simplex virus. Herpes simplex virus infection of the pharynx is closely associated with primary genital herpes, although less frequently associated with a nonprimary first episode or recurrent episodes. Herpes simplex virus is almost always symptomatic when it affects the pharynx.

Disorders of Tonsils and Adenoids

The tonsils and adenoids, which are components of the lymphoreticular system, undergo gradual enlargement until the age of 10 to 12, at which time they undergo a regression through the teenage years. The diseases of tonsils and adenoids most often seen in adolescents are those of chronic or recurrent infection and obstructive hyperplasia. The clinical manifestations of adenoid hyperplasia include mouth-breathing, nasal obstruction, rhinorrhea, hyponasal speech, and otitis media. It does not appear that tonsillar disease has as important a relationship with pathologic processes in the ears or paranasal sinuses as has adenoid disease.

Symptoms from either acute infection or obstruction hyperplasia can affect the tonsils and adenoids. The signs and symptoms of acute adenoiditis include purulent rhinorrhea, nasal obstruction, fever, and otitis media; these findings are very similar to those found in acute sinusitis. In acute tonsillitis, there is sore throat, dysphagia, and tender cervical adenopathy with an associated erythema and exudate on the tonsils (see Chapter 94). Manifestations of adenoid hyperplasia include nasal obstruction with snoring or mouth-breathing, rhinorrhea, and a hyponasal voice. Obstructive tonsillar hyperplasia can present with snoring as well as other symptoms of an obstructive apnea syndrome, restless sleep, dysphagia, and enuresis. A clinical system has been developed to assess the degree of tonsillar enlargement. Lesser degrees of tonsillar hyperplasia may result in obstructive problems, especially in adolescents with craniofacial anomalies.

Initial management in acute tonsillar or adenoid disease is antibiotic therapy. The organisms involved in acute disease include group A beta-hemolytic streptococcus, *Streptococcus pneumoniae, Staphylococcus aureus,* and *Haemophilus influenzae* (see Chapter 94). Chronic disease of the adenoids and tonsils may be complicated by polymicrobial infections, beta-lactamase–producing organisms, and a high antigenic load. Therefore, for recurrent or chronic disease, antibiotics effective against beta-lactamase–producing or encapsulated organisms may avoid subsequent surgical intervention.

Surgical indications for adenoidectomy may be divided into three groups: infection, obstruction, and suspected neoplasia. The infectious indications include chronic or recurrent adenoiditis despite adequate antibiotic therapy, or adenoid hyperplasia associated with recurrent acute otitis media, otitis media with effusion, and chronic otitis media. Obstructive indications for surgery include adenoid hyperplasia with nasal obstruction, sleep apnea, and the presence of cor pulmonale or obligate mouth-breathing that cannot be attributed to other causes. As noted previously, adolescents with craniofacial anatomic abnormalities tolerate mild degrees of adenoid or tonsillar hyperplasia very poorly. Surgical indications for tonsillectomy include recurrent tonsillitis despite appropriate antibiotic therapy or if associated with cardiovascular disease or chronic otitis media, suspected neoplasia, and those symptoms or signs associated with obstruction, including sleep apnea, sleep disturbances, and cor pulmonale, especially if not attributable to other causes. In the preoperative evaluation for either an adenoidectomy or tonsillectomy, a family and personal history should be solicited about any bleeding problems; and for the adolescent about to undergo an adenoidectomy, the presence of a submucosal cleft or velopharyngeal insufficiency should be assessed.

DISORDERS OF THE ORAL CAVITY
Trauma

If the adolescent who presents with fractured teeth has an associated lip laceration, a radiograph should be obtained to rule out tooth fragments within the laceration. When an abrasion or laceration of the chin is sustained through blunt trauma, the health care provider should consider a subcondylar fracture. Other physical findings include swelling and tenderness over the condylar area. A sublingual hematoma should raise the suspicion of a fracture of the mandibular body.

Oral Ulcerative Diseases

Oral ulcerative diseases can be placed into three categories: acute, chronic, and generalized (see Chapter 41). In acute oral ulcerative disease, the lesions are small (less than 1 cm), of recent onset (less than 2 weeks), shallow, and painful. The differential diagnosis includes trauma, recurrent aphthous stomatitis, recurrent labial or intraoral herpes, and herpangina. Causes of trauma may be physical (such as biting one's cheek or abrasion by toothbrush bristles), chemical (e.g., aspirin burn from holding aspirin next to an aching tooth), or thermal (a pizza burn from hot cheese or reverse-smoking marijuana). Recurrent aphthous stomatitis is also known as canker sores or aphthous ulcers. In recurrent aphthous stomatitis the ulcers persist for 1 to 2 weeks, often with a prodrome lasting for a day. There are no signs or symptoms of systemic disease, and there is no vesicular onset. There are three forms: minor, major, and herpetiform aphthae. Nearly two thirds of cases represent the minor form of the disease. The lesions are single or several, well-defined, round to ovoid, 2- to 4-mm erosive ulcers with a yellow-gray membrane and thin, discrete erythematous margins. The sites most frequently involved are the buccal and labial mucous membranes, as well as the tongue, soft palate, and pharynx. Approximately 12% of cases represent major aphthae, which are greater than 1 cm, with deep, raised, rolled borders (see Chapter 41). This form may lead to scar formation, unlike the other two forms. The third form of recurrent aphthous stomatitis presents as multiple lesions in a herpetiform pattern.

Oral herpes simplex virus can present as several syndromes: herpes simplex virus pharyngitis, recurrent herpes labialis (fever blisters), and acute herpetic gingivostomatis. Recurrent herpes labialis is the most common form of recurrent herpes disease. It involves 25% to 50% of the adolescent population. Typically, there is a prodrome of burning or itching followed by an outbreak of vesicles that ulcerate after 2 to 3 days; lesions usually come in crops. The usual course is 5 to 10 days. Vesicle formation is typically on the outer third of the upper or lower lip at or near the mucocutaneous junction. Outbreaks are often associated with febrile illnesses, local trauma or sunburn, or menses. Acute herpetic gingivostomatitis is actually a generalized rather than an acute oral ulcerative disease. It presents as fever, regional adenopathy, malaise, red and swollen gingiva, and the typical pattern of vascular and ulcerative lesions. Multiple small vesicles rupture and form a round or ovoid shallow ulcer. Lesions may appear in crops, always involving the gingiva as well as often involving other mucosal sites, such as the buccal mucosa, lips, and tongue. Acute herpetic gingivostomatitis affects both the anterior and posterior oral pharynx, unlike herpangina.

Herpangina is an acute febrile self-limited viral disease that most commonly occurs in the summer but can affect an adolescent with repeated attacks. There are several 2-mm, discrete, gray-white papulovesicular lesions that rupture to form a shallow ulcer with a distinct erythematous margin. The posterior portion of the mucosa, specifically the posterior soft palate, tonsils, and upper pharynx, is involved. The majority of patients present with fever, anorexia, dysphagia, and sore throat. Coxsackievirus, echovirus, and enterovirus all are associated with herpangina.

When an oral ulcer persists for more than 2 weeks, the differential diagnosis for chronic oral ulcerative disease must be considered. Chronic oral ulcerative diseases may be either painless or painful. The lesions are usually not infectious, with the exceptions of tuberculosis, tertiary syphilis, actinomycosis, histoplasmosis, and herpes simplex in the patient with human immunodeficiency virus infection. Other causes include trauma and neoplasms, the latter being uncommon in adolescents.

Generalized oral ulcerative diseases include syndromes induced by chemicals or drugs, those caused by infections such as herpes or *Candida,* systemic disorders such as inflammatory bowel disease, and those associated with dermatologic disorders, such as erythema multiforme or pemphigus. Contact stomatitis (stomatitis venata) is a localized cellular immune response that begins with mild erythema and progresses to erosive or bullous lesions. It may be caused by mouthwashes, lipsticks, or candy. In stomatitis medicamentosa there is a humoral allergy from systemic administration of a drug; it is more severe and generalized than contact stomatitis. Some potentially offending agents include barbiturates, phenytoin, and antibiotics. Radiation mucositis is a reaction to irradiation of the head and neck; it is exacerbated by the accompanying xerostomia, the effect of radiation on the salivary glands. In cancer chemotherapy, there is a painful mucositis that can be either localized or generalized. Chronic mucutaneous candidiasis is a chronic, often widespread infection involving the skin, nails, and mucous membranes. It is often associated with endocrine autoantibodies and hepatitis.

Treatment of oral ulcer disease includes removal of known etiologic factors, attention to oral hygiene, cleansing mouthrinses (equal portions of 3% hydrogen peroxide and water), and as appropriate, anesthetic mouthrinses and antimicrobial mouthrinses. A commonly used anesthetic mouthrinse includes a mixture of 2% viscous lidocaine, elixir of diphenhydramine, and Kaopectate, in equal portions. A common antimicrobial mouthrinse includes equal potions of elixir of tetracycline, nystatin, and dexamethasone.

DISORDERS OF THE NOSE

The most common cause of epistaxis is mechanical dysfunction of the nose, usually from local trauma or irritation. The vast majority of nosebleeds occur on the anterior aspect of the nasal septum in the Kiesselbach plexus. Males may have a particular predilection to epistaxis with androgenic stimulation of the vessels in the plexus. There are several other potential causes of epistaxis, including blood dyscrasias (see Chapters 52 and 53), an association with menstruation, septal deformity, hereditary hemorrhagic telangiectasia, and juvenile nasopharyngeal angiofibroma. Juvenile nasopharyngeal angiofibroma is the most commonly encountered vascular mass in the nasal cavity, with the usual presentation occurring during the teenage years. The clinical signs and symptoms are those of nasal obstruction and recurrent severe epistaxis; individuals also present with purulent rhinorrhea from secondary sinusitis. The tumor almost always presents in male adolescents and arises from the fibrocartilaginous tissue of the upper cervical vertebrae, with protrusion into the nasopharynx.

There are four major types of nasal obstruction: traumatic, inflammatory, neoplastic, and iatrogenic. If there has been trauma to the nose, the septum must be checked carefully for a hematoma. A hematoma can promote dissolution of the septal cartilage in less than 48 hours because of interruption of circulation to the septum. Inflammation is the most common cause of nasal obstruction; the most frequent condition is the common cold. If nasal obstruction persists for more than 2 weeks, sinusitis or nasal polyposis should be considered; if the symptoms occur in the same season on an annual basis, allergic rhinitis may be the cause.

Allergic rhinitis frequently begins in the adolescent years. The symptoms include clear rhinorrhea, nasal congestion, and nasal or ocular pruritus. On examination, the conjunctiva may be inflamed and the patient may have "allergic shiners." The nasal mucosa is pale blue and edematous with hypertrophied nasal turbinates. The most useful diagnostic procedure is the clinical history. Clinical impression can be substantiated by the demonstration of allergen-specific IgE on skin testing or by radioallergosorbent assay (RAST). Management of allergic rhinitis focuses on maximum symptomatic relief with minimal side effects. Allergen avoidance is very important but often overlooked. Medications include antihistamines, topical nasal corticosteroids, topical nasal cromolyn, and topical vasoconstrictors. Nasal corticosteroids and cromolyn have the fewest side effects, with cromolyn being somewhat better tolerated than corticosteroid treatment. Many patients also benefit from immunotherapy.

There are several other inflammatory disorders in addition to allergic rhinitis. Vasomotor rhinitis is a hyperactive cholinergic response to stimulants such as temperature, a recumbent position, or inhaled irritants. Treatment can be very challenging in these patients. Nasal polyps are associated with persistent nasal inflammation secondary to allergic rhinitis or chronic infections. In the young adolescent, a sweat chloride test is advisable prior to the management of nasal polyps because of the possibility of cystic fibrosis.

Neoplasms that are associated with nasal obstruction include lymphoma (the most common nasopharyngeal malignancy), juvenile nasopharyngeal angiofibroma, rhabdomyosarcoma, and esthesioneuroblastoma, which is an uncommon tumor that generally presents during the teenage years.

Possible causes of iatrogenic nasal obstruction include

prolonged use of topical decongestants (most common) and as a complication of tonsillectomy or adenoidectomy. Rhinitis medicamentosa may not only be a result of prolonged use of topical decongestants but also a side effect from various systemic medications such as β-adrenergic blockers or major tranquilizers. It is important that adolescents not use topical decongestants for more than 3 to 5 days. The examination in rhinitis medicamentosa reveals an edematous, erythematous, thickened nasal mucosa. Management includes systemic antihistamine and decongestant preparations or systemic or topical corticosteroid treatment.

BIBLIOGRAPHY

Bienfang DC, Kelly LD, Nicholson DH, et al: Ophthalmology. N Engl J Med 323:956, 1990.

Bloom JN: Traumatic hyphema in children. Pediatr Ann 9:368, 1990.

Bluestone CD: Modern management of otitis media. Pediatr Clin North Am 36:1371, 1989.

Brodsky L: Modern assessment of tonsils and adenoids. Pediatr Clin North Am 36:1551, 1989.

Havener WH: Synopsis of Ophthalmology, 6th ed. St. Louis, CV Mosby, 1984.

Komaroff AL, Branch WT, Aronson MD, et al: Chlamydial pharyngitis. Ann Intern Med 111:537, 1989.

Lusk RP, Lazar RH, Muntz HR: The diagnosis and treatment of recurrent and chronic sinusitis in children. Pediatr Clin North Am 36:1411, 1989.

McDonald JS: Oral ulcerative diseases. In Paparella MM, Shumrick DA, Gluckman JL, et al (eds): Otolaryngology, 3rd ed. Philadelphia, WB Saunders, 1990.

Myer CM, Cotton RT: A Practical Approach to Pediatric Otolaryngology. Chicago, Year Book Medical Publishers, 1988.

Tongue AC: Refractive errors in children. Pediatr Clin North Am 34:1425, 1987.

CHAPTER 41

Oral Conditions

STEVEN M. ADAIR

The oral cavity can reveal much about the general health, nutrition, diet, activities, and behaviors of adolescents. The dentition of the normal young adolescent can be in transition from primary to permanent teeth at one extreme, or can be one in which all permanent teeth are erupted with the exception of the third molars (wisdom teeth) at the other. By late adolescence, third molars, if present, are usually erupted or impacted. The prevalence of dental caries has diminished greatly in the United States over the past 2 decades, but it remains a significant health problem in certain population groups and for some individuals. During adolescence, prevention of periodontal disease becomes a significant concern.

The factors that predispose adolescents to dental and oral diseases stem from the combination of behaviors, attitudes, and activities that mark the transition from childhood to adult life. Many health care providers find it difficult to motivate adolescents to perform adequate oral hygiene. The lack of knowledge or concern for diet and oral hygiene leads to a caries-prone period during the teenage years for some individuals. Incomplete and infrequent plaque removal, perhaps combined with the stress of adolescence, contributes to the beginnings of periodontal disease. Sports-related activities, especially those unsupervised by schools or other organizations, can contribute to an increase in the incidence of dental trauma. The use of smokeless tobacco and cigarettes produces soft tissue damage, as does oral sexual behavior.

It is beyond the scope of this chapter to provide a comprehensive review of all oral conditions that occur in adolescents. Rather, emphasis is placed on brief discussions of conditions that are common to adolescents and that might be discovered by history and on visual examination. Mention also is made of conditions that although less common and more occult, are associated primarily with the second decade of life.

PERIODONTAL DISEASE

Gingivitis and Periodontitis

Gingivitis and periodontitis are conditions that affect the supporting structures of the teeth. The etiology of periodontal conditions is primarily bacterial. Toxins from bacteria in dental plaque lead to inflammation and breakdown of gingival epithelium and underlying periodontal connective tissue. In most adolescents, the disease progresses no further. Gingivitis is the predominant periodontal problem in this age group. The clinical manifestations include inflammation of the marginal gingiva, edema, loss of surface stippling, and bleeding, either on stimulus or spontaneously (Fig. 41–1). Histologically the lesion is made up predominantly of plasma cells. Gingivitis responds well to debridement of the teeth and improved oral hygiene. Some adolescents are difficult to motivate, and exceptional oral hygiene is just that—the exception rather than the rule. Orthodontic treatment, common in adolescents, contributes to gingivitis by making tooth cleaning procedures more difficult.

Several gingival and periodontal conditions can be identified that occur primarily in adolescents:

1. *Eruption gingivitis.* As a permanent tooth erupts it creates an opening in the overlying gingiva that becomes inflamed. The resultant tenderness may lead to avoidance of oral hygiene in that area, and the partially erupted tooth becomes a "plaque trap." The condition typically resolves spontaneously with continued tooth eruption and improved oral hygiene.

2. *Pericoronitis.* This condition is a special case of eruption gingivitis, typically limited to third molars. As the molar erupts, a flap (operculum) of gingival tissue overlays the crown. The operculum becomes inflamed as a result of food entrapment, swelling, and possible

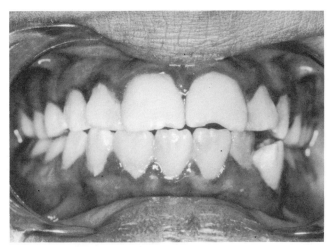

Figure 41–1. Gingivitis in an adolescent. Note inflammation along margins of gingiva and enlargement of interdental papillae.

trauma from opposing teeth. In some cases the inflammation may extend into deeper tissues and require antibiotic treatment. Halitosis often results from the poor local hygiene. Generally, pericoronitis is treated by gentle irrigation and saline mouthrinses. Once the inflammation is controlled, the operculum can be excised or the partially erupted third molar can be extracted.

3. *Puberty gingivitis.* Female adolescents occasionally demonstrate a generalized gingival inflammation and enlargement that results from a combination of local and hormonal factors. The gingival response, including easily stimulated or spontaneous bleeding similar to that seen in pregnancy, is not consistent with the amount of local irritants present. Treatment consists of improved oral hygiene and removal of calculus. Resolution may be slow, and some adolescents may continue to have gingival enlargement until the late teenage years. Remission may leave some fibrotic areas that require surgical recontouring. Puberty gingivitis also may be caused by oral contraceptives, in which case discontinuation or a change in medications generally resolves the condition.

4. *Acute necrotizing ulcerative gingivitis.* This acute infection is recognized by a classic triad of pain, foul breath, and punched-out ulcerative lesions of the interdental papillae (Fig. 41–2). General complaints of malaise, low-grade fever, and lymphadenopathy are often present. Also called trench mouth and Vincent infection, acute necrotizing ulcerative gingivitis results from an altered host-bacterial relationship with *Borrelia vincentii.* Stress is strongly implicated as a contributing factor. The pain is constant and moderate to severe. The foul odor results from necrotic tissue and bacterial accumulation. The interdental papillae, normally pink and knife edged, are blunted and covered by a white pseudomembrane. This disorder is treated initially by careful local debridement. Improved oral hygiene is instituted, and the use of oxygenating agents such as peroxide can help restore the normal balance of oral flora. Antibiotics are not always required but may be helpful in more serious cases. Penicillin or erythromycin are commonly used in doses of 250 mg four times daily for 5 days. Metronidazole can be used for more rapid resolution of acute

symptoms, but it is contraindicated in pregnancy and should not be used with alcohol.

Periodontitis, which is primarily a disease of adulthood, affects perhaps only 5% to 10% of adolescents. In this form of the disease, the gingival attachment to the tooth is lost as the breakdown extends to the periodontal ligament. Gingival pocketing and loss of alveolar bone follow, with loosening and migration of the teeth. It is not clear why some adolescents are susceptible to a progression from gingivitis to periodontitis, whereas in others the bacterial insult is localized to the gingival tissues. The likely explanation is probably related to a changing host response to the bacterial challenge. Except for the inflammation of the gingiva, diagnosis of periodontal disease is made from intraoral radiographs and a periodontal examination using a graduated probe.

Juvenile Periodontitis

Juvenile periodontitis is a condition that occurs in two forms, localized and generalized. The localized form is typically diagnosed in adolescents 11 to 13 years of age, whereas the generalized form affects older adolescents. Untreated localized juvenile periodontitis may progress to the generalized form, or the two may be distinct but related entities.

The localized form has been noted to occur in a familial pattern, with a higher incidence in females and in blacks. Estimates of prevalence are 1.5% to 2% in the United States. It is clinically detectable only by a periodontal probing for loss of gingival attachment levels. Often the gingival tissue looks healthy, and the oral hygiene is reasonably good. Localized juvenile periodontitis is usually diagnosed from radiographs, which demonstrate a typical molar–incisor involvement, mirror-image pattern, with arc-shaped bone loss that progresses rapidly. The cause of localized juvenile periodontitis is believed to be an altered host response to infection by *Actinobacillus actinomycetemcomitans,* perhaps compounded by a deficiency in neutrophil function. The degree of bone loss is much greater than would be expected from the amount of local irritants and gingival inflammation (Fig. 41–3).

Treatment of localized juvenile periodontitis consists of attempting to reestablish the normal balance to the gingival flora with tetracycline. If the localized form is detected early enough, antibiotic therapy alone is usually successful. In more advanced cases, surgical elimination of bony defects and soft tissue pockets is necessary.

Generalized juvenile periodontitis is a more diffuse form of rapidly progressing periodontitis that clinically and microbiologically more closely resembles adult periodontitis. Antibiotic therapy is not as likely to be successful because the lesions of generalized juvenile periodontitis are populated by a variety of microorganisms. Surgical intervention is necessary, and long-term management may require tooth extraction, root amputation, and orthodontic repositioning of teeth.

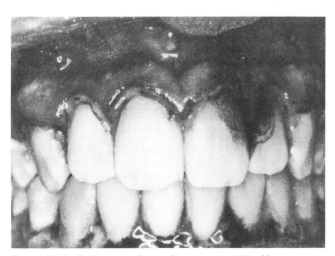

Figure 41–2. Acute necrotizing ulcerative gingivitis. Note spontaneous hemorrhage, cratering, and ulceration of interdental papillae.

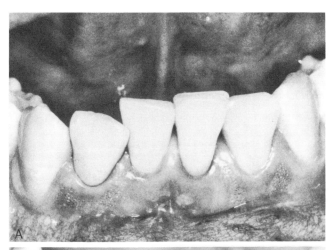
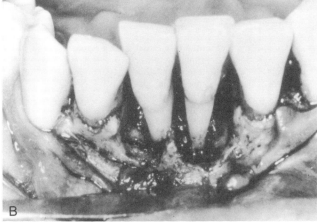

Figure 41–3. Localized juvenile periodontitis. *A*, Note relatively healthy-looking gingiva with little plaque and no calculus. *B*, Reflected full-thickness gingival flap demonstrating loss of supporting bone in same patient. (Courtesy of Dr. M. John Novak.)

Systemic Diseases

The supporting structures of the teeth are susceptible to insults and destruction from a variety of systemic diseases, medications, and host defense abnormalities. Table 41–1 is a list of some of these conditions and the clinical and radiographic findings associated with them.

DENTAL CARIES

Dental caries is a complex, multifactorial process that was pandemic in the United States until recently. Although its prevalence in schoolchildren has decreased dramatically in the past 2 decades, it still constitutes a chronic health problem for adolescents in lower socioeconomic groups and other high-risk groups, such as the medically compromised and developmentally disabled (see Chapter 31).

Etiology and Pathophysiology

Dental caries begins with the colonization of tooth surfaces by adherent bacteria and the production of extracellular polymer chains from the breakdown of sucrose into glucans and fructans. This bacterial plaque becomes populated with aciduric and acidogenic species, especially *Streptococcus mutans*. Intracellular metabolism of carbohydrates produces acids that begin to demineralize the tooth surface. Remineralization occurs, especially in the presence of fluoride, but in caries-susceptible adolescents demineralization predominates. Eventually the enamel surface cavitates and bacteria invade the less-resistant dentin. Thermal, mechanical, and chemical stimuli produce pain. If left unchecked, microorganisms invade the dental pulp. Microabscesses form, and eventually total pulpal necrosis dictates endodontic therapy or extraction. Fortunately, this presentation is increasingly less common among today's adolescents. The primary reason for the reduction in caries prevalence is the widespread availability of fluoride, particularly optimally fluoridated water supplies and fluoride-containing dentifrices. If available in the saliva or from fluoridated hydroxyapatite in the tooth, fluoride alters the dynamics of the demineralization–remineralization phenomenon in favor of enamel surface repair.

Some adolescents are at an increased risk for caries because of poor oral hygiene practices and a diet rich in refined carbohydrates. In addition, a distinct clinical entity known as rampant caries affects a small but clinically significant number of teenagers. This caries pattern is characterized by rapid onset and rapidly progressing caries. Pulpal involvement can occur, with its sequelae of pain and abscess formation. Caries in lower incisors should alert the physician to the possibility of rampant decay.

Chronic caries is a much more slowly progressing phenomenon, in which an adolescent demonstrates new carious lesions every 6 to 12 months. The lesions tend to be smaller, less rapidly progressing, and more manageable than those of rampant decay. Chronic caries is generally controlled by alterations in diet and improvements in oral hygiene. Over-the-counter fluoride mouthrinses are also helpful.

Treatment

Treatment of dental caries is routinely managed by dentists with a variety of restorative techniques. The adolescent dentition, however, presents a number of challenges, such as incomplete eruption, large pulps, malaligned teeth, physiologically or orthodontically shifting teeth, and increased prevalence of gingivitis. These factors often necessitate alterations of standard techniques and the use of long-term temporary restorations, such as stainless steel crowns and pin-retained amalgams instead of cast gold or porcelain crowns. Newer restorative materials that can bond to tooth surfaces are more aesthetic and require less removal of tooth structure.

MALOCCLUSION

In dentistry, the term *occlusion* has a variety of meanings, but generally it refers to the contact and

TABLE 41–1. Systemic and Local Conditions with Periodontal Presentations

CONDITION	CLINICAL MANIFESTATIONS	RADIOGRAPHIC MANIFESTATIONS

Neutrophil dysfunction
  Agranulocytopenia
  Cyclic neutropenia
  Chédiak-Higashi syndrome
  Agranulocytosis
	Onset at puberty or earlier; often accompanied by other chronic/recurrent infections; inflammation ranges from minimal (agranulocytosis) to severe, sometimes with necrotic areas of the gingiva	Involvement of multiple teeth, including primary teeth in agranulocytopenia; bone loss tends to be pronounced and rapid; brief intervals of remission in cyclic neutropenia

Hematologic disorders
  Acute lymphoblastic leukemia
  Anemias
    Sickle cell
    Pernicious
    Thalassemia
    G6PD deficiency
	Diffuse cyanosis with purplish areas of inflammation; pallor; ulceration, necrosis, and enlargement from cell infiltration in acute lymphoblastic leukemia; marked spreading of teeth in thalassemia	Rarefaction of bone in thalassemia; changes in bone trabeculation patterns in anemias; general bone loss, variable in extent

Histiocytoses	Severe gingivitis, loosening of teeth	Alveolar bone loss, "punched-out" lesions
Diabetes mellitus	Consistent clinical findings debatable; gingivitis often reported as a finding	No consistent findings
Papillon-Lefevre	Hyperkeratosis of palms and soles accompanied by severe periodontal disease, acute gingival inflammation; onset can be early (age 2–3 years) leading to loss of primary teeth and, eventually, permanent teeth	Marked bone loss
Hypophosphatasia	Mild to minimal gingival inflammation	Marked bone loss leading to early loss of primary teeth
Idiopathic fibromatosis	Enlargement of attached gingiva and marginal gingiva; pink, leathery, pebbled appearance	No consistent findings; generally no loss of bone
Drug-induced gingival overgrowth (usually phenytoin induced)	Enlargement of marginal gingiva; secondary inflammation possible	No consistent findings
Trisomy 21	Characteristic gingivitis progressing from lower incisors to upper incisors, then molars	Retained primary teeth, delayed eruption of permanent teeth
Pregnancy	Variable, but often displays gradually increasing gingivitis	No consistent findings of bone loss

interdigitation of the teeth when the maxillary and mandibular dental arches are in maximal intercuspation. Very few adolescents demonstrate an ideal occlusion. Disagreement on criteria for normal occlusion has created a wide disparity among epidemiologic studies on the prevalence of malocclusion, ranging from 35% to 95%. Studies with objective criteria determined that approximately 75% of adolescents had some measurable deviation from ideal occlusion.

Etiology

Malocclusion may result from a variety of causes and interactions of causes. The major categories of causes are dental crowding and skeletal growth imbalances. Table 41–2 is a simplified classification of the types of dental crowding. Skeletal causes of malocclusion result from a variety of genetic, epigenetic, and environmental factors, including systemic growth problems, local growth discrepancies of the jaws, oral habits, trauma, surgery, and local infection. Certain syndromes, such as trisomy 21, mandibulofacial dysostosis, craniofacial dysostosis, acrocephalosyndactyly, and others, have craniofacial components that produce malocclusions.

Clinical Manifestations

Most malocclusions are recognized by the resultant discrepancies that are evident in one or more of the three planes of space, combined with a possibility of dental crowding. Suspected malocclusions, if not already

under observation by the adolescent's dentist, should be referred for more detailed evaluation. Criteria for referral include dental crowding, crossbites, high narrow palate, or prominent maxilla or mandible.

Treatment

Treatment varies according to the nature and extent of the problem but generally requires the use of intraoral and extraoral devices to apply forces to the teeth and jaws to redirect facial growth and improve tooth position. These appliances, as noted earlier, compromise oral hygiene and place the adolescent at greater risk for dental caries and gingivitis.

TRAUMA

Dental trauma in adolescents does not occur as frequently as in younger children, but by the midteens the prevalence of such injuries is 15% to 25%. Boys are affected almost twice as often as girls (see Chapter 40).

The causes are varied and include any activities that carry a risk of trauma. Fortunately, most schools require mouthguards for participation in some organized sports, decreasing the incidence of sports-related injuries to teeth. Physical abuse must always be ruled out as a possible cause of trauma to the head.

Clinical Manifestations

The types of injuries sustained by adolescents differ somewhat from those commonly seen in younger chil-

TABLE 41–2. Classification of Dental Crowding

CLASSIFICATION	CAUSE	PREVENTION	TREATMENT
Primary	Genetic; discrepancy between sizes of the teeth and sizes of the dental arches	None	Standard orthodontic treatment. May necessitate extraction of some permanent teeth
Secondary	Environmental: loss of tooth structure from decay and/or early loss of primary teeth; results in drifting teeth and space loss	Prevention of dental caries	Restoration of carious primary teeth as early as possible; regaining lost space and placement of space maintainers, if necessary
Tertiary	Genetic: Presence of third molars and continued growth of mandible into late teens and early 20s	Removal of third molars; prolonged retention of orthodontic correction	Standard orthodontic treatment or re-treatment; tertiary crowding generally refers to relapse of corrected crowding in mandibular incisors.

dren. Denser alveolar bone and completed root formation predispose adolescents to tooth crown fractures, alveolar bone fractures, and an increased likelihood of pulpal necrosis.

Evaluation of dental trauma includes a basic assessment of the teeth and supporting structures. Visual-tactile examination, palpation, evaluation of changes in occlusion, and a radiographic examination are all standard. When the fractured fragment of a tooth crown cannot be found, the physician should examine other oral soft tissues for fragments. Aspiration of a missing fragment should be considered. The adolescent's tetanus status should be reviewed if there is the possibility that an oral wound may have become contaminated.

Traumatic injuries to teeth have been classified by the World Health Organization into four categories: (1) dental hard tissues, (2) periodontal tissues, (3) supporting bone, and (4) gingiva or mucosa.

Crown fractures are classified as complicated or uncomplicated, depending on whether the pulp has been exposed. Pulpal protection or treatment of a recent (less than 24 hours) injury can maintain a vital pulp. Restoration of the crown is managed with contemporary bonding techniques. Fractures of the roots are detected radiographically. The location of the fracture greatly affects the prognosis, with those occurring in the apical third of the root having the greatest likelihood of long-term retention.

Injuries to the periodontal ligament include concussion, subluxation, and luxation. Concussion injuries are not accompanied by displacement or tooth mobility, but the adolescent patient may be sensitive to palpation or percussion of the tooth. Subluxation involves loosening without displacement and often requires splinting. Injury to the periodontal ligament occurs and requires observation and follow-up. Luxation injuries can be intrusive, lateral, extrusive, or avulsive. Luxation injuries are likely to lead to pulpal necrosis because of the interruption of the blood flow to the tooth. These injuries, by definition, involve damage to the periodontal ligament. Lateral luxation and avulsion also may be accompanied by alveolar fractures. Splinting of teeth is required for reattachment of the periodontal ligament, and special pulp therapy is required to prevent the resorption of roots.

In the special case of avulsion, the likelihood of successful replantation is inversely related to the time elapsed before the tooth is repositioned. Instructions should be given to parents or caretakers of the victim to rinse the tooth gently in tap water and reposition it in the socket, using the adjacent teeth as a guide for orientation. If the tooth cannot be repositioned, it should be placed in a container of milk. The adolescent should be referred for immediate dental management. Under no circumstances should the root surface of the tooth be scraped or subjected to disinfecting chemicals. The intent is to maintain viability of the periodontal ligament cells that remain on the root surface. The prognosis for reattachment declines precipitously if the tooth remains out of the socket for more than 30 minutes.

Damage to supporting bone ranges from compression of the socket wall from intrusive or lateral luxation, to fracture of the socket wall or alveolar bone, to fracture of the maxilla or mandible. There is no specific treatment for compression and socket wall fractures. Alveolar bone fractures are manually reduced and maintained by 6-week splinting of the involved teeth. Fractures of the jaws are more involved, may require surgical reduction, and are typically managed by oral surgeons.

Lacerations of gingiva and mucosa require suturing and consideration for antibiotics. Abrasions and contusions generally require observation.

Prevention

Prevention of traumatic accidents requires patient education. The use of mouthguards should be considered for teenagers active in sports, whether school sponsored or not. In fact, several school sports such as baseball, basketball, and soccer do not always require mouthguards. Helmets for bicycling, skating, skateboarding, and similar activities are becoming more acceptable among adolescents today. Inevitably, however, dental trauma will occur and should be managed promptly to reduce the risks of tooth loss and more serious sequelae.

TEMPOROMANDIBULAR JOINT DISORDERS

The articulation between the mandible and the cranium, the temporomandibular joint, is among the most complex in the body. It is a ginglymoarthrodial joint,

TABLE 41–3. Suggested Diagnostic Classification of Temporomandibular Disorders

1. Deviation in form
2. Disk displacement
   2.1. Disk displacement with reduction (upon closing)
   2.2. Disk displacement without reduction
3. Hypermobility
4. Dislocation
5. Inflammatory conditions
   5.1. Synovitis
   5.2. Capsulitis
6. Arthritides
   6.1. Osteoarthrosis
   6.2. Osteoarthritis
   6.3. Polyarthritides
7. Ankylosis
   7.1. Fibrous
   7.2. Bony

With permission from McNeil C, Mohl ND, Rugh JD, et al: Temporomandibular disorders: Diagnosis, management, education and research. J Am Dent Assoc 120:253, 1990.

combining both hinge and sliding actions. The joint consists of the condyle of the mandible and the glenoid fossa of the temporal bone. A dense collagenous connective tissue articular disk (meniscus) is interposed between the bony components, which in turn are covered by avascular fibrous connective tissue with varying numbers of cartilage cells. The joint is enclosed in a fibrous capsule that blends with the disk. A system of ligaments serves to support the joint and possibly to provide neural feedback on mandibular function.

Etiology, Prevalence, and Clinical Manifestations

Temporomandibular joint disorders are a subset of musculoskeletal and rheumatologic disorders. These conditions are viewed as a cluster of related disorders with common features. Pain in the joint and muscles of mastication is predominant, but earaches, headaches, jaw discomfort, and facial pain are common. Other signs include limited jaw opening and joint sounds. Temporomandibular joint disorders in adolescents can be separated into two major categories: (1) internal derangements involving the disk and (2) disorders of the masticatory muscles. The causes are likely to be different, necessitating different treatment options for each. Estimates of the prevalence of temporomandibular joint disorders in adolescents are lacking. The prevalence in adults is variably reported to be 20% to 75% based on signs and symptoms, but these disorders appear to be less common in adolescents.

Unfortunately, knowledge regarding the causes of temporomandibular joint disorders is limited. Table 41–3 is a suggested diagnostic classification. The disorder must first be differentiated from other possible causes of headache or facial pain, including teeth, eyes, ears, nose, sinuses, cranial bones, and masticatory muscles. Screening for temporomandibular joint disorders includes questioning the patient about difficulty or pain with mandibular function, joint noises, headaches, facial pain, and injuries to the joint. A screening examination

consists of palpating the joint during function for clicks, palpation for joint and muscle tenderness, and a thorough dental evaluation. Patients with chronic temporomandibular joint disorders should be considered for behavioral and psychosocial evaluation.

Imaging of the joint is warranted only when the history and clinical examination indicate the existence of a recent or progressive pathologic joint condition. A variety of useful techniques exist, including tomography and, in selected cases, arthrography.

Treatment

Treatment goals for adolescents with temporomandibular joint disorders include (1) reduction of pain, (2) restoration of normal function, (3) reduction of the need for future health care, and (4) a return to a normal lifestyle. The treatment options are consistent with those used to manage musculoskeletal disorders elsewhere in the body. Behavioral therapy, joint stabilization, medication, physical therapy, and the use of occlusal appliances have been helpful in managing temporomandibular joint disorders in adolescents. Pharmacotherapy typically involves analgesics, but muscle relaxants and

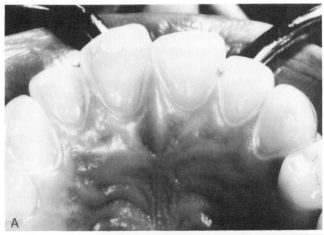

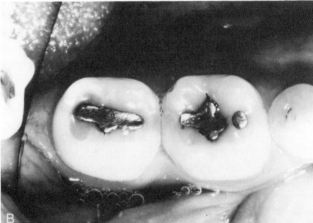

Figure 41–4. Oral findings in bulimia and anorexia nervosa. *A,* Erosion of lingual enamel caused by frequent contact with stomach acid during vomiting. *B,* Erosion of enamel around amalgam restorations gives appearance of fillings growing out of the teeth. (Courtesy of Dr. Ø. E. Jensen.)

antianxiety agents may be necessary in a few instances. Surgery is rarely needed in children and adolescents. The sequence of treatment options begins with the most conservative approaches, adding noninvasive procedures before invasive, irreversible ones.

It is important for adolescents with temporomandibular joint disorders to be educated about the management of their disorder, including habit alteration and proper mandibular function. With a combination of careful diagnosis and conservative treatment, the prognosis for the disorder in adolescents is favorable.

MISCELLANEOUS CONDITIONS

Brief mention should be made of conditions resulting from three behaviors that first become evident in the adolescent years.

Cigarette Smoking and Smokeless Tobacco

In addition to the well-documented effects of tobacco on long-term health, cigarette smoking also creates oral tissue irritation, including generalized erythema of the mucosa, coated tongue, foul breath, and stained teeth. Use of smokeless tobacco can lead to gingivitis, gingival recession, and mucosal hyperkeratosis. Risk of oral carcinoma is increased by both cigarette smoking and the use of smokeless tobacco.

Anorexia Nervosa and Bulimia

The frequent regurgitation in bulimia and even the occasional regurgitation in some anorexics can lead to acid dissolution of the enamel and dentin on the lingual surfaces of the teeth (Fig. 41–4A). This process, known as perimyolysis, creates caries-susceptible sensitive teeth with enamel that flakes off easily. Often the edges of the teeth are sharp, and dental restorations appear to protrude from the teeth (Fig. 41–4B) (see Chapter 60).

Sexual Activity

Oral sexual activity not only leads to the transmission of disease (see Chapters 69 and 75) but also to oral manifestations of numerous conditions:

Herpes labialis—recurrent ulcerations
Condylomata acuminata—lips, gingiva, tongue, palate
Gonorrhea—pharyngitis, tonsillitis, diffuse erythema
Syphilis—chancre, mucous patch, pharyngitis
Acquired immunodeficiency syndrome—periodontitis, *Candida* infections (see Chapter 76)

In addition, palatal hematomas created by negative intraoral pressures may be evident in sexually active adolescents.

BIBLIOGRAPHY

Andreasen FM: Pulpal healing after luxation injuries and root fracture in the permanent dentition. Endod Dent Traumatol 5:111, 1989.

Andreasen JO: Traumatic Injuries of the Teeth, 2nd ed. Philadelphia, WB Saunders, 1981.

Brunelle JA, Carlos JP: Changes in the prevalence of dental caries in U.S. schoolchildren, 1961–1980. J Dent Res 61(special issue):1346, 1982.

Jensen ÖE, Featherstone JDB, Stege P: Chemical and physical oral findings in a case of anorexia nervosa and bulimia. Oral Pathol 16:399, 1987.

Kelly J, Harvey C: An assessment of the teeth of youths 12–17 years. US Public Health Service, DHEW publication No. (HRA)77-1644. Washington, DC, National Center for Health Statistics, 1977.

Leach E: Demineralization and Remineralization of Teeth. Oxford, IRL Press, 1983.

McNeil C, Mohl ND, Rugh JD, et al: Temporomandibular disorders: Diagnosis, management, education and research. J Am Dent Assoc 120:253, 1990.

Novak MJ, Polson AM, Adair SM: Tetracycline therapy in patients with early juvenile periodontitis. J Periodontol 59:366, 1988.

Okeson JP: Temporomandibular disorders in children. Pediatr Dent 11:325, 1989.

Waite IM, Furniss JS: Periodontal disease in children—a review. J Paediatr Dent 3:59, 1987.

Pulmonary Conditions

Maturation of the Respiratory System at Puberty and Related Respiratory System Considerations

GARY MONTGOMERY and HOWARD EIGEN

PULMONARY CONDITIONS

Biologic Maturation of Puberty in Relation to Respiratory System Anatomy and Physiology

The primary function of the respiratory system is to exchange oxygen and carbon dioxide with the circulation and end-organ cells. To accomplish this function, there must be appropriate central neural stimulus for breathing both when awake and when asleep, as well as effective work from the muscles of respiration, unobstructed air flow, and effective matching of ventilation and perfusion. Disorders in any of these areas result in less effective gas exchange and can potentially lead to respiratory failure. An understanding of the anatomy and physiology of the respiratory system as they relate to the growth and development of the adolescent is essential for those who care for teenagers.

Upper Airway

The upper, or extrathoracic, airway includes the middle ear and eustachian tubes, sinuses, nose, mouth, pharnyx, larynx, and upper trachea (see Chapter 40). With growth and maturation, many changes occur in the upper airway that affect the function and susceptibility to disease in adolescents. The position of the eustachian tube changes from 10 degrees to the horizontal axis in infancy to a more vertical position (30 to 40 degrees) in adulthood. This is associated with more efficient drainage of middle ear secretions and a reduced susceptibility to ear infections. The nose and nasal turbinates warm, humidify, and filter air before it reaches the lungs. The nasal mucosa provides about 650 ml of water each day to the air entering the nares, and the air is warmed to body temperature as it passes over the turbinates. Large particulate matter is filtered through nasal hairs. Smaller particles are caught by inertial impaction on the mucous layer of the turbinates

and septum and are then propelled by the cilia, which beat backward toward the pharnyx at which point the mucus is swallowed or expectorated. The turbinates increase in size with the growth of other facial structures and increase the mucosal surface area, thereby acting as radiators to warm and humidify the air. Snorting cocaine or sniffing hydrocarbons (such as model airplane glue) damages the nasal epithelium and septum, resulting in a loss of these protective nasal functions (see Chapter 111). Findings on physical examination may include excoriation, bleeding, and septal perforation.

At birth, the sinuses consist of maxillary antral cavities, 4 to 5 mm in diameter, and a few small ethmoid air cells. By 12 years of age, the maxillary, sphenoid, and ethmoid sinuses have well-defined air spaces, whereas the frontal sinuses, the last to develop, may not pneumatize until well into the second decade of life. All sinus spaces continue to enlarge during adolescence. The physiologic purposes of the sinuses are thought to include insulating the cranial vault, making the skull lighter, and adding resonance to the voice. Adolescents who have allergic rhinitis and asthma have a swollen, boggy mucosa, which can block the sinus ostia, resulting in stasis of mucus and bacterial proliferation, eventually leading to clinical sinusitis. This can also occur in normal hosts as a complication of a upper respiratory viral infection. Indeed, sinusitis should be suspected in any adolescent who has a purulent nasal discharge persisting 10 days after a cold. Maxillary and anterior ethmoid sinus drainage is seen inferior to the middle turbinate, whereas drainage from frontal, posterior ethmoid, and sphenoid sinuses is inferior to the superior turbinate. Persistently swollen turbinates, adenoid hypertrophy, or tonsillar hypertrophy can cause chronic upper airway obstruction. This should be considered in any adolescent with a history of snoring, unexplained fatigue, or falling asleep in class or at work. Such airway obstruction results in obstructive apnea and hypoxia, which can be documented by polysomnography. Acute upper airway obstruction is occasionally seen to result from tonsillar swelling with streptococcal or Epstein-Barr viral infections. Halitosis is sometimes a presenting complaint in adolescents and can cause significant psychosocial morbidity. Common causes include sinusitis, tonsillitis, tooth decay, and tobacco use (smoking or chewing).

The larynx undergoes significant change during puberty (see Chapter 5). There is a rapid increase in vocal cord length, especially in boys, causing the voice to crack, squeak, and change pitch. The larynx also assumes a lower and less anterior position with growth, descending from the level of C-3 in infancy to C-7 in adulthood. With the descent of the larynx, the posterior portion of the tongue follows and can cause obstruction of the larynx in states of altered consciousness. The vocal cords are the narrowest part of the airway in adolescents and adults, in contrast to children less than 8 years of age, in whom the lumen is narrowest at the cricoid cartilage. Therefore, the larynx at the level of the vocal cords is the most common site of obstruction from foreign objects in adolescents. The vocal cords protect the lower airway by laryngospasm and by participation in the cough reflex. These reflexes can be blunted when the sensorium is depressed from alcohol or other drug abuse, resulting in aspiration of oral secretions and vomitus (see Chapter 111). This may cause inflammation of the vocal cords, lower airways, and lungs (aspiration pneumonia). Hoarseness is most commonly caused by overuse or abuse of the voice, such as screaming at an athletic event or concert, and improves in a few days. Chronic hoarseness can be due to vocal cord paresis, laryngeal masses, cigarette or marijuana smoking, or chronic aspiration.

The chest wall bone and muscle structures grow rapidly during the rapid somatic growth spurts of puberty (see Chapter 5). During adolescence there is an increase in chest wall muscle strength with age; it is greater in males than in females. This can be quantitated on pulmonary function tests of maximum voluntary ventilation and maximal inspiratory and expiratory force. Chest wall pain in adolescents is most commonly of musculoskeletal origin and is caused by trauma to the sternocostal joints or ribs or to a strain of the intercostal and pectoral muscles from overexertion in athletics or at a job requiring manual labor. Disorders that affect chest wall anatomy frequently worsen during the rapid growth of adolescence. Scoliosis and pectus excavatum are included in this group and should be followed closely during puberty for changes in the deformity and deterioration of pulmonary function (see Chapter 79). The prognosis is poor for adolescents with muscular dystrophies or severe scoliosis that is left untreated. Death often occurs with severe scoliosis in the fourth or fifth decade of life from progressive alveolar hypoventilation, pulmonary hypertension, and cor pulmonale. The goal of school screening programs is to detect mild curves (less than 30 degrees) prior to the growth spurt, when there are no symptoms, thereby allowing time to look for an underlying cause and establish a plan of management based on the physical, maturational, and cardiopulmonary status of the individual (see Chapter 79). As a general rule, a Cobb angle (a measurement that uses a radiologic method to determine the degree of curvature of a scoliosis) of 90 degrees or more is a prerequisite for significant alveolar hypoventilation. However, abnormalities in lung volumes (forced vital capacity, total lung capacity) are detectable with asymptomatic curves

of 50 to 60 degrees, and reduced exercise tolerance is seen in some patients even with mild scoliosis (less than 35 degrees). In patients with scoliosis, exercise tolerance is often limited by ventilatory factors (see Chapter 79).

Intrathoracic Factors

The lungs continue to grow and mature throughout adolescence, until growth of the thorax is complete, which correlates well with the changes in height that occur during pubescence. These changes are generally completed by 16 years of age in females and 18 years of age in males and have been demonstrated functionally with increased lung volume and anatomically in the growth of the alveoli. The lung volume changes in females are concordant with the increase in height; however, the increase in lung volume in males lags behind the growth in the chest height. This may contribute to the increased incidence of spontaneous pneumothorax in males during adolescence.

Various functional parameters change to different degrees with age, based on whether the function depends on the size of the whole lung (e.g., residual volume, total lung capacity) or on a specific component, such as conducting airways (airway resistance). Certain other values, such as arterial blood gas tensions, ratio of dead space volume:total volume, and ratio of residual volume:total lung capacity, change very little throughout childhood and adolescence. These functional parameters and regression equations for the normal population (reference standards) are detailed elsewhere. Elastic recoil increases throughout adolescence and then declines after about 25 years of age. Disorders or behaviors that result in a premature and excessive loss of elastic recoil include antiprotease deficiency, cystic fibrosis, cigarette smoking, and possibly chronic marijuana use.

The number of segments of conducting airways (to the terminal bronchioles) and their accompanying blood supply is complete at birth. Growth in length and diameter of each segment continues symmetrically until the growth of the thorax ceases. The final length of the conducting airways varies with adult height. It is generally believed that the number of alveoli increases until about 8 years of age, and thereafter it is only the size of each alveolus that increases. However, some investigators have suggested that alveolar number increases until 20 years of age. If this is true, lung damage occurring in adolescence may interfere with the formation of new alveoli and result in fewer alveoli in the adult lung. Whatever the case, it is agreed that alveolar size increases more than alveolar number, and this increase in size continues until growth of the thorax is completed. The size of each alveolus in the adult is relatively constant (250 μ in diameter) regardless of height. In summary, a taller person will have the same number of bronchi and bronchioles as does a shorter person, but the airway diameter is larger and leads to more alveoli that are probably the same size. After growth ceases, pulmonary function is stable for a few years then declines as mechanical properties of the lung deteriorate as part of the aging process.

Bronchial challenge testing in normal individuals has

repeatedly shown that children have more highly reactive airways than do adults, and this reactivity decreases with age. This fact has implications when studying the epidemiology and natural history of diseases such as asthma. This decrease in reactivity may contribute to the belief that some children "grow out" of their asthma, a process that was examined in a long-term study in Australia. About one half of the preschool children with mild episodic asthma became symptom-free by adolescence. However, 60% to 70% of these adolescents had airway hyperreactivity on bronchial challenge testing. In addition, many individuals in this long-term study whose onset of symptoms was in late adolescence or early adulthood actually had episodic symptoms of cough or wheeze in early childhood documented in their medical records, which they did not recall by history. Therefore, it is important to consider a past history of asthma when evaluating "new-onset" respiratory symptoms in adolescents. Boys are more frequently affected with asthma than are girls in childhood (3:1), but because fewer girls improve during adolescence, the sex ratio is 1:1 by adulthood. Exercise-induced asthma often has its onset in adolescence and may present as cough, shortness of breath, chest tightness, wheezing, or presyncope-syncope with exercise. Exercise and bronchial challenge testing are useful in assessing these symptoms objectively (see Chapter 43).

Over the last decade, mortality from asthma in the adolescent–early adult age group has appeared to increase. This disturbing finding has been associated with factors such as inadequate treatment of chronic asthma symptoms, denial of acute symptoms by the adolescent with a subsequent delay in seeking medical care, and inadequate treatment of these exacerbations. Strunk and colleagues described the physiologic and psychological characteristics associated with deaths from asthma in a group of children 8 to 18 years of age. They found a preponderance of psychological risk factors in the asthmatic individuals who died. These results emphasize the importance of carefully considering the role of psychosocial problems in managing patients with severe asthma (see Chapter 43).

A persistent chronic cough in adolescents can cause significant morbidity from school absences, limitation of activity, and social embarrassment. In addition, cough originating from a physical illness can serve as the trigger or initiator of a cough that can be disruptive to relationships at school and at home. Exposure to various environmental pollutants can trigger asthmatic responses (cough or wheezing, or both) in adolescents with hyperreactive airways. Common exposures include cigarette smoke, hair spray, perfume, and paint. Asthma is often the cause of chronic cough, and further study of pulmonary function with bronchial challenge tests may aid in the diagnosis (see Chapter 43). A clinical trial of bronchodilators may also be used for diagnosis and treatment. Chronic cough in the adolescent occasionally results from previously undiagnosed cystic fibrosis, immotile cilia syndrome, or an immune deficiency, especially when associated with recurrent sinusitis or pneumonia (see Chapter 92). Aggressive treatment of these disorders is required to prevent further lung damage.

LOWER RESPIRATORY DEFENSES

The respiratory system has a total surface area exposed to the environment that is 70 times larger than the skin surface area. Each day the lower respiratory tract is exposed to more than 10,000 L of ambient air, which may contain infectious microorganisms and hazardous particles, gases, and chemicals. The respiratory system is developed in such a way that it protects the lungs and circulation from these insults.

The mucociliary elevator is the primary defense mechanism for the lower airways. A thin film of mucus rests on the cilia of the columnar epithelial cells. The cilia beat at a frequency of 1300 times a minute, with the fast phase upward moving the mucus and debris embedded in it out of the lungs and trachea to be coughed out or swallowed. This movement of mucus takes place at a rate of 10 to 20 mm/hour and is greatly augmented by position and coughing. Infections and cigarette smoking cause cilial damage and dysfunction, resulting in stasis of mucous secretions and bacteria, thus increasing the risk of infection. The mucus is secreted by goblet cells in the epithelium and by mucous glands located in the submucosa with their ducts penetrating the epithelium. About 100 ml of mucus is produced daily; however, this varies considerably in conditions such as weather changes, infections, and medication usage. Mucous secretion is mediated by parasympathetic cholinergic fibers, which are blocked by atropine and its derivatives, including various illicit and prescription drugs such as many hallucinogens and opiates, tricyclic antidepressants, and phenothiazines. In addition to the mechanical action of the mucous layer, it is rich in biocidal chemicals and immunoglobulins, including secretory IgA, lysozyme (released from macrophages), interferon, complement, antioxidants, and protease inhibitors (α_1-antitrypsin), all of which participate in the protective response. However, these chemical mediators are also released with exposure to cigarette and possibly marijuana smoke (which contain noxious chemicals, particulate matter, and oxygen radicals), air pollution (acids, oxygen radicals), and occupational hazards (dust and fungi on farms, industrial dust, coal, asbestos, and other chemicals). With this type of stimulus, the abundant chemical mediators released by the lung in its defense can themselves destroy lung tissue, especially with chronic exposure. The adolescent employed in these situations may be starting a lifetime exposure of which he or she is unaware or for complex reasons chooses to ignore. Discussion of potential long-term health problems, as well as appropriate protective measures (e.g., masks) when the occupational history is obtained will help promote a career of healthy habits in the workplace.

Distal airways (terminal bronchioles and beyond) have a nonciliated cuboidal epithelium. Most particles that reach this area are phagocytosed by alveolar macrophages, which then either digest the particle or carry it along the alveolar-bronchiolar surface to the mucociliary transport system. Sighs and coughs create a squeezing mechanism that hastens this movement. In addition, some particle-laden macrophages traverse the interstitial space to travel along lymphatic channels to lymph nodes.

Rarely do the particles get through the nodes to the thoracic duct and the systemic circulation. Other particles that reach the alveoli are sequestered in the lung parenchyma by a tissue reaction, resulting in a calcification sometimes seen on chest radiographs. Such calcifications seen incidentally are most commonly due to exposure to histoplasmosis or coccidoidomycosis; however, tuberculosis and sarcoidosis can also cause calcifications or hilar adenopathy, or both.

The preceding conditions can be classified as nonimmunologic defense mechanisms. The respiratory system also has active immunologic mechanisms for processing specific antigens and developing the classic humoral and cell-mediated immunologic responses against offending microorganisms. Secretory IgA is especially effective in neutralizing viral particles. Immunoglobulin levels are low in infancy and gradually increase so that by adolescence they are stable at the adult levels. It has been proposed that the decrease in respiratory infections with age results from this increase in immunoglobulins, but many other factors may be involved. When one considers the total defense system of the respiratory tract, it is clear that it performs a complex task in protecting one from the daily onslaught of pathogens, and it is rare that it is overwhelmed to the point that a clinical respiratory illness develops.

BIBLIOGRAPHY

American Thoracic Society: ATS Statement Snowbird workshop on standardization of spirometry. Am Rev Respir Dis 119:831, 1979.

Bjure J, Nachemson A: Non-treated scoliosis. Clin Orthop 93:44, 1973.

Bosma J: Anatomic and physiologic development of the speech apparatus. In Towers DB (ed): Human Communication and Its Disorders, Vol 3. New York, Raven Press, 1975.

Cloutier MM, Loughlin GM: Chronic cough in children: A manifestation of airway hyperreactivity. Pediatrics 67:6, 1981.

Cook CD, Mead J, Orzalesi MM: Static volume-pressure characteristics of the respiratory system during maximal efforts. J Appl Physiol 19:1016, 1964.

Davies G, Reid L: Growth of the alveoli and pulmonary arteries in childhood. Thorax 25:669, 1970.

Dickman ML, Schmidt CD, Gardner RM: Spirometric standards for normal children and adolescents (ages 5 years through 18 years). Am Rev Respir Dis 104:680, 1971.

Eigen H: The clinical evaluation of chronic cough. Pediatr Clin North Am 29:67, 1982.

Fairbanks DNF: Embryology and anatomy of the sinuses. In Bluestone CD, Stool SE (eds): Pediatric Otolaryngology, Vol 1. Philadelphia, WB Saunders, 1990.

Martin AJ, McLennan LA, Landau LI, Phelan PD: The natural history of childhood asthma to adult life. Br Med J 280:1397, 1980.

Mellis CM, Phelan PD: Asthma deaths in children: A continuing problem. Thorax 32:29, 1977.

Murray JF: The Normal Lung, 2nd ed. Philadelphia, WB Saunders, 1986, pp 339–360.

Ohashi Y, Nakai Y, Ikeoka H, et al: Increased ciliary beating frequency of nasal mucosa following immunotherapy for allergy. Ann Otol Rhinol Laryngol 98:350, 1989.

Polgar G, Promadhat V: Pulmonary Function Testing In Children: Techniques and Standards. Philadelphia, WB Saunders, 1971.

Proctor B: Embryology and anatomy of the eustachian tube. Arch Otolaryngol 86:503, 1967.

Sears MR: Are deaths from asthma really on the rise? J Respir Dis 8:39, 1987.

Smyth RJ, Chapman KR, Wright TA, et al: Ventilatory patterns during hypoxia, hypercapnia, and exercise in adolescents with mild scoliosis. Pediatrics 77:692, 1986.

Spiropoulos K, Stevens JS, Eigen H: Specificity and sensitivity of methacholine challenge test in children with normal and hyperreactive airways. Acta Paediatr Scand 75:737, 1986.

Strunk RC, Mrazek DA, Wolfson GS, et al: Physiologic and psychological characteristics associated with deaths due to asthma in childhood: a case-controlled study. JAMA 254:1193, 1985.

Tepper RS: Airway reactivity in infants. J Appl Physiol 62(3):1155, 1987.

Thurlbeck WM: Postnatal growth and development of the lung. Am Rev Respir Dis 111:803, 1975.

Wald E: Acute and chronic sinusitis: Diagnosis and management. Pediatr Rev 7:150, 1985.

CHAPTER 43

Lung Diseases

SUSAN L. MILLARD and RICHARD J. LEMEN

RESPIRATORY TRACT INFECTIONS

Upper Respiratory Tract

Upper respiratory tract illness is a frequent occurrence in the adolescent patient. The most common problem is the "common cold." Allergic rhinitis, upper airway involvement of infectious mononucleosis, acute laryngotracheobronchitis and epiglottitis are also discussed in this section.

Viral infections account for most upper respiratory tract infections in adolescents. Rhinovirus, coronavirus, adenovirus, coxsackievirus, and respiratory syncytial virus are usually the culprits. Although the frequency of viral respiratory infections is higher in infants and toddlers than in adolescents, reinfection throughout life is common.

Cold viruses typically infect the upper airways in adolescents. Fever, rhinorrhea, and headache are the usual symptoms. The illness typically lasts 5 to 7 days. On physical examination, the adolescent has a low-grade fever and nasal obstruction with erythematous turbinates and clear, white or purulent nasal drainage. Symptomatic treatment includes rest, antipyretics, and oral decongestants.

In allergic rhinitis, the adolescent does not have a fever or purulent nasal discharge. Adolescents have frequent sneezing and itching of the eyes and nose. The nasal mucosa is pale; a nasal smear contains eosinophils instead of polymorphonuclear leukocytes as is found in infectious rhinitis. Antihistamines are effective for allergic rhinitis.

Infectious mononucleosis is commonly seen in adolescence (see Chapter 93). It is caused by the Epstein-Barr virus (EBV), a member of the herpesvirus family. The virus attacks the oropharyngeal epithelial cells first. It then infects susceptible B lymphocytes within the lymphoid tissue of the pharynx. Sore throat and posterior cervical adenopathy develop after malaise, headache, and nausea. Pharyngitis and tonsillar enlargement may become severe, and steroids may be beneficial in these circumstances.

Acute laryngotracheobronchitis is an infection of the larynx, trachea, and major bronchi most commonly caused by the common cold viruses. Influenza, pertussis, diphtheria, scarlet fever, typhoid fever, and measles are also associated with acute laryngotracheobronchitis (see Chapters 93 and 94). Initial symptoms are often similar to those experienced in viral upper respiratory tract infections. A dry cough with low substernal discomfort or anterior chest pain then develops. The adolescent experiences dyspnea and emesis with coughing. The cough then becomes productive and gradually dissipates. Treatment is supportive. Antibiotics for viral-induced tracheobronchitis do not decrease the incidence of bacterial superinfection.

Pertussis is a bacterial cause of tracheobronchitis and can also be the cause of persistent cough (see Chapter 94). Waning immunity after pertussis vaccination in childhood or inadequate childhood vaccination can result in pertussis infection during adolescence. Erythromycin (estolate form) does not ameliorate the disease but does eliminate nasopharyngeal carriage of this organism. This is an important treatment, especially if there are nonimmunized infants or partially immunized toddlers living at home with the adolescent.

Epiglottitis is also a potentially life-threatening upper airway problem. It is an uncommon diagnosis in adolescents who experience respiratory distress, cough, drooling, and high fever. *Haemophilus influenzae* type B is the causative organism. Maintenance of the airway and intravenous ampicillin or cefotaxime are primary therapeutic measures (see Chapter 94).

Lower Respiratory Tract

The pneumonias are divided into two categories: typical and atypical. Typical pneumonias are caused by *Streptococcus pneumoniae, Haemophilus influenzae*, and *Staphylococcus aureus*. Atypical pneumonias are caused by viruses or *Mycoplasma pneumoniae*. Pneumococcal pneumonia and mycoplasmal pneumonia are the most common types of bacterial pneumonia in adolescents (see Chapter 94). They are considered "community-acquired" pneumonias.

The adolescent patient with pneumococcal pneumonia typically has fever, tachypnea, chills, pleuritic chest pain, a productive cough, and often a preceding viral respiratory tract infection. On auscultation of the chest, isolated crackles may be noted. Chest radiography may reveal a lobar infiltrate. The diagnosis is confirmed by isolation of *Streptococcus pneumoniae* from the blood, pleural fluid, lung aspirate, or cerebrospinal fluid. Nasopharyngeal or throat cultures are not helpful. Rapid methods for pneumococcal capsular antigen detection may be employed. Antigen detection in urine specimens may be available. Coagglutination tests for detection of the capsular antigen in sputum are being developed and tested.

Penicillin is the treatment of choice for pneumococcal pneumonia. Erythromycin is an alternative for adolescents who are allergic to penicillin. The route of administration depends on the severity of the illness. Intravenous penicillin is indicated in adolescents who have complications such as empyema, meningitis, and endocarditis. Asplenia and sickle cell anemia (see Chapter 52) are two other indications for intravenous penicillin G. Pneumococcal infections resistant to penicillin are a potential problem. *In vitro* testing of resistant strains suggests that cefotaxime and ceftriaxone are alternative drugs for these patients (see Chapter 96).

Mycoplasmal pneumonia is insidious in nature. It is typically characterized by headache, sore throat, and a persistent cough. The symptoms are also less severe than the chest radiographic findings. Three typical chest radiographic patterns are seen in mycoplasmal pneumonia: patchy, nonhomogeneous consolidation (35%); peribronchial and perivascular interstitial infiltrates (30%); and homogeneous, acinar consolidations that resemble ground glass (35%). Erythromycin is the treatment of choice.

Less Common Infectious Causes of Respiratory Illnesses

Adolescents may also develop less common types of lower respiratory tract infections. Because such illnesses may be more difficult to diagnose, it is important to obtain a thorough history. A travel or exposure history is necessary, since certain areas of the world are endemic for specific pulmonary diseases. Coccidioidomycosis, for example, is predominantly found in the southwestern United States, whereas histoplasmosis is found in the midwestern and southern United States. Most adolescents with tuberculosis have a history of exposure to tuberculosis. Other less frequently diagnosed pulmonary infections during adolescence are *Moraxella (Branhamella) catarrhalis*, *Legionella pneumophila*, and strains of *Chlamydia psittaci*.

Moraxella catarrhalis was once considered to be a commensal microorganism. It is actually the third most common cause of acute sinusitis and otitis media. It has also been associated with lower respiratory tract infections, especially in previously healthy patients who are on mechanical ventilation. Cefaclor is effective outpatient therapy for *M. catarrhalis* infections.

Legionella pneumophila causes Legionnaires disease. Infection in adolescents is uncommon except in immunocompromised hosts (see Chapters 76 and 92). Pneumonia, however, is a common syndrome in adults. Its severity is variable; some adolescents have mild, influenza-like symptoms, whereas others have severe multisystem disease with gastrointestinal, neurologic, renal, and pulmonary manifestations. Erythromycin is usually effective, but rifampin may be added in serious cases.

Tuberculosis is still a concern among adolescent patients. The incidence of tuberculosis has increased in certain metropolitan and inner city areas of the United States. This increase is in part due to the occurrence of tuberculosis in older adolescents and young adults with AIDS and the possible acquisition of tuberculosis from the increased reservoir of tuberculosis caused by AIDS (see Chapter 76 and section on lung disease in the immunocompromised host.) The American Thoracic Society and Centers for Disease Control do not recommend routine screening of adolescents for tuberculosis unless they belong to certain high-risk subgroups such as Asians, Africans, Latin Americans, American Indians, and Alaskans. The American Academy of Pediatrics, however, suggests that adolescents between the ages of 14 and 16 years should be routinely screened because of a slight increase in incidence during adolescence (see Chapter 25).

The diagnosis of tuberculosis is made by history, chest radiography, skin testing, and cultures. Hilar adenopathy, consolidation, infiltrates, and atelectasis are typical radiographic findings. *Mycobacterium tuberculosis* is best isolated from sputum or gastric aspirates obtained in the morning, before rising. The timing of specimen acquisition is important because respiratory fluids have collected in the stomach overnight and are less likely to be passed through the stomach while the adolescent is still supine and fasting. For cases in which the bacteria have typical antibiotic sensitivities, pulmonary tuberculosis therapy includes isoniazid, rifampin, and pyrazinamide for the first 2 months. Only isoniazid and rifampin are used for the next 4 months. Adolescents who have a positive skin test without evidence of disease or history of previous prophylaxis require preventive therapy with isoniazid for 9 to 12 months.

ASTHMA

Asthma is defined as intermittent, reversible airway obstruction. Approximately 4 to 5 million children and adolescents have asthma; it is the most common chronic lung disorder encountered during adolescence. There is a higher incidence before puberty in males than in females (approximately 2:1 ratio); after puberty the incidence is similar in boys and girls. Some children have improvement in asthma when they become adolescents; the reasons for the improvement or apparent resolution of asthma are uncertain. During the past 10 years, the mortality rate for asthma has increased, whereas mortality rates for most other chronic diseases have declined (see Chapter 42).

Pathogenesis and Physiology

Airway hyperreactivity is the major physiologic problem in asthma, but its etiology is not fully understood. Airway inflammation, airway smooth muscle constriction, and mucous gland secretion all contribute to the airway narrowing.

Several neural and humoral factors have been implicated in both bronchoconstriction and bronchodilation (Fig. 43–1). Bronchoconstriction is most likely mediated through the cholinergic portion of the autonomic nervous system as well as through the release of histamine and leukotrienes. Relaxation of airway smooth muscle

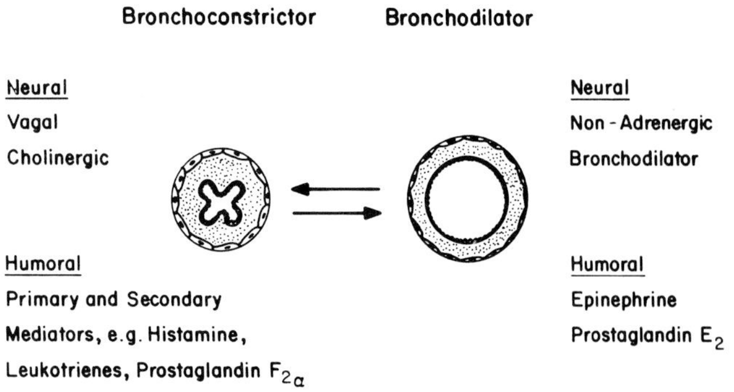

Bronchoconstrictor   Bronchodilator

Neural   Neural
Vagal   Non - Adrenergic
Cholinergic   Bronchodilator

Humoral   Humoral
Primary and Secondary   Epinephrine
Mediators, e.g. Histamine,   Prostaglandin E$_2$
Leukotrienes, Prostaglandin F$_{2\alpha}$

Figure 43–1. The figure shows only the factors that influence smooth muscle tone and control of airway diameter. Whereas acute bronchoconstriction (bronchospasm) in response to environmental stimuli is principally due to smooth muscle contraction, mucosal edema and inflammation play a major role in the airway obstruction of chronic asthma. In particular, the so-called late phase asthmatic response is due to airway inflammation secondary not only to the action of vasoactive and smooth muscle contractile mediators but also to tissue injury resulting from infiltration of cellular elements, e.g., neutrophils, eosinophils, and others. (With permission from Behrman RE, Vaughan VC [eds]: Nelson Textbook of Pediatrics, 13th ed. Philadelphia, WB Saunders, 1989, p 496.)

results from the endogenous catecholamine activity in β-adrenergic receptors. The nonadrenergic, noncholinergic nervous system may also contribute to bronchoconstriction and bronchodilation.

Many stimuli provoke exacerbations of asthma, including viral respiratory infections, exercise, allergens, cold air, pollutants, emotional stress, coughing, and even laughing. The same stimuli that cause smooth muscle contraction may also influence the volume and composition of airway secretions. The mucous glands may hypertrophy, and the goblet cell may become hyperplastic. Mucociliary abnormalities result in the decreased clearance of secretions. Mediators including arachidonic acid metabolites, platelet-activating factor, and histamine potentiate the airway inflammation and increase vascular permeability, leading to edema.

There are at least two phases of asthma: an early phase and a late phase. The early phase is rapid in onset, beginning almost immediately after a specific stimulus, and is characterized by bronchoconstriction of smooth muscle. β-Adrenergic medications and cromolyn sodium are effective during this phase. The late phase occurs 4 to 6 hours later. Nonspecific airway hyperresponsiveness to a variety of stimuli develops and lasts several days or weeks. The accumulation of neutrophils and eosinophils in the lung during this stage may cause airway inflammation. This stage is not inhibited by β-agonists but may be prevented by pretreatment with cromolyn sodium or steroids.

When bronchoconstriction occurs, the caliber of the airways narrows; air turbulence causes wheezing. Wheezing during inspiration indicates more critical airway narrowing than wheezing during expiration. A "silent chest," in which no breath sounds are audible, may indicate that the airways are so constricted that no turbulent airflow occurs.

Airway narrowing reduces airflow during expiration, producing hyperinflation of the lungs and uneven distribution of ventilation. Respiratory distress and hypoxemia ensue because of an impaired ability to exchange gas. As air trapping worsens, ventilation-to-perfusion mismatching increases; greater transpulmonary pressure is required to produce an equivalent tidal volume. Both the work of breathing and the oxygen demand escalate. Increases in ineffective ventilation, secondary to ventilation-perfusion mismatch, and carbon dioxide production require a greater minute ventilation. The respiratory muscles (intercostal muscles, accessory muscles, and diaphragm) are inefficient as a result of hyperinflation. Carbon dioxide retention can develop. If the oxygen demands of the respiratory muscles are greater than the actual supply of oxygen, a metabolic lactic acidosis results.

Clinical Manifestations and Evaluation

CLINICAL MANIFESTATIONS

Asthmatic adolescents often have a dry, hacking, nonproductive cough that may be associated with chest "tightness." The adolescent may complain of coughing or wheezing at night, or both. Symptoms associated with the cough and wheezing include nasal congestion, sneezing, red eyes, abdominal pain, and vomiting mucus during a coughing episode (tussive emesis). The adolescent also may have evidence of allergy such as atopic dermatitis.

EVALUATION

The past medical history for asthma is outlined in Table 43–1. Table 43–2 includes the family and social

TABLE 43–1. Past Medical History: Asthma

Onset and course of asthma
Pneumonia or bronchiolitis during infancy
Difficulty in breathing resulting in
  Previous emergency department visits
  Previous hospitalizations
  Previous intensive care unit admissions requiring intubation or isoproterenol
  Use of inhalers, theophylline, steroids

TABLE 43–2. Family and Social Histories: Asthma

Family history of lung diseases: asthma, cystic fibrosis, emphysema, tuberculosis
Social history of the adolescent

Health habits
Cigarette, marijuana smoking
Sniffing of glue or use of inhalant
Exposure to passive smoking, pets, or smoke from woodburning stove

School history
Attendance
Achievement
Behavior

Social stressors
Death in family
Move
Family illness

histories. Table 43–3 covers the salient parts of the physical examination. The adolescent may be diaphoretic, pale, or even hypoxemic (a PaO_2 of less than 70 mmHg when in room air). A respiratory rate of at least 32/min and a heart rate of more than 120/min indicate significant respiratory distress. Sinus tachycardia is often attributed inaccurately to drug therapy. It is necessary to measure the blood pressure and to look for pulsus paradoxus. The decrease in systolic blood pressure with inspiration is normally less than 10 mmHg. Values over 15 mmHg indicate the presence of a physiologically significant pulsus paradoxus and are associated with significantly reduced pulmonary function.

Laboratory Examinations

During an acute exacerbation of asthma, pulmonary function tests show an increase in residual volume (RV), functional residual capacity (FRC), and total lung capacity (TLC). The RV/TLC ratio is increased. The forced expiratory volume (FEV_1), vital capacity, and peak flow are decreased.

Based on blood gas evaluations, exacerbations of asthma are characterized by three stages: (1) Hypoxemia and respiratory alkalosis occur in the first stage; (2) obstruction worsens, the pH and the PCO_2 normalize, and hypoxemia persists in the second stage; and (3) respiratory acidosis and often metabolic acidosis develop, indicating respiratory failure in the third stage. Retention of carbon dioxide is more likely when the FEV_1 falls to 25% of the predicted value. Thus, a "normal" PCO_2 with tachypnea during an acute asthmatic attack indicates incipient respiratory failure.

In the ambulatory setting, peak expiratory flow measurements can be performed to evaluate the severity of the asthma attack and to determine the response to therapeutic interventions. Three measurements should be taken and averaged. Normal peak flow is based on the patient's height (Fig. 43–2). When a decrease in the peak flow is observed, the adolescent or the parent should contact a physician.

A typical finding on chest radiography is hyperinflation with peribronchial cuffing (Fig. 43–3). Segmental atelectasis secondary to mucous plugging may also be evident. Chest roentgenograms are not required for every adolescent who has asthma but are strongly suggested for the following: (1) adolescents presenting with the first episode of bronchospasm, (2) adolescents who

TABLE 43–3. Physical Examination: Asthma

Acute Manifestations
Speech—full sentences, or phrases only secondary to dyspnea
Signs of respiratory distress
  Orthopnea, inability to recline
  Leaning forward
  Nasal flaring
  Use of sternocleidomastoid muscles
Chest—hyperresonant to percussion, wheezing may or may not be heard

Chronic Manifestations
Clubbing—if present, *not* specific for asthma
Sinusitis

have decreased breath sounds or unequal breath sounds (suggesting the development of a pneumothorax), and (3) adolescents who do not respond appropriately to therapy.

Mild leukocytosis and absolute eosinophil counts greater than 300/mm³ in the peripheral blood may be present during an asthma attack. β-Agonists may also produce a leukocytosis and a mild bandemia. Asthmatics may have elevated immunoglobulin E (IgE) levels. Grossly elevated serum IgE levels (i.e., greater than 1000 mg/ml) may indicate allergic bronchopulmonary aspergillosis (ABPA). Blood samples should be evaluated for IgE antibodies to *Aspergillus* or circulating precipitins of *Aspergillus* antigens, to aid in the diagnosis of ABPA. This disease causes recurrent, severe asthma symptoms and may lead to the development of bronchiectasis.

Differential Diagnosis

Many illnesses present with cough or wheezing, or both. Asthma is the most frequent diagnosis. Many other diagnoses should be considered, including mechanical obstruction, pneumothorax, metabolic causes such as tetany, neurologic causes, trauma, laryngeal abnormalities, and psychosomatic causes. ABPA, as mentioned previously, may present with recurrent wheezing and respiratory distress.

To establish the diagnosis of asthma, baseline and postbronchodilator pulmonary function studies should be performed. These studies are done to demonstrate responsiveness to the bronchodilators. Bronchial provocation tests are also used occasionally. Methacholine or histamine is administered after baseline pulmonary function tests are performed. The adolescent patient is given increasing aerosolized doses of methacholine or histamine until a significant decrease in air flow, the provoking concentration, is observed. A response at a low dose of methacholine or histamine indicates hyperresponsiveness, but a positive test is not diagnostic of asthma. It is correlated with an increased likelihood of asthma, however.

Management

ALGORITHMS

Initiation of bronchodilator therapy is the most important initial treatment for asthma exacerbations. Immediate management is directed at airway smooth muscle relaxation and then treatment of airway inflammation.

The algorithm for home management of the asthmatic is presented first (Fig. 43–4). It is necessary for the adolescent and the parents to be instructed in the proper use of the algorithm. The adolescent and his or her parents should be taught to assess the severity of an attack based on symptoms, respiratory rate, use of accessory muscles, peak flow measurements, color, and mental status.

When the adolescent presents to an emergency de-

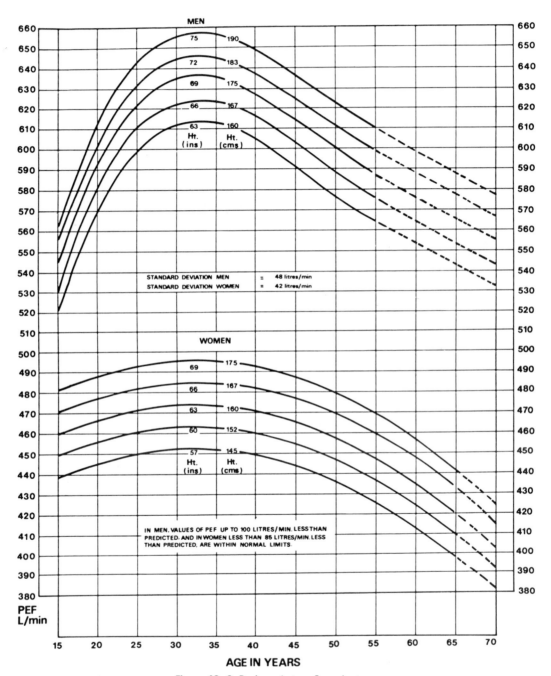

Figure 43–2. Peak expiratory flow chart.

Figure 43–3. An intubated patient with status asthmaticus. Note that the endotracheal tube is at the carina and that severe bilateral hyperinflation is present. The endotracheal tube was subsequently withdrawn 2 cm. A gastrotomy tube is also in place.

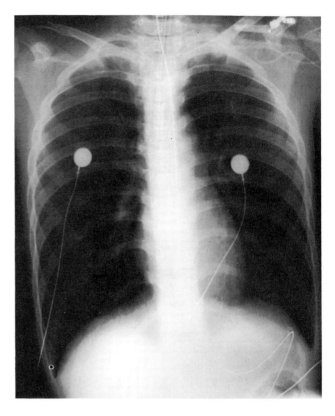

partment, assessment and management should proceed according to the algorithm illustrated in Figure 43–5.

The algorithm intended for the hospitalized adolescent with asthma, illustrated in Figure 43–6, may be used following assessment of the severity of the asthma attack. Hospitalized adolescents require pulse oximetry and peak flow monitoring. Serial arterial blood gas studies may also be required. Moderate to severely ill adolescents with asthma require oxygen. Oxygen must be used during therapy with bronchodilators, since these medications can contribute to hypoxemia through their vasodilator action.

PHARMACOTHERAPY

The selection of therapeutic agents is made on the basis of the severity of the asthma attack. The drugs that are used are outlined in the emergency room and hospital algorithms. For outpatient asthma management, drug selection is based on the severity of the disease. Some adolescents may be treated effectively with few medications. Inhaled steroids or cromolyn sodium may be sufficient therapy for a mild asthmatic attack in conjunction with a β-agonist used on an "as needed" basis. If the patient has more frequent and

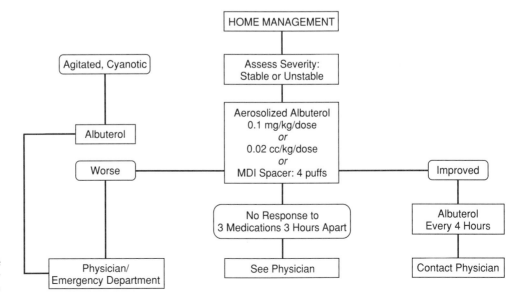

Figure 43–4. Algorithm for home management of asthmatic patient. MDI, metered dose inhaler.

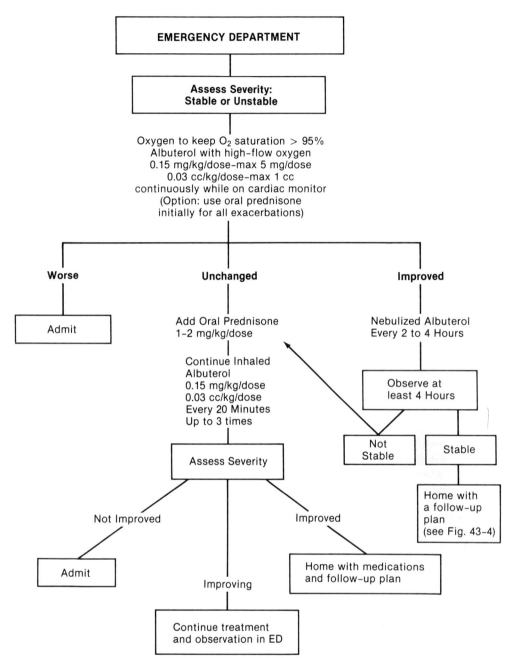

Figure 43–5. Algorithm for emergency department management of asthmatic patient.

severe episodes of asthma, inhaled steroids are used in combination with β-agonists, anticholinergics such as Atrovent, and occasionally theophylline. Theophylline, however, is not routinely used, except for difficult cases.

Many asthma agents have been previously referred to in the algorithms presented earlier. An alphabetical listing of drugs used for asthma with their recommended dosages follows.

Corticosteroids (Table 43–4)

Corticosteroids are administered in various forms, including oral, intravenous, and aerosol routes. For less severe exacerbations in the ambulatory setting, oral prednisone is used in a dose of 0.5 to 2 mg/kg/day in single or divided doses for 3 to 7 days. If the prednisone is taken for less than 7 days, tapering the patient off the

steroids is not necessary. For status asthmaticus, the intravenous route is preferred. Usually, a 2 mg/kg dose of methylprednisolone (Solu-Medrol) is given once, followed by 0.5 to 1 mg/kg/dose intravenously every 4 to 6 hours for up to 5 days. Aerosolized steroid preparations are available in the United States as metered-dose inhalers (MDI). The typical starting dose is 2 puffs two or three times per day for all preparations. Doses of less than 800 µg/day rarely have significant side effects or cause adrenal suppression.

Anticholinergic Medications (Table 43–5)

Two anticholinergic drugs, atropine and ipratropium bromide, are used to treat asthma. The side effects of xerostomia, mydriasis, tachycardia, and abdominal pain

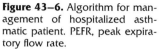

Figure 43–6. Algorithm for management of hospitalized asthmatic patient. PEFR, peak expiratory flow rate.

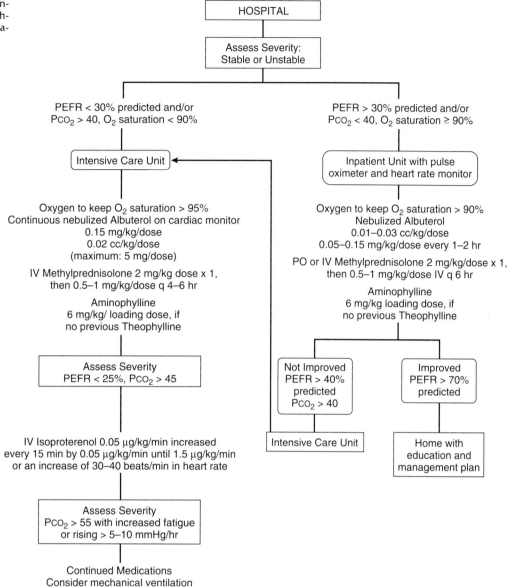

HOSPITAL

Assess Severity:
Stable or Unstable

PEFR < 30% predicted and/or
Pco_2 > 40, O_2 saturation < 90%

PEFR > 30% predicted and/or
Pco_2 < 40, O_2 saturation ≥ 90%

Intensive Care Unit

Inpatient Unit with pulse
oximeter and heart rate monitor

Oxygen to keep O_2 saturation > 95%
Continuous nebulized Albuterol on cardiac monitor
0.15 mg/kg/dose
0.02 cc/kg/dose
(maximum: 5 mg/dose)

IV Methylprednisolone 2 mg/kg dose x 1,
then 0.5–1 mg/kg/dose q 4–6 hr

Aminophylline
6 mg/kg/ loading dose, if
no previous Theophylline

Oxygen to keep O_2 saturation > 90%
Nebulized Albuterol
0.01–0.03 cc/kg/dose
0.05–0.15 mg/kg/dose every 1–2 hr

PO or IV Methylprednisolone 2 mg/kg/dose x 1,
then 0.5–1 mg/kg/dose IV q 6 hr

Aminophylline
6 mg/kg loading dose, if
no previous Theophylline

Assess Severity
PEFR < 25%, Pco_2 > 45

Not Improved
PEFR > 40%
predicted
Pco_2 > 40

Improved
PEFR > 70%
predicted

IV Isoproterenol 0.05 µg/kg/min increased
every 15 min by 0.05 µg/kg/min until 1.5 µg/kg/min
or an increase of 30–40 beats/min in heart rate

Intensive Care Unit

Home with
education and
management plan

Assess Severity
Pco_2 > 55 with increased fatigue
or rising > 5–10 mmHg/hr

Continued Medications
Consider mechanical ventilation

TABLE 43–4. Steroid Preparations

DRUG	METHOD OF ADMINISTRATION	DOSAGE
Beclomethasone dipropionate (Beclovent, Vanceril)	Inhaled	42 µg/inhalation
Triamcinolone acetonide (Azmacort)	Inhaled	200 µg, but only 100 µg delivered (released by inhalation)
Hydrocortisone (Solu-Cortef)	Intravenous	4–6 mg/kg/dose × 1, 2–4 mg/kg/dose q 6 hr
Methylprednisolone (Medrol, Solu-Medrol)	Intravenous or oral	2 mg/kg/dose ×1, then 0.5–1 mg/kg/dose IV q 4–6 hr Duration dependent on clinical course
Prednisone	Oral (5-, 10-, 20-mg tablets)	1 mg/kg/dose q 6 hr for 24 hr, then 0.5–2 mg/kg/day given every morning Duration dependent on clinical course

TABLE 43–5. Anticholinergic Preparations

DRUG	METHOD OF ADMINISTRATION	DOSAGE
Atropine	Solution for inhalation (use injectable form for nebulization, several concentrations available)	0.05 mg/kg/dose per inhalation q 6 hr
Ipratropium bromide	Metered-dose inhaler (18 µg/actuation)	2 inhalations/dose; starting dose is q 6 hr. May be administered up to 2 inhalations/dose q 4 hr

are frequent side effects of atropine. However, since ipratropium bromide is a quaternary derivative of atropine, it does not cross the blood-brain barrier. It therefore has fewer side effects.

These drugs inhibit the binding of acetylcholine to muscarinic receptors. They have a slower onset of action than the β-adrenergic medicines. In the United States, atropine is used in the aerosol form, and ipratropium bromide is available in the inhaler form. The dose for atropine is 0.05 mg/kg every 6 hours. Two inhalations of the ipratropium bromide inhaler may be given every 6 hours or as often as 6 times/day if tolerated by the adolescent. These drugs are used for the management of chronic asthma and are also helpful in status asthmaticus.

β-Adrenergic Agents

Many β-adrenergic agonists are available for the treatment of asthma and include metaproterenol, albuterol, terbutaline, and isoproterenol. Albuterol and terbutaline are selective for β2 receptors and thus have less cardiac side effects. Most of the drugs are available in oral, parenteral, and aerosolized forms. Albuterol offers the most β2 selectivity with the longest duration of action.

In status asthmaticus, aerosolized albuterol can be administered frequently, or even continuously, for relaxation of bronchial smooth muscles. It is as effective as subcutaneous epinephrine, which also has β-adrenergic properties. However, if the adolescent does not respond to the albuterol aerosol, subcutaneous epinephrine may be effective in dilating the airways to allow improved penetration of the albuterol.

Intravenous isoproterenol administered in an intensive care setting with cardiac monitoring is indicated when patients continue to have severe respiratory distress in spite of intensive therapy. Baseline creatine phosphokinase isoenzymes and an electrocardiogram are obtained because of isoproterenol's possible cardiac toxicity. The starting dose is 0.05 µg/kg/minute. The dose is increased every 10 to 15 minutes by 0.05 µg/kg/minute. No further increases are made if the heart rate has increased to more than 180 to 200 beats per minute. The adolescent must be monitored closely for dysrhyth-

mias, hypertension, and elevation of the creatine phosphokinase MB band.

The β-adrenergic agents are listed in Table 43–6.

Cromolyn Sodium

Cromolyn sodium and a newer drug (not yet approved by the FDA), nedocromil sodium, are used to prevent airway inflammation. Cromolyn sodium may inhibit mast cell degranulation by inhibition of cyclic adenosine monophosphate (cAMP) phosphodiesterase or stimulation of guanylate cyclase. Many laboratories are performing studies to understand the mechanism of action for these drugs.

Cromolyn sodium is available in an inhaler form and in a 2% solution (20 mg/2 ml ampules) for nebulization. The solution may be added to β-agonists and atropine. Cromolyn sodium may be given 10 to 20 minutes prior to exercise to prevent exercise-induced asthma. It is also not necessary to stop the medication during asthma exacerbations, using the present drug form. Side effects are very rare, and the drug is well-tolerated by most adolescents.

Theophylline

The mechanism of action of theophylline is not fully understood. Theophylline is a phosphodiesterase inhibitor. The mechanism, as it relates to asthma, may involve adenosine receptors or alteration of calcium flow into the cell. Theophylline is available in various oral forms. Aminophylline is given intravenously for status asthmaticus. Because of the erratic absorption of rectal

TABLE 43–6. β-Adrenergic Agents

DRUG	METHOD OF ADMINISTRATION	DOSAGE
Albuterol	Metered-dose inhaler (90 µg/dose)	2 inhalations/dose (use with a spacer for maximal efficacy)
	Nebulized solution for inhalation (5 mg/ml)	0.05–0.15 mg/kg/dose (0.01–0.03 ml/kg/dose) up to 5 mg every 20 min for 1–2 hr. For severe attacks, 0.5 mg/kg/hr (0.1 ml/kg/hr) by continuous nebulization
Epinephrine (1:1000)	Subcutaneous aqueous preparation (1 mg/ml)	0.01 mg/kg (0.01 ml/kg) up to 0.5 mg (0.5 ml) every 20 min for three doses
Isoproterenol	Intravenous	0.05 µg/kg/min, increased every 15 min by 0.05 µg/kg/min. Max 1.5 µg/kg/min
Terbutaline	Metered-dose inhaler (200 µg/inhalation)	2 inhalations/dose q 4–6 hr
	Subcutaneous	0.01 mg/kg up to 0.3 mg q 2–6 hr
	Intravenous	0.1–1 µg/kg/min

theophylline, this form is not recommended. Theophylline has a narrow therapeutic index of 10 to 20 µg/ml. A drug level of even 7 to 8 µg/ml may have a therapeutic effect (Table 43–7).

The most common side effects are gastrointestinal upset and central nervous system stimulation. Enuresis is an occasional problem that may be secondary to theophylline's diuretic effect. There have been reports of hyperactivity, poor school performance, and behavior problems, but only a few studies have evaluated the psychological and behavioral effects of theophylline. There is, however, a subgroup of individuals with a heightened central nervous system response to these medications. Each adolescent patient placed on theophylline should, therefore, be closely monitored for changes in behavior or school performance. A diet history should be taken because caffeine and other xanthines may potentiate the side effects of theophylline. Because of its narrow therapeutic index, potential side effects, and the availability of more effective medications, theophylline is no longer considered a first-line or "routine" drug to control asthma.

Adolescents who smoke cigarettes may require larger doses of theophylline. Those taking erythromycin or clindamycin may have higher plasma levels of theophylline (see Chapters 39 and 96). Theophylline causes increased metabolism of lithium and antagonizes the effect of propranolol and possibly other β-blockers. It is important to be cautious with use of this drug in adolescents, since it is frequently used in suicide gestures and attempts (see Chapter 101). Finally, its use is contraindicated in adolescents who have seizures (see Chapter 83).

Psychological Issues
(see Chapters 30 and 121)

Asthma is a chronic disease with significant morbidity and mortality. Adolescence is a critical time because of the transition between parental care and self-care and

TABLE 43–8. High-risk Conditions for Death in Asthma

Previous near-death episode requiring resuscitation
Previous episode of respiratory failure requiring ventilation
History of hypoxic seizures with an attack of asthma

developing autonomy. Rebellion may be manifested by problems with compliance (see Chapter 26).

Adolescents may have difficulties with compliance because of a deficit of knowledge about the medications prescribed. They may fear the potential side effects of medications. Adolescent patients may also worry that they will not be able to manage their disease. Adolescents who have asthma require extensive education and knowledge about their asthma and the potential causes of exacerbations to reduce the risk of non-compliance.

The use of a peak flow meter and the direct involvement of the adolescent in discussions about asthma therapy are essential. This is especially important for those adolescents who may have life-threatening exacerbations. High-risk adolescents must be identified so that therapeutic action can be taken even when minor symptoms develop. There are several clues that an adolescent patient is at risk for death secondary to asthma. These are listed in Table 43–8. Identification of these adolescents at risk allows the young person, the family, and the physician to work together in management of the asthma. A management protocol for exacerbations and emergencies should decrease the patient's morbidity and hopefully decrease the risk of death due to this serious disease.

CYSTIC FIBROSIS

Cystic fibrosis (CF) is the most common genetically acquired lethal disease among whites. The disease frequency is approximately 1 in 2000 live births among whites, and about 5% of whites carry the defective gene. It is, however, found in other races, including blacks and Hispanics. The median age of survival has increased from 7 years in 1965 to 26 years in the 1980s. Overall, males have a better prognosis than do females. During adolescence, females may experience a decline in their pulmonary function more often than do their male counterparts.

Mucus accumulation and glandular obstruction in both the respiratory and the gastrointestinal tracts are the hallmarks of this multisystem disease. Bronchiectasis, airway obstruction, hyperinflation, and infection occur in the lungs. Sinusitis and nasal polyps are found in the upper airway (see Chapter 40). Meconium ileus, meconium ileus equivalent, and gastroesophageal reflux occur in the gastrointestinal tract. Malabsorption and glucose intolerance develop as a result of pancreatic disease (see Chapter 62). Cholelithiasis, cirrhosis, and portal hypertension also occur. Vas deferens obliteration causes sterility in most males. Women may have decreased fertility because of thick vaginal and cervical secretions. Metabolic alkalosis and heat injury can occur in cystic fibrosis patients because of increased salt loss with sweating.

TABLE 43–7. Methylxanthines

DRUG	DOSAGE*
Aminophylline (80% anhydrous theophylline)	Loading dose: If theophylline serum concentration is known, for every 1 mg/kg theophylline give 2 µg/ml increase in blood serum concentration If no previous theophylline given, start with 6 mg/kg If previous theophylline was given, start with 3 mg/kg or wait for a serum concentration The usual continuous infusion rates required to obtain a mean steady-state concentration of 15 µg/ml are as follows: Adolescents (9–16 years): 0.8 mg/kg/hr Adults (older than 16 years): 0.5 mg/kg/hr
Theophylline	Orally in nonsmokers 9–12 years: 20 mg/kg/day 13–16 years: 18 mg/kg/day Older than 16 years: 13 mg/kg/day

*Dose frequency depends upon type of medication used and metabolism. Dosing three times a day is preferable to once or twice a day.

Etiology and Pathogenesis

Cystic fibrosis is an autosomal recessive trait. The gene, located on chromosome 7 (discovered in 1989), is 250 kb long. In 70% of cystic fibrosis patients, there is a deletion of three DNA base pairs coding for phenylalanine. This gene product is a protein called the cystic fibrosis transmembrane regulator (CFTR). The defect alters the characteristics of this protein. Data suggest that 30% of patients with CF, however, have a different defect or mutation. Several mutations have already been delineated. This information may explain the diversity of symptoms and differences in disease severity in cystic fibrosis patients.

Other researchers have found that cystic fibrosis airway epithelial cells are relatively impermeable to chloride. Normal epithelial cells transport chloride from the submucosal surface to the mucosal surface actively. This activity controls the quantity and the composition of the respiratory tract fluid and thus affects mucociliary clearance. Researchers have found evidence that CFTR is a chloride channel. Other researchers believe that CFTR regulates the chloride channel. Many centers are examining the cellular and molecular implications of the gene defect and developing potential gene therapies.

Clinical Manifestation and Diagnosis

Cystic fibrosis in older patients may be difficult to recognize if not previously diagnosed. Most adolescents are diagnosed in infancy or childhood as a result of the characteristic lung findings or because of liver and pancreatic problems. The reader is referred to *Nelson Textbook of Pediatrics* for a discussion of the clinical manifestations of cystic fibrosis during childhood. Approximately 10% of patients with cystic fibrosis are diagnosed as adolescents or young adults, because of extremely mild or absent respiratory disease and gastrointestinal problems. Recurrent lung infections, delayed growth at puberty, or failure to thrive may, however, be presenting complaints. Patients with CF may have steatorrhea and carry the diagnosis of encopresis instead of the correct diagnosis of CF-related pancreatic insufficiency. Other presentations include a positive sputum culture for mucoid *P. aeruginosa*, a history of chronic bronchitis or bronchiectasis, or clubbing of the fingers.

Evaluation

Each organ system that may be involved in the disease should be thoroughly evaluated during each visit to a cystic fibrosis center; these visits optimally occur every 3 months. In the physical examination, for example, the adolescent's height and weight should be plotted on standard growth curves (see Chapter 6). Close observation of the patient's growth parameters is necessary to determine whether the pancreatic enzyme supplementation is adequate and whether changes in diet are required. Other general evaluations include examination of skin color for evidence of the pallor of anemia; the extremities, for evidence of clubbing and peripheral cyanosis; and the nares and sinuses, for evidence of polyps.

The pulmonary examination involves more than auscultation for lung sounds. Respiratory rate and chest configuration are important to evaluate, looking for tachypnea and an increase in the anteroposterior chest diameter. This chest deformity occurs because of airway obstruction and gas trapping. It is also necessary to look for accessory muscle use and intercostal and subcostal retractions, which would indicate respiratory distress found in pulmonary exacerbations of CF, for example. During auscultation, it is important to listen for wheezes, inspiratory crackles, or decrease in air exchange. In acute onset of chest pain in a patient with CF, the diagnosis of pneumothorax should be considered. If a pneumothorax is present, there would be decreased or absent lung sounds in the area of the pneumothorax and, possibly, deviation of the trachea.

The abdomen is also an important area in the CF physical examination. Patients with CF may have hepatomegaly or splenomegaly because of portal hypertension. There also may be evidence of a tender mass in the right lower quadrant, which may indicate a meconium ileus equivalent. This problem is secondary to recurrent distal intestinal obstruction, and it occurs in about 10% to 20% of older CF patients.

Laboratory Examinations

The quantitative pilocarpine iontophoresis sweat test is used to establish the diagnosis of cystic fibrosis. Pilocarpine stimulates the sweat glands. Sweat is then collected on a filter paper or gauze for 30 to 60 minutes. The chloride concentration is measured by standard techniques. A positive test result is a sweat chloride concentration of more than 60 mEq/L in a minimum of 50 mg of sweat. The test should be conducted in a laboratory experienced in the performance of sweat tests and should be repeated on a different day to confirm or exclude the diagnosis.

The adolescent who has cystic fibrosis should undergo pulmonary function testing and arterial blood gas or pulse oximetry monitoring annually. Chest radiography and respiratory tract cultures and sensitivities are also performed yearly to follow the course of the disease. On chest radiography, cystic changes and bronchiectasis in the upper lobes are the usual initial findings (Fig. 43–7). As the disease progresses, pulmonary infiltrates with atelectasis and hyperinflation appear. Cystic changes become evident in advanced disease, secondary to the bronchiectasis. Respiratory tract cultures from young CF patients are typically culture-positive for *S. aureus* and *Haemophilus influenzae*. Subsequently, colonization by mucoid *P. aeruginosa* is found in as many as 90% of adolescent CF patients. Colonization with this gelatinous microorganism often correlates with progression of bronchial airway pathology and severity of radiographic changes.

Each year, a complete blood count with platelet count

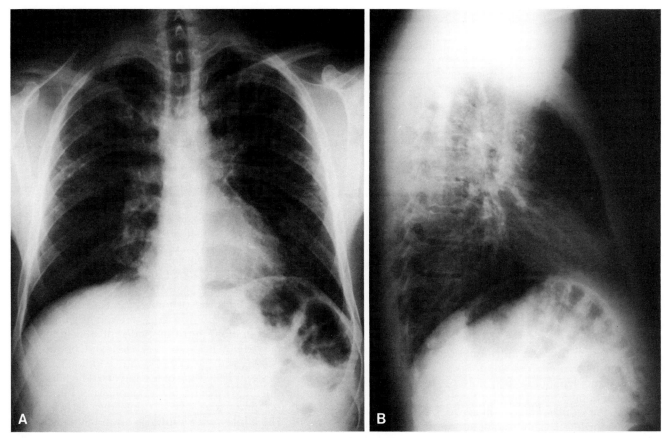

Figure 43–7. Adolescent with mild pulmonary manifestations of cystic fibrosis. Note the bronchiectasis that is especially prominent in the right upper and left upper lobes.

and differential should also be done to detect anemia, leukocytosis, or eosinophilia. Cystic fibrosis patients with ABPA may have eosinophils in their sputum and an elevated serum IgE level. Annual renal function tests should be done to check for abnormalities such as hypochloremia, hyponatremia, and an elevated creatinine. A serum glucose test should also be performed, because the glucose may be elevated if the adolescent patient also has diabetes mellitus.

Liver function tests are also performed yearly. Liver enzymes may be elevated if the adolescent is developing cirrhosis, although the degree of elevation does not correlate with the degree of liver disease. The prothrombin time is an indirect measurement of the vitamin K status. Adolescents who have cystic fibrosis may have vitamin K deficiency because of chronic antibiotic use or decreased vitamin K absorption.

Treatment

Antibiotics, chest physiotherapy with postural drainage, bronchodilators, and pancreatic enzyme supplements are the primary components of treatment. Lung infection therapy is discussed first, followed by nutrition.

Most adolescents take daily oral antibiotics to suppress lung infection. Pulmonary exacerbations are characterized by increased respiratory distress, increased sputum production, anorexia, and decreased exercise tolerance. The adolescent patient may also have a low-grade fever, a decline in pulmonary function and changes on chest radiography. Oral ciprofloxacin is used if the adolescent is healthy enough for ambulatory therapy and has completed his or her growth. Ciprofloxacin is a fluorinated quinolone that has antipseudomonal activity. Research shows that even though there is no significant or sustained bacteriologic response, antibiotics suppress *Pseudomonas* exoenzyme production, which may contribute to the progressive lung injury.

Aerosolized aminoglycosides are often combined with oral ciprofloxacin for treatment of exacerbations. They are also used for long-term therapy. A multicenter clinical study is evaluating the efficacy of large doses of aerosolized tobramycin.

For more serious exacerbations, intravenous antibiotics are indicated. Adolescents are usually treated with an aminoglycoside and a semisynthetic penicillin or ceftazidime. Adolescent patients are typically admitted to the hospital, but recent controlled studies have shown that home intravenous therapy is as effective, as well as less stressful and less expensive, if the adolescent and family are compliant. Home therapy is also advantageous because of possible nosocomial transmission of multiply resistant bacteria and *Pseudomonas cepacia* in the hospital. *P. cepacia* is a bacterium found in approximately 1% of CF patients. Adolescents colonized with this type of *Pseudomonas* are hospitalized more frequently than patients who are not colonized with this organism. Patients with severe pulmonary disease who then develop *P. cepacia* infection generally have a more rapid decline in their health status than do other CF patients.

Chest physiotherapy and postural drainage are used to clear mucus from the smaller airways on a routine basis and especially during pulmonary exacerbations. Coughing is effective only in larger airway mucus clearance. Use of β-adrenergic agents may accelerate mucociliary clearance, and they are also used for CF patients who experience bronchospasm. Theophylline is also used in some patients with bronchospasm.

A high-calorie, high-protein diet is suggested for adolescents who have CF; fats are not restricted. Adolescents are especially susceptible to poor dietary habits (see Chapter 7). Weight loss should be evaluated and discussed with the adolescent, the family, and the dietitian. Weight loss is due most often to worsening disease. If this is observed, nutritional supplementation is important. For example, eggs, vegetable oil, Instant Breakfast, or evaporated milk may be added to milkshakes to increase their caloric content. Fortified milk is made by adding 1 cup of powdered milk to 1 quart of whole milk.

The socioeconomic status of the family should be considered when making nutritional recommendations. Many insurance companies will not pay for vitamins and nutritional supplements such as Polycose or Ensure. Use of supplemental enteral feeds, however, may be required if the adolescent continues to have significant weight loss or fails to gain weight appropriately. Supplementation may be given orally if the adolescent can consume enough volume during the daytime. If the patient does not gain weight, nighttime feedings are given using nasogastric or gastrostomy tubes. Nighttime feedings do not affect the adolescent's daily activities. The nasogastric tube can be placed each evening or the gastrostomy tube can be hidden under clothing. A gastrostomy "button" can also be placed after the gastrostomy site heals. It lies flat against the abdomen and is well tolerated.

Most CF patients require pancreatic enzyme supplementation to prevent malabsorption and failure to thrive. The enzyme dose is based on the specific symptoms of each patient. Patients take the enzymes at the beginning of and sometimes during their meals and also before snacks. CF patients also have problems absorbing fat-soluble vitamins. They are therefore encouraged to take one or two multivitamin pills per day. Daily supplements of 5000 to 20,000 IU of vitamin A, 800 IU of vitamin D, and 200 IU of water-miscible vitamin E are also suggested. Many patients also require vitamin K supplementation.

Adolescents may be resistant to any or all of these therapeutic modalities for many reasons. Use of a nasal cannula for oxygen delivery and gastrostomy tubes are especially problematic. First is the concern for their appearance. This is a significant problem, especially when the patient may already be self-conscious of finger clubbing, hyperinflation of the chest, and chronic cough. Second, the adolescent may have a fear that these therapies signify that the disease is in the terminal stages. The adolescent must understand that the nighttime feedings, for example, are for growth and potentially will decrease the progression of the disease. Third, the adolescent may be engaging in a struggle for control and the development of autonomy. The patient, therefore, wants to make the decisions about his or her treatment and health.

Psychological Aspects

There is no other time in life when it is so important "not to be different" than during adolescence, especially middle adolescence. The adolescent who has CF is different from his or her peers; these differences create major problems for the adolescent. The physicians, nurses, staff, and family must be sensitive to the adolescent's perception of feeling different from peers.

As a result of delayed physical and sexual maturity, the adolescent may look immature and childlike. Adolescents who have CF generally begin puberty about 2 years later than their agemates (see Chapters 56 and 57). The delayed onset of puberty and menarche most often is the result of slower growth (weight gain) resulting from suboptimal nutrition and repeated lung infections. The patient is often very thin and may appear malnourished, with a protuberant abdomen, barrel-shaped chest, and clubbing of the fingers. The adolescent may be ridiculed because of the unpleasant odor of the stools and thus, may avoid using the bathrooms at school. The adolescent with CF is often embarrassed by the loud coughing and the frequent need to expectorate while in class.

Concern about fertility and reproductive issues may place stress on CF patients. Information about fertility and genetics should be given to adolescents and young adults even if previously discussed in childhood. Women who have cystic fibrosis may be fertile (as many as 20%), so contraception should be discussed with sexually active young people. Unlike men, women with CF do not have anatomic reproductive organ abnormalities. However, there is a marked alteration of the cervical mucus, resulting in a thick, tenacious mucus of low volume. The water and electrolyte content of the cervical mucus is low, resulting in absence of "ferning" at midcycle (absent sodium crystallization) and cervical "plugging," which cause a decreased probability of sperm migration. Nevertheless, contraceptive counseling is essential, since, in addition to the usual reasons for contraception, pregnancy in the patient with CF has special risks to the mother and the fetus.

The choice of contraceptive method for the adolescent or young adult with CF must be made based on the individual needs, feelings, and preferences and the physical status of the individual (see Chapter 73). The risk of pregnancy in the CF patient must be balanced against the risk of a particular contraceptive method for that individual. Cystic fibrosis is *not* an absolute contraindication to the use of barrier methods of contraception or to the use of the combined oral contraceptive pill. Modern low-dose pills may be used in select patients with CF, although it is known that gonadal hormones do affect pulmonary secretions and function, pulmonary vasculature and pressure, glucose metabolism, and liver and biliary dysfunction. Clinical evidence of hepatic cirrhosis is a contraindication for the use of oral contraceptives.

The increased risks of pregnancy in the patient with cystic fibrosis demands appropriate counseling. Patients who are pregnant can experience pulmonary deterioration because of elevation of the diaphragm (secondary to the gravid uterus), hypervolemia, increased oxygen requirement, increased nutritional needs, and interference with chest physiotherapy. A female who has CF must understand the risks of having a child and the possibility that she may not survive the baby's formative years.

A male adolescent who has CF should be informed that 95% to 100% of males are infertile; but he should not assume that he is infertile. A semen analysis should be done at approximately 16 to 18 years of age for this reason. The male who has CF is capable of normal sexual functioning. Males with CF, however, lack or have atrophy or obstruction of the vas deferens, epididymis, and seminal vesicles, with subsequent azoospermia. The volume of ejaculate is markedly diminished, and its electrolyte, water, and protein content is abnormal. Other genitourinary abnormalities are increased; the coexistence of absence of the vas deferens and inguinal hernia should alert a physician to a possible diagnosis of cystic fibrosis.

All adolescents, including CF patients, should understand the risks of acquiring sexually transmitted diseases, including hepatitis B and AIDS (see Chapters 65, 75, and 76). The use of condoms should be explained to adolescents with CF because of these concerns.

There are many psychosocial pressures for young people who have cystic fibrosis, including school pressure, college plans, peer pressure, performance expectations, and family issues. Information about the effects of alcohol, cigarettes, marijuana, and other drugs on the adolescent and his or her illness must also be provided. Alcohol ingestion may suppress the cough reflex and has been associated with hemoptysis and gastrointestinal bleeding. The pulmonary toxicities of cigarette and marijuana use should be discussed with the adolescent (see Chapter 44). Adolescents who have cystic fibrosis are also susceptible to the relative effects of passive cigarette smoke (see Chapter 44). The injection of intravenous drugs and their inert ingredients, such as talc, can cause lung injury. The snorting of cocaine or smoking of "crack" cocaine can have direct toxic effects on the nasal mucosa and the lung (see Chapter 111).

Career goals may have to be modified to accommodate the reality of the limitations resulting from the disease. The adolescent may become angry, depressed, or even suicidal when confronted with the potential need to remain physically, socially, and economically dependent on parents rather than being increasingly independent (see Chapter 121). A team approach to the care of adolescents who have cystic fibrosis is imperative to management because of the often complex medical and psychosocial issues.

LUNG DISEASE IN THE IMMUNOCOMPROMISED HOST

Pulmonologists frequently care for immunocompromised adolescents. Lung diseases develop in hosts who lack adequate immunologic defense mechanisms (see Chapter 92). Adolescents may be immunocompromised for a variety of reasons, including malignancy (see Chapter 53), organ transplant, high-dose steroid use, and acquired immunodeficiency syndrome (AIDS) (see Chapter 76). Primary care physicians must be able to identify respiratory disorders when they develop, since many are life-threatening. Because of the wide variety of immunocompromised hosts, this section focuses on pulmonary complications of AIDS.

AIDS-related pulmonary disease is often difficult to diagnose and treat. Travel, pets, employment, and environmental exposures are important historical pieces of information to elicit from the patient. Even though lung disease may be difficult to diagnose, it is a common problem in the AIDS patient.

In a 1984 study of 1067 AIDS patients, 41% had pulmonary complications. Of these patients, 85% were infected with *Pneumocystis carinii*, 17% with cytomegalovirus, 17% with *Mycobacterium avium–intracellulare*, and 4% with *Legionella pneumophila*; 4% had *Mycobacterium* tuberculosis; and 2% had pyogenic bacterial infections. In every febrile AIDS patient, pulmonary infection should be considered. Tuberculosis exposure and previously positive tuberculosis skin tests are important historical points because dormant tuberculosis can become activated when adolescents become immunocompromised secondary to AIDS. Adolescent patients who have AIDS may also have pulmonary disease secondary to Kaposi sarcoma or non-Hodgkin lymphoma (see Chapters 53 and 76).

A thorough physical examination is essential for the diagnosis of lung disease in the immunocompromised adolescent host. For example, a scarlatiniform rash may indicate a streptococcal pneumonia (see Chapter 94); Kaposi papules and nodules would increase the likelihood of Kaposi sarcoma of the lung. Chest radiography, laboratory tests, and diagnostic procedures must be performed rapidly to facilitate the diagnosis and treatment. Sputum is obtained and examined for bacteria, acid-fast bacilli, and fungi. Bronchoscopy with bronchoalveolar lavage (BAL), brush biopsy, or transbronchial biopsy may be required for diagnosis. The etiology may still be elusive. If the condition of the adolescent warrants further investigation, an open lung biopsy may be necessary.

Pneumocystis Pneumonia

Pneumocystis carinii is the most common infectious cause of pneumonia in patients who have AIDS. It occurs in 60% to 70% of the patients and may be an initial manifestation of AIDS (see Chapter 76). *P. carinii* is an extracellular pathogen that has been classified as a protozoan parasite. Recent molecular biology studies suggest that *P. carinii* more closely resembles fungal than bacterial pathogens.

Signs and symptoms of *Pneumocystis* pneumonia are nonspecific and include fever, cough, tachypnea, dyspnea, and hypoxemia. Chest radiographic findings may be normal, even though the adolescent is hypoxic, or they may show bilateral diffuse interstitial or alveolar infiltrates (Fig. 43–8). Total lung opacification often coincides with increasing hypoxemia. More than 90% of patients who have *P. carinii* pneumonia have a decreased arterial oxygen level and an increase in the alveolar-arterial gradient.

The sensitivity for detecting *Pneumocystis* in the sputum can be as high as 90% with the immunofluorescent antibody test and appropriate techniques for collection and handling. Several staining techniques may be performed on BAL fluid or transbronchial biopsies to localize the organisms. The Gomori methenamine–silver nitrate and the toluidine blue O stain are examples. On lung biopsy, foamy exudates are found.

Either trimethoprim-sulfamethoxazole or intravenous pentamidine is used to treat *P. carinii* pneumonia. Trimethoprim-sulfamethoxazole may be given orally or intravenously. Upon diagnosis of AIDS, prophylaxis for *P. carinii* pneumonia should be given. Oral trimethoprim-sulfamethoxazole or aerosolized pentamidine is used for prophylaxis. A high percentage of patients develop side effects from trimethoprim-sulfamethoxazole, which include maculopapular rash, bone marrow toxicity, and fever. Often, patients who have AIDS are also on antiretroviral agents that potentiate the toxic effects on the bone marrow. Pentamidine is the alternative treatment if trimethoprim-sulfamethoxazole side effects occur. Dapsone and pyrimethamine-sulfadoxine are also options.

Mycobacterium tuberculosis and Nontuberculous Mycobacterial Infections

A number of patients who have AIDS develop *Mycobacterium tuberculosis* infection because of defective cell-mediated immunity. Since granulomatous formation does not occur in AIDS patients, the symptoms of *M. tuberculosis* infection are often atypical. Dissemination of the infection occurs more readily than in a nonimmunocompromised host. Also, any adolescent who is diagnosed with tuberculosis should also be suspected of having AIDS, since tuberculosis may be the first manifestation of AIDS.

Extrapulmonary tuberculosis may be present in adolescents with AIDS without lung involvement. When the respiratory system is involved, infiltrates may appear in any portion of the lung. Mediastinal or hilar lymphadenopathy is often seen on chest radiographs. Patients may have night sweats, fever, weight loss, cough, and dyspnea.

Sputum smears from immunocompromised hosts with tuberculosis are less likely to be positive for acid-fast bacilli than those from nonimmunocompromised hosts. Therefore, bronchoscopy with bronchoalveolar lavage or transbronchial biopsy may be required for the diagnosis of *M. tuberculosis* infection. Rifampin-containing regimens are usually effective treatments if the tuberculosis is diagnosed early in the course of human immunodeficiency virus (HIV) infection.

Infection resulting from a nontuberculous mycobacterium is not as easily treated. Patients who have AIDS usually are infected with this type of microorganism late

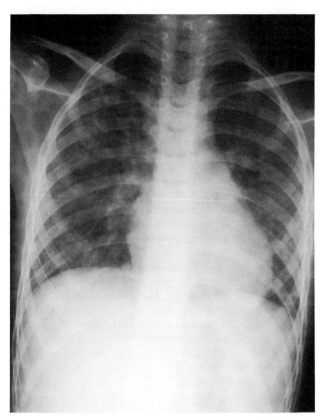

Figure 43–8. A chest radiograph of an adolescent with AIDS who has *Pneumocystis carinii* pneumonia. Note the bilateral interstitial inflitrates.

in the course of the syndrome. *Mycobacterium avium–intracellulare* complex, *Mycobacterium fortuitum*, and *Mycobacterium chelonei* are typical nontuberculous mycobacterial organisms found in AIDS patients. Dissemination of the infection may also be seen.

Chest radiography may reveal adenopathy and infiltrates. Sputum cultures and bronchoscopy with bronchoalveolar lavage are techniques used to make the diagnosis of a nontuberculous mycobacterial infection.

The nontuberculous mycobacteria are well known for their resistance to even multiple-drug therapy. There is no currently effective treatment for these patients.

Other Infectious Causes

Other infectious causes of lung disease are present in AIDS and include cytomegalovirus, Epstein-Barr virus, varicella, *Aspergillus*, *Nocardia*, *Cryptococcus*, and *Candida albicans*. Cytomegalovirus pneumonia, for example, is the second most frequently occurring pneumonia in pediatric AIDS. More common bacterial infections may also be diagnosed in AIDS patients; especially frequent are infections caused by *Streptococcus pneumoniae* or *Haemophilus influenzae*. There is an increased incidence of pneumococcal pneumonia in AIDS patients, owing to B-cell defects secondary to inadequately functioning helper T cells (see Chapter 94). These infections may be fatal even with appropriate antimicrobial therapy.

Lymphocytic Interstitial Pneumonia

Lymphocytic interstitial pneumonia (LIP) may occur in both adolescents and adults but is more common in children. The etiology is unknown, but it may result from an immunologic response of the lung to the human immunodeficiency virus (HIV). Studies have found HIV reverse transcriptase activity in the bronchoalveolar lavage fluid of patients with LIP. Another theory is that Epstein-Barr virus replication occurs in the lung, causing lymphocytic interstitial pneumonia. Epstein-Barr virus genes have been found in lung tissue obtained from a patient with LIP.

Patients have progressive dyspnea and cough. The physical examination may be normal, or crackles may be present upon lung auscultation. Clubbing of the fingers may also be present. Chest radiography reveals interstitial, nodular, or alveolar infiltrates. Bilateral reticulonodular or micronodular infiltrates are seen and are usually more prominent in the lower lobes. In patients with LIP, chest roentgenogram findings are often similar to those in *Pneumocystis* pneumonia.

Laboratory tests are not specific in the diagnosis of LIP, although a peripheral lymphocytosis can occur. This is an unusual finding in most AIDS patients. Arterial hypoxemia is common in LIP patients.

To make a definitive diagnosis of LIP, an open lung biopsy is required. Alveolar septa infiltration with lymphocytes, plasma cells with Russell bodies, and immunoblasts are evident histologically. The specimen also shows nodular aggregates of lymphoid cells with germinal centers.

LIP treatment consists of prednisone and possibly immunoglobulin therapy. Prednisone, 2 mg/kg/day for 2 to 4 weeks, is usually effective. The dose is tapered to 0.5 mg/kg every other day. Steroids are suggested only for those patients who have significant symptoms, such as hypoxemia. Adults with LIP may be at a higher risk for the development of bacterial pneumonia.

Kaposi Sarcoma of the Lung
(see Chapter 76)

Kaposi sarcoma is the most common malignancy complicating HIV infections and occurs most frequently in homosexual or bisexual AIDS patients (see Chapter 32). It is infrequently diagnosed in children and adolescents. The frequency of pulmonary involvement is unknown because often there are no symptoms. Kaposi sarcoma of the lung can affect the parenchyma, the airways, and the pleura. If symptomatic, patients are dyspneic and have a nonproductive cough, hemoptysis, and chest pain. Chest radiography may show parenchymal abnormalities, pleural effusions, or mediastinal and hilar adenopathy. Chemotherapy is the treatment of choice and includes vinblastine, bleomycin, and etoposide. Radiation therapy has also been used. The prognosis for patients with Kaposi sarcoma of the lung is poor. The survival period is approximately 3 to 6 months, although there are reports of patients living several years.

Non-Hodgkin Lymphoma
(see Chapter 53)

Non-Hodgkin lymphoma is another neoplasm occurring in patients who have AIDS. The major cell type in non-Hodgkin lymphoma is the B cell, and the tumors are usually undifferentiated. Chest radiographs are abnormal in fewer than 20% of AIDS patients who have non-Hodgkin lymphoma. The most common chest radiographic findings are parenchymal densities or adenopathy in the hilar, paratracheal, or mediastinal regions. Pleural effusions may also be seen.

Dyspnea, cough, chest pain, fever, and weight loss are the typical symptoms. Diagnosis is difficult because the presenting symptoms are nonspecific, and infectious causes must be ruled out. If a pleural effusion is present, the fluid should be sent for cytology. An open lung biopsy is required to make a definitive diagnosis if there is no pleural effusion.

Chemotherapy for non-Hodgkin lymphoma may cause neutropenia, which enhances the immunologic defects. These patients, therefore, may have infections diseases not commonly seen in AIDS patients, such as invasive *Aspergillus* or gram-negative infections.

PULMONARY MANIFESTATIONS OF SYSTEMIC DISEASES

Connective Tissue Diseases
(see Chapters 50 and 90)

There are few studies of pulmonary manifestations of connective tissue diseases in adolescents. Pulmonary symptoms may be part of the initial connective tissue disease clinical presentation, or respiratory complaints may develop during the course of the illness. The pulmonary symptoms are usually nonspecific, so other organ involvement and specific laboratory tests must be employed to establish the diagnosis. A discussion of connective tissue diseases in general is found in Chapter 90.

SPECIFIC DISORDERS

Juvenile Rheumatoid Arthritis
(see Chapters 50 and 90)

Of all types of juvenile rheumatoid arthritis (JRA), systemic juvenile rheumatoid arthritis (Still disease) is the most common form with pulmonary involvement. Of patients who have Still disease, 4% to 8% also have lung disease. Sixty percent of these patients have pleuritis, pericarditis, or both. Pleural effusions may develop at any time during the disease without symptoms of lung involvement.

Patchy infiltrates, lymphoid bronchiolitis, and lymphoid interstitial pneumonitis are other examples of lung disease seen in JRA. Pleural thickening or small pleural effusions are often seen on chest radiography. Chest radiography may also exhibit interstitial reticular and

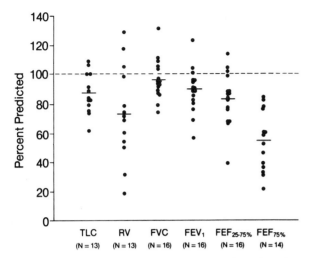

Figure 43–9. Total lung capacity (TLC), residual volume (RV), forced vital capacity (FVC), 1-second forced expiratory volume (FEV_1), maximum midexpiratory flow ($FEF_{25-75\%}$), and forced expiratory flow at 75% of exhaled vital capacity ($FEF_{75\%}$) in patients with JRA, reported as percentage of predicted values based on age, height, and sex. Bars designate the mean for patients with JRA. Individual patient data available from authors upon request. (From Wagener JS, Taussig LM, Debenedetti L, et al: Pulmonary function in juvenile rheumatoid arthritis. J Pediatr 99(1):108–110, 1981.)

nodular infiltrates, transient pneumonitis, and patchy pleural infiltrates. A large percentage of patients have radiographic signs of pneumofibrosis. Less frequent findings are rheumatic nodules and emphysema. Chest radiography should, therefore, be performed early in the diagnostic evaluation of JRA to detect potential lung involvement.

Pulmonary function testing has been studied in JRA patients. In one study, illustrated in Figure 43–9, 16 patients (between the ages of 6 and 18) were examined. Two thirds of the patients with polyarticular arthritis had abnormal pulmonary function tests. One half of the patients with pauciarticular disease had abnormal tests. Decreases in air flow, lung volume, and gas diffusion were found. There was also an abnormal matching of ventilation to perfusion in those patients who could exercise. Sternoclavicular joint and thoracolumbar spine disease may also contribute to the development of restrictive lung disease.

The most common pulmonary manifestations in adult rheumatoid arthritis patients are pleurisy (with or without effusion), necrobiotic nodules, Caplan syndrome (rheumatoid pneumoconiosis), diffuse interstitial disease, and pulmonary arteritis and hypertension. Vasculitis, in general, causes diffuse interstitial inflammation and later fibrosis. Chest radiography shows interstitial changes, especially in the lower lung fields. Microscopically, plasma cells, macrophages, and lymphocytes cause the interstitial destruction. It has been shown that males who have rheumatoid arthritis with interstitial lung disease have a higher prevalence of HLA-B8 and Dw3 antigens than do healthy control subjects. Patients with lung disease have higher serum levels of IgA and IgM. C4 levels are lower in patients with interstitial lung disease than in rheumatoid arthritis control groups. This last observation suggests complement activation.

In addition to the usual treatment regimen for JRA, immunosuppressive therapy is indicated. Physical therapy, especially in adolescents with neck, shoulder, and spine involvement, is also important in maintaining lung function.

Systemic Lupus Erythematosus
(see Chapters 50 and 90)

Pulmonary disease occurs in approximately 20% to 70% of adolescents and adults who have systemic lupus erythematosus (SLE). Pulmonary involvement is more frequent in patients who have the more severe forms of the disease.

In one report of childhood SLE, six of eight patients had pleural effusions at their initial presentation (Fig. 43–10). The effusions are usually bilateral and small, but they may enlarge. They are usually exudative; however, the protein content may not be high if the adolescent has hypoalbuminemia. LE cells, antinuclear antibodies, and elevated levels of DNA-binding antibodies may be found in the pleural fluids. Concomitant infections are common, so microbiologic studies of the pleural fluid are indicated before beginning corticosteroid treatment.

Lupus pneumonitis is a noninfectious disorder causing unilateral or bilateral infiltrates and pleural effusion.

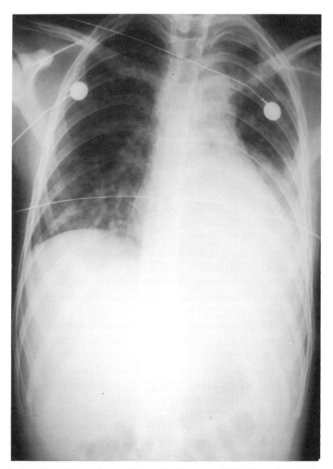

Figure 43–10. A patient with newly diagnosed SLE. Note the cardiomegaly secondary to a pericardial effusion and a left pleural effusion.

The adolescent patient is acutely ill with tachypnea, dyspnea, fever, basilar rales, chest pain, and hypoxia. A lung biopsy reveals vasculitis, interstitial pneumonitis, alveolar hemorrhage, arterial thrombi, and immune complex deposition. Corticosteroids and other immunosuppressive agents may be required.

Pulmonary edema appears on chest radiography in some SLE patients. Typically, fluffy alveolar infiltrates, often more prominent in the perihilar and lower lobes, are found. The specific cause is unknown but may be secondary to uremia, congestive heart failure, aspiration, or infection.

An unusual presentation of SLE is sudden pulmonary hemorrhage, which also can occur in patients known to have SLE. It has a high mortality rate (70% in one series). The pathogenesis is unclear but may be secondary to alveolar hemorrhage. Pulmonary infarction also occurs and may be associated with deep venous thromboses.

General therapy for SLE usually improves the lung findings, but as new pulmonary manifestations occur during the course of the illness, the cause must be identified, if possible. Fever, pleural effusion, and cough, for example, necessitate an evaluation for infection. Besides blood culture, thoracentesis, bronchoalveolar lavage, or lung biopsy may be required to help in the diagnosis, depending upon the patient's presentation. A combination of steroids and antibiotics may be appropriate when infection and SLE are both involved.

Polymyositis and Dermatomyositis
(see Chapter 90)

Polymyositis and dermatomyositis are inflammatory diseases of the skeletal muscle of unknown etiology. They are distinguished by skin involvement (dermatomyositis) or no skin involvement (polymyositis). Since many of the pulmonary problems are common to all categories, the general term, polymositis, will be used here. The presenting complaint in a majority of adolescent patients is weakness of the proximal muscle groups.

Interstitial lung disease may develop secondary to the underlying immunologic abnormalities. Various reports cite a 5% to 30% occurrence of interstitial lung disease. Bibasilar crackles are often heard on auscultation. The chest radiograph shows bilateral interstitial infiltrates, often most prominent in the lower lobes. Pulmonary function tests reveal varying degrees of decreased total lung capacity and diffusing capacities. Steroids and other immunosuppressive agents such as azathioprine, cyclophosphamide, and cyclosporine have been used to treat polymyositis, but there is no specific treatment for the pulmonary complications.

Ankylosing Spondylitis

Ankylosing spondylitis is a chronic inflammatory disease with predominantly large joint, spine, and lower extremity involvement. It is more common in males between the ages of 15 and 30 than in females. HLA-B27 is present in approximately 80% of these patients.

Pulmonary ventilation is typically well maintained in these patients, even though they usually develop progressive limitation of spinal mobility. The thorax is usually fixed at high lung volumes; diaphragmatic movement is not impaired. Over time, the patients may, however, develop chronic infiltrative and fibrotic changes in the upper lung fields.

Mixed Connective Tissue Disease

Mixed connective tissue disease (MCTD) is believed to be a separate connective tissue disease. It has components of other disorders such as systemic lupus erythematosus, juvenile rheumatoid arthritis, polymyositis, scleroderma, and Sjögren syndrome. Pulmonary symptoms occur in about 82% of adults and 40% of children. These symptoms include cough, dyspnea upon exertion, and shortness of breath. Diffuse interstitial lung disease, pleural effusions, and pulmonary hypertension are types of pulmonary disease seen in MCTD. Pulmonary function tests show a restrictive pattern, a decreased carbon monoxide diffusing capacity, hypoxemia, and respiratory alkalosis. These patients usually respond very well to corticosteroid therapy.

Other Granulomatous or Vasculitic Syndromes

Wegener Granulomatosis. This disease is characterized by necrotizing granulomatous vasculitis involving arteries and veins and may initially be confused with Henoch-Schönlein purpura. The disease most frequently affects the respiratory and renal organs (see Chapter 65). Wegener granulomatosis is diagnosed occasionally in adolescents but is more commonly diagnosed in adulthood, especially in the third and fourth decades of life. Ninety-four percent of patients have lung disease. Twenty percent have pleural effusions; approximately 18% have hemoptysis. Characteristic lung findings are multiple, bilateral nodal infiltrates that cavitate. Steroid therapy is usually not successful. Patients have undergone remissions with the use of cyclophosphamide.

Goodpasture Syndrome. This disease is usually seen in adolescent and young adult males. Goodpasture syndrome occurs rarely before age 10 years. It is characterized by pulmonary hemorrhage and glomerulonephritis due to anti–basement membrane antibody disease (see Chapter 65). Twenty to forty percent of patients have renal disease without lung disease; isolated pulmonary involvement is rare. Exertional dyspnea and hemoptysis are common. Microscopic hematuria, anemia, and azotemia may be present. The diagnosis is made by demonstrating the anti–basement membrane antibodies in the serum or in biopsy specimens of the kidney or lung. Pulmonary hemorrhage has a 20% mortality rate, and renal failure has a 75% mortality rate. Corticosteroid therapy, plasma exchange, and immunosuppressive agents may be beneficial.

Henoch-Schönlein Purpura. This is a diffuse necrotizing vasculitis of small vessels that usually develops 1 to 3 weeks after an upper respiratory tract infection. Adults and adolescents are less often affected than are younger children. Pleuritic pain and hemoptysis are the common symptoms in adolescents and adults. Cases of pulmonary hemorrhage associated with the vasculitis have been reported.

Neuromuscular Disorders

DUCHENNE MUSCULAR DYSTROPHY

Duchenne muscular dystrophy presents during childhood, and death often occurs by 20 years of age secondary to pulmonary insufficiency if respiratory support is not provided.

Pulmonary deterioration is a slow process. When the adolescent is ambulatory, pulmonary function is usually normal. The strength of the respiratory muscles, however, is already declining. When the adolescent can no longer walk, vital capacity is decreased and residual volume is increased. Expiratory flow rates also progressively decrease because of the muscle weakness. As an estimate, studies have shown that if the vital capacity is less than 40% of the predicted value, there is severe respiratory impairment. Over 80% of wheelchair-bound patients with muscular dystrophy have severely decreased pulmonary function.

Lung compliance is typically normal until advanced stages of the disease. Respiratory rate is higher and tidal volume lower in these patients than in control subjects. Blood gases and diffusing capacity are usually normal until late in the disease. Pneumonia, cor pulmonale, and atelectasis are complications that occur with deteriorating function. Aspiration results from pharyngeal muscle weakness and inability to handle secretions and food.

No treatment can halt the progression of muscle weakness. Yearly influenza vaccines and routine childhood immunizations are important to prevent pulmonary illnesses such as pertussis, and measles. Chest physiotherapy, inhaled bronchodilators, and intermittent positive-pressure breathing are frequently employed.

MYASTHENIA GRAVIS
(see Chapter 87)

The juvenile form of myasthenia gravis is usually diagnosed in females. Generalized progressive weakness of all muscles is the major problem; approximately one third of patients have respiratory difficulties. Loss of respiratory muscle strength occurs and may include the diaphragm. Vital and total lung capacities decrease, and residual volume increases. If the disease is chronic in nature, pulmonary compliance is decreased.

Acetylcholinesterase inhibitors are used for mild cases, and steroids are prescribed for more severe cases. Steroid therapy is associated with a decline in muscle strength during the early phases of treatment, so pulmonary function should be closely monitored. Cyclosporine, plasmapheresis, or thymectomy may be required for difficult cases.

ANTERIOR HORN CELL DISORDERS

Poliomyelitis results in damage to the anterior horn cells. Patients with bulbar disease typically present with a nasal-sounding voice because the muscles of the soft palate are afflicted. As the bulbar disease progresses, respiratory failure secondary to diaphragmatic and accessory muscle paralyses may develop. Encephalitis may also be seen in bulbar disease, and there is a possibility of seizures, which may also lead to compromised ventilation. Vigilant observation and preparation for potential respiratory compromise are paramount.

GUILLAIN-BARRÉ SYNDROME
(see Chapter 87)

Guillain-Barré syndrome is a demyelinating disease of the peripheral nervous system. It is acute in nature and often is preceded by a recent illness such as mononucleosis. Patients usually have progressive weakness of the extremities, but the disease can ascend to motor neuron levels affecting the respiratory system. Patients may have bulbar and cranial nerve involvement. Respiratory failure may occur secondary to involvement of the diaphragm and accessory muscles of breathing. Adolescents presenting with Guillain-Barré syndrome must be closely monitored with bedside pulmonary function testing; vital capacity measurements lower than twice the predicted tidal volume should alert the physician to intubate the patient and provide mechanical ventilation. The patient should also be intubated if he or she is having difficulty swallowing, since aspiration of secretions is a potential complication. Adolescent patients usually recover from this dramatic syndrome, but reports suggest that plasmapheresis may be beneficial for serious cases.

DRUG–INDUCED PULMONARY DISEASE

Many drugs are known to have adverse effects on the lung. This section discusses some of the more common problems found in adolescent patients. Lung disease secondary to drug toxicity takes many different forms. Several mechanisms are suspected. Pulmonary fibrosis, for example, may develop when disruption occurs between collagenosis and collagenolysis. A type of direct drug toxicity may occur when excessive reactive oxygen metabolites are produced. The exact mechanisms are often unknown or poorly understood.

Anticancer Drugs (see Chapter 53)

Adolescents who have cancer may be treated with drugs toxic to the lungs. Examples are listed in Table 43–9. Bleomycin is highlighted here.

Approximately 4% of all patients receiving bleomycin develop pulmonary disease. Dry cough and exertional dyspnea are symptoms of pulmonary toxicity. On physical examination, bibasilar crackles are heard. The earliest radiographic finding is fine bibasilar infiltrates. Progressive disease results in alveolar interstitial infiltrates. Interstitial pneumonitis, fibrosis, and extensive alveolar damage are usually seen on biopsy findings.

Adolescents receiving bleomycin should be monitored

TABLE 43–9. Anticancer Drugs

Alkylating Agents	*Antimetabolites*
Busulfan	Azathioprine
Chlorambucil	Cytosine arabinoside
Cyclophosphamide	Methotrexate
Melphalan	6-Mercaptopurine
Antibiotics	*Nitrosoureas*
Bleomycin	Carmustine
Mitomycin	

with serial carbon monoxide diffusing capacities. Even asymptomatic patients may have an abnormal diffusing capacity; if the value falls to less than 40% of the pretreatment value, bleomycin therapy is withheld. After a total dose of 400 to 500 units of bleomycin, there is a low incidence of autopsy-proven lung disease. The incidence of fatal toxicity is 1% to 2%. Steroids have been used to treat the disease, but their use is controversial.

Examples of Hypersensitivity Reactions

Hypersensitivity reactions are another common form of drug-induced complications, often caused by hapten-mediated immune response. Bleomycin, nitrofurantoin, sulfasalazine, diphenylhydantoin, carbamazepine, penicillamine, and gold are examples of drugs that can cause a hypersensitivity lung reaction. Bronchoconstriction, mucus hypersecretion, edema, and eosinophilic infiltration occur. Clinically, adolescents present with cough, dyspnea, and fever. The reaction becomes apparent within hours to days after beginning therapy. There is focal patchy consolidation in the periphery of the lung on chest radiography. The first step in treatment is to withdraw the inciting medication. The next step is to treat the symptoms with corticosteroids and β-adrenergic agents.

Drug-Induced SLE

Drugs associated with an autoimmune clinical syndrome similar to systemic lupus erythematosus include hydralazine, sulfonamides, and procainamide. The disease is usually reversible once the drug is withdrawn.

Contraception-Induced Pulmonary Disorders (see Chapter 73)

Pulmonary thromboembolism may occur in adolescents taking estrogens or oral contraceptives, although the incidence at all ages is very low. The use of low-dose pills probably lowers the risk of thrombophlebitis. Pleuritic chest pain, hemoptysis, dyspnea, apprehension, and even respiratory failure are potential presenting symptoms. A chest radiograph may reveal an elevated hemidiaphragm, atelectasis, pleural effusion, hemoptysis, or a decreased vascular pattern on the affected side.

A ventilation-perfusion scan typically reveals that ventilation is normal. The perfusion scan result is abnormal in at least a multiple segmental distribution. These scans are often difficult to interpret, however. The first treatment priorities are basic resuscitative measures and heparinization. Thrombolytic agents are used in massive pulmonary emboli or if shock is present.

Pulmonary Edema
(see Chapters 97 and 111)

Pulmonary edema can occur as the result of various drugs, including heroin and other opiates, cocaine, hydrochlorothiazide, cyclophosphamide, amitriptyline, and terbutaline. Heroin is highlighted here.

Decreased respirations, miosis, stupor, and pulmonary edema constitute a syndrome resulting from the intravenous or intranasal use of heroin. Chest radiography reveals alveolar or interstitial infiltrates. Treatment consists of using the narcotic antagonist naloxone (Narcan) 0.4 to 2 mg intravenously every 2 to 3 minutes (may be repeated two to three times), and supporting ventilation, if required. The pulmonary edema clears within 24 hours, but a restrictive defect with a decreased diffusing capacity may be present. The abnormal diffusing capacity may take 10 to 12 weeks to reverse. If infiltrates persist, a superinfection should be considered.

Heroin also may be diluted with talc, resulting in a foreign body granulomatosis. Chest radiography may be normal or may show diffuse interstitial shadowing to upper zone mass densities. Interstitial fibrosis and pulmonary hypertension may develop.

Marijuana and Narcotics
(see Chapter 111)

Marijuana can cause bronchitis, sinusitis, or rhinopharyngitis. If the marijuana contains a fungus, a chronic granulomatous infection of the lung or allergic bronchopulmonary aspergillosis may develop. Marijuana sprayed with paraquat (a defoliant) causes adult respiratory distress syndrome or pulmonary interstitial fibrosis.

Adolescents who have overdosed on narcotics have slow, quiet breathing, nonreactive constricted pupils, flaccid musculature, cool skin, and bradycardia (see Chapter 97). Cardiopulmonary support and naloxone administration are the primary therapeutic measures.

Vasculitic Complications and Stevens-Johnson Syndrome

Drug-induced polyarteritis nodosa and vasculitic syndromes secondary to sulfonamides are examples of pulmonary vascular abnormalities caused by drugs. In the worst form, sulfonamides are associated with Stevens-Johnson syndrome. Anticonvulsants, penicillin, and barbiturates are other drugs associated with this severe disease.

Bullous erythema multiforme and mucosal lesions are

the hallmarks of Stevens-Johnson syndrome, but one third of the patients have pulmonary involvement. These adolescents have a harsh, hacking cough, and on chest radiography patchy changes are seen. During the acute phase, mortality may be as high as 10%, especially if the respiratory system is involved. Treatment is limited to removing the offending drug and providing supportive care. If the disease progresses, prednisone is often given in the dose of 1 to 2 mg/kg/day. Fluid requirements are high, and hygiene of the skin is important, as in the treatment of burns.

Mediastinal Lymphadenopathy

Mediastinal lymphadenopathy may be seen in adolescents taking phenytoin or methotrexate.

OBSTRUCTIVE SLEEP APNEA
(see Chapter 86)

Adolescents may have a variety of sleep-related problems, including snoring, nightmares, enuresis, and apnea. Obstructive sleep apnea (OSA) is defined as frequent and severe pharyngeal airway obstruction during sleep. Arousals occur during sleep, following the apneic episodes. Adolescents who have OSA snore, are restless during sleep, and frequently are "mouth-breathers."

Etiology and Pathogenesis

OSA occurs when the upper airway collapses during inspiration. During sleep, there is a decrease in the airway-maintaining muscular activity, especially in the rapid eye movement (REM) cycle. Narcotics, sedatives, alcohol, and adenotonsillar hypertrophy contribute to the problem. Morbid obesity is the primary contributing factor for many adolescents who have OSA (see Chapters 49 and 60).

Diagnosis

Enuresis, poor school performance, hyperactivity, morning irritability, and daytime somnolence are symptoms of OSA. Adolescents who have OSA often sit up to sleep. Obese adolescents may sleep on their side. The parents report that the adolescent has pauses in the breathing pattern and then gasps for air. Profuse sweating during sleep may be noted. Systemic hypertension may be present.

A complete blood count may indicate polycythemia, and an arterial blood gas may reveal hypercarbia. A lateral radiographic view of the head in a standard plane provides evaluation of the upper airway dimensions. Fluoroscopy of the upper airway during sleep often identifies the site of obstruction. Since cor pulmonale may occur, an electrocardiogram is indicated.

A polysomnogram is the definitive test for the diagnosis. This study allows quantification of the number of obstructive apneic episodes and indicates the duration and the timing of each episode.

Treatment

Adenotonsillectomy is a major therapy for adolescents who have OSA secondary to adenotonsillar hypertrophy, but it is not without risk. The postoperative course may be difficult, especially if the obstruction is severe. Pulmonary edema may result after removal of the adenoids and tonsils. An endotracheal tube or nasopharyngeal airway may be temporarily required after the surgery to protect the airway. Nasal continuous positive airway pressure (CPAP) is a newer modality that has been effective in adults.

Weight loss is an important intervention for morbidly obese patients, although weight gain frequently recurs after cessation of a strict weight-loss program. A weight-loss program combined with psychotherapy or behavior modification may be indicated (see Chapters 49 and 60).

BIBLIOGRAPHY

Lung Diseases

Barnes PF, Bloch AB, Davidson PT, et al: Tuberculosis in patients with immunodeficiency virus infection. N Engl J Med 324:1644, 1991.

Behrman RE, Vaughan VC (eds): Nelson Textbook of Pediatrics, 13th ed. Philadelphia, WB Saunders, 1987, pp 854–942.

Birkhead G, Attaway NJ, Strunk RC, et al: Investigations of a cluster of deaths of adolescents from asthma. J Allergy Clin Immunol 84:484, 1989.

Hahn DL, Dodge RW, Golubjatnikov R: Association of Chlamydia pneumoniae (strain TWAR) infection with wheezing, asthmatic bronchitis, and adult-onset asthma. JAMA 266:225, 1991.

Kendig EL, Chernick V (eds): Disorders of the Respiratory Tract in Children. Philadelphia, WB Saunders, 1983.

McWilliams B, Kelly HW, Murphy S: Management of acute severe asthma. Pediatr Ann 18:774, 1989.

Murray JF, Felton CP, Garay S, et al: Pulmonary complications of the acquired immunodeficiency syndrome: Report of a National Heart, Lung, and Blood Institute workshop. N Engl J Med 310:1682, 1984.

Murray JF, Mills J: Pulmonary infectious complications of human immunodeficiency virus infection, Part I. Am Rev Respir Dis 141:1356, 1990.

Murray JF, Mills J: Pulmonary infectious complications of human immunodeficiency virus infection, Part II. Am Rev Respir Dis 141:1582, 1990.

Neddenriep D, Schumacher M, Lemen R: Asthma in childhood. Curr Probl Pediatr 19(7):327, 1989.

Ng VL, Gartner I, Weymouth LA, et al: The use of mucolysed induced sputum for the identification of pulmonary pathogens associated with human immunodeficiency virus infection. Arch Pathol Lab Med 113:488, 1989.

Nicklas RA: Perspective on asthma mortality—1989. Ann Allergy 63(2):578, 1989.

Rudolph AM, Hoffman JIE (eds): Pediatrics, 18th ed. East Norwalk, CT, Appleton & Lange, 1987.

Scambler PJ: The cystic fibrosis gene. Arch Dis Child 64:1647, 1989.

Strunk RC: Asthma deaths in childhood: Identification of patients at risk and intervention. J Allergy Clin Immunol 80(3, 2):472, 1987.

Tager IB: Health effects of "passive smoking" in children. Chest 96(5):1161, 1989.

Taussig LM (ed): Cystic Fibrosis. New York, Thieme-Stratton, 1984.

White DA, Matthay RA: Noninfectious pulmonary complications of infection with the human immunodeficiency virus. Am Rev Respir Dis 140:1763, 1989.

Wyngaarden J, Smith L (eds): Cecil Textbook of Medicine; 18th ed. Philadelphia, WB Saunders, 1988.

Pulmonary Manifestations of Systemic Diseases

Baydur A, Gilgoff I, Prentice W, et al: Decline in respiratory function and experience with long-term assisted ventilation in advanced Duchenne's muscular dystrophy. Chest 97:884, 1990.

Behrman RE, Vaughan VC (ed): Nelson Textbook of Pediatrics, 13th ed. Philadelphia, WB Saunders, 1987.

Carroll JL, Taussig LM: Pulmonary disorders. In Stiehm RE (ed): Immunologic Disorders in Infants and Children, 3rd ed. Philadelphia, WB Saunders, 1989; pp 475–502.

Hunt CE, Brouillette RT: Disorders of breathing during sleep. In Chernick V (ed): Kendig's Disorders of the Respiratory Tract in Children, 5th ed. Philadelphia, WB Saunders, 1990; pp 1004–1012.

Mallory GB, Fiser DH, Jackson R: Sleep-associated breathing disorders in morbidly obese children and adolescents. J Pediatr 115:892, 1989.

Parish JM, Shepard JW: Cardiovascular effects of sleep disorders. Chest 97(5):1220, 1990.

Rosenfeld RM, Green RP: Tonsillectomy and adenoidectomy: Changing trends. Ann Otol Rhinol Laryngol 99:187, 1990.

Spagnolo SV, Medlinger A: Handbook of Pulmonary Emergencies. New York, Plenum Medical Book Company, 1986.

Stradling JR, Thomas G, Warley ARH, et al: Effect of adenotonsillectomy on nocturnal hypoxaemia, sleep disturbance, and symptoms in snoring children. Lancet 335:249, 1990.

Tazelaar HD, Viggiano RW, Pickersgill J, Colby TV: Interstitial lung disease in polymyositis and dermatomyositis. Am Rev Respir Dis 141:727, 1990.

Wagener JS, Taussig LM, Debenedetti L, et al: Pulmonary function in juvenile rheumatoid arthritis. J Pediatr 99(1):108, 1981.

Wyngaarden J, Smith L (ed): Cecil Textbook of Medicine; 18th ed. Philadelphia, WB Saunders Co, 1988.

CHAPTER 44

Environmental Conditions, Cigarette Smoking, and Occupational Conditions

MICHAEL D. LEBOWITZ

ENVIRONMENTAL CONDITIONS

There are various environmental influences, irritants, allergens, and infections that can interact with host factors in adolescents to produce different types of acute and chronic obstructive lung disease. Adolescents are considered one of the more sensitive age groups to the effects of these environmental contaminants. This increased susceptibility results from several factors, including the continuing maturation of the lung and respiratory muscles during pubescence (see Chapter 42). Males in particular still have increasing maximum inspiratory pressures during this period. Further, certain upper and lower respiratory conditions can produce greater susceptibility in the adolescent (see Chapter 43). Other host factors are also very important in the etiology of lung disease, including genetic factors (e.g., familial aggregation of allergy), immunologic factors (e.g., B cells, T cells), and biochemical factors (e.g., peptides, antioxidants). The different types of lung disease have their own characteristics in terms of impairment of pulmonary function.

Irritants come from various sources, both indoor and outdoor. Combustion products include nitrogen dioxide, particulate matter, sometimes sulfur dioxide, volatile organic compounds, and trace metals. Building and interior materials emit volatile organic compounds, particulate matter, asbestos, and synthetic fibers. Consumer products emit volatile organic compounds. Outdoor vehicular and photochemically produced irritants include nitrogen dioxide, ozone, volatile organic compounds, as well as others. Bacteria can produce endotoxins that are also irritants. Combustion also releases carbon monoxide and nitric oxide, both of which combine more readily with hemoglobin to change the oxygen dissociation curve. Accidental release of excessive amounts of carbon monoxide leads to hospitalization and a number of deaths each year from asphyxiation.

Several studies have shown a relationship between acute changes in adolescent lung function and asthmatic episodes and a variety of pollutants (particulate matter, nitrogen dioxide, sulfur dioxide, ozone), alone and in combination with meteorologic factors and aeroallergens (see Chapter 43). Acute respiratory changes in children

have been observed during accidents (e.g., chemical spills). In studies of such spills, adolescents were quite seriously affected in terms of both acute illness and sequelae.

A number of studies have shown the influence of air pollutants on respiratory tract illness. Occasionally, epidemics of acute respiratory illness occur in adolescents, a few of which have been associated with environmental factors, including air pollution. Some of these studies have also demonstrated that lung function decreases in adolescents during symptomatic phases of acute respiratory illness, and these decreases are greater during pollution episodes (and in areas of high pollution compared with areas of low pollution). The return to normal function after acute respiratory illness is slower in areas of high air pollution. These effects may lead to chronic changes in adolescent respiratory status, including disease and pulmonary function decrements.

In terms of chronic effects, differences in lung function of adolescents and children in relation to pollutant levels in different geographic areas have been demonstrated by many studies. As an example, one study demonstrated that both photooxidant pollutants and reducing-type pollutants (sulfur oxides and total suspended particulates) can have an effect on pulmonary function in black and white youngsters aged 9 to 13 years. Studies in children and adolescents with chronic lung disease have been performed, which also compared geographic areas. Although these studies did not include pulmonary function measurements, there is a strong correlation between chronic lung disease and impairment of pulmonary function. One study, comparing smelter and nonsmelter towns in Arizona, showed that children's lung function (by age) differs by residence: Children who are exposed to higher particulate matter levels in certain smelter towns have poorer lung function than do children in towns without smelters. Lung growth into adolescence also appears to be affected by the pollution levels (see Chapter 42).

Indoor air pollution, especially that from indoor combustion sources (such as cigarette smoke and cooking stoves that use natural gas) also appears to affect lung function in children. Recent studies have shown that adolescents and children who live in houses with gas stoves or environmental tobacco smoke have poorer lung function than do those who live in houses without these pollutants, controlling for outdoor air pollution levels; these differences appeared to be due to nitrogen oxides or particulates, or both. Other recent studies have also shown increased bronchial reactivity and, in some cases, asthma, in adolescents who live with such exposure (see Chapter 43). Studies continue to show these effects in relation to aeroallergens.

There are various sensitizing allergens that can produce allergic diseases and asthma and can affect lung function. These environmental aeroallergens include pollen, dander, mites, excreta and parts of insects and rodents, molds, amoebae, thermophilic *Bacillus* species, and other proteins. The house dust mite (and its excreta) probably produces more allergic respiratory disorders than does any other aeroallergen. There are a few chemicals in the environment, such as formaldehyde and possibly chromium, that act as allergens as well. There are various chemical sensitizing agents in occupational settings, affecting adolescents as they enter the work force. These types of allergenic exposures have been associated with the development of asthma and even bronchitis (through exaggerated responses to respiratory infections that they may produce), as well as allergic diseases. Viral infections may facilitate sensitization and allergic reactions. Thermophilic *Bacillus* species (and amoebae) are responsible for producing *Legionella pneumophila*, hypersensitivity pneumonitis (see Chapter 43), and humidity fever. *Legionella pneumophila* can even be produced by massive exposures outdoors. Most treatment of allergic disorders appears to focus on the underlying hypersensitivity state, though some disorders require more extensive therapy.

There appears to be a strong environmental effect on increasing asthma in certain situations, sometimes referred to as a "Westernization" influence. In fact, there has been an increase of asthma in individuals with similar genetic backgrounds who have undergone changes in their environment. Examples include Africans who move to urban areas or are introduced to Western fabric that can contain mites, as well as susceptible Kuwaitis in whom asthma developed after Prosopis trees were introduced into their country. These examples illustrate the numerous environmental changes that may also be associated with changing cultures, including increased stress, nutritional deprivation, new exposure to air or work contaminants, new infections, and drug therapies. The phenomena also are representative of the numerous triggers that can provoke asthma attacks. In addition to those previously mentioned, one must include other biologic allergens (e.g., *Bacillus subtilis* in detergents), smoking (active or passive), airborne grain and its contents, and food additives. Contributing factors need study.

Some pollutant classes—such as pesticides, small particles in dry climates, and odoriferous substances—appear to produce allergic responses which are actually irritant responses in the upper respiratory tract. Also, there is a belief by some (such as "clinical ecologists") that there is a state of multichemical sensitivity; this belief is unfounded. There may be states that are more properly referred to as chemical intolerance syndromes, sensory hypersensitivity (e.g., to odors, eye irritants,

skin irritants), mucous membrane states, and a nonspecific "sick building syndrome." These conditions are affected by factors such as atmospheric dryness (or excessive humidity), temperature (cold or hot), and ventilation and wind movement (e.g., draftiness or insufficiency of ventilation, air mixing, fresh air). These classes of problems are currently being studied and discussed.

In summary, it is quite apparent that various environmental influences affect the respiratory health of adolescents, including infectious agents; irritants such as air pollutants, temperature, and seasonal conditions; and allergens. These factors have been known to be important in the outside environment. Recently it has become evident that airborne contaminants are important in the inside environment as well. This is especially critical, since adolescents spend a good deal of time indoors, though they spend more time outdoors than do most other age groups. The ratio of indoor-to-outdoor concentrations is distinct for each pollutant and dependent on many other factors. Furthermore, the amount of exercise, and thus the amount of pollutant received, will vary under different circumstances. Since there is evidence of both acute and chronic effects resulting from exposure to sufficient concentrations of pollutant, and that some of these effects may become irreversible, further evaluation of these effects continues. Both protection of the individual and patient management require that attention be paid to these factors.

CIGARETTE SMOKING

A large amount of information is available on the respiratory effects of smoking cigarettes, but insufficient attention has been paid to adolescents *per se*. In part this is because of the knowledge that most effects of smoking, such as the effect on lung function, occur after some duration of smoking and often result from its cumulative effects. Nevertheless, the onset of most cigarette smoking frequently occurs during adolescence, bringing some respiratory effects with it. The reasons for smoking, and its habituation effects have been studied (see Chapter 38). Some similar effects result from other habituations, such as marijuana and cocaine smoking and alcohol consumption (see further on) and there are also effects from passive smoking on this age group. About 14% of high school teenagers are considered heavy smokers at present; another group of adolescents uses smokeless tobacco. Few of these teenagers are aware of the harm that results from tobacco or from marijuana use. Tobacco, marijuana, alcohol, and cocaine each affect the respiratory system (see Chapter 42), and it is known that tobacco and alcohol, and tobacco and marijuana, used together are synergistic. Smoking other substances, such as crack, would probably be synergistic with these drugs by the nature of the mechanisms involved in producing respiratory effects (see Chapter 43).

It has been assumed, and is now known, that teenagers who have prior respiratory conditions have a greater susceptibility to the effects of tobacco. These conditions include asthma, chronic bronchitis, other serious childhood respiratory conditions, and even atopy (see Chapter 43). Other host factors (some already mentioned) are also of great significance, though they are still being evaluated. It is also known that persons who start cigarette smoking, especially males, are often those with better lung function.

The onset of cigarette smoking almost immediately produces or increases respiratory symptoms in most adolescents. In individuals with few other exposures (e.g., those living in rural unpolluted areas), chronic symptoms are not frequently reported, certainly less than by those in other situations or areas. In almost all smokers, cough and phlegm are signs of the irritation caused by cigarette smoking; these symptoms become chronic with continuation. In individuals with bronchial hyperresponsiveness, sufficient doses of cigarette smoke produce constriction. Asthmatics and persistent wheezers also have increased symptoms. It is assumed that these effects are responsible for the higher rates of nonsmoking individuals and individuals who stop smoking in these groups. Smoking as few as five cigarettes a day for at least 1 year after starting can produce early effects on lung function. We have observed that net decrements in this adolescent–young adult group are about 37 ml in the forced expiratory volume (1 second). We have also seen that individuals who stop smoking cigarettes through their 20s have a type of rebound, so their lung function returns to the same level as nonsmokers. (Later cessation does not have this much beneficial effect.) Cigarette smoking in young asymptomatic individuals has been shown to relate significantly to bronchial hyperresponsiveness, which relates to asthma and bronchitis, as well as to poor lung function.

Marijuana smoking has a much greater effect per cigarette than does tobacco smoking. Presumably, this is mostly due to the depth of inhalation and the length of time the smoke is held in the lungs. A combination of the two types of smoking has synergistic effects at any given time and longitudinally. Although alcohol consumption can lead to chronic obstructive pulmonary disease (COPD) by itself, its effect along with tobacco smoking is quite strong, especially for chronic mucous hypersecretion symptoms and their exacerbations. In addition to decreasing ciliary activity and stimulating mucous secretion (thus also predisposing them to respiratory infections), alcohol produces immunologic changes. It is not known how early this occurs, though by dose it occurs in some heavy teenaged users.

Although there are stronger determinants of lung function in this age group (genetics, early onset of respiratory disease, other causes of an early onset of abnormalities), active smoking, especially if combined with preexisting asthma, other chronic symptoms, or serious acute respiratory illness histories, can produce a significant decrement in function by the end of adolescence. Further, there is a decreased probability of asthma remission and an increased probability of its relapse with smoking.

Passive smoking effects are dose-dependent. With sufficient doses, passive smokers have higher rates of acute respiratory illness and bronchial hyperresponsiveness, a higher incidence of asthma, and poorer lung function. The last entity is almost always significant when accompanied by active smoking and prior lung conditions. Respiratory effects from passive smoking of marijuana do not appear to occur generally. Passive crack smoking, especially large amounts in the very young, appears to produce central nervous system effects that are similar to those seen with active crack smoking. The regular use of cocaine has more of a cardiovascular than a respiratory effect.

OCCUPATIONAL CONDITIONS

There are some basic observations about effects of work exposures on the respiratory system in adolescents: Symptoms in the employed population are about the same as in the general population, and symptoms and disease in workers with occupational exposures increase with age in all individuals. It is also known that smoking and occupational exposures usually produce additive or synergistic effects. We have found that exposed males aged 18 to 44 years have significantly more COPD symptomatology and also that male workers without occupational exposure have about the same symptom and disease rates and lung function as do females (i.e., normal) after controlling for smoking. Although most individuals begin to work during adolescence, the effect of work has not been studied very much (due in part to the difficulties discussed later). A recent analysis conducted in workers aged 15 to 25 years with no ambient exposures showed that occupational dust exposures (not related to smoking) produce little significant symptomatology at that age, except a higher rate of dyspnea in females.

It is known that workers with preexisting conditions, such as asthma and allergy, are much less likely to stay in workplaces with occupational exposures for sufficiently long to be studied. This tendency generates what is called the "healthy workers effect," meaning that only those healthy enough to tolerate the work situation stay in it long enough to be recognized. One could also assume that there is a higher risk for individuals starting employment with lower lung function, unless, as with smoking, they are less likely to start employment when there are significant occupational exposures.

Certain sensitizers have been shown to have more effect on those with atopy, including colophony, the various isocyanates, acid anhydride, animal parts or excreta, and platinum salts. Asthma resulting from occupational exposure, such as that from isocyanates (e.g., toluene 2,4-diisocyanate), can lead to permanent asthma in many sensitized individuals. However, platinum salts are such potent sensitizers that they eventually produce occupational asthma even in nonatopic, nonsusceptible individuals; fortunately, this form of asthma disappears in many of those affected after sufficient time away from the salts. Of interest are the similar effects produced by nitrogen dioxide in grain and missile silos—for example, the increased reactivity seen with indoor pollution exposures. Biologic dusts (such as *Bacillus subtilis*) can lead to hypersensitivity reactions and allergic alveolitis. Similarly, one can develop pigeon breeders' lung, or other similar conditions, of which there are many. The time of onset varies.

Exposure to moldy hay, cotton fibers or endotoxins, and mineral and synthetic fibers is initially irritative to the bronchi and bronchioles; constrictive bronchiolitis and other sequelae may result. (Moldy hay, of course, can lead to farmer's lung in time.) Hypersensitivity pneumonitis and humidifier fever can occur rather quickly also. In general, the textile industry is considered a moderate contributor to chronic conditions (with a slight contribution to acute conditions).

Interstitial pneumonitis can be produced by metallic inhalants, high-tension oxygen, and physical agents (e.g., x-rays and other radiation), sometimes rather quickly. Chemical pneumonitis is not infrequent either, especially as a result of accidental inhalation or ingestion in the workplace. An example of one of these occupational exposures in adolescence relates to cadmium exposure: In one study, the percentage of functional impairment from cadmium in individuals younger than 24 years of age was 17%, or three times that in nonexposed controls. Heavy metals, construction, and agriculture and forestry industries are major contributors to acute conditions. Heavy metals are also moderate contributors to chronic conditions, but the construction and agriculture and forestry industries are considered only slight contributors. Petrochemical and transport industries are considered moderate contributors to acute conditions, but only slight or insignificant contributors, respectively, to chronic conditions, as with manufacturing. Smoke inhalation produces acute bronchitis and edema (and may be accompanied by thermal damage). Such damage, which may occur over a few days, may predispose the affected individual to more severe complications, thus requiring immediate therapy.

Other exposures can, of course, produce restrictive lung diseases (pneumoconiosis, silicosis, and so on) after fairly long periods of exposure. In a cohort study of uranium miners, excess deaths did not occur until after 5 years of employment; it is not even recommended that workers with less than 10 years of exposure be evaluated. However, massive pulmonary fibrosis can occur fairly quickly with very large exposures to silica (as in sandblasting). These are often complicated by tobacco smoking, which can produce an obstructive-restrictive disease, or an industrial bronchitis if the occupational exposure is insufficient to produce disease. Mines and quarries are major contributors to acute and chronic problems.

ACCIDENTS AND INJURIES

It is not known how many recreational and sports injuries are due to hyperventilation syndrome, which is an increase in alveolar ventilation in excess of that required to maintain normal arterial partial pressures of oxygen and carbon dioxide. This condition leads to hypocapnia and possibly respiratory alkalosis and is treated accordingly. The general causes of hyperventilation include psychogenic conditions (acute anxiety, though it can also result from more chronic psychosomatic disturbances), reactions to pain, increased metabolism resulting from exercise (and similarly from increased oxygen consumption), hypoxia itself or

metabolic acidosis, central nervous system lesions, and hormones and drugs.

The major result of injury to the chest or respiratory system occurs through the results of trauma *per se*, such as broken ribs producing pneumothoraces, flailed lung, shocked lung, and resulting adult respiratory distress syndrome. The other major accidental effects on the lungs are through aspiration of water, foreign bodies, or chemicals. Hydrocarbon abuse and substance abuse have become major causes of injury to the respiratory system. Anaphylactic responses to stings or food can also occur. These injuries do not differ much in the adolescent in comparison with the young adult.

Trauma can lead quickly to pneumothorax. If the pneumothorax is sufficient, only minutes separate the onset of complete apnea and ensuing ventricular fibrillation or asystole. If it is sufficiently small or slow, it can lead to atelectasis. Atelectasis may also result from (1) local pressure on parenchymal tissue (e.g., from diaphragmatic hernia), (2) increased intrapleural pressure (often related to exudate, blood, pus, or air in the pleural space), (3) rib fracture and penetration into the parenchyma, or (4) blunt trauma that results in shock lung with edema, leading fairly quickly to respiratory distress syndrome. Often trauma results in a restrictive lung disorder. Trauma can also lead to distention and rupture of the alveoli, which lead to localized emphysema; the emphysema can become generalized if there is lobar or massive atelectasis. Alcohol and other drugs and inhalation of smoke or toxic gases (and chemical pneumonitis) can also lead to edema and respiratory distress syndrome. Treatment of the results of trauma *per se*—pneumothorax, atelectasis, edema, pneumonia, and respiratory distress syndrome—is well defined.

Aspiration can be due to deglutination-regurgitation, debilitation, neural or psychological problems, and accidents. Foreign body aspiration has a fairly distinct clinical picture. Aspiration can lead to pneumonia and obstructive disease (especially emphysema). The results can be suffocation, edema, malformations (including fistulae), and even anaphylaxis. Depending on the foreign body, removal may be recommended. The treatment of the pneumonia is dependent on its severity. Treatment of other outcomes and manifestations (e.g., edema, malformations, anaphylaxis) is fairly typical. However, treatment of emphysematous sequelae and chemical pneumonitis is much more difficult. Some chemical abuse or accidental aspiration—for example, of kerosene or turpentine—can lead to death fairly quickly. Other accidental aspirations (e.g., oily nose drops, other oils and lipids, stearate powder or other powders) have effects related to the substance; pneumonias can be treated as such. (Ingestion of some of these chemicals can also lead to similar effects on the respiratory system through absorption and transport.)

BIBLIOGRAPHY

American Thoracic Society: Health Effects of Air Pollution. New York, American Lung Association, 1978.
Clark DW, MacMahon B: Preventive and Community Medicine, 2nd ed. Boston, Little, Brown, 1981.
Editor: Bronchial asthma and the environment. Lancet 2:786, 1986.

Karvonen M, Mikheev MI: Epidemiology of Occupational Health. Copenhagen, World Health Organization, 1986.

Kendig EL Jr: Pulmonary Disorders, 2nd ed, Vol I. Philadelphia, WB Saunders, 1972.

Lebowitz MD, Burrows B: Risk factor in induction of lung disease: An epidemiologic approach. In Stein TP, Weinbaum G (eds): Mechanisms of Lung Injury. Philadelphia, Stickley, 1986.

Lebowitz MD, Holberg CJ: Effects of parental smoking and other risk factors on the development of pulmonary function in children and adolescents: Analysis of two population studies. Am J Epidemiol 128:589, 1988.

National Research Council: Indoor Pollutants. Washington, DC, National Academy Press, 1981.

Newcomb MD, Maddahian E, Bentler PM: Risk factors for drug use among adolescents: Concurrent and longitudinal analysis. Am J Public Health 76:525, 1986.

Polgar G: Lung development and subsequent function in the adult. In Pulgar G (ed): Pulmonary Physiology, 2nd ed. Philadelphia, Lea & Febiger, 1990.

Surgeon General: The Health Consequences of Smoking: Chronic Obstructive Lung Disease. Washington, DC, US Government Printing Office, 1984.

Weill H, Turner-Warwick M: Occupational Lung Diseases. New York, Marcel Dekker, 1981.

SECTION XII

Cardiovascular Conditions

EDWARD B. CLARK

Those who care for adolescents with normal cardiovascular function, but particularly those who care for adolescents with cardiovascular defects and disease, must be attuned to the special needs of their patients. These chapters address issues of cardiac examination, strategies to identify adolescents at increased risk for sudden death, arrhythmias, late sequelae of congenital cardiovascular malformations, high blood pressure, coronary risk factors, and cardiac involvement from systemic disease as they relate to the cardiovascular health of youth and young adults. Other issues are apparent but so poorly defined that little is known beyond anecdotal data. The field of adolescent cardiology is expanding as we accumulate the knowledge necessary to provide optimal care.

Adolescence represents a major stage in the growth and development of the cardiovascular system from primary morphogenesis through senescence. The heart forms from a muscular tube and through a complex process of septation becomes the four-chambered heart. The next stage of development involves growth and establishment of the control mechanism for cardiovascular function. This phase is completed at about the sixth postnatal month with the maturation of the sympathetic limb of the autonomic nervous system. Other changes include the transition to a coronary circulation, biochemical adaptation for energy production, a switch in contractile proteins, and the transition from cellular hyperplasia to cellular hypertrophy as a response to increased workload.

Puberty, accompanied by rapid growth and sexual maturation, signals another round of dramatic but less well understood changes in the cardiovascular system. As the child becomes an adolescent, heart rate slows, stroke volume and cardiac output increase, and blood pressure rises to adult levels. These changes match the increase in body mass and metabolic demands of the body (see Chapters 5 and 7). With maturation, the adolescent also may begin to establish the cumulative factors that lead to adult-onset cardiovascular disease.

Coronary artery disease and other vascular diseases probably begin during childhood (see Chapters 49 and 67). The risk factors for premature vascular disease and its complications (myocardial infarction, stroke, and hypertension) include the average diet in the United States, which is high in saturated fat; pervasive cigarette smoking; and physical inactivity. Many risk factors that influence the development of coronary artery disease begin as habits and behaviors established during adolescence. These environmental factors are added to genetically determined blood pressure, blood lipids, and predisposition for diabetes mellitus.

Our knowledge about these risk factors is derived in part from primary studies of 40-year-old men. Thus, we do not know with certainty their relationship in adolescents to the development of coronary artery disease. Longitudinal studies in childhood are now in progress, but the results are still 10 to 20 years away.

One of the greatest challenges is to identify adolescents at high risk for coronary artery disease and modify their behavior. There is broad agreement on what is normal but little consensus as to the optimal ways of intervening in the pathogenesis of coronary artery disease without doing physical or psychological harm. There are few proven effective strategies for altering the risk factors for early coronary artery disease.

The cardiovascular system is a primary or secondary target for systemic diseases that affect adolescents (see Chapter 50). Rheumatic fever has recently had a resurgence in the United States, and it continues to be a major disease in developing countries. In developing countries, it is the leading cardiac cause of death in individuals younger than age 45 years and accounts for 25% to 45% of cardiovascular disease in all age groups. Over the last 6 decades, the occurrence of acute rheumatic fever and the development of its cardiac complications have declined markedly in the United States because of an improved scientific knowledge base and societal improvements.

The survivors of childhood cancer have been treated with drugs and radiation that probably have long-term effects on cardiopulmonary function (see Chapter 53). Other systemic diseases such as lupus erythematosus and rheumatoid arthritis affect the heart (see Chapter 90).

Myocardial disease leading to cardiomyopathies is recognized with increasing frequency and accounts for most cardiac transplantation in adolescents. The cardiomyopathy in many of these patients may be an expression of a fundamental abnormality of myocardial formation during embryonic and fetal development. In others, it is the end stage of a viral myocarditis.

For children with cardiovascular diseases, adolescence can be stressful. Most congenital cardiovascular defects are detected by the age of 10 years. Occasionally, however, some abnormalities like atrial septal defect or coarctation of the aorta are noted as the signs and symptoms increase with growth at puberty (see Chapter 47). The diagnosis of a previously unrecognized defect can be particularly disconcerting.

The long-term prognosis of congenital cardiovascular defects varies widely (see Chapters 46 and 47). Each patient is a pioneer, since we have not followed children from surgery at a few years of age through a normal life expectancy. For some, surgical repair returns them to a normal life and a risk level for cardiovascular disease comparable to that of the general population. For others, the future is less clear. Successful open heart surgery is now just beginning to result in sufficient numbers of adult patients to judge long-term prognosis. The late complications of cardiac arrhythmias, residual valvular insufficiency, myocardial dysfunction, and chronic pulmonary vascular damage are threats to long-term survival.

Some children have complicated defects not amenable to surgical repair.

Palliative surgical procedures like systemic shunts and pulmonary artery band have allowed many patients to survive to adolescence. These adolescents may develop late complications during their teenage and young adult years. For those who are cyanotic, persistent hypoxia may delay puberty, slow somatic growth, and produce disfiguring changes in the joints. Adolescents with structural defects may have complications related to increased valvular obstruction, decreased ventricular muscle function, and progressive pulmonary hypertension. Death from the long-term complications of severe congenital heart defects often occurs during adolescence.

The psychosocial effects of congenital cardiovascular defects, diagnostic procedures, and surgical techniques are rarely studied. Profound hypothermia cardiac arrest technique for repair in infants may produce prolonged neurologic dysfunction in the immediate postoperative period. Whereas severe brain injury may be identified during early childhood, subtle manifestations of central nervous system complications may only be recognized late. The best strategy is to carefully monitor these patients throughout their development in childhood and adolescence so as to identify problems early and address them before there is a cascade of consequences.

The initial diagnosis of a congenital cardiovascular defect can be particularly overwhelming. An adolescent may initially experience feelings of sadness, dread, anger, and loss of self. Cardiac catheterization and surgical repair violate the body and can produce a sense of humiliation. These effects can have long-term consequences by altering the adolescent's perception of self and adaptation to adult roles. These psychosocial effects include an influence on sexual identity and development, fear of death, and separation from family. In some, these psychosocial effects may set the stage for a crescendo leading to suicide and suicidal tendencies.

The quality of a young adult life may be adversely affected by the presence of a congenital cardiovascular malformation. The effect is directly related to the severity of the defect, the number of interventional procedures, and external malformations like a chest deformity or persistent cyanosis.

The influence of a congenital cardiovascular defect on an adolescent's intelligence and performance in school is unclear. Heart defects in association with multiple congenital malformations and chromosomal defects often have a central nervous system component. The presence of an isolated heart defect probably does not affect intelligence. However, the attendant complications of prolonged hypoxia and a cerebral vascular bed perfused by blood that has not been filtered through the lungs increase the opportunity for central nervous system injury. Although marked improvement in cardiopulmonary bypass techniques has occurred, there are still complications of embolization, inadequate cerebral perfusion, and biochemical disturbances that may lead to brain damage following cardiac surgery. The long-term sequelae of these events are only now being studied. Some cases of learning and language disorders, mental retardation, seizures, and cerebral palsy are probably related to postnatal events.

The circumstances of an adolescent's cardiovascular disorder can also have a profound effect on his or her family. Parents often experience feelings of despair. They fear the loss of their child, in whom they have a major investment. They are concerned about the consequences of the emotional suffering for their adolescent.

Parents worry about the adolescent's life adjustment, career choices, education, and potential for independence. These fears are often compounded by the parents' own uncertainty about their health, financial situation, retirement, and eventual death. They worry about who will be responsible for their adolescent after their death, particularly if the child has Down syndrome.

Another concern relates to the genetic risk for congenital cardiovascular malformations. Young adults often worry about transmitting the defect to their offspring. Although the overall risk is 3% to 5%, the risk is increased for left and right heart defects and is nearly two times greater for affected women than for affected men. This maternal effect is not well explained but may reflect the transmission of maternal DNA to all children.

Compounding the problem of the cardiovascular health of children is the unavailability of basic health care to nearly 25% of adolescents in the United States. For many, this lack of access is the result of poverty. For others, health insurance that covers dependents is not provided by the employer and is costly, even if the child is insurable. At least one in five children in this country live at or below the poverty level ($12,800 annual income for a family of four), and the number will increase to an estimated one in four by the year 2000. For many other children and young adults with repaired cardiac malformations, the issue is noninsurability. There are an estimated 700,000 adults with repaired cardiac malformations without health insurance, even though the employment records of the survivors of cardiac operations in childhood are excellent. In a recent study, fewer than 50% of adults with a cardiac malformation had seen a cardiologist during the past 10 years. This poignant observation emphasizes the lack of continuity of care of these patients as they mature.

Life insurance is somewhat more available, especially for adolescents who have had successful surgical repair of their defects. Many defects, including atrial septal defect, ventricular septal defect, and pulmonary valve stenosis, are insurable at standard rates; others are insurable at increments up to 50% greater than standard. The availability and rates for insurance coverage vary widely among companies and with the individual company experience.

Employability and career choices may be adversely affected by cardiovascular disability in an adolescent. Because of the increased costs of health insurance to employers, some companies are reluctant to employ patients with a history of heart surgery, a pacemaker, or other preexisting cardiovascular condition. Even the diagnosis of a benign finding such as mitral valve prolapse may alter an adolescent's employability. This is one reason to consider carefully the consequences of labeling mild or trivial abnormalities.

The young men and women with cardiovascular disease or risk factors for the early development of coronary artery disease are a challenge for their pediatricians, family doctors, internists, and cardiologists. The single group in the United States with the least access to health care is 18- to 35-year-olds. For many young women, the only access is through health care provided during pregnancy. For young men, access is often only for treatment of acute illness or injury. The challenge is further compounded by a health care system that does not have an established method for delivering care to them and by an insurance system that may abandon them.

BIBLIOGRAPHY

Allen HD, Taubert KA, Deckelbaum RJ, et al: Poverty and cardiac disease in children. Am J Dis Child 145:550, 1991.

Aram DM, Ekelman BL, Ben-Shachar G, Levinsohn MW: Intelligence and hypoxemia in children with congenital heart disease: Fact or artifact? J Am Coll Cardiol 6:889, 1985.

Boughman JA, Berg KA, Astemborski JA, et al: Familial risks of congenital heart disease assessed in a population-based epidemiologic study. Am J Med Genet 26:839, 1987.

Clark EB: Growth, morphogenesis and function: The dynamics of heart development. In Moller JH, Neal WA, (eds): Fetal, Neonatal and Infant Cardiac Disease. New York, Appleton & Lange, 1990, pp 1–22.

Donovan EF: Psychosocial consideration in congenital heart disease. In Adams FH, Emmanouilides GC, Riemenschneider T (eds): Moss's Heart Disease in Infants, Children, and Adolescents, 4th ed. Baltimore, Williams & Wilkins, 1989, pp 984–991.

Ferry PC: Neurologic sequelae of cardiac surgery in children. Am J Dis Child 141:309, 1987.

Finley JP, Putherbough C, Cook D, et al: Effect of congenital heart disease on the family. Pediatr Cardiol 1:9, 1979.

Hesz N, Clark EB: Cognitive development in transposition of the great vessels. Arch Dis Child 63:198, 1988.

Lentner C: Heart and Circulation; Geigy Scientific Tables. Basel, Ciba Geigy Limited, 1990.

Mahoney LT, Truesdell SC, Hamburgen M, Skorton DJ: Insurability, employability and psychosocial considerations. In Perloff JK, Child JS (eds): Congenital Heart Disease in Adults. Philadelphia, WB Saunders, 1991, pp 178–189.

Mendoza JC, Wilkerson SA, Reese AH: Follow-up of patients who underwent arterial switch repair for transposition of the great arteries. Am J Dis Child 145:40, 1991.

National Cholesterol Education Program: Report of the Expert Panel on Blood Cholesterol Levels in Children and Adolescents. Bethesda, MD, National Heart Lung and Blood Institute, National Institutes of Health, 1991.

Newburger JW, Silbert AR, Buckley LP, Fyler DC: Cognitive function and age at repair of transposition of the great arteries in children. N Engl J Med 310:1495, 1984.

Rubin JR, Ferencz C: Subsequent pregnancy in mothers of infants with congenital heart disease. Pediatrics 76:371, 1985.

Silbert AR, Newburger JW, Fyler DC: Marital stability and congenital heart disease. Pediatrics 69:747, 1982.

CHAPTER 45

Overview of Cardiovascular Evaluation

EDWARD B. CLARK

CARDIAC EXAMINATION*

The normal murmur that many adolescents have must be distinguished from a pathologic murmur indicating a structural heart defect. Yet, not all patients with heart disease have a murmur; cyanotic patients with pulmonary atresia and healthy-looking children with coarctation of the aorta may have no murmur. Thus, the cardiac examination includes what one sees and feels, in addition to auscultation. In addition to blood pressure measurement, the components of the cardiac examination include inspection, palpation, and auscultation.

INSPECTION

Much can be learned from careful observation. Asymmetry of the chest often reflects long-standing enlargement of the heart. Retraction of the suprasternal notch and grooving of the lower rib cage may be caused by vigorous pulling of the diaphragm.

PALPATION

Palpation adds to the examination. Thrills felt over the heart or neck vessels reflect high-velocity blood flow. The cardiac thrust or heave correlates with ventricular enlargement. A palpable pulmonary artery signifies pulmonary hypertension.

An arm and a leg pulse should be palpated simultaneously. A strong brachial and a weak femoral pulse suggest the diagnosis of coarctation of the aorta. A water-hammer pulse may be the clue to aortic insufficiency or another cardiac lesion associated with a wide pulse pressure. The plateau pulse of aortic stenosis can be easily recognized. An enlarged liver correlates with vascular engorgement.

*Adapted from Clark EB: Heart murmurs. In Hoekelman RA, Friedman SB, Nelson NM, Seidel HM (eds): Primary Pediatric Care, 2nd ed. St Louis, MO, Mosby Year Book, 1992, pp 955–956.

AUSCULTATION

The heart sounds relate to the hemodynamic events of the cardiac cycle. The first heart sound is generated by closure of the tricuspid and mitral valves. The second heart sound is produced by closure of the semilunar valves and is particularly important for diagnosis. The first component of the second heart sound (S_2A) is due to aortic valve closure, and the second component is due to pulmonary valve closure (S_2P). The intensity of S_2A and S_2P and their relationship to each other and to respiration provide information about the pressure at which the valves close and about blood flow across the valves. Other sounds such as systolic click of a bicuspid semilunar valve, an opening snap of the mitral valve, diastolic gallop, friction rub, and bruits over intercostal arteries or over an arteriovenous fistula help make an accurate cardiac diagnosis.

TYPES OF HEART MURMURS
(Fig. 45–1)

A heart murmur is caused by turbulent blood flow. The timing, intensity, and location of heart murmurs define the anatomic cause of turbulent blood flow. A thrill is palpable when the murmur is a grade 4 or more in intensity in the grading system of 1 to 6.

An ejection murmur reflects turbulence as blood flows through a narrowed orifice or normal semilunar valve in increased volume. Murmurs arising in the pulmonary outflow tract are best heard in the left second intercostal space. Those arising in the aortic outflow tract radiate to the right second intercostal space.

A pansystolic murmur denotes turbulent blood flow during the isovolemic phase of contraction. Ventricular septal defect (VSD), mitral insufficiency, and tricuspid insufficiency cause such a murmur. The location of maximal intensity distinguishes the murmur of a ventricular septal defect from that of mitral insufficiency. The VSD murmur is heard best along the left lower sternal

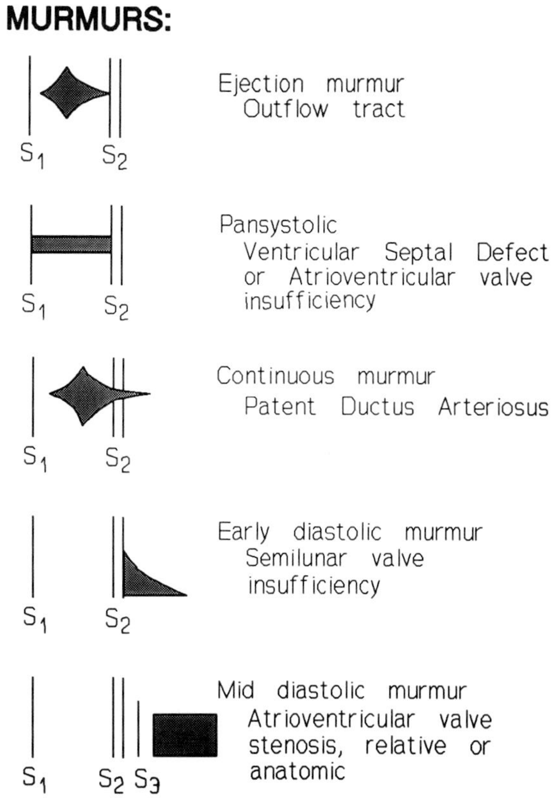

MURMURS:

Ejection murmur
Outflow tract

S_1 S_2

Pansystolic
Ventricular Septal Defect
or Atrioventricular valve
insufficiency

S_1 S_2

Continuous murmur
Patent Ductus Arteriosus

S_1 S_2

Early diastolic murmur
Semilunar valve
insufficiency

S_1 S_2

Mid diastolic murmur
Atrioventricular valve
stenosis, relative or
anatomic

S_1 S_2 S_3

Figure 45–1. Diagram of the five most common types of cardiac murmurs: ejection, pansystolic, continuous, early diastolic, and mid-diastolic. Shaded areas show the timing and intensity of the cardiac murmur in relation to the first (S_1) and second (S_2) heart sounds and third heart sound gallop. (See text for further description.)

border and radiates to the right. A mitral insufficiency murmur is heard best at the apex and radiates to the left axilla. The murmur of tricuspid insufficiency is maximal at the fourth left interspace and varies with respiration.

A continuous systolic and diastolic murmur arises from turbulent flow across a patent ductus arteriosus or another direct connection between high- and low-pressure systems, such as a pulmonary arteriovenous fistula.

An early diastolic murmur begins with the second heart sound and is due to insufficiency of the aortic or pulmonary valve. A high-pitched murmur indicates aortic insufficiency. A low-pitched soft murmur indicates pulmonary regurgitation.

A middiastolic murmur is due to excessive blood flow across the mitral or tricuspid valve. This murmur is heard with a large left-to-right shunt, such as an atrial septal defect, ventricular septal defect, or patent ductus arteriosus.

ASSOCIATED HEART SOUNDS

The second heart sound is particularly important in the diagnosis of congenital heart defects. Normally this sound is split, with the aortic preceding the pulmonary component. The two elements separate on inspiration and fuse on expiration. The louder the pulmonary component and the narrower the splitting, the greater the pulmonary artery pressure. Conversely, delay and diminution of the pulmonary component signify increasingly severe pulmonary stenosis. A wide and fixed split second heart sound occurs with mild pulmonary stenosis and with increased right heart ejection volume, as in the left-to-right shunt of an atrial septal defect.

An early systolic ejection click denotes a bicuspid aortic or pulmonary valve. Clicks can also be heard from a dilated aorta or pulmonary artery. A midsystolic click and a late systolic murmur at the apex characterize the mitral valve prolapse.

An intermittent third heart sound (S_3) at the apex is heard in many normal adolescents; however, a persistent fourth heart sound (S_4) often is pathologic. Persistent S_3 and S_4 gallops reflect blood flow into a stiff ventricle and are often associated with heart failure, myocarditis, or cardiomyopathy.

DIFFERENTIAL DIAGNOSIS: THE NORMAL HEART MURMUR

Most heart murmurs arise from turbulent blood flow in a normal heart. There are four common kinds of normal murmurs:

1. A Still murmur is a short, vibratory, grade 1 or 2 ejection murmur heard over the precordium and is the most common benign murmur. A Still murmur is noted in at least 50% of normal healthy children by the age of 3 or 4 years and may persist into adolescence.

2. A venous hum is a continuous murmur heard above the clavicle when the patient is in the upright position. The murmur disappears when the patient is supine or when the head is turned and the external jugular vein is compressed.

3. A pulmonary souffle is a soft, midsystolic murmur heard in the left second intercostal space (pulmonary area). This murmur is heard in high cardiac output states such as fever, anemia, or hyperthyroidism.

4. A benign peripheral pulmonary murmur is an ejection murmur heard in the left second intercostal space that radiates to both axillae. Most often heard in infants and small children, it represents turbulence of blood flow at the branch point of the main and the right and left pulmonary arteries.

MANAGEMENT

The only management needed in an adolescent with a normal heart murmur is complete reassurance. An adolescent with an organic murmur merits evaluation by a pediatric cardiologist.

BIBLIOGRAPHY

Leon DF, Shaver JA: Physiologic principles of heart sounds and murmurs. American Heart Association Monograph Number 46. New York, The American Heart Association, 1975.

Park MK: Pediatric Cardiology for Practitioners, 2nd ed. Chicago, Year Book Medical Publishers, 1988, pp 9–33.

STRATEGIES TO IDENTIFY LIFE-THREATENING CARDIOVASCULAR DISEASE

A few adolescents die suddenly during athletic contests or sports practice. When sudden death occurs, the primary mechanism is cardiovascular arrhythmia, aortic rupture, or stroke. Naturally, parents, school officials, and students are concerned about identifying those adolescents who are at increased risk for sudden death during vigorous physical activity. Yet, only a small fraction of all adolescents are at risk.

Nearly all teenagers have a physical examination for school attendance, sports participation, summer camp, or employment. Most adolescents have a heart murmur. Therefore, the challenge is to identify those with heart abnormalities that require treatment or those who should be restricted from strenuous sports. This goal must be accomplished without generating anxiety and apprehension, labeling the adolescent as having a disease, producing the perception of being different, or hindering participation in heart-healthy physical activity.

CAUSES OF SUDDEN CARDIOVASCULAR DEATH

The causes of sudden cardiovascular death are relatively few. Hypertrophic cardiomyopathy accounts for the largest proportion of sudden deaths. Presumably, vigorous exercise leads to myocardial ischemia and ventricular tachycardia or fibrillation. Hypertrophic cardiomyopathy can be transmitted as an autosomal dominant trait with variable penetrance and phenotypic expression. In addition, there may be a developmental progression to the disease such that myocardial hypertrophy may not be apparent in childhood or adolescence but may emerge in early adulthood. There is still discussion as to whether treatment by medications, β-blocker or calcium channel blocker, or surgery for obstructive hypertrophic cardiomyopathy improves the patient's prognosis (see Chapter 47).

Congenital coronary artery abnormalities include defects in the origin and course of the arteries supplying the ventricular myocardium. These relatively rare defects include an anomalous origin of the left coronary artery from the pulmonary artery, a single coronary artery, and a coronary artery coursing between the aorta and pulmonary artery. Symptoms are variable, ranging from profound congestive heart failure in infancy to otherwise unexplained sudden death.

Accelerated coronary atherosclerosis is nearly always related to very high cholesterol (>1000 mg/dl) and triglyceride (>2000 mg/dl) levels that occur with homozygous familial hypercholesterolemia (see Chapters 49 and 60). There is usually a strong family history of early heart attacks or angina at younger than 30 years of age.

Patients with Marfan syndrome have connective tissue abnormalities that may lead to aneurysms of the ascending aorta. A dilated aorta may dissect and rupture spontaneously, causing shock and death. Marfan syndrome either may be a spontaneous mutation (15% of cases) or may be inherited as an autosomal dominant trait (85% of cases). The physical features of extreme height, arachnodactyly, and dislocated lenses point to the defect.

Aortic valve stenosis is often progressive with time. A benign bicuspid aortic valve can calcify, resulting in progressive stenosis and increasingly severe obstruction of the left ventricle. The gradual hypertrophy of the left ventricle leads to subendocardial ischemia and the risk for arrhythmias and inadequate cardiac output during maximal exercise.

Hypertension can lead to encephalopathy and stroke. Most patients with hypertension are asymptomatic, but the effects on the target organs, eye, brain, heart, and kidney lead to progressive deterioration in function (see Chapters 48 and 67).

Arrhythmias can lead to sudden death. One widely recognized defect is long QT syndrome, which is characterized by a delay in the repolarization of the ventricular myocardium. This abnormality is recognized on the surface electrocardiogram as a prolonged QT_c interval greater than 0.44 second when corrected for heart rate. The mechanism is episodic ventricular tachycardia triggered by a premature beat. Many patients with long QT syndrome have syncopal episodes and have been treated for an atypical seizure disorder prior to discovery of their rhythm abnormality. Treatment with β-blockers and pacemaker is effective in reducing the risk of sudden death in many patients. Other diseases such as premature degeneration of the conduction system can produce symptoms of syncope for a considerable period of time before sudden death (see Chapter 46).

Each of these abnormalities can be detected by detailed evaluation. However, screening of all adolescents by a pediatric cardiologist is impractical because of cost and the low incidence of sudden unexpected death in otherwise healthy individuals. The cost of cardiac examination, electrocardiogram, chest x-ray film, and echocardiogram for 10,000 students is about $5 million per year. The personnel required are four pediatric cardiologists, four echocardiographers, and a nursing support team. Epstein and Maron estimated that 200,000 competitive athletes must be screened to identify 10 athletes with disease capable of causing sudden death, of whom one would die. The cost of universal screening is prohibitive to all schools and colleges.

Alternatively, a strategy based on a personal and family history and key physical findings allows for effective screening to identify adolescents at greatest risk. Referral can then be directed to the adolescent's physician for appropriate evaluation, or consultation with a pediatric cardiologist can be recommended.

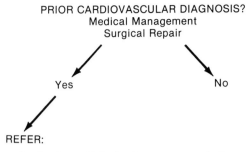

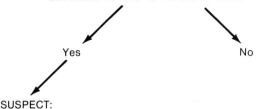

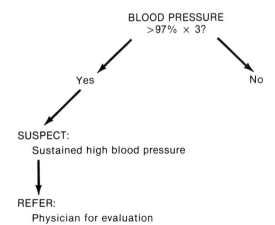

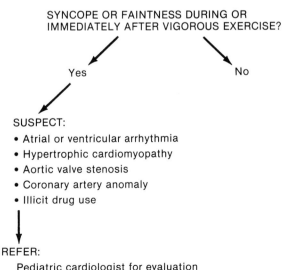

Figure 45–2. Algorithm for identification of adolescents at possible increased risk for sudden death: Previous medical or surgical care of cardiac defect. (See text for details.)

PERSONAL AND FAMILY HISTORY

Adolescents with a previous history of cardiovascular disease either repaired surgically or treated medically should be evaluated by a pediatric cardiologist prior to participation in competitive sports (Fig. 45–2). Many youth with repaired congenital or rheumatic heart defects are capable of full and active interscholastic competition. The vast majority of adolescents with a heart murmur are allowed to participate in sports, and a regular evaluation provides guidance and reassurance to the adolescent, family, and school officials.

Fainting is a common event among adolescents. The vast majority of adolescents faint because of vasovagal phenomena, while standing or in response to a stressful situation. Syncope during or shortly after sustained vigorous exercise is disconcerting and suggests the possibility of an arrhythmia arising spontaneously or may be related to underlying coronary artery anomaly, cardiomyopathy, or drug use (e.g., cocaine) (Fig. 45–3). The cardiac rhythm abnormality may be either an atrial or a ventricular tachyarrhythmia or a bradyarrhythmia, such as sinus node dysfunction with asystole or complete heart block. In each case, there is inadequate cardiac

output and the patient faints and then recovers regular cardiac action (see Chapter 46).

A family history of lethal cardiovascular disease is usually known (Fig. 45–4). Most unexpected deaths in the United States are investigated by a coroner or medical examiner. In the majority of cases, there was an autopsy to define the cause of death. Thus, most families know about family members with Marfan syndrome, hypertrophic cardiomyopathy, or accelerated coronary atherosclerosis, but they may not understand the genetics of an autosomal dominant trait. The history of sudden unexplained death between the ages of 15 and 45 should alert a physician to the possibility of other abnormalities such as arrhythmias caused by long QT syndrome.

PHYSICAL FINDINGS

Elevated blood pressure greater than the 97 percentile for gender, age, and body mass suggests an abnormality in blood pressure control (Fig. 45–5) either secondary

Figure 45–4. Algorithm for identification of adolescents at possible increased risk for sudden death: Family history of early cardiac death or unexplained sudden death. (See text for details.)

Figure 45–3. Algorithm for identification of adolescents at possible increased risk for sudden death: History of fainting. (See text for details.)

Figure 45–5. Algorithm for identification of adolescents at possible increased risk for sudden death: High blood pressure. (See text for details.)

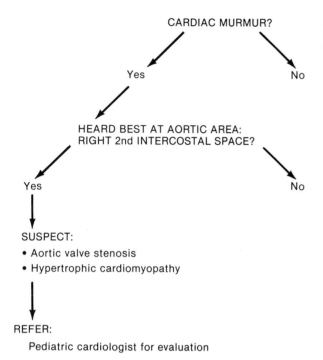

Figure 45–6. Algorithm for identification of adolescents at possible increased risk for sudden death: Cardiac murmur indicative of left ventricular outflow tract obstruction. (See text for details.)

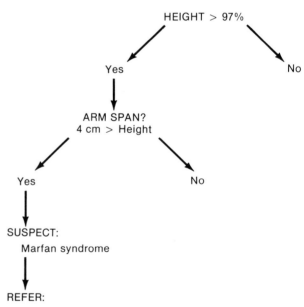

Figure 45–7. Algorithm for identification of adolescents at possible increased risk for sudden death: Phenotypic characteristics of Marfan syndrome. (See text for details.)

to renovascular disease or as an initial manifestation of primary or essential hypertension (see Chapters 48 and 67). However, blood pressure may be more difficult to measure in adolescents with large arms, when blood pressure cuffs do not cover two thirds of the upper arm. Therefore, the most common cause of a high blood pressure measurement is an improperly taken reading. Adolescents with elevated blood pressure should be encouraged to be physically active, as this is one mechanism of reducing blood pressure.

A heart murmur arising from obstruction of the left ventricular outflow tract, from either a hypertrophic cardiomyopathy or an aortic valve stenosis, radiates to the aortic area (Fig. 45–6). This clinical finding, which should alert the physician, includes a systolic ejection murmur heard best in the right second intercostal space. Likewise, height above the 97th percentile suggests Marfan syndrome (Fig. 45–7).

Considering these factors, a series of simple algorithms should allow the identification of at-risk individuals (see Figs. 45–2 to 45–7). There has been, however, no systematic testing of these precepts, and thus, neither the sensitivity and specificity nor the positive and negative predictive values have been defined.

The guiding precept must be to do what is best for the adolescent. It is essential to allow adolescents a full range of activities, sports participation, and maximum exertion without arbitrary restrictions. There is great risk of psychological harm in creating a cardiac cripple by inappropriate limitation of activity. Before denying any adolescent permission to participate in a sport or activity for cardiac reasons, an experienced pediatric cardiologist familiar with the problems of children and youth should be consulted.

BIBLIOGRAPHY

Committee on Pediatric Aspects of Physical Fitness, Recreation and Sports: Cardiac evaluation of participation in sports. Policy Statement of the American Academy of Pediatrics. Evanston, IL, 1977.

Epstein SE, Maron BJ: Sudden death and the competitive athlete: Perspectives on preparticipation screening studies. J Am Coll Cardiol 7:220, 1986.

Maron BJ, Epstein SE, Roberts WC: Causes of sudden death in competitive athletes. J Am Coll Cardiol 7:204, 1986.

McCaffrey FM, Braden DS, Strong WB: Sudden cardiac death in young athletes. Am J Dis Child 145:177, 1991.

Strong WB, Steed D: Cardiovascular evaluation of the young athlete. Pediatr Clin North Am 29:1325, 1982.

CHAPTER 46

Disturbances of Cardiac Conduction and Rhythm

D. WOODROW BENSON, JR.

EVALUATION

Symptom Complexes

The diagnosis of a disturbance of rhythm or conduction may be suggested by specific symptom complexes of chest pain, palpitations, syncope, cardiac arrest, or sudden cardiac death.

Chest pain is a common symptom among adolescents and young adults; it rarely has a cardiac cause. Most chest pain in adolescents is musculoskeletal in origin. Musculoskeletal pain is sharp, brief in duration, and well localized to a costochondral or interchondral junction and can be reproduced by careful palpation. A psychogenic cause, shortly following a stressful event (e.g., death of family member) may frequently be identified (see Chapter 112). Chest pain due to a rhythm or conduction disturbance is usually associated with palpitations.

Palpitations are a symptom complex defined as an unpleasant awareness of the heart beating. Palpitations have been ascribed to a variety of cardiac rhythm disturbances, which include extrasystoles, pauses, and tachycardia. The symptom depends upon the type of rhythm disturbance. For example, a paroxysmal, sustained (seconds to minutes) sensation of rapid heart beating is different from the "flip-flop" sensation of an extrasystole or pause.

Syncope is a transient neurologic disturbance resulting in loss of consciousness and muscle tone (see Chapter 85). *Fainting* is a synonym for syncope. In most cases, syncope results from transient reduced cardiac output leading to cerebral hypoperfusion. If hypoperfusion persists, syncope may be followed by reflex anoxic seizures. Such seizures involve symmetric, tonic-clonic movement and may be associated with incontinence and a postictal state. Syncope is an important diagnostic challenge because the differential diagnosis of syncope and sudden death overlap. Syncope with exertion may precede sudden cardiac death in adolescents.

Cardiac arrest is an episode of absent pulse and apnea with documented ventricular fibrillation or cardiovascular collapse requiring cardiopulmonary resuscitation. Sudden cardiac death is defined as death occurring shortly following these symptoms.

History and Physical Examination

Most adolescents with known or suspected disturbance of cardiac rhythm or conduction have an ostensibly normal heart. This is in sharp contrast with the older patient, in whom rhythm and conduction disturbances may be a manifestation of progressive coronary atherosclerosis or myocardial disease. Thus, adolescents experiencing disturbances of cardiac conduction and rhythm, even life-threatening ones, may have a noncontributory past medical history and physical examination.

An important clue, however, is a family history of rhythm disturbance such as long QT syndrome or unexplained sudden death. Young patients who have had cardiac surgery are particularly susceptible to late-onset cardiac rhythm disturbances (see Chapter 47). For example, bradycardia-tachycardia syndrome occurs commonly following Mustard procedure, and ventricular tachycardia has been noted following surgery for tetralogy of Fallot or double outlet right ventricle. Rarely, the initial sign of cardiomyopathy is a disturbance of cardiac rhythm. Familial neuromuscular disorders, including muscular dystrophy, Friedreich ataxia, and myotonic dystrophy, are associated with disorders of cardiac conduction and rhythm (see Chapters 87 and 88).

The initial evaluation of the adolescent with known or suspected rhythm disturbance should focus on the possibility of underlying heart disease. Even in the absence of obvious underlying heart disease, symptoms should be carefully evaluated for clues to the possible life-threatening nature of the conduction or rhythm disturbance.

Laboratory Techniques

Electrocardiographic studies are especially important in documenting spontaneous occurrences of rhythm disturbance and during provocative studies to evaluate conduction and induce rhythm disturbance.

ELECTROCARDIOGRAM

The electrocardiogram (ECG) remains a fundamental diagnostic tool in evaluating rhythm and conduction disorders. The ECG often establishes a differential diagnosis but may not permit a precise electrophysiologic diagnosis. For example, there are three distinct electrophysiologic mechanisms of supraventricular tachycardia (SVT) that may demonstrate identical ECG features; electrophysiologic studies are necessary to determine the specific type.

ECG recordings from symptomatic patients may be important even when obtained during symptom-free periods. For example, in a patient with a history of paroxysmal palpitations, ECG features of Wolff-Parkinson-White syndrome (WPW) permit inferences that symptoms are caused by orthodromic reciprocating tachycardia, a particular type of SVT.

Evaluation of the ECG should include attention to heart rate and rhythm (i.e., whether they are regular or irregular and the relationship of atrial to ventricular depolarization) even when the heart (ventricular) rate is normal. In addition, the ECG should be examined for the age and heart rate appropriateness of the PR interval, QRS duration, and QT interval (Table 46–1). When QRS duration is prolonged, the specific patterns of bundle branch block or ventricular preexcitation should be determined. The P-QRS relationship should be carefully examined to determine whether first, second, or third degree heart block is present.

LONG-TERM ECG MONITORING

Long-term ECG monitoring may be useful in documenting cardiac rhythm and conduction during symptoms. Long-term ECG monitors are of two basic types: event recorders with short-term memory, and continuous long-term (24-hour) recorders. The latter permit a qualitative analysis of cardiac rhythm during the continuous period of recording. Event recorders are most useful when applied during symptoms but also aid in the measurement of frequency of symptoms.

ELECTROPHYSIOLOGIC STUDIES

An intracardiac electrophysiologic study is a cardiac catheterization using specialized catheters that temporarily pace and record the activity of precise regions in the heart (e.g., atrium, ventricle, and His bundle). Temporary pacing is essential for evaluating conduction and refractory characteristics and testing for tachycardia initiation. The indications for electrophysiologic study in adolescents have not been generally agreed upon, but the ultimate goal of such a study is to permit a precise electrophysiologic diagnosis to be made so as to choose among available pharmacologic, pacemaker, and surgical options.

Electrophysiologic testing should be performed in adolescents with new onset second or third degree AV block to determine the site of the block and the performance of subsidiary pacemakers. All adolescents who have tachycardia with prolonged QRS should undergo electrophysiologic study to differentiate between SVT and life-threatening ventricular tachycardia. Electrophysiologic testing is indicated for adolescents with medically refractory tachycardia or life-threatening symptoms. Electrophysiologic testing may be useful in adolescents with asymptomatic sick sinus syndrome who require drugs that may further depress sinus node function.

A transesophageal electrophysiologic study, in which a catheter is passed down the esophagus to a point adjacent to the left atrium, can be used to evaluate the temporal relationship between atrial and ventricular depolarization and can be used for temporary pacing. The technique is ideally suited for serial evaluation of a patient during drug therapy, for establishing a differential diagnosis of rhythm and conduction disorders, and for testing antiarrhythmic drug efficacy by preventing pacing-induced initiation of tachycardia.

TILT TEST

The tilt test is useful in the evaluation of ostensibly normal adolescents who have recurrent syncope. The goal is to reproduce syncope or near-syncope and document associated heart rate and blood pressure changes. If symptoms are not reproduced, the test result is considered normal. The tilt test is a noninvasive test that may be performed on an ambulatory basis. The name describes the test; heart rate and blood pressure are monitored for 15 minutes in the supine position and during 90-degree upright tilt. If symptoms are not elicited during the baseline state, the tilt is repeated during isoproterenol infusion. As opposed to orthostatic changes, which occur immediately on assuming an upright position, symptoms during upright tilt occur more than 2 minutes after changing position. Among symptomatic patients, three types of response have been observed. The cardioinhibitory response is associated with a dramatic fall in heart rate (maximum RR interval > 6.0 seconds). The vasodepressor response is associated with a fall in blood pressure (mean ≤ 40 mmHg). The mixed response exhibits both heart rate slowing and blood pressure decrease.

SPECIFIC DISTURBANCES OF CARDIAC CONDUCTION AND RHYTHM

Extrasystoles and Escape Beats

Irregularities of cardiac rhythm are common in the adolescent. In addition to sinus arrhythmia, atrial and ventricular extrasystoles and escape beats following pauses are principal causes of an irregular rhythm.

Ventricular extrasystoles result from premature depolarization originating in the ventricle. The basis for concern about ventricular extrasystoles is their possible

TABLE 46–1. Normal ECG Values for Adolescents

Heart rate	60–120 bpm
PR interval	0.10–0.17 sec
QRS duration	<0.09 sec
QT interval	<0.40 sec
Corrected QT interval*	<0.44 sec

*Corrected QT interval = $\dfrac{QT}{\sqrt{RR}}$

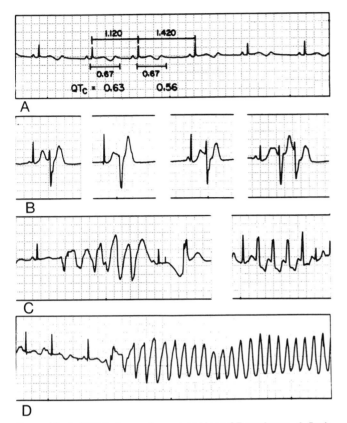

Figure 46–1. ECG features of congenital long QT syndrome. *A*, Both the uncorrected and corrected QT intervals are exceptionally long (>0.44 second). *B*, Multiform premature ventricular contractions (PVCs), couplets, and runs of ventricular tachycardia are present. *C* and *D*, Variation in QRS morphology during ventricular tachycardia is characteristic of torsades de pointes. (See page 348.)

arrest. One approach is ECG documentation that includes a minimum of 24 hours of ambulatory ECG monitoring (Holter monitor). This is critical for determining whether simple or complex ectopy is present. Benign simple ventricular extrasystoles occur commonly in adolescents without other evidence of heart disease. Complex ventricular ectopy is cause for more concern, especially when other manifestations of heart disease are present.

An asymptomatic adolescent with simple ventricular extrasystole and normal physical examination requires no treatment and no restrictions. In contrast, the patient with symptoms of syncope, complex ventricular ectopy, or reduced ventricular function should receive extensive evaluation by a cardiac electrophysiologist. More problematic situations are the asymptomatic patient who has complex ectopy and the symptomatic patient with simple ectopy. Such adolescents should undergo echocardiographic study to assess ventricular function. An electrophysiologic study is indicated for determination of the risk of life-threatening ventricular tachycardia. This is preferable to empirical prophylactic treatment with antiarrhythmic drugs, since there is risk with these therapeutic modalities.

Atrial and junctional extrasystoles are relatively uncommon in adolescents. Atrial extrasystoles are manifested on ECG by a premature atrial depolarization showing a different P wave morphology. Atrial extrasystole may fail to conduct to the ventricles (blocked) or may be conducted with a normal or aberrant QRS. Junctional extrasystole may be difficult to distinguish from atrial extrasystole. The differentiation depends on recognition of the P wave preceding the premature QRS. Treatment is rarely required for these benign rhythm disturbances. As may be true for ventricular extrasystoles, they may serve as an initiating event in patients susceptible to certain types of supraventricular tachycardia (Fig. 46–2).

Slowing and pauses of the sinus rate and escape by the sinus node, as in sinus arrhythmia, or subsidiary atrial or junctional pacemaker result in an irregular cardiac rhythm. These common rhythm disturbances are important to recognize because of their benign outcome; they do not require treatment. Rarely they initiate tachycardia in susceptible patients.

association with underlying heart disease and the risk of sudden death. This concern has developed from clinical experience with older patients who have ischemic heart disease. Clinically significant ischemic heart disease is rare in adolescents, and the precise cause of ventricular extrasystoles in adolescents is unknown.

The prematurity and prolongation of the QRS duration give ventricular extrasystoles a striking electrocardiographic appearance. When ventricular extrasystoles do not reset the sinus node, they are associated with a compensatory pause. This may be helpful in distinguishing them from atrial or junctional extrasystoles. However, in young patients, the compensatory pause is absent when ventricular extrasystoles result in retrograde conduction to the atrium and resetting of the sinus node.

Ventricular extrasystoles may be classified as simple or complex. Simple ventricular extrasystoles occur singly (preceded and followed by a sinus beat) and have a uniform QRS morphology and a fixed relationship (RR interval) to the preceding beat. Complex ventricular extrasystoles have more than one QRS morphology or occur in pairs, triplets, or runs of four or more complexes (Fig. 46–1).

The adolescent with ventricular ectopy should have careful evaluation, emphasizing physical examination and history of presence or absence of syncope or cardiac

Bradycardia

Heart rate varies greatly in adolescents. Therefore, it is difficult to establish a lower limit. A diagnosis of

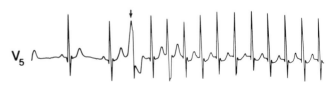

Figure 46–2. Paroxysmal onset of orthodromic reciprocating tachycardia with a ventricular extrasystole (*arrow*). The extrasystole presumably results in conduction to the atrium via the accessory connection and retrograde block in the normal conduction system. After retrograde atrial depolarization, the AV node is not refractory and tachycardia begins.

bradycardia depends upon the adolescent's physiologic state (e.g., temperature), sexual maturity, lifestyle (e.g., athlete versus "couch potato"), and age. The clinical interpretation of the heart rate is also influenced by the cardiac rhythm. For example, a resting heart rate of 50 beats per minute (bpm) in a sexually mature 13-year-old basketball player would not warrant further evaluation. However, a prepubertal, sedentary 13-year-old with the same heart rate should be evaluated for heart block, sick sinus syndrome, or abnormality of physiologic state.

HEART BLOCK

First degree AV block is a prolonged PR interval with 1:1 AV conduction. Second degree AV block is the failure of one or more atrial depolarizations to conduct. Mobitz I block, or Wenckebach conduction, has a periodic prolongation of the PR interval, followed by a shortening of the PR interval. Mobitz II block has abrupt block without PR prolongation. Mobitz I block usually occurs above the His bundle electrogram (HBE) recording site, whereas Mobitz II block occurs below the His recording site (Fig. 46–3). Complete, or third degree, AV block is the failure of atrial impulses to propagate to the ventricle.

First degree block is a relatively common and nonspecific finding. Second degree block is relatively uncommon. Complete heart block may be congenital or postsurgical or may be acquired from myocarditis.

The need for temporary versus permanent pacing is dependent on intrinsic rate, rhythm, site of block, and underlying disease. Most patients with congenital heart block are asymptomatic and do not require a permanent pacemaker unless they have fatigue with activity or syncope. Many patients with postsurgical heart block

recover conduction in the immediate postoperative period, therefore needing only temporary pacing. Those with persistent complete block may require a permanent pacemaker. Many patients with complete heart block and acute myocarditis recover normal conduction with resolution of the inflammatory process.

SINUS BRADYCARDIA

Sinus bradycardia can result from intrinsic abnormality of sinus node function or intraatrial conduction (i.e., sick sinus syndrome, also known as tachycardia-bradycardia syndrome) or from extrinsic influence such as autonomic nervous system tone. Isolated sinus bradycardia may occur in many settings, especially during sleep. In the absence of symptoms, it should be considered normal.

Tachycardia

The upper limit of a normal heart rate also varies. For example, a normal prepubertal 12-year-old may have a resting heart rate of 110 bpm. In contrast, a sexually mature 17-year-old with a resting heart rate of 100 bpm should be evaluated for tachycardia even if he or she is asymptomatic.

SUPRAVENTRICULAR TACHYCARDIA

A supraventricular tachycardia (SVT) involves the atrium, the AV node, or both in its mechanisms. SVT and paroxysmal atrial tachycardia are synonymous. There are three distinct mechanisms that produce a sustained or paroxysmal atrial tachycardia. The natural history and choice of treatment depend on the specific mechanism.

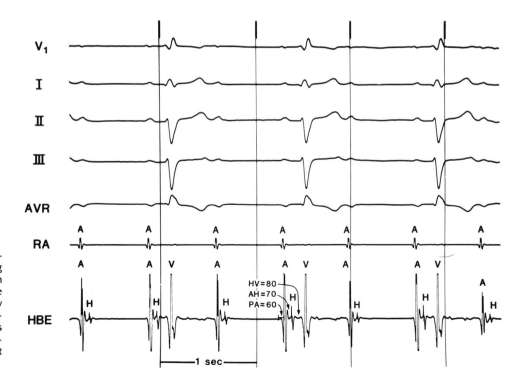

Figure 46–3. Cardiac electrophysiologic recordings during second degree AV block in an adolescent with Kearns-Sayre syndrome. Block occurs below the His bundle electrogram recording site. The HV interval is quite prolonged. The QRS morphology is characteristic of right bundle branch block.

Orthodromic Reciprocating Tachycardia

Orthodromic reciprocating tachycardia (ORT) (see Fig. 46–2) is common and accounts for nearly half the cases of SVT in adolescents. During ORT, antegrade conduction occurs via the normal AV node and His-Purkinje system; thus, the QRS duration and morphology are usually normal. An accessory AV connection serves as the retrograde limb of the reentrant circuit. If the accessory connection conducts in an antegrade direction during sinus rhythm, ventricular preexcitation occurs and is manifested by the presence of delta waves, short PR interval, and prolonged QRS duration (Wolff-Parkinson-White syndrome). When an accessory AV connection is present, but ventricular preexcitation is not present, the accessory connection is said to be concealed.

The pathophysiology of paroxysmal ORT involves two factors. First, the accessory AV connection that supports the tachycardia and permits ventricular preexcitation to occur is a subtle congenital cardiac defect. The second factor is the initiating, or triggering, event; the initiating event occurs as an extrasystole or pause and accounts for the paroxysmal nature of tachycardia (see Fig. 46–2).

Two important variations may occur. Uncommonly, the direction in the reentry circuit may reverse, and during antidromic reciprocating tachycardia (ART) the accessory connection serves as the antegrade limb of the tachycardia, with retrograde conduction occurring via the normal conduction system or a second accessory connection. During ART, the QRS duration is prolonged, as maximal ventricular preexcitation occurs. A second special case is the permanent form of junctional reciprocating tachycardia (PJRT), which is believed to be a variation of ORT, in which tachycardia with a normal QRS morphology occurs incessantly.

Tachycardia due to Reentry Within the AV Node

This is a form of tachycardia believed to arise within the AV node. The tachycardia mechanism results in a regular tachycardia with a normal QRS. On the surface ECG, P waves cannot be distinguished because they are inscribed simultaneously with the QRS. Tachycardia due to reentry within the AV node occurs commonly in older children, adolescents, and adults. This raises the possibility that the capability of the AV node to support reentry is acquired.

During tachycardia it is believed that antegrade conduction occurs in functionally differentiated fibers with slow conduction and a short refractory period and that retrograde conduction occurs in fibers with rapid conduction and a long refractory period.

Primary Atrial Tachycardia

Primary atrial tachycardias arise exclusively within the atria. They may be due to an automatic ectopic focus, but more commonly they are due to reentry. Atrial flutter and atrial fibrillation are examples of the more commonly occurring primary atrial tachycardias. Symptoms are due to the ventricular rate and often a loss of synchronized AV contraction. Primary atrial tachycardias are regularly observed in patients with cardiomyopathy and following surgery for congenital heart disease. Electrocardiographic features may not permit distinction from other SVTs.

The treatment of SVT and the clinical course are dictated by the SVT mechanism and the presence of underlying heart disease. This is the only way of taking advantage of available pacemaker, surgical, or medical options. For all practical purposes, SVT in an adolescent may be a lifelong problem.

Adolescents with frequent episodes of SVT that interfere with their lifestyle should be referred to a pediatric cardiologist who has experience in evaluation and treatment. Although many patients are given drugs to control their episodes, the choice and dose must reflect an understanding of the mechanism of the SVT. The antiarrhythmic drugs have major side effects.

The strategy of medical therapy is aimed at suppression of initiating events (e.g., with quinidine), impairing AV node function (e.g., with digoxin, propranolol, or verapamil), and impairing function of accessory connection (e.g., with quinidine or procainamide). Medically refractory patients should be considered for pacemaker or surgical therapy following thorough electrophysiologic evaluation.

VENTRICULAR TACHYCARDIA

Ventricular tachycardia (VT) is in the differential diagnosis of every patient with a prolonged QRS (> 0.10 second) tachycardia (Fig. 46–4). Ventricular tachycardia arises exclusively within the ventricles, and neither the atrium nor the AV node is required for tachycardia. The link between VT and ventricular extrasystoles has not been well established in the adolescent. One of the goals of evaluation is to discover whether there is a link.

Patients with VT are not a homogeneous group. There is considerable diversity with regard to electrophysiologic mechanism and presence or absence of underlying heart disease. Important distinctions depend on heart rate, QRS morphology (monomorphic versus polymorphic), and duration of episodes (nonsustained versus sustained). In the VT patient, symptoms seem related primarily to the heart rate, the duration of tachycardia, and the presence or absence of underlying heart disease.

All forms of VT require careful and thorough evaluation with cardiac electrophysiologic study and myocardial or skeletal muscle biopsy. An initial goal in evaluation of the adolescent with VT is defining the underlying disease, especially cardiomyopathy and previous history of heart disease. Many aspects of the natural history of VT in adolescents are not known, often because the cause and natural history of the underlying heart disease are not known.

Bundle Branch Block

Ventricular depolarization initiated via the normal conduction system and resulting in an altered QRS configuration is termed aberrancy. The initial step in

Figure 46–4. The standard ECG of regular tachycardia with prolonged QRS. The differential diagnosis would include ventricular tachycardia, supraventricular tachycardia with functional (rate-related) bundle branch block, and antidromic reciprocating tachycardia.

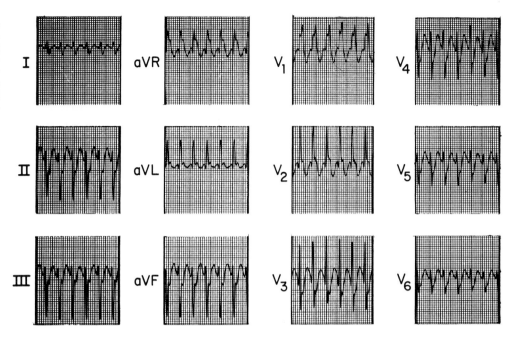

recognizing aberrancy is to observe that the QRS duration is prolonged.

Right bundle branch block (RBBB) results from delay in right ventricular depolarization. This results in sequential (left then right) rather than nearly simultaneous ventricular depolarization. In the adolescent, the electrocardiographic pattern for RBBB includes a prolonged QRS duration (exceeding 100 ms), a dominant R wave in lead V_1, and a dominant S wave in lead V_6. A distinction should be made between RBBB and severe right ventricular hypertrophy. RBBB is commonly observed following surgery for congenital heart disease. Horowitz and colleagues demonstrated that RBBB following cardiac surgery was the result of conduction block at the proximal, distal, or terminal right bundle branch. RBBB is frequently observed in patients with Ebstein anomaly of the tricuspid valve. In contrast, it may be only transiently observed during tachycardia.

The term "incomplete" RBBB describes all ECGs with RSR' morphology and normal QRS duration, although the name implies a conduction system abnormality. However, this is probably a misnomer, since this ECG pattern is commonly observed in patients with atrial septal defect. The ECG becomes normal following surgical treatment, suggesting that the apparent conduction delay was due to dilation of the right ventricle.

Left bundle branch block (LBBB) results from delay in left ventricular depolarization. In adolescents, this conduction abnormality occurs as a functional disturbance at the onset of tachycardia. ECG evidence of LBBB is characterized by prolonged QRS duration, a dominant S wave in lead V_1, and a dominant R wave in lead V_6. LBBB may be associated with normal or left axis deviation. Bundle branch block rarely requires treatment, but in the face of syncope or other symptoms it may signal an underlying depression of the conduction system. The natural history is determined largely by the underlying cause. For example, RBBB following sur-

gical treatment of tetralogy of Fallot is believed to be a static condition.

Preexcitation Syndromes

Preexcitation syndromes result from subtle congenital cardiac malformations. Ventricular preexcitation occurs when the ventricle is depolarized directly from the atrium, bypassing the inherent delay of the AV node. Preexcitation syndromes are noteworthy for the ECG abnormalities produced during sinus rhythm and for their association with paroxysmal tachycardia.

Wolff-Parkinson-White syndrome is a common example. In this case, ventricular preexcitation is the result of fusion of ventricular depolarization through the normal conduction system and an accessory AV connection (previously called Kent bundle). Shortening of the PR interval results from early ventricular depolarization via the accessory connection and is inscribed on the ECG as the delta wave. The accessory connection usually participates in paroxysmal tachycardia (see section on orthodromic reciprocating tachycardia) by serving as the retrograde limb of a reentry circuit.

Preexcitation syndromes may produce life-threatening rhythm disturbance. This may occur when a patient with an accessory AV connection capable of rapid conduction to the ventricles develops atrial fibrillation. The rapid conduction from atrium to ventricle that results during atrial fibrillation leads to a life-threatening situation (Fig. 46–5).

The treatment of preexcitation syndromes is directed toward preventing symptomatic rhythm disturbances. The accessory connections that cause the preexcitation syndromes are congenital anomalies, but their precise cause is not known. Several studies have reported a loss in functional capacity of accessory connections with maturity.

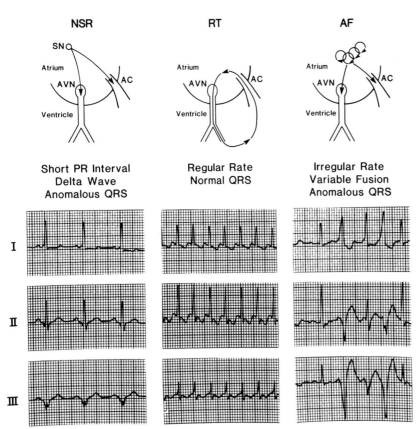

Figure 46–5. ECG features of Wolff-Parkinson-White syndrome. During normal sinus rhythm (NSR), the delta wave and prolongation of QRS duration are the result of fusion of ventricular depolarization via the normal conduction system and the accessory atrioventricular connection (AC). During orthodromic reciprocating tachycardia (ORT), the QRS duration is normal and the tachycardia rate is regular. In contrast, during atrial fibrillation (AF), the rate is irregular and there is variable fusion of ventricular depolarization.

Long QT Interval

The QT interval is an electrocardiographic interval related to age and heart rate (see Table 46–1). The QT interval may be prolonged on a congenital or acquired basis. The incidence of congenital long QT interval syndrome (LQTS) is very low; drug-induced or acquired LQTS is much more common. Syncope and sudden death are risks of a long QT interval. Thus, the goal in the management of the LQTS is prevention of sudden death. In LQTS, sudden death is thought to result from torsades de pointes, a form of ventricular tachycardia showing alternating electrical polarity such that the QRS complexes appear to be twisting around the isoelectric line of the ECG. Thus, prevention or termination of torsades de pointes is the goal of therapy.

ECG features of LQTS include bradycardia, ventricular ectopy, and torsades de pointes (see Fig. 46–1). In acquired cases of LQTS, the QT interval returns to normal upon discontinuance of the antiarrhythmic drug or correction of the electrolyte abnormality. In congenital LQTS, the QT interval can rarely be shortened even though torsades de pointes is prevented.

Congenital LQTS is a single-gene autosomal recessive or dominant condition that may become manifest at any age. Congenital LQTS may be associated with deafness. Torsades de pointes often develops during physical or psychological stress. Death is usually preceded by recurrent syncope.

Drug-induced LQTS may be aggravated by concomitant diuretic therapy. Unfortunately, the relationship between drug dose, QT interval prolongation, and the development of torsades de pointes is nonlinear for most drugs and varies from drug to drug. For example, a modest increase in QT interval produced by low-dose quinidine may lead to the development of torsades de pointes. In contrast, amiodarone-induced prolonged QT or prolonged QT interval induced by hypocalcemia or hypothyroidism rarely leads to the development of torsades de pointes.

It is generally agreed that symptomatic LQTS patients need treatment. In patients with acquired QT interval prolongation, therapy is aimed at removing the cause. A variety of treatments have been proposed for congenital LQTS, including propranolol, mexiletine, propranolol and pacemaker, propranolol and left stellectomy, implantable defibrillator, and cardiac transplant. A consensus is developing that asymptomatic patients with a normal family history need not be treated. The more problematic asymptomatic patients are those with a positive family history for syncope or sudden death.

Isolated Left Axis Deviation

Axis refers to the mean QRS vector. In this context, left axis deviation is present on the ECG in adults with coronary artery disease and following myocardial infarction. However, many adolescents with left axis deviation have a normal heart.

The concept of fascicular block (hemiblock) has been important in ECG interpretation of the left bundle branch, but the anatomic description of fascicular block is overly simplified. The left bundle branch is multifascicular rather than bi- or trifascicular. In the ECG of adolescents, left axis deviation, the principal ECG feature of left anterior fascicular block, is not due to conduction system impairment or block, but rather it is a normal variant. Among patients with congenital heart disease, left axis deviation is commonly observed in tricuspid atresia and atrioventricular septal defect. The ECG features of preexcitation syndromes may mimic left axis deviation. Isolated left axis deviation does not require treatment. The value in recognition of its presence relates to its association with other conditions.

Cocaine-Induced Cardiac Disturbances (see also Chapters 97 and 111)

Cocaine use may precipitate sudden onset life-threatening cardiac events, including myocardial infarction, life-threatening ventricular tachycardia, cardiac arrest, and death. The cardiac consequences may occur following intranasal or intravenous use. Underlying heart disease is not a prerequisite for cocaine-induced problems. The cardiac consequences are not related to massive doses of the drug. Experimentally, cocaine has been shown to increase afterload, potentiate chronotropic response, and potentiate catecholamine-induced rhythm disturbance. Consequently, β-adrenergic antagonists have been advocated as first-line treatment for cocaine-related rhythm disturbances.

Neurally Mediated Syncope

In normal individuals, upright tilt (60 to 90 degrees) results in a reduction in left ventricular volume. Vigorous contraction of the relatively empty left ventricle may activate myocardial sensory receptors that in susceptible individuals initiate an inhibitory reflex, resulting in hypotension or bradycardia, or both. The reduction in ventricular volume during upright tilt is thought to activate vagal afferent fibers (C fibers). Isoproterenol sensitizes these vagal afferent fibers, and β-adrenergic antagonists decrease fiber activity. Bradycardia that occurs during the inhibitory reflex is probably mediated by parasympathetic activation, whereas hypotension resulting from dilation of resistance vessels is due to sympathetic inhibition.

Neurally mediated syncope may result from an inhibitory reflex. There are three approaches to treatment: intravascular volume expansion with mineralocorticoids and salt, beta blockade with specific B_1 antagonists, and α-adrenergic agonists (disopyramide).

BIBLIOGRAPHY

Benditt DG, Benson DW Jr (eds): Cardiac Preexcitation Syndromes: Origins, Evaluation and Treatment. Boston, Martinus Nijhoff, 1986, p 556.

Benson DW Jr: Etiology, prognosis and management of paroxysmal tachycardia in the young. Comp Ther 13:54, 1987.

Benson DW Jr, Smith WM, Dunnigan A, et al: Mechanisms of regular, wide QRS tachycardia in infants and children. Am J Cardiol 49:1778, 1982.

Dunnigan A, Benditt DG, Benson DW Jr: Modes of onset ("initiating events") for paroxysmal atrial tachycardia in infants and children. Am J Cardiol 57:1280, 1986.

Dunnigan A, Benson DW Jr: Disturbances of cardiac rhythm. In Pierpont MEM, Moller JH (eds). Genetics of Cardiovascular Disease. Boston, Martinus Nijhoff, 1986, pp 127–142.

Goldstein MA, Hessleim P, Dunnigan A: Efficacy of transtelephonic electrocardiographic monitoring in pediatric patients. Am J Dis Child 144:178, 1990.

Horowitz LN, Alexander JA, Edwards LH: Post operative right bundle branch block: Identification of three levels of block. Circulation 62:319, 1980.

Isner JM, Estes NAM, Thompson PD, et al: Acute cardiac event temporally related to cocaine abuse. N Engl J Med 315:1438, 1986.

Keating M, Atkinson D, Dunn C, et al: Linkage of a cardiac arrhythmia, the long QT syndrome, and the Harvey "ras"-1 gene. Science 252:704, 1991.

McAlister HF, Kleinentowicz PT, Andrews C, et al: Lyme carditis: An important cause of reversible heart block. Ann Intern Med 110:339, 1989.

Pongiglione G, Fish F, Strasburger JR, Benson DW Jr: Heart rate and blood pressure response to upright tilt in young patients with unexplained syncope. J Am Coll Cardiol 16:125, 1990.

Selbst SM, Ruddy RM, Clark BJ, et al: Pediatric chest pain: A prospective study. Pediatrics 82:319, 1988.

CHAPTER 47

Structural Cardiovascular Defects

KENNETH G. ZAHKA

CONDITIONS OFTEN FIRST DETECTED IN ADOLESCENTS

The referral of an adolescent to a cardiologist is most commonly for the evaluation of a heart murmur, chest pain, syncope, high blood pressure, or arrhythmia. Although most severe heart defects are diagnosed in the first year of life, a few congenital or acquired heart defects are not detected until after puberty. The medical and surgical management of these problems is dictated by the nature and long-term prognosis of the specific defect.

Mitral Valve Prolapse

The clinical association of a late systolic click and murmur with mitral valve prolapse was first described by Barlow and Bosman in 1966. Mitral valve prolapse (floppy mitral valve, or Barlow syndrome) is a common finding in normal adolescents and young adults. The prevalence increases from 0.5% to 2% in school-age children to as much as 20% in the third decade of life, and the condition is approximately three times more common in females than in males. Mitral valve prolapse is less common in later adulthood, suggesting that it resolves in some individuals. Idiopathic mitral valve prolapse is most prevalent in tall, slender young women. In some instances a thorough evaluation of the adolescent with mitral valve prolapse is warranted to exclude the Marfan syndrome or other connective tissue disorders with which it is regularly associated.

Mitral valve prolapse is characterized by a midsystolic click that varies in timing and intensity with position. The redundancy of the mitral valve relative to the systolic volume of the left ventricle determines at what point during systole the click occurs and whether there is mitral regurgitation. Maneuvers that increase the systolic size of the left ventricle (such as deep inspiration or lying down) tend to make the mitral valve "fit" better, diminishing or delaying the prolapse of the valve; the click is heard relatively later in systole or not at all. Maneuvers that decrease left ventricular size (such as the Valsalva maneuver or assuming an upright position) have the opposite effect, shifting the click earlier in systole and possibly inducing mitral regurgitation. The mitral regurgitation murmur associated with mitral valve prolapse begins after the click and may have either a high pitched or a "honking" quality.

The differential diagnosis of a midsystolic click is limited. Mitral valve prolapse must be differentiated from normal splitting of the first heart sound, which is an early systolic, low-frequency sound. Tricuspid valve systolic sounds in patients with Ebstein anomaly are often multiple and tend to be low-pitched sounds rather than clicks. Aortic and pulmonary ejection clicks always occur in early systole and do not have the characteristic changes with position.

Echocardiography confirms the diagnosis of mitral valve prolapse and determines the extent of mitral regurgitation. Individuals with clinical findings of mitral valve prolapse only in the standing position should have echocardiographic imaging done in the standing and the supine positions because left ventricular filling influences function of the mitral valve. Mitral valve prolapse evident only by echocardiography ("silent" mitral valve prolapse) is not clinically important and should be considered a false-positive finding. The electrocardiogram (ECG) is normal in many adolescents with mitral valve prolapse, although as many as 20% have nonspecific T wave changes, most commonly inversion in leads II, III, and aVF. Screening with 24-hour ambulatory ECG monitoring may be required to demonstrate arrhythmias if they exist.

The prognosis of mitral valve prolapse is variable but usually benign. Most adolescents with mitral valve prolapse have minimal thickening or redundancy of this valve. Those with obviously redundant and thickened valve leaflets are at greater risk for complications of bacterial endocarditis, arrhythmias, or progressive mitral insufficiency.

The risk of bacterial endocarditis is related to the extent of the valve abnormality. In individuals without mitral regurgitation, the risk of endocarditis is comparable to that in the general population (0.0046%/year). If mitral regurgitation is present, the risk increases 10-fold to 0.052%/year. Prophylaxis for bacterial endocarditis is warranted in patients with documented mitral regurgitation or in selected adolescents who have particularly abnormal mitral valves by echocardiography.

Atrial and ventricular arrhythmias are more common in adolescents with mitral valve prolapse, possibly related to catecholamine receptor abnormalities. For adolescents with troublesome supraventricular tachycardia, pharmacologic suppression of the arrhythmia is indicated (see Chapter 46). Ventricular arrhythmias are most common in individuals with associated mitral valve regurgitation. In adults with mitral valve prolapse and regurgitation, sudden death is more common; two thirds have ventricular couplets and one third have nonsustained or sustained ventricular tachycardia on 24-hour ambulatory monitoring. These data should be cautiously extrapolated, because there are few specific data available on adolescents with mitral valve prolapse.

Mitral valve regurgitation requiring surgical mitral valve repair or replacement is extremely uncommon in adolescents with idiopathic mitral valve prolapse. Only 4% of men and 1.5% of women with mitral valve prolapse require mitral valve surgery by age 70.

Mitral valve prolapse has been associated with a wide variety of symptoms, including nonexertional chest pain and panic and anxiety attacks. However, in controlled studies, atypical chest pain and panic attacks are no more common in patients with mitral valve prolapse than in control subjects.

Although mitral valve prolapse is a benign finding, some adolescents and their families benefit from the reassurance of a thorough evaluation by a pediatric cardiologist. For those few adolescents who have arrhythmias, treatment should be coordinated by a physician skilled in the management of adolescents with cardiac disease.

Aortic Valve Disease

Congenital malformations of the aortic valve, including bicuspid aortic valve and aortic valve stenosis, constitute approximately 2% to 5% of congenital heart defects. Aortic valve defects can progress, with increasing obstruction or regurgitation through adolescence and young adulthood. Aortic valve disease has one of the highest risks of bacterial endocarditis.

The presenting sign of a bicuspid aortic valve is an early systolic ejection click. This high-pitched, snapping sound is generated as the aortic valve opens, immediately after the first heart sound. The intensity of the click varies little with position or respiration. In some adolescents the click is subtle, and the first sign of aortic valve disease is a harsh systolic ejection murmur or a blowing decrescendo diastolic murmur. The systolic ejection murmur is produced by turbulent blood flow across a stenotic aortic valve, and the diastolic decrescendo murmur indicates aortic regurgitation. The severity of valvular aortic stenosis or regurgitation usually increases gradually over years. In an adolescent previously thought either to be normal or to have an uncomplicated bicuspid aortic valve, the development of a loud stenotic or regurgitant murmur indicates the possibility of acute deterioration of the valve due to bacterial endocarditis.

The auscultatory assessment of the severity of aortic valve disease should be complemented by Doppler-echo and ECG studies. The echocardiogram defines the valve anatomy, demonstrates the degree of left ventricular hypertrophy, and evaluates the presence of associated mitral valve abnormalities, subaortic stenosis, or coarctation of the aorta. Doppler echocardiography measures the velocity and turbulence of the antegrade aortic blood flow and estimates the pressure gradient across the stenotic valve. The presence and severity of aortic regurgitation are determined by Doppler color flow mapping of the regurgitant jet. The ECG is normal in adolescents with a bicuspid aortic valve. Electrocardiographic evidence of left ventricular hypertrophy indicates mild to moderate stenosis.

Medical management of the adolescent with mild aortic valve disease includes prophylaxis for bacterial endocarditis, meticulous dental hygiene, and strategies to reduce atherosclerotic cardiovascular risk factors (see Chapter 49). Participation in competitive sports is individualized by an experienced pediatric cardiologist.

The presence of severe obstruction or regurgitation, especially if associated with any exercise-related dizziness, syncope, loss of consciousness, or chest pain, is an indication for intervention. Balloon valvuloplasty is effective in reducing the gradient in many patients with isolated aortic valve stenosis. If there is associated aortic valve regurgitation or if aortic regurgitation is the primary problem, aortic valve replacement is indicated.

Pulmonary Valve Stenosis

In contrast with aortic valve disease, pulmonary stenosis in adolescents rarely progresses in severity, and, if present, pulmonary regurgitation is asymptomatic. The diagnosis of pulmonary valve stenosis for the first time in an adolescent usually means very mild disease without much increased pressure in the right ventricle.

The typical clinical findings are an early systolic ejection click that is loudest in the supine position during expiration, followed by a harsh systolic ejection murmur that is loudest at the upper left sternal border and radiates to the lungs. The pulmonary component of the second heart sound may be delayed.

The ECG is normal in adolescents with mild pulmonary valve stenosis; the presence of right ventricular hypertrophy suggests either more severe obstruction or an alternative diagnosis. The two-dimensional echocardiogram shows thickening or "doming" of the pulmonary valve and mild dilatation of the pulmonary artery. Doppler studies show the increased velocity and turbulence of the pulmonary artery blood flow and the presence of associated pulmonary regurgitation.

Although easily detected by echocardiography, a small atrial septal defect must be considered in the differential diagnosis of a systolic ejection murmur in the pulmonary area. Extrinsic compression of the right ventricular outflow tract by an anterior mediastinal mass may also produce a murmur and pulmonary artery turbulence. This may also be identified by echocardiography.

The long-term prognosis of untreated mild pulmonary valve stenosis is excellent. Although the risk of bacterial endocarditis is low, bacterial endocarditis prophylaxis is recommended. For adolescents who have moderate to severe stenosis that requires relief of the obstruction, surgical valvotomy has now been replaced by balloon pulmonary valvuloplasty. The long-term follow-up of patients following surgical pulmonary valvotomy shows minimal persistent gradients at the pulmonary valve. Comparable results following balloon valvulotomy are anticipated, although there is a relatively brief duration of follow-up to date.

Atrial Septal Defect

Although it is a congenital condition, the effect of an atrial septal defect varies among individuals and tends to increase with age. In some patients, the left-to-right atrial shunt in early childhood is mild and the physical signs of an atrial septal defect are subtle. As these children become adolescents, the shunt volume increases and the characteristic auscultatory findings become evident. Occasionally chest radiographs obtained for pulmonary evaluation reveal cardiac dilatation.

Atrial septal defects occur most frequently at the ostium secundum in the midportion of the atrial septum at the site of the foramen ovale. Defects at the junction of the right atrium and superior vena cava are termed sinus venosus defects. These defects may be associated with anomalous pulmonary venous return of the right pulmonary veins to the right atrium near the site of the defect. Ostium primum atrial septal defects adjacent to the atrioventricular valves are part of the spectrum of endocardial cushion defects. They are often associated with clefts in the mitral valve and mitral regurgitation. Regardless of the location of the defect, the underlying pathophysiology is similar.

Blood flow occurs across the atrial septal defect from the left to the right atrium. The increased right heart blood flow dilates the right ventricle and pulmonary artery. The magnitude of the shunt is determined by the size of the defect, the compliance of the right and left atria and ventricles, and pulmonary vascular resistance. Although the dominant shunt is left to right, right-to-left atrial shunt may occur during the straining phase of the Valsalva maneuver. Right-to-left shunting may also occur if right ventricular compliance decreases with the development of pulmonary vascular disease.

Atrial septal defect rarely causes symptoms in childhood. In late adolescence and early adulthood, right atrial and ventricular dilatation and dysfunction lead to exercise intolerance and atrial arrhythmias. Pulmonary vascular obstructive disease can develop in the third and fourth decades.

The diagnosis of an atrial septal defect is usually established by physical examination. There is a right ventricular heave or pulmonary artery impulse secondary to the right ventricular and pulmonary artery dilatation and volume overload. The second heart sound is widely split, with minimal variation in the splitting during respiration. Although the flow across the defect itself is silent, the increased pulmonary blood flow gives rise to a systolic ejection murmur at the upper left sternal border that radiates to the lungs. Increased right ventricular filling across the tricuspid valve causes a rumbling middiastolic murmur and a third heart sound.

The electrocardiogram shows right ventricular hypertrophy with a Rsr′ pattern in the right chest leads and a wide, deep S wave in the left chest. The two-dimensional echocardiogram demonstrates the size and location of the defect and the consequent right ventricular and pulmonary artery dilatation. Color flow mapping documents the atrial shunting. Cardiac catheterization is usually not required to diagnose an atrial septal defect.

Surgical closure of atrial septal defect has been performed with outstanding results for nearly 40 years. The recently developed "clam-shell" device for transcatheter closure of atrial septal defects may become an alternative to surgical repair.

Coarctation of the Aorta

In adolescents, coarctation of the aorta is usually discovered following the recognition of systemic hypertension or the observation of decreased intensity of the femoral or pedal pulses. Widening of the pulp space of the teeth on dental radiographs (due to increased blood flow) is also a sign associated with coarctation of the aorta. The obstruction is classically just distal to the origin of the left subclavian artery, although coarctation of the distal thoracic aorta can occur. Collateral circulation develops via the internal mammary and shoulder girdle arteries to supply the body distal to the coarctation.

The chronic pressure overload of the left ventricle proximal arteries leads to left ventricular hypertrophy with eventual left ventricular failure and accelerated atherosclerosis. Coarctation of the aorta is frequently associated with abnormalities of the aortic valve, subaortic area, or mitral valve. A bicuspid aortic valve or subaortic membrane may become hemodynamically significant by young adulthood.

The diagnosis of coarctation of the aorta is made by the documentation of decreased and delayed femoral and pedal pulses with a systolic blood pressure gradient between the arms and the legs. A systolic or continuous murmur, arising from the blood flow through the coarctation or collaterals, is frequently heard over the back in older patients with coarctation of the aorta.

Confirmation of the diagnosis is possible by two-dimensional echocardiographic or magnetic resonance imaging of the aortic arch. Doppler echocardiographic documentation of the continuous blood flow at the coarctation site and the poor pulsatility in the descending aorta can confirm the hemodynamic impact of the obstruction.

When coarctation of the aorta is diagnosed in adolescents, the preferred surgical treatment is excision of the coarctation and end-to-end anastomosis or patch enlargement of the obstruction. Severe perioperative high blood pressure is common in older children. Other complications include abdominal pain and paraplegia. In selected patients, balloon dilatation of a coarctation of the aorta is an alternative to surgery. The long-term efficacy and complications of this approach are unknown.

Persistent hypertension is likely after repair of coarctation of the aorta in adolescence. If it is not caused by recurrent obstruction, hypertension should be treated to avoid the exacerbation of arterial vascular disease.

Cardiomyopathy

Cardiomyopathy is the term used to describe a diverse group of conditions whose common element is abnormal myocardial muscle mass or function. Dilated cardiomyopathy refers to conditions in which the left ventricle is enlarged and left ventricular contractility is impaired. This may be caused by ischemia, metabolic abnormalities, nutritional deficiency, or viral myocarditis. Hypertrophic cardiomyopathy is a disorder characterized by myocardial hypertrophy out of proportion to ventricular afterload. The hypertrophy may be limited largely to the intraventricular septum, or it may involve the entire left ventricle uniformly. The etiology is unknown, although the familial tendency of many cases suggests a heritable disorder of muscle.

DILATED CARDIOMYOPATHY

Dilated cardiopathy presents with symptoms of either congestive heart failure or arrhythmias. Delayed diagnosis is common, and frequently the adolescent has been evaluated for chronic respiratory symptoms due to pulmonary edema or chronic abdominal pain secondary to hepatic distention. Exercise intolerance, paroxysmal nocturnal dyspnea, and orthopnea indicate severely impaired ventricular function.

Findings on physical examination consistent with dilated cardiomyopathy include jugular venous distention, a displaced apical impulse, a third or fourth heart sound, the presence of a mitral regurgitation murmur, and hepatomegaly.

The ECG may show ST-T wave changes, abnormal Q waves, or left ventricular hypertrophy. The echocardiogram documents the degree of ventricular dilatation and dysfunction and associated valvular regurgitation. Evidence for a metabolic defect should be sought by measurement of serum carnitine levels and skeletal muscle biopsy. Serial cardiac enzymes and viral antibody titers for known myocardial pathogens are useful to help exclude an acute myocarditis rather than a chronic cardiomyopathy. Myocardial biopsy assesses the possibility of acute myocarditis.

The treatment and prognosis of dilated cardiomyopathy are determined by its underlying cause. Ischemia due to anomalous origin of the left coronary artery from the pulmonary artery may be reversed by surgical transfer of the coronary artery to the aorta. Some degree of return of myocardial function may be anticipated. Supplementation with carnitine has been advocated as a diagnostic challenge for patients suspected of carnitine deficiency.

Medical management is tailored to the severity of the myocardial dysfunction. The three mainstays of pharmacologic treatment are inotropic support with digoxin, preload reduction with diuretics, and afterload reduction with vasodilators. For patients debilitated despite maximal medical management, cardiac transplantation is an alternative.

HYPERTROPHIC CARDIOMYOPATHY

Localized hypertrophy of the subaortic portion of the interventricular septum (asymmetric septal hypertrophy) is the most common form of hypertrophic cardiomyopathy. This condition occurs sporadically or is inherited as an autosomal dominant trait. Recent studies of familial hypertrophic cardiomyopathy suggest a defective mutation of the myosin heavy-chain gene. The hypertrophy is typically associated with myocardial fiber disarray. The physiologic consequences of the hypertrophy on ventricular systolic and diastolic function are variable. Severely affected patients have severe left ventricular outflow obstruction and impaired diastolic left ventricular filling and relaxation. Obstruction may develop or increase with exercise. Some adolescents, especially early in the course of the disease, have no demonstrable obstruction.

Asymptomatic adolescents with hypertrophic cardiomyopathy are diagnosed by echocardiography prompted by the presence of an affected family member or the incidental finding of a murmur due to subaortic obstruction or mitral regurgitation. Symptomatic adolescents may present with exercise intolerance, dizziness, syncope, angina, or palpitations. Symptoms usually signal severe obstruction and diminished cardiac output with exercise. Atrial arrhythmias, particularly atrial fibrillation, are a problem in adolescents with left atrial dilatation due to outflow obstruction, diastolic dysfunction, or mitral regurgitation. Nonsustained ventricular tachycardia is frequently documented in patients with a history of syncope and is usually treated pharmacologically (see Chapter 46).

β-Blockers, calcium channel blockers, and other negative inotropic agents have been used in the medical management of both asymptomatic and symptomatic patients with hypertrophic cardiomyopathy. There are variable short- and long-term effects of these agents on resting and exercise-induced obstruction, and careful clinical and echocardiographic follow-up is important. Side effects, including severe congestive heart failure, preclude their use in some patients. In patients with severe obstruction or symptoms, surgical septal myectomy or myotomy often dramatically decreases obstruction and improves associated mitral regurgitation. Dyspnea, syncope, and angina are relieved in most patients following surgery.

LATE FOLLOW-UP OF REPAIRED CONGENITAL HEART DISEASE

Advances in cardiac surgery, anesthesia, and postoperative care over the last 3 decades have made repair of most congenital heart defects routine in infancy and early childhood. Extensive experience has been gathered over this period that defines the short- and long-term expectations for these children as they reach adolescence and adulthood.

Atrial Septal Defect

Atrial septal defect was among the first congenital intracardiac defect to be repaired by open heart cardiac surgery. The long-term result of surgical repair of atrial septal defect in childhood is excellent. The right ventricular size returns to near normal, and exercise intolerance or arrhythmias are rare. Occasionally patients, especially those with a sinus venosus atrial septal defect, have bradycardia because of sinus node dysfunction. If repair is delayed until early adulthood, pulmonary vascular disease, atrial arrhythmias, and congestive heart failure may develop, persist, or progress.

Ventricular Septal Defect

Long-term (>30 years) studies have documented the follow-up of surgical repair of ventricular septal defect in large groups of patients. For the majority of adolescents, growth, development, and exercise tolerance are normal following successful closure of ventricular septal defect in childhood. Left-to-right shunts across small residual defects are present in about 10% of adolescents and are not hemodynamically important.

Aortic or mitral valve regurgitation or ventricular dysfunction is unusual immediately after surgery or in the long-term follow-up. Ventricular and atrial arrhythmias are also unusual in adolescents who had uncomplicated ventricular septal defect closure as children. No specific restrictions or daily medications are needed. Bacterial endocarditis prophylaxis is necessary for adolescents with residual ventricular septal defects.

Heart block and pulmonary vascular disease in adolescents require special attention following repair of ventricular septal defect. Complete heart block occurring at the time of surgery requires permanent pacing either in the perioperative period or during follow-up. Although pacemaker and pacing-lead technology has improved over the last 20 years, lead and generator failure or infections are a source of continuing morbidity. Pulmonary vascular disease can often be avoided by repair of large ventricular septal defects in the first 2 years of life. Adolescents with defects repaired later in life may have persistently or progressively increased pulmonary vascular resistance and pulmonary hypertension. Adolescents with mild pulmonary vascular disease are usually asymptomatic. More severe pulmonary vascular disease results in decreased exercise tolerance or overt signs of congestive heart failure.

Tetralogy of Fallot

The pioneering palliative shunt devised by Blalock and Taussig in 1944 and the introduction of open heart, or "direct vision," repair by Lillehei and colleagues in 1955 opened a new era for children with tetralogy of Fallot (a combination of pulmonary stenosis, ventricular septal defect, overriding aorta, and right ventricular hypertrophy). There are now extensive follow-up data on these patients (now adolescents and adults) that define the sequelae of surgical closure of the ventricular septal defect and relief of the right ventricular outflow obstruction.

Studies of postoperative tetralogy of Fallot have documented right ventricular enlargement that is the consequence of several factors including pulmonary regurgitation, tricuspid regurgitation, and a primary right ventricular myopathy. Persistent right ventricular outflow obstruction due to stenosis at the valve annulus, in the main pulmonary artery, or in the branch pulmonary arteries or due to diffuse, severe hypoplasia of the pulmonary arteries poses additional right ventricular load. Severe right ventricular dilatation is associated with diminished exercise tolerance. Symptomatic adolescents with excessive right ventricular volume overload may improve with surgical repair of the tricuspid valve and placement of pulmonary valve prosthesis.

Residual small ventricular septal defects occur in approximately 5% of adolescents with tetralogy of Fallot repaired in childhood. If the defect is sufficiently large to produce symptoms of pulmonary overcirculation and left ventricular volume loading, surgical repair of the residual defect is performed.

Mild aortic regurgitation secondary to aortic annular dilatation is present in 15% to 20% of adolescents and young adults. It is usually not progressive, and aortic valve replacement is rarely required. Left ventricular outflow obstruction due to a subaortic membrane, although rare, should be considered in patients with a harsh systolic ejection murmur that radiates to the neck.

Ventricular arrhythmias, including isolated premature ventricular contractions, ventricular couplets, and ventricular tachycardia, are common following repair of tetralogy of Fallot (see Chapter 46). Several studies have emphasized the relationship between persistent right ventricular hypertension due to unrelieved pulmonary stenosis and the risk of sudden death or ventricular arrhythmias. Ventricular arrhythmias are most frequent in those patients who underwent surgical repair after 10 years of age or in those with severe right ventricular dilatation. In patients without significant heart disease, ventricular bigeminy and couplets may be of limited prognostic significance. In the postoperative period, however, pharmacologic suppression of frequent or more complex ventricular arrhythmias has been advocated. Complete heart block is a rare complication of surgery and usually requires long-term artificial pacing.

Transposition of the Great Arteries

Advances in medical and surgical management have dramatically changed the prognosis of transposition of the great arteries. The first repairs were atrial redirection of blood flow (Mustard and Senning procedures). More recently, an arterial switch operation (Jatene procedure) has been used at many heart centers.

Children who benefited from atrial baffling operations have now reached adolescence and adulthood. In these atrial baffling operations, the aorta and pulmonary artery remained transposed, and the venous inflow was redirected within the atria. This physiologic repair results in fully oxygenated blood in the right ventricle and aorta and poorly oxygenated blood in the left ventricle and pulmonary artery. The anatomic connections of the ventricles and arteries remain abnormal. Although these operations provide excellent relief of hypoxia and in many cases a normal lifestyle, long-term postoperative problems are common.

Atrial arrhythmias due to extensive atrial surgery are

very common and problematic. Sinus node dysfunction with atrial or junctional bradycardia occurs in up to one half of adolescents during follow-up. Resting heart rates between 30 and 40 beats per minute are not unusual and, if associated with dizziness or limitation of exercise, are an indication for permanent pacing. Supraventricular tachycardia or atrial flutter can usually be managed with medications and a pacemaker (see Chapter 46).

Atrial baffle obstruction or leaks usually develop shortly after surgery but may not be clinically evident for several years. Mild or moderate inferior and superior vena caval obstruction is usually well tolerated as a result of the development of venous collaterals. Severe superior vena caval obstruction leads to superior vena caval syndrome with facial and cerebral venous congestion. Pulmonary venous obstruction produces pulmonary edema and chronic respiratory distress. Baffle leaks usually result in pulmonary-to-systemic venous shunting and pulmonary overcirculation.

Right ventricular enlargement is a uniform finding in adolescents following atrial baffle repair of transposition of the great arteries. Right ventricular dysfunction and tricuspid valve regurgitation in adolescents with atrial repair of transposition of the great arteries have physiologic consequences similar to those of left ventricular dysfunction and mitral valve regurgitation in adolescents with normally related great arteries. When systemic ventricular dysfunction and valve regurgitation are severe, they cause exercise intolerance, dyspnea, and fluid retention. This is exacerbated in adolescents with transposition of the great arteries by the limited heart rate response due to sinus node dysfunction.

Medical management of congestive heart failure with digitalis, diuretics, vasodilators, and the insertion of a permanent pacemaker may relieve or improve symptoms. Adolescents with refractory congestive heart failure may be considered for heart transplantation.

Surgical retransposition of the great arteries (arterial switch) is a new procedure in which the basic anatomic defect in transposition is corrected in the first 2 weeks of life. The postoperative outcome for the arterial switch operation is favorable, with evidence of excellent ventricular function, normal rhythm, and a low incidence of obstruction at the pulmonary, aortic, and coronary suture lines. Although continued success through adolescence and adulthood must be documented by careful follow-up, the results from these initial studies are encouraging.

Truncus Arteriosus

Surgical repair of truncus arteriosus in the first months of life has dramatically improved the prognosis of children with this defect. Surgical repair requires, in addition to closure of the ventricular septal defect, the placement of an extracardiac conduit to establish continuity between the right ventricle and the pulmonary arteries. Early repair prevents the development of pulmonary vascular disease and results in normal cardiovascular volume and pressure load. Growth, development, and exercise tolerance are improved.

Extracardiac conduits, including nonvalved tube grafts, porcine valve conduits, and cryopreserved homografts, have complications related to durability of the extracardiac conduit and the problem of fixed conduit size during a period of rapid somatic and cardiac growth. Right ventricular pressure increases over a period of months to years owing to calcification of the conduits and formation of an intimal "peel." Additional right ventricular load due to pulmonary regurgitation is present in all patients with nonvalved conduits and develops in adolescents with degenerating valved conduits.

The timing of conduit replacement is guided by clinical, echocardiographic, and catheterization assessment. Exercise limitation or arrhythmias may prompt surgery in patients with moderate conduit obstruction. Severe obstruction is usually an indication for conduit replacement in all patients with postoperative truncus arteriosus. In adolescents who have reached their adult size, large conduits that tend to minimize the impact of conduit degeneration may be used.

Following surgery, the truncal valve becomes the systemic (aortic) semilunar valve. Although truncal valve stenosis or regurgitation is present in a small proportion of infants, the valve leaflets are frequently abnormally formed. Stenosis or regurgitation due to leaflet thickening or calcification frequently develops in later childhood or adolescence.

Guidelines for truncal valve replacement are similar to those for aortic valve disease; indications include severe obstruction with elevated left ventricular pressure and left ventricular hypertrophy, and severe regurgitation with left ventricular dilatation. In contrast with the adolescent with isolated aortic valve disease, the adolescent with postoperative truncus arteriosus often has the additional problem of abnormal right ventricular loading, which may prompt earlier aortic valve surgery.

Atrioventricular Canal

Repair of atrioventricular canal defects requires closure of the combined atrial and ventricular septal defects and reconstruction of the common atrioventricular valve to form separate mitral and tricuspid valves.

As many as 30% of patients require a second operation for repair or replacement of the mitral valve. The majority of these have moderate or severe regurgitation recognized shortly after operation. However, increasing severity of mitral regurgitation does occur in adolescents, and late reoperation may be required. Tricuspid regurgitation, although common, is rarely clinically evident or troublesome.

Pulmonary vascular disease changes the clinical characteristics and importance of tricuspid regurgitation. In patients with increased right ventricular pressure due to elevated pulmonary vascular resistance, the murmur of tricuspid regurgitation is harsh, holosystolic, and loudest at the lower right sternal border. Fluid retention, hepatic enlargement, and exercise intolerance are evident in these adolescents.

Residual atrial or ventricular septal defects, which are usually small, occur in 10% to 15% of children and rarely require reoperation. Residual ventricular septal defects can be differentiated clinically or by echocardiography from mitral or tricuspid regurgitation. Postoperative left ventricular outflow obstruction occurs most frequently in patients with chordal attachments of the mitral valve to the interventricular septum. Acquired subaortic stenosis due to a discrete subaortic membrane may also develop over a period of years.

Atrial arrhythmias, including atrial tachycardia and atrial flutter, occur primarily in adolescents with moderate or severe mitral regurgitation and left atrial dilatation. Repair of the primary valvular dysfunction in addition to appropriate pharmacologic therapy is effective. Complete heart block is a surgical complication of repair of atrioventricular canal in approximately 5% of patients. Permanent pacing is nearly always required to maintain adequate cardiac output and exercise tolerance.

Persistent Cyanosis and Ventricular Dysfunction

Advances in the medical and surgical treatment of congenital and acquired heart disease have dramatically improved the prognosis for most adolescents with structural or functional heart disease. Adolescents with persistent cyanosis or ventricular dysfunction are a difficult challenge. Defects likely to cause such problems include single ventricle and pulmonary vascular disease (Eisenmenger syndrome).

SINGLE VENTRICLE

Single ventricle occurs in a variety of defects, including tricuspid atresia with hypoplastic right ventricle and double inlet left ventricle with pulmonary stenosis. There is complete mixing of the systemic and pulmonary venous blood flow at either the atrial or the ventricular level, and pulmonary blood flow is limited, leading to cyanosis. Systemic-to-pulmonary shunts usually provide adequate palliation in infancy. Definitive surgery, the Fontan operation, is undertaken in later childhood. In the Fontan operation, the systemic venous return (inferior vena cava, superior vena cava, or right atrium) is anastomosed directly to the pulmonary artery. Other atrial connections (atrial septal defects, tricuspid valves) or arterial connections (shunts, pulmonary valve) must be eliminated to isolate the systemic venous blood from the pulmonary venous blood. Adolescents with low pulmonary resistance, good ventricular function, and a competent mital valve postoperatively are asymptomatic, with normal arterial saturation and good exercise tolerance.

However, right atrial and systemic venous pressures may be elevated as a consequence of pulmonary arterial stenosis, pulmonary vascular disease, or elevated left atrial or left ventricular end-diastolic pressure. Elevated ventricular end-diastolic pressure is found in patients with either ventricular dilatation and dysfunction or severe hypertrophy due to associated subaortic stenosis.

The sequelae of chronic systemic venous congestion include edema, pleural effusion, ascites, and hepatic enlargement and dysfunction. Hypoproteinemia may exacerbate the impact of high venous pressure. Exercise tolerance in adolescents with venous obstruction is abnormal as a result of the combination of decreased cardiac output reserve and impaired pulmonary function from ascites and pulmonary fluid.

The follow-up and management of the adolescent following the Fontan operation are usually dictated by the degree of systemic venous congestion. Those with little evidence of obstruction require no restrictions or medications other than prophylaxis for bacterial endocarditis. A large proportion of adolescents require intermittent or daily diuretics to alleviate edema. Adolescents with severe venous congestion need multiple or high-dose diuretics with potassium supplementation. Careful follow-up of electrolytes, calcium, protein, and renal and hepatic function is important in these symptomatic patients. Exercise intolerance, poor growth, protein-losing enteropathy, and nephrolithiasis are recognized complications of the Fontan procedure and its long-term postoperative management.

Adolescents who are not candidates for the Fontan procedure are managed conservatively. These adolescents usually have limited pulmonary blood flow as a result of either pulmonary artery distortion or pulmonary vascular disease from previous palliative procedures. As a consequence, they are moderately hypoxic and have diminished exercise reserve. Polycythemia is an adaptive response to hypoxia. However, severe polycythemia leads to symptoms related to hyperviscosity, including exercise intolerance, headaches, cerebral infarction, and hemorrhage. Partial exchange transfusion to maintain a hematocrit between 65% and 70% may alleviate symptoms. Iron deficiency should be suspected in the cyanotic adolescent without polycythemia. Prophylactic iron therapy may be needed in females with menorrhagia or in adolescents with inadequate sources of dietary iron.

Bacterial and viral infections in adolescents with single ventricle may be life-threatening. Bacterial endocarditis may occur on systemic-to-pulmonary shunts as well as on the semilunar and atrioventricular valves. The classic signs of endocarditis (petechiae, splinter hemorrhages, Roth spots, Osler nodes, and splenomegaly) may not be present; fever, weight loss, and malaise suggest the diagnosis. Echocardiography may identify vegetation on the valves, but small vegetations near systemic-to-pulmonary shunts may not be imaged. Brain abscess should be suspected in adolescents with fever and central nervous system symptoms or signs. Influenza viral infection, especially with pulmonary complications, is a concern in hypoxic patients, and vaccination is recommended (see Chapter 93).

The cardiovascular complications of single ventricle become evident in the second and third decades. Myocardial dysfunction, dilatation, and atrioventricular valve regurgitation lead to symptoms of congestive heart failure. Treatment with digoxin, diuretics, and vasodilators may be beneficial. Vasodilators must be used with care in severely cyanotic adolescents, in whom systemic vasodilatation may diminish pulmonary blood flow and exacerbate hypoxia.

Atrial arrhythmias, including atrial fibrillation and flutter, are often associated with atrial dilatation. Pharmacologic control of the arrhythmias usually improves symptoms; however, the negative inotropic and gastrointestinal side effects of some agents are problematic. Anticoagulation to diminish the risk of atrial thrombi should be considered in adolescents with chronic atrial fibrillation or flutter.

Isolated premature ventricular beats are common and rarely require treatment. Ventricular tachycardia, especially in patients with ventricular dysfunction, can lead to symptoms, and it should be treated. Sinus node dysfunction or acquired high-degree heart block is treated with permanent pacing.

EISENMENGER SYNDROME

Early recognition and advances in the surgical treatment of congenital heart disease have dramatically decreased, but not eliminated, the development of irreversible pulmonary vascular disease (Eisenmenger syndrome). Pulmonary vascular disease may develop in the first years of life in children with ventricular septal defect, atrioventricular canal, truncus arteriosus, and complex defects with unrestricted pulmonary blood flow. Pulmonary vascular disease develops at a very early age in children with transposition of the great arteries and large ventricular septal defect. It is occasionally seen as a complication of large systemic-to-pulmonary shunts, most typically the Waterston (ascending aorta to right pulmonary artery) shunt.

The natural history of Eisenmenger syndrome is variable, but survival into the third or fourth decade of life is common. Increasing pulmonary vascular resistance leads to severe cyanosis and diminished exercise tolerance. Bacterial endocarditis, arrhythmias, respiratory infections, stroke, and hemoptysis lead to acute exacerbations. Chronic complications include myocardial dysfunction, arrhythmias, and pulmonary regurgitation.

Polycythemia is managed in a manner similar to that in adolescents with cyanosis due to severe pulmonary hypoperfusion. Myocardial dysfunction and atrioventricular valve regurgitation are treated with digoxin and diuretics. Pharmacologic manipulation of the pulmonary vascular resistance with direct vasodilators, calcium channel blockers, or converting enzyme inhibitors may exacerbate hypoxia by lowering the systemic vascular resistance more than the pulmonary vascular resistance. Supplemental oxygen usually does not dramatically improve the arterial saturation, although in selected patients with a documented response it is useful.

Heart-lung transplantation is the definitive treatment for end-stage Eisenmenger syndrome. Difficulties with donor availability, chronic immunosuppression, and complications including bronchiolitis obliterans have made 5-year survival rates disappointing.

Cardiac and major general surgery carry a high risk of intraoperative and postoperative sudden death in adolescents with Eisenmenger syndrome. There is also a high incidence of spontaneous abortions. Death following delivery, even with careful monitoring, is well recognized. The presumed causes of this high mortality rate include acute exacerbation of pulmonary vascular resistance, shifts in intravascular volume, changes in hemoglobin concentration, and systemic or pulmonary emboli.

QUALITY OF LIFE ISSUES

PREGNANCY AND BIRTH CONTROL
(see Chapters 73 and 74)

Pregnancy results in increased total cardiac output, regional cardiac output, systemic venous return, and blood volume and in decreased hematocrit. For adolescents with small ventricular septal defects or other defects with minimal hemodynamic impact, the risk of pregnancy is comparable to that in the general population. Pregnancy following repair of the common congenital heart defects, including atrial septal defect, ventricular septal defects, pulmonary stenosis, and tetralogy of Fallot, is uncomplicated because residual defects are usually minor and ventricular function is normal.

The risk of pregnancy in adolescents with atrial baffle repair of transposition of the great arteries must be considered on an individual basis. Atrial arrhythmias, right ventricular dysfunction, and baffle obstruction limit cardiovascular reserve and compromise maternal and fetal well-being.

Aortic valve disease is usually well tolerated during pregnancy, although the combination of stenosis and regurgitation or severe isolated aortic stenosis is problematic. Associated left heart obstruction, including mitral valve abnormalities or postoperative coarctation of the aorta with mild residual obstruction, may become clinically important as the cardiac output increases during pregnancy. In these adolescents, measurement of upper and lower extremity blood pressure is important as part of the evaluation of hypertension (see Chapters 48 and 67).

Prosthetic heart valves, in the absence of ventricular dysfunction, do not specifically limit a pregnancy. However, warfarin is teratogenic, and anticoagulant therapy should be changed to heparin for the first trimester. Heparin may be reinstituted again just prior to delivery to minimize peripartum hemorrhage.

Although successful pregnancy has been reported in women with Eisenmenger syndrome, complex cyanotic heart defects, and the Fontan operation, the risk of fetal loss, premature labor, and peripartum death is extremely high.

Several general principles apply to the management of the adolescent who has cardiovascular disease during pregnancy. Careful follow-up, involving the fields of obstetrics, pediatrics, and pediatric cardiology, is important in maximizing maternal and fetal health. Clinical evaluation should be supplemented by prepartal and postpartum echocardiographic assessment. Echocardiography may identify ventricular dysfunction before it becomes clinically evident. Iron supplementation is particularly important in cyanotic patients and those with limited cardiovascular reserve.

Many routine cardiac medications, including digoxin and diuretics, either do not cross the placenta or are apparently safe for the fetus. Fetal growth retardation and bradycardia have been observed with chronic maternal propranolol use, although other β-antagonist medications including atenolol have fewer fetal side effects. Quinidine and procainamide are well tolerated and are not known to be teratogenic. The effects of angiotensin-converting enzyme inhibitors and calcium channel blockers on the fetus are unknown. Prophylaxis for bacterial endocarditis is not generally necessary for uncomplicated vaginal or cesarean delivery.

The choice of a contraceptive method for adolescents with heart disease must consider the risk of vascular thrombosis with oral contraceptive pills or infection with intrauterine devices. Oral contraceptives are unsuitable for those with poor ventricular function, unrepaired cyanotic heart disease, pulmonary vascular disease, prosthetic heart valves, or the Fontan operation. The risk of bacterial endocarditis in women with structural heart disease limits the safety of an intrauterine device. Barrier methods have the best compromise of safety and efficacy for adolescents with a contraindication to either oral contraceptives or intrauterine devices (see Chapter 73). In addition to providing effective birth control, they also protect against sexually transmitted diseases that could exacerbate cardiac dysfunction.

Recurrence in Families

The risk of having a child with congenital heart disease has been reported to be between 1.4% and 7.3% for affected fathers and 2.9% to 16.1% for affected mothers. However, many studies are affected by problems of ascertainment bias or incomplete evaluation of the offspring. The latter problem may increase the apparent risk by including children with normal murmurs or decrease the risk by excluding children with possibly "silent" defects such as bicuspid aortic valve.

Furthermore, the risk of recurrence may be high only in certain families in which there is a stronger genetic influence than is usually suggested by the multifactorial model of inheritance. Familial clusters of congenital heart disease have been suggested for pulmonary stenosis and the left heart obstructive defects.

Exercise Restrictions
(see Chapter 81)

Recreational and competitive sports are an important part of the life of adolescents, and the decison to restrict the physical activity of adolescents with heart disease should not be taken lightly. Although established guidelines for participation in competitive sports are helpful, recommendations must be tailored to the individual adolescent's cardiovascular problem and symptoms. These guidelines are not specifically directed toward participation in recreational sports.

The relative contribution of the dynamic and isometric components of a particular activity and the episodic or sustained nature of the exertion affect the adolescent's tolerance of a particular activity. The goal of exercise limitation is to ensure that the demands imposed by exercise will not exceed the adolescent's cardiovascular reserve and lead to dizziness, syncope, arrhythmias, or death. Many adolescents can voluntarily adjust their exercise level to prevent excessive fatigue or dizziness with exercise. Permitting adolescents to adapt their activity guided by their symptoms is effective for many adolescents participating in noncompetitive sports. The demands of competitive sports may not always permit the adolescent voluntarily to limit exertion, and specific restrictions are appropriate for adolescents with limited cardiovascular reserve.

Adolescents with normal ventricular function, normal pulmonary vascular resistance, and mild outflow obstruction or left-to-right shunts may participate in all competitive and recreational activities without restriction. This includes adolescents with small ventricular septal defects, mild pulmonic or aortic stenosis, and many defects following surgical repair. Competitive low-intensity sports, including bowling or golf, are appropriate for adolescents with moderate ventricular septal defect, moderate pulmonary stenosis, mild coarctation of the aorta, mild aortic stenosis, and transposition of the great arteries repaired by atrial baffle surgery.

Competitive sports are usually not advised for adolescents with pulmonary vascular disease, unrepaired cyanotic congenital heart disease, Marfan syndrome, ventricular dysfunction, or moderate aortic stenosis or regurgitation. Treadmill or bicycle exercise testing, ambulatory electrocardiographic monitoring, or stress echocardiography or thallium imaging can provide some reassurance for adolescents, families, and physicians regarding the safety of exercise. However, it is not possible to duplicate the varying dynamic and isometric components of the cardiovascular load of most sports by routine exercise testing.

Recreational sports offer more latitude for participation for the adolescent with heart disease. Some caution and judgment must be exercised by adolescents in choosing and moderating specific activities. Choosing an activity must be guided not only by the cardiovascular load of the activity but also by the consequences of symptoms during exertion. In this regard, swimming, weightlifting, or climbing is inappropriate for adolescents with exercise-induced dizziness or syncope.

Weightlifting, wrestling, and other activities with a high level of isometric load are not advised for adolescents with aortic valve disease, coarctation of the aorta with residual obstruction, or myocardial dysfunction. Adolescents with pulmonary vascular disease have limited cardiac output reserve and become increasingly hypoxic with even low level exertion.

BIBLIOGRAPHY

Chen SC, Nouri S, Balfour I, et al: Clinical profile of congestive cardiomyopathy in children. J Am Coll Cardiol 15:189, 1990.
Gianopoulos J: Cardiac disease in pregnancy. Med Clin North Am 73:639, 1989.
Horneffer PJ, Zahka KG, Rowe SA, et al: Long-term results of total

repair of tetralogy of Fallot in childhood. Ann Thorac Surg 50:179, 1990.

Kron I, Flanagan T, Rheuban K, et al: Incidence and risk of reintervention after coarctation repair. Ann Thorac Surg 49:920, 1990.

Mair D, Hagler D, Puga F, et al: Fontan operation in 176 patients with tricuspid atresia. Circulation 82:IV164, 1990.

McNamara D, Bricker JT, Galioto FM, et al: Cardiovascular abnormalities in the athlete: Recommendations regarding eligibility for competition. Task Force I: Congenital heart disease. J Am Coll Cardiol 6:1200, 1985.

Mohr R, Schaff HV, Puga FJ, Danielson GK: Results of operation for hypertrophic obstructive cardiomyopathy in children and adults less than 40 years of age. Circulation 80:I191, 1989.

Norwood W, Dobell A, Freed M, et al: Intermediate results of the arterial switch repair. J Thorac Cardiovasc Surg 96:854, 1988.

Popp R: Medical progress—Echocardiography (1). N Engl J Med 323:101, 1990.

Trusler G, Williams GW, Duncan KF, et al: Results with the Mustard operation in simple transposition of the great arteries 1963–1985. Ann Surg 206:251, 1987.

CHAPTER 48

High Blood Pressure in Adolescents

EDWARD B. CLARK

Blood pressure, the dynamic force driving blood flow through the body, varies greatly during each day. Transient increases in blood pressure are essential in meeting the metabolic demands of the body, but a sustained increase in blood pressure can lead to premature vascular changes in the heart, brain, and kidneys. Most physicians suspect that the seeds of adult-onset hypertensive disease are sown during childhood. Therefore, abnormalities in blood pressure are of great interest to all who care for adolescents.

Although the highest levels of blood pressure in an adolescent likely correlate with essential hypertension as an adult, data on the long-term outcome in adolescents are only now becoming available. In the Muscatine Iowa Study, 45% of young adults with high blood pressure had also been recorded as having childhood high blood pressure on at least one measurement. Although among individual children there is great variability as to the prediction of adult blood pressure, on a population basis early childhood blood pressure elevations are predictive of risk for future high blood pressure. This important ongoing study and others confirm that regular measurement of blood pressure is an essential part of good primary adolescent health care.

DEFINITION

High blood pressure is the level of systolic or diastolic blood pressure at which there is an unacceptable risk for cardiovascular complications for that individual. Defining that level is difficult because there are no long-term studies relating blood pressure beginning in childhood to vascular disease arising during adult life. Thus, the current definition is statistical and closely correlated with age, gender, physical activity, body size, and sexual maturity.

Primary (essential) hypertension occurs without identifiable pathologic cause and is likely related to genetic factors (Table 48–1). Secondary hypertension is due to chronic vascular, renal, or neuroendocrine causes (see Chapter 67).

This chapter is adapted from Clark EB: High blood pressure in infants, children and adolescents. In Hoekelman RA, Friedman SB, Nelson NM, Seidel HM (eds.): Primary Pediatric Care, 2nd ed. St Louis, MO, Mosby Year Book, 1992, pp 969–975.

DIAGNOSIS

Most adolescents with high blood pressure do not have symptoms. Therefore, recognition requires regular measurements of blood pressure during normal growth and development. The current recommendation is for infants, children, and adolescents to have their blood pressure checked beginning at age 3 and annually thereafter. All symptomatic adolescents, including those evaluated in emergency rooms, hospitals, or critical care units, and high-risk or premature infants should have blood pressure routinely measured.

Blood pressure must be measured in a quiet resting state, since the normative data were gathered under these conditions. The blood pressure cuff must cover more than two thirds of the upper arm, with the bladder positioned over the brachial artery and the sensor (Doppler crystal, oscillometer, or stethoscope) placed over the artery.

Systolic blood pressure is the first sound heard as the cuff is deflated (phase I Korotkoff), diastolic blood pressure is either the muffling (phase IV Korotkoff) or disappearance (phase V Korotkoff) of the sounds. The most frequent explanation for an elevated blood pressure is an improperly taken measurement.

Using the standard blood pressure tables for age, gender, and weight, normal blood pressure is a systolic and diastolic pressure less than the 90th percentile, high normal blood pressure is the average of three or more systolic or diastolic pressure measurements from the 90th to the 95th percentile, and high blood pressure is the average of three or more systolic or diastolic pressure measurements greater than the 95th percentile (see Chapter 25). Note that an adolescent who is taller or heavier than average will have a higher blood pressure than an adolescent of average size. (See Figs. 48–1 and 48–2 for gender-, age-, height-, and weight-corrected systolic and diastolic blood pressures.)

Severe symptomatic high blood pressure (hypertensive crisis) includes evidence of cardiovascular or cerebrovascular malfunction.

Evaluation

Adolescents with normal blood pressure on a single reading require continued annual surveillance (Fig. 48–

3). Those with high normal blood pressure on three consecutive measurements separated by at least 3 days should have three-extremity blood pressure measurements (right arm, left arm, and a thigh) to rule out coarctation of the aorta, urinalysis and quantitative urine culture to rule out chronic urinary tract infection, counseling for dietary salt and weight reduction if appropriate, and more frequent surveillance.

Those adolescents with high blood pressure should have a screening to detect a treatable cause of secondary hypertension (Table 48–2) (see also Chapter 67). The younger the child and the higher the blood pressure, the more likely it is that renal or renovascular disease or other cause of secondary hypertension is present.

Adolescents with symptomatic severe high blood pressure fitting the criteria for hypertensive crisis should have aggressive treatment to reduce blood pressure to safer levels and a thorough diagnostic evaluation to determine the underlying cause (see Table 48–1 and Chapter 67).

Those adolescents who have high normal blood pressure and most children with high blood pressure can be evaluated and cared for in the primary physician's office or clinic. Those adolescents with severe hypertension or a perplexing presentation may wisely be referred to a consultant who has expertise in the diagnosis and management of adolescents. A summary of the approach to such severe and complex cases has recently been written by Balfe and associates.

Associated Signs and Symptoms

When symptoms are present, they are usually associated with either sudden onset or chronic severe elevation in blood pressure. The cardiovascular complications of congestive heart failure and pulmonary edema are often associated with left ventricular hypertrophy on electrocardiogram or an increase in myocardial mass measured from the echocardiogram. Cerebrovascular complications include persistent headache, blurred vision, coma, convulsions, or, rarely, stroke. Retinal vascular changes are evidence of acute and chronic severe hypertension.

ETIOLOGY

The dynamic control of blood pressure occurs through a complex feedback mechanism regulating cardiac output, vascular resistance, and blood volume. A number of pathophysiologic defects are recognized as causes of secondary hypertension (Table 48–2). Renal and renovascular disorders are among the most frequent and most important causes (see Chapters 65 and 67).

Primary (or essential) hypertension has as yet no clearly defined pathophysiologic mechanism(s) but likely has a strong genetic component. This concept is supported by studies showing that high blood pressure tends to occur in families. Studies in experimental animals, together with human studies of blood pressure in twins, of erythrocyte sodium-lithium transport, and of familial patterns of blood pressure response to stress, demonstrate the importance of genetic factors in control of blood pressure.

Identification of youth at risk for primary hypertension is important because elevated blood pressure is one of the risk factors for stroke, myocardial infarction, congestive heart failure, and renal failure in adults.

PSYCHOSOCIAL CONSIDERATIONS

Although it is important to identify adolescents with high blood pressure, it is equally important to avoid erroneous identification as a "hypertensive." The dangers of a false-positive diagnosis include labeling within the family and at school, limiting participation in sports, creating an obstacle to obtaining life and health insurance, losing employment opportunities, and risking the potentially harmful side effects of treatment.

Rigorous diagnosis and care of the severely hypertensive child are essential. Careful evaluation and management of the child with normal high blood pressure are judicious.

MANAGEMENT

The treatment of high blood pressure depends on the cause and degree of elevation. Acute symptomatic severe elevation in blood pressure requires immediate evaluation and treatment. Other forms of secondary hypertension frequently require direct intervention such as surgery for coarctation of the aorta or pharmacologic management for those adolescents with chronic renal disease.

The management of high normal or high blood pressure without an identifiable cause is more difficult. The current recommendation is for conservative therapy: weight reduction if obese, exercise, moderate salt restriction (to approximately 2500 mg/day), and avoiding the use of tobacco, particularly cigarette smoking. There is unanimity on the benefits of dynamic exercise; since isometric forms of exercise such as wrestling and weightlifting may lead to elevation in blood pressure, these activities are more often questioned. The present consensus is that supervised graduated isometric exercise is not harmful and may be beneficial.

Weight reduction is particularly important because tracking data from childhood to adulthood indicates that obesity during childhood is most predictive of obesity

---

TABLE 48–1. A Diagnostic Strategy in the Evaluation of High Blood Pressure

Assess general health: History; physical examination; CBC
Exclude drugs or prior illness: History; physical examination
Exclude coarctation of the aorta: 4-extremity BP
Identify renal causes: Auscultate for abdominal bruits; urinalysis; urine culture; electrolytes; BUN
Assess for end-organ changes: Echocardiogram for left ventricle mass; ophthalmoscopy
Assess vascular disease risk factors: Family history; lipid screen for high-density lipoprotein triglycerides

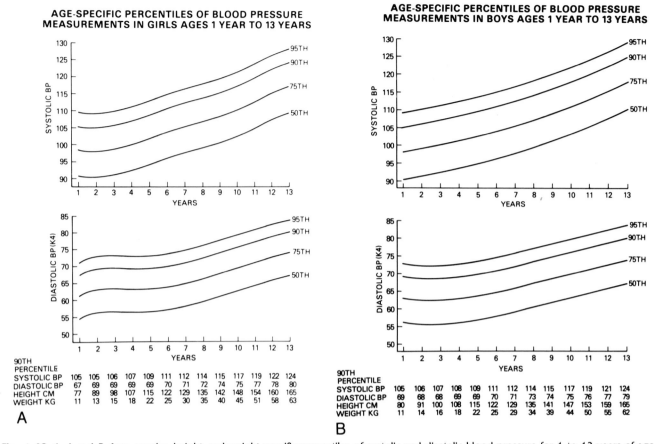

Figure 48–1. *A* and *B*, Age, gender, height, and weight specific percentiles of systolic and diastolic blood pressure for 1 to 13 years of age. (With permission from Task Force on Blood Pressure Control in Children: Report of the Second Task Force on Blood Pressure Control in Children, 1987. Pediatrics 79:1–25, 1987.)

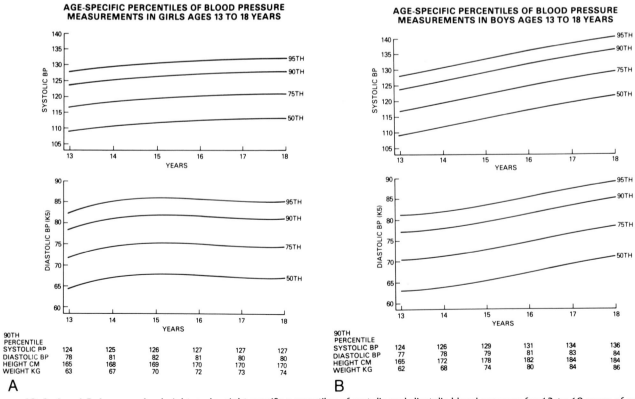

Figure 48–2. *A* and *B*, Age, gender, height, and weight specific percentiles of systolic and diastolic blood pressure for 13 to 18 years of age. (With permission from Task Force on Blood Pressure Control in Children: Report of the Second Task Force on Blood Pressure Control in Children, 1987. Pediatrics 79:1–25, 1987.)

Figure 48–3. Algorithm for identifying adolescents with high blood pressure. (Modified with permission from Task Force on Blood Pressure Control in Children: Report of the Second Task Force on Blood Pressure Control in Children, 1987. Pediatrics 79:1–25, 1987.)

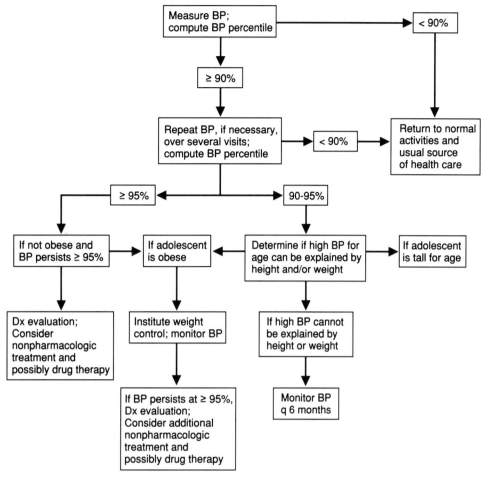

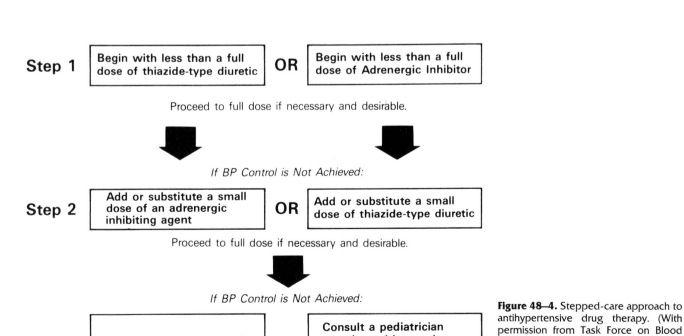

Figure 48–4. Stepped-care approach to antihypertensive drug therapy. (With permission from Task Force on Blood Pressure Control in Children: Report of the Second Task Force on Blood Pressure Control in Children, 1987. Pediatrics 79:1–25, 1987.)

TABLE 48–2. Causes of Secondary Hypertension

RENAL
    Renal parenchymal disease
        Glomerulonephritis
        Pyelonephritis, chronic
        Polycystic kidney
        Connective tissue disease
        Hydronephrosis
        Renal tumors
    Renal vascular disease
        Fibromuscular dysplasia
        Renal arterial obstruction (increased risk in premature
           infants who had an indwelling arterial line)
        Vasculitis
CARDIAC
    Coarctation of the aorta
ADRENAL
    Cortical
        Mineralocorticoid-secreting tumors
        Adrenogenital syndrome
    Medullary
        Pheochromocytoma
NEUROGENIC
    Increased intracranial pressure from a variety of pathologic
        causes
DRUG-INDUCED
    Oral contraceptives
    Amphetamines
    Sympathomimetic amines
    Cocaine, phencyclidine hydrochloride (PCP), illicit drugs,
        licorice

and hence high blood pressure during adulthood. Therefore, strategies designed to prevent the acquisition of excess weight during adolescence may be useful in preventing adult hypertension.

There is a small role for drug treatment because the natural history of blood pressure elevation is obscure, the side effects of lifelong drug treatment are undefined, and the risk of target organ disease is unknown (see Chapter 67). When pharmacologic therapy is necessary, a stepped-care approach has been traditionally used by the pediatrician (Fig. 48–4). Step 1 is usually a thiazide diuretic or adrenergic inhibitor at less than a full dose. Step 2 is the addition of a second drug, gradually increased to full dose. Step 3 is the addition of a third drug, usually in consultation with a physician skilled in treating adolescents with more refractory forms of high blood pressure. Once blood pressure has returned to within the normal range, discontinuing medication is feasible and desirable more often in the young than in older subjects who already have fixed arterial wall changes.

BIBLIOGRAPHY

Balfe JW, Levin L, Tsuru N, Chan JCM: Hypertension in childhood. Adv Pediatr 36:201, 1989.

Burns TL, Lauer RM: Blood pressure in children. In Pierpont MEM, Moller JH (eds): Genetics of Cardiovascular Disease. Boston, Martinius Nijhoff, 1986, pp 305–317.

Gifford RW, Kirkendall W, O'Connor DT, Weidman W: Office evaluation of hypertension. A statement for health professionals by a writing group of the Council for High Blood Pressure Research, American Heart Association. Circulation 79(3):721, 1989.

Lauer RM, Clarke WR: Childhood risk factors for adult high blood pressure: The Muscatine study. Pediatrics 84:633, 1989.

Lauer RM, Anderson AR, Beaglehole R, Burns TL: Factors related to tracking of blood pressure in children. Hypertension 6:307, 1984.

Task Force on Blood Pressure Control in Children: Report of the Second Task Force on Blood Pressure Control in Children, 1987. Pediatrics 79:1, 1987.

CHAPTER 49

Cardiovascular Risk Factors and Prevention

ALBERT P. ROCCHINI

Coronary artery disease has its origins in childhood. Coronary atherosclerotic fatty streaks and fibrous plaques are found at autopsy in many adolescents and young adults. Although the importance of fatty streaks in young people is uncertain, fibrous plaques are an early stage of coronary atherosclerosis. Epidemiologic and clinical studies in adults verified risk factors for coronary heart disease.

These risk factors are high blood pressure, cigarette smoking, lack of physical exercise, increased blood levels of cholesterol, and obesity. Current research on risk factors in children and adolescents is focused on interventions aimed at reducing the risk of coronary heart disease through the earliest establishment of a risk-reducing lifestyle. The following chapter will discuss these risk factors, with a focus on how they affect the development of cardiovascular disease.

HYPERTENSION (see Chapters 48 and 67)

During the past 20 years, it has become increasingly clear that hypertension constitutes a major disease process in adolescents as well as in adults. The incidence of hypertension in the pediatric age group varies from 0.6% to 11%, depending on the age group investigated and the criteria used to define hypertension. Discussion of hypertension, its definition, clinical manifestations, and treatment, is contained in Chapters 48 and 67.

Pathophysiology of Hypertension and Cardiovascular Disease

Hypertension increases cardiovascular risk by altering both cardiac and vascular function and structure. The chronic elevation of arterial pressure causes an increase in myocardial oxygen consumption and an increase in left ventricular wall stress that lead to the development of myocardial hypertrophy. Congestive heart failure can also be associated with either long-standing hypertension or the rapid development of severe hypertension, as observed in adolescents with malignant hypertension. Chronic myocardial hypertrophy is also associated with an increased incidence of cardiac arrhythmias.

Hypertension is also associated with the development of smooth muscle hypertrophy in both large and small arteries. Although the vascular hypertrophy is observed in all organ beds, the changes that occur in the renal, cerebral, and coronary beds are responsible for most of the pathologic consequences of hypertension. In addition to muscular hypertrophy of the systemic arterial tree, hypertension also causes changes in the vascular endothelium that predispose these vessels to the early development of atherosclerosis.

CIGARETTE SMOKING (see Chapters 38 and 44)

If cigarette smoking were eliminated in the United States, there would be an estimated one-third fewer adults with heart disease, 50% fewer with bladder cancer, 85% fewer with chronic obstructive lung disease, and 90% fewer with lung cancer. Although more than 30 million persons in the United States have stopped cigarette smoking in the past 30 years, the prevalence of cigarette smoking has not decreased among adolescents. The majority of adolescents are aware that cigarette smoking is a health hazard, but few believe that it is a threat to their health. Since most adolescents believe they can stop cigarette smoking at will, they do not consider the threat of chronic disease. Thus, adolescents, and particularly female adolescents, represent the largest group of subjects at risk for beginning cigarette smoking (see Chapters 2 and 38).

Pathophysiology

Cigarette smoking increases cardiovascular risk by altering a number of the cardiovascular risk factors. Cigarette smokers have higher serum cholesterol levels and lower levels of high-density lipoprotein (HDL) cholesterol than do nonsmokers. Cigarette smokers have lower blood pressure levels, although it has been found that blood pressure in cigarette smokers rises during the act of smoking. This higher pressure is believed by some investigators to possibly be associated with increased cardiovascular risk.

Treatment

The most effective way of treating cigarette smoking is through its prevention prior to adolescence (see Chapters 36 and 38). Most investigators believe that since the incidence of cigarette smoking is highest among adolescents, it is in this age group that smoking intervention is most critical. Many factors are associated with the teenager's decision to start smoking cigarettes (see Chapters 37 and 38). Although numerous efforts have been made to educate adolescents about the harmful effects of cigarette smoking with the hope that education will lead to avoidance, virtually all studies have come to the same conclusion: education about the harmful effects of cigarette smoking, alone, will not prevent cigarette smoking.

LACK OF CARDIOVASCULAR
FITNESS (see Chapter 81)

Lack of cardiovascular fitness due to lack of physical exercise has been documented by many investigators to be an important cardiovascular risk factor. The effect of exercise training on cardiovascular risk has been studied predominantly in adults. In adults, exercise dilates coronary arteries, decreases triglycerides, increases HDL cholesterol levels, increases cardiac efficiency, decreases blood pressure, and helps maintain a desirable body weight. Exercise level correlates inversely with elevated cholesterol levels, triglyceride levels, and obesity. The changes in triglyceride levels are transitory, returning to pre-exercise levels within a few days following cessation of physical activity. Increased levels of physical activity increase HDL cholesterol, which lowers total serum cholesterol by increased tissue cholesterol clearance and by transporting cholesterol to the liver for breakdown and excretion. Although most physical training studies do show a significant change in the ratio of HDL cholesterol to total cholesterol, there is usually no significant reduction in total serum cholesterol.

Although it is clear that physical activity may be instrumental in improving some of the coronary risk factors in adults, there has been limited information concerning the effects of exercise in children and adolescents. Gilliam and colleagues have shown that after a strenuous 6-week exercise program in 8- to 10-year-old females, there is an increase in HDL levels and lean body mass, whereas triglycerides decrease in two thirds of subjects who had previously confirmed hypertriglyceridemia. Weltman and co-workers have demonstrated that hydraulic-resistance strength training also can significantly improve serum lipid levels in prepubertal boys. Rocchini and co-workers have shown that a 5-month weight-loss program involving caloric restriction and exercise conditioning resulted in a decrease in blood pressure, lipids, and body fat.

More research is needed to delineate the interaction of age, exercise intensity, and coronary disease prevention during childhood. Although there are insufficient longitudinal data available in adolescents relating cardiovascular risk reduction to exercise status, it is prudent to encourage regular physical activity. It may reduce or minimize the development of coronary artery disease during adulthood and may set a pattern for a physically active way of life.

Treatment

An exercise program prescription for an adolescent must include specific instruction for the type, intensity, frequency, and duration of exercise. After an initial 1- to 3-week period of gradually increasing exercise, a goal of 30- to 60-minute sessions three to four times per week is required to maintain cardiovascular fitness. The recommended duration of a particular exercise in a session varies with the type and intensity; for example, walking may be recommended for 30 minutes and jogging for only 15 minutes. Each session should include 5- to 10-minute warm-up and cool-down periods of gentle stretching, walking, or easy jogging. The program must be individualized by considering the type of exercise the adolescent enjoys, the available facilities and equipment, and the assessment of the subject's exercise limitations and capacity. Without guidance, the beginner may exceed his or her physical capabilities and can experience pain, exhaustion, frustration, and ultimately noncompliance to the fitness program.

An exercise program should give specific written instruction for exercise. Presenting the adolescent with an exercise prescription form (Fig. 49–1), complete with his or her data regarding type, frequency, duration, and intensity of exercise, heart rate goals, height, weight, and exercise goals, is a simple and effective method of providing the adolescent with a concise demonstration of expectations.

Not all types of exercise are equally useful for achieving cardiovascular fitness. Activities requiring effort against heavy resistance, such as weightlifting, can cause increased efficiency and hypertrophy of certain muscle groups but do little to improve cardiovascular fitness. To achieve the desired degree of cardiovascular adaptation and conditioning, aerobic exercise is necessary. During aerobic exercise there is a balance between oxygen supply and demand by the muscular tissue. Any activity that can be maintained continuously, is rhythmic, and uses large groups of muscles is aerobic. Activities in which distance, speed, and duration can be specified are recommended, such as vigorous walking, jogging, skating, skiing, aerobic dance, cross-country skiing, bicycling, and swimming.

Monitoring the intensity of the exercise can be done best by taking the pulse and attempting to keep it within a "target zone" for fitness training response. The maximal heart rate is determined by subtracting the patient's age from the number 220. The goal heart rate to obtain a training response is 70% to 80% of this estimated maximal heart rate. For example, a 14-year-old adolescent's average training heart rate would be determined by $(220 - 14) \times 0.75 = 154$ beats/minute.

Despite the reported benefits of regular aerobic exercise training, the initial dropout rate is high. Incentives to continue to exercise include an increase in lean body mass and work capacity. Improved feelings of general

Figure 49–1. An example of an exercise prescription.

Exercise Prescription Form

NAME _____   DATE _____

Measurements: _____
                        HEIGHT   WEIGHT

Activity/Exercise (circle choices)

Walking   Jogging   Aerobic Dancing   X-C Skiing   Bicycling   Roller Skating   Swimming

Other _____   _____

Frequency:

DAY: Mon   Tues   Wed   Thurs   Fri   Sat   Sun

TIME: _____   _____   _____   _____   _____   _____   _____

Duration:

WARM-UP: 5-10 minutes of gentle stretching, walking and slow paced jogging.

ACTIVITY/EXERCISE: 20-60 minutes.

COOL-DOWN: 5-10 minutes of gentle stretching, walking and slow paced jogging.

Intensity:

Count your pulse about five minutes into the ACTIVITY/EXERCISE PORTION of your workout. Find the beat as quickly as possible and count for six seconds. Multiply this number by ten to get your heart rate per minute.

Your maximum heart rate is approximately: _____

Your workout or goal heart rate should be approximately: _____

Heart rate too FAST? Slow your pace down. Heart rate too SLOW? Pick up the pace!!

Remember: There is no such thing as instant fitness. Be patient!! Anything worth having is worth working and waiting for. Go slowly at first. Can you carry on a conversation while exercising? If not, slow the pace until you can. If you miss a few days of your exercise program, get back in to it gradually.

Keep a log of your weekly exercise accomplishments. Increase the duration and intensity of exercise no more than 10% per week.

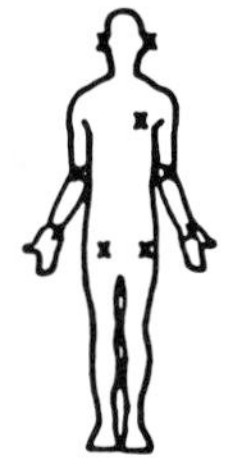

PLACES TO FIND YOUR PULSE

well-being should be explicitly mentioned to the adolescent when the exercise program is presented. Support from family and friends is also important in continued compliance; exercising with a partner may be an incentive to continue to exercise for some adolescents.

LIPIDS (see Chapters 25 and 60)

Epidemiologic surveys show a strong association between plasma cholesterol concentration and the risk of clinically evident coronary artery disease. This finding has been uniform throughout many countries and over a wide range of ethnicity. The Bogalusa, Louisiana, studies suggest that there is a direct link between abnormal lipid profiles in children and the development of atherosclerosis in adults. In a study performed on children, adolescents, and young adults who died from causes unrelated to coronary artery disease, fatty streaks involving the intimal surface of the aorta were present in as many as 61% of patients. The coronary arteries of 29 of 35 (85%) subjects had fatty streaks and fibrous plaques. Raised lesions that progressed to narrow the coronary lumen were also found in the coronary arteries of 6 of the 24 (25%) late adolescent males whose mean age was 19.5 years at death.

The prevalence of lesions in the aorta and coronary arteries appears to vary among gender and race groups. No fibrous plaques were observed in any of the female patients in the Bogalusa study. Fatty streaks in both abdominal and thoracic aortae were more extensive in black subjects than in white subjects. The premortem concentrations of total cholesterol and low-density lipoprotein (LDL) cholesterol in the serum strongly correlated with the extent of aortic fatty streaks. The extent of aortic fatty streaks was inversely associated with the ratio of HDL cholesterol to LDL cholesterol. Higher values for serum triglycerides were also observed in those individuals who had fibrous plaques compared with those who did not. These observations strongly suggest that hyperlipidemia is an important risk factor for the development of atherosclerosis beginning during adolescence.

Pathophysiology

Lipids are insoluble in water and are transported in plasma in protein and phospholipid-coated particles (lipoproteins). Lipoproteins are classified by their ultracentrifugal density, which is related to size. The protein components of lipoproteins are called apoproteins (Table 49–1). Cholesterol is required by nearly every cell for the manufacture and repair of plasma membranes and in certain organs for the production of bile acids and steroids. The sources of cholesterol include dietary cholesterol, intracellular production, and intercellular recycling. Figure 49–2 is a schematic drawing of how the cell regulates cholesterol metabolism.

Some of the cholesterol pool is secreted into the

TABLE 49–1. Physical Properties of Lipoprotein Particles of Human Plasma

LIPOPROTEIN	DENSITY	SIZE (Å)	PROTEIN (%)	CHOLESTEROL (%)	TRIGLYCERIDE (%)	APOPROTEIN
Chylomicron	<0.95	300–5000	2	8	83	A-I, A-II, B-48, C-I, C-II, C-III, E
VLDL	0.95–1.006	300–750	9	22	50	A-I, A-II, B-100, C-I, C-II, C-III, E
LDL	1.006–1.063	200–250	21	46	10	B-100
HDL	1.063–1.021	100–150	33	30	8	A-I, A-II

intestines, either as cholesterol or as bile acid; the remainder of the pool combines with triglyceride to form particles called very low-density lipoproteins (VLDL). These pass into the blood stream, where they are either removed by adipose or muscle tissue, or converted into intermediate density lipoprotein that is quickly converted in the circulation to LDL. LDL is then removed from the plasma by binding to LDL receptors on the liver or other nonhepatic cells that recognize surface apoproteins. LDL is then incorporated into lysozymes and broken down into its constituents.

Cells prefer to use exogenous cholesterol rather than to manufacture it. This preferential usage depends on a negative feedback system in which elevated cholesterol levels reduce cholesterol production by inhibiting the enzyme 3-hydroxy-3-methylglutaryl coenzyme A (HMG CoA) reductase and activate acylcoenzyme A transferase (ACAT), which esterifies cholesterol for storage and inhibits formation of LDL receptor proteins, reducing uptake of cholesterol by the cell. High intracellular cholesterol levels, as occur with a high cholesterol diet, lead to hypercholesterolemia by reducing the disposal of LDL, not by directly increasing cholesterol in the plasma. Reduction of intracellular cholesterol, such as occurs with a low cholesterol diet, ileal bypass, or the use of bile acid sequestrants, leads to up-regulation of the LDL receptor, more rapid catabolism of LDL, and a reduction in the total plasma cholesterol content. However, as the intracellular content of cholesterol falls, intracellular synthesis increases, attenuating the initial lowering.

The cholesterol that passes out of the cell combines with the recycled LDL surface constituents to form nascent HDL particles. In the circulation, these nascent HDL particles bind to peripheral cells, where they take up excess intracellular cholesterol. The apoprotein on the surface of these particles activates the enzyme lecithin cholesterol acetyl transferase (LCAT), which transforms the cholesterol into cholesterol esters. These HDL particles eventually are removed from the circulation by the liver, where the ester is extracted and excreted either as free cholesterol or as bile. Because the formation of HDL cholesterol is the major way in which cholesterol is removed from cells, it has been termed "good cholesterol."

Abnormalities in LDL-receptor development result in

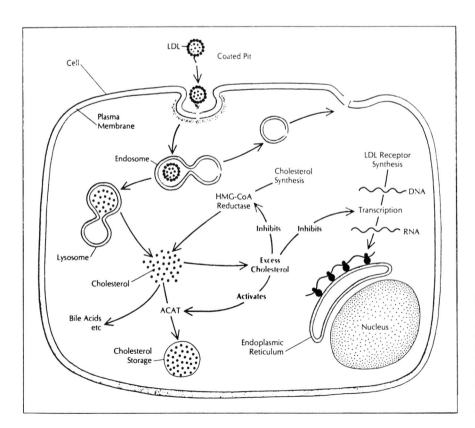

Figure 49–2. Schematic representation of cell regulation of cholesterol metabolism. Abbreviations: LDL, low-density lipoprotein cholesterol; ACAT, acyl coenzyme A transferase; HMG-CoA, 3-hydroxy-3-methylglutaryl coenzyme A. (With permission from Goldstein JL, Brown MS: Familial hypercholesterolemia: A genetic receptor disease. Hosp Pract 20(11):35–46, 1985. Illustration by Irwin Kuperberg.)

TABLE 49–2. Genetic Forms of Hyperlipoproteinemia

DISORDER	PHENOTYPES	MODE OF INHERITANCE	FREQUENCY IN POPULATION
Exogenous hypertriglyceridemia	Type I	Autosomal recessive (?)	Very rare
Familial hypercholesterolemia	Types IIA, IIB	Autosomal dominant	0.1–0.2%
Familial hypertriglyceridemia	Types IV, V	Autosomal dominant	0.2–0.3%
Familial combined hyperlipidemia	Types IIA, IIB, IV, V	Autosomal dominant	0.3–0.5%
Polygenic hypercholesterolemia	Types IIA, IIB	Polygenic	?
Sporadic hypertriglyceridemia	Types IV, V	Nongenetic	?
Broad-beta disease (dysbetalipoproteinemia)	Types III, IV	Autosomal dominant	Rare

one of the common genetic forms of hyperlipidemia, familial hypercholesterolemia. Reduced binding of LDL to the receptors on the cell surface leads to elevated serum LDL concentration, elevated serum plasma cholesterol, and atherogenesis. One half of the normal number of LDL receptors is usually seen in heterozygotes.

Another genetic disease called dysbetalipoproteinemia, or broad-beta disease, has a different molecular basis. In this condition, there is a defect in the metabolism of both intermediate density lipoproteins and chylomicron remnants. In certain patients with this genetic pattern, levels of serum cholesterol and triglycerides are high; individuals with this condition have a high incidence of both coronary artery disease and peripheral vascular disease.

Clinical Manifestations

Table 49–2 summarizes the phenotypic expression, mode of inheritance, and frequency in the population of genetic forms of hyperlipidemia, and Table 49–3 presents the percentiles for cholesterol, triglycerides, LDL cholesterol, and HDL cholesterol. Chapter 60 has further discussion of clinical manifestations and definitions.

Diagnosis

Family history of premature (<55 years of age) coronary artery disease is of prime importance in the initial evaluation of the adolescent patient with hyperlipid-

emia. Other historical features also suggest the presence of hyperlipidemia, as noted in Chapter 60.

Differential Diagnosis (see Chapter 60)

Hyperlipoproteinemia may be either idiopathic or related to medical disorders. The medical disorders that are commonly associated with secondary elevations of lipids include thyroid, renal, and liver disease and diabetes mellitus (see Chapters 55, 59, and 62). Hypercholesterolemia due to elevations of LDL cholesterol commonly occurs in hypothyroidism. Marked elevations of LDL cholesterol, VLDL cholesterol, and triglyceride also occur with nephrotic syndrome (see Chapter 65). Hepatomas, acute intermittent porphyria, and anorexia nervosa are other rare causes of elevated LDL cholesterol concentrations. In biliary obstruction, plasma cholesterol and HDL cholesterol levels can be markedly elevated, but the hypercholesterolemia in biliary obstruction is most commonly due to the presence of an abnormal lipoprotein.

Because the levels of apoprotein B receptors are dependent in part on insulin levels, LDL cholesterol levels may be elevated in diabetes mellitus. With diabetes mellitus, VLDL cholesterol and triglyceride levels are usually elevated as well.

Treatment (see Chapter 60)

The goal of therapy is to reduce the total plasma cholesterol and LDL cholesterol content to less than 180 to 200 mg/dl and 120/dl, respectively, and the LDL-

TABLE 49–3. Lipid Values for Adolescent Atherosclerosis Risk Assessment

PERCENTILE	TOTAL CHOLESTEROL				TRIGLYCERIDES				LDL CHOLESTEROL				HDL CHOLESTEROL			
	5	50	75	95	5	50	75	95	5	50	75	95	5	50	75	95
Age (yr) Sex																
10–14 m	119	158	173	202	32	66	74	125	64	97	109	133	37	55	61	74
f	126	164	171	205	32	60	85	105	68	97	109	136	37	52	—	70
15–19 m	113	150	168	197	32	66	88	125	62	94	—	130	30	46	52	63
f	120	158	176	203	39	75	85	132	59	96	—	137	35	52	—	74
20–24 m	118	159	179	197	44	78	107	165	66	101	118	147	30	45	51	63
f	121	165	186	237	52	96	126	175	70	98	136	151	37	50	60	73

—, n too small to report.
Data from Lipid Metabolism Branch, Division of Heart, Lung and Vascular Disease, National Heart, Lung and Blood Institute: The Lipid Research Clinics' Population Studies Data Book, Vol 1. The Prevalence Study. US Department of Health and Human Services, Public Health Services, National Institutes of Health. NIH Pub. No. 80-1527. Washington, DC, Government Printing Office, 1980.

to-HDL ratio to 3 or less (see Table 49–3). The initial and most important aspect of lipid management is diet.

Weight reduction and exercise are additional effective nonpharmacologic forms of therapy for hyperlipidemia if diet alone is unsuccessful. Obesity-related insulin resistance is associated with increased VLDL triglycerides and the subsequent production of LDL cholesterol. In addition, obesity, through its effects on lipoprotein lipase, is associated with a decrease in HDL cholesterol (Fig. 49–3). Exercise tends to result in weight loss, decrease in percentage of body fat, and increase in HDL cholesterol.

If attempts to modify diet, obesity, and exercise are not effective in lowering lipids, medication may be added to the therapeutic regimen. The initial lipid-lowering agents used in adolescents are bile acid sequestrants that bind bile acids in the intestines to prevent their reabsorption (see Chapter 60).

Course of Illness and Prognosis

Treatment of hyperlipidemia can result in a reduction in coronary-related mortality and regression of atherosclerotic lesions in adults. There are a number of well-conducted long-term studies that outline the efficacy of such treatment. From a dietary standpoint, several controlled dietary studies with clinical end points have been reported. These studies include the Los Angeles Veterans Administration Study, Minnesota Mental Hospital Study, Finnish Diet Study, and Oslo Diet Heart Study. The sample sizes and duration of these studies are not yet sufficient to demonstrate a beneficial effect of lowering cholesterol.

Three non–double-blind studies have been reported that attempted to modify other risk factors in addition to hypercholesterolemia. Two of these studies have demonstrated some substantial improvement in plasma cholesterol as well as in mortality. In the Oslo Heart Trial, 412 hypercholesterolemic male smokers were randomized to a treatment group (cholesterol-lowering diet and efforts to discourage cigarette smoking) and a control group. Compared with the control group, the

treatment group sustained a 13% lowering of plasma cholesterol, and there was a significant reduction in the incidence of both nonfatal and fatal myocardial infarctions. In the United States, the Multiple Risk Factor Intervention Trial tested the efficacy of modifying several risk factors in reducing the incidence of coronary disease in 1200 healthy but high-risk men. Lowering of cholesterol appeared to be related to lower mortality for normotensive smokers with high initial cholesterol values.

A definite beneficial effect of lowering cholesterol is suggested by the Lipid Clinic's Coronary Primary Prevention Trial, a randomized, double-blind, placebo-controlled study involving treatment with a low cholesterol diet and cholestyramine of 3806 hypercholesterolemic men who were 35 to 59 years of age and free of evident coronary artery disease at entry. The 12.6% reduction in LDL cholesterol was associated with a 19% reduction in myocardial infarction and death due to coronary heart disease and a 20% decrease in angina and the need for coronary artery bypass. This study demonstrated the direct and linear correlation between the degree of lipid lowering and the degree of reduction of coronary heart disease death. With regard to the adolescent, little to no data are available on the efficacy of long-term treatment of mild to moderately elevated cholesterol levels to prevent atherosclerosis later in life.

OBESITY (see Chapters 25 and 60)

A study by Becque and co-workers reported that ninety-seven percent of obese adolescents had four or more of the following cardiac risk factors: elevated serum triglyceride levels, decreased HDL cholesterol levels, increased total cholesterol level, elevated blood pressure, diminished maximum work capacity, and strong family history of coronary heart disease.

Pathophysiology

Based on recent research, it appears that the likely mechanism by which obesity increases cardiovascular risk is through its association with hyperlipidemia, hypertension, and glucose intolerance (see Chapter 67). High blood pressure is known to be associated with obesity. Obese adolescents have a blood pressure distribution that is greater than one standard deviation higher than that of the general population (Fig. 49–4), which normalizes with weight loss, especially when the weight loss is combined with physical conditioning.

The mechanisms for high blood pressure in obese adolescents include increased sodium retention, blood volume, and cardiac output (see Chapter 67). The sodium retention may be due to the combined effects of hyperinsulinemia, hyperaldosteronism, and increased sympathetic nervous system (SNS) activity associated with obesity.

The other major cardiovascular risk factor associated with obesity is abnormal plasma lipids. When children and adult subjects are stratified for fatness, there is a direct relationship between lipid levels and obesity.

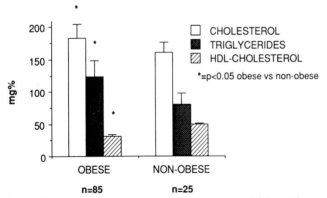

Figure 49–3. The lipoprotein profile of 85 obese and 25 nonobese adolescents (ages 10 to 16 years). Compared with the nonobese adolescents, the obese adolescents have significantly elevated total cholesterol and triglyceride levels and reduced HDL cholesterol levels.

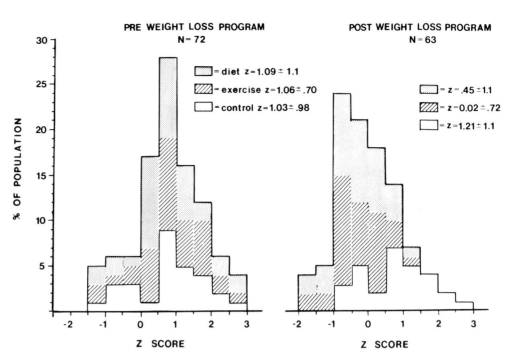

Figure 49–4. Distribution of systolic blood pressure in obese adolescents compared with those rates reported in the Second National Health and Nutrition Examination Survey, before and after a 20-week weight loss program. All values presented are mean ±50. Weight loss groups were designated as Diet (diet and behavior change), Exercise (diet, behavior change, and exercise), and Control (obese control group). (With permission from Rocchini AP, Katch V, Anderson J, et al: Blood pressure in obese adolescents: Effect of weight loss. Pediatrics 82:16, 1988.)

Obesity is the most common cause of hypertriglyceridemia in adolescents who are free from other diseases causing secondary hypertriglyceridemia. In addition, obesity is frequently associated with a significant depression in HDL cholesterol (see Fig. 49–3). Becque and co-workers have demonstrated that, as with blood pressure, lipid abnormalities are markedly improved in obese adolescents following weight loss and that a weight-loss program that incorporates exercise along with calorie restriction produces the most favorable effects on lipids (Fig. 49–5).

Treatment (see Chapter 60)

Treatment modalities involve six fundamental strategies: calorie restriction, anorectic drugs, increased physical activity, therapeutic starvation, bypass surgery, and behavior changes based on social learning therapy. These strategies are limited, produce only modest outcomes, and are so poorly defined that systematic replication has been difficult. For example, group weight loss, or the percentage of weight loss for a total group, frequently is reported without recognizing initial differences among subjects. In addition, many studies report only changes in gross body weight without defining the compositional changes that occur with an adolescent weight reduction program. Data generated in adults suggest that weight loss induced by diet alone results in greater losses in lean body mass than weight loss resulting from diet plus exercise. This is important when caring for adolescents, because in this age group, it is especially important to protect the body cell mass to allow for future growth (see Chapter 6). Data from Rocchini and co-workers suggest that, in the adolescent population, weight loss that is accompanied by a physical

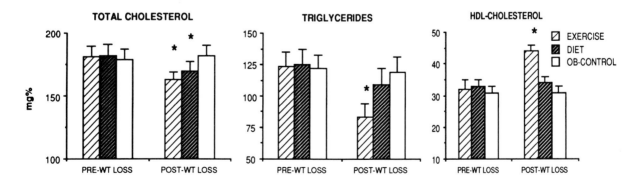

MEAN±SE; *=p<0.01 pre vs post

Figure 49–5. The lipid profile of obese adolescents before and after a 20-week weight loss program. Weight loss, whether or not it is associated with improved exercise conditioning, is associated with a decrease in total cholesterol. However, a weight loss program that incorporates an exercise program is associated with the greatest reductions in cholesterol and triglycerides and the greatest increase in HDL cholesterol.

training program results in a greater loss in fat mass and a greater preservation of lean body mass. In addition, weight reduction as the sole goal of treatment of obesity may be too narrow a focus for adolescents. To interest adolescents, incentives such as increased energy, endurance, fitness, or well-being; decreased fatigue or joint pains; and improved breathing or sports-related skills should be emphasized. These may be more important motivators to lose weight for the egocentric adolescent than for children or adults.

At the University of Michigan, an adolescent weight-loss program has been developed. First, adolescents undergo a thorough history and physical examination. The goal of this examination is to determine any biologic reason for the obesity. Second, the dietary histories of the family and the adolescent are assessed. It is recommended that they meet individually with a dietitian who assesses the adolescent's diet and determines the overall motivation of the family to participate in a weight-loss program. Third, before any adolescent is enrolled in a weight-loss program, he or she should be placed on a trial diet for 2 to 3 weeks. The trial diet in use at the University of Michigan is an introduction to the Problems, Sweets, Snacks, or Fried (PSSF) food contract. The PSSF foods are those that add large amounts of calories to the diet but contain very few nutrients. Adolescents are permitted to continue to eat such items, provided that they agree to record and limit their use to eight such foods weekly.

Initiating the diet by having the adolescent keep the PSSF food contract does several things: (1) The adolescent has control over food choices; (2) the adolescent starts to monitor types of food consumed and portion sizes; (3) overall caloric intake is limited, by decreasing the amount and number of high calorie foods; and (4) the dietitian evaluates the adolescent's motivation to participate in a weight-loss program. If the adolescent is successful with this trial diet, follows the contract, and loses at least 1 to 2 pounds in 2 to 3 weeks, he or she is admitted into the formal weight-loss program. If the adolescent is unsuccessful, the family and the adolescent are counseled. Then they are invited back in 3 to 6 months or sooner if they believe they want to try the program again.

The actual weight-loss program has three components: diet, behavior change, and exercise. During the initial visit, the adolescent is given copies of food records and instructions and is asked to complete a daily food record for 6 days. The caloric requirements necessary for the adolescents to lose 1 to 2 pounds per week are determined by reducing the current level of calories by 500 to 1000 calories per day. An additional 200 calories is subtracted to allow for one PSSF food daily. Adolescent weight reduction diets should not go below 1200 calories per day, because with fewer calories it is difficult to provide adequate vitamins and nutrients to promote normal growth and development (Chapters 6 and 7). Calorie levels should never exceed 2500 calories per day; teenagers will not take the diet seriously if they are allowed too large an intake of calories. An exchange diet is used in the program, since it teaches the adolescent the essentials of good nutrition and involves the adolescent in determining his or her own diet. The

caloric breakdown of the diet should follow the American Heart Association phase one diet (see Chapter 60).

The behavior change components of this program include 1-hour, weekly classes for 20 weeks and then every other week until the adolescent has maintained his or her goal weight for at least 1 month. The classes center around four major elements: nutrition education, record keeping, stimulus control for restricting the external cues that set the occasion for eating, and reinforcement of alternative behavior. The purpose of the behavior change component is to teach the obese adolescent to eat like nonobese people, to become aware of current food habits, and to accept responsibility for his or her eating behaviors. Self-monitoring provides both the adolescent and the nutritionist with the means of assessing progress and behavior change. The behavior therapy program has a built-in reinforcement system (nonfood "points") so that adolescents can maintain their new habits. Each adolescent accumulates points by complying with various components of the behavior program. Parents are encouraged to give positive support and are discouraged from keeping the adolescent's records. The nutritionist monitors parental support closely.

Along with calorie restriction and behavior change, adolescents in this program are encouraged to increase their physical activity levels. Prior to starting the exercise component of the program, all adolescents should undergo an evaluation of physical fitness so that an appropriate exercise program can be developed (see Chapter 81). This is usually accomplished by administering a graded treadmill exercise test in conjunction with a measurement of oxygen consumption. Following the exercise test, all adolescents are enrolled in a 2-week structured exercise class that meets 3 days per week. During this initial 2-week period, the adolescents are instructed in warm-up activities and heart rate monitoring and begin a walking/jogging program. The adolescents are also instructed on exercise record keeping. Following the 2-week class, the adolescents are encouraged to exercise on their own at home, attempting to achieve levels of activity that will consume approximately 500 calories per day. In addition to reinforcing exercise habits and monitoring fitness improvement, the adolescent is expected to attend one structured exercise class per month through the weight-loss program.

BIBLIOGRAPHY

Becque MD, Katch VL, Rocchini AP, et al: Coronary risk incidence of obese adolescents: Reduction by exercise plus diet intervention. Pediatrics 81:605, 1988.

Berenson GS, McMahan CA, Voors AW, et al: Cardiovascular Risk Factors in Children: The Early Natural History of Atherosclerosis and Essential Hypertension. New York, Oxford University Press, 1980.

Berenson GS, Srinivasan SR, Nicklas TA, Webber LS: Cardiovascular risk factors in children and early prevention of heart disease. Clin Chem 34:B115, 1988.

Dayton S, Pearce ML, Hashimoto S, et al: A controlled clinical trial of the high diet and unsaturated fat in preventing complications of atherosclerosis. Circulation 40(Suppl):111, 1969.

Frantz ID, Dawson EA, Kuba K, et al: Minnesota Coronary Survey: Effect of diet and cardiovascular events in death. Circulation 52:4, 1975.

Gilliam T, Katch V: Coronary heart disease risk in children. In Cureton TK Jr, Stull A (eds): Encyclopedia of Physical Education, Fitness and Sports. Salt Lake City, UT, Brighton Publishing, 1980, pp 495–502.

Goldstein JL, Brown MS: Familial hypercholesterolemia. In Stanbury JB, Wyngaarden JB, Fredrickson DS, et al (eds): Metabolic Basis of Inherited Disease, 5th ed. New York, McGraw-Hill, 1983, pp 672–712.

Hofman A: Blood pressure in childhood: an epidemiological approach to the aetiology of hypertension. J Hypertens 2:323, 1984.

Lauer RM, Shekelle RV (eds): Childhood Prevention of Atherosclerosis and Hypertension. New York, Raven Press, 1980.

Leren P: The effect of plasma cholesterol lowering diet in male survivors of myocardial infarction. Acta Med Scand 466(Suppl):1, 1966.

Lipid Metabolism Branch, Division of Heart, Lung and Vascular Disease, National Heart, Lung and Blood Institute: The Lipid Research Clinics' Population Studies Data Book, Vol 1. The Prevalence Study. US Department of Health and Human Services, Public Health Service, National Institutes of Health. NIH Pub. No. 80-1527. Washington, DC, Government Printing Office, 1980.

Miettinen M, Turpeinen O, Karvonen MJ, et al: Effect of cholesterol-lowering diet on mortality from coronary heart-disease and other causes: A twelve-year clinical trial in men and women. Lancet 2:835, 1972.

Newman WP III, Freedman DS, Voors AW, et al: Relation of serum lipoprotein levels and systolic blood pressure to early atherosclerosis. The Bogalusa Heart Study. N Engl J Med 314:138, 1986.

Report of the Second Task Force on Blood Pressure Control in Children–1987. Pediatrics 79:1, 1987.

Riley WA, Freedman DS, Higgs NA, et al: Decreased arterial elasticity associated with cardiovascular disease risk factors in the young. Bogalusa Heart Study. Atherosclerosis 6:378, 1986.

Rocchini AP, Katch V, Anderson J, et al: Blood pressure in obese adolescents: Effect of weight loss. Pediatrics 82:16, 1988.

Rocchini AP, Key J, Bondie D, et al: The effect of weight loss on the sensitivity of blood pressure to sodium in obese adolescents. N Engl J Med 321:580, 1989.

Wall M, Brooks, J, Holsclaw D, Redding G: Health effects of smoking on children. Am Rev Respir Dis 132:1137, 1985.

Weltman A, Janney C, Rians CB, et al: The effects of hydraulic-resistance strength training on serum lipid levels in prepubertal boys. Am J Dis Child 141:777, 1987.

CHAPTER 50

Cardiovascular Aspects of Systemic Disease

J. PETER HARRIS and REGINALD L. WASHINGTON

Cardiovascular dysfunction is a frequent component of systemic disease in adolescents. This chapter will review cardiovascular abnormalities encountered in connective tissue diseases, hematologic and oncologic diseases, endocrinopathies, neuromuscular disorders, and infectious diseases. In addition, acute rheumatic fever is discussed because of an increase in its occurrence in the United States. Most patients with suspected cardiovascular abnormalities should be referred to a pediatric cardiologist for evaluation and therapeutic planning, as part of the multidisciplinary approach to complex systemic disease.

CONNECTIVE TISSUE DISEASES

Juvenile Rheumatoid Arthritis
(see Chapters 43 and 90)

Cardiac abnormalities in juvenile rheumatoid arthritis (JRA) include pericarditis, myocarditis, and, rarely, aortitis leading to aortic valve insufficiency. Cardiovascular complications are the third most frequent cause of death in JRA.

Pericarditis, the most common complication, is detected in 7% to 10% of patients on clinical evaluation, 36% by echocardiography, and 45% at postmortem examination. These figures substantiate the high incidence of asymptomatic pericardial inflammation. Pericarditis is usually seen in the systemic form of JRA, especially during acute flares of systemic symptoms, but may also be encountered in other forms of JRA. Infrequently, pericarditis and pericardial effusion are the presenting manifestations of this disease. The signs and symptoms of pericarditis include precordial pain aggravated by lying supine and breathing deeply, a pericardial friction rub, tachycardia, tachypnea, variably distant heart tones, cardiomegaly on chest roentgenogram, and diffuse ST segment elevation on electrocardiogram (ECG). As pericardial fluid separates the visceral and parietal pericardium, the friction rub may disappear. Therefore, a friction rub is not necessary for the diagnosis of pericarditis. Echocardiography is the most sensitive method of evaluating the pericardial space. As pericardial effusion compresses the heart, signs and symptoms of cardiac tamponade occur, including muffled heart tones, elevated jugular venous pressure, hep-atomegaly, dyspnea, and pulsus paradoxus of greater than 12 mmHg.

A typical attack of pericarditis lasts between 1 and 12 weeks, but inflammation may be characterized by variable exacerbations and remissions. Subclinical and mild episodes of pericarditis often do not require therapy and subside spontaneously. More symptomatic episodes are treated with either aspirin or prednisone, depending on the severity of the inflammation. For an adolescent patient already taking prednisone, a transient increase in steroid dosage often resolves the pericardial inflammation. Pericardiocentesis is necessary for treating cardiac tamponade. Some patients require pericardial stripping.

Myocarditis diagnosed by the echocardiographic findings of decreased ventricular function and cardiomegaly without pericardial effusion occurs in 10% of patients. However, the incidence of clinical myocardial dysfunction is much lower. Myocarditis also occurs most commonly in systemic disease during flare-ups. Myocarditis may cause congestive heart failure. Treatment includes steroids and diuretics, but digoxin should be used cautiously because of the increased frequency of arrhythmias in the setting of myocardial inflammation.

Aortic valvulitis with destruction of valve architecture by rheumatoid granulation tissue occurs rarely in JRA. The valvulitis may lead to progressive aortic valve insufficiency and the need for subsequent aortic valve replacement.

Systemic Lupus Erythematosus
(see Chapters 43 and 90)

Overt cardiac manifestations are seen in 20% of young patients with systemic lupus erythematosus (SLE), and subclinical cardiovascular involvement may be demonstrated in an additional 10% of patients. Cardiovascular involvement includes pericarditis, myocarditis, Libman-Sacks endocarditis, arrhythmias, coronary arteritis, and pulmonary hypertension. The cardiovascular manifestations of lupus are directly related to elevated levels of antiphospholipid antibodies, which serve as a marker of cardiovascular involvement.

Pericarditis occurs in 30% of patients. The clinical picture of pericardial inflammation is similar to that seen in JRA. Pericarditis may be the presenting manifestation and usually occurs during acute systemic disease. Treatment includes nonsteroidal anti-inflammatory agents and corticosteroids. However, in contradistinction to JRA, constrictive pericarditis may follow acute pericardial inflammation. Furthermore, bacterial pericarditis may occur, and pericardiocentesis is necessary if there is any question of infection. As in JRA, occult pericarditis is common.

Subclinical and overt evidence of myocarditis is seen in fewer than 10% of patients with SLE but may be found in as many as 25% at autopsy. In addition to the possibility of congestive heart failure, myocardial inflammation may foster atrial and ventricular arrhythmias. If signs and symptoms of congestive heart failure are present, other factors such as anemia, uremia, and hypertension should be considered in addition to myocardial inflammation. Therapy for lupus myocarditis includes steroids and diuretics, but digoxin should be avoided. Fever, infection, anemia, uremia, and hypertension should also be treated.

Nonbacterial verrucous endocarditis, or Libman-Sacks endocarditis, is characteristic of patients with SLE. These lesions are small, gray or pinkish projections occurring singly or in clumps on the mitral and aortic valves, particularly at the valve annuli and commissures. As the lesions heal, fibrosis and calcification may occur. The verrucae are found in 50% of adult patients at autopsy, but the incidence in young patients with SLE is unknown. Most of the lesions are asymptomatic and are not visualized on echocardiography. Uncommonly, distortion of the left heart valves by large lesions may lead to aortic and mitral regurgitation or stenosis. Embolization and superimposed bacterial endocarditis are unusual complications. In rare instances, valve replacement may be necessary. The verrucae often resolve or become smaller with corticosteroid therapy.

Coronary arteritis may occur in acute SLE, causing myocardial dysfunction, arrhythmias, and rarely myocardial infarction. Coronary arteritis responds to corticosteroids. Accelerated coronary artery atherosclerosis is also a potential complication of SLE and may be a consequence of arterial injury due to arteritis and corticosteroid therapy.

Pulmonary hypertension is a rare cardiac manifestation of SLE and may be a sequela of pulmonary arteritis. Because of its rarity and lack of established pathogenetic mechanism, the efficacy of treatment is unclear.

In addition to the usual caveats of the hazards of pregnancy in a systemic illness, adolescents and young women who have SLE should be warned of the possibility of congenital complete heart block and cardiomyopathy in their offspring.

Ankylosing Spondylitis

Ankylosing spondylitis is an example of HLA-B27–associated spondyloarthritis and enthesopathy. Similar to the course in JRA, myopericarditis may occur in ankylosing spondylitis but in fewer than 5% of patients. The presentation, evaluation, and treatment of myopericarditis are described in the section on JRA. Although valvulitis may lead to progressive and severe aortic regurgitation, aortitis and valvulitis usually are late manifestations of spondylitis. Nevertheless, ankylosing spondylitis should be considered in the differential diagnosis of an adolescent patient presenting with newly acquired aortic or mitral valve regurgitation.

Marfan Syndrome

Marfan syndrome is an autosomal dominant defect in elastic tissue in which the most prominent manifestations are extreme height and long digits. Cardiac manifestations include mitral valve prolapse and, less commonly, aortic valve dilatation. Because medial cystic necrosis of the aorta can result in fatal dissecting aneurysm, adolescents taller than the 97th percentile should be examined for stigmata of Marfan syndrome (see Chapter 45).

Ehlers-Danlos Syndrome

Ehlers-Danlos syndrome, a disorder that is transmitted as an autosomal dominant trait, is characterized by hyperextensible skin and joints, fragile skin, easy bruisability, and poor wound healing. Cardiovascular lesions seen in Ehlers-Danlos syndrome, especially in types I and III, include aortic root dilatation and mitral and tricuspid valve prolapse and regurgitation. Rarely, the pulmonary artery and pulmonary valve annulus may be dilated. A dissecting aneurysm of the ascending aorta, aortic rupture, and a rupture of other large arterial vessels are rare and catastrophic complications of type IV Ehlers-Danlos syndrome. Because of poor vascular integrity and wound healing, cardiovascular surgery has an increased risk.

HEMATOLOGIC-ONCOLOGIC DISEASES

Sickle Cell Anemia
(see Chapter 52)

Adolescents with homozygous sickle cell anemia may have cardiac manifestations secondary to the repetitive sickling process. Adolescent patients with profound anemia (<7 g/dl) have an elevated cardiac output with a shortened circulation time and decreased systemic vascular resistance. Pulmonary flow murmurs are common. The apical middiastolic murmur is due to an accelerated rate of flow across the mitral valve and should not be confused with mitral valve stenosis. Fatigue and dyspnea are due to the anemia and ventilation perfusion abnormalities. In general, the lower the hemoglobin level, the poorer the exercise performance. Cardiomegaly is seen on chest roentgenograms. Echocardiography reveals ventricular and atrial dilatation as well as an increase in ventricular mass. The latter finding may be associated with abnormalities of ventricular filling and relaxation.

Secondary cardiac dysfunction occurs in patients with systemic hypertension from chronic renal disease and cor pulmonale from multiple pulmonary infarctions.

Whether a true cardiomyopathy on the basis of the sickling process occurs is still unanswered. Treatment is outlined in Chapter 52.

Beta-Thalassemia
(see Chapter 52)

Although chronic hypertransfusion programs have improved the prognosis of beta-thalassemia, myocardial iron accumulation leads to congestive heart failure in adolescence or early adulthood. Cardiac dysfunction usually occurs after more than 80 units of blood have been transfused.

An important deposition of iron occurs within the ventricular myocardium, leading to myocardial dysfunction with eventual congestive heart failure. The appearance of congestive heart failure is an ominous sign, with death usually occurring within 1 year despite aggressive anticongestive therapy. Left ventricular hypertrophy is noted on ECG, and mild cardiomegaly is seen on chest roentgenograms. On echocardiography, dilatation of the cardiac chambers is apparent. Complications of excess cardiac iron include pericarditis, arrhythmias, and myocardial failure.

The signs and symptoms of pericarditis are as described in the section on JRA. The attacks are usually brief, lasting only a few days to several weeks, and therapy is generally supportive, but large pericardial effusions often require pericardiocentesis or open pericardial drainage. Constrictive pericarditis may occur.

Arrhythmias include atrial and junctional premature beats, supraventricular tachycardia, atrial flutter, heart block, and ventricular ectopy, including ventricular tachycardia. Arrhythmias likely result from iron deposition in the cardiac conduction system.

Iron chelation treatment may prevent or reverse many of the cardiac complications of iron overload. However, arrhythmias may not be as responsive to chelation as is myocardial dysfunction, and the late introduction of chelation therapy may not change the inexorable course of cardiac hemosiderosis. As in many other chronic diseases of adolescence, noncompliance with the chelation regimen may lead to a further deterioration of cardiovascular function.

Oncologic Disorders
(see Chapter 53)

Although intensive chemotherapy and radiation therapy have markedly improved the survival of young cancer patients, the cardiovascular toxicity of these approaches may lead to both early and late cardiovascular sequelae.

Cardiac toxicity occurs after therapy with the anthracycline antibiotic doxorubicin (Adriamycin). Acute congestive heart failure (occurring within 1 year of the completion of doxorubicin therapy) occurs in as many as 10% of patients. This group of patients generally responds to anticongestive therapy, which may later be discontinued. However, late recurrences of congestive heart failure are not uncommon. Other relatively early cardiovascular manifestations of anthracycline cardiac toxicity include atrial and ventricular dysrhythmias, pericarditis-myocarditis syndrome, and acute hypertensive reactions. With the exception of the arrhythmias, the incidence of these complications is low.

A dose-related decrease in QRS voltage and prolongation of the corrected QT interval (QT interval divided by the square root of the RR interval) have also been described.

A disturbing feature of anticancer therapy is the late development of cardiovascular dysfunction, including abnormalities in contractility and ventricular wall thickness in more than one half of children treated with anthracycline-containing chemotherapeutic agents. The late cardiomyopathic findings occur more than 5 years after the completion of treatment. A small increase in ventricular wall thicknesses in relation to somatic growth suggests a disturbance in myocardial growth and ventricular mass. The consequences of the reduction in ventricular mass and contractility are a decrease in cardiac reserve and the late appearance of potentially irreversible congestive heart failure.

Both early and late cardiac toxicity of the anthracyclines are dose related, but other risk factors include the administration of doxorubicin at an early age (younger than 4 years) and concomitant mediastinal radiation. Because the cardiomyopathic features may not become clinically evident until 15 years after the completion of therapy, continued cardiovascular surveillance is necessary. Other factors that may aggravate cardiac dysfunction include isometric exercise, particularly weightlifting, anabolic steroids (see Chapter 81), growth hormone (see Chapter 56), and alcohol and drug abuse (see Chapter 111).

There is no sensitive method for detecting early cardiovascular changes with the aim of preventing the appearance of a late cardiomyopathy. Current strategies include serial follow-up of corrected QT (QT_c) interval, echo measures of ventricular function and wall thicknesses, gated nuclear angiographic assessment of ejection fraction, and endomyocardial biopsy.

A QT_c interval of 0.44 second or more with no change or an increase in this interval with exercise, a serial decrease in left ventricular shortening fraction, and a reduction in left ventricular ejection fraction to less than 50% all suggest cardiac dysfunction and the potential need for discontinuing anthracycline therapy and instituting enhanced cardiovascular surveillance and intervention. Furthermore, a safe cumulative dose of doxorubicin has not been determined. The previously recommended cumulative dose of 550 mg/m^2 has been reduced to 350 mg/m^2 because of the appearance of cardiac toxicity in patients receiving a total dose between these two values. A prolonged, continuous intravenous drug infusion instead of bolus injections may decrease toxicity.

The cardiac toxicity of the anthracyclines is probably related to free radical formation. Investigators are searching for compounds capable of scavaging free radicals or interrupting the free radical cascade.

ENDOCRINOPATHIES
(see Chapter 55)

Juvenile Hyperthyroidism

The cardiovascular manifestations of juvenile hyperthyroidism include tachycardia, a wide pulse pressure, a hyperdynamic precordium, and a pulmonary flow murmur, all of which resolve with treatment. In adolescent patients with prolonged untreated hyperthyroidism or poor compliance with treatment regimens, mitral regurgitation of variable severity may develop. Mitral regurgitation usually resolves with treatment but rarely can be progressive with the appearance of congestive heart failure, necessitating mitral valve replacement or plication. Whether the mitral regurgitation is related to mitral valve prolapse is unclear. Bacterial endocarditis prophylaxis is recommended for mitral insufficiency.

Atrial arrhythmias including supraventricular tachycardia and atrial fibrillation are common in adult patients but are unusual in adolescents. A mild reversible cardiomyopathy with a paradoxical decrease in left ventricular ejection fraction with exercise may occur in the setting of juvenile hyperthyroidism but is usually subclinical and detected only with echocardiography or other noninvasive measures of ventricular function.

Hypothyroidism

The bradycardia and pericardial effusion that occur in hypothyroidism resolve with treatment. Hypertrophic cardiomyopathy can occur in young patients with hypothyroidism.

Pheochromocytoma

Patients with intermittent and sustained hypertension develop symmetric ventricular hypertrophy from chronic β-adrenergic stimulation. The hypertrophy often resolves following surgical removal of the tumor.

Diabetes Mellitus

Adolescents who have diabetes mellitus often have subtle early increases in left ventricular contractility and mild late decreases in both systolic and diastolic ventricular function. These changes are detected only by echocardiography without clinical expressions. Diabetes mellitus is a risk factor for coronary atherosclerosis. Therefore, adolescent patients who have diabetes mellitus should follow a heart-healthy lifestyle (see Chapters 49 and 60).

Miscellaneous Endocrine Disorders

Adolescent patients with hyperinsulinemia associated with lipodystrophies may develop a hypertrophic cardiomyopathy. Adolescents receiving prolonged courses of corticosteroids and adrenocorticotropic hormone (ACTH) also develop hypertrophic cardiomyopathies secondary to sustained arterial hypertension. Close monitoring of arterial blood pressure in individuals receiving steroid therapy is mandatory.

NEUROMUSCULAR DISORDERS

Duchenne Muscular Dystrophy

Patients with Duchenne muscular dystrophy have sinus tachycardia, left axis deviation, short PR interval, and a characteristic electrocardiographic pattern of tall R waves over the right precordium with an R:S ratio of greater than 1 and narrow deep Q waves (greater than 3 mm) over the left precordium and in the limb leads.

Of adolescents with muscular dystrophy, 15% develop mitral valve prolapse with a variable degree of mitral regurgitation, and 20% develop congestive heart failure with a high mortality rate. Dystrophic cardiomyopathic changes include diffuse loss of myofibers, myofiber splitting, fibrosis, vacuolization, and fatty infiltration. If signs of heart failure are present, anticongestive therapy can be instituted, but the inevitable respiratory insufficiency precludes a satisfactory outcome.

Myotonic Dystrophy

Adolescent patients with myotonic muscular dystrophy frequently have electrocardiographic abnormalities, including prolongation of the PR interval, a wide QRS, and bundle branch block. Progression of conduction abnormalities may lead to sudden death. Arrhythmias range from benign atrial premature contractions to life-altering or life-threatening arrhythmias, such as atrial flutter, atrial fibrillation, and ventricular tachycardia. Mitral valve prolapse is common in this disorder. Rarely, a dilated form of cardiomyopathy may be seen in adolescents. Antiarrhythmic medications have been used to treat the myotonia, but caution should be exercised because of the potential for these agents to aggravate the conduction abnormalities.

Friedreich Ataxia

Cardiomyopathies may be the presenting feature of this disorder, so Friedreich ataxia should be included in the differential diagnosis of a patient presenting with a new myopathy. Concentric myocardial hypertrophy is the leading cause of death in Friedreich ataxia. Dilated cardiomyopathy occurs rarely. Patients with hypertrophic cardiomyopathies are usually asymptomatic until evolution into a dilated form occurs with the subsequent appearance of congestive heart failure. Electrocardiographic findings are also common and include nonspecific ST-T wave changes, a short PR interval, deviations of the frontal plane QRS axis, and precordial QRS abnormalities similar to those seen in Duchenne muscular dystrophy.

INFECTIOUS DISEASES

Lyme Disease (see Chapter 90)

Myocarditis occurs in 4% to 10% of patients infected with Lyme disease during the second, or disseminated, stage. Other manifestations include pericarditis and a reversible depression of left ventricular function on echocardiography, and, infrequently, clinical congestive heart failure. Symptoms of Lyme carditis include substernal chest pain, palpitations, syncope, and dyspnea. Heart block of varying degrees is the most frequent manifestation of Lyme carditis. Lyme disease should be in the differential diagnosis of an adolescent patient with newly diagnosed heart block who lives in an endemic area. Atrioventricular block including complete heart block is usually well tolerated with an adequate and narrow QRS escape rhythm. Rarely, temporary transvenous tracing is necessary if the ventricular rate is inadequate and signs of congestive heart failure are present. The atrioventricular block is usually short-lived and resolves within 1 to 2 weeks. If myocarditis develops, signs of cardiac involvement usually appear 4 to 5 weeks after the initial illness. The appearance of marked prolongation of the PR interval, second degree atrioventricular block, or complete heart block mandates hospitalization with continuous electrocardiographic monitoring. Treatment consists of either intravenous penicillin or oral tetracycline for 10 to 20 days. Whether early therapy with penicillin or tetracycline prevents or modifies the appearance of Lyme carditis is unknown.

Acquired Immunodeficiency Syndrome
(see Chapter 76)

Cardiac disease occurs in two thirds of young patients with acquired immunodeficiency syndrome (AIDS). The abnormalities include ventricular dysfunction with dilated cardiomyopathy, pericardial effusions, and, rarely, endocarditis. Hypertrophic cardiomyopathy progresses to a dilated hypocontractile heart. Acute myopericarditis due to opportunistic pathogens or to the human immunodeficiency virus is the cause of ventricular dysfunction and accumulation of pericardial fluid. A vasculitis may also contribute to cardiac muscle dysfunction and conduction system abnormalities.

Because of the immunologic abnormalities, the exact etiology of myocarditis may be difficult to discern. Cardiac involvement is not limited to the terminal phase of the illness but may be seen in patients at all stages and may present with either an acute or an indolent course. Because of the common accompanying pulmonary dysfunction, clinical detection of cardiac abnormalities may be difficult, and, therefore, serial echocardiographic assessment is recommended.

Electrocardiographic changes are also frequent and include left ventricular hypertrophy, nonspecific ST-T changes, prolongation of the QTc interval, variable heart block, sinus node dysfunction, and ventricular tachycardia. Treatment of myocardial dysfunction includes diuretics and vasodilators, but digoxin should be used with caution.

ACUTE RHEUMATIC FEVER
(see Chapter 94)

Acute rheumatic fever is a delayed nonsuppurative sequela of an upper respiratory tract infection with group A beta-hemolytic streptococci. Since the mean age at diagnosis of acute rheumatic fever in recent outbreaks is 10 years, a substantial portion of afflicted individuals are in the early adolescent age range. Over the past 2 decades, the incidence of acute rheumatic fever has gradually decreased. However, acute rheumatic fever has recurred in recent years, mandating primary and secondary prevention of acute rheumatic fever. Unfortunately, many young physicians have never seen an adolescent who has acute rheumatic fever, and, therefore, recognition may be delayed, with the possible outcome of a larger population with rheumatic heart disease.

Pathogenesis

The pathogenesis of acute rheumatic fever probably represents a form of autoimmunity. A limited number of group A streptococcal strains are associated with acute rheumatic fever. Serotypes M1, M3, M5, M6, and particularly M18 have been associated with recent outbreaks. Mucoid strains of these serotypes may be particularly virulent. These findings again have raised the question of "rheumatogenic" strains of streptococcus as a cause of acute rheumatic fever. A vulnerable host must develop an upper respiratory infection caused by group A beta-hemolytic streptococcus, and, following a latent period of 1 to 6 weeks, acute rheumatic fever with its various manifestations may develop. Host factors may play an important role in the pathogenesis.

There is recent evidence to suggest genetic susceptibility. This evidence includes the distribution of histocompatibility leukocyte antigens, particularly HLA-DR2 in blacks and HLA-DR4 in whites. Furthermore, certain B-cell alloantigens may be present more often in patients with acute rheumatic fever.

Diagnosis

No symptom, clinical sign, or laboratory test is pathognomonic of rheumatic fever. The modified Jones' criteria are a guideline for diagnosis (Table 50–1). The clinical diagnosis of acute rheumatic fever requires either two major criteria or one major plus two minor criteria in addition to evidence of a recent streptococcal infection. Because a complete discussion of the ramifications and vicissitudes of rheumatic fever is beyond the scope of this chapter, the interested reader is referred to the classic monograph entitled "Rheumatic Fever" by M. Markowitz and L. Gordis.

Rheumatic arthritis is common in adolescents. The

TABLE 50–1. Modified Jones Criteria for Diagnosis of Rheumatic Fever

REQUIREMENT FOR DIAGNOSIS	MAJOR CRITERIA	MINOR CRITERIA
Two major criteria *or* One major plus two minor criteria Plus evidence of previous streptococcal infection: Positive throat culture Recent scarlet fever or Antistreptolysin-O (ASO) titer increase	Arthritis Carditis Subcutaneous nodules Erythema marginatum Chorea	Previous rheumatic fever Fever Arthralgia Acute phase reactants First degree atrioventricular block

arthritis involves large joints, in particular the knees, ankles, elbows, and wrists, and is typically migratory, moving from one joint to another. In recent outbreaks, the arthritis has been additive, as new joints were affected before resolution of previous joint involvement. The inflamed joints are exquisitely sensitive to touch. Rheumatic migratory polyarthritis typically clears within several weeks, is responsive to salicylate therapy, and is rarely followed by joint sequelae. The 75% prevalence of polyarthritis in patients with acute rheumatic fever has not changed in the recent resurgences.

Carditis is the most important manifestation of acute rheumatic fever because chronic valve damage may ensue. An old maxim states that rheumatic fever "licks the joints and bites the heart." Rarely, an acute attack of rheumatic fever, but more commonly a recurrence, may be fatal if severe carditis is present. Pancarditis involves the myocardium, endocardium, and pericardium. The diagnosis of carditis requires one or more of the following signs: a new pathologic murmur, cardiomegaly, congestive heart failure, and pericarditis. Although the prevalence of carditis in initial cases of acute rheumatic fever was 40% to 50% in the past, in recent outbreaks, carditis has occurred in 75% of the cases. The onset and presentation of carditis may be insidious, but the frequent occurrence of arthritis in older adult patients cues the practitioner to look for signs of carditis.

The mitral valve is the most common site of cardiac inflammation in rheumatic fever. Mitral regurgitation produces a pansystolic murmur, loudest at the cardiac apex and radiating to the left axilla. Daily auscultation should be performed on any patient suspected of having acute rheumatic fever to search for not only a new murmur of mitral regurgitation but also one of aortic insufficiency. In several cases of pancarditis, a murmur of tricuspid valve regurgitation may also be noted.

In order to avoid underdiagnosis of rheumatic carditis, and at the same time avoid overdiagnosis and erroneous labeling, consideration should be given to prompt referral to a pediatric cardiologist if carditis is suspected. Aortic regurgitation may occur as an isolated feature or in conjunction with mitral regurgitation.

Cardiomegaly with left ventricular and left atrial dilatation signifies myocarditis but may require serial non-invasive assessments with chest roentgenograms and echocardiograms to establish the diagnosis. Congestive heart failure is an uncommon but ominous sign in acute rheumatic fever and, if fulminant, can lead to the adolescent's death. Pericarditis is the least common manifestation, occurring in approximately 7% of patients in the past. Pericarditis usually occurs in association with myocardial and endocardial involvement, and the effusions are rarely large. Detection of a pericardial friction rub can be enhanced by auscultation over the precordium while the patient is kneeling with trunk bent forward and supported by his or her arms.

Other findings that may suggest cardiac involvement include tachycardia with a sleeping pulse rate greater than 100 beats/minute; a decreased intensity of the first heart sound associated with first degree heart block; and arrhythmias that include type I second degree atrioventricular block, junctional rhythm, atrioventricular dissociation, and premature beats. Atrial flutter and fibrillation are rarely seen during the initial bout of acute rheumatic fever. Although these signs are suggestive of carditis, the diagnosis must rest upon one of the four diagnostic signs previously described. The finding of sinus arrhythmia invariably rules out the presence of carditis.

Subcutaneous nodules are small, pea- to marble-sized, hard, painless, nonpruritic, mobile swellings on the extensor surfaces of joints, in the extremities and also along the spine and over the occiput. These nodules are an uncommon manifestation of acute rheumatic fever and usually develop in patients with a long bout of active carditis. Nodules are not pathognomonic of rheumatic fever but also occur in other connective tissue diseases.

Erythema marginatum is also uncommon, particularly in recent outbreaks of rheumatic fever. These skin lesions usually begin as small, pink, slightly raised macules, which then progress to an advancing, erythematous, serpiginous margin that clears in the center. The rash is transient, painless, and nonpruritic and is found chiefly over the trunk and inner aspects of the arms and thighs. The rash has also been reported in drug eruptions and glomerulonephritis.

Sydenham chorea (St. Vitus dance) occurs more commonly in females, has a long latent period of 1 to 6 months following streptococcal pharyngitis, and frequently occurs without symptoms of carditis or polyarthritis. Although less common than cardiac and joint involvement, chorea has been reported in up to one third of patients in recent outbreaks. Because of the long latent period, patients with chorea are usually afebrile and have normal acute phase reactants. Streptococcal antibody titers may also have returned to a baseline level. Chorea is characterized by a gradual onset with changes in behavior such as irritability, impulsive emotional reactions or emotional lability, excitability, and restlessness (see Chapter 87). Involuntary, purposeless, uncoordinated, jerky movements are seen, as well as a deterioration in penmanship, a clumsy gait, less distinct speech, and an overall decrease in fine motor control. Patients are unable to sustain a hand grasp or tongue protrusion. Wrist flexion and finger extension occur upon attempts to hold the arms out straight. Chorea is a self-limited condition with a duration of 3 to 4 months, but, rarely, signs and symptoms may persist for up to 1 year. Consultation with a neurologist is important to rule out other choreiform disorders. Despite the absence of signs of carditis, rheumatic prophylaxis should be instituted, since valvular heart lesions occur in approximately 30% of patients with chorea over long-term follow-up.

The minor Jones criteria are common to many inflammatory disorders and by themselves are not diagnostic of acute rheumatic fever.

Fever is almost always present at the onset of an acute attack and rarely is higher than 104° F, and no characteristic pattern or wide diurnal variations are seen, as in rheumatoid arthritis. Arthralgias may not be used as a minor criteria when arthritis is a major manifestation. Prolongation of the PR interval is commonly seen in acute rheumatic fever but may be seen in many other illnesses, including an isolated streptococcal pharyngitis. Acute phase reactants including the erythrocyte sedimentation rate, C-reactive protein, leukocyte count, and serum gamma globulins are usually elevated during an attack of acute rheumatic fever.

Evidence of a previous streptococcal infection includes a positive throat culture, recent scarlet fever, and an elevated antistreptolysin-O (ASO) titer. The ASO titer is elevated in 70% to 85% of patients. A single value of 500 units is considered an indication of a recent streptococcal infection. A titer of 333 units is of borderline significance, but serial titers may demonstrate an elevation over time. Additional antistreptococcal antibody assays may also be obtained depending on the availability in laboratories. Unfortunately, false-positive results from Streptozyme tests are common, and, therefore, the Streptozyme test should not be used as a sole screening criterion. These antistreptococcal tests indicate only a previous streptococcal infection and alone do not constitute evidence for acute rheumatic fever.

Treatment

It may be necessary to delay therapy for a short period in order to establish the diagnosis of acute rheumatic fever. However, if signs of moderate or greater carditis and, particularly, pancarditis are evident, therapy should be instituted immediately. Even if the throat culture results are negative, adolescent patients with the diagnosis of acute rheumatic fever should receive a single injection of 1.2 million units of long-acting penicillin. Secondary prophylaxis with oral penicillin V at 250 mg bid should be started. Alternatively, adolescent patients can be given 1.2 million units of benzathine penicillin G intramuscularly every 3 to 4 weeks. Patients allergic to penicillin should receive a 10-day course of erythromycin, followed by 250 mg bid or oral sulfadiazine 1 g once a day as secondary prophylaxis. The duration of prophylaxis should be lifelong. Compliance with secondary prophylactic regimens is often difficult in adolescent patients. Therefore, the adolescents should have a thorough understanding of their disease, its natural history, and the need for adhering to the regimens. Frequent encouragement may be necessary.

The choice of anti-inflammatory agent depends upon the severity of the manifestations. Patients with arthritis and very mild carditis as evidenced by a murmur of only slight mitral regurgitation can receive aspirin, 130 mg/kg/day (not to exceed 10 g/24 hours) divided into doses given every 4 hours, aiming for a serum level of 25 to 30 mg/dl. Patients with more than mild carditis should receive oral prednisone, 2 mg/kg/day up to 60 mg/day for 3 to 4 weeks or until a decrease in rheumatic activity is observed. Steroids may then be tapered as aspirin therapy is instituted.

Bed rest is also an important component of therapy. Physical exercise should not be permitted until all signs of inflammation have subsided and the acute phase reactants have returned to normal levels. Tapering of both steroids and aspirin regimens should be done to avoid rebounds, which are common if anti-inflammatory medications are stopped abruptly. Because of the increased incidence of acute rheumatic fever, physicians caring for adolescent patients should become familiar with the manifestations of acute rheumatic fever and should seek consultation from senior physicians who cared for rheumatic patients in the past.

BIBLIOGRAPHY

Alpert BS, Dover V, Strong WB, Covitz W: Longitudinal exercise hemodynamics in children with sickle cell anemia. Am J Dis Child 138:1021, 1984.

Balfour IC, Covitz W, Davis H, et al: Cardiac size and function in children with sickle cell anemia. Am Heart J 108:345, 1984.

Bernstein B, Takahashi M, Hanson V: Cardiac involvement in juvenile rheumatoid arthritis. J Pediatr 85:313, 1974.

Bland EF: Rheumatic fever: The way it was. Circulation 76:1190, 1987.

Cavallo A, Joseph CJ, Casta A: Cardiac complications in juvenile hyperthyroidism. Am J Dis Child 138:479, 1984.

Child JS, Perloff JK, Bach PM, et al: Cardiac involvement in Friedreich's ataxia: A clinical study of 75 patients. J Am Coll Cardiol 7:1370, 1986.

Dajani AS, Bisno AL, Chung KJ, et al: Prevention of rheumatic fever. Pediatr Infect Dis J 8:263, 1989.

Ehlers KH, Levin AR, Klein AA, et al: The cardiac manifestations of thalassemia major: Natural history, noninvasive cardiac diagnostic studies and results of cardiac catheterization. Cardiovasc Clin 11(2):171, 1981.

Englund JA, Lucas RV: Cardiac complications in children with systemic lupus erythematosus. Pediatrics 72:724, 1983.

Fish AJ, Blau EB, Westberg NG, et al: Systemic lupus erythematosus within the first two decades of life. Am J Med 62:99, 1977.

Hausdorf G, Rieger U, Koepp P: Cardiomyopathy in childhood diabetes mellitus: Incidence, time of onset, and relation to metabolic control. Int J Cardiol 19:225, 1988.

Hunsaker RH, Fulkerson PK, Barry FJ, et al: Cardiac function in Duchenne's muscular dystrophy. Am J Med 73:235, 1982.

Jacobs JC: Pediatric Rheumatology for the Practitioner. New York, Springer-Verlag, 1982.

Kaplan EL, Hill HR: Return of rheumatic fever: Consequences, implications, and needs. J Pediatr 111:244, 1987.

Kavanaugh-McHugh A, Ruff AJ, Rowe JA, et al: Cardiovascular manifestations. In Pizzo PA, Wilfert CM (eds): Pediatric AIDS. Baltimore, Williams & Wilkins, 1991, pp 355–372.

Leier CV, Call TD, Fulkerson PK, Wooley CF: The spectrum of cardiac defects in the Ehlers-Danlos syndrome, types I and III. Ann Intern Med 92:171, 1980.

Lipshultz SE, Colan SD, Gelber RD, et al: Late cardiac effects of doxorubicin therapy for acute lymphoblastic leukemia in childhood. New Engl J Med 324:808, 1991.

Markowitz M, Gordis L: Rheumatic Fever. Philadelphia, WB Saunders, 1972.

McAlister HF, Klementowicz PT, Andrews C, et al: Lyme carditis: An important cause of reversible heart block. Ann Intern Med 110:339, 1989.

Miller JJ, French JW: Myocarditis in juvenile rheumatoid arthritis. Am J Dis Child 131:205, 1977.

Nihoyannopoulos P, Gomez PM, Joshi J, et al: Cardiac abnormalities in systemic lupus erythematosus. Circulation 82:369, 1990.

Perloff JK, Stevenson WG, Roberts NK, et al: Cardiac involvement in myotonic muscular dystrophy (Steinert's disease): A prospective study of 25 patients. Am J Cardiol 54:1074, 1984.

Roberts WC, Honig HS: The spectrum of cardiovascular disease in the Marfan syndrome. Am Heart J 104:115, 1982.

Sanyal SK, Johnson WW: Cardiac conduction abnormalities in children with Duchenne's progressive muscular dystrophy: Electrocardiographic features and morphologic correlates. Circulation 66:853, 1982.

Stewart SR, Robbins DL, Castles JJ: Acute fulminant aortic and mitral insufficiency in ankylosing spondylitis. N Engl J Med 299:1448, 1978.

Svantesson H, Bjorkhem G, Elborgh R: Cardiac involvement in juvenile rheumatoid arthritis. Acta Pediatr Scand 72:345, 1983.

Wallace MR, Garst PD, Papadimos TJ, Oldfield EC: The return of acute rheumatic fever in young adults. JAMA 262:2557, 1989.

Westlake RM, Graham TP, Edwards KM: An outbreak of acute rheumatic fever in Tennessee. Pediatr Infect Dis J 9:97, 1990.

Wolfe L, Olivieri N, Sallan D, et al: Prevention of cardiac disease by subcutaneous deferoxamine in patients with thalassemia major. New Engl J Med 312:1600, 1985.

SECTION XIII

Hematologic-Oncologic Conditions

STEPHEN A. FEIG

Adolescence is the bridge between childhood and adulthood. The pubertal changes of growth and sexual maturation are mirrored in the hematologic system by an increase in the normal hemoglobin concentration and red cell volume, especially in males, but there is little direct impact of puberty on white cells, platelets, or procoagulants. Menarche signals an increase in regular blood loss and an increase in the dietary requirement for iron.

Whereas the physiologic correlates of pubescence with hematologic function are modest, the social, psychological, and sexual implications are of enormous importance. The transition from dependent child to independent adult takes place at a different time and pace for each adolescent and must be considered individually in the care of every child with a hematologic disorder or cancer. This issue is complicated by the observation that significant illness may delay or temporarily reverse the process of psychosocial maturation.

Because denial is a fundamental behavior pattern among adolescents faced with morbidity and potential mortality, the physician must first establish a partnership with the patient. This requires the education of the patient with respect to not only the nature of the disease but also the implications of the various treatment options, their risks, and benefits. Most adolescents can conceptualize how they deal with adversity, understand the limits of their tolerance of noxious intrusion, recognize assaults upon their self-image, and evaluate their quality of life; they should, therefore, have substantial input into the planning of their treatment.

Although not all adolescents have complete independence or legal emancipation, their input into the medical decision-making process is essential. To some extent, this can be achieved in the presence of parents (who need similar education), but it also requires private, confidential discussions between the adolescent patient and members of the medical care team. This allows transmission of sensitive information and provides the adolescent patient with the sense that he or she is the focus of attention and has an appropriate measure of control in the decision-making process.

Support groups of peers with the same or similar problems can be beneficial to patients of all ages but may be of unique importance to adolescents. Peers not only may be more in touch with the problems but also may have ready answers to specific questions for which the staff may not have a data base. Some adolescents are reluctant to become involved in such a support group, but many benefit from and enjoy the group once they join.

Hematologic disorders, oncologic conditions, and their treatments impact enormously upon adolescent patients. Issues like alopecia, nausea, vomiting, susceptibility to infection, and time missed from school or social activities must be addressed honestly and sympathetically. Issues such as the risk of teratogenesis from chemotherapy, the genetic aspects of the specific disease, safe sexual practices, pregnancy, and contraceptive options must be explored in confidence and nonjudgmentally. Appropriate goals can be set and attained only in the context of mutual understanding and respect between the adolescent patient and the physicians. Ultimately, the institution of an effective therapy for an adolescent will require the informed consent of the patient to begin treatment and his or her ongoing compliance to see it through.

The care of adolescents has additional implications for those who have been previously treated for a hematologic or oncologic condition. For some adolescents, the condition, its treatment, and restrictions to lifestyle may continue, as in the case of patients with heritable coagulopathies. As the patient matures and as our knowledge of these diseases and their management improves, the patient must be continually reeducated and brought up to date.

Other adolescent patients may have had few early complications of treatment but may be left with substantial long-term sequelae of the disease. For instance, the adolescent patient with hereditary spherocytosis who has undergone splenectomy has a lifelong increased risk of susceptibility to overwhelming sepsis. These individuals must be reminded of this potential risk, the importance of fever, and the need to seek medical attention even though they are no longer anemic.

Cancer survivors are a unique patient population. The successful application of chemotherapy and radiation therapy to childhood cancer is a product of the last few decades. As these patients enter adulthood, they will face a multitude of problems, including

1. job discrimination
2. unavailability of health and/or life insurance
3. potential late effects of cancer therapy, such as cardiac compromise due to anthracyclines, secondary malignancies, substantial neurologic deficits after treatment of brain tumors, and others
4. reproduction issues, such as impaired fertility, the risk of abnormal offspring, and the potential of passing on a heritable susceptibility to cancer

The assessment of these and other issues requires continued longitudinal follow-up of cancer survivors.

It is clear that the treatment of adolescents with hematologic or oncologic conditions is a complex problem that requires substantially more than expertise in medical technology. Optimum management requires a multidisciplinary medical team comprising pediatric and medical specialists, surgeons, radiologists, radiation therapists, and nurses, supported by members of other disciplines, including social workers, dietitians, rehabilitation specialists, prosthetists, physical therapists, occupational therapists, play therapists, school reintegration specialists, psychologists and psychiatrists, and nutritionists. As you read the following chapters, you will find that the recurring theme of multidisciplinary care is central to the successful management of these complex disorders in adolescent patients.

CHAPTER 51

Developmental Overview of Hematology and Oncology

RUTH ANDREA SEELER

BIOLOGIC MATURATION OF PUBERTY IN RELATION TO THE HEMATOLOGIC SYSTEM

Erythrocyte Values

The dramatic physiologic changes of adolescence affect the erythrocyte values primarily for boys because of testosterone stimulation of erythropoiesis (Fig. 51–1 and Table 51–1). Boys aged 12 to 14 years have a mean hemoglobin value of 14 g/dl, which increases 1 g/dl for ages 14 to 18 years, with a further increase of 1 g/dl after 18 years of age. The mean corpuscular volume (MCV) increases from 84 fl at 12 to 14 years of age to 86 fl at 14 to 18 years of age. After 18 years of age, it reaches the adult value of 90 fl. The values for the mean corpuscular hemoglobin (MCH) and the mean corpuscular hemoglobin concentration (MCHC) are the same as those of the adult by 12 years of age. In a study of 1000 adolescents from low-income families, a 1% increase in the hematocrit value for each successive sexual maturity rating (SMR) was noted in males, but not in females (Fig. 51–2).

There are no significant changes in the hemoglobin and hematocrit values and red cell number in females from 12 years of age to adulthood. The MCV shows a gradual increase similar to that seen in males.

Leukocyte Counts and Distribution

The normal ranges printed on hospital laboratory report forms apply to all adolescents because the total white cell count and differential achieve adult values at approximately 8 years of age.

Platelet Counts

Platelet counts are not age related; normal newborns achieve adult values (150,000 to 500,000 mm³) at birth. The introduction of automated blood-counting equipment has generated numerous consultations for thrombocytosis noted as an incidental finding on blood counts performed for other reasons. Platelet counts up to 1 million or more can be seen in numerous viral and bacterial infections, in collagen vascular diseases, postoperatively, with acidosis, and after trauma. Other well-recognized causes for reactive thrombocytosis include hemolytic anemia (especially sickle cell anemia), iron deficiency, Kawasaki disease, and functional and surgical asplenia and hemorrhage. No specific therapy is needed for the thrombocytosis *per se* except therapy (if any) appropriate to the underlying stimulus.

GENERAL APPROACH TO HEMATOLOGIC AND NEOPLASTIC DISORDERS

History

Most adolescents with inherited disorders of hemoglobin and of the coagulation system and with increased susceptibility to infection have been diagnosed in early childhood. Occasionally children with mild bleeding disorders may have escaped diagnosis until menarche or when there is a sports-related trauma with disproportionate bleeding. However, girls with hemorrhagic tendencies or those who are undergoing therapy with anticoagulants may require menstrual suppression or cyclic hormonal therapy to minimize menorrhagia or bleeding from a luteal cyst. The physician caring for a previously diagnosed adolescent patient needs to ascertain from the adolescent what his or her knowledge base is and what his or her attitude toward the chronic disorder is (see section on psychosocial factors).

In adolescents with an established hematologic diagnosis, it is now necessary to determine whether they received any blood products between 1979 and April 1985 that were not treated with heat. If they did, they should be counseled and tested for human immune deficiency virus (HIV) antibodies.

A comprehensive history of the adolescent presenting for health maintenance should include questions about any new or changing symptoms such as lumps and bumps, fleeting but recurring pains, changes in bowel or bladder function or in color of urine or stool, dyspnea on exertion, fevers, night sweats, and nondiet weight loss (see Chapter 25). There are very few malignant or

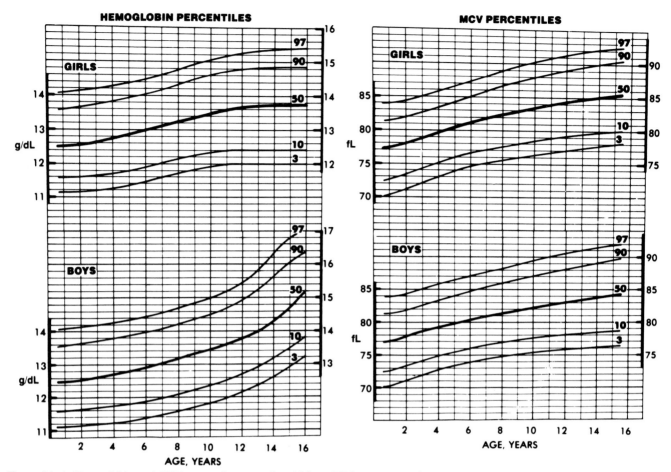

Figure 51–1. Hemoglobin and MCV percentile curves for children. (With permission from Dallman PR, Siimes MA: Percentile curves for hemoglobin and red cell volume in infancy and childhood. J Pediatr 94:26, 1979.)

acquired hematologic conditions discovered on yearly routine visits in asymptomatic adolescents. Most adolescents with these conditions present with symptoms readily recognized by the physician as symptoms of solid tumors or leukemia or other hematologic problems.

The physician should inquire as to the adolescent's routine cancer screening procedures for breast or testicular lesions. It is particularly important that males establish this health habit, as the incidence of testicular tumors far exceeds that of breast malignancies in teenagers (see Chapters 77 and 78).

Physical Examination

Ideally the physical examination is completed no matter what the problem and regardless of apparent good health. For adolescents with known or suspected hematologic disorders, the physician should particularly record the data listed in Table 51–2.

Diagnostic Procedures and Laboratory Testing

COMPLETE BLOOD COUNT

The complete blood count (CBC) is in many respects equivalent to a tissue biopsy, because it representatively

samples the hematopoietic system at that moment in time. The machine-automated differentials are more accurate and reproducible than are those done by technologists because of the greater number of cells (200 to 500) counted. There is no need for differentials to be done manually when the CBC is needed to quantitate the different types of leukocytes. For adolescents who have leukemia, the differential count should be performed by an experienced technician in order to classify blast types and differentiate them from other mononuclear cells. As part of the annual health maintenance visit, healthy adolescents, especially females, should have a hemoglobin or hematocrit determination done in the office.

BONE MARROW

A bone marrow examination should be performed if there is a question of infiltration or storage disorders, leukemia, or inadequate cellular production. Disorders characterized by increased destruction or splenic sequestration of blood cells do not usually require a bone marrow examination for diagnosis. For the erythrocyte disorders, the increased destruction with increased production is usually indicated by an elevated reticulocyte count. There are some transient reticulocytopenias that initially cause confusion, and in these situations a bone marrow examination is usually indicated.

**TABLE 51–1. Changes in Median Hemoglobin
and MCV as a Function of Age**

AGE (yr)		HEMOGLOBIN (g/dl)		MCV (fl)	
		Median	Lower Limit	Median	Lower Limit
12–14	Female	13.5	12.0	85	77
	Male	14.0	12.5	84	76
14–18	Female	14.0	12.0	87	78
	Male	15.0	13.0	86	77
18–49	Female	14.0	12.0	90	80
	Male	16.0	14.0	90	80

With permission from Dallman PR, Siimes MA: Percentile curves for hemoglobin and red cell volume in infancy and childhood. J Pediatr 94:26, 1979.

The bone marrow is usually aspirated from the posterior iliac crest in adolescents. The adolescent deserves a thorough explanation of why the procedure must be done and how it is to be done. The adolescent should be warned that the local anesthetic will not prevent the pain that occurs during the "sucking of the marrow" and that the pain will not last long. Several critical studies have shown that routine bone marrow examination during the remission maintenance phase of chemotherapy in children with leukemia has not contributed to an improved long-term prognosis. Thus, the more newly designed cooperative studies do not require repeated routine bone marrow examinations.

LUMBAR PUNCTURES AND INTRATHECAL CHEMOTHERAPY

The concept of a chemotherapy sanctuary must be explained to and understood by the adolescent patient, or he or she may resent the repeated lumbar punctures. A common mistake is not to wait long enough for the local infiltrative anesthetic to become effective. Most procedures are performed on an outpatient basis and the adolescent can immediately resume normal activities without limitations.

PSYCHOSOCIAL FACTORS

Psychosocial factors in two broad categories of patients need to be considered: (1) Those individuals with inherited or acquired chronic diseases (sickle cell anemia, hemophilia, long-term cancer, and others) who are now experiencing adolescence and (2) those in whom a diagnosis of cancer is established during adolescence (see Chapters 30, 53, and 121).

Chronic disease in youths who have had their disorder diagnosed prior to adolescence is not synonymous with chronic illness or symptomatology. For example, home therapy has made it possible for most adolescents who have hemophilia to view the need for the infusion of coagulation factors as a minor inconvenience. In contrast, more frightening and annoying to many adolescent hemophiliacs and other adolescents with congenital bleeding disorders is that except for the subspecialist, they know more about their disease than do most doctors. These adolescents may become acutely upset by interaction with the house staff in the emergency room or when hospitalized. They become anxious because they believe that they are no longer in control of their disease, something which they have long ago mastered. The same is true for adolescents with sickle cell disease. They are well the vast majority of time, going to school, dating, and doing things other adolescents do. However, when they have a vasoocclusive pain crisis, their perception of pain frequently is not adequately appreciated and treated by emergency room and house staff physicians.

Years previously, when the adolescent's condition was first diagnosed, the parents probably received a very detailed explanation of the hematologic disorder (e.g., sickle cell anemia, hemophilia, cancer, leukemia, risks of chemotherapy and radiation, and so on). However, this information may not have been passed on to the child by the parents as his or her comprehension grew with age. The adolescent needs to take increasing responsibility for his or her own medical care. The physician must assess the adolescent's knowledge of the disorder and teach him or her the signs and symptoms that require prompt medical care and explain why they are important. Many patients lack a clear understanding of the inheritance pattern of their disorder and the risk or nonrisk for their children and grandchildren. The complex issues of compliance and noncompliance are discussed elsewhere in this text (see Chapter 26).

The physician should know and understand the adolescent patient's life goals. Many adolescent patients have not formulated career goals because they did not expect to survive. Some adolescents' goals may be inappropriate to their condition, and the physician should help guide the patient and family in this regard.

Physicians caring for adolescents with chronic hematologic conditions need to be aware that the parents of such patients are frequently overprotective, especially when the adolescent has an inherited disorder, and they may unrealistically limit the adolescent's activities and aspirations.

The physician needs to devote sufficient time exclusively to the adolescent. Some parents may resist this. The younger adolescent may wish to be seen alone but is used to having a parent present and is reluctant to

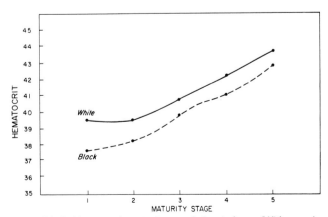

Figure 51–2. Hematocrit-maturity correlation in boys. (With permission from Daniel WA: Hematocrit: maturity relationships in adolescence. Pediatrics 52:388, 1973.)

TABLE 51–2. Physical Signs of Special Importance Related to the Hematopoietic System

ORGAN-SYSTEM	PHYSICAL FINDING	POSSIBLE CAUSE
Height and weight	Disproportionate or rapidly changing percentiles	Growth delay
		Secondary to previous central nervous system irradiation
		Secondary to gonadal failure from chemotherapy
Sexual maturity rating	Failure to progress	Sickle cell anemia
		Severe iron overload
	Accelerated progression	Steroid abuse
		Hormone-producing tumor
Eyes	Scleral icterus	Hemolytic anemia
		Hepatic tumor
	Abnormal ocular motility	Central nervous system or ocular tumor
	Nonconjugate	Amblyopia (only one eye sighted)
Nose	Obstructed air flow or masses	Polyp
		Tumor in nasopharynx
Mouth	Asymmetry of tonsils or soft tissues	Tumor of oropharynx
	Thrush or leukoplakia on lateral border of tongue	AIDS
	Necrotic buccal mucosa opposite lower molars	Precancerous or cancerous lesion secondary to tobacco chewing
	Ulcers of gums	Neutropenia
Lymph nodes	Generalized lymphadenopathy	Leukemia
		Lymphomas, Hodgkin disease, AIDS
	Lymphadenopathy in neck	Leukemia
		Lymphomas, Hodgkin disease
		Metastatic tumor from thyroid or sinuses
	Lymphadenopathy in inguinal area	Tumor of lower extremity or genital region
Skin	Hypo- or hyperpigmented lesions	Neurocutaneous disorder
	Subcutaneous lumps	Neurofibromotosis
	Deeply pigmented moles	Potential melanomas
Breasts	Any masses or asymmetry	Malignancy rare
		Fibroadenomas
Abdomen	Organomegaly	Neoplastic diseases
		Infectious disease
	Masses	Tumors
		Congenital cysts
	Bruits	Vascular tumors
	Dilated superficial veins	Portal or hepatic vein obstruction
	Fluid wave	Ascites, secondary tumor
Spine	Kyphoscoliosis	Vertebral anomaly or bone destruction from tumor
	Sacral dimple	Pilonidal cyst-sinus
	Sacral lump	Lipoma or tethered spinal cord, or both
Testes	Masses	Malignant tumor (see Chapters 53, 66, and 78)
Extremities	Masses in muscle	Soft tissue malignancy
		Hemangioma
	Joint swelling	Hemorrhage, infection, inflammation
	Limitation of internal rotation of hip	Aseptic necrosis from sickle cell anemia
	Asymmetry (atrophy-hemihypertrophy)	Wilms tumor
		Adrenal carcinoma
Neurologic	Asymmetry of reflexes	Central nervous system tumor
	Lack of coordination	Cerebellar tumor

request private time with the physician. Having a hematologic disorder does not protect the young person from the numerous psychosocial issues—drugs, contraception, sexual activity, cigarette smoking, safe sex, and so on—that deserve full attention for all adolescents. The adolescent must be recruited to be a compliant partner in the process of health maintenance and the treatment of illness. Privacy, respect for confidentiality, and sensitivity to the individual needs of the adolescent are essential prerequisites to the establishment of this partnership.

BIBLIOGRAPHY

Altman AJ, Schwartz AD: Malignant Diseases of Infancy, Childhood and Adolescence, 2nd ed. Philadelphia, WB Saunders, 1983.
Dallman PR, Siimes MA: Percentile curves for hemoglobin and red cell volume in infancy and childhood. J Pediatr 94:26, 1979.
Daniel WA Jr: Hematocrit: Maturity relationship in adolescence. Pediatrics 52:388, 1973.
Green DM, Zevon MA, Lowrie G, et al: Congenital anomalies in children of patients who received chemotherapy for cancer in childhood and adolescence. N Engl J Med 325:144, 1991.
Heath HW, Pearson HA: Thrombocytosis in pediatric outpatients. J Pediatr 114:805, 1989.

CHAPTER 52

Hematologic Disorders

DISORDERS OF THE ERYTHROCYTE

CAROLYN L. RUSSO and BERTIL E. GLADER

This chapter focuses on the common anemias seen in adolescents, specifically those resulting from impaired red blood cell production and hemolysis. The important anemias related to leukemia (see Chapter 53) or other causes of bone marrow failure are discussed elsewhere in this text. The reader who wishes more information regarding red blood cell (RBC) disorders should consult one of the excellent hematology texts and reviews in the bibliography.

NORMAL ERYTHROPOIESIS AND RED BLOOD CELL PHYSIOLOGY

RBCs are produced in the bone marrow under the influence of several growth factors, the best known of which is erythropoietin. This growth factor, produced in the kidney, is released into the circulation in response to decreased tissue oxygenation and the need for increased RBC oxygen delivery. The function of erythropoietin is to stimulate differentiation and maturation of early erythroid precursors in the bone marrow. After several intramedullary cell divisions, the RBC is released into the circulation as a reticulocyte (an erythrocyte containing ribonucleic acid [RNA] reticulum). After 1 day as a reticulocyte, the normal RBC ages 100 to 120 days more before it is recognized as old and is removed by the reticuloendothelial system. The function of the circulating RBC is to transport oxygen from the lungs to peripheral tissues; this is accomplished by hemoglobin, which reversibly binds oxygen at different oxygen tensions. Hemoglobin is a tetrameric protein of two α-globin chains and two non–α-globin polypeptides; each globin polypeptide is covalently bound to a heme molecule. In normal children and adolescents, there are three different types of hemoglobin (Table 52–1). Hemoglobin A ($\alpha_2\beta_2$; Hb A) is the major hemoglobin, but there are also small amounts of hemoglobin A$_2$ ($\alpha_2\delta_2$); and hemoglobin F ($\alpha_2\gamma_2$; Hb F). Although fetal hemoglobin (Hb F) is the major hemoglobin of intrauterine life, small levels of Hb F normally persist through adulthood, and in certain pathologic conditions, elevated Hb F levels often occur. The metabolism of the RBC is relatively simple, in that the major metabolic substrate is glucose, which is enzymatically catabolized to lactic acid, thereby generating the adenosine triphosphate (ATP) necessary to maintain cell membrane integrity. Other enzyme reactions generate reducing equivalents that help protect hemoglobin against oxidative injury.

GENERAL APPROACH TO ANEMIA

From a practical perspective, the major causes of anemia include generalized bone marrow failure, hemorrhage, impaired RBC production, and hemolysis. In most cases, the cause of anemia can be identified by the clinical history, physical examination, and data obtained from the following simple laboratory tests: a complete blood count (CBC), including measurement of hemoglobin concentration, hematocrit, RBC number, RBC indices, total leukocyte number, and platelet count; a reticulocyte count as a measure of erythrocyte production; examination of the peripheral blood smear, looking for abnormal RBC morphologic characteristics; and measurement of indirect-reacting serum bilirubin as a marker of increased hemoglobin catabolism (i.e., hemolysis). When evaluating an adolescent for anemia or an RBC disorder, the following questions should be asked:

Does the adolescent have anemia or an RBC disorder? A reliable sign of anemia that is found on physical examination is pallor of the buccal and conjunctival mucous membranes. Paleness of the skin may suggest anemia though this can be misleading because circulatory factors, cutaneous hydration, and fat deposition also can influence skin color. The laboratory definition

TABLE 52–1. Hemoglobin Composition of Normal Red Blood Cells

HEMOGLOBIN	BIRTH (%)	1 YEAR THROUGH ADULTHOOD (%)
A ($\alpha_2\beta_2$)	15–40	96–98
A$_2$ ($\alpha_2\delta_2$)	1	1–3
F ($\alpha_2\gamma_2$)	60–85	0–2

of anemia is a hemoglobin concentration (or hematocrit value) that is more than 2 standard deviations less than the normal mean for the patient's age and sex. In contrast to very young children, in whom normal hematologic values and indices vary considerably as a function of age, normal values in adolescents are similar to those in healthy adult men and women (Table 52–2). Not all RBC disorders are necessarily associated with anemia. For example, adolescents with hereditary spherocytosis often have normal hemoglobin levels and come to the attention of a hematologist only after splenomegaly is found on routine physical examination. In these cases, review of the peripheral blood smear usually reveals spherocytes and polychromatophilia (i.e., young RBCs). Other RBC disorders in which hemoglobin values can be normal include alpha- or beta-thalassemia trait and hemoglobin E (Hb E) or hemoglobin C (Hb C) variants. In each of these conditions, however, the mean cell volume (MCV) invariably is reduced. Thus, to know whether an adolescent is anemic or has a genetic RBC disorder, it is necessary to measure the hemoglobin concentration, determine the MCV, and carefully review the peripheral blood smear for abnormal RBC morphologic characteristics.

Is anemia caused by bone marrow failure? Because of the seriousness of disorders caused by aplastic anemia and leukemia, they must be considered at the outset when presented with an anemic adolescent patient. Both aplastic anemia and leukemia are associated with fever, petechiae, and bruises. However, lymphadenopathy, hepatosplenomegaly, and bone pain, commonly seen in leukemia, are most unusual in aplastic anemia. Laboratory studies to determine whether anemia is due to bone marrow failure (see Chapter 54) must address whether there is also thrombocytopenia, neutropenia, or other leukocyte abnormalities. Bone marrow examination is needed to obtain a definite diagnosis in the face of marrow failure.

Is anemia caused by hemorrhage? The likelihood of recent hemorrhage as the cause of anemia usually is apparent from the medical history and physical examination. Hemorrhage in adolescent females may be the result of heavy menstrual bleeding. However, immediately after bleeding, the hemoglobin level may be normal because the initial response to hemorrhage is vasoconstriction. The hemoglobin concentration begins to decrease only after extravascular fluid enters the circulation, which may not appear until 24 hours after the

initial episode. Reticulocytosis usually is seen 1 to 2 days later, and the maximal reticulocyte response occurs after 4 to 7 days. Anemia following chronic hemorrhage usually presents as a microcytic anemia resulting from iron deficiency.

Is anemia caused by hemolysis? Hemolytic anemia occurs when RBCs are destroyed before their normal demise at 100 to 120 days of age, and marrow erythropoiesis is unable to produce new RBCs at a rate commensurate with their accelerated destruction. Physical findings suggestive of hemolysis include hepatosplenomegaly, jaundice, and scleral icterus. There may be a history of adolescent patients having dark urine. In chronic hemolytic disorders, there may be frontal bossing and maxillary hyperplasia. Characteristic laboratory findings include reticulocytosis (increased RBC production) and hyperbilirubinemia (increased RBC destruction). Chronic hyperbilirubinemia may lead to the development of "early gallstones," occasionally accompanied by a family history of cholecystectomy in young individuals. There also may be a history of splenectomy in some family members.

Is anemia caused by impaired erythropoiesis? The answer to this question is "yes" if there is a low reticulocyte count and no evidence of increased RBC destruction (normal bilirubin levels) and other measured blood parameters are normal. In clinical practice these are very common types of anemia.

ANEMIA FROM IMPAIRED RED BLOOD CELL PRODUCTION

Anemias resulting from impaired RBC production are a consequence of acquired and genetic defects in hemoglobin synthesis or cell division. Iron deficiency is the most common cause of anemia in adolescence.

Iron Deficiency Anemia

Pathophysiology. Iron is necessary for the synthesis of hemoglobin and several other important enzymes. Total body iron status is a balance of the variable dietary intake and gastrointestinal absorption relative to the fixed rate of iron excretion. More than 90% of dietary iron is nonheme iron, but only a fraction of this is absorbed. In contrast, a much smaller portion of dietary iron is heme iron (e.g., meat), though this is more efficiently absorbed (20% to 30%). The average intake of dietary iron for an adolescent is approximately 10 to 12 mg/day, of which about 10% is absorbed, resulting in an intake of 1 to 1.2 mg/day. Average iron losses through skin and in stool are approximately 0.75 mg/day for males and nonmenstruating females. In menstruating females, this loss is increased further, resulting in an average loss of 1.35 mg/day. The iron requirements for growth are 0.5 mg/day for both sexes.

The causes of iron deficiency in adolescents are multifactorial. There are increased iron requirements because the adolescent growth spurt is associated with an increase in blood volume and RBC mass. There may be

TABLE 52–2. Important Red Blood Cell Values in Adolescents

AGE	HEMOGLOBIN (g/dl)	HEMATOCRIT (%)	MCV (fl)
6–12 years	11.5–15.5	35–45	77–95
12–18 years			
Females	12–16	36–46	78–98
Males	13–16	37–49	78–98
Older than 18 years			
Females	12–16	36–46	80–100
Males	13.5–17.5	41–51	80–100

Normal range established by the limits of 2 standard deviations greater than and less than the mean.

decreased iron availability because adolescent diets often do not contain sufficient iron for absorption. There are increased iron losses in adolescent girls as a consequence of menstrual bleeding. Also, in young healthy athletes there may be higher requirements because of increased losses through sweat, physical RBC damage associated with exercise, or hematuria. Moreover, iron balance is affected even further in adolescents who become pregnant. Taken together, it is apparent that the adolescent female, in particular, is extremely vulnerable to becoming deficient in iron. Moreover, pathologic blood loss must always be considered, and any adolescent with iron deficiency anemia, especially males, must be evaluated for occult gastrointestinal bleeding resulting from an ulcer, Meckel diverticulum, polyp, or hemangioma.

Clinical Course. Mild cases of iron deficiency anemia often pass unnoticed; however, more severe anemia interferes with oxygen delivery and can be associated with excessive fatigue or decreased exercise tolerance. The late effects of severe iron deficiency include nonhematologic changes, such as glossitis, koilonychia, (dystrophy of fingernails), and angular stomatitis.

Diagnosis. The first stage of iron deficiency is characterized by reduced iron stores without any hematologic changes. The only laboratory abnormality is a reduced serum ferritin concentration, a predictable marker of tissue iron stores. It has been estimated that 20% to 30% of nonpregnant menstruating females fall into this category of iron deficiency without anemia. A variety of symptoms may accompany this condition such as lethargy. As iron deficiency progresses, a mild normocytic anemia evolves which may respond to iron therapy. Later, as the degree of iron deficiency becomes more severe, this anemia characteristically becomes a microcytic anemia. In addition to reduced serum ferritin levels, typical laboratory findings in iron deficiency anemia include an elevated concentration of free erythrocyte protoporphyrin (a precursor of heme), decreased serum iron levels, and an increased total iron binding capacity (TIBC) with an iron saturation less than 15% (normally greater than 30%).

The major differential diagnosis of hypochromic microcytic anemia includes iron deficiency, a variety of hemoglobinopathies (Table 52–3), and the anemia of chronic disease (see further on).

Treatment and Clinical Outcome. The goal of treatment in iron deficiency is to increase the hemoglobin concentration and also to replenish body iron stores to normal. In addition, a critical aspect of this treatment is the correction of factors responsible for the deficiency state. This includes modifying the diet if necessary and determining whether there is an abnormal source of blood loss.

Oral ferrous sulfate is the iron preparation of choice. Although several other iron salts are marketed with claims for improved palatability, better absorption, or fewer side effects, none of them are therapeutically more effective than ferrous sulfate, and all are more expensive. Ferrous sulfate (300-mg tablets, each containing 60 mg of elemental iron) is prescribed in a dosage that provides 4 to 6 mg of elemental iron/kg body weight each day divided into three doses. Higher iron dosages do not accelerate recovery rate but do cause more side effects. Iron is absorbed best when given between meals; however, this commonly results in significant gastrointestinal distress (nausea, cramping, diarrhea, or constipation). For this reason, it is recommended that the daily iron dosage be gradually increased and divided into three portions taken with meals. This approach is effective for replacing iron, and most importantly, it leads to better compliance. Iron is known to interfere with the absorption of oral tetracycline, which adolescents often take as therapy for acne and sexually transmitted diseases (see Chapters 39 and 75). Hence these medications should be ingested at least 2 hours apart.

The initial hematologic response to iron therapy is an increased reticulocyte count after 5 to 7 days. Subsequently, the hemoglobin concentration begins to increase approximately 0.5 to 1.0 g/dl each week, and regardless of the severity of anemia, it usually takes 6 to 8 weeks to achieve a normal hemoglobin concentration. Once the anemia is corrected, it is essential that full therapeutic doses of iron be continued for 2 to 3 months in order to replenish iron stores. A less than optimal response usually is due to poor compliance (see Chapter 26), a coexistent infection that impairs the marrow response to iron, or ongoing blood loss. An additional reason that the anemia may not respond to iron therapy is an incorrect diagnosis of iron deficiency. It is not uncommon for individuals with thalassemia trait to be treated with iron for months before the proper diagnosis is made.

Iron can be given intramuscularly, but this route of administration has been associated with skin pigmenta-

TABLE 52–3. Laboratory Tests to Differentiate the Cause of Hypochromic Microcytic Anemia

DATA	IRON DEFICIENCY	BETA-THALASSEMIA TRAIT	ALPHA-THALASSEMIA TRAIT	HEMOGLOBIN AE OR EE
MCV (fl)/RBC $\times 10^6$	>13	<13	<13	<13
RBC protoporphyrin	Increased	Normal	Normal	Normal
Serum iron	Decreased	Normal	Normal	Normal
TIBC	Increased	Normal	Normal	Normal
Saturation (%)	Decreased	Normal	Normal	Normal
Serum ferritin	Decreased	Normal	Normal	Normal
Quantitative Hb A$_2$	Decreased	Increased	Normal	Normal
Quantitative Hb F	Normal	Increased or normal	Normal	Normal
Pattern on Hb electrophoresis	A	A	A	AE or EE

tion, tumors in laboratory animals, and allergic reactions, including anaphylaxis, and is therefore not preferred. It can also be administered intravenously. The only indications for parenteral iron are extreme noncompliance in taking oral iron, inflammatory bowel disease (see Chapter 63), and intractable blood loss. Transfusions of RBCs rarely are needed for iron deficiency anemia because the hematologic response to iron is prompt and predictable.

Anemia of Chronic Disease

Anemia is a complication of a variety of chronic disorders. In patients with renal failure (see Chapter 65), a normochromic normocytic anemia exists because of decreased erythropoietin production; this anemia is reversed by the administration of erythropoietin. In other chronic infectious or inflammatory disorders, a mild normocytic to slightly microcytic anemia commonly occurs in association with underlying diseases such as rheumatoid arthritis (see Chapter 90), ulcerative colitis (see Chapter 63), or chronic pyogenic infections (see next subchapter, Disorders of the Polymorphonuclear Leukocyte). In these chronic inflammatory conditions, anemia is related to abnormal iron metabolism, in that marrow macrophages are unable to release iron to developing erythroblasts. Usual laboratory findings in anemia associated with inflammation and infection include a low serum iron concentration, a slightly reduced TIBC, and a relatively normal iron saturation. Characteristically, the serum ferritin concentration is elevated. An additional anemia in this category is seen in the adolescent population with anorexia nervosa (see Chapter 60). In addition to the anemia, neutropenia and bone marrow hypoplasia are seen in this disorder; presumably these cytopenias are due to a deficiency of vital nutrients. The appropriate treatment for all anemias associated with chronic disease is directed at controlling the associated underlying pathologic condition.

Megaloblastic Anemias

Megaloblastic anemias in adolescents are relatively uncommon. Most cases result from folate deficiency. Rarely, vitamin B_{12} deficiency is responsible. Regardless of the cause, megaloblastic anemias are characterized by macrocytic RBCs (an elevated MCV), hypersegmentation of the polymorphonuclear cells, and megaloblastic changes in marrow erythroid precursors.

FOLATE DEFICIENCY

Pathophysiology. Folic acid (vitamin B_6) is an essential cofactor in nucleic acid metabolism. Deficiency of this vitamin causes anemia with megaloblastic changes in hematopoietic precursors. Sources of folate include green leafy vegetables, liver, whole grains, eggs, and yeast. Dietary forms of vitamin B_6 are polyglutamates, whereas it is the monoglutamate form that is absorbed. The conversion of dietary polyglutamates to monoglutamates is regulated by the intestinal enzyme folate deconjugase. Body folate stores last only 3 to 4 months after the vitamin is eliminated from the diet. Insufficient dietary intake is the most common cause of folate deficiency. Less commonly, folic acid deficiency may be a consequence of intestinal malabsorption, increased folate requirements such as those resulting from pregnancy or hemolytic anemias, or impaired folate absorption resulting from drug therapy. Drugs that can cause folic acid deficiency often are used by adolescents, including oral contraceptives and antiseizure medications (phenytoin, phenobarbital), all of which can inhibit intestinal folate deconjugase and thereby lead to impaired folate absorption.

Diagnosis. RBC folate levels, a reasonable marker of body folate stores, is the definitive test because serum folate levels fluctuate widely.

Treatment. Folate deficiency is treated with oral folate replacement, generally 0.25 to 1 mg/day. It is well tolerated and should be used prophylactically in pregnant females and in adolescent patients with chronic hemolytic anemias. The therapeutic response to folic acid is heralded by reticulocytosis in 4 to 7 days, followed by a slower, gradual increase in hemoglobin concentration. In cases of dietary insufficiency or malabsorption, folate should be continued for 3 months after the hemoglobin concentration is corrected. Megaloblastic anemia from impaired absorption of dietary folate (polyglutamate form) responds rapidly to therapy with folic acid (monoglutamate form), and there is no need to discontinue offending drugs such as phenobarbital or phenytoin. Even in adolescent patients with severe malabsorption, folic acid tablets generally correct the anemia. Adolescents receiving folic acid–antagonist drugs (pyrimethamine, methotrexate) occasionally experience megaloblastic anemia as an expected therapy-related consequence of the primary disease being treated.

VITAMIN B_{12} DEFICIENCY

Pathophysiology. Vitamin B_{12} is involved in deoxyribonucleic acid (DNA) synthesis, and when it is lacking, a megaloblastic anemia ensues. Unlike folate, vitamin B_{12} body stores last for years, and therefore dietary deficiency is very rare.

Diagnosis and Clinical Course. The diagnosis is suggested by the discovery of megaloblastic anemia with hypersegmented polymorphonuclear cells, but a definitive diagnosis depends on a reduced serum vitamin B_{12} level. Once the diagnosis of vitamin B_{12} deficiency is established, it is necessary to determine the cause. Meat, eggs, and dairy products are the primary sources of vitamin B_{12}, so a pure vegan can become deficient. Other causes include lack of intrinsic factor (from previous gastric surgery, pernicious anemia) or decreased vitamin B_{12} absorption (from previous ileal surgery, ileal malabsorption). In addition to anemia, patients with vitamin B_{12} deficiency frequently have a peripheral neuropathy affecting primarily the lower extremities.

Treatment. Documented vitamin B_{12} deficiency is treated with monthly intramuscular injections of vitamin B_{12} (100 to 200 µg). The reticulocyte response and increase in hemoglobin following vitamin B_{12} administration are similar to those already described for patients responding to folic acid. In most cases, monthly vitamin B_{12}

injections are continued throughout life. In the rare instance of nutritional deficiency, modification of the diet should obviate the need for ongoing vitamin B$_{12}$ therapy. Administration of folate can correct many of the hematologic abnormalities due to vitamin B$_{12}$ deficiency, though it is unwise to administer folate because it can cause an irreversible exacerbation of the neurologic problems caused by vitamin B$_{12}$ deficiency.

Hypoplastic Anemias

Hypoplastic anemias are characterized by anemia and reticulocytopenia (see Chapter 54). The three major causes of pure RBC aplasia in adolescents include acquired hypoplastic anemia associated with chronic hemolysis, Diamond-Blackfan anemia (DBA), and transient erythroblastopenia of childhood (TEC). The last is a disorder of very young children and does not occur in adolescents.

RED BLOOD CELL HYPOPLASIA WITH CHRONIC HEMOLYSIS

Hypoplastic crises are seen in all types of chronic hemolytic anemia. These crises are recognized because the steady-state hemoglobin and reticulocyte count are reduced, and the magnitude of anemia can be quite severe because hemolysis of circulating abnormal RBCs continues during the period of aplasia. Patients almost always have a concomitant viral illness, which is often due to a parvovirus. RBC transfusions are indicated if there is severe anemia or evidence of cardiopulmonary distress. Usually, only one RBC transfusion is required, since the aplastic period is brief, and reticulocytosis usually occurs within a few days of presentation.

DIAMOND-BLACKFAN ANEMIA

DBA, also known as congenital hypoplastic anemia, is a consequence of the impaired differentiation of developing erythroblasts. It is characterized by a lifelong macrocytic anemia often associated with congenital abnormalities or growth retardation. It may be a genetic disease, since more than one family member is affected in many instances. The diagnosis is suggested by macrocytic anemia, reticulocytopenia, and bone marrow that manifests decreased erythroid precursors. Almost all cases are diagnosed in infancy. RBCs from almost all patients with DBA have a variety of abnormal features (macrocytosis, elevated fetal hemoglobin levels, and increased adenosine deaminase activity) that persist even when the adolescent is older and in clinical remission. The major therapeutic modalities for DBA include corticosteroids and RBC transfusions. Approximately 70% of patients with DBA respond to prednisone (2 mg/kg/day) and are able to maintain a hemoglobin concentration greater than 8 g/dl on a very low dose of prednisone (often as low as 2.5 to 5 mg, one to two times/week). In adolescent patients who do not respond to steroids, RBC transfusions usually are necessary every 5 to 6 weeks to maintain a hemoglobin concentration greater than 7 to 8 g/dl. Deferoxamine chelation therapy is instituted after RBC transfusions are started (see section on beta-thalassemia major). Bone marrow

transplantation with a tissue-compatible sibling has been used successfully in a few selected DBA transfusion-dependent children (see Chapter 54). The prognosis appears to be quite good for most patients with DBA who respond to steroids. Affected females have become pregnant and delivered normal children, though their anemia occasionally is exacerbated during pregnancy. Deaths from iron overload in RBC transfusion–dependent patients and several cases of acute leukemia have occurred in older adolescents with DBA.

HEMOLYTIC ANEMIAS

A useful approach in assessing the cause of hemolysis is to ascertain whether it is due to an acquired extrinsic event or to an inherited intrinsic RBC disorder (Table 52–4). Acquired hemolytic episodes occur in otherwise healthy adolescents who have no underlying disease, or these episodes may be related to other associated pathologic conditions. The vast majority of acquired hemolytic disorders are a consequence of immune-mediated RBC destruction. Whenever acute hemolysis is first recognized, a direct Coombs test must be obtained because autoimmune hemolytic anemia can be life-threatening. Intrinsic RBC disorders that are considered to be the cause of hemolysis can be a consequence of cell membrane defects, alterations in erythrocyte metabolism, or qualitative and quantitative abnormalities of hemoglobin.

Autoimmune Hemolytic Anemia

Pathogenesis. Autoimmune hemolytic anemia (AIHA) results when an individual produces IgG or IgM anti-

TABLE 52–4. Causes of Hemolysis

EXTRINSIC (ACQUIRED)	
Antibody-induced RBC injury	Autoimmine hemolytic anemia (AIHA)
	RBC transfusion reactions
	Associated with drugs (e.g., penicillin)
	Associated with infection (infection with Epstein-Barr virus)
RBC injury due to altered vascular integrity	Vasculitis
	Disseminated intravascular coagulation (DIC)
	Thrombotic thrombocytopenia purpura (TTP)
Mechanical trauma to RBC	Abnormal heart valves
	Insertion of Teflon (polytetrafluoroethylene) cardiac patches
	Hemoglobinuria following "jogging"
Thermal injury to RBC	Associated with severe burns
	Following transfusion of inappropriately heated RBCs
Accelerated RBC splenic removal (hypersplenism)	Any condition with significant splenomegaly (infection with Epstein-Barr virus, malaria, and so on)

INTRINSIC (HEREDITARY)	
Membrane abnormalities	Hereditary spherocytosis
	Hereditary elliptocytosis
Metabolic abnormalities	G6PD deficiency
	PK deficiency
Hemoglobin abnormalities	Sickle cell syndromes
	Thalassemia syndromes

bodies, or both, against his or her own RBCs. The coating of RBC with IgG antibodies, or the IgM-induced fixation of complement (C3), leads to RBC destruction by the reticuloendothelial system.

Diagnosis. Characteristic laboratory features in AIHA include peripheral blood spherocytosis, hemoglobinemia, hemoglobinuria, and a reduced serum haptoglobin concentration. The specific diagnosis of AIHA is confirmed by positive results on direct gamma or complement (C3) Coombs test, or both. In young children, this is an acute process often associated with a viral infection, and the hemolytic episode is self-limited to a few weeks or months. In contrast, AIHA in adolescents is more commonly a chronic disease, and the disorder often is a manifestation of some underlying condition, such as systemic lupus erythematosus or other immunologic problem (see Chapters 90 and 92). Also, frequently there may be an associated immune thrombocytopenia. In cases of AIHA associated with another disease, hemolysis tends to be chronic over months to years, with periodic exacerbations of acute anemia.

Therapy. The management of patients with severe AIHA is extremely challenging. Available therapeutic modalities include immunosuppressive therapy, RBC transfusions, and splenectomy. Immunosuppressive therapy is the mainstay of AIHA treatment and should be started as soon as the diagnosis is made. Prednisone (or parenteral equivalent) is given according to the following dosage schedule: 6 mg/kg/day (days 1 and 2), 4 mg/kg/day (days 3 and 4), and 2 mg/kg/day (for at least 3 to 4 weeks). The onset of a response to steroids is noted by a gradual rise in the hemoglobin concentration and a decrease in the reticulocyte count. Once remission is induced, an attempt should be made to taper and discontinue corticosteroids, though some patients may need low-dose steroid therapy for several months. Whenever possible, this should be given on an alternate-day basis. The Coombs test result may remain positive for months without the presence of clinical hemolysis, but this is not an indication to continue corticosteroid therapy in an otherwise asymptomatic patient. Other immunosuppressive agents (azathioprine, 6-mercaptopurine, and cyclophosphamide) have been used, and on rare occasions they are effective when steroids are not. Usually, however, these drugs are reserved for patients whose conditions are refractory to steroids *and* splenectomy.

RBC transfusions are a critical part of AIHA management; however, this can be a problem because the antibody often is a panagglutinin that reacts with all donor cells, and thus there is no totally compatible blood. In this circumstance, donor RBCs that are known to be compatible with the adolescent patient's major blood group and Rh type should be used and should also demonstrate the least *in vitro* agglutination with the adolescent's serum. Rarely, in the face of life-threatening hemolytic anemia, exchange transfusion may be indicated for the purpose of removing antibody.

Splenectomy often is beneficial because RBCs coated with antibody or complement are removed by the spleen. However, the best time to perform a splenectomy is difficult to identify. Whenever possible, it is most prudent to "tough it out" with steroids and RBC transfusions for at least 6 to 8 weeks. Some believe that splenectomy most commonly should be performed in those individuals who need months of high-dose steroid therapy to sustain a normal hemoglobin concentration or in those who have high RBC transfusion requirements. The results of splenectomy are unpredictable, though a majority of patients have some degree of benefit. More potent immunosuppressive chemotherapy may be needed in patients who do not respond to splenectomy.

Inherited Red Blood Cell Membrane Disorders

HEREDITARY SPHEROCYTOSIS

Pathophysiology. Hereditary spherocytosis (HS) is the most common RBC membrane disorder associated with hemolysis. It is an autosomal dominant condition that results in loss of RBC membrane fragments and the formation of spherocytes. The latter are sequestered and destroyed in the splenic microcirculation, thereby causing chronic hemolysis.

Diagnosis. The diagnosis of HS may be suspected because of anemia, jaundice, splenomegaly, early onset of gallstones, or history of HS in other family members. The anemia in HS is usually mild, with the hemoglobin concentration ranging between 9 and 11 g/dl; occasionally there is no anemia. The peripheral blood smear almost always contains microspherocytes. The reticulocyte count is elevated (5% to 15%), and invariably there is some degree of hyperbilirubinemia. The incubated osmotic fragility test reveals a major population of cells that are markedly fragile when challenged with an osmotic stress.

Clinical Course and Therapy. The definitive therapy for HS is splenectomy, which alleviates the anemia and leads to cessation of the hemolysis. However, since the inherited RBC defect persists following splenectomy, more spherocytes actually are present after surgery, but these cells survive normally without the presence of a spleen. The proper time to perform splenectomy is a matter of some controversy. Our current recommendation is to have the surgery performed when the child is between 5 and 10 years of age, though mild cases may not require splenectomy until adolescence is reached. Pneumococcal vaccine should be given before splenectomy is performed. After surgery, patients are maintained on prophylactic penicillin (250 mg twice daily) for an indefinite period, and they must be educated to seek medical evaluation promptly with febrile episodes. Children and adolescents who appear toxic should be hospitalized for appropriate blood cultures and intravenous antibiotic therapy. Prior to splenectomy children and adolescents may have transient viral-induced "aplastic crises." Also, prior to splenectomy, all children and adolescents should receive prophylactic folic acid (1-mg tablet/day). A long-term complication of chronic hemolysis in many adolescent HS patients is cholelithiasis, though the incidence is minimized if splenectomy is performed before adolescence is reached.

HEREDITARY ELLIPTOCYTOSIS

Hereditary elliptocytosis (HE) is a heterogeneous membrane disorder characterized by elliptocytic erythrocytes. In the majority of individuals, HE is a morphologic curiosity, as there is no hemolysis or anemia. In a fraction of cases, elliptocytes and other fragmented cells are associated with significant hemolytic anemia. In this subset of patients with hemolytic HE, clinical features (splenomegaly) and laboratory tests (increased osmotic fragility) are similar to those seen in HS. From a general perspective, the overall management of hemolytic HE is identical to that described for HS. However, in contrast to HS, the response to splenectomy in hemolytic HE is less complete, and some patients have persistent mild hemolysis, reticulocytosis, and hyperbilirubinemia. Despite this, most patients benefit from splenectomy, and any existing transfusion requirement usually disappears after surgery. However, because of ongoing hemolysis, splenectomized children and adolescents need periodic gallbladder ultrasound examinations to observe for the development of cholelithiasis.

Inherited Red Blood Cell Enzyme Disorders

The two most common RBC enzymopathies associated with hemolysis are glucose-6-phosphate dehydrogenase (G6PD) deficiency and pyruvate kinase (PK) deficiency.

GLUCOSE-6-PHOSPHATE DEHYDROGENASE DEFICIENCY

Pathophysiology. G6PD is an enzyme of the hexose monophosphate shunt that is critical for the protection of the cell membrane and hemoglobin from oxidant injury. Hereditary deficiency of G6PD is the most common RBC enzymatic defect associated with hemolysis, affecting millions of individuals throughout the world. It is a sex-linked disorder occurring primarily in males, though rarely females have significant hemolysis. Approximately 10% of American black males have this enzyme deficiency, but the magnitude of enzyme deficiency in blacks (G6PD A$^-$ variant) is less than in whites (B$^-$ variant) or Asians (Canton variant).

Clinical Course. Acute hemolytic episodes in G6PD deficiency are commonly associated with infections (viral or bacterial) and occasionally occur with certain drugs. In the steady state, adolescents with G6PD deficiency are not anemic and have no clinical or laboratory signs of anemia. Hemolysis in blacks is usually mild and self-limited, but the degree of hemolysis in whites and Asians may be quite severe and occasionally life-threatening. Favism, or the occurrence of massive hemolysis in G6PD deficiency following exposure to fresh fava beans, occurs only in affected Mediterraneans, not in blacks. Clinical features of an acute hemolytic episode include jaundice, fatigue, back pain, and dark urine.

Diagnosis. The diagnosis requires a specific RBC enzyme assay. However, since patients often come to medical attention after the hemolytic episode, and thereafter the most enzymatically severe RBCs have been destroyed, it is often necessary to wait several weeks before there are sufficient numbers of G6PD-deficient RBCs to allow the diagnosis to be made.

Therapy. The only required therapy is an RBC transfusion if the adolescent patient is compromised by the anemia. Folic acid is not needed, and splenectomy has no role in the management of this disorder. It is important to counsel the adolescent patient regarding the potential for hemolytic episodes in the future. In most cases, they will occur with nonspecific infections and are not preventable. In a minority of instances, hemolytic episodes occur after drug exposure (sulfonamide drugs, antimalarial agents); therefore these agents should be avoided.

PYRUVATE KINASE DEFICIENCY

Pyruvate kinase (PK) is a critical glycolytic enzyme that is necessary for erythrocyte production of ATP. The inherited deficiency of PK is an autosomal recessive disorder that varies from a mild hemolytic anemia to a severe disorder requiring regular RBC transfusions. Although it is much less common than G6PD deficiency, it is the most common glycolytic enzymopathy associated with hemolysis. In contrast to G6PD deficiency, hemolysis is relatively constant but is not exacerbated by drugs. If there is associated severe anemia or transfusion dependency, splenectomy is recommended after the child is 5 years of age. In a vast majority of cases, removal of the spleen lessens the severity of the hemolytic anemia and transfusion requirements. Management of children who are splenectomized is identical to that already described for HS. Since hemolysis usually continues following splenectomy, these adolescent patients need to be followed for the development of gallstones.

Inherited Hemoglobin Disorders— Sickle Cell Syndromes

Sickle hemoglobin (Hb S) is found throughout the world, with an increased incidence in central Africa, the Near East, the Mediterranean, and parts of India. Sickle cell trait (AS) is the heterozygous state for Hb S and normal adult hemoglobin (Hb A). Approximately 10% of blacks in the United States are heterozygous for Hb S. Sickle cell anemia (SS disease) is the homozygous state in which a sickle gene is inherited from each parent (Fig. 52–1). Approximately 1 in 400 black infants born in the United States has sickle cell disease. Hb C is a mutant hemoglobin resulting from an amino acid substitution (lysine for glutamic acid) on the sixth position of the hemoglobin β-chain (the same site as the sickle mutation). Hemoglobin SC disease, the heterozygous state for both Hb S and Hb C, is more of a problem and is found in 1 in 2000 black children (one fifth of the frequency of sickle cell anemia). Hemoglobin S–thalassemia is the heterozygous state for both Hb S and beta-thalassemia.

Pathophysiology. Sickle hemoglobin is a consequence of a single base pair substitution in the sickle gene that

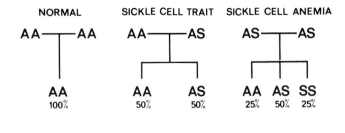

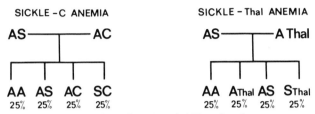

Figure 52–1. Genetics of sickle cell variants.

results in a valine residue replacing glutamic acid at position 6 in the β-globin chain. This single amino acid substitution gives hemoglobin a reduced solubility at different oxygen tensions. The major features of sickle cell anemia result from the fact that deoxygenated Hb S undergoes reversible polymerization, thereby causing RBCs to sickle, adhere to vascular endothelium, and occlude the microcirculation. The major problems in sickle cell disease include anemia, infection, painful sickle crises, organ-specific sickle crises, and chronic problems associated with recurrent sickling. A study in 1981 indicated that 60% of individuals with sickle cell disease survive to be older than 50 years of age.

Diagnosis. The "sickle prep" or sodium metabisulfite test and the hemoglobin solubility test are simple screening procedures for detecting Hb S, though these tests do not unequivocally distinguish the various sickle syndromes. This task is best accomplished by hemoglobin electrophoresis and quantitative measurements of Hb F and Hb A_2. Differences in hemoglobin concentration, MCV, and RBC morphologic features also distinguish between the various sickle syndromes (Table 52–5). The peripheral blood smear in sickle cell disease is characterized by a variety of cell shapes, but mainly there are many irreversibly sickled cells (ISCs), occasionally as much as 30%. Hb SC disease is characterized by numerous target cells, and there may be a few ISCs. Hemoglobin S–thalassemia is characterized by microcytosis and poikilocytosis, but ISCs are not a prominent feature.

Clinical Features and Therapy

Anemia. Anemia (7 to 9 g Hb/dl) is a constant feature of sickle cell disease. There also are intermittent exacerbations resulting from transient viral-induced aplastic crises, infection-related hyperhemolytic crises (characterized by increased scleral icterus), and rare megaloblastic crises from folic acid deficiency (characterized by worsening anemia, reticulocytopenia, and hypersegmentation of neutrophils).

Infection. In very young children with SS disease, infections from *Haemophilus influenzae* and *Streptococcus pneumoniae* are the most serious problems contributing to morbidity and mortality. The risk of life-threatening infections in adolescents is somewhat less than in younger children. The particular infections of concern are caused by the same encapsulated bacteria to which splenectomized children and adolescents without sickle disease are susceptible. In recent years, the incidence of *S. pneumoniae* infections has been reduced by pneumococcal immunization and penicillin prophylaxis (see Chapter 94).

Painful Sickle Crises. Sickling leads to tissue infarction and pain, which clinically characterizes vaso-occlusive crises. Repeated tissue injury ultimately causes organ dysfunction. *In vivo,* vaso-occlusive sickle crises occur with localized hypoxia, acidosis, dehydration, and infection or exposure to cold, or both. However, in a majority of cases, there is no obvious cause for the sickling episode. Localized musculoskeletal or abdominal pain may be the only clinical manifestation, though fever is commonly present. The diagnosis of vaso-occlusive sickle crisis is made on clinical grounds, since there are no changes in any laboratory parameters (number of sickle cells on the blood smear, hemoglobin concentration, leukocyte count, and so on). The differential diagnosis of infarction versus infection is difficult because the clinical presentation is similar in both conditions, and they often occur together. For example, there is no test that clearly distinguishes painful skeletal bone crises from osteomyelitis; both are manifested by bone pain, tenderness, swelling, and fever. Mild vaso-occlusive crises usually are treated at home with increased fluid intake, heat to the affected area, and analgesia (acetaminophen and occasionally codeine). In more severe crises, hospitalization may be indicated for parenteral analgesia (meperidine, 1.5 mg/kg [maximum, 150 mg] every 3 to 6 hours intramuscularly) and intravenous hydration (one-third normal saline with 5% dextrose given at 1½ times the maintenance rate). The issue of drug addiction usually is not a major problem in sickle cell disease, and analgesia should not be withheld because of this concern. Appropriate cultures should be obtained and intravenous antibiotics begun if there is any question of infection. In adolescent patients with painful abdominal crises, chest radiographs are necessary to exclude pneumonia, which frequently causes acute abdominal symptoms. Moreover, in addition to cautious observation, hydration, and analgesia, RBC transfusions or even exchange transfusions to reduce the Hb S concentration to less than 30% may be indicated if abdominal surgery is a possibility. There are increased risks of surgery, necessitating special considerations regarding the conduct of surgery and surgical technique. There is an increased risk of transfusion reactions in patients with sickle cell disease because of gene pool differences between the majority of blood donors and people with sickle cell disease.

Organ-Specific Sickle Crises. Splenic sequestration crises are due to intrasplenic sickling and the sudden pooling of blood in the spleen, thereby leading to hypovolemia and shock. Early in life, children with sickle cell disease have splenomegaly from intrasplenic sickling; after 5 to 6 years of age, repetitive intrasplenic sickling leads to fibrosis and splenic atrophy. Conse-

TABLE 52–5. Hematologic Parameters in Various Sickle Syndromes

	Hb (g/dl)	MCV (fl)	RETICULOCYTES (%)	HEMOGLOBINS PRESENT			
				% S	% A	% F	% C
Normal	12–17	80–100	<2	—	95–98	0–2	—
SS	7–12	92–103	10–25	85–95	—	5–15	—
S-Thalassemia	8–11	60–80	5–15	60–90	5–15	5–20	—
SC	10–12	70–80	3–10	45–55	—	1–4	45–55
AS	12–16	80–90	<2	35–45	55–65	0–2	—
AC	11–16	75–90	<2	—	55–65	0–2	35–45

quently, splenic sequestration crises do not occur in adolescents with sickle cell anemia (but may occur in Hb SC disease and Hb S beta-thalassemia, in which splenomegaly persists).

The acute chest syndromes resulting from infection or infarction, or both, account for a major portion of sickle cell morbidity. The clinical presentation in these patients includes fever, tachypnea, chest pain, and abnormal chest radiographs. The differentiation between intrapulmonary sickle infarction and infection is impossible, and usually they occur together. Proper management includes obtaining appropriate cultures, starting intravenous antibiotics, monitoring arterial blood gases, and administering oxygen. In addition, since these acute chest syndromes can be fatal, the use of RBC transfusions for these patients should be liberal. Moreover, if there is any evidence of pulmonary decompensation, an RBC exchange transfusion often is performed to reduce sickling. It is of note that this acute chest syndrome frequently occurs several days after a patient is hospitalized for an unusually painful abdominal or truncal crisis requiring parenteral analgesia.

Central nervous system sickling causes a variety of neurologic symptoms, including seizures and strokes. RBC transfusions to maintain Hb S at less than a 30% concentration can reverse angiographic abnormalities and prevent recurrence of further strokes; however, sickle-induced central nervous system accidents usually recur when transfusion regimens are stopped. Thus, following a stroke, RBC transfusions must be administered every 4 to 5 weeks indefinitely. Moreover, once a transfusion program is begun, deferoxamine chelation therapy also is instituted (see section on beta-thalassemia major).

Hepatic sequestration crises are characterized by a marked increase in liver size, extreme hyperbilirubinemia, and a fall in hemoglobin concentration. These unusual episodes are self-limited and require no specific therapy.

Priapism occurs as a consequence of sickling within the corpora cavernosa. Prolonged vascular obstruction causes fibrosis, impairment of the erection mechanism, and occasionally, impotence in older adolescent males. The onset of priapism can be spontaneous or associated with sexual activity. Our approach to priapism is to provide hydration, analgesia, and RBC transfusions over 24 hours. If there is no improvement, an exchange transfusion may be needed to reduce Hb S to less than 30%. In older adolescent males, needle aspiration and irrigation of the corpus occasionally is attempted to remove the "sickled sludge" (see Chapters 66 and 78).

Chronic Problems. Growth and development are affected in sickle cell anemia. Young children with sickle cell disease are small for age, but by adolescence most have caught up in height. Puberty is delayed in both boys and girls (see Chapter 4). Cholelithiasis caused by bilirubin stones is common; however, cholecystectomy is indicated only in patients with symptoms. Hyposthenuria, resulting from sickling-induced damage of the loop of Henle, leads to a concentration defect that increases obligate urinary water losses and thereby increases obligate water intake. This must be considered when patients are hydrated for painful crises, since adequacy of fluid replacement cannot be assessed adequately by urinary output alone. Also, the inability to concentrate urine may result in the adolescent's complaining of urinary frequency nocturia and enuresis. Hematuria, resulting from sickling-induced renal damage, usually resolves spontaneously with administration of fluids and rest. It is noteworthy, however, that there is a high incidence of chronic renal failure in adults with sickle cell anemia.

Leg ulcers may be a problem in adolescents and adults with sickle cell anemia. They usually occur around the ankle and can take a long time to heal, often becoming infected, and can be very debilitating. In many cases, RBC transfusions are needed to promote healing.

Ophthalmologic sickling within the retinal vasculature is a serious complication that usually presents in adolescence. These adolescents may have no subjective complaints, since the occluded vessels tend to occur in the periphery. Annual ophthalmologic examinations should be a routine requirement for all adolescents with sickle cell anemia so that this retinopathy can be recognized. Photocoagulation can treat the secondary neovascularization and thereby abort the vitreous hemorrhage and subsequent retinal detachment.

Pregnancy in sickle cell anemia occurs less frequently than in a comparable population not affected by this hemoglobinopathy (see Chapter 74). In all likelihood, this is a result of endocrine failure as a consequence of chronic sickling. In adolescents with sickle cell disease who become pregnant, painful crises often increase in frequency, and cardiovascular stress may lead to cardiac failure. In addition, since the placenta is inordinately susceptible to sickling, a large number of pregnancies end in early miscarriage or premature delivery. Most hematologists recommend regular RBC transfusions throughout pregnancy.

Sickle Cell Trait. Almost all individuals heterozygous for Hb A and Hb S are healthy and have a normal life expectancy. There is no anemia and the RBC morphologic picture is normal. Rare cases of serious visceral sickling have been reported during severe exercise at high altitudes, during flying in unpressurized aircraft, during severe pneumonia, or during general anesthesia. In a review of military recruits, a statistical association was observed between sickle trait and a higher risk of sudden death during basic training. However, whether sickle trait was the actual cause of these deaths remains to be determined. Most hematologists recommend that adolescents with sickle trait be allowed to participate in athletic activities without restrictions. Young adults need to be counseled regarding the possibility that they may bear children with one of the more serious sickle syndromes.

Sickle Beta-thalassemia. This disorder is caused by the inheritance of a sickle gene from one parent and a beta-thalassemia gene from the other parent (see Fig. 52–1). Hb S constitutes 60% to 90% of the hemoglobin, whereas the remainder is Hb F and some Hb A (different mutations of the beta-thalassemia gene can increase or decrease expression of hemoglobin A). The clinical course of Hb S beta-thalassemia usually is milder than SS or SC disease, presumably because of increased Hb F, which inhibits sickling. In contrast to SS disease, patients with hemoglobin S–thalassemia have persistent splenomegaly that does not infarct in early childhood. For this reason, splenic sequestration crises are seen in adolescents and adults. The incidence and complications of pregnancy in Hb S beta-thalassemia are the same as in the general black population.

Hemoglobin SC Disease. The heterozygous inheritance of Hb S and Hb C produces a syndrome that is usually milder than SS disease. Just as with Hb S beta-thalassemia, splenomegaly often persists throughout life without undergoing infarction, and consequently splenic sequestration crises can occur in older children and adults. Vaso-occlusive crises occur and are thought to be due to the higher hemoglobin and blood viscosity in Hb SC disease. Typical obstructive crises (bone pain, abdominal pain) are less frequent, whereas more common problems are related to retinopathy, renal papillary necrosis, and aseptic necrosis of the femoral heads. In women with Hb SC disease, the incidence and complications of pregnancy are the same as in the general black population.

Hemoglobin C Disorders. The heterozygous state for Hb C (AC) is an asymptomatic condition found in 2% of blacks in the United States. Homozygous Hb C (CC) disease is a mild hemolytic disorder found in 0.01% of blacks. Hb C has an electrophoretic mobility identical to Hb E at an alkaline pH but is readily separated and identified at an acid pH.

Inherited Red Blood Cell Hemoglobin Disorders— Thalassemia Syndromes

The thalassemia syndromes represent a heterogeneous group of disorders characterized by a decrease in or lack of production of the α- or β-globin polypeptides of Hb A. Beta-thalassemias result from decreased production of β-globin chains, whereas alpha-thalassemias result from reduced formation of α-globin chains. A consequence of decreased hemoglobin production is anemia characterized by RBCs that are microcytic (decreased MCV) and hypochromic (decreased mean corpuscular hemoglobin). There is also an imbalance in globin chain production because the unaffected (i.e., nonthalassemic) globin chains are produced at a normal rate. In beta-thalassemia major and Hb H disease, this accumulation of normal globin chains injures RBCs and is responsible for the hemolytic component of these disorders.

HOMOZYGOUS BETA-THALASSEMIA (BETA-THALASSEMIA MAJOR, COOLEY ANEMIA)

Pathophysiology. This genetic defect occurs primarily in individuals from the Mediterranean area and, to a lesser extent, in black Africans and Asians. The homozygous state for this disorder results from the inheritance of one beta-thalassemia gene from each parent. The severe anemia is due to both decreased hemoglobin formation (from reduced β-globin chain synthesis) and hemolysis of defective RBCs (from erythrocyte injury caused by accumulation of α-globin chains).

Diagnosis. Common features of this disorder include severe microcytic anemia, reticulocytosis, and numerous nucleated RBCs in the blood (Table 52–6). Circulating RBCs contain Hb F (70% to 90%) and Hb A_2 (5% to 10%), but little or no Hb A (0% to 20%).

Clinical Features. This severe hemolytic disorder appears during the first year of life. In children who are not transfused adequately, common problems include growth retardation from severe anemia, hepatosplenomegaly from hemolysis and extramedullary erythropoiesis, and susceptibility to fractures and facial abnormalities from increased compensatory bone marrow erythropoietic activity.

Therapy and Outcome. Most patients with beta-thalassemia major die unless they receive RBC transfusion therapy. Iron chelation, splenectomy, and bone marrow transplantation are other important therapeutic modalities in this disease.

RBC transfusions are programmed to suppress normal erythropoiesis and maintain a hemoglobin concentration of 10 to 12 g/dl. This approach allows for normal growth during childhood with no physical deformities. Most children treated on such a regimen are able to lead a relatively normal life for 15 to 20 years.

Iron chelation therapy is a critical aspect of care

TABLE 52–6. Hematologic Values in Beta-Thalassemia Disorders

	BETA-THALASSEMIA TRAIT	BETA-THALASSEMIA MAJOR
Hb (g/dl)	9–11	4–7
MCV (fl)	60–75	60–75
Reticulocytes (%)	1–2	2–10
Nucleated RBCs	0	Many
Hb A (%)	90–95	0–20
Hb FA_2 (%)	1–5	60–90
Hb A_2 (%)	4–6	0–10

because the most serious problems of beta-thalassemia major are related to iron overload, a consequence of the RBC transfusion dependency, since the body cannot effectively excrete accumulated iron. The consequences of iron overload often become manifested when there is failure of normal adolescent growth as a result of endocrine failure. Hypogonadism is commonly present and may be treated with estrogens or testosterone replacement therapy. More serious effects of hemosiderosis include cirrhosis, pancreatic failure with insulin-dependent diabetes, and, most importantly, the development of cardiac hemosiderosis as manifested by congestive heart failure and ventricular arrhythmias. The last is now the major cause of death in patients with beta-thalassemia major and usually occurs in the third to fourth decades of life. Chelation therapy with deferoxamine is administered at home with a portable infusion pump. We currently give most adolescents 1.5 to 2 g of deferoxamine subcutaneously or intravenously over 12 hours, 6 nights each week. Also, since compliance is often a problem in adolescents (at a time when ferritin levels often begin to soar), we have used indwelling venous catheters such as the Port-A-Cath. This latter approach has made it possible to improve compliance and give more chelation therapy. Data from the past decade suggest that intensive deferoxamine chelation therapy has a beneficial effect in prolonging life. Active research is in progress to develop effective oral chelating agents.

Splenectomy often has a role in the management of beta-thalassemia major because splenomegaly may cause hypersplenism with a progressive increase in transfusion requirements, which usually decreases after splenectomy.

Bone marrow transplantation has been successfully used in several young children with beta-thalassemia major (see Chapter 54). This approach has been justified because of the fear that currently available chelating agents will not prevent death from iron overload.

Thalassemia Intermedia

Patients with this form of homozygous beta-thalassemia are able to maintain an adequate hemoglobin concentration (7 to 8 g/dl) without RBC transfusions. However, because there is an associated expansion of erythroid bone marrow activity, common problems in these patients include the classic skeletal abnormalities of thalassemia and hepatosplenomegaly from both hemolysis and extramedullary hematopoiesis. Although somewhat controversial, most hematologists believe the management of thalassemia intermedia should be identical to that of beta-thalassemia major (i.e., aggressive RBC transfusions, deferoxamine chelation therapy).

HETEROZYGOUS BETA-THALASSEMIA (BETA-THALASSEMIA TRAIT)

The inheritance of one beta-thalassemia gene is characterized by mild hypochromic microcytic anemia (8 to 11 g Hb/dl), which needs to be differentiated from iron deficiency (see Table 52–3) and beta-thalassemia major (see Table 52–6). Laboratory studies indicate that Hb

A_2 or Hb F, or both, are elevated. This mild anemia occasionally is aggravated by infection and pregnancy; however, life expectancy is normal. No specific therapy is needed, nor is any effective. Individuals with this disease must be counseled regarding the potential for bearing children with homozygous beta-thalassemia.

ALPHA-THALASSEMIA SYNDROMES

Alpha-thalassemia syndromes are seen primarily in Southeast Asians and in blacks. Since α-globin chain synthesis is directed by four structural genes, four clinically different alpha-thalassemia syndromes have been recognized.

Silent Carrier State (Alpha-thalassemia II)

These individuals, who lack one α-globin gene, are hematologically normal and have no clinical problems. Recognition of this entity initially was a result of individuals with the silent carrier state bearing children with Hb H disease (see further on).

Alpha-thalassemia Trait (Alpha-thalassemia I)

These individuals lack two of four α-globin genes, which results in a mild hypochromic microcytic anemia. As seen in Table 52–4, the diagnosis of this disorder is made after excluding the other known causes of hypochromic microcytic anemia. No therapy is needed, and life expectancy is normal. Southeast Asians with this condition need to be counseled regarding the possibility of having a child with Hb H disease or homozygous alpha-thalassemia. The genetic lesion is different in blacks with alpha-thalassemia trait, and, as a consequence, Hb H disease and homozygous alpha-thalassemia rarely ever occur in this ethnic group.

Hemoglobin H Disease

This disorder results from the deletion of three α-globin genes. One parent has thalassemia trait, and the other is a silent carrier for alpha-thalassemia. The decrease in α-globin synthesis leads to the accumulation of β-chain tetramers (i.e., Hb H), accounting for 10% to 20% of the total hemoglobin. Hb H disease is diagnosed by observing a rapidly migrating hemoglobin on electrophoresis. Hb H is relatively unstable and tends to precipitate in RBCs, thereby leading to a moderate hemolytic disorder. RBC transfusions occasionally are needed with exacerbations of the anemia. Life expectancy is normal; however, there may be complications of chronic hemolysis, such as cholelithiasis. As in other chronic hemolytic disorders, folic acid supplementation (1 mg daily) should be given.

Homozygous Alpha-thalassemia (Hydrops)

This disorder, caused by deletion of all four α-globin structural genes, is incompatible with life. Fetuses are aborted early, are stillborn, or, if carried through term, die within the first few hours of life. It is mentioned in this text because this disorder can be diagnosed prenatally. It is of interest that at least two infants with this disorder have done well following intrauterine RBC transfusions followed by regular RBC transfusion therapy after birth, just as for patients with transfusion-dependent homozygous beta-thalassemia.

HEMOGLOBIN E SYNDROMES

Hb E is an abnormal hemoglobin caused by a single amino acid substitution (lysine for glutamate at the twenty-sixth position of the β-globin chain). It is the third most prevalent hemoglobin worldwide. Hb E syndromes can often be confused with thalassemia disorders. Moreover, since Hb E is found almost exclusively in Southeast Asians, it recently has emerged as a common problem in many hematology clinics in the United States. Hb E can be identified by hemoglobin electrophoresis. The heterozygous state (Hb A and Hb E) is characterized by a mild microcytic anemia that is virtually indistinguishable from alpha- or beta-thalassemia trait (see Table 52–3). Homozygous Hb E is very similar to the heterozygous state with minimal if any anemia. It is of importance, however, that the heterozygous state for Hb E and beta-thalassemia (i.e., Hb E beta-thalassemia) is a moderately severe hemolytic anemia often requiring RBC transfusions. The management of patients with Hb E beta-thalassemia is the same as that for thalassemia intermedia.

BIBLIOGRAPHY

Balin NI: Diagnosis and classification of the polycythemias. Semin Hematol 12(4):339, 1975.
Camitta BM, Nathan DG: Anemia in adolescence. 1. Disturbances of iron balance. Postgrad Med 57(2):143, 1975.
Charache S, Lubin B, Reid CD: Management and Therapy of Sickle Cell Disease. Washington DC, US Department of Health and Human Services, Public Health Service, National Institutes of Health, Publication No. 89-2117, September 1989.
Ekert H: Clinical Paediatric Haematology and Oncology. Melbourne, Blackwell Scientific, 1982.
Glader BE: Diagnosis and management of red cell aplasia in children. Hematol Oncol Clin North Am 1(3):431, 1987.
Miller DM, Baehner RL: Blood Diseases of Infancy and Childhood, 6th ed. St. Louis, CV Mosby, 1990.
Nathan DG, Oski FA: Hematology of Infancy and Childhood. Philadelphia, WB Saunders, 1987.
Palla B, Litt IF: Medical complications of eating disorders in adolescents. Pediatrics 81(5):613, 1988.
Platt OS, Rosenstock W, Espeland MA: Influence of sickle hemoglobinopathies on growth and development. N Engl J Med 311:7, 1984.
Rowland TW, Black SA, Kellerher JF: Iron deficiency in adolescent endurance athletes. J Adolesc Health Care 8:322, 1987.
Vichinsky E, Lubin BH: Suggested guidelines for the treatment of children with sickle cell anemia. Hematol/Oncol Clin North Am 1(3):483, 1987.
Whitten CF, Bertles JF: Sickle Cell Disease. New York, The New York Academy of Sciences, 1989.

DISORDERS OF THE POLYMORPHONUCLEAR LEUKOCYTE

LAURENCE A. BOXER

CLINICAL DISORDERS OF NEUTROPENIA

Neutropenia occurs in a wide range of clinical settings, and in this regard normal neutrophil levels should be stratified for age and race. Neutropenia is defined as the absolute decrease in the number of circulating terminally differentiated neutrophils. Individual adolescents may be characterized as having mild neutropenia, with counts of 1000 to 1500 cells/mm^3; moderate neutropenia, with counts of 300 to 1000 cells/mm^3; or severe neutropenia, with counts generally less than 300 cells/mm^3. This stratification may be useful for predicting the risk of pyogenic infections, since only adolescents with severe neutropenia have increased susceptibility to life-threatening infections. Neutropenia does not heighten the susceptibility of adolescents to viral and parasitic infections or to bacterial meningitis. Often, the usual signs and symptoms of local infection, such as exudates, fluctuations, ulcerations, fissure formation, and regional adenopathy, are much less evident in neutropenic than in nonneutropenic individuals because of the lack of cellular constituents.

Neutropenia may accompany hematologic disease, chemotherapy and radiation therapy, infections (including human immunodeficiency virus [HIV]), inflammation, and malignant and nutritional diseases (Table 52–7). Many of these disorders of neutropenia are associated with varying degrees of anemia or thrombocytopenia, or both. In contrast, neutropenia may be the sole hematologic abnormality in conditions such as congenital neutropenia and immune neutropenia, which are the focus of this chapter. Clinically, it is useful to classify the neutropenias pathophysiologically as disorders arising from (1) abnormalities of bone marrow stem cell developments, (2) impaired release of neutrophils from the bone marrow reserve, (3) abnormalities in the distribution of neutrophils between the circulating and marginating pools, and (4) decreased survival of neutrophils in the blood.

CHRONIC NEUTROPENIA

Chronic neutropenia is composed of several different disorders associated with variable clinical presentations.

TABLE 52–7. Clinical Conditions Characterized by and Associated with Significant Neutropenia

PRIMARY HEMATOLOGIC DISORDERS

Abnormalities of bone marrow stem cell development	Aplastic anemia Leukemias Severe congenital agranulocytosis Benign neutropenias Syndrome-associated neutropenias Reticular dysgenesis Cyclic neutropenia Myelofibrosis and myelophthisis Nutritional deficiencies (vitamin B_{12}, folate, copper) Chédiak-Higashi syndrome Lymphoproliferative disease HIV infection

DRUG-INDUCED NEUTROPENIA

Abnormalities of bone marrow stem cell development; decreased survival of neutrophils in the blood	Myelotoxic agents (e.g., alkylating agents) Antimetabolites Hypersensitivity reactions secondary to antibiotics (e.g., penicillins, semisynthetic penicillin, cephalosporins, sulfonamides, quinidine, dilantin, propylthioracil, chlorthiazide, chlorpromazine)

INFECTIONS

Impaired release of neutrophils from the bone marrow reserve; abnormalities in the distribution of neutrophils between the circulating and marginal pools	Sepsis leading to depletion of marrow reserves in neonates, sepsis leading to C5a generation, viral infections, typhoid, paratyphoid, tuberculosis, brucellosis, tularemia, rickettsial infections

AUTOIMMUNE DISORDERS

Decreased survival of neutrophils in the blood	Systemic lupus erythematosus, seropositive rheumatoid arthritis, Felty syndrome, chronic active hepatitis, immune thrombocytopenic and hemolytic anemias, hypogammaglobulinemia, dysgammaglobulinemia, lymphoproliferative disease, Graves disease, Hashimoto thyroiditis, cyclic neutropenia and T8 lymphocytosis, infectious mononucleosis, idiopathic immune neutropenia

HYPERSPLENISM

Decreased survival of neutrophils in the blood	Felty syndrome, Gaucher disease, cirrhosis, sarcoidosis, neoplasms involving the spleen, reticuloendothelial hyperplasia

Adapted from Boxer LA, Morganroth ML: Neutrophil function disorders. Dis Mon 33:683-780, 1987.

For some of these disorders, the clinical presentation may be characteristic, whereas for others it is not.

Pathophysiology. The pathophysiology of most of these conditions has been poorly characterized. Chronic neutropenia occurs because of a defect in the generation and maintenance of adequate numbers of circulating neutrophils. Generally, other hematopoietic cellular elements are present in the peripheral blood in normal to increased numbers. Quite commonly, a peripheral monocytosis is observed; somewhat less often peripheral eosinophilia is present. Bone marrow aspiration and biopsy reveal normal numbers of erythroid and megakarocyte elements; however, the marrow neutrophil precursors are quantitatively normal to decreased, with maturation arrest occurring at variable points in the differentiation and sequence.

Most cases of chronic neutropenia are sporadic, without a family history; whereas in some cases, both autosomal recessive and dominant patterns of inheritance have been ascertained. The cause of chronic neutropenia is not clearly understood, probably in large part because conflicting data result from the underlying heterogeneous nature of the conditions that fall under the rubric of chronic neutropenia.

Clinical Manifestations. Adolescents with the more severe varieties of chronic idiopathic neutropenia may have recurrent infections. Many of these adolescents exhibit neutropenia from birth. This group of patients includes those with severe congenital neutropenia, which is inherited as an autosomal recessive trait in Sweden but occurs sporadically in the United States. Usually the absolute neutrophil count is less than 200 cells/mm³. As a consequence, adolescents with such depressed neutrophil counts are at major risk for severe recurrent bacterial infections, including cellulitis, oral and gingival mucosal inflammation, pneumonitis, liver abscesses, and septicemia. Adolescents with severe congenital neutropenia exhibit variable degrees of monocytosis, eosinophilia, and plasmacytosis. The bone marrow aspirate contains normal to increased numbers of promyelocytes, with markedly reduced bands and segmented neutrophils. On rare occasions, leukemia has developed in adolescents with severe congenital neutropenia.

In adolescents with chronic idiopathic neutropenia of

moderate severity, bone marrow arrest can occur at any stage beyond the promyelocyte. The circulating count in adolescents with symptomatic disease fails to rise when challenged with intravenous corticosteroids, in contrast to the situation in chronic benign neutropenia.

Diagnosis. The onset of severe congenital neutropenia occurs in early childhood, whereas chronic idiopathic neutropenia can occur at any time from early childhood through adolescence. Neutropenic patients often demonstrate listlessness and irritability accompanied by low-grade fevers. These adolescents are afflicted with recurrent aphthous ulcers of the buccal mucosa, lips, tongue, and pharynx, which are often accompanied by tender cervical adenopathy. Many adolescents with severe congenital neutropenia have chronic gingivitis and usually become edentulous during the second decade of life.

Laboratory Evaluation. In adolescents with recurrent bacterial infections or with a family history of neutropenia, obtaining a complete blood count is the first diagnostic step toward establishing a diagnosis. A bone marrow aspirate and biopsy provide insight into the cellularity of the marrow; the adequacy of cell numbers at different stages of myeloid, erythroid, and megakaryocytic maturation; and the orderliness of maturation. The level of maturational arrest of granulopoiesis, if present, provides some indication of the severity of the condition and the relative likelihood of recurrent serious infections. Generally, patients with adequate granulocyte reserve are less likely to experience serious bacterial infection, even if the circulating neutrophil count is less than 300 cells/mm³. For such patients, a bone marrow stimulation test with corticosteroids may prove useful in identifying benign neutropenia in those who are able to raise the circulating neutrophil count twofold.

In situations in which more than one peripheral cell lineage is affected, a bone marrow sample is necessary in order to evaluate the possibility of leukemic or malignant tumor invasion of the marrow space. Other tests that may be useful in ruling out alternative diagnoses include an antineutrophil antibody assay, an antinuclear antibody assay, and antimicrobial serologic assays if specific infections such as hepatitis, Epstein-Barr virus or cytomegolovirus disease, or HIV infections are suspected.

Differential Diagnosis. Chronic idiopathic neutropenia must be distinguished from several primary marrow disorders, including aplastic anemia, leukemia (see Chapter 53), and cyclic neutropenia. A bone marrow aspirate and biopsy allow the physician to establish the diagnoses of aplastic anemia and leukemia. Cyclic neutropenia is characterized by the regular periodic oscillation in the peripheral neutrophil count. In order to exclude this rare disorder, it is necessary to obtain serial blood counts with white cell differential counts twice weekly for 6 to 8 weeks. Other conditions in adolescent medicine that may be associated with chronic idiopathic neutropenia include Schwachman syndrome, myelokathexis, X-linked agammaglobulinemia and dysgammaglobulinemia, and depressed cellular immunity. Other rare disorders associated with neutropenia in adolescent medicine, but with distinctive features allowing separation from idiopathic neutropenia, include cartilage-hair

hypoplasia syndrome, dyskeratosis congenita, and Fanconi anemia. Adults may exhibit neutropenia associated with infiltration of the bone marrow, with functionally suppressive large granular lymphocytes. Both pediatricians and internists will sometimes have difficulty separating the chronic neutropenia related to production defects from immune neutropenia. In the latter case, reliance should be placed upon the presence of antineutrophil antibodies.

Treatment. Careful attention to good hygiene lessens the likelihood of serious bacterial infections. This is a challenge to many adolescents. Regular dental care with prompt restoration of decaying teeth is essential for these adolescents. Furthermore, prophylactic antibacterial agents such as oral trimethoprim-sulfamethoxazole are employed. For febrile adolescents with chronic neutropenia, prompt institution of broad spectrum antibiotic therapy is indicated to guard against the possibility of infection with *Staphylococcus aureus* and gram-negative organisms. When a specific organism is identified as the causative organism of infectious episodes, a specific bactericidal drug may be chosen to initiate antibiotic therapy. The newest and most promising hope for successful medical therapy is the use of hematopoietic growth factors to promote granulopoiesis and thereby elevate the circulating neutrophil count. It appears that adolescents with chronic, severe, and idiopathic neutropenia, as well as cyclic neutropenia, respond to recombinant human granulocyte colony–stimulating factor (GCSF) with a dramatic rise in the peripheral neutrophil count. Other growth factors such as recombinant human granulocyte-macrophage colony–stimulating factor (GMCSF) may similarly prove useful with severe chronic neutropenia; however, GMCSF has more undesirable side effects.

Course of Illness and Prognosis. The outlook for adolescents with chronic neutropenia depends upon the degree of peripheral neutropenia. The prognosis historically has been poor for patients who have severe neutropenia coupled with poor marrow reserve, especially when it has been present from an early age, with many patients dying in the first few years of life. However, with the judicious use of antibiotics and improved supportive care measures, patients with chronic neutropenia are living longer—into adolescence and young adulthood. Although early mortality has been reduced, the morbidity of infectious sequelae and the need for frequent hospitalizations remain major problems. However, the use of recombinant GCSF offers the possibility of treating the underlying problem, with a resultant reduction in the morbidity and frequency of hospitalizations experienced by these patients.

AUTOIMMUNE NEUTROPENIA

Acquired neutropenia may have an autoimmune basis (see Table 52–7). Immune neutropenia occurring without other diseases is uncommon in adults but can occur frequently in children and adolescents. Adolescents with autoimmune neutropenia have severe neutropenia, with counts of less than 200 cells/mm³, that is usually discovered coincidentally during mild infections. Only recently has it been possible to show convincingly that autoimmune antibodies present in the serum in some of these adolescents are responsible for the neutropenia. In some patients, immune complexes are thought to be involved in the neutropenia of adolescent disorders such as systemic lupus erythematosus (see Chapter 90) and drug-induced neutropenia.

Pathophysiology. In some individuals, the antibodies are frequently directed against one of the following neutrophil-specific antigens including NA1, NA2, NB1. Neutrophil antibodies may be of the IgG, IgM, or IgA class, or mixtures of these three classes.

Clinical Manifestations. Adolescents with autoimmune neutropenia can have associated diseases or drug-associated antibodies. They may become acutely ill with autoimmune neutropenia arising from ingestion of a variety of drugs (penicillins, semisynthetic penicillins, cephalosporins, sulfonamides, dilantin, propylthiouracil, chlorothiazide, chlorpromazine).

Diagnosis. A history should be obtained to ascertain exposure to a drug or toxin that is capable of inducing neutropenia, as well as to identify diseases associated with immune neutropenia. A variety of functional and qualitative assays are available for evaluation of the presence of antineutrophil antibodies both directly on the surface of the neutrophil and in the patient's serum. Frequently it is necessary to use more than one assay to verify the presence of antineutrophil antibodies.

Treatment. Treatment of adolescent patients with autoimmune neutropenia consists of the judicious use of appropriate antibiotics for bacterial infections and prednisone therapy for those adolescents with severe neutropenia and recurrent infections. In one half of the reported cases of autoimmune neutropenia, corticosteroid therapy has resulted in a normal neutrophil count. Adolescents with autoimmune neutropenia who fail to benefit from corticosteroid therapy may respond to cytotoxic drugs such as cyclophosphamide, azathioprine, and vincristine. Experience with intravenous gamma globulin therapy in autoimmune neutropenia is limited to only a small number of patients, with variable responses noted. In a few patients, increased margination and shortened blood neutrophil half-times have been demonstrated. The marrow cellularity and maturation of cells are usually normal, which reflects the marrow's ability to compensate for the shortened peripheral blood neutrophil survival. Many adolescents with lupus erythematosus do not have severe enough neutropenia to require therapy.

DISORDERS OF GRANULOCYTE FUNCTION

Neutrophils are the most important phagocytic cell, to defend the host against acute bacterial infections. As such, they form the first line of defense against microbial invasion. During the critical 2- to 4-hour period following invasion by pathogenic organisms, neutrophils must arrive at the site of infection if it is to be contained. In order to be effective and arrive at the site of inflammation, phagocytic cells must adhere or attach to the vascular endothelium near the site of invasion or inflammation, engage in diapedesis through the vessel wall, move in a unidirectional fashion toward the site, and adhere, ingest the offending organism, and activate the biochemical pathways important in intracellular microbial killing. Adolescents with neutrophil disorders may have defects that affect these functional processes (Table 52–8). Chronic granulomatous disease (CGD) is the most common of these rare disorders in adolescence.

Chronic Granulomatous Disease

CGD is an inherited disorder in which phagocytic cells ingest, but do not destroy, catalase-positive microorganisms because the cells fail to generate metabolites that normally kill these microbes. The major clinical and genetic features of CGD are summarized in Table 52–9.

Pathophysiology. The manner in which the metabolic deficiency of the CGD neutrophil predisposes the host to infection relates to the inability of the CGD neutrophil to accumulate hydrogen peroxide (H_2O_2) in the

---

TABLE 52–8. Disorders of Neutrophil Chemotaxis

DEFECTS IN THE GENERATION OF CHEMOTACTIC FACTORS
Familial deficiency of C1r, C2, C4 (classic complement components)
Familial deficiency of C3, C5, properdin
Acquired C3 deficiency (systemic lupus erythematosus, chronic hemolytic anemia, glomerulonephritis, immunoglobulin deficiency)

ENHANCED GENERATION OF NORMAL CHEMOTACTIC INACTIVATORS
Hodgkin disease
Sarcoidosis
Malignancy
Lepromatous leprosy
Cirrhosis

DIRECT INHIBITORS OF THE NEUTROPHIL ITSELF
Immune complex disease (rheumatoid arthritis)
Bone marrow transplantation
C5a generation in plasma (sepsis, hemodialysis, thermal injury)
Wiskott-Aldrich syndrome
Drugs (corticosteroids, tetracycline, amphotericin B, ethanol, antithymocyte globulin)
Juvenile periodontitis (Capnocytophaga)
Hyperimmunoglobulin IgE syndrome
IgA myeloma

INTRINSIC DEFECTS OF NEUTROPHILS
Neonatal neutrophils
Leukocyte adhesion defect
Neutrophil action dysfunction
Chédiak-Higashi syndrome
Specific granule deficiency
Hypophosphatemia
Shwachman syndrome
Glycogenosis Type Ib
Kartagener syndrome
Hyperimmunoglobulin E
Chromosome 7 abnormalities
Zinc deficiency (acrodermatitis enteropathica)
Alcoholism
Increased microtubule assembly

TABLE 52–9. Synopsis of Chronic Granulomatous Disease

Incidence	1 in 1 million; >300 cases reported
Male:female ratio	3:1
Inheritance	X-linked (70%); defective neutrophil membrane-bound cytochrome b Autosomal recessive (30%); defective cytosolic factors (47- and 66-kd proteins)
Carrier state	Seen only in X-linked CGD in mother and sisters—usually asymptomatic, but patient may have lupus-like syndrome or stomatitis, or both
Age of onset	Congenital: first symptoms at <1 year of age, rarely adult onset
Diagnosis	Lack of respiratory burst as measured by NBT test
Clinical manifestations	Recurrent bacterial and fungal infections Sequelae of chronic inflammation (failure to thrive, anemia, hypergammaglobulinemia, hepatosplenomegaly) Obstruction resulting from granulomas
Pathogen	Approximate order of frequency 　No isolate (50%) 　*Staphylococcus aureus* 　*Aspergillus* spp. 　Enteric gram-negative bacteria 　　(*Klebsiella, Serratia, Salmonella*) 　　*Pseudomonas* (often *cepacia*) 　　*Candida albicans* 　　*Nocardia* spp.
Organ affected and clinical effects	Lung: pneumonia (*Staphylococcus aureus, Aspergillus*), abscess, chronic changes Lymph nodes: lymphadenitis (*Staphylococcus aureus*), marked adenopathy Skin and mucous membrane: infectious dermatitis, abscesses, conjunctivitis, persistent rhinitis Liver: hepatic abscess (*Staphylococcus aureus*) Bone: osteomyelitis (*Serratia*) Gastrointestinal tract: stomatitis, esophagitis, gastric antral narrowing, chronic diarrhea, perianal abscess Central nervous system or generalized: sepsis, meningitis Genitourinary tract: obstructive uropathy, cystitis
Prognosis	Variable, death in infancy to middle age

phagosomes containing ingested microorganisms. Hydrogen peroxide, along with myeloperoxidase delivered to the phagosome by degranulation, kills the incorporated microbe. When these organisms gain entrance into CGD neutrophils, they are not exposed to hydrogen peroxide because neutrophils do not produce the hydrogen peroxide, and the hydrogen peroxide generated by the microbes themselves is destroyed by the accompanying catalase. The catalase-positive microbes can multiply intracellularly, be transported to distant sites, and be released to establish new foci of infection. The CGD neutrophils are able to ingest pneumococci and streptococci and kill them because these organisms do not contain catalase. They generate hydrogen peroxide that, together with the myeloperoxidase delivered to the phagosome of CGD neutrophils, kills these bacteria.

The enzyme responsible for the generation of hydrogen peroxide is a reduced nicotinamide adenine dinucleotide phosphate (NADPH)-dependent oxidase that catalyzes the one electron reduction of oxygen to superoxide (O_2^-) and then to hydrogen peroxide. The NADPH oxidase is composed of several subunits, one of which traverses the membrane, completely conducting electrons from the pyridine nucleotide on the cytoplasmic side to oxygen in the external environment. Cytochrome b represents the terminal component of the chain. It appears to bind oxygen, the final electron acceptor (Fig. 52–2). In X-linked CGD, a defective gene codes a defective message for the large subunit of cytochrome b. Most adolescent patients with an autosomal recessive condition lack the 47,000-dalton phosphoprotein.

Diagnosis. Symptoms of CGD usually appear during infancy as the patient begins to suffer from recurrent bacterial and fungal infections. The offending pathogens are almost always catalase-positive bacteria and various species of *Aspergillus* and *Candida albicans*. Adolescents with CGD are also plagued with multiple granulomata, which arise because of the chronic inflammation. The diagnosis of CGD is made by any one of various tests that measure the ability of neutrophils to undergo the respiratory burst in response to surface stimuli. One of the most convenient assays for establishing the diagnosis is the nitroblue tetrazolium (NBT) test, in which the neutrophils are stimulated to undergo the respiratory burst in the presence of NBT. In its oxidized form, NBT is soluble and has a yellow color. When reduced, in cells generating electrons from superoxide, it forms a blue precipitate. CGD cells lack this capacity.

Differential Diagnosis. CGD can readily be distinguished from other phagocytic cell defects by the propensity of affected adolescents to experience infections

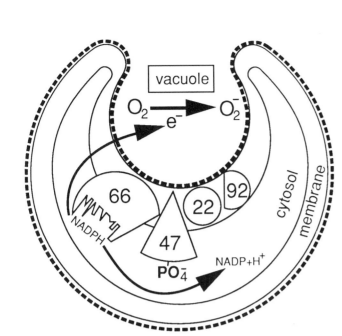

Figure 52–2. The schematic representation of a model of the NADPH oxidase of phagocytic cells. The oxidase consists of an electron transport chain that is interposed between the substrate, NADPH, and the cytosol in the lumen of the phagocytic vacuole. Electrons are pumped across the membrane to reduce oxygen to superoxide. Clearly defined subcomponents of the chain include cytochrome b, with a large β-subunit of 92,000 daltons and a 22,000-dalton α-subunit. There is a 47,000-dalton cytosolic protein that upon activation of the system becomes phosphorylated by a kinase using ATP as a substrate and moves into close association with the cytochrome in the membrane. The proximal molecule could be a flavoprotein with a molecular weight of 66,000 daltons containing the NADPH-binding site. The X-linked form of CGD lacks the cytochrome b, whereas the autosomal forms of CGD most commonly lack the 47,000-dalton protein and less commonly lack the 66,000-dalton protein.

with catalase-positive organisms. Neutrophil motility, adhesion, and degranulation are normal in CGD, a feature that distinguishes it from other phagocyte disorders, such as leukocyte adhesion deficiency and various chemotactic disorders.

Treatment. In the past, the treatment of CGD was largely supportive. In general, antibiotic therapy for the offending organism is indicated, and purulent collections should be drained surgically. Often, empirical therapy with broad spectrum parenteral antibiotics is required while a specific diagnosis is established. Therapy with antibiotics should be continued until the adolescent patient's sedimentation rate returns to normal. The use of prophylactic trimethoprim-sulfamethoxazole has become a mainstay of CGD therapy and has resulted in marked reduction in the frequency of infection. Corticosteroid therapy has proved useful in the treatment of adolescents with gastric outlet obstruction, probably by a mechanism of diminishing the inflammatory state. Finally, interferon-γ has been shown to variably enhance the oxidase response of CGD phagocytes and reduce the number of infections.

BIBLIOGRAPHY

General

Curnutte JT, Boxer LA: Disorders of granulopoiesis and granulocyte function. In Nathan DG, Oski FA (eds): Hematology of Infancy and Childhood, 3rd ed. Philadelphia, WB Saunders, 1987, pp 797–847.

Neutropenia

Bonilla MA, Gillio AP, Ruggeiro M, et al: Effects of recombinant human granulocyte colony-stimulating factor on neutropenia in patients with congenital agranulocytosis. N Eng J Med 320:1574, 1989.

Boxer LA, Greenberg MS, Boxer GJ, et al: Autoimmune neutropenia. N Engl J Med 293:748, 1975.

Bussel JB, Abboud MR: Autoimmune neutropenia of childhood. Crit Rev Oncol Hematol 7:37, 1987.

Hutchinson R, Boxer LA: Disorders of granulocyte and monocyte production. In Benz EJ, Cohen HJ, Furie B, et al (eds): Hematology: Basic Principles and Practice. New York, Churchill Livingstone, 1990, pp 193–204.

Shear NH, Spielberg SP: Anticonvulsant hypersensitivity syndrome. In vitro assessment of risk. J Clin Invest 82:1826, 1988.

Walker RI, Willemze R: Neutrophil kinetics in the regulation of granulopoiesis. Rev Infect Dis 2:282, 1980.

Qualitative Abnormalities

Babior BM, Woodman RC: Chronic granulomatous disease. Semin Hematol 27:247, 1990.

Boxer LA, Morganroth ML: Neutrophil function disorders. DM 33:683, 1987.

DISORDERS OF HEMOSTASIS

JAMES J. CORRIGAN, JR.

HEMOSTATIC MECHANISM

The hemostatic mechanism is composed of the blood vessels, blood platelets, plasma coagulation factors, natural inhibitors, and fibrinolytic factors. The function of the hemostatic mechanism is (1) to provide a hemostatic plug at the site of injury and (2) to ensure that the circulating blood remains fluid. A defective hemostatic mechanism can therefore be the cause of either a hemorrhagic or a thrombotic diathesis.

A series of biochemical and physiologic events is initiated once blood vessel injury occurs. The earliest event produces the platelet plug and is called the primary hemostatic mechanism. At the same time, the coagulation mechanism is activated and produces a fibrin clot. This is called the secondary hemostatic mechanism (coagulation mechanism), which consists of two pathways:

(1) the plasma (or intrinsic) pathway and (2) the tissue (or extrinsic) pathway. The primary and secondary hemostatic mechanisms operate simultaneously. However, separation of these mechanisms is useful for understanding hemostasis, and derangements in one or the other produce a different clinical picture.

Platelets are produced by megakaryocytes in the bone marrow and have a plasma life span of 10 days. Most, and perhaps all, of the coagulation factors are synthesized by the liver. Factor VIII may be the exception, based on the clinical observation that Factor VIII activity increases in adolescents with liver disease. The cell or tissue that is responsible for Factor VIII synthesis is unknown. Factor XII, high molecular weight kininogen, prekallikrein, and Factor XI are called the contact activation coagulation factors. Factors II, VII, IX, and X are the vitamin K–dependent factors, and fibrinogen and Factors II, V, and VIII are the consumption coagulation factors (since they are used up or consumed during the process of clotting).

There are three important, naturally occurring coagulation factor inhibitors found in plasma. Antithrombin III (AT-III) is produced by the liver and is not a vitamin K–dependent protein. It functions to neutralize those activated coagulation factors that have a serine in the active site (e.g., Factors IIa, Xa, IXa, and probably XIa and XIIa). Protein C is synthesized by the liver and is a vitamin K–dependent protein. Protein C must be activated (protein Ca) by a thrombin-thrombomodulin complex. Protein Ca, using protein S as a cofactor, inhibits Factors V and VIII. Protein Ca also enhances fibrinolysis by reducing the activity of plasminogen activator inhibitor. Protein S is synthesized by the liver and by endothelial cells. It is a vitamin K–dependent protein.

The fibrinolytic mechanism is involved with the removal of fibrin by enzymatic proteolysis. It is composed of a precursor (plasminogen) that must be converted to the active enzyme (plasmin) by agents called plasminogen activators. These activators are found in blood, tissues, and body fluids. The plasminogen activators and plasmin are balanced by a set of inhibitors—the plasminogen activator inhibitors and antiplasmins, respectively. Lysis occurs only when the activator content increases or when the inhibitor activity decreases. The lysed fibrin is soluble and can be detected in the blood as fibrinolytic split products or fibrinolytic degradation products.

Clinical Features. Purpura is an all-inclusive term for a group of disorders characterized by purplish or brownish-red discoloration caused by hemorrhages in the tissues. Petechiae are small (pinhead-sized) capillary hemorrhages that usually are not raised. Ecchymoses are bruises or black-and-blue marks; they are caused by larger hemorrhages in the tissues. Thus, purpura ranges from petechial to ecchymotic lesions. However, the term is commonly used to describe bleeding caused by thrombocytopenia, platelet dysfunction, or vasculitis.

A detailed medical history, family history, physical examination, and selected laboratory tests allow the physician to determine if a defective hemostatic mechanism exists, which pathway of the mechanism is impaired, and whether the condition is acquired or inher-

ited. Through these means, the following can be ascertained: the cause of the bleeding or thrombosis (spontaneous or induced), the site of the bleeding (mucous membranes, skin, musculoskeletal), the duration of the bleeding episode (minutes versus hours, easy or difficult to control using local measures), the character of the bleeding (petechiae, ecchymoses, hematomas), family history of a bleeding-thrombotic disorder, drug-induced disease, and any underlying diseases that may be associated with a defect in the hemostatic mechanism.

Laboratory Tests. Laboratory screening tests (Table 52–10) are employed to evaluate the primary and secondary hemostatic mechanisms. There are no reliable screening tests for detection of plasma inhibitor deficiency or vascular diseases.

Since the most common cause of an impaired primary mechanism is thrombocytopenia, the usual first step is to obtain a platelet count and to examine a stained blood smear. The blood smear can be used to estimate platelet quantity and to detect morphologic abnormalities. If the platelet count is normal, a bleeding time can be performed. The bleeding time is the best test for assessing the primary hemostatic mechanism, but it is a measurement mainly of blood platelet function and platelet-blood vessel interaction. An abnormally prolonged bleeding time indicates impaired platelet function. Further *in vitro* studies designed to assess platelet function (e.g., poor adhesion, reduced or no aggregation, and so on) can then be performed.

The screening tests for the secondary hemostatic mechanism include the plasma prothrombin time (PT) and the partial thromboplastin time (PTT). The PT is a measure of the tissue (or extrinsic) pathway and is affected by the levels of Factors II, V, VII, X, and fibrinogen. The PTT is a measure of the plasma (or intrinsic) pathway and is affected by the levels of prekallikrein, high molecular weight kininogen, Factors XII, XI, IX, VIII, X, V, and II, and fibrinogen. Neither test assesses Factor XIII activity; this must be accomplished by using a clot stability test (5M urea or 1% monochloroacetic acid). The thrombin clotting time (TCT) is a measure of the fibrinogen-to-fibrin reaction and therefore is affected by the fibrinogen concentration and inhibitors in the reaction. The PTT, PT, and TCT are useful screening tests for suspected bleeding disorders. They are of limited value in the assessment of hyper-

TABLE 52–10. Screening Tests for Hemostasis

TEST	MEASURES
Platelet count and examination of blood smear	Platelet quantity and morphologic features
Bleeding time	Platelet quality
Prothrombin time (PT)	Factors II, V, VII, X, and fibrinogen
Partial thromboplastin time (PTT)	Factors XII, XI, IX, VIII, X, V, II, and, fibrinogen, prekallikrein, high molecular weight kininogen
Thrombin clotting time (TCT)	Fibrinogen
Clot solubility (5M urea)	Factor XIII
Euglobulin lysis time (ELT)	Fibrinolysis
Fibrinolytic split (degradation) products	Fibrinolysis

coagulability states. Severe and moderate coagulation factor deficiencies can be detected by these tests. Mild deficiencies may give normal results. Further testing may include mixing studies to differentiate between a deficiency and an inhibitor and specific factor assays.

Fibrinolysis is assessed by the euglobulin clot lysis time (ELT) and by the detection of fibrinolytic split products and fibrinolytic degradation products. This test cannot assess hypofibrinolysis. The ELT is a measure of plasminogen activator activity. A short lysis time (<60 minutes) suggests hyperfibrinolysis. The presence of fibrinolytic split products indicates that fibrin or its precursors have been lysed by plasmin. Further studies may include assays for plasminogen activators, plasminogen activator inhibitors, and α_2-antiplasmin.

There are no screening tests for AT-III, protein C, or protein S. Specific functional and protein assays are available.

In the plasma, von Willebrand factor is assessed by functional assays (ristocetin cofactor test, ristocetin-induced platelet aggregation) and immunoprecipitation methods (von Willebrand factor–antigen or protein). A complete discussion of von Willebrand disease follows in the section on coagulation disorders.

HEMORRHAGIC DISORDERS

Disorders of the Primary Hemostatic Mechanism: Platelet and Blood Vessel Disorders

Clinical Features. Adolescents who have defects in the primary hemostatic mechanism present a typical clinical appearance. The most common bleeding symptoms and signs are in the skin and mucous membranes. These adolescents have epistaxis, menorrhagia, and gastrointestinal (GI) and genitourinary hemorrhages. The characteristic types of bleeding are petechiae and ecchymoses. Spontaneous bruises may occur and are usually small (1 × 1 to 3 × 3 cm), superficial, and often multiple. Following injury or surgical procedures, the onset of bleeding is usually immediate and many times can be controlled by local measures such as the use of pressure or ice. In addition, these adolescent patients bleed for a prolonged period from superficial cuts and abrasions.

Platelet and blood vessel disorders are classified as either thrombocytopenic purpura or nonthrombocytopenic purpura on the basis of the platelet count (Table 52–11). The normal platelet count is 150 to 400 × 10⁹/L. Counts less than this range indicate thrombocytopenia from either inadequate production or excessive destruction or removal of platelets.

Inadequate production is almost always due to bone marrow dysfunction, with decreases in the number of megakaryocytes. By contrast, in the thrombocytopenias that result from increased destruction, the megakaryocytes are quantitatively normal or increased.

THROMBOCYTOPENIA

Acquired Disorders

Idiopathic Thrombocytopenic Purpura (ITP). ITP is the most common thrombocytopenic condition in ado-

TABLE 52–11. Platelet and Blood Vessel Disorders

I. Thrombocytopenic Purpuras
  A. *Acquired Types*
    1. Increased destruction or loss of platelets
      (a) Idiopathic thrombocytopenic purpura (ITP)
      (b) Infections
      (c) Immunologic disorders
        (1) Drug-induced (see Table 52–12)
        (2) Autoimmune diseases (e.g., SLE)
      (d) Microangiopathic diseases (e.g., hemolytic uremic syndrome, thrombotic thrombocytopenic purpura, eclampsia-preeclampsia)
      (e) Hypersplenism
    2. Decreased or ineffective production of platelets
      (a) Idiopathic aplastic anemia
      (b) Neoplastic replacement of bone marrow
      (c) Infections
      (d) Chemical agents, drugs, radiation
  B. *Inherited-Congenital Types*
    1. Increased destruction or loss of platelets
      (a) Bernard-Soulier syndrome
      (b) May-Hegglin anomaly
      (c) Familial thrombocytopenia
    2. Decreased or ineffective production of platelets
      (a) Fanconi aplastic anemia
      (b) Other hypomegakaryocytic conditions
II. Nonthrombocytopenic Purpuras
  A. *Acquired Types*
    1. Drug-induced platelet disorders (e.g., aspirin; nonsteroidal anti-inflammatory drugs)
    2. Vasculitis (e.g., SLE, Henoch-Schönlein purpura)
    3. Uremia-induced platelet defects
    4. Hepatic failure–induced platelet defects
  B. *Congenital-Inherited Types*
    1. Platelet defects
      (a) Glanzmann disease
      (b) Storage pool disease
      (c) Platelet release defects
    2. Blood vessel defects
      (a) Ehlers-Danlos syndrome
      (b) Hereditary hemorrhagic telangiectasia

lescence. Clinical manifestations include skin and mucous membrane petechiae, epistaxis, menorrhagia (see Chapter 70), and multiple small ecchymoses. Rarely, there may be central nervous system (CNS) bleeding. There is marked deficiency of circulating platelets in association with adequate numbers of megakaryocytes in the bone marrow. There are two forms of ITP, classified according to the time of clinical onset and the duration of the disease. Acute ITP is of sudden onset, and spontaneous resolution occurs within 3 to 12 months. Chronic ITP is insidious and persists for longer than 12 months. Spontaneous bleeding manifestations are more frequent and generally more severe in acute ITP.

Etiology. The cause of acute ITP is unknown. The disease frequently (70% of cases) is preceded by a respiratory infection. The interval between infection and the onset of purpura is 2 to 4 weeks. Although platelet-bound IgG is present (which may represent immune complexes), specific autoantibodies are lacking in this condition. Chronic ITP, however, is associated with platelet autoantibodies in more than 50% of adolescent patients. Also, a chronic ITP syndrome occurs with other known immunologic diseases, such as systemic lupus erythematosus (SLE) (see Chapter 90), acquired immunodeficiency syndrome (AIDS) (see Chapter 76), lymphomas (see Chapter 53), and Evans syndrome (autoimmune hemolytic anemia with ITP). There is no consistently reliable test for the serologic diagnosis of ITP.

Clinical Manifestations. The onset may be sudden or insidious. The bleeding is typically asymmetric with prominent hemorrhages in and from the mucous membranes. Nosebleeds and uterine bleeding may be severe and difficult to control. The liver, spleen, and lymph nodes are not enlarged. Except for the signs of bleeding, the adolescent appears clinically well.

Laboratory Data. The platelet count is reduced, generally less than $20 \times 10^9/L$ in acute ITP and between 20 and $50 \times 10^9/L$ in chronic ITP. The platelets are large but appear morphologically normal on the blood smear. Tests that depend on platelet function, such as the bleeding time and clot retraction, give abnormal results. The white blood cells are normal, and anemia is not present unless significant blood loss has occurred. The findings on bone marrow examination are normal.

Treatment. Acute ITP has an excellent prognosis, even when no specific therapy is given. Within 9 to 12 months, the platelet count has returned to normal in 90% of adolescents, and relapses are unusual. The decision to begin treatment is based on the severity of the bleeding manifestations irrespective of the platelet count. Simple skin bruising and minor, easy to control mucous membrane bleeding require no specific therapy. Hemorrhages that cause anemia, are difficult to control, or occur in dangerous locations (such as the CNS) are indications for treatment. Therapy may consist of corticosteroids, intravenous gamma globulin, platelet transfusion, and splenectomy. Corticosteroid therapy is associated with the control of the bleeding in 48 to 72 hours in more than 90% of these adolescents. Prednisone is the drug used most often (1 to 2 mg/kg/day, in divided doses). The therapy is continued for 3 weeks. At this point the drug is discontinued even if the platelet count remains low. If thrombocytopenia persists for 4 to 6 months, a second short course of the drug may be given. Infusions of intravenous gamma globulin (IVGG) (Sandoglobulin, Sandoz, Inc.; Gamimune, Cutter Biologicals) have been found to increase the platelet count within 24 hours and may cause remission. The current recommended dose is 2 g/kg given intravenously over 2 to 5 days. IVGG is expensive and must be given by vein. Platelet transfusions are of limited value in ITP. They may be effective in helping to control life-threatening hemorrhage. They provide temporary control of bleeding, but sustained normal platelet counts are not achieved. Splenectomy is reserved for emergency bleeding episodes that are unresponsive to any of the previous therapeutic approaches.

Chronic ITP is defined by the presence of the disease for more than 12 months. The frequency of spontaneous remissions is unknown. Symptomatic patients are treated with a program similar to that for adolescents with acute ITP. However, permanent remissions are unusual. Splenectomy may be curative in 70% to 80% of these adolescents. Adolescent patients who are unresponsive to splenectomy can be treated with corticosteroids or IVGG. It has not been proven that other drugs such as danazol or cytotoxic agents can induce remissions. Adolescents undergoing splenectomy should be warned of the increased risk of overwhelming bacterial infection, should be immunized against pneumococcal and hemophilus polysaccharide, and should be cautioned to seek medical assistance promptly in the event of fever. Some physicians employ antibiotic prophylaxis for asplenic adolescents.

Drug-induced Thrombocytopenia. A number of drugs can cause thrombocytopenia (Table 52–12). The cause can be either an immune-mediated process or a megakaryocyte injury. Treatment consists of removing the offending drug and supportive care. The platelet count usually returns to normal within a few days, but some drugs may cause permanent hematopoietic injury.

Immunologic Disorders. Thrombocytopenia is a frequent manifestation of certain autoimmune diseases (e.g., 20% of patients with SLE; see Chapter 90) and in other immune complex diseases (e.g., serum sickness, bacterial endocarditis, bacterial septicemia). Thrombocytopenia may be an initial clinical manifestation of HIV infection (see Chapter 76).

Microangiopathic Diseases. These diseases have in common small blood vessel injury with microthrombosis in association with hemolytic anemia and thrombocytopenia (not caused by disseminated intravascular coagulation [DIC]). This group includes the hemolytic-uremic syndrome (HUS), thrombotic thrombocytopenic purpura (TTP), and eclampsia-preeclampsia (in pregnant adolescents).

Laboratory Data. Hemolytic anemia is associated with bizarre red cell morphologic features. Many of the red blood cells are contracted and distorted with prominence of burr cells, helmet-shaped forms, and spherocytes (termed *microangiopathic hemolytic anemia*). The platelet count is reduced despite normal numbers of megakaryocytes in the marrow, which indicates excessive peripheral destruction. Tests of the coagulation mechanism usually give normal results. Protein, red blood cells, and casts are present in the urinary sediment, and serious renal damage is reflected by anuria and azotemia (especially noted in HUS and TTP).

Treatment. The management of these diseases consists of red blood cell transfusions for anemia, platelet transfusions for significant bleeding, and dialysis for renal failure. Adolescents who have HUS may benefit from infusions of normal plasma. Recent data suggest that there is a platelet-aggregating substance in the plasma

---

TABLE 52–12. Drug-Induced Thrombocytopenia*

Antibacterial drugs (e.g., chloramphenicol, sulfonamides)
Antirheumatic drugs (e.g., phenylbutazone, indomethacin, gold salts, colchicine)
Anticonvulsants (e.g., diphenylhydantoin, mephenytoin, primidone, ethosuximide, valproic acid)
Cardiac drugs (e.g., digoxin, procainamide, quinidine, methyldopa)
Diuretics (e.g., thiazides, acetazolamide)
Cytotoxic drugs (e.g., methotrexate, 6-mercaptopurine, cyclophosphamide, azathioprine)
Miscellaneous (e.g., heparin, acetaminophen, alcohol, estrogens, allopurinol)

*Note: This list is not all-inclusive.

of HUS patients that may be neutralized by normal adult plasma.

In adolescents who have TTP, plasmapheresis and plasma exchange are reported to be effective in 60% to 79% of these individuals. Corticosteroids and splenectomy are reserved for refractory cases. Heparin therapy does not affect survival or prognosis in these diseases. The termination of pregnancy controls eclampsia and preeclampsia.

Hypersplenism. This condition develops in adolescents who have enlarged spleens secondary to obstructive or increased pressure in the portal or splenic veins. It is manifested as hemolytic anemia, neutropenia, and thrombocytopenia. The treatment of choice is splenectomy in adolescents who have significant thrombocytopenia and bleeding (see risks of splenectomy in section on chronic ITP). Hypersplenic destruction of blood cells may also be seen in inherited storage diseases (e.g., Gaucher disease). Consideration of partial splenectomy should be given in such cases.

Decreased or Ineffective Production of Platelets. Adolescents who have aplastic anemia, neoplastic replacement of the bone marrow, certain infections (e.g., disseminated tuberculosis), or who have been exposed to chemical agents, toxic drugs, and radiation will have thrombocytopenia. Treatment consists of controlling the underlying disease, removal of the toxic material, and supportive care with platelet transfusions for bleeding episodes. Platelet replacement is effective, since the infused cells have a normal circulating life span.

Inherited and Congenital Disorders

Thrombocytopenia. The inherited thrombocytopenias are rare, and most are diagnosed prior to adolescence. These conditions include the Wiskott-Aldrich syndrome (an X-linked disorder with eczema, thrombocytopenia, and immunologic defects), the Bernard-Soulier syndrome (an autosomal recessive disorder with giant platelets and poor platelet adhesion), the May-Hegglin anomaly (an autosomal dominant condition with leukocyte inclusions), and familial thrombocytopenia (an autosomal dominant condition).

NONTHROMBOCYTOPENIC PURPURAS

Acquired Disorders

Platelet Function Disorders. Acquired disorders of platelet function are caused by toxic metabolic products (e.g., in uremia), autoantibodies, immune complexes, fibrin split products, and drugs. The most common acquired defect is caused by drugs. Affected adolescents have prolonged bleeding times and abnormalities in platelet aggregation test results. Treatment consists of removing the underlying cause. Corticosteroids may be helpful in immune-mediated types. Platelet transfusions are rarely needed.

Vascular Disorders. The most common cause of a vascular type of nonthrombocytopenic purpura is Schönlein-Henoch purpura (anaphylactoid purpura). This is an acute inflammatory process of unknown origin involving the small blood vessels of the skin, joints, gut,

and kidney. The centrifugal distribution of the rash and involvement of the legs and buttocks are characteristic especially when combined with arthritis, nephritis, or GI bleeding. Treatment of this self-limited condition is supportive. Corticosteroids have been effective in controlling the painful edema, GI pain, and arthritis but not the skin rash or nephritis. Laboratory test results of hemostasis are normal.

Congenital and Inherited Disorders

Platelet Defects. These are rare causes of nonthrombocytopenic purpura and include Glanzmann disease (impaired platelet aggregation and clot retraction), storage pool disease, and platelet release defects (impaired release reaction). These are autosomal recessive conditions characterized by prolonged bleeding times and various abnormalities in platelet aggregation. Treatment of the bleeding manifestations in these adolescents is difficult. Platelet transfusions are usually required to control significant hemorrhage.

Blood Vessel Defects. Bleeding secondary to defective blood vessels is uncommon in early childhood. They tend to make their appearance in the adolescent period. Disorders such as hereditary hemorrhagic telangiectasia (telangiectasias of the skin, fingers, lips, tongue, GI tract) and Ehlers-Danlos syndrome can cause significant mucous membrane bleeding and bleeding of the skin. All laboratory test results for hemostasis are usually normal in these adolescents. Therapy is supportive.

Disorders of the Secondary Hemostatic Mechanism: Coagulation Disorders

Clinical Features. Adolescents who have defects in the secondary hemostatic mechanism (coagulation mechanism) (Table 52–13) present with ecchymoses and hematomas. Petechiae are not observed. The most common bleeding manifestation is hemorrhage in the deep tissues, especially in the muscles, joints, and skin. Hemarthroses are common in severe cases. These adolescents do not have excessive bleeding from superficial cuts and abrasions. Hemorrhage associated with deep

TABLE 52–13. Coagulation Factor Disorders

I. Acquired Types
  A. Vitamin K deficiency
  B. Consumption coagulopathy
    1. Disseminated intravascular coagulation
    2. Diffuse intravascular thrombosis
    3. Massive localized thrombosis
  C. Parenchymal liver disease
  D. Acquired inhibitors (circulating anticoagulant)
  E. Anticoagulants (iatrogenic)
II. Common Inherited Types
  A. Hemophilias
    1. Hemophilia A (Factor VIII deficiency)
    2. Hemophilia B (Factor IX deficiency)
    3. Hemophilia C (Factor XI deficiency)
  B. Von Willebrand disease

cuts or surgical procedures is characteristically delayed in onset (hours to days) and generally is not controlled by local means. Control of the bleeding is best accomplished by replacement of the deficient coagulation factors.

ACQUIRED CAUSES

Vitamin K Deficiency

Vitamin K is a fat-soluble vitamin that is required for normal hemostasis. The vitamin is involved in the biosynthesis of coagulation factors II, VII, IX, and X and the natural inhibitors protein C and protein S. Vitamin K is found in a wide variety of foods; the highest concentration is in green leafy vegetables. As with other fat-soluble vitamins, bile salts and normal fat absorption are required. Since body stores of the vitamin are limited, a deficiency can occur within a few days in circumstances of reduced intake or absorption. Antagonists of vitamin K (e.g., warfarin) are used as anticoagulants. Vitamin K deficiency beyond the newborn period is seen in adolescents who are anorectic (see Chapter 60), who have restricted oral alimentation (exclusively parenteral hyperalimentation), or who have fat malabsorption or diminished flow of bile (see Chapters 43 and 62).

Signs and symptoms of bleeding include easy bruising, mucosal bleeding (epistaxis, GI bleeding, menometrorrhagia [see Chapter 70]), hematuria, and oozing from puncture sites, cutdowns, and surgical incisions. Intracranial bleeding and hemorrhage into the retroperitoneal space may cause severe morbidity.

Laboratory Findings. The PT and PTT are prolonged. The platelet count and bleeding time are normal. If needed, specific assays for Factors II, VII, IX, and X or laboratory tests for detecting the noncarboxylated protein precursors of the vitamin K–dependent procoagulants can be performed.

Treatment. Adolescents who have severe laboratory abnormalities or clinical bleeding manifestations are treated with parenteral vitamin K. The preparation used is the natural derivative vitamin K (AquaMEPHYTON) (5 to 10 mg subcutaneously). The intramuscular route should be avoided because it can be associated with hematomas and delayed absorption. In most instances, hemorrhage ceases and the PT and PTT return to normal 12 to 24 hours after vitamin K therapy. These tests should be repeated after 24 hours to confirm the correction. If a decrease in bleeding and improvement in the laboratory studies have not occurred, the diagnosis is incorrect, or the patient may have other associated coagulation disturbances.

For the adolescent who manifests significant hemorrhage, fresh frozen plasma (15 ml/kg), in addition to vitamin K, is infused. The plasma provides immediate correction of the coagulopathy for a few hours. Very rarely, a prothrombin complex concentrate may be needed to correct the defect (e.g., Konӯne-HT, Cutter Biologicals, 50 units/kg). These concentrates should be avoided if at all possible, as they are associated with a high risk of hepatitis and can cause thrombosis (especially in adolescents with liver disease).

Following initial replacement therapy with vitamin K, subsequent doses of the vitamin should be given twice to three times weekly if the underlying problem (malabsorption, broad spectrum antibiotic administration, long-term parental alimentation) persists. In adolescent patients with fat malabsorption, an oral water-soluble vitamin K preparation can be employed on a daily basis.

Liver Disease

Coagulation abnormalities are common in adolescents who have liver disease (see Chapter 62); they are estimated to be as high as 85%. The severity of the coagulation abnormality is directly proportional to the extent of hepatic cell damage. The most common mechanism causing the defect is decreased synthesis of the coagulation factors. Less common causes are DIC or hyperfibrinolysis, or both.

Laboratory Findings. Since most of the coagulation factors are produced by the liver, the coagulation screening test results (PTT, PT, and TCT) may be abnormal. Specific assays may be required to differentiate the coagulopathy of liver disease from vitamin K deficiency or DIC, or both.

Adolescents who have liver disease may also have a defective primary hemostatic mechanism from thrombocytopenia.

Treatment. The treatment of the coagulopathy of liver disease consists of replacement with fresh frozen plasma and cryoprecipitates. Fresh frozen plasma (10 to 15 ml/kg) can be expected to temporarily correct all clotting factor defects except that of fibrinogen. For fibrinogen correction, cryoprecipitates are used (four to five bags/10 kg body weight). Since a reduction in the vitamin K–dependent factors is common in acute and chronic liver disease, a trial of the vitamin can be tried. The vitamin can be given orally or subcutaneously in a dose of 5 mg/day for adolescents. An inability to correct the coagulopathy indicates that the coagulopathy may be due to a reduction in one or more of the non-vitamin K–dependent proteins or that the liver is severely impaired and cannot produce the precursor vitamin K proteins.

Inhibitors

Acquired circulating anticoagulants (inhibitors) are endogenous materials (usually gamma globulins) that inhibit the coagulation of normal blood. The anticoagulant may affect coagulation by directly neutralizing a specific coagulation factor or it may act against certain reaction sites in the coagulation mechanism. When the inhibitor acts against a specific factor (such as Factor VIII or Factor IX), the adolescent has a clinical bleeding picture similar to that in the congenital deficiency state. Usually minimal or no bleeding is noted in adolescents in whom the inhibitor is directed toward a reaction site. The most common example of the latter type of inhibitor is the so-called lupus anticoagulant, which was first described in patients with SLE but can be seen in a variety of other diseases. Adolescents who have this type of inhibitor do not have hemorrhagic diatheses.

Circulating anticoagulants are uncommon in otherwise healthy adolescents. They are found in adolescents with SLE, lymphoma, and penicillin and other drug reactions, and as a transient postviral event in normal adolescents.

Laboratory Findings. The PT is normal. The PTT is prolonged and is not corrected by the addition of normal plasma. When the inhibitor is directed against Factor VIII or Factor IX, the PTT in a mixture of patient and normal plasma worsens with incubation. Coagulation factor assays will determine which factor is affected.

The lupus anticoagulant causes a prolonged PTT that is not corrected by the addition of normal plasma and does not worsen with incubation.

Treatment. Adolescent patients with the lupus anticoagulant require no treatment because this inhibitor is not a cause of bleeding. Adolescents with an inhibitor against a clotting factor are difficult to manage and are treated in the same manner as are hemophilia patients in whom an alloantibody develops against Factor VIII or Factor IX. The spontaneous inhibitors that follow viral infections tend to disappear within a few weeks to months. Inhibitors seen with an underlying disease will disappear when the primary disease is treated successfully.

Consumption Coagulopathy

Consumption coagulopathy (Table 52–14) means that intravascular clotting is occurring or has occurred and causes the consumption or utilization of various coagulation factors and blood platelets. Consequences of this process include widespread or local intravascular deposition of fibrin (which may lead to tissue ischemia and necrosis), a generalized bleeding state, and hemolytic anemia.

Consumption coagulopathy is produced by three main processes: (1) DIC, (2) diffuse intravascular thrombosis (DIT), and (3) massive local thrombosis. In DIC, clot-promoting material is infused into the systemic circulation, which activates the coagulation-fibrinolytic mechanisms (e.g., shock, massive tissue damage, certain leukemias). In DIT, there is diffuse and extensive local thrombosis in small to medium blood vessels secondary to vascular damage (e.g., disseminated viral diseases, heat stroke). This process consumes fibrinogen and other clotting factors in the plasma. In massive local thrombosis (e.g., thrombosis of the vena cava, aortic thrombosis), the circulating blood is depleted of coagulation factors. All three conditions produce similar laboratory findings and therefore are classified as the consumption coagulopathies.

Clinical Manifestations. Bleeding frequently occurs from sites of venipuncture or surgical wounds, with associated petechiae and ecchymoses. Tissue thrombosis may involve many organs. Pallor or jaundice, or both, may be present because of anemia. The anemia results from bleeding and, in some adolescent patients, from hemolysis.

Laboratory Findings. The consumption factors (Factors II, V, VIII, fibrinogen) and platelets are consumed by the intravascular clotting process. This results in a prolongation of the PT, PTT, and TCT. The platelets may be significantly reduced. The blood smear shows reduced platelets and the red blood cells may be fragmented, with burr cells and helmet shapes similar to those seen in HUS and TTP. In addition, the fibrinolytic mechanism is activated, which is demonstrated by finding fibrinolytic split products in the blood.

Treatment. The most important component of therapy is the control or reversal of the process that initiated the consumption process. Infection, shock, acidosis, and hypoxia must be treated promptly. In the case of pregnancy-induced DIC (e.g., abruptio placentae), removal of the products of conception will immediately reverse the process. If the underlying problem can be controlled, bleeding quickly ceases and there is improvement of the abnormal laboratory findings. Blood components are used for replacement therapy in patients who have hemorrhage. This may consist of platelet infusions for thrombocytopenia, cryoprecipitates for hypofibrinogenemia or fresh frozen plasma for replacement of other coagulation and inhibitor factors, or both, and packed red blood cells as indicated.

In some adolescent patients, the treatment of the primary disease may be inadequate or incomplete, or the replacement therapy has not been effective in controlling the hemorrhage. When this occurs, the adolescent may be treated with anticoagulants. Heparin is the drug of choice and can be administered on an intermittent or continuous intravenous treatment schedule. Using the intermittent intravenous schedule, heparin is given in a dose of 75 to 100 units/kg every 4 hours. In the continuous schedule, 50 to 75 units/kg is given as a bolus followed by a continuous infusion of 15 to 25 units/kg/hour. The duration and effectiveness of heparin therapy can be judged by serial measurements of the platelet count, partial thromboplastin time, and plasma fibrinogen concentration.

Heparin has been found to be an effective drug in patients with purpura fulminans, progranulocytic leukemia, massive large vessel thrombosis, and pulmonary embolism. Heparin is not indicated and it has been reported to be ineffective in septic shock, snake enven-

---

TABLE 52–14. Examples of Consumption Coagulopathies

I. Disseminated intravascular coagulation (DIC)
  Infection (septic shock; rickettsial, protozoal)
  Shock
  Snake envenomation
  Massive trauma
  Massive head trauma
  Abruptio placentae
  Retained dead fetus syndrome
  Peritoneovenous shunt
  Hemolytic transfusion reaction
II. Diffuse intravascular thrombosis (DIT)
  Infection (disseminated viral)
  Heat stroke
  Vasculitis
III. Localized thrombosis
  Giant hemangioma
  Large vessel thrombosis
  Pulmonary embolism
  Rattlesnake bite

omation, heat stroke, massive head injury, incompatible blood transfusion reaction, amniotic fluid embolism, and abruptio placentae.

CONGENITAL AND INHERITED CAUSES

Hemophilias and von Willebrand Disease

Hemophilia A (Classic Hemophilia). Hemophilia A is caused by a deficiency of Factor VIII activity and is the most common type of hemophilia (80% of patients with hemophilia). It is inherited in an X-linked recessive manner, and 80% of affected individuals have a positive family history of the disease. Patients with hemophilia A and women who are carriers for the disorder have reduced Factor VIII activity but normal plasma levels of von Willebrand protein (in contrast to classic von Willebrand disease in which both levels are reduced) (Table 52–15). The clinical severity depends on the level of the coagulation factor activity in the plasma. Patients with severe disease have less than 1% (less than 1 unit/dl) of normal activity, patients with moderate disease have 1% to 5% (1 to 5 units/dl) of normal activity, and patients with mild disease have 6% to 30% (6 to 30 units/dl) of normal activity. The degree of severity tends to be consistent within a given family.

Clinical Manifestations. Ninety percent of patients with severe disease have had clear clinical evidence of increased bleeding by 1 year of age. Patients with moderate disease rarely have spontaneous bleeding episodes; thus the diagnosis may not be suspected for a number of years. However, most of these patients will be diagnosed by adolescence. Patients with mild hemophilia bleed excessively only after major trauma or surgical procedures. These patients may not be detected until adolescence or adulthood.

The hallmark of severe and moderate hemophilia is hemarthrosis. Hemorrhages into the elbows, knees, ankles, hips, and shoulders cause pain, swelling, and limitation of motion. Repeated bleeding episodes into the joints can produce degenerative changes with subsequent osteoporosis, muscle atrophy, and finally a fixed joint. Muscle hematomas are common and are usually induced by trauma. Spontaneous hematuria is a common but not usually serious complication. Intracranial hem-

TABLE 52–15. Hemophilia A and Classic von Willebrand Disease Laboratory Findings

	HEMOPHILIA A	VON WILLEBRAND DISEASE
Platelet count	N	N
Bleeding time	N	P
Prothrombin time	N	N
Partial thromboplastin time	P	N/P
Factor VIII activity	Low	Low
vWf:Ag	N	Low
vWfR:Co	N	Low
vWf multimers	N	N
RIPA	N	Low

P, prolonged; N, normal; N/P, normal or prolonged; vWf, von Willebrand factor; Ag, antigen (protein); R:Co, ristocetin cofactor; RIPA, ristocetin-induced platelet aggregation.

orrhage and bleeding into the neck constitute life-threatening emergencies.

Laboratory Findings. The PTT is prolonged and the platelet count, bleeding time, and PT are normal. Mixing patient plasma with normal plasma produces correction of the PTT. A specific assay for Factor VIII activity will confirm the diagnosis.

Prenatal Diagnosis. Each male fetus of a mother who carries hemophilia has a 50% risk of having the disease. Prenatal diagnosis is possible through examination of the blood of the male fetus, which can be obtained by fetoscopy at 20 to 22 weeks of gestation. Fetal plasma is assayed for Factor VIII activity. It has recently become possible to identify a fetus with hemophilia by using deoxyribonucleic acid (DNA) polymorphisms in amniotic fluid fibroblasts. Trophoblastic biopsy may permit the diagnosis of hemophilia as early as 10 to 12 weeks of gestation. The family history in pregnant adolescents should always determine if a disorder of hemostasis exists in other family members.

Treatment. Prevention of trauma is an important aspect of care for the adolescent with hemophilia. Aspirin and other drugs that inhibit platelet function must be avoided. Because the patient will be exposed to blood products throughout life, he or she should be immunized against hepatitis B.

When bleeding episodes occur, replacement therapy is essential to prevent pain, disability, or life-threatening hemorrhage. The aim of therapy is to increase Factor VIII activity in the plasma to hemostatic levels (usually greater than 40% activity). This is accomplished by using Factor VIII concentrates. The amount that is infused is determined by the bleeding episode and the subsequent response to replacement therapy. The newer concentrates are heat- or detergent-treated to eliminate transmission of HIV. Most hematomas and early hemarthroses can be treated with one infusion of Factor VIII. Massive hematomas (e.g., in the thigh, pelvis, or retroperitoneum) require more intensive treatment, usually for 2 or 3 days. Oral bleeding (e.g., injuries, lacerations, dental extractions) can be controlled by a single prophylactic infusion of the factor plus the addition of an antifibrinolytic drug for 7 to 14 days. ε-Aminocaproic acid (Amicar, Lederle) is commonly used. Intracranial bleeding and major surgery is treated with infusions of Factor VIII to achieve 100% activity for 7 to 14 days, depending on the need. Desmopressin (DDAVP; Stimate, Rorer Pharmaceuticals) causes an increase in Factor VIII activity in patients with mild hemophilia A. It should be given once every 1 to 2 days and only for minor bleeding episodes such as oral bleeding, dental extractions, and small hematomas. It is ineffective in hemarthrosis and CNS bleeding and for sustaining Factor VIII levels following major surgery. DDAVP cannot be used for prolonged periods because of associated tachyphylaxis.

Home or self-treatment offers optimal management for the adolescent with hemophilia, which allows greater independence and earlier treatment of bleeding episodes, especially hemarthroses. Long-term complications of modern-day therapy include chronic liver disease (perhaps as high as 15% to 20% of patients) and alloimmunization to Factor VIII. Prior to mid-1985, these patients were exposed to HIV. A high proportion are HIV antibody–positive, and overt AIDS has developed in many (see Chapter 76).

Chronic joint disease continues to be a major complication of hemophilia. In the early stages there is proliferative synovitis that progresses to joint destruction and fibrosis. Corticosteroids can help control the synovitis but in most cases will not produce a permanent remission. Other drugs such as nonsteroidal anti-inflammatory agents will give relief of pain and stiffness but will not reverse synovitis. Investigative studies using other drugs (such as D-penicillamine) hold promise, but their efficacy is unproved. Such adolescent patients eventually need synovectomy or, in severe destructive cases, joint replacement.

Factor VIII Inhibitors. Ten to 15% of patients with hemophilia A become refractory to Factor VIII therapy because a circulating inhibitor develops. This inhibitor is an alloantibody against Factor VIII activity. Adolescents who have elevated inhibitor levels are difficult to treat. It is impossible to overpower the inhibitor with massive doses of Factor VIII in most cases. Procoagulant therapy should be avoided, except to treat life-threatening hemorrhage. It has been found that the infusion of prothrombin complex concentrates (Konyne HT, Cutter Biologicals) or activated prothrombin complex (Autoplex, Hyland; FEIBA, Immuno) can bypass Factor VIII in the coagulation scheme and provide hemostasis. However, the activities of the various preparations vary markedly. Porcine Factor VIII (Hyate:C, Porton Products) is effective in some hemophilia A patients with inhibitors. Plasmapheresis followed by an infusion of a large dose of either human or porcine Factor VIII can be employed in life-threatening events but this is of only temporary benefit. Immunosuppressive therapy has been of no value in these patients.

Hemophilia B (Factor IX Deficiency, Christmas Disease). About 12% to 15% of the hemophilias result from Factor IX deficiency. This disease is clinically indistinguishable from Factor VIII deficiency (hemophilia A). It is also inherited in an X-linked manner. Although female carriers can be identified by Factor IX coagulant assays, the detection is more specific when monoclonal antibody or DNA analysis techniques are used. Prenatal detection is difficult.

Laboratory Findings. As in hemophilia A, the PTT is prolonged and the PT, bleeding time, and platelet count are normal. Specific assay is necessary to differentiate the deficiency from hemophilia A and to define the severity of the defect.

Treatment. Factor IX replacement is accomplished by infusions of fresh frozen plasma or a concentrate containing Factor IX. All hemophilia B patients should receive the hepatitis B vaccine. All adolescents with hemophilia B should receive the hepatitis B vaccine.

Hemophilia C (Factor XI Deficiency). Factor XI deficiency is the least common type of hemophilia, being found in 2% to 3% of all adolescents with hemophilia. Factor XI deficiency is transmitted as an autosomal recessive disease that affects males and females. It is seen almost exclusively in Ashkenazi Jews. Only homozygous patients have a bleeding diathesis. Spontaneous bleeding is rare. These adolescent patients may

have epistaxis, hematuria, and menorrhagia; postoperative and post trauma hemorrhage is characteristic.

Laboratory Findings. The PTT is prolonged and the PT, bleeding time, and platelet count are normal. The Factor XI activity level is 1% to 10% (1 to 10 units/dl).

Treatment. The half-life of Factor XI in plasma is between 40 and 80 hours. Replacement therapy is accomplished with fresh frozen plasma.

Von Willebrand Disease. This disease can occur in both sexes and is caused by either underproduction of the von Willebrand protein or synthesis of a dysfunctional protein. The von Willebrand protein contains a platelet adhesive component (called von Willebrand factor); the protein also functions to transport Factor VIII in the plasma. Thus, adolescents have bleeding manifestations because of impaired primary and secondary hemostatic mechanisms. Von Willebrand disease types I and II are autosomal dominant disorders, and type III is an autosomal recessive condition. Type I (classic von Willebrand disease) and type III show reduced Factor VIII activity, reduced von Willebrand protein and function, and normal multimer structure of the von Willebrand proteins on gel electrophoresis. Type II can have normal or reduced Factor VIII activity, normal or reduced von Willebrand protein, reduced von Willebrand factor activity, and a loss of the large and intermediate multimers. Von Willebrand factor activity can be tested by using ristocetin as a platelet-activating agent. Normal platelets aggregate with ristocetin; the aggregation is dependent on the presence of von Willebrand factor in the plasma and platelets.

Clinical Manifestations. Adolescent patients with von Willebrand disease (all types) have epistaxis, bleeding from the gums and after dental extractions, menorrhagia, prolonged oozing from cuts, and increased bleeding following trauma and surgery. Spontaneous hemarthrosis and CNS bleeding are rare.

Laboratory Findings. The bleeding time is prolonged in all of the von Willebrand syndromes. All tests of platelet function are normal except ristocetin-induced platelet aggregation. The platelet count and PT are normal. The PTT may be normal but is usually mildly to moderately prolonged (see Table 52–15).

Treatment. Replacement of von Willebrand factor is accomplished by using fresh frozen plasma or cryoprecipitate. The newer Factor VIII concentrates have inconsistent or no von Willebrand factor and cannot be used in this condition. Cryoprecipitate is the preferred form of therapy for serious bleeding and for preparation for surgery. The recommended dose is two to four bags of cryoprecipitate/10 kg body weight, repeated every 12 to 24 hours as needed. In adolescents with mild to moderate type I disease, minor bleeding manifestations (e.g., epistaxis, menorrhagia) and certain minor surgical procedures (e.g., dental extractions, dilation and curettage) can be treated with DDAVP. Type III disease is severe and does not respond to DDAVP. Hormonal control of menses may be necessary to control serious menorrhagia (see Chapter 70).

Other Inherited Deficiencies. Deficiencies of prekallikrein, high molecular weight kininogen, fibrinogen, and Factors XII, II, V, VII, X, and XIII are very rare. These conditions are inherited in an autosomal recessive manner.

Prekallikrein, high molecular weight kininogen, and Factor XII deficiencies are not associated with a bleeding diathesis. The PTT is prolonged and the PT and bleeding time are normal.

Deficiencies of Factors II, V, VII, and X have a prolonged PT. The PTT is normal in Factor VII deficiency and prolonged in deficiencies of Factors II, V, and X. Bleeding manifestations are treated with fresh frozen plasma or prothrombin complex concentrates, or both, for patients with reduced Factor II, VII, or X.

Factor XIII deficiency shows normal PTT, PT, and bleeding time. A specific test is needed for this factor (clot stability test). Fresh frozen plasma or cryoprecipitate is used for bleeding manifestations.

Fibrinogen deficiency (congenital afibrinogenemia) causes a prolonged PTT, PT, TCT, and bleeding time. The platelet count is normal. Cryoprecipitate is used to treat bleeding manifestations.

THROMBOTIC AND EMBOLIC DISORDERS

Clinical Manifestations and Diagnosis. The mechanism leading to thrombosis consists of vessel injury plus one or all of the following: enhanced platelet adhesion-aggregation, an activated coagulation mechanism, an inactive coagulation inhibitor system, an inactive fibrinolytic mechanism, or reduced blood flow. Arterial thrombosis is dependent on vascular injury. Venous thrombosis generally occurs in low-flow areas associated with either activation of the coagulation mechanism or an impaired inhibitor-fibrinolytic system. In general, vascular occlusive events in children and adolescents have an acute onset. The clinical manifestations reflect organ or tissue injury caused by a lack of or severe reduction in blood perfusion. The diagnosis is made by angiography. Ultrasonography and radionuclide scanning techniques can be employed for screening purposes. Other laboratory studies are rarely helpful in diagnosing a thromboembolic event, except when the event is caused by DIC and in rare patients with inherited deficiencies of the natural inhibitors.

Inherited-Congenital Defects

The formation of a fibrin clot is regulated by a complex inhibitor system that involves AT-III, protein C, and protein S. By regulating clot formation, these proteins prevent spontaneous intravascular coagulation. Reduced plasma levels lead to a propensity to excessive thrombosis. In addition, reduced ability to remove fibrin clots (congenital hypoplasminogenemia and dysplasminogenemia) and the formation of an unusual fibrin clot (certain types of congenital dysfibrinogenemias) allow thrombotic diseases to develop. The thrombotic events affect the venous system; arterial forms are rare. Deep vein thrombosis of the legs, pulmonary embolism, thromboses of the pelvic and mesenteric veins, and sagittal sinus thrombosis are frequent manifestations.

The first thromboembolic event usually occurs at between 10 and 25 years of age (in heterozygous states).

Acquired Causes

Acquired venous thromboembolic disease is noted in adolescent patients in association with the following: estrogen-containing oral contraceptives (see Chapter 73), adolescents with SLE with the lupus anticoagulant, obesity (see Chapter 60), pregnancy (see Chapter 74), prolonged immobilization, as a complication of the chemotherapeutic drug L-asparaginase (see Chapter 53), in DIC syndromes, and as a feature of the rare hematologic condition paroxysmal nocturnal hemoglobinuria.

SUPERFICIAL THROMBOPHLEBITIS

Anti-inflammatory drugs, heat compresses, rest, and elevation of the affected part compose the treatment of superficial thrombophlebitis.

DEEP VENOUS THROMBOSIS-PHLEBITIS

Anticoagulation and, in some instances, thrombolytic agents are used to treat deep venous thrombosis-phlebitis. Heparin anticoagulation should be used in full dosage for 5 to 7 days. In the uncomplicated case and in nonpregnant adolescents, warfarin is begun on day 3 and is continued for 2 to 3 months in those adolescents with proximal venous thrombosis. Heparin should not be discontinued until the warfarin effect is complete; premature discontinuation may lead to an increased thrombotic tendency. Adolescents with thrombosis of the calf vein should be treated with heparin for 5 to 7 days and then either warfarin or subcutaneous heparin for an additional 6 weeks. Acute iliofemoral venous thrombosis has also been treated with thrombolytic drugs, followed by anticoagulation with heparin or warfarin.

PULMONARY EMBOLISM

The adolescent with pulmonary embolism can be treated with either heparin or thrombolytic drugs. The thrombolytic therapy results in a more rapid clinical improvement than does heparin therapy. However, the overall survival and long-term pulmonary function abnormalities appear to be the same in both treatments. If maximal medical management does not produce improvement, embolectomy should be strongly considered.

ARTERIAL THROMBOSIS

Surgical removal of the clot is the treatment of choice in acute arterial thrombosis-embolism. Thrombolytic therapy (via the intraarterial or intravenous route) has been employed successfully in selected patients.

STROKE

Anticoagulation or platelet inhibitor drugs, or both, may be employed. The presence of a hemorrhagic infarct is a contraindication for anticoagulant therapy. It is not known if thrombolytic therapy is beneficial or not.

Treatment

Treatment of thrombotic and embolic disease may consist of anticoagulation, thrombolysis, platelet inhibitors, surgery, or general symptomatic care.

Anticoagulants. Heparin is appropriate initial therapy of most thrombotic-embolic events because of the ease of administration, predictable immediate effect, and rapid metabolism. Heparin does not cross the placenta and can be used throughout pregnancy, if needed. The drug is contraindicated in the following: a recent CNS hemorrhage; bleeding from inaccessible sites; malignant hypertension; bacterial endocarditis; surgery of the eye, brain, or spinal cord; in patients receiving regional or lumbar block anesthesia; and in the rare patient who has a hypersensitivity to the drug.

Heparin can be administered as an intravenous or subcutaneous injection. It is not effective when taken orally, and it should not be given as an intramuscular injection. Heparin can be given as an intermittent or continuous intravenous infusion. Subcutaneous heparin is useful for "minidose" prophylactic dosing and for maintenance after the initial event has been managed.

Heparin can be neutralized immediately with protamine sulfate. However, because of the rapid clearance rate of the drug, most patients can be handled by cessation of the infusion. Complications of heparin therapy include bleeding and, in rare patients, drug-induced (immune) thrombocytopenia. Prolonged heparin therapy may result in osteopenia. The PTT is the clotting test used to assess heparin anticoagulation.

The coumarin derivatives are oral anticoagulant drugs that act by inhibiting the production of the biologically active forms of Factors II, VII, IX, and X, which are the vitamin K–dependent coagulation factors. Warfarin (Coumadin, DuPont Pharmaceuticals) is the drug most often used. Coumarin drugs are contraindicated in essentially the same circumstances as is heparin. The oral anticoagulants cross the placenta and should not be given during pregnancy. Although warfarin is secreted in breast milk, the quantity is insignificant, and the drug can be used by lactating mothers. The PT is the clotting test used to assess warfarin anticoagulation.

Bleeding is the major complication of warfarin therapy. Rare patients may have drug hypersensitivity reactions (skin rash) and skin necrosis. The addition or removal of many drugs in the patient's treatment regimen can have significant effects on oral anticoagulation. For example, the warfarin effect can be enhanced by antibiotics, salicylates, anabolic steroids, chloral hydrate, laxatives, allopurinol, vitamin E, and methylphenidate. Conversely, the warfarin effect can be diminished by barbiturates, vitamin K, oral contraceptives, phenytoin, and other agents. Warfarin-induced bleeding is treated by discontinuation of the drug and the administration of vitamin K.

Thrombolysis. Thrombolytic therapy is the removal of blood clots by enzymatic digestion. This is accomplished by the *in vivo* generation of plasmin through the administration of plasminogen activators such as streptokinase, urokinase, tissue-type plasminogen activator, and others. For this therapy to be effective, the patient must have a relatively fresh clot (less than 7 to 10 days old), the clot must be accessible to the lytic agent, there must be an adequate amount of plasminogen, and the fibrinolytic inhibitors must not interfere with the reaction. Once plasmin is formed, it lyses fibrin. Thrombolytic therapy has been reported to be beneficial in pulmonary embolism, proximal deep venous thrombosis, certain arterial occlusive events, and occluded access shunts. However, there are few published studies on its use in the adolescent age group.

BIBLIOGRAPHY

Comp PC: Heredity disorders predisposing to thrombosis. Prog Hemost Thromb 8:71, 1986.

Corrigan JJ Jr: Hemorrhagic and Thrombotic Diseases in Childhood and Adolescence. New York, Churchill Livingstone, 1985.

Corrigan JJ Jr, Miller DR: Hemostasis. In Miller, DR (ed): Blood Diseases of Infancy and Childhood. St. Louis, CV Mosby, 1989, p 761.

Geddes VA, McGillivray RTA: The molecular genetics of hemophilia B. Transfusion Med Rev 1:161, 1987.

George JN, Nurden AT, Phillips DR: Molecular defects in interactions of platelets with the vessel wall. N Engl J Med 311:1084, 1984.

Harker LA, Slichter SJ: The bleeding time as a screening test for evaluation of platelet function. N Engl J Med 287:155, 1972.

Hathaway WE, Bonnar J: Hemostatic Disorders of the Pregnant Woman and Newborn Infant. New York, Elsevier Science, 1987.

Hilgartner MW, Pochedly C: Hemophilia in the Child and Adult, 3rd ed. New York, Raven Press, 1989.

Hirsh J, Levine MN: The optimal intensity of oral anticoagulant therapy. JAMA 258:2723, 1987.

Kasper CK: Treatment of factor VIII inhibitors. Prog Hemost Thromb 9:57, 1989.

Mannucci PM: Desmopressin: A nontransfusional form of treatment for congenital and acquired bleeding disorders. Blood 72:1449, 1988.

Oster H, Hejtmancik F: Prenatal diagnosis and carrier detection of genetic diseases by analysis of deoyribonucleic acid. J Pediatr 112:670, 1988.

Samama MM: Thrombolytic agents and treatments. Semin Thromb Hemost 13:127, 1987.

Shapiro SS, Thiagarajan P: Lupus anticoagulants. Prog Hemost Thromb 6:263, 1982.

Weiss HJ: Congenital disorders of platelet function. Semin Hematol 17:228, 1980.

CHAPTER 53

Oncologic Disorders

OVERVIEW
JOHN J. HUTTER

The management of cancer and the effects of cancer treatment in adolescent patients must include consideration of the impact of illness viewed within the framework of normal adolescent development. Adolescent oncology patients include long-term survivors of cancer who were treated earlier in childhood, as well as adolescents who are receiving therapy for newly diagnosed cancer. Although there is an overlap between these two groups on many issues, such as the effects of illness on body image and the potential for eventual employment or insurance discrimination, there are also enough differences between adolescent cancer survivors and those receiving cancer treatment to consider these groups separately (see also Chapters 30 and 121).

ADOLESCENTS RECEIVING CANCER THERAPY

The needs of adolescents undergoing cancer treatment are unique enough that many larger cancer treatment centers have developed specialized adolescent programs. The health team providing care for the adolescent with cancer should be both knowledgeable about adolescent issues and comfortable managing adolescent patients. Several unique issues must be considered in the care of the adolescent cancer patient: (1) the patient's understanding of the illness and his or her participation in decision-making regarding treatment options, (2) the effects of protracted periods of cancer treatment that specifically have an impact on adolescent functioning and development, (3) the inclusion of age-appropriate psychosocial support mechanisms, and (4) compliance with cancer therapy.

It is now well accepted that adolescents who have cancer require an explanation of the illness and its treatment that is appropriate to their level of understanding. For adolescents, this includes not only the presentation of precise and accurate medical information but also their active participation in the process of informed consent regarding treatment options (see Chapter 20). For early adolescents, final decisions regarding informed consent and what is best for the patient are usually made by the parents based on medical recommendations and a discussion of options. As the adolescent develops from the standpoint of chronologic age, cognitive abilities and social maturation, he or she assumes increasing responsibility in the decision-making process. Difficulty may occur with an adolescent oncology patient if the parents favor a particular treatment option and the adolescent does not wish to choose this option. In clinical situations in which this decision does not represent a life-threatening emergency, it is best to facilitate discussion between the adolescent and parents and delay decisions until a consensus opinion has been reached based on understanding of the disease and the risks and benefits of alternative treatments.

The prognosis for adolescents with hematologic malignancies and many solid tumors has improved in recent years. Almost all adolescent cancer patients are initially approached with curative rather than palliative intent. Much of the improvement in prognosis is the result of intensive treatment regimens. These intensive cancer treatment protocols usually produce side effects that are acutely unpleasant for the adolescent and may be associated with major disruptions in his or her lifestyle. Side effects of cancer treatment that prove particularly difficult for the adolescent include alopecia, severe nausea, and vomiting. Although methods have been developed for decreasing alopecia by reducing blood flow to the scalp by constriction or cooling, these techniques are not often employed in the management of the adolescent because of (1) decreased effectiveness when multiple drugs are being administered, (2) increased use of infusion chemotherapy rather than bolus administration, (3) concern that sanctuary sites may not be adequately treated, and (4) discomfort associated with scalp hypothermia. Alopecia in the adolescent is managed by the use of wigs and other hair coverings and the assurance that alopecia is almost always transient.

Severe chemotherapy-induced emesis is the side effect that is usually most feared and resented by the adolescent. The coping mechanism of denial that is often strongly exhibited by adolescent cancer patients often keeps them from focusing on the life-threatening aspects of their illness and therapy. Nausea and vomiting, which often occur with ongoing treatment, are constant reminders of the unpleasantness of therapy and may provoke frustration and anger. This may further contribute to noncompliance with therapy if the patient bargains, delays, or refuses treatment that produces severe emesis.

The severity of chemotherapy-induced nausea and vomiting is a function of the type and amount of agent administered. Treatment with Cisplatin, high-dose cytosine arabinoside, or high-dose cytoxan regularly produces severe emesis.

Recurrent severe emesis may result in the conditioned response of anticipatory nausea and vomiting in approximately 30% of patients. Anticipatory nausea and vomiting are characterized by the onset of vomiting concomitant with or prior to actual chemotherapy administration. It may be provoked by repetitive familiar surroundings, such as the appearance of the clinic, and may occur with therapies that do not usually produce emesis. Anticipatory nausea and vomiting are poorly responsive to pharmacologic agents used to control emesis but may be ameliorated by specific behavioral interventions instituted to address this problem.

The physiologic mechanisms of chemotherapy-induced emesis are complex and include a major central nervous system (CNS) component resulting from drug action on the chemoreceptor trigger zone in the area postrema of the medulla. In addition, an intact vomiting center, also located in the medulla, is necessary for emesis to occur. Because of the complexity of the somatic responses of retching and vomiting, it has been difficult to develop uniformly effective therapeutic interventions. Behavioral interventions, such as relaxation techniques and hypnosis, have been shown to be helpful in some adolescents receiving chemotherapy, but approaches to regimens associated with severe emesis usually include pharmacologic agents (Table 53–1). The chemoreceptor trigger zone contains dopamine and muscarinic receptors; thus many pharmacologic agents used for chemotherapy emesis include both dopamine antagonists (phenothiazines, butyrophenones, metoclopramide) and muscarinic blockers (scopolamine). Agents that produce general CNS depression can also be expected to have an effect on chemotherapy-induced emesis. The vast majority of the trials of pharmacologic interventions for nausea and vomiting secondary to cancer therapy

TABLE 53–1. Pharmacologic Agents Used for Chemotherapy-Induced Emesis

Dopamine antagonists
　Phenothiazines
　Butyrophenones
　Metoclopramide
Corticosteroids
　Dexamethasone
　Methylprednisolone
CNS depressants
　Benzodiazepines
　Cannabinoids
　Droperidol
Muscarinic antagonists
　Scopolamine
Serotonin antagonists
Antihistamines*

*Little direct action against chemotherapy-induced emesis but may decrease adverse effects of other agents, for example, dopamine antagonists.

have been conducted in adult subjects, with few studies having been conducted with children or adolescents; therefore, much of the current use of antiemetic agents in adolescents has been determined by extrapolation from the adult studies or by the previous experience of the oncologist. It is important to recognize that some of the adverse effects of antiemetic agents, such as extrapyramidal reactions and anxiety, are more prevalent in younger patients, including adolescents. Antihistamines, such as diphenhydramine (Benadryl) or dimenhydrinate (Dramamine), that are effective in the control of vomiting secondary to motion sickness have little direct effect in reducing chemotherapy-induced emesis. Diphenhydramine is useful, however, in reducing the severity of certain adverse effects, such as extrapyramidal reactions. As chemotherapy-induced emesis is often most severe during the first day of therapy, and the risk of extrapyramidal reactions increases with prolonged use in the adolescent patient, it is advisable to reduce the intensity of pharmacologic antiemetic therapy in many adolescents receiving chemotherapy courses of several days' duration. Preliminary trials using serotonin antagonists to manage emesis secondary to chemotherapy have proved encouraging in that they provide better efficacy and diminished side effects.

Management of the adolescent with cancer requires assessment of both the adolescent's lifestyle and the family dynamics, which have an impact on the care of the adolescent. Whenever possible, flexibility must be allowed in the treatment program so that the needs of the adolescent can be met without compromising medical management. Although adolescents may initially avoid returning to school because of concerns regarding hair loss or other changes in body image, school reentry should be encouraged and facilitated by the health care team. There may be occasions when the adolescent is severely immunosuppressed and the risk of exposure to infection at school may exceed the benefits of attendance, but in general, treatment programs should be planned to minimize school absences and support normal peer relationships. Socialization activities, including participation in athletic and other peer group activities, are important for optimal adolescent development, and deserve attention along with the issue of classroom attendance.

Although it is important for the adolescent to participate fully in receiving information and making decisions regarding treatment, it is also important to remember that the adolescent is a member of a family constellation, upon which he or she is usually dependent for financial and emotional support. Optimal management of the adolescent with a chronic life-threatening illness such as cancer requires assessment of the family dynamics that existed prior to diagnosis to establish optimal support mechanisms for the adolescent patient. Failure to perform this assessment thoroughly and accurately may lead to assumptions that adolescents are more capable of managing their illnesses than is actually the case and can result in compromising the support of the adolescent patient and diminishing compliance with therapy. In addition to the establishment of primary support mechanisms within the adolescent's family, adolescents with cancer often report benefit from participation in activities with other adolescent cancer patients, including socialization activities such as summer camps and more formal peer support group meetings.

It is well recognized that compliance with treatment regimens remains an issue for even life-threatening illnesses such as cancer (see Chapter 26). Studies by Tebbi and co-workers have shown that when adolescents were compared with younger children, lack of compliance with oral chemotherapy regimens was greater in adolescents, approaching 50%. Noncompliance should be suspected when a desired treatment effect is missing. The issue of compliance should be discussed in an open and nonthreatening manner. Factors that may contribute to poor compliance include incomplete understanding of the severity of illness by the adolescent (who is still given independence in treatment administration), the strong coping mechanism of denial present during normal adolescent development, and the patient's wish to be considered normal. Interventions to facilitate adolescent compliance require further investigation, but current approaches include (1) education regarding the illness and its treatment by a supportive member of the health care team; (2) participation of the adolescent in treatment planning, including goal setting and contracts; (3) periodic measurement of drug levels, when available; (4) consideration of parenteral administration of therapy when there is a high risk of noncompliance; and (5) reinforcement of positive behaviors. Caretakers should be aware of their own feelings of anger that may develop when a patient is not compliant. Expressions of anger directed against the noncompliant adolescent are usually counterproductive and should be avoided.

Adolescent sexual maturation must also be considered in the case of the cancer patient. Thrombocytopenia may complicate hematologic malignancy or cytotoxic chemotherapy. Menorrhagia in adolescent girls with cancer may require hormonal suppression to prevent hemorrhage and anemia (see Chapter 70).

Sexual activity is common among adolescents (see Chapter 68). Sexuality should be discussed with cancer patients in confidence and with sensitivity. The adolescent must understand the potential risk of pregnancy and the increased risk of sexually transmitted diseases in the immunosuppressed host. Unsafe sexual practices should be discouraged. Contraceptive options should be offered to diminish the risk of unwanted pregnancy. The teratogenic potential of chemotherapy must be understood by the adolescent patient with cancer.

ADOLESCENTS WHO ARE LONG-TERM SURVIVORS OF CHILDHOOD CANCER

Many pediatric oncology programs have established specific late-effects clinics to follow long-term survivors of childhood cancer through adolescence and into adult life (Table 53–2). Most survivors of childhood cancer are able to complete the normal tasks of adolescent development satisfactorily and can be expected to function capably as young adults. Certainly the effects of

TABLE 53–2. Late Sequelae of Childhood Cancer Treatment

Growth abnormalities
    Regional
    Generalized (short stature)
Second malignancies
Organ damage from previous therapy
    Heart
    Lung
    Hearing loss
    Liver
    Endocrine
    Reproductive
Neuropsychological

therapy that have an impact on body image and the ability to maintain normal activities may be at their greatest during adolescence. Although programs that follow individuals for late effects have been established, participation of adolescents in such surveillance is diminished because of societal mobility, adolescent denial, and lack of insurance coverage by third parties for follow-up services.

Regional abnormalities in skeletal growth are a potential problem for children who have had surgery or radiation therapy, or both, to developing bone. Regional bone growth problems, such as scoliosis, may become clinically more problematic during adolescence when the normal developmental growth spurt occurs. Children who have had paraspinal tumors and those receiving radiation therapy to vertebral bodies are at risk for the development of scoliosis and require careful surveillance during adolescence (see Chapter 79). Modern radiation techniques have reduced, but not completely eliminated, this risk.

Children who have received cranial radiation therapy for CNS tumors and other malignancies are at risk for short stature secondary to growth hormone deficiency (see Chapter 56). Hypothyroidism may also occur in children who have received cranial radiation therapy or radiation therapy to the thyroid gland (see Chapter 55). Abnormalities in endocrine function may not be apparent clinically or detectable by laboratory measurement until several years after completion of therapy or until anticipated pubescence. Children who have received therapy that puts them at risk for endocrine abnormalities should be monitored carefully throughout adolescence. Abnormalities in linear growth have been observed in children with acute lymphoblastic leukemia (ALL) who have received cranial radiation therapy. Physical growth abnormalities in children with leukemia may not be clinically apparent until adolescence and can only partially be explained by growth hormone deficiency.

Children with Hodgkin disease who have been treated with chemotherapy and radiation therapy have at least a 5% chance for the development of a second malignancy, including acute nonlymphocytic leukemia, which has a peak occurrence 5 years after treatment. In addition, Hodgkin disease survivors are at risk for the development of solid tumor malignancies (e.g., CNS tumors, colon cancer, and others), which can begin to appear in adolescence and early adult life. Long-term survivors of bilateral retinoblastoma have a greater than

50% risk of a second malignancy, including the development of osteogenic sarcoma and other sarcomata during adolescence. Osteogenic sarcoma in retinoblastoma survivors may be partly related to prior therapy with chemotherapy and radiation therapy but has also been observed to occur in retinoblastoma patients treated with enucleation only. Fortunately, the risk of second malignancies in children with favorable-risk ALL who are treated with current therapy appears only slightly increased. The risk of secondary leukemias and solid tumors (especially brain tumors) may be greater among children with high-risk ALL who have received more intensive chemotherapy regimens.

Organ damage following cancer treatment is often reversible, but long-term effects after therapy have been observed for many organs, including the CNS, liver, lung, heart, and reproductive systems. Certain toxicities from chemotherapy therapeutic agents are organ-specific. Examples include cardiotoxicity secondary to anthracycline administration and ototoxicity following treatment with cisplatin. These latter toxicities are irreversible and tend to be related to the cumulative dose of the chemotherapeutic agent administered. Anthracycline cardiotoxicity can present as sudden death in adolescents who have received large cumulative doses of anthracycline chemotherapy. The risk for major cardiac abnormalities resulting in sudden death is greatest in patients who demonstrated previous clinical congestive heart failure, but also may occur among children treated with anthracycline who were previously well clinically. The magnitude of this risk has not been completely assessed and indicates the need for prospective follow-up of survivors of childhood cancer. Cisplatin ototoxicity may require intervention with hearing aid amplification when the nerve damage has affected the speech frequencies.

Neuropsychological sequelae are frequently observed in survivors of childhood brain tumors, particularly in infants treated with radiation therapy plus chemotherapy. Current therapy of CNS tumors in children less than 3 years of age emphasizes delayed radiation in an attempt to minimize late CNS effects. Severe neuropsychologic sequelae are fortunately less common in other types of childhood cancer but may occur secondary to neurotoxic chemotherapy as the result of serious CNS infection. Children with ALL who received cranial radiation therapy may also exhibit neuropsychological sequelae that may present in childhood and adolescence as decreased school performance. Adolescent cancer survivors at risk for neuropsychological sequelae may require periodic assessment and specialized education intervention in order to maximize the functional capabilities of the patient.

Cancer therapy may have long-term sequelae with respect to reproductive function. Diminished fertility may result from surgical and radiologic treatments, as well as from chemotherapy. Survivors of cancer are often fertile and should be counseled regarding the potential risk of the teratogenic effects of cancer therapy and potential genetic factors in oncogenesis, if they apply in a specific patient.

BIBLIOGRAPHY

Litt IF, Cuskey WR: Compliance with medical regimens during adolescence. Pediatr Clin North Am 28:3, 1980.
Tebbi C (ed): Major Topics in Adolescent Oncology. Mt. Kisco, NY, Futura, 1987.
Tebbi CK, Cummings KM, Zefon MA, et al: Compliance of pediatric and adolescent cancer patients. Cancer 58:1179, 1986.
Zeltzer L, Kellerman J, Ellenberg L, et al: Psychologic effects of illness in adolescents. II. Impact of illness in adolescents—crucial issues and coping style. J Pediatr 97:132, 1980.

ACUTE AND CHRONIC LEUKEMIAS

BEATRICE C. LAMPKIN, CYNTHIA A. DeLAAT,
and BRADLEY A. GEORGE

Acute lymphoblastic leukemia (ALL), acute myeloid leukemia (AML), and chronic myelocytic leukemia (CML) all occur in adolescents. Accurate incidence and outcome data in adolescents with these diseases are unknown because some adolescents 16 to 21 years of age are treated by pediatricians and others in this age group are treated by internists and family physicians. Nevertheless, the incidence of ALL in patients 10 to 19 years of age has been reported to be 2.3 cases/100,000 individuals/year. The incidence of AML for this age group is less than that for ALL. CML accounts for about 3% of adolescents with leukemia and most commonly is associated with a specific chromosomal abnormality, the Philadelphia (Ph') chromosome.

The prognosis for adolescents with ALL and AML who are treated with intensive chemotherapy appears to be better than that for adults older than 21 years of age but poorer than for children younger than 10 years of age. The prognosis of CML is similar to that in adults.

PATHOPHYSIOLOGY

The etiology of leukemia is unknown, but there are some genetic and environmental factors that have been associated with increased risk of development of the disease. The most frequent association is with Down syndrome, in which there is at least an 11-fold increase in the incidence of acute leukemia. The incidence of both ALL and AML is increased, but the proportion of

Down syndrome patients in whom AML develops in relation to those in whom ALL develops is the same as that in the general population. The presenting clinical features of leukemia in children and adolescents with Down syndrome are no different from those in other ALL patients, but children with AML who have Down syndrome are younger at diagnosis. Other inherited or genetic diseases associated with an increased incidence of leukemia include Bloom syndrome, Fanconi anemia, Kostmann granulocytopenia, Shwachman syndrome, and neurofibromatosis. Congenital hypoplastic anemia, the inheritance of which is not established, also has been associated with an increase in the incidence of leukemia (see Chapter 52). All these diseases are more commonly diagnosed in the younger child than in the adolescent; the type of leukemia that develops is AML. The common denominator for all of these associations appears to be damage or alteration of chromosomes.

PATHOGENESIS

Leukemia develops as a result of clonal expansion of a single cell, the leukemic progenitor. The type of progenitor that expands determines whether ALL, AML, or CML develops. Leukemic cells proliferate in the bone marrow, but the cells also may proliferate in other reticuloendothelial tissues and in other extramedullary sites, such as the central nervous system (CNS), testes, bone, or skin. In adolescent patients with acute leukemia, the expansion of the leukemic cell population in the marrow causes failure either by crowding out the normal marrow progenitor cells or by inhibition of normal proliferation by a substance from leukemic cells. The result is the lack of red cells, platelets, and granulocytes. The exact reason for the ability for leukemic cells within the marrow to replace normal marrow precursor cells is unknown. Until recently, it was thought that leukemic cells proliferate more slowly than do their normal marrow counterparts and that the growth fraction was less. Recent studies indicate that this is a variable phenomenon. Further studies are needed to clarify the cell kinetics of normal and leukemic cells.

CLINICAL MANIFESTATIONS OF ACUTE LEUKEMIA

Clinical manifestations such as anemia, pallor, bruising, petechiae, fever, specific infections or sepsis, and bone pain are common presenting symptoms in adolescents with either ALL or AML. Most adolescent patients with ALL have splenomegaly or hepatomegaly, or both, or lymphadenopathy. Adolescents with AML usually have less organomegaly and bone pain. As expected from the physical findings, most patients with acute leukemia have anemia, thrombocytopenia, and neutropenia at diagnosis. The white blood count (WBC) may or may not be increased. The serum uric acid and lactate dehydrogenase (LDH) levels may be increased, particularly in patients with ALL. Electrolyte abnor-

malities, such as an increase or decrease in potassium or calcium levels, and hyperphosphatemia may also be found, particularly after therapy is started. These findings indicate tumor lysis.

Less common clinical presentations of the acute leukemias will be discussed separately in the sections on ALL and AML, as will the clinical features of CML.

DIFFERENTIAL DIAGNOSIS OF ACUTE LEUKEMIA

In the adolescent with pancytopenia who does not have organomegaly or blasts in the blood, acute leukemia must be distinguished from other clinical conditions, which are listed in Table 53-3. Signs such as an abdominal mass and abnormalities in the peripheral blood smear are helpful in determining what tests are subsequently needed to make the correct diagnosis. For example, in an adolescent with pancytopenia, if the blood smear shows many tear drop cells, thrombocytopenia with large platelets, minimal polychromasia, occasional nucleated red cells, and an occasional immature myeloid cell, the patient most likely has an infiltrated marrow. This might suggest the presence of a solid tumor, leukemic infiltration, myelofibrosis, or granulomas. If, in contrast, the blood smear shows marked polychromasia, spherocytes with great variation in size and shape of red cells, thrombocytopenia, and neutropenia, the adolescent most likely has autoimmune hemolytic anemia. Frequently, in the latter case, the direct Coombs test result is positive. Likewise, in a febrile patient, the presence of many fragmented red cells, thrombocytopenia, marked polychromasia, and myelocytes, but no blasts, in the blood smear should suggest overwhelming infection with disseminated intravascular coagulation (DIC). Hypersegmented neutrophils and macrocytes in the blood smear suggest megaloblastic anemia. A bone marrow aspirate is needed if a diagnosis of a nonleukemic disease cannot be made from the clinical and laboratory findings. Normochromic normocytic anemia, thrombocytopenia, and neutropenia suggest aplastic anemia. A very hypocellular bone marrow biopsy finding confirms this diagnosis. Occasionally a teenager with ALL presents with anemia and clinical manifestations suggestive of rheumatoid arthritis. The diagnosis of leukemia is made by finding abnormal blasts, usually lymphoblasts, in the marrow. Rarely an adolescent presents with anemia, thrombocytopenia, and neutropenia, and the marrow is cellular with a predominance of promyelocytes, but the adolescent does not have leukemia. Instead, the patient has an early

TABLE 53–3. Differential Diagnosis of Acute Leukemia

Aplastic anemia
Marrow infiltration with solid tumor
Autoimmune pancytopenia
Severe megaloblastic anemia
Overwhelming infection
Rheumatoid arthritis
Marrow suppression secondary to drugs, toxins, or infection

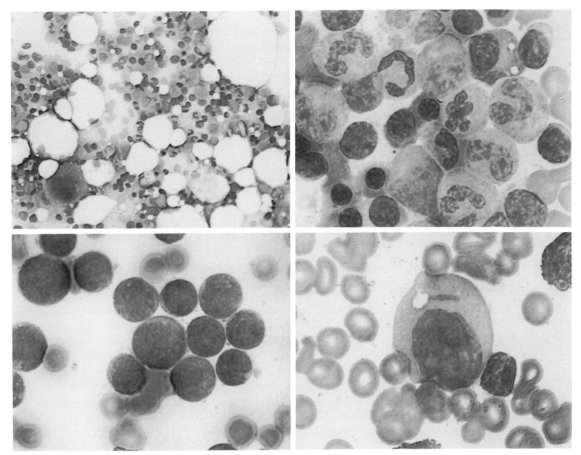

Figure 53–1. Electron micrograph showing blast characteristics. *Left upper panel,* normal marrow (10×). Note the heterogeneous pattern of cells. *Right upper panel,* normal marrow (40×). *Left lower panel,* ALL cells. Note the homogeneous pattern of cells (40×). *Right lower panel,* note large cell with nucleus with multiple nucleoli and abundant cytoplasm with Auer rod. This cell is an abnormal myeloblast (100×).

recovery of the bone marrow, which had been suppressed by a drug, toxin, a preceding viral illness, or an unknown cause. A diagnosis of acute promyelocytic leukemia may be considered in patients with a predominance of promyelocytes, but the diagnosis should not be made unless the blasts show characteristic abnormalities or the characteristic coagulation abnormalities of the disease (see section on acute myelocytic leukemia).

DIAGNOSTIC AND SPECIAL LABORATORY TESTS

Most patients with acute leukemia have abnormal blasts in the blood, and the diagnosis is easily made and confirmed by performing a bone marrow aspiration or biopsy, or both. It is very important for the therapy and prognosis that the type of acute leukemia be diagnosed accurately. The type of leukemia is determined by the characteristics of the blasts stained with Wright or Wright-Giemsa stains (Fig. 53–1). The presence of Auer rods in the cytoplasm indicates that the blasts are associated with AML. Special stains and immunophenotype analysis are helpful in defining the cell type (Table 53–4).

COMPLICATIONS OF LEUKEMIA

CNS infiltration of the meninges or testes may occur with either type of acute leukemia. The incidence of CNS leukemia at diagnosis in patients with ALL is less than 5%, and in patients with AML it is probably about 5%. An additional 5% of children and adolescents with either type of leukemia who are given CNS prophylaxis experience CNS disease, which requires local therapy consisting of either intensive treatment given by a ventricular reservoir or radiotherapy. Systemic chemotherapy is also required. Testicular infiltration may occur in either type of leukemia but is rare in both types at diagnosis. Testicular relapse may occur in patients with CNS disease, as an isolated event, or with bone marrow relapse. The incidence is probably close to 5% in boys with ALL but may be higher in adolescents with ALL. The incidence of this complication appears to be lower in boys with AML but may increase as survival results improve. Therapy requires irradiation of both testes, as well as systemic chemotherapy for both types of leukemia. Ovarian infiltration is an infrequent clinical event. The major complications in acute leukemia are presented in Table 53–5.

ACUTE LYMPHOBLASTIC LEUKEMIA
Morphologic Features and Prognosis

ALL is usually classified according to the French-American-British (FAB) cooperative working group by

**TABLE 53–4. Tests for Confirming the Type
of Leukemia**

SPECIAL STAINS

Positive peroxidase, Sudan black, α-naphthol, or chloroacetate
  esterase stains in cytoplasm of blasts indicate blasts associated
  with AML
Chunky PAS positivity in cytoplasm of blasts indicates
  lymphoblasts

IMMUNOPHENOTYPES OF BLASTS

Surface Antigen	Monoclonal Antibody
B Lymphocyte	
CD10	CALLA
CD19	B4
CD24	BA1
Surface immunoglobulin	Kappa + lambda
T Lymphocyte	
CD2	T11
CD3	T3 (E rosette)
CD5	Leu1
CD7	Leu9
Myeloid	
CD13	My7
CD14	My4
CD33	My9
Other	
CD34	My10

the morphologic criteria of individual leukemic cells. This system was established in the mid 1970s. The different types of leukemia are based on the number and prominence of nucleoli, the amount of cytoplasm present, and the presence of vacuoles. According to this classification system, 80% to 85% of pediatric patients have FAB-L1 morphologic features, 10% to 15% of patients have FAB-L2 morphologic features, and 1% to 3% have FAB-L3 morphologic features. The frequency of ALL characterized by L2 blasts increases with age, and it is often seen in adults. Patients with FAB-L1 have a better clinical outcome than do those with FAB-L2 morphologic features. FAB-L3 morphologic picture is associated with B-cell disease (Burkitt leukemia) and also carries a poor prognosis. There is no correlation between an FAB-L1 or FAB-L2 morphologic picture and immunophenotype.

Clinical Prognostic Factors

The examination of a large number of clinical features has been used as an indicator of prognosis. Poor prognostic indicators include the presence of thrombocytopenia, male sex, black race, presence of a mediastinal

**TABLE 53–5. Major Complications in
Acute Leukemia**

Infection
Side effects of drugs
CNS leukemia
Bleeding
Hyperuricemia
Infiltration of organs (i.e., testes)
Electrolyte imbalance
Anemia

mass or other organomegaly, and presence of CNS leukemia at diagnosis. Another clinical feature that has been associated with prognosis is the time required to induce disease remission. Adolescents in whom remission is not achieved by day 14 of therapy have been noted to have poorer prognoses. Studies of ALL indicate that many of these patient characteristics may be of prognostic significance in adults as well. As treatment regimens have intensified, the significance of these factors may be changing.

The two clinical features that are most strongly associated with outcome are the WBC at the time of diagnosis and age. The higher the WBC at diagnosis, the worse the overall outcome. It has also been noted that infants less than 18 months of age and children older than 10 years of age have a poorer prognosis. Reasons for the higher likelihood of treatment failure in adolescents are not established. It is known that many adolescents present with clinical and biologic features that place them in a poorer prognostic group, such as a higher incidence of T-cell ALL in adolescent males. They also tend to have higher white cell counts and a higher incidence of FAB-L2 morphologic features. Until more information is available to help determine which adolescents are at high risk of relapse, all adolescents should be considered high-risk patients.

Immunophenotype and Prognosis

As indicated in Table 53–4, it is possible to detect various cell surface antigens with monoclonal antibodies that classify leukemic blast cells to T-cell or B-cell origins. The leukemias of B-cell origin can be further subclassified into various stages of differentiation—early pre–B-, pre–B-, and B-cell leukemias. Eighty percent of early pre–B-cell leukemias demonstrate the presence of the common acute lymphocytic leukemia antigen (CALLA or CD-10) on their cell surface. Pre–B-cell lymphoblasts have predominantly the CALLA antigen, but in addition they have heavy chain immunoglobulin (cytoplasmic μ). B-cell lymphoblasts are CALLA-negative, do not have T-cell antigens, and do not contain cytoplasmic μ but have surface immunoglobulin (usually IgM). Early pre–B-cell leukemia appears to have a better prognosis than do the more differentiated pre–B- and B-cell leukemias. Patients with B-cell leukemias have the worst prognosis. The T-cell disease as evidenced by T-cell immunologic markers or E-rosettes accounts for about 15% of ALL and carries a poor prognosis. It is more common in adolescents, and these patients often present with an elevated WBC and a mediastinal mass at the time of diagnosis.

Chromosomal Abnormalities and Prognosis

Chromosomal abnormalities are important in predicting prognosis in patients with ALL. Various translocations and chromosome deletions are associated with a poor prognosis. Leukemic cells that demonstrate a hy-

TABLE 53–6. Template for Therapy of Acute Leukemia

Induction of remission:
CNS prophylaxis
Maintenance therapy
± Reintensification
± Bone marrow transplantation

perdiploidy greater than 50 chromosomes but less than tetraploidy are associated with a better prognosis.

Treatment of ALL

There is no standard treatment protocol for adolescents with ALL (Table 53–6). Many centers now use intensive regimens for treatment of adolescents and young adults because of the poorer prognosis in this disease. Most treatment protocols consist of three phases: an induction phase, a consolidation phase, and a maintenance phase. Steps must be taken to eradicate occult disease from sanctuary sites such as the CNS.

Induction regimens are fairly standard using the following three or four chemotherapy drugs: vincristine, L-asparaginase, and prednisone with or without the addition of daunomycin. Greater than 90% of patients enter remission with standard induction regimens. A complete remission is defined as less than 5% abnormal blasts in the marrow, a normal complete blood count, and no evidence of extramedullary leukemia. Although nearly all patients enter remission, until recently more than half of the adolescents with ALL had recurrence of disease. Because of this, intensive consolidation therapy is now recommended, consisting of administration of different antileukemic drugs that were not used in induction therapy. The consolidation chemotherapy and the schedules by which it is administered are designed to decrease the development of drug resistance by leukemic cells. Maintenance therapy consists of monthly administration of medications. Current recommendations are 2 years of maintenance therapy for girls and 3 years for boys. Recent studies have demonstrated improvement in survival for high-risk groups using a more intensive consolidation therapy followed by reintensification of therapy shortly after maintenance has begun. The reintensification usually reintroduces the medications used in induction and consolidation therapy. Current CNS prophylaxis consists of administration of intrathecal chemotherapy with or without cranial irradiation. Intrathecal chemotherapy has been shown to be as effective as cranial irradiation in low- and intermediate-risk groups for prevention of CNS relapse. The efficacy of such treatment has not been documented in adolescents but is being studied now.

ACUTE NONLYMPHOCYTIC LEUKEMIA (ACUTE MYELOID LEUKEMIA)
Special Clinical Presentations of Acute Myeloid Leukemia
HYPERLEUKOCYTOSIS

Hyperleukocytosis, as defined by a WBC greater than 100,000/mm³, occurs in approximately 22% of adoles-

cents with AML. Many of these patients have headaches and blurred vision; fewer have respiratory distress. Symptoms are secondary to vascular leukostasis and infiltration of the CNS and the lungs. Because of significant mortality from cerebrovascular accidents, AML patients with these findings must be treated as medical emergencies. There is controversy concerning what is the best treatment, but in the authors' experience a double volume exchange transfusion or leukapheresis is preferable. In this manner, blood viscosity is reduced with the cell number, and the risk of metabolic abnormalities is decreased. Since the effect on cell number and blood viscosity is transient, prompt initiation of chemotherapy is required. Adolescents with ALL are much less likely to have CNS or lung complications and rarely need exchange transfusions or leukapheresis.

ACUTE PROMYELOCYTIC LEUKEMIA

Acute promyelocytic leukemia (APL) should be suspected in patients with AML with a predominance of promyelocytes in the bone marrow and a bleeding diathesis or in patients in whom marked bleeding develops shortly after beginning therapy. The bleeding is associated with hypofibrinogenemia, Factor V deficiency, and thrombocytopenia. These coagulation abnormalities have been attributed to release of thromboplastin by promyelocytes, which leads to DIC and secondary fibrinolysis. The use of prophylactic heparin is controversial. Bleeding usually continues until all the circulating promyelocytes are destroyed. A characteristic chromosomal abnormality t(15:17) is found in most adolescents with APL.

CHLOROMAS AND EXTRAMEDULLARY DISEASE OTHER THAN CNS LEUKEMIA

Chloromas are extramedullary solid tumor collections of AML blasts and occur in 2.9% to 13.6% of patients with AML. These tumors most commonly involve the cranium and facial bones and frequently involve the periosteal, perineural, and epidural regions. They receive their name because they exhibit a green color on cut surface, secondary to myeloperoxidase granules in the cytoplasm of the blasts. Rarely these tumors may precede the onset of overt leukemia by many months.

Gum infiltration and leukemia cutis may be seen in patients with acute monoblastic leukemia (AMOL) and acute myelomonoblastic leukemia (AMMOL), and when present, these forms of leukemia should be suspected.

The impact of chloromas, gum infiltration, and leukemia cutis on prognosis is unclear.

Morphologic and Biologic Characteristics of Blasts

Acute nonlymphocytic leukemia is a very heterogeneous group of leukemias. There are currently eight classifications of blasts recognized as being AML (Table 53–7). With the exception of infants with AMOL, who have a worse prognosis, there is no clear association of prognosis with subtype of AML. There is acceptance by most investigators that a WBC greater than 100,000/mm^3 is associated with a poor prognosis.

Biologic characteristics of blasts, such as the ability to proliferate in soft agar, cell kinetics, immunologic phenotype, and karyotype, have also been reported to be associated with prognosis, but the results of these studies have been conflicting. It is likely that most prognostic factors will continue to vary until better methods of therapy are found.

Treatment

As with ALL, the treatment of adolescent patients with AML is very intensive. All induction regimens include cytosine arabinoside (Ara-C), and almost all include an anthracycline, usually daunomycin. Approximately 75% of children and adolescents with AML enter complete remission. In contrast to induction therapy for ALL, it is almost always necessary to induce severe marrow hypocellularity in order to achieve remission.

A complete remission in AML is defined similarly as that for ALL, and, similarly, postremission therapy is divided into consolidation, intensification, and maintenance. As in ALL, it is necessary to use additional therapy beyond the time of remission; however, in contrast to ALL, once consolidation and intensification therapy is given, it is unclear whether maintenance therapy is needed. This question is currently being investigated. One form of very intensive therapy is bone marrow transplantation (BMT) performed when the patient is in first remission for adolescents who have a compatible sibling donor (see Chapter 54). This method of therapy is being compared with very intensive chemotherapy and purged autologous BMT in a current Children's Cancer Study Group protocol. Although recent intensive treatment methods prolong disease-free survival, later relapses occur and long-term prognosis is not established. As in adolescent patients with ALL, adolescents with AML who relapse on therapy or within 1 year of stopping therapy have a poor prognosis, but even some of these adolescent patients may survive with very aggressive therapy.

SUPPORTIVE CARE FOR ALL AND AML

The intensive treatment regimens that are being used in an attempt to increase survival in adolescents with

TABLE 53–7. Types of Acute Nonlymphocytic Leukemia (Acute Myeloid Leukemia)

FAB TYPE	
M$_0$:	Very undifferentiated blasts
M$_1$:	Acute undifferentiated myelogenous leukemia
M$_2$:	Acute differentiated myelogenous leukemia
M$_3$:	Acute promyelocytic leukemia
M$_4$:	Acute myelomonocytic leukemia
M$_{5a}$:	Acute monoblastic leukemia
M$_{5b}$:	Acute differentiated monocytic leukemia
M$_6$:	Acute erythroleukemia
M$_7$:	Acute megakaryoblastic leukemia

acute leukemia require intensive supportive care. With treatment, patients, particularly those with ALL, may experience a tumor lysis syndrome characterized by elevated uric acid levels, hyperkalemia, hypocalcemia, and hyperphosphatemia. This complication must be anticipated prior to institution of chemotherapy. Hydration, alkalinization, and allopurinol (a xanthine oxidase inhibitor that prevents the production of uric acid from xanthine) are indicated to prevent or diminish the severity of tumor lysis syndrome. Serum electrolytes must be monitored closely before and during the initiation of induction chemotherapy.

Adolescent patients may experience long periods of severe neutropenia, which places them at risk for potentially life-threatening infections. Prompt institution of broad spectrum antibiotics is indicated when neutropenic adolescents become febrile. These adolescents are also at risk for the development of viral and fungal infections, especially during periods of intensive chemotherapy. *Pneumocystis carinii* infection poses a significant risk, particularly in adolescents with ALL, even if they are receiving maintenance chemotherapy. All adolescent patients should receive prophylactic trimethoprim-sulfamethoxazole throughout treatment. Adolescent patients frequently require aggressive support with blood products. Most agree that adolescents should receive platelet transfusions to maintain platelet counts of greater than 20,000/mm^3 in order to decrease the risk of spontaneous bleeding. They may also require transfusions of red cells if severe anemia develops during treatment. It is recommended that cytomegalovirus seronegative blood products be used for adolescents who are both cytomegalovirus-seronegative and candidates for bone marrow transplantation, as this virus may be transmitted through blood products and can cause active infections in these immunocompromised patients. Irradiated blood products should be used in intensively treated adolescents to decrease the risk of graft-versus-host disease. Adolescent females can experience significant blood loss from menstrual bleeding when severe thrombocytopenia is present (see Chapter 70). This is most likely to occur during induction or consolidation therapy, and these adolescent patients should receive aggressive support with platelet transfusions. Hormone administration should be used to suppress menses when giving aggressive therapy (see Chapter 70).

Hormonal function may be affected by chemotherapy and cranial irradiation. This may lead to growth failure and changes in the onset of puberty in early adolescents. Cytoxan, which is used in some treatment regimens, is associated with a significant risk of infertility in both males and females. Testicular relapse in males is treated with gonadal irradiation, as well as reintensification of chemotherapy. Infertility and possibly hormonal failure are expected side effects of this treatment.

CHRONIC MYELOCYTIC LEUKEMIA

The majority of children with the classic or adult form of CML are older than 8 years of age. Juvenile CML is seen in much younger children. There is no racial or sexual predilection. CML is an indolent disorder initially but eventually transforms into a "blast phase" that resembles the acute leukemias.

The cause of the malignant transformation of the normal hematopoietic stem cell in CML is unknown. The only environmental factor to be implicated (in a small portion of patients) is ionizing radiation (i.e., survivors of atomic bomb blasts, radiologists, and individuals exposed to radiation for ankylosing spondylitis). There have been no infectious agents associated with CML.

Pathophysiology

Much has been learned about the molecular biology of CML. It was the first human malignancy to be associated with a specific chromosomal abnormality. The Ph′ chromosome is a reciprocal translocation between chromosomes 9 and 22, t(9;22)(q34;q11), and is present in 90% to 95% of cases of CML. The molecular counterpart, a hybrid gene consisting of portions of the break cluster region (bcr) gene and a cellular oncogene (c-abl), can be identified in some adolescent patients who do not have an apparent Ph′ chromosome. The Ph′ chromosome can be identified in neutrophils, monocytes-macrophages, erythrocytes, eosinophils, basophils, megakaryocytes, and their progenitors, which supports the evolution of the malignant clone in CML from a pluripotent stem cell. The Ph′ chromosome can also be identified in small numbers of lymphocytes; however, it is not present in bone marrow fibroblasts or other normal host cells.

Clinical Manifestations of Chronic Myelocytic Leukemia

The hallmark of CML is a marked leukocytosis consisting of immature and mature granulocytes of all types. The average WBC at diagnosis is 250,000 to 350,000/mm^3, with a range of 8000 to 800,000/mm^3. Younger patients tend to have a higher WBC, a higher incidence of extreme leukocytosis (WBC greater than 500,000/mm^3), and an increased percentage of blasts, promyelocytes, and myelocytes when compared with adults. The percentage of myeloblasts and promyelocytes is defined as less than 15% in chronic phase. There is an increase in the absolute numbers of eosinophils and basophils. Most children present with a normochromic, normocytic anemia with an average hemoglobin value of 9 g/dl. The mean platelet count is 500,000/mm^3, with a range of 25,000 to more than 2,000,000/mm^3. Bone marrow examination reveals hypercellularity consisting mainly of increased numbers of granulocytes at all stages of maturation. Myelofibrosis is less common at diagnosis but can develop as the disease progresses. Other laboratory features include elevated serum levels of uric acid, LDH, vitamin B$_{12}$, and its binding protein transcobalamin I. A characteristic abnormality of the white cell population in CML is a decrease in leukocyte alkaline phosphatase (LAP) activity. There have been intrinsic defects identified in the granulocytes of patients

with CML, but for the most part these cells function normally. The natural history of CML in adolescents, as in adults, can be divided into three phases: chronic, accelerated, and blastic.

CHRONIC PHASE

Most patients are diagnosed in chronic phase as a result of an increased circulating WBC. The leukemic cells accumulate in the bone marrow, peripheral blood, spleen, and liver. Symptoms are referable to organ infiltration and hyperproliferation. Nonspecific symptoms of fever, malaise, bone pain, and left upper quadrant fullness or pain are present in most adolescents. An almost universal finding on physical examination is splenomegaly, which may be massive.

ACCELERATED PHASE

The chronic phase of CML lasts for an average of 3 years before evolving into the more aggressive blastic phase. With progression of disease, systemic symptoms return, as does an increase in the WBC with increased numbers of immature cells. This phase of disease is less responsive to chemotherapy. New cytogenetic abnormalities, such as duplication of the Ph′ chromosome, isochromosome 17, or trisomy 8, may be identified. Evidence of extramedullary disease in the meninges, bones, or soft tissues is another indication of acceleration.

BLASTIC PHASE

Some patients may regress to the chronic phase with changes in therapy; however, all adolescent patients eventually undergo blastic transformation. The clinical picture is the same as de novo acute leukemia (greater than 30% blasts in the bone marrow or peripheral blood, anemia, and thrombocytopenia). In the majority of patients (60%), the blasts crisis is myeloid, whereas one third of adolescents enter lymphoid blast crisis.

Differential Diagnosis

The differential diagnosis of chronic-phase CML includes a leukemoid reaction or other myeloproliferative disease. A leukemoid reaction is seen with pyogenic bacterial infections or in autoimmune disorders (see Chapter 90). With leukemoid reactions, splenomegaly is usually lacking, staining of granules with LAP in the cytoplasm of neutrophils is increased, and the Ph′ chromosome is not identified. A bone marrow examination and cytogenetic analysis also help differentiate CML from other myelodysplastic disorders. Rarely, an adolescent patient presents in blast crisis at diagnosis, and again the presence of the Ph′ chromosome differentiates CML from acute leukemia. Occasional adolescents with ALL and a high WBC may present with a Ph′ chromosome in their blasts. These adolescent patients do not have CML, and their disease can be distinguished from CML in lymphoid blast crisis. The bcr-abl protein product is usually a 210-kd molecule in patients with CML and is only 185 kd in patients with ALL.

Treatment

The goal of treatment is to decrease the leukocytosis and to provide symptomatic relief. Conventional therapy does not result in cure of CML, that is, disappearance of the Ph'-positive clone. Because of the extreme leukocytosis present, when initiating therapy, special attention must be paid to the metabolic and viscosity-related complications. Tumor lysis should be anticipated and treated as in the acute leukemias. Leukapheresis or exchange transfusion should be performed simultaneously with chemotherapy in patients with a WBC greater than 200,000/mm³ or symptoms secondary to hyperleukocytosis. The standard approach to management of the chronic phase is single-agent chemotherapy with busulfan or hydroxyurea. These drugs normalize the WBC and provide relief of symptoms but do not delay blast crisis or prolong survival. Busulfan is given intermittently or in low doses to control leukocytosis and can cause marrow aplasia, pulmonary fibrosis, or an addisonian-like syndrome. Hydroxyurea must be administered on a daily basis but has less toxicity. Multiagent chemotherapeutic regimens as used in acute leukemia, splenectomy, or splenic irradiation have not proved of benefit. Adolescent patients in myeloid blast crisis respond poorly to therapy, whereas those with lymphoblastic transformation are more sensitive to chemotherapy.

Interferons—naturally occurring proteins that have antiviral, antiproliferative, and immune and oncogene modulating effects—are active against the leukemic cells of chronic CML. Complete hematologic remissions and, more importantly, suppression of the Ph'-positive clone have been achieved. Both α- and γ-interferon demonstrate activity in CML. Side effects include flu-like symptoms, anorexia, bone pain, and bone marrow suppression.

The only present curative therapy for CML is BMT (see Chapter 54). Survival following allogeneic BMT is 60% when performed in chronic phase, 35% when performed in accelerated phase, and 13% when performed in blast crisis. Patients younger than 30 years of age tolerate transplantation better, and 75% of young patients who undergo transplantation for CML are long-term survivors. The risks of transplantation are death from toxicity or infection, graft-versus-host disease, late toxicities (i.e., sterility), and relapse. If an adolescent has a histocompatible sibling, BMT within a year of diagnosis is the recommended therapy. New approaches with unrelated donor or autologous BMT are under investigation.

Prognosis

The median survival for CML is 3½ to 4 years. Once the disease evolves to blast crisis, there is significantly less response to therapy, and survival averages 3 to 6 months. Attempts have been made to stratify patients into high-risk and low-risk groups according to clinical features. Increased age, spleen size, platelet count, and percentage of circulating blasts have been identified as poor risk factors in adults. Because the only curative therapy is BMT, these prognostic variables are being studied to determine the optimal timing for this high-risk therapy.

BIBLIOGRAPHY

Altman AJ: Chronic leukemias of childhood. Pediatr Clin North Am 35:765, 1988.

Baccarani M, Corbelli G, Amadori S, et al: Adolescent and adult acute lymphoblastic leukemia: Prognostic features and outcome of therapy. A study of 293 patients. Blood 60(3):677, 1982.

Castro-Malaspina H, Schaison G, Briere J, et al: Philadelphia chromosome–positive chronic myelocytic leukemia in children. Cancer 52:721, 1983.

Champlin RE, Goldman JM, Gale RP: Bone marrow transplantation in chronic myelogenous leukemia. Semin Hematol 25:74, 1988.

Crist W, Pullen J, Boyett J, et al: Acute lymphoid leukemia in adolescents: Clinical and biologic features predict a poor prognosis—a Pediatric Oncology Group Study. J Clin Oncol 6(1):34, 1988.

Gaynon P, Steinherz PG, Bleyer WA, et al: Intensive therapy for children with acute lymphoblastic leukaemia and unfavourable presenting features: Early conclusions of Study CCG-106 by the Childrens Cancer Study Group. Lancet 2(8617):921, 1988.

Kantarjian HM, Keating MJ, Talpaz M, et al: Chronic myelogeneous leukemia in blast crisis: Analysis of 242 patients. Am J Med 83:445, 1987.

Lampkin BC, Lange B, Bernstein I, et al: Biologic characteristics and treatment of acute nonlymphocytic leukemia in children. Pediatr Clin North Am 35(4):743, 1988.

Lipshultz SE, Colan SD, Gelber RD, et al: Late cardiac effects of doxorubicin therapy for acute lymphoblastic leukemia in childhood. N Engl J Med 324:808, 1991.

Nachman J, Sather H, Gaynon P, et al: Prognosis of young adults with acute lymphoblastic leukemia (ALL): The Children's Cancer Study Group (CCSG) experience. Presented to the American Society of Clinical Oncology at the 26th Annual Meeting, May 20–22, 1990, Washington, DC.

Ochs J, Mulhern R: Late effects of antileukemic treatment. Pediatr Clin North Am 35:815, 1988.

Poplack DG, Reaman G: Acute lymphoblastic leukemia in childhood. Pediatr Clin North Am 35(4):903, 1988.

Sather HN: Age at diagnosis in childhood acute lymphoblastic leukemia. Med Pediatr Oncol 14:166, 1986.

Sokal JE, Baccarani M, Russo D, Tura S: Staging and prognosis in chronic myelogenous leukemia. Semin Hematol 25:49, 1988.

Talpaz M, Kantarjian HM, Kurzrock R, Gutterman J: Therapy of chronic myelogenous leukemia: Chemotherapy and interferons. Semin Hematol 25:62, 1988.

MUSCULOSKELETAL NEOPLASIA

GERALD ROSEN and JOSEPH MIRRA

Although rare in the general population, tumors of bone and soft tissue origin account for substantial morbidity and mortality in the adolescent age group. In a review of 1890 patients who presented with cancer during the second decade of life at the Memorial Sloan-Kettering Cancer Center during a 20-year period, it was found that the majority of solid tumors in this age group were, with the exception of brain tumors, musculoskeletal in origin (Fig. 53–2). Although this chapter is contained in the section on oncologic conditions, benign processes are included for the purpose of differential diagnosis.

Bone tumors compose 20% to 25% of malignant lesions among adolescents—the second largest group of solid cancers in this age group after brain tumors. Primary musculoskeletal neoplasia is much more common in adolescents than in the general population. In particular, many of the primary bone tumors reach their peak incidence during adolescence, and some of these tumors occur almost exclusively in the second decade of

life. These musculoskeletal neoplasms may be divided into bone tumors and soft tissue tumors. Table 53–8 lists the common bone tumors seen in adolescents. They can be classified as bone-producing, collagen-producing, or cartilage-producing tumors. Fibrous dysplasia produces both abnormal bone and fibrous stroma. Adamantinomas are low-grade malignant tumors that produce a fibrous stroma but also contain some epithelial elements. Although an aneurysmal bone cyst may be of vascular origin, there is a small amount of fibrous stroma, as well as a giant cell component, associated with it. Periosteal osteogenic sarcoma produces some osteoid and thus is classified as an osteogenic sarcoma; however, it produces predominantly cartilage and is frequently confused with chondrosarcoma. In contrast with the majority of chondrosarcomas that occur in adults, the periosteal osteogenic sarcoma and pure chondrosarcomas in adolescents tend to be high-grade malignant lesions. Hemorrhagic and traumatic lesions such as hematomas and myositis ossificans make up the majority of the benign soft tissue tumors seen in adolescents. However, malignant tumors can frequently mimic hematoma, and myositis ossificans can frequently mimic a malignant tumor (Table 53–9).

During the past decade, major advances have been made in the treatment of malignant musculoskeletal neoplasia. Many of these once fatal tumors, the only treatment of which was radical surgery that often required amputation, resulted in death because of a metastatic disease that ranged between 50% and 90%. Through early diagnosis of some of these malignant conditions and rapid institution of multidisciplinary treatment, including chemotherapy, radiation therapy, and surgery, most of these neoplasms are now curable in a majority of patients. However, treatment of many malignant neoplasms requires special consideration regarding the application of these treatment modalities. Because treatment is so complicated and expensive and

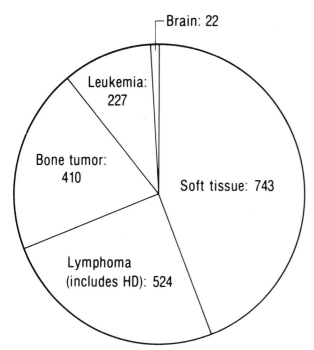

Figure 53–2. Of 1890 patients (some with more than one cancer) between the ages of 10 and 20 years presenting to the Memorial Sloan-Kettering Cancer Center between 1959 and 1979, approximately 40% had tumors of soft tissue origin other than lymphomas and Hodgkin disease. Bone tumors accounted for 22% of the malignancies seen in the adolescent age group. In the second decade of life, leukemia did not make up the majority of neoplastic diseases as it did in the younger pediatric age group. Of the 410 bone tumors seen, approximately 50% were osteogenic sarcoma, and 25% were Ewing sarcoma. The proportion of patients with certain tumors (e.g., benign bone or brain tumors) seen at the Memorial Sloan-Kettering Cancer Center differs from that of the adolescent population at large because of referral patterns to that cancer center for treatment.

TABLE 53–8. Bone Tumors in Adolescents

BENIGN	MALIGNANT
Bone-Producing Lesions	
Stress fracture	Osteogenic sarcoma
Osteoid osteoma	Parosteal osteogenic sarcoma
Collagen-Producing Lesions	
Nonossifying fibroma	Malignant fibrous histiocytoma
Giant cell tumor	Fibrosarcoma
	Adamantinoma
Cartilage-Producing Lesions	
Osteochondroma	Periosteal osteogenic sarcoma
Multiple exostoses	Chondrosarcoma
Enchondroma	Mesenchymal chondrosarcoma
Multiple enchondromatosis	
Chondromyxoid fibroma	
Chondroblastoma	
Tumors of Uncertain Histogenesis	
Aneurysmal bone cyst	Ewing sarcoma
	Primitive neuroectodermal tumor

TABLE 53–9. Common Soft Tissue Tumors in Adolescents

BENIGN	MALIGNANT
Hematoma	Rhabdomyosarcoma
Myositis ossificans	Synovial sarcoma
Neurofibroma	Neurofibrosarcoma
Fibromatosis	Fibrosarcoma
	Malignant fibrous histiocytoma
	Epithelioid sarcoma
	Nasopharyngeal carcinoma

is associated with great morbidity, it is extremely important to arrive at an early and accurate diagnosis. For this reason, it is important to discuss benign as well as musculoskeletal tumors because early, accurate diagnosis is critical for rapid and successful treatment. Since these treatments are intensive and cause substantial side effects, the diagnosis must be specific, and the differentiation of malignant from benign processes must be accurately made.

BONE TUMORS

The benign and malignant bone tumors that are common in the adolescent age group are listed in Table 53–8. As already stated, because of their classification, as well as differential diagnostic considerations in their presentation, it is convenient to divide the benign and malignant bone tumors into (1) those that produce bone, (2) those that produce collagen or contain an abundant fibrous stroma, (3) those that produce cartilage, and (4) miscellaneous tumors, many of which show predominant vascular patterns but do not produce a recognizable background stroma of a single histologic origin.

Most skeletal neoplasms are readily diagnosed by plain roentgenograms. Following basic guidelines, a good skeletal radiologist can usually state with certainty whether a lesion is benign or malignant (Figs. 53–3 and 53–4). Exceptions do exist, and clinical data are essential in interpreting radiologic data. If clinical data indicate a progressive process even in the face of a "benign" roentgenogram, further imaging studies and follow-up are essential. A good rule of thumb for the practicing physician is, "If in doubt, obtain an x-ray," particularly in adolescents who complain of knee pain. The knee is a common site of trauma, but it is also a common site of skeletal neoplasia in adolescents.

Benign Bone-Producing Tumors

STRESS FRACTURE

Benign stress fractures are probably the most common bone "tumor" encountered in adolescents (Table 53–10). They can arise in almost any age group and, as the name implies, are secondary to mechanical stress. They are commonly found in physically active, symptomatic adolescents. Stress fractures can occur spontaneously without abnormal stress because of other underlying bone disease, such as malignant bone tumors, other

benign bone tumors, or severe osteoporosis in immobilized or hypoestrogenic individuals. When there is no underlying disorder, there should be a significant history of stress. Stress does not necessarily mean blunt trauma. However, many malignant bone tumors have a history of trauma to the area of involvement. Stress in those instances has no role in the etiology but merely draws attention to the underlying lesion. Thus, the term *stress fracture* as used here will be confined to stress fractures that occur in otherwise healthy adolescents with healthy bones following strenuous activities.

Stress fractures frequently occur in the tibia or femur in serious athletes, particularly those engaged in jogging and competitive contact sports. "March fractures" involving the metatarsal bones can occur as a result of the trauma of vigorous walking or jogging, as well as other activities, in individuals who do not wear adequate protective footwear. Stress fractures of the lumbar spine also occur in adolescents who engage in the martial arts (judo), as well as in competitive wrestlers. Stress fractures of the anterior surface of the tibia are common in

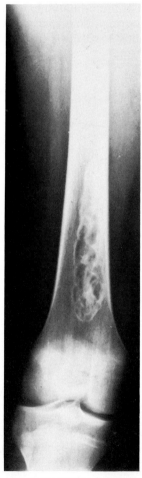

Figure 53–3. The roentgenographic appearance of benign bone lesions includes a regular, well-defined margin that frequently has a rim of sclerosis within the margin of the lesion. In addition, the tumor does not break through the cortex, nor does it produce soft tissue mass as does a malignant tumor. There is no periosteal elevation. This relatively large lesion is a benign nonossifying fibroma. It is seen in the adolescent age group and is discovered during incidental radiographic studies performed for reasons other than symptoms from this lesion, which is usually totally asymptomatic.

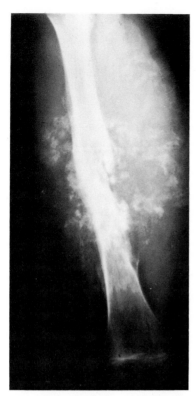

Figure 53–4. The characteristics of a malignant bone lesion include irregular or poorly defined margins within the bone. It is therefore difficult to tell at which points the process begins and ends. In addition, there is usually erosion of the cortex with a soft tissue mass that pushes the periosteum out along with it into the soft tissues. The point at which the elevated or tented periosteum meets the normal contour of the bony cortex is the vertex of what has been called the Codman triangle. The figure demonstrates a fully malignant osteogenic sarcoma as evidenced by the calcifications within the soft tissue mass.

involving the axial skeleton. Lesions identified on bone scan in an adolescent who complains of axial bone pain may be misdiagnosed as metastatic cancer. A careful history often will reveal prior vigorous or unusual physical activity or exercise. Roentgenograms frequently reveal callus formation or bone production around the area of the stress fracture. These fractures are sometimes in characteristic locations, depending on the type of mechanical stress involved. However, because of the bone production, plain roentgenograms frequently do not allow differentiation of a stress fracture from a more ominous bone-producing tumor such as an osteogenic sarcoma. The most helpful diagnostic study is usually linear tomography or computed tomography (CT) scanning. These studies frequently show a fine stress fracture (lucent line) through the area of callus formation, a finding that is usually sufficient to make the diagnosis of stress fracture (Fig. 53–5). A biopsy usually is not necessary once a stress fracture is confirmed by roentgenographic studies. In fact, a biopsy may be misleading because the histologic appearance of an early stress fracture sometimes mimics osteogenic sarcoma. A biopsy would reveal a typical benign stress fracture only if there is extensive callus formation and the stress-inducing event took place at least 3 weeks previously.

When a stress fracture cannot be diagnosed with certainty (lack of lucent line on radiography), osteogenic sarcoma of bone, which is a common malignancy in adolescents, must be considered. The adolescent patient must be followed carefully, and roentgenograms must be repeated. If after 2 weeks of observation, a definite diagnosis of stress fracture cannot be made radiologically, a biopsy must be performed. The importance of the diagnosis of stress fracture is obvious when the differential diagnosis is considered.

OSTEOID OSTEOMA

Osteoid osteoma is a benign bone lesion characterized by pain in the affected area (see Table 53–10). It is usually less than 2 cm and is bone- or osteoid-producing, or both. The tumor itself is frequently referred to as the

female ballet dancers and are secondary to the stress involved in toe dancing.

The most common clinical manifestation of a stress fracture is pain and occasional swelling. Pain is the only symptom in many stress fractures, particularly those

Figure 53–5. A 16-year-old gymnast was referred for the management of a suspected osteogenic sarcoma. She experienced pain and swelling in the medial aspect of her thigh. *A,* A CT scan showed a soft tissue mass that was calcified. Because of her history of being a gymnast and the location of the lesion in the upper diaphyseal portion of the midfemur (in which stress fractures are common), as well as the peculiar pattern of calcification in the soft tissue, a stress fracture with associated callus formation was highly suspected. *B,* A repeat CT scan to look specifically at bone density windows revealed a typical stress fracture in the femur. The adolescent did well with modified activity for several months and is fine 2 years later.

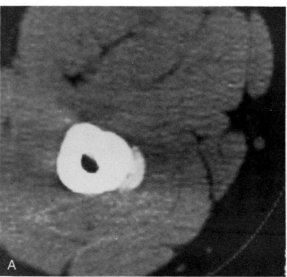
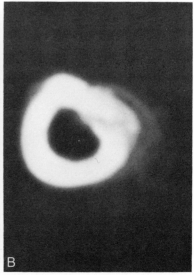

TABLE 53–10. Benign Tumors of Bone

	HISTORY	SYMPTOMS	PHYSICAL EXAMINATION	RADIOLOGIC FINDINGS	BONE SCAN	CT	BIOPSY	TREATMENT	DIFFERENTIAL DIAGNOSIS
Benign Bone-Producing Tumors									
Stress fracture	Physical stress	Pain, occasional swelling	—	Callus formation, location critical	Active	Fracture line	Usually contra-indicated, may mimic osteosarcoma especially if <3 wks duration	Avoidance of stress	Osteosarcoma
Osteoid osteoma	Age: 10–30 years M:F ratio = 2.3:1 No history of trauma	Pain (extremities more than axial skeleton)	Local tenderness	"Nidus" surrounded by sclerotic bone	Active, especially helpful for axial lesions	—	—	Resection, must remove nidus	Osteomyelitis Osteosarcoma
Osteoblastoma	Rare, larger than osteoid osteoma; frequent in spine (post element)	Pain	—	Circumscribed margin	Active	—	Necessary because of large size	Resection; aggressive form may recur locally	Osteosarcoma stress fracture
Fibrous dysplasia	Adolescent; equal incidence in M and F	Pain; swelling (extremities, ribs, skull)	Associated skin lesions in Albright disease	Expansile swelling of dysplastic bony element	Active	—	Rapidly enlarging lesions may indicate sarcomatous degeneration	Resection for monostatic form and for deformity and function correction in polyostotic form	Low-grade osteosarcoma
Benign Fibrous Lesions									
Nonossifying fibroma	M:F ratio = 1.6:1	As with stress fracture	—	Incidental cortical defect, sclerotic borders	—	—	Rarely indicated	None, large lesions with stress fracture may require curettage	—
Osteochondroma	Painless bump, may be multiple	Occasional muscle irritation with exercise	Smooth lump in metaphysis or diaphysis of long bone	Characteristic, must be followed if multiple, because of small potential for malignant degeneration	—	—	Rarely indicated	Remove if painful or disfiguring	Parosteal osteosarcoma

Enchondroma	Rare, usually in older patients	—	—	Usually incidental finding, may be difficult to differentiate from chondrosarcoma, multiple lesions must be followed for malignant degeneration	—	Indicated for large tumors, erosion of inner cortical table or pain	Surgical resection for cosmetic or functional relief	Chondrosarcoma
Chondro-myxoid fibroma	Rare M:F ratio = 1.5:1	Local swelling, indolent pain	—	Well-demarcated, lytic lesion with sclerotic margin	—	—	Curettage	Myxoid chondrosarcoma
Chrondro-blastoma	M:F ratio = 1.7:1	Pain, tenderness	Local swelling	Lytic lesion epiphyseal, internal calcification and sclerotic remnants	—	—	Curettage, wide excision if large, may seed locally or, rarely, to lungs	Giant cell tumor, osteosarcoma
Benign Vascular Lesions of Bone								
Aneurysmal bone cyst		Pain	Local swelling	Expansile, rarely breaks through cortex except with pathologic fractures	—	If large or x-ray appearance not definitive	Curettage may result in excessive bleeding; if surgery impossible, consider radiation treatment; tissue must be examined carefully for evidence of tumor	Telangiectatic osteosarcoma (lytic), malignant fibroma destroying bone, Ewing tumor
Giant cell tumor	M:F ratio = 2:3	Pain from periosteal stretching	Local swelling	Epiphyseal lytic lesion with well-defined border	—	—	*En bloc* resection	Metaphyseal lesion suggests malignant fibrous histiocytoma

"nidus" and can be seen on radiographs to be surrounded by reactive sclerotic bone (Fig. 53–6). This tumor has its peak incidence between the ages of 10 and 20 years with a 2.3:1 male-to-female ratio. The tumor is rare in children younger than 10 years of age and in adults older than 30 years of age.

The majority of osteoid osteomas occur in the long bones of the extremities. The femur and tibia are the most common sites. However, osteoid osteomas can occur in the distal extremities as well as in the axial skeleton. Osteoid osteomas of the spine and pelvis can be the cause of considerable pain, and the diagnosis may not be evident, because plain radiographs of these areas frequently will not reveal a small osteoid osteoma. CT scanning is more useful.

The diagnosis of an osteoid osteoma is usually made based on a history of pain that begins without any apparent trauma. The pain is usually persistent and is worse at night. Classically the pain is relieved by aspirin, and indeed approximately three quarters of patients with osteoid osteomas report such relief. The pain is not related to weight bearing and is not relieved by rest. Indeed, the pain tends to awaken the patient from sleep. Sometimes it is associated with local tenderness, and if the osteoid osteoma is close to a joint space, effusion may result from reactive synovitis. Severe pain resulting in paravertebral muscle spasm can cause scoliosis that typically resolves following removal of the nidus.

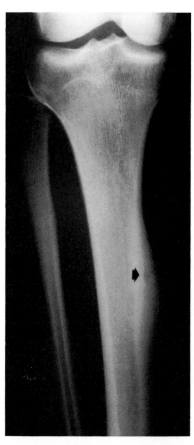

Figure 53–6. An 18-year-old female complained of a painful and tender area in the leg. The pain was worse at night and was relieved by acetylsalicylic acid. Radiographic studies revealed cortical thickening and a small radiolucent nidus (arrow) typical of an osteoid osteoma.

Osteoid osteoma can usually be diagnosed from its characteristic radiographic appearance (see Fig. 53–6). There is reactive bone formation around the nidus and the tumor itself can produce bone, and thus the nidus can appear osteoblastic or dense on the radiograph. Because of its rich blood supply and reactive bone production, this tumor is very apparent ("hot") on bone scans, which are more helpful than plain radiographs in defining a lesion in the axial skeleton.

Because of the pain and tenderness associated with an osteoid osteoma, the differential diagnosis must include osteomyelitis and osteosarcoma.

This lesion can be cured surgically. Treatment is complete resection of the nidus. If the nidus is not completely removed, the lesion and symptoms can recur. However, even if recurrent, an osteoid osteoma is always a benign lesion that does not undergo malignant degeneration.

OSTEOBLASTOMA

Osteoblastoma is a rare bone-producing benign tumor that is almost identical to the osteoid osteoma except in size (see Table 53–10). Bone pathologists have defined the upper limit of size for an osteoid osteoma to be 2 cm, whereas a lesion greater than 2 cm is diagnosed as an osteoblastoma. Osteoblastomas produce rich amounts of osteoid and have the characteristic appearance of a benign tumor on plain radiography. Their margin is usually well circumscribed and their benign nature can usually be determined by radiography. Because of its much greater propensity to occur in the spine, the osteoblastoma is believed to be a different entity than the osteoid osteoma. However, it occurs in the same age group as does osteoid osteoma—that is, predominantly in the second decade of life—and the male-to-female ratio is almost identical to that of an osteoid osteoma, being 3:1. Osteoblastomas do not always produce the characteristic pain syndrome described for osteoid osteoma. Indeed pain may be less acute but just as persistent. Although an osteoblastoma has the typical appearance of a benign tumor on radiographs, a biopsy is indicated because of the large size. As in the osteoid osteoma, an osteoblastoma is "hot" on bone scans.

The differential diagnosis of an osteoblastoma is important because other common tumors, such as osteogenic sarcoma, must be ruled out in the adolescent. Sometimes radiographs are not characteristic, and the differential diagnosis of the sclerotic lesion that produces pain in the adolescent will always include, in addition to a stress fracture, osteogenic sarcoma.

There are what have been termed *more aggressive* osteoblastomas whose differential diagnosis histopathologically from osteogenic sarcoma is not easy.

The osteoblastoma is cured surgically. However, the aggressive osteoblastoma has great local potential for recurrence but does not metastasize. If it does, it is a misdiagnosed osteosarcoma.

FIBROUS DYSPLASIA

The definition of fibrous dysplasia is an unusual intramedullary bone disorder that is characterized by fibro-osseous metaplasia (see Table 53–10). This tumorous condition can arise as a monostotic form, affecting only one bone, or a polyostotic form, with multiple bones involved. There is a distinct clinical form of polyostotic fibrous dysplasia, referred to as the McCune-Albright syndrome, in which patients present with precocious puberty, multiple bone lesions, and abnormal areas of skin pigmentation.

Although it is a rare tumor, fibrous dysplasia occurs with a peak incidence in the second decade of life, and it is rare in individuals older than 30 years and younger than 5 years of age. In the polyostotic form, precocious puberty can be an early manifestation of the disease in the younger child. Girls are affected slightly more than boys, with a male-to-female ratio of 1:1.2. The clinical manifestation of monostotic or solitary fibrous dysplasia is variable, and unless there is pain or swelling that produces a visible or palpable lesion, the disease may be discovered only incidentally when a pathologic fracture occurs.

Fibrous dysplasia can occur in any bone, but the most common sites are the long bones of the extremities, the ribs, and the skull.

The diagnosis of fibrous dysplasia is readily made radiologically. It is important to differentiate atypical lesions from low-grade osteogenic sarcomas.

Polyostotic fibrous dysplasia has been confused with neurofibromatosis because of the pigmented skin lesions associated with the polyostotic variety of McCune-Albright syndrome. However, typical café au lait spots of neurofibromatosis usually have perfectly regular smooth borders ("coast of California"), whereas those of fibrous dysplasia usually contain geographic or irregular borders ("coast of Maine").

Monostotic fibrous dysplasia occurs six times more frequently than the polyostotic form. The tumor is usually totally benign. It is impossible to resect all lesions of the polyostotic form. Polyostotic fibrous dysplasia can produce severe deformities of the skeleton as the adolescent gets older. There is a slight possibility of degeneration of these lesions to sarcoma.

Benign Fibrous Lesions of Bone

NONOSSIFYING FIBROMA

The nonossifying fibroma is a persistent and progressive fibrous cortical defect of childhood that usually becomes manifested during the second decade of life (see Table 53–10). Males are affected more than females, with a male-to-female ratio of 1.6:1. These tumors are usually solitary and totally benign, but they can become symptomatic and are subsequently diagnosed because of an associated stress fracture through the lesion during the adolescent years.

With the exception of pathologic fractures, these lesions are usually asymptomatic and are frequently discovered incidentally when radiographs are obtained for other reasons. Nevertheless, some of these lesions can be of concern because of their large size (see Fig. 53–3). However, the radiologic appearance is characteristic of a benign lesion, having well-defined sclerotic borders.

Usually no treatment is required for nonossifying fibromas, and they rarely need to be biopsied. However, if they appear atypical or become symptomatic, one should be suspicious of a different entity, and a biopsy may be prudent. Occasionally, very large lesions that produce painful stress fractures will require curettage and packing with bone chips.

Benign Cartilaginous Bone Lesions

OSTEOCHONDROMA (BENIGN EXOSTOSIS)

An osteochondroma is a benign cartilage cap protuberance that usually occurs in the metaphyseal or diaphyseal area of the long bones (see Table 53–10). Multiple osteochondromatosis is a hereditary syndrome characterized by multiple osteochondromas. Although they are always benign lesions, there is a very small incidence of malignant degeneration to both chondrosarcomas and osteogenic sarcomas. Malignant degeneration of an osteochondroma, although extremely rare, occurs more frequently in multiple osteochondromatosis than it does in solitary osteochondroma. Although osteochondromas can occur in any bone, they occur much more frequently in the long bones of the extremities. The areas around the knee and the upper humerus are the most common sites.

Osteochondromas are probably developmental abnormalities stemming from cartilaginous nests left behind in the advancing growing bone. However, they become manifest and are usually diagnosed in the second decade of life and therefore are a common bone tumor seen in adolescents.

The usual clinical manifestation of a benign osteochondroma is the production of a palpable, painless smooth bump. Occasionally lesions can produce mechanical irritation of muscle ligaments or tendons during physical exertion and may present as pain or swelling and irritation. Compression of a nerve by a large osteochondroma can also cause pain as a presenting symptom; however, a very smooth characteristic bump can almost always be palpated. These lesions feel characteristic on physical examination because of their smooth contour, and they have a characteristic radiologic appearance as well.

Rarely, because of their eccentrically placed location and variable degree of calcification within the cartilage cap, the radiologic appearance will necessitate including parosteal (or juxticortical) osteogenic sarcoma in the differential diagnosis.

Osteochondromas are benign tumors and usually no biopsy or treatment is necessary. Occasionally removal is required when they produce symptoms of pain or are subject to frequent trauma during physical activity. Sometimes these lesions tend to regress after closure of the epiphysis. Occasionally the lesion will get larger around the time of puberty. In patients with multiple exostoses in particular, periodic follow-up, with physical examination and appropriate x-ray studies, is important.

Osteochondromas that undergo a rapid change in size may require biopsy or removal, or both, not only for cosmetic purposes but also to rule out malignant degeneration.

ENCHONDROMA

Enchondroma is a benign cartilage-producing tumor arising in the intramedullary cavity of the bone (see Table 53–10). Its diagnostic importance is to differentiate it from chondrosarcoma, which it mimics at times, both in its roentgenographic appearance and histologically. It is sometimes difficult to differentiate a benign enchondroma from a low-grade chondrosarcoma. Enchondromas tend to occur in a younger age group. Although the peak incidence of enchondroma is in the third and fourth decades of life, its incidence increases rapidly in the second decade of life. Rare cases have been reported in children younger than 10 years of age. A rare form of multiple enchondromatosis, sometimes referred to as Ollier disease, is more commonly diagnosed in the adolescent age group. It is a developmental disease that usually does not become apparent until adolescence.

Solitary enchondroma can occur in almost any bone of the body. The most common sites include the femur, humerus, and tibia, followed by the short tubular bones of the hands and feet. Less common sites include the ribs, pelvis, and other axial structures.

Most enchondromas are incidentally discovered during radiologic procedures for other reasons. These tumors are painless, and indeed the lack of pain is what differentiates them from low-grade chondrosarcomas. Enchondromas that have a typical radiologic appearance require no treatment (Fig. 53–7). However, atypical findings, such as very large size, the appearance of erosion of the inner cortical table of the bone, thickening of bone cortices, or chronic pain, might prompt a biopsy to rule out less benign conditions.

Multiple enchondromatosis has a higher frequency of morbidity and malignant degeneration to chondrosarcoma. It requires periodic follow-up radiographs with a recommendation that rapidly enlarging lesions be biopsied to rule out malignant degeneration. Additional surgical treatment may be required for cosmetic or functional purposes. Frequently, patients with multiple enchondromatosis require surgery to improve function, particularly when there is multiple involvement of the short tubular bones of the hands and feet. However, this is usually not until later in life and rarely becomes the concern of the adolescent specialist.

CHONDROMYXOID FIBROMA

The chondromyxoid fibroma is a rare, painful benign tumor of bone that is composed of a mixture of fibrous tissue, cartilaginous tissue, and myxoid tissue (see Table 53–10). Its peak incidence is in the second decade of life with a 1.5:1 male-to-female ratio. Its major importance lies in differentiating it from a more malignant tumor, such as myxoid chondrosarcoma.

The differential diagnosis of chondromyxoid fibroma should include that of another lytic tumor—the adaman-

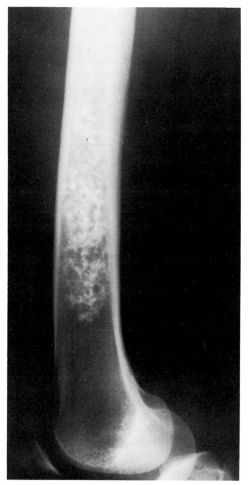

Figure 53–7. An 18-year-old female had a routine radiograph of the distal femur after suffering trauma to the area. An incidentally discovered large lesion in the midfemur was cause for initial concern; however, this lesion with its characteristic appearance of an enchondroma is totally benign. Most enchondromas of bone are painless and are discovered incidentally following radiographic studies that are usually performed for trauma in healthy individuals or bone scans that are performed for staging of patients with malignancies.

tinoma, which is a low-grade malignant tumor that also occurs frequently in adolescents. This tumor requires wider surgical excision for cure and carries with it a worse prognosis than does the benign chondromyxoid fibroma.

Treatment for chondromyxoid fibroma is simple curettage, which usually cures this lesion.

CHONDROBLASTOMA

The chondroblastoma is a benign tumor that is quite characteristic in that it is one of the few tumors with an epiphyseal origin (see Table 53–10). Although chondroblastoma is a relatively rare bone tumor, it occurs almost exclusively during the second decade of life. It occurs most frequently in the proximal humerus and the ends of the femur and tibia, as well as the bones of the ankle. The most common clinical manifestation of the chondroblastoma is pain and sometimes tenderness with slight swelling in the area of the lesion.

The major lesion of concern in the differential diagnosis is the giant cell tumor. It is the only other epiphyseal tumor with a significant occurrence. Giant cell tumors occur in slightly older age groups (peak incidence in the third and fourth decades of life); however, they are not unheard of in adolescents. Extremely rarely, osteogenic sarcomas can occur in an epiphyseal location, and usually those that do are of the rare low-grade variety.

Benign Vascular Bone Lesions

ANEURYSMAL BONE CYST

An aneurysmal bone cyst is a benign vascular tumor that occurs predominantly in the second decade of life (see Table 53–10). Although the majority of aneurysmal bone cysts occur in the long bones, with the lower extremity being more common than the upper extremity, they have also been noted in the pelvis and in other axial locations such as the spine, scapula, and skull. Aneurysmal bone cysts have the characteristic appearance of benign lesions that expand the bone but usually do not break through the cortex. They may, however, be associated with a pathologic stress fracture through the lesion, particularly when they occur in the weight-bearing bones. The predominant signs and symptoms of an aneurysmal bone cyst are pain and swelling in the area. Pain may be acute in onset when the tumor undergoes a spontaneous or pathologic fracture from stress.

The differential diagnosis of an aneurysmal bone cyst includes the possibility of a purely lytic (or telangiectatic) osteogenic sarcoma, a malignant fibrous histiocytoma, or Ewing sarcoma. Therefore, it is important to biopsy these lesions adequately.

Figure 53–8 illustrates a benign aneurysmal bone cyst

of the pelvis found in a 14-year-old girl. Because this tumor was so large and had expanded to the bone it was difficult to differentiate the aneurysmal bone cyst from a malignant soft tissue mass. Biopsy material was obtained with a great deal of bleeding. It was determined that curettage and resection of this aneurysmal bone cyst would be impossible because of the extensive amount of bleeding. Indeed, very experienced surgeons felt that even hemipelvectomy would be necessary in order to get around this lesion, but that it would be almost impossible because of the extensive amount of bleeding that was expected to occur. Therefore, this particular lesion was treated with low-dose radiation therapy. It healed completely over a period of several months (see Fig. 53–8). With the exception of such rare and large tumors, aneurysmal bone cysts can usually undergo complete curettage.

GIANT CELL TUMORS

Giant cell tumors are benign epiphyseal tumors that have a peak incidence in the third and fourth decades of life (see Table 53–10). They make their appearance in the adolescent age group (usually in older adolescents) and seldom occur before that time. The clinical manifestation of giant cell tumor is usually pain. The radiograph is usually characteristic and shows a purely lytic lesion with a well-defined border (Fig. 53–9).

Rarely one encounters a malignant giant cell tumor capable of producing widespread metastases, which should be treated in a manner similar to that for malignant osteogenic sarcomas of bone, with chemotherapy.

Malignant Bone Tumors

MALIGNANT BONE-PRODUCING TUMORS

Malignant bone-producing tumors that are encountered in the adolescent age group include osteogenic

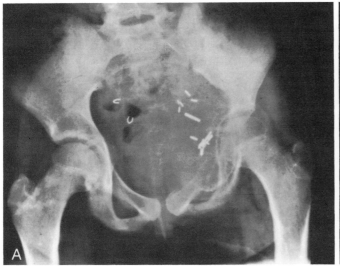 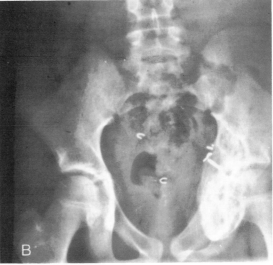

Figure 53–8. *A,* An aneurysmal bone cyst arising from the inner table of the acetabulum in a 14-year-old girl. The straight surgical clips outline the periphery of the lesion in the pelvis. Following biopsy there was extensive bleeding, and it was felt that this lesion was inoperable. *B,* Note the complete healing 6 months after the application of low-dose radiation therapy (24 Gy). Although one prefers to perform surgery and avoid radiation therapy for benign lesions such as this, the clinical situation in this case required radiation therapy, which was totally curative, in a lesion that otherwise would have probably required a hemipelvectomy because of the large amount of bleeding that would have been encountered during any surgical attempt to treat this lesion. If untreated, the adolescent would have sustained a fracture through the lesion and had extensive life-threatening hemorrhage.

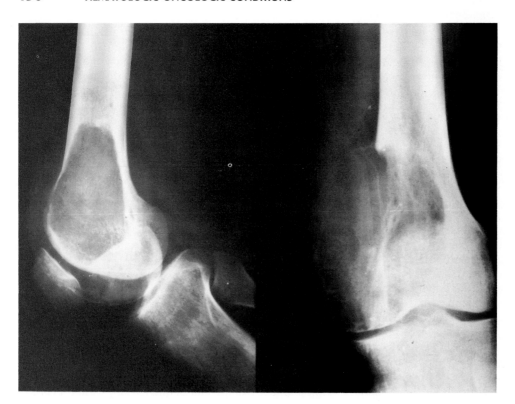

Figure 53–9. An 18-year-old male presented with swelling in the distal femur. Although a malignant bone tumor was suspected, the radiographic appearance was that of a typical benign giant cell tumor as evidenced by the presumed origin in the epiphysis, the relatively sharp demarcated margins of the lesion, and the fact that the soft tissue mass is actually an expansion of the bone with thinning of the cortex rather than erosion through the cortex. This patient was successfully treated with curettage and cryosurgery.

sarcoma and some of its varieties, particularly the juxtacortical or low-grade parosteal osteogenic sarcoma and the periosteal osteogenic sarcoma, which is a high-grade malignancy. Both of the latter tumors originate on the surface of the bone rather than from the central portion of the bone as does the classic osteogenic sarcoma.

Osteogenic Sarcoma

Osteogenic sarcoma is a malignant neoplasm containing malignant spindle cells that produce osteoid or immature bone. Osteogenic sarcoma is the most common bone tumor encountered in the adolescent age group. The classic form of osteogenic sarcoma affects primarily adolescents. The peak incidence of osteogenic sarcoma occurs in girls aged 12 to 13 years and in boys aged 14 to 15 years, corresponding to the onset of the adolescent growth spurt in each gender. Osteogenic sarcoma occurs more frequently in children who have bilateral (familial) retinoblastoma. It occurs in irradiated orbital bones at 1000 times the frequency of that in the normal population and 500 times as often in bony sites distant from the irradiated orbit. It is now well accepted that there is a genetic cause for osteogenic sarcoma in patients who have familial retinoblastoma.

In humans, osteogenic sarcoma is most common in the distal femur, followed by the proximal tibia and the proximal humerus.

The clinical manifestations of osteogenic sarcoma include pain, which is frequently attributed to recent trauma, but the trauma merely calls attention to preexisting small lesions. Swelling occurs relatively late when the tumor has had the opportunity to erode through the bony cortex to produce a soft tissue mass.

Approximately 20% of patients with osteogenic sarcoma have overt pulmonary metastases present at the time of diagnosis. The tumor may present as a pathologic fracture, particularly in certain histologic subvarieties that produce primarily lytic lesions (telangiectatic osteogenic sarcoma). When an adolescent experiences a pathologic fracture without direct or unusually severe trauma, one must suspect a malignant tumor.

Osteogenic sarcoma was dreaded in the past because the disease was lethal in 80% to 90% of adolescent patients, even after radical surgery such as amputation. With modern multidisciplinary approaches—including preoperative chemotherapy, *en bloc* excision of the tumor by an experienced orthopedic oncologist, and continued postoperative adjuvant chemotherapy—most patients with osteogenic sarcoma not only can be cured but also can avoid amputation. Clearly, it is imperative that an early and accurate diagnosis be made.

The diagnosis of osteogenic sarcoma must always be suspected when there is pain and swelling in the distal femur or proximal tibia in an adolescent who denies prior trauma. A radiograph is usually diagnostic, since most osteogenic sarcomas produce visible bone production. Osteogenic sarcoma can produce the classic "sunburst" appearance of radiating rays of calcified osteoid into the surrounding soft tissue (Fig. 53–10). If the tumor is not advanced and has not had time to produce a large soft tissue mass, the finding of a sclerotic bone lesion in an adolescent complaining of pain is suggestive of osteogenic sarcoma. Approximately 60% of patients with osteogenic sarcoma have an elevated serum alkaline phosphatase level. Thus, this finding in an adolescent patient with pain and a sclerotic lesion in any bone is almost diagnostic of an osteogenic sarcoma. Because of the gravity of the diagnosis and the aggressive treatment required, it is extremely important to establish the diagnosis by biopsy of the lesion.

Differential Diagnosis. Rarely, osteogenic sarcoma

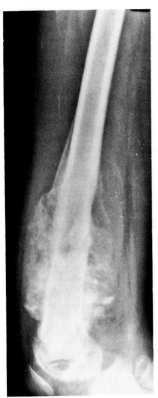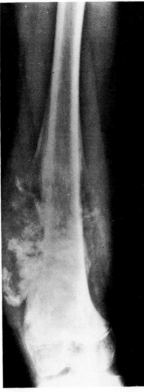

Figure 53–10. The typical appearance of a malignant osteogenic sarcoma in a 15-year-old male. Note the periosteal elevation in the proximal portion of the lesion produced by the soft tissue mass, which has eroded through the cortex. The calcification in the soft tissue is typical of osteogenic sarcoma and in some areas appears to be radiating perpendicular to the femoral shaft ("sunburst" sign). There is mottled sclerosis in the medullary cavity of the bone as well.

can occur in preexisting benign bone conditions, and the initial radiograph of the benign lesion can be misleading. Thus, adolescents with multiple exostosis or osteochondromas may have an enlarging lesion for which degeneration to an osteogenic sarcoma must be considered. An osteogenic sarcoma that is purely lytic can masquerade as an aneurysmal bone cyst. In addition, other malignant bone tumors cannot always be differentiated from osteogenic sarcoma based on the radiologic studies alone. Many primary lymphomas involving bone produce reactive sclerosis and present as a mixed lytic and sclerotic lesion; a biopsy may be necessary to differentiate the type of tumor. This is essential because the treatment for lymphoma of bone is vastly different from the treatment of osteogenic sarcoma. However, with proper treatment, both diseases are now highly curable in the majority of adolescents.

Although Ewing sarcoma is a classic diaphyseal tumor, osteogenic sarcomas can also occur in the diaphysis or midshaft of the bone. Moreover, Ewing sarcoma can occur in the metaphysis, appearing as a lytic osteogenic sarcoma or a malignant fibrous histiocytoma of bone. Fibrosarcoma of bone also may present in a fashion similar to osteogenic sarcoma except that the former is almost always a lytic lesion and does not show sclerosis or bone production (see later discussion).

Myositis ossificans must also be considered in the differential diagnosis of osteogenic sarcoma. It is a benign posttraumatic soft tissue lesion that, although occurring in soft tissues, can be associated with a stress fracture or can appear to be a soft tissue mass emanating from bone.

Treatment. An osteogenic sarcoma should not be treated prior to definitive biopsy. Currently, the majority of adolescents with osteogenic sarcoma of an extremity (no matter how large the lesion) may benefit from limb salvage surgery. Therefore, it is extremely important to plan the biopsy with the help of an orthopedic oncologist so that the biopsy incision is properly placed and does not interfere with or increase the risk of future limb salvage surgery. The current treatment of osteogenic sarcoma must include preoperative chemotherapy; rarely is immediate surgery indicated (Table 53–11). High-dose methotrexate with leucovorin rescue is a unique treatment in that it is extremely effective in about 50% of patients with primary bone tumors, such as osteogenic sarcoma and malignant fibrous histiocytoma. When doxorubicin is used as a single agent in the treatment of osteogenic sarcoma, the dose should be 90 mg/m^2. When used in combination with cisplatin, a lower dose is given. Ifosfamide in high doses seems to be the most effective single agent in the treatment of osteogenic sarcoma, with a response rate of 67% noted in patients with evaluable metastatic disease. It is given with mesna, which is used to protect the bladder from hemorrhagic cystitis.

Although there has been great acceptance of intraarterial chemotherapy, primary tumors respond just as well to intravenous chemotherapy. Besides avoiding the local complications of intra-arterial therapy, the advantage of intravenous chemotherapy is that its ultimate purpose is to prevent pulmonary metastases, and therefore chemotherapy should focus on treating the patient systemically rather than locally. Even if amputation is needed, the adolescent should still undergo preoperative chemotherapy, since the evaluation of its effect on the primary tumor usually will dictate the course of further adjuvant chemotherapy. Furthermore, the adolescent patient's response to preoperative chemotherapy is an important prognostic factor. If the tumor does not respond favorably to preoperative chemotherapy, the prognosis is poor if the same chemotherapy is continued; a change in chemotherapy is indicated. Because most chemotherapeutic agents used for osteogenic sarcoma depend upon renal excretion (and can be toxic to the kidney), adolescent patients with osteogenic sarcoma should have their creatinine clearance determined prior to the start of therapy.

Adolescents with osteogenic sarcoma should have a CT scan of the chest to rule out pulmonary metastases and a bone scan to rule out bone metastases. The finding of small pulmonary metastases at the time of diagnosis may not significantly impair the chance for cure. Follow-

TABLE 53–11. Chemotherapy for Osteogenic Sarcoma

High-dose methotrexate with leucovorin rescue
Doxorubicin
Doxorubicin combined with cisplatin
High-dose ifosfamide with mesna

ing successful preoperative chemotherapy and surgery for the primary tumor, the adolescent patient must eventually undergo thoracotomy to remove any residual metastatic deposits. Thoracotomy should be performed when the initial CT scan of the chest reveals abnormalities, even though the disease may completely disappear following preoperative chemotherapy.

Adolescent patients who have a complete histologic response to approximately 3 months of preoperative chemotherapy require only 4 to 6 weeks of postoperative chemotherapy with the same agents, namely, high-dose methotrexate with leucovorin rescue, ifosfamide, and cisplatin combined with doxorubicin. Following treatment, approximately 75% of patients presenting with osteogenic sarcoma will be cured. Late recurrence of osteogenic sarcoma is usually in the form of delayed pulmonary metastases or local tumor recurrence in the resected primary area.

Approximately half of patients in whom pulmonary metastases develop may be curable. Therefore, following the completion of the initial phase of therapy, adolescents should be followed with frequent radiographs and CT scans of the chest for a prolonged period. After each year of observation passes, the radiologic studies can become less and less frequent until 5 years from the start of treatment, at which time studies can be performed at 6-month intervals.

Adolescents who have had limb salvage surgery are especially prone to late local recurrences. Those with pulmonary metastases especially should be followed carefully because of the possibility of local recurrence. Factors that predispose to local recurrence are large soft tissue masses that do not respond well to preoperative chemotherapy, and the finding of venous invasion at the time of *en bloc* resection of the primary tumor.

There are fewer than 500 adolescent patients who present with osteogenic sarcoma yearly in the United States. The practitioner is urged to identify and consult with an experienced orthopedic oncologist if limb salvage surgery is contemplated.

Other Forms of Osteogenic Sarcoma

Parosteal Osteogenic Sarcoma. Parosteal (or juxtacortical) osteogenic sarcoma is a low-grade osteogenic sarcoma that tends to occur on the surface of the bone. It is more common in the older adolescent, as well as in females. Typically it occupies the posterior metaphyseal surface of the femur but can occur in any bone. It has a peak age incidence of 20 to 30 years. The tumor presents as a painful swelling in the back of the knee and has a characteristic radiologic appearance (Fig. 53–11). The tumor is usually a low-grade malignancy and when confirmed on initial biopsy, definitive surgery is all that is needed.

Periosteal Osteogenic Sarcoma. This variety of osteogenic sarcoma occurs in older adolescents and has a peak incidence between 16 and 25 years of age. Like the parosteal osteogenic sarcoma, it tends to occur on the surface of bones. However, it is more common in males than in females and classically involves the diaphysis of the femur or the upper diaphyseal-metaphyseal region of the tibia.

The tumor presents with the same symptoms of pain and swelling as does an osteogenic sarcoma. However, histologically this tumor is composed primarily of cartilaginous material, and in many instances it is mistaken for a chondrosarcoma. It is a fully malignant tumor, though it tends to metastasize somewhat less frequently than does the classic osteogenic sarcoma. It is somewhat more resistant to chemotherapy.

Periosteal osteogenic sarcoma is treated in a fashion identical to that for classic osteogenic sarcoma, as described previously.

Postirradiation Osteogenic Sarcoma. Patients who have been cured of other malignancies with radiation therapy can experience postirradiation osteogenic sarcoma. This tumor tends to occur at a median time of 10 years after radiation therapy for other malignancies and is a commonly recognized entity. It can occur in bone or soft tissue. The original observation suggested that postirradiation sarcomas tended to occur at a higher frequency when higher dosages of radiation were used for the initial malignancy. It is hoped that the incidence of postirradiation osteogenic sarcoma will become lower as we use lower and lower doses of radiation therapy to treat other disease (e.g., Hodgkin disease; see next subchapter). This trend using lower doses of radiation therapy is made possible through the use of combination chemotherapy plus radiation therapy.

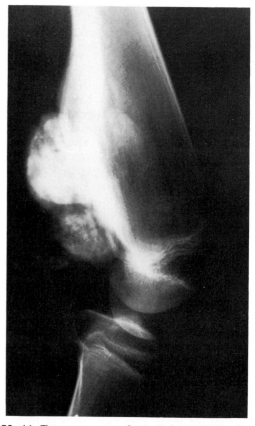

Figure 53–11. The appearance of a typical parosteal or low-grade osteogenic sarcoma arising on the surface of the bone. Although parosteal osteogenic sarcoma reaches its peak frequency in the third decade of life, it also occurs in the second decade of life, as it did in this 14-year-old girl. Although it is a low-grade tumor, treatment requires a radical *en bloc* excision similar to that performed for high-grade osteogenic sarcomas in order to prevent local recurrence.

Postirradiation osteogenic sarcoma is a malignant tumor that was once thought to be an incurable disease, but treatment is as effective as that for classic osteogenic sarcomas with the same chemotherapeutic and surgical considerations as those given to the classic osteogenic sarcoma. However, a postirradiation tumor sometimes represents a more difficult management problem because the tumor is usually located in the axial skeleton in which tissues have undergone radiation therapy. Thus, postirradiation osteogenic sarcoma in patients who have been cured of Hodgkin disease frequently involves the sternum, spine, or the axial skeleton in which radiation therapy was used. It is extremely important to perform preoperative chemotherapy once the diagnosis is established by a biopsy, with the hope of shrinking the primary tumor as much as possible so that radical surgical excision of an axial lesion can be performed. It is hoped that preoperative chemotherapy might alter the dismal prognosis for this rare form of osteogenic sarcoma, which frequently is difficult to control locally with surgery alone.

Malignant Fibrous Histiocytoma of Bone and Malignant Fibrosarcoma of Bone

These entities also occur in the adolescent age group, though unlike osteogenic sarcoma they reach their peak frequency in older adults. These are usually malignant spindle cell sarcomas of bone that differ from the osteogenic sarcoma in that they do not produce enough neoplastic bone or osteoid to classify them as osteogenic sarcomas. Otherwise they behave in the same way as classic osteogenic sarcoma, metastasizing to lung and other bones as late sequelae.

Because of the biologic similarity to osteogenic sarcoma, these tumors are treated in an identical fashion to the classic osteogenic sarcoma. Primary malignant fibrous histiocytomata that we have encountered respond just as well as osteogenic sarcoma and indeed have an excellent prognosis when treated with preoperative chemotherapy and *en bloc* resection.

Chondrosarcoma of Bone

Chondrosarcomas are extremely rare in the adolescent population. Indeed, true chondrosarcomas, which are usually of low-grade malignancy, are rare in patients younger than 50 years of age. They are mentioned here solely because chondrosarcoma, although atypical, is occasionally diagnosed in adolescents. Pure chondrosarcomas encountered in adolescents may be fully malignant tumors and not the low-grade variety found in older adults.

Chondrosarcomas in adolescents are usually aggressive tumors that require pre- and postoperative chemotherapy and surgery, almost identical to that for osteogenic sarcoma.

Low-grade chondrosarcomas are rarely encountered in the adolescent and may represent chondrosarcomatous dedifferentiation of an existing enchondroma in patients with multiple enchondromatosis, as discussed earlier.

Mesenchymal Chondrosarcoma

Mesenchymal chondrosarcoma is a rare tumor that occurs in adolescent patients as a primary tumor of either bone or soft tissue. It can occur in the long bones such as the femur, which is the most common long bone site, but the tumor is more common in the axial skeleton, in which it tends to occur in association with the meninges; these sites are often more common and include the skull and paraspinal areas of the axial skeleton. Because of the degree of the malignancy, soft tissue primary tumors can erode adjacent bones, making it difficult to tell whether the tumor is indeed of soft tissue or bony origin.

The diagnosis of the rare mesenchymal chondrosarcoma is usually made following presenting signs of pain or neurologic symptoms related to paraspinal nerve root compression. Roentgenographic studies usually reveal a soft tissue mass associated with bone destruction. This is a malignant tumor usually composed of small primitive round cells that make up the malignant stroma; these cells sometimes closely resemble those of a Ewing sarcoma of bone. Indeed, mesenchymal chondrosarcomas are treated in a fashion very similar to that for Ewing sarcoma of bone, including preoperative chemotherapy and radiation therapy.

Ewing Sarcoma of Bone

After osteogenic sarcoma, Ewing sarcoma is the second most common malignant bone tumor encountered in the adolescent age group. Ewing sarcoma appears to arise as a primitive mesenchymal tumor. Its histogenetic origin is unknown at this time, though Ewing believed the tumor was of vascular origin because of the amount of vascularity in many of these tumors. Ewing's original paper described this tumor as a "diffuse endothelioma of bone." Ewing was also the first to recognize that this malignant tumor of bone, unlike the more common osteogenic sarcoma, was sensitive to radiation therapy.

Ewing sarcoma reaches its peak incidence during the second decade of life. It occurs in individuals younger than 10 years of age but is extremely rare before the age of 5 years. It is very uncommon in adults, and indeed the diagnosis of Ewing sarcoma after the third decade of life should raise suspicion that one is dealing with a different tumor of bone more common in the older age group, that is, non-Hodgkin lymphoma.

Ewing sarcoma is slightly more common in males than in females, with a male-to-female ratio of 1.4:1. It can occur in any bone in the body but tends to occur in the femur and in the flat bones, such as the pelvis, ribs, and scapula (Fig. 53–12). Classically the tumor was described by Ewing as occurring in the diaphysis of long bones. However, in our experience, Ewing sarcoma can occur in any region of the bone.

Ewing sarcoma presents as pain in the area of the lesion. Although the initial presenting symptom is pain, Ewing sarcoma frequently evolves rapidly into a large mass in the soft tissues as a result of the bony destruction produced by the tumor. The classic history of Ewing sarcoma includes fever, an elevated erythrocyte sedimentation rate, and an elevated white blood cell count.

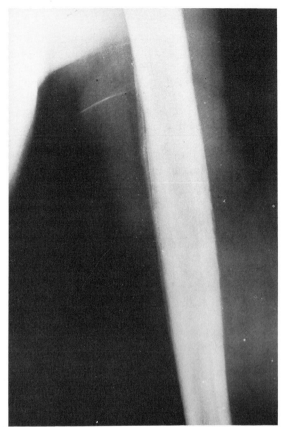

Figure 53–12. Ewing sarcoma of the humerus in a 16-year-old girl. Ewing sarcoma typically is a diaphyseal lesion as shown here. Also note the medial cortical surface of the bone, which shows an "onion skin" appearance produced by the periosteum, which is producing bone as it is being pushed further into the soft tissue by the expanding tumor. There is a mixed sclerotic and lytic lesion in the medullary canal of the bone. Usually Ewing tumors are lytic lesions; however, there can be reactive sclerosis to the malignant process.

In fact, these associated symptoms are rarely found. However, osteomyelitis can present in a fashion similar to that of Ewing sarcoma, and indeed some Ewing sarcomas have been noted to become secondarily infected. When one suspects osteomyelitis, it is necessary that specimens be obtained for culture when necrotic tissue that appears to be pus is encountered on bone biopsy.

A major consideration in the differential diagnosis of Ewing sarcoma (besides osteomyelitis) is primary lymphoma of bone. Lymphomas of bone can appear very similar to Ewing sarcoma histologically. Primitive neuroectodermal tumors, histologically similar to Ewing sarcoma, tend to arise more frequently in the bones or soft tissues of the thorax. Both tumors are treated identically and both carry a similarly poor prognosis if not treated. Because Ewing sarcoma is composed of primitive small round cells, a bone lesion containing Ewing sarcoma could be confused with metastatic neuroblastoma. However, neuroblastoma usually occurs in a much younger age group than does Ewing sarcoma, and metastatic neuroblastoma usually involves bones in a symmetric fashion.

Once the diagnosis of Ewing sarcoma is established, the patient should be evaluated with a bone scan to rule out the presence of bony metastases and with a CT scan of the chest to determine the presence of pulmonary metastases. Patients should undergo staging with bone marrow aspiration, since Ewing sarcoma can involve marrow late in its course (in contrast with primary lymphoma of bone, which tends to involve bone marrow earlier in the course of disease).

The treatment of Ewing sarcoma, like that of osteogenic sarcoma, involves the use of preoperative chemotherapy. Table 53–12 lists the chemotherapeutic agents used for the treatment of Ewing sarcoma. Specific details of treatment have been developed at the Cedars-Sinai Comprehensive Cancer Center. Three weeks after the combination chemotherapy is administered, high-dose cyclophosphamide is given for 2 days. Three weeks later, the first combination treatment is repeated. These drug dosages are very aggressive; however, they produce a very high response rate in primary and metastatic Ewing sarcoma. One week following the start of each chemotherapy course, adolescent patients are monitored with a complete blood count every other day until they recover. If fever develops while the patient is neutropenic, intravenous antibiotic therapy is rapidly instituted and transfusions with packed red blood cells are given to keep the hemoglobin level in the area of 10 g/dl, as are platelet transfusions when indicated. Patients receive a total of 12 treatments (8 with ifosfamide, doxorubicin, and VP-16 and 4 with high-dose cyclophosphamide). There is a 3-week rest period between each treatment.

Following a good response to preoperative chemotherapy by the primary tumor, radiation therapy is applied to the entire bone. Following this, the area of the lesion usually undergoes *en bloc* resection. With precise timing of aggressive therapy—including combination chemotherapy, preoperative radiation therapy, surgical resection, and postoperative adjuvant chemotherapy—approximately 80% to 90% of patients with Ewing sarcoma can be cured. Disease in approximately 10% to 20% of patients proceeds to metastases. Patients with poor prognoses can usually be predicted by their poor response to preoperative chemotherapy. This situation is similar to that found with osteogenic sarcoma following preoperative chemotherapy. Other factors leading to a poor prognosis include very large soft tissue masses (late diagnosis) and the unresectability of the primary tumor, which can lead to a local recurrence after radiation therapy and subsequent late dissemination of disease.

The employment of surgical resection in all patients with Ewing sarcoma will hopefully obviate one of the major long-term iatrogenic sequelae of Ewing sarcoma, that is, postirradiation sarcoma. Surgical resection not

TABLE 53–12. Chemotherapy for Ewing Sarcoma and Primitive Neuroectodermal Tumor

Combination of
Ifosfamide and mesna,
doxorubicin, and
VP-16 (etoposide)
Alternating with single agent:
High-dose cyclophosphamide

only allows lower doses of radiation therapy but also removes much of the irradiated tissue that is at risk for development of a postirradiation sarcoma.

Follow-up for patients with Ewing sarcoma is similar to that used for other malignant tumors—namely, periodic chest CT scans, which are performed more frequently after completing therapy and then less frequently as time elapses. Because the most frequent areas of metastases in recurrent Ewing sarcoma include both the lungs and the bones (particularly the skull and axial skeleton), routine follow-up bone scans are also performed in patients who have completed therapy for Ewing sarcoma.

Primitive Neuroectodermal Tumor

Primitive neuroectodermal tumors are histologically similar to Ewing sarcoma, but on light microscopy the cells tend to show neuroectodermal differentiation such as rosette formation or positive staining for neuron-specific enolase. They tend to occur in the thorax but can occur anywhere in the body. Treatment is identical to that of a Ewing sarcoma.

It was once felt that primitive neuroectodermal tumors had a worse prognosis than did Ewing sarcoma; however, the same principles hold true, and the treatment is the same. Adolescents whose primary tumor completely or nearly completely responds to preoperative chemotherapy have an excellent prognosis, whereas patients in whom there is considerable viable tumor following preoperative therapy have a poor prognosis. The proportion of patients with primitive neuroectodermal tumors who have a poor prognosis under these circumstances is approximately similar to those with the histologic diagnosis of Ewing sarcoma.

SOFT TISSUE NEOPLASMS

Although rare in the general population, soft tissue neoplasms are seen in adolescents. Certain of these tumors tend to have their peak incidence in adolescence, or at least that is when they are recognized. In addition, other malignant tumors that are more common in other age groups, such as rhabdomyosarcoma in younger children and nasopharyngeal carcinoma in adults, represent different histologic and clinical entities when they occur in adolescence. These tumors deserve comment because their treatment in the adolescent patient differs from therapy in the adult (nasopharyngeal carcinoma) or the young child (rhabdomyosarcoma). The common soft tissue neoplasms encountered in the adolescent population are presented in Table 53–9.

Benign Soft Tissue Tumors

Most benign growths that occur in the adolescent patient can be subdivided into three categories: (1) infectious, (2) posttraumatic, and (3) neoplastic. Hemorrhagic, infectious, and traumatic lesions often evolve much more rapidly than do either malignant or benign neoplastic lesions. When taking a history from the patient, the clinician should keep this principle in mind.

HEMATOMAS

The most rapidly evolving lesions in the adolescent are hemorrhagic (i.e., hematoma). It is unfortunate that many adolescents in whom a diagnosis of malignant soft tissue sarcoma is eventually made are considered to have a resolving hematoma over a period of weeks or even months before the correct diagnosis is reached. It should be noted that hematomas usually resolve within a period of a few weeks at the most. If hematomas persist for more than a few weeks, calcifications usually develop in the center of the lesion. However, by this time there is usually a change in the bluish purple skin discoloration to light yellow. The persistence of deep-blue discoloration of the skin in a mass for more than a few weeks is an indication that there may be a malignant tumor. Several of the malignant tumors that occur in adolescents, such as rhabdomyosarcomas, synovial sarcomas, and malignant fibrous histiocytomas, can be very vascular and present with this discoloration. Indeed, when a needle biopsy attempt produces only hemorrhagic material, it can be misinterpreted as a hematoma. If one suspects a malignant tumor because of the persistence of what appears to be a hematoma that is not resolving, an open biopsy is preferred to a needle biopsy to establish a diagnosis.

Infectious lesions are rarely a diagnostic problem, although occasionally a pelvic or deep soft tissue abscess will present as a soft tissue mass. Abscesses may be misdiagnosed on CT scan or magnetic resonance imaging (MRI) since frequently a tumor can have a necrotic center that simulates an abscess.

MYOSITIS OSSIFICANS

Myositis ossificans should be discussed when considering the traumatic lesions other than hematomas that produce mass lesions in the adolescent patient. This entity is an infrequently encountered soft tissue lesion that is often referred to as callus formation in the soft tissues. It is most common in the second and third decades of life in young athletes. Myositis ossificans is caused by trauma to soft tissue.

The most common sites of myositis ossificans are the areas with the most muscle mass, which undergo the most stress, and include the soft tissues of the extremities, gluteus muscles, and occasionally areas within the pelvis that represent a continuation of muscles of the lower extremities. Early pain usually helps differentiate these relatively small masses from malignant tumors, which usually do not produce pain until they reach a much larger size or erode into structures such as bone or impinge on nerves. An early biopsy of myositis ossificans in the absence of a history of prior trauma might lead most pathologists to suspect a malignant tumor, since early myositis contains immature proliferating mesenchyme. As the myositis ossificans lesion progresses and calcification takes place, it becomes more characteristic of a traumatic lesion.

If one strongly suspects myositis ossificans because of

the clinical history, it is prudent to observe the lesion for a period of 2 to 3 weeks until a typical pattern of calcification is seen on either plain radiography or CT scan.

NEUROFIBROMA

Of the developmental lesions encountered in adolescents, the neurofibroma is perhaps the most frequent. Neurofibromas are neoplastic growths that can occur as solitary lesions in the adolescent and always arise from peripheral nerve structures. Although once called benign schwannomas, histogenesis from the Schwann cell has never been established.

Neurofibromas occur in multiple sites in patients with von Recklinghausen disease. It is not practical to excise all the neurofibromas in such patients because these lesions are multiple and usually more occur as the patient grows older. It is important, however, to recognize that approximately 10% to 20% of patients with von Recklinghausen disease will at some point in their life experience malignant degeneration of one of these tumors to a low-grade or intermediate-grade neurofibrosarcoma. For this reason, any patient with multiple neurofibromas in whom there is rapid growth of any single lesion should be a candidate for a biopsy. Likewise, any solitary lump that appears to be a neurofibroma must be biopsied because a benign neurofibroma cannot be ascertained without a biopsy (see subchapter on brain tumors).

BENIGN FIBROMATOSIS

Of all of the benign neoplastic processes seen in adolescent patients, fibromatosis is perhaps the most serious. This lesion represents fibroblastic proliferation and may be referred to as a desmoid tumor, although the clinical entity of fibromatosis is well recognized. It has a tendency to occur in the distal extremities and trunk.

The fibromatosis typically grows in an infiltrating manner and has a tendency to recur if not adequately excised. This can be a crippling disease when it occurs in hand or foot, and after multiple recurrences it can progress locally so that amputation may even be required for ablation. The differential diagnosis of benign fibrosarcoma must always include low-grade fibrosarcoma. The difference between the two tumors consists of only subtle cytologic parameters. After multiple recurrences over 10 to 20 years, low-grade fibrosarcomas can evolve into high-grade fibrosarcomas capable of metastasizing. Because of the tendency of both these lesions to recur locally, and eventually be very destructive in the area of involvement, they are treated by wide surgical excision. Rarely, in locations such as the hand or foot, amputation may be indicated for their control.

Malignant Soft Tissue Neoplasms

RHABDOMYOSARCOMA

Although more common in the pediatric age group, rhabdomyosarcomas present special problems when they occur in the adolescent because they usually have a worse prognosis in this age group. The majority of rhabdomyosarcomas encountered in pediatric patients is of the pure embryonal histologic type, which is exquisitely sensitive to chemotherapy and radiation therapy. Rhabdomyosarcomas that occur in the adolescent frequently have alveolar or pleomorphic histologic characteristics, which when encountered in any age group carry a poorer prognosis. Thus, some rhabdomyosarcomas of adolescence behave more like the resistant sarcomas encountered in the adult population. In addition, many rhabdomyosarcomas occurring in the adolescent population are in an extremity which classically has a worse prognosis (40% to 50% cure rate as compared with 70% to 80% cure rate for the other rhabdomyosarcomas of childhood). A lower cure rate is also seen with pelvic lesions occurring in the adolescent. These lesions usually occur in males and are of paratesticular and prostatic origin. The reason for the apparent poor prognosis in the adolescent is the frequent involvement of regional lymph nodes in both extremities in pelvic tumors. Thus, there is about a 30% incidence of regional node involvement in rhabdomyosarcomas of the extremities and approximately a 50% incidence of involvement of paraaortic nodes in patients with paratesticular, prostate, and perineal primary tumors.

Rhabdomyosarcomas are malignant tumors of striated muscle origin. Next to the tumors of the central nervous system, they represent the most common malignant solid soft tissue tumor in children and adolescents. They can occur in any area in which striated muscle is found, but in adolescents they tend to occur predominantly in the lower and upper extremities, as well as in the paratesticular apparatus. The presenting symptom of this tumor is always a soft tissue mass that is usually painless. Although apparently slow growing early, after a lump has persisted for several weeks or perhaps months it can appear to undergo a rapid growth with discoloration of the skin, resembling a hematoma. The presence of a smaller mass for several weeks prior to this evolution helps differentiate it from a hematoma. Caution at this early stage must be exercised in order not to misinterpret a needle biopsy specimen as a hematoma. However, if diagnostic of a malignant tumor, a needle biopsy may save the patient the morbidity of a surgical procedure. Early surgical excision of these tumors almost always leads to late local recurrences. In addition, the extensive postoperative irradiation required after early nonradical surgery usually leads to late functional complications and, in the case of pelvic lesions, to compromising the amount of chemotherapy that can be delivered postoperatively.

For the preceding reasons, small incisional biopsies (if needle biopsies are not diagnostic) are preferred. Definitive local surgery is delayed until after preoperative therapy. This principle holds true for all soft tissue sarcomas.

After the diagnosis of rhabdomyosarcoma has been established, regional nodes should be dissected. If no disease is present, nothing else need be done for regional treatment. However, if nodes are found to be involved, subsequent radiation should be applied to the regional node-bearing areas proximal to the primary tumor following the completion of chemotherapy. The latter treatment does have significant morbidity in terms of late complications, including the possibility of sterility and rare late radiation complications such as second malignancies. In patients with paratesticular and retroperitoneal primary tumors, approximately half will require late radiation therapy to the paraaortic nodes.

Following surgical biopsy and nodal staging, a CT scan of the lungs should be performed to rule out pulmonary metastases, as should a bone scan to rule out bone metastases, and any other appropriate regional imaging studies to evaluate the primary tumor should be carried out prior to starting preoperative chemotherapy. Figure 53–13 illustrates the current management that we have found extremely effective for the treatment of soft tissue sarcomas in adolescents and adults. Wide local excision of the primary tumor following its shrinkage with chemotherapy and preoperative radiation therapy leads to complete local control in more than 95% of patients (Fig. 53–14).

Rhabdomyosarcomas that occur in the head and neck area (e.g., maxillary sinus) in adolescents behave more like the pure embryonal variety encountered in younger children. Local control can be achieved with radiation therapy alone. Indeed, surgical excision is contraindicated in this area, since it frequently leads to rapid and unusual head and neck nodal recurrences.

Follow-up studies on patients who have completed treatment include periodic chest radiographs, bone scans, and imaging studies, such as CT scans or MRI, of the local area.

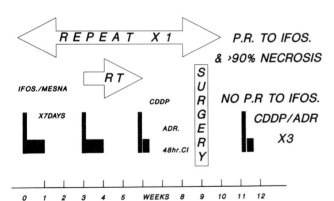

Figure 53–13. The treatment protocol used by the authors for the treatment of spindle cell or adult-type soft tissue sarcomas. High-dose ifosfamide (IFOS.) combined with the uroprotective agent mesna is extremely active in the more resistant adult-type sarcomas. Also active is the combination of cisplatin with a mannitol-induced diuresis combined with doxorubicin (ADR). Preoperative chemotherapy and preoperative radiation therapy (RT) usually lead to dramatic shrinkage of the tumor, which then enables the surgeon to perform *en bloc* surgical resection rather than a radical amputation. Postoperatively, the same chemotherapy the patients had preoperatively is continued if they demonstrate a good response. If they do not, they are given cisplatin combined with doxorubicin without the ifosfamide for adjuvant chemotherapy. This regimen has produced significant tumor regression in more than 75% of patients so treated. We have found that a total of only 6 months of this type of aggressive chemotherapy is more than adequate to cure the majority of the patients who are going to be cured with malignant soft tissue sarcomas. P.R., partial remission.

SYNOVIAL SARCOMA

Synovial sarcoma is a rare soft tissue sarcoma that is encountered in adolescents. The term *synovial sarcoma* is a poor one in that less than 5% of synovial sarcomas actually arise in joint tissues. Indeed this tumor usually arises from soft tissues deep within the muscles, and it is most common in the thigh, leg, and gluteal region. Because the tumor has a high propensity to metastasize as well as to recur locally, its management is similar to that of rhabdomyosarcomas. As in rhabdomyosarcoma in adolescents, the synovial sarcoma can metastasize to regional lymph nodes; however, this occurs at a frequency of only 15%. Therefore regional lymph node dissection before treatment is carried out only if there is suspicion of an enlarged regional node, such as a large inguinal node in a patient with a primary tumor of the lower extremity.

MALIGNANT FIBROUS HISTIOCYTOMA

Malignant fibrous histiocytoma is perhaps the most common soft tissue sarcoma diagnosed in the adult population. It is rare in the pediatric age group; however, it is encountered in older adolescent patients. It is a malignant spindle cell tumor that produces collagen or fibrous tissue. It is similar to a high-grade fibrosarcoma of soft tissue. These tumors can occur in any site of the body; however, they tend to occur in the extremities, as do synovial sarcomas and rhabdomyosarcomas. Their presentation and differential diagnosis are similar to those of rhabdomyosarcoma. The clinical behavior of malignant fibrous histiocytoma and high-grade fibrosarcomas differs from that of rhabdomyosarcoma in that regional lymph nodes are hardly ever involved. Therefore, the treatment and management of malignant fibrous histiocytoma or high-grade fibrosarcoma of soft tissue origin is again similar to that for rhabdomyosarcoma, with the exception that regional lymph node exploration is not performed unless clinically indicated. Following an incisional biopsy and establishment of the diagnosis, patients are treated with preoperative chemotherapy and radiation therapy as shown in Figure 53–13, followed by wide surgical excision and postoperative chemotherapy.

EPITHELIOID SARCOMA

Epithelioid sarcoma is a rare, highly malignant soft tissue sarcoma that occurs predominantly in young adults. The majority of patients with this rare tumor present in their late teens or early 20s, though the tumor has been noted to occur in younger patients. The most frequent primary site is the upper extremity, followed by the lower extremity. The clinical manifestations of this tumor are usually quite similar to those of a small pimple or boil. The tumor usually arises in the subcutaneous tissue and has a benign appearance. However, because of persistence of the lesion, or discoloration from hemorrhage within the tumor, biopsy is frequently performed and the diagnosis made. Because of their relatively small size, surgeons tend to perform local excisions of these tumors. They will always recur follow-

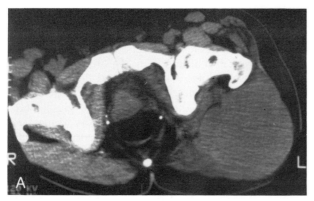
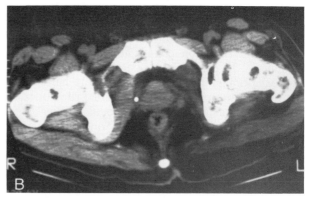

Figure 53–14. A large, malignant, fibrous histiocytoma arising in the gluteus maximus muscle. Note the dramatic complete response to the preoperative chemotherapy as presented in Figure 53–13. Following preoperative therapy, this patient successfully underwent *en bloc* resection of the residual gluteal muscle mass. Histologic analysis of the resected specimen revealed no viable tumor remaining after preoperative therapy, which is an extremely good prognostic sign.

ing local excision with subcutaneous spread, producing satellite lesions. Classically, because of its recognized high malignant potential, treatment for this tumor has been radical amputation. Even with radical amputation, patients are seldom cured. Like the rhabdomyosarcoma, this tumor is unique among adult-type soft tissue sarcomata in that there is a very high propensity for regional node metastases to be present at the time of diagnosis. Approximately 50% of patients presenting with small epithelioid sarcomas have regional node involvement. Regional node dissection must be carried out for this tumor. In upper extremity lesions, which are the most common type, this includes an axillary node dissection. Patients should be treated with preoperative therapy for soft tissue sarcomas as outlined in Figure 53–13. Surgery for these patients might include amputation rather than an attempted wide local excision of the soft tissues.

Even with the aggressive therapies previously outlined, the prognosis for patients with epithelioid sarcoma is still extremely grim, with less than 50% of patients surviving.

NASOPHARYNGEAL CARCINOMA

Nasopharyngeal carcinoma is a common malignancy of older adults, but it does occur as a variant in adolescent patients. Nasopharyngeal carcinoma of adolescence is not always histologically identical to that seen in older adults. Although adolescents with nasopharyngeal carcinomas frequently have an elevated Epstein-Barr virus (EBV) titer, there has been no conclusive proof that EBV plays any role in the etiology of this disease.

The classic manifestation of this tumor, which arises in the nasopharynx, is usually nasal stuffiness, which is persistent and progressive. As the disease progresses, the nose may appear swollen, and in its late stages proptosis may be present. A CT scan will define an abnormal mass in the nasopharynx, which may erode through and involve the maxillary sinus. Biopsy of this area will usually reveal a small cell undifferentiated malignant lesion. The differential diagnosis may be a rhabdomyosarcoma or a lymphoma.

Nasopharyngeal carcinoma in adolescents differs from that in adults in that surgery is rarely needed in the adolescent. The tumor is exquisitely sensitive to radiation therapy, and more than 50% of patients are cured with radiation therapy alone. The course of this disease is to recur first in regional nodes. This tumor is highly sensitive to chemotherapy, particularly with high-dose alkylating agents, and treatment is similar to that for Ewing sarcoma (see Table 53–12). Combination chemotherapy and regional radiation therapy are highly curative. Many of the treatment failures with this tumor have been in patients who have had surgical resection of the nasopharyngeal tumor and part of the maxillary sinus prior to being referred for medical management. Again, as in all solid tumors of soft tissue, initial radical surgery is to be avoided. In this tumor, surgery usually can be avoided entirely, whereas in other tumors, surgery is performed following preoperative therapy. As in rhabdomycosarcomas in this area, the initial use of surgery in this tumor has led to soft tissue and subcutaneous lymphatic metastases in the area of the head and neck, particularly the face, and to multiple recurrences of tumor following the cessation of treatment. If properly managed, the majority of patients with this rare tumor can be cured without the use of aggressive surgery. Late recurrences can include the mediastinal nodes as well as bone metastases, and follow-up studies should consist of chest radiographs and bone scans performed at periodic intervals in patients who have successfully completed therapy.

BIBLIOGRAPHY

Case DR, Enzinger FM: Epithelioid sarcoma: Diagnosis, prognostic indicators and treatment. Am J Surg Pathol 9:241, 1985.

Chawla SP, Rosen G, Lowenbraun S, et al: Role of high-dose ifosphamide (HDI) in recurrent osteosarcoma. Proceedings of American Society of Clinical Oncology, Vol 9, March 1990, p 310 (Abstract No. 1201).

Eilber F, Giuliano A, Eckardt J, et al: Adjuvant chemotherapy for osteosarcoma: A randomized prospective trial. J Clin Oncol 5:21, 1987.

Ewing J: Diffuse endothelioma of bone. Proc NY Pathol Soc 24:93, 1924.

Friend SH, Horowitz JM, Gerber MR, et al: Deletions of a DNA sequence and its encoded protein. Published erratum appears in Proc Natl Acad Sci USA 85(7):2234, 1988; Proc Natl Acad Sci USA 84(24):9059, 1987; unique identifier: 88097427.

Heyn R, Hays D, Lawrence W, et al: Extremity alveolar rhabdomyosarcoma and lymph node spread: A preliminary report from the
Intergroup Rhabdomyosarcoma Study (IRS) II (Abstract). Proceedings of the Annual Meeting of the American Society of Clinical
Oncology, 1984, pp 3 and 80.

Jaffe HL, Lichtenstein L: Non-osteogenic fibroma of bone. Am J
Pathol 18:205, 1942.

Jurgens H, Exner U, Gadner H, et al: Multidisciplinary treatment of
primary Ewing's sarcoma of bone: A 6-year experience of a European cooperative trial. Cancer 61(1):23, 1988.

Link MP, Goorin AM, Miser AW, et al: The effect of adjuvant
chemotherapy on relapse-free survival in patients with osteosarcoma
of the extremity. N Engl J Med 314(25):1600, 1986.

Mirra JM, Gold RH, Picci P, et al: Bone Tumors: Clinical, Radiologic,
and Pathologic Correlations. Philadelphia, Lea & Febiger, 1989.

Rosen G: The current management of malignant bone tumours: Where
do we go from here? Med J Aust 148(8):373, 1988.

Rosen G, Nirenberg A: Neoadjuvant chemotherapy for osteogenic
sarcoma: A five year follow-up (T-10) and preliminary report of
new studies (T-12). In Wagener T, et al (eds): Primary Chemotherapy in Cancer Medicine. New York, Alan R. Liss, 1985, pp 39–51.

Rosen G, Caparros B, Huvos AG, et al: Preoperative chemotherapy
for osteogenic sarcoma: Selection of postoperative adjuvant chemotherapy based on the response of the primary tumor to preoperative chemotherapy. Cancer 49:1221, 1982.

Treuner J, Koscielniak E, Keim M: Comparison of the rates of
response to ifosfamide and cyclophosphamide in primary unresect-
able rhabdomyosarcomas. Cancer Chemother Pharmacol 24(Suppl
1):S48, 1989.

Unni KK, Dahlin DC, Beabout JW: Periosteal osteosarcoma. Cancer
37:2476, 1976.

LYMPHOMAS

WARREN A. McGUIRE

The lymphomas comprise a variable group of proliferative diseases that arise in the lymph nodes or extranodal lymphatic tissues. Lymphoma is the third most
common solid tumor in children and adolescents in the
United States and represents about 10% of childhood
malignant disease in North America. Each year in the
United States there are 13.2 cases per one million
children, divided approximately equally between children with Hodgkin disease and those with non-Hodgkin
lymphoma. The incidence is similar in white and black
children.

In all the lymphomas there is a replacement of normal
lymphoid structure by abnormal cells. The presence of
Reed-Sternberg cells in the appropriate histologic background is diagnostic of Hodgkin disease, whereas in
non-Hodgkin lymphoma there are diffuse or follicular
(nodular) collections of cells that closely resemble normal B or T lymphoid cells at different stages of development. Rarely, these latter tumors may be derived
from histiocytes of the monocyte-phagocyte system.
Because of important differences in the clinical approach
to patients with Hodgkin and those with non-Hodgkin
lymphoma, these two entities are discussed separately.

HODGKIN DISEASE

Hodgkin disease is a malignant lymphoma of unknown
etiology characterized by abnormal giant binucleated
cells (Reed-Sternberg cells) in association with a significantly distorted lymphoid architecture and a heterogeneous cellular infiltrate representing a nonmalignant
reaction to the tumor cells. Although lacking a homogeneous cell population with invasive characteristics,
Hodgkin disease is still considered a malignant process
because the giant cells demonstrate aneuploid karyotypes and produce tumors when transplanted into nude
mice. If left untreated, Hodgkin disease spreads

throughout the lymphatic system and eventually metas-
tasizes to nonlymphoid tissue.

Epidemiology

The incidence of Hodgkin disease has a bimodal age
peak not seen for most other lymphomas. In industrialized countries, including the United States, the early
peak occurs in the middle to late twenties, and the
second peak occurs in late adulthood. One third of
childhood cases present in 5- to 10-year-olds; 60% occur
in the 10- to 15-year-old age group. Its incidence is
greater among males throughout the pediatric age
group. Male predominance is most marked in the first
decade, when the incidence in boys is four times greater
than that in girls; beyond the ages of 10 to 12 the sex
ratio approaches the 55% to 60% male dominance that
is seen in adults.

Etiology

Although the etiology of Hodgkin disease remains
unknown, the search for possible infectious, environmental, or genetic causes has been extensive. Many of
the clinical features of Hodgkin disease suggest an
infectious etiology. Fevers, night sweats, and weight
loss, along with a leukocytosis and an inflammatory
infiltrate in the involved tissues, all may be seen in
patients with Hodgkin disease, as well as in those with
a variety of infectious illnesses. Although many infectious agents, including bacteria, parasites, fungi, and
viruses, have been proposed as the etiologic agent of
Hodgkin disease, none has been conclusively implicated.
Currently, Epstein-Barr virus (EBV) is the most intensively studied. Several large studies have consistently
demonstrated that a prior history of serologically confirmed infectious mononucleosis confers about a three-

fold increased risk of Hodgkin disease. Initial attempts to identify the EBV genome in Hodgkin disease cells were unsuccessful. More recently, however, sensitive molecular biology techniques have demonstrated EBV DNA in 8 of 28 Hodgkin disease samples, and *in situ* hybridization has localized EBV genome to the Reed-Sternberg cells. Whether EBV plays a role in the malignant transformation of the Reed-Sternberg cell or is merely a manifestation of an altered immune system in patients susceptible to Hodgkin disease requires further study.

Initial reports of clusters of Hodgkin disease patients within schools have now been disputed, and more recent studies have demonstrated that exposure to a Hodgkin disease patient at school confers no increased risk of the disease. However, there have been many case reports of the multiple occurrence of Hodgkin disease within the same family. Estimates of increased risk have ranged from threefold for first-degree relatives to sevenfold for siblings of young adult cases.

Pathology

Hodgkin disease is unique among the lymphomas because only a small percentage of cells from the affected tissue are malignant. The vast majority of cells are normal reactive cells, such as lymphocytes, plasma cells, and eosinophils. Reed-Sternberg cells, the malignant cells in Hodgkin disease, may constitute less than 1% of the total cell population. The accurate diagnosis of Hodgkin disease by an experienced pathologist is essential to the proper treatment of the disease. Selection of the proper lymph node for biopsy (i.e., large rather than small; deep rather than superficial; and axillary, cervical, or supraclavicular rather than inguinal) improves the diagnostic success. Proper handling of the specimen, including touch imprints of the fresh lymph node on microscopic slides combined with prompt fixation and thin sectioning (3μ), helps the pathologist to interpret the pathologic material. A review of the slides by an experienced hematopathologist is often desirable because Hodgkin disease is a rare disorder with many subtle variations. When such review is routinely carried out, the diagnosis of Hodgkin disease is confirmed in 85% to 90% of cases. Cases misdiagnosed as Hodgkin disease are most often found to be non-Hodgkin lymphoma or, occasionally, benign adenopathy.

The universally accepted pathologic classification system for Hodgkin disease is the Rye classification, which represents a simplification of the Lukes-Butler classification. This classification includes four groups: lymphocytic predominance, mixed cellularity, nodular sclerosis, and lymphocytic depletion. The histologic subtypes, except nodular sclerosis, represent expression of the inverse relationship that exists between the frequency of lymphocytes and Reed-Sternberg cells. The lymphocytic predominant form of Hodgkin disease is characterized mainly by a proliferation of mature-appearing lymphocytes associated with varying numbers of reactive histiocytes, occasional eosinophils, and rare Reed-Sternberg cells and with essentially no fibrosis. The mixed cellularity type exhibits an intermediate picture of his-

tiocytes, mature neutrophils, eosinophils, plasma cells, and lymphocytes in varying proportions, often with rather numerous and prominent Reed-Sternberg cells. Nodular sclerosis Hodgkin disease is recognized by orderly, dense, collagenous bands of connective tissue that subdivide abnormal lymphoid tissue into cellular nodules. Typical Reed-Sternberg cells are difficult to find, but a larger, variant form of the Reed-Sternberg cell, the lacunar cell, is more frequent. The lacunar cell is so named because imperfect fixation commonly leads to shrinkage of the voluminous, pale-staining cytoplasm, leaving a clear halo around the cell, which then appears as if suspended in an empty lacuna. The lymphocytic depletion form of Hodgkin disease is characterized by a diffuse, disorderly fibrosis and necrosis and a paucity of lymphocytes. Reed-Sternberg cells are usually numerous.

Nodular sclerosis Hodgkin disease is the most common subtype in children, representing approximately 46% of pediatric Hodgkin disease. It is generally a disease of young females, usually localized at diagnosis, and presenting most frequently in the neck and the mediastinum. Mixed cellularity represents approximately 30% of pediatric Hodgkin disease. The lymphocytic predominant form accounts for approximately 16% and frequently presents as localized cervical adenopathy in young males. Lymphocytic depletion is the least common subtype (approximately 6%).

Abnormal mononuclear, binuclear, or multinuclear giant cells found in tissues involved by Hodgkin disease are thought to represent the malignant element of these tumors. The Reed-Sternberg cell, a large cell with a bilobed or multilobed nucleus, prominent nucleoli, and abundant acidophilic cytoplasm, is required to make a diagnosis of Hodgkin disease. However, this cell is not unique to Hodgkin disease, as cells of similar appearance have been reported in infectious mononucleosis, "pseudolymphomatous" adenopathy associated with chronic phenytoin (Dilantin) administration, rubeola, thymoma, and non-Hodgkin lymphoma. The presence of Reed-Sternberg cells is therefore necessary but not sufficient for the diagnosis of Hodgkin disease. In order to make this diagnosis, Reed-Sternberg cells must be accompanied by an appropriate stromal reaction. A mononuclear variant of the Reed-Sternberg cell, called a Hodgkin cell, is also seen in reactive and inflammatory lymphadenopathies and is not sufficient for establishing the diagnosis of Hodgkin disease. However, their presence should encourage a further search for Reed-Sternberg cells.

Before the era of modern therapy, the histopathologic subtype of Hodgkin disease represented an important prognostic variable, with lymphocytic predominant disease having the best prognosis, lymphocytic depletion disease having the poorest, and nodular sclerosis and mixed cellularity types having an intermediate prognosis. However, with current therapy, the prognostic significance of the histopathologic subtype has largely evaporated.

Identification of the cellular origin of Hodgkin and Reed-Sternberg cells has eluded intense investigation and continues to be controversial. Candidates for its precursor have included the B lymphocyte, the T lymphocyte, and the histiocyte (monocyte/macrophage). A new cell type, the interdigitating reticulum cell (IDC), has also been proposed as a candidate for the precursor of the Reed-Sternberg cell. The IDC, which is distributed in thymic-dependent regions of human lymphoid tissues, is thought to be in the macrophage lineage and may function primarily as an antigen-presenting cell to the T lymphocyte. Recently, sensitive immunohistochemical and gene rearrangement studies have suggested that Hodgkin disease is heterogeneous in regard to its cellular origin and that the malignant cells may be of B cell, or T cell, or monocytic derivation. Based on their immunohistochemical studies, Stein and co-workers have proposed that Hodgkin and Reed-Sternberg cells are lymphocytic in origin and that the cell of origin may vary depending on the histologic classification. They have proposed that lymphocytic predominant Hodgkin disease arises from the B lymphocyte system, whereas nodular sclerosing and mixed cellularity Hodgkin disease may be heterogeneous, with their cell of origin being either the B lymphocyte or the T lymphocyte.

Clinical Presentation

Hodgkin disease presents in children and adolescents as a progressive, painless lymph node enlargement. The lymphadenopathy is firm but not hard. The order of frequency of involvement of superficial lymph node groups is cervical (60% to 80%), axillary (6% to 20%), and inguinal (6% to 12%). Splenomegaly is present in slightly fewer than half the patients at the time of diagnosis, and the liver is palpable in one third or more. Evidence of a mediastinal mass or widening of the mediastinum on chest radiograph is found in 20% to 50% of children at diagnosis, and these findings may produce symptoms of cough, dyspnea, or dysphagia or the superior vena cava syndrome. Systemic ("B") symptoms such as fever, malaise, weight loss, and night sweats may be present in as many as 30% of patients at diagnosis and are more commonly seen in advanced stages of the disease. Prognostic significance is attached to the classic B symptoms of unexplained fevers exceeding 38.0°C (101.4°F), unexplained weight loss in excess of 10% of body weight during the preceding 6 months, and drenching night sweats. The fever and weight loss that occur in Hodgkin disease have been attributed to acute phase changes that are produced by interleukin-1. The fever of Hodgkin disease may be intermittent, erratic, recurrent, or sustained. The classic Pel-Ebstein cyclic fever, with intermittent evening temperature elevations alternating with afebrile periods lasting days or weeks, is very rarely seen. Drenching night sweats may occur with or without fever, but the mechanism producing these in the absence of fever is unknown. Pruritus is seen in approximately 15% of adults (particularly in young women with mediastinal nodular sclerosis Hodgkin disease). Although recent evidence again suggests that the presence of pruritus may be of prognostic significance, it is not currently included as one of the B symptoms.

Staging

Once the diagnosis of Hodgkin disease is made, staging is done to determine the location and extent of disease. Accurate staging allows for the rational determination of treatment for individual patients, as well as providing prognostic information. There is strong evidence that Hodgkin disease generally spreads from one adjacent nodal area to another at least until very late in the disease. The Ann Arbor Staging Classification (Table 53–13), adopted at a workshop in Ann Arbor, Michigan, in 1971, is based on this assumption. The elements of the clinical staging of Hodgkin disease are listed in Table 53–14.

The careful questioning of patients regarding systemic symptoms is essential, as their presence or absence plays an important role in prognosis and selecting therapy. Although recent data suggest that night sweats may not be a significant B symptom with contemporary treatment programs or that certain combinations of B symptoms (i.e., fever and weight loss) may be especially important, the presence of any of the three classic B symptoms remains an important factor in defining current treatment.

Baseline laboratory values are helpful in directing further staging investigations. Blood count abnormalities should be evaluated by further hematologic studies and bone marrow examination. However, routine bone marrow aspirate examination and biopsy have an extremely low yield in early-stage patients without B symptoms.

TABLE 53–13. Ann Arbor Staging System for Hodgkin Disease

STAGE*	SUBGROUP	FEATURES
Stage I A or B	I	Involvement of a single lymph node region
		or
	I_E	Single extralymphatic organ or site
Stage II A or B	II	Involvement of two or more lymph node regions on the same side of the diaphragm
		or
	II_E	Localized contiguous involvement of an extralymphatic organ or site
Stage III A or B	III	Involvement of lymph node regions on both sides of the diaphragm
		or
	III_E	Localized contiguous involvement of an extralymphatic organ or site
		or
	III_S	Involvement of the spleen
		or
	III_{ES}	Both extralymphatic organ or site and spleen involvement
Stage IV A or B		Diffuse or disseminated involvement of one or more extralymphatic organs with or without associated lymph node involvement

*A, asymptomatic; B, presence of systemic symptoms (unexplained fever above 38°C, drenching night sweats, unexplained weight loss exceeding 10% of baseline body weight).

TABLE 53–14. Clinical Staging of Hodgkin Disease in Children*

History (including details of fever, weight loss, and night sweats)

Physical examination

Laboratory evaluation
    Complete blood count, platelet count, erythrocyte sedimentation rate, liver and renal function tests (including alkaline phosphatase), serum copper, ceruloplasmin, thyroid function tests (free thyroxine [T_4] and thyroid-stimulating hormone [TSH])

Radiologic studies
    Chest radiograph
    Computed tomography scan of chest, abdomen, and pelvis

Bone marrow aspirate and biopsy

Occasionally useful ancillary studies
    Bilateral lower extremity lymphangiogram
    Bone scan, liver-spleen, and bone marrow scintiscans
    Whole-body ^{67}gallium scanning

*Recommended for all patients.

Liver function abnormalities should prompt further imaging studies and possibly biopsy. An alkaline phosphatase level elevated above that expected for the adolescent's age might be an indicator of bony involvement and should be evaluated by appropriate skeletal radiographs and radionuclide bone scan. Erythrocyte sedimentation rate may provide prognostic information and along with serum copper and ceruloplasmin levels may provide a nonspecific marker of disease activity. In women, however, the utility of the serum copper level is compromised by its elevation in the presence of exogenous estrogens (e.g., with oral contraceptive therapy).

Chest radiograph and chest computed tomography (CT) scan are performed on all patients. Chest CT contributes important information for radiation treatment planning, as well as additional information on pulmonary parenchymal, chest wall, or pericardial involvement. Abdominal CT and liver-spleen scan are less sensitive than surgical staging in defining disease in the liver or spleen. However, these studies may be of use in the patient not undergoing surgical staging. Lymphangiography is more sensitive in defining disease in the retroperitoneal lymph nodes than is CT scan, whereas the celiac axis–porta–hepatis area is better imaged by CT scan. Magnetic resonance imaging (MRI) is currently being evaluated in Hodgkin disease and has potential advantages in detecting chest wall, splenic, and bone marrow involvement. Radioisotope gallium scanning may be especially helpful in evaluating patients for recurrent disease, particularly when other imaging studies demonstrate nonspecific residual soft tissue mass in which the differential diagnosis is fibrosis versus active tumor.

Surgical staging for Hodgkin disease consists of exploratory laparotomy, with attention to both nodal and possible extranodal sites of disease, biopsy of both lobes of the liver, splenectomy, selected abdominal lymph node biopsies, and oophoropexy in selected cases. Ancillary surgical procedures such as appendectomy or cholecystectomy may add morbidity to the operation and are therefore not recommended routinely. Oopho-ropexy, placing the ovaries in the midline posterior to the lower uterine body, is recommended in premenopausal women if there is a possibility that pelvic radiotherapy may be required.

In the past, when radiotherapy was the only curative treatment for Hodgkin disease, staging laparotomy with splenectomy was recommended for all patients. This provided precise information for guiding radiotherapy and gave accurate information for the evaluation of treatment results according to the stage of the patient. However, with the introduction of effective chemotherapy and with better understanding of the potential long-term risks of staging laparotomy, this procedure is no longer routinely recommended. Current indications for surgical staging depend upon treatment options. If therapy will not be altered by pathologic staging, then laparotomy is not justified.

Surgical staging results in a change in clinical stage in at least one third of patients, most frequently with a finding of occult splenic disease. If radiotherapy as the sole treatment modality is contemplated, then careful staging clearly is required. However, if chemotherapy alone or combined with radiation therapy to areas of bulk disease is recommended, then precise staging may not be required. Thus, careful assessment of the potential risks and benefits of surgical staging must be made for each individual patient based on the details of their clinical staging and the therapeutic plan.

Treatment and Results

Hodgkin disease is a curable malignancy and may be successfully treated with radiation therapy, chemotherapy, or combined modality therapy. The choice of therapy must be individualized, taking into consideration the adolescent's age, stage of disease, symptomatology, histopathology, tumor burden, and late effects of therapy. The weighing of each of these factors is a complicated process, and the best results of therapy have been achieved by centers employing a multidisciplinary team of oncologists, diagnostic and therapeutic radiologists, pathologists, and surgeons.

Hodgkin disease is exquisitely sensitive to radiation therapy. Important factors in determining the success of radiation therapy include the radiation dose, the extent of the fields employed, the beams' energy, and the precision of treatment planning. Appropriate radiotherapy involves treatment with megavoltage radiation, ideally using a 4- to 8-MeV linear accelerator. When radiotherapy is the sole modality of therapy, a tumoricidal dose of 3600 to 4400 cGy is required to eradicate Hodgkin disease. Lymphoid regions adjacent to areas of known disease or those that are contiguous via lymphatic channels are treated to full dose. Large fields are designed to treat multiple contiguous lymph node regions. Treatment fields commonly used in Hodgkin disease are listed in Table 53–15.

Combination chemotherapy is also highly effective in Hodgkin disease. The introduction of the MOPP regimen (Mustargen [nitrogen mustard], Oncovin [vincristine], procarbazine, and prednisone) by DeVita and co-workers at the National Cancer Institute was a major

TABLE 53–15. Radiotherapy Fields in Hodgkin Disease

FIELD	DESCRIPTION
Mantle	Cervical, supraclavicular, infraclavicular, axillary, mediastinal, and hilar lymph nodes
Paraaortic	Paraaortic lymph nodes from the level of the diaphragm to the aortic bifurcation, and the splenic hilar lymph nodes in a patient with prior splenectomy
Inverted Y	Paraaortic and splenic hilar lymph nodes, plus the iliac and inguinal-femoral lymph nodes
Subtotal lymphoid irradiation	Combination of mantle and paraaortic fields
Total lymphoid irradiation	Combination of mantle and inverted Y fields

breakthrough in the treatment of Hodgkin disease, producing complete remission in 70% to 80% of patients with advanced stage IIIB and IV Hodgkin disease and long-term cure in more than 50% of patients. Attempts have been made to improve these results or decrease long-term side effects by modifying the MOPP combination or by developing new combination chemotherapy regimens, but to date no combination has been proved conclusively superior to MOPP. Bonadonna introduced ABVD (Adriamycin, bleomycin, vinblastine, and dacarbazine), an alternative regimen that does not demonstrate cross resistance with MOPP. ABVD has been shown to be equivalent in efficacy when compared with MOPP in newly diagnosed patients with advanced Hodgkin disease and is capable of producing a 75% complete response rate in patients who have not responded to MOPP therapy. Although the risk of infertility is less in patients receiving ABVD than in those receiving MOPP, the risk of pulmonary and cardiac toxicities (from bleomycin and Adriamycin, respectively) is greater.

The MOPP/ABV hybrid regimen was developed by Klimo and Connors in Vancouver in order to reflect the Goldie-Coldman hypothesis. This mathematical hypothesis of cellular somatic mutation predicts that the efficacy of treatment of a malignancy is enhanced by the earliest possible introduction and the most rapid alternation of all active agents in a therapeutic program. With the Vancouver hybrid regimen, patients are exposed to seven different chemotherapeutic agents within the first 8 days of treatment (Table 53–16). Preliminary results suggest that this regimen may be at least as effective as MOPP or ABVD therapy alone and less toxic. In comparison with MOPP, the MOPP/ABV hybrid uses one half the total dose of nitrogen mustard and procarbazine, potentially decreasing the risk of leukemogenesis and sterility. Similarly, in comparison with ABVD, the hybrid regimen delivers one half the total dose of bleomycin and 70% of the dose of Adriamycin, thereby potentially decreasing the risk of pulmonary and cardiac toxicity.

Although radiotherapy was the initial cornerstone of therapy for Hodgkin disease, its use in high doses is hampered in children and adolescents who are still growing. The toxic effects of radiotherapy on growth in these patients have led many institutions to recommend combined modality therapy, in which the dose of radiation may be decreased when used in conjunction with effective chemotherapy. This approach was successfully employed by Donaldson and Link at Stanford in the treatment of patients with a chronologic or bone age of 14 years or younger. Patients received six cycles of MOPP plus modified involved field radiotherapy of 1500, 2000, or 2500 cGy, depending on whether the bone age was 5 years or younger, 6 to 10 years, or 11 to 14 years. In the initial 55 children treated, this approach gave a projected survival at 15 years of 89% and a 90% freedom from relapse. Moreover, growth abnormalities were absent, with the standing heights of all patients within 1 to 1½ standard deviations of the mean for their age.

Which patient, then, should receive radiation therapy alone, which one should receive chemotherapy alone, and which one is best treated with combined modality therapy? The answers to this question are still evolving, but certain generalities may be stated. Radiotherapy alone may be optimal treatment for the adolescent or young adult who is fully grown and developed and who has early-stage, favorable disease as determined by thorough clinical and pathologic staging. Such therapy involves high-dose extended-field radiation. The rare patient with stage IA lymphocytic predominant Hodgkin disease arising in a favorable location such as the high right neck or inguinal-femoral region may be a candidate for high-dose involved-field radiotherapy.

Chemotherapy alone has been utilized in children as well as in adults with advanced stage III or IV disease. Follow-up has not been long in these series, but patients with nodular sclerosis subtype or with large mediastinal masses (maximal transverse mediastinal diameter greater than one third of the maximal intrathoracic diameter) are at increased risk for relapse in sites of previous bulky disease when chemotherapy alone has been used. This was also noted in the initial report of the MOPP/ABV hybrid regimen, with 4 of 14 patients who presented with large mediastinal masses failing to obtain a complete remission, and a fifth patient relapsing in the mediastinum after initially obtaining a complete remission.

The majority of children and adolescents with Hodg-

TABLE 53–16. MOPP/ABV Hybrid Regimen for Hodgkin Disease

DRUG	DAY
Nitrogen mustard	1
Vincristine	1
Procarbazine	1–7, inclusive
Prednisone	1–14, inclusive
Adriamycin	8
Bleomycin	8
Vinblastine	8

Rest period: from day 14 to day 28, inclusive.
Cycles repeated every 4 weeks.
Treatment is administered up to a maximum of 8 cycles.
After 6 treatment cycles, and in the presence of persistent disease in one nodal site, administer radiotherapy to the involved site.

kin disease are candidates for combined modality therapy. Most institutions have given at least six cycles of chemotherapy for advanced disease, but currently studies are under way investigating three or four monthly cycles of chemotherapy when combined with radiotherapy in early-stage Hodgkin disease. MOPP chemotherapy has proved effective in terms of disease control, but alternative regimens are being sought for children to try to decrease the incidence of sterility and leukemogenesis that has been associated with MOPP. Other regimens, such as ABVD, may prove to be equally effective and to be associated with less risk of sterility and leukemia. However, the follow-up on patients treated with ABVD is much shorter than on those treated with MOPP, and the ultimate incidence and severity of cardiopulmonary injuries with ABVD are not yet known. The MOPP/ABV hybrid may prove to be both effective and less toxic than MOPP or ABVD alone. In combined modality therapy, it appears that the dose of radiation can be decreased without compromising disease-free survival. In the original Stanford study of combined modality therapy, there was a 97% local control rate with low-dose radiation and six cycles of MOPP, and no difference in local control whether 1500, 2000, or 2500 cGy was administered. Whereas radiation doses in the initial study were based on the patient's age, subsequent studies at Stanford are evaluating a dose of 1500 cGy to areas of original disease for all patients, with a boost to 2500 cGy to sites of initial bulky disease or sites that failed to regress after two cycles of chemotherapy.

Results of modern multidisciplinary treatment of Hodgkin disease indicate that 90% of children who are carefully staged and treated are curable. Even patients with advanced stage III or IV disease have shown a 66% to 100% 5-year survival in different series. However, many questions remain to be answered. The optimal chemotherapy combination with maximal effectiveness and minimal side effects is as yet unknown. The optimal number of cycles of chemotherapy is unknown. It is generally felt that lower stage disease can be treated with fewer cycles of chemotherapy, particularly when combined with low-dose radiotherapy. Investigations of three or four cycles of chemotherapy with or without involved-field radiotherapy are under way for low-stage Hodgkin disease. For advanced stage disease, 6 to 12 cycles of chemotherapy have generally been given, or a minimum of two cycles after obtaining complete remission. The optimal dose and volume of radiation when combined with chemotherapy are still under investigation.

Salvage Therapy

Successful treatment of Hodgkin disease is possible even after relapse, but the chances of success depend upon multiple factors. Patients treated with radiation therapy alone at initial diagnosis have the highest salvage rate when subsequently treated with chemotherapy. Relapse after a chemotherapy-induced remission is associated with a lower salvage rate but is still possible. Patients with more favorable prognoses are those who relapse more than 12 months after achieving complete remission. In one series, 14 of 15 patients whose relapse occurred more than 1 year after MOPP therapy obtained a complete remission when retreated with MOPP, compared with only 5 of 17 patients whose initial MOPP-induced remission lasted less than 1 year. Salvage using non–cross resistant chemotherapy such as ABVD may also be successful, with remission rates between 30% and 60%, depending upon the patient characteristics.

Autologous or allogeneic bone marrow transplantation is another alternative salvage therapy for patients with relapsed Hodgkin disease. Such patients have generally had resistant disease or have relapsed after a chemotherapy-induced remission. Complete responses to the high-dose therapy have been reported in approximately half the patients treated to date, although approximately 50% of the complete responders have relapsed after transplant. However, patients undergoing bone marrow transplant earlier, at a time of minimal disease, have had better results, with as much as a 63% complete response rate and a 77% projected 3-year survival.

Despite the possibility of successful treatment after relapse, this is not 100% successful, and patients should be treated optimally at the time of initial diagnosis in order to maximize the probability of a relapse-free survival.

Acute and Delayed Side Effects of Therapy: The Cost of Cure

Numerous acute and delayed side effects of therapy may occur in patients treated for Hodgkin disease. Attempts to modify or avoid these side effects are a driving force in the development of new treatment strategies for this disease. In patients treated with radiation therapy, acute side effects are relatively mild and may consist of nausea, vomiting, erythema or hyperpigmentation of the irradiated skin, and bone marrow suppression. The severity of the side effects depends upon the total dose and volume of irradiation delivered. Occasionally, patients develop a sensation of "electric shock" radiating down the back and into the extremities upon flexion of the neck (Lhermitte syndrome). This is a self-limited, reversible condition thought to be related to transient demyelination of nerve fibers in the spinal cord.

Acute side effects of chemotherapy include nausea and vomiting, which may be severe with either MOPP or ABVD. These may be severe enough in the adolescent to result in anticipatory vomiting or refusal to continue therapy. Anticipatory vomiting may begin before the adolescent even reaches the clinic and may be ameliorated by diazepam given prior to leaving home or while en route to the clinic. Use of the hybrid MOPP/ABV regimen, with elimination of the emetic dacarbazine (DTIC), is much better tolerated. Hair loss is another major concern for adolescents, with its implications for their body image. Hair begins to fall out within a few weeks of beginning chemotherapy and regrows after the intensity of chemotherapy decreases or treatment is terminated. Ice caps and scalp tourniquets have been used to limit local circulation while the drug is administered, but these may be only partially successful. Wigs are recommended for cosmetic purposes. Pain may occur during peripheral intravenous infusion of certain chemotherapy agents, such as dacarbazine. This may be minimized by further dilution of the drug or by slow intermittent injection into a continuous intravenous infusion. Vesicant medications, such as vincristine and doxorubicin, may cause pain and tissue necrosis if they extravasate into tissues. In such cases, inflammation and ulceration may progress over several weeks, and surgical debridement may be required. Bone marrow suppression, with resultant anemia, thrombocytopenia, and neutropenia, may increase the patient's risk of hemorrhage and infection and, depending upon the severity, may need to be treated with red blood cell or platelet transfusions.

Hodgkin disease patients are particularly susceptible to infections, as a result of both the underlying immunologic deficit inherent in the disease process and the further immune suppression inherent in splenectomy, radiation therapy, and chemotherapy. Because of the T-cell deficiency inherent in the disease process, Hodgkin disease patients are particularly susceptible to a wide variety of infections with nonbacterial agents of low pathogenicity, including *Pneumocystis carinii, Cryptococcus, Toxoplasma, Aspergillus, Candida, Listeria,* and *Nocardia.* They are also at increased risk for developing herpes zoster. However, more than 75% of serious infections in patients with Hodgkin disease are caused by common bacterial pathogens and are related more to the effects of therapeutic maneuvers (splenectomy and chemotherapy) than to a fundamental immune defect. The risk of bacterial infection is increased 10-fold in patients treated with chemotherapy as compared with those treated with radiation alone. The risk of fulminant sepsis and death in splenectomized Hodgkin disease patients, primarily due to *Streptococcus pneumoniae, Haemophilus influenzae,* or *Neisseria meningitidis,* may be significantly decreased by the administration of polyvalent pneumococcal and *Haemophilus influenzae* vaccines prior to splenectomy and the long-term use of prophylactic penicillin or ampicillin therapy. All fevers higher than 38°C (101°F) should be evaluated immediately, and the patient should be placed on vigorous antibiotic therapy.

As cure rates for patients with Hodgkin disease continue to rise, long-term complications of therapy assume a greater role in treatment planning and patient follow-up. The major difference in the evolution of treatment policies between adults and children with Hodgkin disease is due to the late effects of radiation and chemotherapy. Because the toxicity of these therapeutic modalities is greater on growing structures, and because the period of time at risk is longer, potential late effects are particularly important in the treatment of children and adolescents with Hodgkin disease. Impaired skeletal growth in the irradiated field is regularly seen in children receiving 3500 cGy or more. Truncal shortening and decreased sitting height are particularly severe in children irradiated prior to the age of 5 years but may occur in children younger than the age of 14 years. Shortening of the clavicles with a decrase in intraclavicular distance is also seen in children given high-dose irradiation to a mantle field at a young age. Lower doses of irradiation, as are given in combined modality therapy, are less likely to cause significant bone growth disturbance. Growth disturbance is not a significant complication for patients whose bone age is 14 to 15 years or older at the time of therapy. Girls whose breast buds are irradiated in the prepubertal period may subsequently develop hypoplasia of the breasts.

Pulmonary injury, including radiation pneumonitis and paramediastinal fibrosis, may occur secondary to radiation therapy, depending on the total dose, daily fraction size, and volume of lung included in the high-dose irradiated area. The risk of pulmonary injury is greater in patients receiving combined therapy with bleomycin-containing regimens if high-dose radiation is also given. The use of lower dose radiation regimens with multiagent chemotherapy may decrease this risk.

Cardiac injury is also dependent upon radiation dose, volume, and fraction size and may involve either the myocardium or the pericardium. Severe restrictive pericarditis requiring pericardiectomy may occur. There has been an approximately 13% incidence of cardiac injury among children given high-dose mantle irradiation. Adriamycin is known to cause dose-dependent myocardial damage, and the effect on myocardial toxicity of combining this agent with radiation therapy to the mediastinum is an area of much concern and investigation.

Thyroid dysfunction may occur in a high percentage of children who receive neck irradiation. Again, the dose of irradiation is important, with an incidence of thyroid abnormalities as low as 17% in children receiving less than 2600 cGy and as high as 78% in children receiving 2600 cGy or more. Hypothyroidism is the most common abnormality, but thyroid nodules, hyperthyroidism, and thyroid cancer all have been reported in patients treated for Hodgkin disease. Thyroid-stimulating hormone (TSH) and free thyroxine (T_4) levels should be monitored yearly in patients who have received irradiation to the neck, and sustained elevations in TSH levels should be treated with thyroid replacement therapy to reduce stimulation from prolonged TSH elevation.

Gonadal dysfunction is a known complication of both radiation therapy and chemotherapy, particularly in regimens containing nitrogen mustard and procarbazine. Sterility, decreased fertility, and potential gonadal injury following staging and treatment are important issues that must be addressed at the time of diagnosis and prior to therapy. In males, azoospermia, loss of libido, and abnormalities in gonadotropic hormones may occur. In females, delayed menarche, early menopause, and infertility can result. The younger the woman at the time of therapy, the higher the probability of maintenance of regular menses following therapy. For those treated with pelvic irradiation, the technique of oophoropexy, with placement of the ovaries to the midline position, may preserve ovarian function. Combined modality therapy may further impair reproductive potential, but normal pregnancies have occurred even in this group of patients. Hybrid regimens, which increase the number of chemotherapeutic agents while decreasing the total exposure to such agents as nitrogen mustard and procarbazine, may decrease the effects on fertility. However, despite continued normal menses after therapy, it appears that a high percentage of women who have received combined modality therapy in the past have experienced early menopause. Continued menstruation after the age of 35 has been unusual in this group, and it may therefore be unwise for them to delay having their families past this age.

Sterility in males treated with chemotherapy has been an even greater problem. The use of six courses of MOPP therapy has been associated with universal azoospermia, regardless of the age at the time of therapy. Fertility may be maintained in 50% of men if exposure to MOPP is limited to three courses. In general, the hormone-producing cells of the testis are more resistant to the effects of treatment than are the spermatogonia, and the patients generally continue to grow and develop normally. In adult males given ABVD, transient azoospermia or oligospermia may occur in 50% to 60% of patients, but recovery of spermatogenesis has been documented within 18 months of completion of therapy in a high percentage. Sperm storage before chemotherapy is initiated should be considered for the older adolescent and adult male patients; however, it must be understood that 30% to 40% of patients may have primary gonadal dysfunction at the time of diagnosis of Hodgkin disease, and sperm obtained during the acute illness and prior to the initiation of therapy may be of poor quality.

Pregnancy outcomes in girls treated for Hodgkin disease have shown no increase in risk of birth defects. Girls who received abdominal and pelvic irradiation may have an increased risk of premature delivery and small for gestational age babies. It is critical that sexually active adolescents who have been treated for Hodgkin disease understand that they may be normally fertile. The need for birth control counseling may be even greater in this population, as these adolescents may demonstrate a fatalism about infertility and consider their previous therapy as a rationalization for not employing contraceptive measures.

Second malignant neoplasms in children surviving their initial cancer are well recognized. The incidence of second malignant neoplasms in survivors of childhood Hodgkin disease is exceeded only by the incidence in survivors of retinoblastoma. The type and incidence of second malignant neoplasms appear to be related to the intensity of therapy for Hodgkin disease. Those treated with radiation alone have an incidence of less than 1%, increasing to 5% to 7% in those treated with MOPP alone and to 10% when MOPP is combined with radiation therapy. This risk increases with the number of courses of MOPP given. Secondary solid malignancies such as thyroid, bone, or soft tissue sarcomas are seen in patients who were treated with radiation therapy alone, whereas secondary acute nonlymphocytic leukemia and non-Hodgkin lymphomas are seen in patients treated with MOPP alone or in combination with radiation therapy. A 15% incidence of secondary leukemia has been reported when radiation has been given initially and chemotherapy is used as salvage therapy. Second malignant neoplasms have been reported 20 and 30 years after treatment for Hodgkin disease, but the period of greatest risk appears to be the first 10 years following therapy. Thus far, ABVD has not been associated with an increased risk of second malignancies, but because of the possible long latent period, this question is still under study.

As more children and adolescents are cured of Hodgkin disease and other primary malignancies, it becomes encumbent upon the pediatrician and the internist to be aware of the late effects of therapy and to screen patients carefully. As specific anticancer therapy is discontinued and the risk of cancer recurrence diminishes with time, children with cancer are evaluated at less frequent intervals in the oncology center. The patient with symptoms is thus more likely to be evaluated by the primary care provider, particularly if the new problem is not perceived by the patient or family to be related to cancer or its treatment.

The goal of treatment of every child and adolescent with Hodgkin disease is to achieve cure of the disease with a minimum of side effects. Staging and therapeutic decisions must be made with a careful balance of their risks and benefits. Today an adolescent with Hodgkin disease has an approximately 90% likelihood of cure following staging and treatment in a center with expertise in pediatric Hodgkin disease. Such gratifying results require individualization of therapy and the exercise of careful judgment in evaluating the implications of patient age, staging extent of disease, tumor burden, therapeutic options, and the late effects of therapy. Hodgkin disease has become the model of the curable cancer, and further study will be directed toward refining its evaluation and treatment in order to decrease morbidity while maintaining therapeutic success.

BIBLIOGRAPHY

Anagnostopoulos I, Herbst H, Niedobitek G, Stein H: Demonstration of monoclonal EBV genomes in Hodgkin's disease and Ki-1-positive anaplastic large cell lymphoma by combined Southern blot and in-situ hybridization. Blood 74:810, 1989.

Armitage JO: Bone marrow transplantation in the treatment of patients with lymphoma. Blood 73:1749, 1989.

Bonadonna G, Zucali R, Monfardini S, et al: Combination chemotherapy of Hodgkin's disease with Adriamycin, bleomycin, vinblastine and imidazole carboxamide versus MOPP. Cancer 36:252, 1975.

DeVita VT, Jr, Serpick A: Combination chemotherapy in the treatment of advanced Hodgkin's disease (abstr). Proc Am Assoc Cancer Res 8:13, 1967.

Donaldson SS, Link MP: Combined modality treatment with low-dose radiation and MOPP chemotherapy for children with Hodgkin's disease. J Clin Oncol 5:742, 1987.

Feller AC, Griesser H: DNA gene rearrangement studies in Hodgkin's disease and related lymphomas: A contribution to their cellular origin. Recent Results Cancer Res 117:27, 1989.

Green DM, Zevon MA, Lowrie G, et al: Congenital anomalies in children of patients who received chemotherapy for cancer in childhood and adolescence. N Engl J Med 325:141, 1991.

Grufferman SL, Delzell E: Epidemiology of Hodgkin's disease. Epidemiol Rev 6:76, 1984.

Klimo P, Connors JM: MOPP/ABV hybrid program: Combination chemotherapy based on early introduction of seven effective drugs for advanced Hodgkin's disease. J Clin Oncol 3:1174, 1985.

Lukes RJ, Butler JJ: The pathology and nomenclature of Hodgkin's disease. Cancer Res 26:1063, 1966.

Lukes RJ, Butler JJ, Hicks EB: Natural history of Hodgkin's disease as related to its pathologic picture. Cancer 19:317, 1966.

Murphy SB: The lymphomas and lymphadenopathy. In Nathan DG,

Oski FA (eds): Hematology of Infancy and Childhood. Philadelphia, WB Saunders, 1987, pp 1086–1117.

Rappaport H, Strum SB, Hutchison G, et al: Clinical and biological significance of vascular invasion in Hodgkin's disease. Cancer Res 31:1794, 1971.

Staal SP, Ambinder R, Beschorner WE, et al: A survey of Epstein-Barr virus DNA in lymphoid tissues. Frequent detection in Hodgkin's disease. Am J Clin Pathol 91:1, 1989.

Stein H, Schwarting R, Dallenbach F, Dienemann D: Immunology of Hodgkin and Reed-Sternberg cells. Recent Results Cancer Res 117:14, 1989.

Weiss LM, Movahed LA, Warnke RA, Sklar J: Detection of Epstein-Barr viral genomes in Reed-Sternberg cells of Hodgkin's disease. N Engl J Med 320:502, 1989.

NON-HODGKIN LYMPHOMAS

NANCY J. BUNIN

Non-Hodgkin lymphomas (NHL) constitute 10% of pediatric and adolescent malignancies. Lymphomas are the third most common solid tumor of childhood and adolescence and approximately 50% to 60% are NHL. Recent advances in therapy have had a major impact upon the survival rate of children and adolescents with NHL. Cure is now possible for more than two thirds of children and adolescents with NHL and for a larger percentage of patients with limited disease. The current emphasis is on minimizing potential long-term side effects, while maintaining or improving the efficacy of current therapy.

EPIDEMIOLOGY AND PATHOPHYSIOLOGY

The incidence of NHL increases with age, and children older than 10 years of age account for approximately one half of pediatric patients with NHL. However, the peak frequency of NHL is between 7 and 11 years of age. In younger patients, three times as many boys are affected, whereas this predominance is marginal among children older than 10 years of age. The natural history and clinical and histologic features of NHL in adolescence differ substantially from those seen in adults with the disease. These differences may be reflective of differences in immunocompetence. Lymphoid tissue increases rapidly during childhood and exceeds adult size through pubescence, when regression begins. The presentation of NHL in adolescents is generally extranodal, whereas adult NHL generally presents as bulky nodal disease. The histologic features of NHL in adolescents are also much more limited than those seen in adults.

The frequency of NHL differs markedly among countries. For example, in Africa more than 50% of pediatric cancers are lymphomas, generally of the B-cell type. The role of the Epstein-Barr virus (EBV) is unclear in the etiology of these endemic lymphomas; EBV deoxyribonucleic acid (DNA) has been found in almost 95% of these cancers. However, EBV DNA is found in only 15% of the sporadic B-cell lymphomas occurring in Europe and North America.

The risk of NHL is substantially increased in adolescent patients with natural and acquired immunodeficiencies. Adolescent patients with genetically determined immunodeficiencies, such as the Wiskott-Aldrich syndrome, ataxia-telangiectasia, X-linked lymphoproliferative syndrome, and severe combined immunodeficiency, are at increased risk for the development of a lymphoma. Patients who have undergone immunosuppression to prevent organ rejection after solid organ or bone marrow transplantation are also at risk for the development of EBV-associated lymphomas. B-cell lymphomas may also develop in patients with human immunodeficiency virus (HIV) infection. Lymphomas that occur in these populations are generally extremely aggressive and respond to therapy poorly.

CLASSIFICATION

The histologic distribution of NHL in adolescents is different from that in adults. The follicular pattern, observed in almost 50% of adult patients, is almost never found in children and adolescents. NHL in children is virtually always diffuse, and almost all cases can be classified as high grade according to the Working Formulation (Table 53–17). The two most common types of lymphomas are small noncleaved cell lymphomas (SNCL), including Burkitt and non-Burkitt types, and lymphoblastic lymphomas. Each of these composes approximately 40% of the total. Large cell lymphomas are less common, composing 15% to 20% of the total number. True histiocytic lymphomas are extremely rare. The distinction between leukemia and lymphoma can be difficult, but in general, if there are more than 25% blasts present in the bone marrow, the adolescent is

TABLE 53–17. Histologic Classification and Distribution of NHL in Children

HISTOLOGIC FEATURES	IMMUNO-PHENOTYPE	FREQUENCY (%)
SNCL	B	40–50
Burkitt		
Non-Burkitt (undifferentiated)		
Lymphoblastic	T	30–40
Large cell	B or T	15–20

considered to have leukemia. Defining histologic characteristics is extremely important, as adolescent patients with a specific histologic appearance respond better to certain therapeutic regimens.

Immunophenotyping and cytogenetic studies have contributed to our understanding of NHL. Using a panel of monoclonal antibodies, the lymphomas may be designated as either T or B lymphocyte in origin. Almost all lymphoblastic lymphomas are of T-cell origin, with the majority in the mid- to late-thymocyte stage. This is in contrast to T-cell acute lymphoblastic leukemia, which is also common in adolescent males. The majority of these leukemias are in the early- to mid-thymocyte stage. The SNCL are of B-cell origin and express surface immunoglobulin of either heavy chain or κ- or λ-light chain. The majority of large cell lymphomas are B cell in origin, with a smaller number classifiable as being in the late-thymocyte stage and of T-cell origin. The recently described Ki-1 lymphomas appear to be a subset of the large cell type and may be confused with Hodgkin disease because of binucleate tumor cells that resemble Reed-Sternberg cells.

Cytogenetic studies have failed to demonstrate a consistent pattern of translocations in lymphoblastic lymphomas. However, translocations that involve sites of the α– or β–T-cell receptor gene are common and include rearrangements that involve 14q11, 7q34-36, or 7p15. The majority of cases of SNCL have t(8;14), with other translocations, such as t(8;22) and t(2;8), being less common. All of these translocations involve the c-myc oncogene located on chromosome 8, as well as juxtaposition of this gene with sequences from one of the immunoglobulin loci. A specific translocation, t(2;5)(p23;q35), has been associated with the Ki-1 lymphomas, but no oncogene has been associated with this breakpoint as yet.

CLINICAL PRESENTATIONS

Clinical manifestations of NHL in adolescents differ from those in adults. Primary nodal involvement is uncommon at diagnosis. A single primary site may not be apparent when these lymphomas present at an advanced stage. Dissemination may occur from peripheral lymph nodes, thymus, Peyer patches, and Waldeyer ring. NHL in adolescents has a propensity for noncontiguous spread, particularly to the central nervous system (CNS) and bone marrow. In general, clinical features may be related to the extremely rapid growth rate of these high-grade lymphomas.

Small Noncleaved Cell Lymphoma

The most common sites of involvement of SNCL are the distal ileum and cecum. Involvement of the stomach or colon is not seen, in contrast to the disease in adults. Adolescents may present with abdominal pain with a rapidly enlarging mass or symptoms of intestinal obstruction. Intussusception may occur and requires emergency surgical reduction. The disease may be localized within the intestinal wall and be completely resectable, or it

may be diffuse, with massive tumor formation in the mesentery and small bowel. Ascites is common with advanced disease. SNCL may also present as a paraspinal mass, with risk of paraplegia. Bone marrow involvement occurs in up to 20% of patients. CNS involvement may be manifested by cranial nerve involvement, intracerebral disease, or meningeal infiltration.

In the endemic form of SNCL, the abdominal presentation is still the most common, but jaw tumors are more frequently seen in this form of SNCL than in the sporadic form. Jaw tumors are less common in African patients older than 14 years of age, in whom small bowel is the most frequent site of involvement. Bone marrow involvement is less common in the endemic form of SNCL.

Lymphoblastic Lymphoma

The most frequent presentation of lymphoblastic lymphoma is enlarged nodes above the diaphragm with an anterior mediastinal mass. This type of lymphoma should be suspected in an adolescent who presents with rapidly enlarging, painless cervical and supraclavicular lymphadenopathy, wheezing, and respiratory distress. Pleural effusions are common, and pericardial effusion may also occur. Superior vena cava syndrome may be found in association with a large anterior mediastinal mass and is manifested by a swollen, congested face and right arm and enlarged jugular veins, accompanied by tracheal compression and respiratory distress.

Large Cell Lymphoma

There is no consistent presentation of large cell lymphoma. The mediastinum is one of the more commonly involved sites, but unlike in lymphoblastic lymphoma, the clinical presentation and natural history are more typical of Hodgkin disease. Large cell lymphoma grows more slowly than does lymphoblastic lymphoma; patients may have symptoms for many months before seeking medical attention. When adolescent girls present with mediastinal masses, the presence of large cell lymphoma should be considered, in contrast to this presentation in males, who are more likely to have lymphoblastic disease. Bone marrow and CNS involvement are uncommon in patients with large cell lymphoma at the time of diagnosis. Less common sites of presentation include bone and the Waldeyer ring.

DIAGNOSTIC EVALUATION

Lymphomas in adolescents often grow rapidly and require prompt diagnosis and therapy. The diagnosis can often be established by a less invasive method than major surgery. Because these patients may present with respiratory distress or diffuse abdominal disease, extensive diagnostic evaluations and delay may be dangerous. Suggested laboratory and radiographic evaluations are shown in Table 53–18. Laparotomy is recommended only if there is evidence of limited abdominal disease and a complete surgical resection is possible. This may be the case in the adolescent patient who presents with an intussusception. Invasive abdominal surgery or mediastinoscopy is rarely necessary to establish the diag-

**TABLE 53–18. Diagnostic and Staging Studies
for Childhood NHL**

Complete blood count with differential and platelet counts
Serum electrolytes, uric acid, calcium, phosphorus, blood urea
  nitrogen, creatinine, liver function studies (ALT, AST), bilirubin,
  LDH determinations
Urinalysis
Bone marrow aspirate and biopsy
Cerebrospinal fluid cell count, cytologic studies, protein and glucose
  determinations
Chest radiograph and computed tomography (mediastinal
  involvement)
Abdominal ultrasound or computed tomography
Bone scan
Gallium scan (optional)

ALT, alanine aminotransferase; AST, aspartate aminotransferase; LDH,
lactate dehydrogenase.

nosis. Extensive surgery should be avoided in adolescents in whom it is not curative, since therapy may be delayed and morbidity exacerbated by subsequent chemotherapy.

A bone marrow aspirate and biopsy may establish the diagnosis if the bone marrow is involved at presentation. Ascitic fluid in an adolescent with diffuse abdominal disease, or pleural fluid in an adolescent with lymphoblastic lymphoma, usually demonstrates cells in fluid sent for cytologic examination, immunophenotyping, and cytogenetic studies. Biopsy of an enlarged lymph node may be performed under local or general anesthesia if the diagnosis cannot be established with pleural or ascitic fluid or bone marrow. A pediatric anesthesiologist should be readily available when a procedure is attempted on a patient with respiratory compromise.

There are several staging systems used for pediatric and adolescent NHL (Table 53–19). The Ann Arbor staging system, which is commonly used for adult Hodgkin lymphoma and NHL, has little utility in the classification of NHL in children and adolescents. Staging systems used must take into account tumor burden and the propensity for leukemic conversion and CNS involvement. The systems most commonly used in the United States (the one developed at St. Jude Children's Research Hospital [SJCRH] and the one in use in the Children's Cancer Study Group [CCSG]) divide patients into two major groups based upon extent of disease. Adolescent patients with localized disease compose approximately 30% of the total. Adolescents with mediastinal or abdominal disease are considered not to have localized disease because of the propensity for extranodal spread.

THERAPY: GENERAL PRINCIPLES

Combination chemotherapy, improvements in the supportive care required for its use, and the recognition of the need for CNS prophylaxis have greatly improved the outcome of adolescents with NHL. Surgery plays a very limited role and is generally limited to biopsy, unless a complete resection is possible or relief of intestinal obstruction is required.

Prior to the advent of combination chemotherapy,

radiation therapy was the primary therapeutic modality. However, its importance has lessened with the development of intensive combination chemotherapy protocols. Radiation therapy in large volume may limit administration of chemotherapy, and anthracycline cardiotoxicity may be exacerbated when radiation is delivered to the mediastinum. As randomized trials have failed to show an advantage when radiation is added to chemotherapy for NHL, its use is generally reserved for emergency purposes only.

Definitive histologic diagnosis is necessary when treating an adolescent patient with NHL. This was demonstrated in a CCSG study in which therapy was randomized between a 4- or 10-drug regimen for patients with disseminated lymphoma. The 10-drug regimen was more successful in patients with lymphoblastic histologic features, with 76% of patients remaining disease free, compared with only 26% of patients treated with the 4-drug regimen. In contrast, patients with nonlymphoblastic histologic features fared much better with the 4-drug regimen than with the 10-drug regimen.

CNS prophylaxis is important for adolescent patients with advanced disease, as both lymphoblastic lymphoma and SNCL have a propensity to spread to that area. CNS prophylaxis may be accomplished in several ways. Various therapeutic regimens have incorporated CNS irradiation, intrathecal medication, or the delivery of high-dose chemotherapy that attains therapeutic concentrations in the CNS. CNS irradiation is generally reserved for adolescents with CNS disease. Most protocols incorporate a combination of intrathecal medications and high-dose systemic therapy. When adequate CNS therapy is given, CNS relapse is uncommon.

The initiation of therapy in adolescent patients with advanced-stage lymphoblastic lymphoma or SNCL often presents major management difficulties. This is reflective of the extremely rapid growth rates of these lymphomas. Patients with mediastinal lymphoblastic lymphoma may have significant respiratory distress. Immediate symptomatic relief may be accomplished with low-dose radiation—for example, two to three fractions of 200 cGy each. A cervical or supraclavicular lymph node may be shielded during irradiation so that a diagnosis may be made by biopsy when the adolescent is more stable. Lymphoblastic lymphoma is extremely responsive to corticosteroids, and prednisone alone may also result in rapid relief of mediastinal compression. However, this may obscure the histologic diagnosis. If possible, a biopsy specimen or pleural fluid should be obtained prior to the initiation of steroid therapy. Thoracentesis may relieve symptoms related to massive pleural effusions and generally yields sufficient material for diagnosis and special studies. However, the pleural fluid rapidly reaccumulates if definitive therapy is not instituted promptly.

Patients with lymphoblastic lymphoma and those with SNCL are at risk for acute tumor lysis syndrome because of rapid cell turnover. The problem may be present from the outset in patients with SNCL and may be complicated by mechanical obstruction of ureters with tumor masses or renal infiltration by tumor. It is essential that therapy be initiated rapidly in these patients and meticulous attention paid to fluid balance and serum

TABLE 53–19. Staging Systems for Childhood NHL

STAGING SYSTEM	STAGE	DEFINITION
St. Jude Children's Research Hospital	I	Single tumor (extranodal) Single anatomic area (nodal) Excluding mediastinum or abdomen
	II	Single tumor (extranodal) with regional nodal involvement Primary abdominal tumor with or without associated nodes, grossly completely resected Same side of diaphragm: (1) two or more nodal areas, (2) two single tumors with or without nodal involvement
	III	All primary intrathoracic tumors, extensive primary abdominal disease, paraspinal tumors Both sides of diaphragm: (1) two single tumors, (2) two or more nodal areas
	IV	Any of the above with initial CNS or bone marrow involvement
Children's Cancer Study Group	Localized	Single extranodal site, with or without positive regional nodes Limited to nodal sites within one or two adjacent lymphatic regions Abdominal site: gross complete resection
	Nonlocalized	Mediastinal and abdominal sites excluding preceding All other sites and regions

chemistries. Prior to initiation of therapy, intravenous fluid with bicarbonate, to raise the urine pH to 6.5 or more, should be started at approximately 3 to 4 L/m²/day. More fluid may be required to maintain adequate urine output. Uric acid is more soluble in alkaline urine, but alkalinization to a pH greater than 7 may result in precipitation of calcium-phosphate crystals. Allopurinol at fairly high doses should be given prior to initiation of therapy and continued until the tumor lysis has subsided. Diuretics, such as mannitol or furosemide, may be necessary to maintain urine output; in general, the urine output should be at least 80% of the preceding hour's fluid input. A Foley catheter is often necessary to accurately judge fluid balance. During tumor lysis, it is common for potassium levels to rise as intracellular components of the blasts are released. Emergency medications to deal with hyperkalemia should be readily available, and electrocardiographic monitoring may be necessary. The first sign of tumor lysis may be a rise in the phosphate level; this leads to a subsequent decrease in the calcium level. In this circumstance, a phosphate binder may be necessary and may be given through a nasogastric tube. Calcium may be given if the patient becomes symptomatic from hypocalcemia, but it does not need to be given on the basis of laboratory values alone. Hemodialysis may be necessary in the event of mechanical obstruction by tumor, anuria, or metabolic derangements refractory to medical management. Meticulous medical management can prevent permanent renal damage, including death.

THERAPY AND OUTCOME
Localized Disease

Short-term chemotherapy appears to be adequate for patients with localized lymphoma. Shortening of the duration of therapy may minimize some of the potential long-term side effects, such as gonadal dysfunction and cardiotoxicity from anthracyclines. The CCSG has demonstrated that a four-drug regimen—COMP, which contains cyclophosphamide, vincristine, methotrexate, and prednisone—is as effective when administered for 6 months as when given for 18 months. The other major pediatric cancer group in the United States, the Pediatric Oncology Group (POG), used three cycles of CHOP (cyclophosphamide, doxorubicin, vincristine, and prednisone) with oral 6-mercaptopurine and methotrexate as maintenance for 6 months. Radiation therapy was offered in a randomized trial and did not confer any advantages. The elimination of radiation therapy for adolescents with localized lymphomas alleviates potential long-term morbidity as well. The outlook for patients with localized lymphomas with either of these regimens is excellent, with greater than 90% disease-free survival.

Advanced-Stage Small Noncleaved Cell Lymphoma

SNCL responds to a variety of agents, and most current regimens incorporate cyclophosphamide, vincristine, methotrexate in high doses, an anthracycline, and cytosine arabinoside (Table 53–20). The outlook for patients with SNCL has improved dramatically with combination therapy, and aggressive measures for CNS prophylaxis are required. However, certain features are considered to confer a poorer prognosis and mandate extremely intensive therapy. These features include a serum lactate dehydrogenase (LDH) level greater than 1000 U/L, the presence of bone marrow or CNS disease, or widespread abdominal disease (which usually correlates with an elevated level of LDH). The outlook for

TABLE 53–20. Therapy and Results for Disseminated Nonlymphoblastic Lymphoma

GROUP*	THERAPY	DRUGS†	THERAPY DURATION	OVERALL EFS‡	EFS STAGE IV	REFERENCE
CCSG	COMP	CPM, VCR, MTX (IV + IT), PDN	18 months	57%	NS	Anderson et al. (1983)
SJCRH	Total B	CPM, VCR, doxorubicin, MTX (1 g/m²), Ara-C, IT MTX	6 months	60%	20%	Murphy et al. (1986)
SFOP	LMB-0281	CPM, doxorubicin, VCR, PDN, Ara-C, CCNU, 6-TG, MTX (3 g/m²), L-Asp, IT MTX, Ara-C	12 months	64%	19% CNS + 48% BM	Patte et al. (1986)
DFCI	HiCCOM	CPM, VCR, MTX (3 g/m²), Ara-C	2 months	75%	50%	Schwenn et al. (1991)

*CCSG, Children's Cancer Study Group; SJCRH, St. Jude Children's Research Hospital; SFOP, French Pediatric Oncology Society; DFCI, Dana Farber Cancer Institute.

†CPM, cyclophosphamide; VCR, vincristine; MTX, methotrexate; IV, intravenous; IT, intrathecal; PDN, prednisone; Ara-C, cytosine arabinoside; CCNU, lomustine; 6-TG, 6-thioguanine; L-Asp, L-asparaginase.

‡EFS, event-free survival; NS, not stated; CNS, central nervous system; BM, bone marrow.

this group of adolescents has also improved, but those with CNS involvement remain a particularly difficult group to cure. The use of high-dose infusional methotrexate and cytosine arabinoside, combined with frequent intrathecal administration of chemotherapy, may improve the outlook for these adolescent patients. Adolescents without CNS disease now may enjoy up to 80% disease-free survival. Adolescents with CNS disease fare less well, but recent reports demonstrate an improvement over the less than 20% disease-free survival reported previously.

It is apparent that therapy of relatively short duration is all that is required for these adolescent patients. Most relapses occur within 6 to 9 months. These adolescents are now treated on protocols ranging from 2 to 9 months without compromising cure.

Bone marrow transplantation, either autologous or allogeneic, has been used in some instances to intensify therapy for patients with poor prognostic features. However, this is not standard practice, and its use for patients in a first remission is still controversial.

Lymphoblastic Lymphoma

The first significant improvement in disease-free survival for adolescents with lymphoblastic lymphoma was with the LSA_2L_2 regimen designed in the 1970s at Memorial Sloan-Kettering. This is a complex 10-drug regimen, and it has resulted in up to 76% disease-free survival. It is somewhat difficult to administer because of its complexity, and it requires many outpatient visits. Other regimens have been designed that have also proved to be successful and somewhat less cumbersome. Some of these regimens have eliminated agents that may cause sterility (alkylating agents) or cardiotoxicity (anthracyclines), without loss of efficacy (Table 53–21). A recent CCSG study of lymphoblastic lymphoma consisted of a randomized trial of the LSA_2L_2 therapy and a novel therapy consisting of daunomycin, vincristine, cyclophosphamide, prednisone, and L-asparaginase (ADCOMP). Preliminary analysis suggests 76% disease-free survival overall. When the effect of therapy on the outcome of specific age groups is analyzed, however, it appears as if children older than 15 years of age do far less well, with approximately 45% event-free survival. This raises concern regarding the intensity of therapy that this subgroup of adolescents may require, but definitive analysis is lacking. Involved field irradiation has been eliminated without compromising cure. Relapses usually occur more often in the bone marrow or, less commonly, in the CNS than in initial sites of bulk disease.

Therapy for lymphoblastic lymphoma more closely

TABLE 53–21. Therapy and Results for Disseminated Lymphoblastic Lymphoma

GROUP*	THERAPY	DRUGS†	THERAPY DURATION	OVERALL EFS‡	REFERENCE
CCSG	LSA_2L_2	CPM, VCR, MTX, PDN, DNM, Ara-C, 6-TG, L-Asp, CCNU, HU, IT MTX	18 months	76%	Anderson et al. (1983)
SJCRH	X-H	VM-26, Ara-C, VCR, PDN, L-Asp, 6-MP, MTX, IT MTX	24 months	73%	Dahl et al. (1983)
POG	LSA_2L_2	(As above)	24 months	50%	Sullivan et al. (1985)
MSKCC	LSA_2L_2	(As above)	24 months	73%	Wollner et al. (1979)
DFCI	APO	Doxorubicin, PDN, VCR, 6-MP, MTX, IT MTX, CspXRT	24 months	58%	Weinstein et al. (1983)

*CCSG, Children's Cancer Study Group; SJCRH, St. Jude Children's Research Hospital; POG, Pediatric Oncology Group; MSKCC, Memorial Sloan-Kettering Cancer Center; DFCI, Dana Farber Cancer Institute.

†CPM, cyclophosphamide; VCR, vincristine; MTX, methotrexate; IT, intrathecal; PDN, prednisone; DNM, daunomycin; Ara-C, cytosine arabinoside; 6-TG, 6-thioguanine; HU, hydroxyurea; L-Asp, L-asparaginase; CCNU, lomustine; VM-26, teniposide; 6-MP, 6-mercaptopurine; CspXRT, craniospinal irradiation.

‡EFS, event-free survival.

resembles therapy for acute lymphoblastic leukemia than that for SNCL. Therapy is generally given for 18 to 24 months.

Large Cell Lymphoma

Adolescents with large cell lymphoma are commonly treated with protocols for SNCL, and they appear to respond well to such therapy. It is difficult to establish a study for this group of adolescent patients because of the small patient numbers and the diversity of presentations. In general, disease-free survival is approximately 75% when combination chemotherapy is used with effective agents such as cyclophosphamide, vincristine, anthracyclines, methotrexate, and prednisone. Although radiation therapy has been used for bulky disease, it does not appear to improve relapse-free survival unless active residual disease can be documented. This is a difficult issue, as many of these patients are clinically similar to those with Hodgkin disease; a residual mass may be present upon the completion of therapy but usually represents fibrosis and not active lymphoma.

Relapsed Disease

The outlook is poor for adolescents who have a relapse of disease following combination chemotherapy. Bone marrow transplantation is being used as a salvage therapy in many centers. In general, it is successful only in adolescents who have "responsive" disease, that is, those in whom chemotherapy may induce at least a partial remission. Bone marrow transplantation may be performed either with autologous marrow that may be purged of residual lymphoma or with an allogeneic matched marrow. Purging may be accomplished with monoclonal antibodies directed against T- or B-cell antigens or with *in vitro* chemotherapy. Large numbers of pediatric and adolescent patients have not been treated. Thus, the efficacy of transplantation in the management of patients with NHL who have had relapses remains to be proved.

LYMPHOMAS IN ADOLESCENCE: LONG-TERM IMPLICATIONS

The development of combination chemotherapy protocols has become increasingly refined in an attempt to minimize potential long-term effects. Radiation therapy, which can affect bones during a pubertal growth spurt, has generally been eliminated. In addition, the elimination of radiation to the mediastinum in patients with lymphoblastic lymphoma has diminished cardiotoxicity. The duration of therapy has become shorter, which may

result in less exposure to alkylating agents and lessen the possibility of gonadal dysfunction and sterility. Some successful therapies for lymphoblastic lymphoma have eliminated alkylating agents altogether. Although an increased risk of secondary leukemia is reported after treatment of Hodgkin disease, there is less information regarding patients treated for NHL. Shortening the duration of exposure to alkylating agents may decrease this risk.

An adolescent patient with the diagnosis of NHL has an excellent chance of achieving a cure, and advances in therapy may minimize long-term consequences.

BIBLIOGRAPHY

Anderson JR, Wilson JF, Jenkin RDT, et al: Childhood non-Hodgkin's lymphoma: The results of a randomized therapeutic trial comparing a four-drug regimen (COMP) with a ten-drug regimen (LSA₂L₂). N Engl J Med 308:550, 1983.

Cohen LF, Balow JE, Magrath IT, et al: Acute tumor lysis syndrome: A review of 37 patients with Burkitt's lymphoma. Am J Med 68:486, 1980.

Dahl GV, Rivera G, Pui C-H, et al: A novel treatment of childhood lymphoblastic non-Hodgkin's lymphoma: Early and intermittent use of teniposide plus cytarabine. Blood 66:1110, 1985.

Jenkin RDT, Anderson JR, Chilcote RR, et al: The treatment of localized non-Hodgkin's lymphoma in children: A report from the Children's Cancer Study Group. J Clin Oncol 2:88, 1984.

Link MP, Donaldson SS, Berard CW, et al: Results of treatment of childhood localized non-Hodgkin's lymphoma with combination chemotherapy with or without radiotherapy. N Engl J Med 322:1169, 1990.

Magrath IT: Burkitt's lymphoma: Clinical aspects and treatment. In Moladner DW (ed): Diseases of the Lymphatic System: Diagnosis and Therapy. New York, Springer-Verlag, 1983, p 103.

Meadows AT, Sposto R, Jenkin RDT, et al: Similar efficacy of 6 and 18 months of therapy with four drugs (COMP) for localized non-Hodgkin's lymphoma of children: A report from the Children's Cancer Study Group. J Clin Oncol 7:92, 1989.

Murphy SB, Bowman WP, Abromowitch M, et al: Results of treatment of advanced stage Burkitt's lymphoma and B-cell (sIg+) acute lymphoblastic leukemia with high-dose fractionated cyclophosphamide and coordinated high-dose methotrexate and cytarabine. J Clin Oncol 4:1732, 1986.

Murphy SB, Frizzera G, Evans AE: A study of childhood non-Hodgkin's lymphoma. Cancer 36:2121, 1975.

Patte C, Philip T, Rodary C, et al: Improved survival rate in children with stage III and IV B cell non-Hodgkin's lymphoma and leukemia using multi-agent chemotherapy: Results of a study of 114 children from the French Pediatric Oncology Society. J Clin Oncol 4:1219, 1986.

Schwenn M, Blattner S, Lynch E, Weinstein H: HiC-COM: A 2-month intensive chemotherapy regimen for children with stage III and IV Burkitt's lymphoma and B-cell acute lymphoblastic leukemia. J Clin Oncol 9:133, 1991.

Sullivan MP, Boyett J, Pullen J, et al: Pediatric Oncology Group experience with modified LSA₂L₂ therapy in 107 children with non-Hodgkin's lymphoma (Burkitt's lymphoma excluded). Cancer 55:323, 1985.

Weinstein HJ, Cassady JR, Levey R: Long-term results of the APO protocol (vincristine, doxorubicin [Adriamycin] and prednisone) for treatment of mediastinal lymphoblastic lymphoma. J Clin Oncol 1:537, 1983.

Wollner N, Exelby PR, Lieberman PH: Non-Hodgkin's lymphoma in children: A progress report on the original patients treated with the LSA₂L₂ protocol. Cancer 44:1990, 1979.

BRAIN TUMORS

JONATHAN L. FINLAY and RUSSELL WALKER

INCIDENCE

Brain tumors are the most common solid tumors occurring in childhood and adolescence. In frequency, they are second only to leukemias among *all* malignancies in patients younger than 21 years of age. There are approximately 1200 new cases of "pediatric" brain tumors in the United States each year. It is unfortunate that the best national statistics available, from the American Cancer Society, have traditionally analyzed cancer incidence according to the age groups from birth to 15 years of age and from 16 to 34 years of age, making it impossible to gain a complete picture of the relative incidence of brain tumors occurring during adolescence. Nevertheless, by looking at the differing age of onset of individual brain tumors, we are able to recognize certain tumors that are of greater or lesser prevalence during adolescence.

The most common adolescent brain tumor is the supratentorial astrocytoma. The likelihood of high-grade astrocytic tumors, rather than low-grade tumors, increases with age through adolescence into adulthood. Brainstem gliomas, which have a peak incidence in childhood, diminish in frequency through the adolescent years. The incidence of posterior fossa medulloblastoma declines throughout adolescence into adulthood, though it remains the second most common brain tumor during early adolescence. Primary central nervous system (CNS) germinomas represent fewer than 2% of primary brain tumors in childhood and adolescence; nevertheless, they have a peak incidence during adolescence, with a median age of 12 years at diagnosis. Even more rare is the malignant pineal tumor of primitive neuroectodermal origin known as the pineoblastoma; though this tumor is associated with hereditary bilateral retinoblastoma (when it is termed trilateral retinoblastoma), the median age at diagnosis of this tumor is 12 years. Finally, craniopharyngioma, representing about 7% of childhood and adolescent brain tumors, has a peak incidence of diagnosis at 8 to 12 years of age.

ETIOLOGY

The etiology of brain tumors of childhood and adolescence is not known, though both hereditary and environmental factors may play a role in some cases. Hereditary neurocutaneous syndromes (the phakomatoses) are associated with an increased incidence of brain tumors. Cerebral, hypothalamic, or optic gliomas develop in about 15% of children with neurofibromatosis. Children with tuberous sclerosis experience intracranial hamartomas and subependymal giant cell (low-grade) astrocytomas. Von Hippel–Lindau disease is seen in association with retinal angiomatosis and cerebellar hemangioblastoma. Turcot syndrome represents the recognized rare association of malignant brain tumors (medulloblastoma or high-grade astrocytoma) with familial polyposis coli and adenocarcinoma of the bowel. Gorlin syndrome represents the equally rare association of medulloblastoma with the nevoid basal cell carcinoma syndrome. Additionally, some families and identical twins have been reported with multiple cases of brain tumors, suggestive of an inherited relationship.

Environmental factors have also been implicated in the genesis of childhood and adolescent brain tumors. An increased incidence of brain tumors has been reported in the offspring of either mothers or fathers employed in the aircraft industry at or about the time of conception, as well as in the children of workers exposed to petrochemicals. However, other studies have been unable to confirm these associations. There are increasing reports of the development of brain tumors as second cancers in children who have received cranial irradiation either for previous acute lymphoblastic leukemia or for prior brain tumors. The recognized development of high-grade astrocytomas in the site of prior irradiation for a low-grade astrocytoma may reflect a radiation-induced transformation to a higher-grade tumor, but such a transformation can occur without irradiation. Further, it has been suggested that the development of brain tumors in children with acute lymphoblastic leukemia (ALL) might reflect an inherent susceptibility to the development of such tumors in children with ALL; it will be important to see if these brain tumors still arise in the cohort of patients with ALL no longer receiving "prophylactic" cranial irradiation as a routine part of their therapy. It is important to note that the majority of these second primary brain tumors have been reported to arise during adolescence.

CLASSIFICATION

Brain tumors constitute a heterogeneous group of tumors, differing not only in incidence in childhood and adolescence but also in location of origin, pattern of growth and dissemination, clinical presentation, and optimal treatment. In adolescence, as in adulthood (but in contrast to childhood), the majority of brain tumors arise in a supratentorial location. Although the classification of brain tumors remains controversial, and no system is ideal, the World Health Organization (WHO) classification is helpful in clarifying the various subtypes of brain tumor (Table 53–22). The majority of childhood and adolescent brain tumors are neuroepithelial in origin, whereas tumors of nerve sheath or meningeal origin are uncommon.

As the clinical presentation, diagnosis, and treatment differ with each specific histologic diagnosis, this discussion will emphasize the general principles of the approach to the adolescent with a brain tumor.

TABLE 53–22. Classification of Brain Tumors

TUMORS OF NEUROEPITHELIAL TISSUE
Astrocytic tumors
    Astrocytoma
    Anaplastic (malignant) astrocytoma
Oligodendroglial tumors
    Oligodendroglioma
Ependymal Tumors
    Ependymoma
    Anaplastic (malignant) ependymoma
Pineal cell tumors
    Pineocytoma
    Pineoblastoma
Neuronal tumors
    Gangliocytoma
    Ganglioglioma
Poorly differentiated and embryonal tumors
    Glioblastoma
    Medulloblastoma
    Primitive neuroectodermal tumors

TUMORS OF NERVE SHEATH CELLS
Neurinoma

TUMORS OF MENINGEAL TISSUES
Meningioma

GERM CELL TUMORS
Germinoma
Embryonal carcinoma
Choriocarcinoma
Teratoma

Modified with permission from Histological Typing of Tumours of the Central Nervous System. (International Histological Classification of Tumours, No. 21). Geneva, World Health Organization, 1979.

CLINICAL PRESENTATION

The clinical presentation of the adolescent patient suspected of having a brain tumor is determined primarily by the tumor's location. Tumors arising in the midline of the posterior fossa or cerebellum classically present with symptoms of increased intracranial pressure and hydrocephalus resulting from obstruction of the fourth ventricle. Headache is usually bifrontal or diffuse, typically occurring in the morning upon arising. Occasionally, it is abrupt in onset, short-lived, and precipitated by a change in position or by exercise. This type of headache is thought to be due to sudden increases in intracranial pressure, called plateau waves, and lasts 10 to 20 minutes. Lesions in the midline of the cerebellum also cause truncal ataxia, which produces a staggering broad-based gait. Nystagmus and head tilt are other signs indicative of posterior fossa lesions. Brainstem tumors, which infiltrate the brainstem without causing ventricular obstruction, more often show cranial nerve abnormalities and long-tract signs such as spastic gait, hemiparesis, and a Babinski sign. Supratentorial tumors have variable presentations, depending upon the hemispheric location of the tumor and whether or not the cerebrospinal fluid pathways are obstructed. A rapidly growing cerebral astrocytoma will produce focal neurologic deficits or seizures, or both, because of pressure from the tumor and its surrounding edema on contiguous structures. Temporal lobe lesions frequently produce focal seizures or visual field defects. Anterior frontal lesions may be silent until they have grown to considerable size and produce increased intracranial pressure.

A sixth nerve palsy with diplopia may be present because of infiltration of the brainstem by tumor or may be a false localizing sign resulting from traction on the sixth nerve from generalized increased pressure. Personality changes (depression, irritability) or a deterioration in school performance may be the presenting symptoms of a supratentorial tumor in the adolescent.

DIAGNOSIS

The introduction of computed tomography (CT) scans with the administration of iodinated contrast has revolutionized the approach to brain tumors. Ventriculography, electroencephalography, and arteriography are no longer needed, except in rare special circumstances. CT scans not only reveal the size and location of the tumor but also provide information regarding the extent of surrounding edema and the vascularity of the tumor. With the advent of magnetic resonance imaging (MRI) scans and the paramagnetic contrast agent, gadolinium, there has been further refinement in diagnostic capability. MRI has become the screening test of choice in patients suspected of having brain tumors. Its ability to produce images in three planes is extremely helpful in evaluating brainstem lesions and in planning surgical resection. MRI has the further advantage of avoiding exposure to ionizing radiation. In the adolescent patient with a brainstem lesion, MRI scanning is mandatory; it permits differentiation of a cavernous angioma from a glioma, which is not possible with CT scanning.

Examination of the spinal fluid is of value in looking for malignant cells to confirm the diagnosis of leptomeningeal disease and, in the case of the adolescent with a primary CNS germ cell tumor, to determine the presence of tumor-specific markers (alpha-fetoprotein or β-human chorionic gonadotropin [β-HCG]) in the spinal fluid.

Myelography is essential in the assessment of tumor dissemination for those tumors that may seed the spinal fluid; the myelogram may reveal tumor nodules distant from the original tumor site even when the cerebrospinal fluid (CSF) cytologic picture is negative. Seeding of the CSF pathway is most commonly seen in medulloblastoma, primitive neuroectodermal tumors (PNET), and germ cell tumors and is less common with ependymoma and astrocytoma. Recent studies of thin-section MRI scans of the spine with gadolinium suggest that this may become the preferred tool for evaluating disease in and around the spinal cord.

TREATMENT

The treatment of brain tumors in general consists of three modalities: (1) surgery, (2) radiation therapy, and (3) chemotherapy. The general principle of brain tumor surgery is that as much tumor as possible should be removed without any increase in neurologic disability. With the exception of brainstem tumors, there is virtually no tumor that should be treated without a histologic diagnosis. There are certain tumors that arise in vital areas of the brain and, in such cases, only biopsy may be possible. However, it has been shown for both low- and high-grade astrocytomas and ependymomas that the degree of resection is directly related to prognosis. This correlation has likewise been suggested, but not proved for medulloblastoma. There is, however, no role for biopsy in medulloblastoma, as it has been shown that adolescents with these tumors have a worse prognosis than do those who have a partial or complete resection. The cerebellar juvenile pilocytic astrocytoma is usually curable with surgery alone, and there is no role for further therapy even if a complete resection is impossible. The role of resection or biopsy in brainstem tumors remains controversial, but some general statements can be made. There are certain brainstem lesions that have a typical diffuse appearance on MRI scan and are primarily pontine in location. Their MRI appearance may or may not be enhanced with gadolinium. Adolescents with such tumors have been shown to do poorly postoperatively and to have very high grade tumors histologically. The life expectancy among these adolescent patients is usually less than 1 year. There is a subgroup of patients, however, who have tumors located primarily at the pontomedullary junction, which are often dorsally exophytic. These tumors are often of low grade, and surgical resection is beneficial. The location of germ cell tumors, typically in the posterior portion of the third ventricle, renders them difficult to approach surgically. An experienced surgeon is usually able to obtain at least a biopsy so that a definitive diagnosis may be made. Examination of CSF to identify germ cells or tumor-specific markers may obviate the need for biopsy in some germ cell tumors. It is inappropriate to determine the histologic characteristics of a tumor in this location by observing the response to empirical radiation therapy. Recent advances in anesthesia and technology, such as the operating microscope and Cavitron, plus the administration of corticosteroids, have made surgical morbidity manageable and mortality rare.

Much controversy centers around the optimal management of adolescent patients with craniopharyngioma. Some neurosurgeons advocate aggressive surgical resection alone, claiming excellent recurrence-free survival with little or no morbidity from surgery. Others advocate less radical surgical debulking followed by involved-field irradiation for individuals with gross residual tumor. This controversy will remain unresolved until a large multi-institutional collaborative study compares the two strategies for relative efficacy and toxicity. The craniopharyngiomas seen in adolescents have a more indolent clinical behavior and histologic appearance, more typical of the adult pattern than that seen in younger children. Given the deleterious effects of irradiation, even in the adolescent, these authors would favor an observational approach in adolescents with obvious residual tumor, provided that the residual disease does not produce visual or neurologic deficits.

Radiation therapy has been a mainstay of brain tumor treatment for several years. With the exception of the cerebellar juvenile pilocytic astrocytoma, some craniopharyngiomas, and occasionally completely resectable supratentorial low-grade astrocytomas, there are no surgically curable malignant brain tumors commonly seen during adolescence. With the addition of radiation therapy, cure has become possible with some medulloblastomas, ependymomas, and germ cell tumors. In the adolescent patient with high-grade astrocytoma, anaplastic astrocytoma, or glioblastoma multiforme, radiation therapy may extend remissions beyond 1 year. In general, high-grade astrocytomas are treated with a dose of 4500 to 6000 cGy to the tumor and a surrounding 2-cm margin. Tumors that have the potential for dissemination via the CSF should receive radiation therapy to the neuraxis (whole brain and spinal cord) as well.

With increasing recognition of the potentially deleterious effects of irradiation, the approach to low-grade astrocytoma has become controversial. Studies are currently ongoing in the Children's Cancer Study Group and the Brain Tumor Cooperative Group that are designed to ascertain whether longer survival is a result of radiotherapy or is related to the natural history of the particular tumor. Newer techniques for the administration of radiation therapy, such as interstitial brachytherapy for cerebral astrocytomas and hyperfractionated (twice daily) irradiation for brainstem tumors, are under investigation. Improvements in technology are permitting more focused administration of conventional irradiation, with the intent of avoiding needless toxicity to uninvolved brain tissue and maximizing the radiation dose to tumor tissue.

The role of chemotherapy in the treatment of brain tumors has changed markedly over the past 10 years. Initial reluctance to include chemotherapy as a treatment option was due to the impression that the blood-brain barrier would prohibit such agents from reaching the tumor. It was for this reason that the lipid-soluble nitrosoureas were initially introduced for the treatment of brain tumors. However, investigators were subsequently able to demonstrate that the blood-brain barrier is abnormal within tumors and that water-soluble, as well as lipid-soluble, agents are able to penetrate into brain tumor tissue. There are two major consortiums, the Children's Cancer Study Group and the Pediatric Oncology Group, conducting multi-institutional trials of multiagent protocols in patients younger than 22 years of age. Results from these studies indicate that adjuvant chemotherapy combined with surgery and radiation therapy prolongs survival in patients with high-grade astrocytoma as well as advanced stage medulloblastoma. A similar beneficial effect of chemotherapy on the outcome of brainstem gliomas has not been observed.

The agents used in these various protocols vary and include the nitrosoureas, vincristine, platinum compounds, and cyclophosphamide, among others. These agents all have demonstrated some activity in previous trials conducted in children and adolescents with recurrent brain tumors. Since the value of chemotherapy in appropriate tumors has been firmly established, further efforts are now being directed at novel ways of administration. Chemotherapy has traditionally been given during or after radiation therapy. Current investigations are exploring the role of chemotherapy prior to radiation therapy. These studies may be of value in several ways. First, information will be gained concerning the response of specific tumors to particular chemotherapeutic agents. Second, information will be gained about the effect of particular regimens on overall survival. Since irradiation diminishes tumor vascularity, the use of preradiation chemotherapy offers the hypothetical advantage of providing better drug delivery to the tumor than would irradiation after chemotherapy.

Chemotherapy for germ cell tumors may diminish the dose of radiation needed and, for some patients, eliminate entirely the need for radiation therapy. Systemic germ cell tumors are histologically identical to primary CNS germ tumors. They are extremely chemosensitive tumors that may be cured even when disseminated at the time of diagnosis. Although 60% to 80% of adolescent patients with CNS germinomas may be cured by radiation therapy alone, cumulative toxicity often makes the quality of life of the cured adolescent suboptimal. Based on experience with systemic germ cell tumors, protocols have been devised to include chemotherapy prior to irradiation. If complete disappearance of tumor is observed on CT scan, the radiation dose and subsequent morbidity are reduced without an increased risk of relapse. Building on this experience, current protocols at Memorial Sloan-Kettering Cancer Center are intensifying the chemotherapy portion of the treatment with the aim of avoiding radiation therapy altogether.

In recent years, high-dose (marrow-ablative) chemotherapy followed by autologous bone marrow rescue has been applied to the treatment of children and young adults with recurrent brain tumors. Early results are particularly encouraging for patients with high-grade astrocytomas. Pilot studies are now under way using this approach to treat children and adolescents who have newly diagnosed high-grade astrocytomas, administering conventional irradiation following recovery from the high-dose chemotherapy. The utility of other innovative approaches designed to improve the therapy of brain tumors remains to be proved. These approaches include the use of hematopoietic growth factors (cytokines) to stimulate marrow recovery from conventional chemotherapy; biologic agents such as interleukin-2; topical administration of chemotherapeutic or biologic agents with implanted pumps, biodegradable matrices, or the intraarterial approach; and the use of monoclonal antibodies.

PROGNOSIS

The prognosis for the individual adolescent treated for a brain tumor is dependent on three main factors: (1) the histologic features of the tumor, (2) the age of the patient at the time of diagnosis, and (3) the extent of surgical resection. Patients with cerebellar astrocytoma have the best survival (approximately 90%) at 5 years. The 5-year survival rate of patients with germ cell tumors and low-grade supratentorial astrocytomas is 60% to 80%. The 5-year survival rate among adolescent patients with medulloblastoma is 50%; however, late relapses occur, and the 10-year survival rate is only 35%. Recent studies have suggested improved 5-year disease-free survival for medulloblastoma patients; this may reach 70% to 85% for average-risk patients. Among adolescents with high-grade astrocytoma, the 5-year survival rate is less than 35% to 45%, with most studies showing the poorest survival for adolescent patients with

glioblastoma multiforme. The prognosis is even worse for adolescent patients with brainstem tumors, among whom the anticipated 5-year survival rate is less than 20%. Increasing age appears to be a good prognostic feature for brain tumors in general, with the poorest survival usually being seen in the youngest children (less than 4 years of age) having medulloblastoma, ependymoma, or high-grade astrocytoma. Likewise, the Brain Tumor Study Group (BTSG) has reported the best survival among astrocytoma patients aged 15 to 40 years.

SIDE EFFECTS

The treatment of brain tumors has always been complicated by the side effects of the therapy itself, and gains made in diagnosis and treatment are often partially offset by complications of therapy. Each therapeutic modality has unique problems and complications associated with it. Postoperative morbidity has been reduced in recent years because of better localization of the tumor by CT, MRI, and preoperative angiograms, as indicated. The operating microscope has permitted better planes of dissection, with less damage to normal tissues and, accordingly, fewer neurologic deficits.

Radiation therapy has acute, subacute, and chronic side effects. Acute effects occur within hours of a single treatment. An increase in cerebral edema may merely aggravate a focal neurologic deficit or, if severe, may cause cerebral herniation. Corticosteroids may prevent this acute effect of radiation therapy. The radiation somnolence syndrome is a subacute reaction that occurs 4 to 10 weeks following the completion of radiation therapy. The patient may become somnolent, anorectic, and lethargic. Low-grade fever and vomiting may also be present. The symptoms may persist for weeks, but they ultimately resolve completely and spontaneously. The pathophysiology of this syndrome is not known but is believed to result from impairment of myelin synthesis. Occasionally the somnolence is accompanied by focal findings; such patients may be mistakenly diagnosed as having tumor recurrence until the symptoms recede.

Chronic or delayed irradiation damage is the result of radiation necrosis. This usually follows high-dose radiotherapy (doses greater than 5000 cGy). Symptoms appear 6 months to several years following cranial irradiation; symptoms and imaging studies may suggest the recurrence of tumor. The damage may be limited and focal or may progress diffusely; progression may lead to dementia and death. The pathophysiology of delayed irradiation damage is unknown, but there is brain necrosis with hyalinization of vascular structures on histopathologic examination.

An uncommon but worrisome complication of irradiation is the development of a second malignancy in the irradiated field. In addition to second primary brain tumors, thyroid carcinomas have occurred in patients following craniospinal radiotherapy for medulloblastoma. The late occurrence of fibrosarcomas within the brain has been reported.

Endocrine dysfunction may follow irradiation of the hypothalamus and pituitary; such dysfunction includes short stature resulting from growth hormone deficiency, primary or secondary hypothyroidism, hypopituitarism, and hypogonadism (see Chapter 55). Intellectual dysfunction is seen as a sequel to cranial irradiation, and the degree of impairment is directly related to the age of the patient at the time of therapy. Although the most devastating effects are seen in younger children, adverse effects may be seen at all ages.

Chemotherapy for brain tumors also has complications, the nature of which depends on the specific agents used. The most frequent toxicity is bone marrow suppression, though certain agents, such as the platinums and vincristine, may cause nephrotoxicity and neurotoxicity. The nitrosoureas bischloroethylnitrosourea (BCNU) and lomustine (CCNU) may also be responsible for late development of restrictive pulmonary dysfunction.

As the number of surviving adolescents increases, it becomes progressively important to attend to the long-term psychosocial consequences of a brain tumor and its therapy. The adolescent with a brain tumor is, perhaps more than any other cancer patient, more vulnerable to both debilitating and long-lasting adverse impacts upon body image, autonomy, peer relationships, sexuality, education, and future development. The tumor itself may produce permanent and sudden effects upon hearing, vision, intellect, and motor function. Therapy, particularly radiation therapy, can produce more gradual adverse effects upon the same parameters. At radiation doses normally used to treat brain tumors, the hair never regrows completely, as it does in most children who survive cancer. Brain tumor patients frequently are left with thin, sparse, and patchy hair growth—this may leave a far deeper scar upon the psyche of the vulnerable adolescent. Youngsters with brain tumors, particularly adolescents, are a group apart from other youngsters with cancer given their myriad physical and intellectual handicaps. Much more attention must be paid to the psychosocial problems and rehabilitation of the adolescent with a brain tumor.

In conclusion, it is crucial that the adolescent suspected of having a brain tumor be evaluated promptly with appropriate radiologic imaging. When the diagnosis of a brain tumor is established, prompt referral to an experienced neurosurgeon at an institution experienced in the multidisciplinary management of pediatric and adolescent brain tumors is indicated. As with other diseases and other malignancies, the question of referral to a pediatric-adolescent program rather than an adult program for the older adolescent remains controversial, but at best must be individualized, based in part upon the tumor type, but largely upon the level of maturity and independence of the adolescent. Treatment and long-term rehabilitation of the adolescent with a brain tumor require a multidisciplinary team that is attuned to the unique needs of the teenager.

BIBLIOGRAPHY

Allen JC, Bloom J, Ertel I, et al: Brain tumors in children: Current cooperative and institutional chemotherapy trials in newly diagnosed and recurrent disease. Semin Oncol 13:110, 1986.

Allen JC, Kim JH, Packer RJ: Neoadjuvant chemotherapy for newly diagnosed germ-cell tumors of the central nervous system. J Neurosurg 67:65, 1987.

Cohen ME, Duffner PK: Brain Tumors in Children. Principles of Diagnosis and Treatment. New York, Raven Press, 1984.

Duffner PK, Cohen ME, Myers MH, et al: Survival of children with brain tumors: SEER Program, 1973–1989. Neurology 36:597, 1986.

Duffner PK, Cohen ME, Thomas P: Late effects of treatment on the intelligence of children with posterior fossa tumors. Cancer 51:233, 1983.

Epstein F, McGleary EL: Intrinsic brain stem tumors of childhood: Surgical indications. J Neurosurg 64:11, 1986.

Farwell JR, Dohrmann GJ, Flannery JT: Central nervous system tumors in children. Cancer 40:3123, 1977.

Finlay JL, Goins SC, Uteg R, et al: Progress in the management of childhood brain tumors. Hematol/Oncol Clin North Am 1:753, 1987.

Finlay JL, Uteg R, Giese WL: Brain tumors in children. II. Advances in neurosurgery and radiation oncology. Am J Pediatr Hematol Oncol 9:256, 1987.

Gjerris F: Clinical aspects and long-term prognosis of intracranial tumors in infancy and childhood. Dev Med Child Neurol 18:145, 1976.

Sposto R, Ertel IJ, Jenkin RD, et al: The effectiveness of chemotherapy for treatment of high grade astrocytoma in children: Results of a randomized trial. J Neurooncol 7:165, 1989.

Wood JR, Green SB, Shapiro WR: The prognostic importance of tumor size in malignant gliomas: A computed tomographic scan study by the Brain Tumor Cooperative Group. J Clin Oncol 6:338, 1988.

GERM CELL TUMORS

PAUL C. J. ROGERS

Germ cell tumors may arise in the testes, ovaries, and extragonadal sites such as the retroperitoneum and the sacrococcygeal, mediastinal, and pineal regions. These tumors may be of either benign or malignant histologic appearance. Primordial germ cells first appear on the wall of the embryonic yolk sac, and from there they migrate around the hindgut to the genital regions of the developing posterior abdominal wall at which point they become part of the developing gonad. It has been proposed that aberrant migration accounts for the occurrence of germinal cells in the midline sites, giving rise to extragonadal tumors.

After childhood, there is a steep increase in the incidence of both testicular and ovarian cancer in adolescents and young adults. In the 15- to 19-year-old age group, testicular cancer reaches an incidence of 21 cases/1 million population annually, whereas the incidence of ovarian cancer rises to 16 cases/1 million population annually. There appears to be a lower incidence of germ cell tumors in the black population than in the white population.

The oncogenesis of germ cell tumors remains unclear. There are proponents of the theory that the malignant potential of germ cells is under the exogenous control of microenvironmental signals or that somatic cell mutation is the central event in the process of malignant development. A genetic predisposition is possible, as there is an increased risk of germ cell tumors in first-degree relatives. The association of germ cell tumors and congenital anomalies is well documented. Up to 17% of adolescents have associated congenital defects. Recently, an association with leukemia has been shown with 16 patients being described with both conditions. These were predominantly mediastinal tumors and leukemia of megakaryocytic lineage. Germ cell tumors occur frequently in adolescents with gonadal dysgenesis and cryptorchidism. The relationship between gonadal and extragonadal neoplasia and disorders of sexual differentiation is documented but poorly understood. Klinefelter syndrome (47,XXY) is associated with testicular or extragonadal germ cell tumors usually located in the mediastinum or central nervous system.

Tumor karyotype abnormalities have been reported. An isochromosome 12 has been identified in adult germ cell tumors. Abnormalities of chromosomes 1, 3, 6, and 11 have been described. Increased expression of the c-myc and ci-Ki-ras2 oncogenes has been reported in tumor tissue.

PATHOLOGIC FEATURES

Germ cell tumors arise from the primitive germ cell but may differentiate along several lines and be either malignant or benign.

Teratomas most commonly arise in infancy in the sacrococcygeal area, but in adolescence they may present in the ovary or mediastinal area. The teratoma may be mature and benign, immature with a tendency to malignancy, or have malignant components within it. A gonadoblastoma is a benign germ cell tumor that has a mixture of immature germ cells and gonadal sex cord cells that are granulosa, or Sertoli cells. A pure germinoma is a seminoma in the testes, a dysgerminoma in the ovary, or a germinoma in the extragonadal sites. The germinomas are the least aggressive of the malignant germ cell tumors. The other malignant tumors include the yolk sac tumor, also called the endodermal sinus tumor; embryonal carcinoma; choriocarcinoma; and malignant germ cell tumors with mixed histologic features. In younger children, yolk sac tumors are the most common malignant tumors, but in adolescence and young adulthood, embryonal carcinoma becomes more common.

TUMOR MARKERS

Serum tumor markers have proved extremely useful both in diagnosis and in monitoring the response to therapy. Yolk sac tumors secrete predominantly alpha-fetoprotein, choriocarcinomas secrete β-human chorionic gonadotropin (β-HCG), and embryonal carcinomas may secrete either one or both. The half-life of alpha-fetoprotein is approximately 5.5 days; the rate of its elimination can be used to indicate complete resection, and it is the most sensitive marker of relapsing disease. Alpha-fetoprotein levels can be elevated in other disease states, such as hepatic malignancies or in regenerating liver following viral hepatitis.

The β-unit of HCG can be immunologically separated from the α-units and is a sensitive marker of tumors with trophoblastic elements. The half-life of the β-unit is only 45 minutes; therefore, it should rapidly disappear if there is complete removal of the tumors.

Other serum markers that have been used are lactate dehydrogenase (LDH) as a nonspecific tumor marker, neuron-specific enolase (NSE) in germinomas, and placental alkaline phosphatase (PLAP) in some adolescent patients.

PRESENTATION AND DIAGNOSTIC EVALUATION

Ovarian tumors most commonly present with abdominal pain, which may be chronic, but if torsion of the tumor is present, the pain may be acute and severe (see Chapter 70). Slowly progressive abdominal enlargement, constipation, and genitourinary symptoms may be present. Ovarian tumor should be in the differential diagnosis of any abdominal mass presenting in adolescence, and tumor markers should always be requested prior to surgery.

Testicular tumors usually cause a slowly growing, painless mass (see also Chapter 78). A hydrocele may be present. Adolescents should be taught the importance of testicular self-examination. With any germ cell tumor, the physician should palpate for retroperitoneal masses and supraclavicular adenopathy. Extragonadal tumors may present as retroperitoneal masses with increasing abdominal distention. Mediastinal masses can present with shortness of breath and pain. These masses are classically in the anterosuperior mediastinum. Sacrococcygeal tumors may occur in adolescence, but this is relatively rare, more commonly presenting during infancy. A small percentage of tumors arise in the midline of the head and neck. The primary central nervous system germ cell tumors are typically in the pineal or suprasellar region. They may obstruct spinal fluid flow, with resulting symptoms of raised intracranial pressure. Signs of precocious puberty and gynecomastia may be due to the presence of a germ cell tumor.

The pattern of dissemination is the same for all sites, with spread to lungs, liver, regional nodes, and central nervous system. Diagnostic evaluation of germ cell tumors is outlined in Table 53–23.

THERAPY

The approach to therapy is influenced by the site of origin, histologic subtype, and stage of disease. These

TABLE 53–23. Evaluation of Germ Cell Tumors

History
Physical examination
Complete blood count
Liver function tests: BUN, creatinine
α-Fetoprotein, β-HCG, LDH
Radiographic evaluation of primary site, regional disease, and
   metastases; that is, chest radiograph, ultrasound of testes, CT scan
   of abdomen, pelvis, chest, and brain

factors are also of prognostic value. Testicular tumors have a better prognosis than do ovarian tumors, and ovarian tumors have a better prognosis than do extragonadal tumors. The size of the tumor is of significance; large ovarian tumors have a poorer prognosis than do smaller ones. The histologic subtype is important, germinomas having a better prognosis than do other malignant germ cell tumors. Marked elevation of serum markers of alpha-fetoprotein, β-HCG, and LDH have been reported as adverse prognostic features.

Complete resection is the initial aim of treatment and should be undertaken whenever practically possible. When the mass is not easily resectable as a primary approach, initial chemotherapy followed by resection is used. Chemotherapy may result in a complete response that results in the avoidance of surgery in some cases. If residual tumor is seen on radiologic imaging or there continues to be evidence of a raised serum tumor marker of alpha-fetoprotein or β-HCG, repeat (or "second-look") surgery is advocated. Residual mass seen on radiologic evaluation following chemotherapy may not always be tumor but may be fibrotic tissue. Staging of

TABLE 53–24. Staging of Germinal Cell Tumors

		SURGICAL PATHOLOGIC FINDING
Ovarian Tumors		
Stage	I	Growth limited to ovaries
	Ia	Limited to one ovary, no ascites
	Ib	Limited to both ovaries, no ascites
	Ic	Limited to one or both ovaries
		Ascites present with positive cytologic features
Stage	II	Growth involving one or both ovaries with pelvic extension
	IIa	Extension or metastases, or both, to uterus or tubes only
	IIb	Extension to other pelvic organs
Stage	III	Spread to intraperitoneal organs
Stage	IV	Metastases outside the peritoneal cavity
Testicular Tumors		
Stage	I	Local spread
		P1: Confined to testis
		P2: Involves testicular adnexa
		P3: Involves scrotal wall
Stage	II	Confined to retroperitoneal lymphatics
		N1: Microscopic
		N2: Gross involvement without capsular invasion
		N3: Gross involvement with capsular invasion
		N4: Massive involvement of retroperitoneal structures
Stage	III	Beyond retroperitoneum
		M1: Solitary metastasis
		M2: Multiple metastases

P, primary; N, nodes; M, metastasis.

the tumors is important, as this influences the use of adjuvant therapy (Table 53–24).

Ovarian tumors should be resected when feasible. If a tumor is confined to one ovary, conservative surgery with a unilateral salpingo-oophorectomy is recommended. The contralateral ovary should be inspected carefully and any visible abnormality biopsied. A biopsy of the paraaortic lymph nodes and peritoneal washing should be performed at the time of laparotomy. Adjuvant chemotherapy is warranted for ovarian tumors, except for completely resected dysgerminomas and benign or immature teratomas.

Stage I testicular tumors—that is, completely surgically resected tumors—do not need adjuvant chemotherapy. The place of retroperitoneal lymph node dissection remains controversial. It is considered by some to be necessary for staging and to be a therapeutic approach for patients who have stage II disease. However, other authorities believe that if adolescents with stage I disease have a tumor marker that returns to normal after surgery and are under very close observation, it is unnecessary to put them through the morbidity of lymph node dissection, because adolescents who do have a relapse of disease can be treated with chemotherapy. Orchidectomy for a testicular mass should be carried out via a transinguinal resection. Stage I seminomas are treated with prophylactic paraaortic nodal radiation. Stage II and stage III testicular tumors do receive adjuvant chemotherapy. Cure rates in excess of 80% are being reported for all testicular tumors.

Extragonadal tumors are not always as resectable as ovarian and testicular tumors, especially mediastinal tumors. Patients who have malignant nongonadal tumors should receive adjuvant chemotherapy; however, adjuvant chemotherapy to immature teratomas is controversial and may not be necessary for some adolescent patients who have complete surgical resection and tumor markers within normal limits.

Radiotherapy is used for some germinomas and central nervous system tumors.

CHEMOTHERAPY

The platinum-based chemotherapy combinations have proved highly effective in treating malignant germ cell tumors. In 1977, Einhorn described the successful treatment for disseminated testicular germ cell tumors using cisplatin, vinblastine, and bleomycin. Subsequent to

TABLE 53–25. Chemotherapy for Germ Cell Cancer

REGIMEN	DRUG	SCHEDULE	
PVB	Cisplatin	Days 1 to 5	every 3 weeks × 4
	Vinblastine	Days 1 and 2	
	Bleomycin	Begin day 2, weekly × 12	
BEP	Bleomycin	Begin day 2, weekly × 12	
	Etoposide (VP-16)	Days 1 to 5	every 3 weeks × 4
	Cisplatin	Days 1 to 5	

that, etoposide received recognition as a highly effective agent and has generally replaced vinblastine. Recently, cisplatin has been replaced by its analogue carboplatinum with what would appear to be equally effective results. Combination chemotherapy is given over four courses every 3 weeks, as outlined in Table 53–25. Other agents that have shown response in germ cell tumors include cyclophosphamide, doxorubicin, actinomycin D, and ifosfamide. High-dose intensive chemotherapy followed by autologous bone marrow rescue is now being used for very high-risk patients and for patients with relapsed disease. Germ cell tumors are considered to be highly chemosensitive tumors, and the prognosis is generally excellent if appropriate evaluation, therapy, and follow-up are undertaken.

BIBLIOGRAPHY

Arens A, Marcus D, Engelberg S, et al: Cerebral germinomas and Klinefelter syndrome. Cancer 61:1228, 1988.

Bosl GJ, Dmitrovsky E, Reuter V, et al: A specific karyotypic abnormality in germ cell tumors (GCT), Abstract. ASCO 8:131, 1989.

Loehrer PJ, Sledge GW, Einhorn LH: Heterogeneity among germ cell tumors of the testis. Semin Oncol 12:304, 1985.

Lothe RA, Fossa SD, Stenwig AE, et al: Loss of 3p or 11p alleles is associated with testicular cancer tumors. Genomics 5:134, 1989.

Mann JR, Pearson D, Barrett A, et al: Results of the United Kingdom Children's Cancer Study Group's malignant germ cell tumor studies. Cancer 63:1657, 1989.

Nichols CR, Heerema NA, Palmer C, et al: Klinefelter's syndrome associated with mediastinal germ cell neoplasms. J Clin Oncol 5:1290, 1987.

Nichols CR, Roth BJ, Heerema N, et al: Hematologic neoplasia associated with primary mediastinal germ-cell tumors. N Engl J Med 322:1425, 1990.

Sikora K, Evan G, Stewart J, et al: Detection of the c-myc oncogene product in testicular cancer. Br J Cancer 52:171, 1985.

Surveillance, Epidemiology End Results (SEER): Incidence and Mortality Data, 1973–77. NCI Monograph 57, NIH Publication No. 81–2330, June 1981.

Tollerud DJ, Blattner WA, Fraser MC: Familial testicular cancer and urogenital developmental anomalies. Cancer 55:1849, 1985.

Tukstalis DB, Bubley GJ, Donahue JP, et al: Regional loss of chromosome 6 in two urological malignancies. Cancer Res 49:5087, 1989.

Wang L, Vass W, Gao C, et al: Amplification and enhanced expression of the C-Ki-ras2 protooncogene in human embryonal carcinomas. Cancer Res 47:4192, 1987.

CHAPTER 54

Bone Marrow Failure and Transplantation

REGGIE E. DUERST

HEMATOPOIESIS

The bone marrow can be considered an organ of the body that is a fluid suspension of cells functioning within a matrix provided by reticuloendothelial cells. The function of the bone marrow is to produce the cellular components of the blood and lymphoid system for (1) oxygen delivery, (2) neutralization of infections, and (3) balanced hemostasis. The continued production of these cells is sustained by appropriate stimulation of pluripotent progenitor cells (stem cells). The stimuli are provided by reticuloendothelial cells within the bone marrow, mature lymphocytes, and cells located in the kidney (erythropoietin). The colony-stimulating factors (so called for their ability to stimulate marrow cells to produce large clusters or colonies of cells *in vitro*) induce cell division and maturation of stem cells at various stages of differentiation. The ability of the marrow "factory" to produce diverse "products" is a result of the relative amounts of these factors, expression of the corresponding receptor by the stem cells, and the temporal relationship of factor production to receptor expression.

DISORDERS RESULTING FROM FAILURE OF HEMATOPOIESIS

Aplastic anemia is the failure of the bone marrow to produce an adequate number of mature blood cells (see Chapter 52). Causes for aplastic anemia are multiple—the result of congenital disorders manifested at birth or later in life, the result of exposure to infectious agents or toxins, or an acquired disordered immune response that is associated with inhibition of blood cell production. Some of the potential causes of aplastic anemia are listed in Table 54–1 and should be considered during the evaluation of adolescents who have marrow failure.

In 1927, Fanconi described three siblings with constitutional pancytopenia in association with physical abnormalities. Fanconi anemia is characterized by skeletal abnormalities (principally of the upper extremities), generalized hyperpigmentation of the skin, and various renal deformities that are present in approximately one third of patients. The degree of pancytopenia is frequently moderate at diagnosis, with progressive failure of blood cell production. Cytogenetic examination of phytohemagglutinin-stimulated lymphocytes incubated with chromosomal damaging agents reveals excessive breakage and exchange of chromatin in metaphase cells. This disorder is inherited in an autosomal recessive manner. Studies to detect the carrier status of relatives and prenatal diagnosis can be performed with appropriate genetic counseling. Initial therapy for Fanconi anemia is supportive in the form of blood transfusions for anemia, intravenous antibiotic treatment of severe infections and platelet support. Allogeneic bone marrow transplantation can be curative. These adolescent patients are also susceptible to the development of myeloid leukemia, the treatment of which is complicated by poor tolerance of chemotherapy. Similarly, they are very sensitive to standard marrow transplantation cytoreduction regimens, and dosage modification is required.

Shwachman-Diamond syndrome is a constitutional marrow failure disorder in which neutropenia is present in association with exocrine-pancreatic insufficiency (see Chapter 52). The pancreatic insufficiency must be differentiated from cystic fibrosis (see Chapter 43). Neutropenia results in pyogenic skin infections or pneumonia. Pancytopenia may develop in a minority of patients. A similar syndrome has been described by Pearson in which pancreatic dysfunction was associated with anemia and ringed sideroblasts present in the bone marrow. Dyskeratosis congenita is a rare disorder with a diagnostic triad of reticulated hyperpigmentation of the shoulders and face associated with dystrophic nails and mucous membrane leukoplakia. These adolescent patients also present with mild to moderate anemia or

TABLE 54–1. Etiologic Classification of Aplastic Anemia

CONSTITUTIONAL	ACQUIRED
Fanconi anemia	Drugs and toxic chemicals or irradiation
Shwachman-Diamond syndrome	Infectious-viral (hepatitis, parvovirus, varicella, HIV)
Pearson syndrome	Autoimmune
Dyskeratosis congenita	Paroxysmal nocturnal hemoglobinuria
	Nutritional deficiency (e.g., vitamin B_{12}, pyridoxine)
	Pregnancy
	Thymoma

thrombocytopenia, with later progression to marrow failure.

Idiopathic or acquired aplastic anemia is the result of inhibition of marrow function following exposure to various toxins or infectious agents. Severe aplastic anemia is defined by the degree of pancytopenia (anemia, neutropenia, or thrombocytopenia) in conjunction with hypocellular bone marrow. The criteria for severe aplastic anemia are listed in Table 54–2. Drugs that have been associated with aplasia include antibiotics, nonsteroidal anti-inflammatory agents, and phenothiazines. The drugs can directly suppress myelopoiesis, but idiosyncratic or non–dose-related toxicity is frequent. Aplasia has also been reported following exposure to organic solvents such as benzene or toluene.

Although transient suppression of hematopoiesis is not uncommon following infectious illnesses, severe aplasia may result as a consequence of several different viral infections. Medications prescribed during the infectious illness may also contribute to the subsequent aplasia. Aplasia following hepatitis is often severe, with a high rate of morbidity and mortality. The interplay between the viral infection and altered metabolism of drugs used in treating the adolescent with liver dysfunction suggests that the resulting aplasia may be multifactorial. Other viral infections associated with suppression of hematopoiesis include varicella, rubella, cytomegalovirus (CMV), and human immunodeficiency virus (HIV), the etiologic agent of the acquired immunodeficiency syndrome (AIDS) (see Chapters 76 and 93).

Several lines of evidence implicate a disordered immune response as the cause of aplasia in many adolescent patients with acquired aplastic anemia. Humoral factors that inhibit hematopoiesis have been described, and T lymphocytes capable of inhibiting hematopoiesis have been demonstrated *in vitro*. Also, depletion of T lymphocytes from bone marrow suspensions from adolescents with aplastic anemia has resulted in improved growth of hematopoietic cells *in vitro*. Furthermore, immunosuppressive therapy (discussed further on) has been at least transiently effective for approximately one half of adolescents with aplastic anemia. Autologous marrow recovery observed following allogeneic bone marrow transplantation could be a response to the immunosuppressive effects of the marrow ablation regimens.

Paroxysmal nocturnal hemoglobinuria (PNH) is a disorder of the pluripotent hematopoietic stem cell characterized by intravascular hemolysis resulting from increased sensitivity of mature blood cells to complement lysis. The extent of hemolysis is variable and has been related to expression of decay accelerating factor, a normal glycoprotein of hematopoietic cells that inhibits complement lysis. This disease is a clonal disorder with progressive marrow dysfunction manifested as aplasia or malignancy.

Parvovirus has been associated with selective erythroid hypoplasia in patients with underlying hemolytic anemia and congenital or acquired immunodeficiency. The virus infects erythroid progenitor cells and causes their destruction. Adolescent patients who are unable to mount an appropriate immune response are not able to clear the virus, and impaired red cell production persists. Adolescents with hemolytic anemia may require transfusion support until the infection is neutralized, and treatment of the immunodeficient adolescent patient with intravenous immunoglobulin leads to neutralization of the virus with restoration of red cell production. Prolonged pancytopenia has also been reported after parvovirus infection.

DIAGNOSIS

The diagnosis of aplastic anemia is made by documenting pancytopenia in the presence of bone marrow hypocellularity, as already described. In younger patients with skeletal abnormalities, the chromosomal aberrations of Fanconi anemia should be excluded. One should consider testing for complement sensitivity to exclude PNH.

GENERAL THERAPY

Good personal hygiene is important for prevention of infection, and systemic antibiotics are indicated if evidence of infection is found. Transfusion support should be used conservatively as long as marrow transplantation is a consideration (see further on). Bleeding can be minimized in thrombocytopenic adolescents by administration of the antifibrinolytic agent, ϵ-aminocaproic acid.

Allogeneic bone marrow transplantation from a human leukocyte antigen (HLA)-identical sibling donor is the current treatment of choice for bone marrow failure. Prolonged survival without loss of marrow function following transplantation ranges from 60% to 90%, with a better outcome associated with younger patients and those who have not required transfusion prior to bone marrow transplantation. For adolescents without a tissue-identical sibling, immunosuppressive therapy can result in adequate recovery of hematopoiesis to enable long-term survival, though cytopenias may persist. Antilymphocyte or antithymocyte globulin, prepared from sera of horses or rabbits immunized with human lymphocytes, has been used for treatment of adolescent patients without an HLA-identical donor. Use of these antisera was initiated after autologous marrow recovery was observed in allogeneic bone marrow transplant recipients receiving these preparations for suppression of rejection. The response to treatment with these antisera ranges from 35% to 70%. These responses are rarely complete and are frequently not sustained but nonetheless result in improved survival. Forty percent

TABLE 54–2. Criteria for Severe Aplastic Anemia*

LABORATORY EVALUATION	LABORATORY VALUE
Granulocyte count	less than 500/μL
Corrected reticulocyte count	less than 1%
Platelet count	less than 20,000/μL

*Two of three criteria are present and the bone marrow is hypocellular (less than 25% cellular).

to 50% of patients may respond to methylprednisolone, and corticosteroids are often used in conjunction with antilymphocyte globulin to prevent or treat complications of serum sickness. Immunosuppression with high-dose cyclophosphamide (without marrow transplantation) has also been successful. The immunosuppressive agent cyclosporin A has been used with positive effects. Indications for its use alone or in combination with other immunosuppressive agents are unclear at this time. In the past, androgenic steroids were used in the treatment of severe aplastic anemia but are used infrequently at present. Evidence for improved survival of adolescent patients with severe aplastic anemia treated with androgens compared with adolescents receiving supportive care is lacking. The multiple complications produced by androgens, particularly masculinization of female adolescents, and the availability of alternative treatments have led to the decline in their use.

BONE MARROW TRANSPLANTATION

Bone marrow transplantation, like solid organ transplantation, is a form of therapy designed to replace a defective organ system. The organ "system" in this instance is embodied by the diverse functions of the fully differentiated hematopoietic cells. The functions of this system include oxygen delivery by the erythrocytes; direct protection from infection by the granulocytic, monocytic, and lymphocytic cell lineages; and prevention of hemorrhage by platelets, as mentioned previously. In addition, several metabolic and synthetic functions are accomplished by mature blood cells. The latter functions serve bone remodeling, production of inflammatory and coagulation proteins, and catabolism of several potentially toxic products of intermediary metabolism.

Isolated reports of the therapeutic use of bone marrow date to the last century, but the current practice of marrow transplantation began in the 1950s after Thomas documented the safety of intravenous marrow infusion. Mathé, in France, attempted to treat nuclear accident victims with bone marrow transplantation and extended this to several patients with leukemia. Successful transplantation in two infants with immunologic defects at the Universities of Minnesota and Wisconsin in 1968 heralded the expansion of the application of bone marrow transplantation during the 1970s. Allogeneic bone marrow transplantation has subsequently become the treatment of choice for most children with severe immunodeficiency syndromes. Also, allogeneic bone marrow transplantation from a sibling donor matched for the major histocompatibility complex antigens has become the treatment of choice for severe aplastic anemia in children and young adults. Accepted indications for bone marrow transplantation broadened during the 1980s to include treatment of most individuals with leukemia or lymphoma following relapse. The most dramatic increase in the application of bone marrow transplantation involves the use of a patient's own (autologous) bone marrow as the source of replacement

marrow following high-dose chemoradiotherapy for the treatment of malignancy.

The compatibility of donor and recipient cells is determined primarily (but not exclusively) by the HLA system. The genes for these antigens are located on chromosome 6 and are generally inherited as a group (haplotype), one from each parent. The HLA glycoproteins are homologous with immunoglobulin molecules and are defined by serologic typing or specific T-lymphocyte reactivity. Lymphocytes recognize other cells in the context of self-nonself through the HLA system—thus its importance for successful allogeneic bone marrow transplantation.

The treatment administered prior to infusion of the bone marrow is frequently described as supralethal. The prolonged, if not permanent, marrow aplasia that would result if replacement marrow were not provided would result in the death of most adolescent patients from infection or hemorrhage. Destruction of the recipient's marrow is a primary goal in the case of adolescents undergoing bone marrow transplantation for treatment of congenital hematopoietic-immunologic defects or diseases of intermediary metabolism. This destruction must be sufficient to provide "space" or a "niche" for the allogeneic replacement cells so that they will be able to gain a survival advantage over the defective host cells. The host or recipient must also undergo adequate immunosuppression so that the donor cells are not rejected. Successful "engraftment" of donor cells is described as reestablishment of hematopoiesis so that neutrophil production is adequate to prevent bacteremia (approximately 500 neutrophils/μL) and the adolescent does not require frequent transfusions of platelets or red blood cells.

The cytoreductive regimen, or myeloablative therapy, for adolescents with cancer must also be designed with the goal of destroying the adolescent patient's remaining malignant cells. Ideally, the agents chosen are cross-resistant (i.e., any resistance of the tumor cells to these agents is not through a common mechanism), have demonstrated activity against the tumor with steep dose-response curves (large increase in tumor cell death with a small increase in dosage), and have differing nonhematopoietic dose-limiting toxicities. Adolescents undergoing transplantation for Fanconi anemia require an attenuated cytoreduction schedule, as they are very sensitive to the cytotoxic effects of cyclophosphamide and the other agents used for cytoreduction. Total body irradiation (TBI) is employed in the treatment of many patients with malignancies, though regimens using only chemotherapy are increasingly being used. Most centers use fractionated dosing schedules, whereby the irradiation exposure is divided over 2 to 7 days. This is thought to offer improved efficacy, as normal tissues repair radiation damage between treatments, which allows administration of a higher total dosage.

Graft-versus-host disease (GVHD) is the result of immunocompetent donor cells recognizing "transplantation" antigens on host cells. The cytotoxic response by lymphocytes results in dysfunction of several organs. Acute GVHD is defined as occurring during the first 100 days following allogeneic bone marrow transplantation and is manifested by rash, hepatic dysfunction, and diarrhea. The extent of organ malfunction is assessed clinically and assigned a grade of 0 (no GVHD) to IV (extensive involvement of two or more systems). Adolescents undergoing allogeneic bone marrow transplantation receive prophylaxis against development of GVHD in the form of immunosuppressive drugs (cyclosporin A, corticosteroids, methotrexate). T-cell depletion of the donor bone marrow and anti–T-lymphocyte immunotoxins administered to the adolescent patient have also been employed. Chronic GVHD can be manifested in many organs. The involvement usually resembles autoimmune disease, such as scleroderma or sicca syndrome, with prominent histologic features of lymphocytic infiltration or fibrosis of the involved organ, or both. Adolescents with chronic GVHD are also immunosuppressed by the disease process itself. Thus infection becomes the major cause of death in these individuals.

The degree of acute GVHD is predictive for other complications of bone marrow transplantation (e.g., interstitial pneumonitis, infection), subsequent development of chronic GVHD, and a poorer prognosis for individuals undergoing bone marrow transplantation for aplastic anemia. However, adolescent patients undergoing bone marrow transplantation for leukemia who survive the acute complications and in whom chronic GVHD subsequently develops have a diminished risk of recurrent leukemia developing. Thus, the GVHD also provides a graft-versus-leukemia action. Efforts are currently being made to enhance the graft-versus-leukemia effect without increasing the toxicity of GVHD.

Transplantation-related complications can involve any organ system and are associated with the adolescent patient's prior treatment, physical condition prior to the cytoreduction therapy, agents and dosages employed for cytoreduction, and source of replacement marrow (autologous, matched allogeneic, or mismatched allogeneic). Acute cardiomyopathy following high-dose cyclophosphamide therapy and fulminant hepatic failure from veno-occlusive disease of the liver are infrequent but usually fatal complications that occur during or shortly after the cytoreduction regimen. Interstitial pneumonitis associated with CMV infection and GVHD has been a major cause of mortality following allogeneic bone marrow transplantation. It most commonly develops 1 to 2 months after transplantation. The immune systems of most adolescent patients remain suppressed and dysfunctional for months to years whether there is active GVHD or not. These individuals benefit from prophylactic antibiotic therapy and need to be reimmunized following cessation of immunosuppressive therapy. Both males and females have retained fertility following bone marrow transplantation, but sterility is common, particularly after receiving total body irradiation. Sperm-banking can be arranged for mature males, and techniques developed for *in vitro* fertilization may be applicable in the future. Sexual development of prepubertal patients is delayed, and hormonal supplementation is generally required for girls. Testosterone production appears to be affected less often.

The transplantation procedure raises several psychological and ethical questions regarding isolation, compliance with prescribed therapy, and informed consent (for both patient and donor). Adolescent patients can have particular difficulty dealing with the rigorous treatment and isolation from friends and other sources of psychological support when they are struggling with their appearance and identity as well as establishing autonomy. The vulnerability imposed upon the patient by the disease and required treatment conflicts with a natural sense of immortality. These issues can best be addressed before and during hospitalization for transplantation through input from family, friends, and teachers to the multidisciplinary team (i.e., physician, nurse, psychologist, social worker) caring for the adolescent (see Chapter 51).

As already discussed, allogeneic bone marrow transplantation from an HLA-identical, mixed lymphocyte–culture nonreactive sibling is the treatment of choice for severe aplastic anemia. The cytoreduction regimen must provide adequate immunosuppression of the recipient, as many patients can be shown to have T lymphocytes that suppress hematopoietic cells. Cyclophosphamide administered in high dosage over four consecutive days, with or without antilymphocyte globulin or total lymphoid irradiation, is the most common regimen for adolescent patients undergoing transplantation for aplastic anemia. Multiply transfused aplastic anemia patients become sensitized to non-HLA determinants on donor cells and are more likely to reject the transplanted bone marrow. Researchers in Seattle examined the role for donor leukocyte infusions in addition to marrow transplantation for adolescent patients who have received numerous transfusions prior to transplantation (Fig. 54–1). The buffy coat cells provide additional T lymphocytes to counter graft rejection but are associated with an increased incidence of chronic GVHD. Factors that influence outcome positively include younger age of the recipient, lack of prior transfusion, and lack of GVHD.

Patient selection and timing are key for demonstrating the efficacy of any therapy, but they are particularly important for an intensive treatment such as marrow

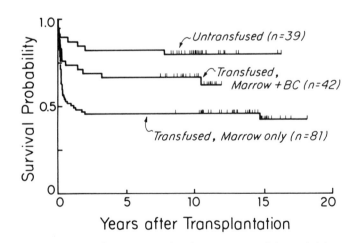

Figure 54–1. Kaplan-Meier product limit estimate of the probability of survival after HLA-identical marrow transplantation, comparing untransfused aplastic patients with transfused aplastic patients receiving marrow only versus those receiving marrow plus buffy coat. All patients received methotrexate for graft-versus-host disease prophylaxis. BC, buffy coat. (With permission from Loughran TP, Storb R: Treatment of aplastic anemia. In Forman SJ [ed]: Bone Marrow Transplantation. Hematol Oncol Clin North Am 4[3]:568, 1990.)

transplantation. Initial efforts to treat adolescent patients who have had multiple relapses of leukemia and are in poor remission status documented the ability to obtain a response following the high-dose therapy in which conventional therapies were inadequate. Subsequent clinical studies have documented the ability to cure 60% to 80% of individuals with chronic myelogenous leukemia (CML) and 30% to 60% of individuals with acute leukemia following allogeneic bone marrow transplantation (see Chapter 53).

Individuals with acute myelogenous leukemia (AML) who undergo allogeneic bone marrow transplantation when in first remission have had an improved disease-free survival compared with those receiving additional conventional therapy. Comparison studies are currently in progress comparing allogeneic (when a sibling donor is available) or autologous bone marrow transplantation with conventional chemotherapy. The potential for cure (following allogeneic bone marrow transplantation in early relapse or second remission) of conventionally treated individuals who relapse must be considered in the analysis. Also, whether or not the autologous bone marrow was treated to reduce or eliminate leukemic cells (see further on) may have an impact on survival for individuals treated in that manner. Acute lymphoblastic leukemia (ALL) in patients less than 18 to 21 years of age can usually be treated successfully with conventional treatment regimens composed of systemic and intrathecal chemotherapy with or without prophylactic irradiation of the central nervous system. Disease-free survival of 50% to 80% can be anticipated for most of these patients. Individuals who relapse (particularly following treatment with current intensive treatment protocols), however, are not effectively treated without high-dose therapy and marrow transplantation. Thus, for individuals with ALL in second or subsequent remission, bone marrow transplantation is the treatment of choice (see Chapter 53). Treatment of these individuals with allogeneic transplantation results in 30% to 60% long-term disease-free survival. The other 40% to 70% of these patients will succumb to leukemic relapse, immediate complications of transplantation, or infection associated with chronic GVHD.

Normalization of hematopoiesis and immune function for individuals with constitutional marrow dysfunction or congenital immunodeficiency syndromes can be attained following allogeneic bone marrow transplantation. This includes diverse diagnoses such as Fanconi anemia, thalassemia, Chédiak-Higashi syndrome, osteopetrosis, Wiskott-Aldrich syndrome, and severe combined immunodeficiency syndrome. Correction of several congenital metabolic disorders (mucopolysaccharidoses, metachromatic leukodystrophy, adrenoleukodystrophy) has also been attempted by allogeneic bone marrow transplantation from normal (or heterozygous) donors. For maximum benefit, children should undergo transplantation before significant symptoms (especially of the central nervous system) develop. These transplants have most often been from unrelated or mismatched donors, as HLA-identical siblings unaffected by the metabolic disorder are not usually available. Future use of gene insertion and autologous marrow transplantation for congenital disorders or malignancies is currently being explored at the basic science level.

As previously discussed, individuals with recurrent or "high-risk" malignancies can benefit from intensive high-dose treatment and bone marrow transplantation. The number of adolescent patients with HLA-identical siblings, however, is limited. The size of families has decreased, and the incidence of divorce and remarriage has increased. As a result, the likelihood of an individual having an HLA-identical sibling has decreased. Except for malignancies involving the hematopoietic stem cells (myelodysplastic syndrome and CML), the patient's own marrow cells are not dysfunctional and can be used as a source of cells with which to reestablish blood cell production. The morbidity of GVHD is largely lacking (though autologous GVHD has been encountered), and immunosuppression to prevent GVHD is not required. However, recurrence of malignancy from cells contaminating the marrow or lack of graft-versus-leukemia can result in failure of this therapy.

The ability of most adolescent patients to be their own marrow donors has dramatically increased the number of individuals undergoing marrow transplantation. These patients must first attain an adequate remission status so that sufficient healthy hematopoietic stem cells can be harvested from the iliac crests. It may not be possible to collect sufficient cells from individuals who have been treated with extensive chemotherapy or irradiation to the iliac crests. Collection of peripheral stem cells by leukopheresis has been successfully employed by several centers as an alternative source of cells for reestablishment of marrow function. Autologous marrow transplantation is being evaluated as the treatment of choice for recurrent or progressive lymphomata, disseminated neuroblastoma, and several other solid tumors that are not effectively treated by current therapies. It is also being evaluated for treatment of individuals who lack an HLA-identical sibling donor and have acute myelogenous leukemia in first or subsequent remission and ALL in second or subsequent remission.

As already mentioned, there is at least a theoretical risk of "autografting" the malignancy one is trying to treat if viable tumor cells contaminate the autologous bone marrow used for reconstitution of hematopoiesis. Thus, several methods have been developed and applied for the elimination of tumor cells from the bone marrow harvested for autologous transplantation. The methods for purging tumor cells from the normal hematopoietic progenitor cells rely on the antigenic differences, differential chemotherapeutic sensitivity, and buoyant density differences of these cells. Monoclonal antibodies produced by hybridoma cells have been isolated that specify antigens differentially (in absolute or relative terms) expressed on tumor cells. These antibodies have been used with complement or conjugated to toxins for selective destruction of contaminating tumor cells. They have also been used with secondary antibody that has been joined to microscopic magnetic beads and flowed past powerful magnets for immunoseparation of tumor cells from the bone marrow. Drugs that have been incubated with bone marrow include activated derivatives of cyclophosphamide, corticosteroids, vincristine, and epipodophylotoxins.

For adolescent patients in whom marrow transplantation is indicated but who lack an HLA-identical sibling and in whom use of their own marrow is not appropriate (e.g., aplastic anemia, myelodysplastic syndrome, mucopolysaccharidoses), alternative sources of replacement marrow include related but not fully matched donors or unrelated individuals who are phenotypically identical at the HLA loci. Computerized marrow donor pools have been established. The HLA typing information of the donors can be compared with that of a potential recipient for identity (or close similarity). Racial and ethnic differences in the frequency of HLA expression cause difficulty in matching an individual whose race or ethnic background is underrepresented in the donor population. If a closely matched donor is identified, confirmatory HLA testing and mixed lymphocyte–culture must be performed. Appropriate efforts are taken to minimize inconvenience or imposition to the donor. However, these efforts do add to delays in proceeding to transplantation. Thus lack of a suitable donor or disease progression while attempting to coordinate a transplantation procedure unfortunately precludes this procedure for the majority of patients seeking an unrelated match. Despite an apparent identity, adolescents who undergo transplantation remain at high risk for graft rejection or severe GVHD and require extended immunosuppressive therapy, factors that reduce the likelihood of a successful outcome when compared with transplantation using an HLA-identical donor.

BIBLIOGRAPHY

Deeg HJ, Klingemann HG, Phillips GL: A Guide to Bone Marrow Transplantation. New York, Springer-Verlag, 1988.

Forman SJ (ed): Bone marrow transplantation. Hematol Oncol Clin North Am 4(3), 1990.

Nathan DG, Oski F (eds): Hematology of Infancy and Childhood. Philadelphia, WB Saunders, 1987.

Santos GW: History of bone marrow transplantation. Clin Haematol 12(3):611, 1983.

Endocrine and Growth Conditions

CHAPTER 55

Endocrine Conditions

MARY L. VOORHESS

THYROID DISORDERS

Disturbances of thyroid gland function are common among children and adolescents. The clinical picture varies from simple thyromegaly found incidentally on routine physical examination to the signs and symptoms of florid thyrotoxicosis. Since virtually every organ system requires appropriate amounts of thyroid hormone for normal operation, excess or deficiency of hormone may have profound pathophysiologic effects. The autoimmune thyroid disorders—Graves hyperthyroidism and chronic lymphocytic thyroiditis—account for the majority of acquired thyroid disorders in teenagers. Findings at presentation depend on the state of thyroid function. Nearly all patients have a goiter, which may be small or large. Girls are affected eight to ten times more often than boys. Many patients have a family history positive for goiter, hyperthyroidism, or hypothyroidism. In autoimmune disease there is a defect in immunoregulation that permits production of antibodies against one or more self-antigens. Probably genetic, immunologic, and environmental factors all are involved in the pathogenesis of disease. The differential diagnosis of teenage goiter is listed in Table 55–1.

Graves Disease

Graves disease is the most common cause of hyperthyroidism in adolescents. It occurs in genetically predisposed individuals of either sex at any age, although it is seen most frequently in adolescent and young adult females. Infiltrative ophthalmopathy and dermopathy may also develop and run a course quite independent of the hyperthyroidism.

PATHOPHYSIOLOGY

Autoantibodies usually of the IgG class are found in affected individuals. Most are stimulatory, but antibodies that are inhibitory to thyroid hormone synthesis and growth have also been found. The hyperthyroidism of Graves disease is caused by antibodies (thyroid-stimulating immunoglobulins) that bind to the thyroid-stimulating hormone (TSH) receptor and stimulate the thyroid gland. They mimic the action of TSH, with resultant hypersecretion of thyroid hormone. The inhibitory, or "blocking," antibodies (TSH-binding inhibitory immunoglobulins) appear to displace TSH binding, resulting

in hypothyroidism. Other anti–TSH receptor antibodies stimulate growth but not function. The presence of HLA-DR3 antigens appears to increase the susceptibility to Graves disease and to be identified with increased relapse rate following medical therapy.

Graves ophthalmopathy appears to be an autoimmune disorder of unclear pathogenesis. It may precede or follow the onset of hyperthyroidism. Even less is known about the cause of Graves dermopathy (pretibial myxedema).

CLINICAL MANIFESTATIONS

Graves disease may develop insidiously over several months or occur quite rapidly, so the clinical presentation is variable. Sometimes the first evidence of a problem is decline in performance and behavior changes noted by school teachers and often attributed to "adolescence." Nervousness, insomnia, palpitations, emotional lability, and large appetite are common. Significant weight loss may occur. Affected adolescents offer complaints of fatigue, muscle weakness, and increased perspiration.

Most adolescent patients have thyromegaly and mild eye prominence. The thyroid gland is usually symmetrically enlarged, smooth, nontender, and soft. If autoimmune thyroiditis coexists, however, the gland may be firm and irregular in contour. Size varies from a small goiter that is barely palpable to visible thyroid enlargement. A bruit caused by increased blood flow often is heard over the gland. Generally the ocular findings in childhood and adolescence are limited to the mild eye prominence or a stare (secondary to retraction of the upper lid and a wide palpebral fissure), conjunctival injection, and increased tearing. Often one eye is affected more than the other. Compared with adults, severe infiltrative ophthalmopathy and progressive exophthalmos are rare in adolescents; dermopathy seldom occurs. The affected area of the skin is brawny and nontender with an "orange peel" appearance. Red or hyperpigmented 5- to 10-mm plaques typically appear over the dorsum of the legs or feet.

Cardiovascular signs including tachycardia, wide pulse pressure, and overactive precordium are common. A systolic murmur is often heard. Tremors of the tongue and outstretched fingers are usually present. Tendon reflexes are brisk. The skin is smooth, warm, and moist.

**TABLE 55–1. Differential Diagnosis of
Goiter in Adolescents**

Autoimmune disorders
    Graves disease
    Chronic lymphocytic thyroiditis
Infections
    Acute suppurative thyroiditis
    Subacute thyroiditis (viral)
Simple goiter
Goitrogens
    Foods
    Drugs
Neoplasia
    Benign: adenoma, cyst
    Malignant
Defects in thyroid hormone synthesis and action
Iodine deficiency

DIAGNOSIS

If the adolescent has exophthalmos, thyromegaly, and clinical evidence of thyroid hormone excess, Graves disease is most likely. Confirmation of this diagnosis involves documentation of abnormally high serum concentrations of thyroxine (T_4), triiodothyronine (T_3) radioimmunoassay, and free T_4 together with suppression of TSH. Thyrotoxicosis associated with increased serum T_3 concentrations but a normal serum T_4 level (T_3 toxicosis) occurs in fewer than 5% of patients. Although the level of TSH receptor stimulatory immunoglobulin (TSI) is high in most patients with Graves disease, routine measurement is usually not performed. Determination of TSI is important when an adolescent with hyperthyroidism is pregnant, however, because the antibody crosses the placenta and may cause neonatal thyrotoxicosis. Measurement of antimicrosomal antibody and antithyroglobulin titers is helpful to diagnose Hashimoto thyroiditis. Sometimes Graves disease and Hashimoto thyroiditis occur together (Hashitoxicosis). Radioactive iodine uptake seldom is necessary. If the gland is nodular, a thyroid scan using iodine-123 or technetium-99m pertechnetate is desirable.

When there are no ocular abnormalities and hyperthyroidism is mild, Hashimoto thyroiditis or subacute thyroiditis may be present. Sometimes these adolescents become hypothyroid after several months if their gland is destroyed by the inflammatory process. When clinical hyperthyroidism is present and both thyroid hormone and TSH concentrations are abnormally high, a diagnosis of TSH-dependent hyperthyroidism or pituitary resistance to thyroid hormone should be considered. If T_3 and T_4 levels are equivocally high, a TRH stimulation test may be necessary to confirm the diagnosis of hyperthyroidism. Because thyroid hormones inhibit the response of pituitary thyrotropes to TRH, hyperthyroid adolescent patients do not have a rise in TSH level.

TREATMENT

Since no specific immunotherapy is available for adolescents with Graves disease, treatment is directed toward reducing thyroid hormone production by antithyroid drugs, subtotal thyroidectomy, or radioiodine ablation. Treatment must be individualized. For example, medical therapy generally requires compliance with drug therapy for at least 1½ to 2 years and should not be initiated if this condition cannot be met. Successful surgery requires a surgeon experienced in thyroid surgery.

The most commonly used antithyroid drugs are propylthiouracil and methimazole. These drugs act by inhibiting the organification of iodine during biosynthesis of thyroid hormone. Propylthiouracil also inhibits the peripheral conversion of T_4 to T_3. Both drugs may have a suppressive effect on the immune system, since a decline in circulating antibody titers has been observed when they are used for therapy for Graves disease. The initial dose of propylthiouracil for adolescents ranges between 300 and 600 mg/day orally in three divided doses every 8 hours. The dose of methimazole is 30 to 60 mg/day orally in three divided doses every 8 hours. Metabolites of the drugs are excreted largely in urine. Propylthiouracil and methimazole cross the placenta and also are found in breast milk.

Response to therapy varies: some adolescents show improvement in 3 to 4 weeks, while those with large glands and significant stores of preformed hormone may not respond for 2 to 3 months. Thyroid hormone levels should be checked every 6 to 8 weeks initially. When a clinical and chemical euthyroid state is achieved, the dosage of propylthiouracil or methimazole can be reduced by one third to one half to maintain thyroid hormone levels in the normal range. Subsequently, adolescent patients should be evaluated every 3 to 4 months. Generally it is necessary to continue drug therapy for a minimum of 1½ to 2 years. Then the medication is slowly tapered and discontinued when drug doses fall to very low levels (25 to 50 mg propylthiouracil daily), and the adolescent patient remains clinically and biochemically euthyroid. Continued thyroid enlargement during therapy suggests that relapse will occur if antithyroid drugs are stopped. Likewise, relapse is highly probable if anti–TSH-receptor antibodies remain elevated at the end of drug therapy. The median time of remission in children and adolescents treated with long-term medical therapy was 4 to 5 years in one study. Thus adolescents treated with propylthiouracil or methimazole for Graves disease may require years of treatment without a guarantee of permanent remission at the end.

Thiourea drugs may cause adverse reactions. The most common side effects are minor rashes that disappear spontaneously and transient leukopenia. Persistent rashes or leukopenia usually can be managed by substituting methimazole for propylthiouracil or vice versa. If significant toxic reactions such as agranulocytosis, drug fever, hepatitis, or lupus-like syndrome develop, therapy must be discontinued. The unpredictable outcome of medical therapy and the risks of reaction to thiourea drugs have led to increased use of radioisotopes for treatment.

β-Adrenergic blockade with propranolol (2.5 to 3.5 mg/kg/day orally in divided doses every 6 to 8 hours) is helpful in controlling the adrenergic findings of restlessness, tremor, palpitations, and perspiration that are present during thyrotoxicosis. When these manifestations have abated, therapy should be discontinued without abrupt withdrawal of the drug, to avoid β-blocker withdrawal syndrome. Use of the drug is contraindicated in asthma. Propranolol alone is not adequate therapy for Graves disease.

After hyperthyroidism is controlled with antithyroid drugs, subtotal or total thyroidectomy performed by a surgeon experienced in thyroid surgery results in minimal morbidity. Hypoparathyroidism and recurrent laryngeal nerve damage occur in fewer than 1% to 2% of patients. Sixty to 70% of patients develop permanent hypothyroidism and require levothyroxine therapy. Recurrence of thyrotoxicosis is rare.

Therapy with pharmacologic doses of iodine-131 is being used with increasing frequency for treatment of adolescents with Graves disease, since medical therapy may fail and long-term follow-up has revealed no apparent increased risk of leukemia and thyroid carcinoma. No genetic damage has been documented. It is the treatment of choice for adolescents who are noncompliant with antithyroid medication, who develop drug reactions, or who are poor surgical candidates. Radioiodine therapy induces a euthyroid state within a few months and is followed eventually by permanent hypothyroidism in most adolescent patients. Treatment of the hypothyroidism that occurs after surgery or radioiodine therapy for Graves disease does not require the frequent medical supervision that is necessary during the use of antithyroid drugs.

Chronic Lymphocytic Thyroiditis

Chronic lymphocytic thyroiditis (Hashimoto thyroiditis or autoimmune thyroiditis) is the most common thyroid disease of adolescence and accounts for most cases of asymptomatic thyromegaly. As many as 1.2% of school-age children have autoimmune thyroiditis (enlarged thyroid and detectable antibodies in the serum). The clinical presentation is variable, ranging from a euthyroid goiter to severe hypothyroidism. Occasionally, affected individuals will have transient hyperthyroidism. As in other autoimmune disorders girls are affected up to eight times as often as boys.

PATHOPHYSIOLOGY

Autoimmune thyroiditis is believed to result from an immunologic abnormality involving both cell-mediated immunity and humoral immunity. An inflammatory reaction occurs, and lymphocytic infiltration replaces normal thyroid tissue. Reactive hyperplasia and fibrosis take place. Antithyroglobulin or antimicrosomal antibodies are present in 90% to 95% of patients with chronic lymphocytic thyroiditis, but they are not specific for the disorder. Some individuals with high antibody titers and no apparent disease may subsequently develop overt thyroiditis. Other antithyroid antibodies also have been detected, including TSH blocking and stimulating as well as thyroid growth-stimulating antibodies. The latter may contribute to thyroid enlargement in some adolescents, and the TSH receptor stimulating antibody may cause the hyperthyroidism seen in chronic lymphocytic thyroiditis.

CLINICAL MANIFESTATIONS

Most adolescent patients are found to have a goiter on routine physical examination and have no symptoms or signs of thyroid dysfunction. The gland is often firm with a granular or pebbly surface. Occasionally nodules are palpable, and the right lobe may be larger than the left. Difficulty in swallowing and local tenderness are rare.

If the inflammatory process has been of long standing, deceleration of linear growth may be observed in young adolescents. Likewise, puberty may be delayed. Severe hypothyroidism is associated with lethargy, cold intolerance, dry skin, constipation, and mild obesity. Menstrual abnormalities and galactorrhea may occur. Rarely adolescents with chronic lymphocytic thyroiditis will have symptoms and signs of transient hyperthyroidism.

DIAGNOSIS

Studies should include measurement of serum T_4, TSH, antimicrosomal antibodies, and antithyroglobulin antibodies. If there are clinical findings consistent with hyperthyroidism, T_3 radioimmunoassay concentrations should also be checked. Since various drugs interfere with thyroid function tests, the physician needs to elicit the medications being taken by the young person to interpret the results. For example, birth control pills increase thyroid-binding globulin levels, raising serum T_4 levels; thus serum free T_4 levels need to be checked (see Chapter 73). Lithium is goitrogenic, and therapeutic doses of lithium carbonate may be associated with elevation of TSH concentrations, but overt hypothyroidism is rare.

Adolescents with chronic lymphocytic thyroiditis may have primary hypothyroidism, compensated hypothyroidism, or mild hyperthyroidism, or they may be euthyroid. The results of thyroid testing in each circumstance are listed in Table 55–2. Rarely TSH response to TRH is required to confirm a diagnosis of hyperthyroidism. Most adolescents also have abnormally high antibody titers (particularly antimicrosomal antibodies) at diagnosis or a few months later. When the thyroid is remarkably asymmetric or nodules are present, a scan should be performed with technetium-99m pertechnetate or iodine-123. The scan shows a spotty pattern of isotope uptake in Hashimoto thyroiditis. If a large cold area is identified, the possibility of adenoma or carcinoma should be considered.

TREATMENT

Adolescents with primary hypothyroidism should be treated with levothyroxine 2 to 3 μg/kg/day orally or a

TABLE 55–2. Thyroid Function in Chronic Lymphocytic Thyroiditis

	T_4	T_3	TSH
Primary hypothyroidism	Low	Low/normal	Elevated
Compensated hypothyroidism	Normal	Normal	Elevated
Hyperthyroidism	Increased	Increased	Undetectable
Euthyroid state	Normal	Normal	Normal

total daily dose of 100 to 200 µg indefinitely. If the adolescent patient is severely hypothyroid, it is appropriate to begin therapy with levothyroxine, 1 to 1.5 µg/kg/day, and increase the dose after 4 to 6 weeks. Patients should have T_4 and TSH levels checked every 3 to 4 months until they are euthyroid and then annually thereafter. A compliant patient seldom needs more than 200 µg/day to maintain a euthyroid state. Adolescents with compensated hypothyroidism also should receive levothyroxine treatment. There is no universal agreement about the need for therapy for adolescents with euthyroid thyroiditis because treatment does not appear to change the natural progression of the disease. Untreated adolescents require regular follow-up studies, however, since compensated or primary hypothyroidism may develop over time. If the goiter is large, treatment of euthyroid adolescents with Hashimoto thyroiditis for 1 to 2 years with levothyroxine usually results in a decrease in its size.

AUTOIMMUNE POLYGLANDULAR DISORDERS

Chronic lymphocytic thyroiditis and Graves disease may occur in association with other autoimmune disorders (Table 55–3). It is particularly important that physicians who care for adolescents with insulin-dependent diabetes mellitus (IDDM) monitor them at diagnosis and annually for autoimmune thyroid dysfunction and autoimmune adrenalitis (see Chapter 59). The prevalence of hypothyroidism or hyperthyroidism in association with diabetes mellitus is 0.3% to 3%, while the prevalence of Addison disease with IDDM is less than 0.03%.

Acute Suppurative Thyroiditis

Bacterial infection of the thyroid gland is rare, perhaps because the gland is encapsulated, making contiguous spread unlikely, and because its high iodine content is unfavorable for bacterial growth. Acute suppurative thyroiditis may occur in association with upper respiratory tract infection or with a congenital pyriform sinus fistula that serves as a route of infection to the gland.

TABLE 55–3. Disorders Occurring in Autoimmune Polyglandular Syndromes

Endocrinopathies
  Addison disease
  Insulin-dependent diabetes mellitus (IDDM)
  Autoimmune thyroid disease
  Acquired hypoparathyroidism
  Autoimmune primary hypogonadism
Some associated conditions
  Mucocutaneous candidiasis
  Pernicious anemia/gastritis
  Alopecia
  Vitiligo
  Malabsorption syndromes
  Chronic active hepatitis
Blizzard syndrome: Addison disease, hypoparathyroidism, mucocutaneous candidiasis (at least two of the conditions)
Schmidt syndrome: Addison disease and thyroiditis
Carpenter syndrome: Schmidt syndrome and IDDM

Staphylococcus aureus, Streptococcus hemolyticus, and pneumococcus are the major pathogens. Anaerobic organisms are frequently found with a pyriform sinus fistula.

CLINICAL MANIFESTATIONS

Clinical manifestations include chills, fever, sore throat, dysphagia, and a painful tender mass in the anterior neck in the region of the thyroid gland. The pain often radiates to the mandible and the ears and is particularly severe on palpation of the neck. Left-sided involvement suggests pyriform sinus fistula.

DIAGNOSIS

Results of thyroid function studies are usually normal. Sonography of the thyroid may demonstrate an abscess. Needle aspiration of the affected area provides culture material for diagnosis and identification of the organisms and antibiotic sensitivities. Barium swallow or fistulography is necessary to identify a pyriform sinus fistula.

TREATMENT

Parenteral, high-dose antibiotic therapy is essential for treatment of suppurative thyroiditis. If a sinus fistula is found, it must be surgically excised to prevent recurrence of disease. Full recovery is expected.

Subacute Thyroiditis

Subacute thyroiditis is a nonsuppurative inflammatory disease probably of viral etiology that usually is preceded by an upper respiratory tract infection. It is more common in adult females than adolescents. The clinical course often includes fever, malaise, and weakness. The thyroid gland is enlarged, smooth, and firm, with pain and tenderness to palpation. Signs and symptoms of mild hyperthyroidism caused by leakage of iodothyronines into the circulation may be noted. In these cases serum T_3 and T_4 levels are increased, and the TSH value is undetectable. Thyroid antibody titers usually are low early in the disease. In contrast with most cases of hyperthyroidism, the 24-hour radioactive iodine uptake is very low, reflecting damage to follicular cells. Patients who are asymptomatic but have these diagnostic findings are said to have "painless thyroiditis."

Subacute thyroiditis is a self-limited disease, but the clinical course may extend from a few weeks to several months. Generally only symptomatic treatment with aspirin or other antiinflammatory drugs is required to relieve the pain and discomfort. If the signs and symptoms of hyperthyroidism are significant during the acute phase of the disease, propranolol will effectively block the adrenergic effects of thyroid hormone excess. If the patient is acutely ill with viral thyroiditis, a brief course of glucocorticoid therapy (prednisone, 0.5 to 1.0 mg/kg/day orally every 8 hours for 1 week followed by gradual tapering of the dose over the next 2 to 3 weeks) usually is helpful. Transient hypothyroidism may develop during the course of the illness and should be treated with levothyroxine. Permanent hypothyroidism is rare after subacute thyroiditis.

Simple Goiter (Colloid Goiter)

Thyroid enlargement that is not associated with inflammation, infection, or neoplasia in a euthyroid individual is called a simple goiter. Generally the adolescent is asymptomatic. Thyroid hormone levels are normal, and thyroid antibodies are negative. The disorder occurs almost exclusively in girls, and often there is a family history of autoimmune thyroid disease.

The course of the goiter is variable. Thyroid growth factors such as TSH, growth-stimulating immunoglobulins, or epidermal growth factor may stimulate thyromegaly. An autoimmune process may be causal. The term *colloid goiter* was originally used to describe the disorder because histologic sections showed enlarged thyroid follicles filled with colloid. Clinical and laboratory studies have replaced biopsy for diagnosis.

Since thyroid function is normal no hormone replacement is necessary. Past reports of reduction in the size of the thyroid gland following thyroid therapy probably reflect the natural history of the goiter.

Thyroid Nodules

Management of thyroid nodules is difficult because one or more nodules may be found in any thyroid disease and there is no definitive study to diagnose malignancy except biopsy.

CLINICAL MANIFESTATIONS

Thyroid nodules are less common in adolescents than adults, but the incidence of carcinoma in nodules is higher, that is, 12% to 15% in adolescents versus 4% in adults. Clinical characteristics that are helpful but nonspecific in evaluating a patient with a thyroid nodule(s) are as follows: a firm solitary nodule suggests neoplasia, but the physical characteristics are poor predictors of malignancy; the risk of malignancy is less in a multinodular goiter than a solitary nodule; exposure to ionizing radiation increases the incidence of both benign and malignant nodules; and common thyroid diseases are not generally associated with thyroid cancer, although there are several reports describing patients with thyroid cancer and autoimmune thyroid disease. Local symptoms such as hoarseness, dysphagia, and obstruction may occur in adolescents with benign multinodular goiters or indicate invasion from thyroid cancer. Slow or rapid growth may occur with a benign or malignant lesion. Lymphadenopathy in the surrounding tissue of the neck suggests malignancy. A history of thyroid cancer in the family raises the possibility of medullary thyroid carcinoma and multiple endocrine neoplasia syndromes.

DIAGNOSIS

Thyroid hormone levels are usually normal in adolescents with a solitary nodule. Functioning nodules causing thyrotoxicosis are rare in adolescents; if present, they should be surgically excised. Sonography, radionuclide imaging, and biopsy are used in the evaluation of thyroid nodules. Sonography can determine the size of the gland and the nodule and can classify nodules as solid, cystic, or mixed solid and cystic. Often micronodules, which are undetectable by palpation, are identified. There are no specific sonographic characteristics that distinguish benign from malignant nodules. A solid nodule is most often benign, but it is more likely to be malignant than a mixed or cystic lesion. The most common isotopes used in scanning the thyroid are iodine-131 and technetium-99m pertechnetate. Nodules are classified according to their ability to take up the isotope: nonfunctioning nodules are "cold," hyperfunctioning nodules are "hot," and normally functioning nodules are "warm." Both cold and hot nodules are most likely benign; most malignant nodules are cold, however. Again, radioisotope scanning cannot distinguish a benign from a malignant nodule.

Fine-needle aspiration biopsy has been used extensively in adults as part of the initial evaluation of thyroid nodules. It provides more direct information than sonography or radioisotope scanning and appears to be an ideal approach to the cystic nodule because it may cure the lesion as well as identify it as benign or malignant. Aspiration biopsy has not been used extensively in adolescents because initial surgical excision is preferred by many pediatric endocrinologists and surgeons.

A trial of suppression of thyroid nodules by treatment with thyroid hormone to differentiate benign from malignant lesions is generally not recommended, particularly if biopsy has not been performed. Malignant tissue may contain TSH receptors and shrink in response to thyroid hormone.

TREATMENT

Lesions that are indeterminate or malignant by needle biopsy require surgical excision. Surgery is advised for cold nodules, particularly if the mass is firm, increasing in size, and associated with lymphadenopathy and other findings suggestive of tumor spread. When biopsy by needle aspiration is not a diagnostic option, excisional biopsy is appropriate for any suspicious solitary nodule. No further surgery is necessary if the mass is benign. If frozen section reveals cancer, total lobectomy should be performed on the side of the lesion, together with near-total removal of the contralateral lobe and excision of regional lymph nodes. Postoperative radioiodine treatment is given to identify and ablate residual functioning thyroid tissue, and metastases. All adolescent patients should be maintained on continuous thyroid hormone to suppress endogenous TSH production and inhibit stimulation of tumor growth.

PROGNOSIS

Fifty percent or more of solitary thyroid nodules are benign cystic or adenomatous lesions. Nearly all malignant neoplasms are carcinomas arising from follicular epithelium or parafollicular cells (C cell). Carcinoma of follicular origin is classified as papillary, follicular, or anaplastic. Carcinoma that is purely or predominantly papillary occurs more frequently in adolescents. Generally it grows slowly and remains localized to the thyroid gland for 20 to 30 years or more. Most papillary carcinomas contain some follicular elements, and metastases, if present, may consist predominantly of the latter. Mortality from thyroid carcinoma during adolescence is limited primarily to medullary carcinoma and anaplastic carcinoma.

ADRENAL DISORDERS

Adrenocortical Insufficiency

Deficient secretion of adrenal hormones results from disease of the adrenal cortex (primary adrenal insufficiency) or from inadequate secretion of adrenocorticotropic hormone (ACTH) by the pituitary (secondary adrenal insufficiency). Primary adrenal insufficiency is usually associated with decrease of glucocorticoids, mineralocorticoids, and adrenal androgens. ACTH deficiency affects glucocorticoids and androgens but does not significantly impair mineralocorticoid secretion, since the prime regulator of aldosterone synthesis is the renin–angiotensin system. The clinical manifestations of adrenal insufficiency may appear acutely (addisonian crisis) or may evolve gradually over many weeks or months. The latter is more common, probably because compensatory increases of ACTH and renin permit the adrenals to produce enough cortisol and aldosterone for daily maintenance. However, when the adrenals are approximately 90% destroyed, compensation fails and a crisis develops that is often triggered by a stressful event. Primary adrenal insufficiency is uncommon in adolescents. The most frequent cause of secondary adrenal insufficiency is prolonged administration of glucocorticoids, leading to suppression of the hypothalamic-pituitary-adrenal (HPA) axis. Causes of primary adrenocortical hypofunction are listed in Table 55–4.

PATHOGENESIS OF PRIMARY ADRENAL INSUFFICIENCY

Primary Atrophy (Addison Disease)

The most common cause (85% to 90%) of primary adrenal failure is autoimmune adrenalitis, a chronic

TABLE 55–4. Causes of Primary Adrenocortical Hypofunction

Autoimmune disease—adrenalitis (Addison disease)
Adrenal infection—bacterial, fungal, tuberculosis
Adrenal hemorrhage
Congenital adrenal hypoplasia—hereditary and nonhereditary
ACTH unresponsiveness
Adrenoleukodystrophy
Congenital defects in cortisol–aldosterone biosynthesis
Glucocorticoid therapy—chronic high dose (causes ACTH deficiency)

process that progresses to atrophy of all three zones of the adrenal cortex but does not destroy the medulla. In two thirds of cases, adrenal antibodies are found in the serum. Affected individuals may also have other endocrine deficiencies from autoimmune destruction of tissue. Adrenal insufficiency caused by infection is rare. Although tuberculosis was a common cause of Addison disease decades ago, it is seldom found now in developed countries. Likewise, adrenal failure from fungal diseases, metastases, and hemorrhage is rare. Postmortem examination reveals the adrenal to be the endocrine gland most commonly affected in acquired immunodeficiency syndrome (AIDS), both by opportunistic infection (50% of cases) and Kaposi sarcoma (12% of cases).

Congenital Adrenal Hypoplasia

Congenital adrenal hypoplasia occurs in two forms: miniature and cytomegalic. In the miniature form the adrenals are normal in structure but are extremely small. The disorder affects both sexes and can be sporadic or autosomal recessive. The cytomegalic form is an X-linked disease affecting only males and is characterized by large vacuolated cells that replace the normal adrenal architecture. The diagnosis of congenital adrenal hypoplasia usually is made in the newborn period because of a severe salt-wasting syndrome. The cytomegalic form is regularly associated with hypogonadotropic hypogonadism in adolescent males, resulting in delayed puberty (see Chapter 57). Glycerol kinase deficiency and congenital dystrophic myopathy may also occur in these patients.

ACTH Unresponsiveness

A rare hereditary disorder, ACTH unresponsiveness, is caused by an ACTH receptor defect in the adrenal and is associated with high ACTH levels, very low glucocorticoid levels, and normal aldosterone secretion. The diagnosis usually is made in childhood.

Adrenoleukodystrophy

Adrenoleukodystrophy is a rare X-linked recessive disorder that is associated with adrenal failure, progressive central demyelinization, blindness, deafness, dementia, and death. Some forms of the disease begin in childhood, while others present in the late adolescent or young adult years.

Congenital Defects in Cortisol-Aldosterone Biosynthesis

See section on congenital adrenal hyperplasia.

PATHOGENESIS OF SECONDARY ADRENAL INSUFFICIENCY

Secondary adrenocortical insufficiency is caused by deficient production of ACTH by the anterior pituitary. It may arise from a disorder of the hypothalamic-pituitary axis but more commonly is a consequence of chronic high-dose glucocorticoid therapy for treatment of nonendocrine disorders.

CLINICAL MANIFESTATIONS

The clinical manifestations of adrenal insufficiency vary according to the stage of the disease. When the adolescent patient has gradual onset of failure, the initial complaints usually are nonspecific, such as anorexia, weakness, and easy fatigue. Later on, weight loss, nausea, abdominal discomfort, alternating constipation and diarrhea, and postural dizziness are common. Irritability, loss of ability to concentrate, and depression may occur. Some adolescents become confused.

When adrenal reserve is expended, often provoked by infection or another stress, acute adrenal failure (addisonian crisis) ensues. This medical emergency is marked by nausea, vomiting, abdominal pain, extreme weakness, dehydration, hyponatremia, hyperkalemia, and shock. Often there is a disparity between the severity of the illness and the marked degree of dehydration and shock in the individual. Of course, adolescents with secondary adrenal insufficiency seldom have electrolyte disturbances.

Hyperpigmentation, especially of exposed skin, buccal mucosa, and pressure points, is a classic finding in long-standing primary adrenal insufficiency. Adrenal androgen deficiency in postpubertal females may lead to loss of axillary and pubic hair. Patchy areas of vitiligo also may be present owing to immunologic destruction of melanocytes.

DIAGNOSIS

Initial evaluation is directed toward defining whether the adolescent has primary or secondary adrenal insufficiency. Hyperpigmented skin together with the classic findings of adrenal failure strongly suggest primary adrenal disease. A history of steroid withdrawal in adolescents who have been on long-term glucocorticoid therapy suggests secondary adrenal failure.

Generally plasma levels of both cortisol and aldosterone are low in primary disease while ACTH is high. The early morning plasma cortisol level is less than 5 μg/dl and ACTH is greater than or equal to 150 to 250 pg/ml. The serum sodium level is low because of inability to conserve sodium, and the potassium value is high because of impaired renal secretion of K^+. Renin production is increased, and there is a low fasting blood glucose level, neutropenia with relative lymphocytosis, and eosinophilia.

Secondary adrenal failure is associated with a normal renin–angiotensin axis. The serum ACTH level is inappropriately low for the subnormal cortisol concentration.

The diagnosis of adrenal insufficiency can be further confirmed by documentation of a blunted cortisol response to ACTH stimulation using cosyntropin (Cortrosyn).

TREATMENT OF PRIMARY ADRENAL FAILURE

Adrenal Crisis

Acute adrenal insufficiency is a medical emergency and must be treated promptly with intravenous fluids using glucose to correct hypoglycemia and saline to correct hyponatremia. Hydrocortisone (hemisuccinate or phosphate) should be given as a bolus of 100 to 150 mg intravenously for adolescents and adults followed by 100 mg/m^2/24 hr administered continuously or in divided doses every 6 hours. As soon as the patient improves, the dose of hydrocortisone can be reduced. Mineralocorticoid therapy is usually not necessary until the daily dose of hydrocortisone is below 75 to 100 mg because of the salt-retaining activity in pharmacologic doses of cortisol. Fludrocortisone (Florinef) should then be added to the therapy. Usually fludrocortisone, 0.05 to 0.15 mg/day in a single oral dose given in the morning is sufficient. The dose should be adjusted based on hydration, serum electrolyte levels, and blood pressure. It is seldom necessary to treat hyperkalemia because serum K^+ levels decrease rapidly when the serum Na^+ concentration is restored to normal and dehydration is corrected.

Maintenance Therapy

Glucocorticoids are best given in a schedule that mimics the normal diurnal pattern of cortisol production, such as 20 mg of hydrocortisone orally in the morning and 10 mg early in the evening. Teenagers seldom need more than a total dose of hydrocortisone of 40 mg/day. Some individuals require a thrice-daily rather than a twice-daily cortisol dosage schedule to control afternoon weakness and fatigue. A mineralocorticoid is generally necessary for treatment of primary adrenal failure to correct aldosterone deficiency even though hydrocortisone has some salt-retaining effect. Fludrocortisone, 0.1 to 0.2 mg, given orally as a single dose in the morning is usually sufficient.

Adequacy of therapy is judged by a decrease in hyperpigmentation, correction of clinical manifestations of cortisol deficiency, and normalization of serum electrolyte and renin levels. During periods of stress the daily dose of glucocorticoid should be increased two or three times the usual maintenance level. When nausea and vomiting occur, parenteral glucocorticoids should be prescribed. The daily dose of mineralocorticoid usually does not need to be increased. All individuals with chronic adrenal insufficiency should wear a Medic-Alert necklace or bracelet.

TREATMENT OF SECONDARY ADRENAL FAILURE

The glucocorticoid regimen for secondary adrenal failure is similar to that described for primary adrenal failure except that mineralocorticoid therapy is seldom required, since aldosterone production is usually preserved. Because ACTH deficiency seldom is complete, the maintenance glucocorticoid requirement usually is one-half the dose for treatment of primary adrenal failure.

Adrenocortical Tumors

Adrenocortical tumors are rare in adolescents. Cortisol-producing adenomas are usually unilateral and pro-

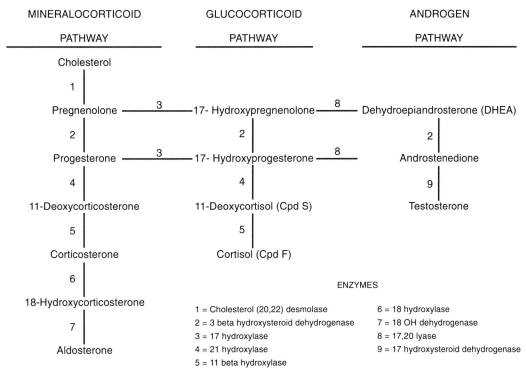

Figure 55–1. Simplified scheme of adrenal steroidogenesis. Congenital adrenal hyperplasia is caused by a specific deficiency of enzyme 1, 2, 3, 4 or 5.

duce only cortisol, so there are no clinical manifestations of sex steroid or mineralocorticoid excess. Most adrenal carcinomas, on the other hand, produce large amounts of all adrenocortical hormones, especially androgens. Primary hyperaldosteronism caused by an adrenal adenoma is exceedingly rare before the third decade but is suggested by the findings of hypokalemia with inappropriate kaliuresis, low upright plasma renin activity, and high plasma aldosterone concentration in a hypertensive adolescent. Nonfunctioning adrenocortical tumors usually are discovered unexpectedly, since there are no clinical manifestations of disease. After the appropriate hormone studies have identified the probable diagnosis of an adrenal neoplasm, abdominal computed tomography (CT) scan, adrenal magnetic resonance imaging (MRI), and sonography are usually effective in localizing the tumor. Adrenal scintigraphy and venography seldom are necessary. Surgical resection is the treatment of choice. It is essential that adolescents undergoing resection of adrenal tumors receive cortisol therapy before, during, and after surgery until the remaining adrenal gland is functioning normally.

Congenital Adrenal Hyperplasia

Congenital adrenal hyperplasia is an autosomal recessive disorder caused by absent or reduced activity of one of the five enzymes required for synthesis of cortisol from cholesterol. The cortisol deficiency is associated with compensatory ACTH excess, which causes the adrenal hyperplasia. Each enzyme deficiency produces characteristic changes in the production of adrenal ste-

roid hormones, their precursors, and their metabolites (Fig. 55–1). These alterations in the usual pattern of hormone secretion are used to diagnose the particular enzyme deficiency and account for the associated clinical findings. When the disorder presents at birth or in early childhood and is associated with total or nearly total enzyme deficiency, the affected individual is said to have a classic form of congenital adrenal hyperplasia. Partial enzyme defects that cause mild endocrine disturbances and are not diagnosed until the teenage or adult years are called the nonclassic (late-onset) forms of congenital adrenal hyperplasia.

The most common enzyme defect is 21-hydroxylase deficiency. Affected individuals have high plasma 17-OH progesterone levels. The disorder is associated with excess production of androgens in utero that causes ambiguous external genitalia in the newborn female. Progressive virilization with advanced somatic growth occurs after birth in both sexes unless treatment with cortisol (hydrocortisone) is initiated. In 75% of cases renal salt wasting occurs because of deficient aldosterone synthesis, and therapy with fludrocortisone is required.

CLINICAL COURSE

Lifelong treatment with hydrocortisone alone or in combination with a mineralocorticoid is necessary. When the diagnosis is made in infancy and excessive adrenal androgen secretion is controlled by adequate cortisol therapy, patients grow and develop normally during childhood. Most female infants require surgery to reduce the size of the clitoris and widen the introitus to prevent urologic problems. To permit adequate sexual activity, further revision of the vagina usually is required after puberty especially in adolescents with the salt-wasting form of the disease in which genital abnormalities are more severe. Females may have delayed menarche or irregular menses, particularly when adrenal androgen production is excessive. It is not clear whether the androgens alter the normal follicle-stimulating hormone/luteinizing hormone (FSH/LH) pattern or have a direct effect on the ovary. Strict medical management usually is required for normal menstruation and for fertility. Successful pregnancies are much more common in females with simple virilizing 21-hydroxylase deficiency than in those with the salt-losing form. Males have normal fertility, but small testes and aspermia have been reported with poor medical regulation. Postpubertal males with inadequate control of androgen secretion also may develop hyperplastic nodular testes because of adrenal rests in the gonads.

Fludrocortisone, 0.1 to 0.2 mg orally once daily, provides sufficient mineralocorticoid therapy for most adolescents with salt-losing 21-hydroxylase deficiency. Measurement of plasma renin activity is used to monitor the adequacy of dosage. Some patients diagnosed as having simple virilizing 21-OH deficiency without salt loss have a high plasma renin activity (indicating some aldosterone lack) and will benefit from mineralocorticoid treatment. This is particularly true in adolescent girls with congenital adrenal hyperplasia who have menstrual disturbances.

Maintenance glucocorticoid therapy is directed toward providing sufficient cortisol for cellular metabolism and also toward suppressing excess adrenal androgen production by inhibiting ACTH secretion. Many physicians prefer to give the largest dose of hydrocortisone at bedtime to inhibit the early morning ACTH surge. There is considerable variation in the glucocorticoid necessary for each individual. The usual replacement dose of hydrocortisone is 20 to 25 mg/m²/day divided into two to three oral doses. Dexamethasone, 0.25 mg given orally twice weekly at bedtime in place of the usual evening dose of hydrocortisone, appears to be helpful in decreasing adrenal androgen levels in adolescents whose androgen levels are difficult to regulate. Measurement of early morning serum 17-hydroxyprogesterone and Δ^4-androstenedione levels should be performed every 6 to 12 months to monitor the adequacy of medication.

Stress doses of glucocorticoid should be used in emergency situations (see section on adrenal crisis).

21-Hydroxylase Deficiency and HLA

Linkage between classic 21-OH deficiency and HLA has been demonstrated with a gene locus between HLA-B and HLA-DR on chromosome 6p. HLA haplotypes can be used in family pedigrees to predict heterozygote carriers and unaffected siblings of index cases. Prenatal diagnosis of congenital adrenal hyperplasia in the fetus at risk is possible in the first trimester by chorionic villus sampling and DNA analysis of genes within the HLA complex. In the second trimester, measurement of hormones in amniotic fluid as well as HLA typing or DNA analysis can be used for diagnosis. There is great interest

in prenatal treatment of 21-OH deficiency by administering dexamethasone to the pregnant mother early in the first trimester in an effort to prevent virilization of the external genitalia of the female fetus. Successful results have been reported in a few cases to date.

Nonclassic (Late-Onset) Congenital Adrenal Hyperplasia

Since the mid 1970s less severe disturbances of adrenal enzyme activity associated with milder endocrine disturbances and absence of genital abnormalities have been identified for 21-hydroxylase, 11β-hydroxylase and 3β-hydroxysteroid dehydrogenase. In fact, nonclassic 21-OH deficiency is reported to be the most common autosomal recessive defect in humans. Linkage of nonclassic 21-OH deficiency to HLA also has been confirmed and is distinct from the classic form.

CLINICAL MANIFESTATIONS

The clinical manifestations of nonclassic 21-hydroxylase deficiencies are variable and are perhaps related to sensitivity to androgens. Some individuals are clinically asymptomatic but have the biochemical abnormality (cryptic congenital adrenal hyperplasia). Others show signs of androgen excess such as premature development of pubic hair, advanced bone age, and linear growth acceleration. Mild to severe acne, amenorrhea or menstrual irregularity, and hirsutism occur in female adolescents. Sometimes the findings mimic polycystic ovary syndrome (see Chapter 70). Males may have acne, early beard growth, enlarged phallus with proportionately small testes, and advanced bone maturation in late childhood. Excess androgen is difficult to identify in male adolescents. There is no abnormality in salt retention in nonclassic congenital adrenal hyperplasia. Girls with nonclassic 3β-hydroxysteroid dehydrogenase deficiency have a clinical presentation similar to that of those with late-onset 21-OH deficiency.

DIAGNOSIS

Diagnosis of late-onset 21-OH deficiency is characterized by elevated baseline plasma levels of 17-OH progesterone (17 OHP) and increased 17 OHP response to intravenous ACTH (Cortrosyn, 0.25 µg IV) compared with normal subjects. HLA genotyping data show a high correlation between late-onset adrenal hyperplasia caused by 21-OH deficiency and HLA-B14 and HLA-Aw33. Patients with nonclassic 3β-hydroxysteroid dehydrogenase deficiency have abnormally high values of 17-OH pregnenolone and dehydroepiandrosterone (DHEA) following Cortrosyn stimulation, while those with nonclassic 11-OH deficiency may have abnormally high values of 11-deoxycortisol (compound S) and androstenedione.

TREATMENT

Treatment with prednisone or dexamethasone is effective in decreasing adrenal androgen production, but the clinical response is variable. A dramatic decrease in hirsutism in female adolescents seldom occurs. Additional experience with treatment of nonclassic congenital adrenal hyperplasia is required before clinical information about the outcome is established.

Withdrawal of Glucocorticoid Therapy

Withdrawal of glucocorticoids after the adolescent has received chronic steroid therapy for a prolonged period of time may be associated with (1) adrenal insufficiency from suppression of the HPA axis, (2) exacerbation of the primary disease for which the glucocorticoid was prescribed, or (3) steroid withdrawal syndrome.

Suppression of the HPA axis depends on the individual patient, the dose and duration of therapy, the drug half-life, the dosage schedule, and the route of administration. Long-acting compounds such as dexamethasone suppress the axis more than equivalent amounts of prednisone or hydrocortisone. Likewise, divided daily doses of drug suppress the HPA axis more than single morning doses. Physiologic replacement with glucocorticoid taken only in the morning usually does not suppress the axis. Alternate-day therapy given early in the morning is usually not associated with significant HPA suppression unless a high dose of medication is prescribed for years. If the patient has a cushingoid appearance, most likely the HPA axis is suppressed. Generally therapy with large doses of prednisone such as 30 mg/day for 1 month or 15 mg/day for 1 year will result in suppression. (Withdrawal after long-term therapy should be very gradual, until recovery of HPA axis function occurs.)

There is no universal agreement about the steps to follow when withdrawing glucocorticoids. If the HPA axis is significantly suppressed, full recovery may take as along as 9 to 12 months. Regardless of the withdrawal plan the physician must be alert to the possibility of acute adrenal insufficiency, particularly during stressful situations. Prudence dictates the use of pharmacologic doses of glucocorticoid (but not mineralocorticoid) during significant stress if the adolescent has received chronic steroid therapy during the past year, even though it is likely that a few adolescents will be treated unnecessarily (see the section on adrenal insufficiency for glucocorticoid dosage).

Following chronic steroid use, the dose of glucocorticoid may be reduced quickly to daily physiologic replacement and the adolescent will be protected from adrenal insufficiency. There may be exacerbation of the underlying disease for which therapy was prescribed, however. Therefore, gradual tapering of glucocorticoid dose is indicated when it is necessary to determine the minimum daily dose that will control the primary disease. When the ultimate goal is discontinuation of steroid therapy and the early morning plasma cortisol level is less than 5 μg/dl, a single morning dose of glucocorticoid in decreasing doses over 3 to 4 weeks or alternate-day therapy, depending on the previous dosing pattern, permits the HPA axis to recover. Glucocorticoid therapy is stopped when the early morning cortisol level reaches normal, signifying a functional HPA axis.

The metyrapone test, or insulin-induced hypoglycemia, occasionally may be indicated to assess adrenal recovery. It is unfortunate that a normal response to these pharmacologic stimuli does not guarantee physiologic responsiveness. Likewise a normal adrenal response to exogenous ACTH or Cortrosyn does not test the integrity of the HPA axis. It is simple and more practical, in most cases, to assume that the adolescent in an emergency situation has cortisol deficiency.

The steroid withdrawal syndrome is an interesting symptom-complex of unknown cause that may follow decreases in steroid dosage or surgical correction of endogenous cortisol excess in Cushing syndrome. The clinical manifestations suggesting glucocorticoid deficiency include low-grade fever, headache, arthralgia, myalgia, nausea, anorexia, vomiting, weight loss, and postural hypotension. They may be present for many weeks even when the adolescent is receiving physiologic or even pharmacologic doses of hydrocortisone. Some physicians have called the disorder "steroid addiction." Successful treatment requires effective psychosocial support and very gradual reduction of exogenous steroids.

Cushing Syndrome

Cushing syndrome results from chronic cortisol excess and is either ACTH dependent or ACTH independent. The source of the increased glucocorticoid is always the adrenal glands except in the case of exogenous steroid therapy. ACTH-dependent Cushing syndrome is caused by excessive pituitary ACTH secretion with resultant adrenal hyperplasia and hypercortisolism (Cushing disease) or secretion of ACTH by nonpituitary tumor with secondary adrenal hyperplasia and cortisol excess (ectopic ACTH syndrome) or exogenous ACTH therapy causing adrenal hyperplasia and hypercortisolism (iatrogenic Cushing syndrome). Non-ACTH-dependent Cushing syndrome results from adrenal tumors or micronodular adrenal disease (primary hypercortisolism) or from chronic administration of large doses of glucocorticoids (iatrogenic Cushing syndrome). Cushing syndrome is rare in adolescents except for the iatrogenic variety.

CLINICAL MANIFESTATIONS

The principal symptoms and signs of Cushing syndrome are listed in Table 55–5. The clinical picture is

TABLE 55–5. Signs and Symptoms of Cushing Syndrome

Weight gain and obesity (often centripetal)
Growth retardation (prior to closure of epiphyses)
Mineralocorticoid effects
   Hypertension, hypokalemia
Protein wasting
   Muscle wasting, thin skin, striae, ecchymoses
   Osteoporosis, hypercalciuria, weakness
Impaired glucose tolerance
Androgen effects
   Acne, hirsutism
Increased susceptibility to infections
Personality changes

quite variable, depending on the length and severity of the cortisol excess. Occasionally the diagnosis is strongly suspected based on clinical findings alone, and at other times detailed laboratory studies are required to establish the diagnosis. Cushing disease and adrenal adenomas are much more common in females, while ectopic ACTH syndrome and adrenal carcinoma are found equally in males and females.

Weight gain and generalized obesity are common presenting factors. When the disease is of long standing, truncal obesity with thin limbs (centripetal obesity) and moon facies are seen. Deceleration of linear growth rate occurs in those patients who have not reached adult stature prior to onset of hypercortisolism. Hypertension and skin changes including fragility, easy bruising, abdominal striae, plethora, and hypertrichosis are present in most patients. The occurrence of weakness and myopathy is variable. Hyperpigmentation is most marked in ectopic ACTH syndrome and absent in primary adrenal disease. When androgen production is increased, oily skin, acne, and hirsutism develop. Clitoromegaly signifies marked hypersecretion of androgen such as occurs with adrenal tumors. Depression is common in Cushing syndrome, and sometimes frank psychosis develops. Osteoporosis, hypercalcemia, and renal stones are less common in adolescents than adults.

DIAGNOSIS

Endocrine Studies

It is unfortunate that there is no simple biochemical test to distinguish those few patients with definitive Cushing syndrome from the majority of individuals who have "cushingoid features" caused by obesity. Most individuals with Cushing syndrome have loss of the normal diurnal pattern of cortisol secretion and excessive 24-hour urinary excretion of corticosteroids. Random or 8 A.M. and 8 P.M. determinations of plasma cortisol levels are of little diagnostic value, however, because most patients with Cushing syndrome have levels within the normal range, whereas stressed or depressed individuals may have high plasma cortisol concentrations.

A simple screening procedure is the overnight dexamethasone suppression test in which the patient takes 1 mg of dexamethasone at 11 P.M. The plasma cortisol level is measured at 8 A.M. the next morning. An 8 A.M. plasma cortisol value of less than 5 μg/dl and an ACTH level of less than 30 pg/ml rules out Cushing syndrome. An 8 A.M. plasma cortisol concentration greater than 5 μg/dl is not diagnostic of Cushing syndrome, however. If an accurate 24-hour urine specimen can be collected, measurement of free cortisol also provides good differentiation of Cushing syndrome from controls. When overnight suppression fails to occur, or urine cortisol excretion is high, further diagnostic studies are indicated.

The second diagnostic step is the 2-day low-dose dexamethasone suppression test in which 0.5 mg of dexamethasone is taken orally every 6 hours for 2 days (eight doses). Plasma cortisol is measured at 8 A.M. on

day 3. Most patients with Cushing syndrome show only partial or no suppression of plasma cortisol levels.

The third diagnostic step is the 2-day high-dose dexamethasone suppression test in which the adolescent takes 2 mg of dexamethasone orally every 6 hours for 2 days (eight doses). The plasma cortisol level is determined at 8 A.M. on day 3. Failure to suppress on the low-dose test combined with suppression to less than 5 μg/dl on the high-dose test is characteristic of Cushing disease. Adolescents who have adrenal tumors (benign or malignant) or ectopic ACTH-producing tumors typically fail to suppress with high-dose dexamethasone because the lesions function independent of ACTH control.

Some patients with Cushing disease or tumors causing Cushing syndrome will have false-negative or false-positive test results. Measurement of 24-hour urinary cortisol levels during the suppression tests may assist with diagnosis. Drugs that induce hepatic enzymes such as phenytoin may increase the metabolism of dexamethasone and alter suppression test results. Obviously if the index of suspicion of disease is high and test results are nondiagnostic, the tests should be repeated.

Serum ACTH levels consistently in the high-normal or moderately elevated range in the presence of hypercortisolism suggest Cushing disease. Normally, ACTH is suppressed when cortisol levels are high. Indeed, Cushing syndrome secondary to adrenal tumor is associated with low ACTH and high cortisol levels. Virilization in an adolescent with suspected Cushing syndrome suggests adrenal tumor (benign or malignant). Measurement of 24-hour urinary 17-ketosteroid excretion together with serum DHEA sulfate and testosterone may be helpful tumor markers.

Generally the corticotropin-releasing factor (CRF), Cortrosyn, and metyrapone tests rarely provide additional information over the standard diagnostic procedure in evaluation of suspected Cushing syndrome. Their use can be reserved for selected cases when diagnosis is difficult.

Nonendocrine Studies

In contrast with simple exogenous obesity, in which growth is generally accelerated, adolescents with Cushing syndrome prior to completion of growth "fall off" the growth curve. Routine blood chemistry results are usually normal. Hypokalemia occurs when there is excessive mineralocorticoid secretion from the adrenals. The white blood cell count generally is elevated because of demargination of white blood cells, while lymphocyte and eosinophil counts are relatively low. Carbohydrate intolerance may develop because glucocorticoids antagonize insulin action and promote glycogenolysis and gluconeogenesis.

LOCALIZATION OF LESION

When pituitary overproduction of ACTH is suspected, CT scan or MRI of the head should be performed. Sometimes no apparent structural abnormality is found, even in a patient who is subsequently found to have Cushing disease. CT of the abdomen is helpful in

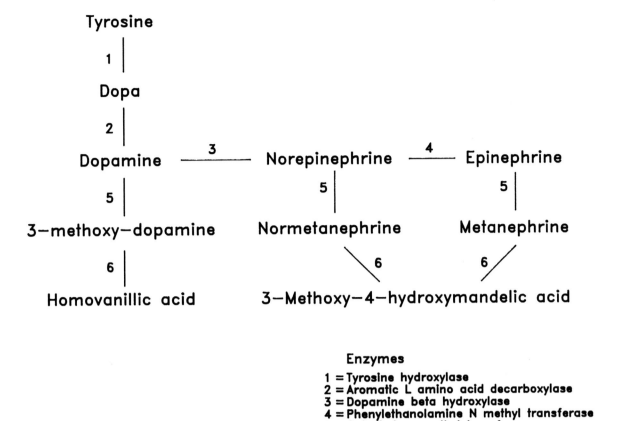

Figure 55–2. Schematic representation of catecholamine synthesis and metabolism.

identifying adrenal tumors. Sonography may provide additional assistance. These imaging studies have largely replaced angiography in identifying an adrenal tumor. Adrenal scanning using radioiodinated contrast material is available in a few medical centers. Its use may be helpful in localizing unilateral adrenal lesions.

Ectopic ACTH-producing tumors are rare in adolescents but have been found in carcinoid tumors of the thymus, in adrenal rest tissue, and in the pancreas. CT scan of the chest may define thymus lesions that are not visible on routine chest radiographs.

TREATMENT

Treatment obviously depends on the underlying cause. Surgical removal of tumor is the best option when possible. Pituitary microsurgery through the transsphenoidal approach is the initial therapy of choice for Cushing disease even when a microadenoma of the pituitary has not been demonstrated by CT scan or MRI. Sometimes the tumor is not visible until surgery. Microadenectomy or removal of part of the central mucous zone of the pituitary corrects the hypercortisolism promptly. Other pituitary functions usually are preserved, and morbidity is low when the procedure is performed by an experienced neurosurgeon. Bilateral adrenalectomy or pituitary irradiation are options if transphenoidal surgery is contraindicated or fails. Use of pharmacologic agents such as cyproheptadine to control ACTH secretion is associated with poor results but may be useful for temporary supportive therapy.

Adrenal adenoma and micronodular disease are treated with surgical excision. Usually the contralateral adrenal is suppressed, so glucocorticoid therapy is required until function is restored. If adrenal carcinomas cannot be fully resected and metastases are present, mitotane is used to control the disease. Metyrapone, ketoconazole, and aminoglutethimide—compounds that inhibit cortisol production—can be used to control the chemical effects of cortisol excess.

Pheochromocytoma

Pheochromocytoma is a rare tumor during the adolescent years. Most commonly it is located in the adrenal medulla, but it can arise from chromaffin tissue anywhere in the body. Bilateral adrenal and multiple tumors may be present. The great majority (90% to 95%) are benign. Familial pheochromocytoma may occur as a single disorder or as part of the multiple endocrine neoplasia syndromes.

PATHOPHYSIOLOGY

Pheochromocytomas arise from cells of the sympathoadrenal system and thus are able to synthesize, store, and release the catecholamines dopamine, norepinephrine, and epinephrine. Figure 55–2 is a schematic diagram depicting catecholamines and their primary metabolites. The physiologic effects of the catecholamines are mediated through adrenergic receptors on the surface of the target cell membrane. The hormone receptor interaction triggers the events that lead to the specific biologic effect of each amine. Norepinephrine stimulates primarily α-adrenergic receptors, causing constriction of blood vessels and a rise in systolic and diastolic blood pressure (see Chapter 67). Epinephrine induces both α- and β-adrenergic receptor activity. The activity of β_1 receptors enhances myocardial contractility, heart rate, and atrioventricular conduction. The β_2 receptors are concerned with bronchodilation and vasodilation. In addition to cardiovascular effects, adrenergic receptor activity mediates basic metabolic processes, including glycogenolysis, lipolysis, and insulin inhibition. The α-adrenergic receptor is blocked selectively by phentolamine or phenoxybenzamine. Propranolol blocks the β-adrenergic receptor.

CLINICAL MANIFESTATIONS

Most clinical manifestations result from the pharmacologic effects of the catecholamines that are released from the pheochromocytoma into the circulation. Since the rate of production and metabolism of amines by the tumor is not constant, the clinical findings vary. Paroxysmal or sustained hypertension usually brings the adolescent to medical attention (see Chapter 67). Orthostatic hypotension may relate to an inability to activate sympathetic reflexes on standing. Headache, sweating, nausea and vomiting, visual disturbances, and weight loss are common. Tremor, tachycardia, and weakness may be noted. Some individuals complain of intermittent abdominal pain and chronic constipation. Acrocyanosis and cool extremities develop when there is pronounced peripheral constriction of blood vessels.

When catecholamine excess and hypertension are severe and of long standing, retinopathy, encephalopathy, and cardiomyopathy with cardiac failure may develop. Abnormalities of glucose metabolism suggest diabetes mellitus. Indeed, pheochromocytoma may also masquerade as essential hypertension, thyrotoxicosis, renal disease, or psychosis. Physicians caring for pregnant adolescents should be aware that pheochromocytomas may first manifest during gestation, labor, or delivery and are associated with high maternal and fetal mortality (see Chapter 74). The tumor also may occur in association with neurofibromatosis, cerebellar hemangiomas, multiple endocrine adenomatosis, Cushing syndrome, and polycythemia.

DIAGNOSIS

Measurement of urinary vanillylmandelic acid or normetanephrine-metanephrine is a satisfactory screening test for a pheochromocytoma. Diagnosis of pheochromocytoma is confirmed by finding abnormally high levels of the catecholamines and normetanephrine-metanephrine or vanillylmandelic acid in a 24-hour urine sample. It is very rare to find normal values of both norepinephrine, epinephrine, and their metabolites when a hormone-secreting pheochromocytoma is present. When paroxysmal attacks suggesting catecholamine release occur and results of analysis of a 24-hour urine sample are inconclusive, measurement of catecholamines in timed urine samples collected during and after an attack will identify whether the episode is associated with catecholamine excess. When an individual is on medication during sample collection, it is very important to be certain the drug will not interfere with the analyses.

Most adolescents with pheochromocytoma also have markedly elevated plasma norepinephrine and epinephrine levels. There is general agreement that a single plasma catecholamine value should not be used as the sole diagnostic test. There is overlap between plasma catecholamine levels among adolescents with essential hypertension and pheochromocytoma. Furthermore, many drugs interfere with the plasma catecholamine assay; adolescent patients whose tumors secrete amines intermittently may have normal values during normotensive intervals; and sample collection technique, emotional stress, and so on affect plasma catecholamine values. Measurement of catecholamines and metabolites in a 24-hour urine sample reflects output over a prolonged period, whereas the concentration of plasma catecholamines can change from minute to minute because of the short half-life of the amines. The use of pharmacologic tests (e.g., tyrosine, glucagon, histamine) to diagnose pheochromocytoma is very seldom helpful and may provoke a hypertensive crisis. False-positive and false-negative results are common. The recently devised clonidine test is also problematic.

LOCALIZATION OF TUMOR

After the diagnosis of a pheochromocytoma has been confirmed by documentation of abnormally high levels of catecholamines and metabolites, studies should be directed toward localization of tumor.

CT scan and MRI will detect tumors with remarkable accuracy. Metaiodobenzylguanidine (MIBG) scintigraphy is particularly helpful for extraadrenal tumors and for metastatic disease, but false-negative results sometimes occur owing to limited tracer uptake by tumor cells. The use of these three techniques has largely eliminated the need for arteriography and venous sampling. As a general rule, patients with a pheochromocytoma should be treated with α-adrenergic receptor blocking drugs before angiography is performed to obviate a hypertensive crisis if there is a sudden release of catecholamine by the tumor.

TREATMENT

The goal of therapy is to correct the excess catecholamine production. Surgical excision of the tumor(s) is the treatment of choice. This should be done as soon as the patient has been prepared for surgery, using α-adrenergic blockade alone or in combination with β-adrenergic blockade. When excision is not possible, pharmacologic agents can be used to inhibit catecholamine synthesis and to establish adrenergic blockade.

PREOPERATIVE TREATMENT

Generally 10 to 14 days of preoperative adrenergic blockade is required to control hypertension and the other physiologic and metabolic consequences of norepinephrine and/or epinephrine excess. This treatment also decreases the potentially serious intraoperative complications, such as hypovolemic shock, that can occur in the absence of adrenergic blockade. The amount of drug required varies from patient to patient and needs to be titrated upward until the desired response is achieved. Phenoxybenzamine (Dibenzyline) is a long-acting oral α-adrenergic blocker that has been used for years for treatment of pheochromocytoma and is usually well tolerated. A starting dose of phenoxybenzamine, 10 to 15 mg every 12 hours orally, should be satisfactory for an adolescent. The daily dose can be increased every 3 to 4 days as necessary. Phentolamine (Regitine), a short-acting adrenergic blocking agent, is particularly effective for intravenous use when acute control of blood pressure is necessary. It is also effective when given orally but has the drawbacks of short duration of action and frequent side effects.

Adolescents whose tumors produce excessive amounts of epinephrine and/or who have serious tachyarrhythmias may require treatment with β-adrenergic blocking drugs. β-Adrenergic blockade should not be prescribed until adequate α-adrenergic blockade has been achieved to protect the heart from unopposed alpha stimulation. Propranolol is an effective drug. The dose should be carefully titrated upward to achieve the desired effect.

INTRAOPERATIVE TREATMENT

There should be careful monitoring of blood pressure and cardiac function from the induction of anesthesia to the end of surgery. With appropriate preoperative preparation intraoperative crisis should be avoided. Parenteral sodium nitroprusside is effective for management of hypertensive episodes, and propranolol can be used for arrhythmias. Hydrocortisone should be available for parenteral use if bilateral adrenalectomy is required.

POSTOPERATIVE CARE

Transient hypertension may be present for 24 to 36 hours postoperatively. Persistent high blood pressure suggests residual tumor or renovascular disease. All patients, regardless of their cardiovascular status, should have repeat measurements of their catecholamines before discharge to be certain the values have returned to normal. Continued long-term follow-up is recommended because the tumor may recur years later. In addition, the patient and family members should be observed for multiple endocrine neoplasia syndromes.

Malignant Pheochromocytoma

Malignant pheochromocytoma is rare (<10%) in adolescents. There are no biochemical features that definitely distinguish malignancy, although dopamine and homovanillic acid levels often are high in malignant pheochromocytomas. The tumor spreads to bone, lymph node, liver, and lung. Malignant pheochromocytoma is generally resistant to radiation therapy and chemotherapy. MIBG therapy may be useful in some patients. Chronic therapy with α-adrenergic blockade and with

α-methyltyrosine (Demser) can be used to control the clinical manifestations of catecholamine excess. Long-term survival for many years is possible.

Multiple Endocrine Neoplasia Syndromes

The multiple endocrine neoplasia (MEN) syndromes are familial disorders characterized by hyperplasia or tumor involving more than one endocrine gland. The disorders are inherited in a mendelian autosomal dominant pattern with variable expressivity and high penetrance. The clinical manifestations may indicate a single gland endocrinopathy for years before multigland involvement becomes manifest. Every adolescent patient with a tumor of one gland should be evaluated regularly for involvement of other endocrine glands. Likewise, family members should be screened. The pathogenesis of the syndromes is not known. Most tumors of the MEN syndromes are derived from cells of the APUD series (*a*mine content, amine *p*recursor *u*ptake and amino acid *d*ecarboxylase activity), so there appears to be a relationship between cell type and tumor.

MEN TYPE 1

MEN type 1 (Werner syndrome or multiple endocrine adenomatosis 1 [MEA1]) is characterized by tumors of the anterior pituitary gland, the islet cells of the pancreas, and the parathyroid glands as well as adenomas of the thyroid gland and the adrenal cortex. Rarely, other neoplasms such as lipomas, carcinoid tumors, and thymomas may be present. MEN type 1 is rare before age 10 and typically begins between 20 and 40 years of age.

Hypercalcemia caused by parathyroid adenoma or hyperplasia is the most common abnormality, especially after age 18 years. The pituitary tumors may be nonfunctional and cause insufficiency or produce growth hormone and cause acromegaly or secrete ACTH or prolactin. Pancreatic tumors may be benign or malignant and secrete insulin, glucagon, or gastrin. Zollinger-Ellison syndrome may develop. Surgical resection is the prime treatment for the tumors.

MEN TYPE 2A

MEN type 2A (Sipple Syndrome or MEA II) is composed of medullary carcinoma of the thyroid, pheochromocytomas, and parathyroid hyperplasia or tumor. Linkage studies using DNA probes have mapped the gene to chromosome 10.

Medullary thyroid carcinoma arises from the C cells of the thyroid gland and is inherited as an autosomal dominant trait. It may occur as a sporadic case (?new mutation), as a familial disorder, or as part of the MEN syndromes. Most often the patient is asymptomatic, and there is no evidence of thyroid disease on physical examination. The C cells of the thyroid and medullary thyroid carcinoma produce the hormone calcitonin. The occurrence of high levels of basal plasma calcitonin or abnormal calcitonin secretion in response to provocative testing with a calcium gluconate infusion or pentagastrin stimulation identifies adolescents with medullary thyroid carcinoma. Total thyroidectomy is the treatment of choice. A careful search for a catecholamine-secreting pheochromocytoma always should be done preoperatively in adolescent patients who have other components of the MEN syndromes so the pheochromocytoma can be removed first. All family members should be screened yearly for medullary thyroid carcinoma when one affected individual is identified. Aggressive screening leads to early diagnosis and reduces the risk of metastatic disease.

MEN TYPE 2B

The major components of MEN type 2B (MEA III) are multiple neuromas, medullary thyroid carcinoma, and pheochromocytoma. Affected adolescents often have a marfanoid habitus without ectopic lentis or aortic abnormalities. Skeletal abnormalities including high palate, pectus excavatum, pes cavus, and dorsal kyphosis are common. Most individuals have mucosal neuromas on lips and tongue as well as numerous gastrointestinal complaints related to alimentary ganglioneuromatosis. The neuromas are not subject to carcinomatous change, and there is no specific treatment for them. Once again, a search should be made for pheochromocytoma and medullary thyroid carcinoma and arrangements made for appropriate treatment and follow-up.

PARATHYROID DYSFUNCTION

There usually are two pairs of parathyroid glands; one pair is derived from the third and the other from the fourth pharyngeal pouches. The latter attaches to the posterior portion of the thyroid capsule, while the pair from the third pouch is positioned near the lower pole of the thyroid. Sometimes accessory or aberrant glands are found adjacent to the thyroid, beneath the sternum or in the mediastinum.

Parathyroid hormone (PTH) is the secretory product of the chief cells of the parathyroid glands. After secretion, it is cleaved into an N-terminal fragment that possesses full biologic activity and a carboxyl terminal fragment that is inactive. The carboxyl terminal fragment predominates in the peripheral circulation and is said to be a good reflection of overall gland activity. Levels of this fragment are usually increased in patients with hyperparathyroidism.

The ionized plasma calcium concentration is the principal regulator of PTH secretion. Diminished calcium concentration increases synthesis and release of PTH, whereas increased levels of ionized calcium inhibit both processes. PTH binds to receptors in bone and kidney and stimulates adenylate cyclase activity, which results in formation of cyclic adenosine monophosphate (AMP). Cyclic AMP mediates intracellular PTH action. PTH induces bone resorption, with release of calcium and phosphorus into extracellular fluid. In the kidney, it causes phosphaturia and increased resorption of calcium and magnesium. It also increases renal excretion of sodium, potassium, amino acids, and bicarbonate. PTH stimulates conversion of 25-OH vitamin D to 1,25 $(OH)_2$ vitamin D in the kidney. The 1,25 $(OH)_2$ vitamin D in turn stimulates intestinal absorption of calcium. Knowledge about these actions of PTH provides a basis for understanding the pathophysiology of hypoparathyroidism and hyperparathyroidism.

Hypoparathyroidism

PARATHYROID HORMONE DEFICIENCY

The de novo diagnosis of hypoparathyroidism is uncommon in adolescence. Congenital absence of the parathyroids such as occurs in DiGeorge syndrome is recognized early in infancy. Idiopathic hypoparathyroidism can develop at any age but is most often manifest between 5 and 15 years of age. Usually it occurs sporadically, but autosomal dominant inheritance has been described. Hypoparathyroidism associated with autoimmune disease and other endocrine deficiencies often begins in childhood. In fact, sometimes the adolescent is believed to have isolated hypoparathyroidism because many years may pass between the appearance of parathyroid deficiency and another endocrine disorder. Damage to the parathyroid glands is a known risk of neck surgery, especially subtotal or total thyroidectomy for treatment of thyrotoxicosis or thyroid cancer. Sometimes the dysfunction is transient owing to edema and compromise of blood supply to the parathyroids, whereas at other times permanent hypoparathyroidism develops and treatment with vitamin D is required. The parathyroids are quite resistant to radiation injury and seldom are destroyed by metabolic disease. Rarely, patients who acquire massive iron deposits from chronic transfusion therapy may have decreased parathyroid reserve.

RESISTANCE OF PTH SYNDROME

In resistance of PTH syndrome the parathyroids secret PTH in normal or increased amounts, but the target cells in bone and kidney show an inadequate response to the hormone. Several types have been described.

Pseudohypoparathyroidism (PHP) Type I

In PHP type I borderline or low hypocalcemia, hyperphosphatemia, and high serum levels of PTH are present. There is a failure of urinary cyclic AMP excretion to rise significantly in response to PTH, suggesting a receptor defect. Affected individuals also have short stature, obesity, round face, short metacarpal and metatarsal bones, subcutaneous and cutaneous calcium plaques, and basal ganglia calcification. Intellect is usually retarded. Hypothyroidism and diabetes mellitus occur with increased frequency.

Pseudohypoparathyroidism Type II

PHP type II is very rare and is characterized by hypocalcemia, hyperphosphatemia, and high levels of

PTH. Affected individuals respond to PTH with an increase in cyclic AMP but no concomitant phosphaturic response, suggesting a postreceptor defect. There are no associated somatic abnormalities.

Pseudo Pseudohypoparathyroidism

Individuals with pseudo PHP resemble those with PHP type I in phenotype but have normal calcium, phosphorus, and PTH levels, together with normal end-organ sensitivity to PTH.

Pseudohypohyperparathyroidism

Patients with pseudohypohyperparathyroidism have renal resistance to PTH but normal bone responsiveness and may have osteitis fibrosa, presumably the result of PTH secretion. A wide spectrum of renal and skeletal end-organ–resistant syndromes are being described.

CLINICAL MANIFESTATIONS

The clinical picture depends on the etiology of the disorder and the chronicity of the PTH deficiency (Table 55–6). Most patients come to medical attention because of neurologic signs and symptoms from the hypocalcemia, including paresthesias, muscle cramps and rigidity, laryngeal stridor, tetany, and convulsions. Chvostek and Trousseau signs may be positive. A prolonged QT interval appears on the electrocardiogram. Central nervous system manifestations include papilledema, dystonia, and nonspecific electroencephalographic changes. Some patients have neuropsychiatric manifestations. Other features include cataracts, dry and thickened skin, scanty hair growth, brittle nails with transverse ridges, and diarrhea. Dental defects are more pronounced when hypoparathyroidism develops early in life. Individuals whose hypoparathyroidism is caused by autoimmune dysfunction may manifest candidiasis, vitiligo, and alopecia areata. Postsurgical hypoparathyroidism is often transient, and the early clinical manifestations are caused by hypocalcemia.

DIAGNOSIS

Hypocalcemia, hyperphosphatemia, and inappropriately low serum PTH concentrations are the biochemical hallmarks of classic hypoparathyroidism. When parathyroid function is normal, hypocalcemia is associated with high, rather than low, serum PTH levels.

TABLE 55–6. Findings in Idiopathic Hypoparathyroidism

Neurologic abnormalities due to hypocalcemia
Prolonged QT interval and abnormal T wave on ECG
Increased intracranial pressure
Mental changes—irritability, paranoia, depression
Cataracts
Ectodermal abnormalities
   Dry and thick skin, ridged and cracked nails, dental defects,
     sparse hair, cutaneous moniliasis, alopecia, vitiligo
Basal ganglia calcification
Diarrhea
Other endocrine deficiencies: adrenal, thyroid, gonadal

Thus, the syndromes of end-organ resistance to the action of PTH are associated with high PTH levels.

The administration of PTH causes a marked increase in urinary excretion of cyclic AMP in normal and hypoparathyroid subjects but not in those with PHP type I. Of course the previously described somatic abnormalities associated with PHP type I are very helpful in establishing the diagnosis. Radiographs will demonstrate the shortened metatarsal and metacarpal lesions and occasionally reveal subcutaneous bone formation and basal ganglia calcification. No specific radiologic features are found in classic hypoparathyroidism. Rarely in long-standing untreated disease osteomalacia is observed, probably related to $1,25(OH)_2$ vitamin D deficiency.

TREATMENT

The goal of treatment in hypoparathyroidism is to maintain normal serum calcium concentrations and avoid chronic hypocalcemia and hypercalcemia. Serum calcium levels should be maintained between 8.5 and 9.5 mg/dl, and urinary calcium excretion below 0.25 mg calcium per milligram of creatinine or 3 mg calcium/kg/ day.

When symptomatic hypocalcemia is present, initial therapy should be directed toward increasing plasma calcium concentrations. Ten percent calcium gluconate, 10 to 20 ml, given slowly intravenously over 10 minutes with monitoring for bradycardia and hypotension, is usually appropriate for acute correction of hypocalcemia. Subsequent intravenous therapy using calcium gluconate at a dose of 50 mg/kg/day diluted in 5% dextrose solution can be given. Serum calcium levels should be measured at least every 12 hours. When symptoms of hypocalcemia are mild, oral elemental calcium 4 to 5 g/day in divided doses every 4 to 6 hours may be prescribed for adolescents. The serum calcium level can be expected to increase by about 0.5 mg/dl for every gram of oral calcium given per day. Calcium carbonate contains 40% calcium by weight and is an appropriate salt to use when large doses of medication are required.

There is no PTH preparation available for treatment of hypoparathyroidism, so vitamin D is prescribed when the diagnosis of hypoparathyroidism is made. Vitamin D therapy is directed toward restoration of normal serum $1,25(OH)_2$ vitamin D_3 concentrations and increasing intestinal calcium absorption. The required maintenance dose of vitamin D varies from person to person and must be individualized to avoid hypercalcemia. It is prudent to begin with a low dose and increase it in a stepwise manner until serum calcium values are in the normal range. Dihydrotachysterol (DHT, structurally similar to 1-OHD) is preferred because of its more rapid onset of action and shorter half-life than vitamin D_3. The usual maintenance dose of DHT is 0.01 to 0.02 mg/ kg/day in a single dose. The onset of the maximal effects is about 2 weeks. Serum calcium and phosphorus levels should be monitored three to four times a week until normal calcium levels are obtained, followed by monthly and then 3-month and ultimately 6-month intervals. Urine calcium excretion should be monitored at every visit after eucalcemia is obtained. Anticonvulsant therapy may increase the requirement for vitamin D, probably because of its effect on 25-OH vitamin D levels.

1,25$(OH)_2$ vitamin D_3 (calcitriol) has a rapid onset of action with duration of activity from a single dose of 3 to 5 days, making it theoretically ideal for treatment of hypoparathyroidism because hypocalcemia and hypercalcemia states can be corrected quite promptly. However, experience has shown rather wide serum calcium fluctuations with its long-term use. Calcitriol is an ideal medication for treatment of transient hypoparathyroidism, however. The starting dose is 1,25$(OH)_2$ vitamin D_3 0.25 µ/day orally. Serum calcium values should be monitored daily. The maximum daily dose required for eucalcemia rarely exceeds 1.5 to 2 µg. When changing from vitamin D_3 to another preparation such as calcitriol it is important to remember that vitamin D_3 has a much longer onset of action than its metabolites and that its duration of action may extend for many weeks.

Some patients require 1200 to 1500 mg of oral elemental calcium supplementation divided in three doses per day in addition to vitamin D therapy for eucalcemia. If hypercalciuria develops, calcium intake should be discontinued and the vitamin D dose decreased or temporarily discontinued.

Primary Hyperparathyroidism

Hyperparathyroidism is uncommon in adolescents. It may occur as familial hyperparathyroidism with autosomal dominant inheritance or as part of the MEN syndromes. Hyperplasia of the parathyroid glands rather than a single adenoma is the rule. Most teenagers are symptomatic at presentation, although routine biochemical screening does identify some adolescents with mild hypercalcemia who are free from symptoms.

CLINICAL MANIFESTATIONS

Signs and symptoms are related to bone, kidney, gastrointestinal tract, central nervous system, and neuromuscular dysfunction. The osteolytic action of PTH leads to bone and joint pain, tenderness, and sometimes abnormal gait. When hypercalcemia is significant, the adolescent has polyuria and polydypsia, renal colic from stone formation (nephrolithiasis), reduced glomerular filtration rate from parenchymal disease, and increased renin production leading to hypertension. Nausea, vomiting, abdominal pain, and constipation are frequent complaints. When the serum calcium level is 15 to 16 mEq/liter, encephalopathy manifested by emotional lability, confusion, impaired memory, depression, and hallucinations is present. Hypercalcemia has a depressant effect on neuromuscular activity, leading to weakness, muscle hypotonicity, and easy fatigue. The adolescent may have difficulty in rising from a squatting position.

DIAGNOSIS

Typically the diagnosis is based on the clinical manifestations and on the finding of hypercalcemia, hypo-

phosphatemia, and increased amounts of carboxyl terminal fragments of PTH (iPTH) on radioimmunoassay. Serum calcium concentrations are often only modestly elevated (11 to 11.5 mg/dl) and may fluctuate on repeated measurement, and iPTH levels may fall in the normal range, making diagnosis somewhat difficult. Hypercalcemia with elevated iPTH occasionally may be found in patients with nonparathyroid tumors that secrete a PTH-like substance and also in patients with secondary hyperparathyroidism associated with chronic renal disease.

Radiographs show bone demineralization, subperiosteal resorption of bones especially in the phalanges, loss of lamina dura on dental films, lytic lesions of the skull, and cysts in the long bones. Nephrocalcinosis and nephrolithiasis may be present. Sonography and CT scan of the neck may identify an adenoma. Few medical centers are able to do selective thyroid vein catheterization to identify the site of the PTH excess secretion.

TREATMENT

Hypercalcemic crisis is rare in teenagers. Emergency treatment consists of vigorous intravenous hydration and sodium diuresis together with low calcium intake and elimination of vitamin D. Parathyroid adenomas are surgically excised. Subtotal parathyroidectomy or total parathyroidectomy with autotransplantation of some of the parathyroid gland into the patient's forearm is used to treat hyperparathyroidism from parathyroid hyperplasia. Patients who have had resection of parathyroid adenomas may have transient hypoparathyroidism for several weeks or months and require treatment as previously outlined.

Secondary Hyperparathyroidism

Secondary hyperparathyroidism may occur in chronic renal disease, intestinal malabsorption disorders, and osteomalacia. The persistent hypersecretion of PTH may produce bone disease of varying degrees of severity.

ENDOCRINE DISORDERS OF THE PITUITARY AND HYPOTHALAMUS

The pituitary gland is composed of two distinct parts: the anterior pituitary or adenohypophysis, which is derived from Rathke's pouch, and the posterior pituitary or neurohypophysis, which forms from an outpouching of the floor of the third ventricle. The pituitary is located in the sella turcica and is separated superiorly from the subarachnoid space by reflections of dura, which form the diaphragma sellae. The pituitary is connected to the hypothalamus by the pituitary stalk, which runs through the diaphragma sellae and is composed of neural elements and the hypophyseal portal vasculature. Releasing hormones secreted by hypothalamic neurons flow down the portal system in the pituitary stalk to the anterior pituitary. In response to the releasing hormones, cells of the anterior pituitary, in turn, secrete their specific tropic hormone, which stimulates activity of target endocrine glands. Since the hypothalamus and the anterior pituitary are outside the blood-brain barrier, there is connection with the systemic circulation. Not only are the topic hormones of the anterior pituitary subject to classic negative feedback regulations, but also they are influenced by the external environment; that is, the light-dark cycle influences ACTH and cold exposure stimulates TSH. Furthermore, the hypothalamus serves as a link between the nervous system and the endocrine system and also controls many other functions, such as temperature, hunger, thirst, and behavior. Thus lesions in the hypothalamus can cause neurologic, endocrinologic, and psychic disturbances. If the pituitary stalk is injured near the hypothalamus, the normal vascular connections to the pituitary can be interrupted, producing hypopituitarism. Expanding intrasellar lesions may encroach on the hypothalamus and cause signs and symptoms of dysfunction (i.e., diabetes insipidus).

Disorders of the hypothalamic-pituitary axis fall into the broad etiologic categories of congenital, tumors, inflammatory or infiltrative lesions, infection, vascular lesions, trauma, radiation induced, and idiopathic. Some of the disorders cause significant endocrinopathy during childhood (e.g., dysgerminomas cause precocious puberty) and are diagnosed during the first decade of life, while others are associated with hypogonadism (Kallmann syndrome) and are not recognized until puberty is delayed.

The majority of hypothalamic-pituitary disorders common to the adolescent years cause disturbances of growth, pubertal maturation, and reproductive function (see Chapters 56, 57, 70, and 78).

Hypopituitarism

DISEASES OF THE ANTERIOR PITUITARY

Clinical Manifestations

The symptoms of hypopituitarism are variable, depending on the specific hormone involved and the progression of disease. Generally, hypopituitarism develops gradually over many months unless it follows hypophysectomy, acute infarction, or trauma, because the destructive process must involve about 75% of the gland before clinical manifestations are evident. Hormone deficiencies often occur in the following order: (1) growth hormone, (2) gonadotropin, (3) TSH, and (4) ACTH. Growth hormone deficiency is suspected when there is deceleration of linear growth during childhood and early adolescence, but its presence is not clinically evident in late adolescence or adulthood. Delayed puberty or secondary amenorrhea in female adolescents and decreased libido and impotence together with decreased beard growth and sexual hair in male adolescents indicate gonadotropin insufficiency. In acute absence of TSH the signs and symptoms of hypothyroidism develop within 4 to 6 weeks; otherwise the onset of clinical findings is very gradual. Signs of ACTH deficiency are subtle because adolescents with hypopituitarism are able to conserve sodium. In fact if hyponatremia is present it probably is caused by water retention rather than sodium loss. Prolactin deficiency does not cause clinical findings except in postpartum necrosis of the pituitary.

In addition to endocrine dysfunction, adolescents with hypopituitarism will have other clinical abnormalities, depending on the basic etiology of the disease (i.e., signs of increased intracranial pressure with a tumor).

Diagnosis

Evaluation of adolescents with suspected hypopituitarism consists of imaging studies of the HPA axis and measurement of pituitary tropic hormones, target gland hormones, or both.

Lateral skull radiography can be used as a screening test for enlargement of the sella turcica and localized erosion of bone, but CT scan, MRI, or both are much more definitive tests. If a tumor is suspected, visual fields also should be examined.

Pituitary insufficiency is present when the target gland hormone concentration is low and the pituitary tropic hormone concentration is normal or low. Thus gonadotropin deficiency in the late adolescent and young adult male is associated with low serum testosterone and low serum LH concentrations. In late adolescent girls and young adult women FSH deficiency is indicated by amenorrhea, immature vaginal cytology, and normal or low FSH. Low free thyroxine concentration combined with a normal or low TSH level indicates TSH deficiency. Although a low early morning plasma concentration of cortisol paired with a normal or low ACTH level suggests ACTH deficiency, ACTH secretory reserve is best measured by the cortisol response to insulin-induced hypoglycemia or to the metyrapone test. Growth hormone reserve is also measured by provocative testing with arginine, insulin, or levodopa (see Chapter 56).

Hormone Treatment in Hypopituitarism

Pituitary hormones *per se* are not used in therapy except when fertility is desired and cyclic therapy with parenteral gonadotropins is prescribed. Otherwise target gland hormones are used. Levothyroxine, 3 to 5 µg/kg/day orally, meets thyroid hormone requirements. Adequate replacement of adrenal glucocorticoids usually is achieved by prescribing hydrocortisone, 20 mg orally in the morning and 10 mg orally at supper time. Patients should be instructed to increase their dose in times of stress and to give parenteral therapy when oral medication cannot be taken. Mineralocorticoid therapy is not usually necessary in treatment of hypopituitarism. Testosterone therapy and estrogen-progesterone treatment requirements are outlined in Chapter 57. Growth hormone therapy is not prescribed after the epiphyses have closed and adult height has been achieved. Replacement of target gland hormones restores the patient to good health, and the prognosis for longevity is excellent if the patient is compliant with appropriate hormone therapy.

EXCESS PITUITARY HORMONE SECRETION

Most pituitary lesions in adolescents cause deficiency of hormones by destruction or compromise of pituitary tissue or by interruption of the hypophyseal-portal circulation in the pituitary stalk. Rarely an adenoma will be identified that secretes excessive amounts of a pituitary hormone. Acromegaly and gigantism occur with excessive growth hormone secretion. ACTH excess causes Cushing disease. Galactorrhea occurs in euthyroid female adolescents with prolactin-secreting adenomas. TSH- and gonadotropin-secreting tumors of the pituitary are extremely rare and are essentially diagnosed only in adults.

Diabetes Insipidus

In diabetes insipidus the kidney is unable to conserve water because antidiuretic hormone (ADH, vasopressin) is not synthesized or is not released from the neurohypophyseal system (central diabetes insipidus) or the kidney fails to respond to ADH (nephrogenic diabetes).

PATHOPHYSIOLOGY

ADH is synthesized in the hypothalamic supraoptic and paraventricular nuclei and is transported along axons in the neurohypophyseal tract in the pituitary stalk for storage in the posterior pituitary. Destruction of the posterior pituitary usually causes only a mild urine concentration defect because adequate amounts of ADH are delivered into the systemic circulation from the pituitary stalk. In contrast, hypothalamic injury with trauma to the supraoptic and paraventricular nuclei or neurohypophyseal damage high in the pituitary stalk most often causes permanent diabetes insipidus.

ADH released into the bloodstream is carried to the kidney, where it conserves water and concentrates urine by altering the permeability of the distal renal tubule. ADH attaches to a specific vasopressin receptor, and its effect is mediated by increased production of cyclic AMP.

Normally ADH secretion is regulated primarily by osmoreceptors located in the supraoptic nuclei and also by changes in blood volume or blood pressure. Increased osmolality and decreased volume stimulate ADH release. Stretch receptors in the left atrium inhibit ADH release during hypervolemia, whereas baroreceptors in the carotid sinus stimulate ADH release during hypotension. In addition to plasma osmolality, blood volume, and blood pressure, other factors can influence ADH secretion. For example, stress, pain, upright position, nicotine, and barbiturates cause increased ADH secretion while recumbent position, alcohol, and phenytoin decrease secretion.

There may be virtual absence of ADH in the presence of hypothalamic destructive lesions such as craniopharyngioma, pinealoma, histiocytosis, granulomatous disease, or head trauma. If osmotic stimuli are impaired, ADH may not be released until plasma osmolality is very high. Sometimes no underlying lesion is found, and the disorder is classified as idiopathic central diabetes insipidus. Most of these cases are sporadic, but vasopressin-deficient diabetes insipidus sometimes occurs in families as an autosomal dominant or X-linked recessive disorder.

Nephrogenic diabetes insipidus is usually diagnosed in infancy. The disease is the result of renal unresponsiveness to ADH, probably caused by a defect in the receptor adenylate cyclase system.

CLINICAL MANIFESTATIONS

The most common clinical manifestations are persistent polyuria, thirst, and polydypsia, which occur day and night. Affected persons generally prefer ice water. When ADH deficiency is severe, fluid intake and output may be 10 to 12 liters or more per day. Urine is dilute, and urine osmolality is below serum osmolality. As long as patients have a normal thirst mechanism and free access to fluids they usually will drink enough to avoid dehydration. Hypernatremia may develop when the osmoreceptor mechanism is defective, the thirst center is defective, or fluids are not available.

Patients who do not empty their bladder frequently enough to keep pace with urine output may develop bladder distention, hydronephrosis, and even renal insufficiency.

Adolescents also may have manifestations of an underlying disease causing the diabetes insipidus, such as increased intracranial pressure secondary to a brain tumor.

DIAGNOSIS

The possibility of diabetes insipidus should be considered in any adolescent with unexplained polyuria and polydypsia. If the adolescent has significant hypernatremia and inappropriately dilute urine that is corrected by administration of ADH, the diagnosis of central ADH-sensitive diabetes insipidus is most likely. Repeated low serum sodium concentrations even in the early morning suggest that the polyuria is caused by excess fluid intake or renal tubular disease. Compulsive water drinkers usually do not drink at night and have no particular preference for ice water, in contrast with patients with ADH deficiency. They may be difficult to differentiate from those with central ADH deficiency, however, because chronic excessive water intake may wash out the renal concentration gradient so urine concentration does not increase significantly with water deprivation.

Water deprivation stimulates ADH release. Restriction of fluid in an ADH-deficient patient results in depletion of extracellular water, rise in plasma osmolality, and weight loss. Before starting a water deprivation test, hypercalcemia, hypokalemia, and renal failure should be excluded. The duration of fluid restriction required for diagnosis depends on the severity of disease, so the patient must be under constant monitoring during the test. Adolescents with severe diabetes insipidus have the potential to develop serious hypernatremia and dehydration when fluids are denied. Likewise, observation prevents adolescents with psychogenic polydypsia from drinking fluids surreptitiously.

Several protocols for water deprivation tests have been devised. A simple test involves fluid deprivation for 7 to 8 hours. The test is started in the morning after a night of unrestricted food and fluid intake and a regular breakfast. Then no food or fluid is given until the test is completed. Body weight, urine specific gravity, and volume are measured at 8 A.M. and every subsequent hour. Serum sodium and urine and serum osmolality are measured before, at noon, and at the end of the test. If weight loss greater than 5% occurs before 8 hours, the test should be terminated.

In adolescents with ADH deficiency or nephrogenic diabetes insipidus, there should be little reduction in urine volume. The urine specific gravity remains less than 1.005, and urine osmolality remains below 150 mOsm/kg. At the end of the test the serum sodium level is greater than 150 mEq/liter, serum osmolality is greater than 290 mOsm/kg, and weight loss is usually more than 5%. Adolescents with partial ADH deficiency may modestly reduce their urine output and concentrate urine, but they never attain normal concentrating ability. Healthy individuals and compulsive water drinkers should attain a urine specific gravity of 1.010 or higher, urine output should decrease, and significant weight loss does not occur. A final urine to serum osmolality greater than 1.5 and/or a change in urine/serum osmolality of 1.0 or more indicates normal ability to concentrate urine. Although theoretically useful, measurement of ADH by radioimmunoassay has not been diagnostically accurate in diabetes insipidus.

An ADH test may be performed at the end of the water deprivation study. Subcutaneous administration of 5 units of aqueous vasopressin or 1 μg of desmopressin will result in reduction of urine output and a greater than 50% rise in urine osmolality in patients with central diabetes insipidus. Adolescents with nephrogenic diabetes insipidus, on the other hand, fail to raise urine osmolality above that of plasma when given ADH.

When a diagnosis of central diabetes insipidus has been established, it is mandatory to study the HPA axis in a search for tumor or the empty sella syndrome.

TREATMENT

The synthetic analogue of ADH, desmopressin, is the preparation most commonly used for treatment of diabetes insipidus caused by ADH deficiency. The medication is administered intranasally through a plastic tube in doses up to 40 μg (0.4 ml) daily for older children and adults. Most patients require desmopressin, 10 μg (0.1 ml), twice daily. The dose must be determined for each patient and adjusted according to the response. Desmopressin administered by nasal spray (rather than rhinal tube) may be used when the required dose is greater than 0.1 ml. Desmopressin is also available for subcutaneous and intravenous use. The antidiuretic dose of desmopressin given by injection is about one tenth of the intranasal dose.

Chlorpropamide has been used to treat patients with partial diabetes insipidus. The drug induces antidiuresis in proportion to its ability to release ADH. A dose of 200 to 500 mg of chlorpropamide once daily is usually effective. Hypoglycemia is a potential side effect of chlorpropamide, but it can be avoided by a regular schedule of eating.

There is no specific therapy for nephrogenic diabetes insipidus. The most useful therapy is chlorothiazides and dietary sodium restriction. Hydrochlorothiazide, 50 to 100 mg/day, and a low sodium diet often will reduce urine output by 30% to 40%. Inhibition of prostaglandin synthesis with ibuprofen or indomethacin has been reported to reduce urine volume and increase urine osmolality. Drug-induced nephrogenic diabetes insipidus may occur in adolescents receiving demeclocycline or lithium, with the defect disappearing when the drugs are discontinued.

Syndrome of Inappropriate Antidiuretic Hormone Secretion

The syndrome of inappropriate ADH secretion (SIADH) is a disorder in which there is increased release of ADH in spite of subnormal plasma osmolality. The classic features include hyponatremia, low plasma osmolality, urine that is less than maximally dilute, urine sodium concentrations greater than 20 mEq/L (unless there is severe sodium depletion), no edema or hypovolemia. The urine usually is more concentrated than plasma. Renal, adrenal, and thyroid function are normal.

SIADH is found in association with disorders of the central nervous system, including trauma, hemorrhage, infections, hydrocephalus, Guillain-Barré syndrome, lupus erythematosus, malignant tumors that may or may not synthesize ADH, stress, and acute psychosis. Drugs such as tricyclic antidepressants, vincristine, and cyclophosphamide may also cause water intoxication.

In addition to eliminating the primary disorder, treatment consists of restricting fluid intake to produce a negative fluid balance. When hyponatremia is marked, parenteral furosemide and saline solution have been advocated as a rapid means of treating patients. The physician must guard against depletion of potassium and other electrolytes.

BIBLIOGRAPHY

Bachrach LK, Foley TP Jr: Thyroiditis in children. Pediatr Rev 11:184, 1989.
Kaplan SA: Clinical Pediatric Endocrinology. Philadelphia, WB Saunders, 1990.
Lifshitz F (ed): Pediatric Endocrinology. A clinical guide, 2nd ed. New York, Marcel Dekker, 1990.
Lippe BM, Landau EM, Kaplan SA: Hyperthyroidism in children treated with long-term medical therapy: Twenty-five percent remission every two years. J Clin Endocrinol Metab 64:1241, 1987.
Mulaikal RM, Migeon CJ, Rock JA: Fertility rates in female patients with congenital adrenal hyperplasia due to 21-hydroxylase deficiency. N Engl J Med 316:178, 1987.
Orgiazzi J: Management of Graves hyperthyroidism. Endocrinol Metab Clin North Am 16:365, 1987.
Robertson GL: Differential diagnosis of polyuria. Am Rev Med 39:425, 1988.
Schteingart DE: Cushing's syndrome. Endocrinol Metab Clin North Am 18:311, 1989.
Speiser PW, LaForgia N, Kato K, et al: First trimester prenatal treatment and molecular genetic diagnosis of congenital adrenal hyperplasia (21-hydroxylase deficiency). J Clin Endocrinol Metab 70:838, 1990.
Winter WE, Maclaren NK: Autoimmune endocrinopathies in pediatric endocrinology. In Lifshitz F (ed): Pediatric Endocrinology. A Clinical Guide, 2nd ed. New York, Marcel Dekker, 1990.

CHAPTER 56

Disorders of Growth

PINCHAS COHEN and RON G. ROSENFELD

The final critical growth period before adulthood occurs during puberty. Linear growth is a sensitive indicator of the health of adolescents, both physically and mentally. It is often during early puberty that previously unrecognized growth disorders become apparent or that previously subtle abnormalities become obvious. Adolescence is often the last opportunity for intervention in the growth process before fusion of the epiphyseal plates occurs.

Puberty and the associated growth spurt are characterized by multiple endocrine and nonendocrine events. Pathology in any one of these processes can be manifested by growth failure. A full understanding of the physiology of normal growth is necessary for the physician to evaluate growth problems. Primarily, one must be able to differentiate between the normal variants of short stature, such as constitutional delay of growth (and puberty), that constitute the majority of cases and other less common conditions. Familiarity with the diagnostic tools available for the workup of these individuals is essential. Bone age determinations and judicious use of pituitary hormone testing and other laboratory tests are among these indispensable tools. Supportive therapy and reassurance are often all that is required, but endocrine therapy, particularly with recombinant growth hormone or with sex steroids, is advocated in certain cases.

PHYSIOLOGY OF GROWTH

Endocrine Regulation of Growth

Although multiple hormones influence growth, the main regulator of postnatal growth is growth hormone (GH). This hormone is secreted in a pulsatile manner from the anterior pituitary as a 22-kd molecule (although other forms may be found). Under normal waking conditions, GH levels are often low or undetectable, but several times during the day, and particularly at night during phase 3 of sleep, surges of GH secretion occur. GH secretion is mainly under hypothalamic control, which in turn is regulated by catecholaminergic neurotransmitters from higher cortical centers. The hypothalamic hormones or growth hormone releasing hormone (GH-RH) and somatostatin stimulate and inhibit, respectively, GH secretion. Many other factors influence this interaction—notably, glucose, which inhibits, and certain amino acids, which stimulate, GH secretion.

Exogenous physiologic and pharmacologic factors are known to stimulate GH secretion. Indeed, some of these agents, which include clonidine, levodopa, and exercise, are used in GH stimulation tests. In plasma the majority of GH is bound to a carrier protein termed *GH binding protein,* which appears to be identical to the extracellular domain of the GH receptor.

In the liver and other target cells, through interaction with its receptor, GH induces the production of somatomedins, or insulin-like growth factors (IGF-I and IGF-II). IGFs are found in plasma bound to a family of proteins called IGF-binding proteins. Both IGFs and their binding proteins are reduced in GH deficiency. The somatomedins, particularly IGF-I/SM-C, are believed to interact with target organs, such as growing cartilage to induce growth; they may also feed back on the pituitary to inhibit GH secretion. This cascade of growth control, known as the somatomedin hypothesis, is summarized in Figure 56–1. It is still uncertain, however, whether all the anabolic actions of GH are mediated by the somatomedins.

Other endocrine factors that are involved in the regulation of growth include thyroid hormone, which is essential for normal linear skeletal growth, and glucocorticoids, which can stunt growth when present in excess (see Chapter 55). Sex steroids, through several direct and indirect mechanisms, can accelerate growth and normally facilitate the pubertal growth spurt. When present in excess at an earlier age, the resulting acceleration of growth is associated with premature closure of the epiphysis and reduced adult height. Parathyroid hormone and vitamin D are essential for normal skeletal ossification, and the absence of, or resistance to, these agents is associated with abnormal growth patterns (see Chapter 55). Nonendocrine factors affecting growth are many and incompletely understood; by far the most important are genetic factors that determine the growth rate, the age of puberty, and the adult height. Psychological and social influences can prevent the genetic potential for growth to be fully expressed. Malnutrition, either through dietary deficiencies or malabsorption or as a manifestation of chronic illness, can interrupt normal growth. It is interesting that GH levels are often elevated in these conditions but somatomedin levels are depressed.

The growth spurt of puberty is regulated by changes in GH secretion and by modulation of GH action, both related to the effects of sex steroids. Puberty is associated with an increase in the number and amplitude of nightly GH surges and a rise in serum IGF-I, both of which parallel the increase in the growth velocity of puberty. The peak height velocity occurs earlier in girls (between sexual maturity stage II and stage III) than in boys (in whom it occurs close to sexual maturity stage IV). Similarly, growth arrest due to epiphyseal fusion occurs earlier in girls. This, and the fact that puberty begins about 6 months earlier in girls, accounts for much of the difference in adult heights between men and women. It is interesting that peak height velocity does not parallel the level of estrogen (which rises later in girls) or testosterone (which rises earlier in boys).

Growth Curves and Growth Patterns

The growth of an individual is a dynamic function of height increment over time. Accordingly, to evaluate growth accurately, one must obtain serial measurements of a child's height and plot them on a growth curve. The accuracy of these measurements is crucial, and it is recommended that specialized devices such as wall-mounted stadiometers be used and that the mean of three measurements be recorded. Nevertheless, even under ideal conditions a measuring error of at least 2 mm is to be expected. The data thus obtained should be plotted on a growth curve and analyzed after a sufficiently long period of time has elapsed between measurements (a minimum of 6 months to 1 year). Growth curves are based on normative population data, and the ones commonly available reflect the North American means compiled by the National Center of Health Statistics of the U.S. Public Health Service. Although some growth curves chart only the 5th to the 95th percentiles of a population, it is preferable to use those that show the standard deviations from the mean or Z score (Figs. 56–2 and 56–3). These types of curves allow a more precise estimation of the degree of short stature when it exists. However, it must be emphasized that such curves are cross-sectional, rather than longitudinal, and are particularly nonrepresentative during puberty, when growth acceleration may normally occur at widely divergent ages. Consequently, it is preferable to perform consecutive measurements of height, which are then used to calculate growth velocity and are plotted on a growth velocity chart (Fig. 56–4). An important additional factor that one needs to take into account when analyzing the growth of the adolescent patient is the sexual maturation and the associated growth spurt; charts are available for comparing the growth of early- and late-developing adolescents. The later the age of puberty and the pubertal growth spurt, the smaller the increase in the observed height velocity that is associated with it. Adolescents with late maturation, however, enjoy a longer period of growth and may achieve a slightly taller adult height (Fig. 56–5).

SHORT STATURE
Definition and Epidemiology

Since height is a normally distributed function, it is simple to provide a statistical definition of "normal

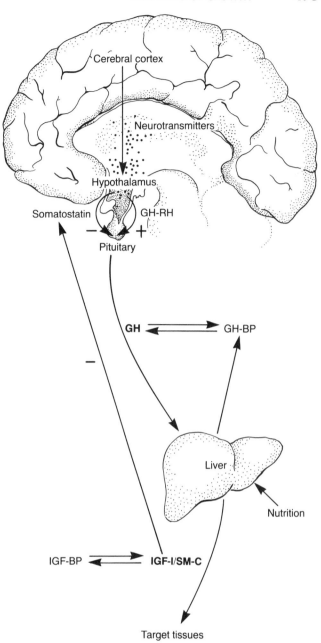

Figure 56–1. Hormonal regulation of growth.

height" as that falling between two standard deviations (Z scores) above and below the mean for each age group. This will include those individuals between the 2nd and 98th percentiles but will exclude approximately 4% of the population, many of whom represent variants of the normal state. Additionally, applying the standards of the North American population to other ethnic groups, particularly Asians and Hispanics, may prove to be an inappropriate screening method for clinically significant short stature. The use of population or disease-specific growth curves (e.g., for Turner syndrome) may overcome this problem. On the other hand, it is important to consider all individuals in the context of the society in which they live and to attempt to avoid using treatment criteria based exclusively on ethnic background.

Text continued on page 500

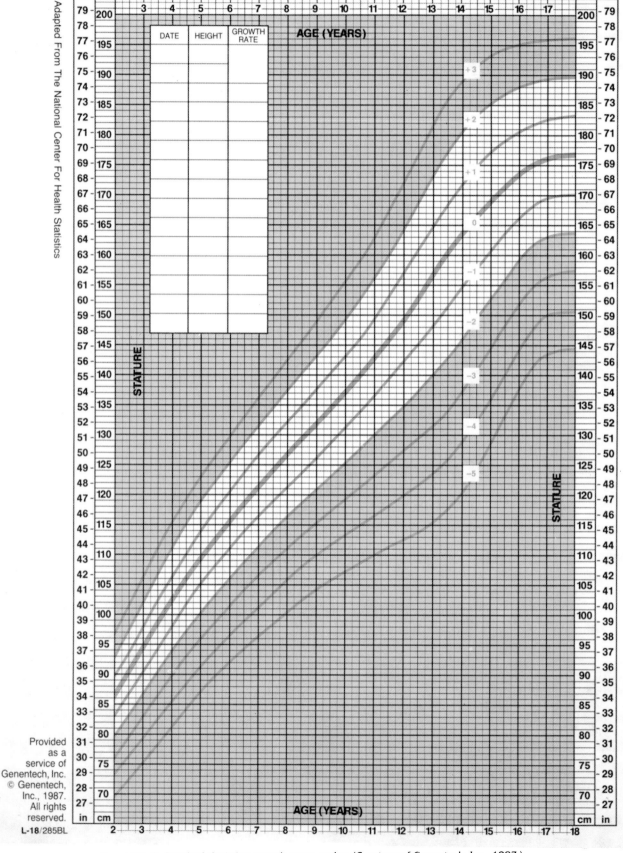

Figure 56–2. Standard deviation growth curve, males. (Courtesy of Genentech, Inc., 1987.)

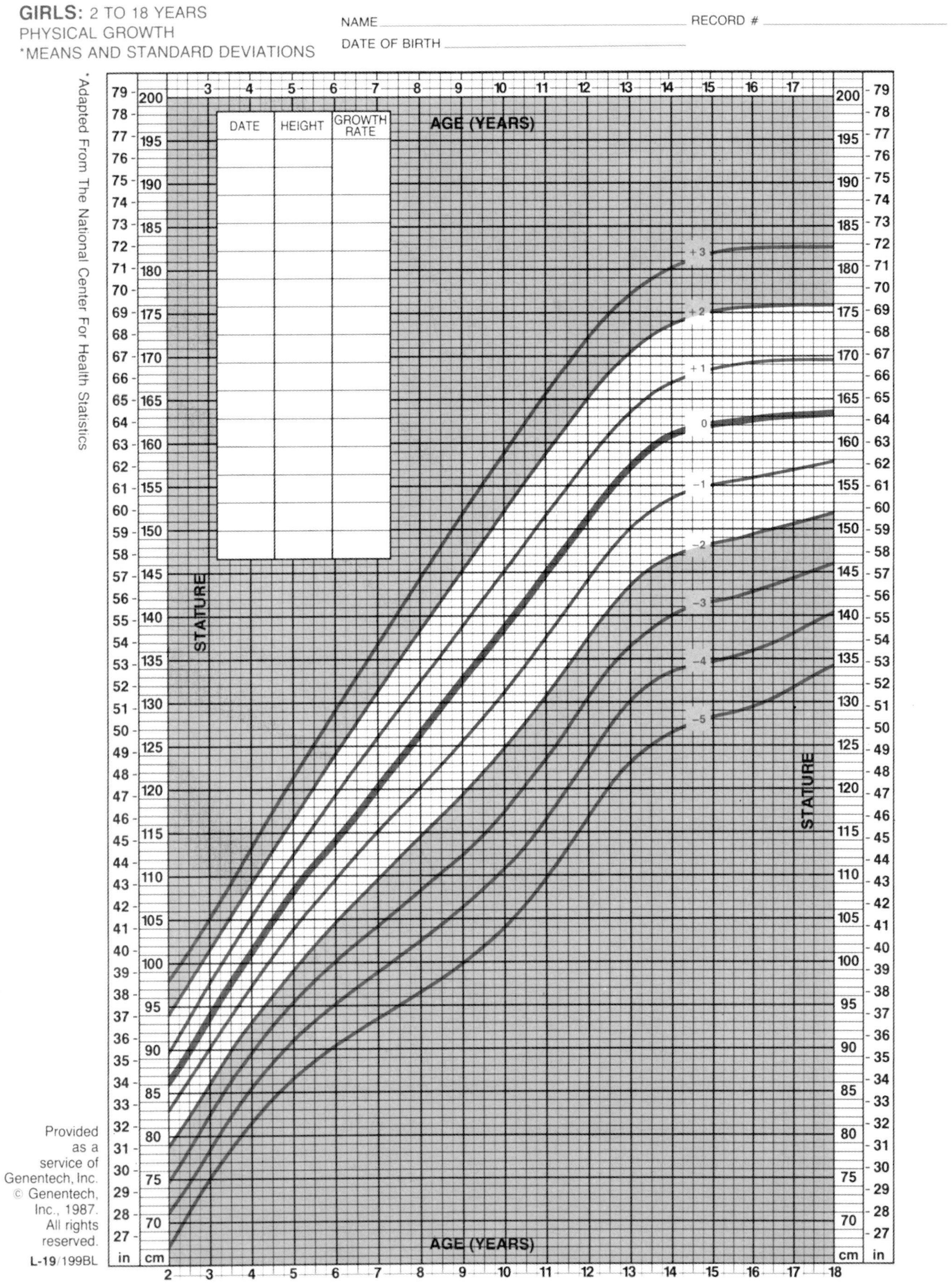

GIRLS: 2 TO 18 YEARS
PHYSICAL GROWTH
*MEANS AND STANDARD DEVIATIONS

NAME _____ RECORD # _____

DATE OF BIRTH _____

Figure 56–3. Standard deviation growth curve, females. (Courtesy of Genentech, Inc., 1987.)

L-19/199BL

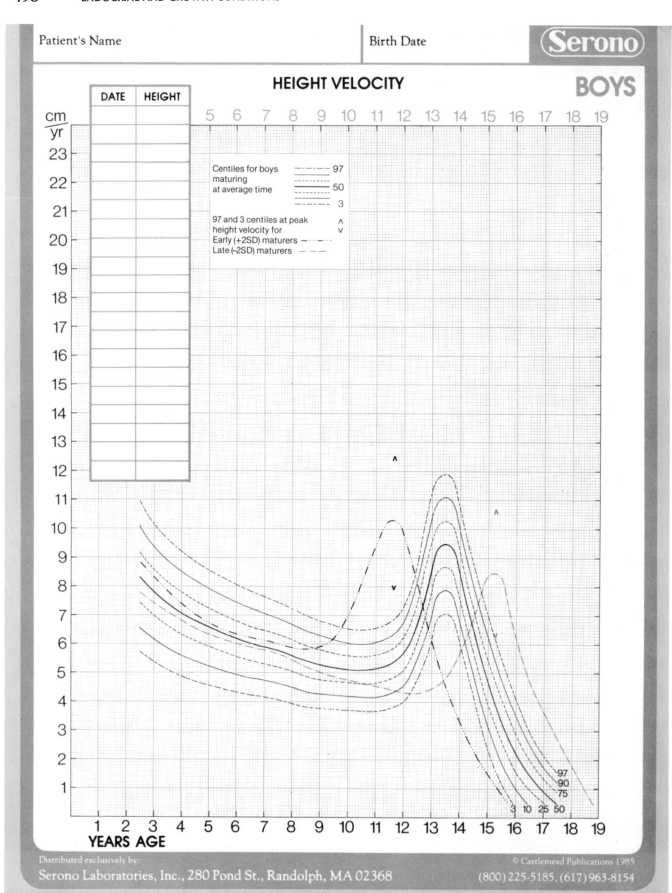

Figure 56–4 *See legend on opposite page*

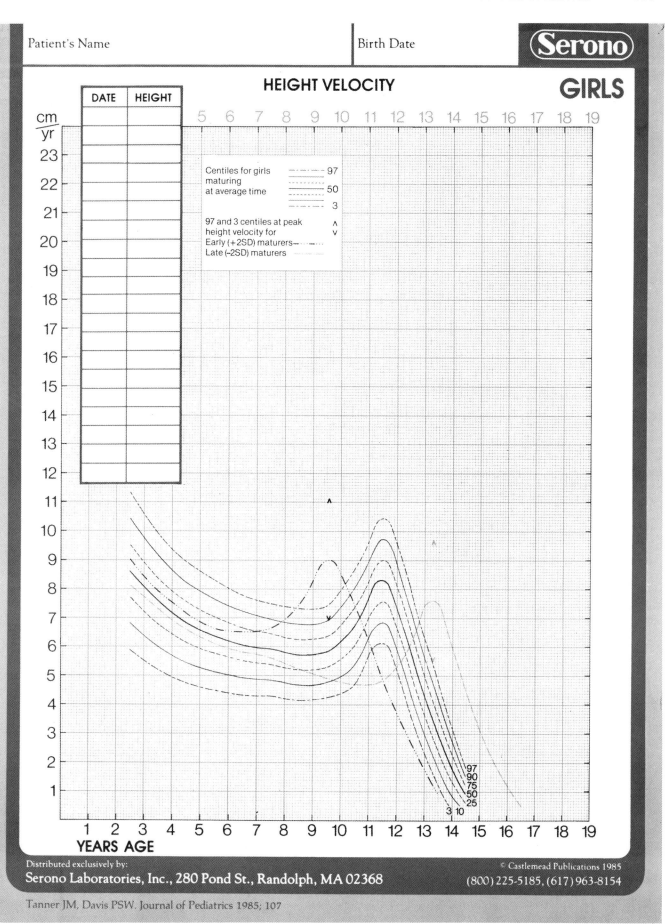

Figure 56—4. Growth velocity curves, males and females. (Courtesy of Serono Laboratories, Inc. © Castlemead Publications, 1985.)

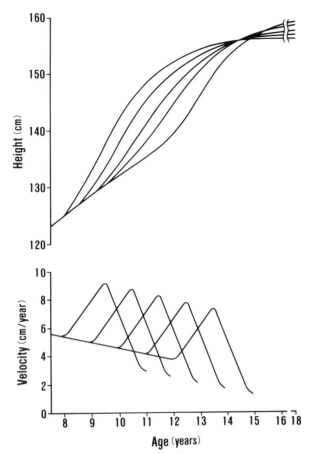

Figure 56–5. Effects of age at puberty on height and growth velocity. The upper part of the figure is a schematic representation of growth curves of five groups of patients. The rightmost curve represents the very late maturers and the leftmost curve the very early maturers. The lower part of the figure is a schematic representation of the growth velocity curves of the same five groups, again with the rightmost peak representing the late maturers and the leftmost the early maturers. Note that all five groups had the same height and growth velocity before puberty, that growth velocity before puberty and the peak growth velocity during puberty decreases with delaying puberty, but that adult height is slightly shorter in the early vs. late maturers. (With permission from Tanaka, Hibi, et al: Acta Paediatr Scand [Suppl] 347:25, 1988.)

Adult Height Prediction

Although short stature is a significant problem at any age, even when it is a transient phenomenon, some emphasis should also be placed on predicting the adult height of an individual. Factors influencing adult height include mean parental height, the patient's current height and sexual maturation rating, the chronologic age, and the bone age. Many methods have been developed for calculating estimated adult height. The initial step in the most easy to use method of predicting adult height is to determine the mean parental height (preferably obtained by direct measurements) and add or subtract (for males and females, respectively) 6.5 cm or 2.5 inches (see Chapter 6). In the absence of chronic illness or endocrine disease, this often provides a fair estimation of the genetic potential. Another simple method that can be easily used in an office setting is the "chart method," which consists of determining the

height percentile (or Z score) of the patient and extrapolating it to the adult height at the same percentile. However, while this method often correlates well with more sophisticated methods when used on normally maturing children, it is highly inaccurate at the time of puberty or when significant pubertal delay or acceleration occurs. One may then use growth curves for early, normal, and late (sexual) maturers. Although the aforementioned methods can provide a low cost and immediate estimate of predicted adult height, when evaluating a child with short stature the use of a bone age radiograph allows for a much more accurate prediction. The most commonly used method for determination of bone age is the Greulich and Pyle (GP) method, which relies on an atlas of left hand and wrist radiographs of healthy children at various ages. Likewise, the simplest and most common method for adult height prediction is the Bayley-Pinneau (BP) method. This method assigns to each bone age a percentage of the adult height that has already been achieved, and the adult height can then be calculated by dividing the present height by the fraction given in the table (see Chapter 6). Different tables are provided for children with bone ages that deviate by more than 1 year from the chronologic age (Table 56–1). The confidence limits of the aforementioned predictions are usually within 2 inches of the actual achieved height and can serve as a basis for family discussions and therapeutic decisions.

Differential Diagnosis

A height greater than 2.5 SD below the mean for age during adolescence can have many causes, including multiple endocrine and systemic disorders (Table 56–2). Of these, the normal variants are by far the most common.

NORMAL VARIANTS

Normal variant short stature (NVSS) can be associated with normal progression through puberty and normal skeletal maturation or with delayed puberty, skeletal maturation, and growth, termed *normal variant constitutional delay* (NVCD). NVSS is a growth pattern representing the genetic potential for growth of that individual and is not associated with any endocrine or systemic pathologic process.

NVSS is often, but not always, associated with a family history of short stature in at least one parent. These patients commonly have normal birth weights, and in the first few years of life their growth pattern usually settles at or just below the 3rd percentile and then follows this percentile with a pubertal growth spurt at a normal age (Fig. 56–6). The adult height achieved by these patients is typically below the 3rd percentile (64 inches or 162 cm for males and 59 inches or 150 cm for females) and is predictable by bone age measurements. Criteria for the diagnosis of NVSS include the exclusion of organic or emotional pathology by history, physical examination, and simple laboratory tests.

NVCD occurs in both sexes, although males are more

TABLE 56–1. Fraction of Adult Height Achieved as a Function of Bone Age

BONE AGE (yr-mo)	GIRLS			BOYS		
	Retarded	Average*	Advanced	Retarded	Average*	Advanced
6-0	0.733	0.720		0.680		
6-3	0.742	0.729		0.690		
6-6	0.751	0.738		0.700		
6-9	0.763	0.751		0.709		
7-0	0.770	0.757	0.712	0.718	0.695	0.670
7-3	0.779	0.765	0.722	0.728	0.702	0.676
7-6	0.788	0.772	0.732	0.738	0.709	0.683
7-9	0.797	0.782	0.742	0.747	0.716	0.689
8-0	0.804	0.790	0.750	0.756	0.723	0.696
8-3	0.813	0.801	0.760	0.765	0.731	0.703
8-6	0.823	0.810	0.771	0.773	0.739	0.709
8-9	0.836	0.821	0.784	0.779	0.746	0.715
9-0	0.841	0.827	0.790	0.786	0.752	0.720
9-3	0.851	0.836	0.800	0.794	0.761	0.728
9-6	0.858	0.844	0.809	0.800	0.769	0.734
9-9	0.866	0.853	0.819	0.807	0.777	0.741
10-0	0.874	0.862	0.828	0.812	0.784	0.747
10-3	0.884	0.874	0.841	0.816	0.791	0.753
10-6	0.896	0.884	0.856	0.819	0.795	0.758
10-9	0.907	0.896	0.870	0.821	0.800	0.763
11-0	0.918	0.906	0.883	0.823	0.804	0.767
11-3	0.922	0.910	0.887	0.827	0.812	0.776
11-6	0.926	0.914	0.891	0.832	0.818	0.786
11-9	0.929	0.918	0.897	0.839	0.827	0.800
12-0	0.932	0.922	0.901	0.845	0.834	0.809
12-3	0.942	0.932	0.913	0.852	0.843	0.818
12-6	0.949	0.941	0.924	0.860	0.853	0.828
12-9	0.957	0.950	0.935	0.869	0.863	0.839
13-0	0.964	0.958	0.945	0.880	0.876	0.850
13-3	0.971	0.967	0.955		0.890	0.863
13-6	0.977	0.974	0.963		0.902	0.875
13-9	0.981	0.978	0.968		0.914	0.890
14-0	0.983	0.980	0.972		0.927	0.905
14-3	0.986	0.983	0.977		0.938	0.918
14-6	0.989	0.986	0.980		0.948	0.930
14-9	0.992	0.988	0.983		0.958	0.943
15-0	0.994	0.990	0.986		0.968	0.958
15-3	0.995	0.991	0.988		0.973	0.967
15-6	0.996	0.993	0.990		0.976	0.971
15-9	0.997	0.994	0.992		0.980	0.976
16-0	0.998	0.996	0.993		0.982	0.980
16-3	0.999	0.996	0.994		0.985	0.983
16-6	0.999	0.997	0.995		0.987	0.985
16-9	0.9995	0.998	0.997		0.989	0.988
17-0	1.00	0.999	0.998		0.991	0.990
17-3					0.993	
17-6		0.9995	0.9995		0.994	
17-9					0.995	
18-0		1.00			0.996	
18-3					0.998	
18-6					1.00	

*Average: Bone age within one year of chronologic age. To determine adult height, divide the height at the time of the bone age by the given fraction.
With permission from Post EM, Richman RA: A condensed table for predicting adult stature. J Pediatr 98:441, 1981.

likely to present to a physician with this condition. A family history of delayed maturation is usually present in at least one parent. The growth pattern typically observed in this condition consists of growth at or slightly below the 5th percentile throughout childhood, with further deviation from the normal growth curve at the time puberty should normally occur (see Fig. 56–6). Puberty develops late in these patients, but when it does it is associated with a nearly normal growth spurt, and the adult height achieved is entirely normal. The diagnosis of NVCD is made by exclusion; Table 56–3 lists the criteria for this diagnosis. After systemic disease has been ruled out by history and physical examination and

pubertal delay documented by careful sexual maturity rating, confirmation of the diagnosis should be made with a bone age measurement and the laboratory tests described later in this chapter. Of these tests, all the results should be normal except those of bone age (which should be delayed) and the IGF-I levels, which may be low for chronologic age (but often not for bone age). Failure to meet all the criteria for the diagnosis should suggest a different disorder, particularly if either puberty or bone age is not delayed. Even "classic" cases require adequate long-term follow-up to ensure continued normal growth velocity and eventual progression through puberty.

TABLE 56–2. Differential Diagnosis of Short Stature in Adolescence

NORMAL VARIANTS
   Normal variant short stature (NVSS) (familial and sporadic)
   Normal variant constitutional delay (NVCD)
   ABNORMAL VARIANTS
   Chromosomal disorders
      Turner syndrome
      Other chromosomal conditions
   Dysmorphic syndromes
   Skeletal dysplasias (primary and secondary)
   Systemic disease
      Malnutrition
      Eating disorders
      Crohn disease
      Other occult chronic disease
   Psychosocial dwarfism
   Endocrine disorders
      Growth hormone deficiency
      Hypothyroidism
      Cushing disease
      Vitamin D–resistant rickets
      Pseudohypoparathyroidism

ABNORMAL VARIANTS

Other causes of growth failure during adolescence may be the result of chromosomal disorders; the most common of these disorders is Turner syndrome (see Chapter 4). This condition is classically caused by a monosomic 45X state, but other abnormalities of the X chromosomes, including partial deletions and mosaic states, may manifest the same clinical findings. Short

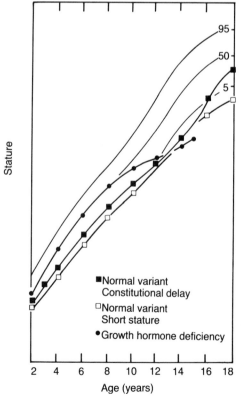

Figure 56–6. Typical growth curves for NVSS, NVCD, and GH deficiency. (With permission from Rosenfeld RG: Evaluation of growth and maturation in adolescence. Pediatr Rev 4:175, 1982.)

TABLE 56–3. Criteria for Presumptive Diagnosis of NVCD

No history of systemic illness
Normal nutrition
Normal physical examination, including body proportions
Height at or below the 3rd percentile but with annual growth rate of at least 3.5 cm/yr
Delayed puberty:
   Boys, failure to achieve G2* by 14 years or P2* by 15 years
   Girls, failure to achieve B2* by 13 years
Normal results of complete blood cell count, erythrocyte sedimentation rate, urinalysis, and chemistry panel
Normal thyroid and GH levels
Delayed bone age (1–4 years retarded)
Normal predicted adult height (boys, >64 inches; girls, >59 inches)

*Tanner sexual maturation stage. G, gonadal; P, pubic hair; B, breast.

stature is the most common finding in Turner syndrome, with primary ovarian failure being the other important feature. Additional findings include typical dysmorphic features (webbed neck, low posterior hair line, increased carrying angle, and other findings) and cardiac and renal anomalies. Nevertheless, short stature may be the only presenting sign in a girl with Turner syndrome, and even this finding may manifest itself only late in childhood. It is, therefore, imperative to consider this condition in the evaluation of any short female. Noonan syndrome is a less common and less well characterized disorder for which no definitive laboratory test exists. It is phenotypically reminiscent of Turner syndrome but may occur in males as well as in females and is characterized by right-sided heart lesions, delayed puberty due to hypogonadotropic hypogonadism, and occasionally mental retardation.

Prader-Willi syndrome is a condition that is usually associated with abnormalities of chromosome 15; it includes short stature, hypogonadism, and obesity (see Chapter 4). Many other conditions of genetic or chromosomal etiology are associated with growth failure but are usually recognized early in childhood and rarely present a diagnostic dilemma to the physician taking care of adolescents. Among these conditions are Down syndrome and other rare chromosomal abnormalities, Russell-Silver syndrome, Seckel syndrome, and Laurence-Moon-Biedl syndrome. Osteochondrodysplasias are a large group of familial disorders ranging from the subtle to the obvious, characterized by well-defined skeletal abnormalities. Increased upper to lower body-segment ratios are useful in distinguishing these conditions from NVSS.

SYSTEMIC DISEASE

Growth failure associated with systemic disease and malnutrition in adolescents is usually characterized by normal or elevated GH but depressed somatomedin levels. During adolescence, these conditions are often associated with delayed puberty (see Chapter 57) as well as a delayed bone age and must be differentiated from NVCD. In developing countries, overt protein-calorie malnutrition is the most common form of malnutrition, but in developed countries, self-induced malnutrition and malnutrition associated with chronic disease are also common. Various kinds of eating disorders (see Chapter 60) frequently have their onset during adolescence and not uncommonly present to the physician as growth stagnation. Anorexia nervosa and bulimia can also be associated with gonadotropin insufficiency and pubertal delay and thus mimic NVCD. Fad diets, macrobiosis, and cholesterol or obesity avoidance regimens can similarly affect growth, without having the behavioral components of anorexia nervosa, especially among boys. Specific mineral deficiencies, especially of iron and zinc, can also be associated with growth delay. Clearly, a good dietary history is essential in the evaluation of short stature.

Gastrointestinal disease may also cause growth retardation, often with few or no appreciable symptoms, usually as a result of malabsorption. Regional enteritis (Crohn disease) commonly manifests growth arrest before intestinal involvement becomes obvious (see Chapter 63); celiac disease, cystic fibrosis (see Chapter 43), and parasitic disease may do the same. Although renal, pulmonary, and cardiac disease severe enough to lead to growth failure are often recognized earlier in life, adolescent patients must be evaluated for occult disease, such as renal tubular acidosis and chronic renal failure (see Chapter 65). Many systemic diseases treated with corticosteroids are associated with growth retardation secondary to the effects of these agents on epiphyseal growth. Of these, asthma, inflammatory bowel disease, and rheumatoid arthritis are the most commonly encountered (see Chapters 43, 63, and 90). Insulin-dependent diabetes mellitus, when not adequately controlled, is associated with depressed somatomedin levels and poor growth; the extreme case of this, Mauriac syndrome, is associated with growth arrest, hepatomegaly, and failure to gain weight. Adequate control of the diabetic state and regulation of the nutritional intake can restore growth rate in diabetics to the normal range (see Chapter 59).

Poverty, depression, and neglect can lead to a form of growth delay referred to as psychosocial dwarfism. This form of growth failure is more common in infancy but has been described in adolescence. Although nutritional factors may play a role in the etiology of this condition, defective GH secretion has also been documented. Psychotherapy and particularly restoration of a normal environment are essential to the management of these cases.

ENDOCRINE ABNORMALITIES

It is helpful to bear in mind that chronic illness frequently tends to retard weight to a greater degree than height, whereas endocrinopathies tend to do the opposite. Endocrine abnormalities account for only about 10% of the cases of short stature; it is, however, imperative to diagnose these children promptly, since adequate therapy can normalize the growth and other abnormalities associated with these disorders (see Chapter 55).

GH DEFICIENCY

Table 56–4 classifies GH abnormalities. Familial GH deficiency displays a variety of hereditary patterns, rang-

TABLE 56–4. Classification of GH Abnormalities in Adolescence

GH deficiency
  Familial
  Sporadic/idiopathic
  Perisellar tumors
  Postinfectious
  Posttraumatic
  Central nervous system irradiation and chemotherapy
GH insufficiency
  Partial GH deficiency
  Neurosecretory dysfunction
Biologically inactive GH
GH resistance (Laron-type dwarfism)

ing from autosomal recessive (type I), to autosomal dominant (type II) and X-linked (type III) (see Chapter 4). Congenital GH deficiency may also be associated with panhypopituitarism and can include abnormal secretion of corticotropin, thyrotropin, vasopressin, or gonadotropins. Congenital GH deficiency is usually recognized early in life, with the constellation of hypoglycemia, small phallus, cryptorchidism, relative obesity, and shortness; if associated with blindness or nystagmus, septooptic dysplasia must be considered. Sporadic GH deficiency can be either idiopathic (most common) or secondary to pathologic processes at the level of the pituitary or hypothalamus. Patients with such disorders are most likely to present at adolescence and represent a critical group of patients that must be differentiated from the normal variants of short stature.

Space-occupying lesions of the brain are the second most frequent cause of GH deficiency. Midline brain tumors and, in particular, craniopharyngioma, are the most common, although many different types of neoplasias can involve the hypothalamic-pituitary area. Craniopharyngiomas are slowly growing, benign suprasellar tumors that infringe mainly on the pituitary and the optic chiasm, and, indeed the most common symptoms of this tumor are growth failure, headache, and visual disturbances. Partial or complete hypopituitarism may develop, and the growth failure may be associated with pubertal delay, thus further complicating the diagnostic picture. Surgery is the treatment of choice for these tumors but is subsequently often associated with varying degrees of hypopituitarism. Other types of brain tumors, infiltrative processes such as sarcoidosis, histiocytosis X, and posttraumatic and postinflammatory conditions all can cause GH deficiency and growth failure.

A growing number of children presenting with GH deficiency and growth failure in adolescence are survivors of malignancies who received central nervous system irradiation and chemotherapy (see Chapters 4 and 53). Children cured of common acute lymphoblastic leukemia represent the majority of this group, since they have often undergone prophylactic irradiation with more than 2000 rad and received intrathecal cytotoxic agents, which may result in clinical symptoms of hypopituitarism years after the primary disease has been treated. Even though the diagnosis of GH deficiency may seem obvious in some of these cases, it is important to perform the full diagnostic workup on these children so that other pituitary deficiencies may be diagnosed as well.

While some short children may successfully pass provocative GH testing, they may respond to GH therapy, nevertheless. Integrated GH levels have been shown to be low in a subset of these children, and the term *neurosecretory dysfunction* (of GH secretion) has been used to describe their condition. Regardless of the cause, children with characteristic GH deficiency display short stature, decreased growth velocity, delayed bone age, and low somatomedin C levels. Failure to adequately secrete GH in two stimulation tests is required for the diagnosis of classic GH deficiency.

Biologically inactive GH is another potential cause of short stature. Patients with this disorder would be expected to have a normal response to exogenous GH, but no convincing cases of this condition have been documented. Laron-type dwarfism is caused by an abnormality of GH receptors and binding proteins and is associated with elevated GH levels with depressed somatomedin levels. This condition can now be diagnosed by assay of the plasma GH binding protein.

Hypothyroidism in childhood is generally associated with poor linear growth (see Chapter 55). Indeed, poor growth and/or delayed puberty (see Chapter 57) may be the presenting signs of chronic hypothyroidism. In adolescents, acquired hypothyroidism is usually caused by Hashimoto thyroiditis (see Chapter 55). It is important to note that hypothyroidism may coexist with GH deficiency and that it may also cause false-negative results on provocative GH testing. It is therefore imperative to consider hypothyroidism as the first step of short stature evaluation.

Glucocorticoid excess, either iatrogenic or due to Cushing disease or primary adrenal hypercortisolism, is associated with attenuation of the growth rate (see Chapter 55). This finding is associated with truncal obesity and the other findings of Cushing syndrome. Congenital abnormalities of bone mineral metabolism, such as vitamin D–resistant rickets and pseudohypoparathyroidism, display classic findings that are generally noticeable prior to adolescence (see Chapter 55).

Diagnosis

Historical features that aid in the diagnosis of short stature include the pregnancy and perinatal history, the growth pattern from infancy to adolescence (for both height and weight), the general medical history, and any symptoms of systemic disease. Particular emphasis should be placed on the review of systems for the presence of neurologic, visual, or gastrointestinal disturbances and any symptom of hypothyroidism. The family history should be probed for parental heights and growth and maturation patterns, as well as for any short stature in the family background. Adequate assessment of the psychosocial and nutritional condition of the adolescent is necessary, as well as an evaluation of the patient's and the family's attitude toward short stature and its treatment.

The complete physical examination should include accurate auxologic measurements of height, weight, arm span, and upper to lower segment ratios and an examination of the thyroid and sexual maturity rating. Any abnormality in the physical examination, especially one suggesting systemic disease or the evidence of dysmorphism, should be carefully noted.

Laboratory evaluation is frequently necessary in an adolescent with clinically significant short stature in whom a systemic disease is not the obvious cause of the growth problem (Fig. 56–7). The presence of occult chronic disease causing short stature can usually be ruled out with a complete blood cell count, erythrocyte sedimentation rate, urinalysis, and blood chemistry panel that includes serum electrolytes, blood urea nitrogen, creatinine, calcium, phosphorus, and alkaline phosphatase. A serum albumin level, as well as beta-carotene or other screening test for malabsorption, should be

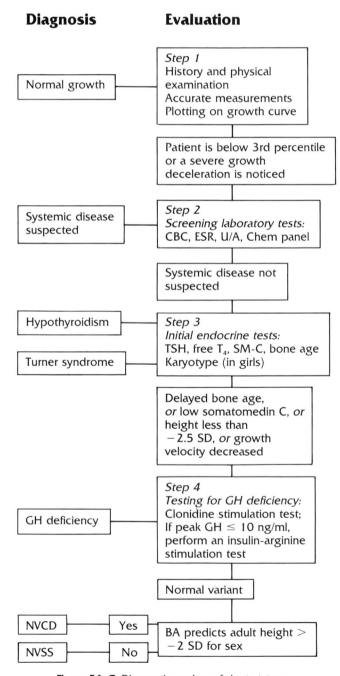

Diagnosis   **Evaluation**

Normal growth — *Step 1* History and physical examination. Accurate measurements. Plotting on growth curve

Patient is below 3rd percentile or a severe growth deceleration is noticed

Systemic disease suspected — *Step 2* *Screening laboratory tests:* CBC, ESR, U/A, Chem panel

Systemic disease not suspected

Hypothyroidism — *Step 3* *Initial endocrine tests:* TSH, free T$_4$, SM-C, bone age

Turner syndrome — Karyotype (in girls)

Delayed bone age, *or* low somatomedin C, *or* height less than −2.5 SD, *or* growth velocity decreased

Step 4 *Testing for GH deficiency:* Clonidine stimulation test; GH deficiency — If peak GH ≤ 10 ng/ml, perform an insulin-arginine stimulation test

Normal variant

NVCD — Yes

NVSS — No — BA predicts adult height > −2 SD for sex

Figure 56–7. Diagnostic workup of short stature.

TABLE 56–5. Diagnostic Findings in the Common Causes of Short Stature

ETIOLOGY	GROWTH VELOCITY	BONE AGE	IGF-I	STIMULATED GH (ng/ml)	PUBERTY
NVSS	Normal to ↓	Normal	Normal to ↓	>10	Normal
NVCD	Normal to ↓	Delayed	Normal to ↓	>10	Delayed
Turner syndrome	Normal to ↓	Normal to ↓	Normal to ↓	>10*	Delayed†
Systemic disease	Normal to ↓	Delayed	Low	>10	Normal to ↓
Classic GH deficiency	Slow	Delayed	Low	<7	Normal to ↓
Partial GH deficiency	Slow	Delayed	Low	7–10	Normal to ↓
GH neurosecretory defect	Slow	Delayed	Low	>10	Normal to ↓

*Adolescent patients with Turner syndrome often have low stimulated GH levels, probably reflecting estrogen deficiency.
†Puberty is delayed, but gonadotropin levels are increased.

performed if intestinal disease is a possibility. Thyroid function can be evaluated by measuring thyroid-stimulating hormone (TSH) and free thyroxine. In girls, a karyotype is obligatory to rule out Turner syndrome, even if no other stigmata exist. A bone age measurement is essential for the diagnostic evaluation and prognosis of all short adolescents, and a SM-C/IGF-I level can provide important insight into the cause of the short stature. The overwhelming majority of children with GH deficiency will have low immunoassayable IGF-I levels. However, IGF-I levels can be low for age in NVCD, when they tend to correlate better with the bone age than with the chronologic age. IGF-I may be low in malnutrition, systemic disease, and hypothyroidism. The clinical use of IGF-I levels is mainly as an adjunct to making a decision on the need for GH stimulation tests. Finally, in the male adolescent suspected of having NVCD and considered for therapy, determination of serum testosterone level is often helpful.

If the adolescent being evaluated is shorter than 2.5 SD below the mean for age and has a low growth velocity and a low IGF-I, GH testing should be performed. In normal adolescents, random, unstimulated GH levels are typically less than 5 ng/ml; therefore, if GH deficiency is suspected, GH should be measured after appropriate pituitary stimulation. Integrated GH levels obtained every 20 minutes for 24 hours or overnight have also been used to diagnose GH deficiency and neurosecretory dysfunction. However, the large variability and the expense of these tests make provocative GH testing the recommended choice. GH screening tests commonly employed include measurement after exercise or after an hour of sleep. Pharmacologic screening tests include obtaining GH levels 30, 60, and 90 minutes after administration of levodopa (250 mg orally for weight less than 30 kg, 500 mg for weight more than 30 kg) or clonidine (0.15 mg/m² orally). Failure to achieve GH levels greater than 10 ng/ml requires the definitive insulin (0.1 U/kg regular insulin, intravenously) and arginine (0.5 g/kg intravenously) stimulation test. On that test, levels of less than 7 ng/ml are diagnostic of GH deficiency, levels of 7 to 10 indicate partial GH deficiency, and levels greater than 10 are considered normal (although neurosecretory dysfunction of GH secretion remains a possibility). Priming the pituitary with estrogen will sometimes augment the GH response to insulin and arginine and is recommended for 1 to 3 days prior to the test in prepubertal adolescents. It is recommended that cortisol levels also be assayed simultaneously with GH levels during the insulin arginine test to rule out pituitary-adrenal axis dysfunction (20 μ/ml is the lower limit of normal for stimulated cortisol). Magnetic resonance imaging of the head is recommended in adolescents with documented GH deficiency to evaluate possible local pathologic processes. Table 56–5 is a summary of the diagnostic findings in the common causes of short stature.

Psychological Aspects

Short stature and growth delay carry with them a great psychological burden, and this is especially true during adolescence. The diminished self-esteem of the short child may be manifest in underachievement in school, even though no organic neurologic or intellectual impairment exists. The small size of these children may cause their parents and other adults to treat them in an overprotective way as if they were younger than their chronologic age, and this in turn may reinforce immature behavior on the child's part. The most severe aspect of the psychological burden of the short adolescent is the impaired interaction with his or her peer group. This is especially true for male adolescents, who consider their disadvantage in sports and athletics to be a major social handicap. The commonly associated pubertal delay can be a further cause of psychological trauma for the teenager who normally would be beginning to interact socially with members of the other sex. Short stature can lead to specific behavioral patterns such as clowning, which can temporarily alleviate the social pressures on the child but may create unhealthy long-term behavior.

The physician taking care of the adolescent with short stature should pay particular attention to the individual psychological adjustments of each patient and provide support and advice. Recommending sports (e.g., soccer, bicycle riding, tennis, golf, and swimming) and activities (music and arts) that do not rely on height is part of the general approach to the care of these patients. Counseling is sometimes indicated.

Management

After the evaluation of short stature has been completed, the physician must balance the needs of the child and the family, the severity of the growth retardation, and the expected adult height in deciding on a therapeutic plan. It is important to appreciate both the potential of growth-enhancing therapy to affect these issues and the cost and possible complications of therapy. For some of the previously mentioned disorders, particularly the normal variants, reassurance and support for the patient and the family, coupled with close follow-up, is all that may be required. On the other hand, for some of the pathologic causes of short stature, as well as for selected severe cases of the normal variants, medical therapy is prudent. In patients with NVSS the exclusion of underlying pathologic processes and the use of supportive therapy constitute the traditional approach to such patients. Recently, however, it has been shown that some of these patients will increase their growth rate with GH therapy, although it is still unclear whether their adult height will be affected. The difficulty in distinguishing these patients from those with "GH insufficiency" or "neurosecretory dysfunction" makes it attractive to consider patients with severe short stature and a slow growth rate candidates for GH treatment even if the patients successfully passed provocative GH testing. The use of such "auxologic criteria" to determine potential candidates for GH therapy remains controversial however, and additional data are required before this can be considered a standard approach.

NVCD is associated with normal predicted adult height, and, in the case of the socially well-adjusted adolescent, reassurance is the most important aspect of therapy, since all these patients will enter puberty eventually and will experience a growth spurt at that time. It is important to note that many of these male adolescents have already (although unknown to themselves) entered puberty if their testicular volume is equal to or greater than 4 ml even if no pubic hair is apparent. Counseling the patient and the family should center around the expected growth that follows puberty. If, however, the teenager feels that he has become so stigmatized by the combination of short stature and sexual immaturity that reassurance alone is insufficient, a course of androgenic steroids should be considered.

Criteria for the treatment of males with androgens are (1) a chronologic age of at least 14 years; (2) height below the third percentile; (3) prepubertal or early G2 stage, with a serum testosterone level below 100 ng/dl; (4) normal thyroid and GH evaluation; and (5) evidence that reassurance alone will not suffice. The therapy most commonly recommended is testosterone enanthate, 200 mg intramuscularly every 3 weeks for four injections. In some patients lower doses of testosterone are sufficient. The great majority of patients so treated are satisfied with this therapy, and their adult height is not compromised. Typically, patients will show signs of pubertal advancement by the time of the fourth injection and linear growth of 3 to 5 inches in the first year, both leading to increased self-confidence. It is important that adolescents continue to be followed regularly after therapy has been completed, to ensure that endogenous puberty has progressed. This can be done by documenting testicular growth and progression of serum testosterone into the adult range (300 to 1200 ng/dl). On those rare occasions when there is no evidence of spontaneous pubertal progression within 1 year after completion of therapy, one should suspect and evaluate for hypothalamic-pituitary dysfunction. Other agents with androgenic effects, such as oral oxandrolone, may also bring about some of these desired responses in NVCD.

Adolescents with Turner syndrome have been shown to benefit from growth-enhancing therapy, and the currently recommended regimen for their management involves initiation of GH regardless of the response to provocative testing. This should be done as soon as they fall below the 3rd percentile and should be continued until the completion of growth. Disease-specific growth curves for Turner syndrome allow the physician to monitor the response to therapy by documenting the adolescent's growth relative to expected growth in Turner syndrome. Recommended GH dosage in Turner syndrome ranges from 0.05 to 0.07 mg/kg/day. Combining GH with low-dose anabolic steroids, such as oxandrolone, enhances the growth response. This may be valuable in older Turner patients but needs to be monitored because of possible virilization and epiphyseal maturation. Estrogen in low doses can be given to these girls if they do not develop advancement of sexual characteristics by the time they reach 14 years of age; cyclic estrogen and progesterone can be substituted at a later time. This treatment does not seem to compromise the height increase obtained with GH and contributes to the general well-being of the patients. Other chromosomal and genetic syndromes do not respond to therapy quite as well and have not yet been adequately studied with regard to GH treatment. Osteochondrodysplasias, however, can sometimes be helped by lower limb–lengthening surgery.

GH deficiency of any type requires GH therapy; and with the unlimited availability of recombinant GH, therapy can be provided to all these adolescent patients. If the diagnosis of classic GH deficiency is made, GH therapy should be started immediately. In the nonclassic forms, however, it is better to carefully document poor growth velocity for 1 year and then to embark on a 6-month trial of GH treatment, at the end of which a decision about further therapy can be made. GH is best given daily, at bedtime, as a subcutaneous injection at a dose ranging from 0.025 to 0.05 mg/kg/day. Some adolescents may develop central hypothyroidism after beginning GH therapy; therefore, thyroid function should be monitored in all patients receiving GH on a regular basis.

When prescribing GH to a GH-deficient adolescent, one must remember that the general public is well aware of some scientific publications on clinical trials of GH in adults. These studies suggested that GH may have an effect on increasing lean body mass in GH-deficient or aging adults and may also have positive effects on skin and bones. Therefore, it is possible that the prescribed GH may be abused by other family members or sold to body builders or people seeking rejuvenation. Every effort should be made to validate the use of the GH by the adolescent patient by examining injection sites and by requesting the return of the empty vials.

Complications of Therapy

Past recipients of human pituitary GH are at risk of acquiring Jakob-Creutzfeldt disease; this is no longer a consideration with biosynthetic GH. Antibodies to GH can occur as a response to some forms of recombinant GH, but it is unclear whether they have any clinical significance. A report of increased incidence of leukemia in GH recipients has been published in Japan, but a subsequent international analysis of the frequency of leukemia in GH recipients placed the risk of developing this disease by GH recipients to be equal to or only slightly above that of the general population. Nevertheless, this remains an important issue to consider and to discuss with adolescent patients and their families. Additional considerations include the local side effects that can be associated with any injectable drug and the possible effects of GH on carbohydrate and lipid metabolism. Slipped capital femoral epiphysis is more common in GH-deficient children and may have an increased incidence with GH therapy. Finally, the cost of GH may be a significant burden on the average family budget, with current costs ranging between $10,000 and $50,000 a year. All the aforementioned considerations should be weighed and discussed before embarking on therapy.

TALL STATURE

Just as for short stature, the normal distribution of height predicts that 2.5% of the population will be taller than 2 SD above the mean. However, the social acceptability and even desirability of tallness (heightism) makes tall stature a much less frequent complaint among adolescents. In North America, it is extremely unusual for boys to seek help regarding excessive height, although in Europe it is somewhat more common. Even in girls tall stature has become more socially acceptable, although tall girls may still ask their physician about ways of curbing their growth rate.

Differential Diagnosis

Table 56–6 lists the causes of tall stature in adolescence. Of these (as was the case for short stature), the normal variant familial or constitutional tall stature is by far the most common cause. Almost invariably, a

TABLE 56–6. Differential Diagnosis of Tall Stature in Adolescence

NORMAL VARIANTS
Familial (constitutional) tall stature
ABNORMAL VARIANTS
Pituitary gigantism
Cerebral gigantism (Sotos syndrome)
Klinefelter syndrome
XYY syndrome
Marfan syndrome
Homocystinuria
Hyperthyroidism
Obesity

family history of tallness can be elicited and no organic pathologic process is present. The child is often tall throughout childhood and enjoys excellent health. The parent of the constitutionally tall adolescent may reflect unhappily on his or her own adolescence as a tall teenager. There are no abnormalities in the physical examination, and the laboratory studies, if obtained, are always negative.

Pituitary gigantism is an extremely rare cause of tall stature, representing the pediatric equivalent of acromegaly. It is caused by a GH-secreting pituitary tumor and is associated with elevated and nonsuppressible GH levels, accompanied by an increase in SM-C/IGF-I. Typical features include disproportionate enlargement of the jaw, the hands, and the feet. Visual field defects and neurologic abnormalities are common. Cerebral gigantism (Sotos syndrome) is an idiopathic syndrome generally associated with mental retardation and seizures. Size is increased at birth; early growth is rapid, but early puberty typically results in a normal adult height. Klinefelter syndrome (XXY syndrome) is a relatively common (1:500 to 1000 live male births) abnormality associated with tall stature, mild mental retardation, gynecomastia, and decreased upper to lower body segment ratio (see Chapter 31). The testes are invariably small, although androgen production by Leydig cells is often at the low normal range. Spermatogenesis and Sertoli cell function are defective and infertility results. XYY syndrome is associated with tall stature and possible behavioral and mental problems. Marfan syndrome is an autosomal dominant connective tissue disorder consisting of tall stature, increased arm span, and decreased upper to lower body segment ratio. Additional abnormalities include arachnodactyly, ocular abnormalities, and cardiac anomalies. Homocystinuria is an autosomal recessive inborn error of amino acid metabolism causing mental retardation when untreated and has many features resembling those of Marfan syndrome, particularly ocular manifestations. Hyperthyroidism in adolescents is associated with rapid growth but normal adult height (see Chapter 55). It is almost always caused by Graves disease and is much more common in girls. Exogenous obesity is a common condition in adolescence (see Chapter 60), and may be associated with rapid linear growth and early maturation; adult height is typically normal.

Diagnostic Evaluation

The purpose of the diagnostic evaluation of tall stature is to distinguish the commonly occurring normal constitutional variant from the rare pathologic conditions. Often, when the history is suggestive of familial tall stature and the physical examination is entirely normal, no laboratory tests are indicated. It is valuable to obtain a bone age radiograph to be able to predict adult height, which serves as a basis for discussions with the family and for management decisions. If, however, the history is suggestive of any of the aforementioned disorders or the physical examination reveals abnormalities, additional laboratory tests should be performed. A SM-C/IGF-I is an excellent screening test for GH excess and can be verified with a glucose suppression test. Laboratory evidence of GH excess mandates magnetic resonance imaging of the pituitary. Chromosome analysis is useful in boys, especially when the upper to lower body segment ratio is decreased or when mental retardation is present. If Marfan syndrome or homocystinuria is suspected from the physical examination, referral to a cardiologist and an ophthalmologist should be made. Thyroid function tests are useful to diagnose or rule out hyperthyroidism when this disorder is suspected.

Management

Reassurance of the family and the patient is the key to the management of normal variant tall stature. The use of the bone age measurement to predict adult height may provide some comfort for them, as will general supportive discussions on the social acceptability of this condition. Although treatment is available for girls and boys with excessive growth, its use should be restricted to patients with (1) predicted adult height greater than 3 SD above the mean (77 inches in men, 72 inches in women) and (2) evidence of significant psychosocial impairment. For the family that strongly favors treatment, a trial of sex steroids is possible. Such therapy is designed to accelerate puberty and epiphyseal fusion and is therefore of little benefit when given in late puberty; therapy is initiated ideally prepubertally or in early puberty. Oral estrogens in various doses have successfully reduced the predicted height of female adolescents by 5 to 10 cm on the average. This is a direct result of the known effects of sex steroids on promoting epiphysial fusion, and therapy must begin, therefore, before the bone age has reached 12 years. Oral ethinyl estradiol at a dose of 0.15 to 0.5 mg/day until cessation of growth occurs has been used successfully in girls. If necessary, a progestational agent can be added after 1 year of unopposed estrogen therapy. In boys, treatment should begin before the bone age reaches 14 years; testosterone enanthate is used at a dose of 500 mg intramuscularly every 2 weeks for 6 months. Although no long-term complications of sex steroid therapy have been clearly documented, short-term side effects are common. These include lipid abnormalities, thromboembolism, cholelithiasis, hypertension, nausea, menstrual irregularities, and acne fulminans. The lack of extensive experience with this form of therapy and the risks involved should be carefully weighed and discussed with the family before beginning therapy.

BIBLIOGRAPHY

Brook CGD, Hindmarsh PC, Stanhope R: Growth and growth hormone secretion. J Endocrinol 119:179, 1988.

Frasier FD: Human pituitary growth hormone therapy in growth hormone deficiency. Endocr Rev 4:155, 1983.

Hintz RL, Rosenfeld RG (eds): Growth Abnormalities. New York, Churchill Livingstone, 1978.

Lee PDK, Rosenfeld RG: Psychosocial correlates of short stature and delayed puberty. Pediatr Clin North Am 34:851, 1987.

Raity S, Kaplan SL, Van Vliet G, et al: Short-term treatment of short stature and subnormal growth rate with human growth hormone. J Pediatr 110:357, 1987.

Rosenfeld RG: Evaluation of growth and maturation in adolescence. Pediatr Rev 4:175, 1982.

Rosenfeld RG: Constitutional delay in growth and adolescence. Semin Adolesc Med 3:267, 1987.

Rosenfeld RG, Hintz RL, Johansen AJ, et al: Three-year results of a randomized prospective trial of methionyl human growth hormone and oxandrolone in Turner syndrome. J Pediatr 111:393, 1988.

Rosenfeld RG, Wilson DM, Lee PDK, Hintz RL: Insulin-like growth factors I and II in the evaluation of growth retardation. J Pediatr 109:428, 1986.

Sorgo W, Scholler K, Heinze E, Teller WM: Critical analysis of height reduction in estrogen-treated tall girls. Eur J Pediatr 142:260, 1984.

Wilson DM, Kei J, Hintz RL, Rosenfeld RG: Effects of testosterone therapy for pubertal delay. Am J Dis Child 142:96, 1988.

Wilson DM, Kraemer HC, Ritter PL, Hammer LD: Growth curves and adult height estimation for adolescents. Am J Dis Child 141:565, 1987.

CHAPTER 57

Delayed Pubertal Development

HOWARD E. KULIN and EDWARD O. REITER

Delayed puberty in the female is defined as the absence of breast development by age 13 or the absence of menses by age 15. For boys, if testicular length does not exceed 2.5 cm by age 14, pubertal development is clearly delayed. By definition, the normal population contains 2.5% of adolescents of both sexes who mature at an age greater than 2 SD from the mean. However, more boys than girls consider such delay a serious concern and seek medical care for diagnosis and treatment. Most of these adolescents have physiologic or so-called constitutional delay in growth and puberty (see Chapter 56). They must be differentiated from patients with true hormonal defects.

A useful classification of the disorders associated with delayed puberty is based on gonadotropin secretion (Table 57–1). This classification relates gonadotropin levels to the stage of sexual differentiation, not to chronologic age. Thus, if normal adult amounts of follicle-stimulating hormone (FSH) or luteinizing hormone (LH) are found in a sexually immature individual, the disorder is considered to be hypergonadotropic.

HYPERGONADOTROPIC HYPOGONADISM

Genetic Gonadal Disease

Gonadal dysgenesis and its variants are clearly the most important and most common causes of hypergonadotropic hypogonadism, especially in girls. A significant proportion of these children may have delayed onset of sexual maturation without the classic somatic stigmata of the condition. The presence of short stature puts these individuals at high risk for partial or complete monosomy of the X chromosome. Others may have gonadal dysgenesis variants that include either an XX or XY karyotype, normal stature, and streak gonads.

Although Klinefelter syndrome is the most common form of male hypogonadism (1:500 males at birth), male adolescents with this genetic syndrome rarely complain of delayed onset of puberty. Because the defect in testosterone secretion is partial in most cases, androgen-related somatic changes are experienced at the appropriate age but may be incomplete (see Chapter 56).

Anorchia

Boys with anorchia constitute the largest group of male adolescents who present with delayed puberty and who have hypergonadotropic hypogonadism. These boys lack anatomically demonstrable or functioning testes, but the appearance of the external genitalia is otherwise normal. Since testosterone is required for development of the external genitalia during early fetal development, testes are assumed to be present during embryogenesis.

Boys with anorchia must be distinguished from boys with bilateral cryptorchidism; the latter group will usually experience normal puberty. However, some boys with bilateral intraabdominal testes have compromised Leydig cell function and may achieve normal testosterone levels only with elevated gonadotropin levels. Increases in FSH and LH levels are usually detectable by age 12 to 13 years in primary gonadal disease.

Gonadal Toxins

The effect of cytotoxic agents, such as cyclophosphamide, has been described as a cause of primary gonadal disease. Testicular and ovarian dysfunction appear to vary with age at onset of drug administration and duration of therapy. Radiation therapy that includes the gonads may also result in primary testicular or ovarian failure. These insults compromise gametogenesis to a greater extent than hormone production, and most patients do not have delayed puberty.

Adolescent survivors of childhood cancers now are receiving increasing attention to the effects of treatment regimens on growth, pubertal onset, and gonadal function. Combination chemotherapy and cranial irradiation for acute lymphoblastic leukemia is the most common circumstance in this regard. Increasing attention is also being paid to the gonadal effects following preparatory regimens (usually chemotherapy and irradiation) for bone marrow transplantation (see Chapter 54).

Enzyme Defects

Individuals with 17α-hydroxylase deficiency usually appear as phenotypically female whether they have XX or XY karyotypes. This enzyme block prevents adequate androgen, estrogen, and cortisol synthesis, which results in failure to virilize *in utero* and in hypokalemia, hypertension, and lack of pubertal development. Unlike the child with testicular feminization, individuals with 17α-hydroxylase deficiency will fail to develop breasts at the

509

TABLE 57–1. Causes of Delayed Adolescence in the Phenotypic Male and Female

HYPERGONADOTROPIC CONDITIONS
Variants of ovarian and testicular dysgenesis
Gonadal toxins (antimetabolite and radiation treatment)
Enzyme defects (17α-hydroxylase deficiency in the genetic male or female and 17-ketosteroid reductase deficiency in the genetic male)
Androgen insensitivity (testicular feminization)
Other miscellaneous disorders
HYPOGONADOTROPIC CONDITIONS
Multiple tropic hormone deficiency
Isolated growth hormone deficiency
Isolated gonadotropin deficiency
Miscellaneous syndrome-complexes (e.g., Prader-Willi syndrome)
Systemic conditions, nutritional and psychogenic disorders; increased energy expenditure
Other endocrine causes: hypothyroidism, glucocorticoid excess, hyperprolactinemia
Constitutional delay in growth and development
EUGONADOTROPIC CONDITIONS: DELAYED MENARCHE
Gonadal dysgenesis variants with residually functioning ovarian tissue
Abnormalities of müllerian duct development
Polycystic ovary disease
Hyperprolactinemia

expected age. Both FSH and LH levels are elevated in this syndrome.

There is also failure to virilize in utero in the genetic male individual with 17-ketosteroid reductase deficiency; breasts may develop at the time of puberty, and thus there may be confusion with incomplete forms of testicular feminization. Pubic hair development in such a phenotypic female adolescent is the result of increased androstenedione production, with conversion to testosterone (and estrogens) at extratesticular sites. LH concentration is increased.

Androgen Insensitivity

The genetic male adolescent with complete insensitivity to androgens (i.e., testicular feminization syndrome) will appear as a phenotypic female adolescent with primary amenorrhea, breast development, and absence of pubic hair. Incomplete insensitivity to androgens produces a clinical picture in which the phenotypic male individual will experience pubertal onset at an appropriate age, but complete androgenization usually fails to occur; gynecomastia, hypospadias, and cryptorchidism are common. The degree of androgen resistance ranges from severe to very mild.

Elevated LH levels reflect resistance to androgens at the hypothalamic-pituitary level. FSH measurements are usually normal, possibly because adequate amounts of estrogen or a nonsteroidal material secreted by the testes (inhibin) participate in its suppression.

Other Disorders

Mumps orchitis produces hypogonadism only after pubertal development is complete. Adolescents with myotonic dystrophy and trisomy 21 may eventually

display some Leydig and germ cell failure in adulthood but not a lag in the onset of sexual maturation. Variable ovarian dysfunction, including marked delay in pubertal onset, has been described in girls with galactosemia.

Girls with primary amenorrhea may have small, unstimulated ovaries with relatively increased gonadotropin levels. These adolescents probably constitute a heterogeneous group, sometimes referred to as having a resistant ovary syndrome. Abnormal or reduced gonadotropin receptors on the gonad are postulated as the primary defect.

Polyendocrine autoimmune conditions may affect the ovary during the course of pubertal development. The onset of sexual maturity may be normal or delayed. Testicular damage by a similar process may occur but is very rare.

HYPOGONADOTROPIC HYPOGONADISM

The presence of low gonadotropin levels in a patient with delayed puberty may be due to a number of different causes. Physiologically delayed puberty is by far the most common type of hypogonadotropic hypogonadism and can be diagnosed with certainty only after excluding other specific disorders.

Multiple Tropic Hormone Deficiency

Children with multiple tropic hormone deficiencies usually have early growth retardation in addition to sexual infantilism. It should be borne in mind, however, that if growth hormone (GH) or thyroid-stimulating hormone (TSH) deficiency, or both, occur relatively late in childhood, the degree of growth retardation may be modest. Hypopituitarism usually results from an idiopathic hypothalamic defect, although tumor or a structural lesion must be excluded (see Chapter 55). Using highly sensitive imaging techniques (e.g., magnetic resonance imaging), anatomic defects of the pituitary gland are being found with increasing frequency.

Lesions of histiocytosis X, tuberculosis, or sarcoidosis may interfere with anterior or posterior pituitary function, or both, by hypothalamic infiltration. Midline developmental abnormalities of the central nervous system (e.g., septo-optic dysplasia) may be associated with a variety of hypothalamic defects. Finally, head and neck irradiation may produce enough cell death to diminish hypothalamic-pituitary function.

Isolated Growth Hormone Deficiency

Patients with isolated GH deficiency will invariably have delayed puberty despite the intact secretion of thyrotropin, adrenocorticotropic hormone (ACTH), and gonadotropins. Most of these patients have idiopathic disease and display early childhood growth failure.

Figure 57–1. The levels of urinary LH ranked according to increasing concentration in 16 subjects (I–XVI) with hypogonadotropic hypogonadism. The levels of urinary FSH and testosterone in these same patients are shown in the middle and bottom panels. The bar represents the mean hormonal measurement with individual determinations indicated by solid dots. The following symbols are used: * = testis size 2.0 to 2.5 cm on the long axis (all others <2.0 cm); C = unilateral cryptorchidism; †† = bilateral cryptorchidism. For comparison, the normal adolescent ranges and the number of individuals included in those normal ranges (in parentheses) are shown in the right panels. It is evident that hypogonadism in this group can exist even with gonadotropin measurements in the late pubertal range. (Reprinted from Santen RJ, Kulin HE: Evaluation of delayed puberty and hypogonadism. In Santen RJ, Swerdloff RS [eds]: Male Reproductive Dysfunction, 1986, p 155, by courtesy of Marcel Dekker, Inc.)

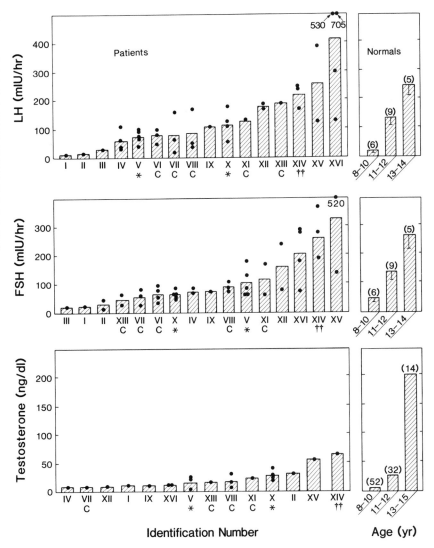

Idiopathic isolated GH deficiency is the most common type of hypopituitarism during childhood and may occur as frequently as 1 in 4000 births. Some patients with constitutional delay in growth and development may have very mild defects in GH secretion that are transiently confined to the physiologic slowing of growth that precedes the pubertal growth spurt.

Isolated Gonadotropin Deficiency

Gonadotropin deficiency without loss of other anterior pituitary hormones results from a number of different genetic disorders. In the subgroup of patients with defects in olfaction (Kallmann syndrome), there is evidence that fetal migration of gonadotropin-releasing hormone (GnRH)–containing neurons from nasal regions into the forebrain is impeded.

Gonadotropin deficiency in this disorder may be variable. In the classic form, both FSH and LH levels are low and no evidence of sexual maturation is apparent. In other forms, sexual maturation begins but then fails to progress in a normal fashion, with resultant incomplete development.

The degree of hormone deficiency in adolescents with isolated hypogonadotropism has been poorly documented because most blood gonadotropin assays are relatively insensitive. Newer serum assay systems should allow delineation of the syndrome-complex as precisely as the quantitation of low gonadotropin levels by radioimmunoassay of urine extracts (Fig. 57–1).

Syndrome-Complexes Associated with Hypogonadotropism

Certain disease complexes, such as the Prader-Willi syndrome, are associated with gonadotropin deficiency. This sporadic condition is associated with hypotonia, obesity, mental retardation, short stature, and adult-onset diabetes mellitus (see Chapters 31 and 56). The degree of hypogonadotropism in this disorder ranges from partial to severe, and some cases of hypergonadotropic hypogonadism have even been recognized.

The Laurence-Moon-Biedl syndrome is characterized by renal abnormalities, retinitis pigmentosa, obesity, mental retardation, and polydactyly. The inheritance is autosomal recessive, and the degree of gonadotropin deficiency is variable. Hypergonadotropism may, in fact, be more common than hypogonadotropism, particularly in males.

The multiple lentigines syndrome has been associated with hypogonadotropism and may involve cardiac defects, urologic abnormalities, short stature, deafness, and autosomal dominant transmission. Additional syndrome-complexes associated with hypogonadotropism include Möbius syndrome, congenital ichthyosis, and cerebellar ataxia.

Systemic Conditions

Any systemic illness that affects growth may cause delayed onset or progression of pubertal development. Renal failure invariably produces marked retardation of growth at any age and must be considered early in the evaluation of delayed puberty. Inflammatory bowel disease and celiac disease are well-described examples of gastrointestinal disorders that may cause a profound degree of growth retardation on a nutritional basis; the latter condition, in fact, may occur only with short stature and pubertal delay in the absence of bowel symptoms (see Chapters 56, 63, and 65).

Recurrent infections and neoplastic disease may be associated with poor growth and delayed pubertal progression. Data from a large group of children with sickle cell disease show increasing deficits in height and weight with age, along with a marked delay in onset of the pubertal growth spurt. Children with cystic fibrosis almost invariably have a delay in pubertal development (see Chapters 43 and 52).

Serious psychosomatic illness, including anorexia nervosa, is usually not difficult to diagnose and may be associated with delayed puberty. Milder forms of psychological problems, however, may be confirmed only by eliminating the possibility of organic disease. Although psychosocial causes of delayed growth have been described primarily in the toddler age group such factors may clearly influence growth at any age, including puberty. Conditions without defined disorders of thought, but which are associated with attaining the thin body image encouraged by Western societies, may result in delayed puberty, the so-called fear of obesity syndrome (see Chapter 60).

It is likely that nutritional insults constitute a common pathway in delaying puberty in many systemic illnesses. The central nervous system mediation of such an insult through suppression of GnRH remains poorly understood. Growth responses and the ability to "catch up" are clearly dependent on the degree and severity of the caloric deficit, as well as on the extrametabolic demands imposed by certain diseases.

Recent interest has focused on the effect of marked energy expenditure on gonadotropin secretion. Most of these data have related to the amenorrhea known to occur in many female long-distance runners. Very clearly, however, vigorous physical exertion in the peripubertal period may have a profound effect on the onset and progression of sexual maturation.

Other Endocrine Causes

Additional endocrine conditions that may cause retarded growth and subsequent delayed puberty are hypothyroidism and glucocorticoid excess (see Chapter 55). The latter may be iatrogenic, and the administration of glucocorticoids for a variety of illnesses is a well-known cause of growth suppression in children.

Although hypothyroidism is classically associated with severe growth delay, signs of puberty may be normal, or even early, in a significant proportion of cases caused by primary thyroid disease. This paradox occurs because FSH and LH may actually be increased (for bone age) in the setting of marked and prolonged hyperthyrotropinemia.

A functional defect in gonadotropin secretion caused by elevated prolactin levels is being recognized with increasing frequency as a cause of delayed puberty. The most common presentation of prolactinoma in the young woman is primary amenorrhea. Gynecomastia is rarely, if ever, present in the male with a prolactinoma.

Constitutional (Physiologic) Delay in Growth and Development

Constitutional factors are by far the most common cause of delayed puberty (see Chapter 56). Most girls with this growth pattern do not seek medical care. Adolescents with this condition represent a variant of the norm; they grew slowly throughout childhood and consequently enter puberty later than usual. There is often a familial tendency to this pattern. These individuals progress through pubertal stages at a relatively normal rate once the process begins.

The major problem in the diagnosis of delayed puberty is the differentiation of patients with physiologically delayed puberty from those with complete or incomplete forms of hypogonadotropic hypogonadism. There is no definitive means of establishing the cause as physiologically delayed puberty other than prolonged observation; the normal pubertal process may occasionally not be initiated until the early 20s.

EUGONADOTROPIC HYPOGONADISM (DELAYED MENARCHE)

Delayed menarche is defined as the normal onset and progression of pubertal development associated with primary amenorrhea. Abnormalities of müllerian duct development account for a large number of these adolescent patients; the defect may involve absence of the uterus, vagina, or both ductal derivatives (Rokitansky-Kuster-Hauser syndrome). Mosaic forms of gonadal dysgenesis may present in this fashion, but gonadotropin levels are usually elevated in these adolescents. Phenotypic female adolescents with androgen sensitivity will also exhibit primary amenorrhea.

There is evidence that polycystic ovary disease may begin during puberty. Thus, adolescents with the Stein-Leventhal syndrome may have secondary amenorrhea or even, on rare occasions, primary amenorrhea (see Chapter 70).

Primary amenorrhea in the presence of galactorrhea

may occur with or without increased prolactin levels. These individuals may have either low or normal levels of gonadotropin production.

CLINICAL PRESENTATION OF THE ADOLESCENT WITH DELAYED PUBERTY

History

The overall pattern of growth during childhood as well as during the pubertal years is an extremely important differential point in evaluating delayed puberty. The majority of children with constitutional delay in growth exhibit a slow growth pattern during childhood with progressive height increments along the lower limits of normal (Fig. 57–2) (see Chapter 56). In contrast, the patient with hypogonadotropic hypogonadism usually has had normal growth during childhood but increments in growth at the time of the expected pubertal spurt have not taken place; hence, growth retardation is a new event with a recently diminished growth velocity. The measurement of growth velocity (in centimeters per

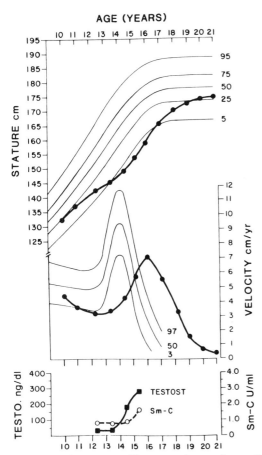

Figure 57–2. Growth pattern and hormone changes in constitutional delay in growth. A typical patient decelerates across growth channels in the late prepubertal year and then catches up in growth. Plasma testosterone and somatomedin-C levels belatedly rise. (With permission from Rosenfeld RL: Clinical review 6: Diagnosis and management of delayed puberty. J Clin Endocrinol Metab 70:559–562, 1990. © by The Endocrine Society.)

year) is helpful in this regard, since the assessment of a child's current growth rate may be more revealing than the plot of height on a conventional (distance) growth chart. If growth retardation is severe (more than 3.0 SD from mean), somatotropin deficiency becomes a strong consideration.

Progression of secondary sex characteristics, as well as the timing of their onset, are important clues in the history. It is crucial to remember that adolescents with partial hypogonadotropic hypogonadism or compensated hypogonadotropism may have the onset of secondary sex characteristics at a normal time, but fail to achieve the normal progression of these physical changes.

The genetic background provides useful information, and attempts should be made to ascertain the time of onset of puberty in siblings, parents, and grandparents of the adolescent patient. Socioeconomic factors may have a marked influence on the time of onset of puberty, occasionally overshadowing genetic influences. The history of any drug ingestion that might be associated with systemic disease is obviously of great importance; cytotoxic agents and glucocorticoids are of particular note in this regard. Heavy marijuana smoking has been reported to cause pubertal delay. Extremes of energy expenditures may influence the pubertal process both in terms of onset and progression of secondary sex characteristics.

A careful review of systems will be helpful in defining any disease states that might be associated with poor growth. In particular, symptoms related to gastrointestinal, cardiac, renal, thyroid, and central nervous system function must be sought. Psychosocial data may be difficult to accrue, and additional social service help in investigating the family setting may be useful. Growth at any time during childhood, and certainly during puberty, may be influenced markedly by psychological factors either directly on secretion of neuroregulatory substances or indirectly through changes in nutrition.

Physical Examination

Adolescents with GH deficiency characteristically have a greater retardation in height than in weight, in contrast with individuals with aberrant psychosocial backgrounds, who usually have greater retardation in weight than in height (see Chapter 56). Eunuchoidal body proportions (arm span greater than height and distance from symphysis pubis to feet greater than from symphysis pubis to vertex of head) appear later in individuals with hypogonadotropism in contrast with the earlier appearance in Klinefelter syndrome.

Some androgenic manifestations (e.g., pubic hair) may reflect adrenal steroid secretion rather than gonadal function. Estrogen effects are monitored by means of breast development, vaginal color and secretions, and uterine size (see Chapters 69 and 77). A careful examination of the central nervous system must be performed and should include tests of olfaction and of peripheral vision. Approximately 80% of boys with Kallmann syndrome exhibit anosmia or hyposmia, and precise quantitation of olfactory threshold is useful. The presence of gynecomastia and galactorrhea should be noted.

Pubertal staging with the additional measurements of breast tissue and testicular size should be obtained. Exact measurement of the length and width of the testes is easily accomplished with a ruler; a length of more than 2.5 cm is a strong indicator of endogenous gonadotropin production. In the boy of pubertal age, the relative disparity between testicular size and other androgenic manifestations such as pubic hair should be noted; testes size usually increases only slightly with the onset of puberty in boys with an XXY karyotype, but pubic hair may be quite advanced.

The disease complexes that include delayed puberty may be revealed by the obesity, short stature, and mild mental retardation of the Prader-Willi syndrome or by the polydactyly and retinitis pigmentosa found in patients with Laurence-Moon-Biedl syndrome (see Chapters 31 and 56). The numerous stigmata of gonadal dysgenesis are among the most significant findings to note. These include an increased number of pigmented nevi, a high-arched palate, low hairline, widely spaced nipples (shield chest), eyelid ptosis, cutis laxa, pterygium colli, shortened fourth metacarpals, heart murmurs, cubitus valgus, nail changes, and deformed ears. Patients with Kallmann syndrome may have a cleft lip, cleft palate, and congenital deafness, in addition to hyposmia or anosmia.

DIAGNOSTIC TESTING

The diagnostic tests to assess the integrity of the hypothalamic-pituitary-gonadal axis are based on the physiologic principles that underlie the process of pubertal maturation. Tests may be used to assess (1) anatomic structure, (2) basal secretion of hormones, (3) dynamic manipulations of the hypothalamic-pituitary-gonadal axis, and (4) miscellaneous aspects. Assistance from a pediatric endocrinologist will frequently be required for a full evaluation.

Anatomic Structure

Imaging techniques allow the assessment of pituitary and hypothalamic structures. Plain skull films will delineate gross sellar enlargement, erosion of bony structures, or calcification. The calculated volume of the sella turcica allows the inferential distinction between a small and a normal pituitary gland.

Computed tomography (CT) scanning and magnetic resonance imaging (MRI) can provide information regarding mass lesions in the pituitary, suprasellar cistern, or hypothalamus; the presence of pathologic calcifications and of increased intracranial pressure may also be noted. These techniques are most helpful in the evaluation of hypogonadotropism in association with deficiencies of other pituitary hormones, especially when craniopharyngioma, pituitary adenoma, or other brain neoplasms are suspected. Despite the sensitivity of current scanners, small hypothalamic lesions may not be visualized yet still result in hypopituitarism. MRI has been particularly useful in delineating heretofore unrec-

ognized anatomic defects of the pituitary, as well as dysplasia of the optic nerves.

Formal visual field testing can detect functional disruption of the optic tracts, chiasm, or nerves. Careful assessment by a trained ophthalmologist can also detect dysplasia of the optic disc, a feature observed in the syndrome of septo-optic dysplasia.

Pelvic ultrasound can sometimes be of assistance in localizing intraabdominal testicular structures in older boys. This noninvasive technique is most useful, however, in detecting the presence or absence of müllerian structures in children who are phenotypically female and sexually infantile or have not progressed in pubertal development to menarche.

The epiphyseal growth centers in the wrists and hands change in response to GH, thyroxine, adrenal androgens, and gonadal steroid levels. In conditions of disordered growth the bone age provides a most useful marker for the degree of hypothalamic maturation.

Basal Hormone Measurements

Despite the improved capacity to measure sex steroids and gonadotropins, methodologic problems of assay sensitivity remain. Levels may vary markedly in a given patient, and, perhaps most importantly, the onset of secondary sex characteristics may occur with relatively small increments in hormones.

Significant increases in the secretion of adrenal sex steroids normally occur by age 7 or 8 years (adrenarche), typified by changes in circulating amounts of dehydroepiandrosterone (DHEA) and its sulfate (DHEAS). Serum DHEA and DHEAS mirror urinary 17-ketosteroid determinations, which are rarely of use in the assessment of delayed puberty. In adolescents with isolated hypogonadotropic hypogonadism, levels of adrenal sex steroids are in the normal range relative to chronologic age. In contrast, the adolescent with constitutional delay has a lag in the maturation of both gonadal and adrenal function (see Chapter 56). This distinction appears to be most useful after the age of 16 years.

Serum estradiol (E_2) determinations in prepubertal girls are so low (usually below the sensitivity of most assays) and the variability within patients so marked that single blood results have a poor correlation with the first increments in gonadal activity. In the rare patient with 17α-hydroxylase deficiency, plasma progesterone and urinary pregnanediol levels will be elevated (as will the mineralocorticoids, desoxycorticosterone and corticosterone). In the adolescent with 17-ketosteroid reductase deficiency, plasma androstenedione and estrone levels will be elevated with relatively small amounts of circulating testosterone detected.

Circulating testosterone can be reliably measured at low levels. However, the first increment in testicular size reflects changes in germinal elements rather than testosterone-producing Leydig cell stimulation. Thus, serum testosterone measurements are usually still prepubertal when the first genital changes appear. Once serum testosterone levels begin to increase during male puberty there is a relatively rapid increment (from 40 to 200 ng/dl) over a 10-month period.

Since diagnostic categories of delayed puberty are based on gonadotropin measurements, these studies are of particular importance in evaluation. Problems with assay sensitivity and the episodic nature of gonadotropin secretion have made precise measurements of blood LH and FSH difficult during the peripubertal period. One convenient means of enhancing the sensitivity of LH and FSH measurements is to concentrate timed 3- to 6-hour urine specimens. With this technique, accurate estimates can be made throughout early childhood as well as during puberty. New immunoassay methods have markedly increased the ability to accurately measure gonadotropins in the blood of prepubertal children.

Episodic or pulsatile secretion of LH (and less so of FSH) also potentially confounds interpretation of single blood gonadotropin measurements used to assess the degree of pubertal maturation. Precise quantitation of integrated LH levels requires either multiple plasma measurements or the assay of timed urine samples. Both methods are highly correlated, provided that the plasma levels are detectable in the particular radioimmunoassay used.

Adolescents who have delayed puberty, low levels of gonadotropins, and a bone age of more than 13 years should be evaluated for a pathologic condition. On the other hand, those individuals with similarly low LH and FSH results but with a bone age of 10 to 11 years are more likely to experience normal sexual maturation. Nevertheless, as shown in Figure 57–3, there is a great deal of overlap in basal gonadotropin values obtained from subjects with constitutional delay of growth and from patients with true hypogonadotropism.

Basal gonadotropins may not be diagnostic in many hypogonadotropic situations. In contrast, however, basal determinations are of great use in the early detection of primary gonadal disease. In the child of late prepubertal age, gonadal dysgenesis may be diagnosed easily by using either blood or urinary specimens. By the age of 11 or 12 years in such girls, urinary gonadotropin measurements have usually reached adult castrate levels. In the boy with primary gonadal disease, FSH and LH levels are also clearly elevated, at least in comparison to the stage of sexual maturity (Fig. 57–4). In the boy with Klinefelter syndrome, gonadotropin increases do not occur until mid puberty.

Basal, followed by serial, gonadotropin determinations are most useful in the assessment of hypogonadotropic adolescents. Urinary measurements are of great value in this regard and aid in separating individuals with physiologically delayed adolescence from those with true hypogonadotropism. Adolescents who are destined to continue through normal puberty will have progressive incremental rises in FSH and/or LH levels in a relatively short period, usually 6 to 12 months. Continued low gonadotropin measurements increase the likelihood of true hormone deficiency (Fig. 57–5).

Dynamic Tests of Hypothalamic-Pituitary-Gonadal Function

Administration of exogenous GnRH allows assessment of the functional capacity of the pituitary gonad-

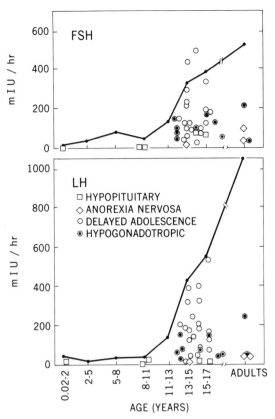

Figure 57–3. Basal urinary gonadotropin results obtained from patients with hypogonadotropism. Hypopituitary adolescents have multiple tropic hormone deficiency, while hypogonadotropic adolescents have decreased amounts of luteinizing hormone (LH) and follicle-stimulating hormone (FSH) only. All the delayed adolescents (n = 20) eventually experienced normal puberty. The dark line represents the mean normal gonadotropin excretion for age. (With permission from Kulin HE: Delayed adolescence: II. Diagnostic studies and treatment. Female Patient 8:48–64, 1983.)

otrophs to release LH and FSH. Two factors influence this response: (1) the number of gonadotropes present and (2) prior exposure of these cells to sufficient amounts of endogenous GnRH. For this reason, the response to a single bolus of GnRH is limited in prepubertal subjects when endogenous GnRH secretion is low. As endogenous GnRH increases in pubertal subjects, the response to exogenous GnRH is enhanced.

Variable increments in LH and FSH have been observed after single injections of GnRH in individuals with hypogonadotropic eunuchoidism, particularly in those with the incomplete forms. Adolescents with physiologic delayed puberty, on the other hand, may exhibit diminished response to GnRH even in the early stages of testicular enlargement. Because of this variability the overlap between normal individuals and those with incomplete hypogonadotropic hypogonadism often makes the acute GnRH test difficult to interpret.

A refinement of the GnRH test that uses an infusion of the releasing hormone and assessment of the early and late LH responses has been employed. A further variation of the GnRH test has used bolus injection of the material before and after a 36-hour period of pulsatile GnRH administration. More sustained stimulation of the gonadotrope and the release of newly synthesized

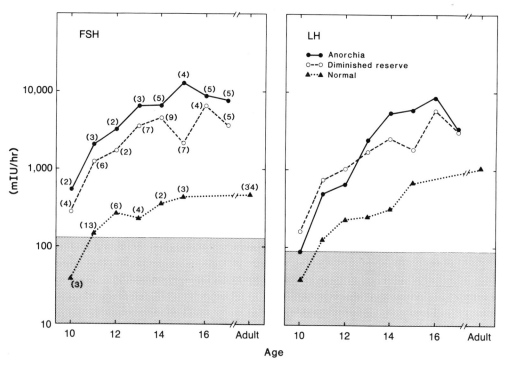

Figure 57–4. Peripubertal change in gonadotropin excretion in 9 anorchic boys, 9 males with diminished testicular reserve, and 31 normal boys. The number of subjects tested at each data point is shown in parentheses on the FSH panel. The shaded areas denote the normal prepubertal range. Note log scale on x-axis. (With permission from Kulin HE, Santner SJ: The assessment of diminished testicular function in boys of pubertal age. Clin Endocrinol 25:283–292, 1986.)

hormone has also been attempted by using single injections of long-acting GnRH agonist. Further experience with the various refinements of the GnRH test is needed, particularly in adolescents with only mild degrees of gonadotropin deficiency.

Responsiveness of the gonad can be determined by administering human chorionic gonadotropin (HCG) and assessing the plasma testosterone increments at various time intervals. While traditional test procedures required daily multiple injections, more recent data indicate that one intramuscular injection of 1500 to 6000 IU is a sufficient stimulus. Plasma testosterone is then measured before and 72 hours after HCG administration. Further experience is needed, however, to ensure the usefulness of any HCG stimulation protocol in differentiating hypogonadotropic adolescents from those with constitutional delay.

Chorionic gonadotropin testing is most useful in the definitive diagnosis of anorchia, since testosterone levels in such adolescents will not increase over prepubertal measurements following stimulation. Testosterone levels may also be increased following HCG administration in boys with diminished testicular reserve. Basal testosterone measurements in such adolescents may be normal for age but only with increased gonadotropins.

Miscellaneous Studies

Determination of serum thyroxine level and measurement of thyroid binding as well as prolactin are always appropriate (see Chapter 55). When height is more than 3 SD from the mean for age, or when growth velocity is reduced, somatotropin provocation tests remain a consideration. Testing the olfactory threshold is useful in adolescent patients presumed to have hypogonadotropism.

Certain genetic tests may provide important information in a number of endocrine diseases, particularly those involving abnormalities of gonadal function. Analysis of the karyotype, determined on blood lymphocytes, skin fibroblasts, buccal mucosal cells, or gonadal tissue may be extremely useful. It is an unusual adolescent patient who requires exploratory laparotomy, but the boy who has a Y-chromosomal cell line and dysgenetic gonads is at a risk for malignant disease; in that setting the dysgenetic tissue should be removed. A testicular biopsy is rarely indicated in the evaluation of delayed adolescence. Receptor studies are needed to confirm androgen resistance.

TREATMENT

Indications

Severe psychological effects may result from a delay in adolescent sexual development. These include the following manifestations:

1. Symptoms of emotional tension, irritability, and depression
2. Psychosomatic complaints (e.g., abdominal pain)
3. Feelings of inferiority with regard to masculinity or femininity
4. Symptoms of overcompensation (e.g., fighting or extreme competitiveness in sports)
5. Regression or withdrawal from peer contact
6. Poor school performance
7. Decreased sports activity
8. Increased school absenteeism
9. Inadequate vocational and educational goals for age
10. Increased parental dependence and parental overprotection as part of overall social immaturity.

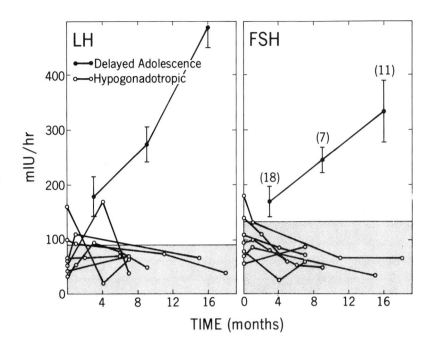

Figure 57–5. Sequential urinary gonadotropin changes following initial referral in 7 boys with hypogonadotropic hypogonadism *(open circles)* and 18 boys with physiologic delay in puberty *(solid circles)*. Results from the patients with physiologic delay were meaned for approximately 6-month intervals of time, with the number of samples at each time interval shown within parentheses of the FSH box. The initial mean ages of the patients in the two diagnostic categories were nearly identical: 14.8 and 15 years. The brackets represent ± 1 standard error, indicating considerable ranges in individual values. The stippled area indicates the prepubertal range. (Reprinted from Santen RJ, Kulin HE: Evaluation of delayed puberty and hypogonadism. In Santen RJ, Swerdloff RS [eds]: Male Reproductive Dysfunction, 1986, p 166, by courtesy of Marcel Dekker, Inc.)

Counseling will be adequate for a few minor symptoms, but marked involvement in any of the above areas indicates a need for hormone replacement therapy as well, regardless of the diagnostic quandaries.

Therapeutic Alternatives

In the absence of a functioning gonad, sex steroid replacement must be provided. In the absence of endogenous gonadotropins or hypothalamic releasing factor however, substances that stimulate the gonad provide alternative therapeutic methods. GnRH has been given on a long-term basis and can induce adult levels of testosterone or estradiol; a frequent drug administration schedule is required, however, because of the short half-life of GnRH analogues.

HCG has long been available as a means of stimulating exogenous androgens in the male adolescent. Multiple weekly injections have usually been employed, but investigations suggest that a single weekly injection of HCG (approximately 1500 IU) may be an adequate growth-promoting regimen. Although it makes good physiologic sense to stimulate endogenous testosterone, there is no clear advantage to initiating puberty by these means. The frequency of injections and the high cost make HCG therapy less than ideal. In addition, boys with hypogonadotropic eunuchoidism associated with bilateral cryptorchidism may have a testicular defect that limits the levels of testosterone that can be stimulated by HCG.

Exogenous androgens and estrogens are preferred for the adolescent patient who needs hormone replacement therapy. A safe and fully effective orally active androgen is not available in the United States. Prompt degradation by the liver necessitates a modification of the testosterone molecule, most commonly methyl or ethyl substitutions in the 17α-position. Such changes may make oral therapy practical, but liver abnormalities appear in a small but significant number of patients so treated.

Esterification of the 17β-hydroxyl group of testosterone is another common modification of the steroid nucleus and provides a slow-release, lipid-soluble depot formulation. One such drug, testosterone undecanoate, is absorbed by intestinal lymphatics and can be administered orally (usually two to three times a day). This material is not available in the United States but is widely employed in Europe.

Most esters of testosterone are given parenterally, and the long-acting cypionate or enanthate is usually administered at intervals of 2 to 4 weeks. Peak levels of testosterone are attained in 24 hours with a duration of action of approximately 2 weeks. These latter substances are the drugs of choice for the replacement of androgens in a boy of pubertal age.

A number of orally active estrogen preparations are available; conjugated equine estrogens (Premarin) are commonly used. Attempts have been made to bypass exposure of the liver, either by intravaginal administration or simply by applying the steroid to the skin. No data are currently available about such regimens in the treatment of the adolescent girl.

As already mentioned, the use of human GH in the treatment of patients with constitutional delay in growth and adolescence remains controversial. A physiologic drop in GH production may occur at the time of the slowdown in velocity just before the pubertal spurt begins. Although exogenous somatotropin may increase height velocity during this period, there is no documentation that final adult height may be influenced by such intervention.

Suggested Therapeutic Approach

The aim of sex hormone therapy for the boy or girl of pubertal age is to promote secondary sex characteristics and normal linear growth. An additional objective in the adolescent with constitutional delay is to speed the pace of hypothalamic maturation.

The secondary sex characteristics of importance in the initiation of puberty are pubic hair and breast development in the female, and increased penile size in the male. Treatment with exogenous androgens also causes an increase in scrotal rugae and pigmentation, but the size of the testes usually remains unchanged. Enlargement of testes during testosterone administration connotes the advance of normal pubertal processes. Pubic hair may appear relatively late in male puberty. It remains unclear what role estrogen plays in the appearance of pubic hair in the female. The appearance of axillary and facial hair and voice change are variable and of little clinical use in following the onset of puberty. Facial hair in the male requires high-dose parenteral therapy and is a late development in the pubertal process.

The primary side effect to be avoided in the initiation of puberty is sex steroid acceleration of bone maturation in excess of chronologic gain. The maturing epiphyses are highly sensitive to estrogen as well as to testosterone, but the usual means of assessing such effects are relatively insensitive ones; that is, the proper interpretation of bone age is dependent on the skill of the person reading the appropriate radiographs, an awareness of the age-related standard deviations of such a measurement, and the fact that it usually takes months for treatment changes to become evident.

The underlying dictum of treatment is to use as little replacement hormone as possible and to realize that remarkably small amounts of steroid are needed to promote growth and the onset of secondary sex characterists. In general, androgen therapy should not be employed before a bone age of 12 to 13 is attained, with greater leeway possible for short-term drug exposures.

Short-Term Trial Therapy with Sex Steroids

Because of diagnostic difficulty in separating normal individuals with physiologic or constitutional delay from some adolescents with specific deficiency disorders of the hypothalamic-pituitary-gonadal axis, a short-term trial of sex steroids may be used (see Chapter 56). This maneuver reduces the psychological effects of sexual immaturity. This type of therapy is quite different from the administration of replacement sex hormones to a patient of pubertal age who is known to be deficient in gonadal function.

In the male adolescent, 50 to 100 mg of testosterone enanthate or cypionate administered intramuscularly every 3 to 4 weeks is appropriate. Depending on patient preference and availability of instruction, the injections may be given by physician, parent, or patient. Therapy is administered for 3 to 4 months and then stopped for a similar period. During the latter interval, the boy is observed for further changes in testicular size and for spontaneous increments in gonadotropin and serum testosterone levels.

Although changes in the first months may be small, many adolescent patients find these advances reassuring enough to let some time pass without additional treatment. Several intermittent courses of low-dose testosterone can be administered until either spontaneous puberty is proceeding or the need for long-term exogenous therapy is confirmed. This regimen has no harmful effect on either the potential for full somatic growth or subsequent testicular function.

When a diagnostic quandary exists in a female adolescent, a similar approach is recommended. A trial of estrogen replacement with continuous daily oral administration of 0.3 mg of Premarin or 5 to 10 µg of ethinyl estradiol is appropriate. The drug should be given for 3 to 4 months and then stopped to allow for observation of further changes in secondary sex characteristics, hormonal (e.g., FSH or LH) levels, or both. Withdrawal bleeding may not occur following the first course, although it may after subsequent trials. If spontaneous sexual maturation does not occur, long-term replacement therapy should be recommended only after several intermittent courses of estrogen.

Long-Term Sex Hormone Replacement Therapy

A somewhat different approach is taken for adolescents in whom the diagnosis of permanent hypogonadism has been made. Such boys will need long-term treatment, and all attempts to duplicate the events of spontaneous puberty should be made. In this regard, careful attention must be paid to somatic growth and corresponding gains in bone maturation (see Chapter 5).

Direct administration of long-acting androgen preparations in the form of testosterone enanthate or testosterone cypionate, 25 to 50 mg intramuscularly every 3 to 4 weeks, is the preferred mode of initial therapy. This regimen is convenient and relatively inexpensive, and hormonal levels can be easily monitored. Gonadal enlargement is usually not seen in those boys with scrotal testes. Remarkably little testosterone is needed to induce considerable change in phallic size, scrotal maturation, and pubic hair.

By the second or third year of treatment, an intramuscular dose of testosterone, 50 to 100 mg every 3 to 4 weeks is appropriate. Over 4 to 5 years, the amount of long-acting testosterone is gradually increased to adult male maintenance levels of 200 mg intramuscularly every 2 to 3 weeks. Bone age monitoring throughout this period is imperative with a view to ensuring that skeletal age does not exceed chronologic age. The amount of testosterone needed to produce facial hair growth varies greatly from person to person; despite the natural desire of some adolescents to achieve this end, the pubertal process must not be speeded up at the risk of excessively rapid bone maturation.

Side effects of long-term androgen treatment are directly related to dosage and duration of therapy. For the male adolescent, the most troublesome event associated with drug administration is gynecomastia (see Chapter 77). This effect is variable and is a result of the fact that testosterone analogues, as well as testosterone itself, can be aromatized in peripheral tissue to estradiol. Significant sodium retention is not a problem.

It is important to remember the differences between initiating puberty and achieving full adult virilization. Libido, like facial hair, is very variable in its relation to a given testosterone level. A heightened feeling of well-being, reported by some adult men whose testosterone levels have been increased from low to normal levels, is not an objective in treating the male adolescent.

Testicular prostheses should be implanted in the agonadal patient in whom the condition is diagnosed in the peripubertal period. Most urologists believe that surgery is easier after some scrotal stimulation by testosterone. For psychological reasons, this aspect of male puberty should not be unduly delayed.

In the female adolescent oral therapy can be used successfully and is recommended. As in virtually all estrogen therapy, the dosage should be the lowest possible that provides the desired effects. There is no convincing evidence that patients with gonadal dysgenesis are more likely to develop endometrial carcinoma; in all hypogonadal individuals, however, dose and duration of therapy are related to endometrial hyperplasia. Also, long-term, unopposed estrogen treatment, even given cyclically, is not recommended, but precise studies of what does constitute the safest method of estrogen treatment in the young person are not available.

It is reasonable to institute replacement therapy with estrogen alone, as occurs normally. Treatment can be started with low daily doses of estrogen (Premarin, 0.15 mg) or ethinyl estradiol (2 to 5 μg) for approximately 1 year. After the initial period of breast and uterine stimulation, the continuous estrogen dose is doubled and continued for an additional 6 to 12 months. Estrogen plus progesterone is then employed cyclically to produce monthly vaginal bleeding. Estrogen is given for the first 25 days of each month, and medroxyprogesterone acetate (Provera, 5 to 10 mg/day) is added for the last 10 to 12 days of the cycle. Alternatively, a combined oral contraceptive–type drug regimen may be prescribed. There is little expected growth retardation with low-dose estrogen replacement, although bone age monitoring is imperative. All efforts should be made to initiate replacement at the expected time of puberty, that is, by the age of 11 to 12 years, using as little sex steroid as possible. There is no convincing reason to use androgens to promote growth in the agonadal female with a sex chromosome anomaly.

BIBLIOGRAPHY

Bourguignon JP: Linear growth as a function of age at onset of puberty and sex steroid dosage: Therapeutic implications. Endocr Rev 9:467, 1988.

Haavisto AH, Dunkel L, Pettersson K, Huhtaniemi I: LH measurements by in vitro bioassay and a highly sensitive immunofluorometric assay improve the distinction between boys with constitutional delay of puberty and hypogonadotropic hypogonadism. Pediatr Res 27:211, 1990.

Krainz PL, Hanna CE, LaFranchi SH: Etiology of delayed puberty in 146 children evaluated over a 10-year period. J Pediatr Endocrinol 2:165, 1987.

Kulin HE: Disorders of sexual maturation: Delayed adolescence and precocious puberty. In DeGroot LJ (ed): Endocrinology. Philadelphia, WB Saunders, 1989, pp 1873–1890.

Lee PDK, Rosenfeld RG: Psychosocial correlates of short stature and delayed puberty. Pediatr Adolesc Endocrinol 34:851, 1987.

Rappaport R, Brauner R: Growth and endocrine disorders secondary to cranial irradiation. Pediatr Res 25:561, 1989.

Rosenfield RL: Clinical review 6: Diagnosis and management of delayed puberty. J Clin Endocrinol Metab 70:559, 1990.

Shalet SM: Treatment of constitutional delay in growth and puberty (CDGP). Clin Endocrinol 31:81, 1989.

Van Dop C, Burstein S, Conte FA, Grumbach MM: Isolated gonadotropin deficiency in boys: Clinical characteristics and growth. J Pediatr 111:684, 1987.

CHAPTER 58

Precocious Puberty

DANA S. HARDIN and ORA HIRSCH PESCOVITZ

Normal pubertal maturation is the result of an integrated neuroendocrine-gonadal axis that becomes active during the third trimester *in utero* and only becomes quiescent after the first year of life, owing to increased sensitivity of the hypothalamic "gonadostat" to negative feedback of sex steroids (see Chapter 4). Thus, throughout most of childhood the amplitude of gonadotropin-releasing hormone (GnRH) is diminished and gonadal activity is minimal. Before the onset of puberty, GnRH secretion once again increases, stimulating follicle-stimulating hormone (FSH) and luteinizing hormone (LH) secretion. These hormones stimulate the gonad to enlarge and produce the sex hormones, which cause the characteristic physical and emotional changes associated with puberty. The occurrence of puberty before the age of 8 years in girls and 9 years in boys is more than 3 standard deviations early compared with average and is considered precocious. Precocious puberty can be classified on the basis of whether or not it is dependent on activation of the neuroendocrine-gonadal axis.

In girls, the characteristic physical findings of puberty begin with thelarche (breast budding) and progress through pubarche (pubic hair development) to menses (see Chapter 5). In boys, puberty is heralded by testicular enlargement, followed by pubarche and growth of the penis. Later, boys develop a deepening voice, penile erections, and ejaculation. In both sexes, puberty can include increased oiliness of the hair and skin, acne, increased perspiration and body odor, axillary hair growth, and emotional or behavioral changes. An increased growth rate, known as the pubertal growth spurt, occurs in both sexes and culminates in fusion of the epiphyses. The physical, secondary sexual changes of precocious puberty are similar to those of age-appropriate puberty.

DIFFERENTIAL DIAGNOSIS

The diagnosis of precocious puberty is made on the basis of clinical findings and laboratory testing (Table 58–1). Each child being evaluated for precocious puberty should have a complete physical examination, including sexual maturity rating (SMR) of breasts in girls and development of pubic hair. Testicular volume, measured by use of the Prader orchidometer, denotes the stage of pubertal maturation in boys and provides important information about the source of the androgen causing secondary sex changes. Penile length (stretched) and penile diameter should be charted. A radiograph of the left hand and wrist to determine bone age provides information about the degree of skeletal maturation caused by increased sex steroids. Children with precocious puberty have pubertal levels of basal LH and FSH, as well as exaggerated LH production in response to GnRH stimulation testing. Based on hormonal and physical characteristics, children with precocious puberty can be assigned to either a gonadotropin-dependent or gonadotropin-independent category (Table 58–2).

GONADOTROPIN-DEPENDENT PRECOCIOUS PUBERTY

Gonadotropin-dependent precocious puberty is also known as central precocious puberty. This is a normal physiologic process that occurs abnormally early. The development of gonadotropin-dependent precocious puberty can be triggered by a mechanism that disrupts the normal hypothalamic-pituitary axis. Such causes can include head trauma, brain tumors, and hydrocephalus. This is especially true in girls younger than 4 years old and in all boys, for whom gonadotropin-dependent precocious puberty often indicates the presence of a central nervous system lesion. Computed tomography or magnetic resonance imaging of the head should be done when gonadotropin-dependent precocious puberty is suggested to exclude neurogenic causes. In most girls older than the age of 4 years, however, a specific cause of gonadotropin-dependent precocious puberty is not found and a diagnosis of idiopathic precocious puberty is made.

The most commonly detected brain lesion in children with gonadotropin-dependent precocious puberty is a benign hypothalamic hamartoma in the floor of the third ventricle. Granules secreting GnRH have been found within the lesion. These growths generally produce no symptoms other than precocious puberty but rarely can be associated with seizures and delays in speech and motor development. A rare syndrome consisting of a triad of hypothalamic hamartoma, precocious puberty, and gelastic (laughing) seizures has been described. This neurologic disorder can progress to include other intractable complex seizures. Because the precocious puberty associated with hypothalamic hamartoma is highly responsive to medical therapy with long-acting GnRH analogues, surgical treatment is not indicated.

I. Complete History
   A. Chronology of secondary sexual development such as menses, breast development, pubic hair, axillary hair
   B. History of growth spurt
   C. History of any behavioral or emotional changes
   D. History of head trauma
   E. Thorough family history (if positive in males, suspect testotoxicosis)
   F. Birth history—history of gender ambiguity
II. Measurement of Height and Weight: Plot results on the growth chart. If possible, obtain prior measurements to assess growth velocity.
III. Complete Physical Examination
   A. Check the patient for dysmorphic features, café au lait spots, or ambiguous genitalia.
   B. Obtain SMR stage of breasts in girls or gynecomastia in boys.
   C. Obtain SMR stage of pubic hair.
   D. Stage axillary hair.
   E. Measure gonad size:
      1. Prader orchidometer in boys
      2. Pelvic ultrasound in girls
IV. Radiography: Obtain radiograph of left wrist and hand for bone age.
V. Diagnostic Laboratory Tests
   A. GnRH stimulation test: Random gonadotropin levels are not useful.
   B. Sex steroid levels:
      1. Estrogen in girls
      2. Testosterone in boys or in virilized girls
   C. Thyroid function tests
   D. Human chorionic gonadotropin level (elevated in tumors such as hepatoblastomas or dysgerminomas)
   E. Prolactin level: Consider checking in boys with markedly tender breasts or girls with galactorrhea.
   F. Adrenal metabolites (dehydroepiandrosterone sulfate, 17-hydroxyprogesterone, 11-deoxycortisol)
VI. Adrenal Ultrasound/Pelvic Ultrasound
VII. Magnetic Resonance Imaging (if available) or Head Computed Tomography

GONADOTROPIN-INDEPENDENT PRECOCIOUS PUBERTY

Gonadotropin-independent precocious puberty, which is also called peripheral precocious puberty, is caused by an abnormality of sex steroid production that does not rely on activation of the hypothalamic-pituitary axis. Excess sex steroids can be exogenous or endogenous, can be produced by either the adrenal gland or the gonad, and can result in either virilizing or feminizing symptoms. Gonadotropin-independent precocious puberty is characterized by either an FSH-predominant pattern or suppressed levels of both FSH and LH in response to GnRH stimulation.

The most common form of isolated premature puberty is premature adrenarche. This condition is secondary to an early increase in adrenal androgen production, resulting in isolated early pubic hair development. There may also be early development of axillary hair, acne, and body odor. Although the precise etiology is unknown, this condition is characterized by dehydroepiandrosterone sulfate (DHEAS) levels that are modestly elevated for chronologic age but not for pubic hair state. In premature adrenarche, boys do not have early genital development and girls are not virilized. No significant growth spurt is associated with this benign condition, and there are no long-term sequelae. Observation for other signs of androgen effects is the only management indicated.

Adrenal enzyme defects (congenital adrenal hyperplasia), in contrast, are characterized by virilization (see Chapter 55). These autosomal recessive conditions result in the build-up of precursors of corticosteroids and mineralocorticoids that have significant androgenic activity. The resulting virilization is usually detected early in girls. In boys, particularly those with milder metabolic defects, the changes may go undetected until the boys show signs of sexual development: penile enlargement, growth spurt, and increase in muscle mass. The absence of testicular enlargement in the presence of obvious androgenic stimulation necessitates the search for an extragonadal source, such as the adrenal gland.

Elevation of the serum concentration of enzyme precursors such as 17OH-progesterone in 21-hydroxylase deficiency, 11-deoxycortisol in 11-hydroxylase deficiency, and 17-OH pregnenolone in 3β-hydroxysteroid dehydrogenase deficiency is characteristic of these conditions. To make the diagnosis of adrenal enzyme defects it is occasionally necessary to measure these adrenal metabolites following stimulation with adrenocorticotropic hormone (ACTH). Therapy consists of carefully monitored glucocorticoid and mineralocorticoid replacement. Inadequately treated congenital adrenal hyperplasia can result in virilization and accelerated linear growth and skeletal maturation.

I. Gonadotropin Dependent (Central Precocious Puberty)
II. Gonadotropin Independent (Peripheral or "Pseudo" Precocious Puberty)
   A. Ingestion of, or exposure to, sex hormones (birth control pills, estrogen-containing makeup, hair creams, or oils)
   B. Adrenal gland
      1. Premature adrenarche
      2. Enzymatic defects
         a. 21-Hydroxylase deficiency
         b. 11-Hydroxylase deficiency
         c. 3β-Hydroxysteroid dehydrogenase deficiency
      3. Tumors: virilizing or feminizing adrenal tumors
   C. Ovary
      1. Tumors
         a. Virilizing: androblastomas, arrhenoblastomas, hilus cell
         b. Feminizing: granulosa-theca cell
         c. Mixed virilizing and feminizing: stromal/luteoma
      2. Cysts
      3. McCune-Albright syndrome
   D. Testes
      1. Tumors
         a. Dysgerminomas
         b. Sertoli-Leydig cell tumors
         c. Leydig cell tumors (may secrete estrogen)
      2. Familial male precocious puberty (testotoxicosis)
   E. Human chorionic gonadotropin–secreting tumors
      1. Hepatoblastomas
      2. Dysgerminomas
      3. Pinealomas
III. Combined Gonadotropin-Dependent and Gonadotropin-Independent Precocious Puberty
IV. Mechanism Unknown
   A. Hypothyroidism
   B. Premature thelarche

Adrenal tumors can produce either excessive androgens or excessive estrogens, but virilizing adrenal tumors are more common than feminizing ones. Markedly elevated DHEAS or testosterone level, or a palpable abdominal mass, suggests an adrenal tumor. Abdominal computed tomography, magnetic resonance imaging, and ultrasonography are the most useful diagnostic modalities, and the treatment of choice is surgical removal with subsequent chemotherapy or radiation therapy, depending on the histopathology.

Gonadal tumors can be either feminizing or virilizing, regardless of sex. Laboratory testing reveals markedly increased estrogen or testosterone levels. Careful radiologic imaging can detect these tumors, and surgical excision is the recommended treatment. Pinealoma or hepatoblastoma may also cause premature sexual development by secreting prolactin or human chorionic gonadotropin.

A rare form of familial gonadotropin-independent precocious puberty, also known as testotoxicosis, can occur in boys. A positive family history can suggest this diagnosis. Premature pubertal development (including testicular enlargement), accelerated linear growth, and advanced skeletal maturation are commonly noted by 4 to 5 years of age. Testosterone levels may be in the pubertal range, although the gonadotropins have a prepubertal pattern. Testicular biopsy reveals Leydig cell hyperplasia, although the precise stimulus for this process is unknown. When these boys reach adulthood there is generally a normal gonadotropin pattern and reproductive capacity; however, cases of defective spermatogenesis have been reported.

Treatment of testotoxicosis remains investigational. Therapy with ketoconazole or combination therapy with testolactone and spironolactone has been moderately successful in slowing the rates of secondary sexual development, linear growth, and skeletal maturation. Ketoconazole interferes with adrenal and gonadal biosynthesis of testosterone. Spironolactone functions as an antiandrogen; its use alone often results in gynecomastia. Testolactone prevents the development of gynecomastia because it is an inhibitor of P450 aromatase, thus interfering with the peripheral conversion of androgens to estrogens.

The McCune-Albright syndrome is also a form of gonadotropin-independent precocious puberty and is characterized by "coast of Maine" café au lait skin lesions, polyostotic fibrous dysplasia, and precocious puberty. In girls, the secondary sexual development frequently occurs in a cyclical pattern in association with ovarian cyst formation and is often manifested by cyclical breast development and vaginal bleeding. Other endocrinopathies including hyperthyroidism, Cushing syndrome, and growth hormone and prolactin excess (see Chapter 55) may also be associated with this condition.

When McCune-Albright syndrome is suggested in a child with precocious puberty, a bone scan to evaluate skeletal lesions should be added to routine testing. The McCune-Albright syndrome, like testotoxicosis, is not responsive to GnRH analogue treatment because it is not gonadotropin dependent. Testolactone therapy is the most effective treatment.

Combined gonadotropin-dependent and gonadotropin-independent precocious puberty occurs when the elevated levels of sex steroid in GnRH-independent precocious puberty trigger secondary activation of the hypothalamic-pituitary axis. The onset of gonadotropin-dependent precocious puberty is associated with significant skeletal maturation, shown by bone age usually greater than 10 years. This condition has been reported in children with congenital adrenal hyperplasia, in association with adrenal or ovarian tumors, or in older girls with the McCune-Albright syndrome. Treatment of the combined types of precocious puberty is aimed at the underlying cause of gonadotropin-independent precocious puberty in combination with GnRH analogue treatment to control the gonadotropin-dependent process.

UNKNOWN MECHANISMS

A poorly understood cause of early sexual development is hypothyroidism (see Chapter 55). A child with this condition usually has decreased rather than increased linear growth. Bone age is frequently delayed. Girls may have large follicular ovarian cysts. There may also be elevations of both prolactin and thyrotropin levels. Although the diagnosis of hypothyroidism should be suspected from the results of the history and physical examination, thyroid function tests should be part of the routine battery of tests for children diagnosed with precocious puberty. Therapy is with thyroid hormone replacement.

Premature thelarche is a benign condition characterized by isolated breast development without evidence of other secondary sexual development and no acceleration of growth rate. Girls with premature thelarche generally have an FSH-predominant (prepubertal) response to GnRH stimulation, whereas girls with classic gonadotropin-dependent precocious puberty have an LH-predominant (pubertal) response. Premature thelarche requires no intervention. However, periodically the child should be monitored for further sexual development because it may be difficult to differentiate premature thelarche from early gonadotropin-dependent precocious puberty.

TREATMENT

The treatment of choice for gonadotropin-dependent precocious puberty is with GnRH agonists, which have been used effectively since 1981. Before that time, therapy was primarily with agents that had inhibitory effects on gonadotropin production, such as medroxyprogesterone acetate, cyproterone acetate, and danazol. Although these agents halted menses and decreased spermatogenesis, they were not effective in preventing premature epiphyseal fusion and thus provided no improvement of final adult height. Other negative features included androgenic side effects and the development of cushingoid features.

Continuous infusions of GnRH inhibit gonadotropin secretion by "uncoupling" the pituitary receptor from further response to GnRH. Because of the short biologic half-life of natural GnRH, longer-acting analogues were developed to ensure continuously high levels of GnRH activity on the pituitary. To date, six long-acting GnRH analogues have been used in the clinical treatment of gonadotropin-dependent precocious puberty (Table 58–3). Each analogue varies in relative potency to natural GnRH and in *in vivo* clearance rate, thus necessitating carefully planned studies to determine the most efficacious dose and route of administration. Inadequate treatment can result in an agonist effect that stimulates, rather than suppresses, gonadotropin release.

Several routes for administration of GnRH analogue have been studied, including daily subcutaneous injection, intranasal administration, and long-acting depot intramuscular injection. Intranasal administration appears to be the least effective route of administration. Most investigators have found that absorption may not be uniform, and effective doses may be 10 to 30 times those used for the same analogues administered subcutaneously. The only side effect reported with intranasal administration is local nasal irritation. However, large dose requirements ultimately have a tremendous impact on the cost of medication.

When adequate doses are used, daily subcutaneous injections of deslorelin, leuprolide acetate, nafarelin, buserelin, and histrelin effectively suppress gonadotropins and sex steroid production. More than 6 years' experience of treatment with deslorelin at 4 µg/kg/day indicates excellent results in halting puberty. Pubic hair and breast development showed no significant progression. Gonadal volume decreased by 50% in both sexes when compared with pretreatment values. The rate of bone age advancement (change in bone age/change in chronologic age) decreased from 2.7 before treatment to 0.5 throughout the 6-year period. Predicted adult height as calculated by the Bayley-Pinneau method increased by 15.9 ± 1.9 cm after 5 years of treatment in 22 children and by 18.0 ± 3.7 cm after 6 years in 10 children.

Depot intramuscular injections provide a constant dose of GnRH agonist over several weeks. Early work with this latest formulation of GnRH agonist demonstrates excellent clinical results. Some researchers have concluded that the suppression of gonadotropin and sex steroid secretions and the reversal of physical maturation are better with intramuscular depot administration of leuprolide than with daily subcutaneous administration of the drug.

Both subcutaneously administered and intramuscularly administered GnRH agonists have been associated with few side effects. There have been reports of local tenderness and erythema, two reported cases of anaphylaxis, and one reported case of cellulitis. The cost of daily and monthly injections ranges from $350 to $400 per month (based on current costs of leuprolide).

Although the long-term implications of GnRH agonist therapy on endocrine and reproductive function have not been systematically studied, there have also been several reports of former GnRH agonist adolescent patients who have become pregnant. Complete reversibility of gonadotropin suppression has been documented once GnRH agonist treatment has been discontinued.

It is very important that patients receive periodic evaluation to assess treatment efficacy. Using a GnRH agonist of low potency, choosing too low a dose, or administration of doses at insufficient frequency may result in failure to induce gonadotropin and sex steroid suppression. In these circumstances, GnRH analogues act as potent stimuli for gonadotropin secretion and clinical symptoms can worsen.

Determination of treatment effectiveness is assessed by sequential physical examinations, measurement of linear growth, and determination of the rate of skeletal maturation. Even with sufficient therapy, secondary sexual development sometimes regresses; but it usually remains unchanged. Pubic hair development often progresses in adrenarcheal children older than 6 or 7 years of age. A reliable method to assess efficacy of gonadotropin suppression includes determination of gonadal size by periodic pelvic ultrasound or measurement of testicular size. With adequate treatment, gonadal enlargement should cease, with gradual return toward prepubertal gonad size. Physical examination and history will generally reveal improvement in such features as behavioral changes, skin oiliness, and acne.

The most readily quantifiable variable related to treatment efficacy is the concentration of gonadotropins and sex steroids. Because gonadotropins are secreted in a pulsatile fashion, random measurements are not diagnostically useful. Documentation of suppressed urinary gonadotropins, or of suppression of the peak gonadotropin responses to GnRH stimulation, along with sex steroid determinations, provides important information and should be used in conjunction with growth and clinical assessments. Basal levels of LH and FSH should fall to prepubertal levels, and the exaggerated response of LH to GnRH stimulation should be suppressed.

In the course of measuring gonadotropins it is important for the clinician to be aware of the type of radioimmunoassay being used. GnRH agonist therapy suppresses FSH and LH β-subunit production but does not appear to suppress production of the α-subunit. If the assay measures the α-subunit, elevated baseline LH levels may not signify inadequate treatment, especially if there is no significant LH response following GnRH stimulation.

The criteria for adequate gonadal suppression remain controversial. Several investigators have considered loss of LH and FSH pulsatility as an indication of adequate

TABLE 58–3. GnRH Agonists Used for Treatment of Gonadotropin-Dependent Precocious Puberty

GENERIC NAME	ROUTE	RELATIVE POTENCY (COMPARED WITH NATURAL GnRH)
Buserelin	Subcutaneous Intranasal	20–40
Nafarelin (Syneril)	Subcutaneous Intranasal	20–30
Leuprolide acetate (Lupron)	Subcutaneous Intramuscular	20–30
Histrelin	Intranasal	140
Deslorelin	Subcutaneous	144
Decapeptyl	Subcutaneous Intramuscular	144

gonadal suppression, while others consider suppression to occur only when LH and FSH levels are undetectable by standard assays. Normal prepubertal children clearly have activity of the hypothalamic GnRH neuron that results in pulsatile gonadotropin secretion and some sex steroid production. However, with current therapy, it is not possible to produce a hypothalamic-pituitary-gonadal axis in gonadotropin-dependent precocious puberty that precisely mimics the prepubertal axis. Although most investigators agree that significant agonist effects from GnRH agonist therapy are detrimental, the level of gonadotropin and sex steroid suppression needed to achieve the desirable growth and skeletal response is still being debated.

BIBLIOGRAPHY

Crowley WF Jr, Comite F, Vale W, et al: Therapeutic use of pituitary desensitization with a long-acting LHRH agonist: A potential new treatment for idiopathic precocious puberty. J Clin Endocrinol Metab 52:370–372, 1981.

Gondos B, Egli CA, Rosenthal SM, Grumbach MM: Testicular changes in gonadotropin-independent familial male sexual precocity: Familial testotoxicosis. Arch Pathol Lab Med 109:990–995, 1985.

Klibanski A, Jameson L, Biller BMK, et al: Gonadotropin and alpha-subunit responses to chronic gonadotropin-releasing hormone analog administration in patients with glycoprotein hormone–secreting pituitary tumors. J Clin Endocrinol Metab 68:81–86, 1989.

Laue L, Kenigsberg D, Pescovitz OH, et al: The treatment of familial male precocious puberty with spironolactone and testolactone. N Engl J Med 320:496–502, 1989.

Manasco PK, Pescovitz OH, Feuillan PP, et al: Resumption of puberty after long-term luteinizing hormone-releasing hormone agonist treatment of central precocious puberty. J Clin Endocrinol Metab 67:358–372, 1988.

Parker KL, Lee PA: Depot leuprolide acetate for treatment of precocious puberty. J Clin Endocrinol Metab 69:689–691, 1989.

Pescovitz OH, Comite F, Hench K, et al: The NIH experience in precocious puberty: Diagnostic subgroups and the response to short-term LHRH analogue therapy. J Pediatr 108:47–54, 1986.

CHAPTER 59

Diabetes Mellitus

MICHAEL P. GOLDEN and DEBORAH L. GRAY

The quality of care that adolescent patients with diabetes mellitus receive has profound implications for their long-term health. Acute, life-threatening complications, such as diabetic ketoacidosis (DKA), often occur as a consequence of psychosocial problems. Chronic microvascular complications, developing during mid- to late adolescence, can lead to severe disability or premature mortality. However, for both physiologic and psychosocial reasons, adolescence is a time during which achievement of metabolic control is often difficult. For these reasons, diabetes mellitus requires the attention of all primary care practitioners who treat adolescent patients.

CLASSIFICATION, EPIDEMIOLOGY, AND ETIOLOGY OF DIABETES DURING ADOLESCENCE

Diabetes presenting before 30 years of age is almost always insulin-dependent diabetes mellitus (IDDM). It is relatively common, with an incidence rate of approximately 1 in 800 adolescents in the United States. By way of comparison, IDDM is three to four times as prevalent as cystic fibrosis or rheumatoid arthritis and equal in frequency to all types of cancer combined. The peak age at onset of IDDM is between 10 and 14 years of age. Interesting epidemiologic characteristics of IDDM include a seasonal variation with increased occurrence in cooler months and a geographic variation with increasing incidence as the distance from the equator increases. These findings suggest an environmental, perhaps infectious, component to the etiology of IDDM, but the nature of that possible component is unknown.

It is clear that autoimmunity is important in the development of IDDM. Figure 59–1 shows a proposed model for the development of clinical symptoms. In a person with a genetic predisposition to IDDM there is the initiation of immunologic abnormalities including development of circulating antibodies to the beta cells and abnormalities in T-cell function. The trigger for these immunologic abnormalities is unknown.

Physiologically there is progressive loss of pancreatic beta cells with concurrent loss of insulin secretory capacity. Initially, decreased insulin secretion can be dem-

onstrated only by measuring first-phase (initial) insulin release in response to rapidly administered intravenous glucose. When 80% to 90% of beta cells are destroyed, acute metabolic decompensation occurs, with fasting hyperglycemia and rapid development of overt clinical diabetes. Future efforts to prevent IDDM will be directed at the period preceding metabolic decompensation when insulin secretory capacity is still adequate to maintain glucose homeostasis.

Non–insulin-dependent diabetes mellitus (NIDDM) is unusual during adolescence and is characterized by significant degrees of insulin resistance, usually associated with hyperinsulinemia. Occasionally, adolescents with a very strong family history of obesity and diabetes present with early diagnosed NIDDM.

Maturity-onset diabetes of the young (MODY) is an inherited autosomal dominant condition, not associated with obesity, in which there are varying degrees of glucose intolerance. Adolescent patients may be asymptomatic and generally are not ketotic. However, they can develop complications and require treatment.

The diagnosis of NIDDM is based on standard diagnostic criteria following an oral glucose tolerance test using 1.75 g glucose/kg up to a maximum of 75 g. To be diagnosed as diabetic, a patient must have (1) a fasting plasma glucose level of 140 mg/dl or more on two occasions or (2) if the fasting glucose level is less than or equal to 140 mg/dl, at least the 2-hour and one other intermediate glucose determination should be greater than 200 mg/dl. Both NIDDM and MODY are unusual in the adolescent age range, and in the remainder of this discussion the focus is on IDDM.

DIAGNOSIS

During the early course of the illness, the typical symptoms are polyuria, polydipsia, and nocturia. Weight loss is variable. Most patients feel well or, retrospectively, may complain of malaise. Diagnosis during this early phase is optimal since a delay leads to progressively more dangerous symptoms, which include increasing weight loss, malaise, and lethargy and which progress with the onset of diabetic ketoacidosis (DKA) to nausea, vomiting, dehydration, somnolence, and eventually coma. During DKA, abdominal pain is common and can be confused with an acute surgical abdomen.

Laboratory diagnosis is generally unambiguous. A random blood glucose level over 200 mg/dl in association

Supported in part by the Indiana University Diabetes Research and Training Center, PHS P60-DK-20542.

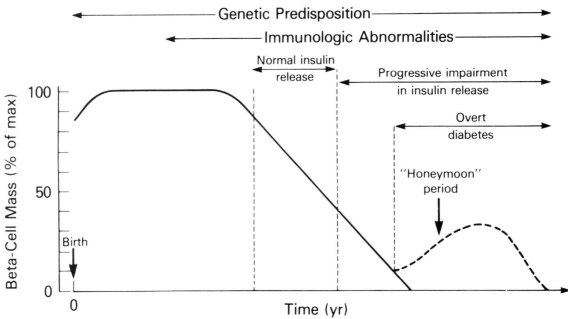

Figure 59–1. Proposed scheme of natural history of beta-cell defect. The timing of the trigger in relation to immunologic abnormalities is unknown. Note that overt diabetes is not apparent until insulin secretory reserves are less than 10% to 20% of normal. (From Sperling MA [ed]: Physician's Guide to Insulin-Dependent (Type I) Diabetes: Diagnosis and Treatment. Alexandria, VA, American Diabetes Association, 1988. Copyright 1988 by The American Diabetes Association. Reprinted with permission.)

with typical symptoms is sufficient to make the diagnosis. Other than for suspected NIDDM, a glucose tolerance test is rarely indicated in adolescents. Glycosuria is almost always detectable, although some adolescents may not be acidotic and urinary ketones may be absent.

DIABETIC KETOACIDOSIS

Diabetic ketoacidosis is a life-threatening condition for which the best treatment is prevention. However, when an adolescent patient has DKA, several basic principles should be followed. First, treatment requires an intensive-care setting with experienced medical and nursing staff and continuous electrocardiographic monitoring and blood pressure determination. Second, there should be careful and frequent reevaluation of both physical and laboratory status. Finally, slow correction of metabolic abnormalities is preferable to rapid correction, as long as there is continual improvement.

The most frequent causes of DKA are diagnosis late in the course of development of symptoms and the omission of insulin, accounting for more than 90% of hospital admissions of adolescents for DKA in our experience. Another cause is chronic poor control in conjunction with another acute illness. Factors that do not induce DKA include overeating, menses, and stress.

On physical examination it is important to evaluate the state of consciousness, with careful documentation of baseline neurologic function. An estimate of the state of hydration is necessary to determine the appropriate fluids. Kussmaul respirations indicate metabolic acidosis. It is important to decide whether abdominal pain is primary or secondary to DKA. Infections must be recognized because they may contribute to insulin resistance and DKA.

Fluid and electrolyte management varies from center to center. Shock should be treated with 350 ml/m² of normal saline intravenously over 20 to 30 minutes. If there are no signs of shock, initial treatment includes intravenous normal saline without glucose. Once the blood glucose level is approximately 300 mg/dl, 5% dextrose is added to the intravenous fluids. Ten percent dextrose can be used if the serum glucose level continues to decline rapidly. Another indication for the addition of dextrose to fluids, even though the serum glucose value is greater than 300 mg/dl, is an insulin infusion rate that has been decreased to 0.05 unit/kg/hour concurrent with a serum glucose level falling at a rate greater than 100 mg/dl/hour.

Insulin is administered by continuous intravenous infusion using a controlled-rate infusion system in a concentration of 0.1 unit/ml in normal saline. An initial bolus of 0.05 to 0.1 unit regular insulin per kilogram is administered if subcutaneous regular insulin has not been given within 4 hours or subcutaneous Lente or NPH insulin has not been given within 12 hours. If subcutaneous insulin has been administered, no bolus is necessary.

Beginning at an insulin infusion rate of 0.1 unit/kg/hour, insulin administration is varied up to 20% per hour in an attempt to achieve a decrease in the blood glucose level of 50 to 80 mg/dl/hour. To provide adequate insulin, the insulin infusion rate should not be reduced to less than 0.05 unit/kg/hour. Unless the adolescent is hypoglycemic, the insulin infusion should not be stopped, since insulin deficiency rapidly leads to metabolic decompensation. Intravenous insulin is continued until the adolescent is rehydrated, the serum glucose level is in the 150 to 250 mg/dl range, and the adolescent can eat.

Fluid therapy should proceed slowly and be carefully monitored. Three categories of fluids should be considered: (1) maintenance, (2) replacement of previous dehydration losses, and (3) replacement of ongoing urinary losses. The maintenance fluid rate is 1500 ml/m²/24 hours. Replacement of dehydration is calculated based on body weight. Most adolescent patients with DKA are at least 10% dehydrated. Rehydration is accomplished evenly over 48 hours. For example, a 40-kg patient (estimated surface area 1.3 m²) requires a maintenance rate of 1950 ml/24 hours or 81 ml/hour. In addition, assuming 10% dehydration, the replacement volume of 4000 ml (10% of 40 kg) is administered over 48 hours; a rate of 83 ml/hour. Total fluid administered is therefore 164 ml/hour. In addition, marked hyperglycemia can lead to osmotic diuresis with excessive urinary fluid loss. If excessive urinary output is preventing adequate rehydration, urine output should be replaced milliliter for milliliter above the maintenance rate. Urinary electrolytes can be used to help in the selection of the replacement solution, or a solution of half-normal saline with 10 mEq/L of potassium chloride can be used empirically. Urinary replacement fluids should not contain glucose. Urine replacement can be discontinued when osmotic diuresis ceases, usually when the glucose value is less than or equal to 300 mg/dl.

Monitoring serum sodium (Na⁺) concentration is important in assessing the degree of hydration and, possibly, in limiting the likelihood of development of cerebral edema. A declining serum sodium concentration may indicate that excess free water is being administered, which is a probable risk factor for cerebral edema. In general, normal saline solution is used for the first 8 to 12 hours of treatment. After that, if the "corrected" serum sodium concentration (corrected Na⁺ = measured Na⁺ + [serum glucose in mg/dl − 100] × 0.016 mEq) is stable and within the normal range, one-half normal saline can be used when dextrose is added to the fluids. The "corrected" serum sodium concentration needs to be calculated (corrected) because of the (apparent) artificial lowering of serum sodium related to the hyperosmolarity of hyperglycemia. If the calculated serum sodium concentration decreases below normal, careful restriction of fluid administration rate is indicated. If hypernatremia develops during initial treatment, one-half normal saline should be used in place of normal saline.

Potassium administration should be started as soon as urine flow is established and hyperkalemia is excluded. If there is no urine production in the first 30 minutes of treatment of DKA, urinary catheterization is indicated. The initial potassium concentration in intravenous fluids should be 30 to 40 mEq/L, with the concentration of potassium adjusted in response to serum potassium and bicarbonate levels. Potassium requirements may exceed 40 mEq/L. In general, potassium is administered as potassium chloride. If the serum chloride level is high or the phosphate is low, one can give half of the potassium as potassium chloride and half as potassium phosphate. A dramatic decrease in potassium can be expected with correction of acidosis, requiring careful monitoring of potassium levels early in treatment.

Rapid administration of bicarbonate is used only for cardiac arrest or shock. With severe acidosis (pH less than 7.1), a slow infusion may be used; the total should not exceed 3 mEq/kg/8 hr. Excessively rapid infusion of bicarbonate can lead to a paradoxical decrease in cerebrospinal fluid pH because carbon dioxide but not bicarbonate crosses the blood-brain barrier.

Frequent laboratory reevaluation is important. To facilitate access to blood, an intravenous heparin lock or, in the case of severe DKA or for DKA complicated by cardiac or pulmonary disease, an intra-arterial catheter should be inserted.

Initial laboratory evaluation should include determination of arterial or venous pH, glucose, electrolytes, blood urea nitrogen, creatinine, calcium, and phosphorus; a urinalysis; and other studies as needed. The serum glucose value should be followed every hour initially and then every 2 hours once a stable and declining pattern is established. Glucose levels can be monitored by glucose oxidase strips with meters for immediate results. Serum electrolyte values are initially monitored every 2 hours. In general, the plasma bicarbonate level may be used to follow the degree of acidosis. The venous or arterial pH is also a useful value.

When the patient is rehydrated and able to resume oral caloric intake, the insulin infusion is discontinued immediately before subcutaneous administration of insulin. In a newly diagnosed adolescent patient, a mixture of regular and intermediate insulin in a total daily dose of 0.5 unit/kg can be given. A typical starting dose includes 55% of the total dose given in the morning and 45% of the total dose given in the evening. The morning dose is then split as 45% regular and 55% intermediate insulin, and the evening dose is split into 50% of each type. In a previously treated adolescent patient, the dose prior to the onset of DKA may be used.

The most common cause of death in DKA among adolescents is severe neurologic dysfunction related to cerebral edema. The typical clinical manifestations of this complication appear several hours to 24 hours after treatment begins. The adolescent with cerebral edema in DKA may have begun to improve and then deteriorates neurologically. The onset can be abrupt or gradual. Signs include increasing confusion and deepening coma, fixed and dilated pupils, or change in respiratory status or other evidence of neurologic impairment. Neurologic evaluation should be performed frequently during the initial phase of treatment, and the adolescent patient should not be left unobserved for more than a brief period. If cerebral edema is suspected, mannitol (0.25 to 0.5 g/kg) should be given immediately and appropriate neurologic and neurosurgical consultation obtained. Treatment at this stage is supportive and frequently not completely successful. The cause of cerebral edema is unknown, although rapid correction of dehydration with fluid overload has been implicated in its pathogenesis.

GOALS OF DIABETIC MANAGEMENT

Therapeutic goals for diabetes management are controversial and still evolving. Much will depend on the results of the Diabetes Control and Complications Trial (DCCT), a multicenter study sponsored by the National

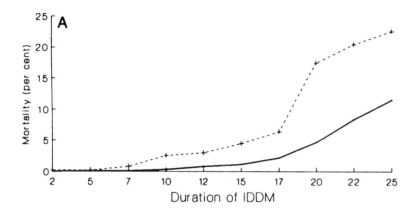

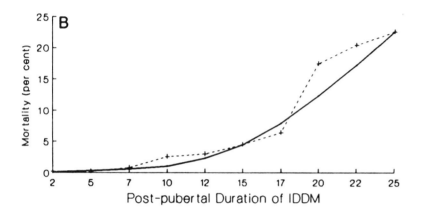

Figure 59–2. Cumulative diabetes-related mortality by duration of insulin-dependent diabetes mellitus (IDDM) *(A)* and postpubertal duration of IDDM *(B)*. Prepubertal *(solid lines)* versus pubertal *(dashed lines)* subjects at IDDM onset. (From Kostraba J, et al: Contribution of diabetes duration before puberty to development of microvascular complications in IDDM subjects. Diabetes Care 12:686, 1989. Copyright 1989 by the American Diabetes Association. Reprinted with permission.)

Institutes of Health designed to evaluate the relationship between metabolic control and development of complications. With the use of currently available intensive therapy regimens, either multiple (three or more) daily injections or continuous subcutaneous insulin infusion (pumps), both adolescents and adults have been randomized into experimental and control arms of this study. Both groups will be followed for 10 years, with progression or development of retinopathy as a principal endpoint. Definitive results relating control to complications are at least several years away.

Until further data are available, most diabetes centers have adopted somewhat similar treatment philosophies. First, adolescents should grow and enter puberty normally. This degree of control should be achievable with all adolescent patients. Occasionally, an adolescent with Mauriac syndrome is seen. These teenagers are in extremely poor diabetic control and present with the triad of growth failure, pubertal delay, and hepatomegaly. Lesser degrees of poor control can result in mild impairment in growth or puberty, and minimal hepatomegaly may accompany moderately poor metabolic control.

Along with ensuring normal growth and development, there is consensus that treatment should eliminate symptoms of hyperglycemia (polyuria, polydypsia, and nocturia) and severe hypoglycemia (changes in level of consciousness). Mild hypoglycemia, treatable with oral carbohydrate, is probably unavoidable and is acceptable if it occurs no more than three to four times per week.

There is less agreement among diabetologists regarding the intensity with which one should strive to achieve normal blood glucose levels. Disagreement results largely from the lack of clear data relating degrees of glycemic control to risk of complications. As mentioned, definitive results of the DCCT will not be available for at least 5 years. Until they are, most diabetologists assume that poor metabolic control accelerates development of complications but that achieving near euglycemia is not practicable in most adolescents. This latter point was clearly demonstrated by the DCCT, in which it has been shown that although some highly motivated adolescents can achieve a significant improvement in metabolic control, an extensive commitment of health care personnel is required. Recent data suggest but do not prove that a metabolic control level characterized by glycohemoglobin levels less than 1.33 times the upper normal nondiabetic limit is associated with a lower risk for complications. This level is achievable in many adolescents and, at this time, seems a reasonable goal.

One factor particularly relevant to developing treatment regimens for adolescents is that the onset of puberty (see Chapter 4) appears to "start the clock ticking" on complications. As seen in Figure 59–2, cumulative diabetes-related mortality begins to increase in direct proportion to the postpubertal rather than total duration of IDDM. Similar findings are seen for retinopathy and nephropathy. How puberty is critical is not clear, but it seems likely that hormonal changes may play a role. Whatever the cause, the onset of puberty does require increased efforts to minimize complications and their effects. This includes, in addition to paying attention to glycemic control, careful monitoring for early, treatable evidence of complications and for factors that contribute to diabetes morbidity. Exemplary management of diabetes includes regular screening and counseling regarding a number of known risk factors.

MONITORING AND TREATMENT OF DIABETES COMPLICATIONS AND RELATED CONDITIONS

Cardiovascular disease is a leading cause of premature death in diabetic patients. The ways in which diabetes mellitus contributes to premature atherosclerosis are not well understood and are probably multifactorial. Peripheral hyperinsulinemia, as occurs with subcutaneous insulin injection, hyperglycemia, and hyperlipidemia all may play a role. Until a method for intraportal or intraperitoneal insulin administration is developed, avoidance of peripheral hyperinsulinemia will depend principally on administration of appropriate insulin doses and on encouraging physical fitness, which increases insulin sensitivity. Appropriate treatment of hyperglycemia is discussed in the section on long-term management.

Hyperlipidemia is a potentially important and treatable risk factor in patients with IDDM. Blood lipid levels should be monitored yearly and should include random total cholesterol and high density cholesterol counts. Desired levels include a total cholesterol concentration under 200 mg/dl and a total–to–high-density cholesterol ratio of less than 4.5. In the presence of hyperlipidemia, fasting triglycerides levels should also be measured.

Unlike in NIDDM, genetic hyperlipidemia is not found with increased frequency in IDDM. Insulin deficiency with suboptimal metabolic control can lead to hyperlipidemia. In such cases, glucose control should be maximally improved before considering other options to treat hyperlipidemia. For all adolescent patients, dietary management is preferable, and a basic hypolipidemic diet is part of the standard American Diabetes Association dietary guidelines taught to all patients. When lipid levels are not in the desired range despite appropriate efforts at improving metabolic control and dietary lipid intake, further dietary modifications are indicated initially. Whereas all adolescent patients are prescribed a "prudent" 200 to 300 mg/day of dietary cholesterol and a relatively high proportion of polyunsaturated fat intake, only for those patients in whom hyperlipidemia is found are these guidelines strongly emphasized. Attempts to limit fat more than this are not likely to be successful among adolescents.

When hypercholesterolemia is not responsive to dietary treatment, pharmacologic therapy should be considered. At this time, HMG-CoA-reductase inhibitors, such as lovastatin, are probably the agents of choice. Long-term side effects are not known because of the recent introduction of these agents. They are, however, strikingly effective in lowering low-density lipoprotein cholesterol and, importantly for adolescents, require single daily dosing. Adolescent patients should be warned about the symptoms of myositis, which include weakness and muscle pain or tenderness, either chronic or acute. Creatine phosphokinase level should be monitored regularly in adolescent patients being treated. Concurrent use of either nicotinic acid or gemfibrozil with HMG-CoA-reductase inhibitors increases the risk of severe myositis, and these combinations should be avoided whenever possible. Recommendations for use of lovastatin include periodic monitoring for development of cataracts, although this has not been a documented side effect in humans.

Cigarette smoking constitutes a major risk factor for macrovascular complications in everyone, and even more so in adolescents with IDDM. Adolescents should be strongly counseled to either stop or not start smoking, and this should be emphasized whenever possible (see Chapter 38).

Hypertension is a serious risk factor for both cardiovascular disease and nephropathy in diabetes mellitus (see Chapter 67). It is more common in adolescents than has frequently been appreciated and must be monitored carefully. Aggressive treatment of hypertension will delay the progression of established renal disease; it has been shown that mild hypertension is often a manifestation of early diabetic nephropathy. Therefore, adolescent patients with blood pressure measurements greater than the 90th percentile for age should be evaluated and usually treated. We give consideration to treating adolescent patients whose blood pressures are consistently greater than 135/85 mmHg. Hypertension may often be labile in its initial stages, and it is not necessary that all blood pressures be elevated to consider treatment. There is no single ideal therapy for all adolescent patients with hypertension in IDDM. In general, however, longer-acting angiotensin-converting enzyme (ACE) inhibitors appear to be the current choice. They are effective antihypertensive agents and retard the progressive decline in renal function when nephropathy is present. Preliminary data suggest that they decrease proteinuria in patients with early diabetic nephropathy. More definitive studies are under way.

As part of screening for diabetic nephropathy (see Chapter 65), measurement of urinary microalbumin by radioimmunoassay is now an accepted measure. A random urine sample for microalbumin should be obtained yearly. If the result is greater than 20 to 30 μg albumin per milligram of creatinine, a 24-hour albumin level should be obtained. Total urinary albumin excretion greater than 30 mg/day is abnormal. Leakage of small amounts of albumin from the kidney precedes established proteinuria measurable by traditional techniques. Whereas fixed macroproteinuria does not respond to improvement in metabolic control, microalbumin excretion does appear to vary with changes in glycemic control and may represent a reversible stage in diabetic nephropathy. Therefore it is important when microalbuminuria is found to intensify metabolic control as much as possible and to make every effort to treat early hypertension. The efficacy of the use of ACE inhibitors to treat microalbuminuria in the absence of hypertension is under study but is not standard practice at this time.

Early nephropathy may also be affected positively by decreasing the amount of dietary protein to the minimum required for growth. Decreasing protein requires an increase in either carbohydrate or fat, either of which may have negative effects. Therefore, these dietary changes should be made carefully and in consultation with an experienced dietitian.

There is no evidence that treatment, other than of hypertension, delays or prevents progression of established diabetic nephropathy to end-stage disease. Renal transplantation is generally preferred to long-term dialysis in young people with IDDM, and the long-term results are increasingly promising.

Diabetic retinopathy develops in a substantial proportion of patients with diabetes, and physicians caring for adolescents are unfortunately likely to see a number of patients with varying degrees of retinopathy during mid- to late adolescence. Whether development of retinopathy can be delayed by optimal blood glucose control will await results of the DCCT trial. It is known that early treatment of preproliferative or proliferative retinopathy with photocoagulation is strikingly effective. Background retinopathy with intraretinal hemorrhages or microaneurysms needs close monitoring. Preproliferative retinopathy and neovascularization with multiple clustered hemorrhages or development of new blood vessels are particularly dangerous and require urgent evaluation and treatment. Because of the varying rates at which retinopathy can develop and the difficulty in appreciating early changes, it is important that all adolescent patients with IDDM of over 5 years' duration have yearly eye examinations by an ophthalmologist who is skilled in the evaluation of individuals with diabetes.

Adolescents with IDDM are at increased risk for other autoimmune diseases, particularly thyroid disease and adrenal failure (see Chapter 55). Hypothyroidism eventually develops in up to 10% of patients with IDDM. Both hyperthyroidism and hypothyroidism are associated with IDDM frequently enough to justify yearly monitoring of thyroid functions. Thyroid autoantibodies should be measured at the time of diagnosis of IDDM. Hypoadrenalism occurs in no more than 1% of adolescent patients with IDDM, and adrenal function should be evaluated only when clinically indicated.

LONG-TERM MANAGEMENT

IDDM is unusual among illnesses in that daily management is completely under the control of the adolescent and his or her family. The physician and diabetes care team can provide excellent education in diabetes management; recommend appropriate, individualized regimens; and by being available for long-term support, provide ongoing education and introduction of appropriate new technology when appropriate. Education, even for adolescents, should include the complete family unit and should be based on appropriate educational principles, taking into account normal variability in development and not pushing too fast or too hard to assume responsibility for all diabetes self-care procedures (see Chapter 9).

Insulin Treatment

Although there is no consensus on exact goals for metabolic control, as mentioned, at puberty the risk for developing complications becomes significant and increases with postpubertal duration of IDDM. Also, the preponderance of evidence is that the risk for complications is related to long-term metabolic control. Therefore, insulin should be adjusted such that glucose levels before meals of between 80 and 140 mg/dl are achieved as often as possible. The limiting factor in achieving euglycemia is the frequency of hypoglycemia. In practice, attempting to maintain almost all glucose measurements under 140 mg/dl results in occasional severe or excessively frequent mild hypoglycemia, or both. Therefore, insulin should actually be adjusted such that the lowest mean glucose value is attained without concurrent severe hypoglycemia (decrease in consciousness) or more than three to four mild episodes (symptoms with no change in consciousness) per week.

Insulin is classified according to species (beef, pork, human), purity, strength, and duration of action (Table 59–1). All insulins now available in the United States are highly purified. Consequently, the incidence of local or systemic insulin allergy and lipoatrophy at the injection site has been greatly reduced. Biosynthetic or semisynthetic human insulins are used most often for routine management. They are least immunogenic and are becoming less expensive. Beef Ultralente has an extended duration of action and has been used to provide a basal insulin level in adolescent patients using an intensified conventional therapeutic regimen. U-100 (100 units/ml) insulin concentration is used almost exclusively in the United States.

From a practical point of view, it is best to learn the properties of a few types of insulins. A mix of human regular and Lente insulin works well for most adolescent patients. Conventional insulin therapy consists of regular insulin combined with Lente insulin given twice daily before breakfast and dinner. Most adolescents require a total daily dose between 0.6 unit/kg/day to 1.0 unit/kg/day, with some exceptions. We initially place adolescent patients on a regimen of 55% of their total insulin dose in the morning and 45% in the evening. The percentages of morning regular and Lente insulin are 45% and 55%, respectively. The evening insulin dose is divided equally. Thereafter, insulin is adjusted according

TABLE 59–1. Types and Characteristics of Most Commonly Used Insulins

INSULIN	ONSET (hr)	PEAK (hr)	USUAL EFFECTIVE DURATION (hr)	USUAL MAXIMUM DURATION (hr)
Animal				
Regular	0.5–2.0	3–4	4–6	6–8
NPH	1–2	4–12	16–20	20–24
Lente	1–2.5	8–14	16–20	20–24
Ultralente	4–8	Minimal	24–36	24–36
Human				
Regular	0.5–1.0	2–3	3–6	4–6
NPH	2–4	4–10	10–16	14–18
Lente	3–4	4–12	12–18	16–20
Ultralente	6–10	?	18–20	20–30

From Sperling M (ed): Physician's Guide to Insulin-Dependent (Type I) Diabetes: Diabetes and Treatment. Alexandria, VA, American Diabetes Association, 1988. Copyright 1988 by the American Diabetes Association. Reprinted with permission.

to target goals and individual response. In general, insulin dose is adjusted based on previous glucose readings averaged over several days: the morning regular insulin dose is adjusted based on noon glucose readings, the morning Lente insulin dose on pre-dinner readings, the evening regular insulin dose on pre-bedtime readings, and the evening Lente insulin dose on 3 AM and pre-breakfast glucose levels.

Other regimens are used for specific problems. For adolescents with elevated pre-breakfast (but normal 3 AM) glucose values, patients can take their combined insulin dose in the morning but take only regular insulin before dinner and Lente/NPH insulin several hours later before bedtime. This delays the peak action of Lente/NPH insulin to coincide with the early morning rise in blood glucose concentration. More recently, we have found that Humulin Ultralente (Eli Lilly, Inc., Indianapolis, IN) is effective in eliminating the early morning rise in blood glucose concentration when given before dinner, thus eliminating the need for a third daily injection.

Two characteristics of adolescence and puberty specifically affect insulin therapy. First, adolescence is a time in which eating and sleeping times may vary greatly on a daily basis. Such variation cannot be accommodated by a traditional insulin regimen. Increased flexibility of lifestyle while maintaining metabolic control is possible using a multidose insulin regimen with three or four injections daily. Very long-acting insulin (animal Ultralente) is combined with regular insulin before breakfast, and regular insulin is given alone prior to the remaining meals or snacks. With this regimen, meals and snacks can be delayed or missed altogether, although careful and frequent blood glucose monitoring is required. This regimen works particularly well for older adolescents and young adults who have widely varying schedules and can benefit from the greater flexibility. Beef Ultralente insulin is used because it is less immunogenic than beef–pork combinations. Human Ultralente insulin does not lend itself as easily to this type of regimen. Insulin is distributed as follows: Ultralente constitutes about 40% of the total daily dose, and regular insulin makes up the remaining 60%, divided equally among the three major meals. An evening snack requires 4 to 6 units of regular insulin, depending on content and size. Adjustments of Ultralente insulin are based on 3 AM and prebreakfast readings. Regular insulin is given according to a sliding scale designed to compensate for every 100 mg/dl of glucose above 100 mg/dl up to 400 mg/dl, with increments of 10% up to a maximum of 50% above the starting dose.

The second important characteristic of puberty is a hormonally mediated decrease in insulin sensitivity. Insulin requirements usually remain fairly constant, between 0.6 and 1.0 unit/kg/day, from about 2 years after diagnosis until puberty. During puberty, insulin requirements increase, and many adolescents require between 1.1 to 1.4 units/kg/day from the onset of puberty until growth is complete. The exact cause of this change is unclear, but increases in growth hormone appear to play a role. After midpuberty, insulin requirements per weight gradually return to prepubertal levels. It is important to note that insulin resistance does not account solely, or perhaps at all, for poor metabolic outcomes during adolescence. Many adolescents maintain excellent control during puberty by appropriately increasing their insulin dose. The adolescent's behavior and emotional state are also important in determining control.

Diet Therapy

The diet is one of the cornerstones of therapy for IDDM. Management is directed toward normalizing plasma glucose levels, maintaining adequate nutrient intake to promote normal growth and development, promoting healthy eating habits, and minimizing the risk of long-term vascular complications. The American Diabetes Association diet is in most common use. Nutrients are distributed as 50% to 55% carbohydrate, 15% to 20% protein, and 30% to 35% fat. Our center has a somewhat liberal attitude toward the use of sucrose, enabling families to incorporate almost all foods favored by adolescents into the dietary plan. We place more emphasis on fat limitation than on sugar limitation. During adolescence, caloric requirements vary considerably and therefore must be individualized to reflect growth, activity, and food habits (see Chapter 7). It is not unusual for athletic adolescents, especially boys, to require far more calories.

Thereafter, calories are adjusted to maintain desirable body weight. Adolescent girls, in particular, need to begin tapering caloric intake before the end of puberty to avoid excess weight gain.

Although these guidelines are useful approximations, a thorough nutritional history by a dietitian well versed in diabetes care is best for determining nutritional requirements. Once requirements are established, calories are distributed over three meals and three snacks to moderate plasma glucose excursions.

Monitoring Metabolic Control

Patient monitoring of blood glucose levels at home is critical to management. Both adolescents and health care providers should use these home records for decisions about insulin therapy. When adolescents are not given appropriate education to respond to their own blood glucose levels, they rapidly decrease the frequency with which they measure their blood glucose. Optimally, blood glucose should be measured before each meal and before the bedtime snack. However, few adolescents test their blood during school. Therefore, decisions about the morning short-acting insulin are based on occasional blood glucose measurements obtained at school or on weekends. When significant changes in the evening long-acting insulin dose are made, blood glucose levels should be monitored at 3 AM to ensure that nocturnal hypoglycemia is not occurring. For the same reason, an occasional 3 AM blood glucose measurement in an adolescent patient who is well controlled is helpful.

Many adolescents do not or cannot monitor themselves as often as recommended. It is important that they be encouraged to test their blood glucose level at different times of the day. Urine glucose measurement is not necessary. Urine ketone measurement is helpful during periods of illness and significant hyperglycemia. Hypoglycemic reactions should be recorded. Occasional (two or three times per week) episodes of mild hypoglycemia are acceptable and probably are unavoidable with good control. Such episodes should not result in changes in level of consciousness.

Glycosylated hemoglobin (HbA_1) is a measure of integrated blood glucose control over the preceding 6 to 12 weeks. This test is an objective means of documenting the previous mean blood glucose level. HbA_1 is a product of a nonenzymatic reaction between glucose and hemoglobin in which the higher the ambient concentration of glucose the greater is the percentage of hemoglobin that is glycosylated. Assays can measure either total HbA_1 ($HbA_{1a} + _b + _c$) or the predominant glycosylated component, which is HbA_{1c}. Assays may have different normative ranges; it is important to interpret the result in view of the laboratory performing the test. For purposes of comparison, therefore, results should be expressed relative to the normal nondiabetic range.

Few adolescents with IDDM of more than 2 years' duration can maintain HbA_1 at or near the normal range. We consider that our adolescent patients are doing well if they are within 1.33 times the upper normal limit for a nondiabetic. For example, if the upper normal limit in a particular laboratory is 7.5%, then 9.9% would indicate very acceptable control. Similarly, an HbA_1 value greater than 1.5 times the upper normal range (approximately 11.2% in the previous example) indicates poor control and the need for significant reevaluation. HbA_1 levels are measured every 3 months, and the results should be communicated to adolescents and their families.

SPECIAL CIRCUMSTANCES

Participation in Sports

In addition to the well-known benefits of exercise, including increased cardiovascular fitness, an increased sense of well-being, and maintenance of normal body weight (see Chapter 81), in IDDM regular exercise offers the specific advantages of lowering blood glucose levels and increasing insulin sensitivity. Insulin requirements may be as much as 30% lower in an aerobically conditioned adolescent than in the same adolescent during sedentary periods. However, exercise can increase the likelihood of hypoglycemia, and exercise must be accounted for by either a reduction in insulin or an increase in food intake, or both, adding food as needed for unplanned activities. An additional 100 to 150 calories of both simple and complex carbohydrates is usually sufficient for an hour of uninterrupted, moderate to vigorous activity. Planned activity, such as an after-school sports program, can be covered by a reduction in insulin dose or a combination of increased food intake and insulin dose reduction. A 10% to 15% decrease in insulin dose for every hour of continuous aerobic activity is generally sufficient. A reduction in insulin dose requires advance planning. For example, sports practice

immediately after school requires a reduction in the dose of morning long-acting insulin. Adolescents should experiment by changing insulin regimens and food intake for activity and monitor their blood glucose closely before, during, and after participation in intensive exercise. The effects of exercise on insulin sensitivity may be prolonged (6 to 8 hours after exercise). Adolescents who engage in unusually prolonged periods of activity are at increased risk for postexercise hypoglycemia during the night. Both increased food intake and decreased dose of evening long-acting insulin can help avoid severe nocturnal hypoglycemia.

Contraindications to exercise are few. However, adolescents should be cautioned against exercise when their blood glucose level is excessively high or ketones are present in the urine. Exercise in the presence of a relative state of insulin deficiency stimulates gluconeogenic pathways, thus elevating plasma glucose level and stimulating ketone body formation. Once the blood glucose level falls below 300 mg/dl and the urine is free of ketone bodies, exercise may be resumed.

Participation in competitive sports should not be restricted because of IDDM. Professional athletes in many sports have had diabetes and often serve as role models. Diabetes does restrict the ability of wrestlers to rapidly lose weight, and that practice should be strongly discouraged. Among recreational sports, many, but not all, physicians believe that scuba diving should be discouraged for adolescents with diabetes.

Illness

Dietary management during illness may be difficult. Liquids containing sugar can be substituted for the usual diet and given at a rate of 20 g of carbohydrate every 1 to 2 hours. Insulin requirements may increase markedly during illness, and meticulous attention to blood glucose and ketone levels is critical. Families should check blood glucose and ketone levels every 4 to 6 hours and provide additional insulin when blood glucose levels exceed 250 mg/dl, particularly if ketonuria is present.

In general, supplementation with short-acting insulin is preferred to a more longer-acting insulin when treating hyperglycemia associated with illness. Additional insulin dosages can be calculated based on 10% to 15% of the total daily insulin dosage as follows: administer 10% of total daily insulin dose as regular insulin when the blood glucose level reaches 250 mg/dl; administer an additional 15% of the total daily insulin dose when ketonuria is also present. When vomiting or other gastrointestinal symptoms preclude usual meals or snacks, a reduction in insulin is needed to lessen the likelihood of hypoglycemia. The intermediate insulin (NPH/Lente) should be reduced to two-thirds the normal dose. Regular insulin should be withheld until the blood glucose value approaches 200 to 250 mg/dl. Then regular insulin is given in amounts of 10% to 15% of total daily insulin based on the absence or presence of ketones, respectively. The presence of vomiting with an elevated blood glucose level and urinary ketones requires that the adolescent be evaluated to rule out DKA. Evaluation is critical if vomiting persists more than 4 to 6 hours or if significant urinary ketones are present.

Pregnancy and Birth Control

Birth control and prepregnancy planning are important considerations for adolescents (see Chapter 73). Risks of an unplanned pregnancy in diabetes mellitus are substantial. The incidence of congenital anomalies among infants of mothers with poorly controlled diabetes is increased. Without careful medical follow-up and excellent metabolic control prior to and during pregnancy, background retinopathy and/or incipient nephropathy may develop. Diabetes, in and of itself, is not a contraindication to the use of birth control pills; these drugs are often the only acceptable and reliable method of contraception for adolescents. When indicated, oral contraceptives with a low progesterone-estrogen dose or progesterone-only formulations are generally best. Patients should receive screening for hypertension and lipid profiles prior to and during birth control use (see Chapters 60 and 67). Finally, young women must be informed about the importance of prepregnancy planning. Because congenital anomalies occur before the eighth to ninth week of pregnancy, good metabolic control before a pregnancy is confirmed is critical.

Drug and Alcohol Use

Drug and alcohol use among adolescents continues to be a problem of national concern (see Chapter 111). Although recent studies show a general decline in drug use among high-school students, alcohol use appears to be increasing. For adolescents with IDDM, alcohol used, even in moderation, can have potentially serious consequences. Although there is usually an initial rise in blood glucose level following alcohol ingestion, it is generally followed by a drop in blood glucose level several hours later. The presence of alcohol in the blood enhances the glucose-lowering effect of insulin and prolongs insulin time action. This enhanced glucose-insulin response may persist for 8 to 12 hours after ingestion and up to 36 hours after heavy consumption. Alcohol also inhibits fuel substrate availability from the liver; that is, it suppresses gluconeogenesis and glycogenolysis. Thus, the normal counterregulatory mechanisms that maintain glucose homeostasis in response to a falling blood glucose value, or fast, are impaired. This significantly increases the risk of hypoglycemia for adolescents with IDDM and is greatest when food intake is restricted or eliminated altogether. Although alcohol predisposes adolescents with IDDM to hypoglycemia, it can be used safely by those who are well controlled.

Adolescents frequently have questions about alcohol and drug use. It is generally advisable to begin to explore the subject by middle adolescence. Many older adolescents will reveal their intent to drink alcoholic beverages if asked about it when parents are not present. Regardless of whether an adolescent expresses an intent to begin drinking, information should be provided that allows the individual to make informed decisions. This means educating adolescents about the effects of alcohol on their health in addition to discussing the social responsibilities of drinking. Guidelines established by the American Diabetes Association include the following:

1. Alcohol should be used only if diabetes is well controlled.
2. Alcohol should be used in moderation—not more than two standard-size drinks once or twice a week.
3. Two standard-size alcoholic beverages can be taken in addition to the regular meal plan. Food should not be omitted or exchanged for alcohol. Alcohol does not require insulin to be metabolized. No additional insulin should be administered.

In addition to the American Diabetes Association guidelines, adolescents should be advised not to skip meals or snacks. They should avoid beverages that are high in carbohydrates (e.g., "light" beer is preferable) and avoid drinking after vigorous exercise or on an empty stomach. Alcohol can mask the early symptoms of hypoglycemia. Hypoglycemia can be avoided by eating shortly before or with drinking. Food should contain complex carbohydrates, protein, and fat to provide available glucose over an extended period of time when counterregulatory mechanisms may be impaired. Hypoglycemia the morning after drinking can be avoided by testing the blood glucose level and eating breakfast at the usual time. Identification should be worn or carried at all times when drinking away from home. Hypoglycemia can easily be mistaken for alcohol intoxication.

Other so-called recreational drugs, including stimulants, depressants, hallucinogens, and marijuana, have a minimal direct effect on glucose homeostasis. However, their use may signal serious psychosocial problems and may contribute indirectly to poor metabolic outcomes. Drugs such as alcohol can cloud judgment and lead to poor decision-making. Moreover, drugs may interfere with the recognition of deteriorating diabetes control or hypoglycemia. Thus, it is important to determine the frequency and amount with which drugs or alcohol are used and make appropriate referrals when abuse may be suspected.

New Therapies

Since IDDM is an autoimmune disease, a number of interventions involving immune suppression have been evaluated. Both cyclosporine and a combination of azathioprine and prednisone have been shown to decrease insulin requirements and to increase the frequency of complete remissions in the early phase of diabetes in some newly diagnosed adolescent patients. However, in all cases the duration of the effect is limited and, once therapy is discontinued, diabetes rapidly recurs. In addition, there are ongoing concerns about the side effects of any immunosuppressive regimen. At this time, immune suppression is experimental and should be implemented only as part of a randomized, blinded therapeutic trial at a center where excellent immunologic monitoring is possible.

Segmental pancreas transplantation in which the entire organ is transplanted has evolved to the state where it is no longer considered experimental under certain circumstances. Technically, transplantation offers a 1-year organ survival rate of up to 80%, with elimination of exogenous insulin requirements in the majority of cases. However, major surgery is required, as is potent immune suppression. For these reasons, pancreas transplantation is principally used for patients who are receiving or have received a kidney transplant, thus already requiring immune suppression. Transplantation for other indications should be considered experimental at this time. Continuous subcutaneous insulin delivery (insulin pumps) has not been found to be acceptable to most adolescents. It requires meticulous attention to self-monitored glucose levels and to the injection sites. Intraperitoneal insulin administration using an implantable pump is under clinical trial. Because it does not incorporate an implantable glucose sensor it is unlikely to be acceptable or safe for adolescents.

PSYCHOSOCIAL CONSIDERATIONS

Because diabetes management is complex and under adolescent and family control, the psychosocial health of the adolescent is critical to the success or failure of treatment (see Chapters 30 and 121). Measures of family and individual psychological and social functioning correlate with metabolic control. Attention to psychosocial issues pays dividends not only in terms of emotional health but also in improving metabolic values. The medical literature on psychosocial issues and diabetes is extensive. Several specific areas are most important to the management of adolescents.

First, an understanding of adolescent cognitive development is necessary to properly guide patients and families in assuming responsibility for the management of diabetes (see Chapters 9 and 11). Self-management tasks range from insulin injections to blood glucose monitoring to adjustment of insulin doses, each requiring a variety of physical, emotional, and computational skills. More complex activities, such as adjusting insulin in anticipation of a change in diet or activity, require the ability to think ahead, an ability usually lacking in younger adolescents and only gradually acquired throughout adolescence. Interestingly, when adolescents with IDDM were surveyed regarding their self-management practices, before age 15 almost no adolescents, but a majority of parents, made decisions as to insulin dose adjustment. After age 15 almost no parents, and only a small percentage of teenagers, did so. Thus, older teenagers were in transition regarding self-management. In general, it is clear that there is no one age at which all adolescents should be expected to assume specific tasks. Rather, families should remain actively involved as long as the adolescent wishes and until he or she demonstrates the consistent ability to safely perform a task. The technical ability to inject insulin, for example,

does not mean that an adolescent patient can do so consistently and reliably without support. For all tasks there should be a gradual transition of responsibility. It is clear that adolescents do best when family members remain actively involved with their diabetes care, particularly when making insulin adjustment decisions, well into late adolescence.

As might be expected, the degree and type of family support strongly affects metabolic control. The more positive the social support network, the better the control. In particular, the ways in which mothers cope with the diagnosis and the extent of the involvement of fathers are key factors. Thus, the diagnosis of diabetes should be treated as a family crisis and family support and, if needed, crisis psychotherapy provided. In particular, active participation by fathers should be encouraged at all stages of care and education.

Varying degrees of psychosocial dysfunction can lead to different levels of impaired metabolic control. Most dramatic episodes occur in those teenagers (frequently but not always girls) who consciously omit insulin in an effort to induce DKA. They do so for a variety of reasons, but all are characterized by repetitive unexplained episodes of severe ketoacidosis or hypoglycemia. The first step in treatment is recognizing that these episodes are not due to any intrinsic metabolic lability. There are no adolescent patients whose diabetes is stable in the hospital but unstable outside the hospital. Rather these adolescents omit insulin or, less commonly, their families do. To treat this situation, one needs to first document that the adolescent does not develop DKA when under supervision. The patient is hospitalized, with the hospital staff administering all insulin and performing all blood glucose monitoring. Insulin should be kept away from the patient so that he or she is not able to surreptitiously administer extra insulin. It is imperative that there be forthright discussion with the adolescent and family about the nature of the problem, followed by appropriate psychological counseling and clarification of the necessity for a responsible adult to directly supervise the administration of insulin. Although this may seem contrary to one's sense of development of autonomy, it is the only safe way to manage these few individuals. Recurrent DKA is life threatening and may result in death. Only after the behavioral nature of the problem is acknowledged can psychotherapy be effective. If this is unsuccessful, child protection avenues may need to be explored to ensure that the minor is receiving adequate medical supervision either in or out of the home.

On occasion, adolescents who have had their ability to induce DKA removed may induce severe hypoglycemia by administering extra insulin. The occurrence of repetitive severe hypoglycemia or a marked unexplained decrease in insulin dose is suggestive of this behavior. Surreptitious insulin administration for the purpose of inducing illness is usually a sign of significant psychosocial dysfunction.

For adolescents who are in poor metabolic control but who take their insulin and do not suffer from acutely life-threatening DKA or hypoglycemia, other approaches must be used. One that has worked is the use of peer groups that meet concurrently with ambulatory visits and emphasize diabetes problem solving based on self-monitoring of blood glucose levels. Whereas problem-solving peer support groups have been shown to aid in improving metabolic control, unstructured social support or so-called rap groups do not seem to be effective. Their development by well-meaning but unskilled staff should be discouraged.

Contrary to some earlier thought, adolescents with IDDM do not engage in more risk-taking behavior than do their peers; in fact, at younger ages they appear to engage in less and even in later adolescence are not less careful. It may be that ego development is delayed in adolescents with IDDM, with consequent delay in developmentally appropriate autonomous behaviors. Overall, it should be appreciated that diabetes does not itself cause psychological dysfunction and that most teenagers with IDDM develop normally.

DIABETES EDUCATION

Patient education is critical to treatment of diabetes. Adolescent patients and families must be able to incorporate multiple facets of a complex treatment regimen into their daily lives. Thus, a primary goal is to teach families how to become effective managers of diabetes.

A multidisciplinary approach is required for recognition of educational programs by the American Diabetes Association and clearly is necessary for good education. Programs that provide a series of organized learning experiences with both group and individual sessions enable group support to be incorporated into programs tailored to a family's particular needs. The content for each series may be sequenced from the simple to the more complex, starting with basic survival skills and ending with algorithms for insulin adjustment.

Education of adolescents with new-onset diabetes and their families may begin with a 3- to 4-day hospitalization, during which time education is focused on basic survival skills, that is, those skills necessary to survive outside the hospital. When geographically and financially feasible, many families can be treated entirely in ambulatory settings in specially designed programs. Initial emphasis is placed on dispelling myths and fears about diabetes, on mechanical skills of insulin administration, on blood glucose monitoring, on treatment of hypoglycemia, and on basic dietary principles. After discharge, frequent contact by telephone is maintained until the intensive outpatient education programs begin several weeks later.

One such outpatient education program lasts 3 full days and meets in groups of six families 1 to 2 months after diagnosis. This delay in more intensive education serves two purposes. It enables patients to begin to incorporate diabetes management into their daily lives and to generate questions. It also increases receptivity to education once patients have had an opportunity to overcome some of the shock of the initial diagnosis that may interfere with learning. The curriculum provides an in-depth discussion of previous topics and adds insulin and dietary self-management, exercise, and psychosocial concerns. For adolescents, topics include managing diabetes around school activities and work, birth control, prepregnancy planning, and complications.

BIBLIOGRAPHY

Amiel SA, Sherwin RS, Simonson DC, et al: Impaired insulin action in puberty. N Engl J Med 315:215, 1986.

Anderson BJ, Wolf FM, Burkhart MT, et al: Effects of peer-group intervention on metabolic control of adolescents with IDDM. Diabetes Care 12:179, 1989.

Diabetes Complications Clinical Trial Research Group: Are continuing studies of metabolic control and microvascular complications in insulin-dependent diabetes mellitus justified? N Engl J Med 318:246, 1988.

Drash AL: Diabetes mellitus in the child and adolescent: Part 1. In Current Problems in Pediatrics, vol 16. Chicago, Year Book Medical Publishers, 1986, p 413.

Drash AL: Diabetes mellitus in the child and adolescent: Part II. In Current Problems in Pediatrics, vol 16. Chicago, Year Book Medical Publishers, 1986, p 469.

Golden MP, Gray DL: Diabetes mellitus in children and adolescents. In Rakel, RE (ed): Conn's Current Therapy 1991. Philadelphia, WB Saunders, 1991.

Golden MP, Herrold AJ, Orr DP: An approach to prevention of recurrent diabetic ketoacidosis in the pediatric population. J Pediatr 107:195, 1985.

Hauser ST, Pollets D, Turner BL, et al: Ego development and self-esteem in diabetic adolescents. Diabetes Care 2:465, 1979.

Ingersoll GM, Orr DP, Herrold AJ, Golden MP: Cognitive maturity and self-management among adolescents with insulin-dependent diabetes mellitus. J Pediatr 108:620, 1986.

Kostraba JN, Dorman JS, Orchard TJ, et al: Contribution of diabetes duration before puberty to development of microvascular complications in IDDM subjects. Diabetes Care 12:686, 1989.

Ramsay RC, Goetz FC, Sutherland DER, et al: Progression of diabetic retinopathy after pancreas transplantation for insulin-dependent diabetes mellitus. N Engl J Med 318:208, 1988.

Rosenbloom AL: Intracerebral crises during treatment of diabetic ketoacidosis. Diabetes Care 13:22, 1990.

Tattersall R: Is pancreas transplantation for insulin-dependent diabetes worthwhile? N Engl J Med 321:112, 1989.

Tattersall RB, McCulloch DK, Aveline M: Group therapy in the treatment of diabetes. Diabetes Care 8:180, 1985.

CHAPTER 60

Nutritional Conditions

ANOREXIA NERVOSA

MICHAEL P. NUSSBAUM

Anorexia nervosa is a disorder in which an individual, usually a white adolescent female, restricts food intake excessively and loses weight markedly below ideal body weight. There is an underlying drive for thinness and an overwhelming fear of fatness that are associated with a distorted body image. The Diagnostic and Statistical Manual of Mental Disorders, Third Edition–Revised (DSM-III-R) diagnostic criteria are listed in Table 60–1. These criteria are important for documentation and comparison studies of different population groups. However, clinicians should recognize that this disorder, especially in adolescents, has subclinical or partial forms. The DSM-III-R recognizes this category as "atypical" or "otherwise unspecified" eating disorders. It has been shown in several epidemiologic studies that there are more adolescents who have subclinical anorexia nervosa than those who meet the formal criteria; for that reason, a subthreshold category has been suggested for the DSM-IV. These adolescents usually have similar underlying psychological characteristics and may need as vigorous treatment as those who meet all DSM-III-R criteria.

PREVALENCE

The prevalence of anorexia nervosa has increased approximately fivefold in the past 30 years. Approximately 1% of white girls between the ages of 16 and 24 years are affected. Rates are increased in higher socioeconomic groups and in middle and late adolescence (peak age of onset between 14 and 18 years of age). There seems to be a spread of anorexia nervosa outside the traditional high-risk groups. More prepubertal girls and boys as well as more adolescent patients from lower socioeconomic groups and outside of industrialized countries are being identified. More males are being diagnosed with anorexia nervosa as the prevalence increases, but males account for fewer than 10% of patients.

ETIOLOGY

There are numerous factors that predispose an adolescent to developing anorexia nervosa, that precipitate its occurrence, and that perpetuate its signs and symptoms once the diagnosis is established. Biologic and genetic, intrapersonal, familial, and sociocultural factors all can play a significant role in the development and maintenance of anorexia nervosa. It is better considered as a final common pathway than as a single disease entity. Furthermore, a biopsychosocial approach to evaluation and treatment is mandatory, since no single treatment modality is uniformly effective.

Biologic and Genetic

Onset is most common as the adolescent emerges from puberty. Increased deposition of adipose tissue during puberty as well as an increased concern about obesity among peers may predispose some adolescents to begin to diet (see subchapter on primary obesity). Hypothalamic dysfunction may also predispose some adolescents to anorexia nervosa. Although many hypothalamic abnormalities are eliminated after weight is restored, some may remain despite weight restoration. Affected individuals rarely have had premorbid hypothalamic function tested. However, reports of retarded growth or amenorrhea prior to the onset of dieting suggest the possibility of a preceding hypothalamic abnormality. Research conducted in 1947 by Keys and colleagues on voluntary starvation in previously normal late adolescent and young adult males demonstrated that subjects developed many of the symptoms observed in patients who have anorexia nervosa. In addition to the physiologic changes of malnutrition, behavioral and cognitive changes also occur. These include hoarding of the little food given to them, hyperactivity, and obsessive thinking about and dreaming of food. Studies have shown increased concordance in monozygotic twins as compared with dizygotic twins. An increased number of cases also are seen among sisters and female relatives of patients with anorexia nervosa.

Intrapersonal

Adolescents with anorexia nervosa often have low self-esteem and high anxiety levels. They tend to be

**TABLE 60–1. DSM-III-R Criteria for
Anorexia Nervosa**

Refusal to maintain body weight over a normal minimum weight for age and height (e.g., weight loss leading to maintenance of body weight 15% below that expected) or failure to make expected weight gain during period of growth, leading to body weight 15% below that expected.

Intense fear of gaining weight or becoming fat, even though underweight.

Disturbance in the way in which one's body weight, size, or shape is experienced (e.g., the person claims to "feel fat" even when emaciated).

In females, absence of at least three consecutive menstrual cycles when otherwise expected to occur (primary or secondary amenorrhea). (A woman is considered to have amenorrhea if her periods occur only following hormone administration.)

introverted, obsessional, and perfectionistic and to have controlling tendencies. They are usually overachievers but have a sense of ineffectiveness; some have associated affective disorders, such as depression. The development of anorexia nervosa can be viewed as an attempt to gain control.

Familial

Normally the adolescent develops independence and autonomy in preparation for separation from the family. Family disturbances preventing this developmental progress have been implicated as a major factor in anorexia nervosa. In many cases, however, the family dynamics are more of a reaction to than a cause of the symptoms. Minuchin and colleagues describe the family pathology of anorexia nervosa in terms of enmeshment, overprotectiveness, rigidity, and lack of conflict resolution. They describe the mother as often controlling and the father as a distant figure in the family. Some patients are only recognized as an "individual" after the illness becomes significant and their need for autonomy and self-determination can no longer be denied.

Sociocultural

The pressures of contemporary society also may contribute to the development of anorexia nervosa. Primarily affected are affluent adolescents from areas of the world in which there is an abundance of food. Anorexia nervosa is most likely to develop in adolescents from a cultural group in which thinness is equated with attractiveness, self-confidence and success. The news media frequently have glamorized anorexia nervosa as a status "in" disease for young women in our society.

Coincident is the increasing sexualization of adolescents, again highlighted by the media. In today's culture, issues of sexuality are not subtle but vivid, not only through mass media promotion of sex and sexual themes, but also through educational programs attempting to prevent AIDS, other sexually transmitted diseases, and unplanned pregnancy. These sociocultural pressures upon the vulnerable adolescent may contribute

to the development of an eating disorder as a defense against the frightening realities of adolescence.

Anorexia nervosa can be viewed as a biopsychosocial developmental arrest. The peak times of onset of anorexia nervosa are after the start of puberty and at the start of a major life separation, such as going away to college or beginning full-time employment. Adjusting to one's body during puberty, coupled with the struggle of independence, may lead to inner conflict. In the older adolescent, issues of separation may lead to family disruption, especially between daughter and mother. That the adolescent is trying to establish control of her own life may not be easily recognized. Among adolescent females in modern society, the ability to diet and lose weight has become an important symbol of control.

Subpopulations of adolescents also appear to be at increased risk for the development of disordered eating. They fall into two groups: one that requires those who have extracurricular activities to be underweight (ballet dancers, gymnasts, male wrestlers) and the other consisting of those who have a chronic medical problem that affects self-image, such as diabetes mellitus and cystic fibrosis. Increased incidence of anorexia nervosa among girls with scoliosis has also been described.

CLINICAL MANIFESTATIONS AND DIAGNOSIS
History

As many as 40% of adolescents who have anorexia nervosa have mild to moderate premorbid obesity. The typical patient is an adolescent female between the ages of 14 and 16 presenting with weight loss, secondary amenorrhea, and denial of problems other than the need to lose weight. Psychological characteristics are listed in Table 60–2. Despite being underweight or even emaciated, she does not see herself as being thin and may believe that certain parts of her body, especially the thighs, the hips, and the buttocks, are too large. Patients restrict calories and food choices so that their diet is monotonous and deficient in energy. A 24- to 72-hour dietary recall and calculation of caloric intake are helpful for assessment. Adolescent patients cut up food into very small pieces and spend more time "playing" with the food than eating it. Some adolescent patients leave the table immediately after eating to go to the bathroom

**TABLE 60–2. Psychological Characteristics in
Anorexia Nervosa**

Distorted body image
Poor self-esteem
Depression
Overachiever, perfectionist
Strong-willed, determined nature
Uncommunicative behavior
Overwhelming sense of ineffectiveness
Distrustful nature
Self-destructive behavior
Difficulty in concentrating
Irritability
Obsessive thoughts about food, eating, and body shape

to vomit. Parents report that the adolescent is exercising frequently and for prolonged periods of time and that he or she becomes irritable if prevented from doing so. They also note that the patient spends less time with friends and is increasingly isolated.

Denial of illness is universal, and hostility to intervention is common. Adolescent patients may admit to feelings of fatness of hips, abdomen, or thighs, while accurately perceiving the body shape of others.

School performance is generally excellent in spite of poor self-image, low self-esteem, and depression. Patients are often perfectionists and have obsessive-compulsive traits. The drive for thinness is an attempt to be perfect in losing weight.

Family dynamics may appear normal initially. The adolescent patient has been the "perfect" child, growing up without any problems. On further questioning, one may find a mother who is enmeshed with the patient. The father is often emotionally distant and plays a minor role in the relationship with his daughter. Other siblings may have had problems, with much attention and family energy directed toward that sibling while little attention is paid to the adolescent patient.

When the girl with anorexia nervosa is first seen, she is extremely concerned that the control she has developed will be lost if she gains weight. Having this control taken away is frightening for the patient because not only does she dread becoming fat again, but also she fears the loss of the secondary gains that the dieting and weight loss have produced.

Early diagnosis and awareness of impending anorexia nervosa may prevent disease progression. Early clues to the diagnosis include dieting associated with amenorrhea, a change in weight goal that the adolescent initially sets for herself, and a feeling of unhappiness once that goal is reached. Abdominal pain, constipation, and bloating are common. Secretive dieting, exercising, vomiting, or laxative use regardless of the patient's weight must be of major concern, especially if the adolescent denies such behavior when it is occurring. Refusing to eat with family or friends and refusal to socialize with friends are signs that there is a significant problem.

Psychological Tests

In addition to the history and structured psychiatric interview, there are several standardized tests to help establish the diagnosis of anorexia nervosa. However, there are a number of adolescents who have atypical anorexia nervosa who do not meet full criteria, but who nonetheless deserve treatment. The Eating Attitudes Test (EAT) developed by Garner and Garfinkel is the most widely used screening test. This 40-item questionnaire measures various symptoms of anorexia nervosa. A shorter version, the EAT-26 emphasizes dieting, food preoccupation, bulimia, and control. These scales are useful in both clinical and research settings. The Eating Disorders Inventory (EDI) is a longer (64-item) testing instrument useful in measuring different psychological traits of adolescent patients with eating disorders. Various other psychological tests are useful adjuncts in

assessing the overall psychological profile of the adolescent, including the Body Shape Questionnaire, Beck Depression Inventory, Borderline Syndrome Index, and the Symptom Check List (SCL-90).

Physical Examination

The physical findings in anorexia nervosa depend on the degree of starvation and the methods used to lose weight. Weight should be measured with the adolescent undressed, except for a gown and underpants, after having voided, because clothing may be used to hide heavy objects, and drinking fluids prior to weigh-in may be used to falsely elevate apparent weight.

The vital signs help differentiate thin but healthy adolescents from those who have significant physiologic adaptation or decompensation from excessive dieting. Bradycardia is most commonly seen, with significant orthostatic increase in pulse on standing. Hypotension with orthostatic changes may also be noted. Hypothermia with oral temperatures frequently less than 36° C is noted. All these changes are responses to starvation and return to normal with improved nutrition and weight gain. The adolescent's height and weight should be plotted on growth charts.

The skin is often dry and scaly with lanugo-type hair on the arms and back; there is little, if any, subcutaneous tissue because of loss of fat. Patients may be shorter in stature than expected based on parental heights and compared with aged-matched control subjects if dieting started at an early age. Cardiovascular examination reveals a small heart and a weak pulse. Abdominal examination is essentially normal except for the easy ability to palpate the abdomen because of the thin, weakened abdominal musculature and the frequent palpation of stool in the left lower quadrant secondary to constipation. Neurologic examination may show proximal muscle weakness or peripheral neuropathy and, in severely emaciated individuals, signs of organic brain syndrome. For example, loss of deep tendon reflexes can occur as well as grossly distorted thinking in which the cachectic adolescent is unable to make decisions about simple daily tasks.

Laboratory Tests

Despite severe malnutrition, many initial screening investigations often are normal (Table 60–3). These results may give a false sense that weight loss is not significant. Hemoglobin is usually normal, though a mild normochromic, normocytic anemia may be seen. White blood cell counts may be low, with lymphopenia the predominant abnormality. The erythrocyte sedimentation rate is normal. Electrolyte levels are usually normal, except if vomiting leads to hypokalemia or a metabolic alkalosis. An elevated blood urea nitrogen may accompany dehydration but may be attenuated by low protein intake. Cholesterol levels are elevated, with an increase predominantly of high-density lipoprotein cholesterol. The urinalysis may show ketones and a high pH. Specific gravity can be elevated or low, depending on whether

TABLE 60–3. Normal Laboratory Findings in Anorexia Nervosa

Hemoglobin
Electrolytes*
Serum protein
Albumin
Vitamin B$_{12}$
Folate
Calcium
Phosphorus
Prolactin

*May be abnormal if there is vomiting or laxative or diuretic abuse.

TABLE 60–5. Abnormal Results of Neuroendocrine Studies in Anorexia Nervosa

LOW	HIGH
FSH	Cortisol
LH	Cholesterol
Estradiol	Endorphins
T$_3$	Serotonin*
Growth hormone	
Somatomedins	
GnRH	
Dopamine	
Norepinephrine	

*Some reports have conflicting results.

the adolescent is dehydrated or water-loaded. Low levels of antidiuretic hormone (arginine vasopressin) may also occur. Hypercarotenemia due to increased intake of vitamin A and carotene from vegetarian diets or due to decreased metabolism of these compounds owing to reduced triiodothyronine (T$_3$) is apparent on examination of the skin.

Other significant abnormalities are listed in Table 60–4. Most significant is ST segment depression seen on electrocardiogram (ECG) during exercise stress testing in 30% of patients. Prolonged QT$_c$, an ECG abnormality that has been associated with fatal ventricular tachycardia in adults with anorexia nervosa, has been reported in 44% of adolescents with anorexia nervosa in one series, but is notably absent in most reports. Cerebral atrophy is observed on computed tomography of the head in more than 50% of cases, presumably due to acute starvation.

Recent research on the etiology of anorexia nervosa centers on neuroendocrinologic dysfunction. The relationship among body weight, food restriction, exercise, hormones, neurotransmitters, and endorphins is complex and is not totally understood. Still debated and unknown is whether the abnormalities of the neuroendocrine axis are a result of malnutrition or a primary abnormality central to the etiology of the disease brought out in a predisposed individual who begins to diet. Abnormalities of neuroendocrine function in anorexia nervosa are enumerated in Table 60–5.

Amenorrhea is central to the diagnosis, basal levels of follicle-stimulating hormone (FSH) and luteinizing

TABLE 60–4. Abnormal Studies Associated with Anorexia Nervosa

Electrocardiogram
  Bradycardia
  Low voltage
Exercise stress test
  Suboptimal response of heart rate, blood pressure, and oxygen consumption
  ST segment depression
Pulmonary function
  Decreased forced expiratory volume in 1 second (FEV$_1$)
Computed tomography of head
  Cerebral atrophy
Ultrasound of pelvis
  Small ovaries
Bone densitometry
  Osteopenia
Gastrointestinal series
  Delayed gastric emptying

hormone (LH) are low, and response to LH-releasing hormone is diminished for LH and exaggerated for FSH. The 24-hour secretory pattern of LH is low, similar to that of prepuberty. Serum estradiol levels are normal to low, as are serum testosterone levels in affected males. Prolactin level is normal.

Thyroid function demonstrates mild depression of T$_3$. Increased levels of reverse T$_3$ are seen and thought to be secondary to malnutrition with decreased peripheral conversion of thyroxine (T$_4$) to T$_3$ as an adaptive mechanism for energy conservation during prolonged periods of catabolism. There is a delayed thyroid-stimulating hormone (TSH) response to stimulation by thyrotropin-releasing hormone (TRH).

Growth hormone (GH) levels initially were reported as high, but more recent research suggests that GH may be low secondary to hypothalamic dysfunction. Disturbances of adrenergic and cholinergic controls result in failure to stimulate release of GH from pituitary stores. Somatomedins are generally low in response to malnutrition.

The serum cortisol level as well as the cerebrospinal fluid (CSF) cortisol level is elevated, and the diurnal secretory pattern of cortisol is lost. Corticotropin-releasing hormone (CRH) levels are also increased in anorexia nervosa, but CSF levels of adrenocorticotropic hormone (ACTH) are decreased.

Studies of serotonin secretion have shown conflicting results. Increases in serotonin have been shown to decrease food consumption and decrease carbohydrate intake. Treatment with cyproheptadine, a serotonin antagonist, might be beneficial (see Treatment section).

Endorphins, which increase following exercise, are extremely elevated in cachectic individuals with anorexia nervosa and may prevent the secretion of gonadotropin-releasing hormone (GnRH), thereby contributing to the amenorrhea. Furthermore, these compounds may account for the highly "addictive" nature of this syndrome. Dopamine and norepinephrine secretion has also been shown to decrease. Both play a role in regulation of LH secretion. It is probable that neurotransmitters and thyroid and adrenal axis hormones play a role in the amenorrhea seen in anorexia nervosa. All return to normal with weight restoration.

Unusual Manifestations

Males with anorexia nervosa account for only 5% to 10% of cases. The psychological symptoms in males may be more severe than those seen in females. Males appear to have more problems with gender disturbances, including a hyperfeminine identification and an increase in ego-dystonic homosexuality.

More prepubertal adolescents are being identified with anorexia nervosa, and they seem to have more problems regarding family issues than body shape disturbances. Anorexia nervosa during adolescent pregnancy can occur. Adolescents with any chronic illness, but especially diabetes mellitus, may be predisposed to anorexia nervosa. They are likely to have problems with self-image and self-esteem in addition to disturbances in development, particularly independence. These patients are difficult to manage because the malnutrition can affect the underlying illness and because weight loss may be due to either the chronic illness or anorexia nervosa.

Differential Diagnosis

Making the diagnosis of anorexia nervosa is usually not difficult. The history and physical examination exclude most illnesses, but in a differential diagnosis one would want to be sure to exclude Addison disease, inflammatory bowel disease (see Chapter 63), hyperthyroidism, diabetes mellitus (see Chapter 59), hypopituitarism, brain tumors (see Chapter 53), and malignancies. Drug abuse (see Chapter 111), specifically cocaine, "crack" cocaine, or other amphetamines, must be ruled out, especially if the adolescent has symptoms of bulimia nervosa (see the next subchapter). Other psychiatric disorders also must be differentiated from eating disorders. These include primary depression (see Chapter 100), manic-depressive disorders, schizophrenia (see Chapter 110), and obsessive-compulsive disorders (see Chapter 105). Once the diagnosis of an eating disorder is made, it is important to differentiate anorexia nervosa from bulimia nervosa and atypical eating disorders.

TREATMENT

Any successful treatment program for anorexia nervosa must be able to manage the medical and nutritional aspects, the individual psychological problems, and the family dynamics. Starvation produces biologically based psychological changes; psychotherapy will not be effective until the severe malnutrition is corrected. Weight restoration must be central to any treatment program. A behavior modification contract between the physician and the adolescent is the most useful tool for enabling the patient to gain weight in a continuous and steady pattern. Furthermore, a written program helps define rules and limits for all treatment team members and prevents the adolescent patient from manipulating the staff in an attempt to avoid weight gain.

A minimum weight gain of 1.2 lb every 4 days has been found to be effective in restoring weight and also reasonable for the adolescent who is extremely anxious about any weight gain and fearful of getting fat and losing control. A slow and steady weight gain is essential if the complications of bulimia and later purging are to

be avoided. Initially, exercise should be prohibited; however, as the patient improves, limited exercise can be used as a privilege for successful weight gain and as a means of improving cardiovascular tone and depression.

All patients and their families should have a psychiatric evaluation. Most adolescent patients need individual psychotherapy, and most families need family or supportive therapy. A combination of individual and family therapy has been found to be most effective although not always possible. All patients benefit from supportive therapy from the treatment team even if they refuse formal psychotherapy. Treatment must focus on improving self-image and self-esteem and helping the patient develop independence.

Criteria for hospitalization include marked emaciation (>20% below ideal body weight), severe bradycardia or dysrhythmias, hypokalemia, neurologic deficits, severe caloric restriction (eating <500 kcal/day), and an inability to gain weight during ambulatory treatment. The need for hospitalization should be individualized, but aggressive management early in the course of treatment may improve the long-term results.

Once in the hospital, modification of eating behaviors is the mainstay of treatment. Nutritional education must be provided as well. The goal of treatment is not to make the adolescent fat but rather to allow her to gain control and achieve a normal weight in a healthy fashion. A weight restoration goal within 10% of mean ideal body weight allows the patient to understand that the treatment team will help to prevent the patient from gaining more than the necessary weight required.

Nasogastric feeding is reserved for those adolescents who are severely emaciated or those who refuse or are unable to gain weight on the behavior modification program. We use slow continuous nasogastric feeding over 24 hours. In severely emaciated patients who have been severely restricting their caloric intake, an initial rate of 1000 to 1200 kcal/day provides enough calories for weight gain and to prevent acute gastric dilatation or overload congestive heart failure. Usually calories can be increased by 150 to 250 kcal every 2 or 3 days. Measuring basal metabolic rate using indirect calorimetry is useful in judging the amount of calories required for each individual. Peripheral alimentation is rarely indicated in nutritional rehabilitation. The gastrointestinal tract is able to function normally (except for gastric atony early in refeeding), and the calories that can be delivered to the stomach or jejunum far exceed that which can be infused into central veins.

The decision to use pharmacotherapy is made on an individual basis, since there is no pharmacologic cure for anorexia nervosa. Depression is often associated with anorexia nervosa and antidepressants are sometimes beneficial, but must be used with caution in the cachectic adolescent. Desipramine is initially started at 50 mg before bed, and the dose can be increased by 50 mg every 3 to 5 days to a maximum of 5 mg/kg. Maximum antidepressant effects may not occur for 2 or more weeks. (This dosage is for patients less than 40 kg.) Before any increase in dosage, an electrocardiogram should be performed to look for signs of impending toxicity: prolongation of the QRS, QT, or PR intervals. Most adolescent patients benefit from a dose of 150 mg;

dosages over 150 mg are not recommended in adolescents. Obsessive-compulsive traits are common, and some patients benefit from drugs such as fluoxetine and clomipramine. Both these drugs are also antidepressants. Fluoxetine is started at a low dose of 10 mg in the morning to reduce wakefulness and can be increased gradually to 60 mg/day. Recent reports suggesting an increased suicide risk for some patients taking fluoxetine underscore the need for close monitoring of patients taking medications. Clomipramine is a tricyclic antidepressant, and the dose and toxicity are similar to those of desipramine. Anti-anxiety drugs such as alprazolam (0.25 mg before meals) are sometimes worthwhile for short-term use to help lessen the adolescent's fear and panic of losing control and becoming fat. However, the addictive potential of this medication should be recognized. Cyproheptadine, a serotonin antagonist, has been used as an appetite stimulant. One study has shown that in doses as high as 32 mg/day it is effective in augmenting weight gain in the patient who desires to gain weight but who has true anorexia. Neuroleptics such as chlorpromazine should always be used with caution and in consultation with a psychiatrist in severely recalcitrant patients after other methods have failed.

Estrogen replacement therapy has been used to induce monthly periods and prevent or reverse osteopenia, but there are no studies that document its effectiveness. Every effort should be made to have the patient gain to within 10% of her ideal body weight before hormonal treatment is initiated, however.

Patient discharge is contingent upon weight gain to within 10% of ideal body weight. A short maintenance phase prior to discharge gives the adolescent much needed reassurance that weight will not continue to increase once he or she has gone home.

Ambulatory management, either as the initial treatment or following discharge, must also be comprehensive and focus on medical, nutritional, and psychological needs. Adolescent patients are seen at least weekly to monitor weight and medical indicators and to provide ongoing nutritional counseling. A behavior modification protocol helps achieve weight goals. The adolescent and the physician set these goals and determine the privileges or restrictions. Parents may have to share responsibility for contract enforcement. This is sometimes difficult or nontherapeutic for some families, whereas for others it helps reestablish appropriate parent-adolescent relationships. The physician provides support while individual or family therapy is maintained based on individual needs.

Group therapy is controversial in the management of anorexia nervosa. It is not a substitute for individual or family therapy but an adjunct for some patients. The individual therapist and the group therapist must have close communication. Self-help groups and groups led by former patients are to be viewed with caution, since change toward improvement is not necessarily a goal of such groups. All therapeutic modalities require concomitant medical and nutritional supervision.

COURSE AND PROGNOSIS

Mortality rates as high as 20% were previously reported in anorexia nervosa. With vigorous emphasis on family and nutritional therapy, mortality has decreased to 2% to 8%.

The prognosis for recovery is variable and not easily defined. A successful outcome must be based on weight restoration without medical complications, return of menstrual function (and presumably fertility), and psychological improvement including a normal body image.

The prognosis improves if the diagnosis and appropriate intervention are made early. Adolescents diagnosed with anorexia nervosa and treated with a developmentally oriented, multidisciplinary approach have an overall success rate of 75% to 85%, with 80% to 90% having a return of menses. As many as 50% of patients may develop bulimic symptoms at some time during their treatment course. Signs of poor prognosis include vomiting, binge eating (see the next subchapter), chronicity, lower minimum weight, failure to respond to previous treatment, and more disturbed premorbid family relationships.

BIBLIOGRAPHY

Bruch H: Anorexia nervosa: Therapy and theory. Am J Psychiatry 139:1531, 1982.
Bunnell DW, Shenker IR, Nussbaum MP, et al: Subclinical versus formal eating disorders: Differentiating psychological features. Int J Eating Disorders 9(3):357, 1990.
Garfinkel PE, Garner DM (eds): The Role of Drug Treatments for Eating Disorders. New York, Brunner/Mazel, 1987.
Gold PW, Gwirtsman H, Avgerinos PC, et al: Abnormal hypothalamic-pituitary-adrenal function in anorexia nervosa. N Engl J Med 314:1335, 1986.
Halmi KA: Behavioral management for anorexia nervosa. In Garner DM, Garfinkel PE (eds): Handbook of Psychotherapy for Anorexia Nervosa and Bulimia. New York, Guilford Press, 1985.
Keys A, Brozek J, Henschel A, et al: The Biology of Human Starvation. Minneapolis, University of Minnesota Press, 1950.
Kreipe RE, Churchill BH, Strauss J: Long-term outcome of adolescents with anorexia nervosa. Am J Dis Child 143:1322, 1989.
Minuchin S, Rosman BL, Baker L: Psychosomatic Families: Anorexia Nervosa in Context. Cambridge, Harvard University Press, 1978, pp 1–73.
Mitchell JE: Psychopharmacology of eating disorders. Ann NY Acad Sci 575:41, 1989.
Neal JH, Herzog DH: Family dynamics and treatment of anorexia nervosa and bulimia. Pediatrician 12:139, 1983–1985.
Nussbaum M, Shenker IR, Marc J, Klein M: Cerebral atrophy in anorexia nervosa. J Pediatr 96:867, 1980.
Nussbaum MP, Blethen SL, Chasalow FI, et al: Blunted growth hormone responses to clonidine in adolescent girls with early anorexia nervosa. J Adolesc Health Care 11:145, 1990.
Weiner H: Psychoendocrinology of anorexia nervosa. Psychiatr Clin North Am 12(1):187, 1989.
Yates A: Current perspectives on the eating disorders: I. History, psychological and biological aspects. J Am Acad Child Adolesc Psychiatry 28(6):813, 1989.

BULIMIA NERVOSA

I. RONALD SHENKER and DOUGLAS W. BUNNELL

Bulimia nervosa is characterized by episodes of binge eating and behaviors to avoid the consequences of overeating, such as self-induced emesis, vigorous exercise, fasting, laxative abuse, and diuretic abuse. Although references to bulimic behaviors can be found in Gull's original description in 1874 of a patient with anorexia nervosa, bulimia and bulimia nervosa were not recognized as distinct disorders until the late 1970s.

In 1979, Russell noted that persons who binge eat and purge frequently exhibited clinical and prognostic features distinct from those persons with anorexia nervosa who attempt to lose weight through food restriction; he suggested that these features constituted an important subgroup of eating disorders. Bulimia nervosa is now recognized as a distinct form of eating pathology with characteristic manifestations (Table 60–6). These criteria include both behavioral and subjective features. The frequency and duration of symptoms distinguish adolescents with bulimia nervosa from other individuals who occasionally overeat and purge. Adolescents who meet the formal diagnostic criteria for bulimia nervosa are substantially different from individuals who only occasionally engage in bulimic behaviors. Preoccupation with shape and weight also differentiate patients with bulimia nervosa from those persons who binge eat and purge occasionally.

PREVALENCE

Controversy concerning diagnostic criteria complicates the assessment of the prevalence and incidence of the disorder. A majority of adolescent and young adult females report dissatisfaction with their weight or shape, but only a minority report episodes of binge eating and self-induced purging. Of this latter minority, only a small subgroup meets formal diagnostic criteria for bulimia nervosa. One estimate in the epidemiologic literature concludes that approximately 8% of adolescent and young adult females and 1% of adolescent and young adult males met the earlier Diagnostic and Statistical Manual of Mental Disorders, Third Edition (DSM-

TABLE 60–6. DSM-III-R Criteria for Bulimia Nervosa

Recurrent episodes of binge eating (rapid consumption of a large amount of food during a discrete period of time)
A feeling of lack of control over eating behavior during the eating binge
Regular episodes of self-induced vomiting, use of laxatives or diuretics, strict dieting or fasting, or vigorous exercise in order to prevent weight gain
A minimum average of two binge eating episodes a week for at least 3 months
Persistent overconcern with body shape and weight

III) criteria for bulimia. Subsequent research using the revised criteria, which include criteria for frequency and duration of binge eating, suggests that the incidence of bulimia nervosa in college-age females approximates 3%. Fewer than 1% of males meet formal criteria for the diagnosis of bulimia nervosa. However, if an adolescent male has an eating disorder, it is more likely to be bulimia than anorexia nervosa.

Patients with bulimia nervosa often develop the disorder during adolescence, but their disorder may not come to the attention of a physician until adulthood. The ratio of females to males who have bulimia nervosa is approximately 10:1, although the incidence in males may be underreported. Although both anorexia nervosa and bulimia nervosa are believed to be disorders of the upper socioeconomic groups, recent research suggests that women of all socioeconomic ranges are susceptible to the illness.

ETIOLOGY

Several models have been described in an attempt to conceptualize the etiology of bulimia nervosa.

Addiction Model

Bulimia nervosa is believed to be a food and behavioral addiction. Treatment emphasizes abstinence, social support, and relapse prevention, similar to the treatment of other addictions, including alcohol and substance abuse (see Chapter 111).

Family Model

The disordered eating of the adolescent is a symptom of a chaotic and underorganized family system. Treatment, therefore, focuses on the identification and amelioration of dysfunctional family interactional patterns. Although methodologic problems have hampered the research in this specific area, it appears that adolescents who have bulimia nervosa are more likely to have a history of childhood physical or sexual abuse than are those who have no history of bulimia nervosa (see Chapters 118 and 119).

Sociocultural Model

Women in Western cultures are subjected to intense and pervasive pressures to change their body shapes. Popular media emphasize the relationship between thinness and success; the dieting industry has capitalized on a nationwide preoccupation with weight loss. Within this social context virtually all females attempt to diet at some point during adolescence. Most fail at their attempts but are able to tolerate this experience without any undue psychological distress. Patients with bulimia nervosa may represent those failures who have resorted to alternative means of attaining thinness.

Cognitive-Behavioral Model

Bulimia nervosa is the behavioral manifestation of irrational thoughts and beliefs concerning shape, weight, dieting, and self-esteem. Treatment focuses on the identification of these dysfunctional beliefs and helps the adolescent develop means of countering these thoughts. Behavioral interventions such as record-keeping, response-prevention, and response-delay aid in reducing the frequency of binge eating. Nutritional guidelines are presented, and the patient is instructed to eat a regular diet. Figure 60–1 presents a schematic representation of the binge-purge cycle from a cognitive-behavioral model perspective.

Psychodynamic Model

Bulimia nervosa represents an attempt to control, avoid, master, or minimize the impact of distressful feelings, impulses, and anxieties. Psychodynamic treatment focuses on the underlying processes, with particular attention to psychosocial developmental features.

CLINICAL SIGNS

Bulimia nervosa has several characteristic features. Table 60–7 lists the clinical signs of bulimia. Although adolescents describe similar symptoms concerning their eating, dieting, and body image, the associated psychological features vary greatly.

Binge Eating

Binge eating is defined as the consumption of a large amount of food in a short period of time. Adolescents often describe a feeling of loss of control during these episodes. It is important to quantify the amount of food ingested in a binge, since it is not unusual for an

TABLE 60–7. Clinical Signs of Bulimic Behavior

Binge eating and food
    Binge eating associated with stress or anxiety
    Guilt associated with eating
    Secretive eating
    Hiding food
    Stealing food
Purging and dieting
    Use of bathroom after meals
    Evidence of vomiting, laxative use, or diuretic use
    Compulsive exercise
    Obsessive dieting followed by binge eating
Body image
    Measuring self-worth in terms of weight and shape
    Weight preoccupation
    Frequent weighing
    Rapid weight fluctuations
Associated symptoms
    Impaired concentration
    Depression

adolescent to consider eating more than was planned as a binge, even though it was an appropriate amount of food. Bulimic patients may consume between 3000 and 7000 kcal per binge. The binge episode often occurs at the same time each day or in response to emotional triggers such as depression, boredom, or anger, and it frequently follows a lengthy period of food restriction. Adolescents may identify particular "binge foods" that are avoided when trying to limit food consumption.

Purging

Patients with bulimia nervosa may use a variety of means of reversing the effects of overeating. Self-induced vomiting is the most common. Adolescents typically induce vomiting with pharyngeal stimulation but may progress to spontaneous vomiting. More drastic means of self-induced vomiting include the use of ipecac syrup. The allegedly cardiotoxic effects of ipecac have caused death in bulimic patients.

Bulimic patients also use laxatives, diuretics, and enemas to rid themselves of food and to alleviate the experience of bloating and fullness. The majority also exercise routinely or excessively to compensate for the binge eating. A minority of patients use exercise as their sole means of purging. Others severely restrict intake following each binge episode. Virtually all adolescent patients with bulimia nervosa are also dieting, and it is within this context of behaviors intended to lose weight that the urge to binge and need to purge usually develop.

Body Image

Adolescents who have bulimia nervosa are preoccupied and dissatisfied with their weight and shape. They feel overweight, even fat, although the majority are of normal weight. This key feature leads to behaviors intended to lose weight or avoid weight gain. Dieting, in turn, appears to create the context for an inevitable loss of control of the restriction, resulting in episodes of binge eating.

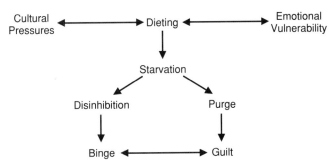

Figure 60–1. Binge-purge regulation model.

ASSOCIATED FEATURES

In addition to the specific eating symptoms, several general psychological symptoms are common. These features, in general, reflect difficulties in the regulation of mood, affect, and impulses that need to be identified before appropriate treatment can occur.

Depression

Patients with bulimia nervosa have significant levels of depression more commonly in their personal and family history than do control subjects. The experience of binge eating and purging may lead to feelings of guilt, remorse, and shame, but depression or dysthymia frequently precedes the onset of the eating disorder, and episodic depression often leads to food binges (see Chapter 100).

Substance Use

Estimates vary regarding the prevalence of substance use in patients who have bulimia nervosa, but there does seem to be an increased risk for addiction. The disease itself is a paradigm of addiction, in which the patient suffers from cravings and engages in addictive behaviors to gratify these cravings only to suffer consequences that cause the cycle to repeat itself. One half of patients with bulimia nervosa have a relative who is alcoholic (see Chapter 111).

Stealing

Some adolescents with bulimia nervosa may engage in shoplifting and stealing that may not be limited to food items. This often impulsive behavior is rare, although a popular conception holds that it is common.

Impulse Control Problems

Patients with bulimia nervosa tend to display difficulties with impulse control, not limited to eating and food, but also involving interpersonal relationships and sexual behavior. A substantial degree of the impulsivity is a response to the bulimia nervosa rather than a preexisting factor. As adolescents who have bulimia nervosa reduce and eliminate their binge eating and purging, they also experience a substantial reduction in their anxiety, depression, and impulsivity. Bulimics may also describe histories of self-destructiveness, including self-mutilation and suicidal behavior.

EVALUATION

History

The initial interview should identify both the specific symptoms of the eating disorder and the adolescent's

TABLE 60–8. Initial Interview

History
Weight history, including highest, lowest, and desired weight
Dieting behavior
Binge eating
Subjective experience of binge and purge
Body image
Scale behavior and exercise
Purging behavior
Personality
Features
Relationship history
Family style and history
Affective disorder
Alcoholism
Eating disorder
Physical/sexual abuse
Cognitive style
General social adaptation
"Willingness" Capacities
To change
To be alone
To have fun
To tolerate anxiety

general psychological functioning. Careful attention should be paid to the most common comorbid psychiatric disorders. The adolescent's motivation for treatment is a crucial feature of the initial presentation. Table 60–8 lists other important areas that should be included in the initial interview.

Standardized Measures

Standardized self-report questionnaires, useful in the initial evaluation and as a means of evaluating treatment progress, are listed in Table 60–9.

Physical Examination

The need for a physical examination, and the process itself, suggests to the adolescent and her or his family that adolescents with this disease may be causing themselves serious bodily injury. During the physical examination, special emphasis should be placed on signs of the consequences of self-induced vomiting. Paramount among these is parotid and submaxillary gland swelling (sialadenosis), which may give a fullness to the face that the adolescent may not realize is self-induced; it is also counter to their desire to appear thin. The knuckles

TABLE 60–9. Standardized Self-report Questionnaires

Eating
Eating Attitudes Test (EAT)
Eating Disorders Inventory (EDI)
Body Shape Questionnaire
General functioning
Beck Depression Inventory
Borderline Syndrome Index
Symptom Check List–90R
Social Adjustment Scale

should be examined for scarring and callus formation, which are caused by forced vomiting (Russell sign). Dentition is at risk for enamel erosion because of acidic stomach contents repeatedly being in contact with the teeth (see Chapter 41). Adolescents with bulimia may have abdominal tenderness or complain of substernal burning. Gastritis, esophagitis, and abdominal pain are frequent findings. Severe vomiting may cause petechiae, especially on the head and face. Subconjunctival hemorrhage is also a manifestation of severe forced vomiting. Chronic constipation and subsequent rectal problems, including rectal prolapse and bleeding, may be present.

As with adolescents with anorexia nervosa, adolescents with bulimia nervosa must be completely undressed when they are examined so that body habitus can be appreciated. The clothed appearance is often deceptively normal. Adolescents with bulimia nervosa may experience marked fluctuations in weight. Menstrual irregularities occur in fewer than one half of patients, and prolonged secondary amenorrhea is unusual (see Chapter 70).

Laboratory Assessment

Recurrent vomiting can cause significant hypokalemic, hypochloremic metabolic alkalosis. Screening laboratory tests should include measurement of serum electrolyte levels, urinalysis, and determination of urine pH. An alkaline urine indicates a significant amount of vomiting; alkaline urine that turns pink when acidified and returns to yellow when alkalized indicates the presence of phenolphthalein, an ingredient in many laxatives abused by adolescents with bulimia nervosa. An elevated serum amylase level indicates significant salivary gland stimulation. A positive result stool guaiac test requires further investigation. Although symptoms of bloating and fullness may be explained by the eating disorder, inflammatory bowel disease can occur as well (see Chapter 63). Thyroid function can be evaluated by determining thyroxine (T_4) and thyroid-stimulating hormone TSH levels. An electrocardiogram (ECG) is indicated as a screening test in the evaluation of the bulimic patient to identify cardiac arrhythmias secondary to hypokalemia or ipecac abuse and also prior to initiating antidepressant medication. Serum emetine levels are positive in patients using ipecac.

DIFFERENTIAL DIAGNOSIS

Anorexia Nervosa versus Bulimia Nervosa

Although these two disorders differ in important ways, many adolescents may present with symptoms of both disorders. As many as one half of patients who have anorexia nervosa develop symptoms of bulimia nervosa. In adolescent patients, mixed and mild symptom pictures are common, and atypical patterns are not unusual (see previous subchapter).

TABLE 60–10. Differences Between Anorexia Nervosa and Bulimia Nervosa

ANOREXIA NERVOSA	BULIMIA NERVOSA
Vomiting or diuretic or laxative abuse uncommon	Vomiting or diuretic or laxative abuse
Severe weight loss	Less weight loss; avoidance of obesity
Slightly younger	Slightly older
More introverted	More extroverted
Hunger denied	Hunger pronounced
Eating behavior may be considered normal and a source of self-esteem	Eating behavior is ego-dystonic
Sexually inactive	Sexually active
Obsessional fears with paranoid features	Histrionic features
Amenorrhea	Menses irregular or absent
Death from starvation/suicide	Death from hypokalemia/ suicide

Table 60–10 presents some of the differences between adolescents who have anorexia nervosa and those with bulimia nervosa. Some adolescents with anorexia nervosa describe episodes of overeating followed by self-induced purging. Others acknowledge that they use purging strictly as a means of weight loss without any episodes of actual overeating. Classically, patients who have bulimia nervosa are not losing weight actively, although they express a wish to do so, and their purging follows clear episodes of binge eating in an effort to avoid weight gain.

Depression

Major affective disorder is the most common psychiatric comorbidity in patients with bulimia nervosa. Although some investigators have argued that bulimia nervosa is actually a variant of affective disorder, the consensus is that these are different disorders sharing many similar features. Patients with bulimia nervosa may report vegetative symptoms of major affective disorder and may describe anhedonia, loss of libido, concentration deficits, and social withdrawal (see Chapter 100).

Personality Disorders

Whereas adolescents with a wide variety of underlying personality disorders can develop bulimia nervosa, only one third of adult patients with bulimia nervosa meet the criteria for the diagnosis of a personality disorder. One should be reluctant to label adolescents with a personality disorder. However, the presence or absence of a comorbid character pathology may affect the patient's response to treatment directed only at the bulimia. Thus, the need for a comprehensive assessment is apparent. Symptom substitution may be averted with such a therapeutic approach (see Chapter 109).

TREATMENT

Psychological Treatment

There are numerous treatment strategies for adolescents who have bulimia nervosa. Although the vast majority of treatment research has employed cognitive-behavioral techniques, the overall findings suggest that any number of different types of treatment can be effective. Many adolescents may improve with relatively short-term intervention, although the majority require ongoing treatment. Most adolescent patients undergo a variety of different treatments over the course of their illness. Treatments such as individual, family, and group psychotherapy may be combined with pharmacologic treatment.

Pharmacologic Treatment

Antidepressant medications, such as imipramine and other tricyclic antidepressants, and newer antidepressants such as fluoxetine (Prozac), although frequently helpful, are not panaceas. The use of antidepressants has been shown to be effective in approximately one third of bulimic patients, as compared with the use of a placebo. After a baseline ECG, a tricyclic antidepressant such as imipramine can be tried at a dose of 3 to 5 mg/kg (up to 300 mg) daily. An increase in dosage should be preceded by an ECG to ensure that the PR interval is not over 0.2 millisecond and the corrected QT interval is not prolonged. The usual procedure is to start with a 50-mg dose at night and increase it weekly by 25 to 50 mg until a clinical response is evident and adequate blood levels are attained. Monoamine oxidase (MAO) inhibitors, such as phenelzine, isocarboxazid (Marplan), or tranylcypromine sulfate (Parnate), can be used (not with tricyclic antidepressants) under the supervision of a psychiatrist. Anticonvulsant medication has been tried in several studies but is of limited use in our experience.

Prevention

It is clear that many adolescents "experiment" with binge eating and purging, although only a minority actually develop the disorder. Educational programs that emphasize acceptance of normal body weight and that outline the risks of binge eating and purging may succeed in preventing adolescents who are experimenting with binging and purging from developing severe disease. Bulimia nervosa in adolescents should be considered a disorder in which only a small proportion of those who demonstrate some symptoms actually meet formal diagnostic criteria for the disorder.

BIBLIOGRAPHY

Casper RC: On the emergence of bulimia nervosa as a syndrome: A historical view. Int J Eating Disorders 2:3, 1983.
Diagnostic and Statistical Manual of Mental Disorders, 3rd ed, revised. Washington, DC, American Psychiatric Association, 1987.
Fairburn CG: Bulimia nervosa. Br Med J 300(6723):485, 1990.
Gull WW: Anorexia nervosa. Trans Clin Soc (London) 7:22, 1874. Reprinted in Kaufman RM, Heiman M (eds): Evolution of Psychosomatic Concepts. Anorexia Nervosa: A Paradigm. New York, International Universities Press, 1964.
Johnson C, Connors ME: The Etiology and Treatment of Bulimia Nervosa: A Biopsychosocial Perspective. New York, Basic Books, 1987.
Russell GFM: Bulimia nervosa: An ominous variant of anorexia nervosa. Psychol Med 9:429, 1979.
Swift WJ, Andrews D, Barklage NE: The relationship between affective disorders and eating disorders: A review of the literature. Am J Psychiatry 143:290, 1986.

OBESITY

MARTHA R. ARDEN

Obesity is defined as excess adiposity, that is, more than 25% of body weight composed of fat in males and more than 30% in females. Measurements of fat rather than weight are more direct determinants of obesity for research, but they have limited usefulness in patient care. Underwater weighing is the "gold standard" for determining the amount of body fat based on density, but it is impractical, as are determinations based on total body potassium content, total body electrical conductivity, and bioelectrical impedance. Near infrared reflectance offers easy noninvasive measurement of body fat but is not widely available. Estimates of fat from measurement of skinfolds at several sites, using inexpensive calipers and published standards, may be used, but the accuracy of this method is dependent on the skill of the examiner (see Chapter 6). A triceps skinfold greater than 18 mm in a male adolescent or 25 mm in a female adolescent is consistent with obesity, but measurements from multiple sites are necessary to accurately assess body composition, since the distribution of fat in the body is not uniform (see Chapter 6). Skinfold determinations are particularly useful in the long-term follow-up of adolescents being treated for obesity, because such measurements can show loss of fat and changes in body composition even when the weight is unchanged, as in the athletic adolescent boy who replaces fat with lean body mass while maintaining a constant weight.

In clinical practice, excessive weight is most commonly used to identify obese adolescents. Appropriate weight is between 90% and 120% of values on standard charts such as those available from the National Center for Health Statistics. More than 120% of average (i.e., more than 20% overweight) corresponds fairly well to the body fat composition definition of obesity. Morbid obesity, which affects fewer than 0.01% of adolescents, is defined as weight more than 100 lb over the normative weight for adolescents over 57 inches tall, or more than 200% of normative weight in those shorter.

For taller and older adolescents, growth charts are not accurate, and normative values can be derived from the Metropolitan Life Insurance Company 1983 Tables, which are indexed by height and frame size. Unfortunately, no well-accepted standards for frame size exist, and individuals are frequently misclassified on the basis of physical appearance.

The body mass index (BMI), defined as the weight (kg) divided by the square of the height (m) [BMI = weight in kg ÷ (height in m)^2], accounts for variations in weight in relation to height and eliminates the need for growth charts (see Chapter 6). It does not accurately reflect obesity at extremes of height in children and adolescents. Percentile values for white adolescents, derived from the First National Health and Nutrition Examination Survey, were published in 1991. The median BMI increases from 18.4 to 22.5 in males and from 18.9 to 21.4 in females from ages 13 to 19 years. The 95th percentile increases from 25.8 to 30.1 in males and 27.9 to 31.3 in females from ages 13 to 19 years. In adults, a BMI exceeding the 85th percentile, which corresponds with 120% of normative values and is associated with increased morbidity and mortality, has been used as a definition of obesity. A similar standard for adolescents has not been determined, however, and the 85th percentile values have not been published.

Obesity can also be defined by the pattern of distribution of fat in the body. The central, or "android," pattern of increased intraabdominal fat, defined by an abdominal-to-gluteal circumference ratio of greater than 0.9 in females and greater than 1.0 in males and resulting in the so-called apple shape, is associated with increased rates of myocardial infarction, stroke, insulin resistance, and mortality. Individuals with a peripheral, or "gynecoid," distribution, with an abdominal-to-gluteal circumference ratio of less than 0.75 in females and less than 0.85 in males, resulting in the so-called pear shape, have a significantly lower risk for these conditions. The pattern of fat distribution does not appear to change when weight is lost.

Obesity can be divided into primary and secondary forms. The former, also called exogenous obesity, is generally due to a combination of too much food and too little exercise. It is, by far, the more common form of obesity in adolescents. Secondary (endogenous) obesity, in contrast, is due to some underlying endocrinologic, genetic, or neurologic cause. The main focus of this chapter is on primary obesity, and unless stated otherwise, the term obesity is used to mean primary obesity.

INCIDENCE

The prevalence of obesity in children and adolescents in the United States is increasing, with the incidence in adolescents estimated at 11% to 19%. More adolescent females than adolescent males are obese; obesity is more common in female adolescents of lower socioeconomic status and in males of higher socioeconomic status. The likelihood of losing weight successfully decreases to less than 5% as the obese individual reaches the end of adolescence.

PATHOPHYSIOLOGY

Obesity is caused by energy intake in excess of energy expenditure. Health care providers must be aware of the various factors contributing to the development and maintenance of excessive body fat so that they can avoid "blaming" the adolescent patient for obesity.

Heredity plays an important role in obesity, but interpretation of human genetic studies is difficult because of strong environmental influences. Approximately 80% of adolescents with obese parents become obese adults, whereas only 14% of adolescents with thin parents become obese. Human studies show good correlation of overweight between parents and their offspring, with the highest correlation occurring during adolescence. An autosomal recessive inheritance of fat distribution patterns has been demonstrated. Studies in Denmark showed a highly significant relationship between the weight of adopted adults and their biologic parents, whereas there was no relationship with the weight of the adoptive parents. Studies of twins also demonstrate the importance of genetic factors, with a much higher correlation of obesity in monozygotic than in dizygotic twins. Studies of BMI of adult identical twins raised separately after birth show intrapair correlation coefficients of .66 to .70, indicating that genetic influences are much more powerful than is the childhood environment in the determination of adult obesity. However, studies suggest the inheritance of a propensity for obesity rather than inheritance of obesity *per se*.

Dietary intake in excess of dietary needs is required for the occurrence of obesity, even when a genetic propensity is present. Increased fat deposition occurs in response to a high-sugar, high-fat diet, which leads to elevated insulin and lipoprotein lipase levels, resulting in storage of fatty acids in adipose tissue. A preference for these foods has been described in obese subjects. The meal pattern also affects energy balance, with the thermic effect of feeding (calories expended during digestion) being higher for several small meals than for one large, isocaloric meal, which is more typically eaten by obese adolescents.

In addition to differences in dietary intake, differences in energy expenditure are found between obese and normal individuals. Food intake may differ by as much as 100% in individuals of the same age, sex, and weight. A reduced basal metabolic rate may be central in the causation of obesity. Although many obese individuals have normal basal metabolic rates, a substantial decrease in metabolic rate has been found in formerly obese adolescents who lose weight, suggesting the presence of a different body weight "set point" that results in a high risk of obesity. One study found the thermic effect of a glucose challenge to be similar in obese and normal-weight adolescent boys, but it was significantly lower after weight loss in the obese group.

Dysfunctional feedback due to abnormal sensory, gastrointestinal, nutrient, or hormonal signals may lead to disrupted nutrient balance and subsequent obesity. This is especially likely in secondary obesity as occurs following encephalitis and other trauma to the hypothalamus. This was thought to be due to damage to a "satiety center," but recent research indicates that the obesity is due to hyperinsulinemia caused by altered autonomic tone leading to stimulation of the vagus nerve. The hyperinsulinemia, in turn, results in hyperphagia and increased lipogenesis. Obesity caused by hypothalamic lesions is eliminated by transection of the vagus nerve or by ablation of the pancreatic beta cells, supporting their key roles in hypothalamic obesity. Elevated insulin levels, which result in deposition of fat, may be the cause of, rather than the result of, obesity. Endogenous opioids, which increase insulin response to meals, may be involved in this pathway. Abnormal sensations of satiety have not been demonstrated in primary obesity, but other hormonal and neural mechanisms do exist.

The fat cell theory, which purports that obesity is due to fat cell hyperplasia in the presence of overfeeding, is not supported by data. Although increases in fat cell number have been documented in infancy and early puberty, it is unclear that obesity results from this hyperplasia.

Psychological factors are important in obesity, but it is difficult to distinguish the causes and effects of obesity in clinical studies. There is no good evidence for the presence of an "obese personality," and there is also no support for theories that cite dependence, lack of impulse control, and inability to delay gratification as causes of obesity. Studies have shown that arousability in response to food cues may be abnormal in obese individuals.

Physical inactivity is associated with high rates of obesity in adolescents with handicaps that restrict their movement, such as meningomyelocele and muscular dystrophy. A direct relationship between overweight and television viewing has been found in otherwise healthy adolescents. In addition to increasing caloric expenditure during and shortly after the activity, exercise increases a muscle's ability to oxidize fatty acids, resulting in decreased fat deposition.

CLINICAL MANIFESTATIONS

In general, there are few clinical manifestations of obesity, other than increased body size with increases in the lean body mass as well as in the adipose tissue. Moderately obese adolescents have an early prepubertal increase in androgens, with advanced linear growth, bone age, and sexual maturation related to the increased lean body mass. Short stature and delayed puberty are unusual and suggest endocrinologic abnormalities causing secondary obesity. There is an increased incidence of hypertension with obesity in the adolescent age group, but spurious hypertension may be due to use of an inappropriately small blood pressure cuff. Physical problems found in more obese adolescents include an increased incidence of pseudogynecomastia and skin problems, including intertriginous candidal infections and irritations from bra straps and other clothing.

Laboratory abnormalities possible in primary obesity include hypercholesterolemia, hypertriglyceridemia, insulin resistance with functional hyperinsulinism, impaired growth hormone release, impaired prolactin release, poor response to thyroid-stimulating hormone with elevated triiodothyronine (T_3), and elevations of cortisol and estrogen levels, with decreased testicular androgens.

DIAGNOSIS

The medical evaluation of the obese adolescent patient is done in order to determine whether any medical problems causing secondary obesity or complications of obesity are present and to recommend a treatment program. This evaluation (Table 60–11) should include a detailed history and physical examination, but extensive laboratory studies are not indicated unless warranted by the results of the examination. An estimation of the basal metabolic rate, which can be done in many hospitals using indirect calorimetry to measure carbon dioxide (CO_2) production and oxygen (O_2) utilization, may be useful in determining an appropriate dietary prescription or in evaluating the obese adolescent who reportedly "doesn't eat a thing."

DIFFERENTIAL DIAGNOSIS

Most overweight adolescents presenting to the physician have primary obesity, but other causes of increased

TABLE 60–11. Evaluation of the Obese Adolescent Patient

HISTORY
Family History: obesity and stature, endocrine problems, psychiatric problems
Past Medical History: serious illnesses, surgery, menstrual history
History of Obesity: abrupt onset vs. chronic history, physical problems or development at time of rapid weight gain, etc.
Dietary History: 24-hour diet recall, review of eating habits including timing and circumstances surrounding mealtimes and snacks, history of previous weight-loss attempts
Social History: family, school, and individual stressors, especially at times of rapid weight gain

PHYSICAL EXAMINATION
Anthropometrics: height, weight, triceps skinfolds
Sexual maturity rating
Vital signs, including blood pressure taken with appropriate-size cuff
Complete physical examination for causes of secondary obesity and complications of obesity

LABORATORY TESTS
Routine screening with cholesterol and triglyceride levels
Endocrine studies *only* if suggested by history or physical examination
Estimate of basal metabolic rate may be helpful

body size or weight and secondary obesity must be ruled out (Fig. 60–2). Many adolescents and their parents consult physicians in the hope that a "physical," easily correctable cause of obesity will be found. The process of determining whether further evaluation is needed is summarized in the algorithm in Figure 60–2. In general, however, if an adolescent appears healthy and his or her growth and sexual development are not delayed, there is little chance of detecting an underlying problem.

In the clinical evaluation of obesity in adolescents, the height curve is often more valuable than the weight curve. Primary obesity is uniformly associated with normal or accelerated growth in stature. Obesity due to an underlying endocrinologic, genetic, or neurologic defect is generally associated with retarded growth in height.

Causes of increased body weight other than obesity include edema, ascites, and intraabdominal masses re-sulting from renal, liver, or neoplastic disease. These conditions are usually easily distinguished from obesity by the clinician. A pregnancy, however, may be missed in the adolescent who denies sexual activity unless a careful examination and human chorionic gonadotropin test are done (see Chapters 69 and 74). Increased muscle mass in athletes may be mistaken for obesity when the weight and height are evaluated, but visual inspection of the adolescent usually quickly reveals that obesity is not present.

A number of genetic syndromes, including Prader-Willi syndrome, Laurence-Moon-Biedl syndrome, Cohen syndrome, and others, are associated with obesity (see Chapter 31). Although most are diagnosed before adolescence, Turner syndrome may present at adolescence with mild obesity, short stature, and delayed puberty (see Chapter 55). Other genetic syndromes and storage diseases that may present with obesity and

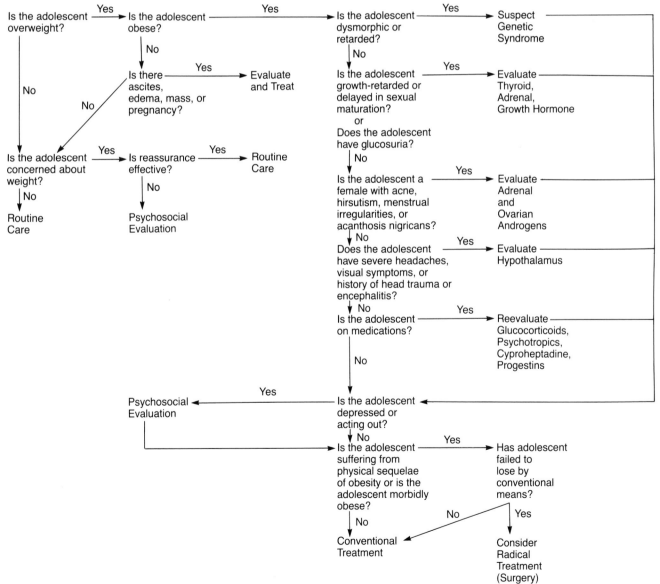

Figure 60–2. Algorithm for differential diagnosis for evaluation of the obese adolescent.

dysmorphic features or developmental delay are described in standard medical genetics textbooks.

Endocrine dysfunction can cause obesity. Hypothyroidism is frequently suspected by parents of obese adolescents, especially when depression or sluggishness is present. Although uncommon, this diagnosis should be suspected in the obese adolescent with growth failure, delayed sexual development, menstrual irregularities, or classic signs of hypothyroidism (see Chapter 55).

Cushing syndrome, caused by excess glucocorticoids, leads to mild to moderate central obesity. Classically, a "buffalo hump" and "moon face" are seen, but striae, hypertension, glucosuria, or short stature may be the only presenting signs (see Chapter 55).

Adolescents who are deficient in growth hormone may present with obesity and height below the third percentile. Insulin excess, due to insulinoma or beta-cell hyperplasia, and pseudohypoparathyroidism are rare causes of obesity that, unlike other endocrine causes of obesity, do not result in growth failure.

Hyperandrogenism may lead to mild to moderate obesity in females. Partial (late-onset or nonclassic) congenital adrenal hyperplasia is a common cause of adrenal hyperandrogenism in females in some ethnic groups, including Hispanics, Italians, Yugoslavs, and Ashkenazic Jews. Hirsutism, acne, menstrual irregularities, and obesity with short stature may be seen, and onset during puberty is common (see Chapter 55). The polycystic ovary syndrome is also associated with hyperandrogenism and obesity, but not all patients present with the classic triad of obesity, menstrual irregularity, and hirsutism. Twenty percent of these patients have normal menses, and 69% have hirsutism (see Chapter 70). The HAIR-AN syndrome of hyperandrogenism, insulin resistance, and acanthosis nigricans (Kahn syndrome) is caused by ovarian overproduction of androgens as the result of stimulation by insulin. Androgen-producing ovarian or adrenal tumors may also be associated with obesity.

Lesions of the ventromedial hypothalamus may cause obesity. These lesions may occur with encephalitis, tumors, or trauma and may present with hyperphagia and rapid weight gain or severe headaches and visual symptoms.

A number of medications may cause obesity. High dose glucocorticoids cause cushingoid obesity, but more subtle, insidious weight gain may occur in adolescents taking steroids for asthma. Obesity may even occur with steroid inhalers or potent topical glucocorticoids. Psychotropic medications, including amitriptyline (Elavil) and phenothiazines, may lead to weight gain. It is particularly important not to attribute weight gain in depressed adolescents to their affective disorder, when medication-induced hyperphagia may be the cause.

TREATMENT (Table 60–12)
(see Chapter 49)

The prevention of obesity in childhood is preferable to its treatment during adolescence, but the data indicate

TABLE 60–12. Treatment of Obesity

Low-Calorie Diet Alone: 1200–1500 kcal/day, with or without exercise
    Balanced caloric reduction (smaller portions)
    Low-fat diets from books (American Heart Association, etc.)
    Calorie or exchange lists from physician
    Commercial programs: Diet Center
    Commercial programs that provide prepackaged meals and no counseling
Exercise Alone: rarely effective, since food intake is often increased and amount of exercise is usually insufficient
Psychiatric
    Behavior modification: TOPs (Teenage Obesity Programs)
    Self-help: Overeaters Anonymous, TOPS (Take Off Pounds Sensibly)
    Individual therapy to deal with feelings about weight
Low-Calorie Diet with Behavior Modification Programs
    Physician supervised: Shapedown
    Commercial: Nutri/System, Weight Watchers, Slender Center
Fad Diets: *these diets provide insufficient nutrients or are nutritionally imbalanced*
Medications: rarely indicated in adolescents
Surgery: morbid obesity only
    Restrictive procedures: gastroplasty
    Malabsorptive Procedures: jejunoileostomy, biliointestinal or duodenoileal bypass
    Vagotomy
    Jaw wiring
    Liposuction

that this is extremely difficult in children of obese parents. One study of the "prudent diet" in infancy did demonstrate significantly lower rates of obesity at age 3 years when compared with historical controls, but much more extensive study of the effects of such a diet must be completed before broad recommendations can be made. The clinician should always examine for the presence of developing obesity during health maintenance visits, providing anticipatory guidance about proper eating and exercise habits (see Chapter 25). In healthy children with obese parents, recommendations for a low-fat diet should be made. Obesity often develops when normal-weight children go through puberty. Such children should receive nutritional education advice about exercise and information on fitness routinely.

The physician and the adolescent must be aware of the difficulty inherent in the treatment of obesity. Therapy can be quite difficult in younger (particularly male) adolescents who are not yet concerned with their appearance. Although weight reduction is more successful in adolescents who are strongly motivated, the success rate of most weight loss plans is poor, and the prognosis for maintenance of reduced weight is even worse.

The most successful attempts at weight loss incorporate parental involvement in a supervised dieting program with nutritional instruction, behavioral modification, social support, and exercise. When a small amount of weight loss is desired, however, simple nutritional education by the physician and advice to exercise may suffice. A low-fat, increased complex carbohydrate diet of 1200 to 1500 kcal/day is more likely to result in long-term weight reduction than a balanced reduction in intake of all food groups.

An aerobic exercise program in conjunction with dieting increases the efficiency of weight loss by reversing the body's reduction of resting energy expenditure that occurs with decreased caloric intake. In addition, exercise to approximately 60% of maximum aerobic capacity results in a prolongation of the postexercise calorie expenditure. Although many obese adolescent boys hope to lose weight by increasing their activity without decreasing food intake, in most cases this method is inadequate to result in significant weight loss.

Psychiatric treatment without diet and activity modification may be beneficial in mildly obese adolescents who are not strongly motivated to lose weight but who need to cope with peer or parental pressure to be thin, or in those whose obesity seems to be strongly related to maladaptive eating habits. Weekly meetings of the Young People's Group of the twelve-step Overeaters Anonymous program may be helpful for older adolescents in need of peer support.

When more weight loss is desired, the physician who is asked for a "diet" should respond with more than a printed calorie or exchange list. Instead, extended dietary, exercise, and behavioral counseling, or a referral to a professional weight reduction program, should be provided. There is currently no regulation of professional weight control programs, but the International Congress on Obesity recommended the following three features: a nutritious and practical diet; safe, regular physical activity; and behavior modification with emotional support. Rather than focusing merely on weight loss, it is preferable to emphasize the improved fitness and sense of well-being that can result from such a program. For example, obese adolescents who have a family history of heart disease could be provided a program such as the one described in Chapter 49.

Behavior modification plans should include specific weight and behavioral goals, emphasizing stimulus control, self-monitoring, cognitive changes, positive reinforcement, and social support. A well-studied adolescent weight-loss program specifically geared to adolescents is Shapedown, a medically supervised diet and behavior program that emphasizes lifestyle changes. The Weight Watchers program may also be suitable for adolescents, but the physician must ensure that the weight goal chosen is suitable for a growing adolescent. Programs such as Nutri/System that provide prepackaged meals are expensive and usually impractical for adolescents who attend school.

Adolescents who are eager to lose weight quickly are often interested in very low calorie diets (VLCD). In a 1989 position statement, the American Dietetic Association cautioned that such diets are *not* appropriate for adolescents. These diets provide 400 to 800 calories of high-quality protein per day, often in the form of a liquid formula. The cardiac dysrhythmias associated with the liquid protein diets popular in the 1970s are not associated with the present formulations. These programs are associated with high dropout rates, however, and high rates of regained weight among those who do complete the program, especially among those who do not have concurrent behavior therapy. Optifast, the largest medically supervised very low calorie diet program, does not accept adolescent patients until they have completed their growth.

Over-the-counter very low calorie diets, such as the Cambridge diet, however, can be purchased and used by adolescents without supervision. In addition, products such as Slim-Fast, which is intended to be used as a supplement rather than a replacement for all food, can be misused by adolescents seeking rapid weight loss. This practice is clearly dangerous for growing adolescents and must be discouraged whenever dieting is discussed.

Fad diets are appealing to adolescents who want quick, easy weight loss, and they should be discussed with all obese adolescents. They are not recommended in adolescents. The very low carbohydrate diets, such as Dr. Atkins' Diet Revolution, Dr. Stillman's Quick Weight Loss Diet, the Scarsdale Diet, and the Woman Doctor's Diet, result in diuresis with rapid weight loss that is difficult to maintain and can lead to dangerous ketosis. The high-carbohydrate diets, such as Dr. Stillman's Quick Inches Off Diet, the Pritikin Diet, and the rice diet, also encourage a nutritionally imbalanced diet that is very difficult to maintain for long periods of time. Other fad diets, such as the grapefruit diet, the Beverly Hills Diet, and the Rotation Diet (first phase), are *not* recommended.

The pharmacologic treatment of obesity is rarely indicated in adolescents, but active research is under way, and safe and effective pharmaceutical approaches to the treatment of obesity may soon be available. The most commonly used medications act centrally to suppress appetite via the catecholamine and serotonin systems. The central nervous system drugs include the amphetamines, fenfluramine (Pondimin), and diethylpropion (Tenuate). Phenylpropanolamine, which is the main ingredient of most over-the-counter appetite suppressants, is probably safe and effective for short-term use, but weight loss will not be maintained unless there is additional behavioral and nutritional treatment.

Thermogenic medications may lead to weight loss by increasing the metabolic rate, but cannot be recommended for use at this time. β-Agonists, such as isoproterenol, have been shown to increase energy expenditure in animal studies and preliminary human studies. In addition, local lipid mobilization from adipose tissue has been demonstrated in obese and lean pigs infused with isoproterenol, suggesting that nonsurgical treatment of obesity in specific areas of the body may be available in the future. Thyroid hormone is not effective in the euthyroid patient, and its use is contraindicated in primary obesity.

Several obesity treatments that affect the gastrointestinal tract are available over the counter and, thus, are frequently tried by adolescents. Candy diet aids containing benzocaine, which numbs the mouth when taken before meals, are widely available, but their effectiveness has not been well studied. Fiber wafers may lead to satiety and decreased intake of high calorie foods, but gastrointestinal distress may occur. "Starch blockers," advertised as a solution to obesity that allows individuals to eat all they desire without weight gain, do not effectively block starch digestion and also may result in significant gastrointestinal distress. Sucrose polyester (Olestra), a synthetic indigestible fat awaiting approval by the Food and Drug Administration for use in food preparation, may significantly decrease caloric intake from fat. Another fat replacement, Simplesse, is available commercially in frozen desserts and other prepared foods. Gastrointestinal medications that seem promising in early studies include tetrahydrolipostatin, a pancreatic lipase inhibitor, and threo-chlorocitric acid, which slows gastric emptying and increases satiety.

Surgical treatment of obesity is reserved for the morbidly obese who are suffering from serious complications of obesity and is thus rarely used in adolescents. Quality of life, however, may be improved, and complications of obesity such as hypertension and sleep disturbances may be reversed. The procedures include restrictive procedures such as gastroplasty ("stomach stapling"), which physically restrict the intake of solid food, and malabsorptive procedures such as jejunoileostomy and biliointestinal or duodenioleal bypass. Combined procedures, with formation of a small gastric pouch and bypass of small bowel, have also been used. The complications of such procedures remain a major problem, with almost half of gastroplasty patients requiring reoperation after 2 to 5 years. The malabsorptive procedures may lead to serious diarrhea, arthritis, nephrolithiasis, cholelithiasis, cirrhosis, and electrolyte imbalances, with 25% of patients incapacitated at long-term follow-up. Despite these drawbacks, surgery may be the only alternative in selected adolescents.

Less frequently used surgical procedures for obesity include vagotomy, which results in slowed gastric emptying and is most effective in conjunction with gastroplasty. Jaw wiring has also been used as a temporary means of decreasing intake of solid foods, but behavior treatment is needed for maintenance of the weight reduction after the wires are removed. Suction lipectomy (liposuction) is a cosmetic procedure that has been used successfully in the treatment of gynecomastia in adolescents. Infection and aesthetic problems such as dimpling are the most common complications, but major complications such as fat embolization, viscus perforation, and shock occur rarely as surgeons become more experienced with the procedure.

COMPLICATIONS AND PROGNOSIS

Complications of adolescent obesity occur during adolescence and adulthood (Table 60–13). Psychosocial complications, including body image disturbance and poor peer relations, contribute to difficulties in achieving normal adolescent development and may lead to low self-esteem. Increased rates of depression have also been found in obese adolescents, with Beck depression inven-

TABLE 60–13. Complications of Obesity

DURING ADOLESCENCE
Psychosocial
  Disturbed body image
  Poor self-image/self-esteem
  Poor family relations: scapegoat and source of embarrassment
  Poor peer relations and social isolation
  Exclusion from activities, especially dating
  Acting out and depression
Medical
  Potentially lethal:
    Obstructive sleep apnea, pickwickian syndrome
    Pancreatitis
    Heart failure from cardiomyopathy
  Less severe:
    Orthopedic: slipped capital femoral epiphysis, coxa vara, Perthes disease, ankle fracture, genu valgum
    Metabolic: gallstones, hypercholesterolemia
    Skin problems: candidal infections, breakdown
    Pseudogynecomastia
    Neurologic: pseudotumor cerebri
  Increased risk of adult obesity
DURING ADULTHOOD
Psychosocial
  Job discrimination
  Others as during adolescence
Medical
  Cardiovascular disease: hypertension, hypercholesterolemia, diabetes mellitus, coronary artery disease, cerebrovascular disease (increased with "android" fat distribution)
  Cancer: endometrial, breast, prostate, colon
  Orthopedic: gouty and degenerative arthritis
  Genitourinary incontinence, male sexual dysfunction
  Surgical: Increased operative morbidity and mortality

tory scores positively correlating with BMI (the higher the weight, the greater the depression). Acting out behavior or isolation may occur.

Medical complications of adolescent obesity include rare, potentially lethal obstructive sleep apnea and pickwickian syndrome, pancreatitis, and heart failure due to cardiomyopathy. Obese adolescents face increased risk of orthopedic problems, including slipped capital femoral epiphysis, coxa vara, Perthes disease, ankle fracture, and genu valgum (see Chapter 79). Exercise intolerance and gallstones are found in obese adolescents and adults, and increased gallbladder volume has been found in obese adolescents without stones. Pseudogynecomastia (breast enlargement due to fat rather than glandular hypertrophy) and skin problems may also be seen. Abnormal cholesterol levels are also more common in obese adolescents, with an increase in BMI being the only factor found to be a significant determinant of increased total cholesterol and decreased high-density lipoprotein cholesterol levels in young men.

The most frequent complication of adolescent obesity, however, is the increased risk of adult obesity. At least 75% of obese adolescents become obese adults. At least 95% of individuals who are obese at the end of adolescence remain obese as adults.

The long-term effects of obesity in adulthood are numerous. Mortality from a number of causes is increased among obese adults. Obesity results in increased rates of hypertension, hypercholesterolemia, and diabetes mellitus, all of which are risk factors for cardiovascular disease that respond to weight loss. The risk of coronary heart disease was found to be positively correlated with the BMI at the age of 18 years in the Nurses' Health Study. Excessive rates of endometrial, breast, prostate, and colon cancer are found in obese individuals. Other complications include pseudotumor cerebri, urinary incontinence, gouty and degenerative arthritis, and dyspnea. Obese men may have increased rates of sexual dysfunction. In addition, complications of surgery, including mortality and pulmonary embolism, are increased among obese individuals.

The other significant complications of obesity are those resulting from its treatment. Low-calorie diets lead to weight loss from both fat and lean compartments. If an individual regains the weight lost, the added weight is usually in the form of fat. As a result, the adolescent patient who repetitively diets and regains weight gradually increases the proportion of body fat and decreases the lean body mass. In turn, the decreased lean body mass leads to a decreased basal metabolic rate. Individuals on very low calorie diets, fasts, and some nutritionally imbalanced diets also risk the possibility of electrolyte imbalances, ketosis, and acidosis. The psychological complications of dietary restriction include feelings of deprivation and mood changes. It has also been suggested that dieting behavior may contribute to the development of anorexia nervosa and bulimia nervosa in adolescents.

The prognosis for the obese adolescent is not good. Even if weight loss is achieved, the maintenance of a lower body weight is extremely difficult. The resting metabolic rate of formerly obese patients is significantly lower than that of individuals of the same weight who were never obese, meaning that lifelong restriction of food intake is required to maintain the lowered weight. In addition, levels of lipoprotein lipase, an enzyme that hydrolyzes triglycerides to form the free fatty acids that are incorporated into adipocytes, increase in relation to the amount of weight lost and possibly enhance lipid storage. If weight loss is not achieved, however, the adolescent faces adulthood with the medical and psychosocial implications of obesity. Because of this, every effort should be made by the practitioner to provide individualized advice, treatment, and referrals to all adolescents who are motivated to lose weight.

BIBLIOGRAPHY

Allon N: The stigma of overweight in everyday life. In Bray GA (ed): Obesity in Perspective, Part 2. New York, Harper & Row, 1975, pp 83–102.
Berland T: Consumer Guide: Rating the Diets. New York, Signet, 1983.
Bouchard C, Tremblay A, Despres J-P, et al: The response to long-term overfeeding in identical twins. N Engl J Med 332(21):1477, 1990.
Bray GA (ed): Obesity: Basic aspects and clinical applications. Med Clin North Am 73(1):1, 1989. (Entire volume provides excellent detailed summary of current research.)
Dietz WH: Prevention of childhood obesity. Pediatr Clin North Am 33:823, 1986.
Gortmaker SL, Dietz WH, Sobol AM, Wehler CA: Increasing pediatric obesity in the U.S. Am J Dis Child 141:535, 1987.
Hammer LD, Kraemer HC, Wilson DM, et al: Standardized percentile curves of body-mass index for children and adolescents. Am J Dis Child 145:259, 1991.
Hammer SL, Campbell MM, Campbell VA, et al: An interdisciplinary study of adolescent obesity. J Pediatr 80:373, 1972.
Lohman TG, Roche AF, Martorell R (eds): Anthropometric Standardization Reference Manual. Champaign, IL, Human Kinetics Books, 1988.
Metropolitan Life Insurance Company: Metropolitan height and weight tables. Stat Bull Metrop Insur Co 64:1, 1983.
Rock CL, Coulston AM: Weight-control approaches: A review by the California Dietetic Association. J Am Diet Assoc 88:44, 1988.
Stunkard AJ, Harris JR, Pedersen NL, McClearn GE: The body-mass index of twins who have been reared apart. N Engl J Med 322(21):1483, 1990.
Weinsier RL, Wadden TA, Ritenbaugh C, et al: Recommended therapeutic guidelines for professional weight control programs. Am J Clin Nutr 40:865, 1984.

HYPERLIPIDEMIA

MARC S. JACOBSON

The derangements of lipid and lipoprotein metabolism are of interest primarily because of their role as risk factors for premature cardiovascular disease. A major public and professional education program, The National Cholesterol Education Program, has resulted in rapidly increasing awareness of the problem and of the need for screening and prevention. This subchapter focuses on screening and treatment of the adolescent for hyperlipidemia. Refer to Chapter 49 for a discussion of cardiovascular risk factors in greater detail.

DEFINITION OF TERMS

Normal Values. Normative data on levels of serum cholesterol, triglycerides, and the lipoprotein subfractions of adolescents in the United States are summarized in Table 49–3. Those below the 75th percentile may be considered desirable or "normal." For total and low-density lipoprotein (LDL) cholesterol, values above the 75th percentile are considered high risk, but risk is actually continuous and gradually rises with rising levels.

Hyperlipidemia. Hyperlipidemia (Dyslipoproteinemia) refers to abnormal circulating levels of lipids (cholesterol and triglycerides), lipoproteins (chylomicrons, very low-density lipoprotein [VLDL] cholesterol, LDL cholesterol, and high-density lipoprotein [HDL] cholesterol), or apoproteins (A-I, A-II, B, C-II, E). These result from underlying genetic abnormalities, from secondary causes such as disease states or drugs, or in response to diet (see Chapter 49).

Atherosclerosis and Arteriosclerosis. These terms refer to the multifactorial pathologic process occurring in the intima and media of arteries that results in luminal narrowing, ischemia, fibrosis, and calcification either with or without thrombosis. The term *atherosclerosis* emphasizes the lipid nature of the problem, whereas arteriosclerosis is a general term for any cause of pathologic arterial plaque formation. In clinical practice, the terms are interchangeable. Both processes result in symptomatic disease when they advance to a state of luminal narrowing of greater than 60%, the particular manifestation being dependent on the site of narrowing.

Phenotype. The classic phenotypic classification of hyperlipidemia (types I to V) is based on the electrophoretic mobility of serum lipoprotein particles described by Fredrickson and colleagues (Table 60–14). It remains a useful scheme for diagnosis despite its limitations of mixing disorders of varying causes and the exclusion of the HDL cholesterol level. Adolescents may commonly present with type IIa or IIb, type IV, or more rarely type III hyperlipidemia. Types I and V are very rare and generally present in childhood. Pancreatitis occurs when the triglycerides are persistently above 500 mg/dl, as seen in types I and V. Atherosclerosis risk is increased when elevations in serum total cholesterol, LDL cholesterol, or triglycerides are found and when levels of HDL cholesterol are depressed, as in types IIa and IIb and in type IV.

PATHOPHYSIOLOGY
(see Chapter 49)

Molecular Basis of Hypercholesterolemia Syndromes

FAMILIAL HYPERCHOLESTEROLEMIA

Familial hypercholesterolemia (FH) (Types IIa and IIb) is caused by a genetic defect in LDL receptor activity. Homozygotes for this condition (incidence of 1 in 1,000,000) have total cholesterol and LDL cholesterol levels in the 700 mg/dl range (e.g., 500 to 1000 mg/dl). As adolescents they demonstrate the onset of angina pectoris and cutaneous xanthomas. The heterozygous form has an incidence of 1 in 500 in the general population and 1 in 100 in subgroups such as French Canadians. Heterozygotes have total cholesterol levels in the 250 to 400 mg/dl range and LDL cholesterol levels in the 160 to 300 mg/dl range. Xanthomas are rarely seen in adolescence, and cardiovascular disease is delayed

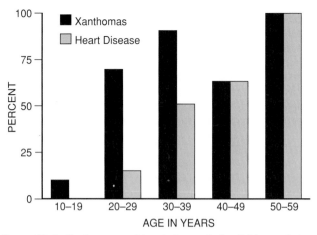

Figure 60–3. Xanthomas and heart disease in familial hypercholesterolemia heterozygotes. (Adapted from Kwiterovich PO Jr: Pediatric implications of heterozygous familial hypercholesterolemia. Screening and dietary treatment. Arteriosclerosis 9:I111, 1989, by permission of the American Heart Association, Inc.)

until the fourth and fifth decades of life in heterozygotes (Fig. 60–3). This defect accounts for up to 5% of the early adult cardiovascular disease in the United States and has served as a model for our understanding of the relationship of LDL cholesterol level to cardiovascular risk.

FAMILIAL COMBINED HYPERLIPIDEMIA

Familial combined hyperlipidemia (FCH) (Types IIa, IIb, IV, and V) is an autosomal dominant disorder that until recently was not diagnosed frequently in the adolescent age group. It results from either or both overproduction and decreased catabolism of VLDL particles. Therefore, it may present with elevated plasma cholesterol or triglycerides, or both, depending on whether the adolescent is obese or ingesting excessive amounts of ethanol, fat, or carbohydrate. FCH may be the most common dyslipoproteinemia in adolescents and probably accounts for as much as 15% of the early cardiovascular disease in adults.

MIXED ENVIRONMENTAL GENETIC HYPERLIPIDEMIA

Mixed environmental genetic hyperlipidemia is a general term for moderate lipid elevations seen in some adolescents on high-fat, high-cholesterol diets. Its mechanisms are less well understood than those of FH and FCH, but there is evidence from animal studies that dietary saturated fat and cholesterol suppress the hepatic LDL receptor in genetically susceptible individuals. This condition is exacerbated by overproduction of VLDL that may be seen in those with excessive caloric or alcohol intake or with sedentary lifestyles. Atherosclerosis risk in this condition is proportional to the elevation in LDL cholesterol level.

TABLE 60–14. Classification of Lipid Disorders

PHENOTYPE	DISORDERS	INHERITANCE	PLASMA APPEARANCE	CHOLESTEROL	TRIGLYCERIDES	ELEVATED LIPOPROTEIN	POPULATION FREQUENCY
I	Exogenous hypertriglyceridemia	Autosomal recessive	Milky	normal to +	+++	Chylomicrons	Very rare
IIa	Familial hypercholesterolemia	Autosomal dominant	Clear	+++	normal	LDL	0.1–0.2%
	Familial combined hyperlipidemia	Autosomal dominant					0.3–0.5%
	Polygenic hypercholesterolemia	Polygenic					?
IIb	Familial hypercholesterolemia	Autosomal dominant	Turbid	+++	+	LDL, VLDL	0.1–0.2%
	Familial combined hyperlipidemia	Autosomal dominant					0.3–0.5%
	Polygenic hypercholesterolemia	Polygenic					?
III	Broad-beta disease (dysbetalipoproteinemia)	Autosomal dominant	Turbid	++	+	Betalipoprotein (SG <1.006)	Rare
IV	Familial hypertriglyceridemia	Autosomal dominant	Turbid	normal to +	++	VLDL	Very rare
	Familial combined hyperlipidemia	Autosomal dominant					0.3–0.5%
	Sporadic hypertriglyceridemia	Not genetic					?
	Broad-beta disease	Autosomal dominant					Rare
V	Familial hypertriglyceridemia	Autosomal dominant	Turbid or milky	normal to +	++	Chylomicrons and VLDL	Very rare
	Familial combined hyperlipidemia	Autosomal dominant					0.3–0.5%
	Sporadic hypertriglyceridemia	Not genetic					?
	Broad-beta disease	Autosomal dominant					Rare

555

Hypertriglyceridemia

In type IV hyperlipidemia, triglyceride levels are elevated in response to diets high in fat and simple carbohydrates. This condition is less common in adolescents than in adults. It is generally seen in conjunction with type II diabetes mellitus. Atherosclerotic risk is moderately elevated.

CLINICAL COURSE

The best single predictor ($r = 0.5$) of adult cholesterol levels in the study of Lauer and colleagues was the cholesterol level in late childhood and early adolescence. The Bogalusa Heart Study also found that cholesterol percentiles track similarly to height and weight percentiles through childhood and adolescence. Therefore, hyperlipidemia discovered in adolescence tends to persist into adulthood if untreated. Since healthy diet habits established early in life may persist, there is a strong argument for screening and treating hyperlipidemia as early as possible (see Chapter 49).

Screening (see Chapters 25 and 49)

It is clear from pathologic data that atherosclerotic lesion formation begins in susceptible populations in childhood and accelerates in adolescence. Newman and colleagues showed that adult risk factors for cardiovascular disease were also associated with lesion formation in adolescents. Preliminary data from a multicenter autopsy series indicate that hyperlipidemia and cigarette smoking are strongly associated with early onset lesions (see Chapter 49). The prevalence of risk factors for atherosclerosis in adolescents is similar to that seen in adults.

Routine screening of all adolescents for cholesterol remains controversial. In general, screening, in the context of well adolescent care (see Chapter 25), is recommended for adolescents who have a family history of premature cardiovascular disease (a parent or grandparent who has had atherosclerosis or suffered a heart attack before 55 years old) or one parent with a high blood cholesterol level (>240 mg/dl). There are also groups of adolescents, as noted in Chapter 49, who have other risk factors for cardiovascular disease: those who have high blood pressure, smoke cigarettes, or eat excessive amounts of foods with fat, cholesterol, and saturated fatty acids. Their screening would be determined by their physicians.

For screening, the adolescent should be afebrile, on his or her usual diet, and taking no medications that affect lipid metabolism (Fig. 60–4). The adolescent should be seated and relaxed for at least 2 minutes before the venipuncture or fingerstick. A total cholesterol level greater than 170 mg/dl on two occasions should be followed by a fasting lipid profile consisting of total cholesterol, triglyceride, and HDL cholesterol. If triglyceride level is less than 400 mg/dl, then the LDL cholesterol level can be estimated using the formula: LDL Cholesterol = Total Cholesterol − HDL Cholesterol − (Triglyceride/5). If the triglyceride or LDL cholesterol level is elevated or the HDL cholesterol level is low (see Table 60–14), a diagnosis of dyslipoproteinemia is made.

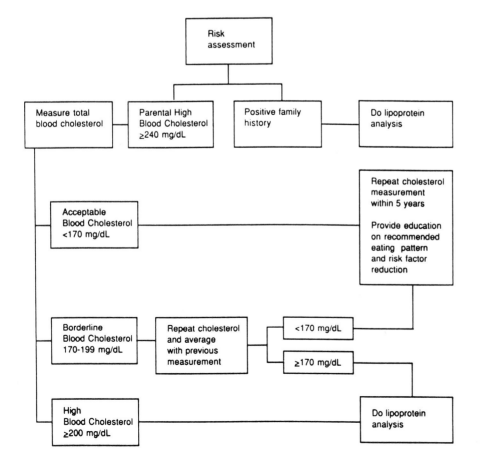

Figure 60–4. Risk assessment. (With permission from NCEP Expert Panel on Blood Cholesterol Levels in Children and Adolescents: National Cholesterol Education Program [NCEP]: Highlights of the Report of the Expert Panel on Blood Cholesterol Levels in Children and Adolescents. Pediatrics 89[3]:497, 1992.)

CLINICAL MANIFESTATIONS

Familial combined hyperlipidemia and mixed environmental genetic hyperlipidemia present with a positive family history of premature cardiovascular disease or hyperlipidemia. Homozygotes for familial hypercholesterolemia are severely affected and manifest disease at an early age. Skin findings are usually seen first, with tendinous xanthomas occurring in the first decade of life (Fig. 60–5). Planar (flat) and tuberous xanthomas of the extensor surfaces of the hands, elbows, and knees; xanthelasma (protuberances on the eyelids); and arcus corneae (a fine white line just inside the iris border of the eye) also appear in the first or second decade of life. Premature coronary artery disease occurs in all homozygotes, with angina reported in about half of such patients by 16 years of age. Other hyperlipidemic patients are asymptomatic as adolescents and present clinically only when screened by family history or blood cholesterol testing

Familial (primary) hypertriglyceridemia type I or V is associated with frequent episodes of acute pancreatitis. Acute abdominal pain in an adolescent may be the first manifestation, but generally these genetic disorders are found at earlier ages when lipemic serum interferes with routine laboratory tests. Triglyceride levels in the 500 to 1000 mg/dl range can result in acute pancreatitis. Strict reduction of dietary fat to 15% of calories is necessary to control these levels and prevent pancreatitis. Conversely, excessive, chronic alcohol intake may lead to pancreatitis, which, in turn, leads to a secondary hypertriglyceridemia. The incidence of hyperlipidemia in patients with acute pancreatitis ranges from 12% to 38%.

DIAGNOSIS

The history should include a family history of cardiovascular disease, xanthomas, xanthelasmas, arcus cor-

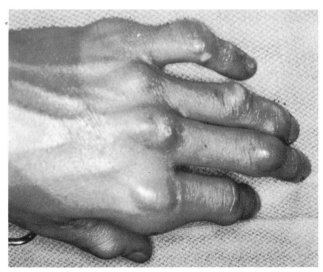

Figure 60–5. Tendon xanthomas of the hand seen over the metacarpal-phalangeal and interphalangeal joints of the fourth and fifth digits in an adult with heterozygous familial hypercholesterolemia. (Courtesy of Dr. Paul Samuel.)

neae, hyperlipidemia, and diabetes mellitus and a complete medical history to rule out secondary causes of hyperlipidemia. Physical examination should focus on signs of hypothyroidism, hepatitis, nephrotic syndrome, connective tissue disease, and other causes of secondary hyperlipidemia (Table 60–15) as well as signs of peripheral lipid deposition.

Laboratory Examination

Blood screening for hypothyroidism and hepatitis is indicated in the adolescent with elevated cholesterol. A primary disorder of lipid metabolism is diagnosed once secondary causes have been ruled out and the elevated values repeated by a reliable laboratory. Apoproteins are difficult to measure and should be used only to support rather than make a diagnosis.

DIFFERENTIAL DIAGNOSIS

Hyperlipoproteinemia may be either idiopathic or secondary to other medical disorders. When hyperlipidemia is discovered, the secondary causes should be ruled out (Table 60–15). These include endocrine, gastrointestinal, renal, and connective tissue disorders; eating disorders; drugs; and other metabolic disorders.

Endocrine Disorders

Diabetes mellitus is a leading cause of hyperlipidemia. Alterations in fat transport and metabolism are known

TABLE 60–15. Causes of Secondary Hyperlipidemia in Adolescence

Endocrine disorders
    Diabetes mellitus
    Hypothyroidism
    Pregnancy, lactation
Gastrointestinal disorders
    Biliary tract obstruction
    Pancreatitis
    Hepatocellular disease
Renal disease
    Dialysis
    Transplant
    Nephrosis
Connective tissue disease
    Systemic lupus erythematosus
    Juvenile rheumatoid arthritis
Dietary disorders
    Excessive consumption of cholesterol,
      saturated fat, or calories
    Anorexia nervosa
Medications
    Oral contraceptive pills
    Corticosteroids
    Thiazides
    β-Blockers
    Isotretinoin (Accutane)
Other metabolic diseases
    Glycogen storage disease
    Acute intermittent porphyria
    Gout

complications of diabetes mellitus. There are several causes for this, including the following:

1. Insulin deficiency causes lipoprotein lipase dysfunction, resulting in elevated plasma VLDL and triglyceride levels and decreased plasma HDL concentrations.

2. Insulin deficiency also results in a state of starvation intracellularly, adipose tissue lipolysis, high plasma free fatty acid concentrations, and increased hepatic VLDL production.

3. Ketoacidosis results in impaired clearance of chylomicrons and VLDL, which results in elevated levels of triglyceride and, to a lesser degree, cholesterol.

4. The diet of some diabetic adolescents is relatively low in carbohydrate and high in fat, saturated fat, and cholesterol, which may result in increased LDL production or decreased clearance.

5. A separately inherited familial form of hypertriglyceridemia or familial combined hyperlipidemia may coexist with insulin deficiency.

Thus, the adolescent diabetic may have elevated levels of triglycerides or cholesterol, or both.

Hypothyroidism is the second most common endocrinopathy associated with secondary hyperlipidemia. Types IIa and IIb patterns are most common, but type III, IV, or V also occurs. The degree of hyperlipidemia correlates with the severity of hypothyroidism. The response to thyroid hormone replacement therapy is usually dramatic and prompt.

Gastrointestinal Disorders

Hyperlipidemia accompanies impairment of bile acid and cholesterol excretion into the bile, as occurs in primary biliary cirrhosis. Plasma cholesterol levels greater than 1500 mg/dl are not uncommon in adolescents with severe liver disease. A characteristic lipoprotein called lipoprotein X is found in these adolescent patients. A similar, less severe type of hyperlipidemia is seen in α_1-antitrypsin deficiency and other hepatocellular diseases, such as hepatitis.

Renal Disorders (see Chapter 65)

Hyperlipidemia can occur in adolescents with renal disease in three circumstances: those undergoing dialysis, those with renal transplant on immunosuppressive therapy, and those with nephrotic syndrome. Each type of hyperlipidemia has a distinct plasma lipoprotein pattern and different pathophysiologic mechanism. In patients undergoing dialysis, a type IV pattern is characteristic. Transplant hyperlipidemia consists of elevated LDL, cholesterol, and a type IIa pattern. Renal transplant patients may also have elevated levels of VLDL triglycerides with a type IV or type IIb phenotype owing to the interaction of increased appetite, obesity, and steroid therapy. The hyperlipidemia of the nephrotic syndrome consists of elevated plasma cholesterol, triglycerides and LDL cholesterol levels and a normal or low HDL cholesterol level. This hyperlipidemia resolves as the edema and hypoalbuminemia clear.

Connective Tissue Diseases

A variety of antibodies have been reported in patients with hyperlipidemia and systemic lupus erythematosus (SLE), juvenile rheumatoid arthritis, nephrotic syndrome, lymphosarcoma, monoclonal gammopathy, and macroglobulinemia. Hyperlipidemia may be the sole manifestation of SLE in adolescents, but more commonly the diagnosis of SLE is suspected from the history, physical examination, and laboratory studies. The hyperlipidemia of SLE in adolescents occurs in two distinct patterns: one attributable to active disease, and the other, in part, due to corticosteroid therapy. The hyperlipidemia of active disease consists of depressed HDL cholesterol and apoprotein A-I levels with elevated VLDL cholesterol and triglyceride levels. The hyperlipidemia that occurs after corticosteroid therapy consists of increased total cholesterol, VLDL cholesterol, and triglyceride levels.

Adolescents with juvenile rheumatoid arthritis have dyslipoproteinemia characterized by low plasma total cholesterol, HDL cholesterol, and LDL cholesterol levels with high VLDL cholesterol and triglyceride levels.

Dietary Disorders

The most common dietary cause of hyperlipidemia is excessive intake of cholesterol, saturated fat, or calories in an individual with genetic sensitivity to these factors. In children with protein energy malnutrition, levels of plasma triglycerides, total cholesterol, and the LDL and HDL subfractions are low. In contrast, patients with anorexia nervosa have a different pattern of hyperlipidemia, consisting of elevated HDL and decreased triglyceride levels, which may be the result of decreased thyroid or increased lipoprotein lipase activity. This pattern has been shown to become more marked with refeeding to within 10% of ideal body weight.

Medication

Oral contraceptives containing estrogen and progestogen exert complex effects on atherosclerotic risk via changes in lipid and glucose metabolism and coagulation (see Chapter 73). Epidemiologic evidence suggests a dose response effect for both hormonal constituents. Estrogens result in high normal plasma triglyceride and VLDL levels; however, in adolescents with a familial form of hypertriglyceridemia, estrogen-containing oral contraceptives can precipitate a massive hypertriglyceridemia and chylomicronemia that can be fatal.

Progestins increase cholesterol and triglyceride levels independent of the effect of estrogen, and some preparations also raise LDL cholesterol and lower HDL cholesterol levels in a dose response fashion, whereas others have an opposite effect. Therefore, measurement of plasma lipid levels may be indicated in adolescents before prescribing oral contraceptive pills and periodically while they are on the medication. Alternative methods of contraception may be needed for those patients who are known to have marked hypertriglyceridemia. The lowest-dose pill that can be used should be prescribed for contraception or menstrual regulation. For the adolescent without familial hypertriglyceridemia, rather than discontinuing oral contraceptives, dietary intervention should be provided when hyperlipidemia is detected.

Corticosteroids have profound effects on lipid metabolism. Administration of corticosteroids results in increases in HDL cholesterol and total cholesterol levels with varied effects on plasma triglyceride levels. Besides the effect on hepatic metabolism, the increased appetite and weight gain in corticosteroid-treated adolescents may also elevate plasma lipoprotein concentrations.

Other drugs that are known to cause hyperlipidemia include thiazide diuretics, β-blocking agents such as propranolol, and 13-cis-retinoic acid (isotretinoin, Accutane). Isotretinoin causes type IV hyperlipidemia by the stimulation of VLDL production and the resultant increase in triglyceride-rich lipoproteins. Thiazides cause elevated VLDL and LDL and depressed HDL concentrations in plasma. β-Blockers cause reduced HDL cholesterol and increased triglyceride concentrations. Therapy with these agents should be avoided, if possible, in adolescents with primary hyperlipidemia. In those without preexisting hyperlipidemia who are receiving chronic therapy for hypertension or other conditions, there should be periodic lipid monitoring. Elevations of 10% to 15% in LDL cholesterol levels should be considered relative contraindications for these medications, and alternatives should be sought. If none is appropriate for a given patient, dietary therapy may be helpful in improving the lipid profile.

Other Metabolic Disorders

Hyperlipidemia may be a dominant feature in patients with type I glycogen storage disease, or glucose-6-phosphatase deficiency. Glycogenolytic and gluconeogenic responses to hypoglycemia in a liver containing abundant glycogen result in elevated levels of serum triglycerides, phospholipids, and cholesterol. Macula halo syndrome, a variant of Niemann-Pick histiocyte storage disease, is associated with hyperlipidemia as well. Hypercholesterolemia with increased plasma LDL levels is seen in patients with acute intermittent porphyria, although the relationship to the primary biochemical defect in this disease is unknown.

Adolescents who are at risk for hypertriglyceridemia related to hyperuricemia include those with renal failure, inborn errors of purine metabolism, anorexia nervosa, and leukemia being treated with chemotherapy.

TREATMENT
Preliminary Steps

Initial treatment of the commonly seen adolescent primary lipid disorders, heterozygous familial hypercho-

lesterolemia, familial combined hyperlipidemia, and mixed environmental genetic hypercholesterolemia, is similar. We attempt to impress upon the family that although the adolescent's risk for cardiovascular disease is increased by the hypercholesterolemia, the adolescent is healthy at present and symptomatic disease is decades away, but that changes in behavior and lifestyle can have a significant impact on the cholesterol levels. We also explain that the purpose of visits with the physician is to maintain health rather than to treat disease.

After addressing the concerns of the family and the adolescent, the clinician should evaluate and treat associated risk factors (see Chapter 49). High blood pressure is an important codeterminant of atherosclerotic risk that should be assessed yearly in the high-risk patient and treated appropriately. The effects of cigarette smoking on accelerating atherosclerosis in adolescents are clear; evidence for the effects of passive smoking is also mounting (see Chapter 44). Therefore, a clear and consistent antismoking message to adolescents and parents is indicated. Finally, although a direct cholesterol-lowering effect has not been demonstrated, a modest amount of aerobic exercise (20 minutes three times per week) is necessary to maintain cardiovascular conditioning and can be an adjunct to dietary cholesterol lowering. Exercise also has a clear role in the management of mild to moderate hypertension and obesity and in lowering of triglyceride levels through changes in insulin and lipoprotein lipase activity. Whether moderate exercise can significantly raise HDL cholesterol levels needs further investigation.

Diet

The dietary treatment of hyperlipidemia is the cornerstone of prevention of atherosclerosis in the adolescent. Experimental data on its safety and efficacy are only now being gathered, so the growth and development of treated individuals should be carefully monitored. The American Heart Association guidelines provide the basic structure of a cholesterol-lowering diet (Table 60–16), but translating these guidelines into food that adolescents will eat is a real challenge.

A practical and highly recommended method is that of substitution. Dietary assessment by food frequency list or a 3-day diet record provides information on the baseline cholesterol, fat, and saturated fat intake for an individual adolescent and highlights the foods that have the highest levels of these nutrients. These identified foods can then be replaced with more healthy foods acceptable to the adolescent and family.

TABLE 60–16. Cholesterol-Lowering Diet*

No more than 30% of total kcal from fat
Cholesterol: 100 mg/1000 kcal
⅓ each
    Saturated fat
    Monounsaturated fat
    Polyunsaturated fat
Adequate kcal for growth

*American Heart Association "Prudent Diet."

Both the saturated fat content and the cholesterol content of the diet must be reduced to obtain and maintain maximum benefit. Although the amounts of cholesterol in chicken, beef, and fish are similar, their effect on plasma cholesterol differs because of their saturated fat content. Shrimp, although rich in cholesterol, have relatively little effect on the plasma cholesterol concentration when eaten in small quantities because they are low in saturated fats. Saturated fat increases the synthesis of LDL cholesterol and decreases LDL cholesterol disposal. Polyunsaturated fat decreases VLDL triglyceride and cholesterol synthesis and the synthesis of apoprotein B. Monounsaturated fat, such as olive oil and peanut oil, can reduce LDL cholesterol when replacing saturated fat in the diet and can also improve the LDL cholesterol–to–HDL cholesterol ratio without increasing plasma triglyceride levels. An increase in the intake of high-fiber foods such as oat bran, beans, and other water-soluble fiber can also lower cholesterol levels. Although the mechanism for these cholesterol-lowering effects has not clearly been defined, increased gastrointestinal loss of bile salt is believed to play a role. Marine or omega-3 fatty acids lower VLDL triglyceride levels primarily by decreasing VLDL synthesis.

For younger adolescents, this method works best when all family members adopt the diet changes. Those adolescents who determine much of their own diet can successfully plan meals with a nutritionist. A good review of this method is presented by Schebendach and Besseler.

Diet modification can be divided into two segments: lowering intake of cholesterol and lowering intake of fat and saturated fat. The guidelines presented in Table 60–17 summarize the steps needed to implement this diet. Lowering of total and LDL cholesterol levels in the range of 10% to 15% can be expected.

Pharmacotherapy

Medications are adjuncts to the management of associated risk factors and diet therapy, not primary therapy. They should be reserved for adolescents with a family history of severe early atherosclerotic disease who have failed to respond in 6 months to dietary

TABLE 60–17. Diet Modification Guidelines

To lower cholesterol intake:
    Eliminate visible egg yolk
    Control portions of meats, fish, and poultry
    Use lowest-fat dairy products
To lower fat and saturated fat intake:
    Reduce visible and invisible fats
    Substitute:
        Unsaturated for tropical oils
        Low-fat for high-fat snacks
        Lean meats for fatty-type meats

therapy under the close supervision of a nutritionist. The medications used in adults (presumably safe and effective in older adolescents) are listed in Table 60–18). They are presented here as a reference guide. Individual practitioners may want to contact specialists caring for more individuals who have hyperlipidemia about pharmacologic treatment.

Nontraditional Therapy

Nontraditional methods that can be considered as adjuncts to the standard therapies are the use of water-soluble fibers and omega-3 fatty acids.

Water-soluble fibers, when they regularly replace saturated fat and cholesterol in the diet (as when a breakfast of bacon and eggs is replaced with a bowl of oatmeal), have a clear cholesterol-lowering effect. Whether addition of fibers such as oat bran or psyllium to the diet without the elimination of other foods can have a pharmacotherapeutic effect is less clear. Experimental evidence suggests that a 3% cholesterol-lowering effect may be seen in persons with hypercholesterolemia who habitually add maximal doses of water-soluble fiber to their diet.

Omega-3 fatty acids, which are present in fish oils, can alter the metabolism of the arachidonic acid series of prostaglandins, thus affecting vascular tone and platelet aggregation as well as triglyceride metabolism. This has been shown experimentally and epidemiologically to lower atherosclerotic risk. Whether clinical trials will show a clear benefit over risk remains to be determined. At this time fish oil capsules are not indicated for adolescents, but an increased intake of fish (particularly

TABLE 60–18. Medications for Hyperlipidemia

TYPE	ACTION	EXAMPLE	DOSE	EXPECTED RESPONSE (LDL CHOLESTEROL)
Bile acid–binding resins	Increase LDL disposal	Cholestyramine Colestipol	Dilute 1 g titrate to 12 g bid	10–25%
Nicotinic acid	Increase LDL disposal Decrease VLDL synthesis	Niacin	Up to 1000 mg tid	10–25%
Antioxidant	Increase VLDL disposal Decrease VLDL production	Probucol	500 mg bid	10–15%
Fibrates	Reduce LDL and VLDL synthesis Increase HDL	Clofibrate Gemfibrozil	500 mg bid–qid 600 mg bid	10–20%
HMG-CoA reductase inhibitors	Increase LDL disposal Reduce LDL/HDL	Lovastatin Simvastatin Pravastatin	20–40 mg qd	20–40%

HMG-CoA, 3-hydroxy-3-methylglutaryl-coenzyme A.

as a substitution for high-fat, high–saturated fat meats and cheese) is recommended.

BIBLIOGRAPHY

Arden MR, Weiselberg EC, Nussbaum MP, et al: Effects of weight restoration on the dyslipoproteinemia of anorexia nervosa. J Adolesc Health Care 11:199, 1990.

Brown MS, Goldstein JL: A receptor-mediated pathway for cholesterol homeostasis. Science 232:34, 1986.

Committee on Nutrition, American Academy of Pediatrics: Indications for cholesterol testing in children. Pediatrics 83:141, 1989.

Godsland IF, Crook D, Simpson R, et al: The effects of different formulations of oral contraceptive agents on lipid and carbohydrate metabolism. N Engl J Med 323:1375, 1990.

Gordon DJ, Rifkind BM: High density lipoprotein–The clinical implications of recent studies. N Engl J Med 321:1311, 1989.

Ilowite NT, Samuel P, Besseler L, Jacobson MS: Dyslipoproteinemia in juvenile rheumatoid arthritis. J Pediatr 114:823, 1989.

National Cholesterol Education Program Report of the Expert Panel on Blood Cholesterol Levels in Children and Adolescents. Pediatrics 89(3)(Suppl):525, 1992.

NCEP Expert Panel on Blood Cholesterol Levels in Children and Adolescents: National Cholesterol Education Program (NCEP): Highlights of the Report of the Expert Panel on Blood Cholesterol Levels in Children and Adolescents. Pediatrics 89(3):495, 1992.

Newman WP, Freedman DS, Voors AW, et al: Relation of serum lipoprotein levels and systolic blood pressure to early atherosclerosis. The Bogalusa Heart Study. N Engl J Med 314:138, 1986.

Schebendach J, Besseler L: Diet therapy. In Jacobson MS (ed): Atherosclerosis Prevention. Monographs in Clinical Pediatrics. London, Harwood Academic Publishers, 1991.

Gastrointestinal Conditions

CHAPTER 61

Acid Peptic Disease

JAMES F. MARKOWITZ

Recent research and pharmacologic discoveries have revolutionized the understanding and treatment of acid peptic diseases. However, data specific to the adolescent with gastritis or peptic ulcer disease are sparse. Data on teenaged subjects are frequently included with those of infants and toddlers in reports of pediatric acid peptic disease, and older adolescents are often included as subjects in adult clinical trials. However, studies specifically designed to delineate the scope and treatment of adolescents with acid peptic problems have not been reported. In this chapter, an attempt is made to extract the pertinent data from available sources and the clinical experience of physicians caring for adolescents with these problems.

NORMAL PHYSIOLOGY

Under normal circumstances the epithelial lining of the stomach and duodenum is exposed to, yet resists, conditions capable of digesting and denaturing dietary proteins. Intragastric hydrogen ion concentrations greater than 150 mmol/L are common during peak acid output, and even during periods of basal acid secretion the gastric pH generally remains 1.5 to 2. Despite rapid neutralization, duodenal pH can also drop to 2 on emptying of the stomach, yet mucosal damage usually does not occur. Injury develops when an imbalance between noxious endogenous or exogenous stimuli and mucosal defenses occurs. Recent advances in delineating the processes underlying this protection of the gastroduodenal mucosa have led to an improved understanding of the pathophysiology of and therapy for acid peptic disease.

Mucosal Defenses

Various anatomic and physiologic factors have been associated with the ability of the gastroduodenal mucosa to resist exposure to noxious intraluminal agents. Bacterial invasion is limited by the bactericidal effects of secreted intraluminal acid. A well-defined mucus layer, together with bicarbonate secreted by the epithelium, protects the mucosa from back-diffusion of hydrogen ion. Mucin may also be important as a scavenger of local oxidants. A rich network of capillaries supplies the mucosa with a continuous supply of oxygen and nutrients to support cellular metabolism. At the same time, this high rate of mucosal blood flow prevents the local accumulation of potentially toxic substances that may have passed through the epithelial barrier.

The epithelium resists injury by a number of mechanisms. The gastroduodenal mucosa has one of the highest proliferative rates in the body. Trophic effects are exerted by a number of hormones, including gastrin, somatostatin, growth hormone, thyroxine, and epidermal growth factor. The relative effects of these hormones in adolescents, as well as how they might change during puberty, have not been investigated. However, regeneration of the mucosa is a relatively slow process (turnover time is estimated at 4 to 6 days), since it requires protein synthesis and cellular mitosis. A more rapid reparative process, reconstitution, has recently been recognized. Reconstitution represents a process by which viable epithelial cells migrate from areas beneath or adjacent to sites of injury to cover denuded areas. This process restores mucosal integrity within minutes of an injury and probably represents a major element of gastroduodenal protection.

A number of endogenous chemical mediators have also been noted to enhance gastroduodenal integrity. Prostaglandins have been the most extensively investigated. These ubiquitous fatty acids are produced locally in the epithelium in response to a variety of luminal irritants. Agents capable of suppressing endogenous prostaglandin production regularly have been shown to be ulcerogenic. Conversely, although exogenous prostaglandin administration is capable of suppressing acid secretion at pharmacologic concentrations, lower doses have demonstrated "cytoprotection" without acid suppression. The mechanism underlying this cytoprotective action remains unclear but appears to be multifactorial. Increased mucus and bicarbonate secretion, maintenance of mucosal blood flow, and strengthening of the cell membrane have all been associated with the cytoprotective effects of prostaglandins in animal models of ulceration. Endogenous sulfhydryl compounds and polyamines have also been demonstrated to impart cytoprotection to the gastroduodenal mucosa in animal studies, but their importance to human mucosal integrity is less well delineated.

Aggressive Factors

The endogenous materials potentially capable of inducing gastroduodenal damage are acid, pepsin, bile acids, and lysolecithin. Under normal circumstances acid and pepsin are elaborated under strict control, thus limiting their noxious potential. The caustic effects of bile acids and lysolecithin are limited to the gastric mucosa. However, the normal antroduodenal pressure gradient and distal propagation of peristaltic motor activity limit the reflux of these materials across the pylorus.

Acid is secreted by the parietal cells of the gastric fundus and body in response to a variety of stimuli (Fig. 61–1). Acetylcholine and gastrin bind to specific membrane-bound receptors and induce acid secretion by raising intracellular calcium. Histamine binds to the H2 receptor and induces acid production through stimulation of adenylate cyclase. Both calcium and cyclic adenosine monophosphate induce intracellular protein kinases, which in turn activate a hydrogen-potassium adenosine triphosphatase, resulting in the active secretion of hydrogen into the lumen. Endogenous antisecretory processes have also been described. In particular, prostaglandins have been shown to bind to cell membrane receptors, resulting in inhibition of intracellular adenylate cyclase and inhibition of parietal cell acid output. Acid secretion is also influenced by gut peptides such as somatostatin and neurotensin. The rate of gastric acid output is therefore fine tuned by the influence of competing messengers.

At least seven different pepsinogens, broadly classified into two immunochemically distinct groups, have been described. Type I pepsinogens are synthesized in chief cells located in the oxyntic glands of the fundus and body of the stomach. Type II pepsinogens are produced in both antral and Brunner glands. Pepsinogen synthesis and secretion appear to be controlled by competing neural, hormonal, and paracrine pathways analogous to those described for acid secretion. At luminal pH below 5, pepsins are formed after cleavage of an N-terminal peptide from pepsinogen, resulting in endopeptidases with proteolytic pH optima around 2 to 3. Pepsins, however, are irreversibly inactivated at pH greater than 6.

PATHOPHYSIOLOGY

The specific pathophysiologic events resulting in acid peptic disease in the adolescent remain to be completely elucidated. Even minor imbalances between protective and aggressive forces in the stomach and duodenum result in pathologic processes. Acid and peptic activity are necessary prerequisites for the development of gastritis or ulcers. However, lesions more commonly develop after changes in mucosal defenses than after acid hypersecretion, since conditions associated with large increases in acid output remain the exception rather than the rule in adolescents.

Gastritis

Gastritis results from a variety of factors including drugs and other toxins, *Helicobacter pylori*, stress, and bile reflux. With the possible exception of bile reflux, all are important causes of morbidity during adoles-

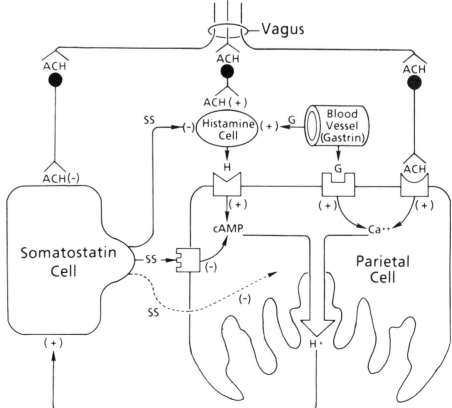

Figure 61–1. Model summarizing the neural, paracrine, and hormonal regulation of gastric acid secretion. Histamine *(H)*, gastrin *(G)*, and acetylcholine *(ACH)* stimulate acid *(H$^+$)* secretion by acting on specific receptors on the parietal cell. In addition, gastrin and acetylcholine release histamine from mucosal stores and acetylcholine inhibits somatostatin *(SS)* release, thus eliminating the restraint exerted by somatostatin on the parietal cell. Somatostatin inhibits acid secretion by (1) inhibiting release of mucosal histamine, (2) binding to somatostatin receptors on the parietal cell that are coupled to inhibition of cyclic adenosine monophosphate *(cAMP)*, and (3) acting within the parietal cell through unknown mechanisms to block gastrin-stimulated acid secretion. There is also feedback stimulation of somatostatin release by secreted acid. (With permission from Schubert ML, Shamburek RD: Control of acid secretion. Gastroenterol Clin North Am 19[1]:1, 1990.)

cence. Atrophic gastritis, common in adults, is not seen in adolescents.

Gastritis is an endoscopic and histologic diagnosis. Described as acute or chronic there is often no evidence to allow accurate determination of the duration of the process. Acute gastritis is used to describe endoscopically apparent erosions with or without hemorrhage. Erosions are usually multiple, small, flat, whitish lesions often surrounded by a red halo. Histologically, erosions do not extend below the muscularis mucosa, but judging the depth of a lesion endoscopically is generally arbitrary. Chronic gastritis often is endoscopically normal, despite the presence of inflammatory cells (both mononuclear and polymorphonuclear) in biopsy specimens. Chronic superficial gastritis is characterized by infiltration of the superficial epithelium by lymphocytes and plasma cells. In chronic diffuse antral gastritis, lymphocyte and plasma cell infiltration involves the entire thickness of the antral mucosa and may be associated with lymphoid follicle formation. Many pathologists further characterize these chronic forms of gastritis as "active" if there is also a polymorphonuclear infiltrate or depletion of mucus in cells of the glandular epithelium.

DRUG INDUCED

A variety of drugs and other agents induce gastric mucosal erosions, hemorrhages, or chronic superficial gastritis. Among adolescents, alcohol, aspirin, and other nonsteroidal anti-inflammatory agents are the usual causes. Gastritis can occur after a single ingestion or after weeks of use.

HELICOBACTER PYLORI

The last few years have witnessed an explosion of information about *Helicobacter pylori* (previously called *Campylobacter pylori*), which has been associated with a chronic, nonspecific, superficial or diffuse antral gastritis. These slender, spiral-shaped, flagellated gram-negative rods are found in the mucus overlying the antral epithelium. Evidence suggests that the bacteria are capable of degrading mucus glycoproteins, leading to increased permeability of the mucus layer and an increase in the back-diffusion of acid. Evidence for the pathogenicity of the organism has been obtained from a number of well-documented, healthy volunteers who ingested the organism and developed acute and/or chronic gastritis.

H. pylori has been identified in 10% to 70% of children and adolescents with primary gastritis and in 0 to 10% of children and adolescents with gastritis secondary to identifiable diseases such as Crohn disease or eosinophilic gastroenteritis. It is also seen in less than 10% of normal antral biopsy specimens. Varying frequencies of *H. pylori* identification in different reports likely represent variations in the distribution of the organism in the environment or unknown host factors. A prospective Toronto study reported seven cases of *H. pylori* in 67 pediatric antral biopsy specimens (10%); a retrospective Cleveland study noted *H. pylori* in 22 of 98 (22%) specimens; and a prospective study from Westchester, New York, identified the organism in 16 of 95 (17%) cases. In contrast, we have identified only 4 cases of *H. pylori* in a prospective study of 185 (2%) consecutive children and adolescents from Long Island, New York, undergoing upper endoscopy. Serologic testing has revealed that antibodies to *H. pylori* increase with age. Only 5% to 10% of teenagers have *H. pylori*–specific serum antibodies, but this prevalence rises to 40% to 60% of adults 50 years of age or older. Intrafamilial clustering has been reported, suggesting that there may be person-to-person spread of the infection.

STRESS INDUCED

Critically ill adolescents are at risk for developing stress-related mucosal damage. Gastritis develops most commonly after severe trauma, after extensive burns, and in adolescents with central nervous system injury or surgery, sepsis, and shock. The pathogenesis underlying these changes is not well understood. Acid is clearly important, since neutralization of the stomach will prevent its occurrence. However, changes in gastric motility may also be important, promoting bile reflux that can further injure the gastric mucosa. Decreased mucosal blood flow and decreased prostaglandin, bicarbonate, and mucus production have also been implicated as contributing factors.

BILE INDUCED

Enterogastric reflux of bile acids (especially deconjugated), lysolecithin, and pancreatic juice can cause gastric mucosal injury. Small amounts of bile reflux are physiologic and not associated with identifiable mucosal change. Although pathologic bile reflux has been associated with previous gastroduodenal surgery, adolescents with intact gastrointestinal tracts and antroduodenal motility disturbances may also develop bile gastritis. Enterogastric reflux usually causes regenerative changes in the glandular epithelium rather than inflammation.

Peptic Ulcer

Peptic ulceration in the adolescent has been the subject of relatively few studies, and the incidence is unknown. Previous estimates based on contrast-enhanced radiographs have been shown to be highly inaccurate. Primary ulcers occur in patients without predisposing causes. Patients with secondary ulcers have underlying disease or have received ulcerogenic medications. Adolescents tend to have primary ulcers. In a recent evaluation of children and adolescents with ulcers, primary peptic ulcers were found in 19 of 23 adolescents but in none of 13 children younger than 10 years of age. Sixty to 75% of both primary and secondary ulcers are found in the duodenum. In one recent report, 83% of gastric ulcers were antral, whereas duodenal ulcers were seen almost exclusively (97%) in the bulb. The male-to-female ratio ranges from 1.5:1 to 4.5:1.

GENETICS

Genetic influences are important in primary, but not in secondary, ulcers. The family histories of many adolescents with ulcers reveal similarly afflicted first- and second-degree relatives. The frequency of family histories positive for ulcer disease ranges from 20% to 63%. These genetic influences are heterogeneous and have been only incompletely characterized. Ulcer patients as a group tend to have high maximal acid output after stimulation by pentagastrin or other stimuli. However, significant overlap exists between ulcer patients and controls. Another marker, high levels of serum pepsinogen I, has been shown to be inherited as an autosomal dominant trait with incomplete penetrance. Hyperpepsinogenemia correlates well with maximal acid output and identifies members of specific kindreds at high risk for duodenal ulcers. In a study of an extended kindred, 40% of those family members with high serum pepsinogen levels developed ulcers, compared with none of those with normal levels. However, many children and adolescents with primary duodenal ulcers do not have high serum pepsinogens despite having a high family incidence of ulcers. Whether these latter families demonstrate the heterogeneity of potential genetic influences or whether their ulcers are due to socioenvironmental factors remains to be evaluated.

HELICOBACTER PYLORI

Despite the fact that *H. pylori* can only be found overlying gastric-type mucosa, increasing evidence from adult populations with recurrent ulcers supports the contention that this organism causes primary duodenal ulcer disease as well as gastritis. If found in the duodenum, the organism invariably overlies areas of gastric metaplasia. In adults with recurrent duodenal ulcers, *H. pylori* has been demonstrated in antral biopsy specimens in as many as 100% of cases. Although there is no direct evidence to implicate *H. pylori* in the development of the actual ulcer crater, indirect evidence that the organism is important in the pathogenesis of duodenal ulcers is accumulating. Bactericidal therapies including antibiotics and bismuth preparations not only result in ulcer healing but also decrease the frequency of ulcer relapse. Moreover, the rate of ulcer relapse is lower than in patients whose ulcers were healed with H2 blockers. In addition, when recurrent ulcers have occurred, evidence for recurrent or persistent *H. pylori* infection has often been documented. However, many *H. pylori*–negative patients with ulcers do exist, especially children and adolescents manifesting their first ulcer. Therefore, the importance of *H. pylori* in the development of duodenal ulcer in the adolescent remains to be determined.

PSYCHOLOGICAL FACTORS

A number of reports suggest links between the development of peptic ulcers and identifiable psychopathology in both adolescents and adults. Many of these studies have been criticized, however, because comparisons were made between patients with ulcers and normal control subjects rather than those with chronic disease. In addition, controlled studies on consecutive patients with ulcers are virtually nonexistent. Recent studies have identified episodes of loss or separation prior to the onset of peptic ulceration. Others have detailed personality traits purportedly more common in children and adolescents with ulcers. A study of 132 adolescents and adults from Sweden, however, does not support the hypothesis that psychological stress is related to the development of ulcers.

CLINICAL MANIFESTATIONS

In adolescents, symptoms do not differentiate gastritis from ulcer disease. Symptoms in adolescents are similar to those in the adult, whereas in young children acid peptic disease is often asymptomatic. Adolescents with primary duodenal ulcers (whether *H. pylori* positive or not) or gastritis have similar frequencies of abdominal pain (80% to 90%), vomiting (20% to 50%), and hemorrhage (either melena or hematemesis, 20% to 40%). Perforation occurs in less than 1% to 2% of cases of primary ulcers but can be noted in 25% to 30% of those of secondary ulcers. On the other hand, stress gastritis is usually painless.

The characteristics of acid peptic pain are quite variable in adolescents. Episodes of pain may be brief or prolonged and may be poorly localized. Adolescents describe their pain as sharp or burning, and at times they may be completely unable to characterize their discomfort. There is also no predictable response to eating. Adolescents with either ulcers or gastritis may have periods of apparent spontaneous remission lasting weeks to months.

Complications arising from acid peptic disease vary. Life-threatening hematemesis and perforation occur in less than 5% of primary ulcers or gastritis, although these complications have been described in 25% to 50% of secondary ulcers. Gastric outlet obstruction related to scarring of the duodenal bulb rarely occurs during adolescence and is more commonly seen in the adult with long-standing ulcer disease.

The most important complication seen in the adolescent is recurrent ulcer disease. Most reports of adolescent patients treated with traditional medical management have noted recurrence rates as high as 50% to 70% following discontinuation of therapy. Although no data allow accurate prediction of which adolescent patients will have recurrences, those with documented hypersecretion and positive family histories appear to be at high risk. So, too, are adolescent patients with *H. pylori* whose infection is not eradicated. It is clear, however, that primary ulcer disease in the adolescent persists into adult life in the majority of cases and that it is in these individuals that many of the complications of acid peptic disease arise.

DIAGNOSIS

Acid peptic disease can be diagnosed most accurately by endoscopy. Outpatient endoscopy is performed with mild intravenous sedation, thus minimizing both risk and cost. However, hospitalization is recommended for the teenager with significant upper gastrointestinal tract bleeding. Direct endoscopic visualization of gastric and duodenal mucosa allows identification of even minor degrees of mucosal inflammation or sources of bleeding (Figs. 61–2 and 61–3). Endoscopy is contraindicated, however, if perforation is suspected.

Mucosal biopsy specimens can also be obtained during endoscopy to aid in the diagnosis of acid peptic disease. A number of reports have documented that there is poor correlation between endoscopic appearance and histology in gastritis. Mucosal changes can be apparent histologically despite a normal endoscopic appearance (Fig. 61–4). In addition, histologic evaluation of the antral mucosa (by Gram, Giemsa, or Warthin-Starry stain), coupled with either direct microbiologic culture of biopsy tissue or identification of urease activity in the biopsy specimen, remains the only generally available method for identifying the presence of *H. pylori* (Fig. 61–5). Urea breath testing using stable radioisotopes remains a research tool, and serologic tests are not yet widely available.

The alternative procedure available for the identification of peptic ulceration is contrast-enhanced radiography. An upper gastrointestinal series can delineate a distinct ulcer crater (Fig. 61–6), but as routinely performed it is rarely sufficiently sensitive to identify the superficial inflammation associated with gastritis. A number of studies have demonstrated that endoscopy identifies about twice as many ulcers as contrast-enhanced radiography. In addition, the frequency of false-positive results with upper gastrointestinal radiography has been reported to be as high as 60% in certain centers. Although double-contrast radiography improves the accuracy of diagnosis in adults, there are minimal data on the use of this technique in adolescents.

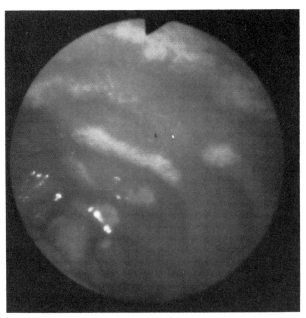

Figure 61–3. Endoscopic appearance of multiple idiopathic ulcers of the duodenal bulb (*Helicobacter pylori* negative) in a 13-year-old girl with abdominal pain.

DIFFERENTIAL DIAGNOSIS

Acid peptic disease must be delineated from the other conditions that cause abdominal pain, vomiting and/or upper gastrointestinal bleeding in the adolescent. These conditions are summarized in Table 61–1. A few conditions may be particularly difficult to differentiate from acid peptic disease. In particular, Crohn disease manifested by antral gastritis, duodenitis, and small apthous ulcerations has been recognized in 10% to 30% of children and adolescents with known Crohn disease. In occasional patients, gastroduodenal involvement represents the only clinically apparent site of Crohn disease. Histologic studies are not particularly helpful in differentiating this condition from peptic ulceration unless a granuloma is present.

Ulcerations also develop as the primary manifestation of the Zollinger-Ellison syndrome. Hypergastrinemia secondary to a gastrin-secreting tumor commonly located in the pancreas or extrapancreatic tissues results in acid hypersecretion unresponsive to normal feedback inhibition. Although multiple ulcerations involving unusual locations such as the esophagus, distal duodenum, or jejunum have been described, 75% of ulcers occur in the duodenal bulb or stomach. The diagnosis of Zollinger-Ellison syndrome requires identification of a fasting serum gastrin value that is usually greater than 1000 pg/ml. These levels increase further after a secretin challenge. Adolescents with atypical ulcer locations or recurrent or intractable ulcer disease should be screened for this rare tumor.

TREATMENT

In most cases, the therapy for acid peptic disease in the adolescent has been extrapolated from clinical ex-

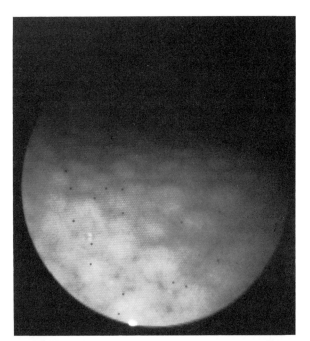

Figure 61–2. Endoscopic appearance of nodular antral gastritis associated with *Helicobacter pylori* infection in a 14-year-old boy with dysphagia.

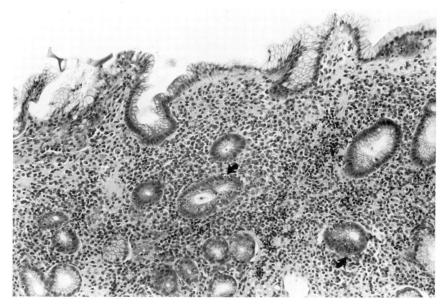

Figure 61–4. Gastric antral biopsy specimen obtained from endoscopically normal tissue in a 15-year-old boy with abdominal pain. Glands of the superficial layer are widely separated by mononuclear cells, and segmented leukocytes can be seen invading the gland epithelium *(arrows)* (hematoxylin & eosin, ×200). (Courtesy of Dr. Ellen Kahn.)

perience and controlled trials in adults. Rarely have specific drug regimens or even dosing requirements been studied in adolescent populations.

Gastritis

The therapy for gastritis is in part dependent on the cause. However, in all cases, maintaining intragastric pH greater than 5 with either neutralizing agents or antisecretory drugs markedly reduces inflammation and promotes healing. Stress-induced changes may require aggressive gastric neutralization until the stress of the underlying disease can be eliminated. Drug-induced gastritis generally improves rapidly after withdrawal of the offending agent. Although misoprostol, a synthetic prostaglandin E_1 analogue, has been shown to be effective in preventing gastritis associated with the use of nonsteroidal anti-inflammatory agents, it has not been shown to be of benefit in treating established inflammation.

Optimal regimens for eradication of *H. pylori* continue to be investigated. Colloidal bismuth subcitrate is bactericidal but eradicates the organism in only 30% of cases if used as a single agent. It is also not yet commercially available in the United States. The substitution of bismuth subsalicylate (Pepto-Bismol) may be effective, but it has not yet been extensively studied. Addition of antibiotics such as ampicillin, amoxicillin, erythromycin, or nitrofurantoin to a course of bismuth appears to enhance clearing rates from the mucosa.

Bile reflux remains the most perplexing form of gastritis to treat. In nonoperated patients, the use of a prokinetic agent such as metoclopramide or cisapride may enhance antroduodenal peristalsis and minimize bile reflux. Antacids and antisecretory agents are often ineffective in controlling symptoms, but sucralfate may be beneficial. The latter agent not only has cytoprotec-

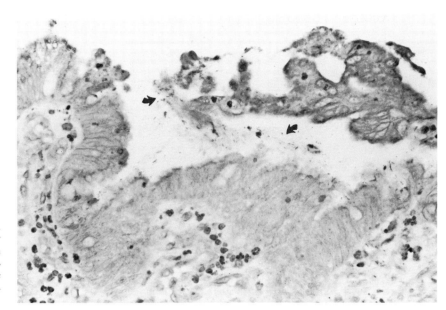

Figure 61–5. Surface epithelium of the gastric antrum obtained from the 14-year-old boy whose endoscopic appearance is shown in Figure 61–2. Curved gram-negative organisms *(Helicobacter pylori)* are easily seen in the mucous layer *(arrows)* (Warthin-Starry, ×500). (Courtesy of Dr. Ellen Kahn.)

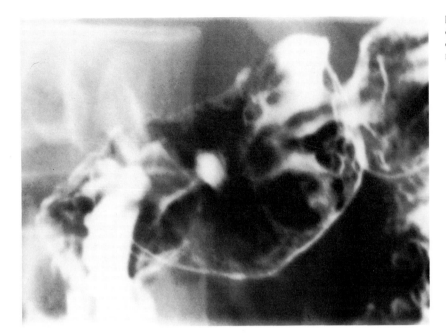

Figure 61–6. Double-contrast barium radiograph of the duodenal bulb from a 14-year-old boy with chronic abdominal pain. A typical ulcer crater with radiating folds is present.

tive effects but also is known to interfere with the interaction between bile acids and the mucosa. At times, however, the symptoms of bile gastritis are so debilitating that surgery designed to divert bile away from the stomach (such as an antrectomy with a roux-en-Y gastrojejunostomy) has been attempted.

Peptic Ulcer

The therapy for peptic ulcers in an adolescent population has not been extensively studied, and often the studies that have been performed do not include routine endoscopic documentation of healing. Therefore, current therapies have largely been extrapolated from adult studies. The agents most commonly used to treat peptic ulcers are listed in Table 61–2. Treatments have traditionally been designed to suppress or neutralize luminal acidity, since it remains well established that ulcers virtually never develop in the absence of acid. However, it has not been established how completely acid must be suppressed for ulcer healing. Newer therapies have increasingly been directed at enhancing mucosal resistance.

Despite the high rate of ulcer recurrences there remain no conclusive data to guide the ultimate duration of therapy. Most commonly employed therapeutic regimens result in ulcer healing in 1 to 3 months. However, with ulcer recurrence, the question of how long to subsequently treat the ulcer remains unanswered. Chronic maintenance therapy has been demonstrated to reduce recurrences and probably should be continued for at least 2 years (the period most commonly associated with recurrence). However, lifelong therapy or surgical intervention may at times have to be considered.

ANTACIDS

Antacids continue to play an important role in the treatment of ulcers. Not only do they relieve pain

TABLE 61–1. Differential Diagnosis of Acid Peptic Disease

Presenting as abdominal pain and/or vomiting:
  Gastroesophageal reflux
  Esophageal motility disorders
  Antral web
  Chronic granulomatous disease
  Crohn disease
  Eosinophilic gastroenteritis
  Gastroduodenal motility disorders
  Food bezoar
  Annular pancreas
  Pancreatitis
  Cholecystitis
  Cholangitis
  Constipation
  Bulemia nervosa
  Pregnancy
Presenting as upper gastrointestinal bleeding:
  Reflux esophagitis
  Esophageal varices
  Mallory-Weiss tear
  Congestive gastropathy associated with portal hypertension

TABLE 61–2. Medications for Peptic Ulcer Disease

Antacids
H_2 receptor antagonists:
  cimetidine
  ranitidine
  famotidine
  nizatidine
Prostaglandin analogues:
  misoprostol
  enprostil
Hydrogen-potassium adenosine triphosphatase inhibitors:
  omeprazole
Anticholinergics:
  pirenzepine
Sucralfate
Colloidal bismuth subcitrate (?bismuth subsalicylate)
Antibiotics

quickly, but when used in sufficient quantities and frequency, they can also maintain intragastric pH at neutral levels. Although ulcers can occasionally be healed by antacid therapy exclusively, the need for frequent dosing and the prevalence of side effects such as severe diarrhea or constipation limits compliance in most adolescents (see Chapter 26). Antacids are therefore generally considered adjuncts to other therapies.

H₂ RECEPTOR ANTAGONISTS

H₂ blockers have become the backbone of modern medical ulcer therapy. These agents inhibit acid production by competing with histamine for binding to the H₂ receptor of the parietal cell. In the United States, cimetidine, ranitidine, famotidine, and nizatidine are commercially available. Although there are wide differences in the relative potencies of these compounds, the recommended dosages for each drug tend to minimize the differences. Durations of action do vary, and the short half-life of cimetidine often limits an adolescent's acceptance of the drug because of the need for frequent daily doses. In addition, gastroenterologists treating adolescents often avoid cimetidine because of the drug's known antiandrogen effects. The potential effect of exposing adolescents to these antiandrogenic properties of cimetidine are theoretically worrisome and have not been well studied.

H₂ blockers have been shown to be effective in relieving symptoms, healing ulcers, and reducing the frequency of ulcer recurrences. Recently published meta-analyses of clinical trials of ulcer healing drugs have demonstrated that a good correlation exists between nocturnal acid suppression and the healing of primary duodenal ulcers. Since daytime acid suppression appears to be much less important, treatment regimens based on single nightly doses of H₂ blockers have become increasingly popular. In general, most studies have demonstrated that 70% to 80% of duodenal ulcers heal after 4 weeks of H₂ blocker therapy. After 8 weeks, over 90% of duodenal ulcers have healed. In contrast, healing of gastric ulcers is more poorly correlated with the degree of acid suppression. On average, only about 60% of gastric ulcers heal after 4 weeks of H₂ blocker therapy, compared with about 85% at 8 weeks and 90% at 10 to 12 weeks.

PROSTAGLANDINS

Synthetic prostaglandin analogues of the E series, misoprostol and enprostil, have been used as both antisecretory and cytoprotective agents in the treatment of gastric and duodenal ulcers. Although the drugs have been shown to be about as effective as H₂ blockers in adults, little experience with these agents in adolescents has been reported. It should be remembered that prostaglandins are contraindicated during pregnancy because of their potential to induce uterine contractions and resultant miscarriages or premature births.

HYDROGEN-POTASSIUM ADENOSINE TRIPHOSPHATASE INHIBITORS

Omeprazole is the only proton pump inhibitor commercially available in the United States. It is currently the most potent antisecretory agent available, but its use has been restricted to treatment of patients with Zollinger-Ellison syndrome, severe reflux esophagitis, or ulcers intractable to more traditional therapies. No specific data for the use of this agent in adolescents are reported. Safety concerns remain about omeprazole, since in animal studies an increased incidence of gastric carcinoids associated with long-term use has been noted. However, no significant adverse effects in humans have yet been reported.

ANTICHOLINERGICS

Agents such as pirenzepine effectively limit acid production by inhibiting the cholinergic-induced rise in parietal cell intracellular calcium. Although anticholinergics are frequently used as adjunctive therapy in adults with recurrent ulcer disease, these agents are only rarely prescribed in adolescents.

SUCRALFATE

Sucralfate is a locally acting sulfated disaccharide complexed to aluminum hydroxide that effectively heals both gastric and duodenal ulcers but does not inhibit acid secretion. Rather, sucralfate binds to the base of ulcers, presumably protecting the underlying mucosa from further damage from acid, pepsin, and bile acids. In addition, sucralfate may also induce cytoprotection by enhancing mucosal prostaglandin production, mucosal blood flow, and mucus and bicarbonate secretion. No systemic effects from this compound have been demonstrated, and the drug is generally well tolerated. However, a short-lived, but intense sense of indigestion occasionally develops shortly after ingesting sucralfate. This side effect can be sufficiently unpleasant to limit the drug's acceptance by adolescent patients.

ANTIMICROBIALS

Given the recent realization that *H. pylori* is nearly universally associated with recurrent peptic ulceration, therapy directed against this organism is playing an increasingly important role in the treatment of the adolescent with ulcers. The regimens described previously for the treatment of *H. pylori* gastritis are also effective in healing peptic ulcers. Although data from adolescent populations have not been reported, adult studies suggest that the frequency of recurrent ulceration is less after bismuth-antibiotic therapy than after healing induced by H₂ blockers.

PSYCHOLOGICAL COUNSELING

Despite the extensive literature suggesting a psychosomatic etiology for acid peptic disease, controlled studies of the efficacy of psychological counseling on the rate of ulcer healing or the frequency of recurrence are rare. A recent study of Swedish adults has demonstrated that the 1-year recurrence rate documented by serial endoscopy is no different for subjects undergoing intensive education and counseling than it was for a comparable control group receiving placebo pills nightly. Both of these groups had significantly higher recurrence rates than a comparable group treated with nightly maintenance therapy with cimetidine.

COURSE

Acid peptic disease is as varied in its course as in its presentation. Drug- and stress-induced gastritis are generally acute and short lived if the offending stimulus can be eliminated. On the other hand, bile-induced gastritis is commonly chronic and debilitating symptoms occasionally require extensive surgery to divert bile away from the stomach. *H. pylori* causes both an acute and chronic gastritis, but therapy can eradicate the organism. The potential for recurrence or reinfection remains high, however.

Peptic ulcers should be considered chronic diseases because of the high rate of recurrence. Perforation and gastric outlet obstruction secondary to deformity of the duodenum occur rarely. Life-threatening hemorrhage is also rare, but more limited hemorrhage is not infrequent. Intractable symptoms or life-threatening complications must frequently be dealt with surgically. Highly selective (parietal cell) vagotomy and/or antrectomy with gastrojejunostomy can result in decreased morbidity for the adolescent patient with a highly intractable, complicated ulcer. The need for such intervention is rare during adolescence but may ultimately be necessary as individuals age.

BIBLIOGRAPHY

Buck GE: *Campylobacter pylori* and gastroduodenal disease. Clin Microbiol Rev 3:1–12, 1990.

Correa P: Chronic gastritis: A clinicopathological classification. Am J Gastroenterol 83:504–509, 1988.

Dooley CP, Cohen H: The clinical significance of *Campylobacter pylori*. Ann Intern Med 108:70–79, 1988.

Feldman M: Mechanisms of gastric acid secretion and its pharmacologic control. Contemp Gastroenterol 1:810–815, 1988.

Howden CW, Jones DB, Peace KE, et al: The treatment of gastric ulcer with antisecretory drugs: Relationship of pharmacological effect to healing rates. Dig Dis Sci 33:619–624, 1988.

Hunt RH (ed): Peptic Ulcer Disease. Gastroenterology Clinics of North America. Philadelphia, WB Saunders, 1990.

Jones DB, Howden CW, Burget DW, et al: Acid suppression in duodenal ulcer: A meta-analysis to define optimal dosing with antisecretory drugs. Gut 28:1120–1127, 1987.

Murphy MS, Eastham EJ: Peptic ulcer disease in childhood: Long-term prognosis. J Pediatr Gastroenterol Nutr 6:721–724, 1987.

Murphy MS, Eastham EJ, Jiminez M, et al: Duodenal ulceration: Review of 110 cases. Arch Dis Child 62:554–558, 1987.

Nord KS: Peptic ulcer disease in the pediatric population. Pediatr Clin North Am 35:117–140, 1988.

Roth SH, Bennett RE: Nonsteroidal anti-inflammatory drug gastropathy: Recognition and response. Arch Intern Med 147:2093–2100, 1987.

Soll AH: Pathogenesis of peptic ulcer and implications for therapy. N Engl J Med 322:909–916, 1990.

Tam PK: Serum pepsinogen I in childhood duodenal ulcer. J Pediatr Gastroenterol Nutr 6:904–907, 1987.

Wolfe MM, Soll AH: The physiology of gastric acid secretion. N Engl J Med 319:1707–1715, 1988.

CHAPTER 62

Diseases of the Liver and Pancreas During Adolescence

JOHN N. UDALL, JR.

Diseases that affect the liver and pancreas during adolescence are myriad. Only the more common afflictions of these organs during adolescence are discussed here; for a more complete presentation of the diseases affecting these organs, the reader is referred to several excellent textbooks of pediatric gastroenterology.

LIVER

Disorders of the liver may be classified according to cause: infectious, genetic or metabolic, toxic or drug-induced, neoplasms, and other conditions that do not fit into one of these categories.

Infections

A variety of infectious agents may cause disease of the liver (Table 62–1). Hepatotropic viruses are one of the more common causes of hepatocellular disease during adolescence; those that have been best characterized are hepatitis A virus and hepatitis B virus (see Chapter 93). It is now estimated that hepatitis A accounts for 20% to 25% of all clinical hepatitis in the developed world. Other viruses that may cause hepatitis include the viruses that cause hepatitis B, C, D, and E. Table 62–2 compares the clinical and the laboratory features of these diseases.

Pathophysiology and Clinical Manifestations. Infection with hepatitis A virus characteristically results in an acute febrile illness with jaundice, anorexia, nausea, vomiting, and malaise. Fulminant infection is rare, and chronic infection is believed not to occur. However, the view that the hepatitis A virus does not cause a chronic form of hepatitis has recently been challenged.

Infection with hepatitis B virus characteristically produces a subacute illness with anorexia, nausea, malaise, and jaundice, although fulminant hepatitis can also occur. Anicteric or asymptomatic infection is common in children and less common in adolescents. Arthralgia or rash, including erythema nodosa, sometimes occurs early in the course of the illness (see Chapter 93). Hepatitis B chronic carrier state with or without chronic liver disease occurs in nearly all those whose infection is acquired perinatally. Chronic carriers, especially those infected at a young age, are at an increased risk of developing cirrhosis or hepatocellular carcinoma in later life.

Infection with parenteral non-A, non-B hepatitis (hepatitis C) accounts for more than 90% of transfusion-associated hepatitis cases worldwide and more than 25% of cases of sporadic hepatitis. Only one third of infected individual patients are icteric, and the majority are asymptomatic. Most infections are acquired from a conventional transfusion and develop between 2 to 26 weeks following the transfusion. Characteristically, the serum transaminases follow a fluctuating pattern, with variable intervals between peaks. Therefore, it may be difficult to define the termination of the acute illness. Although rare, fulminant hepatitis C seems to be more lethal than fulminant hepatitis A or B. The development of chronic hepatitis—persistence of increased enzyme values for 6 months or more—is of far greater concern. This outcome occurs in 50% of persons with transfusion-related non-A, non-B hepatitis.

Infection with the hepatitis D virus requires the helper function of other hepatotropic viruses. The hepatitis D virus can be acquired either as a co-primary infection with hepatitis B or as a superinfection in persons with established hepatitis B infection.

Although more than one agent may ultimately be shown to be responsible for enterically transmitted non-A, non-B hepatitis (hepatitis E), current information strongly suggests that a recently isolated RNA virus is

TABLE 62–1. Pathogens that May Cause Liver Infections

Viral Agents
Hepatitis A, B, C, D, E; cytomegalovirus; Epstein-Barr virus; herpes simplex virus; varicella; adenovirus; rubella and mumps viruses; echovirus; coxsackie B virus; reovirus; Marburg virus; Lassa fever virus; yellow fever virus; Rift Valley fever virus

Nonviral Agents
Bacterial agents
Escherichia coli, Streptococcus faecalis, Proteus vulgaris, Salmonella, staphylococci, Friedlander bacillus, *Pseudomonas, Clostridium welchii, Mycobacterium tuberculosis, Treponema pallidum, Leptospira interrogans*
Nonbacterial agents
Amoebiasis, actinomyces, candidiasis, aspergillosis, cryptococcosis, coccidimycosis, schistosomiasis, malaria, leishmaniasis, *Echinococcus granulosis, Toxocara canis* (visceral larva migrans), liver flukes (*Clonochis sinensis, Fasciola hepatica*)

TABLE 62–2. Hepatitis

FEATURE	A	B	PNANB (C)	D	ENANB (E)
Clinical Presentation					
Age group	Primarily young	All ages	All ages	All ages	Mostly adults
Onset	Abrupt	Insidious	Insidious	Insidious	Abrupt
Incubation period					
Range (days)	15–50	28–160	14–160		
Mean (days)	±30	±8	±50		
Symptoms					
Arthralgia, rash	Uncommon	Common	Uncommon	Uncommon	Common
Fever	Common	Uncommon	Uncommon	Common	Common
Nausea, vomiting	Common	Common	Common	Common	Common
Jaundice	+ +	+ +	+	+ + +	+ + +
Laboratory Data					
Duration of transaminase elevation	Short	Prolonged	Prolonged	Prolonged	
Increased (days)	3–49	35–200	?	?	?
Virus	RNA	DNA	RNA	RNA	RNA
Location of virus					
Blood	Transient	Prolonged	Prolonged	Prolonged	?Transient
Stool	Yes	No	No	No	Yes
Elsewhere	?	Yes	?	?	?
Outcome					
Mortality	Low, 1%	Low 1–3%	Low, 2%	High, 5%	Moderate, ±3%
Chronic hepatitis	No	Yes	Yes	Yes	No
Chronic carrier	No	Yes	Yes	Yes	No
Liver carrier	No	Yes	Possible	?	No
Relapse	Yes	Yes	?	?	?
Transmission					
Oral	+	±	?No	?No	+
Percutaneous	Rare	+	+	+	–
Sexual	+	+	–	+	
Perinatal	–	+	±	–	?
Animal models					
Marmosets	+	–	–		?
Chimpanzees	+	+	+	+	+

PNANB, parenteral non-A, non-B; ENANB, epidemic non-A, non-B.

With permission from Seeff LB: Diagnosis, therapy, and prognosis of viral hepatitis. In Zakim D, Boyer TD (eds): Hepatology: A Textbook of Liver Disease. Philadelphia, WB Saunders, 1990, pp 958–1025.

the major etiologic agent. Clinically, its behavior appears to resemble that of the hepatitis A virus.

Diagnosis. The diagnosis of viral hepatitis is based on the clinical course, elevations of serum bilirubin and liver enzymes, and appropriate serologic testing. The increase in serum bilirubin is mainly conjugated (direct) bilirubin during the early days of jaundice. The levels of bilirubin may reach 10 mg/dl or more and, as the disease progresses, there is a shift from conjugated to unconjugated (indirect) bilirubin. With the onset of jaundice, there is an increase in the urinary excretion of urobilinogen, only to later disappear from the urine when there is complete failure of bile to reach the intestine. During recovery, urobilinogen again appears in the urine in large amounts. Serum glutamic-oxaloacetic (AST) or glutamic-pyruvic (ALT) transaminase levels are elevated early, and their decrease indicates the end of active disease and the beginning of recovery. Serologic testing should include testing of blood for hepatitis B surface antigen (HB$_s$Ag), antibody to the hepatitis A virus (anti-HAV), antibody to hepatitis B surface antigen (anti-HB$_s$), antibody to hepatitis B core antigen (anti-HB$_c$), and antibody to hepatitis C (anti-HCV).

Differential Diagnosis. In the pre-icteric stage, hepatitis can be confused with other acute infectious diseases, with an acute surgical abdomen and with gastroenteritis. Bile in the urine, tender enlargement of the liver, and a rise in serum transaminases are helpful at this stage in distinguishing hepatitis from other diseases. Differentiation from infectious mononucleosis early in the course of the disease may be difficult (see Chapter 93 on mononucleosis). Distinguishing infectious hepatitis from drug-related disease such as accidental or intentional poisonings, prescribed drugs, and anesthetic agents depends largely on the medical history.

Treatment. There is no specific treatment for hepatitis A, B, C, D, or E, but supportive measures may be necessary. Prophylactic immunoglobulin for those individuals exposed to hepatitis A is recommended. Immunoprophylaxis with hepatitis B vaccine and with hepatitis B immune globulin is indicated for persons at high risk of hepatitis B infection, such as physicians and nurses.

Course of Illness and Prognosis. Fulminant hepatitis is rare in individuals less than 15 years of age. The frequency of fulminant hepatitis is greatest for non-A, non-B (hepatitis C), followed by hepatitis A and then hepatitis B. Survival is greatest in hepatitis A, followed by hepatitis B and non-A, non-B (hepatitis C). Fulminant hepatitis rarely may occur with infectious mononucleosis infection.

Among the types of liver disease caused by infectious agents is a syndrome associated with salpingitis referred to as gonococcal perihepatitis or the Fitz-Hugh–Curtis syndrome (see Chapter 75). At least two organisms, *Neisseria gonorrhoeae* and *Chlamydia trachomatis*, have been identified as the etiologic agents in this condition. The condition simulates acute cholecystitis, except that patients with cholecystitis are usually older, whereas those with perihepatitis are usually between the ages of 15 and 30 years. The presentation in a young woman with right upper quadrant abdominal pain may mimic acute viral hepatitis, drug-induced hepatitis, toxic shock syndrome (see Chapter 94), and hepatitis caused by various bacteria, including the treponemes. The patient usually has a mucopurulent cervicitis, uterine and adnexal tenderness on pelvic examination, and an abnormal ultrasound examination of the gallbladder. Treatment is with intravenous antibiotics directed against *N. gonorrhoeae* and *C. trachomatis* (see Chapter 75).

Genetic Diseases

CYSTIC FIBROSIS

The basic defect in this autosomally recessive inherited disease is the deletion of a single trinucleotide codon on the long arm of chromosome 7. Although most patients present with repeated pulmonary infections and failure to thrive, a small percentage of individuals may present with liver or gallbladder disease (see Chapter 43).

Pathophysiology. A number of gross and microscopic hepatic abnormalities have been described in cystic fibrosis (CF). Hepatic steatosis is probably the most frequent lesion. It is found in approximately 60% of CF patients. Fatty infiltration of the liver is also found in prolonged undernutrition; this is of note, because malnutrition is common in CF patients. Biliary fibrosis has been estimated to occur in 25% to 30% of patients dying with CF. Cirrhosis can be present in 5% of patients older than 12 years of age.

Sludge or stones in the biliary tract may lead to obstruction. Impairment of biliary drainage may be important in the pathogenesis of liver disease in CF. Strictures of the distal common bile duct have been found in up to 96% of patients with CF. Pancreatic fibrosis can also lead to partial biliary obstruction by compression of the distal common duct, as can a mucus plug in a shared pancreaticobiliary channel.

By adolescence the gallbladder may be shrunken and hypoplastic, with viscid bile in the lumen. Mucus cysts may also be found in the wall of that viscus. Gallstones occur in about 8% of patients, the risk being greater during adolescence and later.

Clinical Manifestations. Clinical manifestations include hepatomegaly early or a small shrunken liver with spelenomegaly later on. Jaundice is rarely present. End-stage liver disease may also be accompanied with ascites.

Diagnosis. Liver function tests have not proved to be very useful in detecting the presence or evaluating the progress of cirrhosis, because CF does not affect parenchymal cells directly and hepatic function may be well preserved, even in the face of long-standing portal hypertension. Because ultrasonography is not invasive, it is certainly worthwhile and may document portal venous obstruction. A liver biopsy is seldom necessary.

Differential Diagnosis. The differential diagnosis should include α_1-antitrypsin deficiency; liver involvement in α_1-antitrypsin deficiency tends to occur the first few years of life and not during adolescence. However, it is of note that several patients with CF have also had α_1-antitrypsin deficiency. Sclerosing cholangitis may also occur in the teenage years, but in many instances this disease is associated with inflammatory bowel disease (see Chapter 63) or is secondary to another chronic disease process. Wilson disease and chronic active hepatitis should be included in the differential diagnosis. It is of interest that recently liver injury has been noted after the oral and rectal administration of N-acetylcysteine for meconium ileus equivalent in an individual with CF.

Treatment. There is no specific treatment for liver disease secondary to CF other than liver transplantation.

Course of Illness and Prognosis. Liver disease in CF can stabilize or progress to cirrhosis. Approximately 10 patients with CF and hepatic disease have had liver transplants. These patients have had an increase in postoperative morbidity and mortality compared to other patients receiving liver transplants.

WILSON DISEASE

Pathophysiology. Wilson disease is transmitted as an autosomal recessive trait; the gene involved has recently been mapped to the long arm of chromosome 13. The prevalence rate of carriers of this disease (heterozygotes) is approximately 1 in 200. Although the basic effect in Wilson disease has not been elucidated, the pathologic effects in the liver, kidneys, brain, and other organs are considered to be directly related to the accumulation of copper in these organs.

Ingested copper is absorbed in the upper intestine and is rapidly removed by the liver. Once in the liver, the metal may follow one of three courses: (1) it may remain in the liver, bound to a metallothionein as storage copper; (2) it may be incorporated into the serum copper protein, ceruloplasmin; or (3) it may be excreted in the bile, its main excretory route. The defect in Wilson disease does not appear to be at the level of copper absorption or transport. Abnormal copper-binding protein in the liver has been claimed to be the primary metabolic defect. How this leads to toxic accumulation of the metal in other tissues once the protein has become saturated is not clear, unless there is also an excretory defect. One group of investigators speculates that at least part of the defect in copper metabolism in Wilson disease is due to failure to excrete excess copper into bile, which normally occurs via a ceruloplasmin-like protein. Additional studies are necessary to fully elucidate the defect(s) in this disorder of copper metabolism.

An acute hepatitis picture may occur early in the course of Wilson disease. Histopathologically, such an episode is characterized by ballooning degeneration, acidophilic bodies, cholestasis, and infiltration by a few lymphocytes. Biopsies obtained in the precirrhotic stage of Wilson disease reveal nonspecific changes that include focal necrosis, scattered acidophilic bodies, and moderate to marked steatosis. As the disease progresses, there is increasing periportal fibrosis and cholangiolar proliferation, and eventually cirrhosis. Portal inflammation is generally mild to moderate.

Clinical Manifestations. Wilson disease challenges the clinician's diagnostic acumen. Not only may the classic triad of Kayser-Fleischer rings, hepatic cirrhosis, and neurologic dysfunction be absent, but the serum ceruloplasmin level may be normal and not low. The liver slowly accumulates toxic amounts of copper, and any extrahepatic involvement (neurologic, ophthalmologic, renal, and so forth) does not occur until saturation and damage to the liver have occurred first. In one study, investigators reviewed the charts of 25 consecutive patients who were younger than 21 years of age; 18 patients had symptoms at the time of diagnosis, and seven were asymptomatic siblings. From these observations, it is apparent that in Wilson disease the progression to cirrhosis is often insidious.

Approximately 40% of Wilson disease patients present with chronic liver disease, often recognized because of elevations of serum aminotransferases or bilirubin concentrations. However, neuropsychiatric disorders, ranging from subtle personality changes and deteriorating academic performance to clinical depression and even psychosis, may occur. Neurologic symptoms include tremor, rigidity, gait abnormalities, slurred speech, drooling, and inappropriate and uncontrollable grinning (risus sardonicus). Approximately 10% of symptoms are psychiatric and 35% are neurologic. All patients with neuropsychiatric problems have the Kayser-Fleischer ring.

A few patients have their clinical course punctuated by recurring episodes of jaundice resulting from an undiagnosed hemolytic crisis. Such unexplained episodes of hemolysis should always be regarded as a possible sign of Wilson disease. The hemolytic episodes may eventually result in gallstones, which in turn may produce symptoms. Other uncommon presenting problems include hematuria, glycosuria and, in the pediatric patient, acute hepatitis with liver failure, hemolysis, and renal insufficiency (see Chapter 52).

Diagnosis. A low level or an absence of serum ceruloplasmin when serum protein values are normal implies homozygosity or, occasionally, heterozygosity for this disease. In a large series of adult cases, ceruloplasmin values of less than 20 to 22 mg/dl are noted in 95% of homozygotes and in 10% of heterozygotes. Values for serum copper generally parallel the level of serum ceruloplasmin, yet are abnormal (less than 80 μg/dl) in only 50% to 80% of patients. Normal or high values can be found, even in homozygotes for Wilson disease, and therefore this test alone is not diagnostic. The level of copper present in the urine, presumably in the form of amino acid–copper complexes, is usually high in Wilson disease.

Diagnosis of accumulation of copper in the lateral margin of the cornea (Kayser-Fleischer ring) is best made by an experienced ophthalmologist using a slit-lamp examination and is pathognomonic for Wilson disease. However, the presence of Kayser-Fleischer rings is a late finding and may be absent even if liver disease is severe. Nevertheless, every adolescent suspected of Wilson disease should have a slit-lamp examination.

Hepatic copper concentration is the "gold standard" in diagnosing this disease. Hepatic copper values greater than 50 μg/g of dry weight of liver tissue obtained by either percutaneous or open-liver biopsy are considered abnormal. Most patients with Wilson disease have hepatic copper levels greater than 250 μg/g dry weight of liver.

The role of radio-labeled copper in the diagnosis of Wilson disease has its greatest value in those unusual circumstances in which one must differentiate between non-Wilson liver disease with increased urine and liver copper concentrations, and Wilson disease with a normal ceruloplasmin level. However, this test should not serve as a substitute for the important aforementioned laboratory studies except when histologic examination and hepatic copper quantitation cannot be obtained.

Differential Diagnosis. The differential in this disease is the same as noted for CF. In addition, Wilson disease should be distinguished from Indian childhood cirrhosis, non-Indian childhood cirrhosis, and copper poisoning. When an adolescent presents with neuropsychiatric signs or symptoms associated with abnormal liver function studies, Wilson disease should be suspected.

Treatment. D-Penicillamine is the drug of choice. A low starting dose of 250 mg/day is recommended, because rapid mobilization of copper from tissue stores may cause acute hemolysis or deterioration of neurologic functions. Thereafter, 250-mg increments per week may be added until the adolescent is receiving 1000 to 1250 mg/day. Poor compliance because of gastric irritation may be a problem. Pyridoxine should be given to prevent pyridoxal phosphate deficiency.

The quantitative daily urine copper excretion values during treatment are generally one third or less of the pretreatment values after 6 to 12 months of therapy. Daily urine copper excretion values that remain at pretreatment levels should make one suspicious of noncompliance (see Chapter 26). The Kayser-Fleischer rings gradually disappear in most patients after 1 to 2 years of effective treatment.

Adolescents who have Wilson disease must be on a low copper diet, avoiding chocolate, cocoa, mushrooms, liver, shellfish, nuts, and dried fruits. Some investigators have used oral zinc to decrease the absorption of copper. Although zinc may be an effective treatment for Wilson disease, its place among currently available treatments remains disputed.

Course of Illness and Prognosis. The prognosis is excellent if the disease is diagnosed early and the copper deposition in the liver and extrahepatic tissues can be reversed by the aforementioned therapy. When the disease is treated early, there is a reduction in neurologic, psychiatric, and hepatic abnormalities, and some patients become asymptomatic.

Toxic or Drug-induced Injury

Adolescents and young adults are at increased additional risk of drug-induced liver disease because of their experimentation with and abuse of illicit drugs (see Chapter 111). Drug-induced liver disease is generally regarded as rare in children. The reason for the uncommonness of childhood drug hepatotoxicity is not certain. Underdiagnosis and underreporting remain a possibility. Another simple reason is that children take fewer medications, and they are free of many of the factors predisposing to drug hepatotoxicity, such as cigarette smoking and alcohol abuse.

ACETAMINOPHEN

Acetaminophen is increasingly used in suicide attempts (see Chapters 97 and 101). Approximately 10 g produces hepatic necrosis, but the dose actually ingested is difficult to assess because of early vomiting and unreliable histories. Alcohol and barbiturates, by their enzyme-inducing effect, enhance the hepatotoxicity of acetaminophen. Less than 10 g/day may produce significant hepatotoxicity in an alcoholic or someone with underlying liver disease. In severe malnutrition (including patients with eating disorders), toxicity may occur at lower doses because of decreased availability of glutathione (see below and Chapter 60).

Pathogenesis. The electrophilic metabolite of acetaminophen preferentially conjugates with hepatic glutathione. When the glutathione is exhausted, the acetaminophen metabolite reacts with essential cellular proteins, producing hepatic necrosis. Hepatic histology shows centrizonal necrosis, some fatty change, and very little inflammation. Reticulin collapse may be confluent and massive. Adolescents and adults are more susceptible to acetaminophen poisoning than are young children.

Clinical Manifestations. Within a few hours of ingestion, the adolescent becomes nauseated and vomits. Most remain conscious. After approximately 48 hours, recovery seems likely; then the adolescent deteriorates and becomes jaundiced about the third or fourth day, when the liver becomes tender. Serum transaminase levels and prothrombin time are increased. In the more seriously affected, deterioration is then rapid, with signs of acute hepatic necrosis. Myocardial and renal damage and hypoglycemia are prominent.

Long-term (about 1 year) exposure to acetaminophen (within the therapeutic upper limit of 4 g daily) may lead to chronic hepatitis. Underlying liver disease may potentiate the effect; chronic disease is also potentiated by alcoholism.

Diagnosis. If there is a history of acetaminophen ingestion, the severity can be assessed by acetaminophen blood levels, which should always be determined. If the plasma level 4 hours after the ingestion exceeds 300 μg/ml, hepatic toxicity is almost certain; and if it is less than 120 μg/ml, there is no danger. If the acetaminophen level 12 hours after the ingestion exceeds 50 μg/ml, hepatic toxicity is likely; if it is less than 50 μg/ml, there is no danger.

Differential Diagnosis. When there is no history of acetaminophen ingestion and blood levels of the medication are not detectable, other toxins and causes of hepatitis should be considered.

Treatment. The patient should be admitted to the hospital and the stomach lavaged. Charcoal followed in 1 hour by lavage may be useful prior to the use of N-acetylcysteine. Hepatic necrosis occurs insidiously;

therefore, the adolescent's early improvement should not give a false sense of security. Forced diuresis and renal dialysis do not increase the excretion of acetaminophen or its metabolites already bound to tissues. Treatment using N-acetylcysteine is aimed at replenishing hepatocyte glutathione reserves. It may be administered orally or intravenously, but only if it is initiated within the first 10 to 12 hours after acetaminophen ingestion will it influence morbidity and mortality. In malnourished patients, those with underlying liver disease, and those taking enzyme-inducing drugs, the use of N-acetylcysteine should be more liberal. All adolescents who attempt suicide by ingestion of acetaminophen, or any other means, deserve evaluation and treatment of psychosocial issues in addition to medical management.

Course of Illness and Prognosis. The overall mortality for 201 patients admitted to a general hospital was 3.5%. A prothrombin ratio of 20% and hepatic coma are unfavorable prognostic signs. Severity can also be assessed by acetaminophen blood concentrations, as noted above.

Acetaminophen, because of its frequent use by adolescents in intentional overdoses, is the most commonly encountered hepatotoxin in adolescents. There are many other potential prescription and nonprescription drugs and chemicals that cause injury to the liver. The substances of abuse that cause liver damage are addressed in Chapter 111.

The effect of hepatotoxins may in some cases be predictable, whereas in others they may be nonpredictable, or idiosyncratic, allergic, or immunologic. The predictable toxins, such as carbon tetrachloride, toluene, and other solvents, are usually toxic after short exposures and produce characteristic lesions. The nonpredictable toxins, such as chlorpromazine, isoniazid, and erythromycin estolate, do not produce lesions in experimental animals and usually require relatively prolonged exposure before hepatic toxicity is evident. Usually, liver toxicity is manifested by a variable response, from mild elevations of serum transaminases to fulminant hepatitis.

Neoplasms

Primary hepatic neoplasms account for only 0.5% to 2.0% of all pediatric tumors. In a review of the files of the Armed Forces Institute of Pathology of cases received between 1970 and 1986, 345 cases of the nine most common hepatic neoplasms were noted.

Pathophysiology and Clinical Manifestations. The pathophysiology and clinical manifestations depend on the type of tumor. Adolescents with tumors of the liver are commonly asymptomatic, and the tumors may be discovered only as an incidental finding at autopsy or during surgery for a non–liver-related procedure. Symptomatic adolescents, who account for fewer than 10% of patients, may present with episodic abdominal pain, weight loss, vomiting, or diarrhea. Physical findings related to the tumor are usually limited to abdominal distension or a palpable mass in the liver.

Diagnosis. Laboratory findings are usually unremarkable. However, there can be an increase in serum concentrations of lactic dehydrogenase, alkaline phosphatase, and aminotransferases. Increased alpha-fetoprotein values have been reported in some hepatic tumors (hepatoblastomas) but not in others. Imaging studies can be helpful in the diagnosis. Ultrasonography may demonstrate the tumor. Selective arteriography may display a mass and can be used to plan the surgical approach if needed.

Differential Diagnosis. Differential diagnosis includes those tumors listed in Table 62–3.

Treatment. Treatment may be surgical or nonsurgical. Nonsurgical modes of treatment include radiation and chemotherapy.

Course of Illness and Prognosis. The clinical course is dependent on the type of neoplasm and how early it is diagnosed. Adolescent females with liver tumors should avoid using birth control pills for contraception.

Miscellaneous Conditions

OBESITY (see Chapters 49 and 60)

Obesity has been estimated to affect one in three adolescents in the United States. The observation that obesity can cause abnormalities in serum liver enzymes of adults was recognized almost 4 decades ago. Recently, these changes have been documented in adolescents (see Chapter 60).

Pathophysiology. The hepatic damage associated with obesity is caused by fatty infiltration of the liver, which may progress to fibrosis and cirrhosis.

Clinical Manifestations. Obese adolescents with secondary hepatic abnormalities may present with nonspecific abdominal pain and vague right upper quadrant tenderness to palpation. Mildly elevated aminotransferases can occur in association with fatty infiltration of the liver and early fibrosis.

Diagnosis. In one study of 299 obese pediatric patients

TABLE 62–3. Classification of Hepatic Tumors in Adolescents

BEHAVIOR	ORIGIN	NEOPLASM
Benign	Hepatocellular	Focal nodular hyperplasia
		Nodular regenerative hyperplasia
		Hepatocellular adenoma
	Mesodermal	Mesenchymal hamartoma
		Cavernous hemangioma
		Infantile hemangioendothelioma
	Other	Teratoma
Malignant	Hepatocellular	Hepatoblastoma
		Hepatocellular carcinoma
	Mesodermal	Undifferentiated "embryonal" sarcoma
		Embryonal rhabdomyosarcoma
		Angiosarcoma
		Rhabdoid tumor
		Leiomyosarcoma
		Endodermal sinus (yolk sac) tumor
	Other	Teratoma

With permission from Stocker, JT: Hepatic tumors. In Balestreri WF, Stocker JT (eds): Pediatric Hepatology. New York, Hemisphere Publishing, 1990, pp 399–488.

referred to an obesity clinic for evaluation, 16% of the boys and 9% of the girls had elevated levels of serum transaminases. A history of acute or chronic liver disease or transfusion of blood in the past was excluded in all these patients. The highest incidence of liver dysfunction was noted in 12- to 14-year-old boys and 10- to 12-year-old girls.

Differential Diagnosis. Other diseases that may cause fatty infiltration of the liver include diabetes mellitus, cholesteryl ester storage disease, alcoholism, corticosteroids, and hyperlipidemic states.

Treatment and Course of Illness and Prognosis. Treatment is weight reduction. Numerous investigators have shown that the elevated serum transaminases return to normal with appropriate weight reduction.

CHRONIC HEPATITIS

Every type of chronic hepatitis meets certain clinical, biochemical, and histologic criteria. The common types of chronic hepatitis include those caused by hepatitis B; non-A, non-B hepatitis (hepatitis C); α_1-antitrypsin deficiency; cytomegalovirus; rubella virus; Wilson disease; drugs; toxins; alcohol abuse; and autoimmune hepatitis.

Pathophysiology. The pathophysiology depends on the cause.

Clinical Manifestations. Clinically, symptoms range from none to incapacitating exhaustion. Fluctuating jaundice is usual. Features of clinically diagnosable and symptomatic portal hypertension (ascites, bleeding esophageal varices) appear late in the disease.

Diagnosis. Biochemical tests show a variably elevated serum bilirubin level. Serum transaminase values are usually markedly increased and the gamma globulin concentration is also elevated. Hepatic histology shows the features of chronic hepatitis. A common clinical biochemical and hepatic histologic picture has been associated with more than one etiologic agent. Two main types have been identified. One is associated with persistence of hepatitis B infection; the other is associated with a negative result for hepatitis B, but has been termed lupoid or autoimmune because of the association with a positive lupus erythematosus (LE) cell phenomenon in some 15% of patients and with positive serum autoantibodies (see later).

Differential Diagnosis. Differential diagnosis includes the diseases noted above.

Treatment. Treatment is dependent on the cause. Interferon may be helpful in chronic hepatitis caused by the hepatitis C virus. Steroids and immunosuppressive agents may be useful in treating autoimmune hepatitis.

Course of Illness and Prognosis. The prognosis is related to cause and response to therapy.

AUTOIMMUNE (LUPOID) HEPATITIS

As early as 1950, Waldenstrom described an autoimmune-type chronic hepatitis as a disease of young women associated with hypergammaglobulinemia and responsive to corticosteroid therapy. We now know that there are at least three subtypes of autoimmune hepatitis.

Pathophysiology and Clinical Manifestations. Immunologic changes are conspicuous. Serum gamma-globulin levels are grossly elevated. The finding of a (1) positive LE cell test in about 15% led to the term lupoid hepatitis, and (2) antibodies against nuclei, smooth muscle, and mitochondria are also found in a high proportion of patients. Autoimmune chronic hepatitis, or lupoid hepatitis, is not the same as classic systemic lupus erythematosus (SLE), for the liver rarely shows any lesions in classic lupus. Moreover, the smooth muscle antibody and the mitochondrial antibody are not present in the blood of patients with SLE.

Lupoid hepatitis occurs predominantly in young people: one half of patients present between 10 and 20 years of age. Three quarters are female. It is unclear whether the disease can be initiated by acute viral hepatitis, or whether this is simply an intercurrent infection in an adolescent with long-standing chronic hepatitis. Antibody to hepatitis C virus has recently been shown to be associated with some forms of autoimmune hepatitis. Autoimmune hepatitis may remain asymptomatic for months or possibly years before jaundice becomes overt and the diagnosis is made. Although the serum bilirubin level is usually increased, some patients are anicteric. Frank jaundice is often episodic. Rarely, deep cholestatic jaundice is seen. Amenorrhea is usual, and regular menses are a good prognostic sign. However, if menses occur, they may be associated with an increase of symptoms and deepening of jaundice. Epistaxis, bleeding gums, and bruising with minimal trauma are other complaints.

Diagnosis. The adolescent with this disease is often female, of above-average stature, well-proportioned, and healthy-appearing. Spider nevi are virtually always present, occurring frequently on the face, necklace area, and arms. Autoantibodies are important diagnostic markers for autoimmune-type chronic active hepatitis. At least three subgroups can be distinguished serologically. Antinuclear antibodies, smooth muscle antibodies, and liver membrane autoantibodies characterize classic autoimmune-type or lupoid hepatitis. Liver–kidney–microsomal antibodies identify a second type, and antibodies to a soluble liver antigen are present in a third subgroup of autoimmune chronic active hepatitis.

Differential Diagnosis. The differential diagnosis includes those diseases considered in the discussion of chronic hepatitis.

Treatment. It is not surprising that drugs which alter immunologic processes have been used therapeutically in this type of hepatitis, such as corticosteroids with or without azathioprine. The indications for commencing steroids remain ill defined. However, if the adolescent is symptomatic and has very high serum transaminase and gamma globulin levels, and if severe chronic active hepatitis is seen on liver biopsy, steroids are indicated.

Course of Illness and Prognosis. Chronic hepatitis results in cirrhosis with very few exceptions. In a long-term follow-up of patients in the Royal Free Hospital trial of steroid therapy, the 10-year survival for the treated group was 63%, compared with 27% in the control group. Mortality is greatest during the first 2 years, when the disease is most active. Corticosteroid therapy prolongs life, but most patients eventually develop cirrhosis. Esophageal varices are an uncommon

initial finding. Nevertheless, bleeding from esophageal varices and hepatocellular failure are the usual causes of death.

PANCREAS
Acute Pancreatitis

There are a number of infectious agents (Table 62–4) and toxins, particularly alcohol and drugs (Table 62–5), which may cause pancreatitis in adolescents. Congenital abnormalities of the bile ductal system or pancreas may also predispose an individual to pancreatitis. Finally, obstruction to pancreatic flow (gallstones, tumors, and so forth) and systemic diseases (diabetes mellitus [see Chapter 59], hyperlipidemic states [see Chapters 49 and 60], systemic lupus erythematosus [see Chapter 90], and Crohn disease [see Chapter 63]) may be associated with pancreatitis.

Pathophysiology. It is generally agreed that acute pancreatitis is caused by autodigestion of the pancreas as a result of inappropriate activation of pancreatic zymogens to active enzymes within the pancreatic parenchyma. The pathologic changes within the pancreatic parenchyma support this concept, as do animal models of pancreatic inflammation that have similar clinical and morphologic findings. The conditions whereby pancreatic enzymes are activated or the sequence of events required to trigger these events remains uncertain.

Clinical Manifestations. Acute pancreatitis in adolescents can be associated with a wide range of symptoms and complications. As is frequently the case in adults, abdominal pain is the outstanding symptom, but on rare occasions pain may be absent. Typically, pain is sudden in onset, increases gradually in severity, and reaches

TABLE 62–4. Infectious Agents Associated with Acute Pancreatitis

Bacteria
Salmonella typhi
Verocytotoxin-producing *Escherichia coli**
Mycoplasma
Leptospira interrogans
Viruses
Mumps
Coxsackie B
Echovirus
Influenza A
Influenza B†
Varicella†
Epstein-Barr
Rubeola
Hepatitis A
Hepatitis B
Rubella
Parasites
Malaria
Ascariasis (duct obstruction)
Clonorchis sinensis (duct obstruction)

*Associated with the hemolytic-uremic syndrome.
†Associated with Reye syndrome.
With permission from Walker WA, Durie PR, Hamilton JR, Walker-Smith JA, Watkins JB (eds): Pediatric Gastrointestinal Disease. Pathophysiology, Diagnosis, Management. Philadelphia, BC Decker, 1991, p 1216.

TABLE 62–5. Drugs and Toxic Agents Associated with Acute Pancreatitis

Therapeutic Agents
  Definite
    Chlorthiazides
    Furosemide
    Tetracyclines
    Sulfonamides
    Estrogens
    6-Mercaptopurine
    L-Asparaginase
    Valproic acid
  Possible
    Corticosteroids
    Nonsteroidal anti-inflammatory agents
    Methyldopa
    Phenformin
    Nitrofurantoin
    Azathioprine
    Metronidazole

Nontherapeutic (poisons, drug abuse, or overdose)
    Ethyl alcohol
    Methyl alcohol
    Heroin
    Amphetamines
    Organophosphate insecticides
    Acetaminophen overdose
    Iatrogenic hypercalcemia

With permission from Walker WA, Durie PR, Hamilton JR, Walker-Smith JA, Watkins JB (eds): Pediatric Gastrointestinal Disease. Pathophysiology, Diagnosis, Management. Philadelphia, BC Decker, 1991, p 1216.

maximal intensity after a few hours. In a review of pediatric cases from one center; pain was most commonly located in the epigastrium. Other frequent symptoms include anorexia, nausea, and persistent vomiting. Eating was found to be a common aggravating factor of pain and vomiting.

The most frequent physical finding is epigastric tenderness, and this finding is frequently seen with decreased or absent bowel sounds. Abdominal distention, hypotension or shock, low-grade fever, leukocytosis, pleural effusion, ascites, and oliguria may also be present. Thus, pancreatitis simulates an "acute surgical abdomen."

Diagnosis. Serum amylase values are elevated within hours of the onset of acute pancreatitis, and in uncomplicated cases they may remain elevated 3 to 5 days. However, the serum amylase may be only transiently elevated, returning to normal in 48 to 72 hours, even in the presence of continuing inflammation of the pancreas. Contributing to the difficulty of using serum amylase alone as an indicator of pancreatitis is that up to 30% of patients with pancreatitis have a normal serum amylase. A protracted elevation in serum amylase raises the suspicion of a local complication such as a pseudocyst or, alternatively, a pancreatic tumor or macroamylasemia. Sonography of the pancreas enables visualization of the organ without subjecting the adolescent to ionizing radiation or the complications of invasive angiography. Considerable data have been accumulated in support of the argument that sonography is the method of choice in the diagnostic evaluation of any adolescent suspected of acute or chronic pancreatitis. Abdominal computed tomography (CT) should be reserved for difficult cases and situations in which sonography yields unclear information.

Endoscopic retrograde cholangiopancreatography (ERCP) is an invaluable diagnostic tool for the investigation of patients with pancreatic disease. Increasing experience with this technique in adolescents shows it to be a relatively safe and valuable diagnostic and therapeutic procedure in those with pancreatic and biliary tract disease.

Differential Diagnosis. Differential diagnosis includes pancreatic tumors, cholecystitis, cholelithiasis, congenital abnormalities of the pancreatic and biliary tree such as choledochal cysts, stenosis of the bile and pancreatic ducts, annular pancreas, and stenosis of the ampulla of Vater. Peptic ulcer disease, gastritis, and gastroesophageal reflux should also be considered. One group of investigators reported a series of ten adolescents and children with cystic fibrosis who had recurrent attacks of pancreatitis, but no evidence of pancreatic insufficiency.

Treatment. A variety of specific and nonspecific therapeutic approaches have been advocated for acute pancreatitis; some are based on considerations of the pathophysiology of pancreatitis, but most treat disease symptoms and complications. At present, clinicians generally recommend that adolescents fast and insert nasogastric tubes as standard procedures; in adolescents with vomiting or paralytic ileus, this approach seems appropriate. Nonspecific measures designed to reduce duodenal acidification (antacids or histamine antagonists) may be useful for the treatment or prevention of stress ulceration, particularly if gastrointestinal bleeding is present. Other measures designed to reduce secretion of acid or reduce pancreatic flow, which include anticholinergics, glucagon, and vasopressin, are of unproven benefit.

Surgery in adolescents with acute pancreatitis is generally contraindicated. Exceptions include (1) uncertainty of the diagnosis of acute pancreatitis, (2) decompression of obstruction in the main pancreatic ducts or distal common bile duct (congenital or acquired), (3) correction of abdominal complications (e.g., cysts, abscesses), and (4) surgical measures to ameliorate the acute phase of the disease.

Course of Illness and Prognosis. The course of pancreatitis can be protracted. Recurrence and prognosis depend on cause.

Recurrent Pancreatitis

Recurrent pancreatitis is defined clinically as a condition characterized by recurring or persisting abdominal pain, with development of pancreatic exocrine or endocrine insufficiency in some patients.

Pathophysiology. Morphologically, the pancreas shows irregular sclerosis and focal, segmental, or diffuse destruction of exocrine tissue. Frequently, there are deformities of the pancreatic ducts as well as intraductal plugs containing protein or calculi. These changes are considered to be irreversible and progressive, with the exception of obstructive chronic pancreatitis, in which there may be partial or complete restitution if the obstruction is removed.

Clinical Manifestations. The clinical manifestations, diagnosis, and differential diagnosis are similar to those of acute pancreatitis.

Diagnosis. The diagnosis is made by employing the evaluation described under acute pancreatitis. Recurrent bouts of acute pancreatitis establish the diagnosis.

Differential Diagnosis. Differential diagnosis includes hereditary pancreatitis, choledochal cysts, pancreas divisum, familial hypocalciuric hypercalcemia, and sphincter of Oddi dysfunction.

Treatment. Treatment of acute episodes is noted above. Surgery is necessary when pseudocysts are present. Endoscopic retrograde cholangiopancreatography should be seriously considered if surgery is contemplated.

Course of Illness and Prognosis. The course and prognosis are dependent on cause.

Hereditary Pancreatitis

Hereditary pancreatitis was first described in 1952. Early studies raised doubts about the mode of inheritance, but subsequent reports have confirmed an autosomal dominant pattern of inheritance. The degree of penetrance appears to vary according to the pedigree studied. Differentiation from other forms of pancreatitis is usually not difficult, because of the early onset of symptoms and the presence of multiple affected relatives.

Pathophysiology. Most pathologic examinations have been done in patients with long-standing pancreatitis. Nonspecific changes are seen that do not differ from other forms of chronic or recurrent pancreatitis. Gross examination of autopsy specimens reveals a shrunken, fibrotic pancreas, frequently with small proteinaceous plugs and calculi within the pancreatic ducts. Light microscopy reveals extensive interstitial fibrosis, with nearly total acinar atrophy but relative preservation of normally appearing islets. The pathologic features of this disease of the pancreas are considered to resemble those seen in CF (see Chapter 43).

Clinical Manifestations. Males and females appear to be affected equally. Symptoms usually begin at 10 to 12 years of age, and by 20 years of age up to 75% of patients are symptomatic. Symptoms can, however, begin in adulthood. Severe pain due to attacks of acute pancreatitis is the most common first symptom. Pain is frequently initiated by a large meal, alcohol, or stress. The character of the pain is no different from pancreatic pain of any other cause, and is usually accompanied by nausea and vomiting. Spontaneous resolution of acute symptoms generally occurs over a period of 4 to 8 days. Severe hemorrhagic pancreatitis is rare, but if it occurs it is more likely during the first or second acute attack. Between episodes, adolescents are well but usually experience recurrent episodes of pain. The time interval between attacks of pain is variable and may range from weeks to years. Likewise, the intensity of abdominal pain during the attacks varies from mild to incapacitating.

Diagnosis. Hereditary pancreatitis is relatively easy to diagnose when adolescents first present with florid symptoms of acute pancreatitis and there is a strong family history. Routine urine and blood tests are usually normal, unless the adolescent has diabetes mellitus. Serum amylase, lipase, and trypsinogen concentrations may be normal between attacks. Adolescents experiencing acute pancreatitis and those with pancreatic pseudocysts or pancreatic ascites commonly show elevations of serum pancreatic enzymes. Plain radiographs of the abdomen may reveal diffuse or focal pancreatic calcification. Barium contrast studies are insensitive and nonspecific and are no longer used for routine evaluation of chronic pancreatic disease. Abdominal ultrasound and CT may show changes consistent with chronic pancreatic disease. Endoscopic retrograde cholangiopancreatography has been used in the diagnosis and management of adolescent patients with recurrent pancreatic disease.

Differential Diagnosis. Other diseases that should be considered are the same as are noted for recurrent pancreatitis.

Treatment. Treatment of uncomplicated hereditary pancreatitis is usually medical. If a predisposing factor is identified, it may be modified or eliminated by medical or surgical intervention. Attacks of pancreatitis are usually more severe initially, but with an increase in disease duration symptoms become milder. Treatment should be conservative, with bowel rest and restriction of food and fluids by mouth.

Course of Illness and Prognosis. Pseudocysts may occur, and usually arise within the pancreas and frequently communicate with the pancreatic duct. These collections of fluid are not encapsulated within epithelium-lined walls. True epithelium-lined pancreatic cysts are rare. Pancreatic pseudocysts frequently resolve with no management. Those that remain for longer than 6 weeks are unlikely to resolve, and in most instances drainage, either surgically or by needle aspiration, is required. Perforation of a pseudocyst into the free peritoneal cavity produces severe pain and abdominal rigidity because of intense chemical peritonitis, which is often fatal. Emergency laparotomy should be performed with irrigation of the peritoneal cavity and drainage of the cyst if this occurs.

Pancreatic Tumors

Carcinoma of the pancreas is increasing in incidence and affecting a younger population. However, pancreatic carcinoma in children younger than 15 years of age is still considered a rarity.

Pathophysiology. The cause of pancreatic carcinoma is probably multifactorial. The increasing incidence in the adult population suggests that environmental agents may play an important role in the rate of neoplastic transformation. Factors implicated include wine drinking, cigarette smoking, increased consumption of animal fat and protein, ingestion of chemically decaffeinated coffee, and exposure to chemical carcinogens. Genetic predisposition may play a relatively significant role in the occurrence of pediatric and adolescent pancreatic carcinoma.

Clinical Manifestations. The age distribution of pancreatic tumors is equal throughout childhood and adolescence. Of 40 patients, the most frequent presentation was abdominal mass; the most frequent complaint was abdominal pain. In adult patients, the typical description of pain is epigastric, dull, and aching, with radiation to the back. Nausea, vomiting, anorexia, weight loss, and a metallic taste are accompanying symptoms. Although obstruction of the common bile duct occurs frequently in the late presentation of adult carcinoma, causing jaundice in more than 50% of patients, pale stools, dark urine, pruritus, and a distended palpable gallbladder (Courvoisier sign); this constellation is less common in children. Jaundice occurs in only one quarter of pediatric patients, and Courvoisier sign was rarely reported.

Diagnosis. No tumor markers to date can specifically identify or exclude the diagnosis of pancreatic exocrine carcinoma. Some patients do have elevated carcinoembryonic antigen, alpha-fetoprotein, and human chorionic gonadotropin, but these are nonspecific and not consistently present. Widening and distortion of the duodenum with displacement of the stomach on upper gastrointestinal barium series in large tumors involving the head of the pancreas can often be appreciated, but this remains a poor diagnostic screening test.

Diagnosis depends largely on the use of abdominal ultrasonography and CT to visualize a pancreatic mass. The sensitivity and specificity of these investigations exceed 80%. Their limitation in detecting tumor is restricted to small foci of malignancy (less than 2 cm). Endoscopic retrograde cholangiopancreatography, allowing visualization of the pancreatic ductal system, may be sensitive enough to detect even smaller mass lesions, because they often occlude or distort the ductal system.

Differential Diagnosis. Differential diagnosis includes those diseases listed under the differential for acute pancreatitis.

Treatment. Despite the very poor 5-year survival rate for adults, aggressive surgical resection to date is the only form of treatment that has resulted in long-term survival. In adolescents, the more limited experience has tended to support a radical surgical approach to pancreatic carcinoma. Palliative surgery, chemotherapy, and radiotherapy have not been particularly helpful.

However, radiotherapy followed by a "second-look" procedure aimed at radical resection is an alternative in some cases.

Course of Illness and Prognosis. The course and prognosis are dependent on the type of neoplasm and the extent of organ involvement.

BIBLIOGRAPHY

Blustein PK, Gaskin K, Filler R, et al: Endoscopic retrograde cholangiopancreatography in pancreatitis in children and adolescents. Pediatrics 68:387, 1981.

Comfort MW, Steinberg AG: Pedigree of a family with hereditary chronic relapsing pancreatitis. Gastroenterology 21:54, 1952.

Iyengar V, Brewer GJ, Dick RD, et al: Studies of cholecystokinnin-stimulated biliary secretions reveal a high molecular weight copper binding substance in normal subjects that is absent in patients with Wilson's disease. J Lab Clin Med 111:267, 1988.

Kinugasa A, Tsunamoto K, Furukawa N, et al: Fatty liver and its fibrous changes found in simple obesity of children. J Pediatr Gastroenterol Nutr 3:408, 1984.

Lebenthal E (ed): Textbook of Gastroenterology and Nutrition in Infancy. New York, Raven Press, 1989.

Lefkowitch JH, Honig CL, King ME, et al: Hepatic copper overload and features of Indian childhood cirrhosis in an American sibship. N Engl J Med 307:271, 1982.

McDonald GSA, Courtney MG, Shattock AG, et al: Prolonged IgM antibodies and histopathological evidence of chronicity in hepatitis A. Liver 9:223, 1989.

Moran JR, Ghishan FK, Halter SA, et al: Steatohepatitis in obese children: A cause of chronic liver dysfunction. Am J Gastroenterol 78:374, 1983.

Reyes GR, Purdy MA, Kim JP, et al: Isolation of a cDNA from the virus responsible for enterically transmitted non-A, non-B hepatitis. Science 247:1335, 1990.

Schwachman H, Lebenthal E, Khaw KT: Recurrent acute pancreatitis in patients with cystic fibrosis with normal pancreatic enzymes. Pediatrics 55:86, 1975.

Seef LB: Diagnosis, therapy, and prognosis of viral hepatitis. In Zakim D, Boyer TD (eds): Hepatology: A Textbook of Liver Disease. Philadelphia, WB Saunders, 1990, pp 958–1025.

Sherlock S: Chronic hepatitis. In Diseases of the Liver and Biliary System. Oxford, Blackwell Scientific, 1985, pp 280–303.

Stocker JT: Hepatic tumors. In Balestreri WF, Stocker JT (eds): Pediatric Hepatology. New York, Hemisphere Publishing, 1990, pp 399–488.

Walker WA, Durie PR, Hamilton JR, Walker-Smith JA, Watkins JB (eds): Pediatric Gastrointestinal Disease. Pathophysiology, Diagnosis, Management. Philadelphia, B. C. Decker, 1991.

Werlin SL, Grand RJ, Perman JA: Diagnostic dilemmas of Wilson's disease: Diagnosis and treatment. Pediatrics 62:47, 1978.

CHAPTER 63

Inflammatory Bowel Disease

JAMES F. MARKOWITZ and FREDRIC DAUM

Inflammatory bowel disease (IBD) includes both ulcerative colitis and Crohn disease. These idiopathic conditions, characterized by chronic inflammation of the gastrointestinal tract, frequently present during the second decade of life. Ulcerative colitis has been widely recognized for over 100 years. Comprehensive descriptions of Crohn disease date to the 1930s, and even the earliest papers include adolescent subjects. Both conditions result in frequently relapsing, often debilitating symptoms that can interfere with normal growth, sexual maturation, and psychosocial development.

Ulcerative colitis and Crohn disease represent distinct pathologic entities, but in clinical practice, symptoms and signs are often indistinguishable. The two illnesses can usually be distinguished by the extent and depth of the intestinal inflammatory process. Ulcerative colitis is defined by a chronic inflammatory reaction limited to the mucosa and submucosa of the colon. By definition, it is a process isolated to the colon or at times the very terminal ileum ("backwash ileitis"). By contrast, Crohn disease is a chronic, inflammatory reaction that is transmural. Characteristically, Crohn disease can affect any portion of the gastrointestinal tract between the mouth and the anus. Despite these clear-cut differences, however, in practice there is often sufficient overlap when inflammation is restricted to the colon to make differentiation difficult or impossible.

EPIDEMIOLOGY

Incidence and prevalence rates for ulcerative colitis and Crohn disease in adolescent populations have not been determined. In the general population, estimates of the summed annual incidence of both conditions range from 5 to 10 new cases per 100,000 population. Data from the University of Chicago (Figs. 63–1 and 63–2) suggest that 30% to 40% of all cases of both ulcerative colitis and Crohn disease present at between 10 and 20 years of age. This represents a significant number of newly diagnosed adolescents. Since these diseases are rarely fatal, prevalence rates of 10 to 100 per 100,000 of the general population have been estimated. Although the incidence of ulcerative colitis has remained stable over the years, the incidence of Crohn disease inexplicably appears to be increasing worldwide.

A number of factors appear to predispose to the development of IBD. Among children and adolescents with IBD, family studies consistently note that about 15% of patients have similarly affected first-degree relatives, and 30% to 35% have more distant relatives with IBD. Racial and ethnic factors also appear important. Whites are more often afflicted than blacks. Certain ethnic groups, especially Ashkenazic Jews living in North America, also appear to have an increased frequency of IBD. However, in other parts of the world, including Israel, this predilection is much less apparent. Socioeconomic factors do not appear to be particularly important, nor does an urban versus a rural setting. Similarly, studies of HLA or ABO groups have generally not demonstrated any consistent association with either ulcerative colitis or Crohn disease.

ETIOLOGY AND PATHOGENESIS

The cause or causes of both ulcerative colitis and Crohn disease remain elusive. No naturally occurring disease resembling Crohn disease has been described, and attempts at inducing chronic intestinal inflammation by a variety of chemical, infectious, and immunologic mechanisms have not resulted in an appropriate animal model. In ulcerative colitis, the search for an etiology may be closer at hand because a naturally occurring animal model in the cotton-top tamarin has been described.

Investigations on the pathogenesis of IBD focus on mechanisms involved in the regulation of gastrointestinal immune response, including possibly defective suppression of gut-associated lymphoid tissue or immune hyperresponsiveness. The role of inflammatory mediators is also being intensively investigated. Although data exist suggesting that there may be increased macromolecular absorption from the gastrointestinal tract in patients with Crohn disease and their unaffected relatives, no conclusive data linking allergic phenomena with the pathogenesis of Crohn disease have been reported. An infectious etiology for Crohn disease has received renewed attention with the identification of new strains of cell wall–deficient mycobacteria that have been isolated from a number of surgical specimens obtained from patients with Crohn disease. However, serologic studies of Crohn disease populations have not demonstrated any consistent evidence of antimycobacterial antibodies. Theories of psychosomatic etiologies for both ulcerative colitis and Crohn disease have also not been supported by carefully controlled studies.

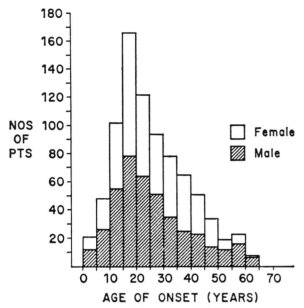

Figure 63–1. Age at onset of ulcerative colitis. (With permission from Rogers BH, Clark LM, Kirsner JB: The epidemiologic and demographic characteristics of inflammatory bowel disease: An analysis of a computerized file of 1400 patients. Chronic Dis 24:747, 1971. Copyright 1971, Pergamon Press.)

CLINICAL FEATURES

Common Symptoms

The symptoms manifested by adolescents with IBD are determined by the site and extent of their intestinal inflammation. Adolescent patients with Crohn disease isolated to the colon may be indistinguishable from those with ulcerative colitis. With extensive or universal colonic involvement, adolescents commonly present with severe cramps and diarrhea. Rectal bleeding can be seen with either form of colitis, but in our experience severe hemorrhage requiring multiple transfusions is more common in ulcerative colitis. Intermittent fevers are common in both diseases. Although acute weight loss is frequent, evidence of long-standing growth failure in ulcerative colitis is unusual at the time of diagnosis. When disease is restricted to the rectosigmoid or left colon, however, weight loss and other systemic symptoms are often absent. In these adolescent patients, a mild increase in the number of daily stools, a change toward a more loose stool consistency, and occasional blood per rectum may be the only symptoms. Tenesmus and urgency commonly suggest active proctitis, which may occasionally be manifested by constipation.

When Crohn disease affects the small intestine, as it does in 75% of cases, symptoms are often different. Patients frequently have cramps, but diarrhea may not be present. Although stools are often positive for occult blood, frank bleeding is less common. By contrast, systemic features, including fevers, are common, as are tender abdominal masses. Dyspeptic features such as nausea, vomiting, or heartburn may arise from Crohn disease affecting the upper gastrointestinal tract or may be the result of partial intestinal obstruction. With extensive small bowel involvement, a decrease in linear as well as ponderal growth is evident on review of old growth records in as many as 80% of cases. In addition, a delay in the onset of puberty or an arrest of ongoing sexual development may occur (see Chapter 57).

A variety of other presentations are often seen in adolescents with Crohn disease. Occasional adolescent patients come to medical attention because of fever of unknown origin. Others are evaluated for short stature and have no identifiable gastrointestinal symptoms. Between 1% and 2% of adolescents present with the acute onset of symptoms indistinguishable from acute appendicitis. The diagnosis is commonly made by the surgeon at the time of exploratory laparotomy when an acutely inflamed terminal ileum is identified.

Extraintestinal manifestations (Table 63–1) occur in both conditions, although they are more common in Crohn disease. Transient arthralgias occur in 10% or more of adolescent patients, while frank, nondeforming, asymmetric arthritis is present in less than 5%. Rashes including erythema nodosum, cutaneous vasculitis, and pyoderma gangrenosum have been described, as have uveitis, spondylitis, and glomerulonephritis. Other "autoimmune" disorders, including chronic active hepatitis and thyroiditis, have also been associated with IBD. The most common extraintestinal manifestations of Crohn disease are chronic perianal fissures and tags, the latter often being confused with external hemorrhoids. These lesions occur in approximately 50% of children and adolescents with Crohn disease. Less frequent, but more debilitating, are perianal fistulae and abscesses. These lesions may be highly destructive and are often resistant to treatment.

Growth Failure

The feature of Crohn disease in the preadolescent and adolescent that most distinguishes it from the adult form is the deleterious effect of the disease on growth and

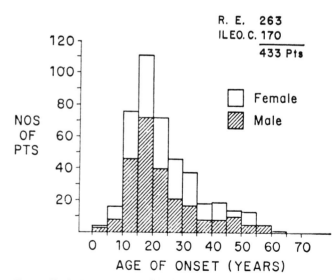

Figure 63–2. Age at onset of Crohn disease. (R.E., regional enteritis; ILEO.C., ileocolitis) (With permission from Rogers BH, Clark LM, Kirsner JB: The epidemiologic and demographic characteristics of inflammatory bowel disease: An analysis of a computerized file of 1400 patients. Chronic Dis 24:750, 1971. Copyright 1971, Pergamon Press.)

**TABLE 63–1. Extraintestinal Manifestations
of Inflammatory Bowel Disease**

Oropharynx
  Aphthous stomatitis
  Gingivitis
  Tonsillitis
Perineum
  Chronic anal fissures
  Hypertrophic anal tags
  Chronic draining fistulae (rectocutaneous, rectovaginal)
  Abscesses
Intra-abdominal
  Abscess (hepatic, splenic, psoas)
  Pancreatitis
  Sclerosing cholangitis
  Chronic active hepatitis (autoimmune type)
  Complicated internal and/or enterocutaneous fistulas
Skin
  Vasculitis
  Erythema nodosum
  Pyoderma gangrenosum
Joints
  Arthralgias
  Nondeforming arthritis
Hematologic
  Thrombosis
Renal
  Nephrolithiasis
  Glomerulonephritis
Eyes
  Uveitis
  Iritis
Systemic
  Fever
  Amyloidosis

sexual development. Although maldigestion and malabsorption of nutrients may play a small role, the primary reason for growth failure in the adolescent with IBD is inadequate nutritional intake. For puberty to progress, and for the expected associated adolescent growth spurt to be achieved, the adolescent with IBD must consume 75 to 90 kcal/kg/day (see Chapter 6). These amounts are often impossible for the adolescent with IBD to achieve. Eating often initiates cramps and diarrhea, resulting in an unconscious avoidance of eating. Many patients also complain of a sense of bloating

or early satiety when they attempt to eat "normal" amounts. Adolescents often consume no more than 60% to 70% of their recommended daily caloric intake but maintain adequate protein intake (see Chapter 7). Micronutrient intakes, especially of calcium and vitamin D, are also commonly inadequate (Fig. 63–3). This deficient dietary intake may precede obvious intestinal symptoms by many months or years. The result is that many adolescents develop nutritional dwarfing, with apparently appropriate weights for heights. These adolescents may fall across more than two or three major percentile curves and frequently manifest complete cessation of linear growth, failure to achieve expected height (Fig. 63–4), or delayed puberty, each with significant psychosocial implications.

Common Signs

PHYSICAL FINDINGS

In the adolescent with mild to moderate ulcerative colitis or Crohn disease, results of a physical examination are often normal. With more active disease abdominal tenderness or localized peritoneal findings can be found. Palpable, mildly tender loops of bowel may be present, especially in the right lower quadrant of the adolescent with ileitis. Varying degrees of subcutaneous wasting occur as nutritional intake, absorption, or both are compromised.

Perianal disease is present in about 50% of adolescents with Crohn disease, half of whom have perianal fissures and tags. Anal fissures are often deep and blue, yet less painful than stercoraceous fissures. Perianal tags can be confused with external hemorrhoids, but the latter lesions are rare in the adolescent (with the exception of the pregnant teenager). Tags are readily distinguished from venereal warts and lymphogranuloma venereum. Approximately 10% of patients with perianal disease have rectal abscesses or chronic draining fistulae.

Laboratory Findings

There are no specific hematologic, biochemical, or serologic laboratory tests for IBD, nor are there any

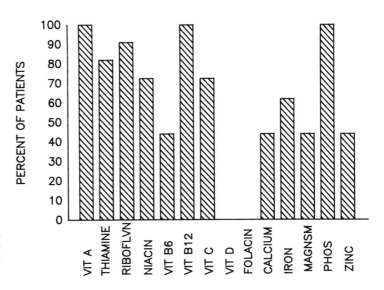

Figure 63–3. Micronutrient intake of children and adolescents with inflammatory bowel disease, expressed as the percentage of patients consuming at least 80% of the recommended daily allowance for each micronutrient.

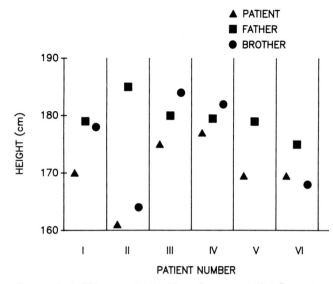

Figure 63–4. Ultimate adult heights of six men with inflammatory bowel disease during adolescence, compared with the adult heights of their brothers and fathers.

reliable blood tests to distinguish Crohn disease from ulcerative colitis. However, routine laboratory tests often reveal typical abnormalities.

Hypochromic, microcytic anemias are common. Anemia due to iron deficiency from chronic blood loss is associated with a low serum ferritin level. However, adolescents with IBD often are anemic, owing to their chronic inflammatory state. In such instances, serum ferritin levels are usually normal. Anemia can also be megaloblastic, secondary to folate or vitamin B_{12} deficiency, when significant lengths of jejunum or terminal ileum respectively are inflamed. Rarely, a Coombs-positive hemolytic anemia is present.

Peripheral white blood cell counts are usually normal but may be elevated during moderate to severe attacks. Characteristically there is a marked predominance of segmented leukocytes (75% to 90%) and band forms. Occasionally, lymphopenia is marked (5% of total white blood cell count). Platelet counts may be elevated but rarely exceed 1 million/cm³. Erythrocyte sedimentation rates are elevated in 60% to 70% of patients. Although fluctuation of the sedimentation rate may reflect changes in the activity of colitis, many patients may have normal sedimentation rates even in the presence of acute, fulminant disease. Sedimentation rates are also poor markers for disease activity in the patient with involvement of the small bowel. Determination of plasma orosomucoid level may be a better measure of inflammatory activity, but this assay is not widely available.

Serum electrolyte values are normal unless there has been pernicious vomiting or diarrhea. Serum protein levels, especially that of albumin, are commonly decreased when disease activity is prominent, reflecting an increase in protein loss across the inflamed mucosa into the bowel lumen. Studies have demonstrated a direct correlation between increased stool α_1-antitrypsin levels and abnormal degrees of enteric protein loss. Except after resection of significant lengths of small bowel, stool fecal fat losses are generally normal. Microscopic examination of the stool, however, often reveals leuko-

cytes, and even normal-appearing stools are positive for occult blood in 50% to 70% of cases.

Contrast-Enhanced Radiographic Findings

Barium studies of the gastrointestinal tract reveal small bowel mucosal irregularity, ulceration, separation of bowel loops, strictures, sinus tracts, or fistulae; double contrast studies may be helpful to detect these changes in mild disease. Care must be taken to differentiate mucosal filling defects caused by nodular lymphoid hyperplasia of the ileum from irregularities secondary to ileal inflammation and pseudopolyps. The terminal ileum is best evaluated by spot films, since mild degrees of inflammation may be otherwise inapparent. An inadequate study is often worse than no study at all; it can lead to misdiagnosis, to otherwise unnecessary testing, and often to repeat radiation exposure.

The radiographic appearance of the colon on barium enema may help differentiate ulcerative from Crohn colitis (Table 63–2). Results of a barium enema study may be misleading, however, since the classic radiographic findings attributed to one form of colitis may be mimicked by the other (Figs. 63–5 and 63–6).

Endoscopic Findings

Endoscopy of the rectosigmoid and colon identifies the gross characteristics of colitis. Classically, ulcerative colitis is described as a distal disease, always involving the anorectum and extending proximally to a variable extent. Crohn colitis is described as frequently sparing the anorectum. However, up to 75% of adolescents with Crohn colitis have anorectal involvement (Fig. 63–7). In the untreated adolescent, patchy inflammation, the

TABLE 63–2. Radiographic Differentiation of Ulcerative and Crohn Colitis

FEATURE	ULCERATIVE COLITIS	CROHN COLITIS
Terminal ileum	Normal	Often irregular or stenotic
Distribution	Diffuse from anal verge proximally for a variable extent	Often skip lesions, cecum and right colon involvement common
Foreshortening	Common	Common
Mucosa	Shallow ulcerations, pseudopolyps	Often deep or longitudinal ulcerations, pseudopolyps, cobblestoning
Fistula/sinus tract	Absent	Variably present
Stricture	Usually absent (if present, suggests superimposed cancer)	Variably present
Toxic megacolon	More common	Less common

Adapted from Daum F: Pediatric inflammatory bowel disease. In Silverberg M, Daum F (eds): Textbook of Pediatric Gastroenterology, 2nd ed. Chicago, Year Book Medical Publishers, 1988.

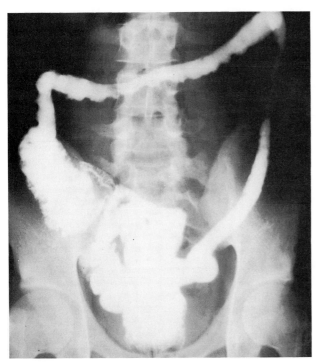

Figure 63–5. Barium enema appearance of ulcerative colitis in a 16-year-old male.

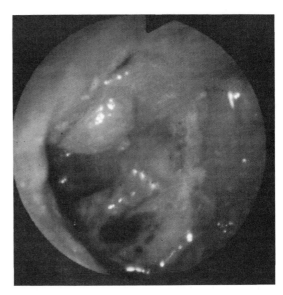

Figure 63–7. Endoscopic appearance of rectum in a 17-year-old male with severe Crohn colitis. Exudate and a fistulous orifice are present.

presence of small, aphthous ulcerations, and distinct skip lesions favor the diagnosis of Crohn colitis. However, treatment may alter the endoscopic appearance of either form of colitis, making endoscopic diagnosis difficult.

Endoscopic visualization of the terminal ileum, in the patient with ileitis, reveals aphthous ulcers, increased

friability, exudate, and nodularity. Endoscopy of the upper gastrointestinal tract may reveal similar findings when Crohn disease affects the esophagus, stomach, or duodenum.

Mucosal Biopsy Findings

Superficial biopsy specimens should be obtained whenever endoscopy is performed, since there is minimal risk and histologic inflammation can be identified even in specimens obtained from grossly normal mucosa. The differentiation of ulcerative from Crohn colitis by mucosal biopsy (Table 63–3) is often difficult. Although certain histologic findings tend to favor one or the other diagnosis, only the presence of granulomas is definitively diagnostic of Crohn disease. Unfortunately, under the best of clinical circumstances, including the use of serial sectioning, granulomas are only found in about 30% of mucosal biopsy specimens obtained from adolescent patients with Crohn disease.

Mucosal biopsy specimens are also indispensable in cancer surveillance in adolescents and young adults with

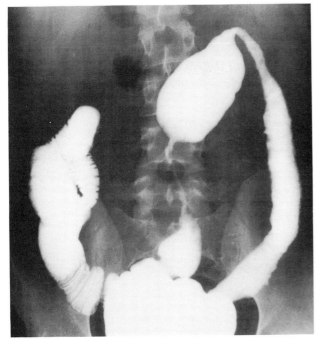

Figure 63–6. Barium enema appearance of Crohn colitis in an 18-year-old male. Note the apparent skip lesion in the distal transverse colon between two stenotic areas.

TABLE 63–3. Differentiation of Ulcerative and Crohn Colitis by Mucosal Biopsy in the Untreated Patient

FEATURE	ULCERATIVE COLITIS	CROHN COLITIS
Inflammation	Diffuse	Patchy
Rectal involvement	Constant	May be spared
Goblet cells	Depleted	Normal
Crypt abscesses	Common	Common
Granuloma	Absent	Common
Signs of chronicity	Present	Present
Lymphoid hyperplasia	Present	Present

Adapted from Daum F: Pediatric inflammatory bowel disease. In Silverberg M, Daum F (eds): Textbook of Pediatric Gastroenterology, 2nd ed. Chicago, Year Book Medical Publishers, 1988.

TABLE 63–4. Differentiation of Ulcerative and Crohn Colitis: Gross Pathology

FEATURE	ULCERATIVE COLITIS	CROHN COLITIS
Distribution	Continuous from rectum	Segmental
Terminal ileum	Normal	Usually abnormal
Foreshortening	Common	Common
Serosa	Normal	Thickened, creeping mesenteric fat
Mucosa	Granular, diffusely involved	Patchy, often cobblestoned, frequent fissuring
Fistula	Absent	Often present
Pseudopolyps	Common	Common
Strictures	Rare (suggests cancer)	More frequent

Adapted from Daum F: Pediatric inflammatory bowel disease. In Silverberg M, Daum F (eds): Textbook of Pediatric Gastroenterology, 2nd ed. Chicago, Year Book Medical Publishers, 1988.

long-standing ulcerative colitis. The risk of developing adenocarcinoma increases with extent and duration of colitis. For adolescents with pancolitis who developed ulcerative colitis during childhood, the relative risk of developing adenocarcinoma has been estimated at 33 to 162 times the general population. For children diagnosed with ulcerative colitis, cancer surveillance must therefore begin during adolescence. Mucosal biopsy specimens of suspicious lesions, or random biopsy specimens obtained every 10 cm throughout the colon, can reveal mucosal dysplasia. Dysplasia noted in areas of severe inflammation may not indicate early malignant transformation, but when seen in areas of quiescent disease the risk for malignancy is quite high.

Gross and Microscopic Pathology

Examination of surgical specimens reveals characteristic changes that differentiate ulcerative colitis from Crohn disease (Tables 63–4 and 63–5, Figs. 63–8 and 63–9). Despite the clear features that distinguish these two disorders, occasionally there is an overlap of histo-

TABLE 63–5. Differentiation of Ulcerative and Crohn Colitis: Microscopic Pathology

FEATURE	ULCERATIVE COLITIS	CROHN COLITIS
Inflammation	Diffuse, mucosal and submucosal	Patchy, transmural
Ulceration	Mucosal	Deep, often into muscularis
Crypt abscess	Common	Common
Granuloma	Absent	Frequently present
Submucosa	Normal	Frequently expanded
Lymphoid hyperplasia	Mucosa and submucosa	Transmural
Neuronal hyperplasia	Absent	Prominent
Serosal fibrosis	Absent	Frequent

Adapted from Daum F: Pediatric inflammatory bowel disease. In Silverberg M, Daum F (eds): Textbook of Pediatric Gastroenterology, 2nd ed. Chicago, Year Book Medical Publishers, 1988.

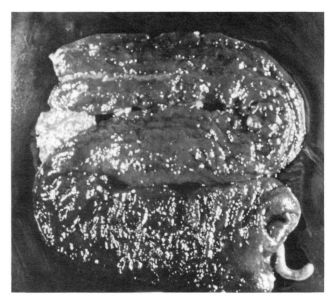

Figure 63–8. Longitudinally opened subtotal colectomy specimen from a 15-year-old girl with ulcerative colitis. Continuous mucosal involvement is present extending from the ileocecal valve (appendix and valve are in the lower right corner of the figure) to the distal margin of resection. (Courtesy of Dr. Ellen Kahn.)

logic characteristics that makes unequivocal differentiation impossible.

DIAGNOSIS

Standard Evaluation

Since the presenting symptoms and signs of IBD are often protean and nonspecific, the diagnosis of either ulcerative colitis or Crohn disease in the adolescent is often difficult. Evaluation requires a thorough history, comprehensive physical examination, and appropriate laboratory studies (Table 63–6). A family history positive for either form of IBD should alert the clinician to the possibility of IBD in the adolescent. Growth records for a number of years prior to the onset of a patient's

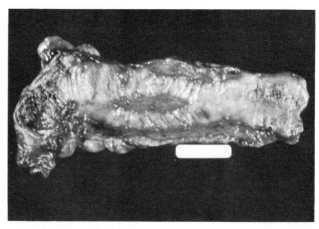

Figure 63–9. Ileo-ascending colectomy specimen from a 16-year-old boy with Crohn disease. A prominent longitudinal ulceration is present. (Courtesy of Dr. Ellen Kahn.)

TABLE 63–6. Evaluation of Inflammatory Bowel Disease

History
Physical examination, including height, weight, anthropometrics, and sexual maturity rating
Growth records (height and weight for age, velocity)
Complete blood cell count, differential, reticulocyte count, erythrocyte sedimentation rate
Electrolytes, serum chemistries (including total protein, albumin)
Serum iron, total iron binding capacity, ferritin
Serum folate, vitamin B_{12}
Stools for enteric pathogens (*Salmonella, Shigella, Yersinia, Campylobacter, Aeromonas*)
Stools for ova and parasite examinations, Charcot-Leyden crystals, white blood cells
Stools for *Clostridium difficile* toxin
Upper gastrointestinal series with small bowel followthrough
Barium enema
Lower flexible sigmoidoscopy or colonoscopy with mucosal biopsies
Esophagogastroduodenoscopy and mucosal biopsy (if indicated)
Nutritional assessment, including bone age

Adapted from Daum F: Pediatric inflammatory bowel disease. In Silverberg M, Daum F (eds): Textbook of Pediatric Gastroenterology, 2nd ed. Chicago, Year Book Medical Publishers, 1988.

symptoms are crucial, since long-standing growth suppression may not be evident on evaluation of an adolescent's current weight for height. Similarly, the history may reveal primary or secondary amenorrhea or arrest of sexual development.

Laboratory evaluation can suggest the presence of an ongoing inflammatory process and enteric protein loss. Stools must be examined for evidence of bacterial or parasitic infection. If there has been recent use of antibiotics, stools should also be screened for the presence of *Clostridium difficile* toxin. Microscopic examination of the stool may reveal leukocytes, while the presence of Charcot-Leyden crystals may suggest an allergic enteritis rather than IBD.

Radiographic studies traditionally have included both an upper gastrointestinal series with small bowel follow through and a barium enema. However, since the introduction of flexible endoscopes, the barium enema has become increasingly unnecessary. Low-grade inflammation is often not apparent even on air contrast barium enema. Endoscopic procedures avoid radiation exposure and allow tissue sampling for pathologic examination, and for many patients they are more comfortable than barium enema. The endoscopic appearance of the rectosigmoid and colon may help differentiate between ulcerative colitis (diffuse mucosal involvement always involving the anorectum) and Crohn disease isolated to the colon (often patchy mucosal involvement with aphthous ulcers and frequent rectal sparing). Full colonoscopy is usually reserved for the adolescent suspected of having Crohn disease whose radiologic examination has been otherwise normal or whose studies reveal atypical findings that require further characterization. In such situations, the ileocecal valve can often be cannulated with the colonoscope, allowing direct visualization and biopsy of the terminal ileum. Full colonoscopy can also be used to differentiate left-sided ulcerative from Crohn colitis or to identify patients with universal ulcerative colitis, a subgroup of patients who are known to have the greatest ultimate malignant

potential. When active perianal disease is present, anoscopy allows better visualization of the anal crypts, the site from which perianal abscesses and fistulae commonly arise. At times, endoscopic examination of the upper gastrointestinal tract is also indicated if symptoms or radiographic studies suggest the presence of Crohn disease in the stomach or duodenum. As discussed previously, biopsy specimens of even normal-appearing mucosa should be obtained whenever endoscopy is performed, since histologic evidence of inflammation or granulomas may be identified.

Nutritional assessment is required on an ongoing basis for adolescents with IBD. Estimates of dietary intake, with analysis for both macronutrients and micronutrients, facilitate optimal management for patients with acute weight loss or long-standing growth suppression. Bone age and anthropometric measures complement the nutritional assessment. Although maldigestion and malabsorption are generally not clinically significant problems, occasional patients benefit from fecal fat studies or stool sampling for pH and reducing substance. Lactose breath hydrogen studies may identify adolescents with lactose intolerance, while dextrose or lactulose breath hydrogen tests may identify those with bacterial overgrowth.

Specialized Laboratory Examinations

A variety of diagnostic studies can complement those obtained as part of the standard evaluation. Abdominal ultrasonography, computed tomography, and magnetic resonance imaging can be helpful in differentiating inflammatory masses from intraabdominal abscesses. These modalities can also be used to direct percutaneous drainage of abscesses. Scintigraphic studies have been used to estimate the extent and severity of mucosal involvement. Scans may also be helpful in distinguishing arthritis from the rare case of osteonecrosis.

DIFFERENTIAL DIAGNOSIS

The differential diagnosis for these conditions in the adolescent varies with the presenting symptoms and site of intestinal involvement (Table 63–7). Most of these can be easily excluded by history, physical examination, and routine laboratory testing. Intestinal tuberculosis and amebiasis are rare in developed countries but common in many third-world areas. These conditions must always be considered if adolescents or their immediate family contacts have traveled to such areas. Enteric infections manifested by abdominal cramps and bloody diarrhea commonly mimic severe colitis. *Giardia lamblia* infection may present as dyspeptic symptoms similar to those of upper gastrointestinal Crohn disease (see Chapter 95), whereas *Yersinia enterocolitica* or *Aeromonas hydrophilia* infection may present as acute ileitis.

The age of the patient is often helpful in diagnosis. The features of IBD in young children can mimic those of allergic enterocolitis, Hirschsprung enterocolitis, or

TABLE 63–7. Differential Diagnosis

DISORDERS AFFECTING THE UPPER GASTROINTESTINAL TRACT
  Gastroesophageal reflux disease
  Peptic ulcer
  Helicobacter pylori gastritis
  Zollinger-Ellison syndrome
  Eosinophilic gastroenteritis
  Intestinal tuberculosis
  Behçet disease
DISORDERS AFFECTING THE SMALL AND LARGE INTESTINES
  Allergic enteropathy, enterocolitis
  Eosinophilic gastroenteritis
  Celiac disease
  Intestinal lymphangiectasia
  Enteric infection (including amebiasis)
  Pseudomembraneous enterocolitis (*Clostridium difficile*)
  Acute appendicitis, appendiceal abscess
  Neoplasms (lymphoma, adenocarcinoma, intestinal polyposis)
  Vasculitis (Henoch-Schönlein purpura, systemic lupus
    erythematosus, hemolytic-uremic syndrome)
MISCELLANEOUS
  Feeding disorders (anorexia and bulimia nervosa)
  Carbohydrate intolerance (lactose, sucrose, sorbitol, xylitol)
  Laxative abuse

Adapted from Daum F: Pediatric inflammatory bowel disease. In Silverberg M, Daum F (eds): Textbook of Pediatric Gastroenterology, 2nd ed. Chicago, Year Book Medical Publishers, 1988.

Henoch-Schönlein purpura, all of which are uncommon in adolescents. Similarly, gastrointestinal malignancies, common in adult populations, are unusual in adolescents.

MEDICAL THERAPIES

The pharmacologic and nutritional therapies of either ulcerative colitis or Crohn disease are primarily supportive, since there are no curative medical treatments. Treatment aims include the suppression of incapacitating symptoms, the promotion of normal growth and sexual development, the control of unavoidable complications, and the avoidance of excessive or inappropriate therapy. Symptoms can rarely be completely eliminated. Adolescents and their families need to understand that treatment of IBD requires a careful balance between sufficient intervention to ensure normal daily functioning and avoidance of overtreatment.

Many different treatments are used in the adolescent with IBD (Table 63–8). Certain therapies are applicable to all patients, whereas others are indicated for specific complications or disease confined to certain sites of intestine.

Nutritional Approaches

One of the keys to the treatment of IBD during the adolescent years is the assurance of adequate dietary intake. Nutritional supplementation to provide adequate macronutrients and micronutrients can be provided orally, enterally, or parenterally and clearly promote normal growth and development. Nutritional modalities can also induce at least temporary suppression of clinical symptoms without additional therapy. However, long-term remission is rarely achieved with nutritional therapy alone.

For the adolescent with mild to moderate symptoms, optimizing dietary intake is important. Daily caloric intake of 70 to 90 kcal/kg/day is generally required to promote normal growth and sexual development in these patients. Oral supplementation of an adolescent's usual diet to achieve caloric requirements results in improved growth; patients unable or unwilling to ingest these amounts can achieve improved growth with long-term (6 to 12 months) nocturnal or repeated courses of short-term (4 to 6 week) continuous nasogastric infusions of either nonelemental or elemental formulae. Supplemental intermittent home parenteral nutrition has also been used. All these techniques allow adolescents to optimize their dietary intake successfully at home for extended periods of time.

For adolescents with more active disease, nutritional support becomes even more important. Complete bowel rest may be required to control intractable symptoms. This can be achieved with total parenteral nutrition or with the continuous enteral infusion of an elemental formula. While promoting positive nitrogen balance, both of these modalities can diminish symptoms associated with Crohn disease of the upper bowel. There may also be a role for bowel rest in certain adolescents with active colitis, but bowel rest does not appear to be as beneficial in the teenager with primarily colonic involvement. In fact, since the colonic mucosa is known to derive metabolic fuels from material in the fecal stream, there is the possibility that providing enteral nutrition to the adolescent with colitis might indeed be therapeutic.

Agents Affecting the Inflammatory Response

CORTICOSTEROIDS

Administered orally, parenterally, or rectally, corticosteroids are capable of suppressing the inflammatory

TABLE 63–8. Medical Therapy for Inflammatory Bowel Disease

Nutrition
  Appropriate dietary intake (with or without supplementation)
  Elemental diet
  Parenteral nutrition
Agents affecting the inflammatory response
  Corticosteroids
  Sulfasalazine
  New salicylates (5-amino salicylates, olsalazine)
  Nonsystemic corticosteroids (beclomethasone, tixocortal pivalate)
Agents affecting the immune response
  Azathioprine and 6-mercaptopurine
  Metronidazole
  Cyclosporine
  Methotrexate
  Intravenous gamma-globulin
Antibiotics
Antidiarrheals
Antispasmodics

response throughout the gastrointestinal tract in both ulcerative colitis and Crohn disease and are standard agents in treatment. Oral prednisone (0.5 to 1.0 mg/kg/day with a daily maximum of 40 to 50 mg) is indicated in adolescents with moderately active disease activity (temperature < 38.5°C, moderate to severe cramps, 6 to 10 loose stools per day with or without blood) and whose ability to perform normal daily activities is impaired. For more severe symptoms, intravenous hydrocortisone (0.5 to 1.0 mg/kg/dose) or methylprednisolone (0.4 to 0.8 mg/kg/dose) given every 6 to 8 hours is useful. Continuous infusion of hydrocortisone may benefit adolescents whose disorder is refractory to the more traditional approach. In one study it was suggested that intravenous administration of adrenocorticotropic hormone in adults with ulcerative colitis is more effective than exogenous corticosteroids in patients not previously treated with steroids, while hydrocortisone remains preferable for those previously treated with corticosteroids. In adolescent patients with severe tenesmus or urgency, rectal corticosteroids, administered as foam preparations or retention enemas, concomitantly with systemic corticosteroids are useful. As remission is achieved, the dosage of corticosteroid is generally continued for 2 to 4 weeks and then slowly tapered by 2.5- to 5.0-mg/day decrements of oral prednisone every 4 to 7 days.

The efficacy of corticosteroids must often be weighed against the adverse effects of these agents. The long-term complications associated with corticosteroid use (e.g., osteoporosis, cataract formation) are well known but are relatively uncommon in adolescents with IBD. Generally more troublesome for the adolescent with IBD, however, are other more immediate side effects. Exogenous corticosteroids interfere with linear bone growth, even in the presence of adequate dietary intake. This effect can complicate the treatment of adolescents with IBD, since the disease may already be adversely affecting growth. Prednisone taken daily for only 7 to 10 days in commonly prescribed dosages (0.3 to 1.0 mg/kg/day) has been shown to impair serum procollagen levels, a postulated marker for linear bone growth. The use of alternate-day dosing regimens has been shown to be beneficial in limiting these effects, while maintaining reduced disease activity. However, in more seriously ill patients unable to tolerate alternate-day dosing regimens, although the anti-inflammatory effects of corticosteroids might be desirous, the coincident suppression of linear growth may limit their usefulness.

The cosmetic side effects of corticosteroids, seen after even a few days or weeks of treatment, are particularly onerous to most adolescents. The cushingoid facies, acne, hirsutism, truncal obesity, and striae that develop as a consequence of corticosteroid therapy are often more difficult for the adolescent to tolerate than the symptoms of IBD. These cosmetic changes are difficult or impossible to avoid or disguise. The potential deleterious effects of corticosteroids on the adolescent's sense of psychosocial well-being cannot be overemphasized. Adolescents and their families must be warned that cosmetic changes will occur, but they must also be taught that all but the striae are generally reversible. Avoidance of foods high in sodium may minimize water retention, but "low-salt diets" are not indicated. Appropriate topical treatments for acne are also helpful (see Chapter 39). Cosmetic effects can best be limited by avoiding excessive doses of corticosteroids.

Poor compliance with corticosteroid treatment is frequent among adolescents and a common cause of "failure" to respond to an adequate regimen of corticosteroids, especially in the patient who does not appear cushingoid (see Chapter 26). Rectal therapy may be particularly disturbing or embarrassing. Enemas must be retained if they are to be useful, but severe proctitis may make retention impossible. Sensitive awareness to these issues from a caring physician and staff significantly lessens the trauma associated with corticosteroid use. This should be of major concern to clinicians treating adolescents with IBD, since patients frequently require multiple courses of corticosteroids to control recurrent flares of disease activity. Adolescents traumatized by their initial exposure often will be highly resistant to another course of corticosteroid therapy.

SULFASALAZINE

Apart from corticosteroids, the primary anti-inflammatory agent used in IBD is sulfasalazine (Azulfidine). The drug combines a sulfa antibiotic (sulfapyridine) with a locally acting anti-inflammatory (5-aminosalicylate) joined by an azo linkage. The 5-aminosalicylate is the active moiety of the molecule, but it must be released by bacterial degradation of the azo linkage once the drug reaches the colon. This restricts the predominant action of sulfasalazine to colonic disease. Studies primarily from adult populations, and widespread clinical experience, have demonstrated that sulfasalazine is effective in inducing remission in mild to moderate attacks of either ulcerative or Crohn colitis. There are also data to suggest that sulfasalazine can maintain a prolonged remission for many patients with colitis. Although occasional patients with Crohn disease of the small bowel appear to benefit from sulfasalazine, its use in these situations remains controversial.

Sulfasalazine (50 to 75 mg/kg/day to a maximum of 2 to 4 g/day in two or three divided doses) will often result in lessened disease activity within 10 to 14 days in mild colonic disease. If no substantial response is seen during this time period, the drug is generally discontinued and alternative therapy instituted. Once remission with sulfasalazine is achieved, the daily dosage can often be reduced to 30 to 50 mg/kg or 2 g/day. Sulfasalazine may need to be continued at least until puberty is completed, although specific studies have not addressed this issue.

Sulfasalazine treatment may rarely be complicated by severe hypersensitivity reactions. About 10% of patients may also experience a reproducible exacerbation of disease activity when on the drug. Headache, gastrointestinal distress, and hemolysis are often dose related and transient. Sulfasalazine inhibits folic acid absorption, but folate deficiency can be prevented by routine concomitant administration of oral folic acid (1 mg/day). Sulfasalazine has also been shown to cause reversible oligospermia, reduced sperm motility, and an increased proportion of abnormal sperm forms. Although this may temporarily prevent conception, these effects are completely reversible 3 months after withdrawal of the drug without adverse effects on subsequent conception. For the most part, however, sulfasalazine is well tolerated and can be used safely for many years.

NEWER SALICYLATES

A number of new agents are currently available in Europe and Canada and are in the advanced stages of clinical trials in the United States. These agents continue to rely on 5-aminosalicylate for their action but have eliminated the sulfapyridine moiety of the sulfasalazine molecule generally responsible for the adverse reations seen with the older agent. These newer salicylates fall into two broad categories. The first group (Asacol, Pentasa, Claversalk) are 5-aminosalicylates whose absorption from the upper bowel is prevented by coating the drug with a variety of polymer coatings resistant to dissolution in the proximal bowel. The second variation, olsalazine sodium (Dipentum), is a dimer of 5-aminosalicylate joined by an azo linkage. Similar to sulfasalazine, this agent's activity requires bacterial cleavage of the azo linkage for optimal anti-inflammatory activity. Both classes of salicylate should theoretically be as effective as sulfasalazine, but the results of ongoing clinical trials are equivocal. A North American multi-institutional study by the Pediatric Gastroenterology Collaborative Research Group had to be discontinued when interim analysis of the data revealed that sulfasalazine was significantly more efficacious than olsalazine in children and adolescents with mild to moderate ulcerative colitis. Further data are required before the ultimate usefulness of these agents will be known.

5-Aminosalicylate has also been released in enema form (Rowasa) in the United States. The rectal administration of this agent has been shown to be effective in distal ulcerative colitis. Although rectal preparations of hydrocortisone (Cortenema, Cortifoam) have been available for many years, the corticosteroid is partially absorbed, systemically active, and capable of inducing adrenal suppression. Rectal 5-aminosalicylate therefore offers an alternative local anti-inflammatory action without the use of corticosteroids.

NONSYSTEMIC CORTICOSTEROIDS

A number of corticosteroids are being investigated for their safety and efficacy in the treatment of IBD. These agents, including beclomethasone dipropionate and tixocortal pivalate, are locally active in the gut but so completely metabolized on first pass through the liver as to effectively have no systemic effects. Agents with these characteristics theoretically would be ideal for the treatment of adolescents with IBD. However, no data are currently available regarding their use.

Agents Affecting the Immune Response

These diverse medications are generally considered more potent drugs than either corticosteroids or salicylates. Although categorized as immunosuppressives, their mode of action in IBD is unknown and their use is controversial and primarily limited to intractable Crohn disease.

AZATHIOPRINE AND 6-MERCAPTOPURINE

The major metabolite of azathioprine (Imuran) is 6-mercaptopurine (Purinethol). These two agents are the most commonly prescribed immunosuppressive agents for adolescents with intractable Crohn disease. The actions of these two agents are generally considered to be the same because of their pharmacologic relationship. However, no studies have directly compared the two drugs. There are also no placebo-controlled therapeutic trials in children or adolescents to support their use. Clinical studies have shown that two thirds of adolescents experience remission of disease and 80% are able to completely discontinue corticosteroid treatment when 6-mercaptopurine is used for at least 1 year. At 6-mercaptopurine doses of 1.0 to 1.5 mg/kg/day (maximum of 75 mg/day), no neutropenia, serious infection, or other untoward reactions are encountered. Side effects reported in adults have included severe allergic reactions and pancreatitis. Concerns about possible carcinogenicity and teratogenicity persist, but fairly extensive adult experience with these agents has not yet demonstrated these adverse consequences.

METRONIDAZOLE

Experience with metronidazole (Flagyl) in adolescents with intestinal or perianal Crohn disease is limited and anecdotal. The mechanism underlying the drug's efficacy in IBD is unknown, but metronidazole has been reported to suppress cell-mediated immunity. We have shown that metronidazole induced remission and had steroid-sparing effects in 13 adolescents with active or steroid-dependent Crohn disease. More than 80% of adults with destructive perianal Crohn disease have a marked degree of healing when treated with metronidazole for more than 2 months with dosages of 20 mg/kg/day (1 to 1.5 g) in three to five divided doses. Discontinuation of metronidazole, however, resulted in reactivation of the perianal disease in two thirds of these patients.

Intolerable side effects, including a peripheral sensory neuropathy that developed in more than 80% of our patients taking metronidazole chronically, may limit its therapeutic role. Although the paresthesias and dysesthesias were entirely reversible, the frequency of these symptoms limited the adolescents' acceptance of this otherwise effective agent. Other troublesome side effects include a metallic taste and frequent complaints of abdominal distress, nausea, vomiting, flushing, or headache after ingestion of alcoholic beverages. These latter effects may have particular relevance in the adolescent.

CYCLOSPORINE

Preliminary clinical experience with cyclosporine in the treatment of IBD has been reported. Studies of fewer than 150 adults with severe refractory Crohn disease and a smaller number of adults with ulcerative colitis have demonstrated significant clinical improvement in 50% to 60% of patients that is often identifiable within 2 weeks of starting treatment. However, many patients experienced relapse within 2 to 3 months while continuing on the drug or shortly after stopping it. No studies of therapy with this drug in adolescents have yet been published. Nephrotoxicity, systemic hypertension, and increased susceptibility to overwhelming viral infection are complications that may be less frequent in patients with IBD than in transplant recipients. Although far from being accepted as standard therapy, cyclosporine and its newer experimental relatives may be therapeutically useful in carefully selected adolescent patients with IBD. Use of this drug should be considered experimental until further experience and extensive clinical trials are completed.

METHOTREXATE

No clinical experience with methotrexate in children or adolescents with IBD exists, although adults with intractable IBD appear to respond to this agent. The drug is known to be hepatotoxic and at the present time cannot be recommended as a therapeutic alternative for adolescents with IBD.

INTRAVENOUS GAMMA GLOBULIN

Anecdotal experience in adolescents and adults with intractable Crohn disease suggests that selected patients may experience marked improvement in their symptoms and sense of well-being following intravenous infusions of gamma globulin. The cost of such therapy is currently prohibitive, however, and until further studies are reported, this therapy should be considered experimental.

Antibiotics

Antibiotics have a major role in the treatment of IBD, although their use is grounded on clinical experience rather than controlled clinical trials. For adolescents with fevers and large inflammatory masses or abscesses, marked reduction in the size and tenderness of the masses can be seen following 7 to 10 days of either oral or intravenous antibiotic therapy. We commonly use a combination of cefoxitin or cefotetan with an aminoglycoside for adolescent patients requiring parenteral therapy. Occasional adolescents may require coverage with ampicillin, clindamycin, and an aminoglycoside, or with imipenem. Oral antibiotics such as tetracycline, metronidazole, or erythromycin can be used to suppress symptoms arising from bacterial overgrowth. Broadspectrum antibiotics have been associated with *Clostridium difficile*–mediated enterocolitis and should be used cautiously. Patients with acute flares of bloody diarrhea should be screened for *C. difficile* toxin if antibiotics (including sulfasalazine) have been prescribed in the previous 3 months.

Symptomatic Agents

Symptomatic agents generally are antidiarrheals or antispasmodics. The former agents include loperamide (Imodium) and opiates such as diphenoxylate (Lomotil) or codeine. Opiates have the potential to induce addiction and should be avoided. The response to loperamide is variable when inflammation is active. The drug, however, does have a more dramatic and predictable effect in reducing ileostomy effluent after subtotal or total proctocolectomy.

Antispasmodics are often prescribed in an attempt to decrease the cramps associated with active IBD but are poorly effective. Anticholinergics must be used with particular caution in patients with colitis, since instances of toxic megacolon have been associated with their use.

SURGERY (Table 63–9)

Ulcerative Colitis

Total proctocolectomy cures ulcerative colitis. However, current practice reserves surgery for cases of severe, refractory disease or developing malignancy. Emergency surgical intervention may be necessary because of acute fulminant colitis, massive intestinal bleeding, free perforation, or toxic megacolon. Indications for elective colectomy are dependence on growth-suppressive doses of corticosteroids, continuous debilitating symptoms despite medical therapy, or both. No longer is growth and pubertal retardation considered a primary indication for colectomy. Normal growth and sexual maturation can usually be achieved by appropriate nutritional therapy if high doses of corticosteroids can be avoided. However, growth failure complicated by unremitting symptoms or corticosteroid dependence will respond to colectomy, and catch-up growth can occur as long as the operation is performed early in puberty before closure of the epiphyses. Surgery performed as prophylaxis for colonic carcinoma seems unwarranted, even in adolescents with disease for more than 10 years. Surveillance colonoscopies with biopsy and flow cytometry studies can reveal changes such as dysplasia and malignancy that indicate when surgery is needed.

Subtotal colectomy with Brooke ileostomy is the initial procedure for most adolescents requiring surgery. Generally there is no need for a mucous fistula. The distal sigmoid, rectum, and anus are left intact. Psychological adjustment to an ileostomy is generally good with adequate preparation. This preparation often re-

---

TABLE 63–9. Indications for Surgery

ULCERATIVE COLITIS
  Intractable disease
  Long-term dependence on growth-suppressive doses of corticosteroids
  Complications (massive bleeding, free perforation, toxic megacolon)
  High-grade dysplasia
  Adenocarcinoma
CROHN DISEASE
  Intractable disease
  Long-term dependence on growth-suppressive doses of corticosteroids
  Complications (massive bleeding, obstruction unresponsive to conservative therapy, recurrent obstruction, abscesses)

quires a team approach, using the expertise of not only the medical and surgical teams but also the enterostomal therapist, mental health workers, and, most importantly, adolescents who have already had such a procedure (see Chapter 27).

The subtotal colectomy specimen is evaluated by an experienced pathologist. Once the clinical diagnosis of ulcerative colitis is confirmed pathologically, the adolescent may then undergo a further procedure to convert the ileostomy to an endorectal pullthrough or ileoanal anastomosis. Adolescents, eager to divest themselves of an ostomy, generally cope well with the subsequent surgery and the aberrant stool pattern that usually persists for months following conversion of a Brooke ileostomy.

Symptomatic antidiarrheal therapy may be needed after an endorectal pullthrough or ileoanal anastomosis. Loperamide, codeine sulfate, or both will usually decrease the frequency of stools sufficiently to allow normal activities. Some teenagers take three loperamide tablets three times a day, while others take somewhat less along with 15 mg of codeine sulfate twice or three times a day. The dosage and the hourly schedule are individualized. Patients generally also take a bulk-forming agent to provide more substance to their stools. Occasional patients require no specific medical therapy postoperatively.

A diet consisting of three meals per day and a limited number of snacks is prescribed to minimize stimulation of the gastrocolic reflex and the number of daily bowel movements. Despite a high frequency of stooling during the first 6 to 12 months, patients ultimately report that their stools are firm. Very few complain of having incontinence or accidents. Evacuation is less frequent when a bathroom is not available (such as in school) and tends to be more frequent when food and beverages are available for frequent snacks. Adolescents generally express satisfaction following one of these operations despite having to adjust for a period of 6 to 12 months to a significantly abnormal stool pattern.

The continent ileostomy, or Kock pouch, which provided an acceptable alternative to permanent ileostomy for many patients in the late 1970s, is rarely performed. Adolescents generally prefer an endorectal pullthrough that allows them to defecate through their anus.

Crohn Disease

Unlike ulcerative colitis, in which surgery is curative, surgery in Crohn disease is recommended only to manage complications unresponsive to medical therapy. However, recurrence of symptomatic Crohn disease is common and can often occur shortly after bowel resection. The recurrence rate in adults with Crohn disease who have had surgical procedures approaches 94%. Recurrence of small bowel Crohn disease is reported to be more frequent after subtotal colectomy and ileorectal anastomosis (43%) than after proctocolectomy (24%). Adults with ileocolic disease often require reoperation and further resection because of recurrence. Still, 10 years later, two of three patients have an intact ileorectal anastomosis, suggesting that a colectomy and ileorectal anastomosis is a useful operation in patients with minimal anorectal disease.

Unfortunately, the transmural nature of Crohn disease and the high rate of recurrence make procedures such as the endorectal pullthrough or continent ileal reservoir ill advised. Therefore, if a total proctocolectomy is required, the resulting ileostomy is permanent. Although a few have required further surgery, all of our adolescent patients who have had proctocolectomy and ileostomy for refractory Crohn disease (many of whom are now in their third decade of life) remain quite satisfied with their lives, either attending school or working on a full-time basis. Their quality of life and growth and development are all vastly improved compared with before colonic resection. Surgery should therefore be considered for adolescents with unremitting, incapacitating colonic Crohn disease.

Ileostomy dysfunction can cause partial obstruction and chronic, voluminous, secretory diarrhea owing to either a fascial ring or recurrent disease at the site of the stoma. In the presence of a fascial ring the examiner is usually unable to insert a finger into the stoma. However, stomal narrowing may not always be obvious by routine examination or by contrast-enhanced radiographs but may be detected by resistance to withdrawal of an inflated balloon catheter that had been advanced 15 to 20 cm beyond the stoma. In such situations, revision of the stoma may be necessary.

As in ulcerative colitis, growth failure in Crohn disease is no longer considered an indication for surgery, unless associated with intractable disease activity or corticosteroid dependence. Intestinal strictures leading to recurrent partial obstruction often require resection, but multiple resections can eventually lead to creation of a short bowel, malabsorption, and inadequate gastrointestinal function. Strictureplasty has been advocated as a safe, efficacious means of eliminating narrowed segments of bowel without resection.

COURSE AND PROGNOSIS

Physical Consequences

Despite the often debilitating effects of IBD, adolescents eventually become fully sexually mature. If the onset of IBD occurs before puberty, patients will often have delayed onset of puberty compared with their parents and siblings. In a study from our group, girls who developed IBD after the onset of puberty had a normal age of menarche of 13.0 ± 1.1 years compared with 12.2 ± 0.8 years for their mothers and 12.3 ± 1.3 years for their sisters. However, among a group of girls who developed IBD before puberty, menarche occurred at 14.6 ± 1.9 years ($p < 0.01$). All did eventually menstruate. However, if growth has been suppressed for long periods of time, full sexual maturation may take place without the usual adolescent growth spurt. Adolescents may not reach their calculated ultimate potential heights, although usually they grow sufficiently to fall within the normal height curves for healthy adults.

Pregnancy (see Chapter 74)

Adolescent girls with IBD have two particular concerns about pregnancy: the effect of a pregnancy on IBD and the effect of IBD on a pregnancy. Pregnancy appears to have little, if any, effect on the frequency or severity of relapse for either ulcerative colitis or Crohn disease. Studies regarding the effect of IBD on pregnancy and outcome are mostly retrospective and indicate that ulcerative colitis and Crohn disease do not substantially alter fertility. Nutritional status might well be the most important determinant of fertility in adolescent girls with IBD, since active disease early in pregnancy is associated with an increased risk of spontaneous abortion. Surgical procedures, including ileostomy and total proctocolectomy with an ileal reservoir, do not pose significant hazards for successful childbirth. Corticosteroids and sulfasalazine used judiciously do not appear to alter the outcome of pregnancy. The use of 6-mercaptopurine or metronidazole during pregnancy is not advised, although there are no teratogenic effects yet described from these medications.

Complications Arising During the Course of IBD

Acute fulminant colitis occurs in both ulcerative and Crohn colitis and is characterized by severe cramps, diarrhea, and fever. Massive bleeding can also occur. Hospitalization, intravenous corticosteroids, and antibiotics are required for treatment. Cyclosporine may also be of some benefit to these patients. Subtotal colectomy and ileostomy may be necessary if the adolescent does not respond to 2 weeks of intensive medical treatment. However, surgery may be required earlier if the patient is deteriorating despite medical treatment. Throughout this period of treatment, patients must be continuously evaluated for the extremely rare, but life-threatening, development of toxic megacolon.

In long-standing Crohn disease, stricture formation or the development of fistulas is common. Strictures arise as collagen replaces elements of the bowel wall, a byproduct of chronic inflammation. Fistulas appear to arise in areas of active inflammation and are not apparently the result of increased pressure in bowel loops partially obstructed by distal strictures. They are frequently associated with the development of inflammatory masses or abscesses. Enteroenteral, enterovesical, and enterocutaneous fistulas are common, but occasionally adolescent patients develop extremely complicated lesions. Closure of fistulas has been described following bowel rest and total parenteral nutrition and treatment with immunosuppressive agents such as 6-mercaptopurine, azathioprine, and cyclosporine. Unfortunately, there is a high frequency of relapse once therapy is discontinued. Surgical treatment may be indicated for complicated lesions but rarely for enteroenteral fistulas.

Long-standing ulcerative colitis is a premalignant condition. The risk of adenocarcinoma of the colon is the same as that of the general population during the first 10 years of disease but increases about 20% per decade with every decade of disease thereafter. Adolescents should therefore be enrolled in a cancer surveillance program that includes frequent complete colonoscopies with biopsies 7 to 10 years after onset of their disease. Patients with Crohn disease appear to be much less at risk for the development of malignancy, and at the present time routine surveillance programs are not advocated. However, malignancies can occur in adolescents and young adults with Crohn disease.

In patients in whom a subtotal colectomy is necessary but who for one reason or another decide to defer restorative surgery, disease activity in the defunctionalized rectal stump can occur. Although drainage usually subsides within a few weeks of surgery, patients may continue to experience the urge to defecate. Passage of blood and mucus per rectum is common, and treatment with corticosteroids or 5-aminosalicylate enemas may occasionally be required. Patients with Crohn disease may develop marked fistulization from the diseased rectal stump, as well as perianal or perirectal abscesses.

Psychosocial Consequences

The psychosocial burden of any chronic illness on normal adolescent functioning can be significant (see Chapters 30 and 121). In one study, 60% of children and adolescents with either Crohn disease or ulcerative colitis manifested identifiable psychiatric disorders, the most common diagnosis being depression. Patients with IBD and short stature and sexual retardation often display maladaptive behaviors similar to those seen in normal children with idiopathic short stature.

Despite early studies suggesting a causal relationship between personality traits, psychopathology, and IBD, current opinion tends to discount psychosomatic theories of etiology. Although adolescents with IBD have been shown to be more compulsive as a group than normal controls and to have psychological styles characterized by depression, withdrawal, anxiety, and frequent somatizing, these traits appear to be at least in part sequelae of having these particular chronic intestinal conditions. Studies from our own patient population suggest that, as a group, adolescents with IBD are less likely to report that they have experienced stressful life events than controls. This suggests that these adolescent patients may have difficulty recognizing and reporting stressful events or that they tend to use denial defenses to cope with stressors. Coping styles in these patients tend to be more rigid and constricted than in healthy controls. These personality traits can make caring for these patients demanding.

BIBLIOGRAPHY

Bayless TM (ed): Current Management of Inflammatory Bowel Disease. Philadelphia, BC Decker, 1989.

Daum F: Ulcerative colitis and Crohn's disease in children. In Bayless TM (ed): Current Therapy in Gastroenterology and Liver Disease, Philadelphia, BC Decker, 1990, pp 291–298.

Daum F: Nutritional support for growth failure in children with inflammatory bowel disease. In Balistreri WF, Vanderhoof JA (eds):

Pediatric Gastroenterology and Nutrition. Aspen Seminars on Pediatric Disease, vol IV. London, Chapman and Hall Medical, 1990, pp 237–243.

Daum F: The use of new drugs in the management of inflammatory bowel disease in children. In Balistreri WF, Vanderhoof JA (eds): Pediatric Gastroenterology and Nutrition. Aspen Seminars on Pediatric Disease, vol IV. London, Chapman and Hall Medical, 1990, pp 186–195.

Kirschner BS: Nutritional consequences of inflammatory bowel disease on growth. J Am Coll Nutr 7:301–308, 1988.

Kleinman RE, Balistreri WF, Heyman MB, et al: Nutritional support for pediatric patients with inflammatory bowel disease. J Pediatr Gastroenterol Nutr 8:8–12, 1989.

Mashako MNL, Cezard JP, Navarro J, et al: Crohn's disease lesions in the upper gastrointestinal tract: Correlation between clinical, radiological, endoscopic, and histological features in adolescents and children. J Pediatr Gastroenterol Nutr 8:442–446, 1989.

CHAPTER 64

Chronic Constipation

MARILYN R. BROWN

DEFINITION AND PATHOPHYSIOLOGY

Constipation, the difficult and infrequent passage of firm stools, occurs in adolescents as well as in younger children. Recurrent abdominal pain and rectal bleeding may develop.

Frequently, constipation in adolescence is a continuation of symptoms that began in early childhood. Chronic constipation often begins with the passage of stools that cause pain. The adolescent responds by trying to withhold the bowel movement to prevent the pain. Withholding leads to hard stools and further pain, and a vicious circle then develops. In the process of withholding, the child learns to squeeze the anal sphincters to keep the bowel movement in when the urge to defecate is felt. Later the child learns to push in an attempt to have the bowel movement but has already learned to tighten the anal sphincters instead of relaxing them. This contributes to inadequate emptying of the sigmoid and rectum.

Encopresis (stool in the underwear) develops as a complication of constipation when the rectal vault is chronically filled with stool. The mental recognition of a sensation of stretch in the rectum normally occurs when stool arrives in the rectum. When the rectum is chronically full, a stretch sensation may not occur, and this leads to the inability of the child to recognize the presence of stool in the rectum. With little or no warning, the anal sphincters may relax and allow the unrecognized passage of stool. Besides not feeling or noticing the encopresis, the child usually does not smell the odor of the stool, which others can readily smell. When this type of constipation and withholding is not treated promptly, the voluntary withholding becomes habitual and involuntary and the youngsters still have problems in adolescence.

DIAGNOSIS

Typical symptoms consist of large infrequent stools with soiling of the underwear daily or for a few days just before a large bowel movement. In small children, the attempt to withhold stool may cause spasm of the sphincters, which is very painful. Behaviors that result from stool withholding that may still be present in the adolescent are hiding of soiled underwear and failure to notice either the passage of small amounts of stool or the odor. As peer-accepted social behavior becomes more important to the adolescent, he or she is more likely to adopt strategies that lead to overcoming these symptoms, and encopresis becomes rare after adolescence.

The only common physical findings are perianal soiling and a rectal vault filled with stool. When abdominal distention and a tight sphincter are present, short segment Hirschsprung disease must be ruled out. When the anal sphincters are lax, spinal cord tumors must be considered.

An abdominal radiograph can be obtained as a means of searching for quantity of stool and bowel dilatation. Studies to diagnose Hirschsprung disease include an unprepared barium enema to look for a transition zone of dilated to normal-size colon, anorectal manometry to look for the absence of the involuntary contraction of the internal anal sphincter secondary to balloon distention of the rectum, and, most importantly, a suction rectal biopsy to look for the absence of ganglion cells and the presence of hypertrophied nerves.

Other causative factors to be considered in constipation include hypothyroidism (see Chapter 55), decreased food intake (see Chapter 60), depression (see Chapter 100), and narcotic abuse (see Chapter 111). Medications that may lead to constipation include anticholinergics, antidepressants, diuretics, anticonvulsants, aluminum antacids, and opioids.

TREATMENT

Treatment of functional constipation is aimed at stimulating a daily soft bowel movement while increasing dietary fiber intake and developing a habitual time of day to have the bowel movement. For mild constipation, increased dietary fiber, stool softeners, or bulk laxatives may be adequate. For a significant problem, the following is recommended:

1. Stimulant or saline laxatives are used in whatever dose needed to result in a daily bowel movement. The dose is given at the same time every day, usually in the evening, to encourage the development of a regular time for the bowel movement. Milk of magnesia works well. Any laxative that is acceptable to the adolescent will work. It usually takes 2 to 3 weeks to determine the dose that works consistently. Rarely, the use of a daily suppository or enema following breakfast or supper may

be necessary to encourage the development of a regular bowel movement.

2. Stool softeners allow a smaller dose of stimulant laxative to be needed. Docusate sodium, mineral oil, psyllium, methylcellulose, soy polysaccharide, bran, and lactulose all are helpful.

3. A daily bowel movement is encouraged until all signs of withholding the bowel movement are gone and a daily bowel movement has occurred for at least a month. Then the laxative is gradually tapered over several months. Depending on the length of time the constipation has been present, medications may be needed for several months to several years.

4. Increased dietary fiber and increased water intake are always encouraged, especially during tapering of the medication.

Once a daily soft bowel movement occurs, recurrent abdominal pain, rectal bleeding, and anal fissure usually resolve.

Fecal impaction was difficult to treat until the development of the Tween-80 (detergent)/Gastrografin (diatrizoate) enema. One or two of these enemas seem to dissolve even large firm masses.

Conditions in which constipation is common include chronic neurologic disabilities (e.g., developmental retardation, spina bifida), anorexia nervosa (see Chapter 60), cystic fibrosis (see Chapter 43), and irritable bowel syndrome (see Chapter 63). Adolescents who are severely retarded often have constipation and may need large amounts of dietary fiber and/or stool softeners (see Chapter 31). Most require regular laxatives or enemas to produce regular bowel movements. Adolescents with spina bifida appreciate a regular bowel continence management program. Continence helps support self-esteem and social acceptance. Management may take the form of daily bisacodyl suppositories, regular enemas, or tactile stimulation to induce stool passage.

Adolescents with anorexia nervosa not infrequently have obstipation with abdominal pain (see Chapter 60). They may have a strong desire to have a regular bowel movement. Large amounts of stool softeners, emollients, fluids, and fiber medications usually relieve sensations of feeling uncomfortable, but stimulant laxatives should be avoided because of their potential to be abused.

Meconium ileus equivalent constipation in cystic fibrosis may be treated with oral Gastrografin, electrolyte lavage solutions, or Tween 80/Gastrografin enema (see Chapter 43). Patients with classic irritable bowel syndrome have recurrent abdominal pain and infrequent passage of loose bowel movements. They often respond well to psyllium or methylcellulose.

BIBLIOGRAPHY

Levine MD: The school child with encopresis. Pediatr Rev 2:286, 1981.

Loening-Baucke VA: Persistence of chronic constipation in children after biofeedback treatment. Digest Dis Sci 36:153, 1991.

Loening-Baucke VA: Factors responsible for persistence of childhood constipation. J Pediatr Gastroenterol Nutr 6:915, 1987.

Lowery SP, Srour JW, Whitehead WE, Schuster MM: Habit training as treatment of encopresis secondary to chronic constipation. J Pediatr Gastroenterol Nutr 4:397, 1985.

Wood BP, Katzberg RW: Tween 80/diatrizoate enemas in bowel obstruction. AJR 4:747, 1978.

Renal and Urologic Conditions

CHAPTER 65

Renal Conditions

JERRY MICHAEL BERGSTEIN

ANATOMY OF THE KIDNEY

In adolescents, each kidney contains approximately 1 million nephrons and averages 12 cm in length and 150 g in weight. The glomerulus (Fig. 65–1), which arises from the afferent arteriole, is a network of specialized capillaries that serves as the filtering mechanism of the kidney. The glomerular capillaries (Fig. 65–2) are lined by endothelial cells with very thin cytoplasm containing many holes (fenestrations). The glomerular basement membrane forms a continuous layer between the endothelial and mesangial cells on one side and the epithelial cells on the other side. The membrane has three layers: (1) a central electron-dense lamina densa; (2) the lamina rara interna, which lies between the lamina densa and the endothelial cells; and (3) the lamina rara externa, which lies between the lamina densa and the epithelial cells. The visceral epithelial cells surround the capillary and project cytoplasmic foot processes, which come into contact with the lamina rara externa. Between the foot processes are spaces or filtration slits. The mesangium (mesangial cells and matrix) lies between the glomerular capillaries on the endothelial cell side of the basement membrane and forms the medial part of the capillary wall. The mesangium may serve as a supporting structure for the glomerular capillaries and probably plays a role in the removal of macromolecules (such as immune complexes) from the glomerulus. This renal microstructure does not change significantly during puberty.

GLOMERULAR FILTRATION

Although the histologic appearance of the glomerulus does not change during puberty, glomerular filtration increases in relation to body size and age (Fig. 65–3). The glomerular filtration rate is commonly estimated by clearance of endogenous creatinine. When the glomerular filtration rate is relatively normal (> 80 ml/minute when body surface area is corrected to 1.73 m²), creatinine clearance approximates inulin clearance. However, as the glomerular filtration rate declines, an increasing proportion of total creatinine in the urine is secreted by the tubules, and creatinine clearance progressively overestimates the actual filtration rate. When serum creatinine exceeds 2 mg/dl, changes in renal function are better monitored by serum creatinine concentration than by creatinine clearance.

GLOMERULAR DISEASES

Clinical Manifestations

Hematuria, proteinuria, or both are frequently the initial clinical manifestations of glomerular disease. Hematuria may be visible to the naked eye (gross), or it may be microscopic (more than five red blood cells per high-power field). Gross hematuria originating in the kidney generally produces brown or cola-colored urine that may contain red blood cell casts; if it originates in the lower urinary tract, the urine is pink to red and may contain blood clots. Gross hematuria may be associated with edema, hypertension, and renal insufficiency in the acute nephritic syndrome, which is frequently seen in adolescents with postinfectious, membranoproliferative, or rapidly progressive glomerulonephritis; lupus erythematosus; or anaphylactoid purpura.

Adolescents with gross hematuria or persistent microscopic hematuria should be evaluated thoroughly to seek an underlying cause for the hematuria. The causes of hematuria are listed in Table 65–1. The evaluation should begin with a thorough history and physical examination followed by the appropriate laboratory studies (Table 65–2). If the studies listed in steps 1 and 2 of Table 65–2 produce normal results, no further studies need be performed despite the lack of a diagnosis because active urinary tract disease has been effectively ruled out. Because of the slight risk for later development of renal disease, the adolescent should undergo an annual reevaluation consisting of history taking, physical examination, blood pressure determination, urinalysis, creatinine clearance, and determination of 24-hour protein excretion. The indications for kidney biopsy and cystoscopy in adolescents with hematuria are listed in Table 65–2.

Protein may be found in the urine of otherwise normal adolescents. Although the upper limit of normal protein excretion is 150 mg/24 hours in sedentary youth, active normal adolescents may excrete as much as 300 mg/24 hours. Thus, dipsticks may detect amounts of protein (albumin) in the urine that are actually within normal limits. Therefore, persistent proteinuria on a dipstick test of $1+$ or greater should be quantitated in a 24-hour urine collection, and its clinical significance interpreted in terms of the amount of daily physical exercise.

The causes of proteinuria are listed in Table 65–3. In the first category—nonpathologic proteinuria—the excessive protein excretion is apparently not the result of

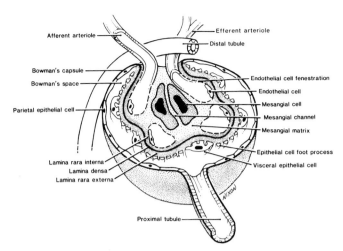

Figure 65–1. Schematic depiction of the glomerulus and surrounding structures. (With permission from Behrman RE [ed]: Nelson Textbook of Pediatrics, 14th ed. Philadelphia, WB Saunders, 1992, p 1324.)

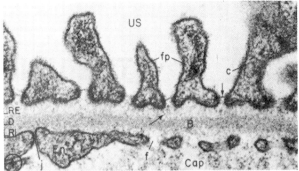

Figure 65–2. Electron micrograph of the normal glomerular capillary *(Cap)* wall demonstrating the endothelium *(En)* with its fenestrations *(f)*, the glomerular basement membrane *(B)* with its central dense layer, the lamina densa *(LD)*, and adjoining lamina rara interna *(LRI)* and externa *(LRE; long arrows)*, and the epithelial cell foot processes *(fp)* with their thick cell coat *(c)*. The glomerular filtrate passes through the endothelial fenestrae, permeates across the basement membrane, and passes through the filtration slits *(short arrows)* between the epithelial cell foot processes to reach the urinary space *(US)* (60,000 ×). (From Farquhar MG, Kanwar YS: Functional organization of the glomerulus: State of the science in 1979. In Cummings NB, Michael AF, Wilson CB [eds]: Immune Mechanisms in Renal Disease. New York, Plenum, 1982.)

a disease state. The level of proteinuria in this category is generally less than 1000 mg/day and is never associated with edema.

Postural (orthostatic) proteinuria is the most common benign cause of dipstick-positive protein excretion in adolescents. Protein excretion may be normal or slightly increased, averaging less than 5 mg/hour, in the supine position. In the upright position, the amount of protein in the urine may increase threefold or more. The proteinuria is usually discovered on routine urinalysis performed on a urine sample collected in the afternoon or evening. Its cause is unknown, and it is not associated with hematuria. The diagnosis is confirmed by obtaining normal supine (first morning void) and abnormal upright timed urine collections.

Proteinuria also may be associated with fever (38.3°C or greater) and vigorous exercise. However, benign proteinuria associated with these circumstances does not exceed 2+ on the dipstick and resolves when the fever abates or after 48 hours of rest.

Pathologic proteinuria may result from either tubular or glomerular disorders. Normal individuals filter large amounts of proteins that are of lower molecular weight than albumin (e.g., hormones, enzymes, light chains of immunoglobulin) across the glomerular capillary wall; these proteins are normally reabsorbed in the proximal tubule. Injury to the proximal tubules results in decreased reabsorption and the loss of these proteins in

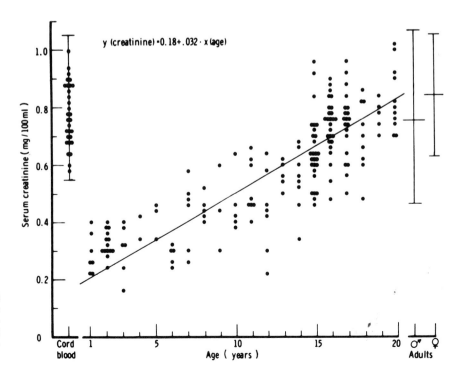

Figure 65–3. The serum creatinine in relation to age. (With permission from McCrory WW: Developmental Nephrology. Cambridge, Harvard University Press, 1972. Copyright © 1972 by the President and Fellows of Harvard College.)

TABLE 65–1. Causes of Hematuria

I. Glomerular Diseases
  A. Recurrent gross hematuria syndrome
    1. IgA nephropathy
    2. Idiopathic hematuria
    3. Alport syndrome
  B. Acute poststreptococcal glomerulonephritis
  C. Membranous nephropathy
  D. Membranoproliferative glomerulonephritis
  E. Glomerular nephritis of chronic infection
  F. Rapidly progressive (crescentic) glomerulonephritis
  G. Goodpasture disease
  H. Anaphylactoid purpura
  I. Lupus erythematosus
  J. Hemolytic-uremic syndrome
II. Infections
  A. Bacterial (including gonorrhea)
  B. Tuberculosis
  C. Viral
III. Hematologic
  A. Coagulopathies
  B. Thrombocytopenia
  C. Sickle cell disease
  D. Renal vein thrombosis
IV. Stones and Hypercalciuria
V. Anatomic Abnormalities
  A. Congenital anomalies
  B. Trauma
  C. Polycystic kidneys
  D. Vascular abnormalities
  E. Tumors
  F. Ureteropelvic junction (UPS) obstruction after trauma
VI. Exercise
VII. Drugs

TABLE 65–2. Evaluation of the Adolescent with Hematuria

STEP 1
(Performed on All Adolescent Patients)
Complete blood count
Urine culture
Serum creatinine
24-hour urine collection for
  creatinine
  protein
  calcium
Serum C3 level
Intravenous pyelogram

STEP 2
(Performed on Selected Adolescent Patients)
DNAse B titer or Streptozyme test if hematuria less than 6 months' duration
Skin or throat cultures when appropriate
ANA
Coagulation studies and platelet count when suggested by history
Sickle cell screen in all black patients
Voiding cystourethrogram (infection, lower tract lesion)

STEP 3
(Invasive Procedures)
Renal biopsy, indications:
  1. Persistent high-grade microscopic hematuria
  2. Microscopic hematuria plus one of the following:
    a. diminished renal function
    b. proteinuria exceeding 150 mg/24 hours
    c. hypertension
  3. Second episode of gross hematuria
Cystoscopy, indication:
  Pink to red hematuria, dysuria, and sterile urine culture

the urine. Such proteinuria rarely exceeds 1 g/24 hours and is not associated with edema. Tubular proteinuria (see Table 65–3) may be seen in inherited and acquired disorders and may be associated with other defects of proximal tubular function, such as glycosuria, phosphaturia, bicarbonate wasting, and aminoaciduria. Tubular proteinuria rarely presents a diagnostic dilemma because the underlying disease is usually detected before the proteinuria is. Asymptomatic patients having persistent proteinuria generally have glomerular, rather than tubular, proteinuria. In occult cases, differentiation between glomerular and tubular proteinuria may be made by electrophoresis of urine. Glomerular proteinuria is the most common cause of proteinuria and results from increased permeability of the glomerular capillary wall. The degree of proteinuria may range from less than 1 g to more than 30 g/24 hours. The constellation of proteinuria resulting in hypoproteinemia, edema, and hyperlipidemia is termed the nephrotic syndrome.

Persistent asymptomatic proteinuria is defined as proteinuria in an apparently healthy individual if it occurs without hematuria and persists for 3 months. The amount of proteinuria is less than 2 g/24 hours, and it is never associated with edema. Causes include postural proteinuria, membranous and membranoproliferative glomerulonephritis, pyelonephritis, hereditary nephritis, developmental anomalies, and "benign" proteinuria.

Evaluation of the adolescent having persistent asymptomatic proteinuria should include urine culture, intravenous pyelography, and measurement of creatinine clearance, 24-hour protein excretion, serum albumin, and C3 complement levels. In individuals with proteinuria of 150 to 1000 mg/24 hours in whom other findings are normal, renal biopsy is not indicated because evidence for a progressive disease is rarely found. Such

adolescents should have an annual reevaluation consisting of physical examination and blood pressure determination, as well as urinalysis and determination of creatinine clearance and 24-hour protein excretion. In-

TABLE 65–3. Classification of Proteinuria

I. Nonpathologic Proteinuria (≤300 mg/24 hours)
  A. Postural (orthostatic)
  B. Febrile
  C. Exercise
II. Pathologic Proteinuria (>300 mg/24 hours)
  A. Tubular (300–1000 mg/24 hours)
    1. Hereditary
      a. Cystinosis
      b. Wilson disease
      c. Lowe syndrome
      d. Proximal renal tubular acidosis
      e. Galactosemia
    2. Acquired
      a. Analgesic abuse
      b. Vitamin D intoxication
      c. Hypokalemia
      d. Antibiotics
      e. Interstitial nephritis
      f. Acute tubular necrosis
      g. Sarcoidosis
      h. Cystic diseases
      i. Homograft rejection
      j. Penicillamine administration
      k. Heavy metal poisoning (mercury, gold, lead, bismuth, cadmium, chromium, copper)
  B. Glomerular (>1000 mg/24 hours)
    1. Persistent asymptomatic
    2. Nephrotic syndrome
      a. Idiopathic nephrotic syndrome
        (1) Minimal-change
        (2) Mesangial proliferation
        (3) Focal sclerosis
      b. Glomerulonephritis
      c. Tumors
      d. Drugs
      e. AIDS

dications for renal biopsy include the development of hematuria, hypertension, diminished renal function, and an increase in proteinuria to more than 1000 mg/24 hours.

Glomerulonephritis

Glomerulonephritis, a histopathologic term signifying inflammation of the glomerular capillaries, may result from two major mechanisms of immunologic injury in adolescents: (1) glomerular localization of circulating or locally formed antigen-antibody immune complexes, or (2) interaction of antibody with glomerular basement membrane antigen *in situ* (antiglomerular basement membrane antibody disease). The inflammatory reaction that follows immunologic injury may result from activation of one or more mediation (complement, coagulation, kinin) systems.

Immunologic injury may stimulate proliferation of the mesangial cells in some (focal glomerulonephritis, Fig. 65–4A) or all (diffuse glomerulonephritis, Fig. 65–4B) glomeruli. Immunofluorescence (Fig. 65–5A) and electron microscopy usually demonstrate that mesangial

proliferation results from immune complex deposition in the mesangium. Immune complexes may also occur in the subendothelial space between the glomerular basement membrane and the endothelial cells, as seen in type I membranoproliferative glomerulonephritis (Fig. 65–5B) and more severe forms of lupus glomerulonephritis, or in the subepithelial space between the glomerular basement membrane and the epithelial cells, as seen in membranous nephropathy (Figs. 65–4C and 65–5C) and poststreptococcal glomerulonephritis.

Crescent formation is sometimes associated with immune complex or antiglomerular basement membrane antibody deposition (Fig. 65–5D) in the glomerular capillary wall. The crescent (Fig. 65–4D) is composed of the proliferating epithelial cells that line the Bowman space, fibrin, and macrophages. Crescents develop in several forms of glomerulonephritis (termed *rapidly progressive*) and appear to result in glomerular obsolescence.

POSTSTREPTOCOCCAL (POSTINFECTIOUS) GLOMERULONEPHRITIS

Poststreptococcal glomerulonephritis is the classic example of the acute nephritic syndrome, which includes

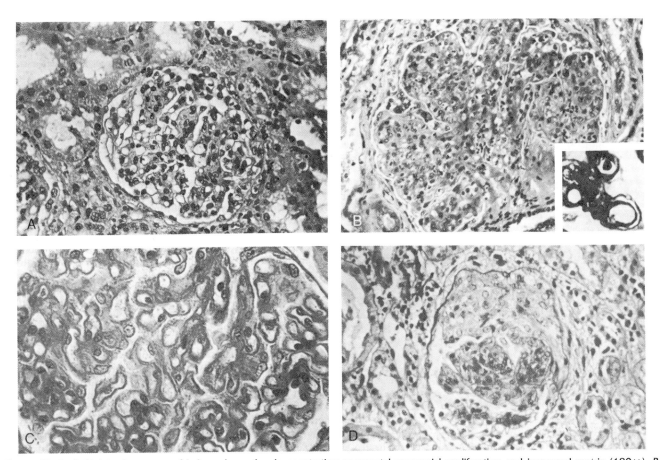

Figure 65–4. *A,* Light microscopy of IgA nephropathy demonstrating segmental mesangial proliferation and increased matrix (180×). *B,* Glomerulus from a patient having type I membranoproliferative glomerulonephritis demonstrating an accentuated lobular pattern, a generalized increase in mesangial cells and matrix, and "splitting" of the glomerular capillary wall *(insert)* (250×). *C,* Glomerulus from a patient having a membranous glomerulopathy demonstrating diffuse thickening of the glomerular basement membrane when cellular proliferation is lacking (400×). *D,* Light micrograph demonstrating a crescent overlying the glomerulus in a biopsy specimen from a child having anaphylactoid purpura glomerulonephritis (180×). (*A, C,* and *D,* With permission from Behrman RE [ed]: Nelson Textbook of Pediatrics, 14th ed. Philadelphia, WB Saunders, 1992, pp 1328, 1331, 1334. *B,* With permission from Kim Y, Michael AF: Idiopathic membranoproliferative glomerulonephritis. Annu Rev Med 31:273, © 1980 by Annual Reviews Inc.)

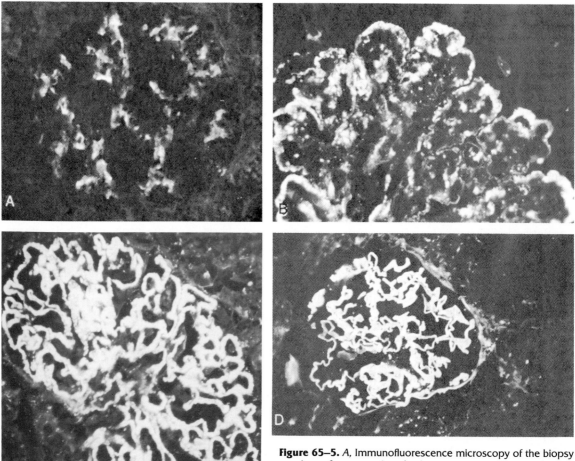

Figure 65–5. *A,* Immunofluorescence microscopy of the biopsy specimen from a patient having recurrent episodes of gross hematuria demonstrating mesangial deposition of IgA (250×). *B,* Immunofluorescence microscopy demonstrating granular deposition of C3 along the glomerular basement membranes and in the mesangium in type I membranoproliferative glomerulonephritis (610×). *C,* Immunofluorescence microscopy demonstrating glomerular basement membrane deposits of IgG in membranous glomerulopathy (250×). *D,* Immunofluorescence microscopy demonstrating the continuous linear staining of IgG along the glomerular membrane as found in diseases mediated by antiglomerular basement membrane antibody (250×). (*A* and *D,* With permission from Behrman RE [ed]: Nelson Textbook of Pediatrics, 14th ed. Philadelphia, WB Saunders, 1992, pp 1329, 1334. *B,* With permission from Kim Y, Michael AF: Idiopathic membranoproliferative glomerulonephritis. Annu Rev Med 31:273, © 1980 by Annual Reviews, Inc.)

(1) the sudden onset of gross hematuria (frequently with red blood cell casts), (2) hypertension (salt and water overload), (3) impaired renal function, and (4) edema (salt and water overload). Although typically associated with streptococcal infection (see Chapter 94), a similar clinical picture may follow infection with coagulase-positive and coagulase-negative staphylococci, *Streptococcus pneumoniae*, gram-negative bacteria, and certain fungal, rickettsial, and viral diseases.

Pathogenesis and Pathologic Features. Acute post-streptococcal glomerulonephritis in the adolescent follows infection of the throat or skin with certain nephritogenic strains of group A beta-hemolytic streptococci. The disease is usually sporadic. In the winter, it commonly results from pharyngitis, whereas in the summer it generally follows skin infection.

Pathologically, the kidneys are symmetrically enlarged. All glomeruli appear enlarged and relatively bloodless and show diffuse mesangial cell proliferation with an increase in mesangial matrix. Polymorphonu-

clear leukocytes are common in glomeruli during the early stage of the disease, and crescents may be found in severe cases. Immunofluorescence and electron microscopy demonstrate lumpy, bumpy immune complex deposits composed of immunoglobin and complement on the epithelial side of the glomerular basement membrane and in the mesangium. These morphologic changes and a depression in the serum complement (C3) level suggest that poststreptococcal glomerulonephritis is mediated by immune complexes.

Clinical Manifestations. Poststreptococcal glomerulonephritis usually presents with an acute nephritic syndrome 1 to 2 weeks after an antecedent streptococcal infection. The severity of the disease may range from asymptomatic microscopic hematuria with preserved renal function to acute renal failure. Depending on the severity of renal involvement, adolescents may experience varying degrees of edema, hypertension, and oliguria. Nonspecific symptoms, such as malaise, lethargy, abdominal or flank pain, and fever, are common. Complications are those of acute renal failure and include volume overload, circulatory congestion, hypertension, hyperkalemia, hyperphosphatemia, hypocalcemia, acidosis, seizures, and uremia.

Diagnosis. Urinalysis reveals hematuria, frequently with red blood cell casts; proteinuria; and possibly polymorphonuclear leukocytes. Although skin or throat cultures may be positive for group A beta-hemolytic streptococci, confirmation of the diagnosis requires serologic evidence of an elevated antibody titer to streptococcal antigen (antistreptolysin O or Streptozyme test) and a depressed C3 complement level.

These laboratory findings, in conjunction with the development of an acute nephritic syndrome after an appropriate latent period, following a streptococcal infection, strongly support the diagnosis of acute poststreptococcal glomerulonephritis, and renal biopsy is not indicated. Biopsy should be considered if acute renal failure or the nephrotic syndrome develops or if decreased renal function, marked hematuria or proteinuria, or a low level of C3 persists for more than 3 months.

The differential diagnosis includes many of the items listed in Table 65–1. Of special concern are systemic lupus erythematosus (SLE) and membranoproliferative glomerulonephritis.

Treatment. Since there is no specific therapy for poststreptococcal glomerulonephritis, the management is that of acute renal failure. A 10-day course of penicillin is recommended to limit the spread of nephritogenic organisms, but it does not affect the natural history of the disease. Specimens should be taken from family members for culture for group A beta-hemolytic streptococci, and if the specimens are positive for these organisms, the affected individuals should be treated.

Prognosis. Complete recovery occurs in more than 90% of patients. Infrequently, the acute phase may be very severe and result in permanent glomerular damage and chronic renal insufficiency. Recurrences are extremely rare.

MEMBRANOUS NEPHROPATHY (GLOMERULONEPHRITIS)

Pathogenesis and Pathologic Features. Pathologically in membranous nephropathy, the glomeruli show diffuse thickening of the glomerular basement membranes without proliferative changes (see Fig. 65–4C). The thickening presumably results from the production of basement membrane–like material by the visceral epithelial cells in response to immune complexes deposited on the epithelial side of the basement membrane (see Fig. 65–5C). In certain areas, this new material may appear as "spikes" on the epithelial side of the basement membrane. These morphologic changes suggest that membranous nephropathy is also an immune complex–mediated disease.

Clinical Manifestations. Membranous nephropathy typically presents as nephrotic syndrome in adults, though it is also a well-known cause of persistent asymptomatic proteinuria. Microscopic hematuria is common, but gross hematuria is rare. The blood pressure and C3 levels are normal.

Diagnosis. The diagnosis is confirmed by renal biopsy. The histologic picture of membranous nephropathy may be seen in association with several other conditions, including SLE, renal vein thrombosis, cancer, gold or penicillamine therapy, and syphilis and hepatitis B infections.

Treatment and Prognosis. Some studies suggest that immunosuppressive therapy may retard progression of the disease. Although the disease may resolve spontaneously in the majority of patients, some may slowly progress over 10 to 20 years to renal failure.

MEMBRANOPROLIFERATIVE GLOMERULONEPHRITIS

The term *chronic glomerulonephritis* implies continuing glomerular injury, frequently leading to progressive glomerular destruction and end-stage renal failure. Membranoproliferative glomerulonephritis is the most common cause of chronic glomerulonephritis in adolescents. The disease seems to have two histologic appearances; whether these truly represent the same or different diseases remains to be determined.

Pathogenesis and Pathologic Features. In type I membranoproliferative glomerulonephritis (the more common form), the glomeruli have a lobular appearance owing to a generalized increase in mesangial cells and matrix (see Fig. 65–4B). The glomerular capillary walls appear thickened and, in some areas, duplicated or split because of interposition of mesangial cytoplasm and matrix between the endothelial cells and glomerular basement membrane. Crescents may be present and, when detected in a high percentage of glomeruli, indicate a poor prognosis. Immunofluorescence microscopy reveals C3 and lesser amounts of immunoglobulin in the mesangium and along the peripheral capillary walls in a lobular pattern (see Fig. 65–5B). Electron microscopy confirms the presence of immune complex–like deposits in the mesangium and the subendothelial region.

In type II disease, the mesangial changes are less prominent than in type I disease. The capillary walls demonstrate irregular ribbon-like thickening caused by the presence of dense deposit material. Splitting of the membrane is rare, but crescents are common. On electron microscopy, the dense deposits appear as a thickening of the glomerular basement membrane in the region of, but distinct from, the lamina densa. Although the deposits are also found in the Bowman capsule, the mesangium, and the tubular basement membranes, their composition is unknown. Immunofluorescent studies show C3, usually with minimal immunoglobulin, along the margin of the dense deposit material.

Clinical Manifestations. The clinical manifestations of types I and II are similar. Although the majority of adolescents present with nephrotic syndrome, initial manifestations include an acute nephritic syndrome, asymptomatic hematuria, or proteinuria. Renal function may be normal to depressed. Hypertension is common, as is a low serum C3 complement level.

Diagnosis. The diagnosis is confirmed by kidney biopsy. The differential diagnosis includes other cause of glomerulonephritis and nephrotic syndrome; SLE and poststreptococcal glomerulonephritis warrant special consideration.

Prognosis and Treatment. Although the outlook for both types of membranoproliferative glomerulonephritis is poor, the prognosis for type II seems worse than that for type I. No definitive therapy exists, but stabilization of the clinical course has been reported in some patients receiving therapy with immunosuppressive (prednisone) or antiplatelet agents.

GLOMERULONEPHRITIS OF CHRONIC INFECTION

Glomerulonephritis has been recognized during the course of a variety of chronic infections in adolescents, including subacute bacterial endocarditis (*Streptococcus viridans* and other organisms), infected ventriculoatrial shunts for hydrocephalus *(Staphylococcus albus)*, syphilis, hepatitis B virus, candidiasis, and malaria. In each condition, the host is infected with organisms of low virulence and is continually seeded with foreign antigen. The host's antibody response, in the presence of high levels of circulating antigen, results in the formation of immune complexes that become deposited in the kidneys and initiate the glomerulonephritis.

The histopathologic findings may resemble poststreptococcal, membranous, or membranoproliferative glomerulonephritis. The clinical presentation is generally an acute nephritic or nephrotic syndrome. The C3 level is frequently depressed.

Eradication of the infection before severe glomerular injury occurs usually results in resolution of the glomerulonephritis. However, progression to end-stage renal failure has been described.

RAPIDLY PROGRESSIVE (CRESCENTIC) GLOMERULONEPHRITIS

The term *rapidly progressive* is applied to those forms of glomerulonephritis in which rapid loss of renal function is associated with crescent formation in the majority of glomeruli.

Pathogenesis and Pathologic Features. Crescents may be found in several well-defined types of glomerulonephritis, such as poststreptococcal, lupus erythematosus, membranoproliferative, and the glomerulonephritides associated with Goodpasture disease, anaphylactoid purpura, polyarteritis, and Wegener granulomatosis. Crescents are located on the inside of the Bowman capsule and are composed of the proliferating epithelial cells of the capsule, fibrin, basement membrane–like material, and macrophages (see Fig. 65–4*D*).

In many adolescent patients having the idiopathic variety of the disease, the cause is unknown, as no evidence for immunologic mechanisms can be detected. Others show antibodies specific for glomerular basement membrane or immune complex deposits on the capillary walls.

Clinical Manifestations. The majority of adolescent patients present with acute renal failure, often with an acute nephritic or nephrotic syndrome prior to the development of renal failure. The disease progresses to end-stage renal failure within weeks to months following onset. In the idiopathic variety, the C3 level is normal.

Diagnosis. The diagnosis is confirmed by kidney biopsy. In addition, appropriate serologic studies (antinuclear antibody, C3, and antistreptolysin O titers) should be obtained to search for defined types of glomerulonephritis.

Prognosis and Treatment. Adolescents having rapidly progressive disease associated with poststreptococcal glomerulonephritis may recover spontaneously. We have had success in treating rapidly progressive lupus nephritis and anaphylactoid purpura nephritis with prednisone and azathioprine. The prognosis is poor for the remaining types of rapidly progressive glomerulonephritis, though some patients have been reported to improve after therapy with combinations of methylprednisolone pulse therapy, immunosuppressive agents, anticoagulants, and plasmapheresis.

GOODPASTURE DISEASE

Goodpasture disease (pulmonary hemorrhage and glomerulonephritis mediated by antibodies reacting with both lung and glomerular basement membranes) should be distinguished from Goodpasture syndrome, which is the clinical picture of pulmonary hemorrhage and glomerulonephritis as may be seen in several disease states (SLE, anaphylactoid purpura, polyarteritis nodosa, Wegener granulomatosis). In some patients, antiglomerular basement membrane nephritis is observed without pulmonary hemorrhage (classified as one of the forms of rapidly progressive glomerulonephritis).

Pathogenesis and Pathologic Features. In most patients, the light microscopic changes resemble rapidly progressive glomerulonephritis. Immunofluorescence microscopy demonstrates a continuous linear pattern of IgG along the glomerular basement membrane, typical of antiglomerular basement membrane antibody (see Fig. 65–5*D*).

Clinical Manifestations. Hemoptysis is usually the presenting symptom, and pulmonary hemorrhage is a potential cause of death. Days to weeks later, the adolescent patient experiences hematuria, proteinuria, and progressive renal failure. The C3 level is normal.

Diagnosis. The diagnosis is suggested by kidney biopsy. Since other diseases may show linear glomerular basement membrane staining for IgG, the diagnosis is confirmed by the demonstration of antiglomerular basement membrane antibody in the circulation.

Prognosis and Treatment. Adolescents surviving the pulmonary hemorrhage commonly progress to end-stage renal failure. Many patients appear to benefit from aggressive immunosuppression and plasmapheresis.

IgA NEPHROPATHY

IgA nephropathy is one of several diseases in which the adolescent may suffer recurrent episodes of gross hematuria. Other diseases include idiopathic hematuria, Alport syndrome, and hypercalciuria. In patients having recurrent episodes of gross hematuria, the hematuria may begin 1 to 2 days after the onset of an upper respiratory infection. This short latent period can usually be distinguished from the 7- to 14-day latent period seen in young individuals in whom poststreptococcal glomerulonephritis is developing. In further distinction from poststreptococcal glomerulonephritis, adolescent patients with recurrent gross hematuria do not have the acute nephritic syndrome.

Pathogenesis and Pathologic Features. By light microscopy, most kidney biopsy specimens obtained from adolescent patients with IgA nephropathy reveal focal and segmental mesangial proliferation and increased matrix (see Fig. 65–4A). In more severe cases, diffuse mesangial proliferation, crescent formation, and scarring may be detected. Immunofluorescence microscopy (see Fig. 65–5A) demonstrates that IgA is the predominant immunoglobulin deposited in the mesangium, but lesser amounts of IgG, IgM, C3, and properdin are common. In severe cases, electron microscopy shows extension of the mesangial deposits onto the capillary walls. The morphologic findings suggest that IgA nephropathy is mediated by IgA-containing immune complexes.

Clinical Manifestations. Patients with IgA nephropathy present with gross or microscopic hematuria. During the course of gross hematuria, renal function usually remains relatively normal, and proteinuria does not exceed 1 g/day. Normal serum levels of C3 help to distinguish this disorder from poststreptococcal glomerulonephritis. The gross hematuria usually resolves within 7 days, but microscopic hematuria may persist between attacks.

Prognosis and Treatment. Despite recurrent episodes of gross hematuria, most adolescents suffer no significant kidney damage, and the disease resolves spontaneously. Progressive disease does develop in 20% to 30% of adolescent patients, in whom a poor prognosis is associated with hypertension, diminished renal function, proteinuria exceeding 1 g/day between episodes of gross hematuria, or histologic evidence of diffuse glomerulonephritis with crescents and scarring. Although controlled studies are lacking, immunosuppressive therapy may be beneficial in progressive disease.

The Nephrotic Syndrome (Nephrosis)

The term *nephrotic syndrome* does not indicate a disease. Rather, as previously mentioned, it represents a clinical picture characterized by proteinuria, hypoproteinemia, edema, and hyperlipidemia that may result from several forms of glomerular injury (Table 65–3). The underlying abnormality in all forms of nephrotic syndrome is an increase in glomerular capillary wall permeability that results in proteinuria. In the nephrotic state, the protein loss usually exceeds 3 g/day and is composed primarily of albumin. Thus the hypoproteinemia is fundamentally a hypoalbuminemia. Edema generally appears in adolescents when the serum albumin level falls to less than 2.5 g/dl.

IDIOPATHIC NEPHROTIC SYNDROME

The idiopathic nephrotic syndrome consists of three histologic patterns: (1) minimal-change disease, (2) mesangial proliferation, and (3) focal sclerosis. Because the cause of the disease is unknown, it remains unclear whether this syndrome is a single disorder with varying histologic features or different diseases having similar clinical manifestations in adolescents. However, prior to treatment, adolescents with nephrotic syndrome should undergo renal biopsy.

Pathologic Features. In minimal-change (nil) disease, the glomeruli appear normal or show a minimal increase in mesangial cells and matrix. Immunofluorescence microscopy shows a normal appearance. Electron microscopy reveals retraction ("fusion") of the epithelial cell foot processes. Most patients with this variety of disease respond to corticosteroid therapy.

The lesion of mesangial proliferative is characterized by a diffuse increase in mesangial cells and matrix. Mesangial deposits containing IgM and C3 may be seen. The majority of adolescents who have this lesion respond to corticosteroids or cytotoxic therapy, or both.

In focal sclerosis, the majority of glomeruli appear normal or show mesangial proliferation. Others, especially those adjacent to the medulla, show areas of scarring (sclerosis) in one or more lobules. The disease is frequently progressive and leads to end-stage renal failure in most patients. Approximately 20% of patients respond to corticosteroid or cytotoxic therapy, or both.

Clinical Manifestations. The initial episode of nephrotic syndrome and subsequent relapses usually follow an apparent viral illness. The disease usually presents as edema, which is initially noted around the eyes and in the lower extremities in which it is "pitting" in nature. With time, the edema becomes generalized and may be associated with weight gain and the development of ascites and pleural effusions. Anorexia, diarrhea, and abdominal pain are common; hypertension is uncommon. During relapse, complications may include an increased susceptibility to bacterial infections and an increased risk of vascular thrombosis.

Diagnosis. Urinalysis reveals proteinuria (3+ or 4+); microscopic hematuria may be present, but gross hematuria is rare. Renal function may be normal or reduced, depending on the intravascular volume. Protein excretion exceeds 3 g/24 hours. The serum cholesterol and triglyceride levels are elevated, the serum albumin level is usually less than 2 g/dl, and the serum calcium level is diminished, primarily from a reduction in the albumin-bound fraction. The C3 level is normal.

Treatment. Edema is controlled with salt and water restriction and diuretic therapy. After confirmation of the histologic diagnosis by renal biopsy, prednisone is initiated at a dosage of 20 mg three times a day. The average response time is 2 weeks; the patient is declared steroid-resistant if proteinuria (2+ or greater) persists after 1 month of treatment.

Five days after the urine becomes free of protein (less than or equal to 1+ on dipstick), the dosage of prednisone is changed to 60 mg taken every other day as a single dose with breakfast. To maintain remission, alternate-day prednisone is continued for 3 to 6 months. After the period of alternate-day therapy, the prednisone may be discontinued abruptly, but intravenous cortisone should be administered during stressful situations such as surgery or severe illness.

Each relapse is treated in a similar manner. If there

TABLE 65–4. Classification of Renal Tubular Acidosis

PROXIMAL	DISTAL	MINERALOCORTICOID DEFICIENCY
Isolated	Isolated	Adrenal disorders ($\downarrow$ A, $\uparrow$ R)*
Sporadic	Sporadic	Addison disease
Hereditary	Hereditary	Congenital hyperplasia
Fanconi syndrome	Secondary	Primary hypoaldosteronism
Primary	Interstitial nephritis	Hyporeninemic hypoaldosteronism ($\downarrow$ A, $\downarrow$ R)
Secondary	Obstructive	Obstruction
Inherited	Pyelonephritis	Pyelonephritis
Cystinosis	Transplant rejection	Interstitial nephritis
Lowe syndrome	Sickle cell nephropathy	Diabetes mellitus
Galactosemia	Lupus nephritis	Nephrosclerosis
Hereditary fructose intolerance	Ehlers-Danlos syndrome	Glomerulonephritis
Tyrosinemia	Nephrocalcinosis	Pseudohypoaldosteronism ($\uparrow$ A, $\uparrow$ R)
Wilson disease	Hepatic cirrhosis	
Medullary cystic disease	Elliptocytosis	
Acquired	Medullary sponge kidney	
Heavy metals	Toxins	
Outdated tetracycline	Amphotericin B	
Proteinuria	Lithium	
Interstitial nephritis	Toluene	
Hyperparathyroidism		
Vitamin D deficiency rickets		

*A, aldosterone; R, renin.

are frequent relapses, resulting in corticosteroid toxicity, or if the patient is steroid-resistant, cytotoxic therapy with cyclophosphamide should be considered.

Course and Prognosis. The majority of patients having corticosteroid-responsive nephrosis have intermittent relapses until the disease resolves spontaneously. The prognosis is guarded for teenagers who fail to respond to corticosteroids. In those who fail to respond to corticosteroid and cytotoxic therapy, the disease is likely to progress to end-stage renal failure.

SECONDARY FORMS OF NEPHROTIC SYNDROME

Nephrotic syndrome may develop during the course of any type of glomerulonephritis but is most common in association with membranous, membranoproliferative, or poststreptococcal glomerulonephritis, lupus erythematosus, chronic infection (including malaria and schistosomiasis), and anaphylactoid purpura glomerulonephritis. Although the development of a secondary nephrotic syndrome may indicate severe glomerular disease, the nephrotic syndrome frequently resolves if the nephritis improves.

Nephrotic syndrome has been described in association with several types of extrarenal neoplasms. In adolescents who have solid tumors, such as carcinomas, the glomerular changes resemble membranous glomerulopathy. The renal involvement is presumably mediated by immune complexes composed of tumor antigens and tumor-specific antibodies. In lymphomas, especially Hodgkin disease (see Chapter 53), minimal-change disease is most commonly found, although proliferative lesions have also been described. In patients having the minimal-change lesion, the nephrosis may develop before or after the malignancy is detected, may resolve as the tumor regresses, and may return if the tumor recurs.

Nephrotic syndrome has developed during therapy with several types of drugs and chemicals. The histologic picture may resemble that of membranous glomerulop-

athy (penicillamine, gold, mercury compounds), minimal-change disease (probenecid, ethosuximide, methimazole, lithium), or proliferative glomerulonephritis (procainamide, chlorpropamide, mephenytoin, trimethadione, paramethadione). Nephrotic syndrome may also develop following parental drug abuse. Heroin is the most commonly abused agent, and focal sclerosis is the most frequent histologic lesion. The prognosis is poor.

Nephrotic syndrome can also develop during the clinical course of acquired immunodeficiency syndrome (AIDS) and is unrelated to the abuse of parenteral drugs. Focal sclerosis is the typical histologic lesion. The course of the disease is marked by rapid progression to renal failure.

TUBULAR DISORDERS

Renal Tubular Acidosis

Renal tubular acidosis (RTA) is a clinical state of hyperchloremic systemic acidosis resulting from impaired urinary acidification (Table 65–4). Three types exist: distal RTA (type I), proximal RTA (type II), and mineralocorticoid deficiency (type IV). A proposed type III was later found to be a variant of distal RTA.

DISTAL RENAL TUBULAR ACIDOSIS (TYPE I)

Pathophysiology. Distal RTA is best described as a deficiency of hydrogen ion secretion by the distal tubule and collecting duct, resulting in a urine pH that cannot be reduced to less than 5.8 despite severe systemic acidosis. The hypokalemia is usually less severe than that found in proximal RTA because less bicarbonate is wasted. Nephrocalcinosis may be present.

Distal RTA may occur as an isolated sporadic disorder or as an autosomal dominant or recessive trait. Distal RTA (secondary) may also develop during the course of several diseases and intoxications involving the distal tubules and collecting ducts (see Table 65–4).

PROXIMAL RENAL TUBULAR ACIDOSIS (TYPE II)

Pathophysiology. Proximal RTA results from reduced proximal tubular reabsorption of bicarbonate, presumably resulting from deficient carbonic anhydrase production or diminished hydrogen-sodium ion exchange. Rather than reabsorbing the normal 85% of filtered bicarbonate, in this condition the proximal tubules may reabsorb only 60%, thus presenting the distal tubule with 40% rather than the usual 15% of the filtered load. Because the distal tubules can maximally reabsorb only 15% of the normal filtered load of bicarbonate, up to 25% may be lost in the urine. As a result, proximal RTA is generally more severe than distal RTA because complete loss of the distal bicarbonate recovery mechanism (which is rare) would waste only 15% of filtered bicarbonate. With urinary bicarbonate loss, the serum bicarbonate level falls until it reaches a level (bicarbonate threshold) at which bicarbonate wasting ceases. At this level (15 to 18 mEq/L), the amount of filtered bicarbonate (serum bicarbonate times glomerular filtration rate) is reduced to an amount that can be totally reabsorbed by the tubules. Because distal tubular acidification mechanisms remain intact, the urine may then be acidified (pH less than 5.5). Flooding the distal tubule with sodium bicarbonate stimulates sodium reabsorption in exchange for potassium, leading to hypokalemia. Contraction of the extracellular fluid volume because of the loss of sodium bicarbonate stimulates chloride reabsorption (resulting in hyperchloremia) and aldosterone secretion (enhancing potassium loss).

Proximal RTA (Table 65–4) may occur as an isolated disorder that is not associated with other disease states or other abnormalities of proximal tubular function. Isolated proximal RTA may be transient, persistent, or sporadic or inherited (autosomal dominant). Proximal RTA may also occur as part of a generalized defect in proximal tubular transport. Called the Fanconi syndrome, this disorder is characterized by glucosuria, phosphaturia, aminoaciduria, and proximal RTA. A primary form of Fanconi syndrome that is not associated with other disease states has been described, showing both autosomal dominant and recessive modes of inheritance. Fanconi syndrome (secondary) may also develop during the course of several inherited and acquired disease states. The classic example is cystinosis, which is an autosomal recessive defect that results from the accumulation of cystine within the lysosomes of the bone marrow, liver, spleen, lymph nodes, kidneys (leading to end-stage failure), fibroblasts, leukocytes, corneas, and conjunctivae. It may present during the first (nephropathic form) or second (juvenile form) decade of life. The initial clinical manifestations of polyuria and polydipsia (concentrating defect), fever (dehydration), growth retardation, rickets, blonde hair and fair skin (diminished pigmentation), and photophobia are much less severe in the form that has its onset later in life. This diagnosis is suggested by detecting cystine crystals in the corneas by slit-lamp microscopy and is confirmed by demonstrating elevated leukocyte cystine content.

Although no definitive therapy exists to prevent intracellular cystine accumulation, a clinical trial with cysteamine is currently in progress.

MINERALOCORTICOID DEFICIENCY (TYPE IV)

Pathophysiology. Mineralocorticoid deficiency results from inadequate production of, or reduced distal tubular responsiveness to, aldosterone. When aldosterone-mediated sodium reabsorption is lacking, hyperkalemia develops. Hyperkalemia suppresses renal ammonia production, resulting in a reduction of ammonium excretion and thus net acid excretion. The result is a hyperkalemic, hyperchloremic acidosis. The urine pH may become acidified (less than 5.5).

Hyporeninemic hypoaldosteronism is a form of RTA that may result from renal diseases associated with interstitial damage and destruction of the juxtaglomerular apparatus (most commonly diabetes mellitus in adolescents); it may also be observed with volume expansion and prostaglandin inhibition. In those conditions, plasma levels of renin and, as a result, aldosterone are reduced; renal function may be compromised. Rarely, type IV RTA may be the result of distal tubular unresponsiveness to aldosterone (pseudohypoaldosteronism); plasma renin and aldosterone levels are elevated, renal function is usually normal, and salt wasting is the rule. This form of RTA may also be observed in adolescent patients with medullary disease and renal insufficiency.

Clinical Manifestations. The clinical manifestations of all three types of RTA include growth retardation, anorexia, constipation, muscle weakness, polyuria, and bone disease. Patients having secondary forms of proximal or distal RTA may present with complaints that are unique to their fundamental disease.

Distal RTA is complicated by hypercalciuria that may lead to nephrocalcinosis, nephrolithiasis, and renal parenchymal destruction. Although the factors producing hypercalciuria are unknown, potential mechanisms include bone breakdown to release calcium carbonate (the carbonate to be converted to bicarbonate in an attempt to control the acidosis) and diminished urinary citrate (which complexes to calcium) levels.

Both proximal and distal RTA may be complicated by osteomalacia in adolescents. Proximal tubular dysfunction may result in phosphaturia and inadequate production of 1,25-dihydroxyvitamin D, whereas distal tubular dysfunction promotes bone disease as a result of hypercalciuria.

Diagnosis. Before considering the diagnosis of the three forms of RTA, other causes of systemic acidosis, such as diarrhea, lactic acidosis, diabetes mellitus, and renal failure, should be excluded. The biochemical features of proximal and distal RTA include low serum bicarbonate and potassium levels in association with hyperchloremia. Mineralocorticoid deficiency RTA is easily detected by the finding of systemic acidosis in association with hyperkalemia. The anion gap in all forms of RTA is generally normal.

Adolescent patients suspected of having proximal or distal RTA should be evaluated by comparing the pH (by pH meter) of the first morning urine specimen

TABLE 65–5. Causes of Interstitial Nephritis

DRUGS	INFECTIONS	DISEASE-ASSOCIATED
	Acute	
Penicillin derivatives	Streptococcal	Sarcoidosis
Cephalosporins	Pyelonephritis	Glomerulonephritis
Sulfonamides	Toxoplasmosis	Transplant rejection
Cotrimoxazole	Diphtheria	Idiopathic
Rifampin	Brucellosis	
Phenytoin	Leptospirosis	
Thiazides	Mononucleosis	
Furosemide	Cytomegalovirus	
Amphotericin B		
Nonsteroidal anti-inflammatory agents		
	Chronic	
Analgesics	Pyelonephritis	Vesicoureteral reflux
Lithium		Nephrocalcinosis
		Prolonged hypokalemia
		Oxalate nephropathy
		Heavy metals
		Radiation
		Obstructive uropathy
		Medullary cystic disease

collected under mineral oil (to prevent the loss of carbon dioxide) with simultaneous measurements of serum electrolytes. In the presence of substantial systemic acidosis (serum bicarbonate less than 16 mEq/L), a urine pH of less than 5.5 supports the diagnosis of proximal RTA, whereas adolescent patients with distal RTA have a urine pH of 5.8 or greater. In individuals who have mild acidosis (serum bicarbonate 17 to 20 mEq/L), ammonium chloride loading may be required to distinguish between the two types. In occult cases, measurement of the fractional excretion of bicarbonate after raising the serum bicarbonate level to normal by intravenous infusion of bicarbonate should be considered. If proximal RTA is detected, other defects of proximal tubular function should be sought (glycosuria, phosphaturia, aminoaciduria). When any form of RTA is confirmed, potential underlying causes (see Table 65–4) should be excluded.

Treatment. The goals of therapy are correction of the acidosis and maintenance of normal serum bicarbonate and potassium levels. Most cases of RTA can be corrected with oral therapy, using citrate (Shohl) solution or sodium bicarbonate tablets. Certain adolescent patients require potassium supplements. Individuals with proximal RTA may also require phosphate and vitamin D. Patients having mineralocorticoid deficiency RTA may need diuretics or polystyrene sulfonate resin, or both, to lower the serum potassium level.

Prognosis. Isolated proximal RTA, though initially more severe than the distal variety, may resolve spontaneously. Isolated distal RTA seems to be a lifelong disease; in some instances, renal failure may develop. However, the prognosis is excellent if the disease is recognized and therapy initiated prior to the development of nephrocalcinosis. Lifelong monitoring of the clinical status and a continuing need for alkali therapy are common.

Mineralocorticoid deficiency RTA may result from obstructive uropathy and usually resolves after correction of the obstruction. In secondary forms of RTA, the ultimate prognosis may depend on the severity of the primary disorder.

Nephrogenic Diabetes Insipidus

Primary nephrogenic diabetes insipidus is a rare, inherited (usually X-linked recessive) disease characterized by complete tubular unresponsiveness to antidiuretic hormone in males (usually presenting in infancy) and partial unresponsiveness in females (which may not present until later in life). Partial or complete nephrogenic diabetes insipidus (secondary) may also be seen in association with disorders that (1) result in loss of the medullary concentrating gradient (acute or chronic renal failure, obstructive and postobstructive uropathy, vesicoureteral reflux, cystic diseases, interstitial nephritis, osmotic diuresis, nephrocalcinosis) or (2) diminish the effect of antidiuretic hormone on the tubules (hypokalemia, hypercalcemia, lithium and demeclocycline therapy).

Bartter Syndrome

A rare form of renal potassium wasting, called Bartter syndrome, is characterized by hypokalemia, normal blood pressure, vascular insensitivity to pressor agents, and elevated plasma concentrations of renin and aldosterone. It typically presents during childhood. Adolescents present with muscle weakness, cramps, or spasms from hypokalemia.

Interstitial Nephritis

Interstitial nephritis is a histopathologic term signifying inflammation between the glomeruli in the areas surrounding the tubules (the interstitium). Acute and chronic forms are recognized, depending on the nature of the inflammatory infiltrate and the presence or lack of edema and fibrosis. Common causes of interstitial nephritis are listed in Table 65–5.

ACUTE INTERSTITIAL NEPHRITIS

Pathogenesis and Pathologic Features. Independent of the cause of the interstitial disease, the interstitial infiltrate is composed of lymphocytes, plasma cells, eosinophils, and occasional neutrophils. The tubules are separated by edema and may show degeneration or frank necrosis. Unless the interstitial nephritis is associated with a glomerulonephritis, the glomeruli are normal.

Clinical Manifestations. In hospitalized adolescents, drugs are the most common cause of acute interstitial nephritis. After a week or so of drug therapy, patients typically present with fever and a maculopapular skin rash. Urine output may be normal or diminished. Increased numbers of eosinophils may be detected in the blood or urine, or in both. Acute renal failure or generalized tubular dysfunction, or both, may result. Other forms of acute interstitial nephritis present a clinical picture resembling acute glomerulonephritis or acute renal failure in association with the clinical manifestations of the initiating disorder.

Diagnosis. The diagnosis is confirmed by renal biopsy, though it may not be suspected prior to biopsy. The differential diagnosis includes other causes of acute nephritis or renal failure.

Prevention. The development of drug-related interstitial nephritis may be reduced by using alternative therapeutic agents when possible (e.g., the substitution of nafcillin for methicillin).

Treatment and Prognosis. After appropriate management of the acute renal failure, withdrawal of possible inciting agents, and treatment of precipitating infection, the acute interstitial nephritis may resolve completely, though residual renal dysfunction is not uncommon. In adolescent patients with severe histologic injury and renal failure, high-dose corticosteroid therapy may result in dramatic improvement.

CHRONIC INTERSTITIAL NEPHRITIS

Pathologic Features. In chronic interstitial nephritis, the inflammatory infiltrate consists of lymphocytes and plasma cells. The edema of the acute form is replaced by interstitial fibrosis. Tubular dilatation and atrophy are widespread. The glomeruli show partial or total sclerosis, presumably resulting from ischemia.

Clinical Manifestations. Chronic interstitial nephritis may result from an occult structural abnormality of the kidneys or lower urinary tract (cystic disease, obstruction, reflux), chronic infection, nephrotoxins, or progression of acute interstitial nephritis. The presenting clinical manifestations may be those of chronic renal failure (nausea, vomiting, pallor, headache, fatigue, hypertension, growth failure) or of the underlying disorder (urinary tract infection, flank mass).

Diagnosis. The diagnosis is suggested by the presence of chronic renal insufficiency in association with a known cause of the disorder; renal biopsy is not usually indicated.

Treatment and Prognosis. The natural history of chronic interstitial nephritis is progression to end-stage renal failure. Whether elimination of infection or cor-rection of reflux or obstruction, or both, will alter this progression is unclear. Avoidance of nephrotoxins prior to the development of end-stage renal failure may result in improvement in renal function.

Toxic Nephropathies. Medications, diagnostic agents (iodinated radiographic contrast media), and chemicals may alter the kidneys directly by reduction of renal blood flow, acute tubular necrosis, or intratubular obstruction or indirectly through induction of an allergic or hypersensitivity reaction in the vessels or interstitium. Common nephrotoxic agents and their clinical manifestations are listed in Table 65–6. The nephrotoxicity is frequently reversible if the noxious agent is removed.

HEREDITARY DISEASES

Diabetes Mellitus

Diabetic nephropathy is a common complication of insulin-dependent diabetes mellitus (see Chapter 59). About 30% to 50% of diabetic individuals will experience this complication approximately 15 years after the onset of diabetes. End-stage renal failure develops 5 to 10 years thereafter. Diabetic nephropathy accounts for 25% of the new cases of end-stage renal failure each year. Although the development of end-stage renal failure resulting from diabetes is rare in adolescence, the early pathologic and clinical manifestations may begin during this period.

Pathogenesis and Pathologic Features. The initial pathologic changes in the kidney include a mild expansion of the mesangium and thickening of the basement membranes of the glomerular capillaries and the tubules. With time, the majority of adolescents experience diffuse mesangial sclerosis (scarring) associated with sclerosis of the arteries and arterioles, tubular atrophy, and interstitial fibrosis. Some adolescents may also experience Kimmelstiel-Wilson nodules in glomerular lobules, fibrin caps within glomerular capillaries, or capsular drops of eosinophilic material on the inside of the Bowman capsule. Hemodynamic injury to the glomerulus, genetic factors, poor glycemic control, metabolic alterations, and biochemical changes in the glomerular basement membrane may be important in the development of the nephropathy.

Clinical Manifestations. The clinical onset of diabetic nephropathy is characterized by the development of microalbuminuria. At this stage, the kidneys may be enlarged and the glomerular filtration rate elevated. Over time, proteinuria increases, sometimes to nephrotic levels, and renal function declines in association with the development of hypertension.

Diagnosis. The diagnosis of diabetic nephropathy is suggested by the detection of proteinuria in a patient who has had diabetes for more than 10 years. Biopsy is usually not warranted. However, it is important to remember that young diabetic individuals may experience other renal disorders, such as minimal-change disease, membranous and membranoproliferative glomerulonephritis, and other forms of proliferative glomerulonephritis. Indications for biopsy include the development of hematuria and the development of

TABLE 65–6. Nephrotoxic Compounds

NEPHROTIC SYNDROME	**RENAL VASCULITIS WITH OR WITHOUT GLOMERULAR CAPILLARY INVOLVEMENT**
Gold salts	
Mercurial diuretics	Hydralazine
Miscellaneous compounds containing mercury	Isoniazid
Paramethadione	Sulfonamides
Penicillamine	Any of the numerous other drugs that may cause a hypersensitivity reaction
Perchlorate	**NEPHROCALCINOSIS OR NEPHROLITHIASIS**
Probenecid	Allopurinol
Tolbutamide	Ethylene glycol
Trimethadione	Methoxyflurane
Nonsteroidal anti-inflammatory agents	Vitamin D
NEPHROGENIC DIABETES INSIPIDUS	**MISCELLANEOUS RENAL MANIFESTATIONS (including proteinuria, hematuria, oliguria, tubular necrosis, and renal failure)**
Amphotericin B	
Demeclocycline	Arsenic
Lithium carbonate	Bacitracin
Methoxyflurane	Cadmium
Propoxyphene	Carbon tetrachloride
FANCONI SYNDROME	Cephaloridine
Cadmium	Cephalothin
Gentamicin	Cisplatin
Lead	Colistin
Lysol	Copper
Mercury	Ethylene glycol
Nitrobenzene	Gentamicin
Outdated tetracycline	Gold salts
Salicylate	Indomethacin
Uranium	Iron
Aminoglycosides	Kanamycin
RENAL TUBULAR ACIDOSIS	Mercury salts
Lithium salts	Mitomycin C
Toluene sniffing	Neomycin
Amphotericin B	Pentamidine
INTERSTITIAL NEPHRITIS WITH OR WITHOUT PAPILLARY NECROSIS	Poisonous mushrooms
	Polymyxin B
Amidopyrine	Radiocontrast agents
p-Aminosalicylate	Streptomycin
Bunamiodyl (papillary necrosis only)	Sulfonamides
Penicillins (especially methicillin)	Tetrachlorethylene
Phenacetin	Vancomycin
Phenylbutazone	Viomycin
Salicylate	
Sulfonamides	
Nonsteroidal anti-inflammatory agents	

nephrotic syndrome or declining renal function in patients with diabetes of less than 10 years' duration.

Treatment. Progression of the nephropathy may be related to poor metabolic control and the development of hypertension. Recent studies suggest that improving metabolic control may delay the progression of the renal disease. Early detection and aggressive management of hypertension are necessary to preserve renal function. Recent studies suggest that angiotensin-converting enzyme inhibitors may be the best choice because they reduce both systemic and glomerular blood pressure and can also reduce the level of proteinuria.

Course and Prognosis. Diabetic nephropathy runs a progressive course to end-stage renal failure. Once end-stage renal failure has developed, transplantation seems to be a better therapeutic option for the young diabetic individual than does chronic dialysis. However, extrarenal complications of diabetes, such as coronary artery disease, may affect survival.

Alport Syndrome

Also known as *hereditary nephritis,* Alport syndrome is one of the most common of several types of hereditary nephropathies occurring in adolescents.

Pathogenesis and Pathologic Features. On light microscopy, the glomeruli initially show an increase in mesangial cells and matrix associated with capillary wall thickening. Progressive changes include glomerular sclerosis, tubular atrophy, interstitial inflammation and fibrosis, and foam cells. Immunopathologic studies generally produce negative results.

In most adolescent patients, electron microscopy reveals nonspecific irregular thinning, thickening, splitting, and layering of the glomerular and tubular basement membranes.

Clinical Manifestations. Adolescents with Alport syndrome present with gross or microscopic hematuria. In individuals with persistent microscopic hematuria, the development of proteinuria indicates the need for a renal biopsy, which establishes the diagnosis.

Besides renal involvement, some patients may suffer sensorineural hearing loss or eye abnormalities, the most frequent of which include cataracts, anterior lenticonus, and macular lesions.

The mode of transmission in most families is consistent with an X-linked dominant trait, although autosomal dominant inheritance has been described. Up to 20% of adolescent patients have no family history of the disease, suggesting a high spontaneous mutation rate.

Diagnosis. The diagnosis is suggested by the clinical manifestations and family history and is confirmed by renal biopsy. Other causes of recurrent episodes of gross hematuria (IgA nephropathy, idiopathic hematuria, hypercalciuria) should be considered.

Treatment. There is no specific treatment for the disease. As renal function deteriorates, hypertension, urinary tract infections, and the manifestations of chronic renal failure will require appropriate therapy. If renal failure develops, transplantation is recommended.

Course and Prognosis. Males with Alport syndrome usually progress to end-stage renal failure, generally in the second or third decade of life, whereas females frequently have a normal life span.

Idiopathic Hematuria

Also known as thin basement membrane nephropathy and benign recurrent hematuria, idiopathic hematuria (a familial, frequently autosomal dominant, disorder) presents as recurrent episodes of gross hematuria in adolescents. Renal function, including calcium excretion, is normal. Renal biopsy specimens appear normal on light and immunofluorescence microscopy. Electron microscopy reveals diffuse thinning of the glomerular basement membranes. The prognosis is excellent, but long-term follow-up is required to exclude Alport syndrome and to monitor the natural history of the disorder.

Sickle Cell Nephropathy

The nephropathy of sickle cell anemia (see Chapter 52) presumably results from sickling in the relatively hypoxic, acidic, hypertonic renal medulla, which leads to vascular stasis, diminished blood flow, ischemia, papillary necrosis, and interstitial fibrosis. Clinical manifestations include gross or microscopic hematuria, a urinary concentrating defect, RTA, and proteinuria. Disease in certain adolescent patients will progress to renal failure.

Cystic Diseases

AUTOSOMAL DOMINANT POLYCYSTIC RENAL DISEASE

Also called *adult polycystic renal disease* because it usually presents in adulthood, this disorder is inherited as an autosomal dominant trait. The genetic defect seems to involve a locus on the short arm of chromosome 16.

Pathogenesis and Pathologic Features. The kidneys are enlarged and show cortical and medullary cysts that appear to be dilatations along various portions of the tubules. The pathogenesis of the "cysts" is unclear. Cysts in the liver are of no clinical significance.

Clinical Manifestations. The disease usually presents in the fourth or fifth decade of life but may be seen in adolescents. Initial manifestations include gross or microscopic hematuria and flank pain. Physical examination reveals enlarged kidneys. Aneurysms of the cerebral circulation may result in intracranial hemorrhage. As the disease progresses, hypertension and renal insufficiency may develop.

Diagnosis. The clinical findings and family history suggest the diagnosis. Because the cysts may be several centimeters in diameter, the diagnosis can usually be confirmed by renal ultrasonography or computed tomography. In occult cases, open renal biopsy may be necessary to confirm the diagnosis.

Treatment. Treatment is supportive. Genetic counseling is warranted.

Course and Prognosis. Clinical problems are rare in adolescence. Individuals with large kidneys should be cautioned about the risks of renal trauma from contact sports. Renal failure may develop but rarely before adulthood.

AUTOSOMAL RECESSIVE POLYCYSTIC RENAL DISEASE

Also called *infantile polycystic renal disease* because it usually presents at or shortly after birth, this rare disorder is inherited as an autosomal recessive trait that may present in adolescents.

Pathophysiology. The kidneys are enlarged and show innumerable cysts throughout the cortex and medulla. Microscopic studies reveal that the "cysts" are dilatations of the collecting ducts. Cysts (actually dilated bile ducts) may be detected in the liver. When they are extensive, they may be associated with cirrhosis; this disorder is called congenital hepatic fibrosis.

Clinical Manifestations. In adolescents, this disorder may present as flank masses, growth failure, a urinary concentrating defect, renal insufficiency, or hypertension.

Diagnosis. The disease is suggested by the detection of enlarged kidneys without radiographic evidence of obstruction or tumor. The diagnosis is confirmed by renal biopsy.

Treatment. Treatment is supportive, including careful management of the hypertension. Genetic counseling is warranted.

Course and Prognosis. Progression to renal failure is usual. In adolescent patients having hepatic fibrosis, cirrhosis may lead to portal hypertension.

MEDULLARY CYSTIC DISEASE

Medullary cystic disease is inherited as an autosomal dominant trait, whereas a similar disorder, juvenile nephronophthisis, is inherited as an autosomal recessive trait. Whether these are separate disorders or the same disorder with variable inheritance remains controversial. Children more commonly have the recessive form, whereas the dominant form is more common in adolescents and adults. The major pathologic finding is cysts in the medulla. As the "cysts" seem to be dilatations of the distal tubules and collecting ducts, some may also be found in the renal cortex. Progressive interstitial inflammation and fibrosis lead to glomerular sclerosis, cortical atrophy, and renal insufficiency. Some adolescents suffer no clinical problems until reaching end-stage renal failure. Others show manifestations of tubular dysfunction such as polyuria and polydipsia (concentrating defect), sodium wasting, and proximal RTA. Red or blonde hair is common. Urinalysis may be normal or show minimal abnormalities. Radiographic studies show small, poorly functioning kidneys. The diagnosis is confirmed by biopsy or nephrectomy if warranted in preparation for transplantation.

SYSTEMIC DISEASES WITH RENAL MANIFESTATIONS

Systemic Lupus Erythematosus

SLE is characterized by fever, weight loss, rash, hematologic abnormalities, arthritis, and involvement of the kidneys, heart, lungs, and central nervous system. The nonrenal manifestations are discussed in Chapter 90. Renal disease is one of the most common manifestations of SLE and may occasionally be the only manifestation.

Pathogenesis and Pathologic Features. Of the several classifications of lupus nephritis, that offered by the World Health Organization (WHO) (which uses light, immunofluorescence, and electron microscopy for diagnosis) is most accepted. In WHO class I, no histologic abnormalities are detected. In WHO class II (also called mesangial lupus nephritis), mesangial deposits containing immunoglobulin and complement are present in some glomeruli; light microscopic features may be normal (class IIA) or show focal and segmental mesangial hypercellularity and increased matrix (class IIB).

WHO class III (also called focal proliferative lupus nephritis) is characterized by mesangial deposits in almost all glomeruli and subendothelial deposits (between the endothelial cells and glomerular basement membrane) in some glomeruli. In addition to focal segmental mesangial proliferation, occasional glomeruli show capillary wall necrosis and crescent formation.

WHO class IV (also called diffuse proliferative lupus nephritis) is the most severe and, unfortunately, the most common form of lupus nephritis. All glomeruli contain massive mesangial and subendothelial deposits of immunoglobulin and complement. All glomeruli show mesangial proliferation on light microscopy. The capillary walls are frequently thickened (resulting from subendothelial deposits), creating the "wire loop" lesion, and commonly show necrosis, crescent formation, and scarring.

WHO class V (also called membranous lupus nephritis) is the least common form of lupus nephritis and, except for mild to moderate mesangial proliferation, histologically resembles idiopathic membranous glomerulopathy.

The transformation of the histologic lesion from one class to another (usually to a more severe class) is common in lupus nephritis, especially in inadequately treated individuals.

Clinical Manifestations. The clinical findings in adolescents who have the milder forms (all class II, some class III) of lupus nephritis include hematuria, normal renal function, and proteinuria of less than 1 g/24 hours. In the more severe forms of lupus nephritis (some class III, all class IV), clinical involvement may include hematuria, proteinuria, and reduced renal function, nephrotic syndrome, or acute renal failure. Strangely, some patients with proliferative glomerulonephritis show no urinary sediment changes, obscuring the renal involvement. Patients with class V disease commonly present with nephrotic syndrome.

Diagnosis. The diagnosis of SLE is suggested by the detection of circulating antinuclear antibodies and is confirmed by demonstrating that these antibodies react with native (double-stranded) deoxyribonucleic acid (DNA). In most patients with active disease, C3 and C4 levels are depressed. In view of the lack of a clear correlation between the clinical manifestations and the severity of the renal involvement, a renal biopsy should be performed in all patients with SLE. The findings will guide the selection of immunosuppressive therapy.

Treatment. The goals of immunosuppressive therapy in SLE are clinical and serologic (normalization of the anti-DNA, C3, and C4 levels) remission, as discussed in Chapter 90.

Prognosis. Aggressive immunosuppressive therapy has dramatically improved the prognosis of SLE, but the disease is controlled not cured. The adolescent remains exposed to the risk of relapse as well as the side effects of chronic immunosuppressive therapy (of special concern are the effects of corticosteroids in girls).

Vasculitis

Vasculitis signifies inflammation of the blood vessels. This may involve the medium- and large-sized vessels (polyarteritis nodosa, Wegener granulomatosis) or the small vessels and capillaries (Henoch-Schönlein purpura).

POLYARTERITIS NODOSA

Systemic features of polyarteritis may include fever, weight loss, rash, arthritis, neuropathy, anemia, and renal disease.

Pathogenesis and Pathologic Features. In most adolescents with polyarteritis, there is no clear cause for the disease, though it has been associated with drug abuse and hepatitis B infection.

Inflammation of the arteries leads to aneurysmal dilatation, best demonstrated by abdominal aortography. Renal biopsy usually reveals a focal segmental necrotizing glomerulonephritis, frequently with crescent formation. Immune deposits are usually lacking.

Clinical Manifestations. Renal involvement may present with hematuria and proteinuria, nephrotic syndrome, or acute renal failure.

Diagnosis. Vasculitis may be confirmed by demonstrating aneurysms in the mesenteric, hepatic, or renal vessels by aortography or tissue biopsy.

Treatment. The disease can usually be controlled with

corticosteroids. In severe cases, the addition of cyclophosphamide is frequently effective.

WEGENER GRANULOMATOSIS

Most adolescents with Wegener granulomatosis present with disease of the sinuses or lungs, but the majority will experience renal involvement. Fever, arthritis, and skin and eye involvement are common. The cause of the disease is unknown. The degree of renal involvement may range from a mild focal and segmental glomerulonephritis with minimal urinary findings to a diffuse necrotizing glomerulonephritis with crescent formation, presenting as nephrotic syndrome or acute renal failure. Immune deposits are usually lacking. Diagnosis is supported by histologic demonstration of granulomas in the respiratory tract or kidneys and by the detection of antineutrophil cytoplasmic antibodies in the serum. Treatment with corticosteroids and cyclophosphamide is usually effective.

HENOCH-SCHÖNLEIN (ANAPHYLACTOID) PURPURA

The typical adolescent patient with Henoch-Schönlein syndrome presents with an urticarial or purpuric rash, or both, on the buttocks and lower extremities, arthritis or arthralgias, and abdominal pain. Intussusception or perforation of the bowel may occur. Evidence for renal involvement is usually detected within 1 month of onset but may not occur until later in the course of disease.

Pathogenesis and Pathologic Features. Although presumably an immune complex–mediated disorder, the precise cause of this disease is unclear. It is a vasculitis of the smallest blood vessels, and perivascular inflammation may be seen in several organs. In the majority of adolescents with renal involvement, the histologic lesion is characterized by a focal and segmental increase in mesangial cells and matrix. A minority of patients show generalized mesangial changes, whereas rare patients have diffuse necrotizing glomerulitis with generalized crescents.

Immunofluorescence microscopy reveals mesangial deposits of IgA, frequently in association with IgG, C3, and fibrin. The predominant deposition of IgA suggests a relationship to IgA nephropathy. Electron microscopy confirms the presence of mesangial deposits and may also reveal deposits along the capillary wall in the subendothelial space.

Clinical Manifestations. Clinical evidence of renal disease develops in approximately 50% of adolescent patients. The majority suffers only mild renal involvement, characterized by hematuria, preserved renal function, and proteinuria of less than 2 g/24 hours. Patients with severe renal involvement are characterized by diminished renal function and heavy proteinuria; these individuals frequently experience the nephrotic syndrome.

Diagnosis. The disease is usually defined by the clinical constellation of rash, abdominal and joint complaints in conjunction with a normal platelet count and C3 level, and the lack of circulating antinuclear antibodies (negative ANA).

Renal involvement is usually mild, and renal biopsy is rarely necessary. Indications for biopsy include diminished renal function, proteinuria exceeding 2 g/24 hours, or the development of the nephrotic syndrome.

Prognosis and Treatment. In most adolescents, the clinical manifestations resolve completely over several months, though microscopic hematuria may persist for more than 1 year. In individuals with severe renal involvement, especially when biopsy shows the morphologic picture of rapidly progressive glomerulonephritis, the ultimate prognosis is extremely poor. Although there is no proof that any form of therapy is effective in adolescent patients with severe renal involvement, we have seen dramatic improvement in some such individuals after treatment with prednisone and azathioprine.

THROMBOTIC ANGIOPATHIES

Hemolytic-uremic syndrome (HUS) and thrombotic thrombocytopenic purpura (TTP) are associated with thrombosis of the microvasculature of the kidneys; renal vein thrombosis involves the larger venous radicles. Whether HUS and TTP are the same disease with varying clinical manifestations or distinct diseases with similar clinical manifestations remains to be determined.

Hemolytic-Uremic Syndrome

Pathogenesis and Pathologic Features. The development of HUS has been associated with bacterial (*Shigella, Salmonella, Escherichia coli, Streptococcus pneumoniae, Bartonella*) and viral infections, endotoxemia, and the use of oral contraceptives. In addition, an HUS-like state has been described in association with SLE, malignant hypertension, preeclampsia, postpartum renal failure, and radiation nephritis. Recent studies have implicated the lack of a plasma factor, which stimulates endothelial cell prostacyclin production in the pathogenesis of the disease. Genetic factors may also play a role. The glomerular lesion is characterized by arteriolar and capillary thrombosis, expansion of the mesangium, and intimal proliferation of the arteries and arterioles. In some individuals, the disease progresses to cortical necrosis.

Clinical Manifestations. HUS is usually preceded by gastroenteritis (fever, vomiting, diarrhea) or, less commonly, an upper respiratory infection. This is followed in 5 to 10 days by the sudden onset of pallor, irritability, weakness, lethargy, and oliguria. Physical examination may reveal dehydration, edema, petechiae, hepatosplenomegaly, and marked irritability.

Extrarenal involvement is being detected with increasing frequency and may include central nervous system manifestations (irritability, seizures, coma), colitis (melena, perforation), diabetes mellitus, and rhabdomyolysis.

Diagnosis. The diagnosis is supported by the findings of microangiopathic hemolytic anemia, thrombocytopenia, and acute renal failure. Urinary findings are surprisingly mild and usually consist of low-grade microscopic hematuria and proteinuria. The severity of the renal involvement is highly variable.

Treatment and Prognosis. Treatment is supportive and includes early dialysis. More than 90% of individuals survive the acute phase, and most recover normal function. Long-term follow-up is necessary.

Thrombotic Thrombocytopenic Purpura

Like HUS, TTP may be associated with a microangiopathic hemolytic anemia, thrombocytopenia, renal failure, and neurologic manifestations. Unlike HUS, the disease occurs primarily in adults and may have widespread organ involvement, focal neurologic manifestations, lack of renal involvement, purpura, intravascular platelet thrombi, and a poor prognosis without treatment. Plasma from patients with TTP may contain a platelet-aggregating factor or antiendothelial cell antibodies. Treatment with plasma exchange and inhibitors of platelet aggregation is effective in many patients.

Renal Vein Thrombosis

Renal vein thrombosis seems to occur in two distinct patterns. In young children, the disease is commonly associated with asphyxia, dehydration, shock, and sepsis. In adolescents, the disease is more commonly associated with the nephrotic syndrome (most frequently membranous nephropathy), cyanotic heart disease, and the use of angiographic contrast agents.

Pathogenesis. The disease presumably begins in the intrarenal venous radicles, spreading in both antegrade and retrograde directions. The main renal vein may not be involved. Thrombus formation is presumably mediated by endothelial cell injury (hypoxia, endotoxin, contrast agents) in conjunction with a hypercoagulable state (nephrotic syndrome); diminished vascular blood flow, which may result from hypovolemia (shock, sepsis, dehydration, nephrotic syndrome); or the intravascular sludging of blood that results from polycythemia.

Clinical Manifestations. The development of renal vein thrombosis may be heralded by the sudden onset of gross hematuria and unilateral or bilateral flank masses. When bilateral, the disease results in acute renal failure.

Diagnosis. The diagnosis is suggested by the development of hematuria and flank masses in a patient with predisposing clinical factors. Most adolescents experience microangiopathic hemolytic anemia and thrombocytopenia. Ultrasonography demonstrates marked enlargement of the involved kidney, whereas radionuclide studies reveal little or no renal function. Although inferior vena cavagrams may be necessary to confirm the diagnosis in occult cases, contrast studies should generally be avoided to minimize the risk of further vascular damage. The differential diagnosis includes other causes of hematuria (especially HUS) or renal enlargement (hydronephrosis, cystic disease, Wilms tumor, abscess, hematoma).

Treatment. In unilateral renal vein thrombosis, therapy is supportive and involves correction of fluid and electrolyte abnormalities and the treatment of infection. Prophylactic anticoagulation to prevent thrombosis in the remaining kidney is unwarranted except, perhaps, in the presence of disseminated intravascular coagulation.

Since bilateral renal vein thrombosis frequently leads to chronic renal failure, consideration should be given to surgical thrombectomy or the use of systemic fibrinolytic agents.

Prognosis. The thrombosed kidney frequently undergoes progressive atrophy, ultimately leaving a small, scarred kidney. Nephrectomy should not be performed in the acute phase and should be performed later only if hypertension or chronic infection develops. The involved kidney may recover function, especially if the thrombosis developed in association with the nephrotic syndrome or cyanotic heart disease.

URINARY TRACT INFECTIONS

Urinary tract infections are far more common in females than in males. They may involve the lower (cystitis) or upper (pyelonephritis) urinary tracts; the latter may be associated with structural or functional abnormalities. Sexually active adolescent females are at greater risk for urinary tract infections than are adolescent females who have not initiated coitus.

Pathogenesis. Most urinary tract infections result from enteric bacteria ascending the urethra. Women with recurrent infections also tend to have an abnormally high vaginal pH, diminished cervicovaginal antibody levels, and increased bacterial adhesiveness to vaginal and uroepithelial cells. Recent studies suggest that the virulence of *Escherichia coli* may correlate with its ability to bind to uroepithelial cells. Binding is accomplished by the adherence of bacterial fimbriae (pili) to specific glycosphingolipid receptors resembling the P blood group on the surface of the uroepithelial cells. These receptors may possess greater density or availability in infection-prone females.

Although the higher frequency of infections in females, as compared with males, has been related to the shorter length of the female urethra, there is no difference in the length of the urethra between females who do and those who do not suffer urinary tract infections. There is also little evidence that distal urethral obstruction plays a role in the pathogenesis of urinary tract infections in females. Urethral dilatation does not reduce the frequency of infection. Interestingly, it does appear that women with recurrent urinary tract infections have pathogenic organisms residing in the distal urethra, whereas commensals are found in females without infection. Bladder mechanisms that prevent infection may include a surface mucin that prevents bacterial adherence to the bladder epithelial cells and complete emptying of the bladder.

The intact vesicoureteral valve-like mechanism protects the kidney from infection by preventing reflux (see Chapter 66). The renal medulla is highly susceptible to infection because of diminished blood flow and the inactivation of complement by tubular ammonia production and because its hypertonic milieu decreases polymorphonuclear chemotaxis and encourages the development of L forms that lack cell walls and are resistant to most antibiotics.

CYSTITIS

Clinical Manifestations. Symptoms of cystitis may include urgency, frequency, dysuria, gross hematuria (hemorrhagic cystitis), and suprapubic and abdominal discomfort. Results on physical examination are usually normal. Therefore, confirmation of the diagnosis requires appropriate laboratory investigation.

Diagnosis. The presence of infection can be suggested by microscopic evaluation of the urine sediment for leukocytes (pyuria) and bacteria. The diagnosis of cystitis is confirmed by a urine culture that is positive for bacteria. Recently, studies in women who have symptomatic infections (as confirmed by suprapubic bladder aspiration or catheterization) indicate that the growth of more than 100 colonies/ml in a "clean-catch" specimen may indicate infection. *In the asymptomatic patient*, infection is suggested by the growth of 100,000 colonies/ml of a single organism, and contamination is indicated by the growth of less than 10,000 colonies/ml of any number of organisms. Cultures containing colony counts between 10,000 and 100,000 colonies/ml should be repeated. *In the symptomatic patient*, especially one with pyuria or bacteriuria, or both, more than 100 colonies/ml is presumed to indicate infection.

Treatment. *Escherichia coli* is the most frequent organism causing cystitis, followed by *Klebsiella, Enterobacter, Proteus, Enterococcus spp.*, and *Staphylococcus epidermidis*. Commonly used agents to which *E. coli* is susceptible include nitrofurantoin, sulfisoxazole, cephalexin, trimethoprim-sulfamethoxazole, and ampicillin-amoxicillin.

The duration of therapy is controversial. Recent studies suggest that short courses of therapy, ranging from one injection of an aminoglycoside or one large dose of amoxicillin or trimethoprim-sulfamethoxazole to 3 days of oral antibiotics, may be effective. However, until sufficient data from clinical studies are available to confirm the efficacy of such short-term therapies, a full 7-day course is recommended. In females, a follow-up culture is unnecessary if symptoms have resolved by the time therapy is completed.

Radiographic Studies. The need for radiographic studies after the first urinary tract infection in a male at any age is clear because of the high frequency of underlying anatomic abnormality. This evaluation should consist of an intravenous pyelogram and a voiding cystourethrogram. Similar studies are performed in females who fail to respond to antibiotic therapy or who suffer recurrent episodes of infection.

Recurrent Infections. Some girls, despite normal radiographic studies, have recurrent urinary tract infections. Such adolescents are candidates for 6 to 12 months of prophylactic therapy with nitrofurantoin or trimethoprim-sulfamethoxazole. If recurrence is related to intercourse, a postcoital dose of antibiotic is usually effective.

Asymptomatic Bacteruria. This condition is usually not treated because it generally resolves spontaneously and rarely leads to symptomatic infection. The exception is during pregnancy, when asymptomatic infection must be treated to prevent complications.

ACUTE PYELONEPHRITIS

Acute pyelonephritis usually results from the reflux of colonic organisms from the bladder to the upper urinary tract. Organisms that reach the upper urinary tract may adhere to the kidney by attachment of their fimbriae to receptors on the uroepithelial cells. The development of pyelonephritis may then be promoted by anatomic or functional ureteral obstruction. Functional obstruction of the ureter may result from paralysis of ureteral peristalsis mediated by products of the infection. Obstruction of the ureter produces pressure-induced changes in the shape of the renal papillae, allowing the ingress of organisms into the renal parenchyma (intrarenal reflux).

Acute pyelonephritis is generally suspected by its clinical manifestations, which include fever, chills, vomiting, flank pain, and enlargement of the involved kidney. Pyuria is usually present; white blood cell casts in the urine, if present, strongly support the diagnosis. Renal function may be diminished if the infection involves both kidneys.

Following the clinical diagnosis of acute pyelonephritis, urinalysis and urine culture should be obtained and intravenous antibiotic therapy should be instituted. Since *Escherichia coli* and gram-positive species are commonly detected, therapy should be initiated with nafcillin and gentamicin. An immediate radiologic procedure (ultrasound, intravenous pyelogram, or diethylenetriaminepentaacetic acid [DTPA] renal scan) should be performed to rule out obstruction. If detected, obstruction must be promptly alleviated.

Antibiotic therapy should be continued for a total duration of 2 weeks. After the fever and toxicity resolve and urine cultures become sterile, the adolescent patient may be switched from an intravenous antibiotic to an appropriate oral antibiotic, on the basis of culture and sensitivity reactions, for completion of therapy. After clinical improvement is obtained, a voiding cystourethrogram should be performed to evaluate the anatomy of the lower urinary tract.

ACUTE RENAL FAILURE

Acute renal failure develops when renal function is diminished to the point that body fluid homeostasis can no longer be maintained. Although oliguria (daily urine volume less than 400 ml/m^2) is common, the urine volume may approximate normal (nonoliguric renal failure) in certain types of acute renal failure (aminoglycoside nephrotoxicity). Thus it remains important to use biochemical studies (blood urea nitrogen [BUN] creatinine levels) in addition to measurement of the urine volume to monitor renal function.

The causes of acute renal failure are listed in Table 65–7. In the first category (prerenal), decreased perfu-

TABLE 65–7. Causes of Acute Renal Failure

PRERENAL	RENAL	POSTRENAL
Hypovolemia	Glomerulonephritis	Obstructive uropathy
Hemorrhage	Poststreptococcal	Ureteropelvic junction
Gastrointestinal losses	Lupus	Ureterocele
Hypoproteinemia	Membranoproliferative	Urethral valves
Burns	Idiopathic rapidly progressive	Tumor
Renal or adrenal disease with salt	glomerulonephritis	Vesicoureteral reflux
wasting	Anaphylactoid purpura	Acquired
Hepatorenal syndrome	Localized intravascular coagulation	Stones
Hypotension	Renal vein thrombosis	Blood clot
Septicemia	Cortical necrosis	
Disseminated intravascular coagulation	Hemolytic-uremic syndrome	
Hypothermia	Acute tubular necrosis	
Hemorrhage	Heavy metals	
Heart failure	Chemicals	
Hypoxia	Drugs	
Pneumonia	Hemoglobin, myoglobin	
Aortic clamping	Shock	
Respiratory distress syndrome	Ischemia	
	Acute interstitial nephritis	
	Infection	
	Drugs	
	Tumors	
	Renal parenchymal infiltration	
	Uric acid nephropathy	
	Developmental abnormalities	
	Cystic disease	
	Hypoplasia-dysplasia	
	Hereditary nephritis	

sion of the kidney results in decreased renal function. The second category includes diseases of the kidney, whereas the third category is composed primarily of obstructive disorders.

Pathogenesis

Prerenal Causes. In these conditions, decreased renal perfusion results from a decrease in the total or "effective" circulating blood volume. Evidence for renal damage is lacking. Diminished intravascular volume leads to a fall in the cardiac output and an increase in renal arteriolar resistance, causing a decline in renal cortical blood flow and the glomerular filtration rate. If hypoperfusion persists, renal parenchymal damage may result.

Renal Causes. The rapidly progressive forms of several types of glomerulonephritis (Table 65–7) are common causes of acute renal failure. Activation of the coagulation system within the kidney, resulting in small vessel thrombosis, may also lead to acute renal failure.

Clinical Manifestations. The presenting signs and symptoms may be modified by the precipitating disease. Clinical findings related to the renal failure include pallor (anemia), diminished urine output, edema (salt and water overload), hypertension, vomiting, and lethargy (uremic encephalopathy). Complications of acute renal failure may include volume overload with congestive heart failure and pulmonary edema, arrhythmias, gastrointestinal bleeding from stress ulcers or gastritis, seizures, coma, and behavioral changes.

Diagnosis. A careful history taking may aid in defining the cause of the renal failure. Vomiting, diarrhea, and fever suggest dehydration and prerenal azotemia, though these symptoms may also precede development of HUS and renal vein thrombosis. Antecedent skin or throat infection suggests poststreptococcal glomerulo-

nephritis. Rash may be found in SLE or anaphylactoid purpura. A history of exposure to chemicals and medications should be sought. Flank masses suggest renal vein thrombosis, tumors, cystic disease, or obstruction.

Laboratory abnormalities may include anemia (with the rare exception of blood loss, the anemia is usually dilutional or hemolytic as seen in SLE, renal vein thrombosis, and HUS), leukopenia (SLE), thrombocytopenia (SLE, renal vein thrombosis, HUS), hyponatremia (dilutional), hyperkalemia, acidosis, elevated serum concentrations of BUN, creatinine, uric acid, and phosphate (diminished renal function), and hypocalcemia (hyperphosphatemia). The urine may contain red blood cell casts and protein (acute glomerulonephritis), white blood cells (infection, interstitial nephritis), or eosinophils (allergic interstitial nephritis). The serum C3 level may be depressed (poststreptococcal glomerulonephritis, lupus nephritis, membranoproliferative glomerulonephritis), and there may be serum antibodies to streptococcal (poststreptococcal glomerulonephritis), nuclear (SLE), neutrophil (Wegener granulomatosis), or basement membrane (Goodpasture disease) antigens. Chest x-ray films may reveal cardiomegaly and pulmonary congestion (fluid overload). In all adolescents presenting with acute renal failure, obstruction should be immediately excluded (and treated, if present) by obtaining a plain x-ray film of the abdomen, renal ultrasound, and a DTPA radionuclide scan; retrograde pyelography may occasionally be necessary to detect occult obstructions. Renal biopsy may ultimately be required to determine the precise cause of the renal failure.

Treatment

Hypovolemia. Since the need for volume replacement may be critical in patients with hypovolemia, the initial physical examination of the adolescent should include careful assessment of the state of hydration. In adolescent patients with hypovolemia, the urine is concentrated (urine osmolality exceeds 500 mOsm/kg H_2O), the urine sodium concentration is usually less than 20 mEq/L, and the fractional excretion of sodium (as determined by using the following equation) is usually less than 1%.

$$\frac{urine\ [Na^+] \div plasma\ [Na^+]}{urine\ [Cr] \div plasma\ [Cr]} \times 100$$

In adolescents with tubular necrosis, the urine is dilute (osmolality less than 350 mOsm/kg H_2O), the sodium concentration usually exceeds 40 mEq/L, and the fractional excretion of sodium usually exceeds 1%.

If hypovolemia is detected, the intravascular volume should be expanded by the intravenous administration of isotonic saline, 20 ml/kg, over 30 minutes. Following this infusion, the dehydrated individual will generally void within 2 hours. Failure to void after this interval indicates that a thorough reevaluation of the patient is necessary. Catheterization of the bladder and determination of the central venous pressure may be helpful. If clinical and laboratory evaluations indicate that the adolescent patient is adequately hydrated, aggressive diuretic therapy may be considered.

Impending Renal Failure. The value of diuretics in preventing the development of anuric renal failure remains controversial. It seems clear that diuretics have no value in adolescent patients with established anuric renal failure. In some oliguric patients, furosemide or mannitol, or both, may increase the rate of urine production without affecting the natural history of the disease that precipitated the renal failure.

In the oliguric adolescent who lacks clinical and laboratory evidence of hypovolemia (and who may have already failed to respond to volume expansion), furosemide may be administered as a single intravenous dose of 2 mg/kg body weight at the rate of 4 mg/minute (to avoid ototoxicity); if there is no response, a second dose of 10 mg/kg body weight may be given. If no increase in urine production is obtained following this dose, further furosemide therapy is contraindicated. A single intravenous dose of 0.5 g/kg of mannitol may be given over 30 minutes in addition to or in place of furosemide. Independent of the response, no additional mannitol should be given because of the risk of toxicity. To increase renal cortical blood flow, dopamine (5 µg/kg/minute) may be administered (if hypertension is not present) in conjunction with diuretic therapy.

Fluid Restriction. If the adolescent fails to produce adequate urine output following volume expansion or the administration of diuretics, daily fluid administration must be restricted to no more than 400 ml/m² (insensible losses) plus an amount of fluid equal to the urine output for the day. Omitting the replacement of insensible fluid losses and urine output will aid in diminishing the expanded intravascular volume in hypervolemic patients.

Hyperkalemia. In acute renal failure, control of the serum potassium level is critical, as the rapid development of hyperkalemia (serum potassium level greater than 6 mEq/L) may lead to cardiac arrhythmia and death.

Procedures to deplete body potassium levels are initiated when the serum potassium level rises to 5.5 mEq/L. To minimize the rate at which the serum potassium level rises, all solutions given to the patient should contain high concentrations of glucose and all foods and fluids should be low in potassium. Gastrointestinal excretion of potassium is enhanced by sodium polystyrene sulfonate resin (Kayexalate); 1 g/kg should be given orally or by retention enema. For best results, the resin should be suspended in 2 ml/kg of 70% sorbitol for oral administration or 10 ml/kg of 20% sorbitol for rectal administration. Resin therapy may be repeated every 2 to 4 hours, the frequency being limited primarily by the risk of sodium overload.

If the serum potassium level rises to greater than 7 mEq/L, emergency measures in addition to Kayexalate must be initiated. The following agents should be given sequentially:

1. Calcium gluconate, 10% solution: 0.5 ml/kg, given intravenously over 10 minutes but discontinued as long as the heart rate is suppressed more than 20 beats/minute from the preinfusion rate
2. Sodium bicarbonate, 7.5% solution: 3 mEq/kg intravenously
3. Glucose, 50% solution: 1 ml/kg, plus regular insulin, 1 unit/5 g of glucose, given intravenously over 1 hour

These measures generally control the serum potassium levels until dialysis can be initiated but must be used only when close monitoring of the heart rate, blood glucose level, and blood pressure can be ensured.

Acidosis. Moderate acidosis is common in renal failure (the result of inadequate hydrogen ion and ammonia excretion) but rarely requires treatment. The correction formula for a pH lower than 7.15 or serum bicarbonate level less than 8 mEq/L is

$$mEq\ NaHCO_3\ required = 0.3 \times weight\ in\ kg \times (12 - serum\ bicarbonate)$$

The remainder of the correction, which should be carried out only after normalization of the serum calcium and phosphorus levels, may be accomplished by the oral administration of sodium bicarbonate tablets or sodium citrate solution.

Hypocalcemia. Hypocalcemia is treated by lowering the serum phosphorus level. Intravenous calcium is used only to treat tetany. To lower the serum phosphorus level, a phosphate-binding calcium carbonate antacid is given by mouth, increasing fecal phosphate excretion. Common agents include Titralac Liquid (starting dose 5 to 15 ml every 6 hours) and Os-Cal 500 tablets (starting dose one to three tablets every 6 hours).

Hyponatremia. Hyponatremia is commonly the result of excessive administration of hypotonic fluids to the oligoanuric adolescent patient. Correction may be accomplished by fluid restriction. When the sodium level falls to less than 120 mEq/L, it may be elevated to 125 mEq/L by the intravenous infusion of hypertonic (3%) sodium chloride using the following formula:

$$mEq\ NaCl\ required = 0.6 \times weight\ in\ kg \times (125 - serum\ sodium\ level)$$

Gastrointestinal bleeding may be prevented with calcium carbonate antacids, which also serve to lower the serum phosphorus level. Alternatively, intravenous cimetidine may be administered at a dose of 5 to 10 mg/kg/day (maximum, 2400 mg/day) every 12 hours in divided doses, or as a continuous infusion.

Hypertension. Hypertension (see Chapter 67) may be the result of the primary disease process or expansion of the extracellular fluid volume, or both. In renal failure, salt and water restriction is critical in hypertensive adolescents.

In individuals who have severe hypertension, the drug of choice is diazoxide. This potent vasodilator must be given by rapid intravenous injection (within 10 seconds) at a dose of 5 mg/kg body weight (maximum dose 150 mg). A fall in blood pressure is usually seen within 10 to 20 minutes. If the fall in blood pressure following the first injection is insufficient, a second injection may be given 30 minutes later. A concomitant injection of furosemide will prevent fluid overload. For less severe hypertension, control of extracellular volume expansion (salt and water restriction, furosemide), β-blockers (e.g., propranolol), and vasodilators (e.g., apresoline) are generally effective.

Seizures. Seizures may be the result of the primary disease process (e.g., SLE), hyponatremia (water intoxication), hypocalcemia (tetany), hypertension, or the uremic state itself. Diazepam seems to be the most effective agent in controlling seizures, but its metabolic products are excreted in the urine and may accumulate in renal insufficiency.

Anemia. Except in the presence of hemolysis (e.g., HUS, SLE) or bleeding, the anemia of acute renal failure is generally mild (hemoglobin 9 to 10 g/dl), is primarily the result of volume expansion (hemodilution) and does not require transfusion. Blood loss from active bleeding should be replaced appropriately, and transfusion over 4 to 6 hours with fresh packed red blood cells (10 ml/kg) can be provided if the hemoglobin level falls to less than 7 g/dl from hemolytic anemia or prolonged renal failure.

Diet. The diet should initially be restricted in protein, sodium, potassium, and water. If renal failure persists beyond 7 days, an oral diet for renal failure or parenteral hyperalimentation with essential amino acids should be considered.

Dialysis. The indications for dialysis include combinations of the following factors: acidosis, electrolyte abnormalities, central nervous system disturbances, hypertension, fluid overload, and congestive heart failure. It appears that the early initiation of dialysis in adolescent patients with a combination of these factors has significantly improved survival from acute renal failure.

Prognosis. The prognosis for recovery of renal function depends on the disorder that precipitated the renal failure. In general, recovery of function is likely following renal failure resulting from prerenal causes, HUS, acute tubular necrosis, acute interstitial nephritis, and uric acid nephropathy. Conversely, recovery of renal function is unusual when renal failure results from most types of rapidly progressive glomerulonephritis, bilateral renal vein thrombosis, and bilateral cortical necrosis.

CHRONIC RENAL FAILURE

Chronic renal failure results from a progressive decline in renal function. Common causes in adolescence include glomerulonephritis, hereditary disorders (Alport syndrome), and anatomic abnormalities (hypoplasia, dysplasia, obstruction).

Pathogenesis. Independent of the cause of renal damage, it appears that once a critical level of renal functional deterioration is reached, progression to end-stage renal failure is inevitable. As renal function deteriorates, compensatory mechanisms develop in remaining nephrons to maintain a normal internal environment. However, when the glomerular filtration rate falls to less than 20% of normal, a complex constellation of clinical, biochemical, and metabolic abnormalities develop, which together constitute the uremic state. The pathophysiologic manifestations of the uremic state are listed in Table 65–8.

Clinical Manifestations. In adolescents in whom chronic renal failure results from glomerular or hereditary diseases, the renal disease is usually detected because of the clinical manifestations prior to the onset of renal insufficiency. However, the development of renal failure may be insidious in individuals who have anatomic abnormalities, and the presenting complaints can be nonspecific (headache, fatigue, lethargy, anorexia, vomiting, polydipsia, polyuria, growth failure). Although the results of physical examination may be surprisingly normal, most adolescents with chronic renal failure appear pale and weak and have high blood pressure. The presence of growth retardation and rickets suggests renal failure beginning in infancy or childhood.

Treatment. The management of the adolescent with chronic renal failure requires close monitoring of the clinical (physical examination and blood pressure) and laboratory status. Blood studies to be followed routinely include determination of the hemoglobin level (anemia), electrolytes (hyponatremia, hyperkalemia, acidosis), BUN and creatinine (nitrogen accumulation and level of renal function), and calcium, phosphorus, and alkaline phosphatase levels (hypocalcemia, hyperphosphatemia, osteodystrophy). Periodic determination of parathyroid hormone levels and bone films may be of value in detecting early evidence of osteodystrophy. Chest x-ray films and an echocardiogram may be helpful in assessing cardiac function. Nutritional status may be monitored by periodic evaluation of the serum albumin, zinc, transferrin, folic acid, and iron levels.

DIET

Although the optimum caloric intake in renal insufficiency is unknown, an attempt should be made to equal or exceed (in adolescents with growth failure) the recommended daily caloric allowance for age. Caloric intake can be enhanced by adding unrestricted amounts of carbohydrate (sugar, jam, honey, glucose polymers; Polycose, Ross Laboratories, Columbus, OH 43216) and fat (medium chain triglycerides oil; MCT Oil, Mead

TABLE 65–8. Pathophysiology of Chronic Renal Failure

MANIFESTATION	MECHANISMS
Accumulation of nitrogenous waste products (azotemia)	Decline in glomerular filtration rate
Acidosis	Urinary bicarbonate wasting Decreased ammonia excretion Decreased acid excretion
Sodium wasting	Solute diuresis Tubular damage Functional tubular adaption for sodium excretion
Sodium retention	Nephrotic syndrome Congestive heart failure Anuria Excessive salt intake
Urinary concentrating defect	Nephron loss Solute diuresis Increased medullary blood flow
Hyperkalemia	Decline in glomerular filtration rate Acidosis Excessive potassium intake Hyperaldosteronism
Renal osteodystrophy	Decreased intestinal calcium absorption Impaired production of 1,25-dihydroxyvitamin D by the kidneys Hypocalcemia and hyperphosphatemia Secondary hyperparathyroidism
Growth retardation	Protein-calorie deficiency Renal osteodystrophy Acidosis Unknown factors Anemia
Anemia	Decreased erythropoietin production Low-grade hemolysis Bleeding Decreased erythrocyte survival Inadequate iron intake Inadequate folic acid intake Inhibitors of erythropoiesis
Bleeding tendency	Thrombocytopenia Defective platelet function
Infection	Defective granulocyte function Impaired cellular immune functions
Neurologic (fatigue, poor concentration, headache, drowsiness, loss of memory, slurred speech, muscle weakness and cramps, seizures, coma, peripheral neuropathy)	Unknown
Gastrointestinal ulceration	Gastric acid hypersecretion
Hypertension	Sodium and water overload Excessive renin production
Hypertriglyceridemia	Diminished plasma lipoprotein lipase activity
Pericarditis and cardiomyopathy	Unknown
Glucose intolerance	Tissue insulin resistance

Johnson, Evansville, IN 47721) to the diet as tolerated by the adolescent.

When the BUN exceeds approximately 80 mg/dl, adolescents may experience nausea, vomiting, and anorexia. These symptoms result from the accumulation of nitrogenous waste products and can be relieved by restricting dietary protein intake to 0.6 to 1 g/kg/24 hours, most of which should consist of proteins of high biologic value, which are primarily metabolized to utilizable amino acids rather than nitrogenous wastes. The proteins of highest biologic value are derived from eggs and milk, followed by meat, fish, and fowl.

Because of inadequate intake or dialysis losses, adolescent patients with renal insufficiency may become deficient in water-soluble vitamins, which should be routinely supplied using preparations such as Nephrocaps. Zinc and iron supplements should be added only after deficiencies are confirmed. Supplementation with fat-soluble vitamins A, E, and K is not required.

WATER AND ELECTROLYTES

Until the development of end-stage renal failure requiring the initiation of dialysis, water restriction is rarely necessary. Most patients with renal insufficiency maintain normal sodium balance with the sodium intake derived from an appropriate diet. Some adolescents whose renal insufficiency is a consequence of anatomic abnormalities may waste sodium in the urine and require dietary salt supplementation. Other individuals who have high blood pressure, edema, or congestive heart failure may require sodium restriction, sometimes in conjunction with aggressive furosemide therapy (1 to 4 mg/kg/day).

In most adolescents with renal insufficiency, potassium balance will be maintained until renal function deteriorates to the level at which dialysis is initiated. However, hyperkalemia may develop in individuals who have only moderate renal insufficiency caused by excessive dietary potassium intake, the development of severe acidosis, or aldosterone deficiency (destruction of the juxtaglomerular apparatus).

ACIDOSIS

Acidosis develops in almost all adolescents with renal insufficiency and need not be treated unless the serum bicarbonate level falls to less than 20 mEq/L. Either Bicitra (1 ml = 1 mEq of base) or sodium bicarbonate tablets (325 and 650 mg; 325 mg = 4 mEq of base) may be used to raise the serum bicarbonate level to greater than 20 mEq/L.

OSTEODYSTROPHY

Renal osteodystrophy commonly develops in association with hyperphosphatemia, hypocalcemia, and elevation of parathyroid hormone levels and serum alkaline phosphatase activity. In general, the serum phosphorus level rises when the glomerular filtration rate falls to less than 30% of normal. Hyperphosphatemia lowers the serum calcium level because of their reciprocal solubility relationship and results in secondary hyperparathyroidism. Hyperphosphatemia may be controlled by enhancing fecal excretion using oral calcium carbonate (an antacid that coincidentally also binds phosphate in the intestinal tract). The usual dosage range is 1 to 4 teaspoons of Titralac or 1 to 4 tablets of Os-Cal 500 with each meal and before bed.

Hypocalcemia may result from hyperphosphatemia, inadequate dietary intake, and decreased intestinal calcium absorption caused by a deficiency in the active form (1,25-dihydroxycholecalciferol) of vitamin D. If the serum calcium level remains low after correction of the serum phosphorus level, oral calcium supplements at a dosage of 500 to 2000 mg/day can be administered.

Vitamin D therapy is indicated (1) in adolescent patients who have persistent hypocalcemia despite reduction of the serum phosphorus level to less than 6 mg/dl and the addition of oral calcium supplements and (2) in adolescents with osteodystrophy, as characterized by elevated serum alkaline phosphatase levels and radiographic evidence of rickets. Therapy may be initiated with one capsule (0.25 μg)/day of the active form of dihydroxyvitamin D (Rocaltrol) or 0.05 to 0.20 mg/day of dihydrotachysterol solution (DHT Oral Solution), which is metabolized to its active form in the liver. The dosage of vitamin D is progressively increased until the serum calcium and alkaline phosphatase levels are normal and healing of the rickets is seen on x-ray film. The dosage of vitamin D should then be reduced to the initiating level.

ANEMIA

Anemia is common in chronic renal failure and is primarily the result of inadequate erythropoietin production by the failing kidneys. However, inadequate dietary intake of iron and folic acid should not be overlooked. In most adolescents, the hemoglobin level will stabilize in the range of 6 to 9 g/dl; transfusion therapy is not indicated, as this would further suppress erythropoietin production. If the hemoglobin level falls to less than 6 g/dl, 10 ml/kg (small volume reduces the risk of circulatory overload) of packed red blood cells should be administered cautiously. Potentially, the problem of anemia will be alleviated with the introduction of recombinant human erythropoietin therapy.

HYPERTENSION

Hypertensive emergencies should be treated with intravenous diazoxide (Hyperstat) as described in the section on acute renal failure. The treatment of sustained hypertension may include a combination of salt restriction (2 to 3 g/day), furosemide (1 to 4 mg/kg/day), propranolol (Inderal, 1 to 4 mg/kg/day), and hydralazine (Apresoline, 1 to 5 mg/kg/day). Newer agents, such as minoxidil and captopril, should be used only in patients whose blood pressure is inadequately controlled on the preceding regimen and should be administered with the guidance of a nephrologist.

DRUG DOSAGE IN CHRONIC RENAL FAILURE

Since many drugs are excreted by the kidneys, their administration to adolescents with renal insufficiency must be altered to maximize effectiveness and minimize the risk of toxicity. The principles of and guidelines for prescribing medications for adolescents in renal failure are summarized in the excellent review by Bennett and associates.

END-STAGE RENAL FAILURE

Dialysis is generally initiated when the adolescent's creatinine level approaches 10 mg/dl, depending on the patient's clinical status, other laboratory studies, and availability of a kidney donor. Hemodialysis remains the standard technique of chronic dialysis. The development of long-term subclavian vein catheters and the creation of arteriovenous fistulae at the wrist have greatly simplified access to the vascular system for hemodialysis. However, the development of continuous ambulatory peritoneal dialysis (CAPD) has revolutionized chronic dialysis so that many young patients now use this technique.

An alternative to CAPD is continuous cyclic peritoneal dialysis (CCPD). This procedure reverses the schedule of CAPD by providing the exchanges at night rather than during the day. The exchanges are performed automatically during sleep by a simple cycler machine. This permits an uninterrupted day of activities, a reduction in the number of connections and disconnections (which should decrease the risk of peritonitis), and a reduction in the time required by the adolescent and parent to perform dialysis, reducing the risk fatigue and "burn-out."

In the treatment of end-stage renal failure in adolescents, the ultimate goal is a successful kidney transplant. The 10-year success rate for human lymphocyte antigen (HLA)-identical sibling transplants approximates 90%, the 10-year success rate for non-HLA–identical living-related donors (usually parents) is 70%, and the 10-year success rate for cadaver-derived kidneys is 50%. Ongoing research into better and less toxic means to prevent graft rejection should improve these statistics.

BIBLIOGRAPHY

Balow JE: Renal vasculitis. Kidney Int 27:954, 1985.
Bennett WM, Aronoff GR, Morrison G, et al: Drug prescribing in renal failure: Dosing guidelines for adults. Am J Kidney Dis 3:155, 1983.
Cameron JS: The treatment of lupus nephritis. Pediatr Nephrol 3:350, 1989.
Chan JCM, Alon U: Tubular disorders of acid-base and phosphate metabolism. Nephron 40:257, 1985.
Couser WG: Rapidly progressive glomerulonephritis: Classification, pathogenic mechanisms, and therapy. Am J Kidney Dis 11:449, 1988.
Holliday MA, Barratt TM, Vernier RL: Pediatric Nephrology. Baltimore, Williams & Wilkins, 1987.
Johnson JR, Stamm WE: Urinary tract infections in women: Diagnosis and treatment. Ann Intern Med 111:906, 1989.
Massry SG, Glassock RJ: Textbook of Nephrology. Baltimore, Williams & Wilkins, 1989.
Neilson EG: Pathogenesis and therapy of interstitial nephritis. Kidney Int 35:1257, 1989.
Reddi AS, Camerini-Davalos RA: Diabetic nephropathy. Arch Intern Med 150:31, 1990.

CHAPTER 66

Urologic Conditions

RICHARD C. RINK, MICHAEL A. KEATING, and MARK C. ADAMS

GENITOURINARY DISORDERS

Although congenital urologic disorders most commonly present in childhood, their diagnosis may be delayed until the second decade of life. Later diagnosis may occur because of atypical, mild, intermittent, or progressive disease. Also, late secondary factors, such as infection or trauma, may result in the identification of previously asymptomatic patients.

Adolescents can also present with acquired urologic disorders that are commonly seen in adults, but occur less frequently in younger children. For example, adolescents are more susceptible to trauma than are younger children because of more vigorous physical activity. As a result, the physician caring for the adolescent must be familiar with urologic problems that affect both younger children and adults.

Symptoms

Adolescents are more likely than younger children to understand their symptoms and communicate them to parents and physicians. However, denial, anxiety, and autonomy-seeking behaviors often influence their communication and presentation to the physician. Self-consciousness, especially with respect to genitourinary anatomy or function, is extremely common among adolescents and greatly affects the patient-physician interaction.

Symptoms related to genitourinary disorders depend on the duration and location of the pathologic condition. For instance, acute obstruction of the kidney or ureter can produce sharp, colicky abdominal pain. High obstruction of the renal pelvis usually produces pain localized to the flank, whereas more distal ureteral obstruction is often characterized by sharp pain localized to the groin with radiation to the scrotum or labia. Adolescents with long-standing obstruction may be asymptomatic but occasionally may complain of vague abdominal or flank pain. Adolescents with previously asymptomatic ureteropelvic junction obstruction may develop intermittent, severe colic after vigorous hydration, most commonly after drinking alcohol; termed Dietl crisis, the pain is related to acute dilatation proximal to an obstruction that becomes exaggerated with diuresis.

Pain related to the genitourinary tract may be accompanied by nausea and vomiting that may be attributed erroneously to a gastrointestinal disorder. Generalized symptoms of vomiting, anorexia, poor growth, and lethargy are occasionally seen in adolescents with severe urologic disease. Adolescents with pyelonephritis often have a continuous ache, which can become severe. Hematuria due to urologic disorders may be microscopic or gross and may occur initially, terminally, or throughout voiding, depending on the degree and location of the bleeding.

Voiding complaints are common and range from irritative symptoms of frequency, urgency, and dysuria to obstructive symptoms such as straining, difficulty initiating a stream, and frank retention. Urinary incontinence and enuresis are also common problems in adolescents. The pattern of wetting, whether it is continual, overflow, stress, or urge related, suggests the underlying cause. Genital complaints of dysuria, urethral discharge, scrotal swelling, discomfort, or pain in boys, although not common, require evaluation.

Unlike children with urologic disorders, adolescents rarely present with a palpable abdominal or flank mass. Beyond an assessment of the abdomen and genitalia, thorough evaluation of genitourinary disorders should include a general physical examination, including sexual maturity rating (see Chapter 5). Measurements of height and weight are necessary to recognize growth retardation that may be related to metabolic acidosis or renal insufficiency. Elevated blood pressure may be associated with renal damage or scarring (see Chapter 67). Careful examination of the spine and a brief neurologic examination are indicated for any patient with voiding complaints or urinary incontinence.

Manifestations During Adolescence of Previously Recognized Conditions

A number of children who have previously diagnosed genitourinary diseases encounter new problems when going through puberty and adolescence. Close follow-up is often required despite a relatively benign clinical condition during childhood. Impaired kidneys that have provided adequate levels of renal function at an earlier age are sometimes overwhelmed by the increase in body mass that occurs with puberty. In addition, alterations in the hormonal milieu can affect changes of the internal and external genitalia. For example, enlargement of the prostate or vagina may alter the urethra and bladder emptying, or the initiation of sexual activity could unmask the functional shortcomings of a previous genital surgery. Finally, and perhaps most importantly, adolescents frequently become noncompliant with self-care, intermittent catheterization, or time-voiding programs (see Chapter 26). Noncompliance with bladder emptying can lead to recurrent urinary infections, the development of reflux, and, in the case of the augmented bladder, bladder perforations. In general, if the patient's genitourinary tract remains functional during puberty, the outlook through subsequent adulthood is usually good.

MYELOMENINGOCELE AND RELATED SPINA BIFIDAS

The internal genitalia of females with myelomeningocele are unaltered, and normal sexual intercourse, fertility, and pregnancy can be expected unless there is some additional anatomic distortion. Affected adolescents, however, do have a 40-fold increased risk of having a child with spinal dysraphism, so that prenatal screening with ultrasonography and alpha-fetoprotein is recommended when pregnancy occurs. Boys with myelomeningocele experience more problems with sexual function. Glandular anesthesia is common, and the capacity for erection and sexual intercourse with ejaculation is variable but often impaired. Fertility is impaired because of retrograde ejaculation as the consequence of neural damage and bladder–sphincter incompetence.

The bladder, the sphincter, or both bladder and sphincter of nearly every child with myelomeningocele are abnormal. Management of children is directed at the preservation of renal function. Later, therapy is directed at attaining urinary continence with careful attention to protection of the kidneys. To this end, a variety of management methods are employed, including intermittent catheterization, anticholinergic medication, and reconstruction of the bladder using portions of the adolescent's bowel. Regardless of the mode of management, the need for chronic surveillance in these children as they enter adolescence cannot be overemphasized.

Puberty represents a special time in development for the genitourinary tract of the child with myelomeningocele or a related spina bifida. Precocious puberty, possibly related to underlying hydrocephalus, occurs frequently, especially in girls (see Chapter 58). The neurologic implications of spinal cord abnormalities are variable and may change during puberty. This is especially true during the height spurt, when the spinal cord may not ascend with the spinal column because of distal fixation due to previous closure or from an unappreciated spina bifida variant. Tethering of the nerves in the region can occur but generally causes few overt symptoms, although the alterations in bladder dynamics and compliance that result have implications for the upper urinary tract. We recommend annual ultrasonographic examination of the kidneys and bladder, as well as periodic urine analysis.

EPISPADIAS-EXSTROPHY COMPLEX

Epispadias generally occurs with exstrophy of the bladder. The corporal bodies of the penis are usually of normal size but are tethered to the pubic bones and base of the bladder, so the penile shaft appears short and stubby. The abnormality is usually corrected at a very early age. However, complete cosmetic normalcy is almost never achieved, and the majority of boys have a very broad, short penis. Despite this, the sexual performance of these boys is normal. In some instances, dorsal curvature of the penis worsens with phallic growth during puberty. When this is severe, secondary surgery to achieve a normal cosmetic appearance and to eliminate any functional problems with coitus can be helpful.

The dynamic characteristics of the bladder with exstrophy (usually surgically corrected in the newborn period) are widely variable, and the prognosis for growth, compliance, and function is unknown. The bladders of some adolescent patients are noncompliant or small and require augmentation to achieve continence. Others have an adequate bladder but equivocal sphincter resistance that results in incontinence. The prostatic growth seen with puberty sometimes supplies enough resistance to allow affected boys to attain continence as they mature sexually. For other boys with exstrophy, however, the increased size of the prostate hampers outlet resistance and bladder emptying. Again, periodic surveillance in each affected child is warranted as he progresses through puberty.

Many children whose bladders have been severely damaged or removed because of exstrophy, tumor, or myelomeningocele have required complex urinary tract reconstructions using intestine as an alternative reservoir for urine. In these cases, segments of bowel, including stomach, colon, and small intestine, have been used to reconstruct the native bladder or create an entire "neobladder." The long-term implications of these types of reservoirs remain undefined, so close surveillance is required. These new bladders (which do not contract normally) provide continence at the cost of chronic urinary retention. The need for intermittent catheterization to empty the reservoir is critical, and noncompliance in the adolescent is common. Perforations of reconstructed bladders are increasingly common: a rate of approximately 7% has been noted in our institution, and we anticipate that number to increase with continued follow-up. In addition, incomplete or sporadic emptying prevents the kidneys and ureters from emptying properly. In the absence of problems, yearly ultrasounds of the kidneys and periodic urine cultures are recommended for surveillance. Management of these complex problems is best coordinated with a pediatric urologist.

FUNCTIONAL DISTURBANCES OF VOIDING

Symptoms

Voiding complaints such as painful urination (dysuria) or involuntary wetting (enuresis) result in several million office visits annually in the United States. Almost one half of the problems encountered in a pediatric urologic ambulatory practice are related to dysfunctional voiding. Many of these patients have urinary tract infections or other secondary organic voiding problems and wetting. However, the vast majority of adolescents with voiding complaints do not have anatomic urologic abnormalities.

Dysuria, frequency, and urgency can result from inflammation of the bladder, urethra, or both. Although less than one fifth of children with such lower urinary tract complaints have urinary infection, adolescents with these symptoms are much more likely to be infected. We have noted frequency and urgency with negative urine culture in adolescents in association with viral cystitis; caffeine, chocolate, and carbonated beverage ingestion; allergic reactions; and seasonal changes. With normal findings on physical examination and urine culture, a full radiographic and cystoscopic examination is not required, and symptomatic treatment of the dysuria alone is indicated. Anticholinergic bladder relaxants (e.g., Bethanacol) or urethral anesthetics (e.g., Pyridium) may be helpful after elimination of all known irritants from the diet.

Hematuria may occur in adolescents as an isolated symptom. When the urine is pink to bright red and associated with irritative voiding symptoms, lower tract infections and idiopathic hypercalciuria should be considered. Tea or cola-colored urine is more likely due to renal causes (see Chapter 65).

The most frequent urologic cause of gross hematuria in the adolescent is cystitis, most commonly in the young female. Viral cystitis, which commonly occurs in children in association with adenovirus infection, is a less likely cause of hematuria in the adolescent. The initial evaluation of hematuria should include urinalysis, urine culture, and appropriate tests for sexually transmitted infections, urine dipstick for protein, and a spot urine determination of the calcium to creatinine ratio (>0.2 denotes hypercalciuria). Radiographic evaluation should include a voiding cystourethrogram (VCUG) and either a renal ultrasonogram or intravenous pyelogram. Cystoscopy in adolescents requires an anesthetic and should only be performed when hematuria is protracted and unexplained or to rule out a specific diagnosis.

Recurrent blood spotting of the underwear is a common complaint in adolescent males and may last for years. This condition, known as urethrorrhagia, is almost always benign and not associated with urologic symptoms, although a urethral diverticulum may present in this way. In females with blood spotting, urethral prolapse should be suspected.

Normal and Abnormal Voiding Patterns

Normal voiding requires urinary sphincter and urinary bladder synergy; as the bladder fills, the sphincter tightens. With voiding, the sphincter relaxes reflexively and the bladder contracts and empties. "Toilet training" is the achievement of voluntary control of the sphincter and bladder mechanism. Dysfunctional voiding in the adolescent results in the loss of synergy after control is established, leading to contractions of the sphincter on voiding. Contractions of the sphincter to prevent wetting that might occur during uninhibited bladder contractions result in detrusor contractions against a closed sphincter that creates a functional bladder outlet obstruction, resulting in extremely high intravesical pressures (up to 200 cm/H_2O). If intravesical pressures exceed urethral closing pressure, urine is released. One half of adolescents will be found to have vesicoureteral reflux under these circumstances. The cause of these contractions is unknown, but no abnormal findings are noted on neurologic examination. Fortunately, these "filling" problems usually resolve by mid-puberty. However, the triad of enuresis, urinary tract infections, and vesicourethral reflux is a recognized symptom complex in adolescents with nonorganic voiding dysfunction. VCUG and renal bladder ultrasound should be done as a baseline evaluation. Treatment is directed toward controlling the uninhibited contractions with anticholinergic bladder relaxants, frequent, timed voiding, and fluid restriction. Urodynamic evaluation is often helpful.

"Emptying" disorders are much more apt to persist into adolescence than voiding dysfunction associated with bladder filling, as just described. These disorders also are much more likely to damage the upper urinary tract and present with urinary tract infection (UTI). A careful voiding history (as well as urinary flow rate) often reveals one of two voiding patterns: a forceful "gushing" stream that suddenly stops, or an intermittent "dribbling" stream. Both of these occur as a result of sphincter contraction during voiding. This learned, voluntary contraction of the external sphincter during voiding results in high intravesical pressures but also poor emptying. The large residual volumes contribute to the high incidence of infection. Vesicoureteral reflux is present in as many as one half of these patients also. A VCUG should be done as well as ultrasonography or intravenous pyelography (IVP). Treatment is more difficult for emptying abnormalities and is directed at achieving sphincter relaxation by biofeedback techniques.

A small number of adolescents with voiding disturbances develop severe detrusor–sphincter dyssynergia, a destructive condition, resulting in a thickened, neurogenic-like bladder. Hydronephrosis, reflux, and UTI commonly accompany this problem. This has been termed the "non-neurogenic–neurogenic bladder." Treatment often requires intermittent catheterization (ICC) and anticholinergic medication. Psychological evaluation may be indicated, because affected adolescents often have underlying emotional problems. These patients often are found to have functional fecal retention, which may itself lead to urinary retention and uninhibited bladder contractions. Constipation must be prevented (see Chapter 64).

Vesicoureteral reflux may resolve spontaneously with treatment of the voiding dysfunction. We recommend surgical correction of reflux if it has not spontaneously resolved by puberty. However, significant voiding dysfunction should be treated first, because surgical antireflux procedures are prone to complications if voiding dysfunction is ignored or unrecognized.

Enuresis

The psychological and emotional impact of nocturnal enuresis on the adolescent can be devastating. Normal family dynamics are often disrupted. The teen often feels guilt and has low self-esteem. Although no single mechanism adequately explains this problem, parents often note that the adolescent is a heavy sleeper. However, sleep disorders are difficult to prove. When bed wetting persists after puberty, a screening renal–bladder ultrasonogram may be helpful.

Although the prevalence of nocturnal enuresis normally declines from 3% at age 12 years to less than 1% at 18 years, awaiting spontaneous resolution is an option that is rarely acceptable to either the adolescent or the parent. An alarm system is a highly successful therapeutic option, considered by many to be the treatment of choice. A urine-sensing device fits inside the underwear or pajamas, and an alarm clips near the shoulder of the nightshirt. This can be quite effective in the adolescent who is motivated to dryness. The results are lasting and medication is avoided. Disadvantages include the time required to achieve success, a high dropout rate, and the need for the parent to sleep near the adolescent, because failure to be aroused by the alarm can result in the rest of the family being awakened and failure of this mode of therapy.

A third option is pharmacologic therapy. Three drugs are currently used. Anticholinergic medication such as oxybutinin (Ditropan), although successful at suppressing uninhibited contractions, is of minimal benefit for the nocturnal enuretic. Imipramine (Tofranil) has been successful in approximately one half of enuretics, although its mechanism of action is unknown. Possible side effects should be explained to the adolescent and family, although they are usually minimal because the dose used is less than that to treat depression (10–75 mg q.h.s.). In addition, high relapse rates make this a less than ideal drug.

Recent work has shown that many bedwetters fail to increase their antidiuretic hormone (ADH) levels at night. Desmopressin acetate (DDAVP), an ADH stimulant, is now available for use in bed wetting. Early trials have noted a success rate similar to the alarm, with only minimal toxicity. Although side effects are uncommon, it does have the disadvantage of being very costly.

URINARY TRACT OBSTRUCTION

With widespread use of routine antenatal and postnatal ultrasonography, many urinary tract disorders resulting in hydronephrosis are diagnosed at an early age, prior to the development of symptoms. Thus, fewer adolescents should present with symptomatic congenital disorders. Children with a previously diagnosed and treated obstructive lesion should have stable urinary tracts by the time they become adolescents, but it is prudent to obtain an ultrasound of the kidneys and bladder at least every 2 years until adulthood. If this study shows decreased growth of the kidneys or increased hydronephrosis, then functional renal studies (IVP, nuclear scan) and cystography may be necessary.

Ureteropelvic Junction Obstruction

Ureteropelvic junction (UPJ) obstruction is the most common congenital obstructive lesion of the urinary tract. It occurs two to three times more often in males than in females, and bilateral disease is present in 10% to 25% of affected patients. UPJ obstruction predisposes the adolescent to renal parenchymal infection, and symptoms such as nausea, vomiting, and vague abdominal or flank pain are common complaints. Older patients with severe renal damage from the obstruction may present with hypertension. Hematuria is common in adolescents with UPJ obstruction, particularly following relatively minor trauma. As previously mentioned, severe intermittent flank pain or colic may suddenly occur, particularly with vigorous hydration. Such patients often have normal radiographic imaging of the kidneys between painful episodes (Fig. 66–1). It is therefore helpful to image the kidneys during the acute episode, in order to demonstrate obstruction.

UPJ obstruction may be caused by intrinsic or, less commonly, extrinsic factors. Smooth muscle is replaced by collagen in the area of the ureteropelvic junction. This results in failure of transmission of peristaltic waves. Ultrasonography reveals marked dilatation of the pelvis and calices without visualization of the ureter. A functional renal study such as an IVP or technetium diethylenetriamine penta-acetic acid (DPTA) scan is necessary for the diagnosis. A voiding cystourethrogram should be performed in search for vesicoureteral reflux.

Surgical correction of UPJ obstruction is indicated for the adolescent who presents with symptoms. Rarely, the obstructed kidney functions so poorly that nephrectomy is required. The results of repair can be excellent and result in improved drainage, stabilization of function,

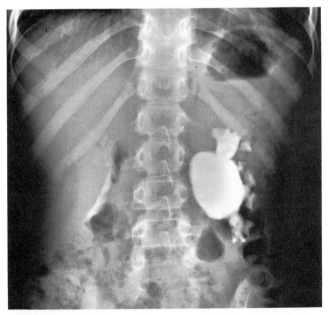

Figure 66–1. Left ureteropelvic junction (UPJ) obstruction. Intravenous pyelography (IVP) done during painful episode reveals dilated pelvis that had not been noted on IVP done when patient was pain-free.

and resolution of symptoms. Postoperative complications are rare.

Ureteral Obstruction

Congenital midureteral obstruction is very rare but may be caused by ureteral valves, polyps, or an aberrant course of the ureter behind the iliac vessels or vena cava.

Ureterovesical junction (UVJ) obstruction, however, is common and is usually due to a distal adynamic segment of ureter (Fig. 66–2). Rarely, true stenosis or valves may be present. The left side is more commonly affected, particularly in males. Although symptoms of infection are most common on presentation, these so-called "primary obstructive megaureters" can also cause hematuria, hypertension, or abdominal pain. Imaging demonstrates a dilated renal pelvis and calices, as with a UPJ obstruction, and also a dilated ureter. IVP may show the typical bulbous distal ureter with a narrow terminal or intramural segment. A VCUG must be obtained to identify reflux if it exists.

Whether or not reflux does exist, obstruction must be searched for, most often by furosemide (Lasix) washout on DTPA scan. This may identify congenital nonrefluxing, nonobstructed megaureters, in which renal function is usually well preserved and surgical correction is not necessary. When obstruction at the UVJ is identified, surgical correction by resection of the distal adynamic segment and reimplantation of the normal, but dilated, proximal ureter is indicated. Adequate reimplantation usually requires tapering or imbrication of the dilated ureter to a more normal diameter. Operative results for obstructive megaureters are generally quite good.

A ureter may also be obstructed distally if it terminates outside the normal bladder location in an ectopic position. Obstruction can be caused by a stenotic ectopic orifice or the passage of the ureter through the bladder outlet sphincter. Ureteral ectopy occurs six times more often in females than in males. Ectopic ureters are usually associated with a totally duplicated collecting system, virtually always with the upper pole moiety, in females. In males, ectopic ureters are more commonly associated with a single collecting system.

An ectopic ureter may completely bypass the bladder sphincter mechanism in females, resulting in continuous wetting despite an otherwise normal voiding pattern. Occasionally, the wetting problem may go unrecognized until adolescence or adulthood. There have been several reports of incontinence developing secondary to ureteral ectopy only after puberty or childbirth. The leakage from ectopic ureters may be worse during the day, especially if the associated upper pole renal segment functions very poorly. An ectopic ureter may open into the vagina, cervix, or uterus, and urinary incontinence may be mistaken for a vaginal discharge.

If an ectopic ureter opens proximally at the bladder neck or in the posterior urethra, incontinence is uncommon. In males, ectopic ureters always enter proximal to the external sphincter and incontinence is rare. Urinary tract infection then becomes the most common presentation of ectopic ureter entering the drainage system proximally, because incontinence is usually not noted but the normal defenses against infection are lacking. In males, epididymitis and prostatitis may occur. This entity should be considered when males who are not yet sexually active develop such infections.

Diagnosis of an ectopic ureter can often be made by renal ultrasonography, during which a dysplastic, hydronephrotic upper pole is usually easily seen. It may be noted indirectly on IVP by displacing the lower pole system laterally and inferiorly ("drooping flower"). If the upper pole system is small, computed tomography (CT) is beneficial. A VCUG demonstrates reflux in 30% of cases.

Appropriate treatment of an ectopic ureter is determined by the function of the associated renal segment. A renal segment that contributes more than 10% of total renal function should be preserved. In up to 90% of cases, however, the associated renal segment does not function well enough to warrant repair and should be removed.

A ureterocele is a cystic dilatation of the terminal ureter beneath the bladder mucosa that causes obstruction (Fig. 66–3). The majority of ureteroceles in adolescents are associated with a duplicated collecting system draining the upper pole renal segment. Such a ureterocele may be situated entirely within the bladder, but often extends to the bladder neck or urethra, where it may prolapse through the urethral meatus. The ureterocele may affect the ipsilateral lower pole renal segment and contralateral kidney by causing obstruction of, or reflux into, those ureters.

Treatment depends on the function of the renal segment drained by the affected ureter. Usually the segment functions so poorly that upper pole heminephrectomy and partial ureterectomy is indicated. This leaves the ureterocele in situ, but decompressed. In the majority of cases, the decompressed ureterocele does not present a problem. However, in at least 25% of cases, persistent infections or reflux mandates bladder surgery

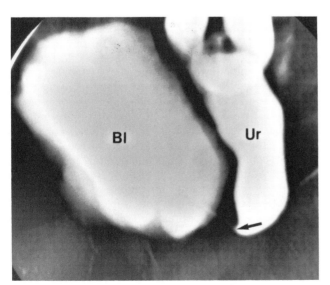

Figure 66–2. Ureterovesical junction (UVJ) obstruction. The beginning of obstruction by an adynamic segment with dilated ureter proximal to the obstruction is seen (arrow). BL, bladder; Ur, ureter.

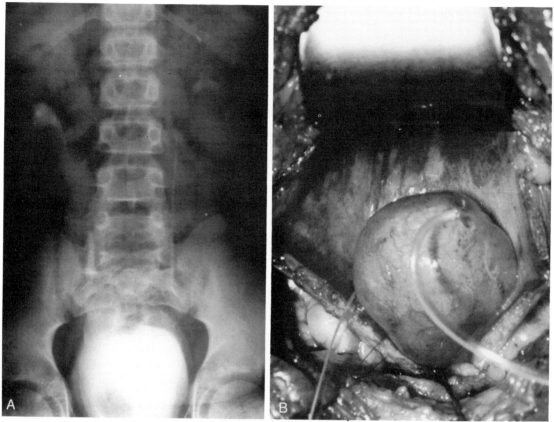

Figure 66–3. Ureterocele. A large filling defect in the bladder is the terminal end of the upper pole ureter of a duplex system. This is the ureterocele. *A*, "Filling defect" in bladder from right upper pole ureterocele on intravenous pyelography. *B*, Large ureterocele with catheter in lower pole ureter.

with resection of the ureterocele and, often, reimplantation of the other ureters.

Bladder and Urethral Obstructions

Congenital bladder outlet obstruction is relatively uncommon, particularly in females. A common cause of bladder obstruction in females is a large ectopic ureterocele extending into the urethra. In males, posterior urethral valves at the level of the verumontanum may cause significant bladder outlet obstruction. Patients with severe posterior urethral valves generally have hydronephrosis on prenatal ultrasonogram or present early in life with renal insufficiency or urinary tract sepsis. Less severe forms of the obstruction, however, may not be diagnosed until adolescence. In such cases, renal and bladder damage is usually minimal. Symptoms may include only persistent wetting or enuresis and, occasionally, cystitis. Anterior urethral valves are much less common than posterior urethral valves, but may also result in obstruction of varying degree. Adolescents who present with either type of valve usually have a mild form of the disease and are generally cured by transurethral resection of the valves alone.

GENITAL ABNORMALITIES

Hypospadias

The past 2 decades have been marked by significant alterations in the management of most genital anomalies, including hypospadias (see Chapter 78). We now prefer to correct these problems in boys between the ages of 6 and 18 months, avoiding problems with genital awareness and toilet training. In addition, the reconstructive surgeon now strives to recreate a normal phallus, a significant deviation from the past, where functional normalcy alone was often the objective and the cosmetic results of surgery could sometimes be worse or no better than the child's preoperative presentation. Nevertheless, because of these historical impressions, many genital abnormalities remain uncorrected.

Adolescents with uncorrected genital anomalies require intermittent assessment at the very least. Peripubertal phallic enlargement can unmask the tethering of dysgenetic fibers and penile curvature (chordee), which might not have been appreciated at an earlier age (Fig. 66–4). In addition, the meatus of some of these boys is intrinsically scarred, does not enlarge as the child grows, and acts as a fixed obstruction. Adolescents who have previously corrected hypospadias require close observation during this transitional period for similar reasons. The cosmetic shortcomings of uncorrected hypospadias

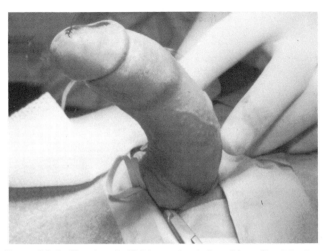

Figure 66–4. Chordee. Artificial erection induced by saline injection and rubber band tourniquet reveals significant penile curvature.

are variable. Many boys with mild distal variants learn to cope with the stigmata of their anomaly, which includes the dorsal-hooded prepuce and flattened ventral glans. However, regardless of its severity, the psychological implications of hypospadias have been well documented and include problems with self-esteem and social interactions. Surgical correction is recommended in most cases.

Priapism

Priapism is persistent painful erections (see Chapter 78). The most common causes in the adolescent include sickle-cell disease (see Chapter 52), leukemia (see Chapter 53), and psychotropic medication (especially phenothiazine and its related congeners). Less common causes include blunt trauma and pelvic tumors. A variable amount of distress is associated with a persistently turgid penis, which is the effect of the stasis of blood in the corpora cavernosa. The glans penis, whose corpus spongiosum is not involved by the disease process, should not be as turgid as it would be with a normal erection.

By the time most boys with a history of prolonged erection with pain are seen by a physician, their penises have become flaccid. These rarely represent true episodes of priapism, but a thorough evaluation of the symptoms, including history, physical examination, white blood cell screen, and sickle-cell screen in black males, is indicated.

Current treatment of priapism is directed at the underlying abnormality; surgery is rarely required. Sickle-cell–related priapism is treated by increasing oxygenization to reverse "sickling" and stasis in the corpora of the penis. Hydration and transfusions usually accomplish this goal. Leukemic priapism commonly resolves after chemotherapeutic treatment of the primary neoplastic process. Finally, any medications known to be associated with priapism should be discontinued. Corporal lavage with epinephrine solution sometimes becomes necessary to counteract the cholinergic effects of medications that caused the priapism. The long-term sequelae of priapism

in the adolescent vary with its duration. Fortunately, permanent corporal fibrosis and impotence are uncommon, regardless of the underlying cause.

Phimosis and Paraphimosis

(see Chapter 78)

Circumcision is now deferred in as many as 50% of newborn males in the United States, owing largely to the American Academy of Pediatrics policy statement in 1974, which cited no medical benefits of circumcision. However, recent evidence suggests that uncircumcised newborn males may be at increased risk of UTIs.

There are some common misconceptions concerning the care of the uncircumcised penis. The foreskin is naturally fused to the glans penis early in development. The gradual sloughing of this layer results in the extrusion of smegma, its breakdown product, and a progressive relaxation of the foreskin. As a result, an inability to retract the foreskin is a common phenomenon in younger males (approximately 10% at 3 years of age), but full retraction of the foreskin should be expected by puberty. In adolescents in whom this is still a problem, the patient should gently retract the foreskin during bathing to loosen the narrowing that occurs naturally at the distal extent of the foreskin in every uncircumcised boy.

In some instances, retraction is impossible, a condition known as phimosis. Ballooning of the prepuce may occur during voiding, and the stasis of accumulated urine beneath the foreskin causes penile irritation, dysuria, and other localized symptoms. With scarring, the opening to the foreskin becomes extremely narrowed, and attempts to gently retract this cicatrix cause pain and should not be pursued. In this case, circumcision should be performed.

Paraphimosis occurs when the foreskin is forcibly retracted behind the glans penis but cannot be returned to its normal resting position. The phimotic collar of the prepuce acts as a constricting ring that compromises blood flow and leads to edema and pain. Fortunately, reduction is usually possible using a combination of traction on the edematous preputial skin and pressure on the glans penis (Fig. 66–5). If this is unsuccessful, immediate surgery is necessary. Circumcision is recommended after an episode of *paraphimosis*.

Buried Penis

Concerns about genital development and phallic size are common for the adolescent and his parents. The typical referral is that of a obese youngster thought to have a small penis. In these instances, a prominent prepubic fat pad causes the more mobile shaft skin to override the corpora of the phallus, giving the penis a concealed or "buried" appearance (Fig. 66–6). Manual compression of the adjacent fat pad usually enables appreciation of the penis that is normally developed and of an average size (Fig. 66–7). Table 66–1 summarizes penile length during adolescence.

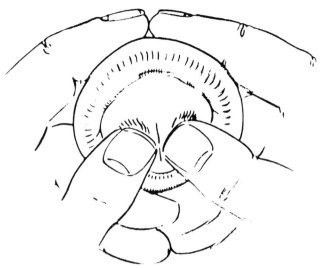

Figure 66–5. Reducing paraphimosis by compressing glans through the paraphimotic foreskin.

Most of these boys require no treatment. The changes in habitus and phallic elongation that occur during puberty usually result in a normal phenotypic appearance. A small group, however, have abnormal development of the investing fascia of the penis, causing it to be truly tethered below the pubis bone. This must be released for penile length to be appreciated. Surgical skin rearrangements in concert with liposuction have been effective.

Urethral Strictures

Urethral strictures in the adolescent are usually the sequelae of urethral trauma, prior urologic manipulation, or the introduction of foreign bodies during sexual experimentation. The duration between the onset of symptoms and the initial insult can be quite variable, and the history of a preceding straddle injury or other perineal trauma is often not well defined. Hematuria and difficulties with the urinary stream are the most common presenting symptoms of a urethral stricture.

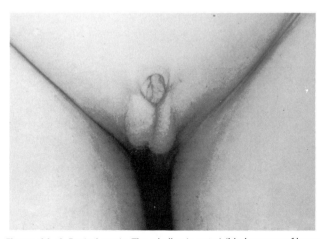

Figure 66–6. Buried penis. The phallus is not visible because of large prepubic fat pad.

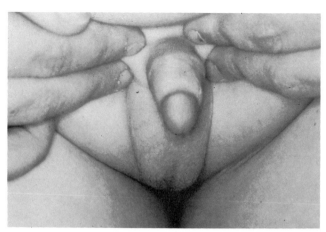

Figure 66–7. Manual compression of fat pad exposes the normal penis.

When stricture is suspected, a cystourethrogram should be obtained. However, problems with catheterization are commonly encountered because of obstruction. No force should be used when difficulty is encountered in attempting catheterization. Instead, the diagnosis of stricture should be confirmed with a retrograde urethrogram or localization at the time of later cystoscopy.

The management of urethral strictures depends on cause, location, and chronicity. Many can be corrected with cystoscopic urethrotomy, but others require open urethroplasty.

UROLITHIASIS

Stones form in the kidney when inorganic crystals coalesce with proteinaceous matrix in the renal calices or pelvis after the concentration of the crystalline substance exceeds its solubility in the urine. Depending on numerous factors, including the substance making up the stone, the nature of the urine being excreted (pH), the presence of infection, and urinary flow rate, they can vary in size from a few millimeters to large, "staghorn" calculi that fill and demarcate the outline of the renal pelvis. Substances such as citrate, magnesium, or polyphosphates appear to inhibit stone formation and are occasionally found in reduced concentration in adolescents with urolithiasis. Most kidney stones in adolescents contain calcium salts (oxalate or phosphate). Struvite (infection-related) stones are composed of magnesium ammonium phosphate or carbonate calcium

TABLE 66–1. Unstretched Penis and Testis Size During Adolescence

AGE (YEARS)	PENIS LENGTH (cm)	TESTIS LENGTH (cm)
8–10	4.2 ± 0.8	2.0 ± 0.5
10–12	5.2 ± 1.3	2.7 ± 0.7
12–14	6.2 ± 2.0	3.4 ± 0.8
14–16	8.6 ± 2.4	4.1 ± 1.0

Adapted with permission from Winter JSD, Faiman C: Pituitary-gonadal relations in male children and adolescents. Pediatr Res 6:126, 1972. © by The Endocrine Society.

phosphate. Patients excreting excessive amounts of uric acid or cystine also have stones composed largely of these substances.

The most common presenting manifestations of stones in adolescents include flank pain, hematuria, and symptoms related to UTI and irritative voiding. As many as one third of adolescents with urolithiasis have an underlying congenital anatomic defect that predisposes to stone formation because of urinary stasis, infection, or both, indicating the need for radiographic evaluation with ultrasonography and a voiding study. Because a metabolic cause can be identified in up to 50% of adolescents with stones, any that are passed or surgically recovered should be chemically analyzed.

Stones composed of calcium constitute a smaller proportion of urolithiasis in adolescents than in adults but remain the most common type in young people. Hypercalciuria is the most common underlying biochemical abnormality. The serum calcium generally is normal in adolescents with hypercalciuria, most commonly due to an idiopathic state of either excessive absorption of dietary calcium from the gut or excessive excretion of renal tubular calcium. In some families, this is an autosomal dominant trait. Distal RTA and furosemide therapy also can be associated with normocalcemic hypercalciuria and urolithiasis (see Chapter 65).

Hypercalciuric, hypercalcemic urolithiasis in adolescents can be the result of hyperparathyroidism, sarcoidosis, hypervitaminosis D, Cushing syndrome, or the mild-alkali syndrome. Adolescents who are immobilized for prolonged periods, as in traction or a body cast, are predisposed to stone formation, as are those with significant gastrointestinal disease. The former is due to increased resorption of calcium from bone as the result of inactivity, whereas the latter is due to excessive absorption of oxalate from the gut. Oxalate stones may also be associated with hyperuricuria, hypocitraturia, or the rare genetic defect primary hyperoxaluria.

Struvite, or infection stones, are relatively more common in adolescents than in adults, particularly in Europe, where they represent the most common type of stone in that age group. These stones are related to infections with urease-producing organisms, including species of *Proteus, Pseudomonas, Providencia, Klebsiella, Serratia,* and, rarely, *Staphylococcus.* Struvite stones are particularly common in obstructive uropathy predisposing to infections. The ammonia formed in such circumstances causes alkalinization of the urine and precipitation of phosphate salts.

Uric acid stones are relatively less common in adolescents than in adults and may be associated with hyperuricemia, hyperuricosuria, chronic excessive fluid losses, or unknown causes. Adolescents with inborn errors of purine metabolism, as well as those with increased purine turnover due to the treatment of myeloproliferative disorders, are at greatly increased risk of stone formation because of excess uric acid production and excretion.

Most patients with classic homozygous cystinuria, an autosomal recessive disorder, produce stones within the first 2 decades of life. Although the tubular defect in this disorder also leads to the excretion of excessive amounts of ornithine, arginine, and lysine, the low solubility of cystine in acidic urine is what causes stones to form.

Urolithiasis in the adolescent should be evaluated by urinalysis and urine culture and determination of levels of serum electrolytes, calcium, phosphorus, uric acid, and creatinine. IVP will delineate renal anatomy and identify radiopaque stones. A 24-hour urine collection for creatinine clearance and excretion of calcium (normal, <4 mg/kg/day), uric acid (normal, <700 mg/day), oxalate (normal, <40 mg/day), and cystine (normal, <100 mg/day) should be performed after treatment. If available, stones should be analyzed.

The treatment of urolithiasis has changed dramatically in the past decade. Many smaller stones (less than 1 cm) pass spontaneously in adolescents and may be allowed to do so if symptoms are not incapacitating and infection is not present.

Although medical management alone rarely dissolves stones, fluid intake should be increased to at least 3 L of fluid daily to dilute the concentration of substances contributing to stone formation in the urine. Thiazide diuretics, which enhance tubular reabsorption of calcium, can be used to treat idiopathic hypercalciuria. Allopurinol enhances tubular reabsorption of uric acid, and bicarbonate increases solubility of cystine. Struvite stones cannot be successfully treated without eradication of the underlying infection. However, removal of as many stones as possible, followed by irrigation of the renal pelvis with hemiacidin, can sometimes result in dissolution of stones.

When surgical treatment is necessary, most stones can be managed with extracorporeal shock-wave lithotripsy (ESWL) or newer endoscopic techniques. Open surgery to remove stones, once the mainstay of surgical treatment, is now rarely indicated.

GENITOURINARY TRAUMA

The kidneys of infants and younger children are more susceptible to trauma because of a more abdominal position and a paucity of surrounding fat. With physical maturation, the kidneys assume a more adult position, where they are better protected by the ribs. Nevertheless, renal trauma does occur in adolescents, often the result of contact sports or automobile or bicycle accidents. In many acute cases, the history is obvious and the presence of hematuria, a flank hematoma, or a palpable flank or abdominal mass will demand further urologic investigation. Two mechanisms, rapid deceleration and severe flexion, can cause severe urologic problems without significant symptoms. Thrombosis of the renal vessels or disruption of the urinary collecting system should be suspected following a history of these types of trauma.

Massive abdominal or flank injuries are not the most common causes of renal trauma. More typically, the adolescent has had one or two episodes of gross hematuria and a recent history of mild to moderate flank or abdominal trauma. These patients are best evaluated with renal and bladder ultrasonography. There is frequently an underlying anomaly, such as a dilated kidney or a tumor that is more prone to trauma and bleeding than a normal kidney. Renal contusions, accounting for 90% of cases of kidney trauma in adolescents as well as more severe renal injuries, can be diagnosed by ultrasonography in most cases.

Serious blunt renal injuries are best managed medically with hemodynamic stabilization and close observation. Surgery is reserved for the patient who cannot be stabilized. Bed rest is recommended for a few weeks or until resolution of the hematuria is noted. Subsequent follow-up of renal function and morphology or changes in blood pressure is required in all but the mildest episodes of trauma. Penetrating injuries of the flank or abdomen that possibly involve the kidney(s) demand surgical exploration for assessment of damage and salvage of the kidney(s), if possible.

Bladder and Urethral Injuries

Severe lower abdominal or pelvic injuries can result in significant trauma to the urethra, bladder, or both. Common signs and symptoms include blood at the urethral meatus, gross hematuria, pelvic instability, a perineal "butterfly" hematoma and, at times, difficulty voiding or urinary retention. A retrograde urethrogram is the initial study of choice when urethral or bladder trauma is suspected. Catheterization of the urethra should not be attempted until a retrograde urethrogram documents patency. Once the urethra is shown to be intact, a catheter can be safely positioned in the bladder and a cystogram obtained.

After some pelvic fractures, urethral disruption and subsequent stricture formation usually occur at the level of the membranous urethra. Here, the fixed urethra is sheared by the movements of the pelvis and its muscular diaphragm at the time of injury. Extravasation of urine can be appreciated on a retrograde study, and attempts at urethral catheterization should be deferred because the catheter may be directed into a false channel and further disrupt the urethra. Instead, suprapubic tube placement is recommended to provide urinary drainage during the acute phases of healing. Although some clinicians have described successful repairs with primary exploration and realignment, excellent results can also be obtained with secondary repair 3 to 6 months after the initial injury. This allows stabilization of the patient, minimizes extravasation of urine and contamination of the pelvic hematoma, and ultimately has less risk of impotence. Suprapubic drainage is usually easily managed by the adolescent until the urethral stricture matures and can be corrected.

Bladder ruptures occur in two forms, intraperitoneal and extraperitoneal, with their anatomic site usually appreciable on cystography. Extraperitoneal ruptures are the more common variety of bladder rupture (80%), and usually occur in association with pelvic fractures that disrupt the bladder wall. Antibiotics to cover likely pathogens and 10 to 14 days of Foley catheter drainage should provide effective treatment of most of these injuries. Intraperitoneal ruptures classically occur in the adolescent with a full bladder who has worn a seat belt during a car accident. This is particularly likely to occur to a driver under the influence of alcohol, because the alcohol causes both diminished and impaired judgment and reaction time. A "blow-out" of the bladder's dome through the overlying peritoneum occurs with sudden impact. Contrast-surrounded bowel loops will be noted on cystography. Urinary extravasation causes extreme peritoneal irritation, and signs of an acute abdomen may be evident on physical examination. Resorption of urine is also commonly reflected in elevations of blood urea nitrogen (BUN) levels. Surgical exploration and repair are indicated for intraperitoneal bladder ruptures.

BIBLIOGRAPHY

Allen TD: Dysfunctional voiding in pediatric urology. International Perspectives in Urology 4:228, 1987.

Heale WF, Weldone DP, Hewstone AS: Reflux nephropathy: Presentation of urinary infection in children. Med J Aust 1:1138, 1973.

Kaplan GW: Hematuria in children. American Urologic Update Series 4:4, 1985.

Kass EJ, Freitas JE, Bour JB: Adolescent varicocele: Objective indications for treatment. J Urol 142:579, 1989.

Keating MA, Duckett JW: Recent advances in the repair of hypospadias. Surg Annu 22:405, 1990.

Koff SA: Evaluation and management of voiding disorders in children. Urol Clin North Am 15:769, 1988.

Koff SA: Pathophysiology of ureteropelvic junction obstruction. Urol Clin North Am 17:203, 1990.

Kroovand RL: Update on outpatient pediatric urology. Dialogues in Pediatric Urology 5:8, 1982.

Kuzmarov IW, Morehouse DD, Gibson S: Blunt renal trauma in the pediatric population: A retrospective study. J Urol 126:648, 1981.

Livne PM, Gonzales ET: Genitourinary trauma in children. Urol Clin North Am 12:53, 1985.

Martin DC, Menck JR: The undescended testis: Management after puberty. J Urol 114:77, 1975.

Noe HN: Complications and management of childhood ureteral stricture disease. Urol Clin North Am 10:531, 1983.

Norgaard JP, Rettig S, Djurhuus JC: Nocturnal enuresis: An approach to treatment based on pathogenesis. J Pediatr 114:705, 1989.

Polinsky MS, Kaiser BA, Baluarte MJ: Urolithiasis in childhood. Pediatr Clin North Am 34:683, 1987.

Reichard SA, Helikson MA, Shorter N, et al: Pelvic fractures in children—review of 120 patients with a new look at general management. J Pediatr Surg 15:727, 1980.

Rink RC, Adams MC, Mitchell ME: Ureteral abnormalities. In Ashcraft KW (ed): Pediatric Urology. Philadelphia, W. B. Saunders Co., 1990, p 125–149.

Vardermark JS II: The acute scrotum: Management with the use of ancillary diagnostic techniques. American Urological Association Update Series. Vol 3. Lesson 17. American Urological Association, 1984.

CHAPTER 67

Hypertension

ALAN B. GRUSKIN and SHERMINE DARBAUGH

Hypertension in the adolescent occurs either as the result of a major life-threatening event such as encephalopathy, heart failure, or renal failure, in association with an underlying disease, or in isolation without other recognizable pathology. This chapter defines and categorizes hypertension. For a clinical classification of hypertension see Chapter 48.

FACTORS INFLUENCING BLOOD PRESSURE CHANGES IN ADOLESCENTS

Normally, blood pressure increases during adolescence in both sexes. Positive correlations have been reported between blood pressure and many variables: age, height, sex, cholesterol index (log HDL cholesterol/total cholesterol) in males, body mass index (log weight − 0.0008 × height), bone age, and sexual maturity scales. It is noteworthy that the blood pressure variability throughout childhood attributed to age or height is eliminated when blood pressures are corrected for the distance between the tops of both the heart and skull (vertex-corrected readings). As blood pressures increase within the normal range, significant positive correlations exist between left ventricular wall thickness, as measured by echocardiogram, and systolic (but not diastolic) blood pressure. Differences have been reported in blood pressures in adolescent populations from various regions within a given country, as well as from different countries. Sexual maturity, rather than chronologic age, should take precedence in determining normal values for an individual adolescent; early maturers experience earlier and larger increases in blood pressure than do late maturers.

Blood pressure levels result from the complex interaction of factors that raise and lower blood pressure when these factors are individually stimulated or inhibited. One or more factors may be involved in hypertensive disorders; often, compensatory factors operate to spontaneously lower blood pressure. An increasing body of data supports the theory that many of these factors are genetically controlled.

EVALUATION OF THE HYPERTENSIVE ADOLESCENT

Persistent hypertension or an acute significant increase in blood pressure require diagnostic evaluation (Table 67–1). Based on the information obtained, laboratory and imaging studies may be indicated. The most likely cause of adolescent hypertension diagnosed in primary care settings is essential (primary) hypertension with or without obesity (see Chapter 25).

In a study at the University of Michigan, a total of 300 adolescents were referred to a preventive cardiology clinic. Approximately 30% did not meet the criteria for hypertension. The remaining adolescents with persistent hypertension had the following diagnoses: (1) essential hypertension, 58% (76% of these adolescents were obese); (2) renal disease, 31% (see Chapter 65); (3) coarctation of the aorta, 6%; (4) endocrine disorders, 4%; and (5) miscellaneous causes, 1%.

In order to make a diagnosis of essential hypertension, blood pressure levels should be persistently elevated for a period of 4 to 8 weeks. Obviously, a diagnosis of essential hypertension, however, is made only after all types of secondary hypertension are excluded. Most forms of secondary hypertension are easy to eliminate by considering the adolescent's history, the findings on physical examination, and readily available laboratory studies: electrolytes, blood urea nitrogen (BUN), creatinine, urinalysis, urine culture, calcium, and phosphorus. Some physicians recommend that a determination of plasma renin activity be included with the initial laboratory studies. If either an abnormally high or low plasma renin activity is found, additional studies are indicated to eliminate secondary forms of hypertension before concluding that the patient has high or low renin essential hypertension. The higher the adolescent's blood pressure, the more important it is to search for secondary forms of hypertension. Renal-related causes of hypertension (including lesions of the renal artery) account for 80% to 90% of cases of secondary hypertension; the remaining cases involve a large number of disorders.

CLASSIFICATION OF HYPERTENSIVE DISORDERS

Secondary Hypertension

These conditions are not presented in order of incidence.

TABLE 67–1. Diagnostic Evaluation of the Hypertensive Adolescent

HISTORY

Symptoms suggestive of secondary forms of hypertension
  Adrenal disorders (cortex)
    Polyuria, constipation, virilization, abnormal genitalia, muscle weakness, ileus, amenorrhea
  Collagen vascular disease
    Rash, fever, arthritis, pain in abdomen and chest, CNS findings
  Hyperthyroidism
    Weight loss, nervousness, heat intolerance, tremors, increased appetite
  Pheochromocytoma
    Palpitations, sweating, headache, weight loss
  Renal disease
    Edema (periorbital upon awakening), polyuria, polydypsia, weight loss, inadequate growth, gross hematuria, urgency, frequency, flank pain, dysuria, enuresis, history of unexplained fevers or urinary tract infection
  Coarctation
    History of murmur
Dietary History:
  Salt craving, excessive intake of calories or sodium
Previous Hospitalization:
  Neonatal: umbilical artery catheters
  Surgical operations
  Trauma to genitourinary tract
Previous Health Care:
  Previous blood pressure measurements
  Growth data: height, weight
  Drugs prescribed
Drug History:
  Illicit drugs, tobacco usage, over-the-counter drugs, alcohol
Lifestyle:
  Stress, level of physical activity
Family History:
  Hypertension, diabetes mellitus, renal and endocrine disorders, premature myocardial infarction, stroke

PHYSICAL EXAMINATION

General Appearance:
  Well or ill, cachectic, obese, cushingoid
Vital Signs:
  Pulse rate (and its persistence over time): four extremities
  Blood Pressure: appropriate sized cuff, take pressures in all four extremities, supine, sitting, and standing pressures
Weight and Height:
  Plot to determine relationships: tall or small for age, obese for age or height
CNS:
  Mental status, gait, focal neurologic findings
Eyes:
  Retinopathy (atherosclerotic or hypertensive), proptosis, papilledema
Neck:
  Thyromegaly, carotid bruit
Lungs:
  Rales, increased work of breathing
Heart:
  Size, murmur, arrhythmia
Abdomen:
  Masses, bruits (particularly flank)
Genitalia:
  Appearance, sexual maturity rating
Joints:
  Arthritis, rachitic changes
Skin:
  Rashes, neurofibroma, café au lait spots, edema
Musculoskeletal:
  Weakness, unilateral limb enlargement

CNS, central nervous system.

BURN-RELATED HYPERTENSION

Trauma from burns probably causes hypertension, although this is disputed. Hypertension in burned patients may be due to anxiety or pain. Other causes of burn hypertension include vasopressor drugs or excessive intravascular expansion—during either initial expansion or mobilization of burn edema after reestablishment of a functional capillary endothelium.

CENTRAL NERVOUS SYSTEM HYPERTENSION

Central nervous system (CNS) disorders cause hypertension by increase in sympathetic outflow, by reflex stimulation of cardiac output, or possibly by stimulation of the renin-angiotensin system (Table 67–2). Treatment for CNS-related hypertension is directed toward the primary disorder. Patients with Guillain-Barré syndrome may continue to have hypertension for months after the neurologic signs disappear as the result of increased activity of the renin-angiotensin system or excessive circulating catecholamines. In adolescents suspected of having intracranial hypertension, controlled and sustained lowering of the blood pressure with nitroprusside is preferred.

COARCTATION HYPERTENSION

Coarctation hypertension is often not recognized until adolescence because of the failure to take blood pressures in all extremities or to document the presence of equal upper and lower extremity pulses. The mechanisms contributing to the hypertensive process include mechanical factors, central sympathetic activation, reset baroreceptors, renal sodium retention, and increased activity of the renin-angiotensin system. Both absolute and relative elevations in plasma renin activity may contribute to the hypertensive process.

Severe and life-threatening hypertension may occur in the immediate postsurgical period following correction of the coarctation. In adolescents who develop the postcoarctectomy syndrome, a predominantly systolic

TABLE 67–2. Nervous System Causes of Hypertension

Anxiety
Cerebrovascular accident
Embolus, hemorrhage, infarction
Collagen vascular disorders
Guillain-Barré syndrome
Dysautonomia (Riley-Day syndrome)
Increased intracranial pressure
Mass lesions, infection
Pain
Poliomyelitis
Trauma
Skull
Spinal cord

TABLE 67–3. Drugs, Toxins, and Heavy Metals Causing Hypertension

Alpha-methyldopa infusion
Amphetamines
Antiemetic infusions
Arfonad (trimethaphan) infusion
Beta blocker withdrawal
Caffeine?
Cigarette smoking?
Clonidine withdrawal
Cocaine
Corticosteroids
Cyclosporine
Guanabenz withdrawal
Imipramine
Lead
Mercury
Methotrexate
Methylphenidate
Minoxidil withdrawal
Oral contraceptives
Reserpine overdose
Spider bite
Sympathomimetic agents (nose drops, cold preparation)

blood pressure elevation occurs 12 to 24 hours after surgery, and a predominantly diastolic blood pressure elevation develops 2 to 4 days after surgery. In its severest form, it is associated with mesenteric arteritis characterized by abdominal pain, fever, leukocytosis, ileus, and, rarely, bowel infarction. These increases have been attributed to a combination of changes in the renin-angiotensin system, increased circulating catecholamines, increased sympathetic outflow, and sodium retention. If begun prior to and continued after surgery, treatment with propranolol may prevent postsurgical paradoxical hypertension. Other drugs used to treat postcoarctation hypertension include metoporol, hydralazine, trimethaphan, nitroprusside, and reserpine. After successful surgical repair, hypertension may occur after a period of years because of progressive restenosis (both anatomic and functional) at the site of surgical repair.

DRUG- AND TOXIN-RELATED HYPERTENSION

A number of drugs, toxins, and heavy metals are associated with hypertension (Table 67–3). Most drugs causing hypertension do so by increasing circulating catecholamines or by stimulating components of the sympathetic nervous system. Hypertension associated with the use of oral contraceptives, cyclosporine, and corticosteroids is discussed later.

HEAVY METAL EXPOSURE AND HYPERTENSION

A direct relationship between hypertension and blood lead levels has been reported in individuals aged 12 to 74 years of both sexes and in black and white patients. Lead levels are higher in black patients and in men than in women and white patients. Chelation studies show that tissue lead is increased in hypertensive individuals. Mechanisms include an increased activity of the renin-angiotensin system and α-adrenergic stimulation. Lowered intakes of calcium are found in adolescents with

higher blood lead levels. Hypertension also results from lead encephalopathy. Chronic mercury poisoning, acrodynia, may be associated with hypertension.

ENDOCRINE HYPERTENSION

Endocrine-mediated hypertension occurs as a manifestation of many endocrine disorders, most commonly with adrenal disease (Table 67–4). Although Cushing disease (see Chapter 55) is more often a result of pituitary rather than adrenal disease, exogenously administered corticosteroids are the most common cause of glucocorticoid-mediated hypertension. The elevated blood pressure and increased blood volume usually occur in the absence of hypokalemic alkalosis and hypernatremia in Cushing syndrome. Although the levels of urinary 17-hydroxycorticosteroids (17-OHCS) and 17-

TABLE 67–4. Causes of Endocrine-Mediated Hypertension

Adrenal gland
  Zona fasciculata syndrome
    Glucocorticoid excess (Cushing syndrome)
      Pituitary-mediated
      Adrenal hyperplasia
      Adrenal neoplasm
      Exogenous glucocorticoid administration
    11β-Hydroxysteroid dehydrogenase deficiency
      Glycyrrhizic acid excess (licorice ingestion)
      Apparent mineralocorticoid excess (Ullrich syndrome)
    Hyperdesoxycorticosteronism (desoxycorticostrerone [DOC] and 19-nor-DOC excess)
      11-Hydroxylase deficiency
      17-Hydroxylase deficiency (Biglieri syndrome)
      Primary DOC excess, adenoma
      Ectopic ACTH syndrome

Primary hyperaldosteronism
  Bilateral (?unilateral) adrenal glomerulosa hyperplasia
  Adrenocortical adenoma, carcinoma
  Glucocorticoid suppressible hyperaldosteronism (autosomal dominant)
  Pseudohyperaldosteronism

Medulla
  Pheochromocytoma
    Adrenal medulla (unilateral 90%, bilateral 5%)
    Extra-adrenal (5%)

Exogenous drug administration associated with catecholamine release
  Antihypertensive
    Alpha-methyldopa
    Reserpine
  Sympathomimetic amines
    Decongestants
    Bronchodilators
  Monoamine oxidase inhibitors (ingestion of high tyramine-containing foods)
Gordon syndrome
Oral contraceptive pills (estrogen-containing)
Hyperthyroidism
Hyperparathyroidism
Hyperpituitarism
  Acromegaly
Ovarian tumors
Neuroblastoma (catecholamine-producing tumors)
Hyperreninism
  Primary hyperreninism
    Juxtaglomerular cell hyperplasia, tumors
    Secondary forms of hyperreninism

ketosteroids are increased in patients with Cushing syndrome, the measurement of 17-ketosteroids is not routinely indicated unless the exogenous features of Cushing syndrome are present. Successful control of blood pressure can be achieved with spironolactone or a standard hypotensive regimen. The simultaneous measurement of peripheral plasma levels of renin and aldosterone in addition to a history and physical examination can be used to differentiate most forms of mineralocorticoid hypertension (Table 67–5).

In some forms of congenital adrenal hyperplasia (11-hydroxylase and 17-hydroxylase deficiency) (see Chapter 55), the defect in steroid synthesis is located at a site that causes excessive production of deoxycorticosterone and results in hypertension. Adrenocorticotropic hormone (ACTH) excess, which stimulates an increased secretion of dexycorticosterone, also causes hypertension. Appropriate treatment with cortisol lowers the blood pressure in patients with adrenal hyperplasia.

In patients with 11β-hydroxysteroid dehydrogenase deficiency, hypertension occurs in conjunction with hypokalemia and a markedly reduced urinary tetrahydrocortisone to tetrahydrocortisol ratio (<1). Spironolactone and triamterine are effective antihypertensive agents for these patients.

Primary hyperaldosteronism (see Chapter 55) is associated with spontaneous hypokalemia in 80% to 90% of patients; administering large amounts of sodium chloride for 4 to 5 days induces hypokalemia in most of the remaining patients. Diagnosis is dependent on the demonstration of inappropriately elevated urinary aldosterone metabolites or blood aldosterone levels in association with suppressed plasma renin activity. In patients with primary hyperaldosteronism, neither sodium chloride loading nor captopril administration lowers aldosterone levels. The differentiation of tumor from diffuse adrenal hyperplasia is critical because the therapy is different. Most adolescents with primary hyperaldostecronism have adrenal hyperplasia rather than adenoma. Most patients with hyperplasia have significantly increased plasma aldosterone levels after being upright for 4 hours; however, adolescents with adrenal adenomas do not experience an increased plasma aldosterone level. Computed tomography (CT), magnetic resonance imaging (MRI), adrenal venous aldosterone sampling, and adrenal iodoscintigraphy [[131]I 6B-iodomethyl-19-norcholesterol (NP-59)] are used to localize adenomas. In patients with hyperplasia, amiloride or spironolactone is usually effective in restoring potassium balance; however, not all patients respond with normalization of their blood pressures. Enalapril maleate has been reported to control both potassium balance and blood pressure.

Glucocorticoid-suppressible hyperaldosteronism is characterized by the hypersecretion of 18-hydroxycortisol and 18-oxocortisol. It is diagnosed either by demonstrating excess quantities of these hormones or by a normalization of the blood pressure after administering small quantities of glucocorticoids to patients with the biochemical features of primary aldosteronism.

Pseudohyperaldosteronism type II (Liddle syndrome) is characterized by hypertension, hypokalemia, and low levels of aldosterone. Thiazide diuretics effectively lower blood pressure in these patients.

Pheochromocytomas, tumors of chromaffin cells that are derived from neural crest cells, are generally unilateral, benign, and localized to the adrenal gland. Tumors can develop anywhere along the sympathetic ganglionic chain. Most pheochromocytomas arising from extra adrenal chromaffin tissue are malignant; these tumors may also be multicentric. Most adolescents have persistent hypertension; relatively few patients experience paroxysmal hypertension with interspersed normal levels of blood pressure. Confirmation of the diagnosis is made by finding either elevated plasma levels of epinephrine or norepinephrine or increased urinary excretion of their metabolites (most often urinary metanephrine) (Table 67–6). Increased plasma renin activity is seen in most patients with pheochromocytoma (see Chapter 55).

The manifestations of hyperkalemic hypertension with normal glomerular filtration rate (Gordon syndrome) also include hyperchlermic acidosis, hyporeninemia, and hypoaldosteronism. Deficiencies in the natriuretic hormone(s) or prostaglandins cause increased sodium reabsorption in the distal tubule, and volume expansion hypertension occurs. Affected patients respond to loop diuretics.

Estrogen-containing oral contraceptives are associated with hypertension due to increased sodium retention and activity of the renin-angiotensin system. As the quantity of estrogen contained in oral contraceptives has been decreased, the incidence of contraceptive-associated hypertension has also decreased (see Chapter 73). In adolescent females, specific blood pressure data on the relationship between oral contraceptive use and blood pressure are not yet available. Increases in systolic and diastolic blood pressures of 14 mmHg and 8 mmHg, respectively, have been reported over the first 5 years of oral contraceptive use.

Pregnancy and preeclampsia should be considered as a cause of hypertension in all fertile females (see later).

Hypertension, characteristically systolic, occurs in approximately 30% of patients with hyperthyroidism (see Chapter 55). The hypertension associated with hyperparathyroidism is often associated with high plasma renin levels and is not believed to be secondary to hypercalcemia-induced renal disease. The degree to which blood pressures fall ifter parathyroidectomy in patients with primary hyperparathyroidism is still unresolved.

TABLE 67–5. Plasma Renin-Aldosterone Profile in Secondary Forms of Hypertension

DISORDER	PLASMA RENIN ACTIVITY	PLASMA ALDOSTERONE
Renal artery stenosis	High	High
Hyperaldosteronism	Low	High
11-Hydroxylase deficiency	Low	Low
11β-Hydroxysteroid dehydrogenase deficiency	Low	Low
21-Hydroxylase deficiency	High	Low
Overtreatment	High	High

TABLE 67–6. Normal Range of Values for Urinary and Plasma Catecholamines

Urine	
Epinephrine	0–35 µg/24 h
Norepinephrine	<550 µg/24 h
Metanephrine	<1.3 mg/24 h
Vanillylmandelic acid	2–7 mg/24 h
Plasma	
Epinephrine	10–55 pg/ml
Norepinephrine	60–400 pg/ml
Dopamine	<100 pg/ml

With permission from Melby J: Clinical review I: Endocrine hypertension. J Clin Endocrinol Metab 69:697–703, 1989. © by The Endocrine Society.

Primary reninism is caused by renin-secreting tumors, benign or malignant, which may be either intrarenal or extrarenal. Most cases of primary reninism occur before 23 years of age. Affected patients consistently experience hypokalemia and have very high levels of plasma renin activity. Localization is accomplished by selective renal angiography or CT scanning. Renin secretion may be either autonomous or responsive to maneuvers that stimulate the renin-angiotensin system. Ectopic renin-secreting tumors, including Wilms tumor, have been reported.

Licorice contains glycyrrhizic acid, which is converted in the liver to a mineralocorticoid-like substance. Therefore, when eaten in excessive quantities, licorice can cause hypertension. The treatment is simply discontinuation of licorice ingestion.

FRACTURE-RELATED HYPERTENSION

Hypertension, which is usually both systolic and diastolic, often develops after adolescents sustain fractures. It has been reported that 12% of casted children and 54% of children placed in traction develop hypertension. Etiologic mechanisms include pain, anxiety, reflex sympathetic nervous system discharge secondary to stretching of nerves, and changes in calcium metabolism associated with immobilization. Although blood pressure elevations are usually mild, elevations to levels leading to hypertensive encephalopathy may occur. When pain medication, sedation, or reductions in traction fail to lower the blood pressure to acceptable levels, antihypertensive medications should be considered.

PREGNANCY- AND POSTPARTUM-RELATED HYPERTENSION

During pregnancy, blood pressure levels fall slightly during the first and second trimesters. During the third trimester, they usually revert to pre-pregnancy levels. Risk factors associated with pregnancy-induced hypertension include primagravida, multiple gestations, family or previous history of preeclampsia/eclampsia, diabetes mellitus, preexisting hypertensive disorders, fetal hydrops, and hydatidiform mole. Preeclampsia is characterized as follows: "new onset" hypertension during the third trimester (blood pressure exceeding 140/90 mmHg when measured twice at least 6 hours apart), "new onset" proteinuria during the third trimester, "new onset" generalized edema during the third trimester,

and a blood pressure increase of 30 mmHg systolic or 15 mmHg diastolic. Preeclampsia usually resolves within 1 to 2 months after delivery and is not indicative of the later development of chronic hypertension. In one study, 12% of patients with severe preeclampsia had renal artery stenosis. Antihypertensive medications are indicated when the diastolic blood pressure exceeds 110 mmHg. Termination of the pregnancy may need to be considered if the adolescent's condition remains severe or worsens severely.

When antihypertensive medications are required during the period of breast feeding, diuretics are best avoided because they reduce milk production. Propranolol, which has the lowest drug concentration ratio of milk to plasma, has not been associated with any adverse effects in suckling newborns. Captopril also has a low milk to plasma ratio. There are insufficient data to make recommendations on the use of calcium channel blockers, vasodilators, and other adrenergic inhibitors in breast-feeding mothers.

HYPERTENSION ASSOCIATED WITH ORGAN TRANSPLANTATION

Hypertension occurs following renal, cardiac, liver, and bone marrow transplantation. Cyclosporine is the major cause of hypertension in patients undergoing cardiac or bone marrow transplantation. The mechanism is renal vasoconstriction and sodium and water retention.

Hypertension that develops in approximately 60% to 80% of patients after cadaveric renal transplantation may be associated with a number of problems and may be the initial finding of transplant rejection (see Table 67–7).

More than 80% of children and adolescents undergoing orthotopic liver transplantation develop hypertension during the perioperative period. Hypertension in liver transplant patients has been attributed to the use of corticosteroids and cyclosporine, and in some patients it has been attributed to an increased plasma renin activity. In combination, these drugs impair the ability of the kidney to adequately respond to the salt and water loading that occurs during surgery. Calcium channel blockers are the most widely used antihypertensive agents to treat this form of hypertension.

METABOLIC DISORDERS CAUSING HYPERTENSION

Diabetes mellitus may result in hypertension secondary to renal disease. Hypercalcemia causes renal impairment and nephrocalcinosis. The mechanism of hypertension in acute intermittent porphyria is unknown.

RENAL-MEDIATED HYPERTENSION

The principal mechanisms causing renal-mediated hypertension are intravascular volume expansion, increased activity of the renin angiotensin system, or both. The increase in extracellular volume either is a result of excessive intake of salt and water when there is a decreasing or low glomerular filtration rate, or is due to an increased reabsorption of filtered sodium. The activity of the renin angiotensin system may be increased absolutely or relatively. The majority of adolescents with acute hypertensive emergencies have renal-mediated forms of hypertension (Table 67–7).

In addition to a history and physical examination, evaluation of patients suspected of having primary renal-mediated hypertension should include urinalysis, blood levels of creatinine and BUN, serum electrolytes, measurements of peripheral plasma renin activity (PRA) and plasma aldosterone, and one or more imaging studies. A voiding cystourethrogram is used to diagnose lower urinary tract obstructive disorders and vesicoureteral

TABLE 67–7. Causes of Renal-Mediated Hypertension

Acute renal failure
    Acute tubular necrosis
    Rapidly progressive glomerulonephritis
Amyloidosis
Chronic renal insufficiency
Cystic disorders
Diabetic nephropathy
Glomerulopathies
    Postinfectious glomerulonephritis (subacute bacterial endocarditis)
    Nephrotic syndrome
    Henoch-Schönlein purpura
    Membranoproliferative glomerulonephritis
Infarction
    Sickle cell, emboli, corticomedullary necrosis
Infection
    Acute and chronic pyelonephritis
Nephrocalcinosis
Nephrolithiasis
Neurofibromatosis
Obstructive uropathy
Postrenal transplantation hypertension
    Acute rejection
    Antirejection therapy
        Corticosteroid
        Cyclosporine
    Acute tubular necrosis
    Chronic rejection
    Intraoperative volume overload
    Lymphocele
    Obstructive uropathy
    Renal artery stenosis
    Recurrence of original disease
Reflux nephropathy
Renal vascular disorders
    Atherosclerosis (inborn errors of lipid metabolism)
    Arteritis
    Congenital renal artery stenosis
    Extrinsic compression
    Fibromuscular dysplasis
    Neurofibromatosis
    Radiation nephritis
    Renal artery aneurysm
    Renal artery fistula
    Thromboembolism (subacute bacterial endocarditis, indwelling arterial catheters)
    Williams syndrome
Systemic collagen vascular disorders
    Systemic lupus erythematosus, periarteritis, Wegener granulomatosis, hemolytic uremic syndrome, scleroderma
Traumatic injury
    Renal artery, parenchymal, perirenal hemorrhage
Tumors
    Wilms, carcinoma, hamartoma, tuberous sclerosis

reflux. Ultrasonography is used to evaluate renal size, to distinguish between solid and cystic masses, to identify large renal scars, and to establish the presence of obstruction. The finding of proteinuria, deformed red cells, or casts suggests a renal parenchymal disorder.

Most adolescents with renal artery stenosis have unilateral disease. Screening tests for renal artery lesions include measurements of peripheral PRA; the 4-hour upright sample may be the best screening test for evaluating PRA in ambulatory adolescents. Of the various radionuclide scans available for diagnosing for renal artery lesions, ^{99m}Tc-DMSA may be the most useful because it also detects regions of scarring and localized ischemia, in addition to evaluating differential renal function. The ^{99m}Tc-DTPA scan can diagnose unilateral main renal artery disease, but it does not detect bilateral or intrarenal disease. If an adolescent with unilateral stenosis is given captopril, perfusion to the affected kidney measured with a ^{99m}Tc-DTPA scan decreases. In adolescents with unilateral renal artery stenosis, the administration of captopril in a dose of 0.7 mg/kg should lower systolic and diastolic blood pressures by 10% and 15%, respectively. However, the value of the captopril stimulation test to measure PRA has been questioned in younger patients. Renal scans with ^{131}I or ^{123}I orthoiodohippurate have been proposed as the best methods to evaluate renal vascular hypertension and renal parenchymal disease.

Renal venous measurements of PRA in combination with digital subtraction (using injections of contrast) or intra-arterial angiography are required to identify adolescents whose renal artery stenoses are surgically correctable. In order to completely visualize the renal arterial system, oblique as well as anterior and posterior radiographs are needed. Blood samples for measuring PRA should be obtained from the inferior vena cava (IVC) above and below the renal veins, from both main renal veins and, if possible, from both upper and lower poles because the arterial lesion may be segmental rather than a main renal artery lesion. The renal vein renin ratio for each kidney is calculated (renal vein PRA minus IVC PRA divided by IVC PRA) and the ratios from the two sides compared. A ratio of less than 1.0 from the contralateral kidney (indicative of renin suppression) and greater than 0.5 from the affected kidney generally predicts a surgical cure. However, if the sum of the ratios from both kidneys exceeds 0.5, either a segmental lesion or improper sampling should be considered. Of note, is the observation that some adolescents with renal artery stenosis have abnormal cerebral angiograms.

Benign and malignant tumors usually cause hypertension by compressing renal vessels. Also, some tumors produce renin. The primary therapy for these tumors is surgical excision. Prior to surgery, renal ablation techniques are used in some cases to selectively infarct regions of the kidney.

Approximately 10% of children and adolescents with renal scars develop hypertension. Affected adolescents have an elevated peripheral PRA and an abnormal DMSA scan. The excretory urogram is also capable of defining renal scars and of differentiating pyelonephritis from other disorders. Treatment options for hypertension caused by unilateral renal disease include partial and total nephrectomy and reconstructive vascular surgery, including *ex vivo* repair, autotransplantation, percutaneous transluminal angioplasty, and drug therapy.

The hypertension associated with acute and chronic glomerulonephritis is primarily due to volume overload; an increased PRA often plays a contributory role. Diuretics are the first class of drugs to consider in treating this group of adolescents; however, other types of antihypertensive drugs are often required. In patients with advanced renal failure, hemodialysis, peritoneal dialysis, or various modifications of continuous arteriovenous hemofiltration (CAVH) are usually needed in order to treat the volume overload component of renal-mediated hypertension.

Volume expansion is the principal mediating factor that causes hypertension in most adolescents with end-stage renal disease. Because excessive activity of the renin angiotensin system often occurs concomitantly, volume depleting maneuvers may aggravate hypertension by further stimulating this system. The current availability of many potent antihypertensive drugs permits effective control of blood pressure in most patients who have end-stage renal disease. For most adolescents, bilateral nephrectomy is not required. However, after bilateral nephrectomy, blood pressure control does improve in some patients with end-stage renal disease, particularly after renal transplantation.

SLEEP APNEA–ASSOCIATED HYPERTENSION

Adolescents who have obstructive pulmonary disease associated with sleep apnea have been reported to have systolic and diastolic hypertension, as well as left ventricular hypertrophy. Etiologic significance has been attributed to reflex adrenergic outflow and to peripheral chemoreceptor-mediated peripheral arteriolar constriction. For adolescents who have obesity-related sleep apnea, weight loss is essential; in those with surgically remedial lesions such as large tonsils and adenoids, corrective surgery is necessary.

VOLUME EXPANSION HYPERTENSION

Volume expansion hypertension is most likely to develop in adolescents who have conditions such as renal failure or who are already volume expanded for other reasons. Transient elevation of blood pressure may follow the rapid or excessive administration of albumin, blood, electrolyte solutions, or plasma. Also, hypernatremia and hyperglycemia may cause intravascular volume expansion and hypertension.

ISOLATED OR PREDOMINANT SYSTOLIC HYPERTENSION

Primary hypertension or hyperthyroidism may present as isolated systolic hypertension. Other disorders causing isolated systolic hypertension include anemia, arteriovenous (AV) fistula (congenital and after placement of AV shunts for hemodialysis), and various cardiac disorders (heart block, constrictive pericarditis, patent ductus arteriosus, and aortic insufficiency).

Primary (Essential) Hypertension

Essential hypertension, with a reported prevalence of 0.5% to 2%, is the most common cause of hypertension in adolescents (see Chapter 48). Most adolescents who have essential hypertension have mild or moderate blood pressure elevations and are asymptomatic; symptomatic or severe hypertension is rarely observed during adolescence. The diagnosis of essential hypertension is important because prolonged, untreated hypertension leads to many complications and an acceleration of the atherosclerotic process.

PREDICTIVE VALUES FOR ADOLESCENT HYPERTENSION FROM TRACKING STUDIES BEGUN PRIOR TO ADOLESCENCE

Of 10,446 children aged 10 to 16 years (7745 whites and 2701 blacks), significant systolic and diastolic hypertension was found in 2.1% and 4.5%, respectively. Of the 2808 adolescents restudied within 3 weeks because their blood pressures exceeded the 70th percentile, significant systolic and diastolic blood pressure persisted in only 0.47% and 0.80%. These data support the conclusion that the prevalence of significant persistant hypertension is low in younger adolescents. An increasing incidence of high blood pressure occurs as adolescents progress through high school and become young adults.

TRACKING OF BLOOD PRESSURE INTO ADULTHOOD FROM CHILDHOOD

Between adolescence and young adulthood, longitudinally obtained blood pressures are not significantly different among American blacks, Mexican Americans, and whites. The higher the systolic blood pressure, diastolic blood pressure, and Quetelet index (100 × weight/height^2) during childhood, the greater the risk for persistence into adulthood. The correlations are more significant for males than for females. For systolic and diastolic blood pressures, correlation coefficients between childhood/adolescence (age 7 to 18 years) and young adulthood (age 20 to 30 years) range from 0.21 to 0.39 and −0.01 to 0.50, respectively (Fig. 67–1). Correlations between blood pressure in adolescents (age 10 years until high school graduation) with those 15 to 17 years later range from 0.25 to 0.51 and 0.19 and 0.45 for systolic and diastolic pressure, respectively. Follow-up of patients who as children had at least one blood pressure measurement that exceeded the 90th percentile revealed that 45% and 40% had high systolic and diastolic blood pressures during young adulthood, respectively. In the children whose systolic and diastolic blood pressure exceeded the 90th percentile at least once, elevations in systolic and diastolic blood pressures were found in 24% and 17%, respectively, after they reached adulthood. These values exceed those expected in adults by 2.4 and 1.7 times normal, respectively.

In a longitudinal study begun in 1960, the prevalence of hypertension (defined as three diastolic pressures exceeding 90 mmHg) was 3.0% and 20.6% for individ-

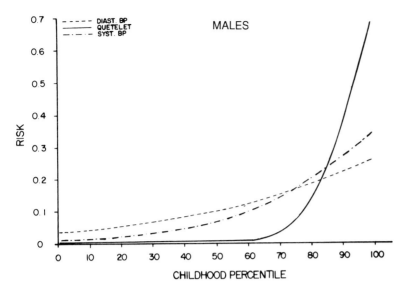

MALES

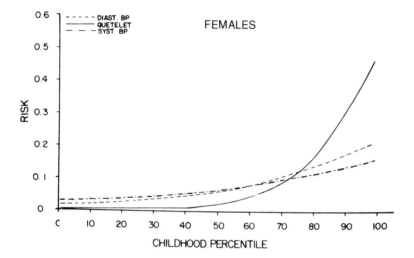

FEMALES

Figure 67–1. Logistic regression curves displaying the probability in 20- to 30-year-old males (top) and females (bottom) for adult systolic and diastolic blood pressures and Quetelet index. A risk of 0.3 indicates that a person, if tracked from adolescence through his or her 20s, has a 3 in 10 chance of having an adult value equal to or greater than the 90th percentile. (With permission from Lauer RM, Clarke WR: Childhood risk factors for high adult blood pressure: The Muscatine Study. Pediatrics 84:633, 1989.)

uals aged 15 to 19 years and 20 to 24 years, respectively. By the time these individuals reached their third and fourth decades, there was an incidence of hypertension in the original 15- to 19-year-old and 20- to 24-year-old groups of 26% and 12%, respectively. Only a small percentage of the original hypertensive group had normal blood pressures. During the first 10 years of follow-up, no treatment was given; after 8 years, a significant number of the patients had already experienced hypertensive-related events. Furthermore, after 16 years, a higher incidence of electrocardiogram (ECG) abnormalities were noted in those patients who were hypertensive at the beginning of the study.

Three conclusions can be drawn from the available blood pressure tracking studies. First, labile hypertension is a common occurrence in prepubertal children and adolescents. Second, there is a significant increase in hypertension toward the end of adolescence. Third, there is a progressive rise in the incidence of "new onset" hypertension throughout young adulthood. Although correlations between adolescent and adult hypertension are reasonably high, not all adolescents with high blood pressure develop chronic hypertension. If an adolescent's systolic blood pressure is repeatedly taken throughout childhood and found to be elevated once,

the risk for that child developing hypertension is twice that of the general population. Multiple, but not single, elevations of diastolic blood pressure are associated with an increased risk for developing adult hypertension. The Quetelet index during childhood positively correlates with young adult blood pressures.

PATHOPHYSIOLOGY

Persistent essential hypertension is thought to evolve through a stage of labile hypertension, which is followed by fixed hypertension. In the initial phase, cardiac output is elevated secondary to an increased pulse rate; also, vascular resistance is within normal limits, although elevated for the degree of increase in cardiac output. The increase in cardiac output is not always found in hypertensive adolescents. The renin-angiotensin system is stimulated and renal vascular resistance is normal. As the disease progresses with age and as the blood pressure becomes fixed, the aforementioned α-adrenergic effects become blunted, the peripheral and renal vascular resistance increases, and PRA falls. It is difficult to distinguish between those factors that might cause essential hypertension and those factors that are secondary to the hypertensive process.

Obesity contributes significantly to the hypertensive process (see Chapter 60). Obese people are more likely to be hypertensive than are lean individuals; also, hypertensives are more likely to become obese than are normotensives. Suggested mechanisms include increased intake of sodium and saturated fats, increased levels of insulin and aldosterone (both of which affect the renal tubular absorption of sodium), altered sex hormone metabolism, increased blood volume, increased activity of the sympathetic nervous system, increased cardiac output, and decreased activity (see Chapter 49).

Calcium transport into cells and intracellular levels of calcium are important modulators of vasoconstriction. Such changes may influence the early phase of primary hypertension. Raised plasma intact parathyroid hormone concentrations, elevated total serum calcium, raised ionized plasma calcium levels and increased serum phosphate levels have been reported in hypertensive adolescents and adults. Also, a reduced dietary intake of calcium may result in hypertension.

Sodium intake clearly plays a role in increasing blood pressure in adolescents when their average sodium intake exceeds the recommended dietary intake by a factor of 6 to 12 (see Chapter 7). The movement of populations from environments of low salt intake to that of a high salt intake is associated with an increased incidence of hypertension. When adolescent offspring of hypertensive parents are subjected to mental stress or a combination of mental stress and 14 days of "salt loading," they experience greater increases in their blood pressure than do adolescent offspring of normotensive parents. Moreover, salt sensitivity is age dependent. After sodium chloride loading, blood pressure increases are lower in those patients who are 10 to 30 years old when these patients are compared to older individuals. Also, a low potassium intake may be of etiologic significance.

Alterations of renal function in adolescents with essential hypertension include decreases in effective renal plasma flow, alterations in intrarenal blood flow patterns, and increases in filtration fraction. The net impact of these disturbances is sodium retention. In order to maintain sodium balance at a level where edema, heart failure, and other complications do not occur, excessive rates of sodium excretion (pressure natriuresis) occur in hypertensive patients. Hyperuricemia, elevated catecholamine levels, decreased kallikrein levels, and prostaglandin activity are also observed in patients with essential hypertension.

Low, normal, or high levels of PRA are found in hypertensive adolescents with primary hypertension. Before concluding that an adolescent with an abnormal PRA has essential hypertension, secondary forms of hypertension associated with an abnormal PRA should be excluded.

Myocardial hypertrophy and decreased cardiac function (measured by echocardiogram or exercise testing) are present in 60% to 80% of hypertensive adolescents at the time of diagnosis. Occasionally, abnormal ECG changes are noted; however, chest radiographs are usually normal. It may be that myocardial hypertrophy develops in response to excessive sympathetic activity prior to the onset of clinical hypertension.

Support for both genetic transmission and environ-mental influences are provided by blood pressure studies of identical and nonidentical twins living together or separately. There are family studies that have shown a progressive increase in the incidence of hypertension when the offspring of nonhypertensive parents are compared with the offspring of one and two hypertensive parents.

TREATMENT STRATEGIES FOR ADOLESCENT ESSENTIAL HYPERTENSION

Treatment strategies for hypertensive adolescents should initially focus on nonpharmacologic therapies (see Chapter 48). In order to lower blood pressure and reduce the long-term risks of hypertension, the physician should consider modifying the following factors: obesity, alcohol intake, hyperglycemia, inactivity, excessive sodium intake, cigarette smoking, and an atherosclerotic diet. Modification of these factors has been shown to independently lower blood pressure or reduce the degree of atherosclerosis. Presumably, their impact is additive when two or more factors are changed. The use of exercise as an antihypertensive therapy must be sustained if it is to be effective. In addition to permitting the adolescent to remain in control of his or her life, convincing the family to participate in nonpharmacologic treatment plans is more likely to produce a sustained benefit. It has been reported in a prospective controlled clinical trial involving adults that a 5-year program combining weight reduction, decreased alcohol intake, and decreased salt intake results in a reduced incidence of hypertension (8.8% versus 19.2% in treated and untreated patients, respectively). An alcohol intake of less than 1 to 2 oz hard liquor per day is recommended for hypertensive adults.

When nonpharmacologic therapy fails, a trial of pharmacologic therapy should be prescribed for hypertensive adolescents. The therapeutic goal should be a normalization of blood pressure. Once blood pressure normalizes for 6 to 12 months, drug therapy may be reduced or discontinued and the response recorded. For those adolescents whose blood pressure immediately rises, antihypertensive drug therapy should be resumed. For those adolescents whose blood pressure remains normal, prolonged follow-up is required because the risk for redevelopment of hypertension is always present. Because many hypertensive adolescents have ventricular hypertrophy, it has been suggested that another goal of therapy ought to be normalization of ventricular size.

It is unfortunate that there have been inadequate clinical trials in adolescents of many of the antihypertensive drugs currently used to treat primary hypertension. There are no long-term studies; however, short-term studies of the use of thiazide diuretics and β-blockers in adolescents report problems similar to those experienced by adults. In hypertensive adults, diuretics and calcium channel blocking agents have been reported to be more efficacious than other classes of drugs in treating black adolescents and adolescents with low renin hypertension. β-Blockers and angiotensin converting enzyme (ACE) inhibitors have been reported to be more efficacious than other classes of drugs in treating whites and patients with high-renin hypertension. The major impact of a sustained lowering of blood pressure in adults has been a reduction in the incidence of stroke. The failure to observe significant differences in the prevention of cardiac events may be due to drug-related effects, which increase lipid levels and alter carbohydrate metabolism. Thus, the use of drugs that are not associated with increased lipogenesis may be advantageous when considering long-term therapy.

TREATMENT OF HYPERTENSION

Nonpharmacologic Therapies for Lowering Blood Pressure

The three components of nonantihypertensive drug therapy for adolescent hypertension are specific treatment for secondary forms of hypertension, recommendations that may lower blood pressure without the use of drugs, and treatment plans that will assist in the prevention of the long-term sequelae associated with hypertension.

SODIUM REDUCTION

Experimental data suggest that the onset of hypertension may either be prevented or retarded in some patients by reducing sodium intake. Approximately 25% of the hypertensive population is salt sensitive. Blood pressure control is clearly improved by sodium restriction in disorders in which salt and water retention contribute to the pathogenesis of hypertension. Blood pressure control appears to be improved in patients with primary hypertension when the dietary intake of potassium or calcium is increased.

WEIGHT REDUCTION

When compared to blood pressures of non-obese, normotensive adolescents, the blood pressures of obese adolescents decrease and increase with decreases and increases in sodium intake, respectively. These changes, which are independent of changes in weight, may be related to changes in the metabolism of insulin, aldosterone, and norepinephrine. Although mild sodium restriction (70 mmol/day) was effective in lowering blood pressure, the sensitivity of blood pressure to changes in sodium intake disappeared when weight loss occurred. In the absence of changes of sodium intake, isolated weight loss also results in a lowering of blood pressure. Although blood pressure often falls to normal before adolescents achieve their ideal weight, a 5% weight loss may lead to a significant and persistent decrease in blood pressure. When obese adults lost 50% of their excess weight, normalization of blood pressure occurred in two thirds of the group. In many obese hypertensive patients, the blood pressure remains normal as long as their weight loss is maintained.

EXERCISE TRAINING

Exercise training programs for adolescents with primary hypertension can lower blood pressure independently of any changes in body weight or skinfold thickness (see Chapters 45 and 48). Systolic and diastolic blood pressures usually decrease after a few weeks of aerobic training. The beneficial impact of exercise on blood pressure usually does not persist when the exercise program is stopped for a few weeks.

Pharmacologic Therapy to Lower Blood Pressure

Pharmacologic therapy is prescribed in order to prevent hypertension-mediated complications and to allow time for diagnosing and treating the underlying disorder. Antihypertensive drugs are indicated in the absence of other forms of effective therapy that control blood pressure chronically. Three groups of drugs are used to treat hypertensive adolescents. The first two groups include diuretics and primary antihypertensive agents. The third group includes those drugs used to treat the multiple disorders that cause hypertension, and will not be considered here. The management of acute hypertensive emergencies and chronic sustained hypertension is discussed below. The prescribed dose should not exceed that which is recommended for adults.

MANAGEMENT OF ACUTE HYPERTENSIVE EMERGENCIES IN ADOLESCENT PATIENTS

The goal of treating acute hypertensive emergencies is to lower blood pressure to levels that preserve blood flow to vital organs and to minimize hypertensive-related complications. The drugs commonly used to treat hypertensive emergencies in adolescents are summarized in Table 67–8. It is recommended that blood pressure be reduced by one third of the total reduction desired in the first 6 hours. The remaining reduction can be

TABLE 67–8. Antihypertensive Agents Commonly Used to Treat Hypertensive Emergencies in Adolescents

DRUG	DOSE	COMMENT
Diazoxide	3–5 mg/kg IV	Can be given as bolus, repeated doses, or as continuous infusion; hypotension, hyperglycemia
Furosemide	1–6 mg/kg IV (at a rate of 4 mg/min IV)	Loop diuretic; use if volume overloaded; ototoxicity
Hydralazine	0.1–0.5 mg/kg IV or IM	Tachycardia, tachyphylaxis
Labetalol	1–3 mg/kg/hr IV	Combined α- and β-blockade
Nifedipine	0.25–0.50 mg/kg sublingually	Calcium channel blocker
Phentolamine	0.1–0.2 mg/kg IV	α-Blockade used to treat pheochromocytoma
Sodium nitroprusside	0.5–8.0 μg/kg/min IV	Metabolic acidosis, orthostatic hypotension, thiocyanate toxicity (>12 mg/dl)

TABLE 67–9. Representative Oral Antihypertensive Drugs*

CLASS AND AGENT	DOSE RELATED TO BODY WEIGHT (INITIAL AND MAXIMUM RECOMMENDED) (mg/kg)	FIXED ADULT DOSE (INITIAL AND MAXIMUM) (mg/day)	TIME BETWEEN DOSES (hours)	TIME TO CHANGE DOSE (days)	SIZE OF TABLET (mg)
α-Adrenergic blocking agents					
Prazosin (Minipress)	30–250 μg/kg (give first dose hs)	1–20	8–12	3	1, 2, 5
Phenoxybenzamine (Dibenzyline)	1–5	20–120	12	2	10
β-Adrenergic blocking agents					
Atenolol (Tenormin) (β$_1$ cardiac blocker)	0.5–2	50–100	24	7	50
Labetalol (Normodyne)	3–10	200–2400	8–12	2–3	200, 300
Metoprolol (β$_1$ cardiac blocker)	1–5	100–450	12–24	7	50, 100
Propranolol (Inderal)	0.5–2	40–320	8–12	3–7	10, 20, 40, 60, 80
Calcium channel blocker					
Nifedipine (Procardia)	0.5–2	30–180	6–8	1	10, 20
Verapamil (Calan)	0.1–0.3	120–480	8	2–3	40, 80
Centrally acting α$_2$-adrenergic agonists					
Alpha-methyldopa (Aldomet)†	1–30	1000–2000	6–12	3–7	125, 250
Clonidine (Catapres)	4–40 μg/kg/day	0.2–2.4	12	3–7	0.1, 0.2, 0.3
Catapres TTS (transdermal patch)					0.1, 0.2, 0.3
Converting enzyme inhibitors					
Captopril (Capoten)†	0.1–6	50–450	8–24	1–3	12.5, 25, 50, 100
Enalapril (Vasotec)†	Unavailable	5–40	12–24	1–3	2.5, 5, 10, 20
Diuretics					
Loop					
Furosemide (Lasix)	1–6	20–320	6–24	0.5	20, 40, 80
Thiazides					
Chlorothiazide (Diuril)	10–20	500–2000	12–24	7–14	250, 500
Potassium-sparing					
Spironolactone (Aldactone)	1–2	50–200	12–24	14	25, 50, 100
Triamterene (Dyrenium)	2–4	200–300	12	7–14	50, 100
Peripheral adrenergic blocking agents					
Reserpine (Serpasil)	0.02–0.07	0.1–0.25	24	14	0.1, 0.25
Guanethidine (Ismelin)†	0.2–1	10–300	24	5–7	10, 25
Vasodilators					
Hydralazine (Apresoline)	0.5–4	40–300	4–8	1–7	10, 25, 50, 100
Minoxidil (Loniten)	0.1–1.5	5–100	8–24	0.25–3	2.5, 10

*Additional agents are available in many classes.

†Increase dose interval by 50% to 100% if renal function is low.

Compiled from The Medical Letter 31:25–30, 1989; Hoffman JIE, Stanger P: Systemic arterial hypertension. In Rudolph AM, Hoffman JIE (eds): Pediatrics, 18th ed. East Norwalk, CT, Appleton & Lange, 1987; Ingelfinger JR: Pediatric Hypertension, Philadelphia, WB Saunders, 1982; and Physicians' Desk Reference, 45th ed. Oradell, NJ, Medical Economics Company, 1991.

achieved during the subsequent 30 to 72 hours. Nitroprusside is recommended for patients who have sustained a significant central nervous system insult, because its use permits ongoing control of fluctuating blood pressures. Otherwise, one of the other drugs listed in Table 67–8 can be prescribed. Because it works quickly and rarely causes problems, sublingual (preferred) or orally administered nifedipine has recently become popular. If an intravenous agent is desired, labetalol is recommended by some clinicians as a preferred antihypertensive drug for the following reasons: it causes both α- and β-adrenergic blockade; it does not cause tachyphylaxis (as does hydralazine); it does not cause severe hypotension (as does diazoxide); and because subsequent antihypertensive therapy often uses sympathetic blocking agents. Diazoxide is preferred by some clinicians. Agents that are rarely prescribed currently to treat acute hypertensive emergencies include alpha-methyldopa, reserpine, and trimethaphan. Patients who have chronic hypertension and who experience sudden elevations in their blood pressure (usually secondary to renal disease) can be treated with sublingual calcium channel blockers, extra doses of hydralazine, one to several doses of minoxidil, or an oral ACE inhibitor. The use of these drugs generally provides adequate, temporary control of blood pressure while other treatments are undertaken (usually salt and water removal).

MANAGEMENT OF CHRONIC HYPERTENSION

Representative orally administered antihypertensive drugs are tabulated in Table 67–9. There is no universally agreed upon approach to chronic drug therapy. Because of the variability in response, the starting dose for antihypertensive drugs should be the lowest recommended dose; dose changes should be made only after the agent has had an appropriate time to become effective. Follow-up blood pressure measurements should be performed with the adolescent both supine and erect in order to diagnose orthostatic hypotension. When selecting antihypertensive drugs for chronically managing blood pressure in adolescents, it is necessary to consider short- and long-term complications, particularly drug-induced changes that may increase the risk of atherogenesis (Table 67–10). Compliance is enhanced by avoiding drugs that affect libido, alter physical appearance or cause prolonged fatigue, can be taken less often, and are affordable (see Chapter 26). The consideration of potential side effects has led to the concept that a lower dose of two or more agents may be more practical than the more traditional concept of reaching a maximum dose before changing or adding other antihypertensive agents. Because of the large number of agents available, it is best for the physician to become familiar with one or two agents in a given class and to prescribe these agents repeatedly. Exceeding the recommended dose does not offer any therapeutic benefit and increases the likelihood of developing side effects.

DIURETICS

Currently, three types of diuretics are used to treat hypertensive adolescents: loop diuretics, thiazides that

TABLE 67–10. Adverse Effects of Oral Antihypertensive Agents

α-Adrenergic blocking agents	
Prazosin	Anticholinergic effects, dizziness, drowsiness, fluid retention, headache, palpitations, priapism, syncope with first dose, vertigo, urinary incontinence
Phenoxybenzamine	Dizziness, faintness, hypotension, lethargy, tachycardia (postural), shock, vomiting
β-Adrenergic blocking agents	
Propranolol	Blood dyscrasia (rare), bradycardia, bronchospasm, congestive heart failure, decreased exercise tolerance, depression, dreams, fatigue, generalized pustular psoriasis, GI disturbances, hallucinations, hearing loss (transient), hypoglycemic symptoms masked, hypotension, laryngospasm, organic brain syndrome, Raynaud phenomenon, serum lipid alterations (decreased HDL, increased triglycerides), skin rashes
Atenolol and Metoprolol	Similar to propranolol but are relatively cardiac selective
Calcium channel blocker	
Nifedipine (Procardia)	Blurred vision, dizziness, dyspnea, constipation, diarrhea, edema, flushing, headache, heartburn, heart failure, hypotension, imbalance, impotence, muscle cramps, nausea, skin rashes, syncope
Centrally acting α₂-adrenergic agonists	
Alpha-methyldopa (Aldomet)	Amenorrhea, "black tongue," blood dyscrasia, bradycardia, colitis, cirrhosis, Coomb's positive hemolytic anemia, decreased mental acuity, edema, GI symptoms, gynecomastia, headache, hepatitis, hepatic necrosis, hypotension, impotence, lactation, loss of libido, lupus-like syndrome, pancreatitis, sedation
Clonidine	Arrhythmias, blurred vision, bradycardia, CNS reactions similar to Aldomet, dry mouth, GI upset, gynecomastia, hallucinations, headache, hyperglycemia, insomnia, rebound hypertension, sedation, skin rashes, weight gain
Converting enzyme inhibitors	
Captropil (Capoten)	Angioedema, anorexia, blood dyscrasia, bronchospasm, cough, hyperkalemia, hypotension, jaundice, laryngospasm, loss of taste, proteinuria, renal failure (if volume depleted, bilateral renal artery stenosis or renal artery stenosis in a solitary kidney), skin rashes
Diuretics (loop)	
Furosemide (Lasix)	Blood dyscrasias, blurred vision, bladder spasm, dehydration, GI symptoms, hearing loss, hyperglycemia, hyperuricemia, hypocalcemia, hypokalemia, hypomagnesemia, hypotension, jaundice, lipid changes (increased LDL cholesterol and triglycerides), metabolic alkalosis, pancreatitis, rashes (including erythema multiforme and exfoliative dermatitis), thromboembolism, tinnitus, vasculitis
Thiazides	
Chlorothiazide (Diuril)	Anaphylaxis, anorexia, blood dyscrasias, depression, dehydration, GI symptoms, hearing loss, hypercalcemia, hyperglycemia, hyperuricemia, hypokalemia, hypomagnesemia, hyponatremia, hypotension, impotence, jaundice, lipid changes (increased LDL cholesterol and triglycerides), pancreatitis, paresthesias, pulmonary edema, rashes (including erythema multiforme and exfoliative dermatitis), vasculitis, vertigo
Potassium-sparing	
Spironolactone (Aldactone)	Amenorrhea, blood dyscrasia, drowsiness, fever, GI symptoms, gynecomastia, hirsutism, impotence, hyperkalemia, hyponatremia, mental confusion, rashes, postmenopausal bleeding, ulcers
Triamterene (Dyrenium)	Anaphylaxis, anemia (megaloblastic), dizziness, dry mouth, fatigue, GI symptoms, headache, jaundice, hyperkalemia, hypokalemia, rashes, renal failure, thrombocytopenia
Peripheral adrenergic blocking agents	
Reserpine (Serpasil)	Angina, arrhythmias, bradycardia, deafness, decreased libido, depression, dizziness, mouth, dull sensorium, dyspnea, dysuria, edema, extrapyramidal tract symptoms, GI symptoms, gynecomastia, impotence, nasal stuffiness, nervousness, nightmares, optic atrophy, rashes, uveitis, weight gain
Guanethidine (Ismelin)	Alopecia, angina, blurred vision, bradycardia, dermatitis, dizziness, dry mouth, dyspnea, edema, hypotension (particularly orthostatic), impotence, inhibition ejaculation, mental depression, nasal congestion, priapism, ptosis, syncope, urinary incontinence, vomiting, weight gain
Vasodilators	
Hydralazine (Apresoline)	Angina, anorexia, blood dyscrasia, conjunctivitis, dizziness, edema, flushing, GI symptoms, headache, hepatitis, hypotension, lacrimation, lupus-like syndrome, palpitations, paradoxical hypertension, paralytic ileus, peripheral neuritis, psychotic reactions, rashes, splenomegaly, urination difficulty, tachycardia
Minoxidil (Loniten)	Lupus-like syndrome, ECG T-wave changes, GI symptoms, hypertrichosis, leukopenia, pericardial effusion and tamponade, pericarditis, rashes, salt and water retention, Stevens-Johnson syndrome, thrombocytopenia

CNS, central nervous system; ECG, electrocardiogram; GI, gastrointestinal; LDL, low-density lipoproteins.
Compiled from The Medical Letter 31:25–30, 1989; Hoffman JIE, Stanger P: Systemic arterial hypertension. In Rudolph AM, Hoffman JIE (eds): Pediatrics, 18th ed. East Norwalk, CT, Appleton & Lange, 1987; Ingelfinger JR: Pediatric Hypertension, Philadelphia, WB Saunders, 1982; and Physicians' Desk Reference, 45th ed. Oradell, NJ, Medical Economics Company, 1991.

act in the cortical segments of the distal tubule, and distal tubular diuretics. The loop diuretics are usually needed to treat significant salt and water retention. This retention may be either due to primary renal disease or secondary to the renal effects of vasodilators.

ANTIHYPERTENSIVE DRUGS

Antihypertensive drugs lower blood pressure by affecting sites that lower arterial resistance or decrease cardiac output. Antihypertensive agents are classified into three groups: drugs that alter sympathetic nervous system function (central nervous system, ganglionic blockade, adrenergic nerve-ending depleting agents, α-adrenergic and β-adrenergic blockade); drugs that are direct vasodilators (including calcium channel inhibitors and minoxidil); and renin angiotensin blockers. Each class offers certain advantages and has its own set of problems. Clonidine is available as a sustained-release dermal patch that needs to be changed once a week. The use of many of the potent vasodilators quickly leads to salt and water retention and is more effective if they are prescribed with a diuretic. Also, because potent vasodilators often cause tachycardia, the simultaneous prescribing of a β-blocking agent may be indicated. Regression of ventricular hypertrophy has been described with the use of diuretics, angiotensin-converting enzyme inhibitors, calcium channel blockers, and sympathetic nervous system inhibitors.

BIBLIOGRAPHY

Dillon MJ: Investigation and management of hypertension in children. Pediatr Nephrol, 1:59, 1987.

Feld LG, Springate JE: Hypertension in children. Curr Probl Pediatr 18:317, 1988.

Gruskin AB, Baluarte HJ, Polinsky MS, et al: Treatment of severe hypertension in children with renal disease. In Strauss J (ed): Acute Renal Disorders and Renal Emergencies. Boston, Martinus Nijhoff, 1984, pp 143–178.

Kahn HS, Bain RP: Vertex corrected blood pressure in black girls. Hypertension, 9:390, 1987.

Laragh JH, Brenner BM, Kaplan NM: Endocrine Mechanisms in Hypertension. New York, Raven Press, 1989.

Loggie JMH, Horan MJ, Gruskin AB, et al: NHLBI Workshop on Juvenile Hypertension. New York, Biomedical International Corporation, 1984, pp 305–334.

Rocchini AP, Key J, Bondie D, et al: The effect of weight loss on the sensitivity of blood pressure to sodium in obese adolescents. N Engl J Med 321:580, 1989.

Sinaiko AR, Gomez-Marin O, Prineas RJ: Significant diastolic hypertension in pre-high school black and white children. The children and adolescent blood pressure program. Am J Hypertens, 1:178, 1988.

Stamler R, Stamler J, Gosch F, et al: Primary prevention of hypertension by nutritional-hygienic means. JAMA 262:1801, 1989.

Task Force on Blood Pressure Control in Children: Report of the second task force on blood pressure control in children. Pediatrics 79:1, 1987.

SECTION XVII

Reproductive Conditions

S. JEAN EMANS

The 1980s witnessed major changes in the field of reproductive health, necessitating new attitudes, skills, and knowledge for the practitioner of adolescent medicine. Despite the spread of human immunodeficiency virus (HIV) infection in the past decade, adolescents are more likely to be sexually active now than they were a decade ago, resulting in unplanned pregnancies, myriad sexually transmitted diseases (STDs), pelvic inflammatory disease (PID), and cervical intraepithelial neoplasia. Other societal trends, such as young women's preoccupation with being thin and their increased participation in athletic activities, have resulted in their experiencing menstrual irregularities, which present a challenge to the practitioner in diagnosis and management.

Each chapter in this section presents new knowledge about female and male reproductive health. In the discussion about adolescent sexuality (Chapter 68), the demographic data and the issues involved in adolescent decision-making are highlighted. The development of sexual identity and the delay or initiation of sexual activity are key concerns for adolescents. Sex education in most schools has been inadequate in providing a balance to the strong and convincing messages from the media, popular entertainment figures, and peers about casual sexual interactions. Simplistic messages of "Just Say No" fail to address the multiple factors associated with the high rates of adolescent pregnancy and STDs in the United States.

Chapter 69 considers screening tests associated with reproductive care. Every office in which adolescent medicine is practiced must have easy, confidential access to pregnancy tests, with results available within minutes. Screening sexually active adolescents for STDs has become a critical part of adolescent medicine. Failing to ask an adolescent female during each routine health visit whether she is sexually active can allow silent cervical infections caused by *Neisseria gonorrhoeae* and *Chlamydia trachomatis* to spread into the upper genital tract in these girls. An increase in abnormal results on Papanicolaou (Pap) smears in adolescent and young adult women associated with the epidemic of human papillomavirus infections is worrisome; the proper procedure for performing Pap screening should be understood by the clinician. Communication with the laboratory that is providing services is crucial, especially since terminology is not yet standardized.

Neuroendocrine changes in adolescence are a transitional stage between the quiescent period of childhood and the ovulatory reproductive capability of the adult woman. The younger the age of the adolescent at menarche, the more rapid the onset of ovulatory cycles, and the more likely the chance of early unplanned pregnancy. Since many adolescents have both ovulatory and anovulatory menses, especially in the first few years after menarche, menstrual irregularity is common. However, apathy is never warranted, because pregnancy and other endocrine disorders can present with similar symptomatology. Chapter 70 discusses amenorrhea and presents an approach for the practitioner to follow, with the goals of excluding a structural, endocrine, or systemic disorder and outlining a treatment course that may include hormonal therapy, weight gain, or rarely surgery. The challenge of knowing when to intervene in treating the hypoestrogenic athletic girl of the 1990s is a special challenge with no controlled trials of estrogen therapy yet undertaken.

Contraception options are still remarkably few for adolescents. Contraceptive research is not a priority for federal funding, and liability risks for companies developing new contraceptive methods sometimes seem insurmountable. Young women and health care practitioners still have significant concerns about the safety of oral contraceptives in spite of increasing evidence that the benefits far outweigh the risks in young women. Since break-through bleeding and other side effects may result in discontinuation of contraceptive pill use by adolescents, practitioners should be knowledgeable about the management of break-through bleeding and a variety of potential problems. Effective counseling is a must, in which the many methods of contraception are clarified and patient management issues are discussed. Norplant, an implantable progesterone product, is a method now under testing in adolescents. With the STD epidemic of the 1980s and 1990s, practitioners must also add condoms when prescribing oral contraceptives. The younger the patient, the more sexual partners she will have in her lifetime and the higher the risk of STDs.

The risks of adolescent pregnancy and parenthood are inextricably associated with sociodemographic factors, including poverty, poor education, unmarried status, nonwhite race, and inadequate prenatal care. STDs, poor nutrition, and, for some adolescents, substance abuse, contribute to the increased incidence of low birth weight (primarily premature) infants and the resultant high neonatal morbidity and mortality rates. Prevention must be directed toward enhancing life options before the first pregnancy occurs. Since maternal and neonatal outcomes can be worse with closely spaced subsequent pregnancies, the long-term involvement of adolescent parents in intervention programs that address contraception, schooling, employment, infant care, and other health issues is needed.

For a variety of sociodemographic, behavioral, and perhaps biologic reasons, sexually active adolescents are particularly vulnerable to STDs. Infections caused by *N. gonorrhoeae* and *C. trachomatis* have significant consequences for the short term, with symptoms and possible hospitalization, and for the long term, with pelvic pain, infertility, and ectopic pregnancy. Screening adolescent girls for *N. gonorrhoeae* and *C. trachomatis* has been routine in many adolescent practice settings for some years, but new approaches for screening young men by first-catch urine samples are promising for the 1990s. The special needs of gay males are also noted in Chapter 32 and in Chapter 76.

Indeed, Chapter 76, which discusses HIV, underscores that the epidemic is already here in many high-risk adolescent populations. Many more men, women, and children will contract acquired immunodeficiency syndrome (AIDS) in the 1990s from individuals infected in the 1980s. The authors of the chapter on HIV, having had firsthand experience with HIV-infected youth and education in high-risk areas, outline a strategy to curtail further spread of this virus: (1) information about HIV infection, transmission, and prevention; (2) education about the purchase and proper use of condoms; (3) education for adolescents to identify their own risk-related behaviors; and (4) skill building to help adolescents with communication and assertiveness about condom use and high-risk behaviors.

Both girls and boys may have breast complaints during adolescence. For adolescent girls, breast masses, infection, pain, and nipple discharge can be sources of concern. The most common breast problem for adolescent boys is gynecomastia. Chapter 77 provides practical up-to-date information on the cause, diagnostic procedures, and treatment of these breast problems.

Books on adolescent reproductive health frequently neglect the many problems of adolescent males. They not only are affected by STDs, resulting in urethritis and epididymitis, but also experience a variety of problems, such as torsion of the testis, hernia, and hypospadias, which require surgery. The need to make a rapid differential diagnosis between epididymitis and torsion of the testis is underscored in Chapter 78. Because recent studies have begun to explore the relationship of varicocele to infertility, approaches to what has often been observed as a benign variant are likely to change to earlier surgical intervention. To date, testicular self-examination has frequently been neglected in school health education classes and practitioners' offices; it should become an important part of adolescent health care.

Practitioners caring for adolescents in the 1990s must have a new knowledge base and new examination skills to be able to offer the diagnosis and treatment of menstrual disorders, strategies to prevent pregnancy, diagnosis and counseling regarding pregnancy, and diagnosis and treatment of common STDs, breast conditions, and male reproductive problems. Educational efforts to teach condom use, avoidance of high-risk behaviors, breast self-examination, and testicular self-examination will require innovative techniques to incorporate instruction into office settings, schools, and community projects.

CHAPTER 68

Normal Sexuality

ESTHERANN GRACE and VICTOR STRASBURGER

Defining normal adolescent sexuality is a challenge because of the variety of culturally acceptable lifestyles and the paucity of research data. This chapter will address the factors known to be involved in an adolescent's decision to initiate sexual activity, the typical sexual behaviors in which they are likely to engage, and the pressures that adolescents encounter to initiate sexual activity.

Reaching responsible sexual decisions is a lifetime task that usually begins during adolescence. Since the expression of adolescent sexuality reflects a variety of psychophysiologic, cultural, and social factors, there is a wide range of normal adolescent sexual behaviors. Awareness of these differences is essential when addressing issues related to sexual behavior with adolescents in an office practice.

The existence of a solitary biologic sex drive that accounts for the onset of sexual activity remains a theoretical concept (see Chapter 13). Rather, the desire for sexual gratification is largely learned and culturally determined. Cultural values (those values that influence how a group views itself and how it is judged by society) are determined by a combination of factors: socioeconomic status, ethnicity, and religion. These values form the group's attitudes toward sexual behaviors, gender identification, and parenthood (see Chapters 32, 73, and 74).

INITIATING SEXUAL ACTIVITY

Adolescents are currently initiating sexual activity at an earlier age than they did in generations past. National data from the National Surveys of Family Growth revealed that in 1988, approximately 53% of females 15 through 19 years of age reported having had intercourse (60.8% of non-Hispanic black, 52.4% of non-Hispanic white, and 48.5% of Hispanics). More adolescent males are sexually active during adolescence than are females for each age group (see also Chapter 2).

The time at which sexual activity is initiated is in part a function of opportunity and partner availability. Dating among adolescents provides the opportunity. Adolescents in general, particularly girls, are monogamous within their dating relationships. The fact that they are monogamous, however, does not mean that they have only one lifetime partner who is chosen during adolescence. The actual number of partners varies. Among

college students surveyed in the late 1980s, the mean number of sexual partners was four by 21 years of age.

Supervised dating usually begins in junior high school with group participation in school activities, for example, dances, sports, clubs. Steady dating early in adolescence has been associated with permissive attitudes and first intercourse at a young age. Adolescents without adult supervision are likely to take advantage of being alone together and follow the normal progression of sexual behaviors.

WHY DO TEENAGERS BECOME SEXUALLY ACTIVE?

Sexual activity during adolescence, particularly during middle and late adolescence, can be considered a normal developmental milestone, a response to biologic drives, a "coming of age" transition, a risk-taking behavior, or a combination of one or more of these factors.

A mature sexual relationship in which the partners can distinguish between true intimacy and genital sexuality and can practice effective contraception is usually achieved by late adolescence (18 to 21 years of age) and for some young persons it may occur later in life. Many reasons have been postulated for the initiation of adolescent sexual behaviors: (1) defining "adult" status, (2) establishing independence, (3) experiencing sensual drives, (4) bolstering self-esteem, (5) satisfying the need for love and intimacy, or a combination of one or more of these factors.

One study of 450 high school and 450 college students followed longitudinally for 4 years determined the following personal and social characteristics of those who initiated coitus compared with those who did not:

1. They were less goal-oriented.
2. They were more tolerant of differing opinions.
3. They were less religious.
4. Their friends' views did not conform to their parents' views.
5. They succumbed to peer pressure.
6. They were more likely to do poorly in school and to experiment with drugs and alcohol.

Another recent survey of 12,600 adolescents (14 to 22 years of age) confirmed the association between the earlier onset of sexual intercourse and drug use (particularly marijuana use) as shown in the previous study. Family relationships have been thought to play a role in the adolescent's sexual explorations. Several studies have identified divorce and poverty as contributing factors to early initiation of coitus. White teenagers in fatherless families were 60% more likely to be sexually active than were those young individuals whose fathers were present. In another study, daughters in white families with female heads of household were more likely to initiate coitus prior to age 15 years and to have multiple partners than were daughters of similar households headed by men. The rates of sexual experience were high for teenagers whose mothers had an unwed pregnancy or early marriage or had divorced and remarried.

Religion may also play a role, although its exact impact is unclear. A 1987 study of 1438 "born-again" teenagers from eight religious groups found that 43% of these young persons had intercourse by 18 years of age. However, those engaging in sexual activity were more likely not to attend church regularly, participate in youth groups, or read the Bible daily.

A 1986 Harris Report found sexual activity to be highest among teenagers whose parents did not graduate from college; teenagers whose grades averaged C, D, or F; and black teenagers. These data reflect the impact of socioeconomic status on adolescent sexual initiation. Social pressure was cited as the prime reason for initiating coitus by 73% of the females and 50% of the males studied.

Television may be another influential determinant of sexual decision-making. Television frequently fulfills the role of sex educator when reluctant parents and inadequate health programs in schools fail to provide teenagers the information they need to make informed sexual decisions. According to a 1986 Harris Poll, a significant minority of teenagers believe that television realistically portrays sexually transmitted diseases (45%), pregnancy and the consequences of intercourse (41%), use of birth control (27%), and individuals making love (24%). Soap operas capture a large percentage of the teenaged female audience. They typically portray sexual relationships as impersonal, emotionless, and exploitive. On those programs, unmarried partners are eight times more likely to have sexual relationships than are married couples, and 94% of all coupling is between individuals not married to each other. Although scientific evidence that television can directly influence behavior is scanty, the National Institute of Mental Health in 1982 noted that American teenagers rate the media third as a major influence on their attitudes and behaviors, superseded only by parents and by their peers.

ADOLESCENT SEXUAL BEHAVIORS

Adolescence is a time of experimentation and of seeking and establishing an identity (see Chapter 9). Gender identity appears to be the consequence of socialization from age 15 months to 5 years. It is during this phase of psychosocial development that the gender preference of the future sexual partner is formed. In the ongoing process of reaching this preference, sexual experimentation with members of the same sex is quite common during early adolescence. Most humans adhere to single gender preference for their sexual partners, but there is a small percentage who engage in bisexual activity throughout their lives.

In the studies of the past 20 years, no significant changes in masturbation practices have been noted among adolescents. Most males are believed to have masturbated to orgasm during adolescence—98% by 18 years of age. About 25% of all heterosexual and 60% of gay males experience mutual masturbation by age 14 years; this is true of 90% of gay males by age 19 years. Most heterosexual males stop mutual masturbation by midadolescence.

A smaller percentage of females are thought to masturbate during adolescence. Adolescent women from lower socioeconomic classes are more likely to prefer premarital coitus than are college-bound teenagers who are more accepting of masturbation. Lesbian females masturbate more frequently than do their heterosexual counterparts, and by age 18 years, both black and white lesbians report a higher incidence of masturbation than do heterosexual women, regardless of socioeconomic status.

Sexual behaviors usually start as distant behaviors, such as holding hands, and then become increasingly close and intimate. Kissing behaviors usually follow holding hands. Petting behaviors usually follow kissing, with above-the-waist petting designated as "light petting," and below-the-waist petting designated as "heavy petting." Younger adolescents are more likely to engage in light petting, with 60% of youngsters younger than 15 years of age admitting to this behavior. In the past 30 years, no differences have been found between the sexes in the amount of light petting in the 16- to 19-year-old age group. Not all adolescent sexual behavior follows the progression from distant to intimate behaviors. Some young persons move directly from kissing behaviors to coital behaviors.

There is a small percentage of otherwise healthy adolescents who rarely if ever experience sexual desire. Because of the persuasive emphasis of sex in the media, these youngsters are constantly reminded of their reduced sexual drive. The mass media, and television in particular, have set idealized standards of physical attractiveness and sexual performance. This degree of physical perfection is rarely achieved by the average adolescent without resorting to extreme measures, such as self-starvation (see Chapter 60), cosmetic surgery, including breast augmentation, and androgenic steroid abuse (see Chapter 81). Failure to transform their bodies into the sexual ideal can precipitate compensatory overt sexual behavior to reassure their fragile self-esteem. The age of the adolescent, partner availability, societal expectations, and parental and peer approval all have an impact on an individual's choice of a sexual partner.

At the time of first intercourse, adolescent females usually seek emotional commitment to the relationship. The majority of these girls perceive themselves to be in love with their partners. Adolescent males do not generally share this concept. They do not require a prerequisite of being in love to justify their sexual activity.

Younger adolescents are often concerned with the status achieved through their dating partner's superficial features (e.g., style of clothes, physical appearance, popularity). Approval by others (peers and parents) is likely to determine their choice of partner. In contrast, older adolescents typically are more independent in their choosing, being less influenced by external approval. They are goal-seeking individuals and expect their partners to share this future orientation. Personality factors are important to late adolescents.

Adolescent males and females typically differ in their stated reasons for choice of partners. Boys stress physical appearance and willingness to engage in sexual activity, whereas girls emphasize personality traits and a need for emotional intimacy within a relationship. The divergent views of the sexes frequently results in confusion on everyone's part, with misinterpretation of sexual behavior for a caring relationship. When uncertainty exists about the sexual interaction, adolescents mimic the sexual behaviors they have witnessed (movies and television). In established relationships, boys tend to defer to their partner's perception of appropriate sexual behaviors. This is in contrast with casual dating ("one night stands") when the boy usually asserts his own sexual demands.

Adolescents engage in sexual behavior when the opportunity presents itself. There is no limit to the availability of times and places. Most teenagers prefer privacy and uninterrupted time. The unsupervised home is a convenient setting. Youngsters take advantage of free afternoons while parents are working, evenings while parents are out, or weekends while parents are traveling. Because of the consistent reliability of the time parents return from work, the afternoon is the preferred time for many teenagers. Babysitting jobs in which the children are nonverbal provide another convenient opportunity. For teenagers living in warm climates, secluded woods and beaches are frequently used.

Older adolescents in college or living independent from parents have access to privacy within their own living arrangements. The parietal rules on entertaining guests in dormitory rooms on most college campuses have been greatly relaxed in the past 15 years. Many school dormitories are now coeducational, with bathrooms the only remaining single-sex restriction. It was hoped that the change in gender segregation would result in a relaxed relationship between the sexes based on normal daily encounters rather than just sexually charged social situations. The observed behavior of college students confirms this rationale. They are more likely to choose partners not living on their dormitory floors. Dormitory mates are considered friends, and for many a sibling-like relationship emerges with its attendant incestual taboos.

ADOLESCENT CONTRACEPTIVE COMPLIANCE

Many adolescents, regardless of their age, are perplexed by their sexual behavior and its apparent spontaneity. As a consequence of their internal confusion, they rarely are prepared with effective contraception when they initiate sexual activity (see Chapter 73). A variety of reasons have been postulated for poor adolescent contraceptive compliance, ranging from psychosocial to economic factors. Despite possessing knowledge of appropriate birth control and having availability of both prescribed and over-the-counter products, adolescents as a group continue to be ineffective users of contraception (see Chapter 26). The adolescent pregnancy rate and incidence of sexually transmitted diseases confirm their noncompliance (see Chapters 74 and 75).

Poor contraceptive compliance is thought to be a result of guilt. Adolescents must accept responsibility for their choice to be sexually active to be effective users of contraception. If guilt is a consequence of their sexual activity, they must deny their control of it ("it just happened"). The situation was beyond their control, and therefore they are exonerated from guilt about not using contraception.

Nevertheless, there is progress in adolescent contraceptive practices. It is unfortunate, however, that many teenagers do not use any method of contraception for the first 6 months of sexual activity, which is the period when 20% of teenage pregnancies occur. Young persons who are likely to use contraception at first intercourse are white, have a mother whose education extended beyond high school and who delayed first coitus until age 19 years, and are living in an intact family. In a sample of black teenagers, the level of socioeconomic status and parents' marital state predicted the first time use of contraceptives.

School-based health clinics have played a role in fostering contraceptive compliance (see Chapter 18). One outcome of peer counseling, particularly in school-based clinics, has been a delay in the onset of first intercourse by female students, with a subsequent reduction in the pregnancy rate. An increase in self-esteem has been credited for this result. The young women felt confident enough in their own identity to say no to their partner's sexual demands. They were willing to risk rejection by the partner and peers. They did not view having a boyfriend—that is, being part of a couple—as essential to their lifestyles. For young women without a strong sense of self, gains within a relationship far outweigh their willingness to risk rejection. The relationship affords them credibility with their peers, relieves the anxiety generated by their dysfunctional families, and ends their loneliness. It is understandable why an adolescent would meet her partner's sexual demands to ensure the continuation of the security the relationship provides her. By teaching young women to use their own inner resources and their community, it appears that the school-based clinics have helped teenagers develop healthier relationships based on mutual respect, not dependency needs.

The expression of normal adolescent sexuality is currently taking place in a world epidemic of potentially life-threatening sexually transmitted diseases, such as AIDS, and adolescent pregnancies. Most believe that educating adolescents about their sexuality should start as early as possible; ideally this education would involve young people and their parents, their health care providers, educators, and other caring and responsible adults.

BIBLIOGRAPHY

Akpom AC, Akpom KL, Davis M: Prior sexual behavior of teenagers attending rap sessions for the first time. Fam Plann Perspect 8:203, 1976.

Blum RW: The State of Adolescent Health in Minnesota. Minneapolis, University of Minnesota, 1989.

Deipold J, Young R: Empirical studies of adolescent sexual behavior. Adolescence 15:53, 1979.

Dryfoos JG, Klerman L: School-based clinics: Their role in helping students meet the 1990 objectives. Health Educ Q 15:71, 1988.

Forrest JD, Singh S: The sexual and reproductive behavior of American women, 1982–1988. Fam Plann Perspect 22:206, 1990.

Garguilo J, Altie L, Brooks-Gunn J, Warren M: Girls' dating behavior as a function of social context and maturation. Dev Psychol 23:5, 1987.

Gordon S, Scales P, Everly K: The Sexual Adolescent, 2nd ed. North Scituate, MA, Duxbury Press, 1979.

Harris L and Associates: American Teens Speak: Sex, Myths, TV, and Birth Control. New York, Louis Harris and Associates, 1986.

Irwin CE, Millstein SG: Biopsychosocial correlates of risk-taking behaviors during adolescence. J Adolesc Health Care 7:825, 1986.

Jessor SL, Jessor R: Transition from virginity to nonvirginity among youth: A social-psychological study over time. Dev Psychol 11:473, 1975.

Mott FL, Haurin RJ: Linkages between sexual activity and alcohol and drug use among American adolescents. Fam Plann Perspect 20(3):128, 1988.

National Institute of Mental Health: Television and Behavior: Ten Years of Scientific Progress and Implications for the Eighties: Summary Report, Vol. 1. Bethesda, MD, National Institute of Mental Health, 1982.

Roscoe B, Cavanaugh L, Kennedy D: Dating infidelity: Behaviors, reasons, and consequences. Adolescence 23:89, 1988.

Thornton A, Camburn D: The influence of the family on premarital sexual attitudes and behaviors. Demography 24:323, 1987.

Update: Kids will be kids. Fam Plann Perspect 20(5):204, 1988.

CHAPTER 69

Reproductive Care in the Office: Screening Methods

FRANK M. BIRO

This chapter includes information on screening methods for reproductive care in the office: the pelvic examination, pregnancy history, Papanicolaou (Pap) smear, and laboratory evaluation of sexually transmitted diseases (STDs). The STD pathogens included are *Chlamydia trachomatis, Neisseria gonorrhoeae, Trichomonas vaginalis,* and *Treponema pallidum.* Additional data on laboratory screening and STDs are found in Chapter 75. Techniques for breast examination are found in Chapter 77; techniques for testicular examination are found in Chapter 78; and testing for human immunodeficiency virus (HIV) is found in Chapter 76.

PELVIC EXAMINATION

Initially, one should establish whether the adolescent prefers to have a family member present during her pelvic examination. For instance, younger adolescents often prefer to have a family member present during the pelvic examination, whereas older adolescents often choose a female nurse. Next, determine the specific positioning of the patient for her examination. Most adolescents prefer a drape over the lower abdomen and knees, and some request that their head be elevated. Then the physician should explain the pelvic examination; explanation may help the adolescent relax and thus avoid discomfort associated with the examination. One investigator found that an important source of anxiety regarding the examination was the adolescents' fear of pain, which was conveyed most frequently from peers. An effective approach would be to describe the physical sensations experienced during the pelvic examination.

After positioning the adolescent and examining the external structures—palpation of the vulvar tissues (including the Bartholin and meibomian glands) and assessment of pubic hair maturity (see Chapter 5) and clitoral size—an index finger is inserted along the posterior vaginal wall. This is useful for several reasons: most adolescents, under guidance, are able to relax their perineal muscles; the cervix can be located; and the speculum can be inserted against the examining finger and away from the sensitive structures along the anterior wall of the vagina. If the adolescent is having difficulty in relaxing, she can be asked to push down as if she were having a bowel movement. The speculum should be lubricated with warm water only, because lubricating gels interfere with cultures and Papanicolaou smears. Following the speculum examination, a bimanual examination is done to evaluate the internal organs of reproduction (uterus, ovaries, and fallopian tubes).

Excess mucus should be removed with a large swab prior to any diagnostic studies (see Chapter 75). After obtaining the cultures, nonculture diagnostic studies (such as *Chlamydia trachomatis* antigen techniques) and Papanicolaou smears are done, and a swab of the posterior vaginal pool is obtained and placed on a slide with a drop of saline. To enhance contrast, one part green food coloring can be added to ten parts saline. Some recommend a second vaginal pool specimen for microscopic examination, with the addition of 10% potassium hydroxide (KOH) solution to lyse epithelial cells and allow improved detection of yeast hyphae. The saline specimen should be examined under the microscope as quickly as possible to ensure continued motility and thus easier detection of *Trichomonas vaginalis.* The presence of clue cells (epithelial cells studded with coccobacilli) may suggest *Gardnerella vaginalis* but is not pathognomonic for *G. vaginalis* infection, as it is also associated with several other potential pathogens, such as *Bacteroides* species, anaerobic peptococci, and *Mycoplasma* species. When discharge containing *G. vaginalis* is mixed with 10% potassium hydroxide, a fishy odor is noted. This is known as a positive "whiff" test. Several excellent photographic atlases for microscopic examination of cervical specimens are available.

PREGNANCY TESTING

Of all reproductive health tests done in the office setting, few have undergone the improvements in sensitivity and convenience as has pregnancy testing (see Chapter 74). Testing is based on the detection of human chorionic gonadotropin (hCG), a glycoprotein hormone that shares α chain homology with luteinizing hormone (LH) and follicle-stimulating hormone (FSH). Additionally, hCG and LH share multiple amino acid residues; this cross-reactivity has contributed to the lower specificities of the immunoassays (see below). Both immunoassays and bioassays have limited applicability in the 1990s, given the lack of specificity (false-positives from several interfering agents such as urine proteins or LH) and relatively poor sensitivity (200 mIU/ml). There are equivalent levels of hCG in blood and urine, regardless of whether there is an intrauterine or ectopic pregnancy.

Currently, the two techniques most extensively used in the office and hospital laboratory are radioimmunoassay and enzyme-linked immunoassay. Radioimmunoassay detects hCG within days of ovulation, and the hCG level doubles every 1.5 to 2.4 days. Human chorionic gonadotropin is compared against two standards: the International Reference Preparation (IRP) and the Second International Standard (2nd IS). Values for 2nd IS are approximately one-half the values of IRP. Because of interlaboratory variability, when serial measurements are necessary (such as in diagnosing ectopic pregnancy), assessment should be performed at the same laboratory. Although radioimmunoassay performed on serum is the most sensitive analytic method, recent studies have questioned the clinical utility of the lower limits of serum radioimmunoassay's sensitivity. A recent study reported a 99.5% concordance between simultaneous urine and serum assays in 871 cases; the urine pregnancy test was correct in three of the four discordant cases. Enzyme-linked immunosorbent assay (ELISA) and immunodiagnostics using monoclonal antibodies are commonly used in the office laboratory and can be used on urine or serum specimens. Additionally, with the improved sensitivity of enzyme-linked immunoassays, more than 95% of ectopic pregnancies will be detected on urine specimens at time of the initial presentation. The average time for detection in intrauterine pregnancy is 10 to 12 days post-conception; there is a question as to when urine tests are positive in ectopic pregnancy.

Serial quantitative hCG assays, transabdominal (and transvaginal) ultrasonography, and serum progesterone assays have revolutionized the approach to ectopic pregnancy. Institutions each define a "discriminatory zone," a minimum value of hCG above which ultrasonography can identify a gestational sac. Despite the fact that ectopic pregnancies generally produce hCG at slower rates than intrauterine pregnancies, a matched pair of sera may not completely exclude (or diagnose) an ectopic pregnancy. This is especially true early in an ectopic pregnancy, particularly prior to development of symptoms, when an ectopic pregnancy may have a normal hCG doubling time (see Chapter 74).

The utility of the home pregnancy test for adolescents remains an unresolved issue. Home pregnancy tests have several limitations. Some manufacturers recommend testing at a time too early in the gestation to obtain reliable positive results, limiting the sensitivity of the method. Additionally, there are technical features in performing these tests that affect the accuracy of results adversely; deviations from test directions were especially noted in those younger than 21 years of age and with less than a high school education. These data suggest that home pregnancy tests may be useful only in a small segment of educated and highly motivated adolescents who are working closely with their health providers (see Chapter 74).

PAPANICOLAOU SMEAR

The screening Papanicolaou (Pap) smear has become a mainstay of preventive gynecologic health care. It is especially important among sexually active adolescents exposed to human papillomavirus because of the association between this virus and cervical neoplasia (see Chapter 75). Pap smear specimens allow the elucidation of changes in cervical cells secondary to inflammation or neoplasia. These cells are obtained through several sampling techniques, including the use of vaginal pool aspirates, plastic and wooden spatula, and the cytobrush. Although the plastic spatula collects more endocervical cells than does the wooden spatula, there is no improvement in the detection of cervical dysplasia using the plastic spatula. When the use of the cytobrush is compared with the use of a cotton swab, significantly more specimens obtained using a cytobrush have good cellular yield. Less-experienced examiners are more likely than are experienced examiners to improve their percentage of specimens with adequate sampling when using the cytobrush. Although the use of the cytobrush adds to the expense of the Pap test, the brush improves the collection of endocervical cells and thus the adequacy of Pap sampling for cytology.

To obtain a specimen from the cervix, the cervix is visualized through a nonlubricated speculum. Cells are obtained from all three areas of the cervix (squamous epithelium, transformation zone, and endocervix), with 360-degree rotation of the sampling instrument. This specimen is then fixed immediately to avoid drying artifacts, and the specimen is sent to the laboratory with appropriate clinical information. There is a considerable false-negative rate of cervical smears (20% compared with paired specimens, 25% to 40% compared with colposcopy and biopsy). Recommendations to improve the relatively poor sensitivity of cervical smears include obtaining paired cervical smears, use of the cytobrush, and cervicovaginal lavage. Despite their shortcomings, cervical smears are an effective tool for cancer detection.

The management of an abnormal Pap smear in adolescents is a challenge. A recent study compared biopsy results with serial Pap smears obtained from 236 women (mean age of 25 years) with atypical, but not necessarily dysplastic smears. Although 25% had biopsy-documented carcinoma intraepithelial neoplasia (CIN), the repeat Pap smear identified only 17% of these patients. The authors concluded that one should not repeat abnormal Pap smears prior to colposcopy and biopsy. This is because of the false-negative rates of Pap smear as noted previously; only a few minimally abnormal cells may represent malignant or premalignant lesions. Conversely, there is controversy regarding a Pap smear that reveals only atypia without any further evidence of HPV on examination, or when associated with a documented STD. Given the limited colposcopy resources, this clinical issue requires further clarification.

There are several current recommendations regarding the interval between Pap smears. Important concerns include the increased rate of abnormal cervical smears noted in recent years (especially among younger women), the natural history of human papillomavirus (HPV) and cervical dysplasia (especially HPV types 16 and 18) (see Chapter 75), and the high rate of false-negative Pap smears. The American Cancer Society and the American College of Obstetricians and Gynecologists have recommended annual Pap smears beginning with the onset of sexual activity (or 18 years of age, whichever occurs first) until the woman has three or more consecutive normal smears. After three normal smears, smears should be obtained at least every 2 to 3 years. However, sexually active adolescents should be considered a high-risk group and should continue to have Pap smears at least annually because of the high rate of exposure to human papillomavirus in sexually active adolescent females (38% as reported by one author) and the rapid progression to dysplasia with some HPV types. Newer techniques of HPV-DNA probing with or without specific HPV typing may modify these recommendations in the future.

DIAGNOSIS OF SEXUALLY TRANSMITTED DISEASES

Chlamydia trachomatis

Chlamydia trachomatis is an intracellular parasite with characteristics of both bacteria and viruses. As noted in Chapter 75, it is highly prevalent in adolescents. Because the organism is intracellular, it can be grown only by cell culture. Although *C. trachomatis* culture technology has become simpler than in the past, it is still expensive ($35 to $45 per culture) and requires careful attention to specimen transport and processing. Other diagnostic techniques to confirm the diagnosis of infection by *C. trachomatis* include detection of pyuria, urethral Gram stains, cervical Pap smears, direct immunofluorescent antibodies, enzyme-linked immunoassay, and nucleic acid probes (see Chapter 75).

Recent data support the detection of pyuria as a less expensive method for detection of STDs in adolescent males. When using urine leukocyte esterase activity, one cannot distinguish between *Neisseria gonorrhoeae* and *C. trachomatis* infections without using other diagnostic tests on urine or on a urethral specimen. The sensitivity of leukocyte esterase (when evaluating results on dipstick of 1+ or greater on a first voided urine) is 72% to 100%, and specificity is 83% to 93% for detection of either *N. gonorrhoeae* or *C. trachomatis*. False-negative results of urine screens are more likely to occur if the individual has voided within 4 hours. A random urine specimen yields comparable sensitivity and specificity if the esterase test results are trace or greater. An additional benefit of urine screens is that a positive esterase test result provides concrete evidence of a possible infection and can serve as an incentive for the asymptomatic adolescent male to undergo further diagnostic testing, which may be somewhat invasive. There are no advantages of urethral Gram stain over urine leukocyte esterase for *C. trachomatis* detection, but the Gram stain is useful for specific detection of *N. gonorrhoeae* (see further on). Endocervical Pap smears have poor sensitivity and specificity for *C. trachomatis* diagnosis.

Cell culture for *C. trachomatis* is still considered the "gold standard," although antigen detection techniques suggest evidence that the sensitivity of culture is approximately 80%. The specificity of culture is 99% to 100%. As noted earlier, there are technical, financial, and transport issues that limit the clinical applicability of cell culture. For instance, specimens must be kept at 4° to 5°C for a maximum of 48 hours prior to culturing. Freezing the specimen decreases the sensitivity slightly. Counterstaining the cultures with fluorescent-labeled monoclonal antibodies improves sensitivity, as does a second passage in culture. Cell culture is the only method that is specific enough for certain clinical situations, such as in legal or criminal cases or for rectal specimens.

Direct immunofluorescent antibody (DFA) tests couple fluorochromes to antibodies specific for *C. trachomatis* antigens. This provides an antigen-detection technique that can be used on clinical specimens directly, as well as an opportunity to assess the adequacy of the clinical specimen. Other advantages of this technique are ease of specimen transportation (since viable organisms are not needed) and greater sensitivity in males as compared with other antigen detection techniques. Two distinct disadvantages of DFA are the variability of results between different laboratories, which may be due to sampling and processing differences, and the technical requirements, which include a fluorescence microscope and observer training. Using a cytobrush may increase the sensitivity of DFA.

Enzyme-linked immunoassay (EIA) as a diagnostic technique for *C. trachomatis* has a comparable sensitivity and slightly lower specificity to DFA in symptomatic adolescent patients. The sensitivity of EIA, however, is only 48% to 75% in the asymptomatic adolescent male (see Chapter 75). Because EIA has an objective end point (optical density or qualitative reaction), there are fewer interlaboratory differences when compared with DFA. Additionally, EIA testing can be batched and automated, which provides a technique for handling a greater number of daily specimens than does DFA.

Preliminary studies on a chemiluminescent nucleic acid probe suggest that the probe has a sensitivity and specificity comparable to the two other antigen detection techniques. More widespread testing is needed to confirm its clinical utility.

The final choice of a specific diagnostic method depends on many factors in a given clinical setting. These include suspected prevalence of *C. trachomatis* in the population (the adolescent age group is generally considered high risk), number of specimens processed daily, local laboratory availability and technical expertise (including transportation factors), and test utilization (a confirmation test should have good sensitivities and excellent specificities).

Neisseria gonorrhoeae

Culture has been the standard for diagnosis of *N. gonorrhoeae* infections, especially in the female. Selective media, such as modified Martin medium, are required to provide enriched media for *N. gonorrhoeae* and to restrict the growth of other saprophytic bacteria in the clinical specimen. With the recent outbreaks of chromosomally mediated penicillin- and tetracycline-resistant gonorrhea, testing for lactamase production alone is inadequate, and laboratories should survey for penicillin sensitivity. Except for epidemiologic considerations, sensitivity testing may be obviated if treatment is with the recommended third-generation cephalosporins (see Chapter 75). Sampling sites may be important considerations. Routine pharyngeal culturing for *N. gonorrhoeae* identifies only an additional 1% of cases in adolescents. The clinician can improve cost effectiveness by utilizing treatment modalities effective for both genital and pharyngeal infections or by culturing the pharynx at the test of cure (see Chapter 75). Gay males, however, should have both urethral and rectal cultures (see Chapter 32).

Alternative diagnostic studies for *N. gonorrhoeae* include antigen detection, urine testing (for pyuria or gonococcal culture), and Gram stains of clinical specimens. Antigen detection techniques, to date, have had poor sensitivities. Obtaining a leukocyte esterase test on first-voided urines has been described in the section on *C. trachomatis*. Urethral Gram stain on symptomatic males has excellent sensitivity (90% to 98%) and specificity (95% to 100%), and culture on first-voided urine has a good sensitivity. Gram stains from urethral specimens in asymptomatic men or from endocervical specimens in women have much lower sensitivities.

Trichomonas vaginalis

The diagnosis of *T. vaginalis* can be difficult in the adolescent patient, especially with the high rate of asymptomatic infection (50% in women, more than 90% in men). Culture has the greatest sensitivity (86% to 97%) but is not widely available, whereas cytology is the least sensitive (34% to 56%), especially in the adolescent who has a negative saline preparation. Fresh saline preparations detect two thirds or more of women infected by *T. vaginalis* (motile, flagellated organisms and the pressure of white blood cells); the sensitivity is greater in symptomatic women or when the vaginal fluid is purulent. A fresh preparation is important because *T. vaginalis* lose their motility when the specimen has cooled to room temperature, as is typical for most protozoa. It has been recommended that if examination of a saline preparation is not routine, it be included for women with a purulent vaginal discharge or when vaginal erythema is present. Colpitis macularis is the most specific clinical manifestation of trichomoniasis but is rarely observed without the use of a colposcope. Additionally, antigen detection techniques include monoclonal fluorescent antibody tests and enzyme immunoassay. Sensitivity of these methods in women is reported to be 80% to 95% with specificity in the upper 90% range; few antigen technique studies have addressed asymptomatic males.

Syphilis

With recent increases in primary and secondary syphilis (see Chapter 75), as well as its association with HIV infection (see Chapter 76), the clinician must continually be aware of the possible diagnosis of syphilis. There are four groups of diagnostic tests currently available: darkfield examination, serologic tests, direct fluorescent antibody tests, and cerebrospinal fluid tests. The first three will be discussed. Because evaluation and follow-up vary by the specific clinical situation, it is important to define pretest probabilities. A single, painless, indurated lesion yields a high probability of syphilis, whereas multiple, painful, shallow ulcers have a low probability. A nonspecific rash on the palms and soles should raise the possibility of the diagnosis of syphilis (see Chapter 75).

The darkfield examination is performed by collecting exudate on a glass slide and examining it under a microscope with a darkfield condenser, looking for motile, corkscrew-shaped organisms. It is highly specific (98% to 99%), but its sensitivity varies with collection technique and the use of recent antibiotics (75% to 95%). Three separate examinations are generally performed prior to accepting a negative result. Darkfield examination is not generally recommended for oral lesions, since *T. pallidum* cannot be distinguished from nonpathogenic treponemes. Specimen collection for the direct fluorescent antibody test is similar, except that the specimen is fixed, labeled with fluorescein conjugated to antibodies to *T. pallidum*, and examined with a fluorescence microscope. This technique can be used for oral lesions.

Serologic diagnosis includes both treponemal and nontreponemal tests. Nontreponemal tests evaluate antibodies to a purified cardiolipin-lecithin-cholesterol antigen, a normal component of many tissues, which is fortuitously positive in most individuals with syphilis. The most commonly used nontreponemal test is the Venereal Disease Research Laboratory (VDRL) test, which like the others becomes reactive during early syphilis infections; the sensitivity of the VDRL has improved in many state laboratories. Sensitivity still correlates with increasing duration of infection (from 40% in infections under 30 days to 96% in infections over 40 days); sensitivity is 100% in secondary syphilis. After adequate treatment, or after more than 1 year of untreated infection, the VDRL titer falls. A fourfold decrease in titer demonstrates adequate therapy, and a similar titer increase suggests relapse or reinfection. Specificity of VDRL varies by health status of the individual, although biologic false-positive results have decreased since utilization of purified antigen. Specificity in healthy subjects is 99.7% but drops to 84% in ill subjects. These false-positive titers occur in autoimmune diseases, hepatitis, tuberculosis, endocarditis, malaria, and infectious mononucleosis.

Treponemal tests include the fluorescent treponemal antibody absorption test (FTA-ABS) and microhemagglutination test for *T. pallidum* (MHA-TP), both of which use whole treponemes or extracts of treponemes as antigen. These tests become reactive during primary syphilis and remain reactive throughout life, except when early treatment aborts an antibody rise. These tests also cross-react with other spirochetal diseases, such as yaws, pinta, leptospirosis, and Lyme disease (the last is negative for the rapid plasma reagin [RPR] test). The FTA-ABS was generally more sensitive than the MHA-TP or the VDRL, when all three were compared in the same population groups, but was slightly less specific (99.2% in healthy subjects, 77.3% in ill subjects).

In a clinical setting of high probability of disease, a positive darkfield examination or VDRL confirms the diagnosis of syphilis, and treatment should be started. If both test results are negative, the VDRL should be repeated in 1 week, and if still negative, in 1 month. In the moderate probability setting, the adolescent should be treated if either the VDRL or the darkfield examination result is positive, whereas syphilis is unlikely if both test findings are negative. Screening for syphilis should be done with the VDRL, and confirmation of positive results made through MHA-TP or FTA-ABS.

Human Immunodeficiency Virus

Screening for human immunodeficiency virus (HIV) is described in Chapter 76.

BIBLIOGRAPHY

Braverman PK, Biro FM, Brunner RL, et al: Screening asymptomatic adolescent males for *Chlamydia*. J Adolesc Health Care 11:141, 1990.

Brown RT, Lossick JG, Mosure DJ, et al: Pharyngeal gonorrhea screening in adolescents: Is it necessary? Pediatrics 84:623, 1989.

Davis AJ, O'Boyle EA, Reindollar RH: Human chorionic gonadotropin in pediatric and adolescent gynecology. Adolesc Pediatr Gynecol 2:207, 1989.

Doshi ML: Accuracy of consumer-performed in-home tests for early pregnancy detection. Am J Public Health 76:512, 1986.

Emancipator K, Cadoff EM, Burke MD: Analytical versus clinical sensitivity and specificity in pregnancy testing. Am J Obstet Gynecol 158:613, 1988.

Fink DJ: Change in American Cancer Society checkup guidelines for detection of cervical cancer. CA 38:127, 1988.

Gilchrist MJR, Rauh JL: Office microscopic examination for sexually transmitted diseases. J Adolesc Health Care 6:311, 1985.

Hart G: Syphilis tests in diagnostic and therapeutic decision making. Ann Intern Med 104:368, 1986.

Jones DED, Creasman WT, Dombroski RA, et al: Evaluation of the atypical Pap smear. Am J Obstet Gynecol 157:544, 1987.

Koss LG: The Papanicolaou test for cervical cancer detection. JAMA 261:737, 1989.

Millstein SG, Adler NE, Irwin CE: Sources of anxiety about pelvic examinations among adolescent females. J Adolesc Health Care 5:105, 1984.

Neinstein LS, Rabinovitz S, Recalde A: Comparison of cytobrush with cotton swab for endocervical cytologic sampling. J Adolesc Health Care 10:305, 1989.

Norman RJ, Buck RH, Rom L, et al: Blood or urine measurement of human chorionic gonadotropin for detection of ectopic pregnancy? Obstet Gynecol 71:315, 1988.

Rosenfeld WD, Vermund SH, Wentz SJ, et al: High prevalence rate of human papillomavirus infection and association with abnormal Papanicolaou smears in sexually active adolescents. Am J Dis Child 143:1443, 1989.

Stamm WE: Diagnosis of *Chlamydia trachomatis* genitourinary infections. Ann Intern Med 108:710, 1988.

Werner MJ, Biro FM: Urinary leukocyte esterase screening for asymptomatic sexually transmitted disease in adolescent males. J Adolesc Health 12:326, 1991.

CHAPTER 70

Menstrual Conditions

NORMAL FEMALE REPRODUCTIVE DEVELOPMENT AND AMENORRHEA

M. JOAN MANSFIELD

DEFINITION OF TERMS

Menarche is the onset of menstruation. It occurs at an average age of 12.8 years in white girls in the United States. *Gynecologic age* is the interval since menarche and is used as a measure of sexual maturation. Almost all pubertal changes are completed by a gynecologic age of 3 years.

Amenorrhea refers to the absence of spontaneous menstrual periods in a female of reproductive age. In the early adolescent, this definition is sometimes inadequate, since there is wide variability in the timing of onset and progression of puberty (see Chapter 5).

Primary amenorrhea is the absence of menarche in a female of reproductive age; that is, (1) delay of menarche beyond 16 years of age (>3 standard deviations), (2) absence of menarche more than 4 years after thelarche (the onset of breast development), or (3) delayed puberty: the absence of thelarche and menarche beyond 13 years of age. The causes of delayed puberty are reviewed in greater detail in Chapter 57.

Secondary amenorrhea is the cessation of menses at any time after menarche. Again, the variability in the pattern of menstruation normally present after menarche makes this condition difficult to define in absolute terms. A 16-year-old with a gynecologic age of 4 years who has had regular 28-day cycles for 2 years should be considered having secondary amenorrhea after missing only three periods. In contrast, a 13-year-old who has experienced menarche within the previous year may not have a menstrual period for more than 6 months and still be normal.

Oligomenorrhea can be defined as menstrual intervals of greater than 45 days. Persistence of oligomenorrhea more than 2 years after menarche should be evaluated.

Although the terms primary and secondary amenorrhea are often used to categorize menstrual abnormalities in adolescence, they are of limited usefulness, since the diagnostic possibilities overlap considerably.

A more useful way of categorizing the menstrual disorders of adolescence is to focus on the source of the dysfunction. Is the problem systemic, hypothalamic, pituitary, or gonadal, or is it due to an abnormal uterus or vagina?

An understanding of the normal physiology of female reproductive development is therefore useful as a basis for the recognition of normal variants and reproductive abnormalities in the adolescent patient.

NORMAL FEMALE REPRODUCTIVE DEVELOPMENT

The reproductive system is functional and active by the end of the first trimester *in utero*. Gonadotropin-releasing hormone (GnRH) is secreted in pulses from the fetal hypothalamus. GnRH causes synthesis and release of luteinizing hormone (LH) and follicle-stimulating hormone (FSH) by the pituitary. Fetal LH and FSH reach a peak by 20 weeks' gestation. In mid–second trimester, negative feedback of estrogen on the hypothalamus and pituitary develops, and the hypothalamic-pituitary-ovarian axis is suppressed by the presence of placental estrogens. With the decrease in gonadotropin levels, the population of oocytes declines throughout gestation. This germ cell atresia continues throughout life. The number of primordial follicles decreases from 2 to 4 million at birth to 400,000 at menarche. Survival of the oocytes requires the presence of two X chromosomes in the gonads. If only one X chromosome is present, as in Turner syndrome, the rate of destruction of oocytes is accelerated, and the ovaries are usually reduced to streak gonads incapable of making estrogen even before birth (see Chapter 55).

Postnatal Development

In the normal newborn, LH and FSH rise in the absence of negative feedback from placental sex steroids. The ovaries often show transient activity in the first 2 years of life, with development of follicles and occasionally sufficient estrogen production to stimulate some breast development. By the middle of childhood,

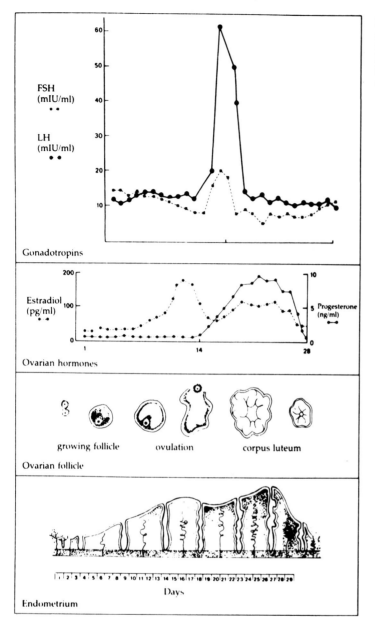

Figure 70–1. Physiology of the normal ovulatory menstrual cycle: gonadotropin secretion, ovarian hormone production, follicular maturation, and endometrial changes during one cycle. FSH = follicle-stimulating hormone; LH = luteinizing hormone. (With permission from Emans SJ, Goldstein DP: Pediatric and Adolescent Gynecology, 3rd ed. Boston, Little, Brown, 1990, p. 115.)

the ovaries are generally quiescent, although small follicles may still be seen on ultrasound examination.

Pubertal Development

With puberty, the hypothalamic-pituitary-ovarian axis reactivates, as described in greater detail in Chapter 4. In the early stage of puberty, LH and FSH are secreted in pulses only during sleep. Later, gonadotropin pulsations occur during waking hours as well. In response to rising gonadotropins, ovarian follicles ripen and produce estrogen. When estradiol levels are sufficient to stimulate growth of the lining of the uterus, menses begin with the cyclic fluctuations in estradiol. Menstrual periods usually begin late in the pubertal process, when the growth spurt is past its peak and breasts are developed to the sexual maturity rating stage 3 or 4 (see Chapter 5). The average menstrual cycle length is 28 days, with a range from 21 to 44 days, although normal adolescents

may experience menstrual intervals of more than 50 days during the first 2 years after menarche. The duration of menstrual flow is normally 4 to 7 days. Menstrual cycles of less than 21 days imply anovulatory bleeding. In a typical ovulatory cycle, the follicular phase lasts 10 to 14 days (Fig. 70–1). In the early follicular phase, during menses, rising FSH levels stimulate a new crop of follicles. By the midfollicular phase, days 5 to 7, a dominant follicle has been established and the others become atretic. This dominant follicle produces rapidly increasing amounts of estradiol that cause proliferation of the endometrium. LH levels exceed FSH levels at this phase of the cycle. Positive feedback of estradiol triggers the LH surge, and the ripe follicle then ruptures, releasing the ovum (ovulation). The remains of the follicle then become the corpus luteum, with a relatively constant life span of 12 to 14 days, giving rise to the luteal phase characterized by high levels of progesterone secreted by the corpus luteum. Under the influence of progesterone, the structure of the uterine endometrium changes from proliferative to secretory. If the ovum is not fertilized, the corpus luteum becomes atretic, progesterone and estrogen levels fall, and the endometrial lining sloughs, resulting in menses. Simultaneously, FSH levels increase, beginning a new cycle.

Adolescent Menstrual Patterns

Whereas negative feedback of estrogen on the hypothalamus and pituitary is present well before birth and continues throughout life, positive feedback (by which rapidly rising levels of estrogen trigger the LH surge required for ovulation) does not develop until middle to late puberty, often several years after menarche. Thus, menstrual cycles in the first few years after menarche are very often anovulatory (see next subchapter).

Cyclic hormone production is usually present in the anovulatory phase of normal female puberty: gonadotropins trigger follicular development and rising estradiol levels, which cause a fall of gonadotropins by negative feedback. Estradiol then in turn declines, and a pattern of regular, although anovulatory, hormonal cycles is established. In pubertal girls even prior to menarche, 28- to 42-day cyclic variations in urinary FSH and LH have been demonstrated. During these periods of physiologic anovulatory ovarian activity in infancy and puberty, the ovaries may be enlarged and multicystic. Ovaries with multiple small cysts can thus be considered to be physiologic in the peripubertal period.

In Widholm and Kantero's study of more than 5000 adolescents, 43% of subjects reported irregular menstrual cycles in the first year after menarche. By the fifth gynecologic year, irregular cycles were present in 20%. Although the majority of young adolescents have fairly regular periods in the first few years after menarche, these cycles are often anovulatory. In a study of 200 normal Finnish girls, Apter found that 80% of the menstrual cycles in the first year following menarche were anovulatory. In the third year, 50% were anovulatory, and by the sixth year, only 10% of the cycles were anovulatory.

Many normal young women have a mixture of ovulatory and anovulatory cycles. For this reason, young adolescents who engage in sexual activity should not rely on relative infertility due to anovulation as a form of birth control; there are reports of adolescents becoming pregnant even before experiencing menarche (see Chapters 73 and 74).

MENSTRUAL IRREGULARITY AND AMENORRHEA

The pattern of menstrual irregularity is a spectrum ranging from frequent or prolonged menstrual bleeding to oligomenorrhea and finally to complete amenorrhea as the disruption of the hypothalamic-pituitary-ovarian axis becomes increasingly severe. The basic questions to be answered in the adolescent with menstrual irregularity or amenorrhea are whether ovulatory cycles are occurring and whether the adolescent is in a normal or low estrogen state.

The most minor perturbation of the normal ovulatory pattern is a short luteal phase lasting less than 10 days. Cycles are shortened to 21 to 25 days. The corpus luteum is short-lived and produces low levels of progesterone. The pattern of marginal follicular development with a prolonged follicular phase and a short luteal phase is common in adolescents and may produce long ovulatory cycles.

With further disruption, the LH surge is finally inadequate to produce ovulation, and cycles become anovulatory. If ovulation is not occurring, but the ovaries are still producing estradiol, persistent stimulation of the endometrium by estrogen may cause hyperplasia and dysfunctional uterine bleeding. Thus, anovulation with continued estrogen production may present as short menstrual cycles, excessive bleeding, oligomenorrhea, or amenorrhea.

If, however, estrogen levels are low as a result of the absence of gonadotropin stimulation or the inability of the ovaries to respond to gonadotropins, the lining of the uterus becomes atretic, and amenorrhea ensues. Adolescent girls who lack estrogen are at risk for the development of osteopenia.

Another common pattern of menstrual irregularity is characterized by lack of cyclicity of hormone production, often in association with excess androgens. In this case, estrogen levels are generally normal to high, but the cyclic fluctuation of estrogen and gonadotropins is lacking. LH levels are higher than those of normal adults and markedly in excess of FSH levels. Androgen production by the ovaries is stimulated by LH, and high levels of both androgens and estrogens result. The clinical picture is often one of hirsutism, obesity, and oligomenorrhea, the classic polycystic ovary syndrome (see next subchapter). However, some adolescents with this LH-predominant pattern of anovulation may not have obvious signs of androgen excess or obesity. These adolescents present simply with a history of persistent menstrual irregularity, usually since menarche. Venturoli found a polycystic ovary–like hormonal and ovarian ultrasound pattern in 35% of 110 adolescents with persistent menstrual irregularity. Longitudinal studies are needed to determine whether some of these adolescents are experiencing a transient adolescent anovulatory phase characterized by LH predominance, which will resolve with further maturation, or whether most or all will develop the more classic picture of polycystic ovary syndrome.

Causes of Menstrual Irregularity

The most common cause of amenorrhea or abnormal uterine bleeding in an adolescent is pregnancy (see Chapter 74). The annual risk of pregnancy in adolescent girls 15 to 19 years of age is 10%. The cumulative risk throughout adolescence is as high as four in ten. Random urinary human chorionic gonadotropin (HCG) screening by enzyme-linked immunosorbent assay (ELISA) technique (see Chapter 69) detects less than 50 mIU/ml HCG and is therefore positive soon after conception, even before the menstrual period is missed. The possibility of pregnancy cannot be ruled out by history, since many adolescents may be unwilling to admit that they are sexually active. Any adolescent who is concerned about menstrual irregularity should have a pregnancy test done promptly. Even if she is not pregnant at that time, she may be communicating that she is concerned about the possibility of pregnancy and in need of contraceptive counseling (see Chapter 73).

Systemic Causes of Amenorrhea

Systemic abnormalities disrupting hypothalamic-pituitary function include endocrinopathies (see Chapter 55), chronic diseases, poor nutrition (see Chapter 60), massive obesity (see Chapter 60), intense exercise (see Chapter 81), stress, and certain drugs. All of these probably interfere with normal GnRH release from the hypothalamus, although the mechanisms of the inhibition are not yet well defined.

The endocrinopathy most typically associated with menstrual dysfunction is hypothyroidism (see Chapter 55). Acquired hypothyroidism due to autoimmune thyroiditis is relatively common during adolescence. These adolescents present with poor statural growth, weight well preserved for height, and either delayed or poorly progressing puberty. Young women who develop hypothyroidism later in adolescence may have excessively frequent periods or amenorrhea as their presenting complaint. Cushing syndrome, either due to rare endogenous cortisol excess or, more commonly, long-term use of higher than physiologic doses of steroids to treat chronic disease, is associated with obesity, amenorrhea, and poor statural growth (see Chapter 55).

Most of the chronic diseases resulting in delayed or interrupted puberty or secondary amenorrhea are accompanied by poor nutrition. In these situations, plotting the adolescent's height and weight on growth charts is often the key to establishing the diagnosis. Adolescents should increase both their height and weight. A fall-off in both height and weight or a failure to gain weight may be the clue to the diagnosis of nutritional insufficiency. Inflammatory bowel disease or other malabsorptive states such as gluten sensitivity may present with pubertal delay or failure of pubertal progression (see Chapter 63). Cystic fibrosis (see Chapter 43), sickle cell disease (see Chapter 52), and poorly controlled diabetes mellitus (see Chapter 59) all can be associated with hypothalamic hypogonadism.

Restriction of caloric intake by dieting is a very frequent cause of amenorrhea in adolescents (see Chapter 60). Amenorrhea frequently begins at the onset of caloric restriction, even before significant weight loss has occurred. Although rapid weight loss or loss of more than 15% of weight is regularly associated with amenorrhea, as many as 30% of adolescents with anorexia nervosa lose their menses at the onset of dieting. Other nutritional inadequacies associated with delayed puberty and menstrual dysfunction include zinc deficiency and possibly iron deficiency anemia.

Obesity can also cause amenorrhea (see Chapter 60). About one half of women who are more than twice their ideal body weight have hypothalamic amenorrhea. Other diagnostic possibilities in the obese patient include ovarian androgen excess (i.e., polycystic ovary syndrome), Cushing syndrome, and genetic syndromes of short stature, obesity, and hypogonadotropic hypogonadism, such as Prader-Willi syndrome.

Intense physical exercise is often associated with menstrual dysfunction (see Chapter 81). Athletic amenorrhea is most common in sports such as running, ballet dancing, skating, and gymnastics, which combine prolonged physical activity with restricted nutritional intake and a focus on a thin physique. However, intense exercise itself independent of nutritional compromise can cause hypothalamic amenorrhea, which resolves with decreased activity alone. The typical school sports activity of up to 2 hours of intramural sports a day does not appear to cause menstrual abnormalities.

Transient or intermittent stress-induced anovulation or amenorrhea is common in young women. Although transient amenorrhea is common in women leaving home, most adolescents maintain fairly regular cycles despite many stressful events in their lives.

Opiates are the drugs most commonly implicated in hypothalamic amenorrhea. Valproate may rarely be associated with irregular menses.

Hypothalamic Lesions

Lesions of the hypothalamus itself are rare causes of amenorrhea or poor progression of puberty. They include mass lesions such as tumors, infiltrative lesions, and damage due to pressure, trauma, or radiation. Hypothalamic tumors most often present with delayed puberty; however, germ cell tumors in the hypothalamus or pineal that secrete gonadotropins may interrupt menstrual cycling. Infiltration of the hypothalamus and pituitary by iron in patients with hemolytic anemias such as thalassemia major that require repeated transfusions can interrupt pubertal progression. Histiocytosis X, another infiltrative lesion that interferes with hypothalamic function, often presents with diabetes insipidus and interruption of pubertal progression. Other rare infiltrative lesions are sarcoidosis, tuberculosis, and central nervous system (CNS) leukemia. Survivors of childhood malignancies who received cranial irradiation may begin puberty early but go on to develop hypogonadotropic hypogonadism in addition to growth hormone deficiency owing to late effects of radiation (see Chapter 53).

Pituitary Amenorrhea

The most common pituitary lesion associated with amenorrhea is a prolactin-secreting adenoma. Prolactinomas typically present with headaches, galactorrhea, and secondary amenorrhea in adolescents or young adults, although a prolactinoma may be manifest early in adolescence with an interruption of pubertal progression prior to menarche. Galactorrhea is not always present in adolescents with prolactinomas (see Chapter 77). Other causes of elevated serum prolactin levels and amenorrhea include drugs (phenothiazines, cocaine, and marijuana), cranial irradiation, and pregnancy. Gonadotropin-secreting pituitary tumors have rarely presented as interruptions of puberty in adolescence. Occasionally adolescents have hypogonadotropic hypogonadism due to acquired pituitary insufficiency following head trauma or without any obvious cause. Empty sella syndrome, in which the pituitary appears compressed by cerebrospinal fluid, is sometimes seen in adolescents with pituitary dysfunction.

Ovarian Amenorrhea

Ovarian failure to respond to pituitary gonadotropins is a relatively common cause of amenorrhea. The common clinical feature is a lack of estrogen effect on breast tissue and vaginal mucosa owing to hypogonadism; the outstanding laboratory finding is serum FSH elevated to postmenopausal levels (hypergonadotropism). Adolescents with gonadal dysgenesis constitute the most common group with ovarian failure and account for 10% to 30% of adolescents with primary amenorrhea. If follicle attrition is complete before puberty, the adolescent with gonadal dysgenesis presents with pubertal delay and has only "streak gonads." If some ovarian tissue remains at puberty, she may have secondary amenorrhea or present with dysfunctional uterine bleeding as she enters early menopause in adolescence. Most women with gonadal dysgenesis have a 45,X or 45,X/46,XX mosaic pattern. Others may have an X/isoX karyotype with a portion of the X chromosome preserved. The majority of adolescents with these patterns of chromosomal abnormalities have short stature and the congenital anomalies of Turner syndrome. Other patients with gonadal dysgenesis have a 46,XX or 46,XY karyotype with a normal prepubertal female phenotype. Small deletions of portions of the X chromosome have been found in some patients with a familial pattern of premature menopause.

Autoimmune ovarian failure is another cause of hypergonadotropic hypogonadism usually presenting as secondary amenorrhea. A lymphocytic infiltration is noted in the ovaries on biopsy, and serum antiovarian antibodies may be present. Some of these patients go on to have other autoimmune endocrinopathies, such as thyroiditis, Addison disease, and diabetes mellitus.

Resistance of the ovaries to FSH has been described as another cause of ovarian failure (Savage syndrome). Ovarian failure is also seen with galactosemia and ataxia-telangiectasia. Viral oophoritis is another cause of ovarian failure. Chemotherapy with agents such as cyclophosphamide may result in ovarian failure, particularly when combined with total body irradiation as preparation for a bone marrow transplant (see Chapter 54).

Other ovarian causes of amenorrhea include ovarian cysts secreting estrogen, persistent corpus luteum cysts, granulosa cell tumors secreting estrogen, germ cell tumors of the ovary secreting gonadotropins, and other neoplasms. In general, ovarian tumors are a rare cause of menstrual irregularity in adolescence.

Congenital Abnormalities of the Reproductive Tract Causing Amenorrhea

In the presence of a normal hypothalamic-pituitary-ovarian axis, amenorrhea may result from abnormalities in the anatomy of the uterus or vagina. An imperforate hymen appears as a dark bulging mass in the vaginal introitus in a patient with primary amenorrhea. A transverse vaginal septum blocking menstrual outflow can be detected by probing the depth of the vagina and visualizing the vagina with a speculum. Adolescents with complete outflow obstruction have normal puberty and primary amenorrhea and often have cyclic abdominal pain and a lower abdominal mass consisting of an obstructed uterus or vagina filled with menstrual fluid. Early diagnosis of outflow obstruction is important, since these adolescent patients may develop severe endometriosis due to retrograde menstruation.

Agenesis of the cervix or the entire uterus causes primary amenorrhea. Congenital absence or abnormalities of the uterus, fallopian tubes, or upper vagina (Rokitansky-Küster-Hauser syndrome) are often associated with congenital abnormalities of the renal system and sometimes with vertebral anomalies.

The patient who is 46,XY but has complete androgen insensitivity presents with primary amenorrhea, normal breast development due to testicular production of estrogen, and scanty or absent sexual hair. Müllerian structures are not present, and the vagina ends in a dimple or short pouch.

Destruction of the endometrial lining following infection or surgical instrumentation of the uterus is a rare cause of secondary amenorrhea.

Oligomenorrhea Due to Androgen Excess

Adolescents who lack cyclicity in the function of the hypothalamic-pituitary-ovarian axis have a history of persistent oligomenorrhea, amenorrhea, or irregular but frequent menstrual bleeding in adolescence. The LH-to-FSH ratio is characteristically greater than 3:1, with frequent high LH pulsations, increased androgens, and enlarged multicystic ovaries. Some of the patients with oligomenorrhea and androgen excess have a history of development of pubic hair and acne in middle childhood, several years prior to the onset of breast development (premature pubarche). In some cases this early appearance of sexual hair followed by progressive hirsutism is due to a mild enzyme defect in the pathway of cortisol production, such as 21-hydroxylase deficiency or 3β-hydroxysteroid dehydrogenase deficiency, which results in androgen excess (see Chapter 55).

Most hirsute adolescents do not have a history of early pubarche but appear to have an "exaggerated adrenarche" with hirsutism, acne, and weight gain appearing during puberty, associated with relatively exuberant levels of adrenal androgen production in the absence of an enzyme block. Chronically elevated levels of androgens can cause progressive hirsutism, acne, and weight gain. Androgens are converted to estrogen in adipose tissue, producing a pattern of noncyclic estrogen production. Perhaps owing to this chronic pattern of sex steroid elevation, these women have frequent high LH pulsations and lower FSH levels. This LH predominance drives androgen production by the ovarian stroma, and ovarian androgen excess results.

The enlarged ovaries with a thickened capsule and multiple subcapsular cysts, which are termed polycystic ovaries, may be the result of ovarian or adrenal androgen excess. Many adolescents have ovarian androgen excess without the histology of polycystic ovaries, thus the diagnosis of benign ovarian androgen excess does not rest on the presence of enlarged ovaries by physical examination or ultrasound testing.

In many of the women with ovarian androgen excess, high levels of insulin are present with insulin resistance. These women may have evidence of the anabolic effects of insulin on physical examination (acanthosis nigricans, upper segment obesity, and thickened digits). Insulin exaggerates ovarian androgen production in the presence of LH, thus contributing to the androgen excess state. Elevated levels of prolactin are associated with adrenal and ovarian androgen excess in a small number of patients presenting with hirsutism. Decreased dopaminergic tone may be the underlying mechanism.

Although ovarian and adrenal androgen-secreting tumors are rare, the diagnosis should be considered in the adolescent with rapidly progressive hirsutism or signs of true virilization (deepening of the voice, male pattern balding, clitoral enlargement). These androgen-producing tumors may be too small to detect on ultrasonography, but markedly elevated androgen levels are the clue to the diagnosis and warrant further evaluation for tumor.

EVALUATION OF THE ADOLESCENT WITH AMENORRHEA OR OLIGOMENORRHEA

The adolescent who presents with amenorrhea or oligomenorrhea should have a careful history and physical examination, including a pelvic examination (see Chapter 69). Persistent menstrual irregularity more than 2 years after menarche should not be presumed to be a normal phase of adolescence. Although some of these patients eventually mature into an ovulatory pattern, others have a persistently anovulatory pattern, which can put them at risk for endometrial hyperplasia.

History

Menstrual history includes dates, duration, and quality of menses recorded as exactly as possible. Menstrual calendars can help clarify vague or conflicting information offered by many adolescents. The presence of symptoms of molimen, such as breast soreness and menstrual cramps, can help establish whether cycles are ovulatory, since anovulatory bleeding usually occurs unexpectedly and is painless. In the course of the review of systems, the adolescent should be asked about current, past, or anticipated sexual activity. The special importance of contraception and pregnancy testing for the patient who is sexually active in the setting of menstrual irregularity should be reviewed. Initial hormonal studies to assess the cause of the amenorrhea are appropriate prior to initiating oral contraceptives in the sexually active adolescent with amenorrhea or oligomenorrhea (see Chapter 73).

Nutritional history includes any changes in weight and any restrictions of diet. A 24-hour food recall is helpful if there is a question of nutritional insufficiency. In the athlete, the number of hours spent per day on the sport and the type of exercise should be determined.

Past medical history should include a search for chronic illness, congenital anomalies, past or present medications, exposure to hormonal medication *in utero*, pattern of growth and weight gain in childhood, and age at appearance of secondary sexual development. Any history of possible androgen excess such as hirsutism or severe acne is important. A history of head trauma, meningoencephalitis, headaches, and visual or other neurologic symptoms should be sought since hypothalamic-pituitary dysfunction may follow major CNS insults. A history of herniorrhaphy as an infant may suggest a possible XY karyotype.

Family history should include endocrinopathies, menstrual irregularities, hirsutism, and age at menarche in family members.

Physical Examination

Physical examination should include current height and weight on the growth chart, which should be updated. Certain congenital anomalies might suggest Turner syndrome or chromosomal disorder. Inspection of the skin for acne, acanthosis nigricans, or hirsutism should be made. Terminal hair on the upper lip, chin, sideburns, upper back, chest, and upper abdomen often implies androgen excess. Hirsutism may be quite minimal in the young adolescent with mild androgen excess. Staging of puberty and measurements of breast size with areolar and glandular tissue dimensions are relevant in the patient whose puberty is incomplete (see Chapter 5). An attempt should be made to express milk from the breasts to check for galactorrhea (see Chapter 77).

The pelvic examination is of special importance in the evaluation of the adolescent with menstrual irregularity (see Chapter 69). Examination of the vaginal introitus gives an opportunity for assessment of current estrogen effect. In the presence of estrogen, the labia minora enlarge, the mucosa becomes thickened and pale pink, and there are clear or white vaginal secretions. This impression can be quantitated with a vaginal smear for maturation index done with a cotton-tipped applicator and fixed with a Papanicolaou fixative. Parabasal cells predominate in the absence of estrogen, and increasing percentage of superficial cells appear with increasing estrogen effect. An enlarged clitoris of greater than 5 mm in diameter of the glans implies exposure to androgen excess. The depth of the vagina should be probed with a gentle one-finger examination and the cervix should be visualized, if possible, using a narrow Huffman speculum in the non–sexually active patient. If the hymenal opening is too narrow for a finger or speculum, a cotton-tipped applicator can be used to assess vaginal depth. If possible, a vaginal-abdominal bimanual examination should assess uterine size and evaluate the ovaries for any possible enlargement. If the hymenal opening is too small to permit a vaginal bimanual examination, a rectoabdominal examination in the lithotomy position permits palpation of the uterus and adnexal areas. An adnexal mass brings up the possibility of a cyst, tumor, or ectopic pregnancy.

Laboratory Testing

Laboratory testing in the adolescent with menstrual irregularity can be focused to some extent based on the differential diagnoses suggested by the history and physical examination. Useful initial screens include a urine beta HCG, serum LH, FSH, prolactin level, and thyroid function tests (thyroxine [T4], total triiodothyronine [T3], thyroid-binding globulin index, and thyroid stimulating hormone). A complete blood count and erythrocyte sedimentation rate screen for chronic illness.

A progestin challenge is a useful initial maneuver to assess estrogen priming of the endometrium in the nonpregnant amenorrheic patient. Medroxyprogesterone (Provera) 10-mg tablets are given daily for 10 days. If the adolescent has adequate endogenous estrogen levels, withdrawal bleeding will occur. If she has no withdrawal, her estrogen state is low. Random estradiol levels are of marginal usefulness in assessing estrogen state, since they fluctuate. A vaginal maturation index provides a better assessment of estrogen effect over time.

Serum LH and FSH levels are very helpful in distinguishing between the general categories of central hypogonadotropic hypogonadism and ovarian failure. If the LH and FSH levels are elevated, the tests should be repeated. If there is persistent elevation of gonadotropin levels, ovarian failure is the likely diagnosis, and tests to determine karyotype and antiovarian antibodies are done next. If LH and FSH levels are normal or low, the focus is directed toward central causes of amenorrhea.

If there is a history of headaches, neurologic symptoms, elevated prolactin level, or unexplained hypogonadotropic hypogonadism, a cranial magnetic resonance imaging (MRI) scan or computed tomography (CT) scan should be considered. If hirsutism or other signs of androgen excess are present or if the LH-to-FSH ratio is persistently in the 3:1 range, suggesting polycystic ovary syndrome, androgen levels should be assessed. Testosterone, free testosterone, and possibly dehydroepiandrosterone sulfate (a primarily adrenal androgen) are useful androgen screening tests.

In the adolescent with androgen excess, the possibility of adrenal enzyme defects can be screened for with an 8 A.M. 17-hydroxyprogesterone and dehydroepiandrosterone test, although the usefulness of a single morning sample in ruling out adrenal enzyme defects remains controversial. Adrenal enzyme abnormalities can be more definitively evaluated with a 1-hour adrenocorticotropic hormone (ACTH) test to look at stimulated adrenal androgen pathways (see Chapter 55).

If questions remain about the pelvic structures despite a pelvic examination or if an adnexal mass is detected, a pelvic ultrasonogram may be helpful.

TREATMENT

The treatment of menstrual irregularity depends on the diagnosis. If the problem is hormonal and not anatomic, the fundamental question is whether the adolescent with amenorrhea is in a high- or low-estrogen state. If the adolescent is exposed to chronically elevated estrogen levels (such as with polycystic ovary syndrome), regular cycling with progestins or combination estrogens and progestins (oral contraceptives) is necessary to prevent endometrial hyperplasia and possible endometrial cancer.

If the patient is to be cycled on medroxyprogesterone alone, there is evidence that 10 mg/day for 12 to 14 days each month is needed to convert the proliferative to secretory endometrium reliably in order to prevent endometrial hyperplasia. In the amenorrheic patient who is sexually active, oral contraceptives are preferable to cycling with medroxyprogesterone (see Chapter 73). Anovulation cannot be counted on as a form of contraception, since many adolescents with menstrual irregularity are intermittently ovulatory.

In the patient with polycystic ovary syndrome, a low progestin oral contraceptive combination such as ethinyl estradiol 35 μg and norethindrone 0.5 mg (Modicon) both lowers androgens and allows regular cycles. Ovarian androgen production is decreased and sex hormone–binding globulin increases on oral contraceptive treatment, so that levels of unbound active androgens are lowered. This can stop the progression of hirsutism in adolescents with polycystic ovary syndrome. Hirsutism is usually not reversed by oral contraceptive treatment, so that hair removal by electrolysis may be desired by some women with polycystic ovary syndrome once androgen control has been optimized. Antiandrogens such as spironolactone can be added if oral contraceptives alone are not sufficient to control hirsutism; however, the long-term effects of using this medication in young women for long periods of time are unknown. Weight control is particularly important in the adolescents with insulin resistance and ovarian androgen excess, since they are at risk for developing type II diabetes mellitus as they get older. Weight loss, although difficult to achieve, can decrease both insulin resistance and androgen production in these patients. Women with polycystic ovary syndrome may have infertility due to anovulation and may need referral for ovulation induction when they wish to become pregnant.

If the adolescent with amenorrhea is estrogen deficient and the underlying problem cannot be corrected, she will need estrogen replacement to protect bone density. It is not clear whether estrogen replacement alone allows the adolescent whose amenorrhea is accompanied by osteopenia to fully recover normal bone density. Bone densitometry is being used in some centers to help quantitate osteopenia in low estrogen states.

Many regimens for estrogen replacement exist. The optimum dose of estrogen replacement in the adolescent has not been established. Estrogen should be combined with cyclic progestins to avoid endometrial hyperplasia. Conjugated equine estrogens (Premarin) 0.625 to 1.25 mg on days 1 to 25 with medroxyprogesterone 10 mg on days 12 to 25 each month is one regimen. Ethinyl estradiol oral contraceptives, 35 µg, are a simple form of estrogen replacement. Estradiol skin patches are another alternative to oral estrogen replacement. If the adolescent has delayed or partially completed secondary sexual development and growth, estrogen replacement is begun at lower doses (i.e., 0.3 mg Premarin daily) to maximize height gain and breast development. The optimal age for beginning estrogen replacement in adolescence has not yet been established. Estrogen replacement should probably be seriously considered by age 16 years in the hypoestrogenic adolescent with hypothalamic amenorrhea and by age 12 to 14 years in the girl with ovarian failure.

BIBLIOGRAPHY

Apter D: Serum steroids and pituitary hormones in female puberty: A partly longitudinal study. Clin Endocrinol 12:107, 1980.

Apter D, Raisanen I, Ylostalo P, Vihko R: Follicular growth in relation to serum hormonal patterns in adolescent compared with adult menstrual cycles. Fertil Steril 47:82, 1987.

Barbieri RL, Smith S, Ryan KJ: The role of hyperinsulinemia in the pathogenesis of ovarian hyperandrogenism. Fertil Steril 50:197, 1988.

Breen JL, Maxson WS: Ovarian tumors in children and adolescents. Clin Obstet Gynecol 20:607, 1977.

Emans SJ, Goldstein DP: Pediatric and Adolescent Gynecology, 3rd ed. Boston, Little, Brown, 1990.

Kaplan SL, Grumbach MM, Aubert ML: The ontogenesis of pituitary hormones and hypothalamic factors in the human fetus: Maturation of central nervous system regulation of anterior pituitary function. Recent Prog Horm Res 32:161, 1976.

Lamarchand-Beraud T, Zufferey MM, Reymond M, Rey I: Maturation of the hypothalamo-pituitary-ovarian axis in adolescent girls. J Clin Endocrinol Metab 54:241, 1982.

McDonough PG: Amenorrhea—Etiologic approach to diagnosis. Fertil Steril 30:1, 1978.

Oherlihy C, Pepperell RJ, Evans JH: The significance of FSH elevation in young women with disorders of ovulation. Br Med J 281:1447, 1980.

Rivkees SA, Crawford JD: The relationship of gonadal activity and chemotherapy-induced gonadal damage. JAMA 259:2123, 1988.

Sherman BM, Korenman SG: Hormonal characteristics of the human menstrual cycle throughout reproductive life. J Clin Invest 55:699, 1975.

Soules MR: Adolescent amenorrhea. Pediatr Clin North Am 34:1083, 1987.

Venturoli S, Porcu E, Fabbri R, et al: Menstrual irregularities in adolescents: Hormonal pattern and ovarian morphology. Hormone Res 24:269, 1986.

Venturoli S, Porcu E, Gammi L, et al: Different gonadotropin pulsatile fashions in anovulatory cycles of young girls indicate different maturational pathways in adolescence. J Clin Endocrinol Metab 65:785, 1987.

Widholm O, Kantero RL: Menstrual pattern of adolescent girls according to chronological and gynecological ages. Acta Obstet Gynecol Scand 14:19, 1971.

DYSFUNCTIONAL UTERINE BLEEDING

JOAN B. WENNING

Menstruation is perceived by most women as a once monthly, self-limited episode of vaginal bleeding, which varies little from cycle to cycle. Concerns related to variations in menstrual flow are common presenting complaints in the first several years of menstruation. Episodes of vaginal bleeding may be perceived as too heavy, too frequent, or too long.

The average blood loss per menstrual cycle should be 20 to 80 ml. Quantitating blood loss historically is difficult. Pad counts are not helpful, as the fastidious woman may change her pad when minimally soiled. An adolescent reporting heavy flow associated with clotting should make the clinician alert, as the clotting suggests that bleeding may be so brisk that the intrauterine fibrinolytic mechanism has not had an opportunity to "turn on." A search for symptoms suggestive of anemia, for example, dizziness and fatigue, may help support a story of heavy menstruation. Determination of hemoglobin and hematocrit levels can be used to help identify the adolescent who requires active intervention rather than education and observation.

The mean duration of normal intrauterine bleeding is 4 to 7 days. Continued bleeding after 10 days should be actively managed. Menstruation can also be characterized by the interval or frequency of flow. The first day of bleeding is day 1 of the cycle, and the interval of flow is always counted from day 1 to day 1. A mean interval is 28 days, with a range of 21 to 44 days (see also subchapter on amenorrhea).

A normal pattern of menstrual bleeding occurs when the endometrium is stimulated by estrogen for a 2-week period, followed by combined estrogen and progesterone stimulation for an additional 2 weeks. Endometrial tissue so stimulated is structurally stable. With a simultaneous withdrawal of estrogen and progesterone, the endometrium regresses, and vasoconstriction with tissue breakdown occurs as a universal event. Endometrial lysosomes and prostaglandins are important mediators of this tissue breakdown. An active fibrinolytic system is present within the endometrium; this is necessary to prevent clot organization and scarring of the uterine cavity. Abnormalities in the steroid hormonal milieu, abnormalities in prostaglandin production, or an underlying coagulopathy conceivably could present as abnormal uterine bleeding (see Chapter 52).

Dysfunctional uterine bleeding may be defined as

abnormal uterine bleeding without a discernible organic uterine or pelvic pathologic condition. In the adolescent girl, anovulation secondary to an immaturity of the positive feedback of estrogen to the hypothalamus is the most common cause (see also subchapter on amenorrhea). The differential diagnosis of dysfunctional uterine bleeding in the young woman includes complications of pregnancy (see Chapter 74), pelvic inflammatory disease (PID; see Chapter 75), disorders of hemostasis, and systemic diseases (Table 70–1). Iron deficiency anemia is felt by some to aggravate dysfunctional uterine bleeding.

In one report of 59 adolescent patients who presented to the hospital with menorrhagia, 19% were found to have a primary coagulation disorder and 7% were found to have other major contributing pathologic conditions. Seventy-four percent were believed to have dysfunctional uterine bleeding, a diagnosis made by exclusion.

The anovulatory adolescent who does not produce progesterone has a structurally unstable endometrium. Continued unexposed estrogen stimulation of the endometrium produces a fragile structure that breaks down randomly in response to fluctuating levels of estrogen. It is this uncoordinated tissue breakdown that produces prolonged episodes of bleeding.

Adolescents will frequently note that anovulatory bleeding is painless and that they have no premenstrual warning symptoms that they are about to bleed. Additionally, the interval of bleeding is often very erratic. It is often this unpredictability of bleeding that is most distressing to a young girl.

TABLE 70–1. Differential Diagnosis of Dysfunctional Uterine Bleeding in the Adolescent Girl

Complications of pregnancy	Threatened abortion
	Incomplete abortion
	Missed abortion
	Ectopic pregnancy
	Molar pregnancy
Pelvic inflammatory disease	Endometritis
	Cervicitis
Blood dyscrasias	Thrombocytopenia
	Clotting disorders
	Platelet disorders (von Willebrand disease)
	Iron deficiency
Endocrine disorders	Hypothyroidism
	Polycystic ovarian disease
	Hyperprolactinemia
	Diabetes mellitus
	Adrenal disease
Ovarian tumor	Functional neoplasm
Uterine problems	Intrauterine contraceptive device
	Endometritis
	Submucous leiomyoma
	Break-through bleeding with oral contraceptive pills
Cervical problems	Cervicitis
	Tumor
	Hemangioma
Vaginal problems	Tumor
	Trauma
	Foreign body
Endometriosis	
Systemic diseases	Systemic lupus erythematosus
	Renal failure
Medications	Anticoagulants
	Platelet inhibitors

Mild unpredictable dysfunctional uterine bleeding usually requires little medical intervention. A complete history and physical examination are always necessary; not uncommonly this will be a young girl's first gynecologic examination (see Chapter 69). Instrumentation of the vagina may not be necessary at the time of this first assessment; examination of the external genitalia and a rectoabdominal examination will often suffice. However, if the adolescent does not respond as expected to a therapeutic regimen, instrumentation of the vagina is then necessary to search for a local cause of bleeding such as a lesion or laceration.

Adolescent and parental education with ongoing review will often suffice until ovulatory cycles become established. Charting of menstrual cycles with the aid of a menstrual calendar is a helpful way of identifying an adolescent whose bleeding has decreased or in whom the situation is worsening.

Laboratory studies should be tailored to each individual adolescent, but initially they should include a complete blood count, including a platelet count. Prothrombin time (PT), partial thromboplastin time (PTT), and bleeding time should be ordered in adolescents with menorrhagia occurring with menarche or causing significant blood loss and anemia. All young patients should be questioned about sexual activity, and β-human chorionic gonadotropin testing performed when pregnancy is suspected (see Chapters 69 and 97). In the sexually active population, endocervical cultures for *Neisseria gonorrhoeae* and *Chlamydia trachomatis* should be performed to rule out cervicitis or endometritis as a cause of abnormal bleeding. It can be 2 to 4 years after menarche that ovulatory cycles become established; if the adolescent has been anovulatory for a prolonged time or if her dysfunctional uterine bleeding is worsening, a hormonal profile including determinations of thyroid-stimulating hormone (TSH), thyroxine (T_4), luteinizing hormone (LH), follicle-stimulating hormone (FSH), and prolactin should be carried out (see subchapter on amenorrhea in this chapter).

Both stress and obesity may prolong the postmenarcheal period of anovulation; therefore, weight loss and stress management may be appropriate subjects to explore with some patients (see also previous subchapter).

Iron supplementation to replenish iron stores should be ordered for all adolescent girls with dysfunctional uterine bleeding, even if this bleeding is mild. The dose should be individualized, with the usual dose being 300 mg orally one or two times daily with meals or food.

Adolescents who have a history of more prolonged, heavier bleeding will require medical intervention. Investigations would include those already noted. In addition to iron supplements, some form of hormonal preparation should be ordered to achieve cycle control if the hemoglobin level is between 8 and 11 g/dl. If the adolescent patient is not bleeding actively, a low-dose progestogenic monophasic oral contraceptive pill can be selected, or a progestogen alone can be used (see Chapter 73). The combined estrogen-progestogen oral contraceptive pill gives more complete cycle control more rapidly than does a progestogen alone. The use of an oral contraceptive pill for three consecutive cycles, followed by a progestogen such as medroxyprogesterone acetate, 10 mg orally once daily on days 14 to 25 of this cycle for three further cycles, will protect against other heavy episodes of bleeding while allowing the adolescent to build up her iron stores and, hopefully, achieve further maturation of her hypothalamic-pituitary-ovarian axis. If spontaneous menses occurs independent of the progestogen therapy after several courses of treatment, it may signal that spontaneous ovulations have become established and would suggest that all therapy could be stopped. A menstrual calendar again is a useful way of prospectively charting the adolescent's response to treatment, and it is a helpful aid to the clinician when trying to decide when to withdraw therapy.

If the adolescent is bleeding actively at the time of presentation, a combination estrogen-progestin oral contraceptive pill can be used aggressively to effect hemostasis. A progestogenic preparation such as Ovral (Wyeth-Ayerst) (norgestrel, 0.5 mg, and ethinyl estradiol, 50 μg) would be an appropriate choice (see Chapter 73). One to two tablets can be given initially, followed by one tablet every 4 to 6 hours until bleeding ceases. Commonly, a very dramatic response to this regimen is seen. When there has been no bleeding for a 24-hour period, the dosage of the pill can be gradually reduced by giving one tablet orally three times daily for 7 days, followed by one tablet orally twice daily for 7 days, followed by one tablet orally once daily for 7 days. A withdrawal bleeding episode should be allowed at this point; however, adolescents and parents should be warned that this will be a heavy but limited episode of bleeding. The progestogenic oral contraceptive pill should then be continued once daily on a cyclic basis for an additional 2 months. If the third withdrawal bleeding episode is normal in duration and amount, cyclic progestogen therapy, as described for mild dysfunctional uterine bleeding, can be used. However, the sexually active girl should continue taking a low-dose oral contraceptive pill (see Chapter 73).

Iron therapy should be always be initiated as part of any treatment regimen. Antiemetic therapy may be necessary, since the high doses of hormonal preparation used frequently produce nausea and vomiting.

The adolescent who is actively bleeding, with a hemoglobin level of 7 g/dl or less, and who is hemodynamically unstable at the time of presentation should be given intravenous estrogen, such as conjugated estrogen (Premarin, 25 mg) every 4 hours (up to three doses) until bleeding ceases. Premarin impedes capillary bleeding through its effects on platelet aggregation, coagulation factors, and capillary permeability. Additionally, estrogen therapy promotes the healing and reproliferation of the endometrium. Estrogen therapy should not be given alone; a progestogenic compound should be given simultaneously to produce stability of the regenerated endometrium. An antiemetic should always be administered prior to intravenous Premarin to minimize the side effects of nausea and vomiting. When the vaginal bleeding has ceased, aggressive use of a combined progestogenic oral contraceptive pill as previously detailed can be undertaken.

Frequently these young women are so hemodynamically unstable at the time of presentation that complete resuscitation requires the administration of blood, which should certainly be undertaken only in extreme situations not only because of concerns about the transmission of hepatitis and the human immunodeficiency (HIV) virus but also because of the risk of isoimmunization of a young woman at the start of her reproductive life.

One study reported on the importance of long-term follow-up of young girls who initially presented with dysfunctional uterine bleeding. They found that 60% of their patients had ongoing difficulties with abnormal uterine bleeding 2 years from the time of their initial presentation. They also found that patients with acute adolescent menorrhagia constituted a high-risk group with an increased incidence of operations, infertility, spontaneous abortions, and impaired reproductive potential.

BIBLIOGRAPHY

Badawy SZA, Ashraf R: Dysfunctional uterine bleeding in adolescent and teenage girls. Adolesc Pediatr Gynecol 3(2):65, 1990.
Claessens EA, Cowell CA: Acute adolescent menorrhagia. Am J Obstet Gynecol, 1:270, 1981.
Reindollar RH, McDonough PG: Adolescent menstrual disorders. Clin Obstet Gynecol 26(3):690, 1983.
Van Eijkeren MA, Christiaens GCML, Sixma JJ, Haspels AA: Menorrhagia: A review. Obstet Gynecol Surv 44(6):421, 1989.

DYSMENORRHEA

JOAN B. WENNING

Pain with menstruation or dysmenorrhea is one of the most common gynecologic complaints for which adolescents seek medical attention. Frequently, the onset of the pain is not associated with menarche but occurs several months to several years following the onset of menstruation. Approximately 50% of women will complain of some degree of menstrual discomfort. It is, however, the young girl who has moderate to severe dysmenorrhea that results in time lost from school who will present in the physician's office.

Dysmenorrhea may be classified as primary or secondary.

PRIMARY DYSMENORRHEA

The pain of primary dysmenorrhea is not associated with a demonstrable pelvic pathologic condition. It has its onset not with menarche but with the onset of ovulatory cycles. The pain is characterized as being intermittent and colicky. Frequently it is felt in the suprapubic region and in the lower back, with pain occasionally radiating down the anterior aspect of the thighs. Associated symptoms can include nausea, dizziness, headache, urinary frequency, and loose bowel movements.

Patients with primary dysmenorrhea have increased uterine muscular activity, which results in increased uterine resting tone and exaggerated uterine contractions. Excessive prostaglandin action stimulates this uterine activity. Patients with primary dysmenorrhea have higher prostaglandin $F_{2\alpha}$ ($PGF_{2\alpha}$) concentrations than do nondysmenorrheic patients, and they have an increased $PGF_{2\alpha}$:PGE_2 ratio. $PGF_{2\alpha}$ causes excessive contractions of uterine muscle probably through the induction of increased myometrial gap junctions. The cause of excessive $PGF_{2\alpha}$ release is unknown but may be secondary to abnormally high levels of plasma estrogen. Vasopressin is also speculated to have a causative role.

The role of the autonomic nervous system and catecholamines in the mechanism of dysmenorrhea is unknown.

EVALUATION

The initial assessment of the young adolescent should include a detailed history and a general physical examination. On abdominal examination, the suprapubic area should be carefully palpated searching for a mass suggestive of hematometra. A pelvic examination must be performed but should be tailored to the girl's age and degree of maturity (see Chapter 69). Instrumentation of the vagina in many instances is probably not necessary. The external genitalia should first be inspected with the adolescent in either a frog-legged or the lithotomy position. The patency of the hymen can easily be established by observation alone. Reexamination of the patient in the knee-chest position allows inspection along the length of the vagina and should be done to rule out an intravaginal septum. If the adolescent is not sexually active, a rectoabdominal examination may be performed in place of the vaginal examination. A bimanual examination is important to assess whether a mass or nodularity is present within the pelvis. If no abnormality is discernible, the diagnosis of primary dysmenorrhea can be made without further studies. Pelvic ultrasonography and diagnostic laparoscopy should not be used as routine adjunctive methods of evaluation.

Treatment of primary dysmenorrhea in the adolescent who is not sexually active is the use of a nonsteroidal anti-inflammatory drug that is a prostaglandin inhibitor. This medication can be given prophylactically at the onset of each menstrual period. Naproxen, mefenamic acid, and ibuprofen are medications that have been shown to provide good pain relief. Sixty to 80% of patients using these agents will experience control of symptoms. These agents inhibit the action of the enzyme cyclooxygenase, thereby blocking the synthesis of prostaglandin. Mefenamic acid additionally blocks the action of prostaglandin at an end-organ level. In theory, therefore, this medication should be slightly more effective in providing pain control. In addition to controlling pain, these prostaglandin inhibitors also control the associated symptoms of headache, urinary frequency, diarrhea, and presyncope. Adverse medication effects frequently reported by patients include gastrointestinal upset, drowsiness, irritability, and dizziness.

If the adolescent discloses that she is sexually active, or if symptom control is not achieved with prostaglandin inhibitors, a low-dose oral contraceptive pill should be administered. The oral contraceptive pill can be used either alone or in combination with a nonsteroidal anti-inflammatory drug. By rendering the endometrium relatively atrophic with a low-dose birth control pill, prostaglandin production can be diminished and dysmenorrhea secondarily relieved (see Chapter 73).

SECONDARY DYSMENORRHEA

Menstrual discomfort that is not relieved by treatment using both a nonsteroidal anti-inflammatory drug and a low-dose oral contraceptive pill requires further evaluation. A diagnostic laparoscopy should be performed to ensure that the diagnosis of primary dysmenorrhea is correct.

Early endometriosis can be found in teenaged adolescents and can produce significant dysmenorrhea. Endometriosis in the young woman frequently does not produce palpable nodularity within the pelvis, and the small lesions of endometriosis are beyond the ability of ultrasound to resolve; therefore, an invasive laparoscopic procedure is justified. Suspicious lesions seen at the time of laparoscopy should be biopsied so that tissue confirmation of the diagnosis can be obtained. Endometriosis can be treated medically with continuous oral contraceptive pill suppression, with danazol, or gonadotropin-releasing hormone analogues. Conservative surgical procedures that can be used include cautery of endometriotic deposits through the laparoscopic or laparoscopic laser ablation of deposits.

If a historical review suggests that pain has been present since the onset of menstruation, and a pelvic mass can be defined on physical examination, an outflow tract abnormality such as a noncommunicating uterine horn must be considered in an adolescent girl. Pelvic ultrasound scanning can be very helpful in defining anatomic structures. If a structural abnormality is defined, appropriate reparative gynecologic surgery must be undertaken. Prior to performing any surgery, pain can be controlled by the use of an oral contraceptive pill on a continuous basis, which would eliminate cyclic withdrawal bleeding.

Since adolescents are currently becoming sexually active at a young age, pain secondary to pelvic inflammatory disease should be included in the differential diagnosis of pelvic pain and dysmenorrhea in young women (see Chapter 75). The history of a prior sexually transmitted disease may be suggestive; however, a diagnostic laparoscopic examination allows a definitive diagnosis of chronic pelvic inflammatory disease to be made.

BIBLIOGRAPHY

Klein JR, Litt IF: Epidemiology of adolescent dysmenorrhea. Pediatrics 68:661, 1981.

Pinsonneault O, Goldstein DP: Obstructing malformations of the uterus and vagina. Fertil Steril 44:241, 1985.

Smith RR: Primary dysmenorrhea and the adolescent patient. Adolesc Pediatr Gynecol 1:23, 1988.

PREMENSTRUAL SYNDROME

JOAN B. WENNING

Premenstrual syndrome (PMS) is defined as a cluster of behavioral, somatic, affective, and cognitive disorders that appear in the luteal phase of the menstrual cycle and that resolve rapidly with the onset of menses. It is a major clinical problem for 30% of women of all ages, with 10% being severely affected. The symptoms may appear shortly after menarche and can be sufficiently disruptive that they have a negative impact on the adolescent's interpersonal and educational life.

The most common physical complaints include bloating, mastalgia, headache, weight gain, clumsiness, increased appetite, and backache. Exacerbations of chronic illnesses such as epilepsy, migraine headaches, or asthma may also be seen premenstrually. Affective symptoms commonly reported include depression, tearfulness, anxiety, irritability, and impaired concentration. Food cravings and changes in libido are also seen in some adolescent patients.

ETIOLOGY

The cause of PMS remains unknown. Psychiatric and endocrine hypotheses have been suggested but have not yet been validated. Theoretical nutritional causes, including altered glucose tolerance, abnormal fatty acid intake, and excessive intake of salt, caffeine, and refined sugars have been suggested but remain unproved. Ovarian hormones (progesterone deficiency, unopposed estrogen production), prolactin, thyroxine, and prostaglandins all have been studied, but there have been contradictory and inconclusive results. Since weight gain and bloating are common symptoms associated with PMS, a fluid-electrolyte imbalance has been theorized by some investigators to be the cause of PMS. Renin-angiotensin-aldosterone, antidiuretic hormone (ADH), prolactin, and estrogen all have been studied and implicated, but causation has not been demonstrated. Increased ADH levels may, however, be involved in some cases of premenstrual edema. An attractive theory is that implicating endorphins. Symptoms of increased endorphin release include agitation and anxiety, whereas features of opiate withdrawal include mood lability, lethargy, and decreased motor activity; these symptoms resemble those noted by patients with PMS. Direct

evidence supporting the endorphin hypothesis remains lacking, however. Some evidence also exists suggesting that alteration in serotonin metabolism may be of etiologic importance.

EVALUATION

Retrospective reporting cannot be relied upon to establish a diagnosis of PMS. Before a definitive diagnosis can be established, daily prospective charting of symptoms must be carried out for at least two cycles. This charting allows the physician to confirm a luteal phase clustering of symptoms and should clearly demonstrate a resolution of symptoms with the onset of menses. Use of a simple numeric scoring system (1 = mild, 2 = moderate, 3 = severe) when recording symptoms allows the physician to select three or four of the most troublesome symptoms to which treatment modalities should be targeted. A lack of luteal phase symptom clustering should prompt a search for another diagnosis, such as major depressive illness.

Lifestyle, dietary, and stress assessments should be part of the evaluation of every adolescent patient, as this may aid in identifying negative factors in her daily routine that the patient may immediately address.

MANAGEMENT

The management of patients with PMS can be challenging. Patient education and stress management training should be an integral part of any treatment program.

Dietary changes include avoidance of caffeine, alcohol, salt, and simple carbohydrates. Regular aerobic exercise has been shown to decrease premenstrual symptoms in some women; therefore, a regular physical activity program should be encouraged.

Treatment with oral contraceptive pills, danazol, and gonadotropin-releasing hormone (GnRH) analogues has been used, with varying degrees of success. The oral contraceptive pill may effect no improvement, symptom worsening, or an improvement in symptomatology. It is unfortunate that it is not possible to predict the adolescent who will benefit from this medication. In double-blind studies, danazol in adults has been shown to decrease mastalgia, anxiety, irritability, and lethargy. It is unfortunate that its side effects of weight gain and androgenic activity limit its use. The recommended dosage is 200 to 400 mg/day. The GNRH analogue induces a menopausal state and is effective in ameliorating symptoms in the majority of patients. This medication is very expensive, however; it is administered by injection and can be used for only a 6- to 9-month period. Its use should be reserved for severely affected patients.

The place of progesterone in the treatment of PMS is unclear. Proponents of the progesterone deficiency theory have adovocated its use, but its benefit over placebo has not yet been demonstrated.

Spironolactone, an aldosterone antagonist, has been effective in decreasing weight fluctuations and affective symptoms in double-blind cross-over studies in adults. A dose of 25 mg by mouth four times daily started 2 to 3 days prior to the onset of symptoms is recommended. Spironolactone should not be used in pregnancy; therefore, it is imperative that a sexually active adolescent be using an effective mode of birth control on a consistent basis if this medication is to be used. Other diuretics have not been found to be better than placebo in alleviating premenstrual symptoms.

The antiprostaglandin agent mefenamic acid (Ponstel) has been shown to alleviate some pain symptoms, such as backache, headache, and breast pain. Doses of 250 to 500 mg orally three times a day have been used from midcycle to menses.

The diagnosis of PMS can be difficult to establish. A clear clustering of symptoms must be demonstrated in the luteal phase of the cycle with a symptom-free interval in the follicular phase. The evaluation of PMS patients should include a complete history and physical review in addition to prospective recording of symptoms. Management strategies should include education, dietary changes, emotional support and drug therapy. Selected drug therapies should be tailored to the adolescent's most troublesome symptoms.

BIBLIOGRAPHY

Kendall DKE, Schnurr PP: The effects of vitamin B$_6$ supplementation on premenstrual symptoms. Obstet Gynecol 70:145, 1987.
Keye WR Jr: General evaluation of premenstrual symptoms. Clin Obstet Gynecol 30(2):396, 1987.
Keye WR Jr (ed): The Premenstrual Syndrome. Philadelphia, WB Saunders, 1988.
Lune S, Borenstein R: The premenstrual syndrome. Obstet Gynecol Surv 45(4):220, 1990.
Massil HY, O'Brien PMS: Approach to the management of premenstrual syndrome. Clin Obstet Gynecol 30(2):443, 1987.

CHAPTER 71

Genital Tract Cysts and Tumors

JOAN B. WENNING

Genital tract tumors are uncommon in children and adolescents. Malignant tumors of the ovary constitute approximately 1% of all types of cancer in girls younger than 15 years of age. In childhood and adolescence, approximately 35% of ovarian masses identified will be malignant.

Nonovarian genital tract tumors are even more rare; one study reported on 55 cases identified in Britain from 1962 to 1987 in girls younger than 15 years of age. Of these cases, 28 were vaginal, 9 were of vulvar origin, 12 were of the uterus, 3 were of cervical origin, and 3 were of nonspecified pelvic origin. Eighty percent of the tumors were sarcomas.

VAGINAL TUMORS

In the first 2 decades of life, malignant tumors of the vagina are usually of mesenchymal origin; rhabdomyosarcomas are the most common. Abnormal bleeding or a protruding vaginal mass are common presenting complaints. Prognosis is dependent on the stage of disease at the time of diagnosis. Treatment is multidisciplinary, including surgery, chemotherapy, and radiotherapy.

Clear cell adenocarcinoma of the vagina is rare in young women, but prenatal exposure to diethylstilbestrol (DES), a medication used to prevent spontaneous abortions in the 1940s to 1970s, has placed many young women at a small increased risk. In DES-exposed women up to the age of 24 years, the risk of developing a clear cell carcinoma of the vagina or cervix is estimated to be 0.14 to 1.4/1000. The average age of disease occurrence in women so exposed is 19 years, with a range of 13 to 31 years. All DES-exposed women should have a gynecologic examination annually beginning at the age of 14 years, or at the time of menarche if this occurs earlier. The examination should include careful palpation of the vaginal walls, as the tumor most commonly involves the upper anterior wall of the vagina. Additionally, cytologic specimens should be obtained from both the cervix and the vagina, and an annual colposcopic examination should be performed. Any identified areas of abnormality must be biopsied. A bimanual pelvic examination should also be performed annually. If a clear cell adenocarcinoma of the vagina is diagnosed, treatment modalities may include surgery or radiotherapy, or both.

Mesonephric duct cysts or Gartner cysts are benign cystic lesions of the vagina that are remnants of the mesonephric duct. Characteristically, they are found in the lateral vaginal walls. These cysts are seen infrequently and require no aggressive management if they are not obstructing the vagina.

VULVAR TUMORS

Malignant tumors of the vulva are rare in young adults, and those that occur are usually sarcomas. The choice of treatment modality should be dictated by the stage of disease at the time of diagnosis and can include both surgical and chemotherapeutic approaches. More commonly seen benign tumors of the vulva include varicosities, lipomas and condyloma acuminata.

UTERINE TUMORS

Uterine tumors are also extremely rare in adolescent patients. Adenocarcinomas, clear cell carcinoma, and sarcomatous lesions have been described. Benign uterine fibroids, or leiomyomas are occasionally detected. These fibroids can be followed clinically, and if they do not demonstrate rapid growth, management should be conservative.

TUMORS OF THE CERVIX

Prenatal exposure to DES places adolescents at an increased risk for the development of a clear cell adenocarcinoma of the cervix. Screening strategies for these patients have been already described.

Because many young adults are becoming sexually active at a young age, it is necessary to reinforce the importance of having regular cytologic smears of the cervix performed. Adolescents who are found to have cellular atypia, cervical dysplasia, or changes compatible with a human papillomavirus infection should be referred for a colposcopic assessment. Some subtypes of the human papillomavirus, including papillomaviruses 16, 18, and 31, are believed to have an oncogenic potential that increases the risk of developing a squamous cell carcinoma of the lower genital tract (see Chapter 75).

OVARIAN TUMORS (see Chapter 97)

Ovarian tumors account for 80% of genital tract tumors in the pediatric age group. Germ cell tumors predominate in patients younger than 21 years of age, whereas epithelial tumors, stromal tumors, and sarcomas are unusual.

Common presenting symptoms include abdominal pelvic pain, vomiting, urinary frequency, and constipation. Occasionally a pelvic mass is unexpectedly found at the time of an annual gynecologic examination. Tumor accidents, including hemorrhage, torsion, or rupture, may precipitate a more acute presentation with a surgical abdomen. Some tumors are hormone-producing; therefore, evidence of increased androgen or estrogen secretion may be seen.

The clinical evaluation of the adolescent in whom an ovarian mass is suspected should include careful abdominal palpation and a bimanual examination. At the time of palpation, the location, size, consistency (i.e., solid versus cystic), mobility, and tenderness of the mass can be defined. Ancillary laboratory tests should include serum alpha-fetoprotein and beta-human chorionic gonadotropin (β-HCG) determinations.

Pelvic ultrasound scanning is a valuable tool that allows precise documentation of tumor size and permits characterization of the internal structure of the mass. Characterizing the mass as cystic, complex, or solid aids the clinician in deciding which adolescents can be managed expectantly over several menstrual cycles and which adolescents require immediate surgical exploration. Benign ovarian tumors, which may appear cystic or complex on ultrasound scanning, include benign cystic teratomas, papillary serous cystadenomas, and pseudomucinous cystadenomas. These tumors require surgical intervention. Appendiceal abscesses, tubal-ovarian abscesses, endometriosis, ectopic pregnancies, and adnexal torsion should also be considered in the preoperative formulation of a differential diagnosis of a complex pelvic mass.

A hemorrhagic corpus luteal cyst or a follicular cyst accident may precipitate an adolescent's presentation to an emergency room with vomiting and abdominal pelvic pain (see also Chapter 97). An ultrasound scan of the pelvis performed at the time of presentation may show either a complex or cystic ovarian mass. Expectant management can be undertaken when both alpha-fetoprotein and β-HCG testing give negative results, and the mass feels mobile, tender, and cystic on physical examination. Disappearance of symptoms and resolution of the mass should be seen over several weeks of observation with serial ultrasound scanning.

Simple ovarian cysts are usually of follicular or corpus luteal origin. In the normal menstrual cycle, a cohort of primordial follicles initially are recruited and begin to pass through a developmental process—preantral follicle to antral follicle, to preovulatory follicle. In the majority of cycles, only one follicle becomes dominant and completes the entire maturation process. The developing preovulatory follicle will appear as a small, simple cystic structure on ultrasound imaging. Similarly, the ovulatory follicle and the postovulatory corpus luteum will appear cystic on scanning. Thus, a simple cyst that is less than 5 cm in maximal diameter most probably is a dominant follicle or corpus luteum and should be seen in an ovulatory female. One would anticipate a spontaneous resolution of such a functional or physiologic cyst over several weeks of observation. If there is no pregnancy, the corpus luteum will undergo a spontaneous luteolysis and the cyst will disappear, being replaced by a corpus albicans.

One must be very careful when reviewing the results of an ultrasonogram with adolescents and their parents. The normal physiology of the menstrual cycle should be reviewed so that the adolescent does not equate the simple functional cyst with a pathologic ovarian tumor. It is unfortunate that not only is an "ovarian cyst" equated with a pathologic condition in the adolescent's mind, but also clinicians frequently perpetuate the patient's concern by repetitively ordering ultrasonograms of the pelvis to follow a simple cyst of less than 5 cm in maximal diameter. If an adolescent girl has regular menstrual cycles and a nontender pelvis on bimanual examination, the finding of a 1- to 5-cm ovarian cyst should be recognized as normal in ovulatory women.

Benign solid ovarian tumors are rare in adolescents, but occasionally an ovarian fibroma will be diagnosed.

Solid malignant germ cell tumors in the adolescent patient include dysgerminoma, endodermal sinus tumor, choriocarcinoma, and gonadoblastoma.

The dysgerminoma is the most common form of malignant germ cell tumor of the ovary. The dysgerminoma is a solid ovarian tumor that occurs bilaterally in 10% to 15% of patients. Presenting complaints may include abdominal pain and abdominal distention. Some syncytiotrophoblastic giant cells may be found within the dysgerminoma. Therefore these tumors may excrete HCG. In the young patient who has not yet had a family, these tumors can be managed with conservative surgery if the tumor is unilateral and well encapsulated. Dysgerminomas are known to be extremely radiosensitive; therefore, adjunctive treatment modalities include radiotherapy and multiagent chemotherapy.

The endodermal sinus tumor is the second most common malignant germ cell tumor of the ovary. Adolescents will frequently present with an abdominal pelvic mass and a complaint of abdominal pain. The average age at presentation is 19 years. This tumor is characterized by the production of alpha-fetoprotein, rapid growth, and extensive intraperitoneal spread. The prognosis for the adolescent with this tumor is often poor, although improved outcomes have been noted recently.

Embryonal carcinoma of the ovary may be diagnosed in the adolescent age group. These tumors may secrete both HCG and alpha-fetoprotein. Approximately one half of patients with this tumor have a hormonal abnormality, including precocious pubertal development, irregular uterine bleeding, amenorrhea, or hirsutism. Treatment modalities include surgery and multiagent chemotherapy. To date, 5-year survival rates have been poor.

Choriocarcinoma is a germ cell tumor of the ovary that differentiates toward trophoblastic structures. This tumor may be mixed with other malignant germ cell elements. These tumors secrete HCG, which is a useful clinical marker that can be used to evaluate a patient's response to treatment. The prognosis for adolescents with choriocarcinoma is poor. Treatment modalities again include surgery and multiagent chemotherapy.

A gonadoblastoma is a rare ovarian tumor that may present as a pelvic mass. This tumor is frequently seen in adolescents with an abnormal chromosomal complement. The prognosis for this tumor is good, and adequate treatment includes bilateral oophorectomy. In the young patient with early-stage disease, consideration should be given to the preservation of the uterus, thus allowing the possibility of a future pregnancy using donor oocytes.

Granulosa and Sertoli-Leydig cell tumors are uncommon ovarian tumors arising from the specialized gonadal stroma. Granulosa cell tumors make up approximately 5% of all ovarian tumors in all age groups. These tumors are estrogen-producing and friable and may be solid or cystic. A 2% to 5% incidence of bilateral disease is reported. Granulosa cell tumors have a low malignant potential; therefore, they potentially can be treated with conservative surgery, preserving a young woman's reproductive potential. Sertoli-Leydig cell tumors account for fewer than 0.5% of all ovarian neoplasms in all age groups but are most commonly encountered in young women. These tumors may produce androgens; therefore, patients can present with clinical signs of masculinization. These tumors have a low malignant potential; therefore, conservative surgery can be undertaken.

Other uncommon ovarian tumors in children are epithelial tumors, which are rare before menarche but may be seen in the adolescent, and metastatic disease, which may present as an ovarian mass.

BIBLIOGRAPHY

Diamond MP, Baxter JW, Peerman CG Jr, Burnett LS: Occurrence of ovarian malignancy in childhood and adolescence: A community-wide evaluation. Obstet Gynecol 71(6):858, 1988.

Disaia PJ, Creasman WT (eds): Germ cell, stromal, and other ovarian tumors. In Clinical Gynecologic Oncology, 3rd ed. St. Louis, Mosby, 1989, pp 417–449.

Disaia PJ, Creasman WT (eds): Management of the female exposed to diethylstilbestrol. In Clinical Gynecologic Oncology, 3rd ed. St. Louis, Mosby, 1989, pp 49–66.

Golladay ES, Mollitt DL: Ovarian masses in the child and adolescent. South Med Jo 76(8):954, 1983.

Haller JI, Bass I, Friedman A: Pelvic masses in girls: An 8-year retrospective analysis stressing ultrasound as the prime imaging modality. Pediatr Radiol, 14:363, 1984.

Kiviat NB, Koutsky LA, Paavonen JA, et al: Prevalence of genital papillomavirus infection among women attending a college student health clinic or a sexually transmitted disease clinic. J Infect Dis 159(2):292, 1989.

Lack E, Goldstein D: Primary ovarian tumors in childhood and adolescence. Curr Prob Obstet Gynecol 11(10):1, 1984.

LaVecchia C, Draper G, Franceschi S: Childhood nonovarian female genital tract cancers in Britain, 1962–1978. Cancer, 54:188, 1984.

Martinez J, Smith R, Farmer M, et al: High prevalence of genital tract papillomavirus infection in female adolescents. Pediatrics 82(4):604, 1988.

Raney R, Sinclair L, Uri A, et al: Malignant ovarian tumors in children and adolescents. Cancer 59:1214, 1987.

CHAPTER 72

Chronic Pelvic Pain

JOAN B. WENNING

Chronic pelvic pain can be a diagnostic dilemma that every clinician treating young women has to address. Frequently these patients are also being seen by a gastroenterologist or general surgeon who has already completed a battery of investigations that failed to define the underlying cause of the chronic pain. Chronic appendicitis, inflammatory bowel disease, chronic constipation, pelvic endometriosis, pelvic inflammatory disease, abdominal pelvic adhesions, and psychosocial factors all have to be included in a differential diagnosis (see Chapters 63 and 64).

At the initial evaluation a detailed history, including a careful characterization of the pain, should be taken. All previous treatments and evaluations must be detailed. Information suggestive of underlying problems or stresses at home or in school should be sought. In addition, symptoms compatible with a depressive illness must not be overlooked. Inquiries should be made in a thoughtful and sensitive manner about ongoing or previous sexual or physical abuse.

A careful abdominal and pelvic examination can aid the clinician in deciding whether a diagnostic laparoscopic examination would be helpful in evaluating the pelvic pain. If it remains unclear as to whether a diagnostic laparoscopic examination should be undertaken, resting the pelvis for several months by using a low-dose oral contraceptive pill on a continuous basis will often help. If the adolescent is free of pain during the time she is on suppressive therapy, this suggests that a pelvic pathologic condition is present, and a diagnostic laparoscopic examination should be performed. If the pain persists unchanged, this may encourage the clinician to defer a surgical procedure until all other evaluations have been exhausted.

A diagnostic laparoscopic examination not only allows the surgeon to visualize the pelvis but also permits a direct inspection of the appendix and the ileocecal area of the bowel. Direct visualization may identify a minimal inflammatory process that is not evident with less invasive testing techniques.

Adolescent patients with chronic pain and no demonstrable organic pathologic condition require continued long-term care so they can continue to function at home and school to the best of their ability. The teaching of stress management and relaxation techniques can, in some instances, improve the quality of life.

BIBLIOGRAPHY

Chronic pelvic pain. Am Coll Obstet Gynecol Tech Bull 129:1, 1989.

Goldstein DP: Acute and chronic pelvic pain. Pediatr Clin North Am 365:573, 1989.

Goldstein DP, deCholnoky C, Emans SJ, et al: Laparoscopy in the diagnosis and management of pelvic pain in adolescents. J Reprod Med 24:251, 1980.

Harrop-Griffiths J, Katon W, Walker E, et al: The association between chronic pelvic pain, psychiatric diagnoses, and childhood sexual abuse. Obstet Gynecol 71(4):589, 1988.

Strickland DM, Hauth JC, Strickland KM: Laparoscopy for chronic pelvic pain in adolescent women. Adolesc Pediatr Gyencol 1:31, 1988.

CHAPTER 73

Contraception

DONALD E. GREYDANUS and DILIP R. PATEL

Providing contraception to the adolescent is an immensely important role. As other chapters in this volume have noted, coital activity is common among today's young people. Millions of teenagers are sexually active, resulting in high numbers of teenaged pregnancies, abortions, and sexually transmitted diseases (see Chapter 2). Although many teenagers do not take active steps to avoid pregnancy (see Chapter 74), there are many youth who will use contraception effectively. Issues of adolescent sexuality, confidentiality, psychosocial issues, reasons for teenaged pregnancy, sexuality education, and other related factors are discussed elsewhere in this volume (see Chapters 9, 20, and 68). This chapter focuses on methods of contraception that are applicable specifically to adolescents (Table 73–1).

The ideal contraceptive method is 100% effective in preventing pregnancy, results in no side effects, can be easily used by the teenager, and is reversible. Although no method except abstinence is "perfect" according to these standards, a number of methods are suitable for youth. It is the responsibility of the health care professional to match the needs of sexually active adolescents with the methods most suitable and acceptable to them.

Despite advances in contraceptive technology (Table 73–2), it must be remembered that such methods are not effective for sexually active adolescents unless they are educated about the existence of such techniques by a sensitive health care professional who has the patience to teach them how to use the method or methods that are suitable for them. In the field of adolescent medicine, the application of contraceptive technology is as important as the method itself.

EVALUATION OF THE ADOLESCENT

Table 73–3 presents a plan for evaluating adolescents for birth control, with suggestions for background questions, history taking. and content of the physical examination. At the end of this initial evaluation, the provider should know whether the adolescent is at risk for pregnancy, wants to prevent pregnancy, is mature enough to understand the consequences of pregnancy and of the method under consideration, and is legally able to assume responsibility for the method.

PREVENTION OF ADOLESCENT PREGNANCY

The various means of preventing adolescent pregnancy will be discussed, with the greatest emphasis on oral contraception and barrier contraception.

Abstinence

A discussion of preventing pregnancy in teenagers should always begin but not end with abstinence. The reasons that youth become sexually active are complex and multiple and include biologic, personal, cultural, and social causes (see Chapter 68). When counseling adolescents about modern contraceptive technology, one should not forget the method with the lowest pregnancy rate—abstinence. Teenagers can be reminded that coital activity is *not* psychologically or physiologi-

TABLE 73–1. Methods of Contraception for Adolescents

Abstinence
Combined birth control pill (estrogen and progestin)
Mini-pill (progestin-only pill)
Barrier methods
  Condoms
  Diaphragm
  Cervical cap
  Vaginal contraceptives (gels, foams, tablets, film, suppositories, other)
  Vaginal sponge
Subdermal implants
  Norplant and Norplant-2
  Capronor
Injectable contraceptives
  Medroxyprogesterone acetate
  Norethindrone enanthate and others
Intrauterine devices
  Progestasert
  ParaGard
Other
  Postcoital contraceptives
  Rhythm method
  Noncoital sexual activity
  Miscellaneous

Adapted with permission from Greydanus DE, Lonchamp DA: Contraception in the adolescent. Med Clin North Am 74:35, 1990.

TABLE 73–2. New Contraceptive Methods

FEMALE	MALE
Postcoital contraceptives designed for regular use	Inhibin (FSH suppression)
Prostaglandin-impregnated tampon	Epididymal function inhibition
Vaccine to prevent pregnancy, which acts on a β-subunit of HCG or human placental lactogen	Combination of androgen and estrogen
Various vehicles for slow release of progesterone	Analogue of testosterone
New progestin IUDs	Immunization
Subdermal progestin implants	Gossypol (male pill developed in China)
Intravaginal ring (with or without estrogen)	
Miscellaneous long-acting injectable contraceptives	
Improved vaginal contraceptives	
Transdermal contraceptive patch	
Mifepristone (RU-486)	

HCG, human chorionic gonadotropin.

With permission from Greydanus DE, Lonchamp DA: Contraception in the adolescent. Med Clin North Am 74:35, 1990.

cally necessary, and postponement of such activity is highly recommended. Counseling may identify why a teenager has decided to become or remain coitally active. There are young persons who will heed the advice for abstinence. However, adolescents who are or who wish to be sexually active will not heed the counselor's advice on abstinence and will seek specific contraceptive information. Thus, it is advisable to start with encouragement for abstinence but to be prepared to proceed to a discussion of other methods (see Table 73–1). Since the risk of pregnancy from a single coital episode is 2% to 4%, reliance on a stern warning "not to do it" with a teenager determined to experiment sexually is not in the overall best interests of either the young person or society.

Oral Contraception (Combined Pill)

The contraceptive pill remains the main medical contraceptive method of sexually active teenagers. Currently there are more than 30 brands available in the United States, consisting of a synthetic estrogen and a synthetic progestogen (Tables 73–4 and 73–5).

The two most commonly used contraceptive estrogens are ethinyl estradiol and mestranol. Mestranol is the methyl form of ethinyl estradiol; it is converted to ethinyl estradiol and undergoes further transformation to estradiol in the liver. Other contraceptive estrogens are known, but ethinyl estradiol will remain the current contraceptive agent of choice for the near future. Synthetic progestogens used in the United States include levonorgestrel, norgestrel, ethynodiol diacetate, norethindrone acetate, norethindrone, and norethynodrel. Other progestins are available in other countries.

Research over the past 20 years has produced effective contraceptives that have a lower hormonal content (commonly referred to as low-dose monophasic contraceptives containing 30 to 35 μg of estrogen), as well as a varying hormonal content during the menstrual cycle

(referred to as triphasic contraceptives [Table 73–5]). Choices for progestin selection are increasing. Progestins likely to be used in new oral contraceptive combination include norgestimate, desogestrel, gestodene, and cyproterone acetate, which is a 17-hydroxyprogesterone and a potent antiandrogenic hormone. Norgestimate,

TABLE 73–3. Evaluation of the Adolescent for Birth Control

BACKGROUND
What is the teenager's age?
What is the motivation for seeking contraception?
Does he or she want to prevent a pregnancy?
Does he or she want a contraceptive method? Who else is aware of his or her decision? If parents are aware, what are their perceptions? If boyfriend or girlfriend is aware, what are his or her perceptions? Are the couple sharing contraceptive responsibility? How? Discuss condom use (see text).
What led to the present visit?
What is his or her current knowledge about contraception? Sex education?
What sexual behaviors are being engaged in?
Will he or she accept a barrier method? Is the female partner an appropriate candidate for using the barrier method?
What concerns does he or she have about oral contraceptives? Discuss any specific concerns.
Can she take the oral contraceptive pill on a daily basis?
HISTORY (FEMALE)
Gynecologic history
   History of abortions, pregnancies, sexually transmitted diseases.
   Menstrual history—menarche, frequency and duration of menses, regularity over the past year, last period, menstrual and perineal hygiene, intermenstrual bleeding, cramps.
Complete medical history and review of systems—particularly attempt to identify the following when considering the use of oral contraception:
   Contraindications.
   Conditions influenced by use of oral contraceptives (e.g., acne, using contact lenses).
   Known drug allergies, current or anticipated use of other medications.
   Cardiovascular risk factors, e.g., lipid disorders, family history of premature heart disease, personal history of smoking, obesity.
   Behavioral or psychiatric problems, alcohol or drug use.
Assessment of adolescent's psychosocial maturation (see Chapter 9).
PHYSICAL EXAMINATION
General physical examination with particular emphasis on the following:
   Height, weight, blood pressure
   Thyroid examination
   Sexual maturity rating
   Breast examination
   Cardiovascular system
   Liver: size, tenderness, stigmata of chronic disease
   Skin: acne, melasma, xanthomata
Pelvic examination: external, by speculum, and bimanual
   Obtain specimens for Papanicolaou smear and tests for *Neisseria gonorrhoeae* and *Chlamydia trachomatis*
   Evaluate for other sexually transmitted diseases
Testicular examination and cultures for sexually transmitted diseases
Laboratory tests—Not routinely performed but should be considered on an individual basis if indicated.
   Complete urinalysis
   Complete blood count
   Liver function tests
   Fasting blood glucose
   Serologic tests for syphilis
   Sickle cell screen if not known
   Serum lipids or lipoproteins

Adapted from Greydanus DE, McAnarney ER: Contraception in the adolescent. Current concepts for the pediatrician. Reproduced by permission of Pediatrics, Vol 65, page 6, copyright 1980.

TABLE 73–4. Some Oral Contraceptives

DRUG	ESTROGEN (μg)	μg/CYCLE	PROGESTIN (mg)	mg/CYCLE
COMBINATION				
Loestrin 1/20 (Parke-Davis)	Ethinyl estradiol (20)	420	Norethindrone Acetate (1)	21
Loestrin 1.5/30 (Parke-Davis)	Ethinyl estradiol (30)	630	Norethindrone Acetate (1.5)	31.5
Levlen (Berlex)	Ethinyl estradiol (30)	630	Levonorgestrel (0.15)	3.15
Nordette	Ethinyl estradiol (30)	630	Levonorgestrel (0.15)	3.15
Lo/Ovral (Wyeth-Ayerst)	Ethinyl estradiol (30)	630	Noregestrel (0.3)	6.3
Modicon (Ortho)	Ethinyl estradiol (35)	735	Norethindrone (0.5)	10.5
Genora 0.5/35 (Rugby)	Ethinyl estradiol (35)	735	Norethindrone (0.5)	10.5
Nelova 0.5/35	Ethinyl estradiol (35)	735	Norethindrone (0.5)	10.5
Norinyl 1 + 35 (Syntex)	Ethinyl estradiol (35)	735	Norethindrone (1)	21
Norethin 1/35 (Searle)	Ethinyl estradiol (35)	735	Norethindrone (1)	21
Nelova 1/35 (Watson)	Ethinyl estradiol (35)	735	Norethindrone (1)	21
Genora 1/35 (Rugby)	Ethinyl estradiol (35)	735	Norethindrone (1)	21
Ortho-Novum 1/35 (Ortho)	Ethinyl estradiol (35)	735	Norethindrone (1)	21
Ovcon 35 (Mead Johnson)	Ethinyl estradiol (35)	735	Norethindrone (0.4)	8.4
Demulen 1/35 (Searle)	Ethinyl estradiol (35)	735	Ethynodiol diacetate (1)	21
Norlestrin 1/50 (Parke-Davis)	Ethinyl estradiol (50)	1050	Norethindrone acetate (1)	21
Ovcon 50 (Mead Johnson)	Ethinyl estradiol (50)	1050	Norethindrone (1)	21
Norlestrin 2.5/50 (Parke-Davis)	Ethinyl estradiol (50)	1050	Norethindrone acetate (2.5)	52.5
Demulen 1/50 (Searle)	Ethinyl estradiol (50)	1050	Ethynodiol diacetate (1)	21
Ovral (Wyeth-Ayerst)	Ethinyl estradiol (50)	1050	Norgestrel (0.5)	10.5
Norinyl 1 + 50 (Syntex)	Mestranol (50)	1050	Norethindrone (1)	21
Ortho-Novum 1/50	Mestranol (50)	1050	Norethindrone (1)	21
Norethin 1/50	Mestranol (50)	1050	Norethindrone (1)	21
Nelova 1/50	Mestranol (50)	1050	Norethindrone (1)	21
Minulet	Ethinyl estradiol (30)	630	Gestodene (0.75)	21
Marvelon	Ethinyl estradiol (30)	630	Desogestrel (1.5)	31.5
Cilest	Ethinyl estradiol (35)	735	Norgestimate (2.5)	52.5

Partly adapted from Med Lett Drug Ther 30:106, 1988.

desogestrel, and gestodene are 19-nortestosterone progestogens chemically related to levonorgestrel. They are antiandrogenic and nonantiestrogenic and have an endometrium-sparing effect. The advantages of these agents may include a decreased incidence of acne vulgaris, weight gain, and amenorrhea in youth when compared with traditional progestins.

Both estrogen and progestin can inhibit ovulation, but when taken together this combination is reliable because of inhibition of follicle-stimulating hormone (FSH) and luteinizing hormone (LH). Combined oral contraceptives act mainly at the level of the hypothalamus and inhibit the hypothalamic-elaborated gonadotropin-releasing hormone (GnRH). This results in suppression of pituitary gonadotropin activities and secondary ovarian suppression. Other effects of the combination oral contraceptive pill include endometrial atrophy, which prevents blastocyst implantation, and cervical mucus thickening, which reduces sperm penetration.

CONTRAINDICATIONS

Clinicians often find the concept of absolute and relative contraindications to the use of oral contracep-

TABLE 73–5. Triphasic Oral Contraceptives

Tri-Norinyl (Syntex)
  Ethinyl estradiol, 35 μg
  Norethindrone, 0.5 mg/day first 7 days, 1.0 mg/day next 9 days,
    0.5 mg/day next 5 days
  Total estrogen dose/cycle: 735 μg
  Total progestin dose/cycle: 15 mg
Triphasil (Wyeth)/Tri-Levlen (Berlex)
  Ethinyl estradiol, 30 μg first 6 days, 40 μg next 5 days, 30 μg next
    10 days
  Levorgestrel, 0.05 mg/day first 6 days, 0.075 mg/day next 5 days,
    0.125 mg/day next 10 days
  Total estrogen dose/cycle: 680 μg
  Total progestin dose/cycle: 1.925 mg
Ortho-Novum 7/7/7 (Ortho)
  Ethinyl estradiol, 35 μg
  Norethindrone, 0.5 mg/day first 7 days, 0.75 mg/day next 7 days, 1
    mg/day next 7 days
  Total estrogen dose/cycle: 735 μg
  Total progestin dose/cycle: 15.75 mg

With permission from Greydanus DE, Lonchamp DA: Contraception in the adolescent. Med Clin North Am 74:35, 1990.

TABLE 73–6. Contraindications to Oral Contraception

ABSOLUTE CONTRAINDICATIONS (ACOG)
  History of thromboembolic disease
  Liver dysfunction
  Undiagnosed uterine bleeding
  Pregnancy
  Breast cancer
  Other estrogen-dependent neoplasias
OTHER STRONG CONTRAINDICATIONS
  Severe hypertension
  Cyanotic heart disease
RELATIVE CONTRAINDICATIONS
  Chorea
  Collagen vascular disease
  Depression
  Drug interactions
  Estrogen-related dermatologic disorders (melasma)
  Lactation
  Retinal disorders
  Severe migraine headaches
  Hyperlipidemia

ACOG, American College of Obstetricians and Gynecologists.
Adapted with permission from Greydanus DE, McAnarney ER: Menstruation and its disorders in adolescence. Curr Probl Pediatr 12(10):22, 1982.

tives useful (Table 73–6). The American College of Obstetricians and Gynecologists notes the following conditions as absolute contraindications to the use of oral contraception: history of thromboembolic or thrombotic disease, liver dysfunction (cholestatic jaundice of pregnancy, jaundice with pill use, hepatic adenoma, carcinoma, or benign liver tumor), undiagnosed uterine bleeding, pregnancy, breast cancer, and other estrogen-dependent neoplasias. Breast cancer and estrogen-dependent neoplasia are unusual in the adolescent population. Table 73–6 lists other absolute and relative contraindications. The relative contraindications are those in which the use of the oral contraceptive produces some risk through the production of side effects; however, the consequences of pregnancy in a teenager may pose even greater risks. Clinical judgment should be exercised in prescribing an oral contraceptive when a relative contraindication is identified.

BENEFITS

Oral contraception is a highly effective, generally safe and acceptable method of reversible pregnancy prevention. The combined oral contraceptive pill has a theoretical failure rate of 0.1 to 0.3, and when taken regularly the pregnancy rate is less than 1/100 women years. Table 73–7 lists the noncontraceptive benefits of oral contraceptives, and a guide to prescribing oral contraception is outlined in Table 73–8.

COMMON SIDE EFFECTS

Oral contraceptive–related side effects are commonly classified as progestin-induced or estrogen-induced (Table 73–9). It is tempting to seek a reduction or elimination of an oral contraceptive side effect by altering the estrogen or progestin ratio. However, it is difficult to predict accurately what side effects are caused solely by any specific contraceptive steroid. Teenagers are often impatient with these side effects and do not tolerate frequent changing of brands as well as adults do.

MANAGEMENT OF COMMON SIDE EFFECTS

Weight Gain

Weight gain associated with fluid retention is caused by estrogen excess, whereas weight gain resulting from increased appetite is caused by progestin-induced appetite. Studies in adolescents have shown no significant weight changes with currently used low-dose formulations. Pregnancy should be ruled out in unexplained weight gain. If the gain appears to be pill-related, a low-progestin oral contraceptive should be tried, and caloric intake should be monitored.

Acne

Acne and hirsutism usually improve with oral contraceptive use. Occasional exacerbation of acne is usually caused by excess progestin. Acne is usually controlled

**TABLE 73–7. Noncontraceptive Health Benefits
of Oral Contraceptives**

WELL-DOCUMENTED, NONCONTROVERSIAL
Protection Against:
Life-threatening diseases
  Ovarian cancer
  Endometrial cancer
  Salpingitis
  Ectopic pregnancy
Diseases affecting quality of life
  Benign breast disease
  Functional ovarian cysts
  Dysmenorrhea
  Iron deficiency anemia

STILL CONTROVERSIAL
Protection Against:
Uterine fibroids
Osteoporosis

With permission from Grimes DA (ed): The Contraception Report, Vol 1, No. 3. Morris Plains, NJ, Emron. 1990.

TABLE 73–8. General Guidelines for Starting Oral Contraception

1. Rule out contraindications (see Table 73–6).
2. Discuss common side effects (see Table 73–9).
3. Strongly urge adolescent to refrain from smoking.
4. Note that effects of long-term (5–6 years) use of oral contraceptives in teenagers are not well-defined.
5. Discuss significant early signs of concern, such as severe abdominal pain, chest pain, headaches, and severe leg pain.
6. Review common drug interactions (see Table 73–11).
7. Review benefits (see Table 73–7).
8. Start 30–35 μg of estrogen-containing combination pills. Combination pills are started on day 1, day 5, or the first Sunday after the start of menses, depending on the pill package. Pill should be taken at about the same time each day, preferably after dinner or at bedtime. Triphasic preparations (Triphasil/Tri-Levlen) are started on day 1 of menses. Prescribe a 28-day pill packet. The use of 21-day pills for teenagers is difficult, as they have to remember to refrain from taking pills for 7 days and then must begin again for 21-day cycle. Generally use a pill with 0.15–1.5 mg/day progestin.
9. An additional contraceptive method is used for the first 7 days of taking oral contraceptives.
10. More than 7 days should not be allowed without the use of the active oral contraceptive between cycles. If one pill is missed, the adolescent should take the missed pill immediately and the next pill at the regular time. If two or more pills are missed, the contraceptive potential is reduced; the adolescent should make up pills and use back-up method. Reevaluate to address compliance and alternatives.
11. Schedule first follow-up visit within 6–8 weeks, then at 3- to 6-month intervals. Blood pressure, weight, and side effects should be noted at follow-up visits. Subsequently, a physical examination, pelvic examination with Papanicolaou test and tests for *Neisseria gonorrhoeae* and *Chlamydia trachomatis* should be performed at least once a year. Clinically applicable tests for human papillomavirus infection may soon be available.
12. If pregnancy is suspected, a pregnancy test should be performed promptly.
13. Oral contraceptives should be discontinued 2–4 weeks before and after elective major surgery requiring bedrest or immobilization.
14. Explore the reasons for teenagers not complying with pill use (e.g., psychosocial issues, side effects). Discuss alternatives if the adolescent wants to continue contraception.
15. Individualize approach to each teenager. Special circumstances (e.g., a recent abortion, postpartum status) require special considerations.
16. Instruct about condom use by the male to provide protection against sexually transmitted diseases.

Partly adapted from Greydanus DE, McAnarney ER: Contraception in the adolescent. Current concepts for the pediatrician. Pediatrics 65:1, 1980.

by antiacne medications (see Chapter 39). For adolescents with acne or hirsutism, an oral contraceptive with low androgenic effects (e.g., Ovcon-35, Modicon) may be useful in controlling the symptoms.

Breast Symptoms

Breast discomfort, fullness, and tenderness result from the effects of estrogen; changing to a lower dose of estrogen may help relieve these symptoms. Early pregnancy and primary disease of the breasts should be considered (see Chapter 77). Benign galactorrhea is occasionally noted in adolescents who are taking oral contraceptives, and some authorities recommend discontinuation of the oral contraceptive, though there is no evidence that the contraceptive induces prolactin-secreting pituitary adenoma.

Break-through Bleeding

Break-through bleeding is the occurrence of vaginal bleeding while the woman is taking oral contraceptives. It is seen commonly with the use of low-dose formulations, especially when doses are missed. Ectopic pregnancy, threatened abortion, pelvic inflammatory disease, and endometriosis should be considered in the evaluation of the adolescent with break-through bleeding. Adolescents should be encouraged to comply with regular use of oral contraception.

Break-through bleeding occurs most frequently in the first one or two cycles. Most midcycle bleeding is self-limited and disappears after one to three cycles of contraceptive use. If treatment is needed, increasing the amount of either estrogen or progestin usually solves the problem—for example, a change to Triphasil, Nordette, or Lo/Ovral. Alternately, 10 to 20 μg ethinyl estradiol daily for the first 7 to 10 days of the cycle can be tried for early-cycle bleeding while continuing the current oral contraceptive.

Oligomenorrhea or Amenorrhea

Oligomenorrhea or amenorrhea is commonly seen in adolescents who are taking progestin-dominant or low-estrogen oral contraceptives. Pregnancy should be excluded through a pregnancy test. Pill-associated amenorrhea in usually transient, and menses may return spontaneously. For persistent amenorrhea in an adolescent who desires menses, changing to a pill with less progestin activity (e.g., Norinyl 1 + 35 to Tri-Norinyl or Lo/Ovral to Triphasil) or to a pill with higher estrogen content (e.g., Norinyl 1 + 35 to Norinyl 1 + 50) may induce withdrawal flow and menses. Also, a small amount of supplemental estrogen (ethinyl estradiol, 20 μg, or conjugated estrogen, 0.625 to 1.25 μg) can be added to the regimen for 21 days for one to three cycles.

Amenorrhea after oral contraceptive use may develop in 1% to 2% of women after discontinuation of the pills; 95% of these individuals are likely to revert to regular periods within 12 to 18 months. The adolescent should be evaluated further if oligomenorrhea or amenorrhea persists (see Chapter 70).

TABLE 73–9. Common Side Effects of Oral Contraceptives

PROGESTIN-INDUCED	ESTROGEN-INDUCED
Alopecia	Cervical ectropion or polyposis, or both
Depression	
Elevated blood pressure (?)	Dysmenorrhea or premenstrual
Fatigue	tension (with or without
Leg cramps	edema), or both
Reduced libido	Elevated blood pressure
Hirsutism	Increased mucoid vaginal
Acne	discharge
Decreased menses	Nausea or emesis, or both
Reduced vaginal secretion	Tender breasts or fibrocystic
Breast regression	breast disease
Weight gain (with increased	Weight gain (with fluid retention)
appetite)	Vascular headaches

With permission from Greydanus DE, Lonchamp DA: Contraception in the adolescent. Med Clin North Am 74:35, 1990.

Nausea and Vomiting

Nausea, vomiting, and gastric discomfort are caused mainly by the estrogen in the pill. These symptoms usually occur early on and resolve over the next 2 to 3 months of oral contraceptive use. Pregnancy and gall bladder disease should be considered. The oral contraceptive should be taken with dinner or at bedtime, and a lower estrogen preparation should be used.

Depression

Symptoms of depression are seen in some women who take oral contraceptives; however, it may be difficult to establish a clear cause and effect association. Possible mechanisms postulated for depression in oral contraceptive users include altered tryptophan metabolism and decreased serotonin levels. In adolescents, environmental causes like interpersonal problems and family dysfunction should be considered. A different preparation may be tried, and some adolescents may benefit from supplemental vitamin B_6.

Eye Symptoms

Rarely women on oral contraceptives experience corneal edema and dry eyes. Women using contact lenses particularly should be made aware of this fact. A decrease in the dose of estrogen may be beneficial. The oral contraceptive should be discontinued if visual symptoms, such as decreased visual activity and blurring, develop. Immediate ophthalmologic evaluation should follow.

Headaches

Oral contraceptives may exacerbate migraine headaches, and severe migraine with ophthalmoplegia or hemiplegia is a contraindication to oral contraceptive use. Any woman who is taking oral contraceptives and in whom headaches develop should be promptly evaluated. An oral contraceptive low in estrogen and progestin can be tried, but serious consideration should be given to discontinuing the oral contraceptive if headaches are exacerbated by pill use. A change to a mini-pill or barrier contraception should be considered.

Vaginitis

Low-dose oral contraceptives do not seem to increase the incidence of *Candida* vaginitis, though colonization may increase. Acute vaginitis is usually controlled by intravaginal antifungal agents. Recurrent vaginitis should be treated more aggressively (see Chapter 75), and the adolescent should be evaluated for other contributing factors, such as the use of antibiotics, diabetes mellitus, and genital tract infection in the male partner.

Early Warning Signs

The development of abdominal pain, chest pain, headaches, eye symptoms, and severe leg pain constitutes early warning of significant oral contraceptive–induced side effects, and prompt and thorough investigation is required.

METABOLIC CHANGES

Diabetes Mellitus and Carbohydrate Metabolism

Low-dose combination oral contraceptives exert minimal effects on carbohydrate metabolism. Oral contraceptives can cause reduced glucose tolerance and increased insulin levels. Both estrogen and progestin seem to have a varying effect on carbohydrate metabolism. There may be an increased risk for glucose intolerance in obese women with a family history of diabetes mellitus. There is no increased risk for the development of diabetes mellitus in otherwise healthy teenagers taking low-dose formulations. Alternative contraceptive methods in a diabetic adolescent should be considered (see Chapters 59 and 65). These methods include the low-dose norethindrone oral contraceptive, the progestin-only pill, or barrier contraception. Careful monitoring of the diabetic teenager who is taking low-dose oral contraceptives is suggested, and the clinician should realize that their use is controversial.

Lipid Metabolism

Levels of serum lipids and lipoproteins are altered by the use of oral contraceptives. Proposed mechanisms for such alterations include enhanced liver synthesis, increased secretion and metabolism of very low density lipoproteins (VLDL), increased low-density lipoprotein (LDL) receptors, and suppression of hepatic endothelial lipase activity. The estrogen component may elevate high-density lipoprotein (HDL) levels, whereas progestin may reduce them. With low-dose preparations, changes are minimal. These effects are usually of no significance in healthy teenagers without the presence of a lipid disorder. Careful history taking should rule out other cardiovascular risk factors.

Biochemical Changes

Oral contraceptive–induced biochemical changes are reflected in altered laboratory values. These changes, however, are of no clinical significance in most adolescents. They are listed in Table 73–10.

CARDIOVASCULAR EFFECTS

Major cardiovascular concerns associated with the use of oral contraceptives are myocardial infarction, vascular thrombosis and thromboembolism, hypertension, and cerebrovascular accidents (hemorrhagic stroke, subarachnoid hemorrhage). The risk of myocardial infarction is low in adolescents. Recent data show that the use of oral contraceptives in individuals who do not smoke cigarettes is not associated with an increased risk of myocardial infarction. Current evidence suggests that there is no increased risk of myocardial infarction in past or current oral contraceptive users. Risk of myocardial infarction seems to increase after 35 years of age

TABLE 73–10. Potential Effects of Oral Contraceptives on the Results of a Selected Group of Laboratory Tests

GROUP	SPECIFIC TESTS AND POTENTIAL ALTERATIONS OF LABORATORY VALUES	
	Increased	Decreased
Carbohydrate metabolism	Fasting blood glucose and 2-hour postprandial insulin level	Glucose tolerance
Hematologic-coagulation	Coagulation factor II, VII, VIII, IX, X, XII; erythrocyte sedimentation rate; fibrinogen; leukocyte count; partial thromboplastin time; plasma volume; plasmin and plasminogen; platelet count; platelet aggregation; and platelet adhesiveness	Euglobulin lysis antithrombin III (total); hematocrit; prothrombin time
Lipid metabolism*	Cholesterol, lipoproteins (pre-β, β, and α); phospholipids, total; total lipids; triglycerides	
Liver function, gastrointestinal tests	Alkaline phosphatase; bilirubin, SGOT, SGPT; cephalin flocculation; formiminoglutamic acid excretion after histidine (urine); γ-glutamyl transpeptidase; leucine aminopeptidase; protoporphyrin, coproporphyrin excretion (urine); uroporphyrin excretion (urine); sulfobromophthalein retention	Alkaline phosphatase; etiocholanolone excretion (urine); haptoglobin (serum); urobilinogen excretion (urine)
Metals	Copper and ceruloplasmin; iron, iron-binding capacity and transferrin	Magnesium; zinc
Thyroid function	Butanol-extractable iodine; protein-bound iodine; thyroid binding globulin; triiodothyronine (serum)	Triiodothyronine resin (serum); free thyroxine
Vitamins	Vitamin A (blood and plasma)	Folate (serum); vitamin B$_2$ (RBC and urine excretion); vitamin B$_6$, vitamin B$_{12}$, vitamin C
Other hormones, enzyme measurements	Aldosterone (blood and urine); angiotensinogen; angiotensin I and II; cortisol (blood and urine); growth hormone; prolactin; testosterone (serum); total estrogens	Estradiol and estriol; FSH (urine), LH (blood and urine); 17-hydroxycorticosteroid excretion (urine); pregnanediol excretion (urine); renin (serum); tetrahydrocortisone
Miscellaneous, laboratory	α$_1$-Antitrypsin; antinuclear antibody; bilirubin; complement-reactive protein; globulins α$_1$, α$_2$; lactate; lupus erythematosus cell preparation; pyruvate; sodium	Albumin; α-amino nitrogen; calcium (serum) and calcium excretion (urine); complement-reactive protein; immunoglobulins A, G, and M

*HDL cholesterol is increased with estrogens and decreased with progestins.
With permission from Hatcher RA, Stewart F, Trussell J, et al: Contraceptive Technology, 1990–1991, 15th ed. New York, Irvington Publishers, 1990.

in women with diabetes mellitus or hyperlipidemia, as well as in those who smoke cigarettes or are obese. Vascular thrombosis, and not atherogenesis, appears to be the principal mechanism in myocardial infarction associated with oral contraceptive use.

Estimates for an increased risk of deep vein thrombosis and pulmonary embolism in women who use oral contraceptives range from no risk to a three-fold increased risk. Although the exact mechanism is not well defined, it is generally agreed that there is an increased tendency toward clotting, which may increase the risk of thromboembolic complications in the presence of other factors, such as diabetes mellitus and prolonged immobilization. It is recommended that oral contraceptives be discontinued 2 to 3 weeks before major elective surgery and 2 to 3 weeks afterward for immobilized adolescent patients, particularly those in long leg casts. Symptoms suggestive of pulmonary embolism in an adolescent taking an oral contraceptive should receive prompt and aggressive medical evaluation.

It is estimated that approximately 1% to 5% of normotensive individuals develop hypertension within weeks to months of starting oral contraceptive use. The risk is increased with age, parity, and obesity. The probable mechanism of action involves the effect of oral contraceptives on the renin-angiotensin-aldosterone system. Blood pressure should be monitored closely, and the oral contraceptive should be discontinued if hypertension is noted. Blood pressure usually returns to normal within 2 to 12 weeks once the oral contraceptive is discontinued. Once blood pressure returns to normal, a low-dose oral contraceptive may be started; if hypertension recurs, another form of contraception should be considered (see Chapters 48 and 67).

The issue of the possible relationship between cerebrovascular accidents and oral contraceptive use remains unresolved, with some studies showing no increase in relative risk whereas others show three- to fourfold increased risk. There is particularly an increased risk of cerebrovascular accidents associated with oral contraceptive use if there is hypertension or cigarette smoking and after the age of 35 years.

The risk of adverse cardiovascular effects developing in otherwise healthy adolescents should be carefully weighed against the potential risks of an unwanted pregnancy. In 15- to 19-year-olds, the mortality rate from pregnancy and childbearing is 11 to 12/100,000 live births. The mortality rate for females aged 15 to 19 years is 1.2 deaths/100,000 oral contraceptive users.

DRUG INTERACTIONS

Oral contraceptives may interact with a variety of other drugs. Table 73–11 provides an overview of such interactions.

TABLE 73–11. Pill Interactions with Other Drugs

INTERACTING DRUGS	ADVERSE EFFECTS (PROBABLE MECHANISM)	COMMENTS AND RECOMMENDATIONS
Acetaminophen (Tylenol and others)	Possible decreased pain-relieving effect (increased metabolism)	Monitor pain-relieving response
Alcohol	Possible increased effect of alcohol	Use with caution
Anticoagulants (oral)	Decreased anticoagulant effect	Use alternative contraceptive
Antidepressants (Elavil, Norpramin, Tofranil, and others)	Possible increased antidepressant effect	Monitor antidepressant concentration
Barbiturates (phenobarbital and others)	Decreased contraceptive effect	Avoid simultaneous use; use alternative contraceptive for epileptics
Benzodiazepine tranquilizers (Ativan, Librium, Serax, Tranxene, Valium, Xanax, and others)	Possible increased or decreased tranquilizer effects, including psychomotor impairment	Use with caution; greatest impairment during menstrual pause in oral contraceptive dosage
β-Blockers (Corgard, Inderal, Lopressor, Tenormin)	Possible increased blocker effect	Monitor cardiovascular status
Carbamazepine (Tegretol)	Possible decreased contraceptive effect	Use alternative contraceptive
Corticosteroids (cortisone)	Possible increased corticosteroid toxicity	Clinical significance not established
Griseofulvin (Fulvicin, Grifulvin V, and others)	Decreased contraceptive effect	Use alternative contraceptive
Guanethidine (Esimil, Ismelin)	Decreased guanethidine effect (mechanism not established)	Avoid simultaneous use
Hypoglycemics (tolbutamide, Diabinese, Orinase, Tolinase)	Possible decreased hypoglycemia	Monitor blood glucose
Methyldopa (Aldoclor, Aldomet, and others)	Decreased antihypertensive effect	Avoid simultaneous use
Penicillin	Decreased contraceptive effect with ampicillin	Low but unpredictable incidence; use alternative contraceptive
Phenytoin (Dilantin)	Decreased contraceptive effect; possible increased phenytoin effect	Use alternative contraceptive; monitor phenytoin concentration
Primidone (Mysoline)	Decreased contraceptive effect	Use alternative contraceptive
Rifampin	Decreased contraceptive effect	Use alternative contraceptive
Tetracycline	Decreased contraceptive effect	Use alternative contraceptive
Theophylline (Bronkotabs, Marax, Primatene, Quibron, Tedral, Theo-Dur, and others)		
Troleandomycin (Tao)	Jaundice (additive)	Avoid simultaneous use
Vitamin C	Increased serum concentration and possible increased adverse effects of estrogens with 1 g or more/day of vitamin C	Decrease vitamin C to 100 mg/day

With permission from Hatcher RA, Stewart F, Trussell J, et al: Contraceptive Technology 1990–1992, 15th ed. New York, Irvington Publishers, 1990; as adapted from Rizack MA, Hillman CDM: The Medical Letter Handbook of Adverse Drug Interactions. New Rochelle, New York: The Medical Letter, 1985.

RELATIONSHIP TO CANCER AND TUMORS

Endometrial Cancer

Combination oral contraceptive use has been shown to have a long-term protective effect against the development of endometrial cancer. Oral contraceptive use for 12 months or longer has been shown to have a protective effect against all major histologic types of cancer, and the protective effect has been shown to persist for at least 15 years after discontinuance of oral contraceptive use. Current evidence indicates that the overall risk is reduced by 50% in "ever users." Although the exact mechanism is not known, it is postulated that progestin exerts an antimutagenic effect on endometrial tissue by inhibiting the synthesis of both estrogen and progestin receptors, and this negates the mitogenic activity of unopposed estrogen.

Ovarian Cancer

A number of studies have reported that the use of oral contraceptives is associated with a decreased risk of epithelial ovarian carcinoma. Oral contraceptive use, even for a period of 3 to 6 months, appears to reduce the overall risk of ovarian cancer up to 40% in "ever

users." Protective effects have been shown for up to 10 to 15 years after discontinuance of the oral contraceptive. The protective effect is increased with duration of use. Suppression of ovulation and suppression of pituitary secretion of gonadotropins have been postulated as possible mechanisms.

Breast Cancer

The true relationship between long-term use of oral contraceptives and causation of breast cancer remains unclear. Studies to date have indicated no increased lifetime risk of breast cancer in oral contraceptive users. However, several recent studies have suggested that an increased risk may exist for certain subpopulations of young women with early or long duration of use. The U.S. Food and Drug Administration and the International Committee for Research in Reproduction recommend no change in the prescription of oral contraceptives as it relates to breast cancer but note that the possible risk for breast cancer in the subgroup of young women on long-term oral contraceptive use remains unclear. Longer term studies are needed before the true relationship between prolonged use of oral contraceptives and risk of breast cancer in women is determined with certainty.

Cervical Cancer

The use of oral contraceptives has been shown to increase the risk of cervical cancer by 1.6 to 3.4 times after 4 to 6 years of use. Although it is possible that oral contraceptives may act as a promoter to increase the risk of cervical neoplasia, confounding factors make the risk assessment difficult. A number of other factors have been associated with cervical cancer, such as age of coital initiation (sexarche), number of sex partners, exposure to human papillomavirus (and possibly other sexually transmitted disease agents; see Chapter 75), and cigarette smoking. Teenagers taking oral contraceptives should be screened regularly by the Papanicolaou screening test, and abnormal cervical cytologic findings should be aggressively managed.

Other Tumors

The risk for the development of liver tumors remains extremely low for otherwise healthy teenagers taking oral contraceptives. The risk of benign liver tumors, particularly hepatic adenoma, may be increased on long-term, high-dose oral contraception in older women. When oral contraceptive use is discontinued, a spontaneous regression of these tumors has been shown to occur. Its clinical significance lies in the fact that these tumors have the potential for spontaneous rupture, causing bleeding. The relationship between hepatocellular carcinoma and oral contraceptive use is not well established. No association between the use of oral contraceptives and the development of pituitary adenomatas has been elucidated. Oral contraceptives do not increase the risk for the development of malignant melanoma.

OTHER ISSUES

The effects of oral contraception on a wide variety of medical conditions have been extensively reviewed in the literature. Oral contraception has not been shown to cause premature closure of epiphyses. Oral contraceptives do not induce urinary tract infections. Teenagers taking oral contraceptives may experience increased benign cervical polyps and may have persistent ectopy (see Chapter 69). Oral contraceptives have been shown conclusively not to produce birth defects.

Thyroid function generally remains normal in oral contraceptive users. Thyroxine (T_4) levels may be increased because of increased binding of globulin, but free T_4 levels are normal. Recent data suggest no increased incidence of cholelithiasis. Oral contraceptive-induced pancreatitis has been rarely reported particularly in women with hyperlipidemia. Liver diseases such as Gilbert disease, Rotor syndrome, hepatitis, and porphyria may be exacerbated by oral contraceptive use. It may also exacerbate acanthosis nigricans, alopecia, spider nevi, erythema nodosum, telangiectasia, and angioneurotic edema and may be associated with the development of chloasma, particularly in dark-skinned

women who are exposed to sunlight. Oral contraceptives have not been shown to exacerbate cell sickling. They have been implicated rarely in a number of conditions, including Raynaud disease, pseudotumor cerebri, chorea, neurofibromatosis, and multiple sclerosis.

Oral contraceptives have been contraindicated in women with systemic lupus erythematosus; however, low-dose preparations are used in some adolescents when the risks of an unwanted pregnancy outweigh the risks associated with contraceptive use. The issue of the protective effect of oral contraceptives against the development of rheumatoid arthritis remains unresolved; however, no adverse effects are noted.

Current evidence indicates no increase in seizures in women on low-dose preparations. Anticonvulsants seem to increase the metabolism of synthetic steroids by increasing conjugation in the gut and enzyme induction in the liver. There is also an increase in the production of sex hormone–binding globulin to which progestin is bound. Thus, there is a potential for lowered efficacy of the oral contraceptive and decreased levels of the anticonvulsant. This may result in an increased risk of pregnancy. Some recommend a high-dose preparation, shortened pill-free interval or a back-up method, especially with break-through bleeding.

Mini-pill (Progestin-only Pill)

Mini-pills, or progestin-only pills (Table 73–12), induce contraception through "secondary" mechanisms, which include altering the endometrium (inhibiting implantation), thickening cervical mucus (inhibiting sperm penetration), increasing movement of the ovum through the oviduct, altering the corpus luteum function, and other mechanisms. Three brands are currently available in the United States: Ovrette, Nor-QD, and Micronor (Table 73–12). Removal of the estrogen results in a reduced risk of thromboembolism, metabolic changes, and hypertension. It may be considered for youth who desire oral contraception but have hypertension, diabetes mellitus, or conditions in which estrogen is contraindicated. Although the combined birth control pill may reduce breast milk volume, the progestin-only pill does not; thus, lactation is not a contraindication to the use of the mini-pill. Some individuals will note improvement in premenstrual tension syndrome and dysmenorrhea while taking the progestin-only pill. One should remember that there is an increased pregnancy rate with this pill: one to three pregnancies/100 woman years of use, particularly during the first 6 months of use. A high rate of break-through bleeding and amenorrhea may limit its

TABLE 73–12. Progestin-Only Contraceptives

TRADE NAME	PROGESTOGEN CONTENT
Ovrette (Wyeth-Ayerst)	Norgestrel, 0.075 mg
Nor-QD (Syntex)	Norethindrone, 0.35 mg
Micronor (Ortho)	Norethindrone, 0.35 mg
Femulen*	Ethynodiol diacetate, 0.5 mg

*Available in the United Kingdom.
With permission from Greydanus DE, Patel DR: Contraceptives. Current Opinion in Pediatrics 2:648, 1990.

TABLE 73–13. Advantages of Condoms

Readily available over the counter
Few side effects (occasional allergy to latex rubber)
Protection from sexually transmitted diseases
Reduced cervical dysplasia
Effective contraception
Improvement in premature ejaculation
Many high-quality types
Allows male to share contraceptive responsibility

With permission from Greydanus DE, Lonchamp D: Contraception in the adolescent. Med Clin North Am 74:35, 1990.

TABLE 73–14. Disadvantages of Condoms (Perceived)

Cost
Religious reasons
Reduced penile sensation
Need for change with each coital act
Refusal of male to accept contraceptive responsibility
Limited recommendation by health care professionals

With permission from Greydanus DE, Lonchamp D: Contraception in the adolescent. Med Clin North Am 74:35, 1990.

use in adolescents. Additional side effects that have been reported include headaches, nausea, and hirsutism. Ectopic pregnancy should be considered if the adolescent becomes pregnant. The progestin-only pill is taken daily without skipping any days. Its use should be avoided in youth who do not take pills regularly, who have irregular menstruation, and who have had history of previous ectopic pregnancy. However, there are some sexually active teenagers who are candidates for this "often forgotten" contraceptive pill.

Barrier Methods

CONDOMS

A number of advantages (Table 73–13) and disadvantages (Table 73–14) to condom use have been identified. Adolescents are often reluctant to use condoms, perhaps because of the failure of society to teach male responsibility regarding sexuality. Pregnancy rates can vary from 3 to 30 pregnancies/100 women years.

Many brands of condoms are available for males mostly of the latex rubber variety. Such condoms can block the transmission of various sexually transmitted disease agents—human papillomavirus, herpes simplex virus, cytomegalovirus, *Chlamydia trachomatis, Neisseria gonorrhoeae,* human immunodeficiency virus (HIV), and others (see Chapter 75). The natural membrane condom, which is made from young lamb cecum, does not block the transmission of HIV or herpes simplex virus and is not recommended for adolescents. Research does note that condoms can lead to a decreased incidence and even regression of cervical dysplasia in the female partner. Condoms coated with spermicides (externally and internally) can offer further protection from sexually transmitted diseases and pregnancy. Recommendations for the use of condoms are outlined in Table 73–15. A brand of female condom (WPC 333, Femshield, Wisconsin Pharmacal, Jackson, WI) is now available. It is a loose fitting polyurethane sheath with two diaphragm-like flexible rings at either end. The inner ring covers the cervix and the outer ring fits against the vulva.

DIAPHRAGM

A number of barrier contraceptives are available (see Table 73–1) to the teenager who is motivated to use this technology. The diaphragm is a rubber cap with a metal spring in its rim. Three types with 11 different sizes are available. The diaphragm is normally kept in place by the pubic bone, the rim spring tension, and the vaginal muscles. The nulliparous young woman usually has excellent vaginal tone and can use the properly fitted diaphragm. Its contraceptive ability results from its potential to block sperm trying to enter the cervix and also from the effects of the added spermicidal cream or jelly. Variable pregnancy rates are noted with the diaphragm (2 to 20 pregnancies/100 women years).

Proper fit and proper technique are essential to maximize the effectiveness of the diaphragm. It is usually placed intravaginally 1 to 6 hours prior to coitus and is left in place 6 to 8 hours after coitus. Additional spermicide is used with further sexual activity. The diaphragm's dome is placed convex to the vaginal opening while the cervix is covered. The female should not feel it once it is in place, and the largest size comfortably placed is prescribed. Most young women do well with the coil-spring diaphragm, whereas the firmer flat-spring type may better suit those with a pointed cervix or an

TABLE 73–15. Recommendations for Use of Condoms

Latex condoms should be used because they may offer greater protection against HIV and other viral STDs than do natural membrane condoms.
Condoms should be stored in a cool, dry place out of direct sunlight.
Condoms in damaged packages or those that show obvious signs of age (e.g., those that are brittle, sticky, or discolored) should not be used. They cannot be relied upon to prevent infection or pregnancy.
Condoms should be handled with care to prevent puncture.
The condom should be put on before any genital contact to prevent exposure to fluids that may contain infectious agents. Hold the tip of the condom and unroll it onto the erect penis, leaving space at the tip to collect semen, yet ensuring that no air is trapped in the tip of the condom.
Only water-based lubricants should be used. Petroleum- or oil-based lubricants (such as petroleum jelly, cooking oils, shortening, and lotions) should not be used because they weaken the latex and may cause breakage.
Use of condoms containing spermicides may provide some additional protection against STDs. However, vaginal use of spermicides along with condoms is likely to provide still greater protection.
If a condom breaks, it should be replaced immediately. If ejaculation occurs after condom breakage, the immediate use of spermicide has been suggested. However, the protective value of postejaculation application of spermicide in reducing the risk of STD transmission is unknown.
After ejaculation, care should be taken so that the condom does not slip off the penis before withdrawal; the base of the condom should be held throughout withdrawal. The penis should be withdrawn while still erect.
Condoms should never be reused.

STDs, sexually transmitted diseases.

TABLE 73–16. Spermicides

REPRESENTATIVE PRODUCTS (BRAND NAMES)	SPERMICIDAL AGENT	COMMENTS
Film:	Contraceptive protection begins 15 minutes after insertion; remains effective no more than 1 hour	
VCF (vaginal contraceptive film)	Nonoxynol-9	Small, thin sheets
Foam:	Contraceptive protection is immediate; remains effective for at least 1 hour	
Delfen, Emko, Koromex	Nonoxynol-9	Aerosol container
Emko Because, Emko Pre-Fil	Nonoxynol-9	Small container
Jellies and Creams:	Contraceptive protection is immediate. When used alone remains effective at least 1 hour; used with diaphragm or cap remains effective at least 6 to 8 hours	
Cream: Conceptrol, Delfen, Koromex Jel, Ortho-Gynol II, Ramses	Nonoxynol-9	Reusable applicator
Koromex Cream, Ortho-Gynol	Octoxynol	Reusable applicator
Gel: Conceptrol Gel, Milex Shur-Seal Gel	Nonoxynol-9	Single-use packets
Suppositories and Tablets:	Contraceptive protection begins 10 to 15 minutes after insertion; remains effective no more than 1 hour	
Encare, Intercept, Koromex Inserts Prevent, Semicid	Nonoxynol-9	

From Hatcher RA, Stewart F, Trussell J, et al: Contraceptive Technology, 1990–1992, 15th ed. New York, Irvington Publishers, 1990.

anteverted uterus, or both. An arching-spring type has a double metal spring in its rim and can be used for those women with poor muscle tone and a posterior cervix. Adolescents often find this type easy to insert because of the leading edge. Diaphragm sizes vary from 55 to 95 mm in diameter, but most nulliparous young women use a 60- to 85-mm size. A size change may occur for various reasons: for example, having vaginismus at first evaluation (especially if virginal), status after a midtrimester abortion, or a 10- to 15-pound weight change. The diaphragm should not be used during menstruation because of anecdotal reports of toxic shock syndrome developing in diaphragm users (see Chapter 94). Recent literature has suggested that females using barrier contraceptives, including the diaphragm, have lower rates of cervical dysplasia.

Contraindications to the use of the diaphragm include severe retroversion, severe anteversion, complete uterine prolapse, allergy to the spermicide or rubber, a short anterior vaginal wall, or perineal tears. A major limiting factor for teenagers is their limited motivation and fear of touching their genitals. Use of the diaphragm has been linked to increased urinary tract infections, possibly because of alteration of vaginal flora (*Escherichia coli* colonization), urethral stasis secondary to urethral obstruction, or spermicidal effects on lactobacilli, or a combination of these factors. Suggested ways to reduce the urinary tract infections that may be associated with diaphragm use include frequent urination, proper diaphragm fit, not retaining the diaphragm for more than 8 hours following coitus, and postcoital antibiotic therapy.

CERVICAL CAP

In 1988, the U.S. Food and Drug Administration approved the Prentif Cavity-Rim Cervical Cap. This is a soft, flexible latex cap that uses suction to fit firmly around the cervix and block sperm. Spermicide is added inside the cap, and the cap is left in place for at least 8 hours after coitus; it can be left in place up to 48 hours before adding more spermicide. The cap is about half the size of a diaphragm. As with the diaphragm, the users must be highly motivated, must not be afraid to touch their bodies, must be willing to plan in advance for sexual activity (which is often not the case with teenagers), and must have proper instruction in its use.

An unusually high failure rate is noted if an improper fitting occurs, if the cap is used irregularly, and if vaginal spermicides are not used. Only four sizes are now available (22, 25, 28, and 31 mm). Approximately 25% to 30% of females are not fitted well with these few available sizes. Contraindications to the use of the cap include adolescents who have cervical laceration, cervical scarring, and a history of toxic shock syndrome.

Some young women find it difficult to insert and remove the cap. Vaginal malodor is a concern for some. Research has noted an increase in abnormal results on Papanicolaou smears during the first 3 months of cap use; thus, adolescents using a cap must have normal results on Papanicolaou smear before the fitting and also 3 months after initial use. Regular Papanicolaou smear screening is recommended for cap users at least once a year. As with the diaphragm, cap dislodgement during coitus can occur, as can pregnancy, especially if the fit is not good. The cap, as with the diaphragm, is most useful for teenagers 16 or 17 years of age and older.

Vaginal Contraceptives

A variety of vaginal contraceptives are available as creams, gels, foams, sponge, tablets, films, and suppositories (Table 73–16). The most common chemical used is nonoxynol-9, which lowers sperm surface tension, causing cell wall breakdown. Other chemicals include octoxynol, phenylmercuric acetate, and ricinoleic acid. The efficacy of vaginal contraceptives can be increased when used with other contraceptive methods. Pregnancy rates vary when they are used alone, from 3 to 21 + pregnancies/100 women years. When used in addition to other barrier contraceptives (e.g., condom, diaphragm, or cap) vaginal contraceptives can provide some protection from sexually transmitted disease microbes including *Candida albicans,* herpes simplex, *Treponema pallidum, Chlamydia trachomatis,* and *Neisseria gonorrhoeae* (see Chapter 75). Other advantages include improvement of dyspareunia and rare allergic reactions, low cost, no need for a prescription, and a reported lower incidence of cervical dysplasia. There is no current evidence linking vaginal contraceptives with resultant birth defects.

There is more complete vaginal coverage with foam. The user must thoroughly shake the can to dispense the spermicide. If vaginal tablets or suppositories are used, the adolescent should allow 10 to 15 minutes for dissolving the tablets in the vagina. The adolescent should be instructed to insert the tablet high into the vagina. Suppositories should be placed near the external cervical os. After coitus occurs, 6 hours or more should pass before bathing or douching. Adolescents should be instructed to add additional vaginal contraceptive if further coital activity occurs.

Vaginal contraceptive film comes in a 2 × 2–inch flat package, with each film containing 72 mg of nonoxynol-9. The film should be inserted into the vagina at least 5 minutes before intercourse and remains effective for 1 hour. Young women should always use vaginal contraceptives with other contraceptive methods and not rely solely on them for effective contraception.

VAGINAL SPONGE

The vaginal sponge is another over-the-counter contraceptive device that is disposable and contains 1 g of the spermicide nonoxynol-9. It is a polyurethane, concave-shaped sponge that has a retrieval loop. Prior to insertion, 2 tbsp of water are added to the sponge; the sponge then swells within the vagina. It can be placed up to 24 hours prior to coitus and is left in place at least 6 to 8 hours after coitus. It inactivates and blocks sperm and offers a method that can be protective during multiple coital encounters over a 24-hour period. Failure rates are comparable to those with the diaphragm, but it is less difficult to use than the cervical cap or diaphragm. It is controversial whether or not parity influences the sponge's failure rate. Problems identified with the sponge include vaginal malodor, vaginal candidiasis, genital pruritus, vulvar rash, and toxic shock syndrome (reported 1 case/2 million users; see Chapter 94). The likelihood of toxic shock syndrome may be increased when the sponge is used during menstruation, if it is left in place more than 24 hours, and if the woman is a vaginal carrier of *Staphylococcus aureus* (see Chapter 94).

Subdermal Implants

Norplant is a levonorgestrel-releasing subdermal reversible contraceptive implant. It consists of six 2.4 mm × 34 mm polymeric silicone (Silastic) capsules, which are inserted subdermally by making a small incision, usually in the inner aspect of the upper arm, with the adolescent under local anesthesia. The capsules release approximately 30 μg of levonorgestrel/day. Norplant provides effective contraception for approximately 5 years, with less effectiveness in obese women. The Norplant-2 system consists of two capsules that are each 44 mm in length. Norplant-2 is effective for 3 years. The cumulative pregnancy rate for users of Norplant at the end of the first year is 0.2 to 0.6/100 women years of use, and the cumulative rate is 1.5 to 3.9 pregnancies over 5 years. Patient acceptance is good. Side effects include irregular menstruation, amenorrhea, weight gain, and headaches. The incidence of ectopic pregnancy is less than with the mini-pill and progesterone-containing intrauterine devices. There is no effect on carbohydrate metabolism, blood coagulation, and liver function. Also, there is no increased incidence of congenital anomalies in subsequent offspring. It is unclear whether adolescents will choose to use this method, which would be ideal theoretically because of removal of factors relating to compliance (see Chapter 26). The need for an incision to place the rods and the possibility that others might see the rods once in place may prove deterrents to the use of this ideal method in adolescents.

Capronor consists of a single biodegradable capsule (available in 2.5-cm and 4-cm sizes) that is inserted subdermally and releases levonorgestrel over a 12- to 18-month period. Benefits include biodegradability, ease of insertion and removal, fewer implants, and cosmetically better acceptance because it is less obvious under the skin.

Injectable Contraceptives

The main injectable contraceptive in the United States is medroxyprogesterone acetate (Depo-Provera), which is given intramuscularly in a dose of 150 mg every 3 months. Its contraceptive mechanisms include ovulation inhibition (by eliminating the midcycle rise of LH), sperm penetration reduction (by thickening cervical mucus), and interference with blastocyst implantation (by endometrial thinning). Its contraceptive efficacy is even better than with combined birth control pill, with pregnancy rates at 0.4 to 0.6 pregnancies/100 women years. The effect of Depo-Provera on blood pressure and lactation is minimal, and it can be used in situations in which estrogen is contraindicated. The most common side effect is irregular menstrual bleeding; most women are amenorrheic 1 year after initiation. A number of other side effects are noted, including nervousness, headaches, nausea, emesis, and weight gain. The Food and Drug Administration has not approved Depo-Provera as a contraceptive agent because of unproven concerns over breast cancer induction and possible congenital malformations. Depo-Provera does seem to cause an increase in breast tumors in some beagle dogs. Depo-Provera is a popular contraceptive agent around the world (especially in China and Latin America), and international studies have not shown it to be harmful. Other long-acting injectable contraceptives under research include norethindrone enanthate and lynestrenol.

Intrauterine Devices

Intrauterine devices (IUDs) are generally not recommended for adolescents because of an increased risk of pelvic inflammatory disease that may result in infertility (see Chapter 75). There is an increased likelihood of expulsion of the device and side effects in a nulliparous teenager. Also, there is a slightly increased risk of ectopic pregnancy among the pregnancies that occur.

Progestasert (progesterone, T-shaped IUD) and ParaGard (TCU-380A) are the two currently approved intrauterine devices marketed in the United States. Progestasert is a progesterone-releasing IUD that must be replaced annually. The vertical stem of the T contains 38 mg of progesterone, which is released into the endometrial cavity at a rate of 65 μg/day. It reduces menstrual blood flow and the incidence of primary dysmenorrhea. ParaGard, a copper-containing IUD with a total of 380 mm² of exposed copper, needs to be replaced every 4 years. Intrauterine devices probably act by inhibition of sperm transport, direct damage to sperm and ova, and resultant failure of fertilization.

Other Forms of Contraception

POSTCOITAL CONTRACEPTIVES

The concept of a "morning after" pill or contraceptive agent is an important one, especially for rape victims and those with sporadic coital activity. A method currently popular is using a birth control pill such as Ovral, which contains 0.5 mg norgestrel with 50 μg of ethinyl estradiol. Two of these tablets are given within 72 hours of coitus and then repeated in 12 hours. It appears to be a safe and effective means of postcoital contraception. Research is being performed to seek other means of postcoital contraception.

RHYTHM METHOD

The avoidance of coitus around the anticipated time of ovulation is a contraceptive method of antiquity. The classic technique is the Ogino-Knaus method (calendar method) in which coital activity is avoided between menstrual days 9 and 18. It is based on the observation that ovulation occurs 14 days before menstruation but also on unproven assumptions that sperm survive in the vagina for 3 to 4 days and oocytes survive up to 24 hours after ovulation. It is unfortunate that teenagers do not use periodic abstinence well because of limited motivation, poor knowledge of their physiology (and anatomy), and the type of menstrual periods many teenagers have—that is, irregular and unpredictable, especially after menarche. Various additional techniques have been developed for the highly motivated, knowledgeable individual who wishes to use periodic abstinence. Teenagers do not use these methods well, and published pregnancy rates vary from 5 to 40 pregnancies/100 women years. Periodic abstinence can be combined with barrier contraceptives or other contraceptive methods to improve efficacy.

NONCOITAL ACTIVITY

Noncoital sexual activity ("safe sex" or "outercourse") includes behaviors such as kissing, hugging, mutual masturbation, sexual massage, and fantasy. These methods are safe, effective, and always available, and such noncoital sexual behavior may provide teenagers with alternatives to sexual intercourse.

MISCELLANEOUS

A variety of other means of delivering progestin and estrogen are being explored. Injectable norethindrone (NET microspheres) has recently been evaluated for its contraceptive efficacy. It has been shown to provide a highly effective contraception for up to 6 months. Microspheres cannot be removed once injected. The transdermal contraceptive patch slowly releases estrogen and progestin in the circulatory system and bypasses the liver. Transdermal patches have been noted to be effective for 7 to 9 days. A progesterone-releasing vaginal ring has also been tested. The silicon rubber ring represents a modification of the vaginal ring and releases levonorgestrel and estradiol. It is placed deep in the vagina for 3 weeks and is then removed for 1 week for menses to occur. The hormones bypass the liver, and the contraception efficacy is close to that of oral contraceptives. It is self-administered, and contraception is readily available. Vaginal rings can be removed during coitus and then replaced. Continuous rings are being developed that could be left in place for 3 months.

Some of the other methods listed in Table 73–2 are either at a research stage of development, are not applicable, or have limited applications in adolescents at the present time.

BIBLIOGRAPHY

Brown KH, Hammond CB: The risks and benefits of oral contraceptives. Adv Intern Med 34:285, 1989.

Derman RJ: Oral contraceptives and cardiovascular risk: Current perspectives. J Reprod Med 34(9):747, 1989.

Emans SJ, Goldstein DP: Pediatric and Adolescent Gynecology, 3rd ed. Boston, Little, Brown, 1990, pp 451–503.

Grimes DA: Reversible contraception for the 1980s. JAMA 255:69, 1986.

Grimes DA (ed): The Contraception Report, Vol 1, Nos. 1, 2, 3, and 4. Morris Plains, NJ, Emron, 1990–1991.

Hatcher RA, Stewart F, Trussell J, et al: Contraceptive Technology, 1990–1992, 15th ed. New York, Irvington Publishers, 1990.

Kulig JW: Adolescent contraception: Nonhormonal methods. Pediatr Clin North Am 36(3):717, 1989.

Mishell DR: Contraception. N Engl J Med 320(12):777, 1989.

Peterson HB, Lee NC: The health effects of oral contraceptives: Misperceptions, controversies, and continuing good news. Clin Obstet Gynec 32(2): 339, 1989.

Shearin RB, Boehlke JR: Hormonal contraception. Pediatr Clin North Am 36:697, 1989.

Upton GV: Lipids, cardiovascular disease and oral contraceptives: A practical perspective. Fertil Steril 53(1):1, 1990.

CHAPTER 74

Adolescent Pregnancy

CATHERINE STEVENS-SIMON and ELIZABETH R. McANARNEY

OVERVIEW

Pregnancy and parenthood during adolescence are associated with significant medical and psychosocial risks for both mother and child. Although once attributed to the physiologic and psychosocial immaturity of the adolescent mother, recent data indicate that the risks associated with adolescent childbearing are not a result of physiologic or psychosocial conditions intrinsic to adolescence (e.g., ongoing maternal growth and reproductive and cognitive immaturity) but rather that adolescent pregnancy is a marker for sociodemographic factors (e.g., poverty, poor education, unmarried status, nonwhite race, and inadequate prenatal care) that increase the risks of adverse pregnancy and parenting outcomes at any age.

RISKS ASSOCIATED WITH ADOLESCENT PREGNANCY

Maternal Risks

If there is an intrinsic biologic risk associated with adolescent childbearing, it is likely to be most evident among young adolescent mothers who conceive prior to their sixteenth birthday. Available data suggest that older adolescents are physiologically mature when they conceive and are at no greater risk for adverse pregnancy outcomes than are sociodemographically similar adults. Although very young pregnant adolescents are at higher risk for the medical complications listed in Table 74–1 than are older pregnant adolescents and adults, recent studies have produced little evidence that these risks are causally related to the physiologic immaturity of the young adolescent mother. Studies controlling for concurrent maternal conditions find no association between young maternal age and the majority of obstetric complications traditionally associated with adolescent childbearing. For example, the risk of pregnancy-induced hypertension has been found to be more closely related to parity than to maternal age, and anemia is better explained by poverty, poor nutritional habits, and late prenatal care than by the effects of maternal age and pubertal growth on iron stores.

Infant Risks

Prematurity (birth prior to the thirty-seventh week of gestation) and low birth weight (less than 2500 g) are the two most common and serious infant risks associated with adolescent childbearing (Table 74–2). Infants born to mothers younger than 16 years of age are more than twice as likely to be of low birth weight than are infants born to older mothers. Because they are small, these infants are nearly three times more likely to die within the first 28 days of life than are infants of older mothers. Despite these alarming statistics, current data fail to support the thesis that these neonatal risks are causally related to maternal physiologic immaturity. One group of investigators reported that when the influences of concurrent low birth weight risk factors were controlled, the incidence of term low birth weight deliveries actually increased as maternal age increased. The results of other studies corroborate these findings and suggest that very young adolescent mothers give birth to smaller babies than do older mothers, largely because they are likely to be smaller and more impoverished than adult mothers. Precocious sexual activity and pregnancy among adolescents are often associated with involvement in other experimental behaviors, such as cigarette smoking and alcohol and drug use. Sexually active adolescents are also at a higher than average risk for acquiring sexually transmitted diseases, particularly chlamydial infections. During pregnancy, adolescents are more likely than adults to be emotionally stressed, to consume a diet of poor quality, and to receive inadequate, late prenatal care. The results of recent studies demonstrate that merely controlling for the main effects, that is, the presence or lack of potentially high-risk maternal characteristics, is inadequate; interactions are also important. For example, the results of several recent studies comparing substance abuse among pregnant adolescents and adults indicate that the adverse effects of cigarette smoking on the fetus increase as the age of the mother increases; thus, controlling only for the number of cigarettes smoked/day does not adequately account for the risk of low birth weight associated with the behavior. Other recently conducted studies show that prompt treatment of sexually transmitted diseases reduces the associated risk of preterm labor; because adolescents enter prenatal care later than do adults and may be less compliant with recommended medical regimens, potentially harmful genital infections may go untreated for a longer time during gestation. If so, the risk of preterm labor associated with sexually transmitted diseases may also increase. Finally, although neither documented dietary deficiencies nor the caloric demands imposed by residual pubertal growth have been shown to be of

**TABLE 74–1. Common Medical Problems
of Pregnant and Parenting Adolescents**

PRENATAL	POSTPARTUM
Small size	Puerperal complications
Anemia	Repeat pregnancy
Pregnancy-induced hypertension	Obesity
Substance abuse	Hypertension
Sexually transmitted genitourinary tract infections	Sexually transmitted genitourinary tract infections
Poor prenatal care	

Adapted with permission from Stevens-Simon C, McAnarney ER: Adolescent pregnancy: Continuing challenges. In Greydanus DE, Wolraich ML (eds): Behavioral Pediatrics. New York, Springer-Verlag, 1991.

sufficient magnitude to retard the rate of intrauterine growth or precipitate preterm labor, there are data suggesting that the anatomic and physiologic changes that accompany the postmenarcheal growth of the reproductive organs could impair the reproductive performance of adolescents and predispose them to preterm delivery.

CONSEQUENCES OF ADOLESCENT PREGNANCY

This section examines the short- and long-term physiologic and psychosocial effects of pregnancy on the growth and psychosocial development of adolescents and their children.

Physiologic Consequences for the Adolescent Mother

Data on the long-term physiologic consequences of adolescent childbearing are minimal. Although it has been reported consistently that adolescent mothers are shorter than adult mothers, it is unclear whether this is a result of the increased levels of gonadal hormones associated with pregnancy, which accelerate the rate of epiphyseal closure and thus permanently stunt growth, or because adolescent mothers mature early and therefore can be expected to be shorter than their later-maturing adult counterparts.

Questions also remain about the effects of pregnancy on the physical health of the adolescent (see Table 74–1). The results of at least one study suggest that adolescent childbearing is associated with a high likelihood of obesity and hypertension later in life; again, further studies are needed to separate the effects of early childbearing and early maturation on the adult habitus of young women who become mothers during adolescence.

Psychological and Social Consequences for the Adolescent Mother

Extensive studies of the long-term psychosocial consequences of adolescent childbearing indicate that early

**TABLE 74–2. Common Medical Problems
of Children of Adolescent Mothers**

Prematurity and its sequelae
Low birth weight
Accidental trauma and poisoning
Sudden infant death syndrome
Minor acute infections

Adapted with permission from Stevens-Simon C, McAnarney ER: Adolescent pregnancy: Continuing challenges. In Greydanus DE, Wolraich ML (eds): Behavioral Pediatrics. New York, Springer-Verlag, 1991.

childbearing profoundly and adversely influences the educational, vocational, and marital experiences of many young persons (Table 74–3). Although it has been demonstrated repeatedly that adolescents who have children obtain less education than does the general teenaged population, school withdrawal and school failure often predate adolescent pregnancy—it is rarely the only reason that young women drop out of high school. Because in many cases school failure apparently leads to dropping out of high school and pregnancy and because academic achievement prior to conception is one of the best predictors of high school graduation following delivery, programs that provide remedial training for young persons at risk for school failure may be effective in preventing adolescent childbearing and enhancing the educational and vocational achievements of adolescent parents.

Longitudinal studies are needed to determine the direction of causality in frequently reported associations. For example, it is not clear whether (1) young women who do not marry and who remain within their parents' home are more likely to graduate from high school because they are relieved of the necessities of supporting themselves financially and the burdens of child care or (2) these young mothers remain at home and postpone marriage because they have career goals in which they value scholastic achievement and a high school diploma over personal independence. Obtaining a clear understanding of the causal sequence is critical for the design of relevant intervention programs.

Even when aptitude scores, socioeconomic status, and educational aspirations are controlled for, early child-bearers obtain less prestigious, poorer paying jobs than do adolescents who delay childbearing; failure to graduate from high school within 5 years of the birth of the first child doubles the risk of welfare dependency 2 decades later. Consequently, the incidence of poverty increases as the age of the mother decreases. It is estimated that approximately one third of mothers who

**TABLE 74–3. Common Psychosocial Problems
of Pregnancy and Parenting Adolescents**

Poverty
Poor education, school failure
Limited vocational opportunities
Marital instability
Social isolation
Depression, stress

Adapted with permission from Stevens-Simon C, McAnarney ER: Adolescent pregnancy: Continuing challenges. In Greydanus DE, Wolraich ML (eds): Behavioral Pediatrics. New York, Springer-Verlag, 1991.

have their first child before they are 17 years of age live below the federal poverty line; this is 2.6 times greater than the poverty rate among women who bear their first child after 20 years of age.

Educational achievement and economic stability have implications for the stability of adolescent marriages and adolescent family life. Most adolescent pregnancies are conceived out of wedlock, and adolescent parents who manage to form a stable relationship with one another are clearly the exception; 17 years after the birth of the first child, only 16% of adolescent mothers in Baltimore remained married to the father of the baby. Although this high rate of separation and divorce has been found consistently among adolescent couples, the etiologic significance of their young age is unclear. Marital instability is a common finding among couples in whom conception occurs prior to marriage, particularly when the out-of-wedlock birth is compounded by the stresses of poverty and financial instability. One study of adolescent couples showed that if the father of the baby was a high school graduate or a skilled laborer, the probability of marital separation within 2 years was 19%; by contrast, if the father was not a high school graduate and was an unskilled laborer, the probability of marital separation within 2 years was 45%.

Finally, the prevalence of depression and other psychiatric symptoms is significantly higher among adolescent mothers than among the general population. In one study of pregnant and parenting adolescents, the incidence of depression was found to be 60%; in another study, 13% of the sample of young women who had given birth before the age of 17 years were found to have been treated for attempted suicide subsequently. Because there are data to suggest that young mothers who are enrolled in postpartum educational and support programs suffer fewer depressive symptoms than do their peers, studies are needed to define the types of psychological disturbances experienced by adolescent mothers so that appropriate preventive interventions can be implemented.

Taken together, these data suggest that maternal age has little direct effect on the long-term psychosocial outcome of poor young women; early childbearing appears to simply hasten the inevitable school failure and leaving high school by the poorest students, whereas young women who are educationally motivated and are not failing in school are apt to graduate from high school and become economically stable regardless of their age at first conception. To reverse this cycle of poverty and failure, it will be necessary to do more than prevent adolescent pregnancies. First, alternative educational and vocational programs are needed for students who are failing in the traditional educational system so that they can obtain dignity and personal satisfaction from pursuits other than parenthood. Second, more must be learned about the personal and societal factors that differentiate the minority of young parents who achieve good outcomes from their less successful peers.

Consequences for the Adolescent Father

Much less is known about the young men who father the children of adolescent mothers; systematic data have been gathered only recently. These data indicate that the father is often 2 to 3 years older than the teenaged mother and is often not a teenager. Clearly, young men who become fathers during their adolescence, like their female counterparts, have significantly more academic and behavioral problems than do their sociodemographically similar, but childless, peers. Although the actual involvement of teenaged fathers with their children has not been systematically studied, information about emotional problems caused by premature parenthood has begun to dispel the common stereotype of the teenaged father as an uninvolved and unaffected bystander. Concerns about vocational, educational, health, and family problems are common and similar to the concerns expressed by adolescent mothers; unfortunately, there are fewer services available to help these young men than are available for the young mothers.

Physiologic Consequences for the Infant

Although the infants of adolescent mothers are smaller at birth than are the infants of adult mothers, this apparently is a result largely of prematurity; infants who survive the neonatal period grow at the same rate as do infants born to older mothers. Nevertheless, infants born to adolescent mothers experience more of the medical problems listed in Table 74–2 than do the infants of older mothers. Even when birth weight is controlled for, the postneonatal mortality rate is approximately twice as high for infants born to adolescents younger than 17 years of age as it is for infants born to older women. The disproportionately high postneonatal morbidity rate is most evident among infants of normal birth weight born to adolescent mothers. Studies indicate that environmental factors (e.g., poverty, overcrowding, and poor health habits), lack of adequate knowledge of child development, and inappropriate childrearing practices and child supervision, rather than the low birth weight of the infants, are responsible for the increased incidence of postneonatal medical problems among infants of adolescent mothers.

Psychosocial Consequences for the Infant

Evidence from a variety of sources indicates that the school-aged children of adolescent mothers exhibit more behavioral problems, score lower on intellectual tests, are more likely to repeat a grade in school, and are more likely to be neglected than are the children of adult mothers who are born into sociodemographically similar environments (Table 74–4). In one study it was reported that 50% of 15- to 17-year-old children born to adolescent mothers had already repeated at least one grade and that 60% were C or D students; grade failure was associated with dropping out of high school and with behavioral problems both in and out of school. Current data suggest that age-related differences in maternal childrearing attitudes and behaviors contribute

TABLE 74–4. Common Psychosocial Problems of Children of Adolescent Mothers

Behavioral problems
Developmental delay
Neglect
School failure and withdrawal

Adapted with permission from Stevens-Simon C, McAnarney ER: Adolescent pregnancy: Continuing challenges. In Greydanus DE, Wolraich ML (eds): Behavioral Pediatrics. New York, Springer-Verlag, 1991.

to the increased incidence of school, behavioral, and emotional problems among the children of adolescent mothers. Studies comparing the parenting behaviors of adolescent and adult mothers have consistently demonstrated that young adolescent mothers reinforce their children's vocalization less and assume a more negative, punitive approach to childrearing than do adult mothers. Furthermore, children who have the advantage of a stable relationship with their father or substantial daily input from other adults do not show the same intellectual deficits as children who are raised primarily by their adolescent mothers. However, it is again important not to mistake association for causality; it is unclear whether the presence of a mature adult in the home has a direct and beneficial effect on child development or whether the same qualities that enable some adolescent mothers to elicit the daily support of others in their environment also make them more nurturing parents.

REPEAT ADOLESCENT PREGNANCY

Repeat adolescent pregnancy (recidivism) occurs commonly; when there is no intensive postpartum follow-up, the prevalence of second pregnancies among adolescents in the year following their first delivery is estimated to be 30%; during the second postpartum year, 25% to 50% of adolescent mothers conceive. Those at highest risk for recidivism are young women who (1) are younger than 16 years of age at first conception, (2) have a boyfriend older than 20 years of age, (3) drop out of school, (4) are below their expected grade level at the time of the first pregnancy, (5) become dependent on welfare after the first birth, (6) have complications during their first pregnancy, and (7) leave the hospital without birth control. Many repeat adolescent pregnancies are planned or at least *not unplanned*. One study showed that 5 years after the delivery of their first child, more than 50% of a sample of single women who explicitly stated that they wanted no more children were not using any kind of birth control. The majority of repeat pregnancies occurs during the 5 years following the first birth; after this, many women who initially became pregnant as adolescents use abortion or voluntary sterilization to control their fertility.

The prevention of recidivism is an important goal because the incidence of low birth weight and prematurity increases, and the likelihood of completing high school, having a job, and being self-supporting decreases with each additional adolescent pregnancy. One study found that among adolescents, the rate of preterm delivery rose from 11% of first births to 21% of second

births to 43% of third births. In another study, a second pregnancy within 2 years of the first adolescent pregnancy was found to be one of the best predictors of the adolescent leaving high school and welfare dependency. Other studies corroborate these dismal findings but suggest that the neonatal medical problems and post-neonatal social problems associated with repeat adolescent pregnancies reflect maternal characteristics that predate the first pregnancy. Data concerning the antecedents of second adolescent pregnancies indicate that the mere prescription of birth control following delivery is not sufficient to prevent recidivism; more intensive postpartum follow-up is needed (see discussion further on).

PATIENT MANAGEMENT

Diagnosis of Pregnancy

Adolescents who are pregnant may present to the health care provider with the same signs and symptoms of pregnancy as do older pregnant women—that is, secondary amenorrhea, breast swelling and tenderness, morning nausea, and weight gain. Other adolescents may complain only of fatigue, headache, abdominal pain, and irregular or scant menstrual bleeding. Still others (those who wish to conceal their pregnancies) may deny both sexual activity and menstrual irregularities and simply request to be seen for an evaluation. Because first-trimester vaginal bleeding occurs in more than a third of adolescent pregnancies, health care providers and young adolescents may fail to consider the possibility of pregnancy. Thus a high index of suspicion is needed to avoid missing the correct diagnosis, and the lack of amenorrhea should never preclude pregnancy testing among adolescents.

When pregnancy is suspected, the adolescent patient should be interviewed about that possibility. A direct approach is preferred. After reaffirming confidentiality (see Chapters 20 and 22), the provider should inquire specifically about the date and normalcy of the last menstrual period, sexual activity, contraceptive use, and the possibility of pregnancy. Abdominal and pelvic examinations should be performed whenever pregnancy is suspected. Examination of the patient is important for dating the gestation, diagnosing and treating concurrent sexually transmitted diseases, and excluding other causes for the patient's symptoms. However, it is unwise to rely on a physical examination for the diagnosis of pregnancy because the characteristic physical signs of pregnancy—a bluish cervix (the Chadwick sign), softening of the cervix (the Goodell sign), and uterine enlargement—take several weeks to develop.

Pregnancy is diagnosed by testing the patient's urine or blood for human chorionic gonadotropin (HCG) (see Chapter 69). Numerous highly sensitive urine pregnancy tests are available, so pregnancy can be reliably diagnosed in the office within 30 days of conception. An earlier diagnosis of pregnancy is possible but may be undesirable because up to a third of these newly implanted ova miscarry. False-positive urine pregnancy test results are rare (1% to 2%) but may be encountered with heavy proteinuria, hematuria, or drug use.

If the initial pregnancy test is performed on a randomly obtained urine sample and gives negative results, other causes of amenorrhea should be excluded (see Chapter 70). If pregnancy is still suspected, the urine pregnancy test can be repeated on a concentrated, first-morning urine specimen, or a serum pregnancy test can be performed. Serum pregnancy tests are more sensitive than are most urine pregnancy tests (usually giving positive results within 10 days of conception) and can also be used to quantify the level of HCG. If test results are negative, the test should be repeated in 7 to 10 days if the patient remains amenorrheic and no other cause is found. A positive pregnancy test result without uterine enlargement should always raise the suspicion of an ectopic pregnancy, especially in adolescent patients who report irregular or abnormal menstrual bleeding or unilateral abdominal or pelvic pain or whose medical histories increase their risk of ectopic pregnancy (e.g., smokers and women who have had pelvic inflammatory disease or who have used an intrauterine device). If the diagnosis of ectopic pregnancy is seriously suspected, a quantitative test for the β-subunit of HCG should be performed immediately and an ultrasound study obtained. Table 74–5 provides guidelines for interpretation. The advice of an obstetrician should be sought if there is any question (see Chapter 69).

When the diagnosis of pregnancy is uncertain, oral contraception should be stopped and the patient instructed to use a barrier method until the diagnosis is made. Home pregnancy tests are expensive, are often unreliable, and may delay appropriate care (see Chapter 69).

Once the diagnosis of pregnancy has been made, the adolescent should be told in private and should be assisted in accepting and understanding the implications. The options should be presented carefully, succinctly, and nonjudgmentally. The risks and benefits of obtaining a therapeutic abortion, relinquishing the baby following birth, and keeping and raising the infant should be discussed with the adolescent in the context of her future career and family plans. Although confidentiality must be maintained, younger adolescents should be encouraged to share the decision-making process with a parent or another trusted adult. If the adolescent seems reluctant to do so, the health care provider should offer to help her inform others of her pregnancy; if the adolescent claims to have no supportive adults, she should be referred to a youth-serving social service agency. After the management decision is reached, follow-up with the appropriate care site should be arranged and a mechanism established to ensure that the adolescent follows through with the agreed upon plan; adolescents who are ambivalent about their decisions often delay or fail to implement the management plan, thus jeopardizing both their own and their unborn child's future health and well-being.

Spontaneous Abortion

It is estimated that approximately 10% of adolescent pregnancies end in miscarriage. Adolescents who have miscarried in the past and who are miscarrying at present should be evaluated by a health care provider; a pelvic examination should be performed to ensure that the miscarriage is complete (no tissue visible in the cervical os and the cervical os is closed tightly). A follow-up visit should be scheduled because adolescents who have miscarried are more likely to conceive again before they are 20 years of age than are their peers who have never been pregnant.

Therapeutic Abortion

The laws governing therapeutic abortion differ from state to state; it is important that health care providers who work with adolescent patients know the laws in their state (see Chapter 20). Health care providers should also be aware of their own feelings about therapeutic abortion; those who strongly oppose this option should refer pregnant patients to neutral sources for counseling.

Approximately 40% of all adolescent pregnancies are terminated by induced abortion, and approximately 33% of all abortions in the United States are performed on women younger than 20 years of age. Teenagers living in poverty are less apt to seek abortion than are their peers living above the poverty level.

Several abortion procedures are available, but the duration of gestation usually dictates the choice of method. A menstrual extraction is the simplest abortion procedure with the lowest risk. It can be performed on outpatients until the sixth gestational week. For gestations of less than 12 weeks duration, abortion is usually carried out by performing a dilation and suction curettage. This procedure also has very low risk and does not require hospital admission. After the twelfth gestational week, hospitalization for dilation and extraction (12 to 16 weeks) or for saline and prostaglandin induction (16 to 24 weeks) is necessary. These two regimens are more costly and carry a higher risk of serious complications especially saline administration. New medical methods for induction of abortion are under investigation in Europe and may soon be available for use early in pregnancy.

TABLE 74–5. Use of Quantitative Serum Human Chorionic Gonadotropin (HCG) and Ultrasound in the Diagnosis of an Ectopic Pregnancy

| ULTRASOUND | QUANTITATIVE SERUM HCG | |
	<6000 mIU	>6000 mIU
No gestational sac visualized	Miscarriage Very early IUP* Ectopic pregnancy	Ectopic pregnancy
Gestational sac visualized	Abnormal IUP Threatened abortion Ectopic pregnancy†	IUP

*IUP (intrauterine pregnancy): the gestational sac is not visible until the serum HCG is greater than 6000 mIU, usually at about 5 to 6 weeks' gestation.
†An ectopic pregnancy may evoke a decidual reaction in the uterus that can be mistaken for a gestational sac.

The physical and psychological consequences of abortion among adolescents are poorly understood; teenagers appear to be at lower risk for complications such as fever and hemorrhage but at higher risk for cervical injury than are adult abortion patients, which raised concern during the 1970s about future cervical incompetence, miscarriage, or preterm labor, or a combination of these factors. The results of recent studies, however, indicate that by using modern techniques to dilate the cervix, there is little or no increase in the risk of subsequent miscarriage associated with a therapeutic abortion; it is less clear whether women who undergo a number of abortions are at increased risk for miscarriage.

Data concerning the short- and long-term psychological sequelae of abortions in adolescents are incomplete. If adolescents are provided with adequate counseling before and after abortion, negative psychological consequences can probably be avoided. Many adolescents who terminate their pregnancies do well; most subsequently use contraception, prevent additional pregnancies, and complete their educations. The reasons for the recurrent use of abortions among adolescents are unclear, but they probably reflect stress, depression, and a chaotic lifestyle rather than simple carelessness. There is no evidence that the procedure is taken lightly at any age.

Prenatal Care

Adolescents who continue their pregnancies should be immediately referred for prenatal care. Comprehensive adolescent maternity programs provide for the nutritional, psychosocial, and educational needs of adolescent mothers, and for reasons not understood, appear to reduce the risks associated with childbearing at this age, particularly when the adolescent mother is less than 15 years of age at conception.

Adoption

Most adolescents who carry their pregnancies keep their babies; approximately 2% to 3% of adolescent mothers relinquish their children.

Postpartum Care of Adolescent Mothers and Their Children

Following delivery, all adolescent mothers should be encouraged to return to their obstetric care site for a 6-week postpartum evaluation; after this visit, primary health care for adolescent mothers can be provided in a variety of settings, including pediatrics, family medicine, and internal medicine practices.

Gynecologic concerns constitute only a small part of the adolescent mother's total health care needs. Studies indicate that young mothers who receive care with their infants at the same visit receive more regular care, are more compliant with contraceptive prescriptions, and postpone second pregnancies for longer periods than do young mothers who receive medical care in other settings. The opportunity to see the same provider as their infant may be optimal for young adolescent mothers; older adolescent mothers may prefer to be seen in a clinic specializing in adolescent medicine, a pediatric practice, a family medicine practice, or an internal medicine practice. In addition to family planning, primary care for adolescent mothers should address common adolescent medical problems and concerns. Blood pressure should be monitored, particularly in young women who had pregnancy-induced hypertension. Expectations for postpartum weight loss should be developed according to the young woman's level of physiologic maturity; it may be physiologically inappropriate for young, still-growing adolescents to return to their pregravid weight. Pediatric providers who elect not to provide primary health care services for adolescent mothers can help reduce the rate of repeat adolescent pregnancies, school failure, and welfare dependency by inquiring about contraceptive use, school attendance, future career and family plans, and symptoms of stress and depression at each well-baby visit. To do so requires only a few additional minutes and demonstrates interest and caring for the adolescent as an individual and a mother. If deficits in contraception or education are identified, or if the young mother is stressed or depressed, the pediatric health care provider can refer her to an appropriate site for care. Young families with multiple social problems may do best if they are cared for in comprehensive adolescent parenting programs. These programs are often extensions of prenatal programs and are designed to meet the global social, psychological, and medical needs of young parents and their children.

The increased frequency of medical and social problems experienced by the infants and children of adolescent mothers emphasizes the importance of observing both their physical and psychosocial development. It is important to identify toddlers who are not responding verbally and children and adolescents who are failing in school before they become discouraged and leave school for a life of delinquency on the streets or early parenthood. Enrolling such children in remedial education programs may be more effective in stopping the transmission of poverty from one generation to the next than enrolling them in programs designed explicitly to prevent adolescent pregnancy, sexual activity, and delinquency. In addition, it is important for health care providers who are caring for the children of adolescent mothers to be aware that young mothers look to them for approval of the way they are caring for their infants. Many teenagers fear that infant symptoms such as skin rashes, mild regurgitation, and sniffles reflect poorly on the mother's caretaking; simple explanations will assist the young mother in gaining confidence and self-esteem as a mother.

BIBLIOGRAPHY

Amaro H, Zuckerman B, Cabral H: Drug use among adolescent mothers: Profile of risk. Pediatrics 84:144, 1989.
Card J, Wise L: Teenage mothers and teenage fathers: The impact of

early childbearing on the parents' personal and professional lives. Fam Plann Perspect 10:199, 1978.

Furstenberg FF, Brooks-Gunn J, Morgan SP: Adolescent mothers and their children in later life. Fam Plann Perspect 19:142, 1987.

Garn S, Lavelle M, Rosenberg KR, Hawthorne VM: Maturational timing as a factor in female fatness and obesity. Am J Clin Nutr 43:879, 1986.

Hardy JB, Duggan AK: Teenage fathers and the fathers of infants of urban, teenage mothers. Am J Public Health 78:919, 1988.

Horwitz S, Klerman L, Kuo H, Jekel J: Intergenerational transmission of school-age parenthood. Fam Plann Perspect 23:168, 1991.

Lee K, Ferguson RM, Corpuz M, Gartner LM: Maternal age and incidence of low birth weight at term: A population study. Am J Obstet Gynecol 158:84, 1988.

McAnarney ER: Young maternal age and adverse neonatal outcome. Am J Dis Child 141:1053, 1987.

McAnarney ER, Schreider C: Identifying Social and Psychological Antecedents of Adolescent Pregnancy: The Contribution of Research to Concepts of Prevention. New York, William T. Grant Foundation, 1984.

McGregor JA: Prevention of preterm birth: New initiatives based on microbial-host interactions. Obstet Gynecol Surv 43:1, 1988.

Stevens-Simon C, McAnarney ER: Adolescent maternal weight gain and infant outcome. Am J Clin Nutr 47:948, 1988.

Zuckerman B, Amaro H, Bauchner H, Cabral H: Depressive symptoms during pregnancy: Relationship to poor health behaviors. Am J Obstet Gynecol 160:1107, 1989.

CHAPTER 75

Sexually Transmitted Disease Syndromes

MARY-ANN SHAFER

Sexually transmitted diseases (STDs) are the most common infections among sexually active adolescents. Of the 20 million cases of STDs reported each year in the United States, 30% occur in adolescents, and more than 50% occur in adolescents and young adults younger than 25 years of age. STDs are linked to the development of pelvic inflammatory disease (PID), and its sequelae of chronic pelvic pain, infertility, and ectopic pregnancy in females and genital cancers in both females and males. Human immunodeficiency virus (HIV) presents new risks to sexually active adolescents, including chronic immunodeficiency-related diseases and death (see Chapter 76).

EPIDEMIOLOGY

The prevalence of most STDs peaks during late adolescence and early adulthood and declines rapidly with increasing age. Table 75–1 gives the prevalence rates for common STD agents in sexually active females, and Table 75–2 gives these rates for sexually active males. In general, *Chlamydia trachomatis* is the most common bacterial STD among adolescents and is frequently asymptomatic. Human papillomavirus (HPV) has recently been recognized as the most common viral STD infection among adolescents. It is estimated that 1% to 10% of women are infected with HPV, with adolescent and STD patients at greatest risk. HPV has been detected by new molecular techniques in 1% to 38% of sexually active adolescents, with younger females at greater risk of infection.

Age is an important factor in the prevalence of STDs; for example, the adolescent-aged cohort (15 to 19 years) experienced the most rapid increase in reported infection during the rapid rise of gonococcal infections that occurred over a 20-year period through 1975. This same adolescent-aged cohort experienced the slowest decline in reported gonococcal infection between 1984 and 1987. Although younger age is clearly identified as a marker for increased risk for STD infections and STD syndromes, the potential contributions by age-related factors such as sexual behavior, contraceptive use, and biologic development of cervical tissue are unknown.

Ethnicity has been associated with STD risk. In the United States, sexually active black adolescents aged 15 to 19 years have higher reported rates of infections with both *Neisseria gonorrhoeae* and *Chlamydia trachomatis* than do sexually active white adolescents. Black adolescent females have ten times the reported rates of gonococcal infections than do white adolescent females; their rates of *Chlamydia trachomatis* infections, secondary syphilis, and PID are also higher. Studies including black, Hispanic, and white adolescent females have shown that black adolescent females have the highest infection rates for cervicitis from *Neisseria gonorrhoeae* (8%) compared with their white (2.1%) and Hispanic (1.4%) counterparts. *Chlamydia trachomatis* infections among females show a similar pattern. The estimated rates of infection according to one study were as follows: black (28%), Hispanic (23%), and white (14%).

The role of contraceptive use and STD infections among sexually active adolescents is complex. Condom use has been repeatedly shown to offer protection from STD infections, including *Neisseria gonorrhoeae*, *Chlamydia trachomatis*, HPV infections, and HIV-related syndromes. In addition to barrier contraceptives, (condoms, diaphragms), spermicides are important for STD prevention. Nonoxynol-9, an ingredient of many commercially available spermicides, causes cell wall destruction by its inherent surfactant-like properties and inhibits yeast *(Candida albicans)*, bacteria *(Neisseria gonorrhoeae, Treponema pallidum, Trichomonas vaginalis)*, and some viruses (herpes simplex I and II, HIV) in *in vitro* studies. The role of oral contraception in the development of STD infections appears to be dependent on the STD agent. For example, the link between yeast (endogenous and sexually transmitted) and higher dosage oral contraceptives has been well accepted. New data considering this relationship in women using low-dose oral contraceptive pills have not corroborated this relationship. The impact of oral contraceptives on the establishment of endocervical infection and the subsequent development of PID remains controversial (see later discussion). Summarizing currently available published data, oral contraceptive use may enhance the establishment of endocervicitis associated with *Chlamydia trachomatis* and decrease the risk for endocervicitis associated with *Neisseria gonorrhoeae*; oral contraceptive users appear to have less severe gonococcal PID and a decreased risk for development of *Chlamydia trachomatis* pelvic infections.

TABLE 75–1. Selected Prevalences of STDs in Adolescent Females (%)

AUTHOR	CLINIC TYPE	N	AGE	S	CT	GC	TV	HPV	HSV	SYP
Saltz et al, 1981	T	100	17.3*	+,−	22	3	16	—	—	—
Golden et al, 1984	T	186	12–17	+,−	10	10	—	—	—	3
Shafer et al,	T	366	13–21	+,−	15	4	8	—	—	—
Bell and Holmes, 1984	D	100	12–18	+,−	20	18	48	4†	2	0
Alexander-Rodriguez and Vermund, 1987	D	285	9–18	+,−	—	18	—	—	—	2.5
Oh et al, 1988	T	102	12–18	+,−	26	10	13	5	2	0
Martinez et al, 1988	T	89	12–19	+,−	37	16	—	13	—	—
Johnson et al, 1989	O	(4201)‡	15–29	−	—	—	—	—	7‡	—

*Mean age.
†Other prevalences for HPV = 18% to 33%.
‡Second National Health and Nutrition Survey sample (7% of total number).
N, number; S, symptomatic; CT, *Chlamydia trachomatis;* GC, *Neisseria gonorrhoeae;* TV, *Trichomonas vaginalis*; HPV, human papillomavirus; HSV, herpes simplex virus; SYP, *Treponema pallidum;* T, teen; D, detention; O, other; +, symptomatic; −, asymptomatic.

ASSESSMENT FOR STDs IN THE WELL ADOLESCENT

The assessment of STDs is an important role of the primary care practitioner. The clinician should incorporate both early detection and treatment strategies into everyday practice. It is the asymptomatic STD infection that the primary care clinician can uniquely affect through office assessment. Interviewing, confidentiality, and pubertal and psychological changes are discussed in Chapters 22, 23, 4 and 5, and 9, respectively. The most critical component of the sexual history is to ascertain whether the young person has ever been sexually active—either volitionally or nonvolitionally. Evaluation of the sexually active adolescent includes a routine physical examination because the presentation of STD syndromes varies widely and includes many organ systems. Table 75–3 includes common signs and syndromes of STDs. Many practitioners prefer to perform a routine pelvic examination at some reasonable time after menarche (2 to 5 years) before sexual activity begins. Others examine all sexually active adolescents, those with complaints at any age, and virginal adolescents at 18 years of age. An introduction to the pelvic examination when young women are asymptomatic is ideal so that they may be taught the typical symptoms and signs of STD infections (see Chapter 69). Testicular examinations should be included at puberty to teach the signs and symptoms of urethritis and to teach self-examination to detect early testicular cancer (see Chapter 78).

TABLE 75–2. Selected Prevalences of STDs in Adolescent Males (%)

AUTHOR	SITE*	N	AGE	S†	CT	GC	SYP
Podgore and Holmes, 1982	O	97	23‡	−	11	2	NA
Adger et al, 1984	T	50	13–20	+,−	32	12	NA
Alexander-Rodriguez and Vermund, 1987	D	2236	9–18	+,−	NA	3	<1
Chambers et al, 1987	T	74	13–21	+,−	30	4	NA
O'Brien et al, 1988	D	91	14–19	−	11	5	NA
Shafer et al, 1989	T,D	435	13–19	−	9	3	NA

*Site of clinic: T, teen; D, detention; O, other.
†S, symptomatic; +, symptomatic; −, asymptomatic.
‡Mean age.
N, number; CT, *Chlamydia trachomatis*; GC, *Neisseria gonorrhoeae*; SYP, *Treponema pallidum*.

Laboratory testing of asymptomatic sexually active adolescents should be routine, since most STDs in adolescents are asymptomatic. Routine laboratory testing in a sexually active healthy female includes (1) endocervical cultures (urethral and rectal as indicated) to look for *Chlamydia trachomatis* and *Neisseria gonorrhoeae* (culture or rapid diagnostic techniques), (2) vaginal sampling for pH and saline and potassium hydroxide preparations to look for common vaginal pathogens (see section on vaginitis further on and Chapter 69), and (3) inspection of the genital skin for lesions. An annual Papanicolaou (Pap) smear should be performed to detect the presence of atypia, dysplasia, and HPV infections (the latter are associated with cervical dysplasia and cervical cancer); (see Chapter 69).

For sexually active adolescent males, an annual genital examination, including inspection of the genital skin for lesions, and screening for urethritis with "first-catch" urinalysis (see section on urethritis) looking for the presence of polymorphonuclear neutrophils (PMNs). Specific diagnostic tests are given in the sections on each syndrome and in Table 75–4 (see Chapter 69).

Laboratory testing for STDs can only be as accurate as the ability of the clinician to ensure correct specimen collection, transportation of the specimen, storage of the specimen, and laboratory identification. All diagnostic tests can lose the ability to identify positives (sensitivity) in the journey from specimen collection to laboratory processing. Cultures are definitive tests that minimize false-negative and false-positive rates. Nonculture tests have a higher potential for false-positive results. False-positive STD tests have obvious important clinical and psychosocial implications. In developing and evaluating the performance of an STD test, it is therefore imperative to generate a test with the lowest possible false-positive rate.

Another important issue in testing involves the variation in performance of a test, depending upon the prevalence of the infection in the population studied. For example, if 250 men were screened for urethritis by test "X" using the culture as the "gold standard" in both a high-prevalence (20%) and a low-prevalence (5%) population, the test performance could vary as shown in Table 75–5. Positive and negative predictive values (i.e., the likelihood that a positive or negative result is *true* in a certain population) vary with prevalence. It is important that the clinician using nonculture

TABLE 75–3. Common Signs and Syndromes of Sexually Transmitted Diseases

ORGAN SYSTEM	SIGNS	SYNDROMES	STD AGENT
Skin			
Generalized or localized: conjunctival, oropharyngeal, perineal	Rash: pain, pruritus, macular, papular, vesicular, ulcers, edema, erythema	Generalized: AIDS, syphilis, hepatitis Localized: conjunctivitis, oropharyngitis, vulvovaginitis proctitis, warts	Generalized: SYP, HIV, Hep B Localized: CT, GC, HSV, yeast, HIV, HPV
Bone	Erythema, edema, joint pain	Arthritis	GC, ? CT
Gastrointestinal			
Liver	Right upper quadrant tenderness (±) jaundice	Hepatitis, perihepatitis	GC or CT (Fitz-Hugh–Curtis), Hep B
Anorectum	Tears, excoriations, tenderness; mucoid, purulent bloody discharge; rash	Warts Proctitis Trauma	HPV, SYP CT, GC, HSV, SYP Enteric organisms
Genitourinary			
Urethra	Edema, excoriations, erythema, discharge; vaginal discharge (±)	Urethritis Vulvitis Vaginitis	CT, GC, HPV, TV Yeast, HSV, HPV, TV (See "vaginitis" in text)
Epididymis	Scrotal edema, tenderness	Epididymitis	CT, GC
Vagina	Abnormal malodorous discharge, tenderness, edema, erythema	Vulvovaginitis, bacterial vaginosis	Yeast, TV, GV, anerobes
Cervix	Mucopurulent discharge, erythema, edema, friability, abnormal results on Pap smear	Endocervicitis, ectocervicitis	CT, GC, TV, yeast, HSV (SYP, HPV have cervical lesions—not true cervicitis)
Uterus	Abnormal bleeding, uterine tenderness	Endometritis	CT, GC, anaerobes, other
Fallopian tubes	Cervical motion tenderness often associated with cervicitis and endometritis	Endometritis, salpingitis (PID)	CT, GC, anaerobes, other
Lymphoid tissue	Localized lymphadenopathy, generalized lymphadenopathy	Local STD infection AIDS	Most STDs HIV

SYP, *Treponema pallidum;* HIV, human immunodeficiency virus; Hep B, hepatitis B; CT, *Chlamydia trachomatis;* GC, *Neisseria gonorrhoeae;* HSV, herpes simplex virus; HPV, human papillomavirus; TV, *Trichomonas vaginalis;* GV, *Gardnerella vaginalis;* STDs, sexually transmitted diseases.

techniques be appraised of the performance profile of the test and the prevalence of the condition in the population tested. It is also critical that the reputation of the quality control of the laboratory be known and monitored appropriately, since some tests, such as fluorescent antibody screening for *Chlamydia trachomatis,* require specific equipment and training to ensure correct identification of diagnostic inclusions (see Chapter 69).

CLINICAL SYNDROMES

Syndromes comprise a constellation of clinical symptoms and signs associated with an infection with one or more STD agents (Table 75–6). The most common lower genital tract infections in women include vaginitis, cervicitis, PID, and urethritis. Men commonly present with urethritis, epididymitis, and proctitis. Both men and women can experience hepatitis, perihepatitis, and conjunctivitis. STD syndromes are the clinical presentations of STD infections. Specific STD agents will be discussed within the section on their respective syndromes. In addition, selected STD agents are referred to by syndrome and diagnosis in Table 75–4.

Vaginitis

Vaginitis is a syndrome characterized by an inflammatory response of the vaginal mucosa following exposure to an external chemical irritant or STD agent, such as yeasts, trichomonads, and bacterial vaginosis-associated bacteria. Although some do not consider bacterial vaginosis an "inflammatory" infection of the vaginal mucosa, and therefore not a true vaginitis, it will be included in the following discussion. Table 75–7 includes information on the three most common forms of vaginitis caused by *Candida albicans, Trichomonas vaginalis,* and *Gardnerella (Haemophilus) vaginalis.*

CANDIDA ALBICANS VAGINITIS

More than 500 species of yeast have been isolated from humans; 90% are pathogenic and 50% are associated with genital infections. *Candida albicans* has been isolated from the vagina in 2% to 40% of women. Most authors estimate that approximately 20% of women in their reproductive years have asymptomatic colonization with *Candida albicans* and that as many as 75% of women will have at least one symptomatic infection with *Candida albicans* during their lifetimes.

The addition of potassium hydroxide to vaginal secretions demonstrates yeast in mycelial and hyphal forms. Three laboratory methods to differentiate various strains of *Candida albicans* have recently been developed: (1) the Resistogram, which evaluates differences in tolerance to preselected chemicals, (2) killer toxin factors, and (3) biochemical characteristics, which identify strains by their reaction to specific biochemicals.

The exact mechanisms for pathogenic activity are not clear, but the following factors have been related to the development of symptoms: medications (antibiotics and higher dose oral contraceptives), adherence capabilities

TABLE 75–4. Selected Sexually Transmitted Diseases

NAME	COMMON SYNDROMES	DIAGNOSIS	COMMENTS
Neisseria gonorrhoeae: (Gonorrhea) gram-negative diplococci Treatment: see Table 75–9*	*Uncomplicated:* conjunctivitis endocervicitis pharyngitis proctitis urethritis *Complicated:* Disseminated gonococcal infection (DGI) Pelvic inflammatory disease	*Female: cervicitis* endocervical culture, Gram stain (sensitivity varies with experience of viewer) *Male: urethritis* Gram stain (gram-negative intracellular diplococci and polymorphonuclear cells) culture	Many asymptomatic infections in females and males; rapid diagnostic test available Screen all adolescents who have suspected *Neisseria gonorrhoeae* infections for syphilis
Chlamydia trachomatis: (Chlamydia) Treatment: see Table 75–9*	*Uncomplicated:* conjunctivitis endocervicitis urethritis proctitis *Complicated:* Pelvic inflammatory disease (pharyngitis?)	*Female: endocervicitis* mucopus >30 PMNs/high-power field on Gram stain or endocervical friability or endocervical culture (+) or antigen detection test (+) *Male: nongonococcal urethritis* negative gonococcal culture *or* Gram stain ≥4 polymorphonuclear cells/oil immersion (mean of 5 high-power fields × 1000×) and no gram-negative intracellular diplococci urethral culture (+) antigen detection test (+)	Many asymptomatic infections in females and males; most common cause of cervicitis in adolescent females and urethritis in adolescent males
Treponema pallidum Treatment: see Table 75–12*	*Primary:* chancre *Secondary:* generalized skin rash, especially palms and soles; Early, late, latent *Tertiary:* rare in adolescents	*Primary:* treponemes on dark-field study *Secondary:* Venereal Disease Research Laboratory (VDRL) test or rapid plasma reagin test (RPR), confirmed by fluorescent treponemal antibody absorption test or microhemagglutination-*Treponema pallidum*	Rate has recently doubled in teenagers; screen with VDRL test or RPR if contact history, diagnosis of any STD or in population with high syphilis rate
Herpes simplex virus Treatment: see Table 75–12*	Genital herpes: primary (systemic) recurrent (local) vulvovaginitis cervicitis proctitis penile lesions urethritis oropharyngitis	Based on symptoms and signs at presentation Herpes simplex virus culture with fluorescent antibody	Infection in adolescents often primary disease
Human papillomavirus Treatment: see Table 75–14	*Condyloma acuminatum:* visible genital skin wart Subclinical human papillomavirus: invisible flat condyloma occur anywhere in anogenital tract	*Condyloma acuminatum:* visible on genital skin Subclinical human papillomavirus: pretreatment of area with 3% acetic acid wash; colposcopic examination: dense, white areas (biopsy) Human papillomavirus: DNA detection (hybridization techniques) Pap smear: for screening only (koilocytosis)	*Disease by type:* Benign genital warts types 6, 11 Anogenital neoplasia types 16, 18, 31, 33, 35 *Condyloma acuminatum:* Liquid nitrogen: pain on application Podophyllin: systemic toxicity; teratogenicity precludes use on mucosa and during pregnancy Trichloroacetic acid: Safe with mucosa and pregnancy; local sensitivity Subclinical human papillomavirus: Refer all adolescents with visible warts for evaluation and treatment of possible subclinical human papillomavirus

*STD Treatment Guidelines, Centers for Disease Control, 1989.

TABLE 75–5. Example of a Screening Test's Performance Variance between High- and Low-Prevalence Populations for a Sexually Transmitted Disease "X"

		POPULATION	
		High Prevalence	Low Prevalence
Total Number (N) Tested		250	250
Prevalence N (%)*		50 (20%)	13 (5%)
Test Results:			
TP (True positive)	FP (False positive)	45 | 5	12 | 5
FN (False negative)	TN (True negative)	5 | 195	1 | 232
Performance			
Sensitivity (%)	= TP/(TP + FN)	90%	90%
Specificity (%)	= TN/(TN + FP)	98%	98%
Positive predictive value (%)	= TP/(TP + FP)	90%	71%
Negative predictive value (%)	= TN/(TN + FN)	98%	99.6%

*Using "gold" standard test, i.e., culture.

of the organism, and diseases such as diabetes mellitus and acquired immunodeficiency syndrome (AIDS). Genital *Candida albicans* can be transmitted by sexual activity. Natural protection from the development of symptomatic infections exists in several forms. Normal vaginal bacterial flora provide a milieu that is not supportive of the establishment of candidiasis. In contrast, antimicrobial agents can alter the normal bacterial flora, allowing *Candida albicans* to flourish, with little competition for nutrients from the normal vaginal inhabitants. A humoral antibody response (IgM, IgG) has been described with candidal infections. Cellular elements of the immune system, such as phagocytic cells, PMNs, and monocytes may limit the infectivity of the *Candida*. Cell-mediated immunity is an important aspect of defense from *Candida*. Clinical characteristics and treatment regimens are outlined in Table 75–7.

TRICHOMONAS VAGINALIS

Trichomonas vaginalis is a flagellated protozoan that is sexually transmitted in humans and causes vaginitis.

Trichomonas vaginalis colonizes the genital organs of both sexes.

The prepubertal vagina is not hospitable to the growth of *Trichomonas vaginalis*; in the child *Trichomonas vaginalis* probably originates in the urinary tract or possibly from sexual abuse. Most women who have a genital tract infection have a urinary tract infection with *Trichomonas vaginalis*. It has been established that about one third of asymptomatically infected women become symptomatic within 6 months. Several factors have been identified in assisting the establishment of or exacerbating *Trichomonas vaginalis* infections in females, including menses, pH changes, hormonal influences, and changes in the normal flora of the vagina. It is, therefore, recommended that asymptomatic females with *Trichomonas vaginalis* infections be treated. Although more than 75% of the female partners of men with *Trichomonas vaginalis* infections are found to be infected, less than one half of the male partners of women with infections are infected, and most of these infected males are asymptomatic.

The pathogenesis of human trichomonal infections has yet to be delineated precisely. *Trichomonas vaginalis*

TABLE 75–6. Common Syndromes Associated with Sexually Transmitted Disease Agents

	FUNGAL PROTOZOAL		BACTERIA						VIRAL			
SYNDROMES	CA	TV	CT	GC	MY	SYP	GV	HD	HPV	HSV	Hep A, B	HIV
Urethritis	X	X	X	X	X	—	—	—	X	—	—	—
Epididymitis	—	—	X	X	?	—	—	—	—	—	—	—
Proctitis	X	—	X	X	—	—	—	—	—	X	—	—
Vulvitis	X	—	—	—	—	—	X	—	—	X	—	—
Vaginitis	X	X	—	—	?	—	X	—	—	—	—	—
Cervicitis	X	X	X	X	—	—	—	—	—	X	—	—
PID (endometritis, salpingitis)	—	—	X	X	?	—	?	—	—	—	—	—
Genital ulcers	—	—	—	—	—	X	—	X	—	X	—	—
Genital warts	—	—	—	—	—	X	—	—	X	—	—	—
AIDS	—	—	—	—	—	—	—	—	—	—	—	X
Hepatitis/perihepatitis	—	—	X	X	—	X	—	—	—	—	X	?
Cervical neoplasia	—	—	?	—	—	—	—	—	X	X	—	—

CA, *Candida albicans*; TV, *Trichomonas vaginalis*; CT, *Chlamydia trachomatis*; GC, *Neisseria gonorrhoeae*; MY, *Mycoplasma* spp, SYP, syphilis; GV, *Gardnerella vaginalis*; HD, *Haemophilus ducreyi*; HPV, human papillomavirus; HSV, herpes simplex virus, type 2; Hep A, B, hepatitis A and B; HIV, human immunodeficiency virus; PID, pelvic inflammatory disease.

TABLE 75–7. Clinical Profile of Common Causes of Vaginitis from Sexually Transmitted Diseases

PROFILE	NORMAL	CANDIDAL VAGINITIS	TRICHOMONAL VAGINITIS	BACTERIAL VAGINOSIS
Microbe	Normal flora; lactobacillus	*Candida albicans,* other yeast	*Trichomonas vaginalis*	*Gardnerella vaginalis,* anaerobes, other
Vulvovaginal discomfort*	—	Mild to marked pruritus	Moderate to severe	Mild
Vaginal mucosa	—	Erythema, edema	Can have marked erythema, edema not inflammatory	Not true inflammatory vaginitis, i.e., "vaginosis"
Discharge				
quantity	Varies	Scant to moderate	Increased	Increase (slight)
quality	Nonhomogenous	Clumped to adherent	Purulent, frothy	Watery
color	Clear, white	White	Yellow to green	White, gray
odor	None	None	odor	Fishy with 10% potassium hydroxide
pH	≤4.5	≤4.5	≥5	≥5
Cervix	Normal	Can cause cervicitis (columnar epithelia relatively immune)	Can cause cervicitis	—
Microscopy				
Sodium chloride	Epithelia, occasionally polymorphonuclear neutrophils, lactobacilli	Few polymorphonuclear neutrophils	Polymorphonuclear neutrophils; motile trichomonads	Few polymorphonuclear neutrophils, clue cells, few lactobacilli
Potassium hydroxide	Negative	Yeast, mycelia, pseudohyphae	—	—
Gram stain	Normal flora, occasional polymorphonuclear neutrophils	—	—	Few lactobacilli, mixed flora includes *Gardnerella vaginalis,* anaerobes
Treatment	None	Clotrimazole (intravaginal) 100 mg daily for 3 or 7 days	Metronidazole 2 g orally for one dose	Metronidazole 500 mg orally twice daily for 7 days

*With symptomatic disease.

Adapted with permission from Holmes KK: In Holmes KK, Mardh PA, Sparling PF, Wiesner PJ (eds): Sexually Transmitted Diseases, 2nd ed. New York, McGraw-Hill, 1990, p 527.

attaches to squamous epithelial cells of the vagina, with columnar epithelia appearing to be relatively resistant to infection. It is therefore more efficacious to obtain specimens from the vaginal mucosa (squamous) rather than the endocervix (columnar cells) when diagnosing *Trichomonas* infection. *Trichomonas vaginalis* causes an acute inflammation of the mucosa with increased, often frothy, copious yellow and green vaginal discharge. There is no actual invasion of the mucosa itself. On microscopic examination, PMNs are abundant in the discharge. This phagocytic cellular activity is the predominant cell response to *Trichomonas vaginalis,* and PMNs have been shown to kill the organism. To date, other immune system mechanisms, such as humoral immunity and cell-mediated immunity, have not been proved to have major roles in the human defense against infection with *Trichomonas vaginalis.*

Clinically, symptoms appear within a few days to 1 month after apparent exposure. Symptoms include increased vaginal discharge (50% to 75%), genital pruritus (23% to 82%), dysuria (30% to 50%) and, in a small number of women, pain in the lower abdomen (up to 12%). The diagnosis is confirmed with the identification of motile flagellated organisms on microscopic examination of vaginal secretions in both symptomatic and asymptomatic females (see Chapter 69). Such wet mount examination correctly identifies *Trichomonas vaginalis* in 40% to 80% of cases. Pap smears are accurate in the diagnosis of *Trichomonas vaginalis* in approximately 60% to 70% of cases, with culture in anaerobic condi-

tions yielding the best recovery rate. Currently, immunofluorescent antibody and enzyme-linked immunoassay tests for *Trichomonas vaginalis* have been developed and are being evaluated, with early results producing sensitivity rates greater than 90%. Common clinical findings in *Trichomonas vaginalis* vaginitis and treatment regimens are found in Table 75–7.

BACTERIAL VAGINOSIS

Controversy continues to surround bacterial vaginosis, including its name, pathogenesis, clinical presentation, treatment, and its relationship to complications. Gardner and Dukes first suggested its existence in 1955, describing a vaginal infection, without the presence of vaginitis, with either *Trichomonas vaginalis* or *Candida albicans,* which was associated with the presence of a small gram-negative organism *(Haemophilus vaginalis,* now called *Gardnerella vaginalis).* The syndrome has undergone several name changes, which reflect our evolving understanding of its cause and pathogenesis: *Haemophilus vaginalis* vaginitis, nonspecific vaginosis, and, currently, bacterial vaginosis. The most recent term, *bacterial vaginosis,* represents the current understanding of the syndrome in that vaginal epithelial inflammation is not a major component of the clinical presentation; it probably is the interaction of several microorganisms that results in the clinical symptoms and signs attributed to the syndrome.

The exact prevalence of the syndrome is difficult to

determine accurately because it is not a reportable disease, and a specific definition of the syndrome for diagnosis is not accepted by everyone. Although there is strong evidence to support the sexual transmissibility of the organisms associated with bacterial vaginosis, these microorganisms have also been isolated from virginal females. However, the bacterial vaginosis–associated microorganisms are reportedly found most frequently among sexually active females. It has been reported that as many as 40% to 60% of adolescent girls attending adolescent clinics for reproductive health examinations have bacterial vaginosis.

Bacterial vaginosis appears to be a result of the replacement of the normal bacterial vaginal flora with the vaginosis-associated organisms and their subsequent interactions, which changes the vaginal microbiologic and biochemical vaginal milieu. The suggested pathogenic bacteria include *Gardnerella vaginalis*, genital mycoplasmas, and anaerobes (*Peptostreptococcus* spp., *Bacteroides* spp., *Mobiluncus* spp.). The presence of these organisms causes a change in the composition of the vaginal fluid so that there is a decrease in the number of lactobacilli, and therefore lactate, and an increase in organic products such as succinate and putrescine (among others), which are most likely responsible for the odor associated with typical vaginal secretions.

Three of the four criteria put forth by Amsel are required for the diagnosis of bacterial vaginosis: (1) a homogeneous, uniformly adherent white vaginal discharge; (2) a vaginal pH greater than 4.5; (3) positive "whiff" test, that is, the release of a "fishy" amine odor when the vaginal secretion is mixed with a solution of 10% potassium hydroxide on a glass slide (one drop of discharge to one drop of potassium hydroxide); and (4) the presence of "clue" cells under microscopic examination of vaginal fluid (at least 20% of the epithelial cells present/field). Gram staining vaginal fluid can be useful to determine the change in the microbiologic shift and should show a decrease or lack of lactobacilli and an increase in the number of gram-variable coccobacilli (*Gardnerella vaginalis* or *Bacteroides* spp.). Culture of the vaginal fluid usually does not assist much in the immediate diagnosis of the syndrome. Table 75–7 describes the clinical presentation and treatment regimens. Treatment of asymptomatic women with bacterial vaginosis remains controversial.

Cervicitis

Cervicitis might be considered the female equivalent of male nongonococcal urethritis. Incidence data in adolescents are not available (beyond those reported for the recovery of *Chlamydia trachomatis*, and *Neisseria gonorrhoeae*) because of the problems associated with diagnosis. The embryonic development of the cervix results in the prepubertal ectocervix having columnar epithelial cells, with the transition zone between "immature" columnar cells and "adult" squamous cells well out on the ectocervical surface. With age, the transition zone and the columnar cells regress to within the cervical os in adulthood. Squamous epithelia are more resistant to infection than are columnar cells. *Chlamydia trachomatis* and certain types of *Neisseria gonorrhoeae* have a predilection for infecting columnar cells. Adolescent females have vestiges of columnar cells on the ectocervix. Therefore, the increased incidence of infection from these organisms in this population may result from this anatomic vulnerability.

Although there are numerous reported causes of both infectious and noninfectious cervicitis (Table 75–8), the main causes of endocervicitis include *Chlamydia trachomatis*, *Neisseria gonorrhoeae*, and herpes simplex virus. In attempting to assess the presence of cervicitis, two factors must be considered. First, adolescent females have more columnar epithelia on the cervix as a normal part of development, and this "ectopy" is often difficult to differentiate from an inflamed cervix. Second, it is important to differentiate between cervicitis and vaginitis, as they are often found together.

The hallmark of endocervicitis is the presence of "mucopurulent cervicitis." Although one group has established criteria for the clinical diagnosis of mucopurulent cervicitis, the criteria are often difficult for the inexperienced clinician to reproduce. Endocervicitis is diagnosed in the presence of mucopurulent endocervical discharge (yellow or green discharge from the os on a white swab against a white background), edema and erythema of ectopic tissue (determined most accurately by colposcopy), and friability (easy bleeding induced by touching affected tissue with a swab) and the presence of greater than 30 PMNs on a Gram-stained smear of the endocervical secretion on oil immersion. Mucopu-

TABLE 75–8. Reported Causes of Cervicitis

MICROBIOLOGIC			OTHER
Bacterial	**Viral**	**Protozoal**	
Chlamydia trachomatis	Herpes simplex virus	*Trichomonas vaginalis*	Autoimmune
Neisseria gonorrhoeae	Cytomegalovirus	Others	Malignant
Calymmatobacterium granulomatis	Adenovirus		Physical
Treponema pallidum	Human papillomavirus		Trauma
Mycoplasma tuberculosis			Chemical
Gardnerella vaginalis			Irradiation
Enterobacteriaceae			
Group B streptococcus			
Haemophilus spp.			
Streptococcus aureus			
Mycoplasma hominis			
Ureaplasma urealyticum			

Adapted with permission from Paavonen J, Stamm WE: Lower genital tract infections in women. Infect Dis Clin North Am 1:188, 1987.

rulent endocervicitis is most closely correlated with the presence of *Chlamydia trachomatis,* though *Neisseria gonorrhoeae* is probably also related. Herpes simplex virus is associated with ulcerative lesions on the cervix, especially in the presence of external genital lesions.

In addition to the Gram stain for determining the presence of PMNs, culture or rapid diagnostic testing for specific microbial antigen detection can confirm the diagnosis. The sensitivities of nonculture techniques vary according to the specimen source, gender of the adolescent, presence of symptoms, and the microbe. Most tests have not been studied in detail in a number of populations differing by gender and by symptoms. To date, however, the sensitivity for the chlamydial enzyme immunoassay test for females is greater than 95%, and for males, it is approximately 70% (see Chapter 69). *Chlamydia* fluorescent antibody sensitivity rates for females is about 70%; the gonorrheal enzyme immunoassay test sensitivity in males is 93%. Cervical cytologic assessment (Pap smear) and colposcopy can also be used as adjunctive tests in the confirmation of cervicitis. Examination of the sexual partner may provide additional information about the cause of the infection. Treatment is directed toward the common etiologic factors—*Chlamydia trachomatis* and *Neisseria gonorrhoeae;* the diagnostic and treatment regimens are outlined in Tables 75–4 and 75–9, respectively.

Pelvic Inflammatory Disease

PID, along with its sequelae of infertility and ectopic pregnancy, is one of the most important conditions among young women of reproductive age. Almost one half of the estimated annual 1 million cases of acute PID occur in women younger than 25 years of age. The rate of PID, based on hospital discharge summary data, was 292 in 100,000 hospitalized women aged 15 to 19 years in 1987. This rate underestimates the actual risk for PID in this age group, since only 50% of 15- to 19-year-old females have ever been sexually active, and many others have intercourse only intermittently. It is the *adolescent* female that is at greatest risk for the development of PID compared with all other women when adjustments are made for sexual activity.

Although age is the strongest predictor of risk for PID, the importance of the individual contributions of the biologic development of the genital tract and the behavioral factors that place the adolescent at increased risk for PID is unknown. Ethnic differences in risk for PID are shown at all age groups of women in their reproductive years, including adolescents. The ratio of nonwhite:white cases of PID in 15- to 19-year-old females is 2.5:1. However, after adjusting for sexual activity, the ethnic prevalence for PID risk disappears.

Contraception has been shown to both increase and decrease the risk for PID and its sequelae. This relationship is dependent upon the type of contraception used. For example, barrier methods used in combination with a spermicide, such as nonoxynol-9, decrease the risk of PID by offering protection from transmission of STDs during intercourse. In contrast, intrauterine devices (IUDs) increase the overall risk for PID by a factor

of 2 to 5. The IUD establishes local endometritis. It has been suggested that the infection spreads to the fallopian tubes from the inflamed endometrium. The risk for PID appears to vary with the type of IUD used. The Dalkon shield has been associated with particularly severe PID. IUDs with attached strings may provide bacteria increased access to the endometrial cavity. Data on the role of oral contraceptives and PID have been confusing. Currently, most studies support the concept that oral contraceptives offer at least some protection from PID.

The timing of the menstrual cycle has been linked to the development of acute PID. Cases resulting from both *Neisseria gonorrhoeae* and *Chlamydia trachomatis* have been shown to occur significantly more frequently within the first week after the onset of menstruation. It has been postulated that the loss of the protective cervical mucous plug, the presence of the rich nutrient environment provided by the menstrual blood, and retrograde menstrual flow into the fallopian tube itself may enhance the growth and ascension of potential pathogens through the endocervix to the fallopian tube. However, additional factors must play a role in the menses link to PID, since the occurrence of PID not associated with *Chlamydia trachomatis* or *Neisseria gonorrhoeae* does not appear to be related to the menstrual cycle.

Other risk factors for PID include a prior history of PID caused by *Neisseria gonorrhoeae,* a history of multiple sexual partners, vaginal douching, and STD infections. Finally, there may be biologic factors that place the adolescent female at risk for PID.

PID is polymicrobic, which affects its treatment and prevention. The causative agents are numerous and are often present in a variety of combinations. In the United States, *Neisseria gonorrhoeae* is isolated in 30% to 50% of cases, *Chlamydia trachomatis* is isolated in 25% to 40% of cases, and a number of anaerobes and facultative aerobes have been identified in samples from the fallopian tubes in 25% to 50% of females with acute PID. Specific microorganisms linked to infection in the fallopian tubes include *Chlamydia trachomatis, Neisseria gonorrhoeae,* mixed anaerobic bacteria (*Bacteroides* spp., *Peptostreptococcus* spp., and *Peptococcus* spp.), and facultative bacteria (*Gardnerella vaginalis, Streptococcus* spp., *Escherichia coli,* and *Haemophilus influenzae*). In addition, the role of the genital mycoplasmas is unclear in the development of PID. Of recent interest is the possible association of the organisms related to the bacterial vaginosis syndrome and PID. *Bacteroides* spp., *Peptostreptococcus* spp., and *Mobiluncus* spp., as well as α-hemolytic streptococci, have been related to both PID and bacterial vaginosis, suggesting that a lower genital infection with bacterial vaginosis organisms may occur prior to upper tract infection.

PID is established through the exposure of the vagina and endocervix to potentially pathogenic organisms via sexual activity, the canalicular spread of the organisms through the endocervix along the endometrial mucosa and finally to the fallopian tube itself, and ultimately leakage of infected material onto peritoneal surfaces through the fimbriated end of the fallopian tube. It is estimated that 10% to 20% of women with endocervical infections with either *Neisseria gonorrhoeae* or *Chla-*

TABLE 75–9. Treatment Regimens for Gonococcal and Chlamydial Infections*

GONOCOCCAL INFECTIONS
Uncomplicated Urethral, Endocervical, or Rectal Infections
*Recommended Regimen**
Ceftriaxone: 250 mg intramuscularly, one dose
        PLUS
Doxycycline: 100 mg orally twice daily for 7 days†
Alternative Regimen
When patient cannot take ceftriaxone:
  Spectinomycin: 2 g intramuscularly, one dose (followed by doxycycline)
Proven non–penicillinase-producing *Neisseria gonorrhoeae* strain
  Amoxicillin: 3 g orally with 1 g probenecid once (followed by doxycycline regimen)
In *pregnancy* or when patient cannot take tetracycline-doxycycline
  Erythromycin base or stearate: 500 mg orally four times daily for 7 days
      OR
  Erythromycin ethylsuccinate: 800 mg orally four times daily for 7 days

Pharyngeal Gonococcal Infection Only
Recommended Regimen
Ceftriaxone: 250 mg intramuscularly once
Alternative Regimen
When patient cannot be treated with ceftriaxone:
  Ciprofloxacin: 500 mg orally once (repeat culture in 4 to 7 days since experience with this regimen is limited)
In pregnancy, see CDC STD Treatment Guidelines, 1989
Disseminated Gonococcal Infection (DGI)
Hospitalization is recommended for initial therapy and to evaluate for evidence of endocarditis or meningitis
Recommended Regimens
Ceftriaxone: 1 g intramuscularly or intravenously every 24 hours
      OR
Ceftizoxime: 1 g intravenously every 8 hours
      OR
Cefotaxime: 1 g intravenously every 8 hours
Alternative Regimens
Patients allergic to β-lactam antibiotics
  Spectinomycin 2 g intramuscularly every 12 hours
If gonococci proved to be penicillin-sensitive, change to
  ampicillin 1 g every 6 hours (or equivalent)
Recommended Treatment Course
Compliant patients with uncomplicated disease may be discharged 24 to 48 hours after all symptoms resolve and may complete the *total* of 1 week of antibiotic therapy with:
Cefuroxime axetil, 500 mg bid
      OR
Amoxicillin, 500 mg with clavulanic acid
      OR
Ciprofoxacin, 500 mg twice daily *if not pregnant*
Adult Gonococcal Ophthalmia (nonsepticemic)
Recommended Regimen
Ceftriaxone 1 g intramuscularly once
Recommended Adjunct Management
Irrigation of eyes, ophthamologic consultation, and evaluation for concurrent chlamydial infection should be performed

GONOCOCCAL INFECTIONS *Continued*
Treatment of Other Syndromes, Follow-up, and Partner Management
Evaluation or treatment, or both, for concurrent chlamydial infections.
Treatment regimens for other sites, including meningitis, endocarditis, and treatment of infants and children is described elsewhere (Treatment Guidelines, CDC, 1989)
Partners within the last 30 days should be contacted and evaluated for both gonococcal and chlamydial disease and treated; condoms should be used
Follow-up of patients should occur 4 to 7 days after treatment, and definitive diagnostic tests should be performed when possible to assess test of cure and encourage safer sexual practices, including condom use
All patients with gonorrhea should be tested for syphilis
Treatment for pelvic inflammatory disease is outlined in Table 75–11
CHLAMYDIAL INFECTIONS
Uncomplicated Urethral, Endocervical, or Rectal Infection
Recommended Regimens
Doxycycline 100 mg orally twice daily for 7 days
      OR
Tetracycline 500 mg orally four times daily for 7 days
  (may have decreased compliance because of four times daily protocol)
      AND
Ceftriaxone 250 mg intramuscularly once
Alternative Regimens
Erythromycin base or stearate: 250 mg orally four times daily for 7 days
      OR
Erythromycin ethylsuccinate: 800 mg orally four times daily for 7 days
Additional alternative when erythromycin is not tolerated
  Sulfisoxazole: 500 mg orally four times daily for 10 days
In pregnancy, may use erythromycin base: 500 mg orally four times daily for 7 days; and ceftriaxone 250 mg intramuscularly once
      OR
Erythromycin ethylsuccinate: 800 mg orally four times daily for 7 days
Partner Management
If there has been sexual contact within 30 days of onset of symptoms, partners should be tested and treated, or treat when testing not available
Treatment regimens for acute pelvic inflammatory disease are described in Table 75–11
Epididymitis (*Neisseria gonorrhoeae* or *Chlamydia trachomatis* most likely cause in heterosexual male <35 years)
Recommended Regimens
Ceftriaxone 250 mg intramuscularly once
      AND
Doxycycline 100 mg orally or intramuscularly twice daily for 10 days
      OR
Tetracycline, 500 mg orally four times daily for 10 days

Adapted from Centers for Disease Control: STD Treatment Guidelines. Washington, DC, U.S. Dept. of Health and Human Services, Public Health Service, 1989. (Other alternative regimens in pregnancy are outlined in CDC document also.)
*Most patients with incubating syphilis (seronegative and no signs) may be cured by any regimen containing β-lactams (e.g., ceftriaxone) or tetracyclines.
†Tetracyclines alone are no longer considered adequate therapy for gonococcal infections but are added for treatment of coexisting chlamydial infection; tetracyclines are contraindicated during pregnancy.

---

mydia trachomatis will experience acute PID. The reasons for the ascension of infection in some women and not in others is not well understood, but it is likely a combination of host, organism, and environmental factors acting individually or in concert to enhance the establishment of PID.

The short-term complication of most concern in acute PID is the development of a tubo-ovarian abscess (TOA), which occurs in up to 16% of cases. The abscess is the result of infected material leaking from the fim-

briae onto the surface of the ovary and causing an inflammatory mass and abscess complex involving both the fallopian tube and the ovary. It is estimated that 3% to 15% of TOAs rupture, creating a surgical emergency. However, fertility may still be possible; a conservative approach is recommended when surgery is necessary.

Perihepatitis (Fitz-Hugh–Curtis syndrome) develops in 5% to 20% of women with acute PID. Perihepatitis has traditionally been associated with gonococcal infections. However, both *Neisseria gonorrhoeae* and *Chlamydia trachomatis* can be causative agents. Classically, perihepatitis presents with acute pleuritic right upper quadrant pain, which radiates from the shoulder to the back. Although two thirds of affected individuals experience the onset of pain with the abdominal pain of acute PID, the remainder of individuals may experience the onset of right upper quadrant pain for up to 2 weeks after the resolution of the lower abdominal pain of salpingitis. The diagnosis of perihepatitis is likely in the young woman with acute PID, right upper quadrant pain, and a normal ultrasound examination of the gallbladder (see Chapter 62).

In Swedish studies, common long-term sequelae of acute PID include ectopic pregnancy in 5%, involuntary infertility in 21%, and chronic pelvic pain, pain with intercourse, and pelvic adhesions in another 21% of individuals. Ectopic pregnancy has increased by a factor of 4 between 1970 and 1983 in the United States. It is the leading cause of maternal death in the first trimester of pregnancy and in large part results from tubal damage secondary to acute PID. PID caused by *Chlamydia trachomatis* is most closely associated with ectopic pregnancy. Infertility is another long-term sequela of PID. Fallopian tube factor infertility may be responsible for up to one third of the estimated 2 million cases of female infertility. The risk factors associated with infertility following PID are tubal obstruction, a nongonococcal cause (especially *Chlamydia trachomatis*), repeated episodes of PID, hospitalization for PID, an erthrocyte sedimentation rate of more than 15 mm/hour when PID is diagnosed, and the type of contraceptive used.

Only 65% of patients with presumed PID (based on the traditional symptoms and signs of acute PID, such as lower abdominal pain, vaginal discharge, cervical motion tenderness, and uterine and adnexal tenderness) have been shown to have PID verified by laparoscopy. Other conditions that can present with similar signs and symptoms include cystitis, cholecystitis, pyelonephritis, acute appendicitis, mesenteric lymphadenitis, ectopic pregnancy, intrauterine pregnancy, septic abortion, ovarian tumor, ovarian cyst with or without torsion, hemorrhagic ovarian cyst, severe constipation, and traumatic injuries to the abdominal organ. Since the use of the laparoscope is not always practical for all cases of suspected PID, the diagnosis is dependent upon eliciting risk factors from a careful history taking and performing an examination, including a pelvic examination. Many of the signs associated with the diagnosis are "subjective" findings, such as abdominal tenderness and cervical motion tenderness. It is therefore useful for the clinician to base the diagnosis of acute PID on reasonable guidelines, which are outlined in Table 75–10.

When possible, direct cultures or rapid diagnostic tests for *Chlamydia trachomatis* and *Neisseria gonorrhoeae* should be performed. Examination of, and specimen culture from, the male partner or partners can aid in the diagnosis of PID. A rapid urine or serum pregnancy test should be performed as part of the work-up and for efficacious and safe medical diagnostic and treatment regimens. Ultrasound can be helpful in the diagnosis of an intrauterine or an ectopic pregnancy and in the determination of an inflammatory mass or abscess.

TABLE 75–10. Clinical Criteria: Diagnosis of Acute Salpingitis (Pelvic Inflammatory Disease)

All three of the following should be present:
1. Lower abdominal tenderness
2. Cervical motion tenderness
3. Adnexal tenderness (unilateral or bilateral)

PLUS

One of the following should be present:
1. Temperature $\geq 38°C$
2. White blood cell count $\geq 10,500/mm^3$
3. Purulent material obtained by culdocentesis
4. An inflammatory mass present on bimanual pelvic examination or sonography, or both
5. Erythrocyte sedimentation rate >15 mm/hour
6. Evidence of the presence of *Neisseria gonorrhoeae* or *Chlamydia trachomatis*, or both in endocervix:
   Gram stain reveals gram-negative intracellular diplococci
   Monoclonal antibody to *Chlamydia trachomatis* positive
7. Presence of ≥ 5 polymorphonuclear neutrophils/oil immersion field on Gram stain of endocervical discharge

Adapted with permission from Sweet RL: Pelvic inflammatory disease and infertility in women. Infect Dis Clin North Am 1:199, 1987.

Treatment is begun as soon as the diagnosis is made and is designed to be broad-based and to preserve fertility. The Centers for Disease Control recommendations are found in Table 75–11.

The management of PID in the adolescent includes the use of diagnostic criteria as guidelines, "overdiagnosis" of PID to begin early treatment and prevent sequelae, broad spectrum antibiotic treatment, careful reassessment of the patient in 48 to 72 hours to confirm the diagnosis and course, and management of the sexual partner or partners.

Urethritis

In males, sexually transmitted urethritis is traditionally classified as gonococcal and nongonococcal. Nongonococcal urethritis is most often associated with *Chlamydia trachomatis* or *Ureaplasma urealyticum*. Twenty percent to 50% of males diagnosed with gonococcal urethritis have a concomitant infection with *Chlamydia trachomatis*. Although *Chlamydia trachomatis* is responsible for 30% to 50% or more of the cases of nongonococcal disease, *Ureaplasma urealyticum* has been found in 10% to 40% of cases. In addition, approximately 20% to 30% of cases of nongonococcal urethritis are associated with organisms other than *Chlamydia trachomatis* and *Ureaplasma urealyticum*, including *Trichomonas vaginalis*, yeasts, viruses (herpes simplex virus, HPV, adenovirus), and possibly *Bacteroides* spp. and *Mycoplasma genitalium*.

The syndrome of urethritis is the most common presentation of infection with *Neisseria gonorrhoeae* in males. Approximately 2 to 6 days after exposure to *Neisseria gonorrhoeae*, symptoms of dysuria and urethral discharge develops. The characteristic discharge associated with *Neisseria gonorrhoeae* is described as copious and purulent. However, the spectrum of discharge includes "scant" and "mucoid," which is considered the classic description for discharge associated with urethritis caused by *Chlamydia trachomatis*. Sexual transmis-

TABLE 75–11. Treatment Regimens for Acute Pelvic Inflammatory Disease

RECOMMENDED INPATIENT REGIMENS
1. Cefoxitin: 2 g intravenously every 6 hours
OR
Cefotetan:*   2 g intravenously every 12 hours
PLUS
Doxycycline: 100 mg intravenously every 12 hours
Use intravenously for minimum of 48 hours after patient improves
After discharge, continue doxycycline, 100 mg orally twice daily to complete 10- to 14-day course
OR
2. Clindamycin: 900 mg intravenously every 8 hours
PLUS
Gentamicin: 2 mg/kg intravenously or intramuscularly in one loading dose, followed by a maintenance dose of 1.5 mg/kg intravenously every 8 hours in patients with normal renal function
Use intravenously for minimum of 48 hours after patient improves
After discharge, doxycycline, 100 mg orally twice daily for 10 to 14 days total
OR
Continue clindamycin 450 mg orally four times daily to complete a 10- to 14-day course as an alternative

RECOMMENDED OUTPATIENT REGIMENS
1. Cefoxitin: 2 g intramuscularly
PLUS
Probenecid: 1 g orally
OR
2. Ceftriaxone: 250 mg intramuscularly or equivalent cephalosporin
PLUS
Doxycycline: 100 mg orally twice daily for 10 to 14 days
OR
Tetracycline: 500 mg orally four times daily for 10 to 14 days

RECOMMENDED ALTERNATIVES FOR PATIENTS WHO DO NOT TOLERATE DOXYCYCLINE OR WHO ARE PREGNANT
Erythromycin: 500 mg orally four times daily for 10 to 14 days (based on limited clinical data)

MANAGEMENT OF SEX PARTNERS
As in any STD, partners should be evaluated for STD and treated empirically for *Neisseria gonorrhoeae* and *Chlamydia trachomatis* infection

---

*Other cephalosporins, such as ceftizoxime, cefotaxime, ceftriaxone, provide adequate gonococcal coverage; other facultative gram-negative aerobic and anaerobic coverage may also be used in appropriate doses.

From Centers for Disease Control: STD Treatment Guidelines. Washington, DC, U.S. Dept. of Health and Human Services, Public Health Service, 1989.

---

sion roles are gender-specific. After one sexual exposure to a partner infected with *Neisseria gonorrhoeae*, approximately 20% of males will experience urethritis. In contrast, the male to female transmission rate approaches 50%, though studies controlling for the number of sexual exposures are not available.

The pathogenesis of *Chlamydia trachomatis* urethritis is not well understood. It may take days to weeks after sexual exposure before urethral symptoms appear. Many urethral infections are asymptomatic. One study reported that 9% of asymptomatic sexually active adolescent males screened through cultures were shown to have urethral infections caused by *Chlamydia trachomatis*.

The diagnosis of urethritis in males is based on the clinical findings of dysuria or urethral discharge, or both. On examination, the urethral meatus may be inflamed and edematous. The urethral discharge may be present spontaneously or present only after stripping the urethra (three times).

Laboratory evaluation of urethritis begins with Gram staining the sample obtained by placing a small urethral swab at the meatal os and then by rolling the swab tip on a glass slide. The Gram-stained preparation is then examined under oil immersion for the presence of 4 PMNs or more/field (urethritis): the finding of PMNs accompanied by intracellular diplococci is consistent with urethritis caused by *Neisseria gonorrhoeae*; the finding of PMNs without intracellular diplococci is diagnostic for nongonococcal urethritis and is usually considered to be synonymous in young men with *Chlamydia trachomatis* urethritis until proved otherwise.

The sensitivity of predicting urethral infection caused by *Neisseria gonorrhoeae* by Gram staining is greater than 95% among symptomatic males and decreases to 70% among asymptomatic males with urethritis caused by *Neisseria gonorrhoeae*. Access to laboratories that process *Neisseria gonorrhoeae* is readily available, whereas few laboratories can provide chlamydial culture services. In addition, cultures are costly, and the results are not immediately available. Recently, several immunoassays that detect antigen have become available to diagnose *Neisseria gonorrhoeae* and *Chlamydia trachomatis* urethritis using specimens from urethral secretions and urine sediment. However, confirmation of suspected gonococcal infections through cultures allows the opportunity for antibiotic resistance testing. Currently, nonculture techniques, such as enzyme immunoassays, are being evaluated in populations of males and females in whom there is low prevalence of STDs, as well as in asymptomatic males and in specimens of first-void urine sediments. The clinical diagnosis by STD agent is reviewed in Table 75–4.

Treatment of urethritis in males is outlined in Table 75–9. In gonococcal disease, treatment is dictated by several factors, as addressed in the Centers for Disease Control's Treatment Guidelines, 1989: (1) the spread of antibiotic-resistant *Neisseria gonorrhoeae*, including penicillinase-producing gonococci, tetracycline-resistant gonococci, and strains with chromosomally mediated resistance to multiple antibiotics; (2) the high frequency of infections caused by *Chlamydia trachomatis* in persons with gonorrhea; (3) recognition of the serious complications of infections caused by *Neisseria gonorrhoeae* and *Chlamydia trachomatis*; and (4) lack of a fast, inexpensive, and highly accurate test for infection caused by *Chlamydia trachomatis*.

In regard to complications, approximately 3% of individuals with nongonococcal urethritis experience epididymitis (see Chapter 78).

Proctitis (see Chapter 32)

Anorectal-colonic infections include a host of diseases involving the lower gastrointestinal tract from the anal opening to the lower colon (colitis, proctocolitis). In a manner similar to the transformation of tissue types from the ectocervix to the endocervix, the tissues of the lower gastrointestinal system change from squamous epithelia in the anal canal to squamocolumnar epithelia at the junction between the anus and the rectum to columnar epithelia in the rectum. Susceptibility to infection as well as clinical presentation of STD infections vary with the location in the lower gastrointestinal tract in which infection occurs. For example, lesions in the anus and at the anorectal juncture may be more painful than those in the rectum because the anorectal juncture is highly innervated. Most anorectal infections are associated with anal intercourse among gay men. However, women have STD-related gastrointestinal conditions as well, though infections caused by *Neisseria gonorrhoeae* are often asymptomatic and associated with concurrent endocervical gonorrhea.

Sexually transmitted agents associated with lower gastrointestinal disease include *Neisseria gonorrhoeae, Chlamydia trachomatis* (oculogenital and lymphogranuloma venereum strains), *Treponema pallidum,* and herpes simplex virus. In addition, other microorganisms have been shown to be sexually transmitted among homosexual men, including enteric organisms such as hepatitis A, *Shigella, Giardia, Entamoeba,* and *Campylobacter.* Anorectal symptoms of infection include mucus or blood in the stools, cramping and loose stools, anal pruritus, and pain with defecation, resulting in tenesmus and constipation. Mucopurulent anal discharge (with or without blood) is a variable finding. Examination by anoscopy shows an erythematous and friable mucosa with ulcers and mucopurulent discharge. Assessment includes a sexual history to elicit the previous occurrence of anal intercourse; number and gender of sexual partners; condom use; history of prior STD infections—including urethritis, hepatitis, and syphilis; and other unusual infections that may be associated with immunodeficiency disease. In females, additional information about pelvic infections, contraception, and endocervicitis should be elicited. Appropriate genital, rectal, and stool specimens for culturing enteric bacteria and parasites, as well as *Chlamydia trachomatis, Neisseria gonorrhoeae,* should be taken. Syphilis serologic tests are indicated. Treatment is dependent upon the organism responsible for the infection, and regimens are outlined in Table 75–9.

Genital Ulcer Syndromes

Genital ulcers are present in infections with herpes simplex, *Treponema pallidum,* chancroid, and lymphogranuloma venereum. Donovanosis (granuloma inguinale) is a genital ulcer disease as well, but it is very rare (22 cases reported in the United States in 1987). Although an ulcer is itself a nonspecific sign of genital infection, classic findings by syndrome are presented in Table 75–12 in an effort to assist in the differentiation of ulcers by cause.

The clinical assessment of all individuals with a suspected STD ulcerative lesion should include a careful physical examination (including a pelvic examination in the female), noting the presence and characteristics of adenopathy, as well as the characteristics of the lesion itself. In addition, diagnostic testing for the two most common causes of STD ulcers—syphilis and herpes—should be performed. As in all STD infections, more than one STD agent may be present. Diagnosis and treatment are outlined in Table 75–12.

There is recent evidence that the prevalence of syphilis, in particular, has been increasing, especially among inner-city youth, and this increase may be related to high-risk sexual behaviors associated with the current crack cocaine epidemic. In addition, clinical research has reported some findings that indicate that a genital ulcer, such as the syphilitic chancre, may actually facilitate the transmission of HIV (see Chapter 76). For example, HIV target cells such as macrophages and activated lymphocytes are found in the base of a genital ulcer. The adolescent who is not infected with HIV and who has an STD genital ulcer such as a chancre may be at increased risk for acquisition of HIV if exposed. In addition, the HIV-infected adolescent who has a genital ulcer containing HIV with its target cells is potentially a more efficient transmitter of HIV to an uninfected partner during sexual contact. Therefore, syphilis is important not only because of its own disease potential in the adolescent and the female adolescent's offspring but also because it potentially increases the risk for HIV transmission. Screening for syphilis should be performed in all adolescents who have an STD infection and in high-risk adolescent groups, such as drug abusers and youth who exchange sex or drugs for money.

Genital Warts: Human Papillomavirus Infections

HPV infections may be the most common sexually transmitted infections among adolescents and young adults. It is estimated that there are more than 1 million persons affected annually with genital warts, and the number of visits to physicians for treatment of genital warts increased by 400% in males and 700% in females between 1966 and 1984. Although the problem of genital warts appears to be one of epidemic proportions, it is the link between HPV and the development of genital carcinoma that is most worrisome.

A definitive prevalence of HPV infection is not possible for several reasons. First, HPV infection is not a reportable disease. Second, the infection has a spectrum of clinical expression from obvious visible genital warts on the external genitalia to subclinical infection on the female cervix that is invisible to the unaided eye, making it impossible to define prevalence on clinical examination alone. Finally, there are a number of diagnostic techniques with varying sensitivities and availability to the practitioner that do not necessarily correlate with the presence of clinical disease. Tissue culture techniques to isolate the virus are not available at this time. With these constraints, it has been estimated that HPV infections have been identified as follows: 1% by gross clinical inspection; 1% to 10% by Pap smear; 10% to 27% by colposcopy; 1% to 38% by HPV deoxyribonucleic acid (DNA) detection; and 40% to 80% by polymerase chain reaction (PCR). Among adolescent females in one San Francisco–based study, 15% of the young women screened had HPV identified by HPV DNA hybridization techniques. Little information is available on males, but one study demonstrated that 8% of males between the ages of 16 and 35 who underwent screening had evidence of HPV DNA.

TABLE 75–12. Genital Ulcer Syndromes

	HERPES SIMPLEX	SYPHILIS (PRIMARY, SECONDARY)	CHANCROID	LYMPHOGRANULUM VENEREUM (LGV)
Agent	Herpes simplex virus (HSV)	*Treponema pallidum*	*Haemophilus ducreyi*	*Chlamydial trachomatis* LGV serovars
New cases*	~250 to 500,000	35,147	4998	303
Incubation (days)	2 to 7	12 to 40	3 to 40	20 to 40
Primary lesions	Vesicle	Papule	Papule-pustule	Papule-vesicle
size (mm)	1 to 2	5 to 15	2 to 20	2 to 10
number	Multiple, clusters, (coalesce ±)	Single	Multiple (coalesce ±)	Single
depth	Superficial	Superficial or deep	Deep	Superficial or deep
base	Erythematous, nonpurulent	Sharp, indurated, nonpurulent	Ragged border, purulent, friable	Varies
pain	Yes	No	Yes	Yes
Lymphodenopathy	Tender, bilateral	Nontender, bilateral	Tender, unilateral, may suppurate, unilocular fluctuance	Tender, unilateral, may suppurate, multilocular fluctuance
Laboratory diagnosis	Smear (Pap) Tzanck preparation: multinucleated cells (sensitivity low) Cell culture (sensitivity varies with stage of disease) Direct immuno-fluorescence stain	Dark-field microscopy, Serology: RPR, VDRL; FTA-ABS, MHA-TP	Culture	Complement fixation, immunofluorescent antibody serologic tests
Treatment†	Primary genital: acyclovir: 200 mg orally five times daily for 7 to 10 days or to resolution Recurrent: most do not benefit	Benzathine penicillin G: 2.4 million U intramuscularly or if penicillin allergy: tetracycline: 500 mg orally four times daily for 15 days, if not pregnant	Erythromycin base: 500 mg orally four times daily for 7 days or Ceftriaxone: 250 mg intramuscularly	Doxycycline 100 mg orally twice daily for 21 days

*New cases in United States in 1987.

†Centers for Disease Control: STD Treatment Guidelines. Washington, DC, U.S. Dept. of Health and Human Services, Public Health Service, 1989. Screen and treat all partners and encourage use of condoms.

RPR, rapid plasma reagin; VDRL, Venereal Disease Research Laboratory; FTA-ABS, fluorescent treponemal antibody absorption; MHA-TP, micro-hemagglutination–*Treponema pallidum*.

Adapted with permission from Hook EW: Syphilis and HIV infection. J Infect Dis 160:530, 1989.

Risk factors for HPV infection parallel other STDs and include multiple sexual partners, lack of condom use, sexual intercourse with an infected partner, pregnancy, an altered immune system, and age less than 25 years.

HPV infections are caused by a virus that belongs to

TABLE 75–13. Types of Human Papillomaviruses and Their Clinical Expression

TYPE	DISEASE
1, 2, 4, 10	Verruca plantaris and plana (deep plantar and palmar warts)
2, 4, 29	Verruca vulgaris (common warts)
19 to 25, 36, 46, 47, 50	Epidermodysplasia verruciformis
6, 11, 42, 54	Anogenital condyloma acuminatum
6, 11, 16, 18, 30, 31, 33, 34, 35, 39, 40, 42, 43, 45, 51, 56, 58	Cervical intraepithelial neoplasia or cervical carcinoma, or both

Adapted with permission from Moscicki AB: In Schydlower M, Shafer MA (eds): AIDS and Other Sexually Transmitted Diseases. State of the Art Reviews in Adolescent Medicine. Philadelphia, Hanley and Belfus, 1990, pp 451–469.

the Papovaviridae family and the *Papillomavirus* genus. Although defined as a very common infection by a variety of DNA detection techniques, it develops into clinically apparent disease in a limited number of infected individuals. Clinical expression ranges from visible warts to inapparent subclinical disease detectable only by colposcopy and biopsy.

More than 60 different types of HPV have been recently identified. More than one third of these types have been associated with anogenital infection. The HPV types are outlined according to clinical expression in Table 75–13. Those types associated with the development of cervical intraepithelial neoplasia or cervical carcinoma, or both, are most important.

Clinically, HPV is expressed as condyloma acuminatum (visible genital wart) and as condyloma planum (subclinical papilloma infection that is not visible to the naked eye). HPV infection can occur in any location in the anogenital area of both men and women and can take either or both forms, that is, condyloma acuminatum or condyloma planum. In women, the vulva, vagina, cervix, and perianal areas are commonly involved, whereas the penis, scrotum, urethra, and perianal areas can be affected in men.

Evidence for the diagnosis of HPV infection can be obtained through a careful sexual history that indicates a high risk for exposure, as well as close visual inspection, cytologic examination by Pap smear, and colposcopy with directed biopsy for histologic examination. A history of multiple sexual partners, exposure to an infected partner, and a history of previous lesions, as well as current lesions identified on visual inspection, and an abnormal Pap smear (females) indicate possible risks not only for HPV infection but also for the more serious complication of HPV-associated dysplasia or carcinoma.

Although the Centers for Disease Control recommend annual Pap smears for women who have had condyloma acuminatum, many experts who care for adolescents recommend referral for colposcopy for the adolescent female under the following conditions: (1) an abnormal Pap smear, (2) condyloma acuminatum in the patient or partner, and (3) high-risk sexual behavior (such as multiple sexual partners using little or no barrier protection, especially condoms). For example, approximately one half of women with cervical condyloma acuminatum also have had cervical subclinical papilloma infection identified after colposcopy. Referral for colposcopy is not currently recommended for those individuals who have no lesions and were found only to have evidence of HPV on DNA screening tests (see further on). Colposcopy is undertaken after the external genitalia, vagina, and cervix are generously bathed in a solution of 3% acetic acid to visually enhance HPV lesions. In males, the penis, scrotum, and perianal areas can also be soaked in the acetic acid solution prior to examination.

Using colposcopy, the most common HPV lesion is described as being well circumscribed, with slightly elevated white epithelia within the transformation zone of the cervix, and extensions of satellite lesions beyond the transformation zone itself. Although not always present with infection, the characteristic vascularity is described as coarse punctate vessels ("warty vessels"). Other patterns of vascularity have been described as well, including mosaic patterns similar to those found in carcinoma in situ. Since it is difficult for even the most expert colposcopist to differentiate HPV changes from atypical metaplasia or even neoplasia, the colposcope should be used to direct the biopsy of suspicious lesions.

Although the colposcopic examination may be more sensitive (30% to 80%) in detecting the presence of HPV infection when compared with the Pap smear (30% to 50%), the Pap smear is the most common screening test for subclinical HPV infection in women. The koilocyte—a mature squamous cell with characteristic perinuclear clearing, irregularly dense marginal cytoplasm, and a pyknotic nucleus—is traditionally associated with HPV infection, though there are recent indications that such findings are not restricted to HPV infection alone. It is estimated that 5% to 13% of women with abnormal cytologic findings that are consistent with possible HPV infection will have lesions that will progress to higher grade neoplasia; types 16, 18, and 31 are thought to progress at a higher rate than type 11. Therefore, though the finding of koilocytosis is not definitive of HPV infection, it does indicate the necessity for colposcopy and biopsy.

Recently, a number of ribonucleic acid (RNA)-DNA hybridization techniques to detect HPV infection have been developed with sensitivities from 70% to 90% (Southern blot, Dot blot). Although they perform within an acceptable sensitivity range for screening for infection, the presence of HPV is not necessarily associated with clinical disease. For example, the meaning of the presence of HPV when risk factors and clinical disease are lacking is unclear at this time. Although a Food and Drug Administration (FDA)-approved DNA hybridization kit is commercially available (ViraPap; Bethesda Research Laboratories, Gaithersburg, MD) that can detect and differentiate among HPV types 6, 11, 16, 18, 31, 33, and 35, routine screening for low-risk asymptomatic young women is not currently recommended without signs of clinical disease. Such techniques are being used for the most part within research settings to study women with and without clinical disease and the potential progression from simple uncomplicated infection with HPV to clinical disease and even carcinoma.

Treatment of HPV is governed by the location, clinical expression, and extent of disease (Table 75–14). The overall rationale for early detection and treatment of clinical disease is to prevent progression to carcinoma. Location is important because it has been determined that infection of the metaplastic cervix may increase the oncogenic potential as much as 1000 times, compared with infection of the vulvar epithelia. Expression of disease is also important because subclinical papillomavirus infection may be more recalcitrant to treatment than the condyloma acuminatum lesion. Finally, the extent of disease plays a role in the choice of treatment, as extensive multicentric disease may be more resistant to traditional approaches to uncomplicated disease and may require multiple modalities.

TABLE 75–14. Treatment Regimens for Human Papillomavirus*

TYPE	REGIMEN	COMMENTS
Condylomata acuminata (visible warts)	Liquid nitrogen 25% podophyllin	Pain on application Systemic toxicity, teratogenicity (unsafe pregnancy)
	Trichloroacetic acid (TCA, 85%) Laser Interferon	Safe with mucosa and pregnancy; local sensitivity
Subclinical papillomavirus infection	Refer for TCA, 5-fluorouracil, cyrotherapy, laser	Refer all patients with visible warts for colposcopy for possible subclinical human papillomavirus

*Therapy may be dictated by location of lesion, that is, cutaneous versus epithelial.

Data from Moscicki AB: HPV infections: An old STD revisited. Clin Pediatr 6:12, 1989 and Moscicki AB: In Schydlower M, Shafer MA (eds): AIDS and Other Sexually Transmitted Diseases. State of the Art Reviews in Adolescent Medicine. Philadelphia, Hanley and Belfus, 1990, pp 451–469.

BIBLIOGRAPHY

Adger H, Shafer MA, Sweet RT, Schachter J: Screening for *Chlamydia trachomatis* and *Neisseria gonorrhoeae* in adolescent males: Value of the first catch urinalysis. Lancet 1:944, 1984.

Alexander-Rodriguez T, Vermund SH: Gonorrhea and syphilis in incarcerated urban adolescents: Prevalence and physical signs. Pediatrics 80:561, 1987.

Amsel R, Totten PA, Spiegel CA, et al: Nonspecific vaginitis. Diagnostic criteria and microbial and epidemiologic associations. Am J Med 74:14, 1983.

Bell TA, Holmes KK: Age-specific risks of syphilis, gonorrhea, and hospitalized pelvic inflammatory disease in sexually experienced U.S. women. Sex Transm Dis 11:291, 1984.

Berg AO, Heidrich FE, Fihn SD, et al: Establishing the cause of genitourinary symptoms in women in a family practice. JAMA 251:620, 1984.

Brunham RC, Paavonen J, Stevens CE, et al: Mucopurulent cervicitis—the ignored counterpart in women of urethritis in men. N Engl J Med 311:1, 1984.

Cates W: Teenagers and sexual risk taking: The best of times and the worst of times. J Adol Health 12:84, 1991.

Centers for Disease Control, Division of Sexually Transmitted Disease: Sexually Transmitted Diseases Statistics, 1985. Washington, DC, U.S. Department of Health and Human Services, Public Health Service, 1987.

Centers for Disease Control: STD Treatment Guidelines. Washington, DC, U.S. Department of Health and Human Services, Public Health Service, September 1989.

Chambers CV, Shafer MA, Adger H, et al: Microflora of the urethra in adolescent males: Relationships to sexual activity and nongonococcal urethritis. J Pediatr 110:314, 1987.

Chernesky MA, Mahony JB, Castriciano S, et al: Detection of *Chlamydia trachomatis* antigens by enzyme immunoassay and immuno-fluorescence in genital specimens from symptomatic and asymptomatic men and women. J Infect Dis 154:141, 1986.

Golden N, Hammerschlag M, Neuhoff S, Gleyzer A: Prevalence of *Chlamydia trachomatis* cervical infection in female adolescents. Am J Dis Child 138:562, 1984.

Holmes KK: Lower genital tract infections in women: Cystitis, urethritis, vulvovaginitis and cervicitis. In Holmes KK, Mardh PA, Sparling PF, Wiesner PJ (eds): Sexually Transmitted Diseases, 2nd ed. New York, McGraw-Hill, 1990, pp 527–545.

Hook EW: Syphilis and HIV infection. J Infect Dis 160:530, 1989.

Jacobson L, Weström L: Objectivized diagnosis of acute pelvic inflammatory disease. Am J Obstet Gynecol 105:1088, 1969.

Johnson RE, Nahmias AJ, Magder LS, et al: A seroepidemiologic survey of the prevalence of herpes simplex virus type 2 in the United States. N Engl J Med 321:7, 1989.

Kaufman RD, Wiesner PJ: Nonspecific urethritis. N Engl J Med 291:1175, 1974.

Krockta WP, Barnes RC: Genital ulceration with regional adenopathy. Infect Dis Clin North Am 1:253, 1987.

Martinez J, Smith R, Farmer M, et al: High prevalence of genital tract papillomavirus infection in female adolescents. Pediatrics 82:604, 1988.

Mindel A: Prophylaxis for genital herpes: Should it be used routinely? Drugs 41:319, 1991.

Moscicki AB: HPV infections: An old STD revisited. Clin Pediatr 6:12, 1989.

Moscicki AB: Genital human papillomavirus infections. In Schydlower M, Shafer MA (eds): AIDS and Other Sexually Transmitted Diseases. State of the Art Reviews in Adolescent Medicine. Philadelphia, Hanley and Belfus, 1990, pp 451–469.

Moscicki AB, Palefsky J, Gonzales J, Schoolnik GK: Human papillomavirus infection in sexually active adolescent females: Prevalence and risk factors. Pediatr Res 28:507, 1990.

O'Brien SF, Bell TA, Farrow JA: Use of a leukocyte esterase dipstick to detect *Chlamydia trachomatis* and *Neisseria gonorrhoeae* among asymptomatic adolescent male detainees. Am J Public Health 78:1583, 1988.

Oh MK, Feinstein RA, Pass RF: Sexually transmitted diseases and sexual behavior in urban adolescent females attending family planning clinic. J Adolesc Health Care 9:67, 1988.

Piot P, Plummer FA: Genital ulcer adenopathy syndrome. In Holmes KK, Mardh PA, Sparling PF, Wiesner PJ (eds): Sexually Transmitted Diseases, 2nd ed. New York, McGraw-Hill, 1990, pp 711–716.

Podgore JK, Holmes KK: Asymptomatic urethral infections due to *Chlamydia trachomatis* in male U.S. military personnel. J Infect Dis 148:828, 1982.

Quinn TC, Stamm WE, Goodell SE, et al: The polymicrobial origin of intestinal infections in homosexual men. N Engl J Med 309:576, 1983.

Saltz GR, Linnemann CC, Brookman RR, Rauh JL: *Chlamydia trachomatis* cervical infections in female adolescents. J Pediatr 98:981, 1981.

Schachter J, Pang F, Parks RM, et al: Use of Gonozyme on urine sediment for diagnosis of gonorrhea in males. J Clin Microbiol 23:124, 1986.

Shafer MA: Pelvic inflammatory disease in the adolescent female. In Adolescent Medicine: State of the Art Reviews, Vol 1., Philadelphia, Hanley and Belfus., 1990, pp 545–564.

Shafer MA, Blain B, Beck A, et al: *Chlamydia trachomatis*: Important relationships to race, contraceptive use, lower genital tract infection and Papanicolaou smears. J Pediatr 104:141, 1984.

Shafer MA, Moscicki AB: Sexually transmitted diseases. In Hendee WB (ed): The Health of Adolescents. San Francisco, Jossey-Bass, 1991, pp. 211–249.

Shafer MA, Schachter J, Moscicki AB, et al: Urinary leukocyte esterase screening test for asymptomatic chlamydial and gonococcal infections in males. JAMA 262:2562, 1989.

Sweet RL: Pelvic inflammatory disease and infertility in women. Infec Dis Clin North Am 1:199, 1987.

Weström L: Incidence, prevalence, and trends of acute pelvic inflammatory disease and its consequences in industrialized countries. Am J Obstet Gynecol 138:880, 1980.

Wolner-Hanssen P, Svennson L, Mardh PA: Laparoscopic findings and contraceptive use in women with signs and symptoms suggestive of acute salpingitis. Obstet Gynecol 66:233, 1985.

Wolner-Hanssen P, Krieger JN, Stevens CE, et al: Clinical manifestations of vaginal trichomoniasis. JAMA 261:571, 1989.

Zelnik M, Kantner JF: Sexual activity, contraceptive use and pregnancy among metropolitan teenagers 1971–1979. Fam Plann Perspect 12:230, 1980.

CHAPTER 76

Acquired Immunodeficiency Syndrome and Human Immunodeficiency Virus–Related Syndromes

MICHELE D. KIPKE and KAREN HEIN

Acquired immunodeficiency syndrome (AIDS) is rapidly becoming one of the leading causes of death among adolescents. As of 1988, it was the sixth leading cause of death among 15- to 24-year-olds in the United States. Although adolescents, aged 13 to 21 years, represent only 1.2% of the total number of cases, the number of adolescents diagnosed with AIDS is doubling every 14 months. The number of reported cases greatly underestimates the potential threat to adolescents, since reported AIDS cases do not include adolescents who are infected with the human immunodeficiency virus (HIV) and are asymptomatic, nor does it include infected adolescents whose symptoms do not meet the specific criteria for AIDS. The number of reported cases similarly does not include young adults who were infected as teenagers, but who became symptomatic during their 20s. Given the long period of latency between infection and the onset of symptoms (mean of 11 years), many individuals 20 to 24 years of age with AIDS are likely to have been infected as teenagers. Finally, this number does not include adolescents who are not infected but who are engaging in risk-related sexual and drug use behaviors and are at high risk for infection.

This chapter provides a review of the epidemiology of AIDS and HIV infection among adolescents and explores some of the factors that put adolescents at increased risk for HIV infection. Strategies for conducting a risk assessment, HIV testing of adolescents, clinically managing HIV-infected adolescents, and developing interventions for prevention and risk reduction are also presented.

EPIDEMIOLOGY

Prevalence of AIDS

As of October 1991, 2292 adolescents, 13 to 21 years of age, have been diagnosed with AIDS in the United States. A breakdown of cumulative reported cases indicates that adolescents with AIDS are primarily male (80%) and minority youth (58%). Overall, nearly 80%

of these individuals were infected through sexual exposure or intravenous drug use; 19% were infected through exposure to HIV-infected blood or blood products; and 4% were infected through undetermined exposure. Heterosexual contact was the most frequent route of transmission among females, accounting for 50% of the cases.

A more complete analysis of cases among adolescents, aged 13 to 21 years, reported by January 1988 indicates that there are significant differences in sex ratio, ethnicity, and reported risk behaviors between adolescents and adults, as well as among adolescents from different locales. When compared with adult cases, there was a greater proportion of females (14% versus 7%) and minorities (53% versus 38%) and heterosexually acquired cases (47% versus 22%) among adolescents with AIDS. These differences were even greater for adolescent cases reported in New York City, in which the ratio of male-to-female adolescent cases was 3:1, compared with 7:1 among New York City adults and 15:1 among adults in the United States excluding New York City. Minority groups predominated among the adolescents (58%) and adult cases (55%) in New York, which differed from the rest of the country, in which 60% of the affected individuals were white. Heterosexual transmission was more common among New York City adolescents (15%) than among New York City adults (8%) or adolescents in the rest of the United States (8%). Heterosexual transmission accounted for 52% of New York City adolescent female cases compared with 21% of New York City adult female cases. Nationwide, hemophilia is the leading risk factor for AIDS among younger adolescent males. In New York City, only 11% of male cases were transfusion-related. Figure 76–1 summarizes these differences in transmission routes for children, adolescents, and adults.

Rates of HIV Infection

It is not known how many adolescents are infected with HIV; however, available seroprevalence data from population-based studies indicate that the number is

711

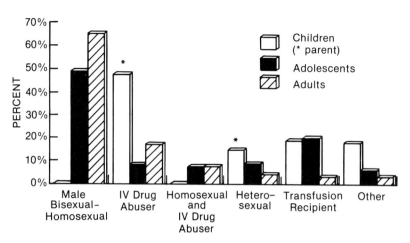

Figure 76–1. Percentage of AIDS cases in the United States. (Adapted from Vermund SH, Hein K, Gayle HD, et al: Acquired immunodeficiency syndrome among adolescents. Case surveillance profiles in New York City and the rest of the United States. Am J Dis Child 143:1220, 1989.)

substantial. The Department of Defense, which requires HIV testing as part of its admissions procedures to military service (see Chapter 29), reported a seroprevalence rate of 10.3 in 1000 among New York City applicants of all age groups. Of the New York City applicants who are 21 years of age and younger, the seroprevalence rate was 3 in 1000. The Job Corps similarly requires mandatory testing of all entrants in residential sites. The rate among Job Corps entrants, aged 16 to 21 years, was 3.9 in 1000 applicants nationwide, with significantly higher rates among minority youth: 7 in 1000 among black youth and 2.4 in 1000 among Hispanic entrants compared with 1.4 in 1000 among white entrants. In a center serving runaway and homeless youth, 6% of the 16- to 21-year-olds and 16% of the 18- to 21-year-olds were seropositive. Rates of infection among the newborns of teenaged mothers in New York City have been increasing at alarming rates. From May 1979 to May 1988, a total of ten teenaged mothers gave birth to seropositive infants. By comparison, 88 teenaged mothers gave birth to seropositive infants from May 1988 to June 1989. The rate of HIV infection increased with the mother's age, from 1 in 1000 among 15-year-olds to 1 in 100 among 19-year-olds in an analysis from May 1988 to May 1989. In an anonymous seroprevalence study of patients at a hospital in the Bronx, the rates were 27 in 1000 among patients 15 to 24 years of age.

Another group of adolescents at high risk for HIV are adolescents who have been infected with other sexually transmitted diseases (STDs) (see Chapter 75). One STD clinic in Baltimore reported seroprevalence rates ranging from 22 in 1000 among 15- to 19-year-olds to 36 in 1000 among 20- to 24-year-olds. Rates among college-aged students seeking health services at 17 college campuses were 1 in 500, with positive results from 5 of the 17 college campuses located throughout the United States.

These findings suggest that HIV infection is spreading silently but rapidly among sexually active adolescents, particularly youth living in urban settings in which seroprevalence rates are high.

FACTORS ASSOCIATED WITH RISK

A number of factors put adolescents at increased risk for HIV infection, including their physiologic development and the high prevalence of risk-related sexual and drug use behaviors and STDs among adolescents. Adolescents who live in areas in which there is high viral prevalence may also be at particularly high risk for infection given the increased probability of their being in contact with an infected sexual partner or partner in drug use. The following provides a brief review of the factors placing adolescents at increased risk for infection.

Physiologic Development

The time of infection relative to the stage of physiologic development may play a role in the susceptibility to infection and the natural history of disease progression. Physiologic changes in adolescents that could modulate both the infectivity and natural history of HIV include (1) developmental differences in the immune system that are associated with changes in the number of lymphocytes and macrophages at various pubertal stages and (2) changes in the adolescent female genitourinary tract that affect the size and position of the squamocolumnar junction of the cervix, possibly exposing more columnar cells directly to all agents causing STDs, including HIV (see Chapter 75). The incomplete menstrual patterns, with frequent anovulatory cycles, and the vaginal, ovarian, and cervical function of adolescent females may put them at even greater risk than the young adult female for complications from STDs, such as gonorrhea, and by analogy, possible HIV infection.

Sexual Activity

Unprotected sexual intercourse is the most prevalent risk behavior among adolescents. There are three types of sexual intercourse that are associated with HIV transmission: vaginal, oral, and anal. Studies on HIV transmission suggest that receptive anal intercourse (see Chapter 32) may be a more efficient means of transmission than vaginal intercourse, which, in turn, may be more efficient than oral intercourse. Latex condoms, when used with spermicidal lubricant, have been found to be an effective barrier against STDs, including HIV. Thus, adolescents who consistently use condoms during intercourse (vaginal, oral, and anal) are at less risk for infection than are adolescents who do not use condoms during intercourse (see Chapters 73 and 75).

The current trend is for increasingly younger teenagers to become sexually active (see Chapter 2). There is also evidence to suggest that some risk-related sexual behaviors are more prevalent than others. For example, oral intercourse may be practiced more frequently among high school students than vaginal intercourse, and anal intercourse appears to be practiced by as many as 10% to 26% of adolescents. For some adolescents, anal intercourse is perceived to be an activity that preserves one's virginity and protects females from becoming pregnant. Adolescent males who engage in same-sex intercourse, particularly receptive anal intercourse, may be at particularly high risk for infection given the high prevalence of HIV infection among gay and bisexual males (see Chapter 32). The prevalence of homosexual activity to orgasm among contemporary adolescent males is estimated to range from 17% to 37%.

Despite the protection associated with condom use, few adolescents consistently use condoms during vaginal intercourse, and even fewer report using condoms during oral and anal intercourse. Although 75% of adolescents may use some form of contraception, as few as 15% report using condoms. Younger adolescents are even less likely than are older teenagers to use contraception, and they are more likely to be sporadic and ineffective in their contraceptive use. Black adolescents are more likely to report having never used contraception or to have used it inconsistently when compared with white adolescents (see Chapters 2 and 73). However, increased attention and education regarding the advantages of using condoms, may be effective in encouraging some adolescents to use condoms. Data from a recent survey suggest that rates of reported condom use (at least intercourse) more than doubled between 1979 and 1988 among 15- to 19-year-old males.

Multiple sexual partners also increases the adolescent's risk for coming into contact with the virus, and older partners may be more likely to be infected than younger partners. In one survey, 39% of male and 17% of female young adults (18 to 24 years) reported having three or more partners in the last year. Male partners of heterosexual female adolescents are usually 2 to 3 years older, and male partners of gay male adolescents are on average 7 years older.

Sexual abuse has been reported to put adolescents at risk for HIV infection. It is estimated that at least 3% of all teenagers have experienced some form of sexual abuse, and more than half of all rape victims are adolescent females (see Chapters 118 and 119). In addition to the fact that many of these encounters may have resulted in HIV transmission, sexual abuse is associated with increased and compulsive sexual activity that could secondarily put abused adolescents at increased risk for infection.

Taken as a whole, these data indicate that the majority of adolescents are engaging, or will engage at some point in their teenaged years, in sexual behaviors that could result in HIV transmission. Some adolescents may be at greater risk than others, for example those who are having unprotected intercourse at younger ages and with multiple and older partners in geographic areas with a high seroprevalence of HIV infection.

Sexually Transmitted Diseases

STDs have been found to be highly correlated with and predictive of HIV infection, which itself is sexually transmitted. This has led some investigators to use STDs as a surrogate marker for behaviors associated with HIV infection. Infection with an STD may also make a person more susceptible to HIV infection, particularly diseases associated with genital ulcers, which provide access for HIV entry through the barrier usually provided by intact skin. Thus, STDs are important factors associated with the risk for HIV transmission and infectivity.

STDs are a major cause of morbidity among sexually active adolescents. Rates of STDs among adolescents have increased since the 1950s, despite the availability of antimicrobial treatments. Prior infection with an STD would suggest a higher probability of infection with HIV. The increased incidence of syphilis, chancroid, and congenital syphilis has been associated with HIV (see Chapter 75).

Drug Use Behaviors

Drug use significantly increases the risk for HIV in adolescents for two reasons: (1) the sharing of needles during intravenous drug use effectively transmits the virus and (2) drug use often increases sexual desire and decreases inhibitions, thus reducing the likelihood that adolescents will use risk reduction techniques (see Chapter 111). The prevalence of intravenous drug use among adolescents is thought to be relatively low. Survey data, however, indicate that a sizable percentage of adolescents are using drugs that can be injected intravenously (e.g., cocaine, heroin, amphetamines, steroids). In a 1988 survey, approximately 12% of high school seniors reported having used cocaine; 8% had used cocaine in the past year, 3% were currently using cocaine, and 1% had used heroin. These numbers are likely to grossly underestimate the prevalence of drug use and intravenous drug use among adolescents, since the survey did not include adolescents who had dropped out of school before their senior year. These adolescents are more likely to use and inject drugs than are teenagers who remain in school. Even if individual teenagers do not inject drugs intravenously, they may become infected through sexual contact with persons who do.

There is also a substantial number of adolescents who use substances (e.g., alcohol, marijuana) that may impair their judgment, thus reducing the likelihood that they will employ safe sex practices or increasing the likelihood that they will accept intravenous drugs when offered and share needles when injecting. More than 90% of adolescents in the United States use alcohol before graduating from high school, and two thirds of high school seniors reported drinking in the prior month. Approximately 5% of high school seniors use either alcohol or marijuana daily (see Chapter 111). In a survey of incarcerated adolescents 16 to 17 years of age, alcohol consumption (48%) and drug use (10%) frequently occurred before or during intercourse; 17% of the sample reported prior infection with an STD.

Service providers increasingly report that addiction to crack cocaine is highly associated with risk-related sexual behaviors, particularly "survival sex," or the exchange of sex for crack or money to purchase crack, food, or shelter. Crack use has recently been found to be associated with HIV infection among adolescents seen at an outpatient clinic in New York City. The Centers for Disease Control (CDC) has noted that cities reporting high levels of crack use are also reporting dramatic increases in STDs, including syphilis and gonorrhea. Additional risk may be associated with adolescents who inject heroin to help them "come down" from the crack cocaine high.

Homeless and Runaway Youth

Homeless and runaway youth are at particularly high risk for HIV infection (see Chapter 33). It is estimated that between 730,000 and 1.3 million youth run away from their homes each year. About one fourth of these adolescents are thought to be homeless, with no permanent residence or adult support. According to recent literature, largely based on shelter or agency clients, homeless youth are a varied, diverse population. Usually, their ages start at about 13 years, though an increasing number of even younger children have been reported, some as young as 9 years old. Recent reports suggest that homeless and runaway youth suffer from multiple problems, including high rates of STDs and mental health, alcohol, and other drug problems. In a study of 97 12- to 17-year-old homeless and runaway adolescents in Los Angeles, illicit drug use was reported by the majority of teenagers; one quarter reported intravenous drug use at least once, and nearly half were reportedly abusing alcohol. Almost all of these adolescents (92.3%) had had sexual intercourse, though only half of the sexually active teenagers reported using a condom during their last sexual encounter involving intercourse. An analysis of runaway and nonrunaway youth aged 12 to 24 years who were seen at an outpatient medical clinic in Los Angeles revealed that 84% of the runaways reported intravenous drug use compared with only 3.7% of the nonrunaway youth. More than half of the sample (57.3%) reported intercourse prior to 10 years of age. Sexual and physical abuse was more prevalent among the runaway youth, and a higher percentage of runaways (26% versus 2%) reported that they had engaged in street prostitution or "survival sex."

CARING FOR ADOLESCENTS AT RISK FOR OR INFECTED WITH HIV

As more adolescents become infected with HIV, there is an urgent need for services to care for their medical and psychosocial needs appropriately. Existing services, which were developed primarily for children and adults with AIDS, do not address the unique needs of adolescents. Strategies must therefore be developed to identify and link high-risk adolescents with systems that will provide comprehensive care, that is, risk assessment, preventive interventions, and psychosocial services before they become infected, or counseling and medical services for early diagnosis and treatment of HIV-related diseases.

Risk Assessment

The risk of an adolescent contracting HIV infection can be assessed by performing a complete, confidential evaluation of risk-related sexual and drug use behaviors and a medical history. The information obtained during a risk assessment can be used to (1) identify and triage high-risk adolescent youth into appropriate services and (2) tailor interventions for prevention and risk reduction to the needs of a particular adolescent. Information collected during a risk assessment is used to determine the need for HIV testing and medical and psychosocial services. Sample questions for performing a risk assessment with adolescents are provided in Table 76–1.

HIV Testing

HIV testing has become an increasingly important diagnostic tool as treatments become available for asymptomatic HIV-positive individuals. HIV testing of adolescents, however, still raises unique ethical, legal, psychological, and social questions with respect to confidentiality, disclosure, and discrimination (see Chapter 20), particularly since most currently available HIV testing services are not directed to the specific needs of adolescents. HIV testing should never be performed without prior consent or adequate counseling before and after testing. Counseling prior to the test may be extended over several sessions and should provide adolescents with information about AIDS and the HIV antibody test to help them make an active, informed choice about testing. Adolescents should have the same right to confidentiality about HIV-related medical information as do adults. Few states have specific laws regarding HIV testing for minors, but all states permit minors to be tested for STDs without parental consent or knowledge. Specific recommendations for HIV testing of adolescents are presented elsewhere.

Clinical Management

Adolescent-specific health care and counseling services are only sporadically available. Although there is

TABLE 76–1. Sample Risk Assessment

SEXUAL BEHAVIORS

1. Do you do any of the following with a boyfriend or girlfriend: hugging, kissing, touching, rubbing bodies, masturbation?
2. Has anything ever happened to you sexually that hurt or scared you?
3. Has anyone ever forced you to do something sexually that you did not want to do?
4. Have you ever been involved with someone sexually and had vaginal, oral, or anal intercourse (define each form of intercourse)? If the answer to this question is yes, then finish answering the questions in this section.
5. How old were you when you first had vaginal, oral, or anal intercourse?
6. With how many different partners have you had vaginal, oral, or anal intercourse?
7. With how many different partners have you had vaginal, oral, or anal intercourse during the past month?
8. Approximately how many times have you had vaginal, oral, or anal intercourse?
9. How many times have you had vaginal, oral, or anal intercourse during the past month?
10. How old are the people with whom you have intercourse?
11. How old was the first and the last person with whom you had intercourse?
12. Have you ever had intercourse with a person who injects drugs or "shoots-up"?
13. Have you ever had intercourse with a male who has had intercourse with another male?
14. Have you ever had intercourse with a person who is infected with the virus that causes AIDS or who has AIDS?
15. Have you ever had intercourse in exchange for money, drugs, food, or a place to sleep or live?
16. Do you drink alcohol or take drugs before or while you are having intercourse?

CONTRACEPTION AND PREGNANCIES

17. Have you ever used a method of contraception or birth control? If the answer is yes:
    a. Which of the following methods have you used: oral contraceptives, diaphragm, intrauterine device (IUD), condom, withdrawal, rhythm, other?
    b. How often do you use each method?
    c. Did you use any form of birth control the last time you had sexual intercourse?
    d. Do you ever use condoms when you have oral intercourse?
18. Have you ever been pregnant? If so:
19. How many times have you been pregnant?

20. How old were you when you became pregnant?
21. Have you ever had an abortion? If the answer is yes:
    a. How many abortions have you had?
    b. How old were you when you had the abortion or abortions?
    c. Have you ever had a miscarriage? If so:
    d. How many miscarriages have you had?
    e. How old were you when you had the miscarriage or miscarriages?

SEXUALLY TRANSMITTED DISEASES

22. Has a doctor ever told you that you had a sexually transmitted disease (also called venereal disease [VD])? If the answer is yes:
    a. What sexually transmitted disease or diseases did you have? (List them.)
    b. How old were you when you had the sexually transmitted disease or diseases?
    c. What treatments were you given? (How were they administered? If pills, what did they look like?)
    d. Have you ever had sexual intercourse with someone who has had a sexually transmitted disease?

DRUG USE BEHAVIORS

23. Have you ever used any of the following: alcohol, cigarettes, marijuana, crack cocaine, cocaine, heroin, amphetamines, other? If the answer is yes:
    a. At what age did you begin using each drug?
    b. How have you used each drug (smoked, "snorted," injected)?
    c. Approximately how often have you used each drug?
    d. How many times have you used each drug in the past month?
    e. Have you ever injected heroin or cocaine (or a mixture of the two called a *speedball*)? If so:
    f. How old were you when you started injecting a heroin-cocaine mixture?
    g. During the past month, how many times have you injected a heroin-cocaine mixture?
    h. On the average, how many times a day do you inject a heroin-cocaine mixture?
    i. else? If so:
    j. Who do you share your "works" with (stranger, friends, relative, lover)?
    k. How often do you share your "works"?
    l. Do you clean or sterilize your needles before you use them? If so:
    m. How do you clean them?
    n. Do your friends ever use any of the following: alcohol, cigarettes, marijuana, crack cocaine, cocaine, heroin, amphetamines, other?

a growing literature about the natural history of HIV infection among children and adults, little is known about the progression of HIV infection in adolescents. A new challenge is that of children who have developed AIDS through congenital infection and who are entering adolescence. The natural history of HIV infection from congenital infection is that all such children develop AIDS by 10 years of age. Therefore, there are some children in whom infection develops early in life and others who are asymptomatic until school age. Those who are school age when they become symptomatic most likely begin therapy and start having major medical problems from the infection during early adolescence.

The following are suggested guidelines for evaluating and treating HIV-infected adolescents.

STAGING CLASSIFICATION

Clinical management of HIV-infected adolescents begins with a staging evaluation that involves eliciting symptoms characteristic of HIV-related infections or AIDS and assessing immunologic function. Information collected during the medical history, physical examination, and laboratory assessment are used to stage the progression of HIV infection. This classification, in turn, is used to determine the risk of disease progression and is the basis for choosing the most appropriate course of treatment. Several classification systems have been developed for staging HIV-seropositive young children and adults, including the CDC's pediatric and adult classification of HIV-AIDS and the Walter Reed staging classification for adults. No criteria have been developed specifically for the classification of adolescents. Thus, a combination of classification criteria should be used to stage HIV infection and AIDS in adolescents.

MEDICAL HISTORY

A medical history should assess prior medical treatments or illnesses that may be HIV-related. The time at which transmission occurred might be determined by assessing symptoms characteristic of acute HIV seroconversion illness, which includes mononucleosis-like symptoms of fever, malaise, and lymphadenopathy. A medical history for adolescents should include (1) sexual and menstrual history, including a screening history for pregnancy; (2) use of contraception in females and males; (3) prior illnesses (e.g., STDs) and treatable infectious diseases that may become reactivated in the presence of HIV infection (e.g., tuberculosis); (4) drug use behavior; (5) hospitalizations; (6) history and sources of medical psychiatric care; (7) history of blood transfusions and receipt of blood products, particularly if prior to 1985; (8) immunizations; (9) medications; (10) allergies, especially to medications; (11) family medical and psychiatric history; and (12) psychosocial history, including living situation, family and peer supports, education and work status, past and present depression and anxiety, and prior and present suicidal thoughts and attempts.

PHYSICAL EXAMINATION

A complete physical examination should be performed to identify HIV-related signs and symptoms, with particular attention to (1) vital signs, including weight and loss of weight; (2) general examination, including nutritional status and appearance of skin; (3) lymphadenopathy (location, number, size, consistency of lymph nodes); (4) head, ears, eyes, nose, and throat examination, including a fundoscopic examination and an oral examination; (5) lung examination seeking evidence of pneumonia; (6) abdominal examination seeking masses or hepatosplenomegaly; (7) examination of genitalia, including sexual maturity rating of secondary sexual characteristics; (8) a pelvic examination and Papanicolaou (Pap) test for sexually active females; (9) cultures of vaginal discharge or penile discharge; and (10) a neurologic examination, including a mental status examination (neuropsychological testing should be performed if neurologic involvement is suspected).

LABORATORY ASSESSMENT

Laboratory evaluation should be performed in all symptomatic and asymptomatic adolescents when they are HIV-seropositive (baseline) and then at regular intervals (follow-up) to assess the stage of infection and to monitor shifts in immunologic functioning.

Baseline Assessment

Studies have begun to describe changes in immunologic markers that signal disease progression, notably decreases in T-helper lymphocytes; the T4 cells or the CD4+ cells. Although the prognostic value of any particular test has not been fully established, there is evidence that the simultaneous shifting of several markers is highly significant. The test with the greatest prognostic significance at present is the measurement of T cells, especially CD4+ cells, and the helper-to-suppressor (T4-to-T8) ratio. Although T-cell subset levels do not always correspond precisely to the clinical stage of disease, in general, the lower the CD4+ count and the lower the T4-to-T8 ratio, the greater the likelihood of clinical immunodeficiency (at present or in the near future). A CD4+ count of less than 500 cells/mm³ indicates abnormal immune function and indicates the need for antiretroviral therapy. The risk of different opportunistic infections also varies with the level of CD4+ cells. The risk of recurrent varicella zoster (shingles) infection, tuberculosis, and atypical syphilis increases with a level of CD4+ cells less than 250 to 350 cells/mm³. The risk of *Pneumocystis carinii* pneumonia appears greatest at less than 200 CD4+ cells/mm³. The CDC has therefore recommended that prophylactic therapy be used against *Pneumocystis carinii* pneumonia when the CD4+ count is less than 200 cells/mm³. Measurement of CD4+ cells should therefore be performed at baseline to determine the degree of immune competence and continuously to monitor changes in immune functioning.

HIV antibody testing (both enzyme-linked immunoassay [ELISA] and Western blot) should be performed to determine which antibody bands are present. The loss of antibody to p24 antigen has been shown to correlate with disease progression. Elevations of p24 antigen and β₂-microglobulin have also been shown to correlate with virus activity. These tests are not yet commercially available.

A complete blood count (CBC) will assess anemia, lymphopenia, neutropenia, and a decreased number of platelets. The erythrocyte sedimentation rate (ESR) may be elevated. A complete chemistry panel (SMA-20) should also be performed to determine whether there is decreased albumin from malnutrition-malabsorption; increased total protein (from an increased immunoglobulin fraction); increased blood urea nitrogen (BUN); creatinine, or potassium; decreased serum bicarbonate (HIV renal involvement) or increased liver enzymes (chronic hepatitis).

HIV infection has been associated with a rapid progression of cervical neoplasia, supporting findings on Pap smears in females. Assessment of sexually active females and males with vaginal discharge or penile discharge should also include a wet preparation, Gram stain, gonorrhea cultures, and screening for *Chlamydia trachomatis* (see Chapter 75). Titers for syphilis, hepatitis, rubella, toxoplasmosis, and cytomegalovirus should also be analyzed, as these diseases can be reactivated in HIV-positive adolescents. A tuberculin skin test (purified protein derivative; PPD) with anergy panel should be performed to evaluate for tuberculosis and to assess cell-mediated immunity. A baseline chest x-ray film should also be obtained for comparison if respiratory symptoms develop. A pregnancy test should also be performed.

Follow-up Assessment

Asymptomatic adolescents with normal immune systems (CD4+ count greater than 500/mm³) can be followed medically at 3-month intervals with routine blood work (CBC and SMA-20). Monitoring of the CD4+ cell count should be performed every 4 to 6 months to assess changes in immunologic function and to determine when medical interventions are appropriate. In addition, a Pap smear should be performed every 6 to 12 months in sexually active females, as well as a serologic test for syphilis at least every year or if symptoms of an STD appear in sexually active adolescents. A PPD and anergy panel should also be performed every 12 months in infected adolescents.

Symptomatic adolescents and asymptomatic adolescents with abnormal immune functioning (CD4+ count less than 500/mm³) require monthly follow-up visits for physical examination and repeat laboratory assessment. Patients who are on drug protocols will also require more frequent visits (e.g., zidovudine [AZT] requires bimonthly monitoring of CBC and blood chemistry during the first 2 months of use).

Clinical Manifestations

HIV infection causes a broad spectrum of disease manifestations and a varied clinical course in adolescents. Infection with HIV ranges from an acute febrile illness, similar to the infectious mononucleosis syndrome, to an asymptomatic chronic carrier state, to the severe immunodeficiency and AIDS characterized by opportunistic infections and malignancies. Little is known about the natural history of HIV infection in adolescents—what proportion of teenagers will become symptomatic quickly and die within months after becoming infected (one of the patterns of very young children) or the proportion who will remain asymptomatic for many years. A high level of suspicion should be maintained, particularly with the following clinical manifestations: persistent oral candidiasis; generalized lymphadenopathy; hepatosplenomegaly; recurrent diarrhea; recurrent bacterial, parasitic, and fungal infections; opportunistic infections; malignancies; encephalopathy; cardiomyopathy; and hepatic, renal, or other organ system involvement.

Treatment

Many of the complications associated with HIV can also be suppressed. The following provides a description of available treatments.

ANTIVIRAL MEDICATIONS

Results from a national clinical trials program indicate that early treatment with ZVD is effective at delaying the onset of AIDS and advanced-stage AIDS-related complex among participants with fewer than 500 CD4+ cells/mm³ at entry into the study. The results do not prove whether or not overall length of survival will be affected by this treatment or even whether ZVD will confer a long-term reduction in the incidence of AIDS or advanced-stage HIV infection. However, the findings confirm that ZVD, when used in a total daily dose of 500 mg, can delay disease progression in asymptomatic HIV-infected individuals with fewer than 500 CD4+ cells/mm³. Clinical trials are currently evaluating other

promising antiviral agents, such as dideoxyinosine (DDI) and dideoxycytidine (DDC). However, doses were determined for adults or young children, not teenagers who have different pharmacodynamic patterns from other age groups for other classes of medications.

PROPHYLAXIS

There have also been recent advances in the prevention of *Pneumocystis carinii* pneumonia, the opportunistic infection that affects 80% of patients with AIDS. Until recently, most studies focused on preventing relapses. More recently, efficacy has been proved for primary prophylaxis during the asymptomatic period in HIV-infected individuals, those with an abnormal immune system (CD4+ count less than 200/mm³). The role of aerosolized pentamidine and other drugs that are used in secondary prophylaxis of *Pneumocystis* pneumonia in early intervention strategies is now being investigated. Although children have had less adverse reactions with trimethoprim-sulfamethoxazole (Bactrim) than have adults, it is unknown how adolescents will respond.

IMMUNIZATIONS

Although there is a theoretical risk of activation of HIV from immunization (resulting from stimulation of lymphocytes) and a decreased antibody response to immunizations in these immunocompromised patients, the following immunizations are recommended to prevent infections commonly found among HIV-seropositive patients: *Haemophilus influenzae* B, pneumococci, tetanus, influenza, measles, rubella, and hepatitis B.

STRATEGIES FOR PREVENTION AND RISK REDUCTION

The primary strategy available for curtailing the further spread of HIV infection among adolescents is prevention. At this time, all adolescents, regardless of risk, need to learn how to protect themselves from HIV infection by preventing or modifying HIV risk-related behaviors. This may require that they develop or refine specific decision-making, assertiveness, and communication skills for prevention and risk reduction. Suggested components of a prevention and risk reduction program include (1) information about HIV infection, transmission, and prevention; (2) instruction and demonstration on how to properly use and purchase condoms; (3) information to help adolescents identify their own risk-related behaviors; and (4) instruction and role play exercises to help the adolescent develop the communication and assertiveness skills needed for negotiating condom use with a sexual partner and resisting peer pressure to engage in risk-related behaviors. These strategies were recently evaluated in community-based settings in New York City and were found to be effective in increasing adolescents' knowledge about HIV and AIDS, and building assertiveness and communication skills for negotiating HIV prevention and risk reduction.

The following provides a description of these components.

AIDS Education

Providing basic information about HIV infection, transmission, and prevention should constitute the first component of any prevention and risk reduction program. The information discussed should be simple, specific, and presented in a straightforward manner. It should include a discussion about the differences between AIDS and HIV infection and high- and low-risk behaviors while attempting to correct misconceptions about transmission through casual contact. Adolescents should be encouraged to either abstain from or delay intercourse or practice "safe sex" by using condoms during sexual intercourse. Adolescents should be encouraged to discuss their thoughts and feelings and ask questions. Throughout this discussion, adolescents' sexual behaviors and sexuality should be discussed in a positive light, to promote a healthy sexual identity. Gay and lesbian adolescents are likely to require special attention with respect to AIDS education (see Chapter 32). The challenges faced by gay and lesbian youth differ dramatically often from those of heterosexual youth. In many cases, the stigmatization of being identified as homosexual can have a number of negative consequences, including ostracism, violence, and expulsion by peers and families; self-destructive behavior, such as substance abuse or suicide attempts; prostitution or dangerous sexual activities; and feelings of isolation, alienation, and confusion. All these consequences are likely to directly influence their ability to prevent or reduce their risk for HIV infection successfully. In these instances, referrals should be made to supportive, caring, and nonjudgmental mental health professionals who will assist these youth in the process of exploring sexual feelings, thoughts, and fantasies.

Avoidance of pregnancy among adolescents at risk for HIV infection should be stressed (see Chapter 73). The risk of HIV transmission from mother to infant is in the range of 20% to 40%.

Enhancing Risk Perception

Adolescents are not likely to change their risk-related behaviors unless they perceive themselves to be at risk for infection. Although studies have revealed that adolescents are aware of the high-risk activities associated with HIV transmission, a very low percentage report actually modifying their sexual behaviors because of their concern of acquiring HIV or AIDS. Immature cognitive development and concrete thinking may make it difficult for some teenagers to understand the future consequences of their current behaviors (see Chapter 9). After describing behaviors associated with risk, adolescents should be encouraged to examine their own sexual and drug use behaviors and estimate their own risk; for example, they are not at risk if they are not engaging in sexual intercourse or intravenous drug use; they are at moderate risk if they use latex condoms during intercourse; they are at high risk if they are engaging in unprotected intercourse. If, after this exercise, adolescents indicate that they want to lower their risk for infection, they should be encouraged to develop practical and specific strategies for risk reduction—that is, engage in alternative "safe sex" activities, such as hugging, kissing, touching, and masturbation or begin consistently using condoms during intercourse, or a combination of these behaviors.

Instruction and Demonstration on Proper Use of Condoms

All adolescents, regardless of their prior sexual experiences, need to know that latex condoms with non-oxynol-9 spermicide are effective at reducing the risk of HIV infection through sexual intercourse. There is some degree of risk associated with condom use if the condoms were to break, leak, or fall off. This is likely to occur when condoms are used properly. Adolescents should be provided the opportunity to talk about, examine, and learn how to use condoms properly. A demonstration should take place using a model of a penis. Both males and females should be encouraged to practice proper condom use on the penis model.

Decision-making, Communication, and Assertiveness Skills

Adolescents may require some assistance in building problem-solving, communication, and assertiveness skills for avoiding risk-related behaviors and situations associated with these behaviors—that is, deciding whether or not to abstain from or delay intercourse and discussing prevention with a boyfriend or girlfriend before initiating sexual intercourse. Communication and assertiveness skills are likely to help adolescents feel more comfortable when initiating a discussion about prevention or communication with a sexual partner about the need to use condoms. Group discussions and role play exercises can be developed to help adolescents learn how to (1) clarify a partner's request and intention, (2) refuse to engage in risk-related behaviors, (3) state the need for HIV prevention, (4) propose alternative low-risk activities (e.g., hugging, kissing, masturbation), and (5) pregnancy prevention.

SUMMARY

Studies of HIV seroprevalence and reported cases of AIDS document that the epidemic now includes adolescents. The impact of the epidemic extends beyond those currently infected to include those at risk as well as those not at risk whose thoughts and actions are motivated by the fear of AIDS. HIV-infected adolescents require extensive medical and psychosocial services.

Some adolescents will lose a parent, relative, or friend to AIDS, and these adolescents will similarly require special services and psychological counseling. Other low-risk youth will become frightened unnecessarily or irrationally fearful from inaccurate information about routes of transmission. Thus there is an immediate need for the development of methods for providing all adolescents with accurate, age-appropriate, and culturally relevant information and interventions for prevention and risk reduction; identifying high-risk adolescents and triaging them to different levels of care and risk reduction counseling; and providing ongoing medical and psychosocial treatments. All primary health care and service providers who work with youth should become knowledgeable about HIV in order to incorporate methods of assessment, referral, and treatment into their practice. This is particularly critical given that the number of adolescents affected by the AIDS epidemic will continue to increase to the end of this century.

BIBLIOGRAPHY

Brooks-Gunn J, Boyer CB, Hein K: Preventing HIV infection and AIDS in children and adolescents: Behavioral research and intervention strategies. Am Psychol 43(11):958, 1988.

Centers for Disease Control: Guidelines for prophylaxis against *Pneumocystis carinii* pneumonia for children infected with human immunodeficiency virus. MMWR 40:1, 1991.

Gayle HD, Keeling RP, Garcia-Tunon M, et al: Prevalence of the human immunodeficiency virus among university students. N Engl J Med 323:1538, 1990.

Kipke MD, Futterman D, Hein K: HIV infection and AIDS during adolescence. Med Clin North Am 74(5):1149, 1990.

Miller H, Turner C, Moses L: AIDS: The Second Decade. Washington, DC National Academy of Science, in press.

Novello A: Report of the Secretary's Work Group on Pediatric HIV Infection and Disease. Washington, DC, Dept. of Health and Human Services, 1988, pp 17–20.

Jean Garrison (ed): Adolescents and AIDS. J Adolesc Health Care 10:1S-69S, 1989.

Hein K: Mandatory HIV testing of youth: A lose-lose proposition. JAMA 266:2430, 1991.

Hein K: Risky business: Adolescents and human immunodeficiency virus. Pediatrics 88:I1052, 1991.

Surgeon General's Follow-up Workshop on Children with HIV Infection and Their Families: Washington, DC, Department of Health and Human Services (HRSA), updated recommendations, 1990.

CHAPTER 77

Breast Disorders

ROBERTA K. BEACH

Breast concerns are common during adolescence. Underlying fears about physical attractiveness, emerging sexual identity, and being normal typically add to the teenager's anxiety. The majority of teenagers will have minor or self-limiting episodes of signs and symptoms. A few will have significant conditions requiring diagnostic evaluation. Pathologic conditions are closely related to age, and though most disorders in adolescence are benign, one in nine women will experience breast cancer later in life. This chapter presents the most common breast symptoms occurring in adolescents.

ANATOMIC CONSIDERATIONS

The female breast is a modified apocrine gland that undergoes rapid growth at puberty, achieving adult form between the ages of 11 and 19 years (see Chapter 5). The breast consists of 15 to 20 separate wedge-shaped lobes. Each lobe is drained by one excretory duct, which opens on the nipple and branches peripherally into the lobules and acini that form the milk glands. The milk glands are surrounded by dense fatty connective tissue (stroma), which accounts for most of the breast mass. A superficial layer of adipose tissue between the mammary glands and skin gives the breast its smooth, rounded contour. Fibrous bands (Cooper ligaments) extend from the skin to underlying pectoral muscle, providing some support (Fig. 77–1). A sweep of glandular tissue (the axillary tail of Spence) may extend from the upper outer quadrant into the axilla. During puberty and pregnancy this tissue may enlarge, mimicking an axillary tumor. The swelling spontaneously regresses when the hormone surge abates. The pigmented areolae contain sebaceous glands (Montgomery tubercles), which enlarge during pregnancy and lactation. The tubercles are sensitive to hormone changes and may become activated during puberty, resulting in a self-limited episode of discharge that resolves in 3 to 5 weeks. The nipples extend above the areolae and contain the minute openings of the lactiferous ducts (Fig. 77–2). Occasionally the nipples may be inverted (which can be surgically corrected if they are severely abnormal) or depressed (they may project after puberty or on stimulation). The mammary gland becomes secretory in response to pituitary prolactin hormone at the time of parturition, producing colostrum the first few days followed by milk.

The male mammary gland is similar in structure to that of the female, including the lactiferous ducts, from embryologic development to puberty. Postpubertal changes are slight, unless hormone imbalance causes hypertrophy (gynecomastia).

BREAST EXAMINATION

Examination of the breasts should become a regular part of physical assessment starting from the time of breast budding, usually around 9 to 12 years of age. The examination provides an excellent opportunity for education and reassurance. Indications include the routine well-teenager physical, the annual gynecologic examination, the initial family planning visit, or any time symptoms are present.

Breast assessment includes history, inspection and palpation, and discussion. The patient history should include breast symptoms, family history of breast disorders, medications or drugs the adolescent is currently taking, menstrual history, and specific risk factors such as prior radiation therapy involving the chest. During the physical examination, sensitivity to the adolescent's modesty can be expressed through tactful use of gowns and drapes accompanied by an explanation of the importance of the examination.

Technique may vary with different examiners. If symptoms are present, inspection and palpation in full sitting (or standing) and supine positions are recommended. For routine assessment of asymptomatic teenagers, examination in just the supine position is sufficient. Inspection in the sitting (or standing) position is performed with the adolescent's arms at her side, then with arms stretched up over her head, and finally with hands on her hips and arms tensed to contract the pectoralis muscles. In the supine position, the adolescent places one arm under her head for examination of the ipsilateral breast, then reverses her arms for the opposite breast. Palpation is performed with the fat pads of the examiner's middle three fingers using firm but gentle pressure. Several methods may be used to systematically palpate the entire circumference of the breast from axilla to sternum. The breast may be palpated in concentric circles (starting either at axilla or nipple), may be divided into spokes of a wheel and palpated along each spoke, or may be palpated in horizontal or vertical strips across all quadrants (Fig. 77–3). Lastly, the nipple is pressed to detect masses or discharge.

Breast inspection should note sexual maturity rating

Figure 77–1. Internal anatomy of the breast (sagittal section).

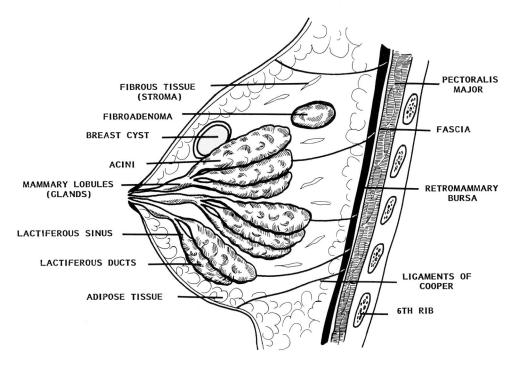

FIBROUS TISSUE (STROMA)
FIBROADENOMA
BREAST CYST
ACINI
MAMMARY LOBULES (GLANDS)
LACTIFEROUS SINUS
LACTIFEROUS DUCTS
ADIPOSE TISSUE
PECTORALIS MAJOR
FASCIA
RETROMAMMARY BURSA
LIGAMENTS OF COOPER
6TH RIB

(see Chapter 5); symmetry; size; shape; skin findings such as excoriation, dimpling, retraction, or redness; and any pattern of venous engorgement. Palpation detects masses, pain, and lymph node enlargement. Normal adolescent breast tissue may feel nodular (especially just prior to menses), grainy, or dense. The inframammary ridge, a prominent oblong of firm tissue felt at the lower edge of both breasts in girls with large breasts, is also normal. Any findings should be diagrammed on the adolescent patient's record, along with appropriate measurements.

Any notable features, including minor anomalies and normal variations, should be discussed with the adolescent. She may be anxious about the same findings whether she has mentioned them or not. Using the breast examination as an educational opportunity increases both the adolescent's comfort and her knowledge.

Teaching Breast Self-examination

The breast assessment provides an appropriate time to teach the adolescent breast self-examination (BSE).

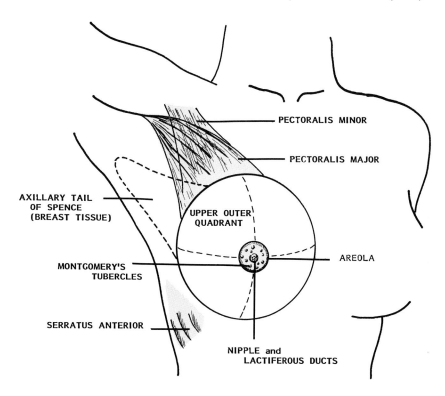

PECTORALIS MINOR
PECTORALIS MAJOR
AXILLARY TAIL OF SPENCE (BREAST TISSUE)
UPPER OUTER QUADRANT
AREOLA
MONTGOMERY'S TUBERCLES
SERRATUS ANTERIOR
NIPPLE and LACTIFEROUS DUCTS

Figure 77–2. External anatomy of the breast with major muscle groups.

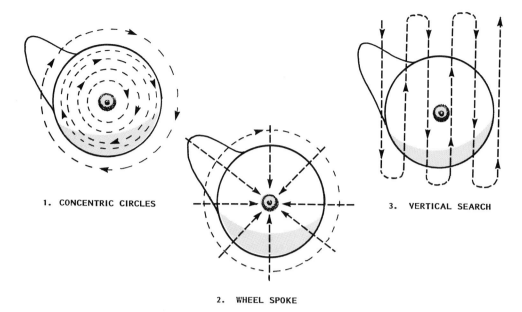

1. CONCENTRIC CIRCLES

2. WHEEL SPOKE

3. VERTICAL SEARCH

Figure 77–3. Three methods of palpation during breast examination (shown on right breast with axillary tail). The entire area from midaxilla to sternum and from clavicles to base of breast should be palpated.

Many teenagers informally check their breasts anyway, as evidenced by hospital studies that show that about 80% of breast masses in adolescents are self-detected. Besides detection of lesions, other advantages of BSE include (1) demystification of female sexual development, (2) familiarization with the feel of normal breast glandular tissue, (3) early formation of lifelong health habits, and (4) promotion of a sense of responsibility for self-care. Questions have been raised about the cost-effectiveness and reliability of BSE in any age group, especially adolescence. Concerns center on poor compliance, low yield, the risk of increasing anxiety, and the added medical costs of office visits or biopsies for benign lesions. Most adolescent specialists feel the benefits outweigh the disadvantages and encourage caregivers to teach routine self-examination.

Adolescents who are especially suited for learning BSE include older teenagers who are cognitively mature enough to appreciate the long-term health benefits, those at higher risk because of family history or personal risk factors (e.g., chest irradiation), and teenagers of any age who express interest. Instructions should cover the following: when to perform the examination (at the end of each menses), how to perform the examination (in the shower or lying down, using the same method of palpation as used by the caregiver), when to seek medical advice (for lumps lasting more than a month, nipple discharge, or symptoms of infection), and an education sheet or pamphlet for the adolescent to take home. Learning is enhanced by observing the patient perform a practice self-examination and by using inexpensive silicone breast models with sample lumps for demonstration.

Common Benign Variations

During breast examination, several benign conditions may be noted and discussed with the adolescent.

Athelia. This is the lack of either nipple (athelia) or breast (amastia). It is a very rare congenital anomaly usually associated with other chest wall deformities (e.g., the Poland syndrome).

Polythelia. Supernumerary nipples, the most common congenital breast anomaly, with an incidence of 0.2% to 0.5%, may appear anywhere along the milk line from axilla to thigh. Associated aberrant breast tissue is rare, but if it is present, there may be swelling and discomfort during pregnancy or lactation. An association with renal and other anomalies is reported. Surgical removal may be advised for cosmetic reasons.

Hypomastia (Small Size). Final breast size is determined primarily by heredity. There are no normal standards for breast size, and aesthetic preferences change with time and culture. Augmentation mammoplasty with silicone gel implants should be delayed until the age of legal consent and even then is controversial. Adverse surgical effects include potential interference with breastfeeding, scarring, and capsule formation, resulting in hard or misshapen breasts. Rarely lack of development may be due to a congenital lack of glandular tissue, destruction of tissue by radiation therapy or inadvertent biopsy of a breast bud, severe malnutrition, genetic disorders (gonadal dysgenesis), or endocrine disorders (congenital or late-onset adrenal hyperplasia) (see Chapters 55 and 60).

Macromastia (Large Size). Simple macromastia (mammary hyperplasia) is also hereditary and may be associated with intertrigo, breast or back pain, postural problems, and intense psychological distress. Reduction mammoplasty may be undertaken once breasts reach mature size (sexual maturity rating [SMR] 5). Surgical consultation should include a thorough discussion of outcomes, complications, and effects on future breastfeeding.

Massive Macromastia (Virginal or Juvenile Breast Hypertrophy). Explosive, sudden breast growth resulting from end-organ hypersensitivity to normal levels of gonadal hormones is a rare condition occurring at puberty or occasionally during pregnancy. The growth may be bilateral, unilateral, or segmental. The breast tissue does not regress; hence, treatment consists of reduction mammoplasty as soon as rapid breast growth stabilizes (which may be before SMR 5). Hormone suppression with antiestrogenic drugs such as tamoxifen has been recommended. Although not curative, it may be useful for 6 months or more prior to surgery to control excessive growth and for 6 to 12 months after surgery to reduce recurrences.

Asymmetry. Unequal rates of breast growth are normal during puberty. About 25% of women have persistent visible asymmetry. A careful examination should rule out abnormal asymmetry caused by one underdeveloped (hypotrophic) or overdeveloped (hypertrophic) breast or by general body hemihypertrophy. Asymmetry can also be a sign of giant fibroadenoma. Surgical reduction or augmentation can be performed for cosmetic correction in severe cases.

Nipple Excoriation. Excessive friction from clothing can cause scaling excoriation of the nipple and areola ("jogger's nipples"). The differential diagnosis includes psoriasis, seborrheic dermatitis, atopic dermatitis, and eczema. Intraductal carcinoma (Paget disease) is extremely rare in young women.

Areolar Hair. Noticeable areolar hair, hereditary in some women, is benign. Repeated plucking can result in ingrown hairs and potential infection, so clipping should be advised if the teenager desires removal.

In general, cosmetic breast surgery for benign conditions should be considered with great caution. Complications, poor cosmetic outcomes, and especially the loss of the ability to breastfeed are significant risks that the adolescent may not fully appreciate at the time but may deeply regret later.

BREAST MASSES

The discovery of a breast lump causes great anxiety because of the inevitable fears of cancer. Almost one half of women of reproductive age will have palpable breast lumps on a careful examination; hence, teenagers commonly present with a self-identified lump. Pubertal breast budding, which usually occurs between 9 and 12 years of age, may be unilateral at first. Parents may be concerned about a "tumor" on the child's chest. A breast bud must never be biopsied, since removal will terminate any future breast growth. Most breast masses in adolescence are benign (Table 77–1), with the great

TABLE 77–1. Breast Masses in Adolescent Females

MOST COMMON	RARE
Benign fibroadenoma	Lymphangioma
Breast cyst	Hemangioma
LESS COMMON	Neurofibromatosis
Giant (juvenile) fibroadenoma	Dermatofibromatosis
Virginal (juvenile) hypertrophy	Papillomatosis
Breast abscess	Papilloma sarcoidosis
Lipoma	Nipple adenoma
Hematoma	Nipple keratoma
MALIGNANT POTENTIAL	Mammary duct ectasia
Adenocarcinoma	Intraductal granuloma
Invasive ductal carcinoma	Galactocele
Intraductal papilloma	Metastatic disease
Cystosarcoma phyllodes	Other

majority being either fibroadenomas or simple cysts. Cancerous lesions can occur (approximately 150 cases annually in American women younger than 25 years of age), and tend to grow more rapidly and be more malignant than in older women; the diagnosis is often missed or delayed. Any persistent palpable breast lump requires careful evaluation.

The basic office approach includes a history of how and when the lesion was discovered, the progression of size, presence of pain, and relationship of symptoms to menstrual cycle. A past history of breast problems, family history of breast diseases, and any associated factors of trauma or drug use should be determined. Pregnancy should be ruled out in any adolescent girl who has breast symptoms. A breast examination—noting the location, size, margins, mobility, and tenderness of the lesion—should be performed. The lesion should be measured and its location and dimensions recorded in the medical chart. In most cases, the adolescent patient should be seen again 1 week after her next menses. At that time, the lesion is remeasured, and the diagnosis is based on the second examination.

Fibroadenomas

Benign fibroadenoma is the most common breast tumor in adolescence, accounting for 70% to 95% of lesions in biopsy studies.

Pathophysiology. The cause of fibroadenoma is unknown, but it is presumed to result from abnormal sensitivity of breast stroma to estrogens, which may explain why the lesion is found most often in young women or postmenopausal women who are on estrogen replacement therapy. The histologic appearance varies among lesions but usually includes increased stromal cellularity, fibrosis, and epithelial hyperplasia.

Clinical Manifestations. The classic appearance of benign fibroadenoma is a single, nontender, firm, rubbery, well-demarcated mobile lesion less than 5 cm in the upper outer quadrant of the breast. It usually grows slowly. In 10% to 13% of adolescent patients, multiple lesions in one or both breasts may be found. An unusual variant is the giant juvenile fibroadenoma, which grows rapidly to 6 cm or more (Fig. 77–4).

Diagnosis. The presumptive diagnosis is based on the history and physical findings as described. Definitive diagnostic procedures include imaging studies, cytologic findings on aspiration, or biopsy. Mammography is of minimal use in teenagers because the breast tissue is too dense for accurate interpretation. Ultrasonography or needle aspiration of fluid can differentiate a solid tumor from a cyst (Fig. 77–5). Current ultrasound technique does not reliably differentiate between benign and malignant solid tumors, though the use of high-frequency transducers and geometric analysis has improved accuracy. Fine-needle aspiration, a method of obtaining cellular material for cytologic examination, is a major advance in the management of palpable breast lesions. It has an accuracy rate in predicting malignancy of 70% to 98% and is equally reliable in all age groups. In recent studies of young women less than 35 years of age, the sensitivity in predicting malignancy was 37%

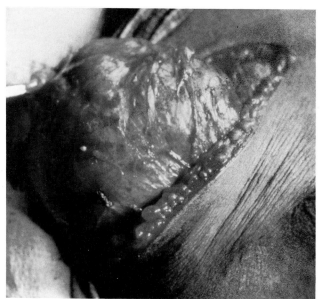

Figure 77–4. Giant juvenile fibroadenoma removed from a 13-year-old girl. (With permission from Beach RK: Routine breast exams: A chance to reassure, guide and protect. Contemp Pediatr 4(10):70, 1987.)

for clinical examination, 55% for mammography, and 78% for fine-needle aspiration. In clinical settings in which cytologic examination by fine-needle aspiration is not available, the evaluation of a suspicious mass requires excisional biopsy.

Differential Diagnosis. *Breast cysts* are the second most common mass in teenagers (see further on). *Giant fibroadenomas,* though benign, may cause breast atrophy and should be excised. *Virginal hypertrophy,* especially if segmental, may be confused with a rapidly growing tumor. *Lipomas* may be large, firm, and encapsulated. *Cystosarcoma phyllodes,* which can be either benign or malignant, presents as a large, firm mass sometimes accompanied by skin retraction or necrosis. Venous engorgement of the overlying skin may occur from rapid tumor growth. Malignant forms are more common in adolescents than in older women. *Intraductal papilloma* usually presents as a unilateral cylindrical mass under the areola, often with bloody nipple discharge. Most are benign, but an infiltrating malignant variant is known. *Adenocarcinoma* presents as a hard, nonmobile, nontender, indurated mass (see Table 77–1).

Treatment. If the examination is consistent with benign fibroadenoma, it is safe to observe the lesion for 2 to 3 months. If the lump persists or enlarges rapidly, a definitive diagnosis is needed. In experienced referral centers, negative results on cytologic examination with fine-needle aspiration could justify continued observation for many months. Otherwise, surgical excision biopsy provides both resolution and definitive diagnosis of the mass. Since the delay in diagnosis of breast cancer in young women is well documented, cytologic confirmation of apparently benign fibroadenomas is essential if these adolescent patients are to be managed conservatively as recently advocated. There is no proven relationship between fibroadenoma and later breast cancer.

Breast Cysts

Fluid-filled breast cysts, the most common cause of painful breast lumps in adolescence, are more frequent in office practice than in biopsy studies. They may mark the onset of progressive symptoms of "benign breast disease" (discussed further on), especially in teenagers with a positive family history.

Pathophysiology. The cyst forms from terminal ducts and acini. Cyst fluid differs from normal serum by the strikingly high amounts of dehydroepiandrosterone sulfate and androsterone sulfate contained therein. The serous fluid collects and regresses because of poorly understood relationships with hormone fluctuations, neuroendocrine effects, and drug metabolite pathways. Although the data are conflicting, progesterone deficiency in the luteal phase, hyperestrogenism resulting from high levels of unbound estradiol, and high evening levels of prolactin production have all been found in women with cystic breast disorders.

Clinical Manifestations. The classic finding is a single tender, soft, spongy, mobile mass. Pain and size are greatest just prior to menses and subside thereafter. Also common are multiple cysts, or a painful "thickening" without well-defined borders, and diffuse nodular lesions. It is unusual for teenagers to experience the chronic lumpy breasts or recurrent cystic lesions called benign breast disease, which more typically affects women in the middle decades.

Diagnosis. If the tender lump regresses after menses, the diagnosis is confirmed. A persistent or enlarging lesion needs definitive diagnosis after 3 months. Breast ultrasonography, if available, is the best noninvasive means of differentiating a cyst from a solid tumor. Simple needle aspiration of serous fluid will also confirm a cyst. Cysts in teenagers do not require biopsy.

Differential Diagnosis. The primary concern is to

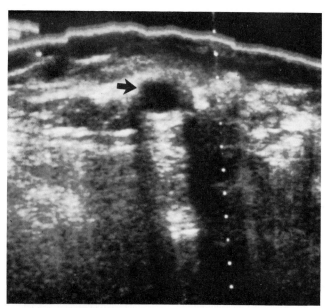

Figure 77–5. Ultrasonogram showing breast cyst *(arrow).* (With permission from Beach RK: Routine breast exams: A chance to reassure, guide and protect. Contemp Pediatr 4(10):70, 1987.)

differentiate a benign cyst from a solid tumor (fibroadenoma or the other causes of breast mass listed in Table 77–1). A breast abscess (see section on breast pain) will also be tender, but signs of inflammation will be present.

The diagnosis best used for a teenager with multiple recurrent painful cysts is not clear. The current literature on the breast is filled with a confusion of terms (fibrocystic disease, cystic mastitis, and mammary dysplasia among others), a confusion of symptoms (pain, swelling, cysts, nodularity), and a confusion of significance (the boundaries of normal cyclic physiologic change versus breast disease). Many authors now recommend that the term *benign breast disease* be used to cover all these conditions, but when or if the term should be applied to teenagers is controversial. Using descriptive diagnoses (e.g., recurrent cyst) and avoiding the label *disease* would be prudent.

Treatment. Simple cysts require only observation or needle aspiration of fluid if they are very large and painful. Reassurance and mild analgesics (e.g., acetaminophen or ibuprofen) are appropriate. Oral contraceptives lessen the incidence of breast cysts and are often recommended for adolescents. Severe recurrent symptoms have been effectively treated with danazol, bromocriptine, and tamoxifen, but significant adverse effects (including nausea, headaches, and severe depression) require caution. High cost and a disappointing relapse rate after drug therapy are also limiting factors.

Course and Prognosis. Spontaneous regression of individual cysts is typical, with one half resolving in 2 to 3 months. Progression to chronic recurrent symptoms with advancing age is possible, especially if there is a strong family history. The relationship of benign breast disease to an increased risk of future breast cancer is unclear.

Malignant Breast Masses

Breast cancer is unusual in adolescents, with malignant lesions accounting for fewer than 1% of biopsied lesions. Fewer than 100 published cases in children aged 3 to 19 years have been reported in the literature, some of which were in male children. Nationally it is estimated that about 150 cases of breast cancer occur annually in American women younger than 25 years of age; hence, more vigorous case reporting would be a helpful contribution to the literature.

Pathophysiology. About one half of reported malignancies in young patients are adenocarcinomas (primarily infiltrating ductal carcinoma), with the rest being secretory carcinomas (of the mammary lobules), malignant cystosarcoma phyllodes, metastatic sarcomas, secondary malignancies of leukemia and lymphoma, and other uncommon types.

Clinical Manifestations. More than 90% of malignant lesions in younger patients present as breast masses. The typical lesion is hard, nontender, indurated, relatively immobile, and fixed to the underlying tissue. It is usually unilateral, solitary, and located in the upper outer quadrant. If the lesion is advanced, other findings may include skin or nipple retraction, *peau d'orange* skin, venous engorgement (cystosarcoma phyllodes),

edema, or lymphadenopathy. In metastatic disease, systemic symptoms such as chest pain, back pain, arm or leg swelling, pleural effusion, or hepatomegaly may be found.

Diagnosis. Cytologic examination by fine-needle aspiration or by biopsy is used for diagnosis. As noted previously, neither mammography nor ultrasonography is reliable in this age group. Unfortunately, the diagnosis is often delayed in younger women, resulting in advanced disease and a poorer prognosis compared with older patients. Any solid tumor that fails to regress within 3 months requires cytologic examination by fine-needle aspiration or excisional biopsy. In the small number of studies available, adolescents with breast malignancies did not appear to have any specific predisposing risk factors, such as family history, that might otherwise raise suspicion.

Treatment. The treatment is based on histologic features and the stage of disease, as in older patients. Without lymph node involvement or metastases, conservative surgery is the treatment of choice, including wide excision (lumpectomy), segmental mastectomy, or simple mastectomy. Radiation therapy is used following surgery to minimize recurrences. Breast reconstruction following mastectomy is especially important for adolescents. For advanced disease, radiation, chemotherapy, hormone therapy (tamoxifen), and immunotherapy may be used in addition to surgery.

Prognosis. In the past, the prognosis has been poor for younger patients because of delayed diagnosis and the aggressive nature of some types of malignancies. With earlier diagnosis, the prognosis should be similar to that for adult patients. Favorable indicators include small tumor size (less than 2 cm), secretory histologic type, positive estrogen receptor status, lateral (versus medial) location, and lack of lymphadenopathy, nipple involvement, or metastases. Five-year survival rates range from 100% for noninvasive carcinoma *in situ,* to 90% for stage I (tumor less than 2 cm), to 75% for stage II (tumor less than 5 cm), and then to progressively worsening rates for invasive or metastasized lesions.

NIPPLE DISCHARGE AND GALACTORRHEA

Nipple discharge can be present in both adolescent girls and boys. It is almost always galactorrhea (inappropriate lactation), usually caused by prior pregnancy (females), drug use, or neuroendocrine disorders such as pituitary prolactinoma or thyroid disease.

Pathophysiology. The production of colostrum and milk is controlled by pituitary prolactin, which is influenced by a wide variety of physiologic pathways mediated by prolactin-releasing or prolactin-inhibiting factors. Termination of pregnancy, whether by delivery or by induced or spontaneous abortion, results in postpartum milk production for several weeks to several months. Numerous drugs (Table 77–2) stimulate low levels of prolactin secretion, primarily through dopamine receptor blockade or catecholamine depletion. Use of illicit "street" drugs, estrogens, and antidepressants

TABLE 77–2. Drugs Associated with Breast Symptoms

ILLICIT OR ABUSED DRUGS	PRESCRIPTION MEDICATIONS
Amphetamines	Chlordiazepoxide
Marijuana	Chlorpromazine
Meprobamate	Cimetidine
Opiates	Diazepam
Codeine	Digoxin
Heroin	Fluphenazine
Morphine	Haloperidol
HORMONES AND RELATED DRUGS	Isoniazid
Bromocriptine	Mesoridazine
Estrogens	Methyldopa
Human chorionic gonadotropin	Perphenazine
Methyltestosterone	Phenothiazines
Oral contraceptives	Reserpine
Tamoxifen citrate	Spironolactone
ANTICANCER DRUGS	Thiethylperazine
Busulfan	Thioxanthenes
Vincristine sulfate	Tricyclic antidepressants
	Amitriptyline
	Imipramine
	Trifluoperazine hydrochloride
	Trimeprazine tartrate

is most common in teenagers. The list of possible neuroendocrine causes is extensive. Prolactin-secreting pituitary tumors (prolactinomas, pituitary adenomas) are the most frequently reported pathologic entities in adolescent males and females. Hypothyroidism in adolescent girls is not an uncommon cause of elevated prolactin. Unusual causes include neurogenic stimulation of the breast or chest wall (nipple manipulation, jogging, crutch-bearing), severe psychogenic stress, and rare hormone-secreting tumors of the ovaries, testes, or adrenal glands.

Clinical Manifestations. Galactorrhea classically presents as a milky discharge expressed from both nipples by firm squeezing. However, it may be unilateral or bilateral, intermittent or persistent, and readily expressed or difficult to observe even with firm "stripping" of the milk ducts. Occasionally breast tenderness will be present. Rarely the discharge will not be galactorrhea but rather a bloody discharge or serous fluid of variable color (see further on). Purulent discharge indicates mastitis.

Diagnosis. The clinical objective is to determine the cause of the galactorrhea. A careful confidential history should document the date of last menses and any possibility of recent pregnancy or abortion. A thorough history of drug use (oral contraceptives, prescription or nonprescription medications, and street drugs) should be obtained. A review of any neuroendocrine symptoms (e.g., headache, visual disturbance, oligomenorrhea) should be elicited (see Chapter 70). The physical examination includes a full breast examination, documentation of discharge, and any neurologic or endocrine signs.

Laboratory studies will depend on clinical suspicions. A glass slide of the discharge can be stained for fat globules to confirm galactorrhea if the diagnosis is in doubt. If serous fluid is found, a Papanicolaou (Pap) smear can be sent for cytologic examination to rule out abnormal cells. A serum human chorionic gonadotropin

(HCG) titer, which remains positive (> 25 IU) for 2 to 4 weeks following termination, may confirm a recent pregnancy. Tests for prolactin level and thyroid-stimulating hormone (TSH) should be obtained. A drug screen, luteinizing hormone (LH), and follicle-stimulating hormone (FSH) may be helpful. Hyperprolactinemia strongly suggests a pituitary tumor, for which computed tomography (CT) or magnetic resonance imaging (MRI) scans are indicated. When hyperprolactinemia or neuroendocrine signs or symptoms are present, consultation with specialists is advised for further evaluation.

Differential Diagnosis. *Intraductal papilloma* is associated with unilateral bloody or rarely black nipple discharge from one duct. Adolescent patients with this condition should be referred for surgical consultation. *Duct ectasia* produces a serous fluid of variable color (clear, yellow, gray, brown, or green). The condition is almost always benign and self-limited, but a Pap smear of the fluid is performed for reassurance to detect rare malignant cells. *Montgomery tubercles* on the areola occasionally produce benign whitish discharge for a few weeks during puberty or during pregnancy and lactation.

Treatment and Clinical Course of Galactorrhea. The approach to treatment depends on the underlying cause. Postpartum galactorrhea requires observation only. It usually resolves within 2 to 3 months after induced or spontaneous abortion. After term delivery (when the mother is not breastfeeding), it may persist 6 months or longer, especially if there is continued manual expression by the adolescent or her sexual partner. If galactorrhea is drug-related, the adolescent should be instructed to stop using any illicit drugs. With prescription medications, the adolescent patient may be offered reassurance, or alternate drugs may be tried. Drug-induced galactorrhea resolves within 2 to 3 months after drugs are discontinued. For most pituitary adenomas, bromocriptine therapy is now the treatment of choice, with surgery reserved for large or persistent tumors, even though bromocriptine therapy also may be used for large or persistent tumors. Patients with elevated prolactin levels require intensive follow-up until a cause is identified. Many will eventually be found to have a pituitary tumor.

If prolactin levels are normal and no drug history can be elicited, management of persistent galactorrhea is problematic. Boys should still be evaluated for pituitary lesions. Girls with amenorrhea deserve further evaluation for both pituitary lesions and the polycystic ovary syndrome (see Chapter 70). Girls who are menstruating regularly can be followed with annual prolactin level determinations to rule out a slow-growing adenoma. In general, if the entire work-up is normal, adolescent patients are followed annually with repeat prolactin level determinations. Normal prolactin levels usually indicate a benign prognosis. Often the galactorrhea resolves spontaneously and no cause is ever identified. Adolescents should be instructed not to stimulate the breasts by manual expression.

BREAST PAIN

Breast pain (mastodynia or mastalgia) is one of the most common breast symptoms mentioned by teenagers.

It affects 30% to 40% of women in their reproductive years, and in 8% of these women it is severe enough to interfere with activity. It is usually physiologic, but breast masses, inflammation, or underlying chest wall pain should be considered. Breast pain is one of the earliest signs of pregnancy, which may be the girl's unexpressed worry and reason for the visit.

Pathophysiology. The cause of physiologic breast pain is not known. Hypersensitivity to normal levels of estrogen and progesterone is usually postulated, but recent studies suggest it may be an abnormality of lipid metabolism mediated by prolactin. The same drugs associated with galactorrhea (see Table 77–2) can cause breast pain, including exogenous hormones, antidepressants, phenothiazines, and many street drugs. Progesterone deficiency has not been confirmed as a cause. The role of dietary methylxanthines (caffeine, tea, cola, chocolate) is controversial, with small studies and anecdotal evidence indicating a relationship unconfirmed by large-scale studies.

Clinical Manifestations. The classic syndrome includes cyclic breast swelling, tenderness, and engorgement that begin in the luteal phase of the menstrual cycle, peak a few days prior to menses, and resolve rapidly after onset of menstrual flow. Noncyclic mastodynia is less common in adolescents and may indicate a drug association.

Diagnosis. The history should include the pattern of pain, the relation to menses, the possibility of pregnancy or drug use, and recent trauma or muscle strain. A careful breast examination will rule out masses, nipple discharge, inflammation, or abscess, and will detect pain that actually arises from the pectoral muscles or chest wall. Laboratory studies are not usually needed, except for a pregnancy test and perhaps a prolactin determination in severe, persistent cases. If the examination produces normal results, the presumptive diagnosis is based on history.

Differential Diagnosis. Cyclic mastodynia is physiologic and benign. Noncyclic mastodynia may be drug-related or the precursor to galactorrhea. Breast masses, especially cysts, may present with pain. Chest wall pain may arise from pectoral muscles, intercostal spaces, or costochondral junctions. Sports, weight-lifting, trauma, or the Tietze syndrome (postviral inflammation of localized costochondral junctions) are common causes. Breast inflammation presents with the classic signs of swelling, heat, tenderness, and erythema; an abscess may be palpable (see further on).

Treatment. Mild cyclic breast pain is a normal physiologic condition. Most adolescents will respond to adequate reassurance, mild analgesics, and the use of a supportive brassiere. If illicit drug use is implicated, the drugs should be stopped. Many treatments have been advocated for severe symptoms. Recent extensive literature reviews conclude that bromocriptine, danazol, and tamoxifen are effective in older women, but they are associated with significant side effects and have not been studied in adolescents. Evening primrose oil and dietary fat restriction are probably effective in reducing symptoms. Use of vitamin E and diuretics and limitation of salt or methylxanthines have not been adequately evaluated in women with cyclic mastalgia.

Cause and Prognosis. Cyclic breast pain is usually benign and self-limited. It may be the precursor to later benign breast disease (a syndrome of nodularity, cysts, swelling, and pain) in some women.

BREAST INFECTIONS

Adolescent breast infections, progressing from cellulitis to mastitis and abscess formation, have potentially serious consequences and require prompt treatment.

Pathophysiology. Breastfeeding is the most common cause of mastitis in adolescents, typically occurring 2 to 4 weeks postpartum. Engorgement, milk stasis, and cracked nipples contribute to bacterial spread. Nonlactational infections may result from trauma, cracked nipples, or cutaneous spread of infection from acne pustules, ingrown areolar hairs, folliculitis, or other skin lesions. *Staphylococcus aureus* is present in 80% to 90% of breast infections in teenagers. A wide variety of other aerobic and anaerobic organisms can be involved, including *Pseudomonas, Streptococcus,* and *Escherichia coli.*

Clinical Manifestations. Breast pain is the initial symptom. Localized erythema, tenderness, and warmth follow, usually adjacent to the areola. Edema, induration, and possibly a mass may be noted. A palpable fluctuant abscess is a late-stage finding, often accompanied by fever, leukocytosis, and regional adenopathy. Because of the anatomy of breast tissue, significant deep infection may be present with only minimal surface signs.

Diagnosis. The history and physical findings will usually confirm the diagnosis. Purulent drainage should be cultured. For lactational infections, examination of the milk may reveal abnormally high leukocyte and bacterial counts. Because of the presence of skin bacteria, a midstream milk specimen is required for culture.

Differential Diagnosis. Although infection is usually self-evident, other considerations include contusion, hematoma, and fat necrosis from trauma, superficial phlebitis of the skin (Mondor disease), and duct ectasia with nipple discharge (nonpurulent).

Treatment. A vigorous course of broad spectrum antibiotics that are effective against *Staphylococcus aureus* (e.g., dicloxacillin or a cephalosporin) should be initiated early and continued until all signs and symptoms resolve, which may take 4 weeks or more. Repeat examinations to confirm resolution are essential. If significant cellulitis is present, intravenous antibiotics should be considered initially. If a fluctuant abscess is found, the adolescent should be referred for surgical incision and drainage. Office drainage should not be attempted, since the abscess is often deep and difficult. In lactational infections, unless there is purulent nipple discharge, breastfeeding should continue in order to prevent abscess formation and preserve milk supply.

Course and Prognosis. If treated early, full resolution may be expected. If only partially treated, 50% of these infections will recur. The most common cause of recurrence is inadequate length of antibiotic treatment or abrupt discontinuation of breastfeeding in lactating adolescents. Complications of untreated mastitis include tissue necrosis, extensive parenchymal destruction, and rarely septicemia.

GYNECOMASTIA

Gynecomastia may be defined as any palpable mammary development in the male. A lump in the breast is just as anxiety-producing for boys as it is for girls. Transient pubertal gynecomastia occurs in up to 70% of boys at SMR 2 to 4, peaking around age 14 years (see Chapter 5). However, gynecomastia before puberty or after growth is complete requires careful evaluation for underlying disorders.

Pathophysiology. Since the male mammary gland is anatomically similar to the prepubescent female's, including lactiferous ducts and stroma, hormone stimulation can cause hypertrophy. The precise cause of pubertal gynecomastia is unknown, but it may relate to temporary hormone imbalance in biologically active estrogens, to the ratio of testosterone or androstenedione to estradiol, or to end-organ sensitivity. Persistent or later-onset gynecomastia may be induced by a wide variety of drugs (including most of those given in Table 77–2) or by hormone-secreting tumors or other endocrinopathies.

Clinical Manifestations. The classic presentation of pubertal gynecomastia is a 12- to 14-year-old boy with a unilateral, tender breast lump found on self-examination, which is subareolar, firm, discoid, and 2 to 3 cm in size. Bilateral growth, concurrent or sequential, is also common. Rarely the growth may enlarge beyond the areola to resemble a SMR 3 female breast. Very rarely galactorrhea may be present, usually related to drugs or self-manipulation. Breast enlargement in an older adolescent male who has finished growing (SMR 5) is not a normal variant and requires thorough evaluation.

Diagnosis. The clinical evaluation should differentiate normal pubertal events from any underlying disorder. Any history of drug use (especially marijuana) or symptoms of systemic illness should be elicited. Examination of the breast, testicles, liver, and thyroid should be documented. Healthy pubertal males with otherwise normal examinations do not require laboratory studies. Otherwise, the work-up depends on the suspected diagnosis.

Differential Diagnosis. The list includes transient pubertal gynecomastia, persistent physiologic gynecomastia, drug-induced gynecomastia (see Table 77–2), adipose tissue (in obese males), hormone-producing tumors (testicular, pituitary, adrenal, pulmonary, Hodgkin disease), liver disease, thyroid disorders, renal disease, and Klinefelter syndrome. However, by incidence, drug use, Kleinfelter syndrome, and testicular tumors are most likely.

Treatment. If other causes are ruled out, treatment of pubertal gynecomastia consists of reassurance, explanation of the natural course of the condition, and psychological support. The condition should be explained as a "temporary imbalance of hormones during puberty" and the adolescent should be assured that he is not becoming a female. Advise the adolescent that street drugs will aggravate the condition. For very large or persistent growth, surgical reduction is recommended. Hormone therapy has not been adequately evaluated.

Prognosis. Transient pubertal gynecomastia resolves within 2 years. Only a few cases persist to adulthood.

BIBLIOGRAPHY

Ashley S, Royle GT, Corder A, et al: Clinical, radiological and cytological diagnosis of breast cancer in young women. Br J Surg 76:835, 1989.

Beach RK: Routine breast exams: A chance to reassure, guide and protect. Contemp Pediatr 4(10):70, 1987.

Emans SJ, Goldstein DP: The breast: Examination and lesions. In Emans SJ, Goldstein DP (eds): Pediatric and Adolescent Gynecology, 3rd ed. Boston, Little, Brown, 1990.

Erickson R, Shank C, Gratton C: Fine needle aspiration biopsy. J Fam Pract 28(3):306, 1989.

Fornage BD, Lorigan JG, Andry E: Fibroadenoma of the breast: Sonographic appearance. Radiology 172:671, 1989.

Frisell J, Eklund G, Nilsson R, et al: Additional value of fine needle aspiration biopsy in a mammographic screening trial. Br J Surg 76:840, 1989.

Goodwin PJ, Neelam M, Boyd NF: Cyclical mastopathy: A critical review of therapy. Br J Surg 75:837, 1988.

Greydanus DE, Hofmann AD: The thorax: Disorders of the breast. In Hofmann AD, Greydanus DE (eds): Adolescent Medicine, 2nd ed. East Norwalk, CT, Appleton-Lange, 1989.

Greydanus DE, Parks DS, Farrell EG: Breast disorders in children and adolescents. Pediatr Clin North Am 36(3):601, 1989.

Griffith JR: Virginal breast hypertrophy. J Adolesc Health Care 10:423, 1989.

Harris VJ, Jackson VP: Indications for breast imaging in women under age 35 years. Radiology 172:445, 1989.

Kopans DB, Meyer JE, Sadowsky N: Breast imaging. N Engl J Med 310:960, 1984.

Leung AKC, Robson WL: Polythelia. Int J Dermatol 28(7):429, 1989.

McSweeney MD, Egan RL: Breast cancer in the younger patient. Results Cancer Res 90:36, 1984.

Neinstein L: Galactorrhea. In Neinstein L: Adolescent Health Care, 2nd ed. Baltimore, Urban and Schwarzenberg, 1990.

Rohn RD: Galactorrhea in the adolescent. J Adolesc Health Care 5:37, 1984.

Sainsbury JRC, Nicolson S, Needham GK, et al: Natural history of the benign breast lump. Br J Surg 75:1080, 1988.

Schwartz GF: Benign neoplasms and inflammations of the breast. Clin Obstet Gynecol 25:373, 1982.

Schydlower M, Imai WK, Stafford EM, Getts AG: Breast disorders. In Strasburger VC (ed): Basic Adolescent Gynecology. Baltimore, Urban and Schwarzenberg, 1990.

Wang DY, Fentiman IS: Epidemiology and endocrinology of benign breast disease. Breast Cancer Res Treat 6:5, 1985.

CHAPTER 78

Male Reproductive Conditions

EFSTRATIOS DEMETRIOU

PHYSICAL EXAMINATION

A genital examination is part of a complete physical examination of a male adolescent. The genitalia should be examined with the patient supine, following examination of the abdomen, and standing after the remainder of the examination has been completed. The latter allows for better appreciation of a varicocele or hernia. Clothing should be removed from the genital area.

The size of the penis and testicles and the quantity and distribution of the pubic hair are noted, and sexual maturity ratings (SMRs) are determined (see Chapter 5). External lesions such as folliculitis and pubic lice or nits are noted next. The inguinal area is palpated for adenopathy or hernias. Enlarged or tender nodes may indicate malignant or, more commonly, infectious conditions of the genitalia.

The penis is then inspected, and superficial lesions are noted. The size and location of the urethral meatus are noted. The meatus should be separated with the thumb and forefinger and inspected for mucosal lesions (ulcers and warts) (see Chapter 75). Appropriate microbiologic studies should be initiated if there is any urethral discharge. If present, the foreskin should be retracted to exclude phimosis, balanitis, and other lesions of the glans and the urethral meatus. The shaft of the penis is inspected for abnormal lesions. The urethra should be "stripped" or "milked" and urethral secretions sent for microbiologic evaluation.

The scrotum and its contents are examined next. The skin is inspected for abnormalities. If the cremasteric reflex is to be tested, this should be performed prior to palpation of the testes, since such palpation can induce a reflex retraction of the testes that might not be appreciated. The testes are palpated between the thumb and first two fingers. Their size, shape, symmetry, consistency, and position within the scrotum should be noted. The normal testis is firm and freely mobile. A hard area within the substance of the testis is considered neoplastic until proved otherwise. The presence of tenderness, nodularity, and masses should be determined. Masses should be transilluminated to determine whether they are solid or cystic. The epididymis is palpated between the thumb and forefinger. It begins along the upper testicular pole and extends toward the lower pole along the posterior aspect of the testis.

The spermatic cord is palpated along its entire course by rolling it between the index finger and the thumb. A varicocele may be palpated, and in many cases it may be visualized with the patient in the upright position. A finger is inserted through the scrotal skin into the inguinal canal to evaluate for an inguinal hernia. A "pulse" will be palpated during a cough or a Valsalva maneuver if a hernia is present.

Examination of the prostate is then performed if indicated by the history. The patient may be positioned in the lithotomy position, or standing and bent over the end of the examining table, or in the lateral prone position. A lubricated, gloved finger is inserted into the rectum, with the pad of the finger facing the anterior rectal wall. The normal prostate is the size and shape of a chestnut and has a firm and elastic consistency. Tenderness, bogginess, and induration should be noted.

The physical examination provides an excellent opportunity for teaching the adolescent as well as reassuring him. Explaining each portion of the genital examination as it is performed increases the adolescent's knowledge about his body and usually diminishes anxiety. Testicular self-examination can be demonstrated at this time.

Testicular Self-examination

Because testicular cancer has an excellent overall prognosis, early detection is extremely important. No cost-effective screening test exists; therefore, testicular self-examination (TSE) is the only way of detecting testicular cancer at an early stage.

Recent surveys indicate that young men are ignorant of their risk for developing testicular cancer. In one study of college athletes, 87% were almost completely unaware of their risk, and only 10% had been taught TSE, 5% by their physicians. A survey of primary care physicians and surgeons found that only 18% routinely taught TSE to adolescent patients.

Instruction regarding TSE should be incorporated into the routine health care visit beginning in midpuberty (see Chapter 25). Once an adolescent male is informed that the most frequent cancer in his age group is testicular cancer, his curiosity will usually be piqued. Adolescents are instructed to roll each testicle between the thumb and the tips of the first three fingers until the entire surface has been covered. They are told that the testicles should feel round and smooth, similar to hard-boiled eggs. Lumps, irregularities, change in size of the testis, or a heaviness should be reported to a physician. The examination should be performed monthly, preferably while in the shower. TSE should be reviewed at every subsequent routine health care visit. Printed materials reviewing TSE are available from the American Cancer Society.

SCROTAL DISORDERS

Scrotal Masses

Scrotal masses are commonly encountered in adolescents. They may represent a potentially life-threatening malignant tumor or, in the case of testicular torsion, may pose a threat to future testicular function. They also may produce considerable anxiety for the male patient who is concerned about his masculinity. It is, therefore, important that practitioners have a basic understanding of the conditions that present as a scrotal mass in adolescents and be familiar with their evaluation.

EVALUATION

The differential diagnosis of a scrotal mass is shown in Table 78–1. It is helpful to first consider whether the mass is painful or painless. A painful scrotal mass requires prompt evaluation. If pain is present, its location, radiation, and onset (sudden or gradual) and history of previous episodes should be noted. The presence of dysuria, urethral discharge, underlying genitourinary pathologic condition, or systemic symptoms such as fever or vomiting and history of sexual activity or trauma should be determined. A change in testicular size or a sensation of heaviness may suggest a neoplastic process.

It is important to determine whether the mass is part of or separate from the testis. A mass within the testis is likely to be a tumor. Clear transillumination suggests a structure filled with translucent fluid, such as a hydrocele or spermatocele. Pain that is diminished when the scrotum is elevated (positive Prehn sign) is suggestive of orchitis or epididymitis. Epididymitis is further suggested by the presence of polymorphonuclear leukocytes

**TABLE 78–1. Differential Diagnosis of
Scrotal Masses**

PAINFUL SCROTAL MASSES
Testicular torsion
Torsion of testicular appendages
Acute epididymitis
Orchitis
Incarcerated inguinal hernia
Testicular trauma
Idiopathic scrotal edema
Henoch-Schönlein purpura

PAINLESS SCROTAL MASSES
Varicocele
Hydrocele
Spermatocele
Epididymal cyst
Testicular tumors
Extratesticular tumors
Inguinal hernia

in the urine or urethral discharge. Urethral culture for *Neisseria gonorrhoeae* and culture or rapid test for *Chlamydia trachomatis* are indicated in such adolescents. In patients with a history of genitourinary disease, a midstream urine specimen should be examined for pyuria and bacteriuria and cultured for urinary pathogens. A blood leukocyte count is often not helpful diagnostically since both testicular torsion and epididymitis can produce an elevated white blood count.

Radionuclide testicular scanning and color Doppler ultrasonography are useful in the evaluation of the acute scrotum in order to reduce unnecessary surgical exploration. If the history and physical examination strongly suggest testicular torsion, prompt surgical exploration is indicated; diagnostic studies should not be used to confirm this clinical diagnosis. These procedures may be used to confirm the absence of torsion in cases in which the diagnosis is not readily evident.

Radionuclide scanning requires injection of technetium-99m sodium pertechnetate intravenously, followed by serial imaging of its uptake by the testes. The appearance of radionuclide in each hemiscrotum is a direct function of its blood supply. In acute testicular torsion, there is decreased uptake, whereas epididymoorchitis and torsion of the testicular appendages demonstrate normal or increased uptake. Studies have demonstrated the accuracy of the radionuclide scan to be 86% to 100%. The scan should be interpreted in light of the patient's clinical course. False-negative results may occur following spontaneous detorsion and in very early torsion. False-positive results may occur in the presence of a hematoma, abscess, hydrocele, necrotic tumor, or hernia overlying the testes.

Color Doppler ultrasonography is a recently developed imaging technique that is capable of evaluating blood flow *and* anatomy. Color images representing blood flow are superimposed on real-time, gray-scale ultrasound images; correlation of perfusion data with anatomy can thus be achieved.

High-resolution ultrasonography is the imaging modality of choice for most other scrotal pathology; it is the procedure of choice in evaluating patients with a painless scrotal mass or trauma. The ability of ultrasonography to reliably differentiate intratesticular from extratesticular pathologic features as well as cystic from solid masses is the basis for its important role in the diagnostic evaluation of such patients. A palpable mass within the testis represents a malignant tumor until proved otherwise and mandates prompt surgical exploration. Most malignant tumors have decreased echogenicity or have a mixed pattern of decreased and increased echogenicity compared with benign testicular tissue. Following trauma, rupture of the tunica albuginea, a hematocele, or a hematoma can be detected with a high degree of accuracy.

TESTICULAR TORSION

Testicular torsion is a urologic emergency that requires prompt evaluation and surgical intervention if the gonad is to survive. Although torsion can occur at any age, it is most common during the teenage years. In one large series, 65% of cases occurred between ages 12 and

18 years. Increased testicular size and physical activity, often combined with an underlying structural anomaly, account for its high incidence in this age group.

Pathophysiology. Affected testes in adolescents are associated with anomalies of suspension that allow them to twist within the tunica vaginalis (in contrast with those in the neonate, in which the entire spermatic cord twists). In most individuals, the testicle is attached to the epididymis and posterior scrotal wall (Fig. 78–1). In those with the "bell clapper" deformity, the most commonly recognized anomaly, the tunica vaginalis surrounds the testicle and extends above it to the distal portion of the spermatic cord. The testicle lies transversely and, lacking its normal attachment to the scrotal wall, is able to twist relative to the cord, resulting in obstruction of the vascular supply. The mesorchium joining the testis to the epididymis may also be very loose, allowing it to twist between the epididymis and testis. Both anomalies are usually present bilaterally.

The initial effect of testicular torsion is obstruction of venous return. Secondary edema and hemorrhage of the testicle occur, followed by compromised arterial blood flow. The degree of testicular damage depends on the degree and duration of ischemia. Animal studies reveal that spermatogenic cells are damaged after 4 hours of ischemia; hormone-producing Leydig cells are more resistant, demonstrating complete destruction after 10 hours or more of ischemia.

Clinical Manifestations. Classically, the onset of pain is sudden. There may be a history of similar pain in the past that resolved spontaneously. The pain is located over the affected hemiscrotum but may also be over the inguinal area and lower abdomen and may be associated with nausea and vomiting. Erythema and swelling of the involved hemiscrotum may be absent initially but are invariably present later. As many as 10% of affected adolescents may have swelling without significant pain.

Diagnosis. On physical examination, uniform testicular and epididymal tenderness and swelling are present. When the patient is examined while standing, the af-

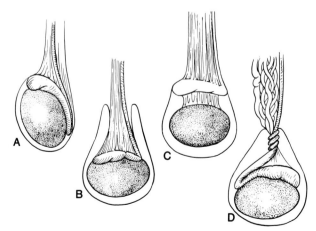

Figure 78–1. *A,* Normal intrascrotal anatomy. *B,* Suspension anomaly: abnormally high attachment of tunica vaginalis with horizontal testicular lie. *C,* Suspension anomaly: long mesorchium with horizontal testicular lie. *D,* Suspension anomaly with testicular torsion. (From Stillwell TJ, Kramer SA: Intermittent testicular torsion. Pediatrics 77:908, 1986. Reproduced by permission of Pediatrics.)

fected testicle is often elevated and lying in a transverse position within the scrotal sac. A palpable twist of the spermatic cord may be present. The epididymis may be found in an anterior rather than in the normal posterolateral position. The uninvolved testicle is often found with its axis in a horizontal plane as well. Elevation of the scrotum does not relieve the pain (negative Prehn sign), and the swollen testicle does not transilluminate. The cremasteric reflex is usually absent.

If testicular torsion is strongly suspected clinically, the patient should undergo immediate surgical exploration. Surgery should also be performed in the event of equivocal findings if a nuclear scan or color Doppler ultrasound scan cannot be immediately performed. A radionuclide scan is appropriate in an adolescent for whom the diagnosis is unclear, and for confirmation of the diagnosis of another scrotal disorder; it demonstrates decreased isotope uptake with testicular torsion. Color Doppler ultrasonography often demonstrates decreased pulsations to the affected testicle.

Differential Diagnosis. Other disorders that should be considered in the differential diagnosis of the acute scrotum are listed in Table 78–1. The classic features that help differentiate testicular torsion from acute epididymitis and appendiceal torsion (the other most common causes of acute scrotal pain in adolescents) are listed in Table 78–2.

Treatment. External manual detorsion may be attempted by an experienced individual while the patient is being prepared for surgery; if successful, strangulation can be relieved more quickly. Surgery, however, is the only definitive treatment. Both testicles should be explored, detorsion of the affected testicle accomplished, and nonabsorbable sutures used to affix the testicle to the scrotum. If the testicle is necrotic, it should be removed, and a prosthesis can be inserted at a later time. Because an ischemic testis can result in autoimmunization, with destruction of spermatogonia on the unaffected side, many surgeons will remove a testis of questionable viability to decrease the risk of later infertility.

Clinical Course and Prognosis. Most clinical series report testicular viability approaching 100% if detorsion is achieved within 6 hours, with a sharp fall-off to about 20% at 10 to 12 hours; after 24 hours the chances of viability are almost nil. Long-term sequelae include diminished testicular volume in two thirds of affected individuals and abnormalities of semen quality in one half to two thirds. These findings emphasize the need for prompt diagnosis and treatment.

TORSION OF TESTICULAR APPENDAGES

Torsion of the testicular appendages can also cause acute scrotal pain that is often confused with that of testicular torsion. Its peak incidence is in early adolescence, earlier than that of testicular torsion.

Pathophysiology. There are four testicular appendages, all representing vestigial structures: the appendix testis (hydatid of Morgagni), the appendix epididymidis, the paradidymis (organ of Giraldés), and the vas aberrans (organ of Haller). The appendix testis accounts for 92% of all appendiceal torsions. It is a small, oval,

TABLE 78–2. Differential Diagnosis of the Acute Scrotum in Adolescents

CHARACTERISTIC	TESTICULAR TORSION	TORSION OF TESTICULAR APPENDAGE	ACUTE EPIDIDYMITIS
Age	Early adolescence	Preadolescence to early adolescence	Late adolescence, young adulthood
Pain			
Onset	Sudden	Sudden or gradual	Gradual
Location	Testes, groin, abdomen	Upper pole of affected testis	Epididymis, then entire testis
Prior episodes	Common	Uncommon	Uncommon
Fever	Uncommon	Uncommon	Common
Dysuria, urethral discharge	Rare	Rare	Common
Involved testis			
Position	High in scrotum, horizontal, rotated	Normal (vertical)	Low riding, vertical
Tenderness	Diffuse, no change with elevation	Tender, palpable appendage; becomes diffuse	Epididymis initially; becomes diffuse; relieved with elevation
Contralateral testis	Often in horizontal position	Normal (vertical)	Normal (vertical)
Pyuria	Unusual	Unusual	Common
Blood flow	Decreased	Normal or increased	Increased

Adapted with permission from Haynes BE, Bessen HA, Haynes VE: The diagnosis of testicular torsion. JAMA 249:2522, 1983. Copyright 1983, American Medical Association.

pedunculated structure attached to the upper pole of the testis or to the cleft between the testis and the epididymis. The appendix epididymidis, a pedunculated structure that is attached near the head of the epididymis, accounts for 7% of cases.

Clinical Manifestations. The sudden or gradual onset of pain is the presenting complaint. Generally mild to moderate, it can be severe in some cases. It is usually localized to the upper pole of the testis, although initially it can begin in the inguinal area or lower abdomen. Nausea and vomiting are rarely present, and a history of similar pain is uncommon.

Diagnosis. Physical findings include localized tenderness and a firm, tender nodule at the upper pole of the testis. The cyanotic appendage may be seen through the scrotal skin (blue dot sign). Erythema and edema of the scrotal skin and a secondary hydrocele are also frequently seen.

Often, classic signs are not present on examination, and torsion of an appendage must be distinguished from testicular torsion. Color Doppler ultrasonography will indicate increased flow to the area around the involved appendage, and a radionuclide scan will show normal to mildly increased uptake.

Differential Diagnosis. For the differential diagnosis, see Tables 78–1 and 78–2.

Treatment. Appendiceal torsion can be managed without surgery in most cases, if the possibility of testicular torsion can be eliminated. Pain can be treated with an analgesic; for persistent or severe pain, surgical removal of the appendage relieves the discomfort.

Clinical Course and Prognosis. Symptoms usually subside within a few days. There are no long-term sequelae, and fertility is unaffected.

ACUTE EPIDIDYMITIS

During early and middle puberty, acute epididymitis is less common than testicular torsion and torsion of the appendix testis, but it becomes the most common cause of an acute scrotum.

Pathophysiology. There are three major pathogenic processes that produce epididymitis. The most common mechanism in adolescents is retrograde migration of sexually transmitted microorganisms from the urethra, through the vas deferens, to the epididymis. The most common organisms are *Neisseria gonorrhoeae* and *Chlamydia trachomatis*. The second major mechanism, relatively uncommon in adolescents, involves the reflux of infected urine via the vas deferens to the epididymis, usually in the presence of obstructive abnormalities or following urinary tract surgery or instrumentation (see Chapter 66). Typical urinary pathogens include *Escherichia coli*. Finally, the least common mechanism is hematogenous spread of microorganisms to the epididymis as a result of systemic disease due to *Mycobacterium tuberculosis*, *Brucella*, pneumococci, meningococci, *Haemophilus influenzae*, cryptococci and other fungi, and viruses, including mumps virus and enterovirus.

Clinical Manifestations. Presenting symptoms are scrotal pain and swelling. The pain usually develops gradually over hours or days but may also be abrupt in onset. It may initially be localized to the area of the epididymis and then generalize to the entire testis. There is usually a history of recent sexual activity, dysuria, or urethral discharge, alone or in combination. Most adolescent patients are afebrile and are nontoxic even if they have a fever.

Diagnosis. On examination, the tender, swollen epididymis is in its normal posterolateral position in relation to the testis. Early in the course of the disease the testis is relatively uninvolved. As the disease progresses, a reactive hydrocele may develop, and the infection may spread to the testis, resulting in an epididymoorchitis and making clinical assessment more difficult. Elevation and support of the scrotum often relieve the discomfort (positive Prehn sign). The cremasteric reflex is usually present. Bilateral involvement may occur.

Urethral secretions should be sampled prior to the adolescent's submitting a specimen for urinalysis; a urethritis may otherwise be missed because white blood cells and bacteria have been washed away during urination. White blood cells on Gram stain confirm urethritis. The presence of gram-negative intracellular diplococci or positive studies for *N. gonorrhoeae* or *C.*

trachomatis will confirm the etiologic agent. For those with no evidence of urethritis, a midstream urine specimen should be submitted for urinalysis and Gram stain. Pyuria and bacteriuria strongly suggest coliform epididymitis, and the urine should be cultured for urinary pathogens in such circumstances.

When the diagnosis is uncertain, a urologic consultation should be sought. A radionuclide scan or color Doppler ultrasound scan is useful and will show normal or increased flow to the involved testis. If uncertainty remains, it is safest to perform surgical exploration to exclude testicular torsion.

Differential Diagnosis. For differential diagnosis, see Tables 78–1 and 78–2.

Treatment. Antibiotic therapy is the mainstay of treatment for epididymitis. Most patients can be treated with oral antimicrobials, but hospitalization and parenteral antibiotic therapy are indicated if the patient appears toxic or has an underlying urologic anatomic abnormality. For epididymitis of presumed sexually transmitted origin, ceftriaxone, 250 mg given intramuscularly, followed by a 10-day course of tetracycline hydrochloride, 500 mg po qid, or doxycycline, 100 mg po bid, for at least 10 days, provides satisfactory treatment for infection due to either *N. gonorrhoeae* or *C. trachomatis*. Those adolescents with presumed coliform epididymitis should be started, pending culture reports, on an antimicrobial agent effective against urinary pathogens, such as trimethoprim-sulfamethoxazole, 160/800 mg po bid, amoxicillin, 500 mg po tid, or cephalexin, 500 mg po qid, for 10 to 14 days. The tetracyclines also provide adequate therapy for most urinary tract pathogens.

Ancillary therapy includes bed rest, scrotal elevation with a towel, oral analgesics, and scrotal support when ambulatory. Bed rest with scrotal elevation helps ensure adequate lymphatic drainage of the infected epididymis. When epididymitis is due to a sexually transmitted pathogen, the adolescent patient's sex partner(s) should be treated.

Clinical Course and Prognosis. Adolescent patients with sexually transmitted epididymitis require posttreatment cultures; those with coliform epididymitis should be evaluated for structural urinary tract pathology with an intravenous pyelogram (IVP) and voiding cystourethrogram. Neoplasia should be considered if symptoms have not resolved in 10 to 14 days because epididymitis may be the presenting symptom in some adolescents with testicular cancer.

The literature reports numerous complications due to epididymitis, including abscess formation, testicular infarction, chronic pain, testicular atrophy, and infertility in older patients. Complications appear to occur relatively infrequently in adolescents, however.

ORCHITIS

Pathophysiology. Acute orchitis is an inflammation of the testis. Orchitis can develop as a result of three mechanisms: ascending infection through the vas deferens and epididymis to the testis; metastatic spread of bacteria, viruses, parasites, and fungi via the blood or lymphatic vessels; and trauma. Epididymoorchitis is managed in the same manner as acute epididymitis,

described previously. Any bacterium causing septicemia can, on occasion, produce pyogenic orchitis. Traumatic orchitis may be the result of lowered resistance of injured tissue to bacteria, or a granulomatous reaction due to proteins from extravasated sperm following trauma or surgical procedures. Isolated orchitis is much less common than epididymoorchitis and most commonly is due to viral infection including mumps, echovirus, coxsackievirus, varicella, influenza, dengue, Epstein-Barr virus, and arbovirus.

Clinical Manifestations. Mumps orchitis is a highly incapacitating but self-limited disease. It occurs most often in postpubertal males; one recent study found that 30% of those older than 10 years of age with mumps developed orchitis, but this percentage is high because orchitis is more likely to be reported to physicians than is uncomplicated mumps. Onset of orchitis usually occurs 4 to 6 days after the onset of parotitis but can occur without parotid involvement. In one series, 84% had preceding parotitis, and 3% had parotitis concurrent with orchitis.

Diagnosis. Symptoms can vary from mild testicular pain and swelling to severe pain and swelling accompanied by nausea, vomiting, lower abdominal pain, fever, and chills. Both testes are involved in about one third of cases. The diagnosis can be made with reasonable certainty only when there is concurrent or recent parotitis. A radionuclide scan or color Doppler ultrasound can rule out other conditions.

Differential Diagnosis. For differential diagnosis, see Table 78–1.

Treatment. Treatment consists of bed rest, scrotal support, and analgesics. Some urologists recommend surgical drainage of a reactive hydrocele in severe cases.

Clinical Course and Prognosis. Symptoms subside in 7 to 10 days. Atrophy of the involved testis occurs in more than half of all cases. Degenerative changes have been observed in the clinically uninvolved testis. Sterility is an infrequent sequela. There may be an increased risk of testicular cancer in those who develop testicular atrophy due to mumps orchitis.

INGUINAL HERNIA

Although the majority of indirect inguinal hernias are diagnosed in the first year of life, they may occasionally present during adolescence.

Pathophysiology. An indirect inguinal hernia develops if the processus vaginalis remains patent after birth. An intraabdominal structure entering the processus vaginalis produces a hernia. Incarceration occurs when its contents cannot be easily reduced into the intraabdominal cavity; strangulation occurs when bowel within the hernia becomes ischemic or gangrenous. The spermatic cord can also be readily compressed between the margin of the external inguinal ring and herniated bowel, obstructing the venous return of the involved testicle and producing edema, ischemia, and pain.

Clinical Manifestations. An adolescent with inguinal hernia usually presents with a painless swelling at the external inguinal ring or extending for a variable distance medially and downward into the scrotum. Sometimes the mass will be evident with vigorous coughing or straining at stool. An incarcerated hernia can present with the additional symptoms of abdominal pain, vomiting, and painful scrotal swelling; these symptoms intensify as the hernia contents and involved testicle become ischemic.

Diagnosis. A normal testis is palpated below the hernia. If the hernia is not visible or readily palpable, having the patient strain as the examiner manually compresses the abdomen results in a palpable "pulse" of intraabdominal contents. The hernia is usually reduced spontaneously or with manipulation. When an incarcerated hernia produces acute scrotal pain and swelling, a radionuclide scan or color Doppler ultrasound study may be necessary to distinguish it from other conditions.

Differential Diagnosis. For differential diagnosis, see Table 78–1.

Treatment. An inguinal hernia in an adolescent will not resolve spontaneously. Herniorrhaphy is mandatory because of the risk of incarceration. Initial management of an incarcerated hernia with no signs of strangulation involves an attempt at nonoperative reduction. A hernia that cannot be reduced, or one whose contents may be strangulated, requires prompt surgery.

Clinical Course and Prognosis. Testicular atrophy may complicate a small percentage of uncomplicated hernia repairs. Infarction of the testicle occurs in about 2% of adolescents with incarcerated hernia. Intestinal resection is required in 1% to 8% of cases owing to bowel infarction.

TESTICULAR TRAUMA

Because of its mobility and position, scrotal injury is relatively infrequent.

Pathophysiology. Blunt trauma during athletic activities resulting in the crushing of scrotal contents against the pubic bone is the most common mechanism of injury. Blunt trauma due to violence, motor vehicle accidents, or falls also occurs, as do penetrating injuries.

Clinical Manifestations. There is sudden onset of marked pain, swelling, and discoloration following trauma. Scrotal injury can result in testicular rupture, hematocele, testicular hematoma, posttraumatic epididymitis and orchitis, scrotal hematoma, scrotal urinoma, and delayed infection.

Diagnosis. Examination of urine and urethral secretions, as well as diagnostic imaging studies with real-time or color Doppler ultrasonography, and radionuclide scanning are useful in evaluating an acute scrotal injury. Real-time ultrasonography is useful in diagnosing hematocele, rupture of the tunica albuginea of the testis, scrotal hematoma, intratesticular hematoma, and traumatic epididymitis and orchitis.

Differential Diagnosis. The differential diagnosis includes testicular torsion and epididymitis (see Table 78–1). Patients with these conditions often attribute their symptoms to an episode of minor trauma.

Treatment. A ruptured testis requires prompt surgical exploration. Necrotic and devitalized seminiferous tubules should be debrided and the tunica albuginea closed primarily. Large, expanding hematoceles should be explored and drained. A large scrotal hematoma is an indication for prompt exploration of the testis and spermatic cord.

Clinical Course and Prognosis. Conservative management with ice and elevation should be avoided, since it may result in ischemic necrosis and atrophy, prolonged discomfort, and secondary infection. Early surgical exploration and repair increase the chances of preserving testicular long-term viability and function and decrease the incidence of ischemic necrosis and abscess formation.

ACUTE IDIOPATHIC SCROTAL EDEMA

Although accounting for as many as one third of cases of acute scrotal swelling requiring hospitalization in childhood, acute idiopathic scrotal edema is unusual after puberty. The etiology of this disorder remains unclear; an allergic mechanism has been postulated. It presents with sudden onset of unilateral or bilateral erythema and edema of the scrotum and minimal, if any, pain. The erythema may extend to the perineum and anterior abdominal wall. A normal testis, epididymis, and cord structure can be palpated. Urinalysis results are normal. Although the diagnosis is made on clinical grounds, a radionuclide scan or color Doppler ultrasound study will show normal testicular perfusion. No treatment is necessary, and symptoms subside in a few days.

HENOCH-SCHÖNLEIN PURPURA

Adolescents may occasionally be affected by Henoch-Schönlein purpura–related vasculitis of the scrotal skin, epididymis, testis, or spermatic cord, resulting in painful scrotal swelling. In patients with other manifestations of the disease, the diagnosis can be made clinically; if necessary to rule out other conditions, a radionuclide scan or color Doppler ultrasound study can be performed, which will be normal.

VARICOCELE

A varicocele is a dilated and tortuous pampiniform venous plexus surrounding the spermatic cord. Prevalence in postpubertal males is between 10% and 15%.

Pathophysiology. Varicoceles occur primarily on the left (95%) because of the differences in venous drainage. The pampiniform plexus drains into the internal spermatic veins bilaterally, but the left internal spermatic vein is 10 cm longer than the right one and joins the left renal vein at a more acute angle, resulting in elevated pressure and dilation of the left pampiniform plexus. A right-sided varicocele may be secondary to venous crossover, situs inversus, or venous obstruction.

Reduced sperm counts, decreased sperm motility, and abnormal sperm morphology have been reported in about 50% of adult males with varicocele and may be due to elevation of intrascrotal temperature caused by venous dilatation, decreased testicular blood flow, or reflux of venous blood containing steroids and catecholamines. Testicular biopsies performed on infertile males with varicocele reveal histologic abnormalities in both testes, with the most pronounced lesions in the involved testis. Similar, though less severe, changes have been reported in adolescents undergoing varicocele ligation. Serum luteinizing hormone (LH), follicle-stimulating hormone (FSH), and testosterone levels are generally normal, although studies, including at least two in adolescent boys with varicocele, have demonstrated an exaggerated response of FSH and LH to gonadotropin-releasing factor infusion, indicative of testicular dysfunction.

Clinical Manifestations. Varicoceles usually become clinically evident during puberty. Most are asymptomatic and are found on routine examination. Adolescent patients may complain of a dull ache or fullness in the scrotum.

Diagnosis. Examination should be performed with the patient standing. A large varicocele is visible on inspection. A smaller varicocele is enhanced by a Valsalva maneuver. Palpation reveals the classic "bag of worms" sensation along the length of the spermatic cord. Testicular size should be measured using volumetric plates. Studies of pituitary-gonadal function and semen analysis may be indicated in adolescents with significant loss of testicular mass or in young adults with infertility. A left varicocele found prior to puberty or persisting in the supine position, or a right varicocele should prompt a search for venous obstruction by tumor or other abnormalities.

Treatment. Surgical repair of a primary varicocele during adolescence has been recommended if there is associated genital discomfort, significant testicular volume loss, abnormal semen analysis, or abnormal gonadotropin-releasing hormone stimulation test result. Although it is not known whether varicocelectomy during adolescence will prevent infertility, repair in infertile adults has been reported to improve semen quality and fertility. Following varicocelectomy in the adolescent with small testis, 70% show catch-up growth to equal the other testis. Percutaneous occlusion of the internal spermatic vein is an alternative to surgery being used by some experts.

Course of Illness and Prognosis. The most important complication of a varicocele is infertility. Prevalence in men with primary infertility is 19% to 41%, although many with abnormal sperm characteristics are fertile. It is reasonable to counsel adolescent patients and their parents regarding possible infertility whenever a varicocele is palpated.

HYDROCELE

A hydrocele results from fluid accumulation within the tunica vaginalis. It is most common in infancy but may occur later in childhood and adolescence.

Pathophysiology. Most pediatric hydroceles are primary (idiopathic) and communicating; a patent processus vaginalis allows fluid to enter from the peritoneal cavity. A hydrocele that appears in adolescence is usually idiopathic but sometimes may be secondary to epididymitis, orchitis, testicular torsion, trauma, or a testicular tumor.

Clinical Manifestations. Most hydroceles are asymptomatic, although some adolescent patients may complain of a scrotal mass or scrotal heaviness.

Diagnosis. A hydrocele appears as a cystic mass anterior to and separate from the testicle. It may become so large and tense that the testicle cannot be palpated adequately. In patients with a patent processus vaginalis, a hydrocele may disappear in the supine position. A hydrocele will transilluminate brightly. Ultrasonography is helpful in equivocal cases and establishes that the testicle is normal.

Differential Diagnosis. Other disorders that present as a painless scrotal mass are listed in Table 78–1.

Treatment. Treatment of idiopathic hydrocele is not required, unless it is causing discomfort or cosmetic problems. Surgical hydrocelectomy may be recommended in such cases; aspiration and sclerotherapy is another treatment option.

SPERMATOCELE

Spermatoceles are sperm-containing cystic dilatations of the efferent ductules that connect the rete testis to the head of the epididymis. They are usually located above and posterior to the testis at the head of the epididymis and may be bilateral and multiple. They are usually less than 1 cm in diameter but can attain a diameter of 8 to 10 cm. They are distinct from the testes and usually transilluminate. Ultrasonography can be used to confirm their extratesticular location and cystic structure. Surgical excision usually is not required but may relieve discomfort or embarrassment.

EPIDIDYMAL CYST

Clear fluid-containing cysts may develop in the epididymis. They have been reported to occur with greater frequency in those exposed to diethylstilbestrol *in utero*. Their evaluation and management are similar to those for spermatoceles.

TESTICULAR TUMORS (see Chapter 53)

Although testicular cancer in adolescents is relatively rare, its incidence increases during and after puberty and peaks between the ages of 20 and 34 years, when it is the most common carcinoma. Its annual incidence ranges from 2 to 3 per 100,000. The incidence in blacks is significantly lower. In 1989 there were 5500 new cases and 500 deaths due to this disease, which underscores the curability of these tumors.

Pathophysiology. Classification of neoplasms of the testes is based on that devised by Dixon and Moore (Table 78–3). Ninety-six percent of all primary testicular tumors in adolescents arise from germinal cells and are malignant; they are further classified as either pure seminoma (40%) or nonseminomatous tumors. The latter include pure embryonal carcinomas (15% to 20%), teratomas (5% to 10%), pure choriocarcinomas (1% to 2%), yolk sac tumors (1%), and germinal cell tumors of more than one histologic type (30% to 40%), consisting of various combinations of the first four cell types. The presence of *any* histopathologic nonseminomatous element renders a tumor as a nonseminoma. The distinction between seminoma and nonseminoma is important in staging and management. Seminomas me-

**TABLE 78–3. Pathologic Classification
of Primary Testicular Neoplasms**

I. Germinal Cell Tumors
  A. Tumors of one histologic type
    1. Seminoma
    2. Embryonal carcinoma
    3. Teratoma
    4. Choriocarcinoma
    5. Yolk sac tumor
  B. Tumors of more than one histologic type (may demonstrate
    two or more of the histologic types listed above)
II. Non–Germinal Cell Tumors
  A. Specialized gonadal stromal neoplasms (Leydig cell tumors,
    Sertoli cell tumors, granulosa cell tumors)
  B. Gonadoblastoma
  C. Miscellaneous neoplasms
    1. Adenocarcinoma of the rete testis
    2. Neoplasm of mesenchymal origin
    3. Adrenal rest tumors
    4. Adenomatoid tumors

Adapted from Einhorn LH, Crawford ED, Shipley WU, et al: Cancer of the testes. In DeVita VT, Hellman S, Rosenberg SA (eds): Cancer: Principles and Practice of Oncology. Philadelphia, JB Lippincott, 1989, pp 1071–1098.

tastasize through regional lymphatics to retroperitoneal, mediastinal, and supraclavicular lymph nodes and are very sensitive to radiation. Nonseminomas metastasize via lymphatic and hematogenous routes (especially to lungs and liver) and are resistant to radiation therapy.

Nongerminal cell tumors arise from major elements of testicular stroma, the Leydig and the Sertoli cells, and account for 3% to 4% of all primary testicular tumors. About 10% are malignant and metastasize via regional lymphatics.

The etiology of germinal cell tumors is unknown. Several factors are known to predispose to their development. Approximately 10% of all testicular tumors develop in previously undescended testes. Both a unilateral cryptorchid testis and the contralateral normally descended testis are at risk, suggesting that an underlying defect may predispose to both maldescent and tumor development. The effectiveness of orchipexy in reducing the risk of malignancy has not been established. Other predisposing factors include mumps orchitis and childhood inguinal hernia.

Clinical Manifestations. The most common presentation of a testicular neoplasm is a painless, hard, smooth, nontransilluminating, unilateral testicular mass. Approximately 40% of adolescent patients complain of a dull ache or a sensation of heaviness in the scrotum, inguinal area, or lower abdomen. A secondary hydrocele may be present. Occasionally adolescent patients present with acute scrotal pain and swelling due to sudden hemorrhage within the tumor. Back pain due to retroperitoneal lymph node metastases, and bone pain due to osseous metastases, are occasional presenting symptoms. A prominent abdominal mass or inguinal or supraclavicular adenopathy may also be present in metastatic disease. Nongerminal cell tumors may secrete androgens or estrogens that may result in precocious puberty, gynecomastia, or feminization.

Diagnosis. If physical examination is equivocal, ultrasonography can reliably determine whether the mass is intratesticular or extratesticular. Once the mass has been determined to be intratesticular, additional studies are required. Germ cell tumors often secrete biologic markers that can be detected in blood. Alpha-fetoprotein is commonly excreted by embryonal carcinomas and yolk sac tumors. Pure seminomas never elaborate alpha-fetoprotein, and its presence implies presence of non-seminomatous elements in the tumor. The beta subunit of human chorionic gonadotropin is most often secreted by choriocarcinomas and embryonal carcinomas and rarely by pure seminomas. Both markers are used to detect metastases following orchiectomy and to monitor response to therapy. Serum lactic dehydrogenase may be a useful measure of tumor bulk.

Surgical exploration completes the diagnostic evaluation. Inguinal orchiectomy establishes a pathologic diagnosis, determines the extent of and provides treatment for local disease, and is curative if disease is confined to the testis.

For seminomatous disease, stage I refers to tumor confined to the testis, stage IIA to minimal retroperitoneal infradiaphragmatic involvement, stage IIB to bulky lymphatic metastases below the diaphragm, stage III to tumor involving lymphatics above the diaphragm, and stage IV to extralymphatic metastases. For nonseminomatous disease, stage I refers to tumor confined to the testis, stage IIA to microscopic retroperitoneal adenopathy with five or less involved nodes, stage IIB to retroperitoneal adenopathy that is grossly evident or with more than five involved nodes, and stage III to metastases to lymph nodes above the diaphragm or to other viscera (lung, liver, bowel) (see Chapter 53).

Differential Diagnosis. For differential diagnosis, see Table 78–1.

Treatment. Seminoma is exquisitely sensitive to radiation and usually presents at an early stage. Adolescents with stage I and early stage II disease are treated with orchiectomy followed by radiation to the subdiaphragmatic lymphatics and ipsilateral groin. Patients with advanced stage II, stage III, and stage IV disease are treated with orchiectomy and combination chemotherapy that includes cisplatin; some are treated with post-chemotherapy radiation to areas of bulk disease and, occasionally, surgical excision of bulk disease.

Adolescents with stage I nonseminoma are treated with either orchiectomy and retroperitoneal lymph node dissection or orchiectomy alone coupled with close observation; treatment with combination chemotherapy or radiation therapy is instituted if relapse occurs. Early stage II disease is treated with orchiectomy and retroperitoneal lymph node dissection followed by combination chemotherapy at first relapse, or chemotherapy may be given initially. Late stage II and stage III disease are treated with chemotherapy followed by surgical excision of significant tumor masses. Additional chemotherapy is given if surgical specimens reveal viable cancer.

Course of Illness and Prognosis. Untreated testicular cancer is highly malignant and often rapidly fatal. Seminoma currently has an excellent prognosis, with an overall cure rate for all stages of over 90% at 5 years. Patients with stage I disease have a 95% to 97% cure rate, and those with early stage II disease have an 85% to 90% survival rate. Cure rates close to 85% have been reported for stages IIB, III, and IV disease.

Cure rates of 60% to 70% can be expected from

orchiectomy alone in stage I nonseminomatous disease. Addition of retroperitoneal lymph node dissection increases cure rates to 85% to 90%. Chemotherapy with or without tumor-reductive surgery can cure 80% to 85% of those with advanced (stages IIB and III) disease.

With the success of newer treatment, long-term complications have emerged, including the possibility of gonadal dysfunction. Retroperitoneal lymph node dissection often results in ejaculatory dysfunction, loss of orgasm, or impotence. Azoospermia often follows treatment with vinblastine, bleomycin, and cisplatin, agents commonly used in the therapy for testicular cancer, although studies suggest that sperm count and quality recover within 2 to 3 years of treatment in approximately half of patients. Finally, radiation therapy may result in germ cell depletion and hypogonadism due to damage of the uninvolved testicle if proper shielding techniques are not utilized.

Pretreatment sperm-banking preserves reproductive potential. Unfortunately, pretreatment analysis of semen reveals suboptimal quality in 50%, including reduced sperm count and poor motility, which may preclude sperm-banking. Collection of multiple ejaculates can increase the total number of sperm available for banking.

EXTRATESTICULAR TUMORS

Although most extratesticular masses are cystic, some are solid. Approximately 60% of solid masses originate in the spermatic cord; the remainder are from the epididymis and the scrotal tunic. Tumors originating in these structures account for 7% of all intrascrotal neoplasms. Malignancy is common (occurring in 24% of epididymal neoplasms, 31% of spermatic cord tumors, and 59% of scrotal tunic neoplasms); most are sarcomatous. Lipomas of the spermatic cord and adenomatoid tumors of the epididymis are the most common benign neoplasms.

Solid paratesticular tumors do not transilluminate. Ultrasonography can confirm their extratesticular location and solid structure. All should be surgically explored, with the exception of a painful epididymal mass, which may be treated expectantly as epididymitis with antibiotics and followed.

Cryptorchidism

Cryptorchidism refers to a testis that has failed to descend to its usual location in the scrotum. Cryptorchid testes may be abdominal; canalicular, located between internal and external inguinal rings; or ectopic, located away from the normal pathway of descent. They are found in 3% to 4% of term newborn male infants. Most testes descend over the first 4 to 6 months of life but seldom afterward. Cryptorchidism is present in 0.8% of adolescents.

Pathophysiology. Histologic abnormalities in undescended testes appear by 2 years of age and affect primarily the seminiferous tubules. There is conflicting evidence as to whether the Leydig cells are affected. It is uncertain whether these histologic changes reflect a primary defect or are secondary to the cryptorchid state. Similar changes are found in the normally descended testis in unilaterally cryptorchid individuals. The prevalence of infertility in unilateral cryptorchidism is 30%.

Clinical Manifestations. Most affected individuals are asymptomatic, and the undescended testicle is incidentally noted during physical examination. Bilateral cryptorchidism is associated with several hypogonadal disorders that present with delayed puberty during adolescence.

Diagnosis. Careful physical examination should be performed to distinguish cryptorchid from retractile testes. Examination is performed while the patient is relaxed in a warm room; the patient is examined in the standing, squatting, and recumbent positions. Valsalva maneuver and pressure applied to the lower abdomen facilitate palpation of a retractile testis. When the testes are not palpable despite these maneuvers, magnetic resonance imaging (MRI), computed tomography (CT) scan, or laparoscopy may be used to determine their location. The most accurate test is the MRI, and the CT scan has a fair accuracy.

Differential Diagnosis. Cryptorchid testes must be distinguished from retractile and absent testes. Retractile testes are located in the scrotum but withdraw into the inguinal canal or abdomen with minimal stimulation; this is the result of an exaggerated cremasteric reflex that is weak or absent at birth but develops during childhood. They should be suspected in cases in which testes were palpable at birth but became nonpalpable later. They adopt a permanent scrotal position during early adolescence, require no surgical intervention, and are not associated with any of the complications associated with true undescended testes. About 5% of nonpalpable testes are entirely absent, most commonly because of an earlier vascular accident.

Treatment. Surgery, the treatment of choice, preserves testicular function and allows easier examination of the testis for malignancy. Orchiopexy should be undertaken as early as possible, preferably at 9 to 15 months of age. Testicular prostheses may be placed in the affected hemiscrotum after puberty to produce a cosmetically acceptable result when a testis is atrophic or absent.

Course of Illness and Prognosis. Complications of cryptorchidism include infertility, malignancy, testicular torsion, and the possible psychological effects of an empty scrotum. Infertility is the rule in adults with untreated bilateral cryptorchidism. Early surgery increases the potential for fertility, although studies show that of those with bilateral cryptorchidism treated in childhood, 42% were azoospermic and 31% oligospermic. Of those with unilateral cryptorchidism treated in childhood, 15% were azoospermic and 30% oligospermic. Surgery in infancy may improve these figures.

The risk of malignancy in undescended testes is 10 to 40 times that in descended testes. There is no evidence that orchiopexy protects from later malignant change, although testes undergoing malignant change may be recognized earlier if they are placed in the scrotum. Adolescents with a history of undescended testes should be made aware of their increased risk for testicular cancer and should be taught testicular self-examination.

PROSTATITIS

Prostatitis is the term used to describe a poorly defined syndrome of inflammation of the prostate. It is relatively common in adults but occurs infrequently in adolescents. It can be divided into four subcategories: acute bacterial prostatitis, chronic bacterial prostatitis, nonbacterial prostatitis, and prostatodynia. Nonbacterial prostatitis is the most frequently encountered prostatitis syndrome in young men; acute bacterial prostatitis is also sometimes seen. Chronic bacterial prostatitis, the most common cause of recurrent urinary tract infection in men, is rarely seen in adolescents. Prostatodynia occurs primarily in men ages 20 to 45 years.

Pathophysiology. Causative organisms in bacterial prostatitis are *E. coli* and other urinary tract pathogens, and occasionally *N. gonorrhoeae*. In the preantibiotic era, approximately 15% of patients with gonococcal urethritis developed prostatitis, but this rarely occurs today (see Chapter 75). The etiology of nonbacterial prostatitis is unknown, but *Chlamydia trachomatis, Ureaplasma urealyticum,* and *Trichomonas vaginalis* have been implicated.

Pathogens may reach the prostate by several routes, including ascending urethral infection, reflux of infected urine into the prostatic ducts that empty into the posterior urethra, invasion by rectal bacteria by either direct extension or lymphatic spread, and hematogenous infection. Ascending spread of microorganisms introduced by sexual activity, and reflux of infected urine associated with an indwelling catheter, are probably the primary routes of infection in younger men.

Clinical Manifestations and Diagnosis. Adequate laboratory examination is important in accurately differentiating the causes of prostatitis; it includes Gram stain and culture of urethral discharge for *N. gonorrhoeae* and *C. trachomatis,* and microscopic examination and culture of urine samples obtained using the four-glass urine technique. Four specimens are obtained: the first-voided 10 ml of urine (urethral specimen), midstream urine (bladder specimen), expressed prostatic secretions (EPS) following prostatic massage, and the first-voided 10 ml of urine after prostatic massage (prostatic specimen). The microscopic appearance of the EPS should be compared with the spun sediment of the three urine samples in order to localize the site of the inflammatory response. All four specimens should be cultured for urinary pathogens. The diagnosis of prostatitis is confirmed if the number of white blood cells found on smear of the EPS or in the sediment of the prostatic urine specimen significantly exceed those of bladder and urethral urine specimens.

Acute bacterial prostatitis is associated with fever, chills, and pain in the lower back and perineum. Prostatic inflammation may produce dysuria, frequency, urgency, and urinary retention. The prostate is markedly tender, swollen, firm, and warm on rectal examination. Because of the risk of bacteremia, only one rectal examination should be performed if the diagnosis is suspected. White blood cells and bacteria are present in greatest numbers in EPS secretions and the prostatic urine specimen; culture of these fluids is positive for the causative organism.

Chronic bacterial prostatitis is an indolent, relapsing disease with occasional acute exacerbations. Clinical manifestations are variable. Sometimes asymptomatic bacteriuria is found incidentally; other patients complain of varying degrees of irritative voiding symptoms and pelvic discomfort. The prostate is frequently normal on examination but may be tender, firm, and boggy. Inflammatory cells are present in greatest numbers in EPS secretions and the prostatic urine specimen. Causative organisms are similar to those for acute bacterial prostatitis.

The adolescent patient with nonbacterial prostatitis has no history of urinary tract infection. Except for sterile cultures, the clinical and laboratory findings are similar to those in chronic bacterial prostatitis.

Adolescent patients with prostatodynia complain of pelvic pain, prostatic tenderness, and occasionally of irritative voiding symptoms but have no history of urinary tract infection; no inflammatory cells are seen in the EPS, and culture results are negative. The etiology of this disorder is unknown.

Differential Diagnosis. In those with persistent symptoms without evidence of inflammation in the EPS, interstitial cystitis, bladder tumor, prostatic obstruction, bladder calculus, detrusor-sphincter dyssynergia, and herniated vertebral disk should be considered.

Treatment. Hospitalization and intravenous ampicillin and an aminoglycoside are indicated for the adolescent with acute prostatitis who is toxic or has concurrent underlying disease. For the less toxic patient, trimethoprim-sulfamethoxazole, ampicillin, or doxycycline may be administered orally for 4 weeks. The highest cure rates for chronic bacterial prostatitis have been achieved using trimethoprim-sulfamethoxazole for 4 to 6 weeks; doxycycline, minocycline, erythromycin, carbenicillin, and cephalexin have also been used. Discontinuation of therapy will often lead to reinfection; continuous suppressive therapy with low doses of trimethoprim-sulfamethoxazole has proved useful in such circumstances. Nonbacterial prostatitis may be treated with a tetracycline or erythromycin; anti-inflammatory agents such as ibuprofen provide good relief of pelvic pain and urinary discomfort for many patients.

Course of Illness and Prognosis. Acute prostatitis responds well to adequate antibiotic therapy. Once a common complication, prostatic abscess is rare today; chronic bacterial prostatitis is an infrequent complication. Treatment of chronic bacterial prostatitis improves symptoms and sterilizes the urine; however, recurrences are common following discontinuation of therapy, so the adolescent should be prepared by the practitioner for prolonged therapy. Treatment of nonbacterial prostatitis is also difficult; a chronic course with intermittent symptoms is often seen. The relationship of prostatitis to infertility is controversial.

PENILE DISORDERS

Hypospadias (see Chapter 66)

Hypospadias occurs in 1 in 150 male births. There is familial clustering: the risk of occurrence is 8% if an individual's father is affected, 14% if a sibling has the condition, and 21% if two family members have hypospadias.

Pathophysiology. The cause of hypospadias is unknown but appears to be multifactorial. It results from failure of, or delay in, ventral fusion of the urogenital folds in utero.

Clinical Manifestations. Hypospadias may present as a ventrally displaced urethral meatus on the distal penile shaft or, in more severe forms, with the meatus opening on the shaft or perineum. The ventral prepuce is deficient, and the dorsal prepuce appears hooded and flaplike. Hypospadias is often associated with some degree of ventral curvature of the penis (chordee) that is most apparent during erection. In severe cases, chordee makes sexual intercourse difficult or impossible. Chordee may occur without coexisting hypospadias.

Diagnosis. The displacement of the urethral meatus and the presence of a hooded prepuce is usually obvious. Chordee is often overlooked or its severity underestimated, particularly when the penis is observed in the flaccid state. An adolescent with mild, uncorrected hypospadias should be queried regarding the presence of curvature with erections. The severity of the defect is best described by the position of the urethral meatus and the location and severity of the chordee. Upper urinary tract anomalies are infrequent, and radiologic studies are unnecessary. A utricle (diverticulum of persistent urogenital sinus origin) is found in 11% to 14% of cases and may be associated with recurrent infection; urinalysis and urine culture may be indicated periodically. Undescended testes and inguinal hernia are commonly associated with hypospadias.

Treatment. The objective of surgical correction is to straighten the penis and form a urethral extension with the new meatus as close as possible to its normal site, thus permitting a forward-directed urinary stream and normal sexual intercourse. The optimal time for surgical repair is from 6 to 18 months of age; a complete repair is usually accomplished as a single procedure. Cosmetic surgical repair of previously uncorrected mild hypospadias may be performed in an adolescent. Surgical correction is also indicated for the adolescent with an associated chordee. Routine circumcision should be avoided prior to corrective surgery in boys with hypospadias.

Clinical Course and Prognosis. Problems in healing following surgery may result, requiring reoperation. When repair is performed by experienced surgeons, excellent cosmetic and functional results can be obtained.

Balanitis, Posthitis, and Balanoposthitis

Balanitis refers to inflammation of the penile glans, posthitis to inflammation of the penile prepuce, and balanoposthitis to inflammation of both.

Pathophysiology. These disorders may be caused by trauma, exposure to irritants, or bacterial or fungal infection or may be a manifestation of a systemic illness, such as psoriasis and diabetes mellitus. They are much more common in uncircumcised males, particularly in those with phimosis. The prepuce normally harbors beneath it smegma (desquamating epithelial cells, glandular secretions, and *Mycobacterium smegmatis*) and provides a warm, moist culture medium predisposing to infection.

Clinical Manifestations and Diagnosis. Candidal balanitis is often seen among adolescent males. It is usually sexually acquired from an infected female partner (see Chapter 75). It is generally self-limited in circumcised men, but in those who are uncircumcised, diabetic, or immunocompromised, severe infection can develop. Typical symptoms include itching, edema, and burning of the glans. Small pustules or papules that rupture and leave superficial, erythematous erosions are seen on the glans or coronal sulcus. Satellite lesions may be present. The organisms may be demonstrated by potassium hydroxide preparation and cultured readily. Occasionally, an adolescent may develop a hypersensitivity reaction to a partner's monilial infection, with transient penile burning and redness shortly after intercourse but without actual infection.

Bacterial balanitis almost always occurs in uncircumcised males. Poor hygiene with smegma buildup and excess urinary moisture are contributory. It is caused by an overgrowth of various organisms that are normally present. Signs and symptoms include small, red erosions on the glans or undersurface of the prepuce; exudate, edema, and erythema of the glans and prepuce; and pain. If untreated, a gangrenous phase may occur.

Treatment. Candidal balanitis usually responds to cool bathing with Burow solution and application of a topical antifungal agent. Sex partners should be treated. Those with persistent or recurrent infections should be evaluated for underlying disease. Bacterial balanitis is treated with local cleansing, exposure to air, bathing with Burow solution, and topical antibiotics. Systemic antibiotics are useful for more advanced infections.

Clinical Course and Prognosis. Most episodes respond promptly to the measures previously described; good hygiene usually prevents recurrences. Secondary phimosis often complicates bacterial balanitis. Circumcision is indicated as treatment for recurrent balanitis and secondary phimosis.

Phimosis and Paraphimosis

(see Chapter 66)

Phimosis refers to a tight or adhered prepuce that cannot be retracted over the glans. It may be congenital or secondary to infection or trauma. Phimosis is physiologic at birth, but by school age the foreskin is retractable in 90% of uncircumcised males. Symptomatic phimosis presents with a thickened distal ring of foreskin that cannot be retracted. It can cause discomfort with voiding or sexual activity. The treatment of choice is circumcision.

Paraphimosis occurs when a phimotic prepuce has been retracted behind the coronal sulcus and cannot be reduced back over the glans. Edema, pain, and vascular compromise can occur. The edema is decreased by treatment with cold compresses. It may then be reduced by lubricating and then applying firm pressure to the glans, with countertraction on the foreskin. In the extremely rare case of irreducible phimosis, a dorsal slit or emergency circumcision is necessary. Elective circumcision is indicated after the edema has subsided.

Pearly Penile Papules

Pearly penile papules are small, raised, pearly or gray-white papules 1 to 3 mm in diameter found on the corona of the penis. They are very common, with a prevalence of 15% to 20% in adolescents and young adults. Histologically, they are formed of dense connective tissue. They may be mistaken for condylomata acuminata. Adolescents should be reassured that these papules are normal and require no treatment.

Sebaceous Cysts

Sebaceous cysts are frequently found on the scrotal skin. They rarely cause symptoms, although they may be of concern to some adolescents. They are filled with a white, keratinous cheesy material. Incision and expression of the contents are curative, although treatment is indicated only for larger, more cosmetically noticeable lesions.

Penile Allergic Contact Dermatitis

Allergic contact dermatitis of the penis and scrotum is often very dramatic because the skin is thin and highly vascular. Secondary exposure to a sensitizing agent evokes pruritus, erythema, vesiculation, and edema. Sensitizers include *Rhus* catechols, which produce poison ivy dermatitis; vulcanizing accelerators (used in rubber manufacture), antioxidants, and lubricant jellies from condoms; and agents acquired during sexual contact, including douches, spermicides, and feminine sprays.

Treatment includes avoidance of the sensitizing agent. Symptoms may be treated with oral antipruritic agents and topical steroids. Severe symptoms may require oral steroid therapy. Those with condom dermatitis can use condoms manufactured from animal intestines, although such condoms do not protect from human immunodeficiency virus (HIV) (see Chapter 76).

Priapism (see Chapter 66)

Priapism is a prolonged, painful, involuntary erection unassociated with sexual stimulation. It is most common in young adults but does occur in adolescents.

Pathophysiology. Primary, or idiopathic, priapism involves pathologic tumescence in the absence of any contributing medical illness and is the most common form of priapism. Secondary priapism occurs as a result of preexisting pathology. Hematologic disorders (see Chapter 52), primarily sickle cell disease, are the most common cause in adolescents. Sickle cell trait, thalassemia, leukemia, polycythemia, and macroglobulinemia have also been implicated. Drug-induced priapism is common in adult populations and may also occur in adolescents. Alcohol, marijuana (see Chapter 111), and antihypertensive and antipsychotic medications are most commonly involved. Central nervous system lesions, spinal cord trauma, certain local and systemic infections, neoplastic disease, and renal dialysis have also been implicated. Regardless of cause, priapism is caused by inflow of blood to the penis in excess of outflow capabilities. This can be due to an imbalance between neural stimuli, a mechanical obstruction to venous outflow, or both.

Clinical Manifestations and Diagnosis. Adolescents generally present with a painful, persistent erection. Significant delay in seeking care often occurs as a result of embarrassment. Time elapsed since onset of symptoms, presence of predisposing illness, recent use of medications, and previous occurrence of symptoms should be determined. On examination, the corpora cavernosa are firm and may display discoloration due to tissue ischemia. The corpus spongiosum is unaffected, so the glans is nonturgid. Signs of urinary retention should be sought. A careful general physical examination and laboratory evaluation are directed toward uncovering any condition that may precipitate priapism.

Treatment. Initial therapy includes maintenance of adequate oxygenation and hydration. Sedative and analgesic agents may be of comfort to the patient and produce detumescence. Other measures include bed rest and application of ice to the groin. Treatment of specific medical causes of priapism should be promptly undertaken.

A urologic consultation should be obtained promptly (see Chapter 66). Some success with intravenous ketamine, infiltration of the base of the penis with lidocaine or bupivacaine, and spinal anesthesia has been reported. If such measures fail, aspiration and irrigation of the corpora cavernosa with normal saline are performed. If detumescence cannot be maintained, surgical shunting, usually between the distal corpus cavernosum and glans, is indicated.

Course of Illness and Prognosis. Impotence is the most common complication but is rare in adolescents; adolescents are less likely to experience impotence than are adults. The longer the interval from onset of erection to detumescence, the greater the risks of tissue damage and residual impotence. Fibrosis and gangrene of the penis are other complications sometimes seen in priapism.

Impotence

Impotence is the inability to achieve or sustain penile erection of sufficient rigidity for sexual intercourse. It is common in adult men with medical problems and increases in prevalence with advancing age. It is occasionally encountered in the older adolescent and young adult. It is generally underdiagnosed because of the reluctance of patients and physicians to discuss sexual dysfunction.

Pathophysiology. Neurogenic causes include spinal cord trauma, multiple sclerosis, and peripheral neuropathy due to alcoholism or diabetes mellitus. Endocrine causes include hyperprolactinemia, hyper- and hypothyroidism, and decreased androgen levels owing to hypogonadism. Psychogenic impotence may be caused by sexual performance anxiety, relationship conflict, sexual inhibition, past history of sexual abuse, conflict over sexual preference, and fear of pregnancy or sexually transmitted disease. Vasculogenic causes of impotence include atherosclerotic or traumatic pelvic arterial occlusive disease and incompetency of the corporal venoocclusive mechanism of the penis. Impotence may also be a side effect of histamine (H_2 type) receptor antagonists, antipsychotics, antidepressants, and some antihypertensive medications.

Clinical Manifestations and Diagnosis. The initial evaluation of the impotent patient includes a careful medical (including use of prescription and nonprescription drugs), psychosocial, and sexual history, physical examination, and laboratory testing to differentiate psychogenic from organic impotence. Features suggesting primary psychogenic impotence include an acute onset related to a specific event and a history of normal erections on awakening and with masturbation. In contrast, progressive loss of erectile ability, with consistent changes in rigidity or ability to sustain erections, is suggestive of an organic cause. A psychological history should include inquiries regarding the adolescent patient's relationship with his partner, economic or social stresses, symptoms of affective disorders, and history of psychopathology. Underlying risk factors for vascular disease, previous pelvic trauma, surgery, irradiation, known neurologic disease, concomitant changes in bladder and bowel function, and use of alcohol and other medication should be identified. The physical examination includes a careful evaluation of endocrine, neurologic, and vascular systems as well as examination of the penis. Laboratory tests should screen for diabetes mellitus, hyperlipidemia, thyroid dysfunction, hyperprolactinemia, and hypogonadism. More detailed evaluation can be undertaken at a multispecialty sexual dysfunction clinic and may include psychometric testing, nocturnal penile tumescence testing, various types of vascular testing, and specialized neurologic examinations.

Treatment, Course of Illness, and Prognosis. Treatment and prognosis depend on the cause of the impotence. Appropriate medical therapy is indicated for underlying endocrine disorders. Behaviorally oriented sex therapy has been successful in 35% to 80% of those with psychogenic impotence, although long-term studies suggest a substantial rate of recurrence. Intercavernosal self-injection of vasoactive drugs is particularly helpful in those with neurogenic impairment and vascular insufficiency. Patients with psychogenic impotence may also be candidates for this form of therapy. Vascular surgery may be successful in selected individuals. Penile prostheses have proved helpful for individuals with organic or psychogenic impotence refractory to other treatments. Vacuum constriction devices, which suction blood into the penis and produce an erection, have recently been introduced for the treatment of organic impotence.

MISCELLANEOUS DISORDERS

Hematospermia

Blood in the ejaculate is known as hematospermia or hemospermia. It is uncommon in adolescence, and its etiology is unknown. Tuberculosis was once the most common cause, but most recent studies suggest that isolated hematospermia is rarely associated with systemic disease. Hematospermia in adolescents is most likely secondary to inflammatory conditions such as prostatitis and epididymoorchitis, particularly those caused by a sexually transmitted organism.

The adolescent who seeks medical attention for this complaint may experience considerable anxiety but should be evaluated with the knowledge that significant disease is unusual. If he is otherwise asymptomatic and results of genital examination, urinalysis, and diagnostic studies for sexually transmitted diseases are negative, no further evaluation is necessary. Urologic consultation may be indicated for severe or persisting bleeding. Differential diagnosis includes external penile trauma and bleeding from the female genital tract. The natural history of the condition may include recurrences over a period of weeks to months and ends in spontaneous resolution.

Diethylstilbestrol Exposure

Between 1940 and 1972, a synthetic nonsteroidal estrogen, diethylstilbestrol (DES), was prescribed to pregnant women in the United States to treat or prevent pregnancy-related problems; over this period, an estimated three to six million women and their offspring were exposed to DES. Less research has been conducted on the male offspring of DES-exposed mothers, and the results have been more contradictory. Although studies of DES-exposed males have disclosed an increased incidence of epididymal cysts, testicular atrophy, cryptorchidism, and abnormal semen analyses, one recent study found no relationship between DES exposure and cryptorchidism in male offspring. Unlike the situation in exposed female offspring, there has been no evidence to date for an increased potential of genital tract malignancy in male offspring.

BIBLIOGRAPHY

Coldiron BM, Jacobson C: Common penile lesions. Urol Clin North Am 15:671, 1988.

Edelsberg JS, Surh YS: The acute scrotum. Emerg Med Clin North Am 6:521, 1988.

Einhorn LH, Crawford ED, Shipley WU, et al: Cancer of the testes. In Devita VT, Hellman S, Rosenberg SA (eds): Cancer: Principles and Practice of Oncology. Philadelphia, JB Lippincott, 1989, pp 1071–1098.

Goldenring JM: Teaching testicular self-examination to young men. Contemp Pediatr 2(July):73, 1985.

Kass EJ: Adolescent varicocele: Current concepts. Semin Urol 6:140, 1988.

Krane RJ, Goldstein I, Saenz de Tejada I: Impotence. N Engl J Med 321:1648, 1989.

Paola AS, Kahn SA: Clinical evaluation of scrotal masses: An overview. Hosp Pract 24:255, 1989.

Schick RM: Scrotal imaging. Hosp Pract 20:142, 1985.

Stewart C: Prostatitis. Emerg Med Clin North Am 6:391, 1988.

Walsh PC, Gittes RF, Perlmutter AD, Stamey TA: Campbell's Urology, 5th ed. Philadelphia, WB Saunders, 1986.

Yealy DM, Hogya PT: Priapism. Emerg Med Clin North Am 6:509, 1988.

Musculoskeletal Conditions

CHAPTER 79

Orthopedic Conditions

G. PAUL DeROSA

This chapter focuses on non–sports-related orthopedic conditions in adolescents. Conditions that will be discussed are those that occur frequently, those that incite considerable anxiety in adolescents or their parents, and those that can lead to significant disability if overlooked. The chapter is divided into anatomic areas for ease in identification and reading. With rare exception, fractures and dislocations resulting from trauma are not covered in this chapter (see Chapter 80).

UPPER EXTREMITY

Most conditions involving the upper extremity are present early in the adolescent's life, for example, congenital pseudarthrosis of the clavicle, brachial plexus (obstetric) palsies, and the like. The one problem that increases in severity and frequency during adolescence is dislocation of the glenohumeral joint. Most commonly, the humeral head dislocates anteriorly and inferiorly beneath the coracoid process of the scapula. Less common are true posterior dislocations caused by direct force applied to the anterior surface of the shoulder or by a fall onto the outstretched upper extremity. Even less common are inferior dislocations, in which the arm is in the position of full abduction, or luxatio erecta position. Any dislocation may produce stretching of the neurologic components of the brachial plexus, although this is very rare. More commonly, the only neurologic complication is an area of hypesthesia over the deltoid muscle caused by a neurapraxia of the axillary nerve.

Voluntary dislocation of the shoulder is a significant adolescent problem. Frequently, there is no history of antecedent trauma, and the intentional dislocation or subluxation is usually painless. The best approach to adolescents with voluntary dislocation of the shoulder is a careful examination, both clinically and radiographically. Neurologic causes predisposing to dislocation, such as muscle wasting atrophy secondary to a syringomyelia, must be ruled out. Once neurologic causes for the dislocation are ruled out, the best treatment is counseling the adolescent and the parents about the risk of pain and arthritis if such behavior continues. Emotional and behavior problems frequently accompany voluntary dislocation of the shoulder; psychological counseling is the treatment of choice for these individuals. Surgical results in voluntary dislocation of the shoulder are uniformly dismal.

SPINE

With school screening for spinal deformity, much attention has been generated about scoliosis and kyphosis in the adolescent. The argument over school screening and its cost effectiveness continues.

Scoliosis

Scoliosis is defined as a lateral curvature of the spine, usually associated with rotation of the vertebrae around their vertically oriented axes. This rotation almost always involves the movement of the posterior elements of the vertebrae toward the concavity of the curve. The term *idiopathic* scoliosis most likely should be replaced by *familial*, because in as many as 80% of new cases one or both of the parents demonstrate a positive forward bending test. In adolescent idiopathic (familial) scoliosis, there is no primary structural abnormality in the vertebrae. The cause most likely is multifactorial and probably includes subtle central nervous system dysfunction, genetic predisposition, and other factors as yet unidentified.

The prevalence of scoliosis in the population is approximately 4% to 5%. Scoliosis is divided into infantile, juvenile, and adolescent types. The infantile type presents before the age of 3 years. Juvenile onset scoliosis (presenting between the ages of 3 and 9 years) and adolescent type (onset at 10 years or older) progress less rapidly than the infantile type of scoliosis.

DIAGNOSIS

The diagnosis of idiopathic scoliosis is simple and rests on five specific physical signs. These are easily detected by examining the adolescent who is undressed from the waist up (girls may retain their brassiere) and standing with back to the examiner, feet together, and head up and looking straight ahead (Fig. 79–1). The arms are relaxed and hanging at the sides. The examiner looks for (1) asymmetric shoulder levels; (2) prominence of a scapula; (3) unequal distance from the arms to the trunk, or an unequal waist line; and (4) a palpable lateral curving of the spine. Next, the adolescent is asked to bend forward from the waist with the arms dangling

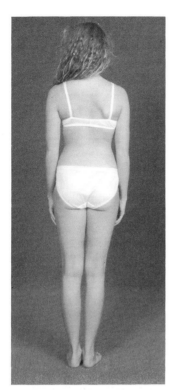

Figure 79–1. Adolescent female with obvious deformity of the spine. Notice the prominent right scapula.

loosely, the so-called forward bending test of Adams. In this position, the most reliable sign is an asymmetric prominence of one side of the chest wall or lumbar region (Fig. 79–2).

All adolescents with an abnormal screening examination require follow-up. Measurement with a scoliometer of the displacement of the scapula from horizontal or forward bending will detect those with curves significant enough to require a standing anteroposterior (AP) radiograph of the entire spine from the occiput to the sacrum to detect possible spinal anomalies. A standing lateral radiograph of the spine will reveal the normal cervical lordosis, thoracic kyphosis, and lumbar lordosis and the relationship of the lowest lumbar vertebra to the first sacral segment, as well as the defect of spondylolisthesis, if present. A thorough physical and neurologic examination as well as a radiographic confirmation is essential for all adolescents who have scoliosis in order to identify any lesions that may accompany this physical sign. For example, adolescents with painful scoliosis should be suspected of having an intraspinal neoplasm until proven otherwise, since familial scoliosis is painless.

The medical significance of scoliosis depends on the location and magnitude of the curve. Thoracic curves that exceed 60 degrees have been shown to produce restrictive obstructive pulmonary disease with subsequent cor pulmonale. If these curves approach 90 degrees, it has been shown that these adolescent patients, when followed into adult life, have a significant increase in mortality rates. Curves in the thoracolumbar and lumbar regions do not affect pulmonary function as much as do thoracic curves, but they do have the

propensity for causing increasing low back pain in adult life. It is best to attempt to restrict a curve to less than 30 to 40 degrees if at all possible. Additionally, the larger the curve, irrespective of its location, the greater is the cosmetic deformity.

TREATMENT

Once the diagnosis of familial or idiopathic scoliosis is confirmed, follow-up is necessary. It is most appropriate for pediatricians and family physicians to continue to follow those adolescents who do not need active treatment. This would include those with curves less than 25 degrees, as measured by the Cobb method (Fig. 79–3). Curves that are progressive or are greater than 25 degrees or both, should be referred to an orthopedic surgeon who is knowledgeable in the treatment of these conditions.

At present, the only proven effective methods of treating progressive scoliosis are a surgical operation and an orthotic device (brace) (Fig. 79–4). Neuromuscular stimulation is still in the experimental phase and has not yet been tested over time, as have bracing and surgery. Spinal manipulation, traction, exercise programs, megavitamin therapy, specific diets, and so on have never been shown to be effective in altering the natural course of scoliosis and, in fact, may be harmful by allowing relentless curve progression to occur under the false assumption that "something is being done for the patient."

Each curve in each adolescent patient should be treated as an individual problem. The greater the sexual immaturity of the adolescent at time of diagnosis *and* the greater the magnitude of the curve, then the greater is the risk of progression. Irrespective of the initial curve, scoliosis tends to progress most rapidly during the growth spurt, during sexual maturity rating stage 2

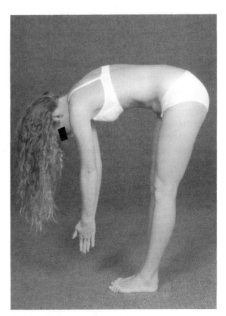

Figure 79–2. The patient in Figure 79–1 is now doing the forward bending test. The right thoracic cage is more prominent than the left, giving a positive screening test for scoliosis.

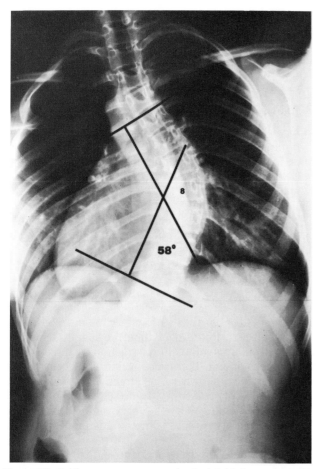

Figure 79–3. The measurement method of Cobb for scoliosis. The observer selects out those vertebrae that are making one continuous arc. A line is drawn across the top of the top vertebrae in that curve, and a line is drawn across the bottom of the bottom vertebra of that curve. Perpendiculars are erected to those lines, and the angle of intersect is taken as a measure of the degree of scoliosis.

or 3 in females and 3 or 4 in males. Adolescents should be monitored frequently (up to every 3 months) to assess the progression of the curve until after peak height velocity has been reached. Some curves, particularly those greater than 40 to 50 degrees, may continue progressing at variable rates throughout life and are most likely to require surgical intervention. However, even a curve of less than 30 degrees can continue to progress beyond skeletal maturity and into adult life. Those curves between 30 and 40 degrees may be braced effectively to halt the progression of the curve, which is the primary treatment goal.

Kyphosis

Abnormal kyphosis may be defined as an excessive roundback of the thoracic spine. It is measured by the method of Cobb from the superior end plate of the most tilted upper thoracic vertebra, usually T-1 or T-2, to the inferior end plate of the most tilted lower vertebra, usually T-12, on the standing lateral radiograph. The values for normal thoracic kyphosis vary from 20 to 45 degrees.

Excessive kyphosis, or hyperkyphosis, has a propensity to become rigid and may be progressive beyond adolescence into adult life. A rigid hyperkyphotic spine may cause back pain, easy fatigability, pulmonary compromise, and cosmetic deformity. Rarely, if ever, does it cause neurologic compression of the spinal cord. The prevalence of kyphosis in school screening is approximately 4%. The clinical examination is much like that for scoliosis, but the forward bending is viewed from the side (Fig. 79–5).

There are two types of hyperkyphosis seen in the adolescent population. One is postural roundback, which has excessive curvature but no vertebral changes. The distribution of this type is about equal between the sexes. The second type, more common in boys than in girls, is Scheuermann disease, which is defined as hyperkyphosis with structural vertebral changes, including greater than 5 degrees of anterior wedging of at least two consecutive vertebrae. End plate irregularities of the superior and inferior bodies and intervertebral disc space narrowing are often seen (Fig. 79–6). In contrast with postural roundback, which is usually painless, up to 40% to 50% of adolescents with Scheuermann disease complain of localized back pain. Although initially described by Scheuermann as a lumbar deformity, it is seen most frequently in the midthoracic and thoracolumbar regions. Although the etiology is uncertain, a probable cause is relative osteopenia or structural insufficiency of the vertebral end plates. This is most likely related to rapid overall skeletal growth, which allows micro- and macrocompression of the vertebral bodies.

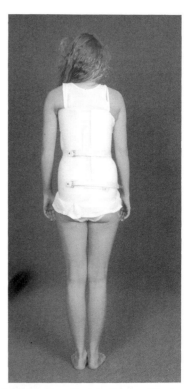

Figure 79–4. Adolescent patient in Figures 79–1 and 79–2 in a thoracic-lumbar-sacral orthosis (TLSO) for prevention of progression of her scoliosis deformity.

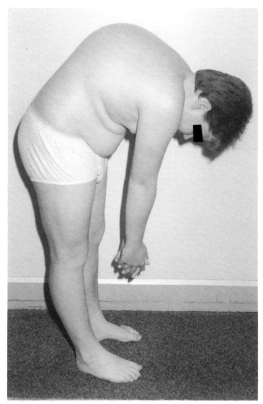

Figure 79–5. This 17-year-old male demonstrates a significant roundback deformity on the forward bending test.

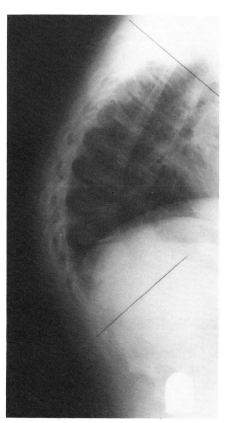

Figure 79–6. Standing lateral radiograph of patient in Figure 79–5, demonstrating the severe degree of deformity (Cobb measurement angle, 80 degrees) with irregularity of end plates. This is best classified as a thoracic Scheuermann deformity.

TREATMENT

The treatment for mild hyperkyphosis consists of either observation or hyperextension thoracic exercises (Fig. 79–7). For curves not larger than 70 degrees, an orthotic device plus an exercise program is appropriate. The type of orthotic device is usually either low profile or the full Milwaukee brace. One of the prerequisites for treatment with a brace is flexibility. A lateral supine radiograph with a firm bolster placed at the apex of the curve demonstrates the amount of flexibility in the kyphotic spine. If the spine is flexible, than an orthotic device may be prescribed with good success. If the kyphosis is rigid and is in excess of 70 degrees, surgical correction of the deformity may be required. Since the growth plates of the thoracic vertebrae are among the last in the spine to close (at about 17 years of age in females and 19 years in males), orthotic treatment may be successful even though the remainder of the patient's skeleton is nearly mature.

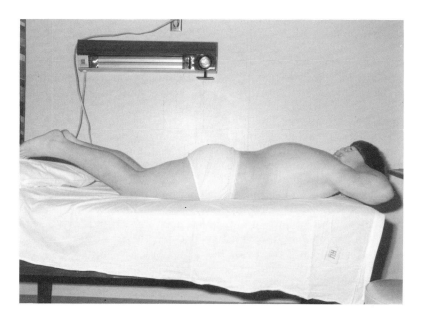

Figure 79–7. Same patient as in Figures 79–5 and 79–6, demonstrating the hyperextension exercises that reduce the kyphosis by a significant degree.

A second indication for surgical correction is short, sharply angulated kyphosis, regardless of magnitude. This type is likely to progress or to become painful in adult life. Surgery to correct and stabilize this severe deformity is a safe and reasonable treatment.

Spondylolisthesis

Spondylolisthesis (from the Greek *spondyl,* meaning back, and *olistheros,* to slide forward) refers to a forward slipping of one vertebra upon the other. It has been subclassified into several types: (1) dysplastic; (2) isthmic; (3) degenerative; (4) traumatic; and (5) pathologic. Only the first two are commonly found in adolescents. Both result from a lesion of the pars interarticularis of the posterior vertebral arch. In the dysplastic variety, the pars interarticularis becomes elongated, whereas in the isthmic type, a fracture occurs, most likely a stress fracture or fatigue fracture, which subsequently fails to heal. The vertebral articulation is weakened, and the superior articular facet of the caudad vertebra cannot prevent the forward slippage of the inferior articular facet of the cephalad vertebra, which lies posterior to it.

Spondylolisthesis is most common at the lumbosacral junction and occurs with progressively decreasing frequency at the L-4, L-3, L-2, and L-1 areas. It is rarely seen in children younger than the age of 5. The isthmic fatigue fracture known as spondylolysis occurs in about 5% of the population of the United States. Most of these heal satisfactorily, but some progress to spondylolisthesis.

The pars interarticularis fatigue fracture results from forced extension or forced rotation of the lumbar spine and is therefore common in young gymnasts and football players (especially interior linemen, who withstand significant forces when they stand to block on pass plays). In the isthmic type, there is a positive familial history in 15%; and spina bifida occulta at the involved vertebral level is seen in one third of cases. The dysplastic type is less common but is associated with positive family history in about one third of the cases. Conservative care is usually satisfactory for the isthmic variety, whereas the dysplastic variety responds best to surgical stabilization.

Spondylolisthesis is one of the most common causes of back pain in adolescence. The signs and symptoms may include low back, buttock, and thigh pain, which rarely goes below the knee; tight hamstrings; postural deformity with hyperlordosis; and in severe grades, a palpable "step-off" at the lumbosacral junction. In addition, there can be weakness and hypesthesia of the lower extremities and abnormalities of gait. The diagnosis is confirmed by means of plain radiographs, including standard AP and lateral views, to include obliques, to best visualize the pars interarticularis (Fig. 79–8). In adolescent patients with spondylolisthesis and low back pain, radiographs of the entire thoracic and lumbar spine should be obtained, since scoliosis is associated with this condition about 40% of the time.

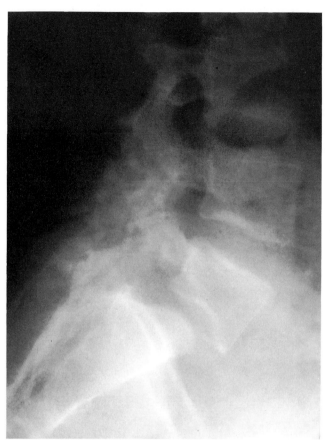

Figure 79–8. Standing lateral radiograph of the lumbar spine of a 15-year-old girl with back pain, demonstrating forward slipping of the vertebral column L-5 on the sacrum. This would be classified as a grade II spondylolisthesis because of its severe forward slip.

TREATMENT

Once the diagnosis of spondylolisthesis has been made, even those patients who are asymptomatic should be followed. There is a small but definite risk of increased forward slipping, particularly before the age of 15 years. The risk of progressive slip appears to be independent of the initial magnitude of the slip, and it is more likely in the immature spine with dysplastic changes and in the child whose sacrum is more vertically oriented than usual (increased "slip angle"). The author's preference for following these patients is to take standing lateral radiographs at 6-month intervals until the adolescent has reached skeletal maturity. This is needed to document nonprogression. If progression is seen, then stabilization is recommended. Nonoperative treatments of symptomatic spondylolisthesis include limiting activities, bed rest, analgesics, and even a trial of immobilization in a plaster of paris cast or an orthotic device. Acute spondylolysis or a fracture of the pars interarticularis may be seen following trauma. This demands immobilization and usually heals in 3 months.

Unfortunately, conservative treatment does not often succeed in patients with chronic types of painful spondylolisthesis. Therefore, the indications for surgical stabilization are (1) refractory pain; (2) progressive slipping, demonstrated by standing lateral radiographs; (3)

severe deformity (greater than 50% slip relative to the adjacent vertebra); and (4) significant gait disturbance unsuccessfully managed by bracing. The surgical treatment most often consists of a bilateral transverse process spinal fusion from the vertebra that has slipped forward to the sacrum. About 95% of patients are asymptomatic and are able to return to an active life, including athletic activities, after surgery.

Back Pain in Adolescents

Although the incidence of back pain in adolescents is far lower than that in the adult population, it is more likely to be caused by a major pathologic lesion than by chronic muscular or ligamentous strain or degenerative changes. Although spondylolisthesis is the most common cause of low back pain in adolescents, it is essential to consider that any child complaining of back pain may have a tumor (neoplasm), infection of the spine, or herniated disc. Such lesions have the potential to produce permanent neurologic deficit and spinal destruction unless promptly diagnosed and treated. In the absence of anatomic defects such as these and muscular or ligamentous strain, functional or psychosomatic causes of back pain must be considered.

However, as is emphasized in other chapters of this book, the diagnosis of a psychosomatic or functional condition should not be made merely on the basis of negative "organic" findings in an adolescent. One must search for possible explanatory factors such as depression, anxiety, or unresolved conflict at home, at school, or with peers. In the absence of such data, the clinician should continue to monitor the physical examination and selected laboratory studies and make an ongoing assessment of psychosocial factors. Referral to a psychologist or psychiatrist for treatment of back pain, based on the absence of organic findings, rarely proves useful. Such referral is better made on the basis of worries, fears, anxieties, or conflict uncovered during the biopsychosocial evaluation (see Chapter 113).

TUMORS

Tumors of the spine or the neural axis usually present with pain that is constant in nature, associated with involuntary muscle spasm, rigidity of the spine on attempted motion, and neurologic deficit. This deficit may include weakness, sensory deficit, foot deformity, or interference with bowel and bladder function and control. Once the diagnosis of a tumor has been established, prompt surgical treatment is indicated.

INFECTIONS

Back pain caused by infection of the spinal column is most likely due to diskitis (infection in the intervertebral disk space). Vertebral osteomyelitis occurs most commonly in adults, but diskitis results from a hematogenous seeding after a bacteremia, with the primary focus of infection usually being in the respiratory or urinary tract. The most common site of occurrence is in the lumbar region, and the most common causative organism is *Staphylococcus aureus*. The clinical presentation consists of back pain, commonly with pain radiating into the hip or leg. Occasionally cases present as isolated abdominal pain or simply as an inability to walk. Physical signs include tenderness to percussion over the involved area of the spine and involuntary muscle spasm. The plain films reveal the diskitis only after symptoms have been present for at least 2 or 3 weeks. Initially, they reveal only disk space narrowing, later followed by irregularity or erosions of the end plate with or without a soft tissue mass in the adjacent area. Bone scans and soft tissue scans yield positive findings much earlier in the course of the illness than do plain films.

Treatment of diskitis consists of rest with or without a body cast, depending upon the amount of pain and spasm. The author's preference is to administer antibiotics, but this is not universally accepted. Failure to improve clinically (continued symptoms, elevated white blood count and erythrocyte sedimentation rate) within 2 weeks necessitates aspiration of the disk space and the administration of intravenous antibiotics. Treatment should be continued until the sedimentation rate returns to normal.

Vertebral osteomyelitis can occur in adolescents, especially in those who are frequent intravenous drug users (see Chapter 111). The infection presents with signs and symptoms quite similar to those of diskitis, but radiographs show erosion and collapse of vertebral bodies. The treatment is markedly different. When osteomyelitis of the vertebral body is suspected, needle biopsy must be performed to obtain material for culture. Blood cultures are positive in 50% of cases. Bed rest and immobilization in a cast are appropriate. If the adolescent fails to respond to these treatments, open surgical biopsy with anterior spinal fusion may be indicated.

HERNIATED DISK

A herniated disk is an uncommon cause of back pain in adolescents. The presenting clinical picture is much like that of the adult counterpart, with low back pain and radiculopathy. The pain radiates through the distribution of the specific nerve root. Trauma is usually not an antecedent event. There is decreased range of spinal motion with muscle spasm. With significant neurologic involvement and nerve root compression, the changes classically seen are muscle weakness, atrophy, sensory loss, and reflex diminution. Plain radiographs usually show no abnormality; the diagnosis is best established by computed tomography, myelogram, or magnetic resonance imaging. The treatment of herniated disk disease in the adolescent population consists initially of bed rest and administration of analgesics for a period of 2 to 3 weeks. An exception to this is the patient with a progressive neurologic deficit, who should have prompt surgical decompression with removal of the offending disk material. Another indication for surgical treatment is failure to respond to an adequate trial of conservative therapy. Surgical treatment classically involves a small laminotomy incision and excision of disk material.

BACK STRAIN

Individuals who are obese (see Chapter 60) or inactive, or both, frequently experience chronic muscular or ligamentous strain and low back pain. This is a diagnosis of exclusion, since there are no anatomic defects. The pain is nagging but tolerable, usually intermittent, and rarely radiating. It responds best to muscle stretching and strengthening exercises, weight reduction, and alteration of activities, which are continued until the patient is symptom free.

FUNCTIONAL BACK PAIN

A common cause of back pain in adolescents is functional disturbance, including somatoform disorders such as somatization disorder or conversion reaction. These adolescents may present with bizarre somatic pain patterns. The results of the physical examination, including a meticulous neurologic examination, often reveal inconsistent or nonphysiologic findings with no objective findings of pathology. The results of laboratory and radiographic studies are normal. The adolescent with functional back pain almost always shows disproportionate disability and an unusual affect in addition to the bizarre somatic pattern. The approach to the diagnosis, as mentioned previously, must not be the mere exclusion of organic etiology. In the biopsychosocial model, significant positive psychosocial factors must be identified before a psychosomatic cause can be considered. The treatment consists of attention to the psychosocial problems not only of the adolescent but also of the family (see Chapter 113).

HIP

The syndromes that are most common in the adolescent period are Legg-Calvé-Perthes disease and slipped capital femoral epiphysis.

Legg-Calvé-Perthes Disease

Avascular necrosis of the femoral head was first described in 1909 independently by Arthur Legg of the United States, Jacques Calvé of France, and Georg Perthes of Germany; in the orthopedic literature, it most commonly bears the name of Perthes disease. The disease has an incidence of approximately 1 in 2000, with males outnumbering females by approximately four to one. There is no predilection for right or left side, and 10% to 15% of cases are bilateral. The peak incidence is between 5 and 6 years of age, but an increasing number of 10- to 12-year-olds are being seen with Perthes disease.

ETIOLOGY

The specific cause of the presumed avascular necrosis is unknown. In some cases, there may be a genetic predisposition or an association with trauma, recurrent synovitis, and a retarded bone age. Because Perthes-like changes can be produced in laboratory animals by increasing the intracapsular pressure above venous outflow pressure for 8 to 10 hours, the theory has evolved that venous congestion may be an etiologic agent.

PATHOLOGY

Five sequential phases of avascular necrosis occur, classified as (1) prenecrosis; (2) necrosis; (3) revascularization; (4) reossification; and (5) remodeling. During the prenecrotic stage, there is interference with blood flow that may be related to trauma of the arterial supply, increased intra-articular pressure, hypercoagulability, and thrombosis. Venous occlusion may also be a primary factor. During the next phase, the resulting necrotic involved bone of the femoral epiphysis undergoes micro- and macrofractures and ceases to grow. In severe cases, a cyst may form within the femoral epiphysis and metaphysis. The amount of femoral head necrosis has been variously classified by Catterall, Thompson, and Salter.

The revascularization stage is initiated as the dead bone is resorbed and replaced with granulation tissue and cartilage. Concurrently, the cartilage model that has been deposited in the area of the previously dead bone begins to reossify. This reossification may take as long as 18 months to 3 years to complete (Fig. 79–9).

The final stage is remodeling, during which there may be gradual improvement in the congruity of the hip joint. The natural history of Perthes disease is a protracted course lasting 1 to 4 years. The femoral head always heals by revascularization, but it almost always has some residual deformity. In spite of this, most adolescent patients have a good long-term prognosis and do not experience significant pain or loss of motion. The older the child is at the time of diagnosis, the more likely that the result will be poor.

DIAGNOSIS

Diagnosis of Perthes disease is based upon the clinical symptoms and signs and radiographic examination. The clinical picture includes (1) a limp; (2) pain, which may be referred to the anterior thigh or rarely is present in the anterior lateral hip area; (3) loss of motion, particularly internal rotation in the prone position and abduction in the flexed position; (4) atrophy of the thigh and buttock muscles; and (5) tenderness to palpation over the joint (synovitis). Radiographic findings depend upon the stage of the disease process and the extent of femoral head involvement. The key to a good prognosis is congruity between the healing femoral head and the acetabulum.

TREATMENT

The goals of treatment in Perthes disease are to prevent subluxation of the femoral head from the acetabulum, to preserve the sphericity of the femoral head, and to maintain good muscle function to allow for a normal gait once the lesion has healed. Early treatment consists of obtaining and maintaining a full range of non–weight-bearing motion. This is best achieved by

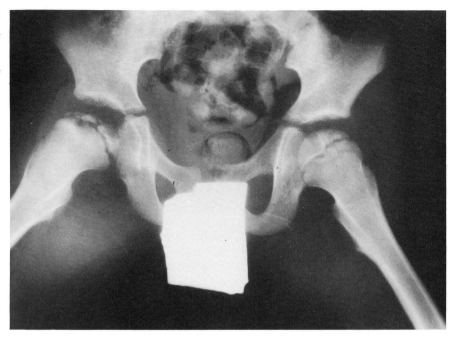

Figure 79–9. A frog pelvis radiograph of a 10-year-old boy with healing Perthes disease of the right hip. Notice the reossification of the cartilaginous femoral head from separate islands of centers of ossification. Remodeling will occur throughout the rest of growth of this young adolescent boy.

bed rest, often combined with traction of the limb in order to unload the hip.

Once the adolescent patient is comfortable and has an improved range of motion, definitive treatment may begin. This definitive treatment is dependent upon the severity of the head involvement and the chronologic age of the patient. The severity is usually such that at least two thirds to three fourths of the femoral head is involved. The object of the modalities of treatment is avoidance of weight bearing, maintenance of motion, or use of an operative technique of placing the femoral head deep within the acetabulum via either femoral osteotomy or acetabular osteotomy.

Occasionally, adolescent patients with Perthes disease are first seen during the stage of reossification and already have a somewhat flattened, subluxed femoral head. Many authors believe that in these cases it is best to wait until complete healing has occurred before attempting a salvage procedure such as (1) the reshaping of the femoral head (i.e., cheilectomy), (2) a valgus osteotomy to put the rounder part of the femoral head up into the acetabulum; or (3) pelvic osteotomies to make the acetabulum large enough to contain the entire femoral head.

Slipped Capital Femoral Epiphysis

Slipped capital femoral epiphysis (SCFE) may develop as either an abrupt or a gradual displacement of the femoral neck from the femoral head. The slipping occurs through the growth plate. The term is somewhat a misnomer, since the head is actually contained within the acetabulum by the acetabular contour; therefore, the femoral neck displaces anteriorly and slightly superiorly. The incidence has been reported as approximately 1 in 50,000 population, with a 2:1 to 3:1 male-to-female ratio. It almost always occurs in adolescents or preadolescents, hence its other name, adolescent coxa

vara. The likelihood of occurrence of bilateral slipped epiphyses is 40% in the author's series.

ETIOLOGY

Because a single, specific causative agent has not been identified, it is probable that most adolescents develop this condition from a combination of factors. These factors may include the fact that the physis is weaker during the adolescent growth spurt; trauma (the rate of occurrence is higher in the United States in spring and summer months); an inflammatory or autoimmune process; hormonal factors, particularly those conditions affecting growth hormone or changes in estrogen or testosterone balance; a proposed intrinsic defect in the growth plate; the angle at which the growth plate is aligned to the pelvis; and an increased body mass and obesity. More than 50% of the patients are classified as obese, and many of these same patients are taller than the 90th percentile in height. Lastly, genetic factors may play a role, since approximately 4% of patients with slipped capital femoral epiphysis have a positive history in their family.

SIGNS AND SYMPTOMS

In adolescents, 5% to 10% of slipped epiphyses seem to occur as the result of an acute, sudden event (e.g., a baseball player sliding into second base, experiencing pain in the hip and thigh and subsequent inability to bear weight on the extremity). These are classified as acute slips and most likely represent a traumatic displacement through a weakened growth plate. Frequently, a careful history reveals that these patients have had nagging thigh or knee pain for several months prior to the catastrophic event.

Physical examination reveals painful motion in all ranges, with marked limitation of internal rotation and abduction. The pathognomonic sign of any slipped epiphysis is obligatory external rotation as the hip is moved into flexion.

More commonly, the presenting symptoms are subacute. The adolescent complains of a mild intermittent pain with a limp. Occasionally, there are complaints of weakness in the involved lower extremity. The symptoms may have been present for an extended period of time, even for a year in some cases. The third category of slipped capital femoral epiphysis is an acute superimposed upon a chronic slipped epiphysis. The age range at time of presentation of all three types is from 9 to 17 years, or at closure of the upper femoral growth plate.

All adolescents with any signs or symptoms referable to the hip should be suspected of having a slipped capital femoral epiphysis until proved otherwise. The earliest radiographic sign of subtle slips is widening of the growth plate with mild osteopenia of the proximal femur when compared with the uninvolved side. Usually, minimal displacement has occurred in these early signs. Biplanar

views are essential to the diagnosis of slipped epiphysis, as frequently it cannot be easily detected on the AP film. Frog-leg AP pelvis views are acceptable, but a better appreciation for the degree of slip can be obtained by ordering a cross-table lateral x-ray film, sometimes called a true lateral or a "shoot-through" lateral (Fig. 79–10). In chronic slipped epiphyses, remodeling changes of the inferior aspect of the neck of the femur may be seen. These remodeling changes are due to the displacement of the femoral head stripping the periosteum of the femoral neck and the formation of new bone by the stripped periosteum.

CLINICAL SIGNIFICANCE

The significance of slipped epiphysis includes the potential for further slipping, for interruption of the vascular or the nutritional supply to the bone of the upper end of the femur, and for development of pre-

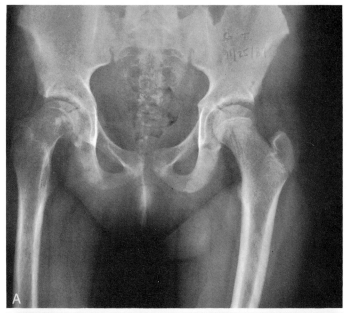

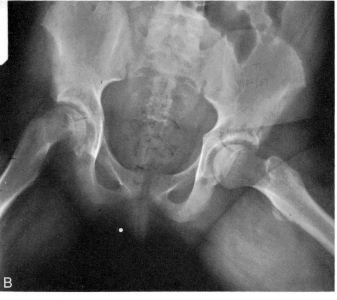

Figure 79–10. AP *(A)* and frog lateral *(B)* radiographs of an adolescent demonstrating a slipped capital femoral epiphysis. Note the displacement of the right femoral head relative to the neck of the femur.

mature degenerative osteoarthritis of the hip. Any hip with an identified slip, either acute or chronic, must be considered at risk for further slipping, and as such, treatment is extremely urgent. The adolescent should not be allowed to walk but should be placed in recumbent or sitting position and transported directly to a qualified orthopedist's care.

Complications of the disease process are avascular necrosis of the femoral head and chondrolysis. Chondrolysis is a condition in which the cartilage of the femoral head and acetabulum degenerates, producing joint narrowing, stiffness, contracture, pain, and limping. It may be idiopathic but also has been associated with severe slips and with trauma to the articular surface experienced during therapeutic maneuvers.

TREATMENT

The objective of treatment for slipped capital femoral epiphysis is to prevent further slipping. In cases of acute slipping or acute on chronic slipping, an additional objective is to correct the slip to the severity at the pre-acute phase so as to minimize the risk of avascular necrosis or chondrolysis. If the slip is minimal (grade I), simple *in situ* fixation of the slip either by insertion of pins or by bone graft epiphysiodesis is the treatment of choice. A less useful alternative is prolonged immobilization in a hip spica cast. In chronic slipped epiphysis of severe degree, there may be need for corrective osteotomy. Because of the external rotation deformity of the femur, varus deformity of the hip, and loss of flexion, any corrective osteotomy must take these facts into consideration to produce a more congruous hip joint. The intent of any treatment for slipped epiphysis is to (1) prevent further slipping; (2) realign the leg for normal weightbearing; (3) minimize the risk for avascular necrosis and chondrolysis; and (4) minimize the risk for late degenerative changes. The most important considerations regarding slipped capital femoral epiphysis are to have a high index of suspicion for this entity in any adolescent with a limp or who complains of hip, thigh, or knee pain; to confirm or rule out the diagnosis immediately with the use of appropriate biplanar radiographs; and once the diagnosis has been made, to promptly refer the adolescent for orthopedic treatment without allowing him or her to bear weight on the affected limb.

KNEE

Pain in the knee, especially the anterior aspect of the knee, is very common in adolescents. Although the patellofemoral joint, the tibiofemoral joint, or the surrounding soft tissues are most often the source of the disorder, it is critical to remember that major hip disease, such as slipped capital femoral epiphysis, Perthes disease, and tumors about the hip, may frequently present with referred pain to the medial aspect of the knee. It is imperative in all adolescents who have a complaint of knee pain with normal physical examination of the knee that a proper examination of the hip, including appropriate radiographs, be obtained.

Patellofemoral Problems

(see Chapter 82)

The patella is the largest sesamoid bone in the body. The main mechanical function of the patella is to increase the lever arm of the quadriceps knee extensor muscle group. It also functions to centralize the pull of the quadriceps and to resist compression of the quadriceps tendon as it passes over the knee joint, to protect the anterior knee as a bony shield, and to bear weight during kneeling or knee walking. The posterior surface of the patella that articulates with the femur contains the thickest articular cartilage in the body. This thick cartilage covers the subchondral bone, which is richly innervated by pain fibers. The forces across the patellofemoral joint can be extreme. For instance, in stair climbing, with the knee flexed at 60 degrees, a force equivalent to three and one-half times body weight is exerted on this joint by the pull of the quadriceps. During a deep knee bend, more than seven times body weight is transmitted to the posterior aspect of the patellofemoral joint.

The major patellofemoral problems seen in adolescents are related to malalignment and instability. Symptoms of malalignment and instability include pain, particularly when climbing stairs or during knee bends, intermittent giving way, or "buckling," of the knee, crepitus over the patellofemoral joint, occasional swelling, and a feeling of stiffness, or "catching," in the knee. True locking of the knee (i.e., inability to fully extend or flex the knee) is rare with patellofemoral joint disease and more often is a sign of tear of the meniscus.

Patellofemoral pain is probably caused by either increased intraosseous pressure or subchondral bone microfracture. The latter results from increased pressure on one side of the patella, usually the lateral side, due to lateral tracking of the patella secondary to malalignment during flexion and extension of the knee. This lateral tracking may be the result of soft tissue laxity; a high riding patella (patella alta), which is secondary to tightness of the rectus femoris; increased valgus at the knee (knock knees); or femoral anteversion, which also can increase the lateral quadriceps vector of force.

Positive signs of malalignment include atrophy of the vastus medialis oblique part of the quadriceps, tightness of the rectus femoris or the iliotibial band or both, high-riding patellae, increased knock knee, anteversion, pronated and valgus feet, pain on palpation of the retropatellar facet, and crepitation and pain on compression of the patella against the femoral trochlea.

Frequently, the term *chondromalacia* is used in patellofemoral disorders. Chondromalacia is a pathologic diagnosis meaning fibrillation and fragmentation of the retropatellar articular cartilage. It is the result of chronic overuse and excessive pressure. The increased lateral pressure syndrome responds best to a program of exercises designed both to stretch the tight rectus femoris and iliotibial tract and to strengthen the quadriceps muscle, especially the vastus medialis obliquus. Isometric exercises with the knee at or near full extension are more appropriate than isotonic exercises through a full range of motion, since less patellofemoral loading occurs in the last 10 degrees of full extension; so these would best be summed up as "stretching and strengthening" exercises.

Patellar Subluxation or Dislocation

Patellofemoral subluxation or dislocation or both may be the result of isolated traumatic episodes or simply severe malalignment over a period of time. The condition most commonly occurs between the ages of 10 and 25 years, with a peak incidence at age 15. It is four times more common in girls than in boys. Patients with this subluxation usually show the signs of increased lateral pressure and have positive "apprehension" sign (Fairbank). This sign is elicited by attempting to displace the patella laterally. A positive result is a marked increase in the adolescent's apprehension, often to the point that the adolescent will grab the examiner's hand. As in the malalignment syndrome, patellofemoral subluxation frequently responds to an exercise program, using the same principles of stretching and strengthening. If an adequate exercise program is not successful, then surgical realignment procedures may be appropriate. The surgical procedures are complex; they involve muscle balancing procedures and may also include realignment of the attachment of the patellar tendon to the tibial tubercle. Lastly, if excessive genu valgum (knock knee) is present, it may need to be corrected prior to any soft tissue procedure done around the infrapatellar tendon.

Internal Derangement of the Knee

Internal derangement of the knee refers either to a torn meniscus or torn cruciate ligament or to a loose body within the knee joint. Meniscal tears are usually the result of trauma and present with a history of locking, giving way, pain, and intermittent swelling. With advancements in arthroscopic surgical procedures, partial meniscectomy and in frequent cases repair of the meniscus produce better long-term results than total meniscectomy.

A loose body in the knee joint may be the result of a small articular surface fracture, but often no history of trauma can be elicited. Synovial chondromatosis produces multiple loose bodies. A loose body in the knee joint produces intermittent symptoms of instability, pain, swelling, and locking of the knee, similar if not identical to those of meniscal disease. When loose bodies are identified, they should be removed to prevent damage to the articular surfaces.

Osteochondritis Dissecans

This unusual lesion is commonly seen on the medial femoral condyle (Fig. 79–11). It is probably caused by single or repeated trauma to the partially flexed knee, which results in a compression fracture due to impingement either of the facet of the patella or of the tibial spine, and is therefore seen more commonly in active

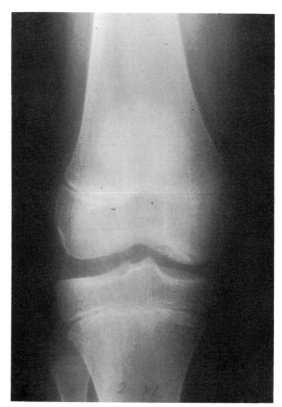

Figure 79–11. AP radiograph of the knee of a 16-year-old boy with an osteochondritis lesion of the medial femoral condyle. Notice the radiolucent line within the femoral condyle, outlining the large fragment. It is in continuity with the femoral condyle and did not become displaced during treatment.

or athletic adolescents (see Chapter 80). Osteochondritis (osteochondrosis) dissecans is more common in boys than in girls, and the condition is frequently bilateral. Often the lesion is asymptomatic, but it may present with poorly localized knee pain, mild effusions, and even symptoms of giving way or locking. In most cases, the cartilaginous articular surface remains intact, although partial or complete detachment of an osteochondral fragment may occur. A free fragment in the knee joint produces symptoms of repeated locking, giving way, pain, and effusion.

The treatment for lesions without loose fragments consists of activities restricted to the patient's tolerance level. Healing may be expected in a period of 3 to 4 months. If healing does not occur, a period of immobilization of the knee is appropriate. If there is any question of a fragment being loose in the knee joint, arthroscopic examination is appropriate. Small loose fragments should be removed from the knee joint, whereas large fragments with significant bony component should be replaced into their osseous beds and secured with some type of internal fixation.

Osgood-Schlatter Disease

This disorder, an osteochondrosis of the tibial tuberosity, is generally related to activity. It is described in greater detail in Chapter 80.

FOOT

Flatfeet

There are few anatomic aberrations that incite as much parental anxiety as do flatfeet. The most common flatfoot is the flexible or physiologic type. These feet are easily detectable because they are mobile, have excellent muscle strength, and are uniformly painless unless the deformity is severe. The patients present with low or incomplete medial longitudinal arch of the foot (Fig. 79–12). During weight bearing, the heel appears to be in slight increased valgus. When the adolescent stands on tiptoe, the arch is restored, and the heel returns to neutral or goes into slight varus.

Radiographs taken of the foot while weightbearing show the flattening of the longitudinal arch (Fig. 79–13) and an increase of the talocalcaneal angle on both the AP and the lateral projections. The talus becomes more vertically aligned because of lack of support from the os calcis, which is in valgus.

Frequently, the family has been to numerous doctors when the child was younger, and most likely the adolescent was treated with "orthopedic shoes," medial heel wedges, arch supports, and so forth. It should be remembered that the "corrective" shoe is a misnomer. The shoe will not correct the foot in any way; the foot will deform the shoe. It simply prolongs shoe wear, prevents ligament overstretching, and relieves mild symptoms, such as aching in the longitudinal arch. If the symptoms are mild to moderate, formal orthotic devices to give support to the talus medially and prevent the os calcis from going into valgus may be necessary.

Although there are numerous surgical procedures for the correction of the hypermobile flatfoot, the only indication for surgery is severe, uncorrectable deformity or pain that is not relieved by the use of appropriate foot orthotic devices. If, however, the foot is rigid, this should be considered a pathologic flatfoot, and care must be taken to look for an etiologic factor in this rigid flatfoot, such as neuromuscular disease, tarsal coalition, infection of the foot, rheumatoid arthritis, bony cyst, or tumor in and about the foot.

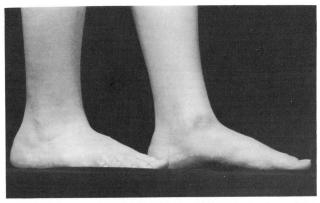

Figure 79–12. Photograph of a 10-year-old boy who had complaints of mild fatigue pain in the longitudinal arch of his foot. He demonstrates relaxed physiologic flatfeet.

Tarsal Coalition

The most common nonneuromuscular cause of pathologic flatfoot in the adolescent is a tarsal coalition, in which two or more of the tarsal bones are united either by a bony bar or by a fibrocartilaginous bridge. The result is frequently a rigid flatfoot, associated with spasm of the peroneal musculature. The cause of the coalition is probably incomplete separation of the mesenchymal anlage of the tarsal bones during fetal development. The bar is most likely cartilaginous in infancy, and as the cartilage ossifies, less motion is available, causing the foot to become more rigid. The most common locations for bars are the calcaneonavicular joint and the talocalcaneal joint middle facet (Fig. 79–14). Much less common are talonavicular and calcaneocuboid bars. Rarely, more than one coalition exist in the same foot. Bilaterality is common. There is often an autosomal dominant inheritance pattern.

The effect of a coalition is decreased motion of the hindfoot, particularly the ability for the os calcis to move into valgus and varus and the talus to move into plantar flexion and dorsiflexion. These complex motions are necessary when one walks over uneven terrain. It is postulated that the coalitions cause increased stress at

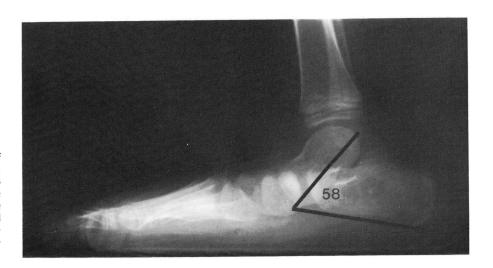

Figure 79–13. Standing radiograph of an adolescent complaining of foot pain. Notice the talocalcaneal angle of 58 degrees is significantly greater than the norm of 20 to 40 degrees and that the long axis of the talus is plantar flexed relative to the long axis of the metatarsals. This is a classic finding of physiologic flatfoot.

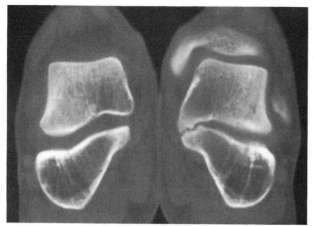

Figure 79-14. A computed tomography (CT) scan through the hindfoot of a patient complaining of pain in the left foot and loss of subtalar movement. There is an osteocartilaginous bony bar in the area of the middle facet of the subtalar joint on the left foot.

other joints and thereby cause early degenerative changes. This is consistent with the observation that most individuals with coalitions do not become symptomatic until adolescence. However, many coalitions never become symptomatic.

When a painful and rigid foot is seen, appropriate x-ray films are needed for diagnosis. It may be necessary to obtain computed axial tomograms or special axial projections on ordinary film to detect the talocalcaneal coalitions. The calcaneonavicular bar is best detected on an oblique view of the midfoot and hindfoot (Fig. 79-15).

The usual treatment of tarsal coalitions is to make the foot symptom free by using nonsteroidal anti-inflammatory drugs, applying a short leg cast for a period of

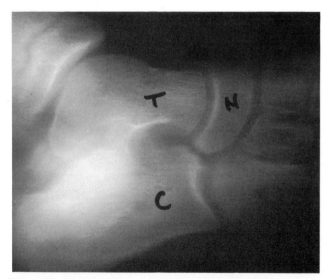

Figure 79-15. This 12-year-old patient presented with midtarsal foot pain and limited motion. Oblique radiograph of the hindfoot reveals an osteocartilaginous tarsal coalition between the anterior beak of the os calcis and the navicular. (N, navicular; C, calcaneus; T, talus.) The osteocartilaginous bone was removed surgically, and the extensor digitorum brevis muscle was interposed as a tissue graft to prevent reformation of the bar.

time, or using orthotic devices. These rarely produce lasting relief, and so most cases require surgical intervention. In those adolescents with no significant degenerative changes and who are still skeletally immature, surgical excision of the bridging bone with interposition graft material, such as fat or muscle, is the best treatment available. If, however, the adolescent is near skeletal maturation and the bar is sufficiently large, especially in the subtalar joint, then further fusion of the hindfoot may be necessary (triple arthrodesis).

Cavus Feet

A cavus deformity of the foot is one in which there is an excessively high medial longitudinal plantar arch. This is associated with dorsiflexion of the calcaneus and with an equinus supinated and varus deviation of the forefoot relative to the midfoot. This type of foot pattern is frequently seen in neuromuscular diseases, such as myelodysplasia, poliomyelitis, Friedreich ataxia, and Charcot-Marie-Tooth disease (hereditary motor and sensory neuropathy). It also may be a sign of intraspinal neoplasm. A much less common cause is familial idiopathic cavovarus feet; therefore, an adolescent presenting with cavovarus feet needs a careful evaluation both orthopedically and neurologically, and a careful family history must be obtained to find out whether other family members are so afflicted.

Once the neurologic basis is confirmed, then treatment is aimed at correcting deformities to establish a foot flat gait that is pain free. In late adolescence and in early adulthood, this may require triple arthrodesis of the hindfoot to achieve correction and lasting stability.

Foot Pain

METATARSALGIA

Frequently, adolescents with one or more unusually prominent metatarsal heads on the plantar aspect of the feet complain of pain in the distal metatarsal region. The discomfort is easily relieved by use of pads or bars placed across the sole of the shoe. The insert should be positioned just proximal to the metatarsal heads. When the metatarsalgia is recalcitrant to such treatment, consideration should be given to a shortening metatarsal osteotomy, which allows more even distribution of weight bearing across the metatarsal heads.

STRESS FRACTURES

Adolescents who subject their feet to prolonged walking and running may develop fractures of the shaft of the bone, predominantly the second and third metatarsals. If an adolescent who has begun a running exercise program or high-impact aerobics program complains of foot pain, one must suspect a stress fracture. It may be difficult to demonstrate the stress fracture on routine radiographs; however, technetium bone scans can detect the area of increased uptake long before there is radiographic evidence of callus formation.

Treatment consists of restricting the activities until the symptoms subside. In some individuals, walking plaster of paris or fiber glass cast may be necessary to help relieve symptoms.

FREIBERG INFRACTION (DISEASE)

A curious affliction called Freiberg infraction (disease) is avascular necrosis of the head of the metatarsal. It most frequently involves the second metatarsal, which is the longest and most rigid of the metatarsal bones. The infraction can also occur in the third and fourth metatarsal heads. The presentation of Freiberg infraction is one of pain and tenderness, usually with minimal swelling over the involved metatarsal head. This produces a noticeable limp.

The findings on radiograph are typical of avascular necrosis, namely sclerosis, irregularity, and what appears to be collapse of the metatarsal head (Fig. 79–16), but these changes may not appear until weeks following the onset of pain.

Treatment is symptomatic and consists of restriction of activities, including the application of a short leg walking cast or the use of a metatarsal pad in the shoe, which is sometimes required for several years. If pain is more severe than suspected, relief from weight bearing may be appropriate. The majority of cases are usually self-limiting and will ultimately revascularize, leaving the metatarsal head minimally deformed, but usually restoring nearly full function.

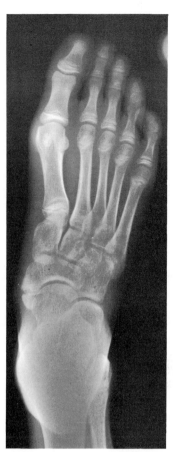

Figure 79–17. AP view of the foot of a 15-year-old girl with complaints of pain upon strenuous activities and weightbearing over the medial aspect of the midfoot and hindfoot. She demonstrates a nonunited ossicle to the tarsonavicular. She had pain and discomfort from shoe wear against the prominent ossicle. This was relieved with surgical excision of the ossicle and medial beak of the navicular, with replantation of the tibialis posterior tendon.

TARSONAVICULAR BURSITIS

An accessory ossicle just medial to the tarsonavicular may be present in 10% of the population. It may not present as a separate ossicle, but rather as a large hypertrophic medial projection of the tarsonavicular (Fig. 79–17). This becomes painful owing to overlying bursitis or strain of the attachment of the posterior tibial tendon at that point. Frequently, there is an associated mild relaxed flatfoot. If the bony prominence causes symptoms of pressure from the shoe counter, then surgical excision of the ossicle with plication of the tibialis posterior tendon may be indicated for chronic pain syndromes.

SEVER SYNDROME

This is an uncommon lesion, usually occurring in adolescent boys ages 10 to 12. It ordinarily involves pain on the posterolateral aspect of the os calcis and is intensified by exercise. It is described in greater detail in Chapter 80.

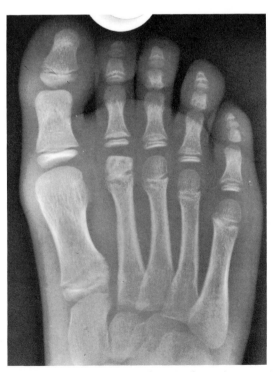

Figure 79–16. Patient complaining of anterior foot pain was a catcher on his baseball team. Radiograph reveals typical sclerosis with mild collapse of the second metatarsal head. This is classic Freiberg infraction.

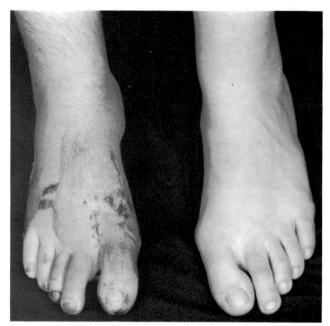

Figure 79–18. AP photograph of a 16-year-old girl who had bilateral hallux valgus. She is 2 months postoperative treatment on the right side and awaiting operative treatment on the left.

Hallux Valgus

This condition, which is extremely common in adults, is rarely seen in young children but has increasing severity in adolescents. The great majority of cases are caused by congenital or developmental abnormalities in the first ray, particularly the first cuneiform and metatarsal regions. A deviation of the first metatarsal medially into varus is the pathologic disorder in most cases, with subsequent adaptive valgus angulation at the metatarsophalangeal joints. This is usually secondary to soft tissue bowstringing or muscle imbalance with powerful overpull of the adductor hallucis. Pointed-toed or ill-fitting shoes draw attention to the deformity because of pressure over the bunion but do not cause it. Hallux valgus is more than just a cosmetic deformity; it is the occurrence of a painful bursa over the medial aspect of the head of the first metatarsal. Unless extremely severe, the deformity does not interfere with function of the great toe during walking.

Not infrequently, the discomfort is so disabling that surgical intervention is indicated. Each individual foot must be assessed as to the bony architecture and muscle balance or lack thereof, and treatment should be aimed at restoring muscle balance and the anatomy of the metatarsals to nearly normal, that is, the angle between the first and second metatarsal rays should be significantly less than 8 degrees. The procedure of choice is to balance muscles around the first ray by detaching the adductor hallucis from the lateral sesamoid and rerouting it into the neck of the first metatarsal through a drill hole. A proximally based first metatarsal osteotomy, either closing wedge or a concentric domed osteotomy, can correct for the intermetatarsal malalignment (Fig. 79–18).

BIBLIOGRAPHY

Bradford DS: The surgical management of patients with Scheuermann's disease: A review of 24 cases managed by combined anterior and posterior spine fusion. J Bone Joint Surg 62A:705, 1980.

Crosby EB, Insall J: Recurrent dislocation of the patella. J Bone Joint Surg 58A:9, 1976.

Hensinger RN: Spondylolysis and spondylolisthesis in children. American Academy of Orthopaedic Surgeons Instructional Course Lectures 32:132, 1983.

Jacobs B: Diagnosis and natural history of slipped capital femoral epiphysis. American Academy of Orthopaedic Surgeons Instructional Course Lectures 21:167, 1972.

Lawson JP: Symptomatic radiographic variants in extremities. Radiology 157:625, 1985.

Linden B: Osteochondritis dissecans of the femoral condyles. A long-term follow-up study. J Bone Joint Surg 59A:769, 1977.

Mosier KM, Asher M: Tarsal coalitions and peroneal spastic flatfoot. A review. J Bone Joint Surg 66A:976, 1984.

Scoles PV: Pediatric Orthopaedics in Clinical Practice. Chicago, Year Book Medical Publishers, 1982, pp 93–102.

Staheli LT: Shoes for children: A review. Pediatrics 88:371, 1991.

Weinstein S, Zavala DC, Ponseti IV: Idiopathic scoliosis: Long-term follow-up and prognosis in untreated patients. J Bone Joint Surg 63A:702, 1981.

CHAPTER 80

Sports Injuries and the Osteochondroses

JAMES G. GARRICK

A listing, much less a discussion, of common sports injuries encountered in adolescents is beyond the scope of this chapter. We have chosen, rather, to briefly outline a triage scheme for managing the injured athlete, to discuss the physician's role with the athlete and the injury, and to describe in some detail a group of problems, idiosyncratic to the adolescent athlete—the osteochondroses—and their relationship to sports and recreational activities. The management of chronic knee pain and acute ankle injury is addressed in Chapter 82.

TRIAGE OF SPORTS INJURIES

(see Chapter 81)

It would be ideal to arrive at a precise diagnosis, incorporating the exact anatomic structure involved, the precise amount of damage, and its importance in relationship to a specific athletic activity. Unfortunately this is often not possible at the first encounter; it is usually not necessary to providing informed, appropriate medical care.

Aside from the rare, life-threatening injury, there are only a few common sports injuries requiring early, specific diagnosis and urgent management. Although closed viscus injuries such as a ruptured spleen or kidney do occur in sports, their diagnosis and treatment differ little whether the injuries occur on the football field or, much more commonly, as the result of vehicular trauma.

Fractures and dislocations require some urgency in their management. The treatment of virtually all these injuries embodies the same general principles: evaluation of neurovascular integrity distal to the injury and immobilization and support until definitive treatment is available. The dictum "splint it as it lies and get help" is medically sound. Fortunately, the most common of these injuries are relatively minor, involving the fingers, and with appropriate gentle, in-line traction, can be reduced and splinted immediately. Shoulder dislocations (see Chapter 79), another common sports injury, can also often be managed acutely with traction applied by the patient utilizing the "clasped hand" method. Elbow, knee, and ankle fracture dislocations present with obvious deformity, require emergent definitive treatment, and, if accompanied by neurovascular compromise, merit immediate attempts at gentle in-line traction and reduction.

However, in sports, life- or limb-threatening injuries are the exceptions rather than the rule. The typical acute sports injury is a sprain, strain, or contusion, none of which requires an immediate, precise diagnosis to guide appropriate early management. Indeed, treatment consisting of rest, ice, focal compression, and elevation is not only appropriate but definitive for virtually all these acute athletic injuries (see Chapter 82).

The decision needs to be made as to whether an orthopedic referral is necessary. Almost without exception, those conditions requiring such a referral fulfill at least one of the following criteria:

1. Rapidly occurring and obvious swelling
2. A "pop" or "snap" heard at the time of injury
3. Obvious deformity
4. Inability to move the injured part
5. Evidence of neurovascular compromise
6. Evidence of instability (whether by history or examination)

Thus, the anterior cruciate ligament tear—exceedingly difficult for the inexperienced examiner to document—will be referred to the orthopedist appropriately by virtue of the obvious swelling within a few hours, the "pop" heard at the time of injury, and the sense of instability experienced by the adolescent. Likewise the adolescent with a nondisplaced or minimally displaced ankle fracture will be referred by virtue of the rapid onset of swelling of the ankle and the adolescent's unwillingness to move or bear weight.

For the physician interested in pursuing the topic of sports injuries in more depth, a number of texts are available, three of which are listed in the bibliography of this chapter.

INTERACTIONS WITH THE INJURED ATHLETE

Few activities in medicine offer greater potential for a truly positive physician-patient relationship than that of supervising the treatment of the injured athlete. The sports injury is an obvious problem in need of a solution. For the serious young athlete, forced cessation of sports participation may be the most threatening problem he or she has ever faced (see Chapters 81 and 82). Successful treatment of the adolescent's problem, even if it is accompanied by surgery or prolonged rehabilitation, if approached properly, will be appreciated by the adolescent and his or her family.

This positive outcome—indeed, successful treatment of the adolescent's sports injury—can be achieved only if the physician recognizes the importance of sports participation among his or her adolescent patients. All too often, in a zealous effort to protect the young patient, the physician falls prey to the antisports bias. Appropriately concerned with reports of crippling knee injuries, anabolic steroid use, harmful dietary practices, and psychological stresses associated with athletic participation (see Chapter 81), the physician may view the athletic injury as an excuse to remove the adolescent from this potentially harmful environment. Organized sports participation may well be the safest activity available to the teenager outside the classroom. Even the most hazardous interscholastic sport, football, is safer than spending a comparable amount of time behind the wheel of an automobile. Successful management of the injured athlete requires three additional factors: communication, goal-setting, and education.

Communication

First, the athlete must be apprised of the significance of the injury in the context of the sport. The majority of sports injuries are of negligible long-term medical significance. Unlike juvenile diabetes mellitus (see Chapter 59), or rheumatoid arthritis (see Chapter 90), or even pregnancy (see Chapter 74), the vast majority of athletic injuries do not have lifelong consequences. However, a medically insignificant injury can have negative effects on sports participation by the adolescent. For example, the mildly sprained wrist of a 13-year-old girl gymnast, the Osgood-Schlatter disease of a Little League catcher, or the thigh contusion in a football player all are self-limiting conditions in which a complete recovery can be expected. More important, however, they all require some limitation of athletic participation by the adolescent during treatment, and this must be clearly described to the athlete.

Minimizing the extent of the injury, based on its lack of medical severity, will destroy the athlete's confidence in the physician's judgment. Telling the gymnast that her sprained wrist is "a minor injury that should be well in a few weeks" may be medically correct but is an inappropriate comment to be made to an adolescent who now faces time off that will not only halt skill acquisition, but also result in a perceptible deterioration of conditioning and technique. It is better to acknowledge these facts and further note that continuing to work out with the symptomatic wrist not only will encourage the use of improper techniques, but also may well lead to an injury of greater significance.

Parents and coaches must also be apprised of the athlete's condition. The fact that many adolescent athletes are accustomed to seeking medical care for their athletic injuries independently or with their coaches does not absolve the physician of the medical-legal responsibility for obtaining permission to treat the ado-

lescent (see Chapter 20). Parents and especially coaches must be told of any limitations of the adolescent's activities personally. The athlete cannot (and should not) be expected to convey medical information to either his or her coaches or parents. More often than not the athlete is unwilling to tell the coach that he or she cannot practice or is unable to compete. Any limitations should be conveyed directly by the physician to the coaches or the parents, either by a phone call or written note sent by mail, not delivered by the athlete.

Working directly through the coaches also relieves the pressure perceived by the athlete to continue participation for the "good of the team." Whether real or imagined, the pressure is there, and part of the physician's duty is to protect the athlete.

Goal-setting

Athletes are accustomed to setting and achieving goals. Thus, treatment of their injuries should be organized into a series of steps measured by the attainment of realistic goals. Although the ultimate goal with any injury is the return to full participation, that should not be the only goal, since it allows no feedback regarding interim progress. For example, for the adolescent with an ankle sprain, the interim goals are cessation of active swelling, alleviation of swelling, restoration of normal motion, ability to walk without a limp, reestablishment of normal strength, ability to run without pain or a limp, and the execution of the maneuvers necessary for sport participation.

Setting goals at the onset of treatment also keeps the physician out of the athlete's "time-trap." The first question posed by most injured athletes is, "When can I play again?" An answer expressed in any dimension of time is not only inappropriate but probably erroneous. If the physician says "2 weeks," the athlete will return either in 1 week and think the physician assessed the problem incorrectly, or in 3 weeks and believe that it was treated inadequately. It is better to answer with a series of functional goals that must be first attained. The athlete will have no difficulty in understanding the necessity of regaining strength or the need to be able to walk without a limp before trying to run.

Education

Education is an important part of injury management because sometime in the future the athlete will probably be reinjured. Education will help the athlete assess and initially manage future injury problems, often minimizing severity and time loss of time. Every athlete should know that the appropriate initial treatment for any acute injury is relative rest, ice, compression, and elevation (R.I.C.E.) (see Chapter 82). These simple steps, initiated at the time of injury, can decrease disability by days or even weeks. What better time to teach this lesson to the adolescent than during the treatment of an acute injury?

Depending on the activity, overuse (i.e., gradual onset) injuries may occur as commonly as those of the acute variety. In the treatment of overuse injuries, it is essential to determine the cause. These injuries are usually the result of "training errors," the euphemism for trying to do too much too fast. Thus, a careful history of the activities and events surrounding the onset of the injury is necessary. Once it has been established that the problem occurred during activity alterations, such as, for example, beginning to practice the tennis serve for 2 hours rather than 1 hour a day, abruptly increasing daily running distance from 1 to 4 miles, or tripling the time spent working on the vault in gymnastics, it should be obvious to both physician and the adolescent that there may be a relationship between the changes in activity and the symptoms.

While the athlete with an overuse injury is being treated and returned to full athletic participation, a lesson can be taught. One can demonstrate that a more gradual approach to perfecting the tennis serve, increasing the running mileage, or acquiring additional skills in vaulting results in the attainment of these athletic goals without being reinjured and that, if the athlete had approached attaining these goals gradually in the first place, the original injury might have been prevented.

OSTEOCHONDROSES (see Chapter 79)

The osteochondroses are a group of idiopathic conditions characterized by disorderliness of endochondral ossification, including both chondrogenesis and osteogenesis, in areas of previously normal growth, that result in radiographic changes and symptoms in the growing adolescent. Because these signs and symptoms are often associated with physical activity, the conditions are often considered "sports injuries" of the overuse variety.

The osteochondroses have been described at more than 50 anatomic sites and include conditions with significant, long-term orthopedic consequences such as tibia vara (*Blount* disease) and Legg-Calvé-Perthes syndrome; acute, activity-threatening problems such as osteochondritis dissecans of the knee and elbow; and primarily radiographic observations associated with overuse injuries in the young athlete (Sever disease).

Clinical confusion surrounding these conditions stems from two factors: (1) They are named after the individual(s) who first described them with eponyms that impart the status of "disease" to problems of minor significance (e.g., Osgood-Schlatter disease, Freiberg disease); and (2) by definition they are associated with radiographic abnormalities that encompass the spectrum from "normal variations" to "crippling," most of which are not seen with enough frequency to allow the clinician certainty in either ignoring or acting on them. Anatomically, they can involve articular, nonarticular, or physeal surfaces. The conditions appear to be the result of pressure, as with humeral condylosis (Panner disease) or tension (Osgood-Schlatter disease) on an epiphysis.

Duthie and Houghton have characterized the osteochondroses and note that common denominators among these conditions seem to include (1) that few of the conditions can be attributed to any single etiologic agent; (2) that some degree of trauma is required to cause the disturbance in bony architecture observed on radiograph; and (3) that, in some instances, this "trauma" may be normal stress on abnormally developing bone (as in non–sports-related occurrence).

In adolescents, the osteochondroses generally occur during the growth spurt. With the exception of Freiberg disease (second metatarsal head), the conditions are more common in boys than in girls. They are rarely seen in black children and adolescents.

Duthie and Houghton speculate that during growth the rapidly dividing osteogenic cells are hypersensitive to trauma, with mild ischemia encouraging mesenchymal stem cells to differentiate into less metabolically active fibroblasts rather than osteoblasts. This effect may be heightened by the delayed appearance and maturation of growth centers (seen in males), resulting in a relatively "immature" epiphysis challenged by the demands of supporting a larger and heavier body.

From a clinical standpoint there are two important issues: (1) Does proper management require any more than treating the symptoms? and (2) What is the long-term prognosis? Implied in these questions is a determination of the importance of the "abnormal" findings on x-ray films. In some of the conditions, such as Scheuermann kyphosis, x-ray findings not only mandate treatment but also provide some insight into the ultimate prognosis.

Articular Osteochondroses

The major problem associated with primary osteochondroses is the potential for permanent deformation of not only the involved articular surface but also the other bones articulating in the joint, resulting in degenerative arthritis. Thus, the major goal in the treatment of these conditions is to minimize epiphyseal deformity.

PRIMARY ARTICULAR OSTEOCHONDROSES

Primary articular osteochondroses occur with initial involvement of articular and growth cartilage. Omer has characterized these conditions as having three stages based on radiographic findings. Initially the intra-articular and periarticular soft tissues are thickened owing to edema. The second stage is characterized by irregularity of the contour of the epiphysis, with the subcortical zone of rarefaction being thinned; the epiphysis may appear to be completely fragmented. The third, or repair, stage is characterized by replacement of the necrotic tissue. Since during this phase the structural support of the necrotic bone is compromised, the articular surface may become flattened and compressed.

The disorderliness of the epiphysis as seen on x-ray films is not a reliable prognostic sign. The destruction and subsequent repair process usually require 2 to 3 years, during which rather striking abnormalities on x-ray films persist. A better guide to prognosis is the duration of symptoms. As a general rule, the longer the symptomatic period, the longer the period of protection.

Treatment of these conditions involves protection of the affected articular surface from inordinate pressure, followed by the gradual resumption of activities. Protection is adequate if the adolescent remains symptom-free despite activity. The avoidance of symptoms must be continued through the activity-resumption phase as well.

Osteochondrosis of the Metatarsal Head (Freiberg Disease, Freiberg Infraction)

This condition is described in greater detail in Chapter 79. This section will focus only on sports-related issues.

The treatment goal is the absence of pain. This almost always involves some attenuation of athletic activities. It does not, however, necessarily mean the complete cessation of sports involvement. A soccer player, for example, may be symptomatic while playing as a forward but pain-free as a goalkeeper. Likewise, continued participation in gymnastics may produce pain, whereas competitive diving may not. If activity attenuation and metatarsal padding do not result in pain-free activity, surgical intervention may be necessary. This usually involves only the removal of osteochondral loose bodies but may, in some recalcitrant cases, involve the resection of the deformed metatarsal head as well.

Osteochondrosis of the Capitellum of the Humerus (Panner Disease)

This condition is seen almost exclusively in boys prior to puberty. The primary symptom is pain, usually accompanied by the inability to fully extend the elbow comfortably. Radiographs reveal fragmentation of the entire capitellum. It should be noted that Panner disease is a distinct entity not to be confused with osteochondrosis dissecans of the capitellum, commonly known as "Little Leaguer" elbow, which is discussed further on.

Treatment is aimed at alleviation of pain. During the acute phase this may include the use of a sling or posterior splint for a few weeks. Subsequently activities are graduated to allow freedom from discomfort. Because complete regeneration of the epiphysis may require from 1 to 3 years, treatment may result in a significant compromise in certain athletic activities for a prolonged period of time. Thus, even though the condition may begin before puberty, it can still affect the performance of the pospubertal adolescent. Those activities in which the upper extremities are used as "weight-bearing appendages" present at least a theoretically enhanced level of danger; thus, gymnastics, wrestling, and weightlifting all should be approached with caution. Likewise, throwing activities, such as baseball, may place inordinate pressure on the lateral side of the elbow and should be considered with caution.

This condition usually has a generally benign course and results in minimal or insignificant deformity of the adult capitellum. Repeated trauma to the regenerating epiphysis can, however, result in appreciable deformity and disability.

SECONDARY ARTICULAR OSTEOCHONDROSES

Secondary articular osteochondroses are the result of epiphyseal necrosis and, if long-standing or progressive, may affect both osteogenesis and chondrogenesis. Legg-Calvé-Perthes syndrome is the classic example of this condition. However, because Legg-Calvé-Perthes syndrome is frequently not associated with sports participation, it is discussed in detail in Chapter 79.

OSTEOCHONDROSIS DISSECANS

Osteochondrosis (osteochondritis) dissecans is a group of conditions of unknown origin that share in common the separation of an abnormal ossification area within an epiphysis covered by articular cartilage. Pappas, considering chronologic and skeletal ages, radiographic appearance, symptoms, and prior treatment, has classified these conditions into three categories, the first two of which present during early to late puberty. Such categorization applies to the various anatomic locations where this condition is found and offers diagnostic and prognostic guidelines.

Category I includes children through the age of early puberty (skeletal ages of 11 years for girls and 13 for boys). Although many times these adolescents present with activity-related aching pain or swelling caused by effusion, this condition may also be identified on radiographs taken for other reasons. If the symptoms have been present for more than a few days, examination may reveal muscle atrophy and weakness as well as limitation of motion. At this age there is a higher incidence of bilateral involvement. The prognosis for healing in this group is excellent.

Treatment of patients in category I is aimed at alleviation of the symptoms and usually involves some (temporary) attenuation of the symptom-producing athletic activities. During this period of decreased activity the adolescent should be placed on a comprehensive rehabilitation program aimed at reestablishing normal strength, endurance, and flexibility. The employment of such a program not only enhances the likelihood of an ultimate safe return to sporting activities but also occupies the idle time created by the temporary decrease in athletic activities.

Category II includes girls with a skeletal age between 12 and 20 years and boys between 14 and 20 years (sexual maturity rating of 3 to 5). Although x-ray films of young people of these ages may reveal open physes, their contribution to longitudinal growth is in its terminal phase. Like those in category I, these adolescent patients usually appear with complaints of pain and swelling. Occasionally the symptoms appear abruptly with little provocation and are accompanied by a sudden loss of motion ("locking"). Such circumstances demand a more aggressive management, because they often signify detachment of a fragment of the joint surface.

Although the "minor trauma" often associated with the repetitive actions of athletic activities has not been documented as the "cause" of these conditions, the association is often evident in the clinician's office. Thus, osteochondrosis dissecans affecting the knee or the ankle is often associated with running and jumping sports such as soccer or basketball, whereas the elbow is most frequently affected in association with throwing or weight-bearing activities such as baseball or gymnastics, respectively. Although this relationship may represent nothing more than an indication of intolerance of a diseased joint to the forceful, repetitive actions demanded by athletic endeavors, it cannot be ignored because the primary goal of treatment is the absence of symptoms. Treatment must, therefore, include the cessation of specific athletic activities.

Patients with category II and III osteochondrosis dissecans lesions should be referred to an orthopedic surgeon. Surgical intervention may be necessary depending on the integrity of the fragment or the continuity of the overlying articular cartilage. Such determinations often require radioisotope, arthrographic, or arthroscopic examinations. The indications for the various treatment options (drilling, fixation, or removal) are not always clear.

If surgical options are not employed, then the treatment requirements are similar to those for category I patients, that is, avoidance of symptom-producing activities and initiation of a comprehensive rehabilitation program.

Category III includes patients older than 20 years of age with closed physes and a sexual maturity rating of 5. Symptoms in this group are more often sudden in onset, heralding detachment of the necrotic fragment. If the fragment has not separated, x-ray films usually reveal a zone of lucency located between the sclerotic nidus of bone and the equally sclerotic base of the crater. It is the author's opinion that this category represents an asymptomatic problem arising in childhood or adolescence that becomes symptomatic in young adulthood.

Early orthopedic referral is particularly important in category III osteochondrosis dissecans. Although there are case reports of successful reimplantation of a fragment that has become a loose body, reestablishment of fragment viability appears much more likely if the condition is identified and treated prior to complete separation.

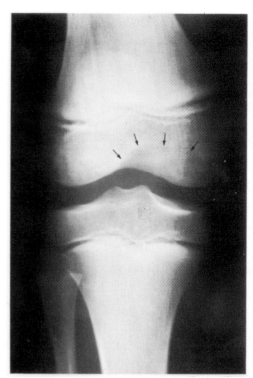

Figure 80–1. Osteochondrosis dissecans of the knee, poorly seen on standard anteroposterior radiograph.

Osteochondrosis Dissecans of the Knee (Femur)

Osteochondrosis (osteochondritis) dissecans most frequently involves the knee and, in 75% of cases, the medial femoral condyle (Figs. 80–1 and 80–2). Osteochondrosis dissecans can also involve the weight-bearing portions of either femoral condyle (10% each) or the anterior intercondylar groove or patella (5%). Since this is often a non–sports-related condition, it is discussed in greater detail in Chapter 79.

Osteochondrosis Dissecans of the Ankle (Talus)

Osteochondrosis dissecans of the talus involves either the superolateral or the superomedial aspect of the articular surface. The diagnosis of these lesions is complicated by the fact that these locations are also often the sites of fractures associated with ankle sprains that are frequently not identified on initial radiographs. By the time the condition is identified, the initiating ankle injury may have been forgotten by the adolescent. Thus, what appears to be osteochondrosis dissecans may in reality be an ununited intra-articular fracture.

This differentiation has important treatment implications. If it can be established that the lesion is osteochondrosis dissecans, it should be treated symptomatically, that is, by prohibiting only those activities that result in pain or swelling. If, however, it can be established that the condition is an ununited fracture and purely the result of trauma, then non–weight-bearing, cast immobilization is the most appropriate treatment.

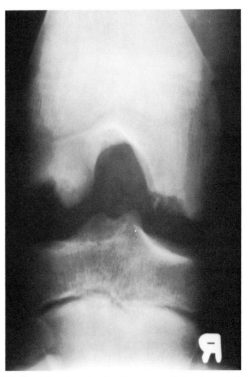

Figure 80–2. Osteochondrosis dissecans of the knee, obvious on "tunnel view" radiographs (same knee as in Fig. 80–1).

The identification of osteochondrosis dissecans of the talus is also complicated by the fact that, as in the knee, the lesion can be overlooked easily on standard radiographs (Fig. 80–3). The usual ankle x-ray series includes anteroposterior (AP), lateral, and "mortise" views, the last being an AP view with the leg internally rotated 15 to 20 degrees. All are usually taken with the ankle relaxed in a position of comfort, usually plantar-flexed. These projections place the posterior, rather than the superior, dome of the talus in profile. If this condition is suspected, it is helpful to obtain mortise views with the ankle in three positions (maximal plantar flexion, neutral, and maximal dorsiflexion), thus profiling most of the superior aspect of the talus, where the condition is likely to occur.

Adolescents with this condition usually present in one of two ways: with the gradual onset of aching pain and swelling in the ankle or with an ankle "sprain" that has continued to be symptomatic in spite of adequate treatment and rehabilitation. Although the sharp, impingement-type pain associated with loose body formation is sometimes encountered, the actual displacement of a loose body is rare because of the more constrained architecture of the ankle.

Osteochondrosis Dissecans of the Elbow (Capitellum)

Depending on the sport involvement of the adolescent, this condition is often considered as one of the variants of little leaguer or gymnast elbow. The condition usually involves the central or lateral aspect of the capitellum, which is that portion of the joint subjected to the most pressure with upper extremity weight-bearing or throwing activities.

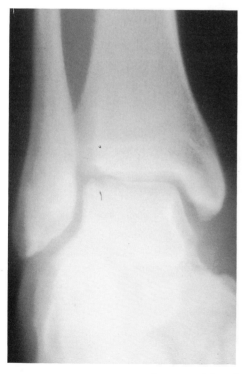

Figure 80–3. Osteochondrosis dissecans of the talus.

The usual presentation is one of activity-related, aching pain and swelling. During the examination, if a slight valgus force (i.e., gently increasing the carrying angle of the elbow) is applied while flexing and extending the elbow, one can often elicit pain at a specific point in the range of motion. This is presumably caused by the head of the radius coming in contact with the lesion.

Adolescents with osteochondrosis dissecans of the elbow seem to present for treatment later in the course of their disease than those with the condition in other anatomic sites. Perhaps this is because of the fervor and intensity with which gymnastics and baseball pitching are approached, or perhaps it is because these activities are often accompanied by more benign elbow discomfort. X-ray films often reveal well-developed lesions at the time of the first visit to a physician.

From a purely medical standpoint, osteochondrosis dissecans of the elbow is treated in the same manner as this condition is elsewhere in the body. Unfortunately, from the adolescent's perspective, the activity limitation necessary to alleviate the symptoms often means avoidance of the sport (gymnastics or baseball pitching). This hiatus of a year or longer usually means that the gymnast will never return to his or her previous level of accomplishment. Thus, with the diagnosis of this condition, some effort should be made to immediately channel the athlete into a related but less "elbow-intensive" activity, such as diving for the gymnast or playing the infield for the baseball pitcher.

Nonarticular Osteochondroses

Nonarticular osteochondroses occur at sites of tendon or ligament attachment to growth cartilages (apophyses), which in turn develop bony centra (like an epiphysis) and grow by apposition. Excessive force (tension on the attached tendon or ligament) may result in disorderly growth and in local irregularity or prominence. Complicating the diagnosis of these conditions is the fact that apophyseal irregularities on radiographs are very common in growing children and adolescents. Thus, such irregularities must be combined with symptoms for a "disease" to exist.

Treatment of these conditions is also primarily symptomatic. However, because of the insidious onset of nonarticular osteochondroses, adolescents with these problems have often been symptomatic for weeks or months prior to being seen by the physician. The activity alterations resulting from even minimal symptoms often result in a loss of muscular strength and flexibility. Thus, treatment must include rehabilitation to reestablish both strength and flexibility of the involved muscles.

Although difficult to document epidemiologically, all of the "traction osteochondroses" seem to be more prevalent during periods of rapid growth. We describe this to athletes and parents as the "bones outgrowing the muscles," and indeed these conditions do seem to be associated with a relative loss of flexibility of the involved muscles. Such an explanation seems to make it easier for the athlete to accept the need for the stretching and strengthening program, even if there is not actually a cause and effect relationship.

Osteochondrosis of the Tibial Tuberosity (Osgood-Schlatter Disease)

Osgood-Schlatter disease is the most well recognized of these conditions. Although the nidus for this apophysis forms at about age 7, the condition is usually not seen until early puberty, when through traumatic overuse adolescents sustain either microtearing of the fibers of the attachment of the quadriceps tendon from the epiphysis or partial separation of the physis. It is much more common in males than in females and occurs during the growth spurt. Adolescents present with activity-related pain well localized to the region of the tibial tuberosity. As with other overuse injuries, the symptoms are usually ignored until they result in compromised athletic performance or are present with the activities of daily living. Thus, when the athlete presents to the physician he or she is often limping and has a grossly swollen and exquisitely tender tibial tuberosity. Occasionally the local reaction is so severe as to suggest the presence of an infection, fracture, or tumor.

Radiographs often show foci of ossification in the distal portion of the patellar tendon or fragmentation of the apophysis (Fig. 80–4). Although such changes are also associated with an increased prominence of the tibial tuberosity, they usually bear little relationship to the severity of symptoms. A badly fragmented tibial apophysis raises concerns about the strength of the attachment of the tendon and the quadriceps mechanism. Ruptures or avulsions of the tendon are exceedingly rare, partially owing to the fact that only a portion of the tendon inserts into the apophysis, the remainder inserting directly into the tibia.

Temporary avoidance of symptom-producing activi-

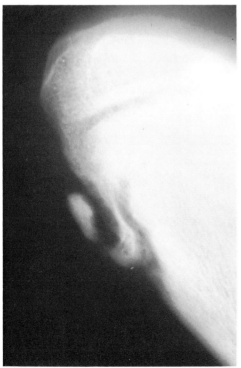

Figure 80–4. Ossification in the distal portion of the patellar tendon or fragmentation of the apophysis.

ties, the application of ice, and the administration of nonsteroidal anti-inflammatory medications constitute the immediate treatment for this condition. Intralesional corticosteroids have no place in treatment. Quadriceps strengthening and stretching exercises should be initiated as soon as they can be accomplished painlessly. Athletic activities can be resumed when they can be accomplished comfortably and both the strength and the flexibility of the quadriceps are equal to the uninjured side. Local trauma to the now-prominent tibial tuberosity can be avoided by the use of a donut-shaped pad over the affected area. Although the condition generally becomes quiescent once the proximal tibial growth plate closes, surgical excision may be required of ossicles in the infrapatellar tendon that fail to unite with the underlying tibia.

Osteochondrosis of the Patella (Sinding-Larsen Syndrome)

This condition might be viewed as Osgood-Schlatter disease of the patella, since the entire patella is actually an epiphysoid bone. The condition is characterized by fragmentation of the inferior aspect of the patella and is treated similarly to Osgood-Schlatter disease.

Osteochondrosis of the Medial Epicondyle of the Humerus (Little Leaguer Elbow)

The medial epicondyle of the humerus is the site of attachment for not only the medial collateral ligament of the elbow but also the common flexor tendon. Thus, the traction producing this osteochondrosis is both passive, from valgus forces applied to the ligament, and active, from muscular activity. Although the ossification center appears between ages 6 and 9 years, the clinical problem is usually not manifested until early puberty.

The condition presents most commonly as activity-related pain and localized swelling over the medial epicondyle in young baseball pitchers. Radiographs may reveal widening of the apophyseal line and fragmentation, but most often simply reveal enlargement of the apophysis. Treatment is symptomatic and generally less prolonged than that for osteochondrosis of the articular surface of the capitellum (Panner disease).

Osteochondrosis of the Calcaneus (Sever Disease)

The traction apophysis to which the Achilles tendon is attached appears between ages 5 and 12 years. The clinical condition is usually seen in boys 10 to 12 years old who are involved in running sports such as soccer and, to a lesser extent, football or basketball. Surprisingly, the condition is less frequent than might be expected in young cross-country running participants (perhaps because they are relatively few in number).

The mechanism of injury is chronic strain of the attachment of the Achilles tendon to the os calcis epiphysis. Thus, the athlete presents with heel pain on the inferior, posteroinferior, or posterolateral aspect of the calcaneus. The calcaneus is usually tender and occasionally swollen. Often the young athlete attributes his or her symptoms to pressure from the shoe. Radiographs are of little value because of the myriad normal configurations of the calcaneal apophysis.

In addition to local treatment, twice daily Achilles tendon stretching exercises, and strengthening exercises directed at the calf musculature, the use of a small (⅜ inch) heel lift in the shoe is often helpful. Most cleated athletic shoes (e.g., soccer and football) have a flat heel, unlike the raised heel found in the running or all-purpose athletic shoes worn for daily activities. Thus, during athletic participation, the Achilles tendon and the attached apophysis are subjected to more stretch and tension than what they normally experience. A heel lift relieves some of this tension.

Osteochondroses of the Vertebrae (Scheuermann Disease)

The irregularity of the superior and inferior borders of the vertebrae, narrowing of the disk space, wedging of at least 5 degrees of one or more vertebrae, and an increase beyond normal (25 to 40 degrees) of the kyphosis present in a growing adolescent with osteochondroses of the vertebral bodies generally result in painful roundback. Although more common in boys than in girls, it is not generally associated with activity. It is described in greater detail in Chapter 79.

BIBLIOGRAPHY

Bradford DS: Vertebral osteochondrosis. Clin Orthop 158:83, 1981.
Brower AC: The osteochondroses. Orthop Clin North Am 14(1):99, 1983.
Duthie RB, Houghton GR: Constitutional aspects of the osteochondroses. Clin Orthop 158:19, 1981.
Garrick JG, Webb DW: Sports injuries. Philadelphia, WB Saunders, 1990.
Micheli LJ (ed): Pediatric and Adolescent Sports Medicine. Boston/Toronto, Little, Brown, 1984.
Omer GE: Primary articular osteochondroses. Clin Orthop 158:33, 1981.
Pappas AM: Osteochondrosis dissecans. Clin Orthop 158:59, 1981.
Siffert RS: Classification of the osteochondroses. Clin Orthop 158:10, 1981.
Sullivan JA, Grana WA (Ed): The Pediatric Athlete. Park Ridge, IL, American Academy of Orthopedic Surgeons, 1990.

CHAPTER 81

Sports Medicine

ROBERT A. PENDERGRAST, JR., and WILLIAM B. STRONG

Several trends have been evident in recent years: (1) an increased number of young people are participating in organized sports, (2) an increased number of women are participating in previously male-dominated sports, and (3) there is a societal preoccupation with professional sports. These trends influence the practice of adolescent sports medicine in the physician's office.

The physician involved in adolescent sports medicine has at least three major responsibilities. The first is to advise adolescents, parents, and coaches on the development of sports programs that are based upon the principle of maximizing enjoyment and satisfaction for all adolescent participants. The second is the prevention of catastrophic events (severe injuries with lifelong morbidity), and the third is the treatment and rehabilitation of injured athletes. The focus of this chapter is on organized athletic activity rather than on casual recreational activity.

DEVELOPMENTAL PERSPECTIVES

Biologic Issues

The progression of linear growth and pubertal development and their variations according to chronologic age have been reviewed in previous chapters (see Chapters 4 and 5). Participants in adolescent sports activities should be grouped according to their size and maturational level rather than by their chronologic age. For example, the skeletal muscle mass of a late-maturing 15-year-old boy is considerably less than that of his early-maturing classmate. This variation in normal development may place the late-maturing 15-year-old boy at increased risk for injury if he were to play with more mature 15-year-olds. Thus, it is important to include sexual maturity ratings (SMR) as a standard part of the preparticipation athletic examination (see Chapter 5). During the phase of most rapid skeletal growth, usually at SMR 3 to 4, the young person is at particularly high risk for injury to the growing ligaments and to the epiphyses. Specific orthopedic injuries related to rapid adolescent growth are covered in the other chapters in this section.

The physiologic maturity of the neuromuscular system is generally complete by late childhood. Even though children can be taught a variety of sports-related motor skills, not all adolescents are able to integrate fundamental neuromuscular skills into complex motor activi-

ties demanded by certain athletic events. Adolescents who are limited in their neuromuscular skills should be directed to activities in which they can succeed, rather than to sports that make them feel incompetent and for which they do not have the requisite skill.

Cardiopulmonary capacity and maximal oxygen uptake increase during adolescence. Adolescents, unlike younger children, demonstrate an effect of training on cardiopulmonary capacity beyond that expected from growth alone. After the age of peak growth velocity, athletic training is associated with increased maximal oxygen uptake. Prior to puberty, training is likely to have little effect on aerobic capacity.

Some women athletes experience amenorrhea. The exact cause is unknown but may be associated with generally poor nutritional status or weight loss, or both. The emphasis on the pursuit of thinness among ballet dancers, gymnasts, and long-distance runners can be associated with deficient nutrition even without the development of anorexia nervosa (see Chapter 60). Adolescent women athletes who are amenorrheic may experience decreased bone mineralization, which may not be totally reversible with the resumption of normal menses and nutrition. The most appropriate therapy is to improve nutritional intake and temporarily decrease the intensity of the exercise; the usefulness of supplemental estrogen remains unproved.

There has been concern that serious or permanent harm to the developing breasts of the female could result from athletic activities. There is no evidence that there is any increased incidence of traumatically induced breast abscesses or other serious breast disease in young women participating in competitive athletics. Discomfort due to excessive motion of the breast during jogging or with other physical exercise can hinder young women from participating in fitness activities. These symptoms can be minimized by the use of specially designed sport bras that minimize vertical displacement of the breast by utilizing a fabric that is only minimally elastic and that pulls the breasts close to the body (see Chapter 77).

Adequate nutrition for the developing adolescent athlete is of importance. "Health foods," especially protein supplements and amino acids, are potentially harmful to the growing adolescent athlete. The diet for an adolescent athlete should be the same as for a nonathletic adolescent, that is, the American Heart Association Prudent Diet (see Chapter 49). Adolescents participating in strenuous physical activity require an increased intake of water and calories, but additional food supplements are not necessary. Calcium and iron supplementation may be valuable.

Iron deficiency anemia, as well as iron deficiency without anemia, has been associated with reduced exercise capacity. Supplemental iron can reverse these changes and can lead to improved athletic performance even in iron-deficient athletes who are not anemic. The growing adolescent, because of rapidly increasing red cell mass, requires adequate iron intake. A discussion of adolescent nutrient requirements, physical activity, and performance can be found in Chapter 7.

The adolescent with a single paired organ must take special precautions. Although he or she may be capable of vigorous physical activity, there is risk for loss of the remaining organ. The adolescent who has a single kidney should not participate in collision sports. Adolescent males who have a single testicle should be advised to wear a protective cup during collision sports but should not be excluded from any sports. Protective glasses should be strictly enforced for young people who have uncorrectable poor vision in one eye, the most common paired-organ defect.

Psychosocial Issues

A primary task of adolescence is that of establishing independence from the family of origin and developing one's own unique identity (see Chapter 9). The need to become competent and master skills can be fulfilled, in part, by participation in athletic events. It is generally believed that competence in athletic activities can be an enhancement to adolescent self-esteem.

As young people make independent choices about the use of their time and their energy, many will choose organized athletics as a means of expressing their identity and competence. If this philosophy is consistent with those of their families, there usually is no major conflict between them and the family. Structured family times together, during which time parents and siblings attend athletic events, can be a positive experience for all involved. However, if all the family's interests are centered on the adolescent athlete, while the needs of siblings are ignored, problems may arise. There are situations in which the adolescent disagrees with the family regarding the value of participation in sports. In some families the adolescent may believe the sport is important, but the family may not, and in others, the reverse may be true.

Chronically ill adolescents may be able to master athletic events with adaptation for their specific chronic illness or disability. For example, adolescents who have diabetes mellitus need to learn about balancing exercise and their ongoing nutritional and insulin regimens. Modification of the rules for winning and decreasing the level of competitiveness may be necessary for some disabled young people in order to decrease their sense of failure and helplessness. Progress has been made in this area, especially for mentally handicapped individuals, since the first Special Olympics were held in Chicago in 1968.

Many adolescents discontinue athletic participation each year. This is an area of current research. Although the reasons are not entirely clear, some young people may find the necessity of employment, changing interests, increasing academic demands, or time constraints more important than their participation in athletics. There are young people, however, who are superior athletes who "burn out" as the increasing demands of athletic performance exceed the self-perceived competence of the young person. Unfortunately, the burn-out syndrome may be accompanied by depression, anxiety, and signs of psychological stress (see Chapter 100).

CLINICAL SPORTS SYNDROMES

Both orthopedic and cardiac conditions related to sports participation have been covered in their respective sections in orthopedics and cardiology (see Chapters 46, 79, 80 and 82).

Exercise-Induced Bronchospasm

Management of exercise-induced bronchospasm is a problem for the adolescent athlete and the physician (see Chapter 43). Adolescents complaining of cough, dyspnea, or wheezing with exercise may have significant exercise-induced bronchospasm but in the office may be completely asymptomatic and have normal peak expiratory flow. If the physician has any doubt about what is happening, a trial of medication is warranted. (Medications prohibited and allowed by the International Olympic Committee are listed in Table 81–1). A β-adrenergic agent given by metered-dose inhaler (albuterol, metaproterenol) immediately before exercise is the treatment of choice. Oral agents are not nearly as effective and are associated with more side effects. Inhaled cromolyn sodium is slightly less effective when used alone but may be useful as a second medication if β-adrenergic inhalants are not effective alone. Adolescents who have exercise-induced bronchospasm should

TABLE 81–1. Asthma and Stimulant Medications Prohibited and Allowed in 1990 by the International Olympic Committee

PROHIBITED	ALLOWED
Albuterol (oral)	Aminophylline (theophylline)
Caffeine*	Inhaled β-agonists
Ephedrine	Bitolterol
Isoetharine HCl	Metaproterenol
Isoproterenol	Salbutamol (albuterol)
Metaproterenol (oral)	Terbutaline
Phenylephrine	Cromolyn sodium
Phenylpropanolamine	Inhaled corticosteroids
Propylhexedrine	
Pseudoephedrine	
Corticosteroids (oral)	
Terbutaline (oral)	

*Caffeine is considered a stimulant at levels sufficient to give 12 μg/ml in urine.

For additional information, the US Olympic Committee provides a drug control hotline (1-800-233-0393).

Adapted from Hulse E, Strong WB: Preparticipation evaluation for athletics. Pediatrics in Review 9:173, 1987. Reproduced by permission of Pediatrics.

be given a specific prescription for warm-up exercises prior to participation in the athletic event. This should include vigorous exercise 45 minutes to 1 hour prior to the event, consisting of either exercise to the point of inducing mild wheezing or several consecutive 10-second sprints. Either activity should induce a refractory period for the event itself.

Fluid and Electrocyte Disturbances

Fluid and electrolyte problems are common concerns. The physician's chief concern is the prevention of acute or chronic dehydration. Loss of body water through sweating can exceed 1 L/hour/m^2 of body surface area. It is not sufficient to rely on the thirst response to replace losses occurring during an athletic event. Coaches and athletic trainers should monitor the body weight of each athlete before and after practices and games and ensure that 16 ounces of water is replaced for each pound of body weight loss during exercise. An adolescent athlete who loses 2% to 3% of body weight through acute water loss during exercise is at increased risk for heat-related injury, including circulatory collapse. For most purposes, water alone is a sufficient rehydration fluid. However, hypotonic fluids containing small concentrations of sugar and electrolytes may enhance water absorption. Most commercially available "sports drinks" should be diluted with water to reach a suitably low osmolality.

The use of salt tablets during athletic activity should be strongly discouraged. Only small amounts of sodium and chloride are lost in the large volumes of water lost through sweat. Adolescent athletes who are already at risk for dehydration should not aggravate the condition by ingesting hyperosmolar solutions or salt.

Another area of concern for fluid imbalance is that of the adolescent wrestler who is attempting to "make weight"; this often involves intentional dehydration prior to an event to allow the wrestler to compete in a lower weight class. Extreme fluid restriction or laxative and diuretic use is employed by some young athletes and may lead to acute and chronic dehydration. Besides increasing the adolescent athlete's risk for heat-related injury, dehydration also reduces endurance and athletic performance, defeating the adolescent's purpose for weight loss. Athletes as well as coaches should be warned of the danger and futility of this practice. In addition, it gives the wrong message to the athlete that "being in shape" and "winning" are more important than the young person's health.

Central Nervous System Injuries

Central nervous system injury may be identified during the preparticipation examination or during an athletic event itself. Catastrophic cervical spine injuries are rare, but it is estimated that 20% of high school football players experience concussions during each season. The "concussion syndrome" is defined as any temporary impairment of neurologic functioning immediately fol-

lowing a blow to the head. This definition does not require loss of consciousness as part of the syndrome.

Recommendations regarding the management of concussions are based largely on "expert opinion" rather than on empirical data. If the preparticipation examination reveals a history of concussion during the previous athletic year, but the athlete is currently asymptomatic neurologically and cognitively, he or she should be allowed to participate in sports. During an athletic event, any concussion with symptoms lasting longer than 15 minutes should result in removing that player from participation for the duration of the game. Any player removed from a game because of a concussion should have a neurologic evaluation prior to returning to play. Any athlete who has persistent neurologic or cognitive symptoms from a previous concussion should not be allowed to return to play in contact sports because of the risk of fatal cerebral edema following another blow to the head.

Performance-Enhancing Substance Use

The use of chemical substances or ergogenic aids to enhance athletic performance should be condemned at all levels of sports at all ages; their use is particularly problematic in adolescents because of the serious health risks involved. A variety of stimulant medications are abused, including caffeine and amphetamine derivatives. Excessive doses of these medications can be associated with hypertension, other adverse cardiovascular effects, and seizures. It is also hypothesized that these medications contribute to increased aggressiveness on the playing field, perhaps leading to injuries as a consequence of risk taking.

Anabolic steroids are also used very commonly among athletes, and recent data indicate a trend toward decreasing age at first use of anabolic steroids. The International Olympic Committee on Drugs banned the use of anabolic steroids in 1976, and the American College of Sports Medicine published a position paper against

TABLE 81–2. Potential Adverse Effects of Anabolic Steroids

HEPATIC
Impaired excretory function
Peliosis hepatis
Benign and malignant tumors
CARDIOVASCULAR
Hypertension
Decreased high-density lipoprotein cholesterol
Myocardial changes (animal studies)
ENDOCRINE/REPRODUCTIVE
Impaired glucose tolerance
Oligospermia, decreased testicular volume
Menstrual irregularities, virilization
Premature epiphyseal closure
Acne, temporal hair recession
PSYCHOLOGICAL
Euphoria during period of use
Aggressive behaviors
Increased libido
Mood swings

SPORTS PARTICIPATION HEALTH RECORD

This evaluation is only to determine readiness for sports participation. It should not be used as a substitute for regular health maintenance examinations.

NAME _____ AGE _____(YRS) GRADE _____ DATE _____

ADDRESS _____ PHONE _____

SPORTS _____

The Health History (Part A) and Physical Examination (Part C) sections must both be completed, at least every 24 months, before sports participation. The Interim Health History section (Part B) needs to be completed at least annually.

PART A — HEALTH HISTORY:
To be completed by athlete and parent

 1. Have you ever had an illness that: YES   NO
    a. required you to stay in the hospital? ____ ____
    b. lasted longer than a week? ____ ____
    c. caused you to miss 3 days of practice
       or a competition? ____ ____
    d. is related to allergies?
       (ie, hay fever, hives, asthma, insect stings) ____ ____
    e. required an operation? ____ ____
    f. is chronic? (ie, asthma, diabetes, etc) ____ ____

 2. Have you ever had an injury that:
    a. required you to go to an emergency room
       or see a doctor? ____ ____
    b. required you to stay in the hospital? ____ ____
    c. required x-rays? ____ ____
    d. caused you to miss 3 days of practice
       or a competition? ____ ____
    e. required an operation? ____ ____

 3. Do you take any medication or pills? ____ ____

 4. Have any members of your family under age
    50 had a heart attack, heart problem, or
    died unexpectedly? ____ ____

 5. Have you ever:
    a. been dizzy or passed out during or after
       exercise? ____ ____
    b. been unconscious or had a concussion? ____ ____

 6. Are you unable to run 1/2 mile (2 times
    around the track) without stopping? ____ ____

 7. Do you:
    a. wear glasses or contacts? ____ ____
    b. wear dental bridges, plates, or braces? ____ ____

 8. Have you ever had a heart murmur, high
    blood pressure, or a heart abnormality? ____ ____

 9. Do you have any allergies to any medicine? ____ ____

10. Are you missing a kidney? ____ ____

11. When was your last tetanus booster? _____

12. **For Women**
    a. At what age did you experience your first menstrual
       period? _____
    b. In the last year, what is the longest time you have
       gone between periods? _____

EXPLAIN ANY "YES" ANSWERS _____
_____
_____
_____

I hereby state that, to the best of my knowledge, my answers to the above questions are correct.

Date _____

Signature of athlete _____

Signature of parent _____

PART B — INTERIM HEALTH HISTORY:
This form should be used during the interval between preparticipation evaluations. Positive responses should prompt a medical evaluation.

 1. Over the next 12 months, I wish to participate in the
    following sports:
    a. _____
    b. _____
    c. _____
    d. _____

 2. Have you missed more than 3 consecutive days of partici-
    pation in usual activities because of an injury this past year?
    Yes _____ No _____
    If yes, please indicate:
    a. Site of injury _____
    b. Type of injury _____

 3. Have you missed more than 5 consecutive days of participa-
    tion in usual activities because of an illness, or have you had
    a medical illness diagnosed that has not been resolved in
    this past year?
    Yes _____ No _____
    If yes, please indicate:
    a. Type of illness _____

 4. Have you had a seizure, concussion or been unconscious for
    any reason in the last year?
    Yes _____ No _____

 5. Have you had surgery or been hospitalized in this past year?
    Yes _____ No _____
    If yes, please indicate:
    a. Reason for hospitalization _____
    b. Type of surgery _____

 6. List all medications you are presently taking and what condi-
    tion the medication is for.
    a. _____
    b. _____
    c. _____

 7. Are you worried about any problem or condition at this time?
    Yes _____ No _____
    If yes, please explain: _____
    _____
    _____
    _____

I hereby state that, to the best of my knowledge, my answers to the above questions are correct.

Date _____

Signature of athlete _____

Signature of parent _____

Figure 81–1. Preparticipation examination form. (Courtesy of American Academy of Pediatrics.)

Part C – PHYSICAL EXAMINATION RECORD

NAME _____ DATE _____ AGE _____ BIRTHDATE _____

Height _____   Vision: R _____/_____, corrected _____, uncorrected _____

Weight _____   L _____/_____, corrected _____, uncorrected _____

Pulse _____ Blood Pressure _____ Percent Body Fat (optional) _____

	Normal	Abnormal Findings	Initials
1. Eyes			
2. Ears, Nose, Throat			
3. Mouth & Teeth			
4. Neck			
5. Cardiovascular			
6. Chest and Lungs			
7. Abdomen			
8. Skin			
9. Genitalia - Hernia (male)			
10. Musculoskeletal: ROM, strength, etc.			
a. neck			
b. spine			
c. shoulders			
d. arms/hands			
e. hips			
f. thighs			
g. knees			
h. ankles			
i. feet			
11. Neuromuscular			
12. Physical Maturity (Tanner Stage)	1. 2. 3. 4. 5.		

Comments re: Abnormal Findings: _____

_____

_____

PARTICIPATION RECOMMENDATIONS:

1. No participation in: _____

_____

2. Limited participation in: _____

_____

3. Requires: _____

_____

4. Full participation in: _____

Physician Signature _____

Telephone Number _____ Address _____

American Academy of Pediatrics

Figure 81–1 *Continued*

their use in 1987. Despite these statements, most adolescents are still unable to identify the adverse affects of anabolic steroids (Table 81–2), and many are still encouraged to use them by their coaches.

Recent estimates indicate that at least 500,000 adolescents in the United States are using anabolic steroids; approximately 20% of current steroid users are obtaining these drugs legally by prescription from their physicians. Most are obtained, however, on the black market and are distributed locally through health clubs, gymnasia, and other athletic facilities. As many as one of three adolescents using anabolic steroids take them primarily for the purpose of enhancing their personal appearance rather than improving athletic performance. The use of steroids is more prevalent among male athletes, especially football players and weightlifters, but a small proportion of steroid users are not participating in any organized athletics. When combined with proper diet and strength training, anabolic steroids may cause an increase in muscle strength and lean body mass. They do not have any effect on aerobic capacity.

Anabolic steroids affect many organ systems adversely (see Table 81–2). Impaired hepatic excretory function and jaundice have been identified, as well as peliosis hepatis, and both benign and malignant hepatic tumors. These drugs are also associated with an increased atherogenic profile, including impaired glucose tolerance and insulin resistance, decreased high-density lipoprotein cholesterol fraction, hypertension, and cardiomyopathy in animal studies. Changes in the reproductive system include oligospermia and decreased testicular volume due to steroid-induced suppression of gonadotropin production. These reproductive effects seem to be reversible in adults, but it is unknown what their long-term effects are on the developing gonadal system of adolescents. Prolonged use also leads to premature epiphyseal closure, possibly shortening ultimate adult height. Psychological effects of anabolic steroids include increased libido, mood swings, aggressive behaviors, and a euphoria similar to that of other drug-induced states. There is both anecdotal and epidemiologic evidence that superpharmacologic doses of anabolic steroids are extremely addictive both physically and psychologically.

PREPARTICIPATION EXAMINATION

Examination of the adolescent athlete prior to sports participation, the preparticipation examination (PPE) (Fig. 81–1), has several specific and somewhat limited goals. Currently there are no national guidelines for preparticipation examinations, and examination requirements vary within states. The efficacy of the PPE remains untested.

Most authorities do not believe that this is the most appropriate time for a complete health assessment (see Chapter 25).

The major goals of the PPE are (1) to detect preventable causes of catastrophic or life-threatening events, (2) to detect previous and incompletely rehabilitated injuries that can predispose to further musculoskeletal injury, and (3) to direct young athletes into sports or positions within a given sport that minimize the individual risk of injury and maximize opportunity for athletic excellence. The essential and often forgotten first step in reaching this last goal is an overall assessment of the young athlete's size and level of physical maturity (SMR) in the context of the sport or position to which he or she aspires. For example, the late-maturing or small athlete may be best to play an extra year on the "B" team rather than on the varsity team.

The superior type of PPE is the group or station examination. In this format, a large group of athletes move individually between stations that are staffed by physicians, nurse practitioners, physical therapists, and athletic trainers whose specific task is to evaluate one area of the body or one particular organ system. At the end, the record of each athlete is reviewed by a physician who makes recommendations or referrals. Group examination has the potential benefit of promoting interagency cooperation among schools, health professionals, and medical societies.

TEAM PHYSICIAN

The team physician has an important role not only in the on-site recognition and treatment of significant sports-related injuries but also in the establishment of guidelines and policies for the maintenance of a safe athletic program. Functions include (1) cooperation with coaches and referees to ensure strict enforcement of safety rules, (2) assessment of the safety of the physical environment in which athletic events occur, and (3) assessment of the appropriateness of protective equipment. These concerns should be brought to the attention of coaches and referees regularly. The team physician can provide guidelines for training for coaches and athletic trainers concerning warm-ups, stretching, first aid, and prevention of dehydration. He or she is also in a position to ensure the presence of an emergency medical system and back-up for serious injuries.

BIBLIOGRAPHY

American College of Cardiology: 16th Bethesda Conference, Cardiovascular abnormalities in the athlete: Recommendations regarding eligibility for competition. J Am Coll Cardiol 6:1186, 1985.
Braden DS, Strong WB: Preparticipation screening for sudden cardiac death in high school and college athletes. Phys Sports Med 16:129, 1988.
Goldberg L, Bents R, Bosworth E, et al: Anabolic steroid education and adolescents: Do scare tactics work? Pediatrics 87:283, 1991.
Hulse E, Strong WB: Preparticipation evaluation for athletics. Pediatr Rev 9:173, 1987.
Johnson M: Anabolic steroid use in adolescent athletes. Pediatr Clin North Am 37:111, 1990.
Larsson Y: Physical performance and the young diabetic. In Boileau RA (ed): Advances in Pediatric Sport Sciences, Vol 1. Champaign, IL, Human Kinetics Publishers, 1984.
Linder CW, DuRant RH, Seklecki RM, et al: Preparticipation health screening of young athletes. Am J Sports Med 9:187, 1981.
Nelson MA: Medical exclusion from sport. Adolescent Medicine. State of the Art Reviews 2:13, 1991.
Primos WA, Landry GL: Fighting the fads in sports nutrition. Contemp Pediatr 6:14, 1989.
Rowland TW: Iron deficiency and supplementation in the young endurance athlete. In Bar-Or O (ed): Advances in Pediatric Sport Sciences, Vol 3. Champaign, IL, Human Kinetics Publishers, 1989.
Smith NJ: Food for Sport. Palo Alto, CA, Bull Publishing, 1976.
Squire D: Female athletes. Pediatr Rev 9:183, 1987.

CHAPTER 82

Management of Common Sports Injuries

ALBERT C. HERGENROEDER

The physician who cares for adolescent athletes or for adolescents who play sports should develop comprehensive approaches to specific injuries. Understanding the mechanism of the injury, the diagnostic possibilities, and the treatment options is essential. The primary physician should consult a sports medicine specialist depending on the injury and its severity, and the experience of the primary physician. A physical therapist should be involved in the rehabilitation of many sports injuries. The purpose of this chapter is to review the basic principles of managing chronic and acute musculoskeletal injuries using patellofemoral dysfunction as an example of the former and ankle sprain as an example of the latter.

PATELLOFEMORAL DYSFUNCTION

(see Chapter 79)

Patellofemoral dysfunction (PFD), also referred to as the patellofemoral pain syndrome, is an overuse injury to the extensor-decelerator mechanism of the knee that is characterized by anterior knee pain. PFD is the most common injury seen in sports medicine clinics and with ankle sprains is the most common injury diagnosed in children and adolescents. Approximately 25% to 40% of adolescents have knee pain consistent with PFD; the rate is higher in athletes. The majority of such injuries are diagnosed as Osgood-Schlatter disease, patellar tendinitis, or chondromalacia patellae. PFD is a general term that includes several diagnoses that share a similar mechanism of injury: exercise in combination with lower extremity biomechanical forces results in repetitive injury to the patellofemoral joint or its stabilizing structures.

Mechanism of Injury

Patellofemoral disorders can be classified according to cause, such as acute or repetitive trauma, patellofemoral dysplasia, osteochondritis (osteochondrosis) dissecans, and synovial plicae (Table 82–1). These categories are not mutually exclusive. For instance, repetitive trauma (which for some adolescents is simply going up and down stairs or walking) can exacerbate pain in any patellofemoral disorder. Categorizing the causes of PFD does not necessarily imply a different treatment approach for each category, since there is considerable overlap in rehabilitation of injuries in certain categories. The focus of this discussion is the etiology, evaluation, and treatment of chronic anterior knee pain due to PFD. For information on subluxation, dislocation, and other acute injuries to the patellofemoral joint the reader is referred to Chapter 79.

The stability of the patella in the femoral groove is a function of the bony and soft tissue dynamic and static stabilizers of the patellofemoral joint (Fig. 82–1). These stabilizers include the patella, the femur, the tibia, the iliotibial band, the quadriceps, the hamstring muscles and tendons, patellar retinaculum, patellofemoral and patellotibial ligaments, fat pads, and bursae. In the normal state they function to maximize patellofemoral contact and provide a broad surface over which to distribute the forces on the patellofemoral joint. This force distribution is a function of the shape of the femoral groove and the patella, the position of the patella, and the function of the stabilizers. The forces on the patellofemoral joint are depicted in Figure 82–2. The vastus medialis generates a force that pulls the patella medially and is countered by the lateral static stabilizers (lateral patellofemoral and patellotibial ligaments and the lateral retinaculum) and lateral dynamic stabilizers (vastus lateralis and iliotibial tract). The vastus lateralis generates a force that pulls the patella laterally and is countered by the vastus medialis and medial static stabilizers (medial patellofemoral and patellotibial ligaments and the medial retinaculum). The rectus femoris and vastus intermedius create a force that pulls the patella in a direction parallel to the femur. The net force vector pulls the patella in a direction roughly parallel to the rectus femoris. Abnormalities in any of these structures may result in suboptimal force distribution and subsequent injury to the extensor-decelerator mechanism of the knee.

Both intrinsic and extrinsic factors contribute to PFD. Intrinsic factors include the static and dynamic stabilizers mentioned previously and malalignment of the adolescent's lower extremity. Extrinsic factors include the forces to which the patellofemoral joint are subjected as determined by the type, duration, and intensity of exercise. Many patients with the clinical diagnosis of chondromalacia patellae have no arthroscopic evidence of damage of the patellar cartilage, suggesting that

TABLE 82–1. Classification of Patellofemoral Disorders

1. Trauma (conditions caused by trauma in the otherwise normal knee)
   A. Acute trauma
      1. Contusion
      2. Fracture
         a. Patella
         b. Femoral trochlea
         c. Proximal tibial epiphysis (tubercle)
      3. Dislocation (rare in the normal knee)
      4. Rupture
         a. Quadriceps tendon
         b. Patellar tendon
   B. Repetitive trauma (overuse syndromes)
      1. Patellar tendinitis ("jumper's knee")
      2. Quadriceps tendinitis
      3. Peripatellar tendinitis (e.g., anterior knee pain of the adolescent due to hamstring contracture)
      4. Prepatellar bursitis ("housemaid's knee")
      5. Apophysitis
         a. Osgood-Schlatter disease
         b. Sinding-Larsen-Johanssen disease
   C. Late effects of trauma
      1. Posttraumatic chondromalacia patellae
      2. Posttraumatic patellofemoral arthritis
      3. Anterior fat pad syndrome (posttraumatic fibrosis)
      4. Reflex sympathetic dystrophy of the patella
      5. Patellar osseous dystrophy
      6. Acquired patella infera
      7. Acquired quadriceps fibrosis
II. Patellofemoral dysplasia
   A. Lateral patellar compression syndrome
      1. Secondary chondromalacia patellae
      2. Secondary patellofemoral arthritis
   B. Chronic subluxation of the patella
      1. Secondary chondromalacia patellae
      2. Secondary patellofemoral arthritis
   C. Recurrent dislocation of the patella
      1. Associated fractures
         a. Osteochondral (intraarticular)
         b. Avulsion (extraarticular)
      2. Secondary chondromalacia patellae
      3. Secondary patellofemoral arthritis
   D. Chronic dislocation of the patella
      1. Congenital
      2. Acquired
III. Idiopathic chondromalacia patellae
IV. Osteochondritis dissecans
   A. Patella
   B. Femoral trochlea
V. Synovial plicae (anatomic variant made symptomatic by acute or repetitive trauma)
   A. Medial patellar ("shelf")
   B. Suprapatellar
   C. Lateral patellar

With permission from Merchant AC: Classification of patellofemoral disorders. Arthroscopy 4:236, 1988.

chronic anterior knee is not related to the pathologic diagnosis of chondromalacia patellae. That is not to say that damage to the cartilaginous surface of the patella cannot cause chronic knee pain. Rather, the clinical diagnosis of chondromalacia patellae manifested as crepitus of the patella with knee flexion and extension and patellar facet tenderness is not synonymous with patellar cartilage damage on arthroscopy. Peripatellar pain might be secondary to subchondral bone injury without necessarily causing cartilage damage. One author identified peripatellar soft tissues, specifically the medial and lateral retinacula, as sites of pain in patients with patellofemoral pain.

Emphasis is now placed on patellofemoral malalignment as the principal cause of anterior knee pain in the young athlete. Patellofemoral malalignment consists of preexisting abnormalities of the patellofemoral articulation, soft tissue support of the patellofemoral joint, and malalignment of the lower extremity. Examples of patellofemoral malalignment are patella alta, femoral anteversion, external tibial torsion, pronation, genu varum and genu valgum abnormalities, and vastus medialis and lateralis weakness. Since these intrinsic factors affect the distribution of forces at and stability of the patellofemoral joint, they should be assessed in an adolescent who has PFD. However, the presence of biomechanical abnormalities cannot predict whether PFD will occur. One author reported that no single anatomic variant related to the patellofemoral joint correlated with any specific type of PFD in a group of track and field athletes and recreational joggers. Others reported that the majority of 112 patients with PFD had normal patellofemoral and long bone alignment, although malalignment was assessed only by inspection of the patellofemoral joint at rest and not with measurements such as Q-angle. They emphasized the potential role of decreased hamstring and quadriceps flexibility in some cases of PFD. Another group of authors reported no difference in Q-angle, joint mobility, genu valgum, and femoral anteversion in 446 13- to 17-year-old male and female students with and without PFD. They related the presence of anterior knee pain to athletic participation, highlighting the role of extrinsic factors (exercise) in the development of PFD.

In fact, the most frequent cause of PFD is training error and *not a specific biomechanical abnormality*. In the adolescent's history, it is common to link the onset of knee pain to some change in training. For the adolescent who has Osgood-Schlatter disease, the onset of tibial tuberosity pain may be related to the onset of a new activity but frequently follows a period of rapid height increase.

In summary, chronic anterior knee pain due to PFD is the result of a complex interaction of factors including the adolescent's lower extremity alignment and growth, the status of the static and dynamic stabilizers of the patellofemoral joint, and the forces to which the patellofemoral joint are exposed. There is no specific biomechanical abnormality or anatomic variant that predicts whether PFD will develop or the type of PFD that may develop. Training errors leading to overuse of the patellofemoral joint are the most important factors that predate the onset of PFD.

History

An adolescent who has PFD complains of anterior knee pain. This pain can be acute, as in the case of an adolescent who attempts vigorous and prolonged exercise without adequate training and develops the sudden onset of unilateral or bilateral knee pain associated with swelling. There is often no specific traumatic episode

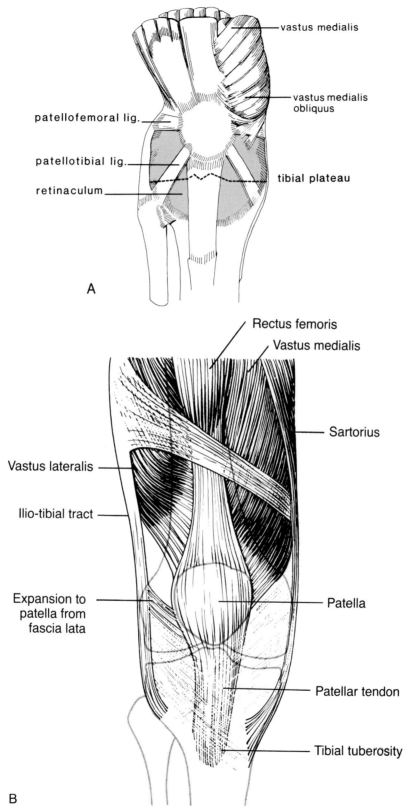

Figure 82–1. Static and dynamic stabilizers of the patellofemoral joint (see text). (*A*, With permission from Hughston JC, Walsh WM, Puddu G: Patellar Subluxation and Dislocation. Philadelphia, WB Saunders, 1984, p 10. *B*, With permission from Ficat RP, Hungerford DS: Disorders of the Patello-Femoral Joint. Baltimore, Williams & Wilkins, 1977, p 16.)

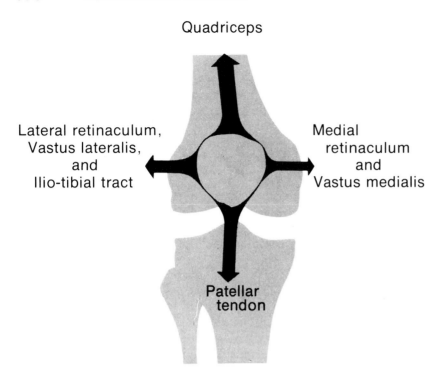

Quadriceps

Lateral retinaculum,
Vastus lateralis,
and
Ilio-tibial tract

Medial
retinaculum
and
Vastus medialis

Patellar
tendon

Figure 82–2. Forces in the frontal view on the patella with quadriceps contraction. (With permission from Ficat RP, Hungerford DS: Disorders of the Patello-Femoral Joint. Baltimore, Williams & Wilkins, 1977, p 15.)

during the sporting event that caused the symptoms, but rather a gradual onset of pain and stiffness.

More commonly the adolescent presents with weeks to months of pain, sometimes described as being "just underneath the knee cap." Swelling is not a common finding. Initially the pain occurs within a day after exercise. The pain is often made worse by going up and down stairs. If the symptoms are ignored and the exercise continues, the pain will appear progressively earlier in exercise. In the worst cases, the pain is present throughout exercise and even with normal activities of daily living. Some adolescents complain of pain and stiffness when arising after sitting for an extended time, referred to as the "theater sign." Others complain of "popping" or "snapping" when they arise from sitting, which can be a manifestation of a pathologic synovial plica. Some patients complain of the knee "giving way." If the adolescent actually falls because the knee was unstable and subsequently had swelling, then intraarticular pathology such as meniscal tears or anterior ligament insufficiency should be considered. However, more commonly the knee loses its fluid motion and the knee feels unstable, but the adolescent does not fall and there is no subsequent pain or swelling. This history is consistent with PFD.

Some well-conditioned athletes present with a 2- to 3-week history of pain that followed a change in their training. For instance, they may have abruptly started running hills or steps, longer distances, at a faster pace, on a harder surface, or with different shoes.

The adolescent with Osgood-Schlatter disease presents with pain over the tibial tuberosity that can be very debilitating (see Chapters 79 and 80). One study described 68 adolescent athletes of an average age of 13 years whose pain had caused them to stop training for an average of 3 months and had limited training for an average of 7 months. It is not uncommon for the adolescent to have been told that these are growing pains or that there is nothing that can be done and that they simply have to stop playing sports. This erroneous advice can be devastating to the adolescent athlete.

Some adolescents may report patellofemoral pain following a period of immobilization from another injury. For instance, the adolescent may have been placed on crutches for several days following an ankle injury and may favor that leg for the next week while recovering from the ankle injury. The adolescent's vastus medialis obliquus muscle will atrophy within days of being on crutches; it will atrophy even further as that leg is favored.

Physical Examination

In order to assess the bulk and tone of the quadriceps muscles, the flexibility of the quadriceps and hamstring muscles, and the lower extremity alignment, the adolescent should be examined in gym shorts or in a hospital gown. An adequate examination cannot be performed while the adolescent is wearing pants. The adolescent should also remove his or her shoes; the shoes should be inspected for wear pattern, especially if the shoes are older.

Excess pronation can contribute to PFD by increasing force dissipation to the knee. Pronation is manifested as a heavier wear pattern on the medial sole of the shoe. The adolescent's gait should be assessed both in shoes and barefoot. Abnormal foot anatomy, abnormal biomechanics, and abnormal patellar tracking should be noted. Limb lengths should be measured; a limb length discrepancy greater than 2 cm is abnormal. A useful maneuver to detect functionally significant limb length discrepancy is the "magazine test," in which a magazine is placed under the shorter leg. If the adolescent feels more balanced when standing on the magazine, a functional limb length discrepancy exists, and the adolescent may benefit from a shoe insert that would partially correct the discrepancy. If a limb length discrepancy is noted, evaluation for scoliosis should be done.

With the adolescent actively contracting the quadriceps muscle, the bulk and tone of the vastus medialis muscle should be assessed. The vastus medialis obliquus muscles must be inspected as well as palpated. Although the bulk may appear normal, the diminished tone compared with the contralateral side may indicate insufficiency on the affected side. A decrease in bulk or tone of the vastus medialis muscle is consistent with decreased dynamic medial stability of the patellofemoral joint. This vastus medialis insufficiency, especially of the vastus medialis obliquus, plays an important role in some cases of PFD, as either a primary or a secondary factor causing inadequate medial stability. However, decreases in vastus medialis muscle bulk and tone are not demonstrable in all patients with PFD.

The peripatellar region should be palpated for tenderness of the retinacula, patellar tendons, and medial and lateral patellar facets. Tenderness can be present at one or more sites. One author reported that 38% of patients referred with a diagnosis of PFD had no tenderness on examination.

In patellar tendinitis, the pain occurs along the patellar tendon; in chondromalacia patellae, the pain is on the undersurface of the patella. The undersurface of the patella is assessed best by displacing the patella laterally with the knee in full extension and palpating the lateral facet of the patella and repeating the maneuver medially.

Mobility of the patella should be assessed with the adolescent's knee flexed to 45 degrees and medial and lateral pressure applied (Fig. 82–3). Adolescents who have a previous history of patellar dislocation may become apprehensive with this maneuver and may tighten the quadriceps muscle to prevent any further displacement. Adolescents with recurrent patellar subluxation may have increased mobility in the affected knee with this maneuver compared with the movement of the other patella.

Flexibility of the hamstring muscles should be assessed; hamstring tightness has been associated with PFD. Likewise, flexibility of the quadriceps muscles should be evaluated, because quadriceps muscle inflexibility leads to increased compressive forces of the patella. However, the association of demonstrable decreased flexibility in the hamstring and quadriceps muscles in some cases of PFD does not explain the mechanism by which the interaction of hamstring and quadriceps inflexibility leads to PFD. Quadriceps muscle flexibility should be assessed with passive knee flexion and hip extension, since the rectus femoris muscle originates proximal to the hip joint and is a hip flexor as well as a knee extensor. After the physician focuses on the patellofemoral joint, the remainder of the knee examination should be completed to detect other causes of knee pain, including meniscal and ligamentous injuries that give rise to joint effusion or an unstable knee joint.

Radiologic Evaluation

Many investigators recommend that radiographs be used routinely in the evaluation of PFD. Considering the range of patellofemoral disorders outlined by Merchant, routine radiographs are indicated in some cate-

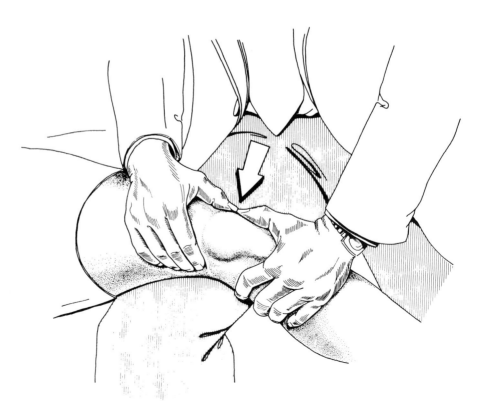

Figure 82–3. Testing for patellar hypermobility. (With permission from Hughston JC, Walsh WM, Puddu G: Patellar Subluxation and Dislocation. Philadelphia, WB Saunders, 1984, p 31.)

gories, especially those related to acute trauma, chronic subluxation, and osteochondritis dissecans. However, routine radiographs are usually not indicated in the initial assessment of chronic PFD for most adolescents unless a disorder likely to be evident on radiograph is being considered. In this instance, radiographs are confirmatory rather than diagnostic. Osgood-Schlatter disease, for instance, is a clinical diagnosis, yet many adolescents receive radiographs as part of the evaluation. The x-ray findings do little to change the adolescent's management. Radiographs are more likely to be of value in the patient with chronic PFD who is showing no improvement after 6 weeks of rehabilitation, yet has been compliant with exercise, and relative rest.

Treatment

Regardless of the adolescent's lower extremity alignment, PFD is an overuse injury of the decelerator-extensor mechanism of the knee associated with inflammation and some loss of flexibility, strength, and endurance of that mechanism. The treatment of PFD, in principle, is similar to the treatment of other overuse injuries. The treatment goals are to reduce the inflammation and restore the flexibility, strength, and endurance of the injured structures. Approximately 80% of adolescents with PFD have a satisfactory improvement with a conservative rehabilitation program as suggested.

Reduction of Inflammation. Ice should be applied directly to the sites of inflammation for 10 to 15 minutes as often as possible, but this is rarely accomplished more than twice a day. Ice should be applied after exercise, never before; exercise should be avoided for at least 1 hour after ice is applied. One indication for using nonsteroidal anti-inflammatory medication is pain with routine activities of daily living. Some adolescents with relatively acute PFD characterized by pain and swelling may benefit from electric galvanic stimulation (EGS).

TABLE 82–2. Walk-Run Program

Stretch before and after.

Ice after.

Do not do isometric or other restrengthening exercises immediately before.

Day	Run	Walk
1, 2	—	5 min
3, 4	—	10 min
5, 6	—	15 min
7, 8	—	20 min
9, 10	5 min	15 min
11, 12	10 min	10 min
13, 14	15 min	5 min
15	20 min	—

If you have pain at any point during the program, rest a day and then start again one level back.

When you begin running (day 9), run first then walk.

If the athlete has been in significant pain or not exercising for a long period of time, then consider starting with 5–10 minutes of walking, increasing one minute per day up to 20 minutes. Then start the walk-run program.

With permission from Garrick JG, Webb DR: Sports Injuries: Diagnosis and Management. Philadelphia, WB Saunders, 1990.

TABLE 82–3. Hamstring Stretch

Purpose:
To lengthen or maintain length of hamstring muscles (back of thigh)

Techniques:
Stand with feet pointing straight ahead
Position feet shoulder-width apart
Keep knees straight
Slowly bend forward
Stop at point of discomfort
Hold 6–10 seconds
Straighten up by bending knees first
Repeat 5 times

Warning:
Don't bounce
Don't bend past the point of discomfort

Relative Rest. Most adolescents who have PFD are able to walk pain-free. For those who cannot, aggressive reduction of inflammation is indicated. Immobilization by casting or by using a knee immobilizer may be associated with reduction in pain, but is also associated with atrophy and loss of flexibility of the patellar stabilizer muscles, which prevents improvement of the flexibility, endurance, and strength of the extensor-decelerator mechanism of the knee. Adolescents who have a prominent, tender tibial tuberosity benefit from an Osgood-Schlatter pad, which protects the site from direct trauma. Adolescents whose pain is worsened by walking up and down stairs should avoid stairs as much as possible until that activity is pain-free. Once the adolescent is walking pain-free, then he or she may attempt a walking-running program similar to the one outlined in Table 82–2.

Flexibility. Hamstring and quadriceps muscle stretching (Tables 82–3 and 82–4 and Figs. 82–4 and 82–5) should be initiated as long as these exercises are pain-free. The stretches should be held for 20 to 25 seconds and repeated 3 or 4 times before and after other exercise. The adolescent should feel a dull stretch, but no sharp pain (which would indicate that the muscle is

TABLE 82–4. Quadriceps Muscle Program

1. Quadriceps Stretching:
   While standing and holding onto a support, pull toes up and straight behind you. Hold the stretch for 20 to 25 seconds. Repeat 3 or 4 times. Stand erect and don't overflex the knee.

2. Quadriceps Isometric Strengthening:
   Straight leg quad sets.
      Sit long-legged, contract quads (pull the kneecap toward you). Squeeze hard. Hold for 6 seconds. Ease off. Relax 4 seconds. Repeat 10 times. Attempt 5 to 10 sets of 10 repetitions throughout the day.
   Bent knee quad sets.
      Sit in chair. Push your heel down into ground. Hold for 6 seconds. Relax 4 seconds. Repeat 10 times. Attempt 3 to 5 sets of 10 repetitions throughout the day.
   Bent knee quad isometric.
      Sit in chair. Cross involved leg behind the other leg. Push forward with involved leg and resist with the other leg, allowing no movement. Hold for 6 seconds. Relax 4 seconds. Repeat 10 times. Attempt 3 to 5 sets of 10 repetitions throughout the day.

3. Repeat quadriceps stretching.

4. Ice massage painful area for 8–10 minutes.

Figure 82–4. Hamstring stretch (see text and Table 82–3). *A*, Passive stretching. *B* and *C*, Active hamstring stretch using the quadriceps (resting and stretched positions, respectively). (Hamstring stretching is generally to be avoided with anterior cruciate ligament deficiency.) (With permission from Garrick JG, Webb DR: Sports Injuries: Diagnosis and Management. Philadelphia, WB Saunders, 1990, p 220.)

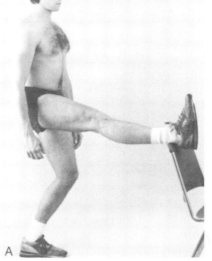

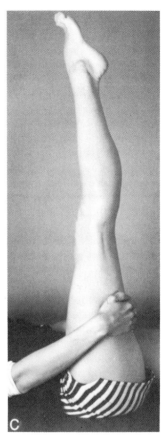

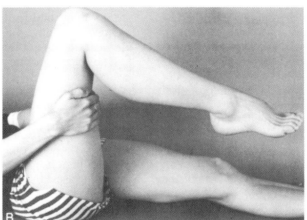

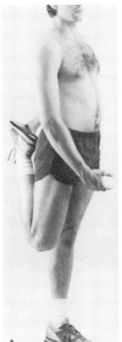

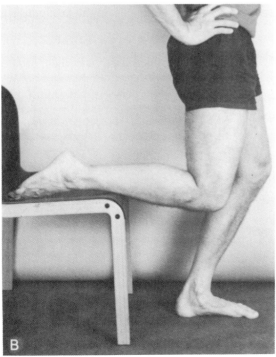

Figure 82–5. Quadriceps stretch (see text and Table 82–4). *A*, The foot is held with the opposite hand to prevent "cheating" by abducting the hip. The patient is told to emphasize extending the hip rather than flexing the knee. The stretch should be felt in the anterior aspect of the thigh, not the knee. *B*, The chair stretch is used when the knee cannot be flexed far enough to allow grasping the foot. (With permission from Garrick JG, Webb DR: Sports Injuries: Diagnosis and Management. Philadelphia, WB Saunders, 1990, p 219.)

being stretched excessively). Initially, some patients are too sensitive to stretch the quadriceps without pain. The adolescent should wait until the inflammation has decreased to the point at which he or she can stretch pain-free.

Strength. Initially, quadriceps muscle strength, especially vastus medialis obliquus muscle strength, can be increased by doing "quad sets" (isometric quadriceps contractions). Ten maximal contractions at one time should be attempted and repeated 5 to 10 times daily. The adolescent should try the quad sets in the physician's office to ensure that the exercise can be done properly. Patients whose muscles are too tender to do an adequate quad set may require a portable electrical muscle stimulator unit, which the adolescent can assist, to initiate quadriceps muscle contractions.

Endurance. Cycling and riding a stationary bike are excellent ways of increasing the strength and endurance of the quadriceps muscles. Initially the adolescent should cycle at 60 to 80 revolutions per minute (rpm) for 15 to 20 minutes with very little resistance. As they improve, the duration and intensity of the workouts can be increased. The adolescent should be fitted to the bike by adjusting the seat and handlebar height, since PFD can be worsened by cycling if the cycle is inappropriate for the patient.

Bracing. Some adolescents may benefit from a neoprene patellar stabilizing brace. One approach is to use the brace for patients who are not improving with rehabilitation and who have abnormal patellar tracking. Many of the braces are bulky and impractical, but they should provide patellar stability.

Referral

Unless the physician is able to teach the adolescent the rehabilitative exercises for PFD, the adolescent should be seen by a physical therapist. Those adolescents who have mild to moderate PFD may need only one session with the therapist to learn the program. Those with severe pain need more aggressive therapy, requiring several visits, and may benefit from an electrical muscle stimulator (EMS) unit at home. Those who have intractable pain may benefit from biofeedback in conjunction with an EMS unit. Referral to a sports medicine specialist is indicated if there is doubt about the diagnosis or if the adolescent is not improving at 8 to 12 weeks and is following the treatment plan correctly. Surgery for chronic PFD should be considered only in adolescents for whom an aggressive rehabilitation program has failed and in whom the PFD is significantly limiting their sports participation.

ANKLE SPRAINS

Ankle injuries are the most common acute musculoskeletal injury affecting adolescent athletes. Approximately 10% to 30% of all musculoskeletal injuries are ankle injuries, and 25% of playing time lost by athletes is due to ankle injuries. Basketball players have the highest rate of ankle injuries, followed by football players and cross-country runners.

Mechanism of Injury

Eighty-five per cent of ankle sprains are inversion injuries (Fig. 82–6). In inversion injuries the three lateral ligaments that support the ankle joint are vulnerable: the anterior and posterior talofibular ligaments and the calcaneofibular ligament (Fig. 82–7). During inversion, once the muscle restraints have been overcome, the force of the fall is translated primarily to the ligaments, especially the anterior talofibular ligament. The anterior talofibular ligament is the first ligament injured in inversion. If the force of the inversion continues, the second ligament injured is the calcaneofibular ligament, and finally, in severe sprains, the posterior talofibular ligament may be torn. The process may stop at any point and result in one, two, or three ligaments being torn. Only in the most severe injuries, with talar dislocation, are all three ligaments torn.

The other primary mechanism of ankle sprain is eversion, accounting for 15% of ankle injuries (Fig. 82–8). In general, these are more severe than inversion injuries because of a higher rate of fractures and disruptions of the ankle mortise, leading to instability. All but the mildest eversion ankle injuries should be evaluated by an orthopedic surgeon. The deltoid ligament is the most common ligament injured (Figs. 82–8 and 82–9). In some cases, the adolescent cannot describe the mechanism of injury, and the examiner must proceed assuming that a variety of mechanisms of injury may have occurred.

Differential Diagnosis

The most likely structure to be damaged in an ankle injury depends on the mechanism of injury and the stage

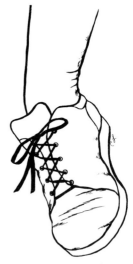

Figure 82–6. Inversion ankle injury. (With permission from Hergenroeder AC: Diagnosis and treatment of ankle sprains: A review. Am J Dis Child 144:809–814, 1990. Copyright 1990, American Medical Association.)

Figure 82–7. Lateral ligament complex of the ankle. (With permission from Hergenroeder AC: Diagnosis and treatment of ankle sprains: A review. Am J Dis Child 144:809–814, 1990. Copyright 1990, American Medical Association.)

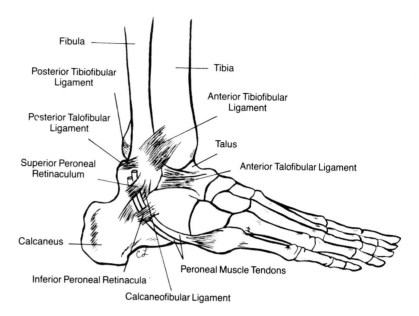

Fibula

Posterior Tibiofibular Ligament

Posterior Talofibular Ligament

Superior Peroneal Retinaculum

Calcaneus

Inferior Peroneal Retinacula

Tibia

Anterior Tibiofibular Ligament

Talus

Anterior Talofibular Ligament

Peroneal Muscle Tendons

Calcaneofibular Ligament

of sexual maturation of the adolescent. In the adolescent with open epiphyseal plates, ligaments are stronger than the epiphyses, so epiphyseal injury may occur before a ligamentous sprain. Most ankle injuries involve only ligaments. However, fractures of the talus, lateral and medial malleoli, or base of the fifth metatarsal; epiphyseal injuries; peroneal tendon subluxation; and tibiofibular syndesmosis injuries can complicate an ankle sprain. These injuries most often are diagnosed at initial presentation but should be suspected in those adolescents who show no improvement in pain, swelling, and weight bearing at 3 to 4 days into treatment. At this point further diagnostic studies should be initiated or the adolescent should be referred to an orthopedist. Indications for immediate referral include

1. Fracture (structurally significant, as opposed to a small avulsion fracture)

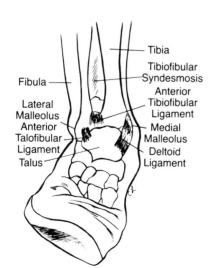

Figure 82–8. Eversion ankle injury. (With permission from Hergenroeder AC: Diagnosis and treatment of ankle sprains: A review. Am J Dis Child 144:809–814, 1990. Copyright 1990, American Medical Association.)

Tibia

Tibiofibular Syndesmosis

Anterior Tibiofibular Ligament

Medial Malleolus

Deltoid Ligament

Fibula

Lateral Malleolus

Anterior Talofibular Ligament

Talus

2. Obvious deformity
3. Evidence of neurovascular compromise
4. Wound penetrating into the joint space
5. Sudden locking of the ankle
6. Suspicion of a grade III strain (tendon rupture)
7. Syndesmotic injury

The majority of inversion sprains can be managed by the primary physician who has adequate experience in the management of musculoskeletal injuries in adolescents either in an emergency or sports medicine setting.

Physical Examination

The examination during the immediate postinjury period may be limited by swelling, pain, and muscle spasm at and around the injury site. The examination should assess for those conditions that require immediate referral.

Inspection should focus on obvious deformity and vascular integrity. Point tenderness over a bone suggests a fracture. Tenderness along the peroneal tendon posterior to the lateral malleoleus suggests a peroneal tendon subluxation. Assessment of the adolescent's gait is important; the adolescent who can walk without pain is unlikely to have a fracture or instability of the joint. If the joint has diffuse swelling and tenderness, then a radiograph is imperative, since the physical examination will be of limited value. Pain confined to the area anterior and inferior to the lateral malleolus, along the joint line in an adolescent who can weight bear, suggests that no fracture has occurred. The physician should use discretion in ordering a radiograph in this circumstance. However, if swelling and decreased range of motion are present, then a radiograph is indicated. Also, because of the possibility of an epiphyseal injury, radiographs are indicated in skeletally immature adolescents except in the mildest injuries.

When swelling is either stabilized or resolved (2 to 3 days), the adolescent should be reevaluated, since the

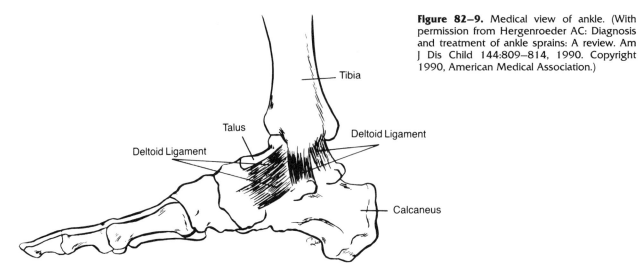

Figure 82–9. Medical view of ankle. (With permission from Hergenroeder AC: Diagnosis and treatment of ankle sprains: A review. Am J Dis Child 144:809–814, 1990. Copyright 1990, American Medical Association.)

second examination may be more useful than the first in trying to pinpoint areas of tenderness. Pain-free active range of motion of the ankle should be assessed, including dorsiflexion and plantarflexion and abduction and adduction, along with resisted range of motion for these movements. If range of motion is limited because of pain, muscle strength testing can be done from the neutral position rather than the extremes of range. This will help distinguish pain due to muscle injury or weakness from pain due to the position of the ankle.

The ankle should be palpated for bony and ligamentous tenderness. It may be difficult to distinguish between rupture of the anterior talofibular ligament and calcaneofibular ligament or between the anterior talofibular ligament and the anterior tibiofibular ligament. Finally, using passive range of motion, joint instability should be assessed. Palpable and visible displacement of the foot more than 4 mm out of the mortise is consistent with tear of the anterior talofibular ligament and the anterior joint capsule, a positive anterior drawer sign (Fig. 82–10). Asymmetry of drawer signs may be more useful than using the 4 mm criterion. In the acute state, edema and muscle spasm may prevent such displacement even with a tear of the anterior talofibular ligament. In the subacute or follow-up stage, the anterior drawer test is more useful. However, a positive anterior drawer sign in an asymptomatic adolescent with no history of ankle trauma is not indicative of ankle instability.

Adduction of the heel, the "talar tilt" (Fig. 82–11), is used to assess instability. However, because in normal uninjured ankles the degree of tilt can be from 0 to 23 degrees, it may be more useful in subjects with chronic ankle instability and recurrent ankle sprains.

The clinical classification of injury severity is confusing because there are several grading systems based on the number of ligaments injured or the severity of the ligamentous injury. The following are guidelines for grading injuries to the lateral ligament complex:

1. Mild, grade I—minimal functional loss, mild effusion, local tenderness, and mild pain to stress testing
2. Moderate, grade II—moderate functional loss with difficulty in walking and toe raising, diffuse tenderness, and moderate joint effusion
3. Severe, grade III—functional disability due to tendon rupture with marked tenderness and large joint effusion and marked decreased range of motion; crutches are required

It is likely that many adolescents who have grade I injuries do not present to physicians or they may present after some delay if symptoms persist. Clinically it is difficult to differentiate grade II from grade III ligamen-

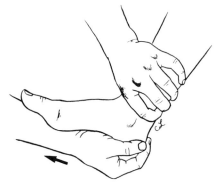

Figure 82–10. Anterior drawer test for ankle instability. (With permission from Hergenroeder AC: Diagnosis and treatment of ankle sprains: A review. Am J Dis Child 144:809–814, 1990. Copyright 1990, American Medical Association.)

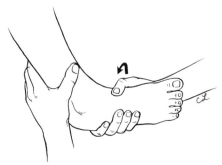

Figure 82–11. Talar tilt test for ankle instability. (With permission from Hergenroeder AC: Diagnosis and treatment of ankle sprains: A review. Am J Dis Child 144:809–814, 1990. Copyright 1990, American Medical Association.)

tous injuries. One approach is to treat all lateral ankle ligament injuries with early mobilization and air stirrup and not to do a primary repair on the first inversion injury. If obvious instability or deformity is present, then surgery is indicated.

Radiologic Evaluation

Indications for radiograph include

1. Rapidly expanding hemarthrosis
2. Obvious dislocation
3. Eversion injuries
4. Point tenderness along the talus, medial and lateral malleoli, fifth metatarsal, or proximal fibula
5. Inability to bear weight

The radiologic evaluation should include anteroposterior (AP), lateral, and mortise views. A radiograph may not be necessary in an adolescent who can walk with minimal discomfort and who has tenderness and swelling confined to an area anterior and inferior to the lateral malleolus with full range of motion. The threshold for radiographic examination of sexually immature adolescents with ankle injuries should be low because of potential epiphyseal injury. The value of stress films in the diagnosis of ankle instability is questionable. Joint instability should be determined on the basis of history and physical examination, rather than with radiographs.

Treatment of Uncomplicated Sprains

In routine sprains, the goal of treatment is to limit disability. Successful treatment is not measured merely by the absence of pain but also by return of full range of motion, strength, and proprioception. The immediate phase of treatment should be designed to limit the amount of swelling, stabilize the joint, and promote early range of motion to prevent muscle atrophy. The rehabilitative phase, which overlaps the immediate treatment phase, should be designed to return the ankle to full function.

Immediate Treatment—Early Mobilization and Air Stirrup

Adolescents who, within 36 hours following an injury, apply treatment according to the RICE (*rest, ice, compression, elevation*) mnemonic have a more rapid rehabilitation than those who do not.

Rest. Relative rest was discussed previously under patellofemoral dysfunction. If the adolescent cannot walk in a heel-toe gait without pain, crutches and instructions on appropriate usage are required until he or she can walk without pain.

Ice. Ice should be applied directly to the ankle for 20 minutes at a time, every 2 hours, if possible, during the first 1 to 2 days. Icing for longer than 20 minutes should be discouraged. Ice should be placed in a plastic bag and applied to the skin. The bag should not be put in a towel, since the towel will insulate the ankle and not promote cooling. Icing should continue until the swelling has disappeared. For athletes who present with marked swelling and muscle spasm, EGS is indicated. This will accelerate the treatment program by promoting more rapid resolution of edema.

Compression. Compression is directed to keeping fluid out of the joint space. Felt adhesive (¼ inch, cut in the shape of a horseshoe) should be placed along the medial and the lateral joint lines. An elastic tube stockette should be applied distal and proximal to the ankle joint. An elastic wrap will suffice but is not optimal. The felt and tubing are removed for icing and then replaced by the adolescent. The tubing and horseshoe pads are worn for the first 2 to 3 days until the swelling of the ankle has decreased. An air stirrup (available through medical supply houses) that allows pain-free dorsiflexion and plantarflexion but stabilizes the ankle against accidental inversion or eversion should be used (Fig. 82–12). Casting of uncomplicated sprains is not indicated.

Elevation. The affected leg should be elevated as long as possible until the swelling has stabilized.

Rehabilitation

A scheme for rehabilitation following a routine ankle sprain is depicted in Figure 82–13. By using the early mobilization program, the rehabilitation process begins immediately by limiting swelling and promoting pain-free range of motion. As soon as possible, Achilles tendon stretches are initiated (20 seconds per stretch,

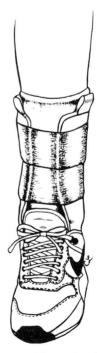

Figure 82–12. Air stirrup used for acute ankle injuries. (With permission from Hergenroeder AC: Diagnosis and treatment of ankle sprains: A review. Am J Dis Child 144:809–814, 1990. Copyright 1990, American Medical Association.)

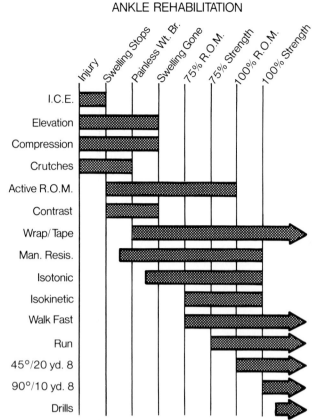

Figure 82–13. Ankle rehabilitation. Man. Resis., manual resistance; R.O.M., range of motion; Wt. Br., weight bearing. (Adapted with permission from Garrick JG: A practical approach to rehabilitation of the ankle. Am J Sports Med 9:67, 1981.)

three or four stretches before and after exercise). After the swelling stabilizes (usually within 48 hours), the adolescent can improve range of motion by tracing the letters of the alphabet for 4 minutes while the toes are in warm water, followed by 1 minute in ice water, repeating this warm-cold cycle four times. This technique is called "contrast bathing." It is crucial, however, that the adolescent knows to stop the contrast bathing if swelling of the ankle worsens. Contrast bathing may be indicated for the athlete who needs to return quickly to participation. Most adolescents can return to participation soon without the contrast bathing by simply using ice until the swelling resolves.

Once the adolescent can walk pain-free, he or she starts toe and heel walking, 5 minutes each, 1 to 2 times a day, to strengthen the ankle plantarflexor and dorsi-flexor muscle groups, respectively. Isometric ankle muscle strengthening can be initiated early in the rehabilitation, followed by specific resistance exercise using large rubber bands or an isokinetic machine. The latter might be used in better-trained athletes but is not needed for most recreational athletes. To retrain kinesthetic function to the ankle, the adolescent balances pain-free on the injured foot for 5 minutes with the eyes closed and then practices toe raises with the eyes closed while holding on to a stationary object for 2 to 3 minutes.

Another way of improving kinesthetic sense is with a "wobbleboard" (a board that balances on a round object). After the adolescent has achieved 75% range

of motion and strength, he or she starts a walk program over several days. When the adolescent is pain-free, running and sharp turning exercises can be initiated. These exercises can increase to sharper angles over several days progressively, if range of motion and strength continue to improve. If the adolescent remains pain-free, he or she can return to activity. Athletes who have ankle sprains are less likely to reinjure the ankle if they wear high-top shoes and tape the ankle.

Chronic Ankle Instability

Chronic ankle instability, in many cases, results from one of three factors, alone or in combination: (1) loss of range of motion, (2) loss of muscle strength, and (3) loss of proprioception. The described rehabilitation program is designed to avoid these causes of persistent ankle instability. If an adolescent patient presents with recurrent ankle sprains, then the three areas need to be assessed clinically and rehabilitation of any deficiencies accomplished. Involving a physical therapist in this rehabilitation is usually indicated. If sprains or signs of instability continue in spite of a concerted rehabilitation program, then mechanical instability or internal derangement, such as with a chondral fracture, needs to be ruled out and referral for surgery considered.

BIBLIOGRAPHY

Antich TJ, Randall CC, Westbrook RA, et al: Evaluation of knee extensor mechanism disorders: Clinical presentations of 112 patients. JOSPT 8(5):248, 1986.

Brostrum L: Sprained ankles, I. Anatomic lesions in recent sprains. Acta Chir Scand 128:483, 1964.

Brostrum L: Treatment and prognosis in recent ligament ruptures. Acta Chir Scand 132:537, 1966.

Brostrum L, Leljedahl S-O, Lindvall N: Sprained ankles: Arthrographic diagnosis of recent ligament ruptures. Acta Chir Scand 129:485, 1965.

Fairbank JC, Pynsent PB, Van Poortvliet JA, Phillips H: Mechanical factors in the incidence of knee pain in adolescents and young adults. J Bone Joint Surg [Br] 66:685, 1984.

Ficat RP, Hungerford DS: Disorders of the Patello-Femoral Joint. Baltimore, Williams & Wilkins, 1977.

Freeman MAR: Instability of the foot after injuries to the lateral ligament of the ankle. J Bone Joint Surg [Br] 47:669, 1965.

Garrick JG: The frequency of injury, mechanism of injury, and epidemiology of ankle sprains. Am J Sports Med 5:241, 1977.

Garrick JG, Webb DR: Sports Injuries: Diagnosis and Management. Philadelphia, WB Saunders, 1990.

Henry JH (ed): Patellofemoral problems. Clin Sports Med 8:153, 1989.

Hergenroeder AC: Diagnosis and treatment of ankle sprains: A review. Am J Dis Child 144:809, 1990.

Hughston JC, Walsh WM, Puddu G: Patellar Subluxation and Dislocation. Philadelphia, WB Saunders, 1984.

Hunter-Griffin LY (ed): Athletic Training and Sports Medicine. Park Ridge, IL, American Academy of Orthopaedic Surgeons, 1991.

James SL, Bates BT, Osternig LR: Injuries to runners. Am J Sports Med 6:40, 1978.

Merchant AC: Classification of patellofemoral disorders. Arthroscopy 4:235, 1988.

Rubin JG, Witten M: The talar-tilt angle and the fibular collateral ligaments: A method for the determination of talar tilt. J Bone Joint Surg [Am] 42:311, 1960.

Steiner ME, Grana WA: The young athlete's knee: Recent advances in injuries to the young athlete. Clin Sports Med 7:527, 1988.

Neurologic Conditions

CHAPTER 83

Epilepsy and Seizure Disorders

GIUSEPPE ERBA and ROBERT G. ZIEGLER

Epilepsy is the term used to describe recurrent paroxysmal events (seizures) due to self-activation of cerebral cortex and gray matter. The seizure manifestations vary according to the location, anatomic connections, and functions of the centers and pathways activated within the central nervous system (CNS). Consequently, an "epileptic seizure" may trigger in part or in its entirety the motor system, the sensory system, the autonomic system, the limbic system, or all of these, often in succession.

In contrast with many diseases of the CNS that are related to aging, epilepsy is predominantly a condition of youth. Epileptic seizures are always a symptom of an underlying disorder: a postinflammatory or posttraumatic scar; a malformation (vascular, glial, or neuronal); a tumor (often benign); or an intrinsic (idiopathic) disorder, presumably due to faulty neurotransmission. The last condition is genetically transmitted and is responsible for the "seizure threshold" of the individual. Although the symptoms of the disorder may not be apparent, any type of epilepsy during the first 2 decades will produce consequences that may be felt throughout life. Loss of control, which makes epilepsy so difficult to accept, is a particularly sensitive issue in adolescents struggling for competence and autonomy. Regaining control is so important that denial may be used to cope with the sense of helplessness, disappointment, or anger, which, in turn, can complicate medical cooperation. Although only recurrent seizures originating within the CNS should be called "epilepsy," any type of seizure disorder, irrespective of etiology (syncopal, metabolic, psychogenic), can be equally disruptive and requires diagnostic investigations and vigorous treatment. Therapeutic intervention varies according to the cause, and a basic understanding of how the various epileptic seizures originate and propagate allows the primary physician to initiate treatment with one of the major anticonvulsants. Thus, the first issue to be addressed in treating a seizure disorder is the differential diagnosis. Once the presence of epileptic seizures is established, the cause should be sought and, if identified, removed when possible. When the cause remains undetermined, prevention of the symptoms is the main objective. Consultation with a specialist in the field becomes necessary only in special and resistant cases.

It is important that physicians treating adolescents who have epilepsy be sensitive to the psychosocial consequences of this condition and be prepared to discuss with the patient and the family the etiology, the genetic aspects, the various remedies, and the undesirable side effects of medications. The potential limitations imposed by this disorder are most often transient. If a young patient faces the necessity of curbing important daily activities such as sports or driving, he or she may react with discouragement, rebellious and noncompliant behavior (see Chapter 26), or depression (see Chapter 100). Academic performance may drop. The treating physician is the first source of counseling and support that may preserve the adolescent's self-esteem and encourage effective coping. Should the medical therapy fail after the initial attempts, the adolescent and his or her family should be made aware that specialized centers are available for more in-depth investigations and alternative treatment (i.e., surgery). Providing education and information and sharing the plans of management both are important supports and facilitate coping with the disease and the adolescent's adaptation to treatment. The bond established between the physician and the adolescent facilitates success in the lifelong challenge of this disorder.

CLASSIFICATION

Epilepsy is best classified by referring both to the underlying condition (idiopathic or symptomatic) and to the extent of the CNS involvement (partial, unilateral, or bilateral; diffuse or generalized). The epilepsies are also classified according to the phenomenology (petit mal or grand mal epilepsy) or topography of the epileptogenic area, defined as the part of the cortex in which the seizure manifestations originate (e.g., temporal lobe epilepsy, frontal lobe epilepsy, and so on), or by the presumed mechanism (e.g., centrencephalic or cortical-reticular epilepsy). This represents an attempt to identify the CNS structures (cortical and subcortical) primarily involved during the paroxysmal event (ictus) and to define pathways of spread. Until the basic pathophysiologic mechanisms are established, the various "epileptic syndromes" are grouped according to composite criteria that take into consideration the likely pathogenesis, the findings in the electroencephalogram (EEG) and neuroimaging, the type of ictal manifestations, and the clinical characteristics (age at onset, course, and prognosis).

Classification of Epileptic Seizures

Since the manifestations of epileptic seizures are predictable according to their origin within the CNS, the

TABLE 83–1. International Classification of Epileptic Seizures

I. PARTIAL SEIZURES (seizures beginning locally)
  A. Simple partial seizures (consciousness not impaired)
    1. With motor signs
      a. focal motor without march
      b. focal motor with march (jacksonian)
      c. versive
      d. postural
      e. phonatory (vocalization or speech arrest)
    2. With somatosensory or special-sensory symptoms
      a. somatosensory (e.g., tingling)
      b. visual (usually simple hallucinations, e.g., light flashes)
      c. auditory (e.g., buzzing)
      d. gustatory-olfactory
      e. vertiginous
    3. With autonomic symptoms or signs (epigastric sensations, pallor, sweating, flushing, piloerection, pupillary dilatation)
    4. With psychic symptoms (disturbance of higher cortical functions)
      a. dysphasic
      b. dysmnesic (e.g., déjà vu, jamais vu)
      c. cognitive (e.g., dreamy states, distortion of sense of time)
      d. affective (fear, anger, etc.)
      e. illusions (perceptual distortions such as micropsia, macropsia, hyperacusis)
      f. structured hallucinations (e.g., music, scenes)
  B. Complex partial seizures (with impairment of consciousness)
    1. Beginning as simple partial seizures and progressing to impairment of consciousness
      a. with no other features
      b. with features as in I.A.1–I.A.4
      c. with automatisms
    2. With impairment of consciousness at onset
      a. with no other features
      b. with features as in I.A.1–I.A.4
      c. with automatisms
  C. Partial seizures secondarily generalized
    1. Simple partial seizures evolving to generalized seizures
    2. Complex partial seizures evolving to generalized seizures
    3. Simple partial seizures evolving to complex partial seizures to generalized seizures
II. GENERALIZED SEIZURES (bilaterally symmetric and without local onset)
  A. Absence seizures
    1. Impairment of consciousness only (simple absence)
    2. With mild clonic components (e.g., eye blinking)
    3. With atonic components
    4. With tonic components
    5. With automatisms
    6. With autonomic components
    7. Compound forms
  B. Atypical absence (with some retained consciousness, with stronger atonic or myoclonic components, e.g., head-nodding)
  C. Myoclonic seizures (myoclonic jerks, single or multiple)
  D. Clonic seizures (body jerks, usually more rhythmic and more prolonged than myoclonic seizures)
  E. Tonic seizures
  F. Tonic-clonic seizures
  G. Atonic seizures (also called "astatic" = loss of postural tone)
III. UNCLASSIFIED EPILEPTIC SEIZURES due to
  A. Inadequate or incomplete information
  B. Lack of proper category in present classification
IV. ADDENDUM—Epileptic seizures occurring under unusual circumstances
  A. Isolated seizures. They occur unexpectedly without apparent provocation.
  B. Situation-related seizures. Attacks precipitated by environmental or internal factors, i.e., menstrual cycles, sleep-waking cycle, fatigue, alcohol, stress. This includes "reflex seizures" triggered by sensory stimulation, e.g., photosensitive seizures, startle seizures.
  C. Prolonged or repetitive seizures: status epilepticus, e.g., frequent repetitive seizures without complete recovery between attacks or prolonged seizures (usually more than 20 minutes)
    1. Convulsive status epilepticus
      a. partial (e.g., jacksonian; epilepsia partialis continua)
      b. generalized (e.g., tonic-clonic status)
    2. Nonconvulsive status
      a. absence status (also called petit mal status, electrical stupor)
      b. fugue states (e.g., prolonged complex partial seizures with automatic behavior and amnesia)

With permission from Commission on Classification and Terminology: Proposal for revised clinical and electroencephalographic classification of epileptic seizures. Epilepsia 22:489–501, 1981.

first and most important step is taking an accurate history. The symptoms experienced by the individual and the signs and behavior described by witnesses are crucial for understanding the origin and mode of spread of the ictal discharges in the CNS. This information is relevant when selecting the anticonvulsant(s) for symptomatic treatment or when considering other therapeutic options such as the eradication of the epileptic process by surgery.

The International Classification of Epileptic Seizures

(Table 83–1) offers a compendium of all known seizure types grouped according to the initial symptoms and the functional characterization of the cerebral cortex or other area of the brain where the initial discharges are presumed to originate. It makes a clear distinction between partial seizures (synonymous with *symptomatic* and *cortical*) and generalized seizures (often synonymous with *idiopathic*) in which the whole brain is involved from the start. The various subgroups defined by this classification have proved to be of practical value and have stood the test of time. However, concepts evolve and changes gradually occur. For instance, the term *aura* is now synonymous with *simple partial seizure*, since the initial stereotypic and conscious experiences represent the onset of the attack. They are highly specific to the site of origin of the electrical discharge. To illustrate: Initial motor manifestations, somatic sensations, auditory, gustatory, or visual hallucinations indicate that the seizure begins, respectively, in the motor cortex, parietal cortex, superior temporal gyrus, orbital frontal or mesial temporal cortex, or occipital cortex. Cognitive or psychosensory aura, such as sense of unreality, déjà vu and jamais vu phenomena, and formed, stereotyped hallucinations or distorted perceptions, suggest that the attack originates within the temporal lobe cortex or adjacent regions where memory traces are stored. Involvement of the limbic cortex (mesial-temporal, cingulum, and orbital-frontal) elicits affective symptomatology or sensations within the gastrointestinal tract and autonomic system. After the initial subjective phenomena, the attack may progress to visible manifestations, which can be motor (clonic movements, jacksonian march, versive movements, dystonic posturing) or autonomic (pupillary dilatation, piloerection, or flushing). Such manifestations imply activation of adjacent areas of the cortex. Often, when the original discharges progress to involve the limbic system or the cortex of the contralateral hemisphere, consciousness is usually impaired, now identified as *complex partial seizure*. Frequently there are motor or speech automatisms. These consist of specific patterns of learned behavior for which the subject retains no memory. Further spread triggers a *secondarily generalized seizure*. All partial seizures may progress to secondarily generalized seizures by propagating to all other cortical regions and to subcortical centers. If they do so very rapidly, the initial portion of the attack (partial seizure) can go unnoticed and the seizure may be erroneously classified as primary generalized.

Classification of the Epilepsies and Epileptic Syndromes

Epilepsy is a symptom complex, always the expression of underlying disorder, but not a disease in itself. Therefore, it cannot be classified according to the underlying cause. Lesions of different nature may result in seizure manifestations that are indistinguishable clinically and electrically. Conversely, the same etiologic factor may produce a variety of seizure types, depending on its location in the CNS. For practical purposes, the localization and extent of the underlying pathology are more important than its nature.

The classification of the epileptic syndromes provides broad definitions of the main types of epileptic disorders identified so far, based on clinical observations and currently accepted principles of epileptogenesis. This classification of the epilepsies has been periodically revised and is likely to continue to change in the future. The one presented in Table 83–2 is the most recent version and, so far, the most comprehensive. It makes a distinction between two main groups: the localization-related and the generalized syndromes. Each is subdivided into idiopathic, those without apparent underlying structural lesion, and symptomatic, those due to a focal or diffuse disease. Each group is characterized by typical interictal and ictal EEG patterns and by the presence or absence of neurologic deficits and findings on neuroimaging. Many syndromes have a characteristic age at onset, evolution, and prognosis (see Table 83–2).

It is generally accepted that forms of *idiopathic epilepsy* are related to an intrinsic disorder of regulatory mechanisms (i.e., neurotransmitters). Predisposing genetic factors play a major role in this condition, which shows a predilection for younger individuals. Since idiopathic epilepsy usually involves widespread neuronal systems, it leads, as a rule, to "generalized" seizures.

The most typical varieties of primary generalized seizures (absence, tonic-clonic) occur in the idiopathic forms of epileptic syndromes; whereas generalized seizures associated with encephalopathies, either due to known disease or "cryptogenic," are likely to present more atypical manifestations (atonic, myoclonic, tonic seizures).

Epilepsy is defined as partial or localization-related when it results from focal (acquired) brain disease and expresses itself as partial seizures. An exception to this is a group of age-related partial epilepsy syndromes that, despite the partial seizures and the focal EEG findings, are not associated with any known underlying focal pathologic condition and appear to be genetically determined. The prototype of such idiopathic partial epilepsy syndromes is the *benign epilepsy of childhood with rolandic spikes*. Epileptic syndromes thought to be associated with bihemispheric encephalopathy, either due to known disease or cryptogenic, are classified as generalized epilepsies, within the symptomatic or cryptogenic group, if they cause generalized seizure manifestations or as undetermined syndromes if the manifestations are both partial and generalized.

The latest version of the classification of the epilepsies also includes a group of special syndromes in which the seizures are triggered by specific modes of activation, such as changes in body temperature, metabolic disturbances, hormonal variations, or drug withdrawal. As a result, syndromes previously not considered to be a form of epilepsy, such as febrile convulsions and alcohol withdrawal seizures, along with other special syndromes such as catamenial epilepsy, startle epilepsy, and reading epilepsy, have been included, mainly because they have seizure patterns, EEG abnormalities, and predisposing genetic traits in common with the more classic epileptic syndromes.

TABLE 83–2. International Classification of Epilepsies and Epileptic Syndromes

1. LOCALIZATION-RELATED (FOCAL, LOCAL, PARTIAL) EPILEPSIES AND SYNDROMES
   1.1 Idiopathic (with age-related onset).
      a. Benign childhood epilepsy with centrotemporal spike
      b. Childhood epilepsy with occipital paroxysms
      c. Primary reading epilepsy
   1.2 Symptomatic. This category comprises syndromes of great individual variability
      a. Temporal lobe epilepsies (amygdalo, hippocampal, lateral posterior temporal, opercular insular)
      b. Frontal lobe epilepsies (supplementary motor, cingulate, anterior polar, orbitofrontal, dorsolateral, motor)
      c. Parietal lobe epilepsies
      d. Occipital lobe epilepsies
      e. Chronic progressive epilepsia partialis continua of childhood
      f. Syndromes characterized by seizure with specific modes of precipitation
   1.3 Cryptogenic presumed symptomatic, but etiology is unknown. Defined by seizure type (see Table 83–1), clinical findings, anatomic localization
2. GENERALIZED EPILEPSIES AND SYNDROMES
   2.1 Idiopathic (with age-related onset, in order of age at appearance)
      a. Benign neonatal familial convulsions
      b. Benign neonatal convulsions
      c. Benign myoclonic epilepsy in infancy
      d. Childhood absence epilepsy (pyknolepsy, petit mal)
      e. Juvenile absence epilepsy
      f. Juvenile myoclonic epilepsy (impulsive petit mal)
      g. Epilepsy with grand mal seizures (GTCS) on awakening
      h. Other generalized idiopathic epilepsies not defined above
      i. Epilepsies with seizures precipitated by specific modes of activation
   2.2 Cryptogenic (idiopathic/symptomatic, in order of age at appearance)
      a. West syndrome (infantile spasms)
      b. Lennox-Gastaut syndrome
      c. Epilepsy with myoclonic-astatic seizures
      d. Epilepsy with myoclonic absences
   2.3 Symptomatic
   2.3.1 Nonspecific etiology
      a. Early myoclonic encephalopathy
      b. Early infantile epileptic encephalopathy with suppression burst
      c. Other symptomatic generalized epilepsies not defined above
   2.3.2 Specific syndromes: Epileptic seizures may complicate many disease states. Under this heading are included those diseases in which seizures are presenting or predominant feature
      a. Inborn errors of metabolism
      b. Progressive myoclonic epilepsies with specific pathology
3. UNDETERMINED EPILEPSIES AND SYNDROMES
   3.1 With both generalized and focal features
      a. Neonatal seizures
      b. Severe myoclonic epilepsy in infancy
      c. Epilepsy with continuous spikes and waves during slow-wave sleep
      d. Acquired epileptic aphasia (Landau-Kleffner syndrome)
      e. Other undetermined epilepsies
   3.2 Without unequivocal generalized or local features
4. SPECIAL SYNDROMES
   4.1 Situation-related seizures
      a. Febrile convulsions
      b. Isolated, apparently unprovoked epileptic events
      c. Seizures related to other identifiable situations, such as stress, hormones, drugs, alcohol, or sleep deprivation

Adapted from Commission on Classification and Terminology: Proposal for revised classification of epilepsies and epileptic syndromes. Epilepsia 30:389–399, 1989.

DIAGNOSTIC APPROACHES

History

This should include

1. A search for all predisposing factors, including family history of paroxysmal disorders (fainting, migraine, epilepsy, other neurologic disease); birth history; developmental history; febrile convulsions in early life; significant head trauma or disease that may have caused cerebral injuries; previous history of loss of consciousness; and alcohol or drug abuse, sleep habits, and other physical or emotional stressors.

2. A description of the actual seizure(s). This should be accurate, factual, and objective, based on the adolescent's rendition as well as on reports from direct and reliable witnesses. It should focus on the modalities of onset and early manifestations, when the seizure is still partial simple or complex, rather than on the impressive, but predictable phenomena of the late phase when the seizure is generalized. A description of the seizure and any incontinence or loss of consciousness all should be included in the history.

3. An account of the circumstances surrounding or immediately preceding the event (sleep deprivation, drug intoxication, prodromal symptoms). This is helpful in ruling out seizures of extracerebral origin.

4. A brief psychosocial history, which should detail level of education, school progress, social adjustment

and behavior, interpersonal relationships, and family dynamics.

Examination

A thorough assessment of the cardiovascular and pulmonary systems (see Chapters 42 and 45) is necessary in all adolescents with a history of loss of consciousness. Orthostatic hypotension should be ruled out by measuring blood pressure in the reclining and standing positions. Examination of the skin and the eyes is necessary to exclude neuroectodermal syndromes. Auscultation of the neck, orbits, and skull is appropriate to exclude bruits. While obtaining a complete neurologic assessment, the examiner should pay attention to soft signs. Asymmetries of limb posturing, pronator drift, or facial asymmetry may be the only subtle evidence of hemiparesis. Left-handedness and difference in nailbeds or other signs of hemiatrophy may be the only indications of cerebral lesions acquired during the first year of life. Similarly, tightening of one or both heel cords may indicate cerebral palsy. Ocular signs are important and should include peripheral visual fields of each eye by confrontation. This may reveal quadrantanopic or hemianopic defects otherwise inapparent because patients compensate easily for deficits acquired early in life.

Laboratory Diagnosis

ELECTROENCEPHALOGRAPHY

The EEG is the best tool for measuring cerebral excitability. Interictal recording can display diagnostic patterns of abnormalities such as the three-per-second spike and wave complexes, pathognomonic for idiopathic generalized epilepsy. Hyperventilation triggers such abnormality and has become part of the routine EEG procedure. The frequency of the spike-wave complexes is significant. Spike-wave complexes at a rate greater than three per second are usually associated with normal background activity and idiopathic generalized epileptic syndromes of later onset (e.g., juvenile myoclonic epilepsy), whereas the slower variety is usually an indicator of a coexistent encephalopathy. It tends to be replaced by polyspike discharges in sleep, and is associated with multiple seizure types.

Random focal spikes in one area of the surface EEG indicate a chronic process of local epileptogenesis as a result of a brain injury, leading to a form of partial epilepsy. Focal abnormalities of the background activity may reflect more extensive damage or surrounding inhibition. Because of the connectivity of the nervous system and the configuration of the cortical gyri, focal spikes may be displaced on the surface EEG at a distance from their site of origin. Independent multifocal spikes in one or both hemispheres are indicative of diffuse chronic encephalopathy with epileptic potential, if background activity is also abnormal. In contrast, spike discharges with inconsistent, widespread distribution or focal spikes in the central regions with a tendency to shift from side to side represent the EEG correlate of idiopathic epileptic syndrome, with benign prognosis. In such cases the frequency and extent of the EEG discharges are deceptively high, but the background activity and organization are normal.

Intermittent photic stimulation normally induces changes of the posterior cerebral rhythms that depend on the frequency of stimulation (driving). In individuals with a genetic predisposition to have convulsions, it may elicit generalized polyspike-wave discharges (photomyoclonic response), which may be associated with body jerks (photoconvulsive response). This may be the only abnormality in the interictal EEG and represents an important landmark of certain familial idiopathic generalized epileptic syndromes (e.g., juvenile myoclonic epilepsy).

NEUROIMAGING

Computed tomography (CT) has an important role in the diagnosis of the epileptic syndromes. Abnormalities have been reported in 50% of patients with the Lennox-Gastaut syndrome. Large structural malformations (e.g., porencephaly), hamartomas (e.g., tubers), or neoplasms, especially if calcified, are easily detected with this technique. However, the atrophy or subtle cortical malformations that represent the underlying pathology of most partial epilepsies are best detected with magnetic resonance imaging (MRI). All adolescents with partial seizures and a focal EEG, with normal or questionable findings on CT scan, should have an MRI scan. Certain neoplastic lesions of the mesial temporal region and hippocampal sclerosis can be clearly visualized only with this technique, partly because of their proximity to bony structures.

Differential Diagnosis

A careful review of the circumstances surrounding a seizure disorder is necessary to rule out attacks that may be of extracerebral origin. Adolescents are prone to having a tonic or tonic-clonic seizure in the context of vasovagal syncope. It is important to document that fainting and dimming of vision occurred prior to the loss of consciousness and that the face was pale as the result of hypotension. Adolescents can be exquisitely sensitive to specific triggers such as the sight of blood, venipuncture, or intense pain.

Adolescents with the first generalized seizure and a history inconsistent with syncope require immediate attention. A thorough physical examination and history with the adolescent and the family are in order. They should be accompanied by complete blood count and chemistry to rule out blood dyscrasias, hypoglycemia, and electrolyte imbalance, and a drug screen. Prior to initiating any treatment, an EEG should be obtained, in both the waking and the sleep states. The study should include hyperventilation and photic stimulation. The patient should be instructed to abstain from stimulants and to be at least partially sleep-deprived prior to the test. If the study reveals interictal abnormalities consistent with a form of idiopathic generalized epilepsy, the adolescent should be treated accordingly, without need for further investigation. An EEG pattern suggesting focal or diffuse underlying encephalopathy requires symptomatic treatment with anticonvulsants and further investigations (CT, MRI scan, and lumbar puncture) in search of the underlying cause.

Simple partial seizures may be difficult to differentiate from the prodrome of a migraine attack, especially if the headache component is inconspicuous. Perceptual distortions such as micropsia, macropsia, or hyperacusis as well as the tingling and weakness of hemiplegic migraine are indistinguishable from cortical epileptic phenomena. The distinctive feature is the tendency toward impairment of consciousness in epilepsy, whereas during a migraine attack the adolescent has heightened awareness. The apprehension of the adolescent with the migraine is justified and should not be confused with the sense of fear and impending doom characteristic of an affective aura in temporal lobe epilepsy.

The transitory impairment of consciousness during an absence seizure and a complex partial seizure may be very similar, especially if both are accompanied by automatisms. By definition, absence seizures are never preceded by experiential phenomena as in a simple partial attack. They begin and end abruptly, and they are never followed by the confusional state characteristic of a complex partial seizure. The interictal EEG abnormalities confirm the diagnosis.

Physicians treating adolescents with idiopathic generalized epilepsy should be aware that loss of consciousness during absence seizures may no longer be complete as the patient grows older. Similarly, the interictal EEG abnormalities may become less diagnostic or the EEG may normalize after puberty. This is a normal evolution for certain forms of generalized epilepsies. Also, the description of the subjective experiences by the adolescent patient may be misleading. Bright students who have moved from home to college may describe phenomena and experiences during incomplete absence states very reminiscent of the psychic auras in simple partial seizures. This may induce the new treating physician to favor anticonvulsants such as carbamazepine, which is not effective for absence seizures. Awareness of the past history and previous EEG abnormalities should avoid this mistake. If EEG findings are dubious and the seizures appear resistant to treatment, a psychogenic seizure disorder should be considered. These develop *de novo* in adolescents as well as in adolescents who already have a clearly established seizure disorder.

EPILEPTIC SYNDROMES

Partial (Localization-Related) Epilepsies Characterized by Partial Seizures

Pathophysiology. The underlying pathologic condition of these forms of symptomatic epilepsy can be either very discrete or diffuse within one hemisphere. A discrete lesion generates the elementary manifestations of a simple partial seizure with symptoms appropriate for the function of that cortex. Extensive lesions or diffuse pathology within one or both hemispheres are usually accompanied by significant neurodeficits and behavioral abnormalities. The presence of a multifocal pathologic condition is also likely to generate a wide variety of seizure manifestations, both partial and generalized, since multiple epileptogenic zones may act independently or synchronously.

Underlying Mechanisms. More than a century ago, John Hughlings Jackson postulated on purely clinical grounds the existence of motor cortical centers and proposed that an epileptic seizure was the result of abnormal excessive discharges of nerve cells. This concept was subsequently confirmed by electrical stimulation of the brain. The refined electrophysiologic, biochemical, and neuropharmacologic techniques that developed during the last 3 decades have demonstrated that individual elements of an epileptic neuronal aggregate undergo typical and rather stereotyped changes that reflect transitory alterations of membrane activity. Intracellular recording of cortical neurons in various experimental models of epilepsy indicates that the typical feature of this abnormal behavior is recurrent paroxysmal depolarization shifts (PDSs) of the resting membrane potential. PDSs result from a summation of excitatory postsynaptic potentials (EPSPs) mediated either by an excitatory neurotransmitter (i.e., glutamate) or by nonsynaptically activated ionic conductances across the membrane, which produce a Na^+ inward current responsible for the membrane depolarization. Unlike normal action potentials, which are single events immediately followed by postexcitatory hyperpolarization, PDSs are the result of repetitive action potentials during transient depolarization. These synchronous bursts emanating from groups of individual neurons within the "epileptogenic zone" give rise to pronounced extracellular field potentials that are recorded in the EEG as interictal epileptic spikes. The same mechanisms that promote the restoration of the resting membrane potential after a normal action potential control the abnormally bursting neurons of the epileptogenic focus during interictal periods. These mechanisms are provided by inhibitory postsynaptic potentials (IPSPs) released by gamma-aminobutyric acid (GABA) generated at the GABA-ergic terminals of local basket cell interneurons. Such terminals end on the soma and basal dendrites of pyramidal cells and trigger K^+ or Cl^- transmembrane hyperpolarizing currents, which interfere with the synchronous bursting activity. Whenever a pyramidal cell generates an EPSP, the recurrent axon's collaterals activate the network of basket interneurons so that excitation is always modulated by recurrent inhibition. The same dual influence is also represented in the epileptogenic focus, in which the hyperexcitable center is surrounded by a population of hyperpolarized neurons. It has been suggested that interictal spike activity may be instrumental in maintaining this area of surrounding inhibition, preventing the propagation of the epileptic discharge that leads to a seizure. Transition from the interictal equilibrium to ictal state is due at least in part to a failure of these intrinsic inhibitory mechanisms.

TEMPORAL LOBE EPILEPSY

Temporal lobe structures, particularly the mesial cortex, are highly epileptogenic. The pyramidal cells of the hippocampus are particularly vulnerable to anoxic or toxic damage, and the complex cytoarchitectonics of the region can be easily disrupted by neuronal migration defects. This area frequently can be the site of malformations or low-grade glial tumors that, despite a very benign course, may be responsible for refractory epileptic disorders. Superficial contusions of the cortex due to trauma can leave a cicatrix with the same effect.

Simple or complex partial seizures originating in the temporal lobe frequently begin in childhood or adolescence. There is often a history of a difficult delivery or prolonged febrile convulsions in infancy. A familial history of seizures is common. Psychic, autonomic, olfactory, and gustatory auras are the landmark of the simple partial seizures typically seen in this condition. When the attacks originate within the amygdalohippocampal complex (mesiobasal, limbic, rhinencephalic cortex), rising epigastric sensations with nausea or emotional experiences, most frequently fear, are particularly common. Visual or auditory illusions and hallucinations as well as a sense of depersonalization frequently occur at the onset of a temporal lobe seizure originating within the lateral cortex. Memory processes can also be disturbed at the onset of the ictus, leading to temporal disorientation, dreamy state, a flashback, or a sense of familiarity: déjà vu if the experience is visual; déjà entendu if the experience is auditory; or jamais vu if the experience suddenly feels unfamiliar. About one half of the adolescent patients do not report any aura because there is amnesia for it or because impairment of consciousness is present from the onset. Many patients tend to "lose" their aura or their ability to report it over the course of years. Because of the diagnostic value of such phenomena, it is important to ask the adolescent specifically whether these aura ever occurred. Many patients are unable to describe it in detail but recognize without hesitation that an unusual and stereotyped experience occurs at the onset of the seizure. These subjective phenomena are usually of brief duration, although quite distinct and intense, and may be reported simply as "dizziness" or "numbness."

Seizures with a simple partial onset may evolve into a complex partial seizure with impairment of consciousness and automatisms. Proof of such evolution usually requires the confirmation of witnesses, and it is pathognomonic. Automatisms represent patterns of learned motor behavior performed during the attack while the subject is amnestic for the event. Automatisms can be of the oro-alimentary type (lip-smacking, chewing, gulping), mimetic (facial expression of fear, bewilderment, vacant stare, discomfort, smiling), gestural (repetitive movements of the hands and fingers, tapping, rubbing, picking on clothing), ambulatory (walking or running), or vocal or verbal (humming, coughing, or repetitive, stereotyped short sentences). Various types of automatisms can occur during the same seizure. Complex partial seizures often begin simply with motor arrest, a vacant stare, and unresponsiveness. Propagation of ictal paroxysms to the frontal cortex causes motor phenomena typical of that region, such as head and eye deviation, posturing, and eventually secondary generalization. After a complex partial seizure there is always a period of confusion and disorientation during which the patient may become inappropriately defensive and combative, especially if restrained. Often this is mistaken for aggressive and violent behavior, but such behavior is not purposeful or directed. Complex partial seizures and secondary generalization may be precipitated by emotional stress, fatigue, or sleep deprivation.

Diagnosis. The exact and full sequence of the ictal symptoms and the information derived from interictal EEG recordings are essential for the diagnosis. The EEG may show no abnormalities; asymmetry of the background activity; or temporal spikes, sharp waves, or slow waves, which are unilateral or bilateral and synchronous but also independent. These findings are not always confined to the temporal region. Sphenoidal electrodes inserted deeply in the infrazygomatic region and recording mesial and inferior-temporal activity in proximity of the foramen ovale have been a very useful addition for the detection and lateralization of hippocampal abnormalities. In addition to scalp EEG, intracranial recording (epidural and subdural electrodes, implanted depth electrodes) may allow better definition of the intracranial distribution of the interictal abnormalities. Ultimately, the diagnosis is established by extracranial or intracranial recording of ictal events.

Selective cognitive deficits on neuropsychological testing and asymmetries or focal anomalies in neuroimaging studies when concordant with the EEG findings validate the diagnosis. MRI is particularly accurate in detecting subtle asymmetries in the area of the hippocampus (mesial temporal sclerosis) and indolent, noncalcified lesions not clearly demonstrable on CT scanning.

Treatment. The treatment of choice is carbamazepine. Unfortunately, a number of patients develop allergic reactions or tolerate this medication only at a dose insufficient to control the condition. The addition of a benzodiazepine, especially clorazepate (Tranxene), is helpful in a few cases. However, the benefit is usually transient. Diphenylhydantoin and barbiturates (particularly primidone) can be almost as effective as carbamazepine but may cause cognitive and behavioral disturbances. Other antiepileptic drugs such as valproate and acetazolamide (Diamox) are less effective but can be considered as add-on medications. The burden of having temporal lobe epilepsy can be devastating for an adolescent. Complex partial status epilepticus is known to precipitate episodes of psychosis, and repetitive complex partial seizures may lead, in the long run, to significant personality changes, particularly depression. Because of the high success rate after temporal lobectomy in well-selected candidates, refractory cases should be identified and considered for surgery as soon as possible.

FRONTAL LOBE EPILEPSY

Owing to the large representation of motor functions in the frontal lobes, simple partial seizures with motor expression are common in this form of epilepsy. Their manifestations depend on the side and topography of the area involved.

Clinical Manifestations

Motor Cortex. When the epileptogenic zone is located within or in proximity to the rolandic gyrus, the ictus begins with clonic activity in muscle groups contralateral to the hemispheric focus. Hand and face are more frequently involved because they have wide cortical representation. Propagation of the discharge along contiguous areas of the precentral gyrus gives rise to a jacksonian march, characterized by gradual involvement of additional muscle groups. This may become bilateral. Transient paralytic phenomena (e.g., Todd paralysis) are not uncommon following motor excitatory clonic seizures, especially if these were severe or prolonged. However, motor inhibitory attacks are infrequent as a solitary manifestation of a seizure. Usually there is sensory loss or dysesthesia associated with the inability to move.

Lateral (Premotor) Cortex. Focal lesions involving the frontal convexity give rise to motor manifestations that reflect the function of the supplementary motor and premotor cortex, primarily concerned with bilateral synergistic movements. Activation of the frontal eye field causes contralateral head and eye deviation (versive seizure); involvement of the supplementary motor area is likely to be accompanied by vocalization (phonatory seizures) or speech arrest and asymmetric posturing of the limbs (fencing–focal tonic seizure). Involvement of the frontal operculum is likely to cause inability to speak (salivation, laryngeal symptoms, autonomic symptoms) while consciousness is retained (speech arrest–aphasic seizure). The pattern of seizures originating in the anterior frontopolar region includes forced thinking or conscious contraversive movements of the eyes and head, followed by loss of contact, axial clonic jerks, and falls. The widespread connections of the frontal cortex with the contralateral lobe via callosal pathways and with the diencephalic centers greatly facilitate the rapid evolution of a partial motor seizure into a bilateral attack. In generalized seizures of frontal origin, the tonic component is always predominant over the clonic phase.

Mesial and Orbital Cortex. The mesial (cingulate) and orbitofrontal cortex belong to the limbic system. Therefore, seizures originating in this region are not different from those described in mesial temporal lobe epilepsy. Common features of the orbitofrontal region are olfactory hallucinations, whereas in the cingulate region, changes in mood and affect are prominent. Another confounding element in the differential diagnosis is the sensory auras reported by some patients with frontal lobe epilepsy (FLE). However, these subjective experiences usually consist of somatic sensations, different from those reported in temporal lobe epilepsy (TLE).

Diagnosis. FLE is more difficult to diagnose, and its course is more severe than is that of TLE. Ictal motor manifestations are usually sudden, can be brief but violent, are predominantly tonic, and often cause injuries. They are often repetitive and generalize quickly. Episodes of status epilepticus are frequent. Unless there is an underlying structural anomaly detectable on neuroimaging, the localization of the focus on surface EEG recording is often made difficult by the rapid generalization of the discharges. Invasive monitoring is often necessary to identify the site of origin, especially if located on the orbital or mesial cortex.

Treatment. Phenytoin (PHT) is the drug of choice because of its specific effect against the tonic phase of maximal electroshock seizures and the propagation of a focal discharge. Treatment with other major antiepileptic drugs (benzodiazepines, barbiturates, valproate) is often unsatisfactory. Methsuximide (Celontin) may be effective, but often only transiently. Seizures of frontal lobe origin not only are more difficult to treat pharmacologically than are temporal lobe seizures but also do not respond as favorably to surgical resection. When sudden drop seizures are the prevalent symptoms, the condition is very disabling, and anterior or total callosotomy may be the best alternative, especially in case of bilateral disease or of a unilateral structural lesion that cannot be removed because it is located in an area of essential cortex.

PARIETAL LOBE EPILEPSY

Seizures originating in the parietal lobe are relatively infrequent and may lead to sensory-motor manifestations similar to those seen in FLE. However, they are predominantly somatosensory, with features more frequently described as numbness or dysesthesia (tingling, pins and needles sensation, feeling of electricity), rarely painful, and referred to body parts with the largest cortical representation (i.e., the hand, arm, face, and tongue). Facial sensory phenomena may occur bilaterally. The initial somatosensory symptomatology may spread in a jacksonian manner (simple partial sensory seizure). It may also evolve into a complex partial seizure if the discharge propagates to other regions such as the temporal lobe. Involvement of the cortical association areas at the parietal-occipital-temporal junction may lead to visual distortions or formed hallucinations, severe vertigo, or disorientation in space, particularly if the focus is in the nondominant hemisphere. Seizures in the dominant parietal lobe result in a variety of receptive and conductive language disturbances. Tonic posturing of the limb, inability to move, or rapid secondary generalization with loss of consciousness may occur, just as in FLE, especially if the epilepsy has been of long duration.

Diagnosis. EEG localization, especially if the focus resides in the paracentral lobule, may require intracranial recording.

Treatment. Treatment is the same as that for FLE.

OCCIPITAL LOBE EPILEPSY

An epileptogenic focus near the primary visual cortex usually, but not always, causes simple partial seizures characterized by elementary visual sensations, such as flashing lights, colored or dark spots, and, less frequently, negative phenomena such as loss of vision. As a rule, these symptoms are referred to the contralateral eye field but can spread to the entire field. Perceptual illusions and visual distortions (micropsia or macropsia) may mimic the onset of a migraine attack. Often there is head and eye deviation or rapid forced eye movements. Not infrequently the direction is ipsilateral to the focus because of callosal spread. When ictal manifestations begin with the appropriate sensory phenomena, the diagnosis is relatively simple. However, depth electrode studies have demonstrated that the pattern of spread from the occipital cortex can vary among individuals and between seizures in the same individual. A focus in the temporo-occipital junction often originates typical complex partial seizures, although the origin is extratemporal. As a result, a sizable number of patients with interictal occipital spike foci in the EEG and with demonstrable pathologic findings in the same region may exhibit the same seizure manifestations as those of TLE. We followed an adolescent with arteriovenous malformation of the occipital pole who for years experienced attacks of classic migraine and complex partial seizures preceded by the same visual aura, in whom both seizures and migraine subsided following surgical removal of the malformation. Another adolescent with rare generalized grand mal seizures exhibited periods of prolonged nausea with anorexia and weight loss, in association with complex partial seizures without visual aura. The underlying pathologic condition was a porencephalic cyst of the occipital lobe secondary to perinatal vascular occlusion. Surgical resection of the atrophic cortex at the margin of the cyst produced only temporary relief of the symptoms. Her attacks did not become controlled until she underwent a temporal lobectomy that removed residual atrophic cortex extending along the mesial aspect of the temporal lobe.

Methods of diagnosis and treatment for simple and complex partial seizures of occipital origin are not different from those for the other symptomatic partial epilepsies. However, if the medications fail, surgical resection is not always a viable alternative unless a visual field defect is already present.

DIFFUSE HEMISPHERIC (MULTILOBAR) EPILEPSIES

Although extensive lesions of one hemisphere are more likely to occur at an earlier age, the effects persist in adolescence. Extensive pathologic conditions, such as a large porencephalic cyst or multilobar atrophy due to vasculitis, meningoencephalitis, collagen disease, or Rasmussen encephalitis, usually are associated with multiple epileptogenic foci. As a result, seizures are of mixed type, including absence-like attacks, simple complex partial seizures, and focal motor seizures. Secondary generalization and status epilepticus are frequent events, especially when the frontal lobe is involved. Rapid generalization and sudden drop attacks may occur. If medications fail and if contralateral hemianopsia and hemiplegia are already present, these adolescents may be candidates for subtotal hemicorticectomy or hemispherectomy (see section on surgical treatment), both highly successful surgical interventions, when indicated. If the use of the contralateral hand is preserved and if speech is retained on the side of the lesion, mapping of the eloquent areas of the cortex by direct electrical stimulation or by subdural grid implantation may be necessary to tailor the cortical resection and minimize neurologic loss.

SYMPTOMATIC EPILEPSIES WITH BIHEMISPHERIC INVOLVEMENT AND MIXED MANIFESTATIONS

Bihemispheric pathologic conditions may result from severe anoxic or traumatic insults, meningoencephalitis, congenital anomalies, or neurocutaneous syndromes (bilateral Sturge-Weber disease, tuberous sclerosis, and so on). The etiology may remain unknown (cryptogenic forms). Such conditions are likely to be acquired prenatally or in infancy and tend to become symptomatic at an early age. They are usually accompanied by behavioral, cognitive, and neurologic deficits. However, these encephalopathies are not progressive. The seizure disorder is the most prominent feature, characterized by both partial and generalized attacks with atypical manifestations. It seems that the anatomic and physiologic substrata leading to the typical manifestions of a grand mal seizure in the idiopathic epilepsies are perturbed by the acquired encephalopathy, so the manifestations become unusual, less predictable, and less responsive to pharmacologic treatment. Diffuse encephalopathies often involve the frontal lobes. The widespread connections of the premotor cortex and its proximity to the supplementary motor area may produce rapid secondary generalization, which may mask the partial onset and produce brief tonic (or myoclonic) seizure manifestations.

The Lennox-Gastaut syndrome is the prototype of such disorders. Because the pathologic features are diffuse and the seizure manifestations are predominantly generalized, these syndromes are classified among the generalized epilepsies.

Generalized Epilepsies and Syndromes

Pathophysiology and Underlying Mechanisms. The same basic mechanisms described for partial seizures apply to generalized seizures; however, diffuse neuronal systems become activated at once, resulting in bilateral, synchronous discharges in the EEG and generalized manifestations.

Idiopathic generalized seizures should be viewed as a dysfunction of physiologic regulatory mechanisms, leading to exaggerated (paroxysmal) events. In the nervous system a balanced interaction between two elementary phenomena, excitation and inhibition, is essential for optimum level of functioning. Impulses delivered at excitatory synapses (EPSPs) are necessary for promoting activity but need to be modulated by an appropriate degree of inhibition (IPSPs). Excitatory and inhibitory networks are ubiquitous and strictly interrelated. Traditionally, epileptic seizures are viewed as an expression of excessive excitation. However, the various types of ictal manifestations seen in the generalized epilepsies can be interpreted as paroxysmal events that involve both of these opposed but complementary systems, although either one can be affected to a different degree or in a different sequence.

The role of inhibition in the context of increased cortical excitation is especially prominent in the pathogenesis of generalized spike-and-wave discharges in the EEG that accompany absence seizures. Electrophysiologic studies correlating intracellular recording with surface EEG have demonstrated that the first component of the complex (the spike) corresponds to cellular membrane depolarization (EPSP), whereas the slow wave corresponds to hyperpolarization (IPSP). The net result of this diffuse phenomenon, consisting of rhythmic, repetitive, brief excitatory states alternating with inhibitory states of longer duration, is an interference with normal cortical functions. This leads to the predominantly negative phenomena of an absence seizure (motor and speech arrest, inability to comprehend, loss of consciousness). Certain predisposed individuals with generalized epilepsy and spike and waves in their EEG may show a prevalence of either the slow components (inhibitory) or the spikes (excitatory). Shifting states (i.e., waking versus sleep) can also alter the morphology of the discharges and consequently cause various types of seizures in the same individual. This concept sheds some light on why the same patient with generalized epilepsy may exhibit absence seizures in wakefulness and grand mal seizures in sleep and why absence seizures in childhood may be replaced by grand mal seizures during adolescence. The wide spectrum of epileptic manifestations seen in generalized epilepsy reflects the many possible ways bilateral synchronous spikes combine with the slow wave components in the EEG. The rhythmic muscle jerks seen during 3-second spike waves of a myoclonic absence are an example of how excitatory impulses can coexist with a state of motor and cognitive arrest. The single body jerk of a myoclonic seizure represents a more powerful excitatory impulse correlated in the EEG with a burst of spikes, immediately aborted by a bout of slow waves. A tonic seizure derives from a sustained excitatory discharge due to summation of excitatory potentials during neuronal "recruitment" at cortical and subcortical levels. This phenomenon is characterized in the EEG by a train of sustained polyspikes. The same mechanism may lead to a grand mal seizure. This consists of the tonic phase, followed by a clonic phase characterized by groups of polyspikes (muscle contractions) alternating with periods of slow waves (muscle relaxation). The neuronal substrates and electrophysiologic mechanisms of atonic seizures (simply a loss of axial muscular tone) are not known. It can be speculated that the underlying mechanism is a massive activation of motor inhibitory cortical-subcortical pathways, another example of how the normal organization of the CNS serves as a substratum for pathologic mechanisms, leading to various types of epileptic phenomena.

IDIOPATHIC GENERALIZED EPILEPTIC SYNDROMES

These primary forms of epilepsy are classified in the idiopathic group because they are not accompanied by any known structural abnormality of the CNS. Similarly, the interictal EEG is usually normal.

CHILDHOOD ABSENCE EPILEPSY (PETIT MAL, PYKNOLEPSY)

This is a generalized nonconvulsive epileptic syndrome. Absence attacks typically appear during school age in children with strong genetic predisposition but who are otherwise normal. Simple absences can be very frequent, but in most patients they are easily controlled with medication. However, in a number of instances, absence attacks are resistant, especially if associated with myoclonic, tonic, or atonic components (see Table 83–1). This condition is more frequent in girls than in boys. Generalized tonic-clonic seizures (GTCSs), or grand mal attacks, may appear at puberty, particularly in sleep or upon awakening. Absence attacks tend to become less frequent or to remit with age, whereas if absence attacks persist during adolescence, consciousness may no longer be totally abolished. In this case, the adolescent may have the perception of having a seizure and be aware that his or her ability to function is suddenly impaired for a brief period of time. Often young adults with petit mal epilepsy report quick "lapses," which are not otherwise detectable unless documented by EEG. These atypical manifestations of absence epilepsy can be easily misdiagnosed or dismissed, depriving the patient of the proper care (see section on differential diagnosis).

Diagnosis. The diagnosis of petit mal (absence) epilepsy often can be established during an office visit by asking the patient to hyperventilate. This maneuver triggers three-per-second spike waves in the EEG, often accompanied by the signs of an absence seizure. If these are not clinically apparent, the EEG will reveal the unmistakable marker of this condition, either spontaneously or after provocative procedures (hyperventilation, sleep, methohexital injection). The interictal EEG is otherwise normal.

Treatment. Ethosuximide (Zarontin) remains the drug of choice in simple absence epilepsy. However, this type of epilepsy in adolescence is best treated with valproate because of the likely association of GTCS, which can be facilitated by ethosuximide. If valproate is not tolerated, Zarontin can be easily combined with phenobarbital or phenytoin in one single dose given at bedtime. Benzodiazepines such as clonazepam (Klonopin) should be used as a last resort in resistant cases. Acetazolamide (Diamox) or another carbonic anhydrase inhibitor can be helpful, although it may be effective only for a limited period of time. Petit mal epilepsy is, in general, a relatively benign condition. However, when it persists or begins in adolescence, it is unlikely to resolve spontaneously and may be relatively refractory to medical treatment. Absence epilepsy is not easily tolerated in this age group because of the social embarrassment and the limitations imposed by this condition, especially the inability to obtain a driver's license.

JUVENILE ABSENCE EPILEPSY

The distinction of this syndrome from the previous one is justified by the age at onset, during puberty, and by the sporadic occurrence of absence seizures, whereas GTCSs are frequent and often associated with myoclonic manifestations. The method of diagnosis and treatment is not different. Spike-wave discharges in the EEG are often faster than 3 cycles per second (CPS), and response to therapy is usually favorable.

JUVENILE MYOCLONIC EPILEPSY (IMPULSIVE PETIT MAL)

This form of epilepsy has been described by Janz and typically starts in otherwise normal adolescents, with a strong familial predisposition. This is in contrast with other forms of myoclonic epilepsies of earlier onset often accompanied by encephalopathy. Seizures are characterized by brief, bilateral, single or repetitive myoclonic jerks, mostly in the arms. Single body jerks occur without apparent loss of consciousness but may cause some patients to fall suddenly. They are more likely to occur shortly after awakening in the morning. When the jerks become repetitive, there may be clouding of consciousness and the episode may culminate in a GTCS. This is more likely to occur in the context of sleep deprivation or other stressful circumstances. The association with absence seizures is rare.

Diagnosis. The diagnosis is easily established by the characteristic clinical history and by the typical EEG findings. The involuntary spilling of orange juice at the breakfast table may be the clue to the diagnosis. Otherwise the condition may remain undiagnosed until the first GTCS occurs. Since this disorder may be inherited, the search for a positive family history, particularly photosensitive epilepsy, is important. The interictal and ictal EEG shows rapid, generalized, often irregular spike-wave and polyspike-wave discharges with no consistent correlation between EEG spikes and body jerks. These individuals are highly photosensitive, and intermittent photic stimulation, particularly at the frequencies of 15 to 17 stimuli per second, triggers polyspike–slow wave discharges. Persistent photic stimulation may lead to repetitive body jerks and to a GTCS. Unlike absence epilepsy, hyperventilation usually does not activate the EEG discharges.

Treatment. The drug of choice is valproate, which is effective against both the minor and the major seizures and photosensitivity. Phenytoin and carbamazepine prevent the major attacks but not the myoclonic jerks. The benzodiazepines can be extremely effective in controlling myoclonic activity, especially after sleep deprivation (e.g., after a party). When given in such circumstances, they may avert a major attack. Juvenile myoclonic epilepsy is unlikely to remit spontaneously but responds well to appropriate drug treatment, which may be required for life. Overall, the condition is well tolerated, and it imposes few limitations. Myoclonic epilepsy is not a contraindication to driving, although the photic sensitivity may pose an additional risk. In most cases, it can be demonstrated in the EEG laboratory that the response to the sensitive frequencies can be significantly reduced or abolished during monocular stimulation. This information is of practical value to the patient who can be instructed to close one eye whenever body jerks occur while driving in adverse circumstances.

EPILEPSY WITH GENERALIZED TONIC-CLONIC SEIZURES ON AWAKENING

The tonic-clonic seizures of grand mal epilepsy often represent an evolution of the absence seizures of petit mal epilepsy. They may also be associated with myoclonic seizure disorders. Otherwise, the onset of this form of epilepsy occurs most frequently during the second decade of life. Sleep has a facilitatory effect. Often, the patient is made aware of having had an attack by waking up with a sore tongue, strained muscles, or a headache or by the realization of having been incontinent. The GTCSs also occur frequently upon awakening or in the evening prior to falling asleep. Seizures may be precipitated by sleep deprivation or other stressful circumstances. Genetic predisposition with photosensitivity is frequent. If other seizures are associated, they are mostly of the absence or myoclonic type, but, unlike in the previous two syndromes, the predominant manifestations are GTCSs. Daytime attacks are infrequent and should be prevented by prescribing the appropriate medication to minimize the disruption in the life of a young individual. Unnecessary admissions to hospital emergency departments should be avoided when the diagnosis has been clearly established, since the attacks are self-limited. Peer acceptance and preservation of self-esteem are crucial for an adolescent, and the interplay of seizures with these issues should be addressed with sensitivity.

Diagnosis. The interictal EEG may be normal or may show one of the patterns of idiopathic generalized epilepsy, most likely synchronous spike-wave discharges of the fast variety.

Treatment. Any of the major anticonvulsants can be effective. Barbiturates and phenytoin present the advantage of a single dose at bedtime, which facilitates compliance. If GTCSs consistently occur at night, there is no contraindication to driving, although the patient should be made acutely aware of the additional risk that follows sleep deprivation. Idiopathic GTCSs, by definition, are not preceded by any aura but may start with a crescendo of myoclonic jerks or may be preceded by a period of mental confusion. Educating adolescents and family permits prompt recognition and prevention by the immediate administration of a benzodiazepine. This may abort an impending major attack.

CRYPTOGENIC (IDIOPATHIC AND SYMPTOMATIC) GENERALIZED EPILEPSIES

These forms of symptomatic epilepsies with mixed seizure manifestations of partial and generalized type are usually caused by bihemispheric pathologic conditions, which may result from severe anoxic or traumatic insults, meningoencephalitis, congenital anomalies, or neurocutaneous syndromes (bilateral Sturge-Weber disease, tuberous sclerosis, and so on) or from an unknown cause (cryptogenic forms). These encephalopathies become symptomatic at an early age and may be accompanied by behavioral, cognitive, and neurologic deficits, but the seizure disorder is the most prominent feature. Typically this consists of various seizure types, both partial and generalized with atypical manifestations. The

Lennox-Gastaut syndrome is the prototype of such disorders. Because the pathologic condition is diffuse and the seizure manifestations are predominantly generalized, these syndromes are classified among the generalized epilepsies.

Lennox-Gastaut Syndrome

Defined as epileptic encephalopathy with slow spike and waves by Gastaut, this condition represents a response of the brain to a variety of diffuse and focal insults and may evolve from a previous epileptic syndrome (e.g., infantile spasms). Less frequently it may strike children with previously normal development for no apparent reason (cryptogenic forms). In such cases, the onset is subacute, and seizures of increasing severity are accompanied by a decline in cognitive functions and by slowing of motor responses mainly as the result of prolongation of reaction time and mental processes. The encephalopathic picture correlates with diffusely slow background in the EEG and frequent spike-wave discharges of the slow variety (less than three per second). These are often accompanied by the subtle manifestations of an incomplete absence seizure and loss of postural tone (atonic seizure). This may be partial (head drop seizure) or repetitive (head-nodding seizure). If there is a fall, this may be followed by a period of akinesia (astatic-akinetic seizure). Tonic seizures are always present, at least in sleep. They are typically characterized by flexion of the head and trunk and hyperextension of the extremities and frequently cause severe injuries. Myoclonic seizures, complex partial seizures, and generalized tonic-clonic attacks are also present in various combinations. Status epilepticus is a common event (stuporous states with myoclonic activity, tonic and atonic seizures). In adolescents and younger adults with this syndrome the most frequent epileptic manifestations are the tonic seizures. They usually occur as sporadic events during sleep but may also occur in rapid succession for periods of hours or even days (tonic status epilepticus). This condition has a long course, marked by exacerbations of seizure activity associated with decline in the level of functioning and relative remissions. The prognosis is variable but usually poor. Contrary to the infantile spasms (West syndrome) of earlier onset, the cryptogenic forms of Lennox-Gastaut syndrome do not necessarily have a better outcome than do symptomatic cases.

Diagnosis. Despite the severity of the condition, the family history is usually negative for epilepsy. The history of intractable mixed seizure types, particularly drop seizures during the daytime and tonic seizures in sleep, along with intellectual retardation and slow spike and waves in the EEG are the landmarks for the diagnosis. Multifocal spike discharges are not infrequent. During sleep the slow spike-wave pattern is replaced largely by generalized polyspike discharges.

Both tonic and atonic manifestations are accompanied by the same decremental changes in the EEG, followed by a generalized fast discharge of increasing voltage. Minor tonic seizures may involve mainly the facial musculature (eyes wide open and fixed, drooping of the jaw) with minimal stiffening of the body without a fall.

Unless the EEG is monitored, this minor variety of tonic seizures may not be recognized. If they occur in rapid succession for long periods, the severe mental changes and delayed motor responses may lead to the erroneous diagnosis of acute psychosis.

Neuroimaging shows underlying structural lesions in the symptomatic cases and mild symmetric bilateral atrophy in the majority of the cryptogenic ones.

Treatment. The Lennox-Gastaut syndrome is notoriously difficult to treat medically. The medication of choice for the tonic seizures is phenytoin and for the various types of daytime seizures is valproate. The benzodiazepines, particularly clonazepam, may be helpful but have limited use because of the sedative side effect. These patients often appear oversedated, usually as a feature of the syndrome rather than an effect of the medication. Polypharmacy is usually required for the prevention of the multiple seizure types. Yet, this does not usually control the minor motor seizures and does not prevent episodes of status epilepticus. These patients have to wear protective helmets, and because of the disabling psychomotor delay, they can function only in sheltered environments. In a small percentage of cases, at least the daytime seizures remit spontaneously after puberty. In the others, management is mostly supportive. If violent tonic seizures persist, surgical treatment (callosotomy) can be considered, but it is not likely to be successful.

OTHER FORMS OF IDIOPATHIC SEIZURE DISORDERS

Isolated Convulsive Seizures

Tonic-clonic convulsions may occur as isolated phenomena in patients without an epileptic disorder who never develop a chronic epileptic syndrome. These events can be classified as reactive seizures on the assumption that unusual circumstances have triggered the attack in an otherwise normal individual. The precipitating circumstances often remain obscure. If results of the neurologic examination, neuroimaging, and EEG are normal, there is no need for treatment, since in the majority of cases, the seizures do not recur. However, as a precautionary measure, it is advisable to discourage the patient from driving for a reasonable period of time.

Primary Partial Epilepsies

Benign childhood epilepsy with centrotemporal spikes is a form of epilepsy that typically starts and ends before puberty. Its benign course does not interfere with the behavior and normal development of young individuals. Typical of this condition are partial sensory-motor seizures affecting the face areas and causing speech paralysis, salivation, and clonic movements with retained consciousness. Secondary generalization occurs mostly at night. Both are easily prevented with moderate amounts of anticonvulsive medication (carbamazepine, phenytoin, phenobarbital). About one half of the patients have only one seizure, and it is reasonable not to treat this condition after the first attack. There is no known underlying pathologic condition for this form of seizure disorder. Intellectual functioning is normal or above normal, and the neurologic examination is invariably unremarkable. The family history is often positive, implying an idiopathic hyperexcitability of the rolandic cortex, which is genetically transmitted and whose clinical expression is limited to prepubertal age. The EEG presents focal spike discharges with a widespread distribution over the rolandic and midtemporal regions of one side or both sides independently. These interictal discharges are greatly activated by sleep, and their lateralization may change from side to side over the years. The EEG abnormalities are striking, compared with the benign clinical course, and may persist for some years after the epileptic manifestations either have spontaneously remitted or have been controlled. It is usually not necessary to protract treatment throughout adolescence even if the EEG remains abnormal. It is not unusual that an EEG obtained for other reasons may display the pattern of centrotemporal spikes in adolescents who have been totally asymptomatic.

NONEPILEPTIC PAROXYSMAL DISORDERS

Syncope

This paroxysmal disorder is characterized by attacks of loss of consciousness with loss of motor control caused by brain ischemia (see Chapter 85). Syncope may lead to secondary epileptic phenomena, mimicking a GTCS. Therefore, this common disorder is often confused with epilepsy. A genetic predisposition to convulse may play a role. It is most helpful in the differential diagnosis to obtain a positive family history of fainting and a past history of autonomic hypersensitivity or dysfunction such as migraine, vertigo, motion sickness, or near fainting. However, the most revealing part of the evaluation is a detailed history of the circumstances surrounding the event and a description of the attack. In young individuals, syncope is usually vasovagal and can be triggered by psychogenic stimuli, which often can be very specific (the sight of blood, venipuncture, visits to the dentist's office), or by physical stimuli (a sudden unexpected pain, micturition, coughing, Valsalva maneuver). Adolescents may be embarrassed to admit this sensitivity, so careful taking of the history is necessary. The "passing out" may be almost instantaneous, but usually the subject recognizes the prodromal symptoms and expects the attack and may try to abort it.

Orthostatic hypotension mechanisms are next in order of frequency. Cardiac syncope, peripheral neuropathies, and familial dysautonomia are uncommon in this age group. The prodromes are stereotyped and consist of malaise, vertigo and dizziness, blurring, and fading of vision before the loss of postural tone. Reports by direct witnesses that the patient looked pale and limp during the period of loss of consciousness are useful confirmatory data.

Not infrequently the attack may progress to a brief generalized tonic spasm, occasionally followed by a few clonic contractions, especially if the patient is held in the upright position. There may be incontinence.

Postictally, the adolescent may feel exhausted but is alert. The differential diagnosis includes atonic seizures, GTCS, and simple partial seizures. Important clues are the brevity of the attack, the lack of injuries during the fall, the fall preceding the tonic rigidity, the lack of postictal confusion and combativeness, and the fact that the prodromal symptomatology never progresses to a complex partial seizure with automatisms. The identification of the triggering mechanism and the history of similar near-syncopal attacks are pathognomonic for the condition. Investigations to rule out orthostatic hypotension and cardiac arrhythmias may be warranted. The results of interictal EEG and neurologic examination are normal. The diagnosis can be confirmed by reproducing the circumstances leading to an attack during EEG monitoring in the laboratory. When the attempt is successful, the EEG will show diffuse slowing during the initial stage of limpness with bradycardia or brief asystole, whereas it will become isoelectric during the tonic phase.

Hyperventilation

This is a very common condition in adolescence and is usually induced by stress, anxiety, and other emotional stimuli. The acid-base and electrolyte imbalances caused by prolonged periods of deep breathing lead to marked neuromuscular changes such as paresthesias, muscle twitches, and spasms. Decreased cerebral perfusion due to vasoconstriction is responsible for lightheadedness, depersonalization, blurring of vision, and loss of consciousness. Unlike in epileptic attacks, the symptoms occur gradually and are slow in progression.

The deep breathing with characteristic heaving of the chest, the typical carpopedal spasms, the perioral paresthesias, and bilateral tingling of the fingertips are points of importance in the differential diagnosis. The facial twitching induced by secondary hypocalcemia may be distinguished from clonic seizures by demonstrating that the symptoms can be relieved by rebreathing exhaled air.

The interictal EEG is normal. During hyperventilation it shows diffuse slowing with no epileptiform abnormalities during the typical symptomatology.

After the cause is identified, no treatment is required except counseling. The adolescent can be reassured and advised to breathe in a paper bag during the attacks.

Migraine

Epilepsy and certain forms of migraine share many features, and the definition of boundaries between the two conditions is not always clear (see Chapter 84). For instance, a classic migraine attack starting with lights or scotoma, especially if referred to the contralateral hemifield, or with hemisensory loss, paresthesias, and weakness on one side of the body can be mistaken for a simple partial seizure of occipital or parietal origin followed by postictal headache. Similarly, the visual distortion (micropsia or macropsia) or the accentuated behavior and amnesia of confusional migraine attacks can be interpreted as partial seizures or fugue states of temporal lobe origin. The headache may be absent in migraine, especially in young individuals (acephalgic migraine), and the incidence of epileptiform EEG abnormalities and true epileptic seizures is high in patients with migraine. In addition, true epileptic seizures can be precipitated by migraine so that the pathophysiologic distinction between the two disorders becomes even less clear.

The main distinguishing features to be used in the differential diagnosis are the following:

1. The slow speed of progression of the migraine prodromal symptoms (minutes, as opposed to seconds in partial seizures).

2. A typical "fortification scotoma" is never reported in an epileptic attack.

3. Consciousness tends to become impaired early and subjective description is somewhat vague in epilepsy, whereas migrainous patients remain acutely aware and able to give an accurate account throughout the attack.

4. The headache represents an evolution of the prodromal symptoms in migraine, whereas it occurs after loss of consciousness and a secondary GTCS in epilepsy.

Despite the similarities, preventive therapy for the two conditions is different, although dual treatment combining antiepileptic drugs with antimigraine medications is indicated when GTCSs are triggered by an attack of migraine.

Narcolepsy and Cataplexy

The disorders of sleep organization usually manifest themselves in adolescence (see Chapter 86). Because of the hallucinatory experiences of narcolepsy and sudden loss of postural tone in cataplexy, the differential diagnosis with an epileptic seizure disorder may be considered. Other sleep disorders such as sleep walking or the Kleine-Levin syndrome, consisting of behavioral disturbances, episodic hypersomnia, hyperphagia, and hypersexuality in adolescent boys, may raise the same questions. An accurate history emphasizing the lack of motor and postical phenomena during the narcoleptic loss of consciousness and the presence of precipitating factors (e.g., laughter) in cataplexy are usually sufficient to clarify the issue. In dubious cases, the altered rapid eye movement (REM)–non-REM sequence demonstrated by sleep EEG studies will establish the diagnosis.

Psychogenic Seizures (see Chapter 112)

Psychogenic seizures remain a diagnosis of exclusion. However, their presence should be considered in adolescents whose seizures have atypical features, in those with an established seizure disorder who suddenly de-

velop a new presentation, and in those instances in which a new seizure disorder in an adolescent does not respond to usual trials of medication. Psychogenic seizures can occur in diverse types of adolescents, ranging from those with serious developmental or familial stressors to relatively well functioning young persons.

The diagnosis requires the use of simultaneous EEG and videotape recordings, sometimes associated with saline and sodium methohexital (Brevital) injections, and careful observation. All attempts are warranted to firmly establish the diagnosis. Neuropsychological testing is a pertinent aspect of the diagnostic workup, since 66% of patients treated by us had a learning disability. Adolescent, parent, and family psychiatric interviews play an important role in the course of the diagnostic workup in order to reveal hidden developmental or familial stressors. There is no one typical psychiatric presentation, diagnosis, or feature (including la belle indifference) that is pathognomonic. The simultaneous recording of the behavioral event with normal EEG on videotape establishes the diagnosis. It also provides the treatment team with convincing evidence to be used with the parents and the adolescent patient, when indicated, to begin the psychoeducational treatment approach that has been described for adults.

TREATMENT

Pharmacologic Treatment

Because epileptic seizures are so unpredictable, prevention is based on the chronic use of antiepileptic drugs (AEDs). An ideal AED should control all seizure activity, be given once daily, and cause no undesirable side effects. When starting treatment with a new anticonvulsant, it is important to know the side effects. Those that are dose-related should be measured against the benefits and should be tolerated only at a minimum. Allergic reactions of a mild nature can often be managed without complete withdrawal of the medication. Idiosyncratic reactions require immediate withdrawal.

Blood Level. The aim of optimal treatment is to establish the lowest maintenance dose necessary to achieve control of the epileptic seizures. It is important to remember that this may be lower than the amount required to reach the recommended "therapeutic blood level." The range of plasma concentration defined as "therapeutic" for each medication represents a statistical average, below which the majority of patients in whom the drug is effective may relapse and above which signs of toxicity may appear. When assessing the effectiveness of a drug in resistant cases, the blood concentration can be pushed to levels beyond therapeutic range, if tolerated, while carefully monitoring the clinical response. Whenever possible, blood levels should be obtained consistently at trough point.

For greatest effectiveness, the plasma concentration of an AED should be as constant as possible throughout 24 hours. The ability to maintain a relatively constant blood level depends on the drug's half-life (the time required for the plasma concentration to decline by 50% after reaching steady state). The half-life for each AED depends on the characteristics of the drug (rate of absorption, distribution in body tissues, biotransformation, and excretion) (Table 83–3). Each of these phases is subject to change under different circumstances and is also affected by the interaction with other drugs. Some understanding of the pharmacokinetics specific to each AED is essential to setting therapeutic strategies and to maximizing effectiveness (Table 83–4).

Absorption. Different preparations of the same drug may have different bioavailabilities, and therefore serum concentrations may vary significantly without changing the daily intake if the brand medication is changed to a generic or if one generic is switched to another generic. Intramuscular administration of an AED does not present particular advantages over other routes and is actually contraindicated in the case of PHT (Dilantin). PHT is a weak acid, soluble only in alkaline medium, that will precipitate crystals when injected in tissue at a physiologic pH of 7.4. For acute needs (i.e., immediate loading, inability to take medication orally), the intravenous administration is the route of choice. Rectal administration (when feasible) is a very practical, rapid, and effective alternative.

Distribution. Following absorption, the circulating AED is bound to proteins, mostly albumins, to a degree that is characteristic for each drug. Blood levels measure the total (bound and unbound) drug concentration. Only the free fraction can enter the active sites and is responsible for the therapeutic as well as the nontherapeutic side effects of the drug. The determination of the free fraction, especially of Dilantin, may be important when two AEDs with high affinity for albumin (e.g., valproic acid and Dilantin) are given together. Since they compete for protein-bindings, the free fraction of Dilantin may increase and cause signs of toxicity, despite no changes in the daily intake and in the total plasma concentration. Similarly, adolescents who have hypoalbuminemia are at risk for developing toxicity at a given total drug serum concentration. Most AEDs are lipid-soluble, a property that explains their affinity for the phospholipids in the CNS and for adipose tissue. As a result, obese individuals accumulate large amounts of AEDs outside the active site. This does not affect the steady state of the drug after such compartments are filled but may require a larger loading dose when the drug is started and may prolong the total elimination time when the drug is discontinued.

Biotransformation. Biotransformation of most AEDs occurs in the hepatic microsomal oxidative system (cytochrome P-450) and converts the parent drug into inactive metabolites for excretion. In some cases, the first oxidated metabolite is also an active antiepileptic compound (e.g., phenylethylmalonamide from primidone and 10,11-epoxide from carbamazepine). Competition for the hepatic oxidative system slows breakdown and increases the plasma concentration of both the parent drug and the early metabolites, the epoxides. The latter may be primarily responsible for the teratogenic effects. Therefore, the use of multiple anticonvulsants is particularly contraindicated in adolescents who have seizure disorders and are at risk of becoming pregnant. In the majority of cases, the oxidated metabolites undergo conjugation so that they can be excreted by the kidney. Hepatic failure decreases the rate of inactivation or conversion into active metabolites, resulting in increased serum concentration of the parent drug. The hypoalbuminemia often associated with hepatic failure represents an additional risk for toxicity.

Excretion. Some AEDs can be excreted in the unconjugated form and can be almost entirely eliminated directly through the kidney (acetazolamide, bromide, and trimethadione). Other AEDs (phenobarbital, primidone, ethosuximide) are partially eliminated by direct renal excretion. Renal disease may cause rising serum concentrations of these drugs (see Chapter 65). Hemodialysis has little effect on serum concentration of lipid-soluble AEDs (Dilantin) but removes a significant quantity of water-soluble drugs such as those directly excreted in total or in part by the kidney. In contrast, plasmapheresis may remove a significant quantity of PHT. Therefore, the appropriate amount of drug should be supplied to the bath to prevent seizure exacerbations after this procedure.

Pharmacokinetics. With a certain daily dose, irrespective of the route of administration, the plasma concentration depends primarily on the enzymatic processes of biotransformation and the half-life of the drug. When the enzyme system is not saturated, the rate of biotransformation varies directly with the concentration of the drug. When absorption is increased, biotransformation accelerates and the blood concentration increases proportionately (first order enzyme kinetics); but when the enzyme system is saturated, the rate of biotransformation remains the same. Therefore, the blood concentration increases disproportionately (zero order enzyme kinetics). PHT (Dilantin) usually follows the predictable pattern of first order kinetics when administered at a dose of 4 to 12 mg/kg/day, but changes to zero order kinetics when given in higher dosage. This phenomenon is accompanied by an apparent increase in the elimination half-life and leads to gradually rising blood levels until signs of drug toxicity occur. Unfortunately, it is not possible to predict exactly when this threshold is reached, because many factors influence biotransformation, including competition for the same enzyme system by other drugs.

Steady State. After establishing the appropriate maintenance daily dose and starting the administration, it is important to know that there is a delay prior to reaching steady state (drug absorption = elimination rate). This corresponds to five times the half-life of the drug. The same process occurs in reverse when the drug is discontinued after reaching steady state. This is intuitive, since the serum concentration drops to 50% after one half-life, to 25% after two half-lives, and virtually down to 0% after five half-lives. To eliminate such delay (when therapeutic plasma concentrations are needed immediately), a loading dose is necessary. Experiments in adult human volunteers have indicated that the loading dose for Dilantin is approximately 1000 mg, about twice the daily maintenance dose. The loading dose for intravenous phenobarbital is estimated at 10 to 20 mg/kg but has been less extensively studied. The same principles apply when the dosage of an individual drug is changed. Because of this delay, several days should elapse before the clinical effects are assessed. Serial determinations of

TABLE 83–3. Characteristics of Most Commonly Used Antiepileptic Drugs

DRUG NAME	ACTION	SEIZURE TYPE	ACTIVE METABOLITE	TOLERANCE	DRUG INTERACTION	COMMON SIDE EFFECTS
Acetazolamide [Diamox] 125 and 250 mg tab 500 mg SR caps Powder (IV inj) Generic: interchangeable	Carbonic anhydrase inhibitor and blockade of ion transport	Absence All others as second-line drug	—	High (3–6 mo) Most effective when given intermittently	None	Drowsiness Paresthesias Hyperventilation ↑ Micturition ↑ Thirst (transient) Teratogenicity
Carbamazepine (CBZ) [Tegretol] 200 mg tab 100 mg chewable tab 100 mg/5 ml susp Generic: different bioavailability	Class 1	Partial (especially temporal lobe origin) GTCS	10,11-epoxide	Moderate (autoinduction)	Blood levels decreased by PB and PHT; increased by propoxyphene; erythromycin increases free fraction of VPA and PB	Drowsiness, blurred vision, diplopia, dysequilibrium, leukopenia, gastrointestinal distress, hepatic failure
Clonazepam (CZP) [Klonopin] 0.5 mg tab 1 mg tab 2 mg tab Generic: interchangeable	Class 2–1	Myoclonic Absence (as second-line drug) Mixed minor motor seizures	—	High	Potentiates sedative action of ethanol, barbiturates, antihistamines, psychotropic drugs, analgesics Combination with VPA may result in absence status Plasma level may be decreased by PB and PHT	Sedation, ataxia Behavioral disturbances (hyperactivity in children), drooling
Clorazepate dipotassium [Tranxene] 3.75 mg tab 7.5 mg tab 15 mg tab Generic: interchangeable	Class 2	Partial, especially complex GTCS	N-desmethyl diazepam (rapid conversion)	Moderate to high (autoinduction)	Potentiates sedative action of ethanol, barbiturates, antihistamines, psychotropic drugs, analgesics	Similar to clonazepam but milder
Ethosuximide (ESM) [Zarontin] 250 mg capsules 250 mg/5 ml syrup	Class 3	Absence	—	—	—	GI distress Inability to concentrate Hiccups Headache Psychosis Bone marrow depression
Phenobarbital (PB) 15 mg tab 30 mg tab 60 mg tab elixir Parenteral preparation Generic: interchangeable	Class 2–1	Partial GTCS	—	—	Decreases plasma level of CBZ, PHT, digoxin, isoniazid, propranolol, phenylbutazone, coumarin Facilitates accumulation of other drugs, oxidated metabolites (teratogenicity) Metabolism inhibited by VPA	Decreased cognitive function, sedation, hyperactivity in children, depression, teratogenicity (indirectly through accumulation of epoxides etc.)
Phenytoin (PHT) [Dilantin] 30 mg and 100 mg capsules 50 mg chewable tab 30 and 125 mg/5 ml susp Parenteral preparation (IV inj) Generic: different bioavailability	Class 1	Partial GTCS	Inactive metabolite arene oxide (teratogenic) First-order kinetic metabolism at low concentration, zero order at high concentrations	—	↓ Absorption by Ca-based antacids With polytherapy, plasma concentration may vary owing to reciprocal enzyme induction and competition for protein binding sites Free fraction increased by VPA Plasma concentration increased by chloramphenicol, cimetidine, dicumarol, disulpheran isoniazid Decreases effectiveness of oral contraceptives	Gingival hyperplasia Hirsutism, coarse facial features Acneiform eruption Peripheral neuropathy (asymptomatic) Nystagmus, diplopia, Ataxia Decreased mental functions (plasma level > 30 µg/ml) GI distress Hepatic failure Pseudolymphoma Hypocalcemia Osteomalacia ↑ Metabolite of vitamin K Teratogenicity (arene oxide)

TABLE 83–3. Characteristics of Most Commonly Used Antiepileptic Drugs *Continued*

DRUG NAME	ACTION	SEIZURE TYPE	ACTIVE METABOLITE	TOLERANCE	DRUG INTERACTION	COMMON SIDE EFFECTS
Primidone (PRM) [Mysoline] 50 mg tab 250 mg tab 250 mg/5 ml susp Generic: interchangeable	Class 2–1	Partial GTCS	Phenylethylmalonamide (PEMA) Phenobarbital	—	Decreases plasma level of CBZ, PHT, digoxin, isoniazid, propranolol, phenylbutazone, coumarin Facilitates accumulation of oxides (teratogenicity) Metabolism inhibited by VPA	Same as for PB
Trimethadione (TMO) [Tridione] 150 mg chewable tab 300 mg capsules 40 mg/ml solution	Class 3	Absence Myoclonic-atonic	Dimethadione	?	—	Blurred vision in bright light Sedation High teratogenicity
Valproic acid/ Divalproiex sodium (VPA) [Depakene, Depakote]	Class 2–1	Idiopathic Myoclonic GTCS Absence	Diene triene metabolites (inactive but teratogenic)	—	Free fraction increased by coadministration of PHT, CBZ, salicylates, phenylbutazone Increases plasma level of free CBZ and PHT and of total PB	Toxicity, GI distress Sedation, ataxia Tremor Hair loss Increased appetite, weight gain Hepatotoxicity Pancreatitis Encephalopathy (hyperammonemia without hepatic dysfunction) Inhibition of platelet aggregation (risk of hemorrhage); thrombocytopenia; megaloblastic anemia Teratogenicity (spina bifida)

TABLE 83–4. Therapy Using Antiepileptic Drugs

DRUG NAME	HALF-LIFE (hrs)	PEAK TIME (hrs)	TIME TO REACH STEADY STATE (hrs)	PROTEIN BINDING	LIVER ENZYME INDUCTION	ADULT DOSE (mg/kg/d)	THERAPEUTIC PLASMA LEVEL (µg/ml)	STARTING DOSE (mg)	NUMBER DAILY DIVIDED DOSES	WITH-DRAWAL
Acetazolamide [Diamox]	10–12	2–3	40–48 (2 days)	90%	—	8–30	10–14	Same	qd/tid	Abrupt
Carbamazepine (CBZ) [Tegretol]	12	2–6	70–72 (3 days)	70–90%	+ + Self-induction	15–25	5–12	Gradual ↑ ⅓–½ maintenance	qid	Gradual
Clonazepam (CBZ) [Klonopin]	24–48	1–2	150 (6 days)	40–80%	—	0.03–0.3	20–80	Low; gradual ↑	bid	Very slow
Clorazepate dipotassium [Tranxene]	24–48	1*	150 (6 days)	?	?	0.7–1.0	1–2	7.5 bid	bid/tid	Very slow
Ethosuximide (ESM) [Zarontin]	40–60	2–3	240	Negligible	—	10–30	40–100	250 hs Gradual ↑	qd/bid	Abrupt
Phenobarbital (PB)	96 (4 days)	6–18	(3 weeks)	60%	+ + +	2–4	15–40	90 hs	qd	Gradual
Phenytoin (PHT) [Dilantin]	24	3–12 Variable	(5 days)	90%	+ +	3–8	10–20 or more	Loading	qd (hs) or bid	Gradual
Primidone (PRM) [Mysoline]	12	2–4	150 (3 days)	Negligible	+ + +	10–20	5–15	125 hs Gradual ↑	qid	Gradual
Trimethadione (TMO) [Tridione]	240* (10 days)	?	?	Negligible	?	20–60	500–1200	300 bid	bid/tid	?
Valproic acid/divalproex sodium (VPA) [Depakote, Depakene]	12–14	3–8	150(3 days)	90%	—	10–20 (monotherapy) 30–60 (polytherapy)	50–100	Gradual	qid	Gradual

*Valve refers to active metabolites.

plasma concentration are helpful in these circumstances. The issue is complicated further by the presence of other AEDs. Therefore, simultaneous drug changes should be avoided.

Frequency of Antiepileptic Drug Administration. In order to prevent undesirable side effects at peak levels and the risk of breakthrough seizures at trough serum level concentration, the interval between doses should be approximately equal to the elimination half-life. Therefore, the daily maintenance dose of AEDs with a half-life of 24 hours or longer (e.g., phenytoin [Dilantin] and ethosuximide [Zarontin]) can be administered in a single amount once daily, preferably at bedtime. Medications with a faster rate of absorption and elimination require multiple fractionated doses. More frequent administrations decrease the difference between peak and trough levels after each dose. This can be totally eliminated by continuous intravenous infusion. Adolescents are less compliant when a drug regimen requires taking the medication frequently (see Chapter 26). Therefore, the medication should be prescribed at the longest possible intervals that provide sufficient protection at trough blood levels after each single dose and avoid peak drug levels causing toxicity.

Classification of Antiepileptic Drugs. Based on present knowledge, three main classes of AEDs are identified (see Table 83–3).

Class 1. These medications prevent the tonic phase of maximal electroshock (MES)–induced seizures by acting on the sodium channels. The prototypes are phenytoin (Dilantin) and carbamazepine (Tegretol). Despite their structural differences, these two drugs reduce focal as well as generalized sustained repetitive firing (SRF) of neurons at the onset of a focal or a generalized seizure at therapeutic concentration. Barbiturates and benzodiazepines have similar effects but at supratherapeutic concentrations. Therefore, they are useful in acute situations such as status epilepticus but are not ideal for chronic administration.

Class 2. These compounds have more than one mechanism and share the properties of Class 1 AEDs, that is, they block SRF by increasing sodium channel inactivation. This class includes drugs such as benzodiazepines, barbiturates, and valproate, which increase inhibition by acting on the chloride channels situated on the GABA-a receptors.

Class 3. AEDs in this class selectively prevent pentylenetetrazol (PTZ)-induced seizures. The prototype is ethosuximide (Zarontin), and this class includes the less commonly used trimethadione (Tridione). The mechanism of action of these drugs appears very specific but is still poorly understood. These compounds act on calcium channels and currents, both important for the presynaptic release of neurotransmitters. However, whereas other drugs (PHT, barbiturates, benzodiazepines) have a nonselective effect on calcium influx and tend to require supratherapeutic concentrations, class 3 drugs have a specific effect on calcium currents mediated by the small T channels in the thalamic neurons at therapeutic concentrations. They all are effective against petit mal epilepsy.

It is important to remember that one drug may affect more than one membrane mechanism and that ulti-

mately the excitatory or inhibitory result depends not on a single change in membrane activity but rather on complex circumstances that include the type of synapses, neuronal pathways, and connections in which such changes take place.

Monotherapy is highly recommended to avoid cumulative side effects and other less conspicuous but not less important drug interactions that affect blood levels reciprocally. This is mostly the result of induction of oxidative enzymes in the liver. Most important, the accelerated metabolism causes an increase of the epoxide derivates that are responsible for other major side effects, including teratogenesis and idiosyncratic reactions. The use of multiple anticonvulsants is acceptable only in complex cases in which different types of seizures coexist.

Surgical Treatment

It is estimated that at least 80% of childhood epilepsies remit or are controlled by medication. Assuming that this figure is correct, the life of a substantial number of adolescents is going to be affected by a refractory form of this condition. For many of these cases, surgery may be the answer. The outcome reported by most centers has been very gratifying: more than two thirds of patients undergoing temporal lobectomy become seizure-free or almost seizure-free. The success rate is even higher for the few patients who qualify for hemispherectomy. The success rate is lower and the results are less predictable for extratemporal resections. The rate of improvement after palliation surgery (callosotomy) to alleviate the most severe seizure types remains uncertain. Patients who do not improve are usually not any worse after surgical intervention than they were before.

Since TLE is by far the most common form of partial epilepsy, anterior temporal lobectomy is the most frequently performed operation. The key to successful surgery is a rigorous selection of the candidate. This requires an elaborate array of assessments and special diagnostic procedures that include both noninvasive and invasive methods of investigation. These services can be provided only in specialized centers. The process of selection involves

1. Comprehensive clinical evaluation, including the psychosocial aspects of the disorder.

2. Extensive EEG reviews and long-term monitoring with videotape and EEG until a number of actual seizures are recorded. If information from scalp and sphenoidal recordings is not satisfactory and the patient is still a candidate for surgery, monitoring may have to be repeated with invasive electrodes (subdural strips, grids, depth electrodes).

3. Psychometric testing and careful neuropsychological assessment. These identify areas of strength and weaknesses in cognitive functions.

4. CT scanning and MRI with volumetric studies of the hippocampal region.

5. Intracarotid amobarbital injections (Wada test) to

study hemispheric lateralization for language and memory.

6. Monitoring of the EEG from the exposed brain during the operation (electrocorticography).

Preoperative mapping of cortical functions by direct electrical stimulation of the cortex is often necessary to localize essential areas not to be removed at operation.

The indications for resective surgery are:

1. The identification of a discrete, unilateral focus of seizure origin.

2. Intractability. This is defined as seizures persisting after at least 1 year of medical treatment by an experienced neurologist, in which all major primary AEDs are utilized either singly or in combination, with adequate documentation of plasma levels.

3. Potential for a tangible improvement in the quality of life if seizures are controlled. This delicate issue has to be carefully and compassionately addressed by the treating physicians and the evaluating team on a case-by-case basis.

Intractable cases in which a unilateral focus cannot be demonstrated may benefit from disconnection of the major interhemispheric commissure (callosotomy). This does not remove any tissue responsible for seizure activity and aims mainly at controlling the most severe seizures (palliation surgery). Indications for callosotomy are (1) multifocal, bilateral, or nonlocalized seizures with frontal preponderance, especially those with tendency to generalize secondarily; and (2) tonic-atonic seizures (drop attacks) that occur in the context of the Lennox-Gastaut syndrome.

The issue of potential loss of cognitive abilities with surgery should be addressed by the health care professionals when considering these alternatives. Information available in this area is less clear and often contradictory, partly owing to the fact that surgical procedures, even a standard anterior temporal lobectomy, vary from center to center and from case to case, especially with respect to the extent of the hippocampus removed. Cognitive deficits, especially in the area of learning and memory, are often found preoperatively in patients with intractable complex partial seizures, especially if the epileptogenic zone is located in the dominant hemisphere. Certain specific deficits tend to be magnified by anterior temporal lobectomy. However, a right temporal lobectomy is often followed by improvement of some functions, whereas statistically significantly lower scores are expected on verbal subtests after a left (dominant) lobectomy. The degree of loss can be predicted to an extent, depending on the accuracy of the presurgical evaluation. In well-selected cases, cognitive losses are minor or insignificant and are compensated largely by the benefit of seizure relief.

Affect and behavior can be greatly influenced by intractable epilepsy. In these areas, changes following surgery are less predictable. Whereas adolescents qualifying for hemispherectomy may show great behavioral improvement when made seizure-free by the intervention, affective and psychiatric disorders may persist or worsen after temporal lobectomy. Therefore, adolescents undergoing this type of intervention require psychiatric attention prior to and after surgery.

Callosotomy is usually performed in two stages. First, the anterior two thirds callosotomy is performed, then the disconnection is completed if seizure control is still inadequate. The first stage is usually well tolerated, whereas complete callosotomy carries the risk of severe neuropsychological and cognitive disabilities, including the split brain syndrome.

The adolescent and his or her relatives and friends should be aware of the potential risks as well as the potential benefits. The health care team evaluating the risk-to-benefit ratio should consider the following factors: the probability of relief of seizures, the adolescent's preoperative level of cognitive functioning, the anticipated possible cognitive changes that may affect the adolescent's life and career ambitions, and the degree of support available to the adolescent should the surgery not relieve the symptoms.

MANAGEMENT OF THE ADOLESCENT WITH EPILEPSY

Sexual Development

Any type of epilepsy, particularly TLE, can have a direct or indirect effect on hormone secretions of the hypothalamic-pituitary-gonadal axis. For instance, it is well established that tonic-clonic seizures and complex partial seizures, particularly those originating in the temporal lobe, cause significant increase in prolactin levels within minutes of the attack. Given the role of the hippocampus in seizure generation, it is conceivable that the connections between this structure and the hypothalamus are responsible for this effect. Considering the frequency of complex partial seizures in certain individuals, this may constitute a contributing factor to the high frequency of anovulatory cycles in these patients and the low fertility rate attributed to patients with epilepsy.

It is a generally accepted notion that estrogen lowers seizure threshold, whereas progesterone "protects" against seizure activity. The periodic surge of epileptic activity in catamenial epilepsy coincides with the rapid fall of estrogen and progesterone serum levels toward the end of the menstrual cycle and follows the midluteal phase during which these two hormones reach high blood concentration and fewer seizures occur. Increased frequency of seizures is also noted during anovulatory cycles when no ovum is produced and progesterone concentration remains low. Such effects may not be immediately obvious in adolescents with epilepsy, but knowledge of the consequences that this condition may have on sex hormone regulation later in life warrants particular caution.

The neuropharmacologic effects of chronic treatment with AEDs should also be given careful consideration. Enzyme-inducers such as phenobarbital, primidone, phenytoin, and carbamazepine increase the metabolism of sex steroid hormones and stimulate sex hormone–binding globulin (SHBG) production. SHBG binds 41%

of the circulating testosterone and 30% of estradiol. When the availability of this protein is increased, the concentration of the unbound hormones decreases. The low serum concentration of unbound testosterone found in males with long-standing epilepsy has been considered to be responsible for the hyposexuality reported by young men who have this disorder. Therefore, treatment with AEDs in adolescence should be as conservative as possible. Preference should be given to non–enzyme-inducer drugs such as valproate and benzodiazepines, and the use of multiple drugs should be minimized.

There is no specific contraindication to the use of oral contraceptives, although the overall effect may have to be assessed on an individual basis. Failure rates in preventing pregnancy have been higher in patients with epilepsy than in the general population, probably because of the faster liver metabolism of steroid hormones induced by AEDs. For adolescents who have epilepsy, the dose of hormones necessary for contraception should be adjusted according to the individual need. The frequency of breakthrough bleeding is a good indicator that the dose is not sufficient. Although the interaction between epilepsy, especially TLE, and hormones of the hypothalamic-pituitary-gonadal axis is well established, the mechanisms involved are still unclear and the reports on the psychosocial effects (changes in fertility, sexuality, and so on) are often contradictory. However, the consequences on the lifestyle and well-being of young patients with epilepsy may be significant and long lasting, so that the surgical approach, especially in the case of TLE, may be preferable to prolonged and heavy use of antiepileptic agents.

Pregnancy

In women of childbearing age who are being treated for epilepsy, pregnancy should be planned in advance in order to reduce exposure of the fetus to AEDs, especially during the first trimester. Therefore, it is important to offer birth control counseling to all sexually active teenagers treated for this condition. A number of clinical reports in the last 2 decades have pointed out that the use of certain AEDs in pregnancy is associated with increased rate of congenital malformation in the fetus. Experimental studies in animals indicate that virtually no AED is exempt, if given in sufficiently high dosage. More recent experience, corroborated by the results of longitudinal controlled studies, has demonstrated, however, that current practices of prescribing AEDs, particularly avoidance of polypharmacy, and monitoring of blood levels have decreased the risk of teratogenic effects to a nonsignificant level. It appears that the factor mainly responsible for fetal malformation is the high serum concentration of the first oxidated metabolites of major AEDs. Therefore, circumstances that facilitated the oxygenation of the parent drug and that may interfere with further biotransformation, such as the coadministration of two or more AEDs, should be avoided. Thus, the first rule to be strictly observed during pregnancy is monotherapy.

In addition, the chosen drug should be prescribed at the lowest effective serum concentration. Certain medications such as Tridione, known to be associated with a high rate of stillbirth and congenital malformations, should never be prescribed to women of childbearing age, although they still may be of value in male patients. If valproic acid (VPA) is the drug of choice, alpha-fetoprotein levels should be monitored throughout pregnancy because of the increased risk of spina bifida associated with this medication.

Physiologic changes in drug pharmacokinetics occur during pregnancy, namely AED blood levels tend to decrease, requiring adjustment of the dose in order to prevent seizure breakthrough. A rebound effect, with signs of toxicity, should be expected after delivery. This is probably caused by changes in absorption and increased biotransformation rate due to activation of the endothelium reticulum, but also may be due to decreased compliance for fear of teratogenicity. Careful clinical monitoring and counseling are highly recommended. Patients should be advised that whereas the occurrence of partial seizures is of no consequence, GTCS should be prevented. They pose a far more concrete risk of fetal damage than the potential, but remote, teratogenicity of AED.

Psychosocial Aspects

It is important to note that some physicians tend to overestimate the importance of medical concerns and underestimate the importance of psychosocial concerns in comparison with parents or educators. Adolescents with seizures face the same developmental tasks as normal adolescents. In addition, they must assimilate the meaning of having epilepsy within the context of living a normal life and fulfilling personal, familial, and societal expectations. A variety of studies suggest that the degree to which adolescents understand their illness and its treatment, as well as their perceptions of themselves, is correlated with the adolescents' overall sense of well-being.

The foundation for managing epilepsy is laid down by early interactions between the child and the family. If the burden of achieving a positive adaptation is poorly completed by the child and family, it reappears as the adolescent confronts the challenges of young adulthood: establishing an intimate relationship, managing job or school applications, and achieving independence from the family. Adolescence is a time during which the early coping strategies of the child are challenged. A child's sense of autonomy and competence is an essential component of self-esteem. If there have been problems in these areas during middle childhood, they will be exacerbated in adolescence.

Poor adaptation in youngsters with epilepsy often reflects both poor seizure control and the presence of other family problems and stressors. Earlier patterns of denial, avoidance, minimalization, and lack of effective emotional communication or problem solving resurface while coping with epilepsy and, in turn, complicate the adolescent's ability to handle the new demands of the adolescent era. Previous studies have stressed the greater vulnerability of epileptic children to both anxiety and dissatisfaction with themselves.

IMPORTANCE OF COMMUNICATION

For those adolescents who face the onset of seizures during their teenaged years, as well as those youngsters whose seizure patterns are complicated by the emergence of a new form of epilepsy (e.g., from absence to grand mal), reactions to epilepsy are magnified. The need for open communication and discussion is underlined by the impact of secrecy in the creation of a negative self-image. In one study, those youngsters who were the most neurologically normal often had the most negative self-image and social adjustment. They also worried about the effect of their problem on the family. The better their seizure control was, the less discussion took place. Their handicap was invisible. However, those adolescents who had a seizure in public demonstrated a better adaptation than those who continued to fear having a seizure outside of the home, with all of its implications. This fear of stigma or self-revelation often mirrors the family's experiences and problems with self-esteem. The more the family or parents fear the revelation of their adolescent's underlying medical "defect," the more likely the adolescent carries a similar fear. As a result, the early referral for psychosocial education and support can minimize the impact of these issues on adolescents. These patients and their families often benefit from a counseling intervention in which the normal "stock-taking" about a serious event is facilitated. Issues of overprotection and restrictiveness within the family are no less likely in the second decade than they were in the first. The parents need as much help and support as does the adolescent.

Because an adolescent's sense of well-being comes from a sense of pride in his or her new physical development, positive psychological health is related to feeling healthy. Adolescents who have seizures have many struggles. Adolescents are proud of a job well done and want to be able to use their competence to establish further their sense of being able to manage on their own. They assess and compare their abilities against those of their peers. As a result, feelings of social isolation, peer acceptance, and worries about normalcy can be typical concerns of young people who have epilepsy.

Adolescents require information about whether their epilepsy will affect their participation in sports or tasks like driving. It is important to be able to reassure them that vigorous exercise does not affect levels of AEDs nor is there much likelihood that a seizure will be precipitated by the vigorous exertion of competitive sports. Adolescents who have epilepsy face the uncertainty of how their seizures may affect more demanding school functions, the reactions that may arise from friends and employers (issues of stigma), and the adolescent's own concerns. Another major area of concern is the fatigue caused by medication, which affects their school or work performance.

Adolescence is the period during which the most experimentation occurs. Therefore, the potential complications of drug and alcohol misuse require open discussion. Reports that seizure threshold may be lowered by certain drugs (marijuana, cocaine) and the epileptogenicity of alcohol along with its additive side effects to anticonvulsants warrant attention. Issues of emerging sexuality may be confused by the adolescent's sense of being "defective" or by potential cosmetic side effects of medications that affect attractiveness or sexual function, a topic rarely discussed. In addition, adolescent females whose seizure control may vary with their menstrual cycles need further support. The lessened effectiveness of birth control pills due to enzyme induction or other hormonal effects should also be openly discussed.

Even when seizures are not a major burden, the fact that poor information and misinformation still exist (like the belief that adolescents could swallow their tongue, that they could die during a seizure, that epilepsy is contagious) should remind us of the importance of discussion. Especially when there has not been good familial communication, opportunities for confusion abound. Without psychosocial support, poor communication increases the likelihood that the adolescent's own repressed or poorly understood feelings will complicate his or her strategies for dealing with teachers, peers, or employers when they have to discuss their epilepsy.

COMPLIANCE (see Chapter 26)

Compliance with the medical regimen is important. The net result of familial difficulties that do not prepare the adolescent to assume an increasing role in self-care and in accepting the meaning of having seizures is often expressed through noncompliance. There is some suggestion that noncompliance is an indicator of both poor psychological adjustment and disturbed patterns of communication within the family. The feelings expressed through noncompliance can range from anxiety to reactions of anger or helplessness. In one study, it was found that when financial distress of the family is combined with inability of the adolescent to assume responsibility, the likelihood of noncompliance is approximately four times as great as that in comparison groups. In many adolescents, noncompliant behaviors can remind us of their need for autonomy and their wish "not to depend on anything," including their medication. Ironically, after comparing control groups with youngsters affected by chronic illness (diabetes or epilepsy), those with epilepsy were found to be more dependent than those with diabetes or control subjects. These issues highlight the degree to which the adjustment of adolescents who have epilepsy depends upon a continued need for discussion and periodic medical follow-up.

EMPLOYMENT

Preparation for vocational or educational goals begins during middle adolescence. Adolescents who have seizures face more complex questions than do adolescents without seizures because of their fears about employers' reactions as well as the way in which stigma plays a role in the job market. In addition, their assessments of their readiness for independent functioning as well as their competence influence what they are willing to undertake. In spite of all these obstacles, however, long-term job performance and adjustment to work among adolescents with well-controlled epilepsy are good. There is, however, greater unemployment and underemployment in those with epilepsy when compared with the general population, as a result of cognitive and personality variables. Significant problems are found, for the most part, in those adolescents whose seizures had an earlier age of onset, longer duration, and greater severity as well as those with intelligence quotient (IQ) scores below normal limits. In one study, both social contacts (73%) and employment (71%) were the most frequently cited complaints of patients in this group. However, a significant positive effect has been reported in both job duration and employer satisfaction when family counseling is implemented.

EDUCATION

As in issues of employment, adolescents with epilepsy often function quite well in school. Poor school function is an indicator of poor psychological adjustment, family problems, or learning complications. When school function appears impaired, it warrants investigation. In a study of university students with epilepsy, although 50% still had seizures, their intelligence and attitude permitted an optimal adjustment.

School function in adolescents with epilepsy is most affected by the possible presence of attentional problems or learning disabilities. The possible side effects of medications should be reviewed for their impact on learning. Attentional problems should be ruled out. Attentional factors that impede performance can weigh as heavily as academic disabilities on the overall adjustment of the adolescent. The use of neuropsychological testing can be crucial in establishing this diagnosis as well as unveiling potential learning impairments (see Chapter 99).

Awareness of the cognitive side effects of some AEDs should be shared with adolescents and their parents. Their reports can be as useful as teacher checklists and periodic cognitive testing. In this fashion, problems related to the side effects of certain medications can be part of the risk-benefit discussion that occurs as part of the treatment of seizures. Educational supports and treatment strategies, including the use of psychostimulants and other medications, should be utilized, when warranted, because these drugs are as effective in adolescents with seizures as in those without. Fear of increased likelihood of seizure with psychotropic drugs should not prevent this treatment when it proves to be beneficial for learning.

PSYCHIATRIC COMPLICATIONS

Psychogenic seizures (pseudoseizures) may occur during adolescence. The adolescent who has epilepsy may be responding to a developmental or family crisis. In some of these adolescents, significant personality disorder is already present. In those without these complications, often a supportive and educational intervention as well as help with solving the crisis minimizes the presence of pseudoseizures; the others usually require long-term intensive psychotherapy involving the family. Adolescents whose first presentation is pseudoseizures pose a diagnostic challenge that may take some time to

clarify. In this group, the precipitant for the development of this pattern appears to be the combination of head trauma associated with a high anxiety level in the family that is actively communicated to the adolescent. Once the diagnosis is made and the family thoroughly reassured, the symptom usually subsides.

Other complications interfering with positive outcome include depression, personality disorder, and psychotic-like states (see Chapters 100, 109, and 110). Depressive disorders in children or adolescents may not necessarily reflect the impact of seizures *per se,* but a coincident vulnerability to depression (see Chapter 100). While taking the history, it is important to determine if a first-degree relative has a history of an affective disorder. In addition, the tendency to depression may be exacerbated by treatment with certain AEDs (i.e., barbiturates, but not carbamazepine).

In a small percentage of cases, patterns of thought distortion, overtly psychotic thinking, or other major forms of mental illness exist. Psychotic-like states are not infrequently precipitated by status epilepticus, especially in predisposed individuals. Persistent psychosis has been reported in about 7% of patients with epilepsy, although this association and other interictal personality or psychiatric disorders continue to be a source of debate in adolescents and adults alike. The potential psychotic side effects of certain AEDs such as ethosuximide (Zarontin) as well as the psychotic-like states induced by rapid withdrawal of some anticonvulsants should be considered as well.

LONG-TERM OUTCOME

Long-term outcome is most impaired in those adolescents whose epilepsy is poorly controlled or who suffer from other handicaps. If there are attendant developmental delays or handicapping conditions (especially impairment of language skills) or if the condition is a major preoccupation because of poor seizure control, the family must find ways of supporting and managing both the adolescent's condition and the related demands that challenge the adjustment of the entire family. Adolescents whose seizures have been poorly controlled show poorer adjustment in family relationships, vocational outlook, and ability to deal with their disorder.

Uncontrolled epilepsy may unleash a cascade of negative events for an adolescent. Driving is prohibited. The impact of the probability of a seizure during key social events often prompts withdrawal or isolation. Dating is impeded. Personality development is distorted by the use of psychological defenses that often interfere with the best possible adjustment to reality and to the choices the individual may face. For all these reasons, if therapy with AEDs fails, alternative treatment (i.e., surgery) should be considered as early as possible. However, assessment and prevention of the psychosocial complications are essential for a good outcome, irrespective of the modality of treatment. For those who survive the impact of chronic uncontrolled epilepsy with positive psychological coping mechanisms and good adjustment within the family, outcome continues to be positive when their seizures are controlled by surgery.

For those whose prior individual and family adjustment were poor, adjustment to living, even when they become seizure-free, often continues to be poor.

BIBLIOGRAPHY

Commission on Classification and Terminology: Proposal for revised clinical and electroencephalographic classification of epileptic seizures. Epilepsia 22:489, 1981.

Commission on Classification and Terminology: Proposal for revised classification of epilepsies and epileptic syndromes. Epilepsia 30:389, 1989.

Dodrill CB, Batzel LW, Wilensky AJ, Yerby MS: The role of psychosocial and financial factors in medication non-compliance in epilepsy. Int J Psychiatry Med 17:143, 1987.

Earl WL: Job stability and family counseling. Epilepsia 27:215, 1986.

Hodgman C, McAnarney ER, Myers G, et al: Emotional complications of grand mal epilepsy. J Pediatr 95:309, 1979.

Margalit M, Heiman, T: Anxiety and self-dissatisfaction in epileptic children. Soc Psychiatry 29:220, 1983.

Scheuer ML, Pedley TA: The evaluation and treatment of seizures. N Engl J Med 323:1468, 1990.

Ziegler R: Impairment of control and competence in epileptic children and their families. Epilepsia 22:339, 1981.

Other General References

Engel J Jr: Seizures and epilepsy. Contemporary Neurology Series No. 31. Philadelphia, FA Davis, 1989. (An updated and comprehensive review of the pathophysiology, classification and treatment of currently identified epileptic syndromes and other seizure disorders.)

Goldblatt D, Devinsky O (eds): Behavioral aspects of paroxysmal disorders. Semin Neurol 11(2), 1991. (Useful and extensive review of the phenomenology and behavior associated with various epileptic syndromes.)

Goldblatt D, Spencer SS (eds): Epilepsy. Semin Neurol 10(4), 1990. (The entire issue is devoted to the classification, diagnosis, medical management, and surgical treatment of various forms of epilepsies.)

CHAPTER 84

Headache

DEWEY K. ZIEGLER

Headache is one of the most frequent symptoms, having been found to affect 90% to 95% of all individuals. In community studies it has been found that at least half of the adolescent population admit to some type of headache. Approximately 30% give a history of "severe" headache at some time, and 4% to 7% give a history of migraine more narrowly defined. However, only approximately 20% of adolescents and young adults who suffer headaches have consulted physicians.

Headache appears to be prevalent in all cultures and populations studied, although there remain interesting differences in the degree of prevalence. For example, compared with the United States or Great Britain, headache appears to be less frequent in the People's Republic of China. In the 15- to 24-year-old age group of the population of China, severe headache was found in only 2% to 3%. The equally interesting question of whether prevalence varies with occupation or income level remains controversial. Studies from Great Britain report comparatively uniform prevalence of migraine over widely varying socioeconomic groups. One study from China, however, reported half the prevalence in rural as compared with urban populations in both young and older adults.

ACUTE HEADACHE

The acute headache presents problems quite different from those of chronic, continual, or frequently recurring headache. Sudden headache may be a part of a wide variety of syndromes. Although all these diagnostic entities must be considered in patients seen in emergency departments or doctors' offices with acute headache as an isolated symptom, fewer than 5% will be suffering from a condition other than migraine, tension-type headache, or some variant thereof. This is especially true in adolescents, since several entities producing acute headache (e.g., brain tumors and cerebrovascular disease) are more common in advanced adult years.

The pain of headache occurs in the distribution of the trigeminal nerve and the high cervical nerve roots. Why pain occurs in these areas is in most cases unknown. Structural abnormality of the central nervous system pain pathways (which include the thalamus and reticular formation of the brainstem) is vary rare. It is speculated that these areas in idiopathic headache syndromes receive inappropriate stimulation. The throbbing nature of headache has in the past suggested pain derived from the walls of arterial vessels. This may be the source of pain in some pain syndromes (e.g., febrile headache) but probably is not in others (migraine), as discussed later. Pain receptors occur also in muscles and tendons. Stimulation, usually mechanical, of these structures in the neck can cause pain referred to the head.

Headache with Acute Systemic Disease

Headache commonly occurs during the course of the common cold, influenza, and other acute infections (see Chapters 93 and 94). Such headache is usually not referred to any specific region of the head, is constant and not episodic, and frequently is coincident with fever. Nausea and vomiting are rarely present. The symptom characteristically disappears with subsidence of the viral infection, although occasionally it may linger for weeks or even months. In some of these adolescents, spinal fluid examination reveals a small number of lymphocytes, rarely more than 100, suggestive of meningoencephalitis.

Headache Secondary to Exogenous Agents

After excessive indulgence in alcohol, headache is well known ("hangover"). There usually is no problem in diagnosis; pain is generalized, frequently throbbing, and usually not associated with nausea. Hangover may be indistinguishable from migraine. Headache may occur in other withdrawal states and as a reaction to the abuse of other drugs (e.g., marijuana or cocaine) (see Chapters 97 and 111).

Subarachnoid Hemorrhage

This event, common in adolescents, characteristically has an explosive onset with extreme headache, usually maximal in the occipital areas, as the most common manifestation. Accompanying nuchal rigidity is the rule. Often there are varying degrees of impairment of higher functions, from confusion to deep coma. Concomitant intracerebral bleeding may also occur, producing a variety of focal neurologic deficits—hemiplegia, aphasia, and visual field deficit.

Subarachnoid hemorrhage occurs rarely in more subacute forms productive of a less cataclysmic event. These adolescents may have a persistent occipital headache, usually of sudden onset.

The most common source of bleeding, particularly in the young, is ruptured cerebral aneurysm, and local signs of such a lesion are of great importance in the differential diagnosis. A common site of such aneurysms is the proximal portion of the anterior cerebral artery, often with resultant pressure on the third cranial nerve. Various degrees of third nerve deficit are then apparent—ptosis, lateral deviation of the eye, or pupillary dilatation.

Subarachnoid hemorrhage may more rarely result from any pathologic process that prolongs bleeding time or disturbs the clotting mechanism. A variety of diseases and medications, notably anticoagulants, can have this effect (see Chapter 52).

It is important to make an early diagnosis of subarachnoid hemorrhage so that appropriate therapy can be instituted. The differentiation from acute migraine is often difficult. The most important clues to the diagnosis of subarachnoid hemorrhage are (1) nuchal rigidity, (2) presence of neurologic abnormalities, (3) absence of a history of similar acute episodes (there will be a history of migraine, however, in a certain percentage of adolescents with aneurysm), and (4) presence of some alteration of consciousness. This differentiation is particularly difficult in the adolescent, since the first attack of migraine commonly occurs in these years. Some points of differentiation between meningeal irritation caused by an accumulation of blood and migraine are illustrated in Table 84–1.

If a reasonable possibility of subarachnoid hemorrhage is present, computed tomography (CT) scan of the head and lumbar puncture should be performed. The latter procedure should be done even if the CT result is negative because occasionally the CT findings may be negative in the presence of early hemorrhage or small amounts of blood.

The clinician must weigh the likelihood of subarachnoid hemorrhage in each acute headache episode. Obviously the prevalence of recurrent headache is such that these diagnostic tests cannot be performed in all cases of acute headache.

TABLE 84–1. Migraine Attack vs. Subarachnoid Hemorrhage

	MIGRAINE	SUBARACHNOID HEMORRHAGE
Onset	Often rapid but rarely abrupt	Usually abrupt
Site of pain	Usually maximal in frontal or temporal region	Maximal in occipital region
Warning (visual)	Frequent	Absent
Accompanying nausea or vomiting	Usual	Uncommon
Nuchal rigidity	Rare	Common
Scalp tenderness	Frequent	Rare
History of similar attacks	Usual	Uncommon

Encephalitis and Meningitis

These entities produce severe headache, rarely of the abrupt onset seen in subarachnoid hemorrhage or migraine. Usually the diagnosis is suspected because of the presence of many systemic signs of infection, somnolence and confusional states, and, often, focal signs of cerebral dysfunction. Such signs clearly mandate a complete blood count, spinal fluid examination, and an electroencephalogram (EEG). The diagnosis is revealed by the characteristic spinal fluid profiles (presence of more than five white blood cells and elevated protein). With bacterial or fungal meningeal infection, cerebrospinal fluid glucose is depressed. With encephalitis, diffuse focal slow abnormality on the EEG is seen in more than 90% of the cases.

Acute Sinusitis

Often cited as the cause of headache, sinusitis is rarely the culprit. When it is, systemic signs of infection are always present—fever, leukocytosis, and elevated sedimentation rate (see Chapters 40 and 43). There is usually marked tenderness to percussion and pressure over the affected sinuses (usually frontal or maxillary). These signs indicate the necessity of sinus x-ray films, which confirm the diagnosis by showing opacity of one or more sinuses and occasionally a fluid level. Chronic sinusitis is a rare cause of headache.

Acute Ophthalmic Conditions

Optic neuritis, a not uncommon ophthalmic syndrome, is often painful, but the pain is rarely of truly abrupt onset and is restricted to a localized area—retroorbital and unilateral. It is invariably accompanied by diminution of vision on the painful side. In approximately half the patients, the optic disk is swollen in the affected eye. There may be tenderness of the globe to touch.

Optic neuritis is of unknown cause in more than 50% of the cases, especially in the young. In multiple sclerosis, it is the first event in approximately 15% of cases and occurs during the course of the disease in about half the cases (see Chapters 87 and 88). It also can occur in the various forms of vasculitis, occasionally in other diseases, and as the result of a wide variety of toxins (e.g., heavy metals or herbicides). Diagnostic tests for these entities often need to be performed.

Conjunctivitis, chorioretinitis, and uveitis all can cause headache, but the diagnoses are not difficult because pain is persistent and localized and eye pathology is apparent. Contrary to lay opinion, refractive errors do not commonly give rise to significant headache unless clearly related to severely impaired vision.

Acute Psychiatric States

In adolescents, as in adults, headache may be part of a syndrome of an acute psychosis or neurosis. In psychosis, headache is expressed often as part of a delusional system, with comments by the adolescent such as "Something is influencing my brain" or "Something is growing in my head." In such cases, the symptom often responds to neuroleptic drugs. In neurosis, headache is often part of an acute anxiety state with the usual signs of tachycardia and sympathetic nervous system overactivity.

CHRONIC OR RECURRENT HEADACHE

Increased Intracranial Pressure

Headache of this cause is constant in more than 90% of cases and often overlies the site of the lesion. Recurrent vomiting without nausea is common in the advanced stages. Focal neurologic abnormalities and papilledema are usually, but not universally, present. Increased intracranial pressure can be due to bleeding or infection irritating the meninges (as mentioned previously), space-occupying lesions, or obstructive or nonobstructive hydrocephalus. Hydrocephalus may be secondary to previous meningitis, subarachnoid hemorrhage, or injury.

Increased pressure occurs in the absence of structural pathology in the entity known as benign intracranial hypertension or pseudotumor cerebri. This condition is more frequent in youth than in older age groups. It is often a manifestation of some systemic disease (e.g., endocrine abnormality). For unknown reasons it occurs more frequently in females and is often associated with obesity, use of tetracycline, vitamin A, or other drugs, and menstrual irregularities. Imaging of the brain often shows small ventricles. Spinal fluid pressure is over 200 mm H_2O and may be as high as 400 mm H_2O, with frequent fluctuations from day to day. Adolescent patients usually respond to repeated drainage of spinal fluid with lowering of the pressure. The condition is usually self-limited, but if it does not respond promptly to lumbar puncture, a variety of other therapeutic maneuvers may be tried, although their effectiveness is still in doubt. These include prednisone and hyperosmolar agents such as glycerol, acetazolamide, and mannitol. If increased pressure does not respond to these therapies, there is danger of damage to optic nerves, with subsequent optic atrophy. Visual fields and visual acuity should be checked at intervals, the frequency depending on visual symptoms. If visual fields become impaired, the adolescent may need a surgical procedure such as lumbar thecoperitoneal shunt or incision of the sheath of the optic nerve to prevent permanent damage.

Metabolic States

Although hypoglycemia *per se* is not a common single cause of headache, a mild degree often precipitates attacks in patients who are headache prone. Headache also is common in a variety of endocrine and electrolyte disorders—notably, in patients undergoing dialysis, in whom the symptoms may well be due to fluctuations in electrolyte levels (see Chapter 65). In mild degrees of cerebral hypoxia, and after exposure to carbon monoxide, headache occurs in over half the cases. A wide variety of medications have headache as a side effect, for example, phenothiazines, tricyclic antidepressants, and antihypertensives (see Chapter 67). With vasodilators and other drugs with cardiovascular actions, this adverse effect may occur in 10% of patients. The frequency of this adverse effect increases with increased dosage.

Headache occurs in hay fever in about half the cases. How important allergic phenomena are in the genesis of recurrent headache is controversial. There have been reports of patients sensitive to certain substances who are helped by desensitization or, in the case of food allergies, by elimination diets. Probably in fewer than 10% of adolescents with recurrent headache are allergies an important cause.

Adolescents habituated to the use of excessively large amounts of analgesics (e.g., acetaminophen) may suffer a paradoxical perseveration or even increase in headache, despite continued use of the drugs. A similar phenomenon occurs even more prominently with excessive use of ergotamine. Such individuals need to be withdrawn from the drug, often a difficult process psychologically. Withdrawal from caffeine in individuals habituated to large amounts also often produces severe headache.

Posttraumatic Headache

A variety of headache syndromes may follow head trauma. The major or only manifestation of subdural hematoma is headache in 10% to 25% of cases. More common as a posttraumatic syndrome is headache that is constant and associated with a variety of other symptoms—fatigue, memory disturbances, and nervousness. Adolescents are less subject to this syndrome than are older adults and more likely to experience resolution in 2 to 3 weeks. In many cases, medicolegal matters related to an accident may prolong posttraumatic headache. Recurring severe, generalized headache occurs in a small percentage of individuals after head trauma and may have no relation to the severity of the head injury. On occasion, this headache may have most of the characteristics of migraine.

Also common is the persistent head pain, usually greatest in the occipital and neck regions, following sudden acceleration and deceleration of the body occurring in motor vehicle accidents, also often with medicolegal implications (whiplash injury). Such patients usually have tenderness of the paraspinal muscles in the cervical area and complain of pain on passive movement of the head. There are often complaints of many other nonspecific symptoms (e.g., fatigue, blurring of vision).

Inflammatory Vasculitides
(see Chapter 90)

In disseminated lupus erythematosus, headache occurs in at least 50% of patients. Usually the symptom is not clearly episodic and not associated with nausea, vomiting, or prodromata. Disseminated lupus affects primarily women; it is more frequent in young adults than in adolescents. The disease is manifested by a variety of other clinical phenomena (e.g., rashes, arthralgia, fever, and lymphadenopathy). Common laboratory findings are leukopenia, elevated sedimentation rate, anemia, abnormal liver functions, and often the presence of a variety of antibodies in the serum. Headache is a major manifestation of giant cell arteritis, but this disease is extremely rare in adolescents.

Migraine

Migraine, a common disease in adolescents, is characterized by five primary symptoms: (1) recurring episodes of limited duration, (2) nausea and often vomiting during attacks, (3) unilateral pain, (4) photophobia during pain, and (5) warning symptoms (usually visual) preceding the pain. Also characteristic of attacks are diarrhea, vasoconstriction of extremities, and exacerbation of the pain by exercise. How many of these features are required for the diagnosis of migraine is controversial. Periodicity, at least at some time during the life course, is necessary for the diagnosis, however. A constant headache lasting for weeks or more cannot be called migraine.

Although it is known that migraine is frequent, its actual prevalence is debatable. The more conservative estimates give figures of 2% to 10% in the United States population, but some studies have reported higher frequencies. It is at least twice as common in women as in men. Onset is very frequent in childhood but equally frequent in adolescence and early adulthood. Life history is extremely variable; some individuals have rare attacks (e.g., one or two per year), others more frequent (several per month). There are often long periods of spontaneous remission. In about 10% of female sufferers, attacks regularly cluster around the time of menstrual periods and often disappear during pregnancy. There is often a history of precipitation by a wide variety of stimuli, including emotional stress, sleep loss or excessive sleep, ingestion of certain food substances (notably chocolate or red wine), blows on the head, flickering or brilliant light, strong odors, excessive exertion, and sexual intercourse.

There probably is no single cause of migraine. There is frequently a strong family history of severe headache, but it is not known what the inherited predisposition might be. The importance of cerebrovascular dysfunction in migraine is debatable. It has been proved that pathologic cerebrovascular events occur during the aura of migraine. Cerebral blood flow is diminished at this time. Recent work, however, has shown that in these patients diminution of blood flow occurs initially in the occipital area and the phenomenon travels anteriorly over the head at a slow rate, strongly suggestive of a primary neuronal depressive process ("cortical spreading depression"). Whether cerebral blood flow is abnormal in migraine without aura remains controversial. That significant vascular phenomena occur in migraine is supported by the fact that it is a risk factor (although

of debatable magnitude) for subsequent stroke. The mechanism of the pain, as discussed previously, is not known; it probably is not due to dilatation of extracranial vessels.

Since there is no laboratory or other objective test diagnostic of migraine, some clinicians have increased the number of clinical diagnostic features necessary for the diagnosis to include, for example, autonomic nervous system phenomena during the attack and history of severe headaches in family members.

Warning symptoms (aura) are probably the least common of the generally accepted criteria. Warnings of attacks occur at some time in approximately one third of migraine patients. The fraction of migraine attacks associated with aura varies markedly. In some patients such attacks are rare, in others they are the rule. The aura is usually visual, described by the patients as "spots," "lights," or "jagged lines," often colored. They characteristically precede the headache by a few minutes to an hour and are often associated with a variety of types of impairment of vision—commonly a hemianopia, less commonly a partial central scotoma, and rarely cortical blindness. With onset of headache, these phenomena usually disappear, although photophobia during the attack is characteristic of migraine. The visual aura of migraine attacks frequently occurs without subsequent headache. Auras lasting for hours are of a less well-defined nature characterized by altered emotional states, depression or euphoria, or difficulty in thinking.

Other specific neurologic phenomena occur with considerably less frequency than does the visual aura of migraine. Of these, paresthesias are the most common. They tend to be stereotyped, beginning in the hand, progressing proximally up the arm, with frequent involvement of the ipsilateral side of the face. Unilateral weakness usually of mild degree can also occur in relation to an attack but in not more than 0.5% of cases. Usually only the upper extremity is affected. Hemiplegia also occurs rarely; one variety is familial.

There are many other variants of migraine, defined by the neurologic deficits that occur. They include ophthalmoplegia, confusion, coma, syncope, and loss of vision in one eye. None occur in more than a fraction of a percentage of all migraine patients. All these rare variants of migraine are more prevalent in children and adolescents than in adults.

Another rare variant of migraine is associated with multiple neurologic deficits—cranial nerve dysfunction, vertigo, ataxia, and depressed state of consciousness—all presumably due to brainstem dysfunction. This latter syndrome has been called basilar migraine or Bickerstaff syndrome, after the physician who first called attention to it. Children with migraine occasionally suffer episodes of abdominal pain thought to be "migraine equivalents."

Most of these uncommon phenomena occur, as noted, within a brief interval preceding the attack and disappear with the onset of headache; the deficit, however, may last several hours. Rarely it may be permanent, presumably the result of a cerebral infarction. Recent studies with magnetic resonance imaging have documented unsuspected small lesions, probably infarctions, in some migraine patients.

The relationship of seizures to migraine is a complex

one. In children and adolescents, the occurrence of seizures in individuals with migraine is more common than in control subjects. One case has been described of migraine with aura culminating in status epilepticus.

Tension-type Headache

More common than migraine are headaches that are not unilateral and not accompanied by nausea or vomiting and usually not by photophobia. Such headaches are often accompanied by involuntary contraction of frontalis or cervical paraspinal muscles. These muscles are often tender to pressure. Partially for this reason such headaches have been called in the past "muscle contraction" headache. The most recent classification labels them tension-type. It is, however, not known to what degree the inappropriate muscle contraction is a primary phenomenon and to what degree it is secondary to head pain of unknown cause. Electromyograms of neck and scalp muscles have not shown a consistent increase in involuntary contraction specific to a certain headache syndrome.

With these headaches the pain is often long lasting and described as pressure-like or band-like. Aura is absent, as is nausea, during the attack. Frequently there seems to be a close connection between this type of headache symptom and stressful life situations. This link between emotional disturbance and headache seems particularly strong in younger patients. Increased psychological distress has been found in adolescent headache sufferers as compared with headache-free control subjects. Increased stress within the family and other environments has been associated with increased reporting of a variety of other pain syndromes in adolescents.

Although the association of specific personality types with recurrent headache has remained a controversial point in adults, in children and adolescents there have been more consistent reports of correlation of headache history with depression, anxiety, poor self-confidence, fearfulness, and type A personality. Whether, however, such personality qualities in early years are specific to migraine or to another headache syndrome or are a nonspecific result of recurrent pain remains as controversial an issue in adolescents as it is in adults.

In adolescents, as in adults, it is often difficult to distinguish tension-type headache episodes from common migraine (i.e., migraine without aura). Some have held that it is a mistake to assume that the two are distinct entities and have taken the position that there is a continuum depending on severity—with migraine at the most severe end and tension at the least severe. It is certain, furthermore, that a large percentage of adolescents with typical migraine also suffer from another less severe headache without migrainous features but without clear relationship to stress.

Chronic Daily Headache

It is common for patients to suffer periods of daily headache that seem to have no consistent relation to emotional stress or muscle contraction. Usually such headache is described as dull, generalized, and of moderate severity. The location is usually bifrontal or occipital. There may be aching or tenderness of cervical paraspinal muscles as occurs in tension-type headache, but to a lesser degree. Etiology is unknown. Adolescent patients who have or have had typical migraine also frequently develop such headache.

Cluster Headache

This distinctive headache syndrome, unlike migraine, is strikingly more common in males than in females. It occurs in adolescence but is rare before the third decade. The pain is invariably unilateral, retro-orbital, brief in duration (usually less than 1 hour), and of extreme severity. There is no aura, and nausea and vomiting rarely occur. Attacks are often accompanied by congestion of nares and injection of the conjunctiva on the side of the headache. Occasionally ptosis on the affected side occurs. Unlike migraine, similar headache in relatives is not the rule. Attacks characteristically occur with great frequency during a limited period of time (days or weeks), with these "clusters" often separated by long headache-free intervals. This entity is quite clearly not related to migraine. The pathophysiology is unknown, but most involve the trigeminal nerve or its nucleus because of the pain distribution.

Cervicogenic Headache

Disease of the cervical spine is a common cause of head pain in later life but is rare in adolescents except as a transient phenomenon following trauma. When such headache does occur, it is usually precipitated by head movement. A type of headache simulating migraine and originating in the cervical area and possibly deriving from soft tissue has recently been described. It is also rare in adolescents.

Temporomandibular Joint Dysfunction

Generalized head pain may rarely result from various abnormalities of the temporomandibular joint. In such cases, localized pain is elicited by wide opening of the jaws, and there is usually tenderness to pressure over the joint. It is not uncommon for pain of this origin to simulate other types of headache.

TREATMENT

There are two aspects to the treatment of headache: (1) treatment of the symptom, both as an acute and chronic phenomenon, and (2) in patients with intermittent attacks, prophylactic treatment for prevention of future attacks.

General Aspects of Treatment

In the majority of headache episodes the pain is often not of great severity and responds to small doses of over-the-counter drugs—aspirin, acetaminophen, or ibuprofen. It is important that adolescents be taught the potential side effects of these commonly used medications. Occasionally gastric ulceration is produced by chronic use of large doses of aspirin. Such long-term large doses of aspirin or acetaminophen can also result in nephropathy or hepatic dysfunction. It is particularly important for adolescents not to develop a habit of taking these medications. Specific limits to the amounts used should be set, and patients should be warned of the exact dangers of overuse. Adolescents who have been taking these medications in large amounts should have kidney and liver function checked. In addition to these dangers, when analgesics are taken in large amounts on a daily basis, they seem to lose effectiveness and frequently result in paradoxical increase in headache. Overuse of analgesics also decreases the effectiveness of prophylactic medications (discussed later).

A combination of analgesics with sedatives (e.g., butalbital with aspirin or acetaminophen) is commonly prescribed for relief of the milder headache episodes. In some patients the sedative seems to potentiate the analgesic action, but there is danger of habituation. These compounds should not be used regularly by younger patients.

MIGRAINE ATTACKS

Occasionally the progression of a migraine attack can be aborted by use of appropriate medication at the onset of the aura before pain occurs. A variety of drugs, discussed later, have been reported to do this (e.g., propranolol, verapamil, ergotamine). Usually, however, the aura is so brief that the attack progresses, and the following measures are indicated. The adolescent and his or her family should be included in the discussion of the use of medication for headache.

Decrease of Stimuli. The patient should be in a quiet dark environment. Most will demand this, but some adolescents of a particularly obsessive and driving personality type will wish to "tough it out," carrying on normal activities as best they can. In addition to being painful, this course of action is particularly inadvisable if medication is prescribed. Several of the medications for the acute migraine attack have sedative action that diminishes mental and sensory acuity, with resultant errors at school and work, danger of falling, or accidents while driving or using equipment.

Antiemetic Medication. The prevention of nausea and vomiting is a prime objective of treatment, since these symptoms often intensify the pain and prevent absorption of medication from the stomach. A variety of antiemetics are suitable (e.g., metoclopramide, trimethobenzamide, prochlorperazine), the dosage varying with severity of symptom and weight of the patient. Because nausea often occurs early in the attack, medications available by suppository are particularly useful. It is often helpful to have patients take an antiemetic early in the attack.

Analgesics. For severe headache episodes, the more potent analgesics may be necessary. These include codeine, oxycodone, propoxyphene, and pentazocine. These compounds are commonly used in preparations in which they are combined with aspirin or acetaminophen. In addition to their analgesic effect, these medications produce varying degrees of alteration of emotional states, sedation, and slowing of bowel function. The amount prescribed must be carefully limited, and the adolescent and the family should be advised that the medications should be used only for severe pain and should not be taken regularly. The personality of the adolescent should be considered in determining the risk of overuse of these drugs. The possibility of the adolescent's obtaining these drugs from more than one physician must also be kept in mind.

Very rarely, more potent opiates (e.g., meperidine or hydromorphone parenterally) may be needed for an adolescent who has had a prolonged, extremely painful attack that has not responded to other medications. The use of these potent opiates carries the definite and important risk of the adolescent patient becoming psychologically dependent on this treatment for subsequent attacks. Usually a habituation rather than a true addiction develops.

Vasoconstrictor Medication

Ergotamine. This drug is available in tablet, suppository, sublingual, and inhaler forms. Ergotamine also is most useful when taken early in the migraine attack and in sufficient doses (e.g., two tablets of an oral ergotamine-caffeine preparation). Occasionally more can be prescribed for a single attack. Inhalation delivers the drug extremely rapidly, and suppository with slightly less speed. Adolescents and their families should be informed of the emetic properties of this drug and of the vasoconstrictive actions when used to excess. Strict limits on the amount used per week or month should be set to avoid ergotism, manifested by symptoms of vasospasm of arteries in extremities, viscera, and brain. Habituation to ergot, with paradoxical chronic headache, has been described.

Dihydroergotamine. Given intramuscularly or intravenously, 0.5 mg is effective in terminating attacks in some patients. The danger of vasospasm with this drug is less than that with ergotamine, but nausea is frequent. Nausea can be controlled by simultaneous use of an antiemetic.

Isometheptene. This compound is a milder vasoconstrictor than ergotamine. It is available in capsule form in combination with the sedative dichloralphenazone and acetaminophen. Two capsules at onset of attack are recommended. The precautions listed under ergotamine and acetaminophen must be observed.

Sedative Medication. Mild sedation enhances analgesia and induces sleep, which is desirable because it terminates many migraine attacks. Patients often need a large amount of sedative medication to induce sleep, and a dose should be repeated if sleep does not occur with the initial dose. As in use of analgesics and ergotamine, patients must be instructed as to the limitation of amounts to be used. The danger of habituation should again be specifically stressed.

Prophylactic Treatment

General Management. After it is determined that there is little chance that a headache is caused by structural disease of the brain, adolescents and their families should be reassured strongly on this point. Many patients come to physicians not because they need treatment but because they fear the presence of a brain tumor or some other serious disease; these fears are often not voiced in the initial history. After such reassurance, some current knowledge about migraine and tension-type headache can be shared, particularly with older adolescents. It is helpful to explain that there is no single cause of headache, but rather that there is probably interplay of several etiologic factors of unknown degree—genetic, biologic, and psychological. It is often reassuring to point out that a large percentage of the population (at least in the United States) has at some time or other suffered from headache, and of these, a sizable number from severe headache. It is also wise to state that treatment, even if successful, should not be thought of in terms of permanent total "cure," since headache often recurs, but it can be successfully treated a second time. The acceptance of this approach, however, is dependent on the adolescent's and the parents' personalities. Inevitably some individuals (or their families) believe that there must be one definable "cause" and will continue to seek that physician who will discover and eradicate it.

For those adolescents whose headaches have many characteristics of the migraine, it is advisable next to discuss some aspects of lifestyle that lower the threshold to migraine attacks:

1. Missing meals. Although the laity vastly overemphasizes the prevalence and importance of hypoglycemia, modest reductions in blood sugar, as noted previously, can definitely precipitate attacks in the migrainous individual. Adolescents should be advised not to omit meals (especially breakfast), and if dietary intake is minimal for some period, meals should contain more protein than carbohydrate.

2. Regular sleep. In some adolescents, loss of sleep precipitates attacks. Conversely, some individuals who have migraine headaches may awaken with an attack after a particularly long night's sleep. This sequence of events occurs characteristically with a long Friday night's sleep followed by "weekend headache." Adolescent patients should be told to try to keep the number of sleep hours fairly uniform.

3. Foods. Approximately 10% of migraine patients of all ages have attacks precipitated by certain food substances. Those most consistently implicated are chocolate, sharp cheeses, red wine, and monosodium glutamate; adolescents who have migraine headaches should avoid these foods. Occasional individuals have headache that seems to be related to excess use of caffeine.

It becomes apparent with certain adolescents—after a careful interview concerning the circumstances surrounding headache, the daily schedule at work or school, and their home environment—that migraine attacks are occurring in the context of severe depression or anxiety (see Chapters 100, 102, 103, and 104). Many such individuals are urgently in need of counseling or formal psychiatric care. In one community study, depression, as measured by the Zung self-rating depression scale, was significantly correlated with disabling or severe headaches in almost all age groups. In intractable constant headache in particular, "masked depression" must be considered (see Chapter 100).

Medication. A decision must be made jointly by the adolescent, family, and physician as to whether a program of prophylactic daily medication, in an attempt to prevent headache recurrence, is in order. The first variable that must enter into this decision is the frequency of the headache. A headache that occurs two or three times a year rarely demands prophylactic treatment; with this history the patient usually sees the physician only for reassurance. On the other extreme, headaches several times a week always demand such treatment trials. For frequencies between these extremes the probability of patient compliance, the side effects of medication, and the possibility of aborting severe attacks by use of early treatment instead of daily prophylactic treatment all must be considered in the decision. For young people in particular, an effort should be made to avoid the recommendation of long courses of medication. Once use of prophylactic medication is elected, the following medications are those that have been of demonstrated benefit.

β-Adrenergic Blocking Agents. Several of these substances have been reported successful in prevention of headache; the one in most common use and the only one currently approved by the U.S. Food and Drug Administration for this purpose is propranolol. The effective dosage varies markedly; the majority of patients respond to 80 to 120 mg daily, either in divided doses or in a once-daily dose using a sustained action preparation. To avoid side effects, treatment should be begun with a small dose. Several other drugs of this series (those lacking sympathomimetic activity) have also been reported effective. There is no evidence that any one of this group is more effective than another. The major limiting side effects of these medications are bradycardia, hypotension, and fatigue (not true sedation), all varying markedly from one individual to another. A degree of impotence (reversible) also can occur. These drugs should not be given to adolescents with active asthma because they can exacerbate attacks.

Tricyclic Antidepressants. Amitriptyline and nortriptyline are the most used drugs of this group for headache prophylaxis. The average daily dose of amitriptyline for this purpose is 25 to 100 mg, which is below the usual antidepressant dose. There is great variation in the degree of patient therapeutic response and tolerance of side effects. Anticholinergic symptoms can occur—commonly dry mouth and occasionally urinary retention. Sedation, the usual major limiting side effect, may aid certain patients (e.g., those with insomnia).

Calcium Channel Blocking Agents. In controlled studies, diltiazem, verapamil, nifedipine, and nimodipine all have shown efficacy in headache prophylaxis.

Side effects are usually minor; constipation is the chief one. Cardiac arrhythmias and hypotension, however, can rarely occur. Calcium blocking agents and β-adrenergic blocking agents prescribed together increase slightly the frequency of cerebrovascular side effects.

Methysergide. Of the variety of pharmacologic properties possessed by this drug, the antiserotonin and vasoconstrictive ones are thought to account for its effectiveness in migraine prophylaxis. Occasionally patients develop unpleasant affective or sensory symptoms when given this drug. It should not be given for more than 5 months without a "vacation" period off the drug, since cases of visceral fibrosis (peritoneal, pleural) have occurred with long-term use, and it is not recommended for adolescents younger than 16 years. The usual dose is 2 mg three times daily.

Nonsteroidal Anti-inflammatory Agents. Aspirin in small doses on a daily basis has been reported to be prophylactic against migraine. Naproxen has also been reported effective in average doses of 250 to 500 mg twice daily. Irritation of the gastric mucosa with symptoms of epigastric distress is the common side effect of this group of drugs; activation of peptic ulcer can occur. Bleeding time is prolonged, and bleeding from various sites is another rare complication. An additional risk is nephropathy if these agents are used steadily in large amounts.

Monoamine Oxidase Inhibitors. These agents are currently not commonly used for headache prophylaxis but can be tried in stubborn cases. If used, adolescents must be warned that exposure to certain vasoconstrictor amines (e.g., in cold remedies and in various foods) must be avoided because the impaired metabolism of the amines by the drugs can result in hypertension.

There is little knowledge concerning the comparative efficacy of the aforementioned agents in headache prevention, or whether one is superior to another in a specific form of headache. One placebo-controlled study did find amitriptyline and propranolol approximately equally effective in migraine when weekly headache scores were compared. Most studies have been carried out on migraine, but amitriptyline has been reported effective in tension headache. Certainly the less episodic the headache, the less chance of success with medication prophylaxis. β-Adrenergic blocking agents are useful in prevention of anxiety attacks, and it is therefore reasonable to use them in adolescents who suffer from this symptom in addition to migraine. Amitriptyline has, as noted, antidepressant and sedative effects and is therefore helpful when depression or insomnia is present. Nonsteroidal anti-inflammatory agents are particularly helpful if musculoskeletal disorders seem related to the headache (e.g., if areas of tenderness occur or if there is marked pain in head movement). Calcium channel blocking agents have the advantage of having few side effects. Balancing the risks of side effects may help select appropriate patients.

Two of these agents in combination, furthermore, may well be more effective, at least in some patients, than any single one. Side effects also, however, are additive. There is little systematic knowledge concerning efficacy of such combinations.

If success is achieved in prevention of headache at-tacks, the question of duration of treatment arises. Headache, and migraine in particular, has a markedly variable life course. Many individuals have long periods of remission. It is advisable, therefore, to prescribe gradual reduction in prophylactic medication after adolescents have had a period of absent or markedly diminished headache; such a period varies with the duration of the period that the patient has suffered from migraine and the severity of attacks.

There is no evidence that any of these agents are age-specific (i.e., that they are more or less effective in youth). Adolescents are somewhat less in danger of side effects because temporary adverse events (e.g., hypotension) are less productive of permanent damage.

Nonpharmacologic Prophylaxis. A variety of behavioral therapies have been tried for prophylaxis of headache in adolescents as well as in adults. These have included training in progressive muscle relaxation, imagery, stress reduction training, and self-hypnosis. Evaluation of results is difficult because of the variation of techniques, the variation of criteria for headache diagnosis, and the variation of controls. Most studies of the young have not separated adolescents from younger children. In general, improvement has been frequent and has been correlated with several environmental factors.

Biofeedback treatments are those in which there is provision of a visual or auditory signal as to the degree of the patient's success in altering some physiologic variable presumably related to headache. Most literature refers to the use of surface electrodes recording degrees of relaxation of underlying muscle contraction, usually frontalis or cervical paraspinal muscles. Success in elevating skin temperature of the hands has also been reportedly correlated with headache prevention. Whether use of biofeedback gives results superior to training in muscle relaxation or other kinds of nonpharmacologic treatment remains uncertain. Patients who respond are those with the most characteristics of tension-type headache, but success has also been reported in common migraine and migraine with aura. Frequency of headache has been the characteristic most modified. Treatment results overall with these nonpharmacologic methods seem to be better in children and adolescents than in adults.

TENSION-TYPE HEADACHE

Over-the-counter analgesics often control this type of headache. Adolescents must be cautioned, however, to avoid taking large amounts of these medications daily because of previously described risks.

Some patients with tension headache respond to prophylactic amitriptyline in doses used for migraine. Whether this is due to direct action on pain centers or relief of an underlying depression is unclear. In some, tender "pressure points" in the scalp and the posterior head and neck region have been described, with improvement occurring by anesthetizing these spots with small amounts of parenteral lidocaine.

As noted previously, patients with tension-type headache are thought to be the best subjects for nonpharmacologic treatment (i.e., training in relaxation and biofeedback). There are reports of particular benefit in children and adolescents. Individuals with obvious psychological disturbances may need formal psychiatric care. However, clinicians themselves are advised to treat adolescents with presumed psychosocial problems causing headaches, because referral to mental health treatment can be construed as indicating that the pain is not being taken seriously.

CLUSTER HEADACHE

The acute attack of cluster headache is brief and therefore usually does not respond to oral medication. Inhalation of oxygen, 4 to 5 L/minute, is markedly beneficial in some attacks. Ergotamine is helpful in others; when rapid absorption is needed, rectal or inhalation routes can be used. Occasionally patients respond to anesthetizing of the sphenopalatine ganglion by intranasal drops of anesthetic.

For termination of the series of cluster headache, the corticosteroids are the most generally useful medication. A large initial dose is usually required (e.g., 60 mg prednisone daily), with a rapidly decremental dosage over the subsequent 3 to 4 weeks. Some patients respond to a brief course of daily ergotamine (with care to avoid more than 10 mg/week), and some to methysergide in doses used for migraine. Occasionally recurrent cases have responded to maintenance doses of lithium carbonate in usual doses of 300 mg three or four times daily.

In intractable cases, surgical procedures have been tried. These include partial destruction of the trigeminal nerve and division of the nervus intermedius. There are, however, conflicting reports as to the long-term usefulness of these procedures.

For the rare variety of cluster headache that becomes chronic without periods of remission, indomethacin in doses of 50 to 250 mg daily has been reported as a specific therapy.

BIBLIOGRAPHY

Cunningham MA, McGrath PJ, Latter J, et al: Personality and behavioral characteristics in pediatric migraine. Headache 27:16, 1987.

Duckro PN, Cantwell-Simmons E: A review of studies evaluating biofeedback and relaxation training in the management of pediatric headache. Headache 29:428, 1989.

Hockaday JM: Basilar migraine in childhood. Dev Med Child Neurol 21:455, 1979.

Johnson RH: Beta-blockers in the management of migraine. In Zanchetti A (ed): Advances in Beta-Blocker Therapy. Proceedings of the Second International Symposium. Princeton, NJ, Excerpta Medica, 1982, pp 194–212.

Krabbe AA: Cluster headache: A review. Acta Neurol Scand 74:1, 1986.

Linet MS, Stewart WF: Migraine headache: Epidemiologic perspectives. Epidemiol Rev 6:107, 1984.

Morgenlander JC, Wilkins RH: Surgical treatment of cluster headache. J Neurosurg 72:866, 1990.

Nattero G: Menstrual headache. Adv Neurol 33:215, 1982.

Solomon GD: Comparative efficacy of calcium antagonist drugs in the prophylaxis of migraine. Headache 25:368, 1985.

Waters WE: Migraine: Intelligence, social class and familial prevalence. Br Med J 2:77, 1971.

CHAPTER 85

Syncope and Dizziness

DEWEY K. ZIEGLER

SYNCOPE

Syncope can be defined as abrupt loss of consciousness of brief duration, accompanied by loss of postural muscle tone, and without obvious cause, such as a blow on the head. Such disturbance of consciousness is the result of temporary impairment of function of the central portion of the pons and medulla oblongata—specifically, the anatomic structure known as the reticular activating system.

Causes

A wide variety of adverse events can cause temporary dysfunction of this area. Causes can be divided into five types: cerebral ischemia, anemia, seizures, metabolic abnormality, and psychosomatic conditions.

CEREBRAL ISCHEMIA

The vast majority of syncopal episodes are of this type, which includes all pathophysiologic processes by which the brain is temporarily deprived of adequate blood supply. This deprivation may be the result of episodic hypotension, cardiac disturbances (usually arrhythmias), or arterial disease. Combinations often occur.

Episodic Hypotension

Syncope of this cause occurs when the adolescent is upright (orthostatic hypotension). It can occur in normal adolescents whose usual blood pressure is low when they are ill (e.g., with fever or hyponatremia, or during inadequate fluid intake), are stressed by extreme environmental heat, or stand for a prolonged period. Syncope of this type is often preceded by some sensations of apprehension (presyncope).

The levels of blood pressure that induce syncope vary greatly, depending primarily on the normal blood pressure for that person. In general, children and adolescents are more resistant to symptoms from intermittent hypotension than are the elderly.

Orthostatic hypotension with resultant syncope can also be induced by various medications, such as β-adrenergic blockers, calcium channel blockers (or other antihypertensive agents), tricyclic antidepressants, or phenothiazines.

Emotional stimuli are a well-known cause of vascular syncope, particularly in the adolescent. Commonly included in this category are pain and the apprehension of pain (vasovagal attacks). Hypotension is usually the major component of the cerebral ischemia that causes such spells, although bradycardia and, occasionally, cardiac arrhythmias also occur.

Many illnesses affecting the central or peripheral nervous system can also cause episodic hypotension. Long-standing diabetes (with autonomic nervous system derangement) and Shy-Drager syndrome, however, occur in older patients and are rare in adolescents.

Episodic Cardiac Disturbances (see Chapter 46)

Syncope occurring in the context of pain or emotional disturbance is the result of varying degrees of hypotension and cardiac rhythm disturbances. Occasionally, in adolescents noxious stimuli can produce "pale" syncope, associated with temporary cardiac arrest. This syndrome, however, is more typical of infants and small children. In these episodes there is often a diphasic response, with the heart rate and arterial pressure showing a transient increase before decreasing, with resultant symptoms.

Many types of structural abnormalities of the heart or arteries impair cardiac output to the degree that temporary cerebral ischemia and therefore syncope are produced. Most of these conditions cause numerous other symptoms and are therefore not diagnostic problems. These include aortic stenosis, myocardial infarction, subclavian steal syndrome, and dissecting aortic aneurysm—all rare in adolescents. Valvular heart disease and atrial myxoma resulting in impaired cardiac output are also extremely rare causes of unexplained syncope. Pulmonary hypertension and pulmonary embolus can result in syncope, but these diagnoses are usually made with ease.

In certain individuals, stimulation of the carotid sinus (e.g., by a tight collar) produces cardiac arrhythmia, hypotension, or both. The frequency of occurrence of a sensitive carotid sinus tends to parallel that of vascular disease, such as hypertension and coronary disease, and is therefore rare in adolescents. Not all those with a sensitive carotid sinus suffer syncopal attacks.

Various stimuli to the viscera can result in reflex cardiac dysrhythmia or temporary cardiac arrest, with simultaneous or subsequent hypotension and syncope. These syndromes include the following:

Micturition Syncope. Syncope of this type characteristically occurs at the end of micturition and is more common in men, probably because of an orthostatic component.

Defecation Syncope. This rare event occurs after straining at stool. There may be more than one component to the syncope—stimulation of vagus afferents in the bowel and a marked increase in intrathoracic pressure, with secondary impaired venous return and cardiac output. It can be a complication of sigmoidoscopy, and electrocardiographic abnormalities have been demonstrated during manual dilatation of the anus.

Swallow Syncope. This reflex event, also rare, usually occurs secondary to swallowing a substance of extreme temperature. Syncope secondary to glossopharyngeal neuralgia is a similar phenomenon.

Cough Syncope. Syncope of this type generally occurs only after prolonged coughing. The mechanism is probably one of impaired cardiac output and reduced arterial pressure secondary to the markedly increased intrathoracic pressure.

Effort Syncope. A group of young adolescents has been identified as having abnormalities on the electrocardiogram (ECG) consisting of increased atrioventricular (AV) conduction times, which were thought to be a result of excess vagal activity (vagotonia). Some of these adolescents experienced syncope on extreme exertion—specifically, weightlifting. Episodes stopped on discontinuance of these activities. Increased intrathoracic pressure may play a part in this syndrome, as it does in cough syncope. The significance of the ECG findings remains questionable, because other asymptomatic adolescents were demonstrated to have similar changes.

Arterial Disease

Intermittent ischemia of the brainstem with resultant dysfunction of the area crucial to the maintenance of consciousness—the reticular activating system—occurs with vertebrobasilar artery diseases. It is rare in adolescents. Probably the most common causes in this age group are the inflammatory arteritides and AV malformations, including the abnormal network of arterial vessels known as moyamoya disease (which can result in occlusion of major arterial trunks). Other symptoms of brainstem or occipital lobe dysfunction almost invariably occur in addition to syncope (e.g., visual field disturbances, ataxia, and cranial nerve disturbances).

ANEMIA

The brain depends on normal flow of blood with adequate oxygen-carrying capacity. Anemia can therefore be a contributing cause of syncope. Almost invariably, however, unless the anemia is extremely severe, it is not the sole cause but is additive to hypotension or cardiac dysfunction, which are the primary processes.

SEIZURES (see Chapter 83)

Although usually manifested by some type of movement, seizures can be characterized by episodic akinetic states, with arrest of consciousness and loss of muscle tone. There is probably more than one type of such attack. (The differential diagnosis from vascular syncope is discussed later.) The diagnosis of such cases is complicated by the fact that the paroxysmal electrophysiologic discharge of the brain during a seizure can induce marked cardiac dysrhythmia.

METABOLIC DISTURBANCES

Severe disturbances of electrolytes, particularly hyponatremia, can be contributory causes of syncope in those of all ages. The underlying disease, however, is usually apparent. "Functional" hypoglycemia (as opposed to insulin-induced hypoglycemia) can also be contributory, but it is rarely a primary cause of episodic syncope. In episodes of impaired consciousness secondary to mild or functional hypoglycemia, there is not usually complete loss of consciousness. Conversely, complete loss of consciousness generally occurs only with marked degrees of hypoglycemia. With syncope resulting from hypoglycemia, the onset is usually insidious, and there is more than momentary loss of consciousness.

PSYCHOSOMATIC CONDITIONS

In psychosomatic states no neurophysiologic abnormality can be found. Hyperventilation is one of these conditions. While experiencing feelings of anxiety, the adolescent hyperventilates, blows off carbon dioxide, and may have a syncopal episode. Other psychosomatic conditions include conversion (see Chapter 112) and malingering. The diagnosis of these states is often extremely difficult; this problem occurs frequently in adolescents. The following diagnostic features can help in identification of "pseudosyncope":

1. If falls occur, the body usually does not strike any object or sustain injury.
2. Spells are often characterized by more than just the apparent loss of consciousness and include fluttering of the eyelids, clutching of the head, or dramatic movements of the extremities—"swooning." There is often evidence of a considerable degree of response to the examiner and environment during apparent unconsciousness. Seizure-like phenomena can occur, and the differentiation of complex partial seizures from these pseudoseizures is often difficult.
3. Spells can often be initiated and terminated by suggestion.
4. During the apparent loss of consciousness there may be flaccidity of muscles in the presence of vigorous opposition, of an organized form, to passive movements by the examiner.
5. Consciousness is often disturbed or impaired for extended periods.
6. Immediate and rapid recovery occurs when the adolescents think they are unobserved.

Differential Diagnosis

The most frequent diagnostic problem in adolescents is differentiating vascular syncope from seizures. The usual distinguishing features of these two conditions are summarized in Table 85–1.

Syncope caused by a drop in blood pressure or bradycardia is heralded by an unpleasant feeling, described by patients as faintness (presyncope), and often by sympathetic nervous system discharge, with resultant diaphoresis, nausea, and pallor. Some syncopal states of cardiovascular cause, however, are of abrupt onset. With seizures, loss of consciousness often occurs with no warning. When there are preceding subjective phenomena (aura) they often consist of olfactory sensations, usually of an unpleasant nature. Various affective states also occur, also usually unpleasant (e.g., depression, apprehensiveness, anxiety), but occasionally euphoria is experienced. These phenomena are sometimes difficult to differentiate from the sensation of faintness that precedes syncope of vascular origin. Usually lacking in seizures, however, is the desire to lie down.

Vascular syncope is generally accompanied by flaccidity without any motor phenomena; occasionally, a few myoclonic jerks occur, particularly if circulation does not return promptly. Only when cerebral hypoxia-anemia is more prolonged does tonic extension of the arms and legs occur. Rarely, cerebral anemia can cause episodes indistinguishable from those of epilepsy.

In complex partial seizures of the akinetic variety, there is frequently some minimal type of movement (e.g., of the face or fingers), although this is not true of generalized seizures characterized by akinesia (drop attacks). Confusion after seizures is usually present to some degree; it is generally minimal to absent after cardiovascular syncope.

If the diagnosis is not clear, it may be clarified by other maneuvers:

1. 24-hour ECG.
2. Examination with the adolescent's head tilted in the up position. Individuals are positioned and kept at a 60- to 70-degree tilt on a tilt table, with ECG monitoring. The recommended duration of tilt varies from 20 to 30 minutes or until symptoms, ECG abnormalities, or hypotension occurs. Syncope is accompanied by marked bradycardia, hypotension, or both (see Chapter 47). The head tilt test has reproduced syncope in a high percentage of healthy, elderly persons, but produces symptoms only extremely rarely in healthy young men. A recent modification of the test involves the intravenous infusion of isoproterenol, 1 μg/minute for 5 minutes, using graded infusion rates to 5 μg/minute. This increases the sensitivity of the head tilt test while only minimally reducing its specificity. Bradycardia and vasodilation are thought to be produced through the stimulation of central mechanoreceptors.

3. Carotid sinus pressure. When this test is used the pressure exerted should be mild, and each side should be tested separately. As with syncope of other causes, syncope results from bradycardia and/or hypotension produced by a reflex mechanism. Sensitive carotid sinus as a cause for syncope occurs primarily in elderly adults who have accompanying vascular disease, and is rare in adolescents.

Tilt testing and pressure on the carotid sinus should be done only with ECG and blood pressure monitoring, and emergency equipment should be immediately available, because cardiac arrhythmia or arrest can occur. At the first indication of syncope, hypotension, or bradycardia, the maneuver should be discontinued.

4. Electroencephalogram (EEG). If no cardiovascular abnormalities are found, and if there is a reasonable possibility of a seizure, an EEG should be obtained. The optimal method of study is over a prolonged period (e.g., 24 hours), with simultaneous EEG, ECG, and video monitoring, so that any syncopal episode may be observed and correlated with an EEG or ECG abnormality. This monitoring helps determine whether reported episodes of syncope are seizures or pseudoseizures.

A note can be made, finally, of diagnostic probabilities. As previously noted, many of the cardiovascular causes of syncope occur in the context of diseases of the elderly and are rare in adolescents. These include myocardial infarction, atherosclerotic arterial disease (carotid), aortic aneurysm, Shy-Drager syndrome (multiple system disease), and sensitive carotid sinus. Of cardiovascular causes, the only one common in adolescents is situational syncope—that is, syncope elicited by pain or emotion (vasovagal attacks). Reflex attacks elicited by internal stimuli (e.g., micturition, swallow) are rare at all ages. Adolescents are also more resistant to the hypotensive side effects of drugs than the elderly. Seizures, however, are frequent in all age groups, and particular attention should therefore be given to the possibility of atypical seizures in adolescents as a cause for recurrent loss of consciousness. Frequently, the cause of syncope remains obscure. Adolescents with syncope deserve medical follow-up because of the high likelihood of recurrence and the need to monitor potential progression of symptoms.

Management

In those adolescents in whom syncope recurs only with definite stimuli, such as from severe pain or emo-

TABLE 85–1. Seizures Versus Syncope

FEATURE	SEIZURES	CARDIOVASCULAR SYNCOPE
Warning	Complex sensory or psychological states	Feeling of faintness and desire to lie down
Behavior during unconsciousness	Often staring facial expression; often no loss of muscle tone; usually some type of involuntary movement	Always loss of postural tone, often with fall; eyes closed; movement rare
Recovery from unconsciousness	Confusion common for several minutes, or longer	Usually prompt recovery in minutes, with no confusion
Stimuli preceding unconsciousness	Usually nothing predictable	Commonly, pain, apprehension, vagal stimuli, extreme emotion
Urinary incontinence	Common	Rare
Posture preceding event	No specificity; occur when standing, sitting, or recumbent	Usually with standing

tion, there is no specific treatment, except to avoid the precipitating stimuli. They can be warned to heed premonitory symptoms (e.g., a feeling of faintness) and to lie down immediately.

Adolescent patients in whom syncope is demonstrated by 24-hour ECG to be correlated with transient cardiac arrhythmias probably need more extensive cardiac study. The use of various medications and a pacemaker needs to be considered. These subjects are discussed elsewhere (see Chapter 46).

If syncope recurs, with no demonstrable cause, and seizures and pseudosyncope are ruled out, two measures need to be considered:

1. Study of cardiac physiology in a manner similar to that in patients in whom cardiac dysrhythmia has been demonstrated. Follow-up studies of patients with syncope of unknown cause have revealed, as previously noted, a small number with sudden death, possibly because of cardiac arrest in the course of a dysrhythmia. This event, however, is probably a rarity in adolescents.

2. Therapeutic trial of anticonvulsants. Occasionally, seizures occur that are indistinguishable from syncope of vascular causes. Sometimes this occurs because the adolescent patient was completely amnesic for the episode, and there were no witnesses. In others, the phenomenology of the seizure was actually indistinguishable from that of vascular syncope, and the EEG was normal. In some adolescents subsequently proven to have seizures, even the EEG recorded from the scalp during the episode was nondiagnostic. In cases of recurrent syncope, therefore, in which extensive investigation has revealed no cause, it is reasonable to carry out a therapeutic trial with a standard anticonvulsant in adequate dosage. The prompt cessation of episodes suggests the diagnosis of seizures.

DIZZINESS

Dizziness is a term of great ambiguity. It generally refers to a sensation of altered position in space. Episodes of dizziness, or vertigo, are common at all ages, and they occur in many types of pathophysiologic states.

Causes

True vertigo occurs from a disturbance of the vestibular system. The pathologic process may affect the eighth cranial nerve itself, the vestibular nucleus in the brainstem, or, more rarely, the central connections of the vestibular system, primarily in the temporal lobe of the cerebrum. The result is a subjective feeling of turning, or of the environment turning at varying degrees of speed and severity. Another clue to the diagnosis of true vertigo is the precipitation of increased symptoms by rapid movements of the head. When severe, vertigo from any cause is often accompanied by nausea, vomiting, or both. There are strong connections of the vestibular system with the cerebellum, particularly its midline (vermis), which controls posture. Dizziness caused by vestibular system malfunction therefore often

results in instability of varying degrees when sitting, standing, or walking, and nystagmus also occurs. The common causes (some rare in adolescence) are discussed below.

Exogenous Toxins. Alcohol is the most frequently used toxin that affects the vestibular system, and alcohol intoxication is the most common cause of vestibular cerebellar dysfunction that results in ataxia, dysarthria, and vertigo (see Chapter 97). Phenytoin in excessive amounts can adversely affect the vestibular system and result in vertigo.

Motion Sickness. Motion sickness affects those of all ages, and in markedly varying degrees. It can occur when someone is traveling in any type of moving conveyance or is turning rapidly. It can also occur in susceptible individuals when they are stationary but the environment appears to be moving—for example, watching moving objects on a large screen. It is mentioned here because it is a common cause of vertigo, even though the cause is obvious.

Benign Positional Vertigo. Certain normal persons of all ages can experience a sensation of marked vertigo on rapid change in body-head position. Such sensations can occur on rapid turning, lying down, or sitting up. The symptoms are brief, usually lasting less than a minute, and often follow head injury or viral infection. Nystagmus is occasionally seen as a transient phenomenon.

Vestibular Neuronitis. With this syndrome, during a viral infection or shortly thereafter, the subject abruptly develops true vertigo of varying degrees of severity. Fever, myalgia, and headache are frequently present, and some adolescent patients have drowsiness or other signs of an encephalopathy. Nystagmus is usually prominent and is most striking on head movement. There is occasionally leukopenia resulting from the primary viral infection. As in other viral infections, lymphocytes are found in the cerebrospinal fluid. Recovery usually occurs in a few days or weeks but can be prolonged. As in Menière disease, there is often a definite directional component to the symptom—that is, movement of the head in one direction produces maximal vertigo and movement of the eyes in one direction also produces maximal nystagmus.

Menière Disease. In this condition, caused by the presence of increased fluid in the semicircular canals, vertiginous episodes are the rule. Almost all adolescent patients also complain of tinnitus, and there are varying degrees of hearing loss, usually unilateral and reversible in the early stages. Nystagmus occurs during the attack. Various tests of the acoustic-vestibular system help confirm the diagnosis; these include caloric testing, audiometry, and rotational tests. This disease is uncommon in adolescents.

Multiple Sclerosis. Not infrequently, a transient episode of vertigo is the first manifestation of multiple sclerosis, a disease that can have its onset in adolescence, although the peak ages of onset are in the third and fourth decades (see Chapters 87 and 88). Episodes of vertigo are also common later in the course of the illness. The vertigo results from a lesion in the brainstem, and often there are other neurologic symptoms referable to that area—diplopia, ataxia, and paresthesias, or weakness of an extremity. Early in the disease, the patient may show neurologic abnormalities not suggested by the history, such as early spasticity (as evidenced by hyperreflexia and Babinski signs). The following are confirmatory laboratory test results: (1) elevated gamma globulin levels in the cerebrospinal fluid (CSF) productive of oligoclonal bands; (2) abnormality of visual and/or brainstem evoked potentials; and (3) irregular areas of periventricular abnormality seen on magnetic resonance imaging (MRI) studies of the head. Any or all of these may be absent early in the disease.

Acoustic Neuroma. This tumor is a slowly growing intracranial neurofibroma. The first signs and symptoms are hearing loss and tinnitus. When the lesion enlarges, it can compress the trigeminal and facial nerves. Episodic vertigo sometimes occurs. It is rare in adolescents, but patients of all ages with neurofibromatosis are at high risk for developing the lesion.

Ischemia of Brainstem. Again, as in multiple sclerosis, other signs and symptoms of brainstem dysfunction commonly occur in this syndrome. Because the posterior cerebral arteries supply the occipital lobes, episodic disturbances of visual function, commonly hemianopic visual field disturbances, may also occur. This syndrome is extremely rare in adolescence, because almost all cases result from atherosclerotic disease of the vertebrobasilar circulation, a disorder of late adult life. An exception is a variety of migraine (see later).

Intramedullary Space-Occupying Lesions of the Brainstem. These include tumors, vascular malformations, and syringomyelia. All are rare causes of dizziness in adolescents and are almost invariably associated with one or more signs and/or symptoms of brainstem dysfunction accompanying the vertigo (e.g., spasticity, ataxia, nystagmus, ophthalmoplegia, hypalgesia of face). Episodic dizziness is rarely the sole finding.

Seizures. Episodic vertigo without disturbance of consciousness is rarely the manifestation of paroxysmal EEG discharges and is therefore a seizure phenomenon (see Chapter 83). The origin of the seizure is usually the temporal lobe. In such cases, attacks are very brief and are often accompanied by a history of a more frequent type of seizure (e.g., tonic-clonic). This diagnosis should be confirmed by demonstrating the occurrence of the paroxysmal EEG discharge during the vertiginous episode. Response to a therapeutic trial of anticonvulsants is also diagnostic. These seizures have no age predilection.

Migraine. An uncommon cause of vertigo in adolescence is the aura of an attack of migraine. The diagnosis is clarified by the nature of the accompanying headache. It is of interest that, in children, episodic vertigo may alternate with migrainous attacks. A specific migraine syndrome is associated with vertigo, ataxia, cranial nerve abnormalities, and syncope (basilar migraine—discussed previously). This syndrome seems to be more common in children and adolescents.

Various conditions that are not vertigo may be described by the patient as "dizziness" and include the following:

1. Faintness caused by episodic cerebral ischemia. Vasovagal syncope and preceding presyncope occurring from the many possible causes, a common symptom in adolescents, has been discussed in the section on syncope. This may initially be described by the adolescent patient as dizziness. On questioning, however, the adolescent usually aids in ruling out vertigo by giving one or more of the following clues: (1) the sensation is described as one of "lightheadedness" or "about to faint or pass out"; (2) episodes do not occur in the recumbent position, and the symptom can be quickly relieved by lying down; (3) episodes are precipitated by specific stimuli (discussed under syncope; e.g., pain, emotion, cough); and (4) there is no sensation of a moving environment.

2. Ataxia. Episodic vertigo is frequently accompanied by ataxia, but the latter can occur without vertigo in disturbances of the cerebellum. Careful questioning ascertains that the adolescent patient, during the episode, lacked the true sensation of turning, even though unsteadiness of gait was present.

3. Brief disturbance of consciousness. Partial complex seizures with altered states of awareness are often described by adolescent patients as spells of dizziness. As noted earlier, however, true vertigo is rarely a manifestation of seizure.

4. Anxiety episodes. Frequently, such attacks are initially described as dizziness. The features of true vertigo are absent; usually, adolescents admit to symptoms of hyperventilation or to the subjective feelings of nervousness and often to the precipitation of dizziness by certain emotionally charged situations. Symptoms of this type are characteristically more long-lasting than episodic.

Chronic, undefinable states of other types are often also described as dizziness. Patients may describe their heads as feeling full or unusual in other ways. These symptoms are frequently seen in the setting of psychological disturbance or as descriptors of headache. On careful questioning, such symptoms almost invariably lack the major hallmarks of true vertigo—episodic in nature and exacerbated by head movement.

Evaluation

In the adolescent with dizziness, a careful history should help rule out the states that are not vertigo. Blood pressure in the recumbent and upright positions should be measured to rule out orthostatic hypotension. If there are signs of systemic illness accompanying vertigo, CSF examination may reveal a small number of lymphocytes characteristic of viral infection. If attacks recur, audiometry and labyrinthine testing should be carried out to look for findings of Menière disorder, and MRI scans of the head should be obtained to search for the lesions of multiple sclerosis or acoustic neuroma. The possibility of multiple sclerosis also indicates the need for CSF examination. If brainstem lesions are a possibility, brainstem-evoked potentials may be valuable. Occasionally, cerebral angiography is necessary, especially when there is a possibility of vasculitis. Electroencephalography is also indicated if seizures are a possibility.

Management

Treatment focuses on the causative condition. If the attack is self-limited (e.g., motion sickness, vestibular neuronitis), symptomatic relief is usually obtained by the use of various over-the-counter medications, such as Dramamine or meclizine. These may temporarily have to be used in large doses, and patients must be warned of drowsiness as a side effect. When the diagnosis of vertiginous episodes is doubtful, a therapeutic trial with one of these agents is often useful as a diagnostic maneuver.

REFERENCES

Syncope

Almquist A, Goldenberg IF, Milstein S, et al: Provocation of bradycardia and hypotension by isoproterenol and upright posture in patients with unexplained syncope. N Engl J Med 320:345, 1989.

Glick G, Uyu PN: Hemodynamic changes during spontaneous vasovagal reactions. Am J Med 34:42, 1963.

Haslam RHA, Jameson HD: Cardiac standstill simulating repeated epileptic attacks. JAMA 224:887, 1973.

Ikeno T, Shigematsu H, Miyakoshi M, et al: An analytic study of epileptic falls. Epilepsia 26:612, 1985.

Kapoor WN, Karpf M, Wieand S, et al: A prospective evaluation and follow-up of patients with syncope. N Engl J Med 309:197, 1983.

Kushner JA, Kou WH, Kadish AH, Morady F: Natural history of patients with unexplained syncope and a nondiagnostic electrophysiologic study. J Am Coll Cardiol 14:391, 1989.

Lukash WM, Sawyer GT, Davis JE: Micturition syncope produced by orthostatism and bladder distention. N Engl J Med 270:341, 1964.

Sapire DW, Casta A: Vagotonia in infants, children, adolescents and young adults. Int J Cardiol 9:211, 1985.

Ziegler DK, Lin JTY, Bayer WL: Convulsive syncope: Relationship to cerebral ischemia. Trans Am Neurol Assoc 103:1, 1979.

Dizziness

Baloh RW: Dizziness, Hearing Loss and Tinnitus: The Essentials of Neurotology. Philadelphia, FA Davis, 1984.

Drachman DA, Hart CW: A new approach to the dizzy patient. Neurology 22:323, 1972.

Harker LA, Rassekh C: Migraine equivalent as a cause of episodic vertigo. Laryngoscope 98(2):160, 1988.

Harrison MS, Ozsahinoglu C: Positional vertigo. Arch Otolaryngol 101:675, 1975.

Lanzi G, Balottin V, Fazzi E, et al: Benign paroxysmal vertigo in childhood: A longitudinal study. Headache 26:494, 1986.

Schuknecht HF, Kitamura K: Vestibular neuritis. Ann Otol Rhinol Laryngol 90(Suppl):78, 1981.

CHAPTER 86

Sleep Disorders

RICHARD SATRAN

An expanding body of information concerning sleep disorders has developed. Initially, much of this information was derived from the results of sleep studies in the neonate and adult, but with a greater focus on adolescent medicine, more attention has been devoted to sleep needs and disturbances in this age group. These developments have occurred because of increased interest in sleep medicine and the use of all-night polysomnography in sleep laboratories.

In any consideration of sleep and sleep disturbances, reference is frequently made to sleep stages and other physiologic observations. Sleep may be divided into two types, active, or rapid eye movement (REM) sleep and slow-wave sleep (non-REM). The time spent in REM and non-REM sleep, as well as total sleep time, varies with age. Slow-wave sleep is classified into four stages, based on electroencephalographic criteria. Stage I sleep, or drowsiness, is characterized by a decline in the amount of alpha activity and desynchronization of the occipital rhythm, as well as by mild central-parietal slowing. Stage II sleep is highlighted by the presence of vertex transients and recurrent sleep spindles. Delta sleep, or stage III and stage IV sleep, consists of high-voltage slow potentials and associated spindles. Stages III and IV are differentiated by the amount of slow-wave activity present.

During each of the five or more sleep cycles, delta sleep gradually decreases. Each slow-wave cycle is followed by progressive lightening of sleep and ultimately by a period of REM activity. The duration of REM sleep increases during each successive sleep cycle so that approximately 100 minutes is spent in REM sleep each night. Most dreaming occurs during REM, especially in the early morning hours. In addition, heart rate and respirations become irregular. Muscle tone as monitored by the electromyogram is greatly reduced. The presence of rapid eye movements can be detected by the appropriate placement of canthal leads.

Sleep disturbances of adolescents may be discussed from the perspective of the 1979 Classification of Sleep and Arousal Disorders. This classification includes disorders of initiation and maintenance of sleep (insomnias), disorders of excessive sleep, disturbances in sleep-wake schedules, and dysfunctions related to sleep stages or partial arousals, known as parasomnias.

The sleep needs of adolescents and their sleep characteristics have been studied by several workers. There do not appear to be gender-related differences in sleep, and the most dramatic developmental change in sleep is the decrease in slow-wave sleep (stages III and IV) during puberty. Sleepiness in the normal adolescent occurs frequently and may be related to societal or peer factors. Nevertheless, as observed by Carskadon and Dement, a gradual reduction in the amount of time spent in sleep appears to be the dominant factor. Concern for increased sleep need and dissatisfaction with sleep quality have been noted in studies carried out in high-school and college students.

Analysis of sleep disturbances begins with a thorough history. Often, parents, roommates, and/or bed partners must be interviewed to secure necessary historical data. In addition to a detailed elaboration of the chief complaint, a longitudinal history of sleep problems and a review of past medical and psychological history are essential. Finally, the use of medications and sleep hygiene must also be considered.

TYPES OF DISTURBANCES

Insomnia

As may as 20% of adolescents may experience insomnia on an acute or chronic basis. In most cases the origin of the complaint reflects the psychological stress of this period of maturation. In some situations, excessive napping may play a role in the difficulty experienced in initiating nocturnal sleep. Disruptive sleep conditions may be responsible for the problem. Drugs, particularly alcohol, may result in sleep disruption. Excessive daytime sleepiness may be a consequence of working more than one job, in addition to having a shortened sleep time.

An analysis of the factors responsible for the insomnia and the use of appropriate psychological and/or medical therapy are necessary.

The usual advice concerning sleep hygiene consists of stressing the avoidance of all naps during the day and retiring to bed only when the desire for sleep occurs. It must be emphasized that bed should not be used for reading or watching television. If sleep is not achieved within 10 to 15 minutes, it is often helpful for the adolescent to get up and not return until drowsiness occurs. The wake-up time each day should be regulated.

Excessive Daytime Sleepiness

Beyond the sleepiness that occurs in adolescence as a consequence of insufficient sleep, narcolepsy and sleep apnea have most often been associated with excessive daytime sleepiness. Parkes and Lock have studied the genetic aspects of narcolepsy and parasomnias.

NARCOLEPSY

Narcolepsy is a chronic disorder that usually has its onset in late childhood or adolescence. Its exact cause is unknown. Those who have this problem are subject to constant sleepiness and irresistible sleep attacks, which may be delayed in some instances by physical activity. Repetitive, sedentary, stereotyped tasks heighten the tendency for the sleep attack. These recurrent attacks often subject the adolescent to significant psychological stress.

It is estimated that 80% of narcoleptics have associated cataplexy. Cataplexy, or brief loss of muscle tone, may be associated with weakness of the facial or limb musculature and sudden falling to the ground. Consciousness is maintained. The cataplectic attack is often triggered by an emotional stimulus, such as laughter or a slap on the back. Those having narcolepsy may also experience sleep paralysis or hallucinations on falling asleep or awakening.

Narcoleptics, as a consequence of their excessive sleepiness, usually exhibit short sleep latencies and early onset REM sleep, which can be documented by the use of the Multiple Sleep Latency Test. In this test the subject is allowed to nap five times at 2-hour intervals. Twenty minutes are granted for sleep onset and a total of 10 minutes of sleep is permitted.

Familial cases of narcolepsy have been reported, and the mode of inheritance is considered to be autosomal dominant. It has been observed that almost everyone having narcolepsy is HLA-DR2 positive. Therapy for narcolepsy consists of well-timed naps, which may be successful in ameliorating symptoms. Increased sleep time as well as naps may also be effective. Drugs used for the reduction of narcoleptic symptoms include methylphenidate and pemoline. Imipramine has been used to treat cataplectic symptoms. Long-term psychological support of the adolescent and the use of medication are essential. The hazards of driving must be stressed.

SLEEP APNEA SYNDROME

Sleep apnea syndrome, another cause of excessive daytime sleepiness, can also occur in adolescents. Daytime sleepiness, snoring, and periodic prolonged respiratory pauses are the usual symptoms. In these cases there is usually impairment in school performance as well as psychological difficulties, which stem from being unable to remain awake in class, perform adequately, and successfully participate in examinations. Usually the cause is secondary to airway obstruction related to enlarged tonsils and adenoids. Potsic has suggested that the decline in tonsillectomy and adenoidectomy is related to the increased incidence of airway obstruction. At earlier ages sleep apnea is usually found to be related to craniofacial anomalies. Down syndrome can cause similar symptoms.

Although the diagnosis of obstructive sleep apnea can often be made on clinical grounds, there are situations in which the possibility of central apnea has to be considered. Polysomnography and consultation with an otolaryngologist are warranted.

DELAYED SLEEP PHASE SYNDROME

Another cause of excessive daytime sleepiness in adolescence is the delayed sleep phase syndrome. Characteristic morning sleepiness coupled with poor performance at school and behavioral difficulties may result from an inability to initiate sleep at socially acceptable or customary times. This tendency of some adolescents to go to bed and fall asleep later than their peers often begins in early childhood, at which time the problem may be regarded as insomnia. These adolescents have difficulty in arising in the morning, and they perform poorly early in the day. They may be continuously late in getting to school. Their efficiency usually improves later in the day as they become more wide awake. As a group they tend to sleep longer on weekends and have been found to have increased REM sleep. Psychological tests often reveal significant features of hypochondriasis and depression.

The diagnosis of this condition can usually be made from the history and the use of sleep logs. Excessive sleepiness can be confirmed by the use of Multiple Sleep Latency Tests. A resetting of the sleep schedule can be achieved by delaying sleep onset by 3 hours each day, as described by Thorpy and associates. They used sleep deprivation and advancing the sleep time of their adolescent subjects to preclude their having to sleep during the day.

Parasomnias

Parasomnias include nightmares, night terrors, sleepwalking, and enuresis.

Nightmares are experienced at all ages and occur any time during the night. They are usually associated with REM sleep. The unpleasant vivid dreams, when they are recalled, are frequently characterized by fears of pursuit, personal injury, and death. Withdrawal of certain drugs, notably alcohol and sedatives, may trigger nightmares. In adolescence a frequent cause is emotional stress. Repetitive nightmares are best explored by a review of potential areas of life stress and anxiety before treatment is begun.

In contrast with nightmares, night terrors (pavor nocturnus) occur after sleep onset during the first part of stage III or IV slow-wave sleep. The onset of the terror is heralded by an abrupt crying out, followed by symptoms of confusion, panic, and extreme apprehension. Unlike the nightmare there is little, if any, recollection of the event. Part of the clinical picture is an intense autonomic response with rapid heart rate, increased respiration, sweating, and pupillary dilatation. In milder forms of night terror, some subjects experience relatively minor physiologic effects and leave their beds and move about (sleepwalking). The cause of night terrors is unknown, but in most cases a familial tendency can be documented. Often, the episode may occur in the setting of intercurrent illness. Many people with night terrors exhibit some type of psychological illness, which should be investigated if episodes are frequent. Treatment with imipramine and benzodiazepines has been found to be useful.

At times it may be difficult to separate a parasomnia from epilepsy. Often, repeated observations, neurologic consultation, and prolonged electroencephalographic recordings, including telemetry, are necessary to help clarify diagnosis.

OTHER PROBLEMS

Panic Attacks

Panic attacks may be diurnal or nocturnal and are viewed as a type of anxiety disorder. In addition to chronic anxiety there may be associated depression. Alterations in sleep during classic psychotic depression include early onset REM sleep, increased REM density, and increased time spent in REM sleep. Hauri and colleagues studied a group of patients ranging in age from 18 to 60 years and found that nocturnal panic attacks occurred in 8 of 24 patients. Most of the events took place during the transition from stage II to stage III sleep. Generally, the patients as a group exhibited more limb movements during stage II sleep. Some panic attacks occurred during a hypnic body jerk as the patients were dozing, and after the panic attack the subjects usually had difficulty in returning to sleep. Panic attacks did not appear to occur in the setting of REM sleep. The memory and emotional content of the event was usually fragmentary.

Enuresis

Nocturnal enuresis usually occurs in childhood but may persist into adolescence. In some the problem is habitual or recurrent. A family history of this problem is often encountered, and sometimes there are other associated sleep disorders. At one time enuresis was thought to be prevalent only during slow-wave sleep, but repeated studies have shown that it may also occur during REM sleep. Enuresis may be either primary or secondary. Primary enuresis occurs frequently in children in whom a family history may be present, in addition to associated abnormalities in urinary tract function and/or bladder control. Often, bladder overload or infection may be the cause of symptoms (see Chapter 66). In adolescence enuresis may occur in the setting of sleep apnea syndrome. Secondary enuresis is considered to be the result of impaired adjustment in coping with life stresses. In primary enuresis, bladder training exercises can be used, as well as conditioning devices involving the use of bells or buzzers to awaken the subject. Because of the psychological factors associated with secondary enuresis, psychotherapy is often part of the treatment regimen. Imipramine is a drug that has been used in the management of enuresis in the older child or adolescent. Similarly, oxybutynin chloride has been noted to be effective. Tricyclic antidepressants, including imipramine or desipramine, may be helpful for short courses of therapy, but long-term treatment with these agents is not advised.

CONCLUSION

Some of the more common sleep disturbances in adolescence have been reviewed. Often, the event is transient and easily forgotten. Conversely, there may be significant alteration in the health and behavior of those adolescents with recurrent or chronic sleep disorders. As a consequence of heightened interest in sleep medicine, more precise evaluation, diagnoses, and appropriate treatment are now possible.

BIBLIOGRAPHY

Carskadon MA, Dement WC: Sleepiness in the normal adolescent. In Guilleminault C (ed): Sleep and its Disorders in Children. New York, Raven Press, 1987, pp 53–66.
Fournier JP, Garfinkel BD, Bond A, et al: Pharmacological and behavioral management of enuresis. J Am Acad Child Adolesc Psychiatry 26:849, 1987.
Hauri PJ, Friedman M, Ravaris CL: Sleep in patients with spontaneous panic attacks. Sleep 12:323, 1989.
Kales A, Soldatos CR, Kales JD: Sleep disorders: Insomnia, sleepwalking, night terrors, nightmares and enuresis. Ann Intern Med 106:582, 1987.
Lugaresi E, Cirignotta F: Hypnogenic paroxysmal dystonia: Epileptic seizure or a new syndrome? Sleep 4:129, 1981.
Mattison RE, Handford HA, Vela-Bueno A: Sleep disorders in children. Psychiatr Med 4:149, 1987.
Parkes JD, Lock CB: Genetic factors in sleep disorders. J Neurol Neurosurg Psychiatry (Suppl) 101, 1989.
Potsic WB: Sleep apnea in children. Otolaryngol Clin North Am 22:537, 1989.
Sleep Disorders Classification Committee, Association of Sleep Disorders Centers: Diagnostic classification of sleep and arousal disorders. Sleep 2(1):1, 1979.
Thorpy MJ: Classification of sleep disorders. J Clin Neurophysiol 7:67, 1990.
Thorpy MJ, Korman E, Spielman AJ, Glovinsky PB: Delayed sleep phase syndrome in adolescents. J Adolesc Health Care 9:22, 1988.

CHAPTER 87

Inflammatory Conditions Affecting the Central and Peripheral Nervous Systems

JAMES F. BALE, JR.

The disorders discussed in this chapter are grouped together as inflammatory conditions of the nervous system. Although the disorders affect varying regions of the neuraxis, they share several pathophysiologic, clinical, and therapeutic features. All appear to be mediated by aberrant humoral or cell-mediated immune responses, and several of the disorders have strong epidemiologic associations with antecedent infections. However, with the exception of rheumatic fever, these disorders have not been linked with a single, specific causative factor. All the disorders present diagnostic and therapeutic challenges.

MULTIPLE SCLEROSIS

Multiple sclerosis (MS) is an important inflammatory condition causing long-term neurologic disability in late adolescence and early adulthood. The fundamental pathologic abnormality in MS is a white matter lesion, or plaque, that occurs in the periventricular white matter, optic nerve, brainstem, or spinal cord. Plaques vary in size, number, location, and temporal course, features that contribute directly to the multifocal, episodic nature of MS. The presentation in adolescents is described in greater detail in Chapter 88.

GUILLAIN-BARRÉ SYNDROME

Guillain-Barré syndrome (GBS), an acute, demyelinating polyneuropathy, accounts for a substantial proportion of all polyneuropathies among adolescents. Although many issues regarding the pathogenesis of GBS require further clarification, GBS appears to reflect an aberrant immune response initiated against peripheral myelin. Adolescents constitute approximately 15% of patients with GBS, with an attack rate of 0.2 to 0.5 case per 100,000 population.

Pathophysiology

The pathologic features of GBS consist of focal demyelination and inflammation of peripheral nerves. Demyelination typically occurs near the junction of the anterior and posterior roots of the spinal nerves and involves the myelin lamellae deposited by Schwann cells. Schwann cell bodies are unaffected, whereas axons can be damaged in severe GBS. Macrophages, the predominant inflammatory cells, invade nerve fibers and ingest myelin that otherwise appears normal when studied by electron microscopy. In some studies, sera from patients with acute GBS induce demyelination when inoculated into the peripheral nerves of experimental animals.

GBS has a strong epidemiologic association with antecedent infection, and a more tenuous relationship with immunization and prior surgery. Of the 1034 patients identified in 1978 and 1979 by a United States GBS surveillance study, 67% had a prior respiratory or gastrointestinal illness, 5% had surgery, and 4.5% had received an immunization within the 8 weeks prior to the onset of GBS. The remainder had no identifiable precipitating factors. Infectious agents linked with GBS include cytomegalovirus (CMV), the Epstein-Barr virus (EBV), varicella-zoster virus, enteroviruses, the hepatitis viruses, *Mycoplasma pneumoniae,* and *Campylobacter jejuni.* The herpesviruses EBV and CMV, common infections among adolescents, contribute to approximately 20% to 25% of GBS cases. In adults with acquired immunodeficiency syndrome (AIDS) and polyradiculopathy similar to the GBS, CMV can be detected within peripheral nerves.

Clinical Manifestations

GBS develops 1 to 3 weeks after the antecedent infection. As summarized in Table 87–1, the characteristic features of GBS consist of progressive motor weakness—symmetric but variable in severity—and areflexia (loss of tendon reflexes). The usual adolescent patient initially experiences leg weakness (distal more than proximal), which may ascend or simultaneously involve the arms, truncal musculature, or cranial nerves. Weakness involves the upper extremities initially or, more severely, in only 5% to 20% of patients. Approximately 50% of patients with GBS have facial weakness (cranial nerve VII), often bilateral. Cranial nerve IX, X, XII,

TABLE 87–1. Clinical and Laboratory Features of Guillain-Barré Syndrome

Features required for diagnosis:
  Progressive motor weakness of more than one limb
  Areflexia (loss of tendon jerks)
Features strongly supportive of the diagnosis:
  Clinical features
    Progression—90% reach nadir by 4 weeks
    Relative symmetry of weakness
    Mild sensory involvement
    Cranial nerve involvement—50% have facial weakness
    Recovery—most recover functionally
    Autonomic dysfunction (bladder or bowel dysfunction unusual)
    Absence of fever at onset of neuritic symptoms
  Cerebrospinal fluid
    CSF protein level is elevated or rises after the first week of symptoms
    CSF cell count usually below 10 mononuclear leukocytes/mm^2
  Electrodiagnostic features
    Most (80%) have impaired nerve conduction (slowing or block)
    Conduction studies may not be abnormal until several weeks into the illness

Modified with permission from Asbury AK: Diagnostic considerations in Guillain-Barré syndrome. Ann Neurol 9(Suppl):1–5, 1981.

III, IV, or VI (listed in decreasing order of involvement) can also be affected, leading to dysphagia, weakness of the tongue, or ophthalmoplegia.

Other features compatible with GBS include autonomic dysfunction (hypertension, postural hypotension, tachycardia, or other arrhythmias) and mild sensory symptoms or signs. Some patients have prominent sensory loss with areflexia, and blurred disk margins resembling papilledema can occasionally be identified. By contrast, features such as asymmetric weakness, bladder or bowel dysfunction, a sharp sensory level, and prominent fever are not suggestive of GBS.

GBS has several clinical variants, with the Fisher syndrome among the most prominent. This disorder, characterized by ophthalmoplegia, areflexia, and ataxia, begins abruptly and involves the central and peripheral nervous systems. Relapsing or chronic demyelinative polyneuropathies share clinical and pathophysiologic features with GBS, but are usually considered as distinct clinical entities.

Diagnosis

The diagnosis of GBS requires the presence of progressive motor weakness of more than one limb and areflexia. Cerebrospinal fluid (CSF) findings that support GBS consist of an elevated protein level after the first week of symptoms and 10 or fewer mononuclear leukocytes/mm^3 (the albuminocytologic dissociation). However, most adolescents have a normal CSF protein level during the initial few days of the illness, and occasionally patients with GBS have CSF mononuclear leukocyte counts as high as 50/mm^3. The CSF protein level peaks 3 to 5 weeks after the onset of symptoms. Other routine laboratory studies are usually normal.

Approximately 80% of patients with GBS have abnormal electrophysiologic studies, consisting of slowed nerve conduction velocities (an electromyographic feature indicative of demyelination), increased distal laten-

cies (another sign of impaired nerve conduction), and abnormal F-wave responses. The latter, an evoked response that reflects the integrity of afferent and efferent motor nerve arcs, can be abnormal early in the course of GBS. By contrast, nerve conduction velocities often remain normal during the first week of GBS.

The differential diagnosis of GBS includes disorders of the brain and spinal cord, and several conditions affecting the peripheral nerves or the neuromuscular junction (Table 87–2). Although many of these conditions can be identified on historical or clinical grounds, some adolescent patients require further laboratory or neurodiagnostic investigation. These studies may consist of analyses for toxins (e.g., urine screens for heavy metals or porphyrin metabolites) or magnetic resonance imaging (MRI) of the spine, brainstem, and cerebrum. Because of the strong association of GBS with infectious pathogens, serologic studies for EBV or *Mycoplasma pneumoniae*, urine and buffy coat cultures for CMV, and stool cultures for *Campylobacter jejuni* should be considered.

Treatment and Prognosis

The therapy for GBS consists largely of supportive care. Respiratory failure, the most serious complication, develops in approximately 10% to 20% of adolescent patients with GBS and should be managed with intensive monitoring and ventilatory support. Several studies have suggested that plasmapheresis reduces the duration of GBS-associated weakness and improves long-term outcome, particularly among children and adolescents and those who have respiratory failure. Response to plasmapheresis tends to be more favorable when plasma exchange is initiated within 7 days of the onset of symptoms. Patients may also improve after intravenous gamma globulin. Corticosteroids do not have a beneficial effect in acute GBS but may be beneficial in those with relapsing inflammatory polyneuropathies.

GBS reaches maximum severity within 4 weeks of onset in 90% of cases, and the duration of hospitaliza-

TABLE 87–2. Differential Diagnosis of Acute Symmetric Weakness

Central nervous system
  Stroke (bilateral)
  Hysteria
  Transverse myelitis
  Compressive myelopathy
Peripheral nervous system
  Polio-like disorders (usually asymmetric)
  Toxic neuropathy (e.g., heavy metals, drugs)
  Diphtheria
  Tick paralysis
  Porphyria (can cause facial diplegia)
  Lyme disease
Muscle or neuromuscular junction
  Botulism
  Acute, severe myasthenia gravis
  Inflammatory myopathies
  Metabolic muscle disorders

Modified with permission from Evans OB: Guillain-Barré syndrome in children. Pediatr Rev 8:69–74, 1986. Reproduced by permission of Pediatrics.

tion averages 35 to 45 days. Most adolescent patients recover completely, although convalescence typically lasts several weeks. Approximately 2% to 5% of patients die from complications of GBS, and 10% to 25% of the survivors experience permanent motor disabilities of variable severity. Children and adolescents and those whose weakness develops slowly have a more favorable long-term prognosis.

BELL PALSY

Bell palsy refers to an acute idiopathic paralysis of the seventh cranial (facial) nerve. Adolescents account for approximately 10% of cases of Bell palsy, and females outnumber males by 2:1. Bell palsy may represent an immunologic response to an antecedent infection or a direct virus-induced neuritis. Direct inspection of the involved seventh cranial nerve frequently reveals edema, whereas signs of inflammation or ischemia are less prominent.

Clinical Manifestations

More than 95% of adolescent patients with Bell palsy have unilateral (right side equivalent to left side) facial paralysis of variable severity and cannot smile, wrinkle the forehead symmetrically, or close the eyelids tightly. Patients often experience facial discomfort localized to the ear as a prodromal event. On the involved side, the palpebral fissure is widened, the blink reflex is lost, and the nasolabial fold becomes flattened. Approximately 50% of adolescent patients have altered taste sensation, whereas hyperacusis, indicating weakness of the stapedius muscle, or decreased tear formation occurs less frequently.

Diagnosis

Acute, acquired facial paralysis can complicate several other disorders, including otitis media (with or without mastoiditis), craniocerebral trauma, Lyme disease, diabetes mellitus, hypertension, neoplasms, pseudotumor cerebri, or connective tissue disorders. These disorders can usually be excluded by a detailed history and physical examination.

Routine laboratory studies, including CSF analysis, are usually normal in adolescents with Bell palsy. Mild elevations of the peripheral white blood cell count may be seen; rarely, adolescent patients have CSF pleocytosis. Because of the epidemiologic association of Bell palsy with several infectious agents (e.g., EBV, varicella-zoster virus, respiratory viruses, Lyme disease), cultures or serologies for infectious pathogens should be considered. Electrophysiologic studies that assess the function of the facial nerve frequently reveal abnormalities after 72 hours, which may assist in determining the prognosis for recovery.

Treatment and Prognosis

Corticosteroids or surgical decompression have no proven benefit in Bell palsy. Most adolescents with Bell palsy recover spontaneously and completely. However, adolescent patients with Lyme disease and facial paralysis should be treated with antibiotics (amoxicillin, doxycycline, or ceftriaxone). Approximately 10% of adolescents with Bell palsy have recurrent paralysis or a family history of the disorder.

MYASTHENIA GRAVIS

Myasthenia gravis (MG), an immunologically mediated disorder of the neuromuscular junction, causes episodic or progressive skeletal muscle weakness. Children and adolescents with MG, so-called "juvenile myasthenia gravis," constitute 10% to 15% of all MG patients. Females are more commonly affected.

Pathophysiology

Most adolescent patients with MG possess antibodies directed against the acetylcholine receptor, a glycoprotein composed of several subunits. These antibodies, primarily of the IgG1 and IgG2 subclasses, appear to disrupt the function of the acetylcholine receptor. Pathologic studies of muscle from MG patients reveal quantitative and qualitative abnormalities of the acetylcholine receptors, and electron microscopic studies indicate that most patients with MG have destructive changes within the neuromuscular junction that appear to be immune-mediated.

Although the role of acetylcholine receptor antibodies in MG has been elucidated, the events that induce the antibodies have not been fully characterized. Preceding antigenic stimulation, such as a recent viral infection, could participate by generating cross-reacting antibodies or by fostering the production of autoantibodies. Immunogenetic factors may also be important, because certain HLA types (e.g., HLA-B8) are overrepresented in some groups of MG patients. The role of immune processes in MG is further supported by the association of thymoma and MG (usually in older adults) and the presence of nonspecific immunologic abnormalities in MG patients.

Clinical Manifestations

Most patients with juvenile MG experience the insidious onset of weakness of the ocular, facial, and oropharyngeal muscles. Ptosis, unilateral or bilateral, and diplopia are the usual initial complaints. The adolescent's face is less expressive, the voice frequently changes, becoming hoarse or weak, and weakness of chewing or swallowing may develop. These signs fluctuate, tending to worsen late in the day or during times of increased fatigue, stress, or intercurrent infection.

Generalized muscle weakness may be absent initially,

but most adolescent patients subsequently lose stamina and experience fluctuating or slowly progressive weakness. Abrupt onset, with generalized weakness, proximal weakness (limb girdle myasthenia), or respiratory distress is less common. Rarely, acute bulbar paralysis and respiratory failure can be the initial manifestations of MG.

Neurologic examination usually reveals ptosis and weakness of the facial or extraocular muscles. The pupils, as well as the funduscopic examination, are normal. Fatigability of systemic muscles can be demonstrated by repetitive maneuvers, such as repeated deep knee bends, or by maintenance of posture against gravity. Fatigability can be assessed semiquantitatively by recording how long the adolescent can maintain an upward gaze or elevate a limb against gravity. Deep tendon reflexes are normal or hyperactive.

Diagnosis

The Tensilon test (2 mg of edrophonium chloride intravenously, followed by 3 to 5 mg if the adolescent does not respond and has no untoward muscarinic side effects) generally results in an abrupt improvement in strength, such as resolution of ptosis or improvement in an obviously paretic extraocular muscle. A positive response supports but does not confirm the diagnosis of MG, because positive responses can occasionally be observed in other conditions, such as polymyositis or brainstem processes. Atropine (0.01 mg/kg) should be available, because some patients can experience severe muscarinic effects (e.g., bradycardia or airway compromise).

Acetylcholine receptor antibodies can be detected in the sera of most adolescent MG patients with severe generalized disease, with the titers roughly paralleling the clinical severity of MG. Adolescents with MG have normal nerve conduction velocities and normal-appearing muscle action potentials, but typically have a decrement in the amplitude of the muscle action potential when subjected to repetitive stimulation at three to five stimuli per second.

Treatment and Prognosis

Almost all adolescents with MG respond, at least temporarily, to cholinesterase inhibitors. Pyridostigmine bromide (Mestinon) can be initiated at a dose of 30 or 45 mg orally every 4 hours and then titrated to the response of the patient (total daily dose of approximately 7 mg/kg). An optimum dosage schedule allows the patient to participate in normal activities without substantial muscarinic (diarrhea, abdominal cramps, excessive salivation) or nicotinic (weakness) side effects. Mestinon overdose can induce generalized weakness that mimics that of myasthenic crisis.

Prednisone, an important component of MG therapy, can be initiated when adolescents relapse during Mestinon therapy. One approach is to begin daily prednisone at a dose of 2 mg/kg and then reduce the dose to an every-other-day regimen in the range of 1 to 2 mg/kg

when the adolescent patient stabilizes. Because adolescent patients may worsen during the initiation of daily prednisone, hospitalization should be considered. The goal of corticosteroid therapy is to maintain muscle strength while limiting side effects. Azathioprine or cyclosporine also has a potential beneficial role in MG.

Adolescents with MG also improve after thymectomy. The response tends to be most favorable in patients within the first year of diagnosis, in patients with thymic hyperplasia or thymoma (a rare occurrence in juvenile MG), and in patients with high antibody titers. Some studies have suggested that the timing of thymectomy does not greatly influence long-term outcome, and that thymectomy should be reserved for more severely involved adolescent patients.

Because of their potential to induce neuromuscular blockade and exacerbate symptoms of MG, certain medications should be avoided in. myasthenic adolescents. These include several antibiotics (aminoglycosides, tetracyclines, clindamycin), certain cardiotropic drugs (lidocaine, quinidine, procainamide, propranolol), psychotropic drugs (lithium, chlorpromazine), and the anticonvulsant phenytoin. These drugs may exacerbate known MG or unmask subclinical MG.

The long-term prognosis of adolescents with juvenile MG remains favorable. MG remits spontaneously in 20% to 25% of affected individuals and improves or remits in many adolescents who undergo thymectomy. Nonetheless, 5% to 10% of MG patients die as a direct consequence of their disease. Children and adolescents with MG, particularly females, have an increased risk of hyperthyroidism, and seizures may occur more frequently in juvenile MG patients.

SYSTEMIC LUPUS ERYTHEMATOSUS (see Chapter 90)

Systemic lupus erythematosus (SLE), an autoimmune disorder that affects numerous tissues, produces neurologic or psychiatric complications in 50% or more of adolescent patients with the disorder.

Pathophysiology

Pathologic studies reveal CNS abnormalities in many patients with SLE-induced neurologic signs or symptoms. These abnormalities include focal or multifocal CNS hemorrhages or infarctions of varying sizes, perivascular inflammation or gliosis, and atrophic changes. Although many patients have destructive changes within cerebral vessels (fibrinoid or hyaline degeneration), few autopsied patients have actual CNS vasculitis.

In a review of the autopsy materials of 50 patients with SLE, embolic brain infarction and CNS infections were relatively common. Sources of emboli appeared to be cardiac and included endocarditis, valvulitis, and mural thrombi. In addition, several patients had clinical or pathologic evidence of thrombotic thrombocytopenic purpura (TTP), typically as a preterminal event. These observations suggest that SLE-associated cardiac lesions and TTP play major roles in the pathogenesis of SLE-induced neurologic complications.

Autoantibodies against certain CNS antigens may participate in the pathogenesis of SLE-induced neuropsychiatric complications. Antibodies that are cytotoxic to a neuroblastoma cell line have been detected in the CSF of patients with CNS lupus, and serum antibodies against ribosomal P proteins appear to correlate with the presence of SLE-induced psychosis. These observations suggest that autoantibodies may induce CNS dysfunction directly through cytotoxic effects or by interfering with critical neuronal functions.

Clinical Manifestations

Adolescent patients with SLE are at risk for numerous neurologic complications caused by SLE directly or as a consequence of systemic complications (e.g., severe hypertension or uremia) or anti-SLE therapy. Seizures, generalized tonic-clonic or partial, are the most frequent neurologic complication, affecting as many as 40% of adolescent SLE patients. Seizures can be the initial manifestation of SLE, can occur during acute exacerbations of the disease, or can be secondary to hypertension, uremia, or intercurrent CNS infection.

SLE can affect the entire neuraxis, including the cerebral cortex, basal ganglia, spinal cord, and peripheral nerves. Chorea, a manifestation of extrapyramidal involvement, occurs more commonly in adolescent patients with SLE and may predate other signs or symptoms of the disorder. Adolescents with SLE can have various neuropathies, involving the cranial nerves (typically CN III, IV, or VI) or peripheral nerves, either individually or as a Guillain-Barré–like disorder. Hemiplegia, quadriplegia, or signs indicative of myelopathy can also occur.

Adolescents with SLE experience psychiatric disturbances that can mimic those of affective disorders or schizophrenia (see Chapters 100 and 110). Specific abnormalities include depression, irritability, confusion, visual or auditory hallucinations, and suicidal ideation. SLE-induced psychiatric complications, particularly psychosis, may be difficult to differentiate from the psychobehavioral complications of corticosteroid administration or uremia.

Diagnosis

No currently available neurodiagnostic study is specific for SLE. Adolescents with SLE can have nonspecific abnormalities when studied by electroencephalography, CT, or MRI. CT findings range from diffuse sulcal enlargement to infarction or hemorrhage. MRI may reveal lesions of white matter. The CSF may be normal or may show modest lymphocytosis or protein elevation, and anti-DNA antibodies may be detected in the CSF in some adolescent patients. Adolescents with SLE may also have oligoclonal IgG bands and an elevated CSF immunoglobulin index, indicating synthesis of immunoglobulins within the CSF.

Treatment and Prognosis

Seizures that occur in the absence of systemic signs of SLE can be treated with anticonvulsants (e.g., carbamazepine or valproic acid) specific for the seizure type. Adolescent patients with chorea may respond to haloperidol in initial doses of 0.25 to 0.5 mg twice daily.

Corticosteroids should be used for adolescent patients who have more severe CNS disease (e.g., with dementia, psychosis), particularly when other systemic signs of SLE, such as nephritis, are present. No single therapeutic regimen has gained universal acceptance. Prednisone can be initiated at a daily dosage of 1 to 2 mg/kg and continued on a daily basis until a beneficial response occurs. Nonresponders may benefit from short-term therapy with higher doses of prednisone or pulse therapy with intravenous methylprednisolone. Others may require cyclophosphamide or azathioprine.

SYDENHAM CHOREA

Sydenham, or rheumatic, chorea remains the most commonly identified cause of acute or subacute chorea in children and adolescents. Although the association of chorea with childhood rheumatic fever (see Chapter 50) has been recognized for nearly two centuries, medical science has made only modest progress in determining the pathogenesis of the disorder.

Pathophysiology

Sydenham chorea represents a postinfectious complication of group A β-hemolytic streptococcal pharyngitis (see Chapter 94). Alterations in central dopaminergic function are assumed to cause chorea. Neuropathologic changes in Sydenham chorea are nonspecific, consisting of a mild vasculitis or modest neuronal degeneration of the cerebral cortex or basal ganglia.

Genetic factors appear to influence the risk of chorea following streptococcal infection and to enhance the risk of rheumatic fever in general. From 2% to 15% of adolescent patients with Sydenham chorea have a first-degree relative who also had chorea. Moreover, a family history of rheumatic disease is identified in 25% to 35% of adolescent patients with Sydenham chorea.

Clinical Manifestations

The incidence of Sydenham chorea peaks in preadolescents between the ages of 7 and 10 years. Adolescents with onset after the age of 12 years constitute approximately 15% to 20% of the cases of Sydenham chorea. Among patients with onset between 11 and 17 years of age, females outnumber males by nearly 2:1.

Sydenham chorea typically begins 1 to 6 months after streptococcal infection and usually appears without other concurrent signs of rheumatic fever. The movement disorder begins insidiously, and affected individuals initially appear restless or irritable and may be misinterpreted as having a behavior problem. As the disorder progresses, chorea—irregular, rapid involuntary movements—becomes more pronounced, typically affecting the face and upper extremities. Chorea is unilateral in approximately 20% of adolescent patients.

Physical signs, in addition to chorea, frequently include facial grimacing, dysarthria, emotional lability, and an inability to sustain hand grip or tongue protrusion. Approximately 10% of adolescent patients with Sydenham chorea exhibit encephalopathic signs, such as personality change or disorientation, and approximately 5% have altered deep tendon reflexes or substantial unilateral weakness. Other neurologic abnormalities, such as headache or convulsions, occur infrequently.

Diagnosis

The diagnosis of Sydenham chorea rests largely on the clinical features of the disorder and on the absence of other causes of chorea, such as systemic lupus erythematosus, oral contraceptive use, drug ingestion, hyperthyroidism, familial chorea, or Huntington disease. Laboratory studies are generally not helpful. A modest proportion of adolescent patients with Sydenham chorea have elevated antistreptolysin O (ASO) titers, but these titers usually decline to undetectable levels by the time chorea appears. Anti-DNase B levels persist for longer periods and have some diagnostic usefulness. Many adolescent patients have nonspecific abnormalities when studied by electroencephalography.

Treatment and Prognosis

Most adolescents with Sydenham chorea have mild symptoms and require no therapy. Chorea usually disappears within 5 to 15 weeks of onset. Approximately 15% to 20% of adolescent patients have severe chorea that limits daily activities, affects behavior or school performance, and leads to weight loss and substantial disability.

Several medications appear to benefit adolescents with severe chorea. Haloperidol, in initial doses of 0.25 to 0.5 mg twice daily, may reduce chorea and allow resumption of normal activities. Patients may also respond to chlorpromazine, at a dose of 300 to 400 mg/day, or to valproic acid, using 15 to 25 mg/kg/day divided into two or three doses.

Although chorea gradually resolves, cardiac valvular disease (see Chapter 47) appears subsequently in approximately 25% to 30% of adolescent patients with Sydenham chorea. Adolescents with Sydenham chorea require penicillin prophylaxis. Some adolescent patients have mild neurologic or psychological residua. Chorea recurs at least once in nearly 20% of adolescent patients, but multiple bouts are unusual. Women with a prior history of Sydenham chorea have a slight risk of recurrence during pregnancy (chorea gravidarum) or with oral contraceptive use (see Chapters 73 and 74).

OTHER DISORDERS

Neuromyelitis optica, or Devic syndrome, a rare demyelinating disorder that involves the optic nerves and spinal cord, affects adolescent patients at an average age of 18 years. Individuals with the disorder experience unexplained visual loss (optic neuritis), usually bilateral, and spinal cord dysfunction (transverse myelitis) within an 8-week period. Signs of cord dysfunction consist of weakness, bladder or bowel dysfunction, and a sensory level. The disorder frequently represents a variant of multiple sclerosis but may also occur as a postinfectious encephalomyelitis.

Laboratory abnormalities in Devic syndrome usually consist of an abnormal CSF profile with an elevated total protein content and a lymphocytic pleocytosis. Adolescent patients may have oligoclonal IgG bands and an elevated IgG index, findings that support multiple sclerosis as the underlying disorder. CT studies are usually normal, whereas MRI studies may reveal abnormalities of cerebral white matter (usually on T_2-weighted images) or spinal cord. In adolescent patients with acute transverse myelitis, spinal MRI or myelography should be considered emergently to exclude a compressive myelopathy.

Although no uniform therapeutic approach has been established for Devic syndrome, some adolescent patients may benefit from corticosteroid therapy. Most adolescents with the disorder have long-term sequelae of variable severity, and, although possible, complete recovery is unusual.

Postinfectious encephalomyelitis usually occurs in young children but may also occur in adolescents. Neurologic features usually begin 1 to 3 weeks after a nonspecific illness and can consist of seizures, ataxia, multifocal neurologic deficits, papilledema, or altered consciousness. Several infectious agents, such as the Epstein-Barr virus, viruses responsible for childhood exanthems, and *Borrelia burgdorferi* (Lyme disease) have been linked with encephalomyelitis.

Laboratory abnormalities can include an elevated erythrocyte sedimentation rate, elevated peripheral white blood count, or, occasionally, thrombocytosis. The CSF often shows a modest leukocytosis, and the protein or IgG content can be elevated. CT studies reveal abnormalities in approximately two thirds of adolescent patients, whereas MRI studies usually disclose multifocal white matter lesions.

Adolescent patients with postinfectious encephalomyelitis may respond dramatically to a short (7- to 10-day) course of daily corticosteroids, using intravenous methylprednisolone or oral prednisone. There appear to be no reliable predictors of steroid responsiveness, and an equal number of adolescent patients improve spontaneously. Relapses can occur, and approximately 15% of adolescent patients ultimately develop multiple sclerosis.

Several other rare inflammatory conditions, such as Wegener granulomatosis, polyarteritis nodosa, and Behçet disease, can be associated with neurologic complications in adolescents. In general, these disorders tend to induce multifocal neurologic signs or symptoms, including ataxia, seizures, cognitive dysfunction, brainstem signs, peripheral neuropathy, and motor deficits. Certain conditions (e.g., Behçet disease) produce a meningoencephalitis.

Approximately 25% to 50% of patients with Wegener granulomatosis have neurologic involvement. Adolescents with this condition typically have respiratory tract vasculitis, usually in association with glomerulonephritis and arthralgias. Neurologic complications consist of cranial neuropathies (usually of cranial nerves II, III, IV, and VI) and peripheral neuropathies. Diabetes insipidus or focal lesions of the brain or spinal cord occur less commonly.

Polyarteritis nodosa, a disorder associated with widespread vasculitis, produces neurologic complications in approximately 50% of affected adolescent patients. Both the central and the peripheral nervous systems can be involved. CNS complications consist of seizures, encephalopathy, and stroke, whereas signs of peripheral nervous system dysfunction include sensory loss and distal weakness.

Behçet disease, a rare condition in children or adolescents, is frequently associated with keratitis, uveitis, aphthous ulceration, arthritis, and erythema nodosum. Neurologic complications include headache, meningoencephalitis, ataxia, paralysis, sensory abnormalities, and seizures.

All these disorders present diagnostic and therapeutic challenges. Some adolescent patients may respond to corticosteroids, using a regimen similar to that outlined for systemic lupus erythematosus. Other adolescents may require antimetabolite therapy with drugs such as cyclophosphamide or azathioprine. In certain disorders, such as polyarteritis nodosa, neurologic involvement contributes substantially to the morbidity and mortality of affected adolescents.

BIBLIOGRAPHY

Adelman DC, Saltiel E, Klinenberg JR: The neuropsychiatric manifestations of systemic lupus erythematosus: An overview. Semin Arthritis Rheum 15:185, 1986.

Ammann AJ, Johnson A, Fyfe GA, et al: Behçet syndrome. J Pediatr 107:41, 1985.

Asbury AK: Diagnostic considerations in Guillain-Barré syndrome. Ann Neurol 9(Suppl):1, 1981.

Devinsky O, Petito CK, Alonso DR: Clinical and neuropathological findings in systemic lupus erythematosus: The role of vasculitis, heart emboli, and thrombotic thrombocytopenic purpura. Ann Neurol 23:380, 1988.

Duquette P, Murray TJ, Pleines J, et al: Multiple sclerosis in childhood: Clinical profile in 125 patients. J Pediatr 111:359, 1987.

Engel AG: Myasthenia gravis and myasthenic syndromes. Ann Neurol 16:519, 1984.

Evans OB: Guillain-Barré syndrome in children. Pediatr Rev 8:69, 1986.

Guillain-Barré Syndrome Study Group: Plasmapheresis and acute Guillain-Barré syndrome. Neurology 35:1096, 1985.

Kurtzke, JF: Epidemiologic contributions to multiple sclerosis: An overview. Neurology 30:61, 1980.

Moore PM, Cupps TR: Neurological complications of vasculitis. Ann Neurol 14:155, 1983.

Nausieda PA, Grossman BJ, Koller WC, et al: Sydenham chorea: An update. Neurology 30:331, 1980.

Rodriquez M, Gomez MR, Howard FM, Taylor WF: Myasthenia gravis in children: Long-term follow-up. Ann Neurol 13:504, 1983.

CHAPTER 88

Multiple Sclerosis

ANDREW D. GOODMAN

The most common chronic demyelinating disease of adolescents is multiple sclerosis (MS). MS is an immune-mediated disorder characterized by demyelination and scarring of white matter pathways that recur in more than one central nervous system (CNS) location over time. Historically, the eponyms Devic, Schilder, and Baló were associated with the demyelinating conditions of neuromyelitis optica, progressive diffuse sclerosis, and concentric sclerosis, respectively. There is no convincing evidence that these are distinct entities, but they may describe severe variants of MS and other myelin diseases that can occur in adolescents.

PATHOLOGY AND PATHOPHYSIOLOGY

Grossly, there are multiple grayish, hardened lesions, "plaques," distributed throughout the CNS white matter. Their predilection for periventricular regions is unexplained. Microscopically, individual lesions are typically centered around venules within white matter. Within plaques there is a loss of myelin and oligodendrocytes (the myelin-forming cells of the CNS) but relative sparing of axons and neurons. Perivenular cuffing by T and B lymphocytes, macrophages, and edema are seen in acute lesions but give way to astrocytic proliferation (scar) and axonal degeneration ("sclerosis") in chronic lesions. Most cases show various activities between these extremes in different lesions. On electron microscopy, macrophages can be seen stripping myelin from axons. Various abnormalities in circulating lymphocyte subsets or mitogenic responsiveness suggest underlying immunologic abnormalities. Over the years, neuropathologists have noted the similarity of these findings among patients who are biopsied and those who come to autopsy despite the marked heterogeneity of their clinical courses.

The mechanism underlying the signs and symptoms of MS is still incompletely understood. Various elements of lesion composition probably contribute to conduction delay or block through white matter pathways. Among these factors may be edema, soluble mediators of inflammation, myelin breakdown itself, astrocytic scarring, and axonal degeneration. All these could be involved to different degrees in a given adolescent patient in lesions of varying ages or severity. An exacerbation of symptoms often accompanies elevation of body temperature from endogenous or environmental sources, because heat further disrupts conduction through demyelinated areas.

Causative Factors and Pathogenesis

Most epidemiologic studies have found a gradient of incidence ranging between 50 and 150 in 100,000, with those in latitudes farthest from the equator showing the highest rates. Furthermore, studies of persons migrating between high- and low-incidence areas indicate that the risk of MS appears to be acquired by the age of 15. These observations have been taken to implicate environmental and age-related factors in the cause of this disease.

There is mounting evidence that immunogenetic mechanisms operate in MS. Several genetic markers are more prevalent in MS patients than in the general population. Among these are the immunoglobulin (Ig) Gm allotype, α_1-antitrypsin phenotype, T-cell receptor α-chain repertoire (chromosome 14), T-cell receptor β-chain repertoire (chromosome 7), histamine sensitivity, and HLA-DR2, particularly (chromosome 6). In the United States, whites have a higher risk of MS than blacks, Native Americans, or Asians.

A widely held hypothesis is that viral infection(s) occurring during childhood or adolescence in the immunogenetically susceptible individual triggers an ongoing (but fluctuating) autoimmune process with the CNS white matter after a variable period of clinical latency. Several characteristics of MS immunology implicate autoimmunity as the pathogenic mechanism:

1. Its similarity to experimental allergic encephalomyelitis, an autoimmune demyelinating disease
2. Peripheral immune dysregulation, including T-cell subset and functional abnormalities and impaired suppression of the autologous mixed lymphocyte and B-cell responses
3. Central nervous system immune abnormalities, including the lymphocytic infiltrate and oligoclonal B- and T-cell repertoire in cerebrospinal fluid (CSF)
4. Clinical response to immune-modulating therapies

DIFFERENTIAL DIAGNOSIS

The principal conditions in adolescents included in the differential diagnosis of demyelinating disease include idiopathic optic neuritis, acute disseminated encephalomyelitis, inherited leukodystrophies, and neurologic manifestations of collagen vascular disease (see Chapter 90). The former two entities are distinguished from MS by their monophasic course, involving the optic nerve alone or showing more diffuse brain and spinal cord involvement. The underlying pathogenic mechanisms are unknown but may be similar to those in MS.

The leukodystrophies are the result of inborn metabolic errors of myelin metabolism. Metachromatic leukodystrophy, the most common, is an autosomal recessive disorder that is distinguished clinically from MS by the involvement of peripheral nerves, causing ataxia and relatively early progressive intellectual deterioration (usually a late phenomenon in MS, when it occurs). Only the juvenile form of metachromatic leukodystrophy presents during adolescence. The diagnosis can be confirmed by the presence of metachromatic bodies in peripheral nerve biopsy and by low levels of fibroblast arylsulfatase A, the enzyme that catalyzes conversion of sulfatide to cerebroside in myelin.

Adrenoleukodystrophy and adrenomyeloneuropathy are sex-linked disorders that may become apparent during adolescence. Neurologic deterioration accompanied by adrenal dysfunction distinguish them clinically from MS. The diagnosis can be confirmed by the presence of very long-chain fatty acids in peripheral blood.

Collagen vascular diseases such as systemic lupus erythematosus (SLE) and Sjögren syndrome may present with multifocal CNS involvement that can mimic MS (see Chapter 90). These conditions should be ruled out by the usual clinical and laboratory criteria before making the conclusive diagnosis of MS.

CLINICAL MANIFESTATIONS

Because of the highly variable location, severity, number, and progression of demyelinated plaques, the clinical manifestations of MS are protean. The most common presenting symptoms in adolescents are sensory, including visual symptoms (central scotoma or diplopia) and impaired sensation in approximately 60% (Table 88–1). Furthermore, one third to two thirds of adolescents with isolated optic neuritis eventually develop MS. Motor weakness, gait incoordination, and bladder or bowel dysfunction tend to be uncommon early symptoms. Sexual dysfunction may occur but is generally not a presenting complaint. These symptoms may occur alone or in combination. Behavioral and cognitive changes can occur as isolated symptoms but are generally later findings and are not as prominent as in more rapidly progressive disorders, such as the leukodystrophies.

The ratio of females to males with MS is approximately 1.7:1 in adolescents. There is a steep increase in the onset of MS symptoms during the second decade of life, beginning at 0.3 per 100,000 below the age of 10 years and rising to almost 6 per 100,000 by age 20. This has been a consistent finding in areas of relatively high incidence throughout the world. For example, in northern countries, such as Denmark, the incidence rises

TABLE 88–1. Initial Clinical Features of Multiple Sclerosis

CLINICAL FEATURE	PERCENTAGE OF PATIENTS WITH FEATURE
Sensory symptoms (pure)	26
Optic neuritis	14
Diplopia	11
Motor symptoms (pure)	11
Gait disturbance	8
Blurred vision	6
Cerebellar ataxia	5
Combined sensory and motor symptoms	5
Optic neuritis and other CNS signs	3
Transverse myelitis	3
Vestibular symptoms	2
Sphincter dysfunction	1

With permission from Duquette P, Murray TJ, Pleines J, et al: Multiple sclerosis in childhood: Clinical analysis of 125 patients. J Pediatr 111:359, 1987.

rapidly after 10 years of age, with one third to one half of individuals with MS exhibiting symptoms by 20 years of age.

DIAGNOSIS

There is no single diagnostic test which is specific for MS. Rather, the diagnosis is based on the clinical syndrome, supplemented by confirmatory laboratory data. Clinical grounds for the diagnosis of MS include a history of multiple episodes or chronic progression of neurologic symptoms and physical examination findings of neurologic dysfunction in more than one CNS location. Because these are not always apparent, electrophysiologic or neuroimaging data suggesting multiple CNS lesions and CSF immunoglobulin abnormalities indicative of an ongoing immunologic process within the CNS may be helpful in confirming the diagnosis.

Electrophysiologic Studies

Electronic signal averaging permits the recording of low-amplitude potentials from scalp electrodes evoked by visual (checkerboard pattern reversal), auditory (multiple clicks), or somatic sensory stimulation (electric shocks). The objective of these studies is to demonstrate abnormalities in latency of conduction through myelinated sensory pathways that were not detectable from the clinical examination of the patient, but they are less sensitive than imaging or CSF studies.

Neuroimaging Studies

Although computed tomography (CT) of the head is more readily available, magnetic resonance imaging (MRI) is the imaging modality of choice in the diagnosis of MS. Its diagnostic usefulness involves the identification of one or more lesions within periventricular white matter in the brain or spinal cord that are not apparent on clinical grounds alone and the exclusion of other neuropathology. The abnormalities detected on MRI are a result of the prolongation of T_1 and T_2 relaxation times, which depend on the tissue-specific content of hydrogen nuclei (protons). These changes in relaxation times may relate to increased free water content because of the instability of the blood-brain barrier in an inflamed area, an increase in neutral lipids from myelin breakdown products, or decreased myelin lipid content itself. Certain paramagnetic compounds such as gadolinium–diethylenetriaminepenta-acetic acid (DTPA) are now used to enhance imaging of acute lesions with blood-brain barrier breakdown.

Cerebrospinal Fluid Analysis

Analysis of the CSF is indicated in all adolescents suspected of having MS. The CSF protein level is moderately elevated, rarely exceeding 100 mg/dl, and CSF lymphocyte concentrations rarely exceed 50/mm³. CSF immunoglobulin abnormalities occur in more than 90% of adolescents with clinical MS, including both quantitative elevations and qualitative changes in oligoclonal bands.

Because the amount of IgG in the CSF is small in comparison to blood, a quantitative assessment of blood-brain barrier integrity should be included with any evaluation of CSF immunoglobulin to determine whether the increase is caused by leakage of proteins from blood into the CNS or from a traumatic lumbar puncture. Two widely used indicators of intrathecal IgG synthesis are the IgG index (Link) and the IgG synthetic rate (Tourtellotte). The former is abnormal (>0.7) in 93% and the latter is abnormal (>3 mg/day) in 96% of patients with a definite diagnosis of MS.

Oligoclonal banding (OCB) describes a pathologic pattern of discrete bands rather than the homogeneous smear found in the characteristic region for IgG on an electrophoresis gel of concentrated CSF stained for protein. The standard interpretation of this phenomenon in MS has been that the IgG present in each band in the CSF is the homogeneous product of a single, active, plasma cell clone present in the CNS. OCB is not specific for MS and has been described in various other inflammatory conditions (e.g., SLE, syphilis, subacute sclerosing panencephalitis [SSPE], HIV infection) of the nervous system.

CLINICAL COURSE AND THERAPY

The clinical course of MS is variable. In most adolescents, the disease first is manifested as well-delineated exacerbations and remissions, with complete or nearly complete recovery of function. Some adolescents continue with minimal disability, but in many the degree of improvement decreases after each exacerbation. Often, a chronic phase of slowly progressive worsening develops over a period of many years. Adolescents tend to be spared from the inexorably but slowly progressive disease (usually myelopathy) characteristic of MS that is first manifest in the third or fourth decade of life. A small number of adolescents have a severe, rapidly progressive form, which may be terminal within 1 or

TABLE 88–2. Treatment Directed at Underlying Immunopathology of Multiple Sclerosis

CLASS OF DRUG	PHARMACOLOGIC AGENT(S)
Anti-inflammatory	Pulse corticosteroids (prednisone, methylprednisolone, adrenocorticotropic hormone [ACTH])
Immunosuppressive	Cytotoxic drugs (azathioprine, cyclophosphamide)

more years of onset and may include some cases previously thought to be Schilder or Baló disease.

There is no definitive cure for this illness, but treatment consists of the use of pharmacologic agents (Table 88–2) and symptomatic management (Table 88–3). Typically, pulses of high-dose corticosteroids (intravenous methylprednisolone, 500 to 1000 mg daily for 4 to 5 days) are given to adolescents with acute exacerbations early in the course of the disease to shorten the time to clinical remission, but these do not alter the long-term outcome of MS. If neurologic signs and symptoms become progressive, cytotoxic agents (cyclophosphamide) may be added to halt this process, although no treatment has been completely successful. These regimens are best administered by clinicians experienced in their use.

Spasticity of sufficient severity to be treated may respond to baclofen at an initial dose of 5 mg three times a day, increasing to 40 to 80 mg/day. Side effects include sedation, lightheadedness, and fatigue; abrupt withdrawal can be associated with seizures or hallucinations. Although bladder dysfunction is less commonly seen in adolescents than in adults with MS, a regimen that includes intermittent self-catheterization, propantheline, or both may be required.

Neurologic abnormalities usually reach maximum severity days to weeks after onset and then resolve gradually over the course of several weeks. More than 50% of adolescents experience a relapsing course, with a second relapse within 3 years of the initiation of symptoms. As many as one third of adolescents with MS have a progressive course, but onset in adolescence confers a slightly more benign prognosis than later onset.

Several recently developed immunotherapeutic strategies offer hope for the future treatment of immune-mediated demyelinating disease. These focus on altering

TABLE 88–3. Symptomatic Management of Multiple Sclerosis

SYMPTOM	PHARMACOLOGIC AGENT(S)
Spasticity	GABA-ergic drugs (baclofen, diazepam)
Tremor	Clonazepam, Mysoline
Seizures	Phenytoin, carbamazepine
Pain	Carbamazepine, phenytoin, antidepressants
Fatigue	Amantadine, pemoline
Depression	Tricyclic antidepressants, fluoxetine
Emotional lability	Amitriptyline
Bladder dysfunction	Oxybutynin, imipramine, prazosin, self-catheterization

GABA, Gamma-aminobutyric acid.

elements of the trimolecular complex of immune recognition—the T-cell antigen receptor, the histocompatibility (HLA) molecules, and the target antigens.

The identification of the oligoclonal nature of the intra-CNS autoimmune T-cell response in experimental allergic encephalomyelitis (EAE) and MS patients could lead to a highly specific immunotherapy. This might be accomplished by administration of a peptide or cellular vaccine containing epitopes of the oligoclonal antigen-specific T-cell receptors found in the CNS to cause the immune system of an affected individual to suppress the activity of those T cells bearing the autoimmune receptor types.

Two additional immunomodulators, β-interferon and copolymer (Cop) I, are currently undergoing clinical trials after showing promise in the treatment of early MS in preliminary studies. β-Interferon suppresses immune reactivity by down-regulating cell surface expression of HLA molecules essential to antigen recognition. Cop I is a synthetic analogue of myelin basic protein (MBP), a constituent of CNS myelin that may be an important autoantigen in MS. Although the mechanism of the demonstrated inhibitory effect of Cop I in EAE is unclear, it appears to inhibit an autoimmune reaction to MBP by triggering a suppressive idiotype–anti-idiotype antibody network. Another mechanism of its activity might be through the stimulation of endogenous β-interferon production.

BIBLIOGRAPHY

Duquette P, Murray TJ, Pleines J, et al: Multiple sclerosis in childhood: Clinical analysis of 125 patients. J Pediatr 111:359, 1987.

Goodman AD, McFarlin DE: Multiple sclerosis. Curr Neurol 7:91, 1987.

Hallpike JF, Adams CWM, Tourtellotte WW (eds): Multiple Sclerosis. Baltimore, Williams & Wilkins, 1983.

Matthews WB, Acheson ED, Butchelor JR, Weller RO (eds): McAlpine's Multiple Sclerosis. London, Churchill Livingstone, 1985.

McFarlin DE, McFarland HF: Multiple sclerosis. N Engl J Med 307:1183, 1982.

Morell P: A correlative synopsis of the leukodystrophies. Neuropediatrics 15 (Suppl):62, 1984.

Warren S, Cockerill R, Warren KG: Risk factors by onset age in multiple sclerosis. Neuroepidemiology 10:9, 1991.

Youl BD, Kermode AG, Thompson AJ, et al: Destructive lesions in demyelinating disease. J Neurol Neurosurg Psychiatry 54:288, 1991.

CHAPTER 89

Biochemical and Molecular Markers

CRAIG L. HYSER

Biochemical and molecular markers of diagnostic importance are known for several neurologic disorders encountered in adolescents. This discussion focuses on those conditions that can presently be distinguished by specific testing, as well as on those in which biochemical and molecular genetic investigations are likely to yield clinically relevant results in the future.

NEUROMUSCULAR DISORDERS

Dystrophin Deficiency Myopathies

The concept of dystrophin deficiency myopathies, or Xp21 myopathies, has recently emerged. These disorders are characterized by a deficiency of the muscle protein dystrophin. They result from mutations that affect the dystrophin gene, whose locus is within the X chromosome region Xp21. A clinical spectrum of myopathies is represented, including typical childhood-onset Duchenne muscular dystrophy, the more benign Becker muscular dystrophy, manifesting female carriers of the abnormal dystrophin gene, adolescents with nonprogressive muscle disease presenting with cramps or myalgias, and adolescent patients with isolated elevations in serum creatine kinase levels. Given this clinical heterogeneity, dystrophin deficiency should be considered in any adolescent with an undistinguished myopathy, particularly if there is a family history compatible with X-linked recessive inheritance or if the adolescent patient is male. The diagnosis can be made by DNA analysis of the dystrophin gene and by analysis of dystrophin protein in muscle biopsy specimens.

Myotonic Dystrophy

Myotonic dystrophy (MyD) is inherited as an autosomal dominant disorder. The gene has been localized on chromosome 19 through recombinant DNA techniques. This most common of the muscular dystrophies is notable for its variability in severity and age at onset. As such, it may sometimes be difficult to determine whether an at-risk adolescent has inherited the gene. Although no definitive test exists, DNA polymorphisms closely linked to the MyD gene can be used to track the gene through a family. This indirect method must suffice until the underlying genetic defect is known.

Metabolic Myopathies

Application of biochemical techniques to the study of muscle tissue has led to the identification of specific defects underlying several muscle diseases. Because they often present in adolescents, the glycolytic and lipid metabolic defects associated with exercise intolerance, cramps, and myoglobinuria are of significance. The most frequently encountered of these are myophosphorylase deficiency (McArdle disease) and carnitine palmitoyl-transferase deficiency. More rarely implicated are defects of the glycolytic enzymes phosphofructokinase, phosphoglycerate kinase, phosphoglycerate mutase, and lactate dehydrogenase.

Periodic Paralyses

Hypokalemic and hyperkalemic periodic paralyses are autosomal dominant disorders characterized by episodic weakness. The causes of these disorders are unknown, but they are probably related to dysfunction of the muscle cell membrane. They can be readily diagnosed, however, by observing hypokalemia or hyperkalemia during a bout of weakness. Because adolescent patients do not always present during acute attacks, provocative tests relying on measures to raise or lower the serum potassium level may be necessary. Provocative testing is performed with simultaneous monitoring of the serum potassium level, the adolescent patient's strength, and the electrocardiogram (ECG).

Myasthenia Gravis

Myasthenia gravis (MG) results from antibodies directed against the nicotinic acetylcholine receptor (AChR) at the neuromuscular junction. These anti-AChR antibodies are found in nearly 90% of adolescent patients with generalized MG and in about 75% of adolescent patients with restricted ocular MG. AChR antibodies are essentially specific for the disease. The titer of AChR antibody, however, does not necessarily correlate with disease severity.

Hereditary Sensory and Motor Neuropathies (HSMN)

Several genetic disorders of the peripheral nervous system are included under the acronym of HSMN (also called Charcot-Marie-Tooth disease, or peroneal muscular atrophy). These disorders are the most frequent cause of peripheral neuropathy in adolescence. Classification of these disorders has been problematic because of considerable overlap of clinical, genetic, electrophysiologic, and neuropathologic features. Linkage studies using classic and molecular genetic markers are helping to clarify this issue, and certain subtypes of HSMN are now delimited by their linkage to loci on chromosomes 1, 17, or X. Of the HSMNs, however, only Refsum disease (HSMN type IV) is defined by a distinct biochemical marker.

Refsum disease is an uncommon autosomal recessive disorder that is characterized by retinitis pigmentosa, ichthyosis, and hearing loss, in addition to a peripheral sensorimotor neuropathy. The disorder results from impaired α-oxidation of branched-chain fatty acids and can be diagnosed by demonstrating elevated serum phytanic acid levels. It is important to identify this condition, because treatment by dietary restriction of phytol intake and plasma-pheresis can improve neurologic function.

Acute Intermittent Porphyria (AIP)

AIP is an autosomal dominant disorder of heme biosynthesis caused by a deficiency of the enzyme porphobilinogen (PBG) deaminase. It is discussed with neuromuscular disorders because acute or subacute peripheral neuropathy is a common feature of AIP attacks, along with mental and gastrointestinal disturbances. Attacks of AIP generally commence after puberty and may be precipitated by various factors, such as drugs, alcohol, infection, stress, or poor nutrition. During an attack, an adolescent patient's urine may turn pink or reddish brown because of the presence of porphyrins, and quantitative analysis reveals elevated levels of the heme precursors porphobilinogen and δ-aminolevulinic acid. AIP can be specifically diagnosed by demonstrating reduced erythrocyte PBG-deaminase activity. Recognition of AIP is vital, because specific therapeutic measures such as glucose or hematin administration may curtail acute attacks, and avoidance of precipitating factors can prevent future ones. Counseling family members is also important. The gene carrier state can be identified by determining erythrocyte PBG-deaminase activity or by DNA analysis with PBG-deaminase gene probes.

MOVEMENT DISORDERS AND ATAXIAS

Huntington Disease

This autosomal dominant disease was the first genetic disorder whose chromosomal location was determined by recombinant DNA techniques without prior knowledge of the gene product. The Huntington disease gene has been localized to the tip of the short arm of chromosome 4 (4p16.3) but has not yet been isolated, and the gene product remains unknown. There is no biochemical marker that can separate adolescent patients with Huntington disease from those with other movement disorders, but linked DNA markers can be used to identify gene carriers in families in which Huntington disease is known to be present.

Wilson Disease (see Chapter 62)

Wilson disease is an autosomal recessive condition resulting from an inborn error of copper metabolism. Wilson disease often presents in adolescents with various signs and symptoms, including tremor, chorea, dystonia, dysarthria, and behavioral abnormalities. The diagnosis can be made by finding excessive copper excretion in the urine (cupriuria), a reduced serum copper concentration, and a decreased level of the copper protein ceruloplasmin. Copper deposition in the cornea produces the characteristic Kayser-Fleisher ring. The basic defect in Wilson disease is unknown. It is not caused by a primary molecular defect of ceruloplasmin, because the ceruloplasmin gene has been shown to reside on chromosome 3, and that for Wilson disease is on chromosome 13. It is important to diagnose this potentially devastating condition, because it can be treated by measures to lower the body copper level.

Friedreich Ataxia

Friedreich ataxia is an autosomal recessive disorder that usually presents in the first or second decade. Characteristic findings include ataxia, nystagmus, dysarthria, sensory loss, areflexia, and skeletal abnormalities. Atypical presentations are common, and it may sometimes be difficult to distinguish a case of Friedreich ataxia from the larger group of hereditary ataxias. A number of metabolic abnormalities were proposed and later rejected as the cause of Friedreich ataxia. The disease gene, however, has been localized to chromosome 9 by molecular genetic techniques. This represents a major step toward identifying the underlying defect, as well as developing accurate DNA diagnostic testing.

LEUKODYSTROPHIES AND LIPIDOSES

A number of disorders of lipid metabolism can be diagnosed specifically. These should be considered when an adolescent presents with progressive neurologic deterioration, especially when multiple systems are involved.

Adrenoleukodystrophy

This X-linked recessive disorder results from defective β-oxidation of very long-chain fatty acids (VLCFA). Adolescent patients with adrenoleukodystrophy (ALD) may develop visual loss, optic atrophy, dysarthria, dysphagia, deafness, gait abnormalities, seizures, and dementia. A phenotypic variant of ALD, adrenomyeloneuropathy (AMN), is characterized by progressive spastic paraparesis and peripheral neuropathy. Clinical manifestations may be seen in female carriers of the ALD-AMN gene. In addition to neurologic abnormalities, adolescent patients may display overt signs of adrenal insufficiency, and the adrenocorticotropic hormone stimulation test usually reveals adrenal insufficiency in males. Definitive diagnosis is possible by finding elevated VLCFA levels in plasma and cultured skin fibroblasts. Detection of female carriers and prenatal diagnosis can also be accomplished by VLCFA determination. The gene responsible for ALD-AMN has been localized on the distal long arm of the X chromosome, but has not been isolated. Polymorphic DNA markers closely linked to the gene can be used for carrier testing.

Metachromatic Leukodystrophy

Adolescent onset may be observed with the juvenile and adult forms of metachromatic leukodystrophy (MLD). Adolescent patients often present with personality changes or deterioration in school performance. Gait abnormalities, ataxia, dysarthria, dysphagia, spasticity, and peripheral neuropathy can develop. The late-onset varieties of MLD, like the infantile form, are autosomal recessive disorders of myelin metabolism characterized by a deficiency of the enzyme arylsulfatase A. Diagnosis is possible by assaying arylsulfatase A activity in urine, leukocytes, or cultured skin fibroblasts. The heterozygous state can also be identified. The cause of the enzyme deficiency and the mechanisms underlying the phenotypic variation of MLD are not known precisely, but the technique of cloning the arylsulfatase A gene should facilitate further investigations of these issues.

Hexosaminidase Deficiency

Hexosaminidase deficiency was originally described as infantile encephalopathy, or Tay-Sachs disease. A spectrum of neurologic syndromes has been found to result from the enzyme deficiency. These may present at any age and with various features, including dementia, seizures, ataxia, spasticity, dystonia, and motor neuronop-

athy. The deficiency state can be identified by measuring hexosaminidase activity in serum, leukocytes, or skin fibroblasts. Hexosaminidase is composed of α and β subunits. The genes for both subunits have been isolated, providing the foundation for exploring the molecular basis for these disorders.

Gaucher Disease

Gaucher disease is an autosomal recessive condition caused by a deficiency of the enzyme glucocerebrosidase. Type 3, or the subacute neuronopathic form of Gaucher disease, has its onset in childhood or adolescence. Neurologic features include dementia, ataxia, spasticity, myoclonus, seizures, and supranuclear ophthalmoplegia. The associated presence of hepatosplenomegaly or bony lesions should suggest the diagnosis, which can be confirmed by demonstrating reduced glucocerebrosidase activity in leukocytes or fibroblasts. The gene for glucocerebrosidase has been cloned.

PHAKOMATOSES

Neurofibromatosis Type 1

The gene for neurofibromatosis type 1 (NF1), or von Recklinghausen disease, has been localized to the long arm of chromosome 17 (17q11.2). To date, the gene has not been isolated, and the cause of this autosomal dominant disorder remains unknown. Diagnostic testing in NF1 families is possible, however, using polymorphic DNA markers that are closely linked to the NF1 gene.

Tuberous Sclerosis

Genetic linkage studies indicate that this autosomal dominant disorder may be heterogeneous. Initial studies indicated that the tuberous sclerosis gene resided on chromosome 9, but more recent data suggest linkage to chromosome 11 markers as well. The biochemical defect responsible for tuberous sclerosis is unknown, and preclinical testing with DNA markers is not feasible until the issue of the genetic heterogeneity has been clarified further.

BIBLIOGRAPHY

Chamberlain S, Shaw J, Wallis J, et al: Genetic homogeneity at the Friedreich ataxia locus on chromosome 9. Am J Hum Genet 44:518, 1989.

Dyck PJ, Thomas PK, Lambert EH, Bunge R (eds): Peripheral Neuropathy, 2nd ed, Vol 2. Philadelphia, WB Saunders, 1984.

Engel AG, Banker BQ (eds): Myology. New York, McGraw-Hill, 1986.

Goldgar DE, Green P, Parry DM, Mulvihill JJ: Multipoint linkage analysis in neurofibromatosis type 1: An international collaboration. Am J Hum Genet 44:6, 1989.

Hayden MR, Robbins C, Allard D, et al: Improved predictive testing for Huntington's disease by using three linked DNA markers. Am J Hum Genet 43:689, 1988.

Hyser CL: Recombinant DNA approach to neurogenetic disease. In Joynt RF (ed): Clinical Neurology, Vol 4. Philadelphia, JB Lippincott, 1989, pp 1–17.

Johnson WC: The clinical spectrum of hexosaminidase deficiency diseases. Neurology 31:1453, 1981.

Moser HW, Moser AE, Singh I, O'Neill BP: Adrenoleukodystrophy: Survey of 303 cases: Biochemistry, diagnosis, and therapy. Ann Neurol 16:628, 1984.

Rowland LP: Clinical concepts of Duchenne muscular dystrophy. The impact of molecular genetics. Brain 111:479, 1988.

Scriver CR, Beaudet AL, Sly WS, Valle D (eds): The Metabolic Basis of Inherited Diseases. New York, McGraw-Hill, 1989.

Rheumatologic Conditions

CHAPTER 90

Collagen Vascular Disorders

DAVID M. SIEGEL

JUVENILE ARTHRITIS

Epidemiology

In adolescents, chronic, noninfectious arthritis occurs in different forms, collectively known as juvenile arthritis. Other names used for this illness include juvenile rheumatoid arthritis (JRA), juvenile chronic arthritis (JCA), and Still disease. JRA should apply only for adolescents having a positive rheumatoid factor and Still disease only for adolescents with the systemic onset form of the illness. The overall prevalence of juvenile arthritis is between 0.2 and 1.0 case in 1,000 children and adolescents. In this chapter the different subtypes of juvenile arthritis are discussed, with particular emphasis on issues relevant to adolescents (Table 90–1).

Types

PAUCIARTICULAR ARTHRITIS

The most common chronic arthritis in adolescents is the pauciarticular form, affecting fewer than five joints and accounting for about half of all cases. The age of peak onset of this subtype in adolescents occurs between 12 and 16 years. The most frequently affected joints are the larger lower extremity joints, predominantly the knee, but also including the ankle or hip. Sites of recurrent synovitis ordinarily appear within the first 6 months of illness. The pattern of the affected joints is asymmetric. Systemic symptoms such as fatigue and signs such as weight loss or rash are not characteristic of pauciarticular disease; these adolescents generally report feeling well, with the exception of the inflamed joint(s).

TABLE 90–1. Types of Juvenile Arthritis

Pauciarticular arthritis
Females
With antinuclear antibody (ANA)
Without ANA
Males
With HLA-B27
Without HLA-B27
Polyarticular arthritis
With rheumatoid factor (RF)
Without RF
Systemic onset

Those caring for younger children recognize that pauciarticular arthritis also occurs in girls around the age of 2 years who experience exacerbations and remissions of the arthritis (without consistent precipitants), but who do not usually develop progressive or destructive joint disease. The presence of antinuclear antibody (ANA) in these girls represents a marker for increased risk of uveitis or iridocyclitis, which is unrelated to the extent of joint activity. Despite the onset of joint disease in childhood, inflammatory eye disease may appear years later, during adolescence. Nodules or serositis are not generally seen in these adolescent patients.

Male adolescents with pauciarticular arthritis generally present in early puberty and have HLA-B27 antigen. These adolescent patients can experience a destructive and progressive arthritis involving such joints as the hips, knees, and ankles. Sacroiliac inflammation is very common in these young men. Although almost all adults (80% to 90%) with ankylosing spondylitis have HLA-B27, only between 10% and 20% of adolescents with peripheral arthritis and positive HLA-B27 go on to develop vertebral involvement. Such patients also have a propensity for enthesopathy (inflammation at the tendinous insertions into bones), and can present with painful heels.

Physical examination of adolescents with pauciarticular arthritis reveals warm, tender, painful joints, particularly on movement with limited motion. There may be muscle wasting, such as quadriceps atrophy in cases of knee involvement. Paradoxically, the extremity with the affected joint tends to be longer than the unaffected side because of the increased blood flow resulting from the chronic synovitis and consequent accelerated bone growth. This length discrepancy usually normalizes after an extended period of remission, with the unaffected side catching up. By late adolescence significant leg length discrepancy is not usually a problem, although compensatory orthotics may have been necessary when the adolescent was younger.

The long-term prognosis in most of these adolescents is good. About half have a total remission by young adulthood, without sequelae. Another 25% have some minor disability such as a mild joint contracture, with the remaining 25% having more significant and persistent problems. There are no specific laboratory tests for this condition; a positive HLA-B27 has been reported in approximately 36% of all patients with pauciarticular arthritis and in up to 60% of males. Characteristically there are normal hemoglobin, hematocrit, and white blood cell (WBC) values, whereas the erythrocyte sedimentation rate (and platelet count) is normal or mildly elevated. At disease onset x-ray films may reveal soft tissue swelling and joint effusions, but erosions, subchondral cysts, and joint space narrowing are rare. In the presence of HLA-B27, however, sacroiliac involvement as seen on x-ray film is common.

Because pauciarticular disease involves the large joints, and at onset only one joint is affected, this is a form of (monarticular) juvenile arthritis (JA) in which the diagnosis might be delayed because of the consideration of other disorders. These include septic arthritis, traumatic arthritis, Legg-Calvé-Perthes disease, and toxic synovitis of the hip (see Chapter 79).

Arthrocentesis is an essential diagnostic procedure, particularly in monarticular disease in adolescents, for identifying septic arthritis. Although inflammatory joint fluid can show a moderately elevated WBC count (2000 to 75,000/mm³) and an increased proportion (>50%) of polymorphonuclear leukocytes (PMN), an infected joint usually shows a WBC count that is greater than 100,000/mm³ and PMNs greater than 75%. In addition to the WBC count in the aspirated fluid, other parameters useful in distinguishing a septic joint from the synovitis of juvenile arthritis include the following: (1) glucose level (depressed in infection, normal in arthritis); (2) Gram stain (which may reveal organisms in fluid from a septic joint, but show only leukocytes in JA); and (3) bacterial culture of the fluid. Bacterial infection of a joint also results in the breakdown of hyaluronic acid in the joint fluid and a decrease in viscosity. An acutely inflamed joint in an adolescent with JA, however, may manifest the same loss of synovial fluid viscosity.

A particular example of septic arthritis in adolescents deserving separate comment is gonococcal arthritis. An adolescent who has disseminated *Neisseria gonorrhoeae* infection may suffer from two types of arthritis. The organism can infect primarily the joint space, with bacteria (intracellular gram-negative diplococci) evident on microscopic examination of the synovial fluid and in culture. This presentation is similar to that seen in other cases of septic arthritis. There is, however, a syndrome of a sterile inflammatory joint disease associated with gonococcal infection, and the fluid can be indistinguishable from that of JA. The physician caring for adolescents must be cognizant of this syndrome and seek out consistent findings of rash, urethritis, cervicitis, and concomitant sexually transmitted disease (STD) to make the correct diagnosis (see Chapter 75).

POLYARTICULAR ARTHRITIS

Polyarticular disease is found in about 30% of the young people who have juvenile arthritis. It is characterized by symmetric arthritis involving five or more joints, usually appearing within the first 6 months of the illness. Affected joints commonly include the small joints of the hands and feet, as well as the wrists, elbows and, less commonly, larger joints. The pattern of involvement is usually symmetric (different from the pauciarticular group), but, similar to the pauciarticular group, these adolescents do not usually experience systemic symptoms. The exception is the subgroup of approximately 10% to 15% of patients with juvenile arthritis who have a positive rheumatoid factor (RF+) and are predominantly adolescents. The median age of onset is 12 years (as opposed to 3 years for the RF-negative polyarticular group) and more females than males are affected (as with the RF-negative group), but the joint disease is progressive and destructive, very similar to that seen in adults with rheumatoid arthritis. There is a strong correlation between the presence of high titers of RF and the development of subcutaneous nodules. The usual course of RF-negative disease, on the other hand, includes exacerbations and remissions, with the long-term prognosis being good for most adolescent patients.

As in all types of juvenile arthritis, there are no specific diagnostic studies for polyarticular disease. Adolescents who are RF-negative may have a normal hemoglobin concentration and WBC count, whereas the erythrocyte sedimentation rate (ESR) and platelet count are usually elevated. X-ray films are initially normal, although adolescents who are RF-positive typically go on to develop erosions, cysts, and loss of joint space. Arthrocentesis is not usually performed in these adolescents, because multiple joints are involved, thus making a septic process unlikely. In addition, these adolescents seem otherwise well, and their presentation is not clinically consistent with that of multiple bacterial joint infections. The ANA is positive in 20% to 25% of RF-negative adolescents who have polyarticular disease, but in 75% of those who are RF-positive. Other disorders in which polyarthritis occurs, such as viral infections (see Chapter 93), acute rheumatic fever (see Chapter 50), and Kawasaki disease, are associated with systemic or "toxic" symptoms, unlike polyarticular disease.

SYSTEMIC ONSET ARTHRITIS

Systemic onset juvenile arthritis, or Still disease, presents in the most dramatic fashion of the three types of arthritis with regard both to clinical and laboratory manifestations. Although this is generally a disease of young children, occasionally late adolescents and young adults develop this condition, and it is referred to as adult onset Still disease. The illness typically begins acutely with daily, late afternoon fever spikes (to 40°C or higher), with the temperature being normal early in the day. While febrile, the adolescent experiences myalgias, arthralgias, fatigue, irritability, and the classic Still rash characterized by pale pink (salmon-colored), 1- to 2-cm, nonpruritic, evanescent macules. Mild friction on the skin often precipitates a local area of rash (Köebner phenomenon). These adolescents appear acutely ill and "toxic" while their temperature is elevated, but often seem only mildly uncomfortable when they are afebrile. Physical findings can include generalized lymphadenopathy, hepatomegaly, splenomegaly, pericarditis, and pleuritis, but only occasionally is arthritis present at the onset of the disease.

A marked anemia is seen with systemic onset disease (hematocrit of 20% to 30%), as well as significant leukocytosis (20,000 to 80,000 WBC/mm³) and thrombocytosis (500,000 to 1,000,000 platelets/mm³). The ESR is usually elevated, often to levels of 100 mm/hour or higher. The ANA and RF are generally negative in these adolescents, and x-ray films may reveal some soft tissue swelling at onset, but no bony destruction or other lesions. As with the other forms of juvenile arthritis, this is a clinical diagnosis with consistent but not absolutely confirmatory laboratory results. For example, liver enzyme abnormalities, observed in up to 85% of adolescents with Still disease, are often helpful in the differential diagnosis.

Important considerations in the differential diagnosis of adolescents who have systemic onset JA include bacterial sepsis, acute viral illness, malignancy, and systemic lupus erythematosus. Young children and adolescents may be hospitalized and treated presumptively with antibiotics at the onset of their illness prior to proper diagnosis. The initial laboratory studies are consistent with infection, but negative cultures and the evolution of the rash and serositis make the correct diagnosis more apparent.

Systemic symptoms comprise much of the initial presentation but usually fade with time and treatment as polyarthritis develops. Small and large joints can be affected, and erosive disease in multiple, usually symmetric, joints is seen. More commonly, however, these adolescents have alternating periods of remission and exacerbation. When affected at a young age, it is usual to see cervical spine inflammation and eventual fusion (frequently C-2 to C-3 and C-3 to C-4), as well as micrognathia, which has a high association with the cervical spine involvement. Rarely, acute airway compromise may occur as a result of acute cricoarytenoid joint involvement. Temporary tracheostomy may be required in these patients in addition to a course of acute corticosteroid therapy.

Management

Management of adolescents who have juvenile arthritis consists of medication (systemic and/or intrarticular), physical therapy, psychological therapy and, in some patients, orthopedic surgery. Nonsteroidal anti-inflammatory drugs (NSAIDs), which inhibit prostaglandin synthesis and thereby decrease joint pain and swelling, as well as fever (in systemic onset disease), are useful in all three subtypes. Although aspirin has traditionally been the first choice of treatment for juvenile arthritis, this is no longer true for various reasons. The alleged association of Reye syndrome with the use of aspirin in the treatment of influenza or varicella is cause for concern, and the shorter half-life and consequent need for more frequent dosing makes salicylate therapy less appropriate than use of the newer NSAIDs. The Centers for Disease Control have documented an increased incidence of Reye syndrome in young people with juvenile arthritis who are exposed to salicylates. Tolmetin sodium and naproxen sodium have been approved for adolescents and are generally effective in controlling joint symptoms and the fever seen in systemic onset disease. Tolmetin is given at a dose ranging from 20 to 40 mg/kg/day (in three divided doses, up to a maximum of 1200 mg/day) and is available as 200-mg tablets and

400-mg capsules. The latter can be opened and used as "sprinkles" for those adolescents who cannot swallow pills. Naproxen is given twice daily at a dose ranging from 10 to 30 mg/kg/day, to a maximum of 1000 mg/day. Naproxen is available in several tablet sizes (250, 275, and 500 mg), and is now also available as a suspension (125 mg/5 ml). On occasion, individual patients, particularly with resistant fevers, may require higher doses of these drugs. With older adolescents the physician has a wider array of NSAIDs from which to choose, just as in adult patients. Predicting the clinical response to a given NSAID is impossible, and trials of different preparations at different doses are often necessary to establish effective therapy.

All these drugs carry the potential risk of gastric erosion and ulcer formation. Ingestion with food is an important precaution, and adolescents are less prone to ulcerogenesis from these medications than are older adults. When gastrointestinal intolerance is a significant concern, one should consider enteric-coated aspirin or diclofenac (Voltaren—an enteric-coated NSAID). Less common, but still serious, is the occurrence of nephritis in adolescent patients who take NSAIDs regularly.

Long-acting or disease-modifying agents are appropriate in adolescents with progressive disease; these include gold salts (intramuscular) or oral gold, methotrexate, cyclophosphamide, azathioprine, hydroxychloroquine, penicillamine and, more recently, cyclosporine. These drugs should be used with consideration of their various toxicities and the generally favorable natural history of most subtypes of juvenile arthritis in adolescents.

Systemic corticosteroids can be very effective in low doses as adjunctive therapy to NSAIDs, but should be given as short-term treatment whenever possible because of long-term pituitary-adrenal suppression caused by superphysiologic doses of corticosteroids. Such suppression results in some degree of immunodeficiency, osteoporosis, growth retardation, amenorrhea, and impaired stress response. Additionally, the adolescent on long-term corticosteroids must contend with the distressing complications of worsened acne vulgaris, truncal obesity, and upper posterior thoracic fat pad accumulation. These latter conditions are particularly distressing to some adolescents who are concerned about their body image. If adolescents follow the adult Still disease pattern, most have chronic disease with erosive arthritis, especially of the wrists; there may be a need for prolonged high-dose steroids and disease-modifying agents.

Joint aspiration is of diagnostic and therapeutic value in the management of adolescents with juvenile arthritis. The adolescent who presents with an acutely swollen, red, warm, and tender joint without any previous arthritis should have the joint aspirated and the fluid examined and cultured for bacterial infection. An adolescent who has known arthritis (pauciarticular or polyarticular) with a joint that is persistently swollen and limited in motion should have the fluid aspirated and a steroid preparation instilled into the joint space. I recommend the use of triamcinolone acetonide (40 mg/ml) mixed with 1% lidocaine; the dose depends on the size of the joint and the degree of inflammation (usually 40 to 60 mg). Frequent intraarticular injections

TABLE 90–2. Noncollagen Vascular Diseases in the Adolescent with Musculoskeletal Complaints

DIAGNOSIS	SYMPTOMS	SIGNS	LABORATORY AND X-RAY FINDINGS	MANAGEMENT
Hypermobility syndrome	Arthralgias; often seen in those involved in dance or gymnastics	Hyperextensibility of at least three of the following: thumb, wrist, metacarpo-phalangeals, elbows, knees, back	Normal	NSAIDs; reassurance
Chondromalacia patellae (patellofemoral pain syndrome)	Painful knees, rarely with swelling; locking or giving way of knees	Full range of motion in joints; pain and crepitus with patellar "scrubbing"; sometimes quadriceps weakness	Normal	Quadriceps and adductor strengthening; NSAIDs
Fibromyalgia	Arthralgias, myalgias; fatigue, restless and nonrestorative sleep; headache; abdominal pain	Tender points; full range of motion in joints; full muscle strength	Normal	Tricyclic medications; NSAIDs; physical therapy; reassurance

are not recommended, because this might lead to atrophy of cartilage and surrounding soft tissue. The general guideline is no more than three injections in a given joint annually.

Although treatment with medication is important to control pain and inflammation, it is essential to combine this with aggressive physical and occupational therapy. Without consistent range-of-motion and muscle-strengthening exercises, contractures and muscle atrophy develop and produce serious sequelae, even in cases of early remission. Occupational therapy is directed toward skills necessary for independent living, particularly important for the adolescent who is in the process of individuating and separating from the family.

Joint replacement surgery is necessary when cartilaginous and bony destruction result in significant limitation of motion and/or persistent pain. Timing of the surgery is important, because later bone growth will necessitate early prosthesis revision. Thus, the growth plates should be closed before joint replacement is undertaken. Prosthetic surgery is usually delayed until sexual maturity rating 5 is attained, but must be fit into the other important life transitions that are occurring.

The psychological impact of juvenile arthritis is similar to that of other chronic diseases. The adolescent is particularly preoccupied with physical adequacy and the development of joint dysfunction and disfigurement, even if temporary, can be distressing. Steroid therapy and/or persistent disease activity (particularly the systemic type) can cause growth failure and pubertal delay, further compounding the coping difficulties. Additionally, the entire family is affected by the illness, because a disproportionate amount of time and emotional and material resources are redirected to the chronically ill family member. More detailed discussion of these issues and recommendations for management are presented elsewhere in this text (see Chapter 30).

Other Conditions with Musculoskeletal Symptoms

There are several disorders that occur during adolescence that are frequently mistaken for juvenile arthritis, and these deserve a brief description (Table 90–2). Polyarthralgia in adolescents without objective arthritis, preceding trauma, or acute illness can present a diagnostic dilemma; hypermobility syndrome is one consideration. These adolescents display hyperextensibility of their joints (double-jointed) and there is often a family history of similar symptoms and findings. Diffuse joint aching without swelling, warmth, erythema, or tenderness is reported by these adolescents but, unlike juvenile arthritis, the time of least discomfort is in the early morning, prior to regular physical activity. Because of the extreme joint range of motion, these adolescents often excel in activities in which flexibility is an asset, such as gymnastics, ballet, and basketball, and often are highly valued members of teams at school. Ironically, their vigorous participation in these sports results in significant discomfort by the end of the day. Although somewhat predisposed to sprains and strains, these adolescents are otherwise healthy, without x-ray or laboratory evidence of abnormality.

The diagnosis of hypermobility syndrome is made on physical examination by the finding of at least three of the following five hyperextensible articulations (and the lack of any other abnormalities): (1) extension of the wrist and metacarpal phalanges so that the fingers are parallel to the dorsum of the forearm; (2) passive apposition of the thumb to the flexor aspect of the forearm; (3) hyperextension of the elbows (≥ 10 degrees); (4) hyperextension of the knees (≥ 10 degrees); and (5) flexion of the trunk with the knees extended so the palms rest on the floor.

The prevalence of hypermobility syndrome in the general population has been reported to be from 4% to 7%. Of 262 patients referred to our Pediatric Rheumatology Clinic between 1979 and 1981, 5.7% were found to have the hypermobility syndrome accounting for their joint symptoms. Management of this condition includes reassurance and NSAID or enteric-coated aspirin therapy. Maintenance of good muscle strength is protective in case of injuries resulting from the joint hyperextensibility. Rarely do the adolescents have to discontinue their preferred level of physical activity.

Chondromalacia patellae (also referred to as patellofemoral pain syndrome; see Chapters 79 and 80) is a condition that presents as chronic knee pain, infrequently with episodes of knee swelling. These adolescents also experience sensations of the knee locking (especially when flexed) or suddenly giving way when extended. This may present as difficulty in negotiating stairs, particularly descent. Adolescents may also report resistance to knee extension after prolonged sitting (the theater sign). Physical examination reveals externally normal-appearing knees, but active quadriceps contraction by the adolescent (with the knees extended) and consequent movement of the patella proximally against resistance (by the examiner's hand forcing the patella distally) results in palpable crepitus and exquisite discomfort for the adolescent. This maneuver has been referred to as the avoidance test because, after going through the procedure once, adolescent patients avoid another such examination. Physical examination may also detect quadriceps weakness, a decrease in muscle bulk (as measured by thigh circumference), and patellar laxity. Laboratory studies are normal, and x-ray films of the inferior surface of the patella only rarely show irregularities (and are not indicated). Arthroscopic visualization of the ventral patella can be diagnostic, but is not necessary in establishing this diagnosis. Management includes quadriceps and adductor strengthening exercises and NSAID therapy. Most adolescents can continue their maximum level of desired activity.

Fibromyalgia syndrome (sometimes referred to as fibrositis) can show generalized pain and arthralgias, myalgias, abdominal pain, headaches, and chronic fatigue. It most commonly affects older adolescents and young adults (especially women). A key point in the history for making this diagnosis is the adolescent's (or parent's) report of restless sleep and the sense of inadequate rest on arising in the morning. Although joint symptoms can be prominent in the history, the physical examination uncovers no arthritis, but discrete (approximately 1 cm in diameter) areas of tenderness can be found bilaterally in the supraclavicular, suprascapular, infrascapular, occipital, elbow, iliac crest, greater trochanter, and medial knee regions (tender points). Not every adolescent has involvement in all of these areas. These points are not only tender locally, but can also produce a radicular pattern of pain similar to the myalgias and/or arthralgias the adolescent has been experiencing. In the case of radicular symptoms, these soft tissue tender areas are called trigger points. Diagnostic criteria for fibromyalgia syndrome stipulate a minimum of 11 out of 18 possible tender points associated with widespread body pain. Adolescents may present with fewer than 11 tender points. Laboratory studies, x-ray films, and even histologic specimens from the tender point areas are normal.

Management requires regular and supportive contact with the adolescent and family and is directed at correcting the sleep disorder, the often associated depression, and the chronic pain. Tricyclic medications to restore adequate stage IV sleep are used, and NSAIDs can help alleviate the arthralgias and myalgias in some adolescents. Regular, nonstrenuous physical activity can also be beneficial.

Finally, the possibility of somatization resulting in joint pain, often referred to as psychogenic rheumatism, must be considered (see Chapter 112). Adolescents who are depressed, undergoing psychological stress, trying to avoid what they consider an unpleasant activity (especially school), or coming from a dysfunctional or somatization-prone family can present with disabling joint symptoms (see Chapters 100 and 103). Perceptive interviewing with the adolescent and family and solicitation of observations from school personnel, often result in a picture of psychological maladaptation consistent with this diagnosis. Obviously, the physical examination, laboratory studies, and x-ray films are all normal; the latter two are best avoided when the diagnosis is apparent at the initial examination.

SYSTEMIC LUPUS ERYTHEMATOSUS

Epidemiology and Etiology

Systemic lupus erythematosus (SLE) is a multiorgan system disease with an extremely varied presentation. The underlying pathology in all patients centers around the production of autoantibodies (anti–double standard DNA, or anti-dsDNA) with a direct effect on target organs and the formation of immune complexes, leading to dysfunction caused by deposition in other involved organs, usually the kidney. The incidence of SLE in adolescents has been estimated to be 0.6 in 100,000, with an overall 5:1 predominance of females to males. This ratio describes the disease after puberty; in prepubertal populations the female-to-male ratio is only 3:1. In addition, black, Puerto Rican and, to some extent, Asian young women are at greater risk for the development of SLE than are their white counterparts. The peak age of onset of SLE is in the second and third decades, making this condition particularly relevant to those physicians caring for adolescents.

In addition to sex and age, other risk factors for the development of SLE have been identified or are under investigation, and include the following:

1. Genetic factors. In one series, 10% to 20% of children and adolescents with SLE had affected first-degree relatives, increasing to 27% when aunts and uncles were included. Interestingly, 57% of monozygotic twins are concordant for SLE.

2. HLA associations have been reported, particularly at the A1, B8, and DR3 loci.

3. Drugs such as hydralazine, procainamide, isoniazid, phenytoin (and other anticonvulsants), and chlorpromazine have been associated with the onset of a positive antinuclear antibody (ANA) test and an SLE-like illness.

4. Sun exposure has been found to be a risk factor.

5. Sex hormone abnormalities, which seem to result in stronger and longer lasting estrogenic and weaker androgenic effects, have been found in adolescents with SLE. These may explain why pubertal females are at higher risk for the development of SLE.

Various immunologic abnormalities have been found in adolescents with SLE. This area continues to be one of intensive investigation in regard to the causes of and primary therapy for SLE. Lymphopenia is a common complication of SLE, that results from a decrease in various lymphocyte subpopulations, including CD4 (helper-inducer) and T8 (suppressor) cells. There seems to be concurrent stimulation of B-cell production, leading to an imbalance in these lymphocyte populations and perhaps to the activation of B-cell production of autoantibodies, so prevalent in adolescents with SLE.

Clinical Features

SLE is a multisystem disease, although an individual adolescent patient may manifest only limited involvement. Common to almost all adolescents with SLE are the general symptoms of weight loss, anorexia, malaise, and fatigue. Fever is common, but may be a sign of underlying infection.

The most common symptoms are related to the skin and joints. The typical malar or butterfly rash is present over the cheeks and the bridge of the nose and is usually maculopapular, with fine scale and an erythematous hue. In some adolescents, only a slightly reddened macular eruption is seen, similar to a localized, mild sunburn.

Occasionally, these lesions ulcerate, crust over, and become hyperpigmented or hypopigmented during healing. Other areas of rash include infarcted areas (frequently nail beds), particularly on the hands. Mucocutaneous ulcers occur on the lips, buccal mucosa, gingiva, and palate. The external cutaneous lesions are often photosensitive, although some adolescents also experience exacerbation of other (noncutaneous) disease symptoms when exposed to excessive ultraviolet irradiation. The mucocutaneous lesions of discoid lupus are not photosensitive, because they are inside the mouth and nose. Alopecia (characterized by thinning and/or patchy hair loss) or breaking of the frontal hairs so that the hair over the forehead is short has been reported in 22% to 55% of adolescent patients with SLE.

Musculoskeletal complaints are common with myalgias, arthralgias, and arthritis seen in 65% to 100% of adolescent SLE patients. This can result in morning stiffness and contractures, but erosive disease with permanent deformity is unusual. Although the muscles may be painful and apparently weak, myositis (elevated enzyme levels, and abnormal biopsy findings) is rare. Severe deformity of the hands, with subluxations of the fingers and reversible ulnar deviation, does occur (Jaccoud arthritis). Raynaud phenomenon, with its color progression in the digits from white to blue to red, accompanied by pain and often swelling, is secondary to vasospasm and can precede the full development of SLE by years.

There are a number of other organ system complications seen in SLE.

Pulmonary Effects. These occur in 19% to 73% of cases. Pleuritis is the most common finding, but interstitial changes can occur. Pulmonary hemorrhage is an acute life-threatening process reported in adolescents (see Chapter 43).

Cardiac Effects. These occur in 17% to 91% of cases.

Pericarditis is common, but massive effusions and tamponade are unusual (see Chapter 50). Myocarditis with ventricular dysfunction, congestive heart failure, and conduction abnormalities are all seen, and occasionally a noninfectious verrucous endocarditis involving the mitral, aortic, or tricuspid valves can develop (Libman-Sacks endocarditis).

Gastrointestinal Effects. These occur in 19% to 36% of cases. Esophageal dysfunction, pancreatitis, spontaneous bacterial peritonitis, retroperitoneal fibrosis, hepatomegaly, protein-losing enteropathy, and mesenteric arteritis with bowel perforation have all been reported.

Renal Effects. Renal disease (see Chapter 65) affects from 20% to 90% of adolescent patients with SLE, and is often a major source of morbidity. The mechanism of injury is the deposition of immune complexes (immunoglobulin and complement) in the mesangial areas and glomeruli. The type and extent of renal disease are variable, and the World Health Organization (WHO) has established a standardized classification based on light and electron microscopy and immunofluorescent staining. The six types are shown in Table 90–3, and morbidity and mortality are correlated with increasing renal pathology class. Hypertension is a complication of the renal disease, and patients may develop nephrotic syndrome.

Central Nervous System Effects. These occur in 17% to 59% of cases, and involvement can be subtle or dramatic. If mild cognitive and affective disorders detected by neurophysiologic testing are included, the highest estimate of involvement is 75%. Vasculitis has been implicated as the cause, but has been challenged on the basis of more recent information. Antineuronal antibodies and anticardiolipin antibodies have also been implicated. Manifestations can range from acute cerebral infarction to minor behavioral changes. Other symptoms include headache, seizures, visual disturbances, chorea, transverse myelitis, pseudotumor cerebri, psychosis, and depression. Some of these symptoms can also result from high-dose steroid exposure, but each of these can be caused by SLE vasculitis alone.

Laboratory Studies and Diagnosis

Several laboratory studies are useful in evaluating the adolescent for SLE, but the ANA test has become the standard screening procedure. Antinuclear antibodies are present in 96% to 100% of adolescent patients with

TABLE 90–3. World Health Organization Classification of Lupus Glomerulonephritis

CLASS	FEATURE
I	Normal glomeruli
II	Pure mesangial nephritis
III	Focal segmental glomerulonephritis
IV	Diffuse proliferative glomerulonephritis
V	Membranous glomerulonephritis
VI	Advanced sclerosing glomerulonephritis

Adapted with permission from Baldwin DS, Gluck MC, Lowenstein J, et al: Lupus nephritis: Clinical course as related to morphologic forms and their transitions. Am J Med 62:12, 1977.

SLE, and represent various IgG and IgM antibodies to various nuclear antigens. The test is reported as a titer (1:80 being the lowest titer usually considered significant) and the appearance of the cell is also classified (rim, homogeneous, nucleolar, speckled), sometimes helping to distinguish between the various conditions in which the ANA is positive. The lupus erythematosus (LE) cell test is time-consuming and highly dependent on the skill of the technician, limiting its usefulness. Antibodies to native or double standard DNA (anti-dsDNA) are present in approximately 50% of adolescent patients with SLE; because they are specific to SLE they can, when present, help confirm the laboratory diagnosis. The level of anti-dsDNA is also associated with the risk for nephritis and is a reflection of overall disease activity. Antibody to Sm antigen (anti-Sm) is also specific to SLE, but is present in only 30% to 40% of adolescent patients. Other antinuclear element antibodies found in these adolescents, but not specific to SLE, are anti-RNP (35%), anti-Ro (SS-A; 30% to 40%), and anti-La (SS-B; 15%). The latter two are most prevalent in Sjögren syndrome (70%), but in pregnant adolescents with SLE and anti-Ro there is an increased risk of congenital complete heart block in the newborn.

The erythrocyte sedimentation rate (ESR) is elevated in 94% to 100% of cases but is more useful as a confirmation of diagnosis than as a predictor of disease exacerbation. Anemia (50% to 80%), leukopenia (20% to 70%), and thrombocytopenia (10% to 43%) are common, as is a Coombs-positive hemolysis (20% to 80%). Detection of increased circulating immune complexes (C1q) and depression of complement levels (CH50, C3, C4) are indices of active disease. A relatively new and important finding in SLE is the presence of a group of antiphospholipid antibodies (particularly anticardiolipin antibody), that lead to the prolongation of the partial thromboplastin time (PTT), uncorrected by addition of human plasma—the lupus anticoagulant, *in vitro* and cause various thromboembolic complications *in vivo*. This is particularly true in pregnant adolescents, in whom placental thrombosis and insufficiency lead to recurring miscarriage and fetal losses. The presence of anticardiolipin antibody has not been associated with other particular clinical or laboratory findings (e.g., hemolytic anemia, recurrent central nervous system events, chorea, venous and arterial thromboses). The diagnosis of SLE is made when at least 4 of 11 clinical and laboratory criteria are observed serially or simultaneously (Table 90–4).

Management

The treatment of SLE varies with the extent of the illness. Some adolescents experience only mild photosensitivity and arthralgias and can be treated with topical ultraviolet light blockers and with salicylates or other NSAIDs. These adolescents must be monitored for progression of their disease. Most adolescents experience other manifestations of SLE (as outlined above) and, in these cases, corticosteroids remain the mainstay of therapy. Prednisone, beginning at 1 to 2 mg/kg/day, provides immunosuppression, but may require augmen-

tation with azathioprine (1 to 3 mg/kg) or pulse cyclophosphamide. Consideration of the latter must include discussions with both the male and the female adolescent about subsequent infertility and the development of later malignancy. The risk of infertility is 50% overall for females (adolescents, approximately 25%, and women older than 30 years of age, 75%). The risk of developing acute myelogenous leukemia is approximately 10% after receiving 30 g or more of cyclophosphamide.

During acute exacerbations (such as sudden CNS or renal involvement), pulse steroid therapy (30 mg/kg/day of methyl prednisolone for 3 days) can be superimposed on the maintenance regimen. Plasmapheresis has also been used when other modalities have failed, but without clear efficacy. Thrombocytopenia can be effectively treated with intravenous gamma globulin. If skin and/or joint involvement is predominant, hydroxychloroquine (5 mg/kg/day) can be helpful. Adolescent patients must be monitored for the many side effects of long-term steroid use and an alternate-day schedule should be used when possible. Other aspects of management include regular physical therapy and addressing the financial and emotional challenges and stresses placed on the adolescent patient and family by this unpredictable chronic illness (see Chapter 30).

JUVENILE DERMATOMYOSITIS
Epidemiology and Etiology

Juvenile dermatomyositis (JDMS) is an inflammatory myopathy characterized by vasculitis with involvement of the skin and muscle. JDMS shares many features with polymyositis (PM)—the latter is an adult illness that usually lacks the typical dermatologic manifestations of JDMS. This discussion focuses on JDMS, because this is most likely to be encountered in adolescents. The overall incidence (of JDMS and PM) has been reported as between 1 and 3.2 in 1,000,000 annually among whites and 7.7 in 1,000,000 annually among blacks. Among adolescents in the United States, JDMS is 10 to 20 times more likely to occur than is PM. Girls are more likely (2:1) to develop JDMS than are boys. As with other rheumatologic disorders, certain HLA loci seem to predominate; in the case of JDMS these are HLA-DR3 and HLA-B8.

The causes of JDMS are not completely understood, although studies have shown a high association between disease onset and complement fixation titers to coxsackie-B2 and -B4 viruses, as well as a higher incidence of JDMS during the summer and fall (the same seasons as coxsackie infections). Pathophysiologic studies have shown vasculitis in the capillaries, venules, and small arteries of the skin, and in the gastrointestinal tract, muscles, fat, and small nerves. Vascular occlusion and perivascular atrophy are seen on muscle biopsy.

Clinical Features and Diagnosis

Characteristic in children and adolescents who have JDMS are skin and muscle involvement. A skin rash

TABLE 90–4. 1982 Revised Criteria for Classification of Systemic Lupus Erythematosus*

CRITERION	DEFINITION
1. Malar rash	Fixed erythema, flat or raised, over the malar eminences, tending to spare the nasolabial folds
2. Discoid rash	Erythematous raised patches with adherent keratotic scaling and follicular plugging; atrophic scarring may occur in older lesions
3. Photosensitivity	Skin rash as a result of unusual reaction to sunlight, by patient history or physician observation
4. Oral ulcers	Oral or nasopharyngeal ulceration, usually painless, observed by a physician
5. Arthritis	Nonerosive arthritis involving two or more peripheral joints, characterized by tenderness, swelling, or effusion
6. Serositis	Pleuritis—convincing history of pleuritic pain or rub heard by a physician or evidence of pleural effusion *OR* Pericarditis—documented by ECG or rub or evidence of pericardial effusion
7. Renal disorder	Persistent proteinuria greater than 0.5 g/day or greater than 3+ if quantitation not performed *OR* Cellular casts—may be red cell, hemoglobin, granular, tubular, or mixed
8. Neurologic disorder	Seizures—in the absence of offending drugs or known metabolic derangements (e.g., uremia, ketoacidosis, or electrolyte imbalance) *OR* Psychosis—in the absence of offending drugs or known metabolic derangements (e.g., uremia, ketoacidosis, or electrolyte imbalance)
9. Hematologic disorder	Hemolytic anemia—with reticulocytosis *OR* Leukopenia—less than 4000/mm^3 total on two or more occasions *OR* Lymphopenia—less than 1500/mm^3 on two or more occasions *OR* Thrombocytopenia—less than 100,000/mm^3 in the absence of offending drugs
10. Immunologic disorder	Positive LE cell preparation *OR* Anti-DNA: antibody to native DNA in abnormal titer *OR* Anti-Sm: presence of antibody to Sm nuclear antigen *OR* False-positive serologic test for syphilis known to be positive for at least 6 months and confirmed by *Treponema pallidum* immobilization or fluorescent treponemal antibody absorption test
11. Antinuclear antibody	An abnormal titer of antinuclear antibody by immunofluorescence or an equivalent assay at any point in time and in the absence of drugs known to be associated with "drug-induced lupus" syndrome

*The proposed classification is based on 11 criteria. For the purpose of identifying patients in clinical studies, a person shall be said to have systemic lupus erythematosus if any 4 or more of the 11 criteria are present, serially or simultaneously, during any interval of observation.

With permission from Tan EM, Cohen AS, Fries JF, et al: The 1982 Revised Criteria for the Classification of Systemic Lupus Erythematosus. Arthritis Rheum 25:1274, 1982. Reprinted from the ARTHRITIS AND RHEUMATISM journal, copyright 1982. Used by permission of the American College of Rheumatology.

most commonly occurs as a mild swelling of the eyelids, which have a light violaceous hue, telangiectasia, and scaling (the so-called heliotrope rash). An erythematous maculopapular eruption can also appear over the extensor surfaces of the arms and legs and in a V distribution over the chest. The scaly, erythematous-violaceous, slightly papular lesions over the interphalangeal joints, elbows, knees, and malleoli in those with dermatomyositis are known as Gottron sign. The rash over the interphalangeal joints can become thickened, smooth, and shiny; this is then referred to as Gottron patches or papules (or collodion patches). These rashes can precede or follow the myositis by months. In the more insidious onset form of the illness, the rash can be accompanied by gradual arthralgia and difficulty walking. The acute onset form of the disease is typified by sudden fever, severe muscle weakness, and the appearance of the rash.

The muscle involvement is primarily proximal, with difficulty in walking or in arising from a supine position (Gower sign). This can lead to confusion of the diagnosis with Duchenne muscular dystrophy in younger patients. Neck flexor, masseter, and soft palate dysfunction can

also sometimes be noted as a nasal-sounding voice. Muscle pain and tenderness may be present, especially early. Clinically significant cardiac involvement (e.g., arrhythmia, congestive heart failure, high-grade heart block) is unusual, occurring in fewer than 5% of adolescent patients. Interstitial or alveolar fibrosis is also seen in JDMS, but is unusual (<5%). Gastrointestinal complications, including dysphagia and abdominal pain, have been reported in 25% of adolescent patients, whereas bowel perforation is a severe problem (but rare). Arthritis is reported in about 25% of cases.

Although these findings are likely to resolve with time and treatment, calcinosis is a frequent (one third of adolescents) complication later. Unfortunately, this deposition of calcium in soft tissue and tendons persists after all the muscle and rash findings have gone into remission. Subcutaneous collections often ulcerate through the overlying skin, and adolescent patients are at risk for superinfection. Attempts to excise these collections often stimulate further calcification because of the trauma of surgery. Debulking of large calcific masses, using a dental drill to avoid trauma to the surrounding soft tissue, has worked well. The complications of calcinosis and flexion contractures are likely to be encountered during adolescence and early adulthood (Table 90–5). Earlier aggressive treatment has resulted in lower mortality and a good functional outcome in 80% of adolescent patients. Some adolescents have significant morbidity (fibrosis and contractures), however, and some die from their disease.

The diagnosis is made on the basis of the typical rash, proximal muscle weakness, and demonstration of one or more of the following: (1) increase in the creatine phosphokinase (CPK) or aldolase enzyme level; (2) abnormal muscle biopsy; and (3) an abnormal electromyogram (EMG).

The ESR may be increased, but not invariably, and is not as consistent a finding as elevation in the muscle enzyme levels. The ANA can be positive but the presence of other autoantibodies (dsDNA, ENA, RNP, anti-Sm, and Jo-1) is not significantly associated with JDMS. Skin biopsy reveals poikiloderma, perivascular lymphocytes and histiocytes, and a striking vasculopathy with small vessel thrombosis. EMG can be useful in confirming the diagnosis (fibrillation potentials at rest and short-duration, low-amplitude polyphasic potentials with volitional contraction), and muscle biopsy reveals group atrophy of fibers at the periphery of the fascicle, disruption of myofibrils, central nuclear migration, prominent nuclei, and basophilia. None of these changes are unique to JDMS, and the typical clinical features are more specific.

Treatment begins with oral corticosteroid therapy, although the appropriate dose is still debated. Initial high-dose therapy (2 mg/kg/day of prednisone, or 3 days of intravenous pulse steroids, 1 g/day), with tapering after symptoms and enzyme levels have returned to normal, can be used. Alternatively, to avoid the myopathy that can occur with prolonged (4 to 6 months) high-dose steroid therapy, 0.2 to 0.5 mg/kg/day of prednisone can be given effectively in all but the most severely affected adolescents. Immunosuppressive therapy with methotrexate and azathioprine can be added in resistant cases; recent trials of cyclosporine have been encouraging, although not yet rigorously evaluated. Physical therapy to preserve range of motion where joints and tendons have been affected is also important. Unfortunately, chelation therapy for the calcinosis has not been successful. Colchicine has been used to treat the secondary effects of the crystal deposits causing local inflammation, and apparently has long-term benefit.

SCLERODERMA

Epidemiology

Scleroderma, which means "hard skin," is composed of a spectrum of illnesses ranging from localized skin pigment changes to severe and disfiguring involvement of an extremity, with diffuse internal organ involvement. Although unusual in children under the age of 10 years, approximately 7.2% of all cases develop in those between the ages of 10 and 19 years. There is a female predominance for developing scleroderma, but no familial clustering of the disease has been noted. The

TABLE 90–5. Features of Juvenile Dermatomyositis

Rash and swelling of eyelids—violaceous, scaly, telangiectatic (heliotrope)
Rash over dorsum of interphalangeal joints—initially scaly and erythematous (Gottron sign); then thickened, shiny, smooth (Gottron patches)
Arthralgia, myalgia, proximal muscle weakness, muscle tenderness
Fever
Arthritis, calcinosis, contractures (later)
Elevated CPK and aldolase levels; increased ESR

overall incidence in those of all ages has been reported to be between 4.5 and 12.0 new cases in 1,000,000.

Types

LOCALIZED SCLERODERMA

Localized scleroderma involves two conditions, linear scleroderma and morphea. Although these can be distinguished by the presence of linear lesions in the former and by circular, plaque-like, or guttate lesions in the latter, these descriptive distinctions are not significant or useful. These diseases present with cutaneous plaques or linear bands, often beginning as an erythematous or violaceous skin discoloration that can become either depressed or raised. The affected areas are thickened, waxy, and eventually hyperpigmented. The lesions are smooth, shiny, hairless, and bound to underlying structures (hidebound). Sclerodactyly refers to digits with tight, shiny skin, prominent knuckles, and atrophy of muscle and subcutaneous fat. With localized scleroderma there is always the potential for atrophy of underlying structures, including fat, muscle, periosteum, and bone. In addition, there is often disturbance of growth in the affected area, with limb foreshortening and hypoplasia of the facial bones and skull when overlying skin lesions are present (as in coup de sabre lesions). It is the location and depth of the skin involvement that determines the functional and/or cosmetic loss.

SYSTEMIC SCLEROSIS

Progressive systemic sclerosis (PSS) is more typical of adult onset scleroderma, but can present during adolescence. PSS is subdivided into two types: (1) diffuse cutaneous—symmetric, widespread skin involvement, with rapid progression and early visceral involvement; and (2) limited cutaneous—symmetric but restricted skin involvement, with a long delay in the appearance of internal manifestations and an association with CREST (calcinosis, Raynaud phenomenon, esophageal hypomotility, sclerodactyly, and telangiectasia). In both types the earliest finding is often Raynaud phenomenon, which may present months or years before any obvious skin lesions become apparent. This intermittent spasm of small arterioles in the fingers and toes is manifested acutely by three progressive phases: (1) pallor or white coloration of the distal digit, representing occlusive spasm of the vessel; (2) cyanosis as a result of partial spasm and deoxygenated blood; and (3) erythema or hyperemia, which is the result of reactive dilatation of the vessel. These represent the classic white, blue, and red color progression of Raynaud phenomenon and are seen in 75% of adolescent patients with PSS. Digital pitting and/or the loss of toe and finger pads secondary to ischemia and infarction are seen in those with severe and persistent Raynaud phenomenon. Limited disease is 75% anti–centromere antibody–positive and has a 5-year survival rate of 80%. Diffuse disease is 30% anti–SCL70-positive and has a 5-year survival rate of about 10% to 25%.

Joint symptoms can have three major causes. Overlying scleroderma can cause the contracture of joints in the absence of any synovial inflammation, whereas true monarthritis or polyarthritis can occur in adolescents with scleroderma or PSS. Finally, myositis similar to that seen in dermatomyositis can occur, and manifest secondarily as decreased range of motion in joints.

Esophageal dysmotility is commonly seen in adolescents with PSS, and is also found in those with localized disease. A barium swallow confirms involvement in those having difficulty swallowing and the sense of food feeling "stuck on the way down." In localized scleroderma the changes may not be permanent, although in PSS the abnormality usually persists. The remainder of the bowel can be affected, usually with hypomotility that includes dilatation of the duodenum and jejunum and sacculations of the small bowel and colon caused by intermittent atrophy of the muscularis (this is particularly seen in PSS). Adolescents with this condition may experience bloating, cramping, diarrhea, or constipation.

Adolescents who have systemic disease can also have pulmonary fibrosis with impaired gas exchange and decreased vital capacity and symptoms of dyspnea and/or bronchospasm (see Chapter 43). Myocarditis and pericarditis may be seen early in PSS and can also be causes of dyspnea (see Chapter 50). The pulmonary fibrosis can lead to pulmonary hypertension and eventual right heart failure, and myocardial tissue is often replaced with interstitial fibrosis as the disease progresses (see Chapter 43).

Perhaps the most devastating systemic complication of scleroderma is renal involvement. This can be gradual and progressive or it can be acute, with malignant hypertension and rapid deterioration resulting from vasoconstriction with fibrosis and with intimal obstruction of the small arteries and arterioles of the renal cortex. The malignant hypertension phase of the disease seems to be associated with an increased secretion of renin and angiotensin (see Chapter 67).

Finally, subcutaneous calcifications, especially of the distal finger pads, extensor surfaces of the forearms, and about the knees and elbows, are seen in patients with scleroderma. The CREST syndrome is a confined form of systemic disease (Table 90–6).

Laboratory Studies

There are no specific diagnostic laboratory studies available that can confirm the presence of scleroderma.

TABLE 90–6. Features of Scleroderma

LOCALIZED FEATURES	SYSTEMIC FEATURES
Cutaneous plaques and/or linear bands; initially erythematous, then thickened, hardened, smooth, shiny, hyperpigmented	Raynaud phenomenon—complicated by digital pitting and infarction, if persistent
Contractures	Contractures
Sclerodactyly	Sclerodactyly
Arthritis	Arthritis
Atrophy of underlying fat, muscle, periosteum, bone	Esophageal dysmotility
	Bowel hypomotility
	Pulmonary fibrosis
	Renal fibrosis
	Calcinosis
	CREST syndrome

Raynaud phenomenon can be an isolated finding, or it may indicate localized or systemic disease. A complete blood count may reveal chronic anemia and urinalysis may reveal nephritis. The serum creatinine, blood urea nitrogen, and muscle enzyme (CPK, aldolase) levels should be measured serially.

Rheumatoid factor (RF) can be positive in 25% to 35% of adolescent patients and may persist, especially when synovitis is present. Antinuclear antibody (ANA) is usually positive, especially in PSS, and about 25% of adolescents have anti-RNP activity. Anticentromere antibodies (ACA) occur in approximately 50% of adolescent patients with PSS, but are found in 90% of those with CREST syndrome. Anti–SCL-70 antibodies are found in 75% of all patients with limited scleroderma and in about 33% of those with diffuse PSS. Tissue biopsy is diagnostic for scleroderma. Cell-mediated and general immune function in scleroderma patients are normal, except as compromised by therapy (e.g., by immunosuppressive agents).

Management

Localized scleroderma tends to progress over 3 to 4 years from the time of appearance of the first lesion(s) and then stabilizes without cutaneous progression. Lesions may often lose their hyperpigmentation and can become more pliable and less hidebound. In PSS, the natural course of the illness is generally characterized by a gradual progression of organ involvement and subsequent disability. Early and aggressive therapy may alter the usual deteriorating course.

Management of adolescents with scleroderma depends on the extent of the illness but focuses on physical therapy, primary chemotherapy, and psychological assessment and intervention. Contractures resulting from linear banding, sclerodactyly, and/or synovitis is common and requires early and regular physical therapy to preserve range of motion, muscle strength, and functional capacity. As in all of the collagen-vascular disorders therapy of the primary disease process is less than satisfactory, because the primary mechanism of the disease is unknown.

Painful and disabling arthritis, or myositis, can be treated with NSAIDs. Raynaud phenomenon is managed with careful attention to maintaining the warmth of the extremities and involves the use of vasodilating agents, such as calcium channel blockers (e.g., nifedipine, verapamil). Drugs directed toward decreasing platelet aggregation (e.g., salicylates, dipyridamole) have been tried without consistent benefit. General skin care is advisable and includes the use of hydrophilic base creams, limited sun exposure, and avoidance of local irritants, but it is unclear whether these measures moderate the progression of the illness. Systemic corticosteroids can be used during periods of acute inflammation (such as "sausage digits"), but are only recommended for short-term use. Immunosuppressive agents such as azathioprine and cyclophosphamide have also been used, with variable success. Penicillamine is the most consistently useful drug for both localized and systemic disease, perhaps because it interferes with the cross linking of collagen. With gradual increasing of the dosage to 10 to 15 mg/kg body weight/day, long-term treatment can often be maintained, and should be instituted in patients with significant involvement.

The psychological impact of a chronic and disfiguring illness on a developing adolescent and family is discussed elsewhere in this text (see Chapter 30), and should receive the highest priority in the total management of these adolescents. The family and school must be involved in supporting and (when necessary) adapting to the needs of the adolescent patient.

LYME ARTHRITIS

A relatively recent addition to the differential diagnosis of arthralgia and arthritis in the adolescent is Lyme borreliosis, or Lyme arthritis. Representing a range of symptoms and organ system involvement, Lyme disease results from infection with the spirochete *Borrelia burgdorferi,* an *Ixodes* tick–borne organism found in *I. dammini* in the northeastern and midwestern United States, in *I. pacificus* in the western U.S., in *I. ricinus* in Europe, and in *I. persulcatus* in Asia. Over 14,000 cases have been reported to the Centers for Disease Control since 1982, 90% of which have come from Massachusetts, Rhode Island, Connecticut, New York, New Jersey, Wisconsin, and Minnesota. The infection rate of *I. dammini* with *B. burgdorferi* in some endemic areas has been found to be more than 50%. The preferred host for the tick is the white-tailed deer.

The clinical manifestations of Lyme disease vary with the time since inoculation by the tick, beginning with stage 1 of early infection, in which 60% to 80% of adolescents develop the characteristic rash, erythema migrans, sometimes associated with fever, fatigue, myalgias, arthralgias, and regional lymphadenopathy. The rash begins as a red macule or papule at the site of the tick bite and expands to form a large annular erythema with a bright-red outer border and partial central clearing. As the disease progresses into the second stage of early infection, the rash gradually fades over 3 to 4 weeks (regardless of treatment), and further symptoms of malaise, fatigue, headache, stiff neck, and migratory arthralgias and myalgias can develop. Although usually absent during stage 1, antibody titers to *B. burgdorferi*

develop in most patients during stage 2 (this rise in antibody titer can, however, be blunted if early antibiotic therapy is instituted). Other problems that can develop during late stage 2 and stage 3 include unilateral or bilateral facial palsy and peripheral neuritis or meningitis (15% to 20%); varying degrees of atrioventricular block (4% to 8%); keratitis (4%); and subtle encephalopathy with memory impairment, somnolence, or behavioral changes (4%).

The most common stage 3 clinical manifestation is large-joint arthritis affecting the knee. This asymmetric mono- or oligoarthritis usually consists of intermittent episodes lasting several weeks, although adolescents are at greater risk for more prolonged arthritis (4 to 5 months) than are younger children. In the presence of HLA-DR4, boys are at particularly high risk for chronic joint inflammation (more than 1 year). Destructive synovitis with contractures and erosions is not typical of Lyme arthritis.

Clinical diagnosis of Lyme borreliosis can be made early with the finding of the rash or a definite tick bite in the setting of consistent signs and symptoms. In those patients without these findings, IgG and IgM antibodies to the spirochete can be helpful in the appropriate clinical context. It must be kept in mind, however, that standardization of both the immunofluorescent assay (IFA) and the enzyme-linked immunosorbent assay (ELISA) is still poor, and such factors as antibiotic treatment and infection with other spirochetes (such as *Treponema pallidum*) interfere with accurate interpretation of the results. Most laboratories consider a titer of 1:256 or more as positive. The current development of a polymerase chain reaction detection of the organism will greatly improve serologic diagnosis.

Treatment varies with the time of diagnosis. Early recognition of the disease provides the option of oral antibiotics with tetracycline, penicillin V, or amoxicillin for 10 to 30 days, whereas the patient for whom the diagnosis is late (or who has persistent or recurrent symptoms following an initial course of oral antibiotics) requires parenteral therapy with ceftriaxone or penicillin G for 2 to 3 weeks. When present, the arthritis is treated with nonsteroidal anti-inflammatory drugs (NSAIDs), although intraarticular steroid preparations may be necessary in cases of prolonged inflammation. Unlike in the other rheumatologic illnesses, prevention is possible in Lyme disease by wearing long-sleeved shirts and long pants and the judicious use of tick repellents such as permethrin or deet.

BIBLIOGRAPHY

Allen RC, Gross KR, Laxer RM, et al: Intraarticular triamcinolone hexacetonide in the management of chronic arthritis in children. Arthritis Rheum 29:997, 1986.

Biro F, Gewanter HL, Baum J: The hypermobility syndrome. Pediatrics 72:701, 1983.

Cassidy JT, Levinson JE, Bass JC, et al: A study of classification criteria for a diagnosis of juvenile rheumatoid arthritis. Arthritis Rheum 29:274, 1986.

DeHaven KE, Dolan WA, Mayer PJ: Chondromalacia patellae and the painful knee. Am Fam Pract 21:117, 1980.

Goldenberg DL: Fibromyalgia syndrome. An emerging but controversial condition. JAMA 257:2782, 1987.

Jacobs JC: Pediatric Rheumatology for the Practitioner. New York, Springer-Verlag, 1982.

Lacks S, White P: Morbidity associated with childhood systemic lupus erythematosus. J Rheumatol 17:941, 1990.

Pachman LM: Juvenile dermatomyositis. Pediatr Clin North Am 33:1097, 1986.

Reveille JD, Bartolucci A, Alarcon GS: Prognosis in systemic lupus erythematosus. Arthritis Rheum 33:37, 1990.

Rosenberg AM: Advanced drug therapy for juvenile rheumatoid arthritis. J Pediatr 114:171, 1989.

Singsen BH: Scleroderma in childhood. Pediatr Clin North Am 33:1119, 1986.

Steere AC: Lyme disease. N Engl J Med 321:586, 1989.

Szer IS, Taylor E, Steere AC: The long-term course of Lyme arthritis in children. N Engl J Med 325:159, 1991.

Wolfe F, Smythe HA, Yunus MB, et al: The American College of Rheumatology 1990 criteria for the classification of fibromyalgia. Report of the Multicenter Criteria Committee. Arthritis Rheum 33:160, 1990.

SECTION XXI

Infectious Conditions

CHAPTER 91

Developmental Overview

VINCENT A. FULGINITI

In this section and throughout this text are chapters that address specific issues of infectious diseases in adolescents. This overview places these issues in perspective.

Developmentally, the adolescent has reached a peak of immunologic function (see Chapter 92). If adolescents have had adequate medical care prior to adolescence, they will have received the recommended immunizations and most likely will have escaped infection with pertussis, diphtheria, tetanus, measles, mumps, rubella, and poliomyelitis in childhood. Generally, 90% to 95% of immunized adolescents remain protected from many of these diseases for the remainder of their lives, because that is the range of effectiveness for most of these vaccines. If unexposed to these diseases, the 5% to 10% who remain unprotected because of primary vaccine failure never experience them. However, if adequate immunization levels are not maintained, miniepidemics can (and do) occur, and this group of susceptible adolescents may suffer from measles, rubella, and mumps, in particular.

Developmentally, most adolescents have a fully functioning immune system that has responded to the antigens in the various vaccines and has rendered them immune to other infections, based on an adequate response to minor or even asymptomatic infections during infancy and childhood. The peak of immunologic responsiveness is manifested by rigorous, secondary, recall responses to exposure to most infectious agents. This immunologic memory either protects the adolescent totally from recurrence of infectious diseases (e.g., measles) or results in milder or localized infection (e.g., streptococcal pharyngitis). However, some infectious agents may become clinically apparent for the first time (or recur) in adolescence (e.g., Epstein-Barr virus infection as infectious mononucleosis or as recurrent chronic fatigue syndrome).

To demonstrate how a single pattern of disease may ablate this somewhat idealistic picture of a protected adolescence, the increasing frequency of measles virus infection in the adolescent age group can be examined. Since the development of an effective live virus measles vaccine in 1963, a group of adolescents has moved through childhood susceptible to measles for various reasons: (1) they did not receive vaccine; (2) they received vaccine but were "primary vaccine failures" (i.e., they were among the 3% to 5% of individuals who did not respond to vaccine with an adequate immune response); or (3) they had no exposure to the disease

(secondary to the reduction in frequency of measles following massive efforts at immunizing most of the population). This group of unprotected adolescents reached high school, college, and other group settings. Miniepidemics of measles have occurred in these adolescents, infecting a large proportion of susceptible individuals. The disease has often been severe, and deaths were recorded in adolescents and young adults during these outbreaks. From 1980 to 1987, this pattern of disease prevailed. By 1989 and 1990, the peak incidence of measles occurred in children of preschool age because of inadequacies of the health care system to reach this age group. However, it is now apparent that a very high proportion of school-aged children are protected; thus, in the future, we anticipate a lower incidence of disease in the adolescent age group.

To ensure that this is achieved, all recommending bodies support the concept of a two-dose regimen for measles virus immunization. Today, live measles virus vaccine, usually given as a combined measles-mumps-rubella vaccine, is administered to 15-month-old infants routinely, and a second dose of vaccine is recommended for those entering school (the recommendation of the Centers for Disease Control, Advisory Committee on Immunization) or just prior to puberty (the recommendation of the American Academy of Pediatrics' Committee on Infectious Diseases). This two-dose regimen is intended to provide protection for adolescents and young adults and, when fully implemented, will help prevent a recurrence of the miniepidemics of the early 1980s.

Physicians who care for adolescents should inquire about the adolescent patient's measles vaccine status and ensure that a second dose is given to those who have received only a single dose. It is also recommended that colleges and other institutions in which there are groups of adolescents and young adults institute a policy of ensuring that those who require a second dose receive it.

The increase in the frequency of measles reminds us that adolescents and young adults may also be susceptible to other contagious diseases, such as rubella and mumps. In 1989 and 1990, a marked increase in the incidence of rubella was observed, validating this assumption. Because measles is more contagious than these other viral infections, outbreaks of measles usually occur prior to the onset of outbreaks of mumps and rubella. Most authorities recommend that the combined measles-mumps-rubella (MMR) vaccine be used, instead of just measles vaccine, to ensure protection against all three diseases. Thus, the use of MMR in the two-dose protocol is recommended.

Poverty and its consequences leave some adolescents susceptible to various other infectious illnesses. Growing numbers of adolescents are homeless, or live in conditions other than "at home" with their families. These individuals often fail to enter the traditional health care system or receive fragmentary, emergency care, rather than planned, preventive health care. The potential for suffering from transmissible and environmental infections in this group is obviously high.

Furthermore, there are some unique susceptibilities of adolescents and young adults. Epstein-Barr virus (EBV) infection (see Chapter 93) can occur during adolescence. Chronic fatigue syndrome, probably caused largely but not exclusively by a viral infection, is particularly prevalent in this age group (see Chapter 93). When toxic shock syndrome was first described, many of those affected were adolescents who used tampons during menstruation. Although the use of highly absorbent tampons has decreased, this toxic disease still affects this age group (see Chapter 94).

Currently, the greatest risk to adolescents, if they engage in a lifestyle that includes promiscuous sexual activity, homosexual encounters, or drug and substance abuse, is infection with human immunodeficiency virus (HIV) and the subsequent development of acquired immunodeficiency syndrome (AIDS). These conditions are discussed in the reproductive health section (see Chapter 76) but shall be commented on here because of their importance during adolescence and young adulthood. Some adolescents have been infected by HIV because of receiving contaminated blood products in the past; these include young people who have hemophilia and those who required multiple transfusions in childhood for conditions that required surgery (e.g., cardiac surgery). The virus, dormant for a period, then becomes manifest as AIDS usually during adolescence and young adulthood, marring what would otherwise be a healthy time of life. Other blood-borne infectious agents, transmitted by infected needles used by those who abuse drugs, include the various hepatitis viruses and cytomegalovirus.

The environment and habits of adolescents also contribute to an increased risk of exposure to certain infectious diseases. The rise in sexually transmitted diseases, other than HIV infection, is a direct consequence of early sexual activity among some young people. Gonorrhea, syphilis, chlamydial infections, herpes simplex infection, human papillomavirus infection, and other diseases that primarily involve the genital tract have increased in frequency and severity among this group. When coupled with poor access to health care, either because the adolescent doesn't seek care early or because of poverty, these diseases may exert a greater toll than they should, given the availability of adequate treatment of most conditions.

Immunologically, primary immunodeficiency is a rarity in adolescence, simply because this group of diseases manifests in childhood and the more severe forms result in death prior to adolescence. With improvement in treatment for some of these disorders, however, individual patients survive to adolescence and present to physicians for continuing care. Secondary immunodeficiencies do occasionally occur in adolescents as a first manifestation of disease (see Chapter 92).

Some "childhood" diseases still present during adolescence. For example, pertussis may affect this age group because adolescents are beyond the period when the vaccine is routinely given and the disease itself is milder once the airways have grown in size. Adolescents may therefore have mild forms of pertussis, often diagnosed only as "bronchitis" or as a severe upper respiratory infection. A more detailed discussion of this disease is presented in Chapter 94. Other childhood diseases can affect adolescents, such as streptococcal infection and *Haemophilus influenzae* infection (see Chapter 94).

Mycoplasma pneumoniae causes pneumonia more frequently than other organisms in the school-aged population. During adolescence, this is the predominant causative pathogen in the development of pneumonia. All aspects of infection with *M. pneumoniae* are discussed in Chapters 43 and 94.

Chapter 96 presents the choices of antimicrobial agents for infections that are encountered in adolescents. The discussion ranges from general considerations about the susceptibility of infectious agents to the various antimicrobials that can be used. Empiric therapy for suspected infections and specific therapy for identified infectious agents are outlined.

Adolescence provides an opportunity for physicians to identify particular susceptibilities to infection and to counteract them with preventive measures, including vaccine administration. Physicians also have the opportunity to diagnose specific infectious diseases and their cause and to intervene with therapeutic measures. Information about susceptibility and infection enables the physician to select the appropriate preventive or therapeutic strategy.

Physicians must be aware of the unique features of infectious diseases in this age group, and must respond to their adolescent patients appropriately. A history must be obtained to identify susceptibilities, to recognize high-risk behaviors, and to detail immunization status. The physical examination must be appropriate to the age group, with adequate examination of such sites as the entire skin surface and the genital tract. Some physicians may have to "retool" themselves for gynecologic and male genital examinations and should familiarize themselves with the procedures for obtaining proper specimens for identifying of pathogens common in this age group, but that are rarely encountered in their younger patients (e.g., herpesvirus, HIV).

With adequate information and skill in the appropriate diagnostic and therapeutic techniques, physicians can have a significant and positive effect on the health of their adolescent patients.

It should be noted that the infectious conditions included in this section have been carefully selected and are those for which adolescents have a particular likelihood of acquisition because of their habits or particular susceptibility (e.g., Epstein-Barr virus infection, toxic shock syndrome, *Mycoplasma pneumoniae* infection, Rocky Mountain spotted fever) and conditions that providers may fail to consider in adolescents because they are generally regarded as childhood diseases (e.g., infection by *Haemophilus influenzae* or *Bordetella pertussis*). If there are no major differences in a given infectious disease in adolescents as compared with children or adults, then that condition is given less emphasis or is not included. The reader is referred to the relevant pediatric, internal medicine, or infectious disease textbook. Chronic fatigue syndrome, the cause of which is uncertain, is discussed under viral infection (see Chapter 93).

This section does not contain all the information in this textbook regarding infectious diseases. Recommen-dations regarding routine immunizations are contained in the well adolescent care chapter (see Chapter 25). Information on sexually transmitted diseases (sexually transmitted disease syndromes, AIDS, and infection with HIV) is included in the section on reproductive conditions (see Chapters 75 and 76). Infections in pulmonary conditions are discussed in Chapter 43. The discussion of hepatitis is found in the section on liver and pancreatic disease (see Chapter 62). Therefore, some infectious conditions are discussed in other sections of this text because we believe that practitioners of adolescent medicine would be most likely to seek such information in those chapters.

CHAPTER 92

Immunologic Aspects of Adolescence

ROBERT L. ROBERTS and E. RICHARD STIEHM

During adolescence the immune system is usually functioning at maximum efficiency. Measures of immune competence, such as the ability to produce specific antibodies, mount a delayed hypersensitivity response, and contain bacterial infections, are operating at highest adult capacity. The thymus gland reaches its greatest absolute weight at puberty and then begins a slow involution. The frequent infections experienced in early childhood and prescribed immunizations provide a wide spectrum of specific immunoglobulins and memory cells to protect against infection. Until fairly recently, children with severe congenital immune defects did not survive until adolescence; early recognition and advances in medical treatments have now allowed many of these children to reach adulthood.

The many hormonal changes accompanying puberty have important physiologic effects on the immune system and accentuate the differences in the immune response of males and females (see Chapters 55 and 57). Males are more likely to have a primary immune defect, partly because of the X-linked inheritance pattern responsible for many of these disorders. Women have higher levels of immunoglobulin than men, reject allografts more rapidly, and are less susceptible to most viral and bacterial infections. Another consequence of this greater immune responsiveness in females, however, is their higher incidence of autoimmune disease; women are almost ten times more likely to develop systemic lupus erythematosus than men and four times more likely to develop rheumatoid arthritis (see Chapter 90).

Social factors also affect the immune status of adolescents. Close contact with individuals from diverse geographic areas, such as in boarding schools, dormitories, colleges, military academies, and camps, exposes the adolescent to new pathogens for which they may have no specific immune defense. Sexual experimentation puts them at risk for an array of sexually transmitted diseases (see Chapter 75), and infectious mononucleosis (see Chapter 93) may be transmitted by saliva exchanged in intimate relationships.

Currently, the most significant danger to the adolescents' immune system in many parts of the world is exposure through sexual contact or intravenous drug use to the human immunodeficiency virus (HIV), the agent that causes acquired immune deficiency syndrome, AIDS (see Chapter 76). Although adolescents (13 to 21 years) account for only 1.2% of the total number of AIDS cases in the United States, AIDS is increasing faster in this age group than in any other segment of the population. Indeed, a large percentage of young adults who now have AIDS acquired the infection as teenagers. The high-risk behavior characteristics of this age group continue to put them at risk for HIV infection, despite the best educational efforts.

In this chapter we focus on deficiencies in the immune system occurring in adolescents that make them susceptible to infection or malignancies. The excessive activity of the immune system that may lead to autoimmune disease or allergies is discussed elsewhere in this text (see Chapter 90). The clinical and laboratory features of suspected immunodeficiency are discussed, and the specific immunodeficiencies encountered in adolescents are reviewed. Treatment of these diseases is also summarized.

IMMUNODEFICIENCY IN ADOLESCENCE: OVERVIEW

Immunodeficiencies may be either primary or secondary. A secondary immunodeficiency occurs in individuals with a previously normal immune system who, as a result of another medical condition, have a temporary (or permanent) deficiency of one of the limbs of the immune system, which increases their susceptibility to infection. Secondary immune deficiencies are more common than primary deficiencies (Table 92–1). The causes of secondary immunodeficiency are apparent by the time most patients reach adolescence; therefore, the identification of an immune defect in a previously healthy adolescent may foreshadow the diagnosis of a malignancy or chronic infection.

The initial diagnosis of a primary immunodeficiency in adolescence is also less likely than a secondary one, because most patients with primary immunodeficiency (80% to 90%) have already been identified in infancy or early childhood. However, there are patients with chronic granulomatous disease (CGD), common variable immunodeficiency (CVID), and hyperimmunoglobulin E (HIE) syndrome in whom the initial diagnosis is not made until adolescence or early adulthood.

Table 92–1. Causes of Secondary Immunodeficiency in Adolescence

CAUSATIVE FACTOR	EXAMPLES
Hereditary and metabolic diseases	Chromosome abnormalities
	Diabetes mellitus
	Malnutrition, vitamin and mineral deficiencies
	Cystic fibrosis
	Protein-losing enteropathies
	Nephrotic syndrome, uremia
	Sickle cell disease
Immunosuppressive agents	Radiation
	Immunosuppressive drugs
	Corticosteroids and anabolic steroids
Infectious diseases	Viral infections (HIV, measles, varicella, cytomegalovirus, Epstein-Barr virus)
	Acute bacterial disease
	Severe mycobacterial or fungal disease
Infiltrative and hematologic disease	Histiocytosis
	Sarcoidosis
	Hodgkin disease, lymphoma
	Leukemia
	Myeloma
	Agranulocytosis and aplasia
Miscellaneous	Burns, surgical trauma
	Splenectomy
	Cocaine abuse
	Lupus erythematosus
	Chronic active hepatitis

DIAGNOSIS OF IMMUNODEFICIENCY

Many of the clinical features of immunodeficient patients are listed in Table 92–2. Recurrent or persistent respiratory infections are a common finding in many adolescent patients. The infections do not respond to antibiotics, or recur as soon as antibiotics are discontinued. There is often a history of persistent otitis media in infancy and of chronic sinusitis and bronchitis as the child matures. By adolescence, permanent lung damage may have already occurred in the form of bronchiectasis or pneumatoceles (common in adolescent HIE patients). Respiratory infection must be distinguished from respiratory allergy, which is usually associated with a clear, nonpurulent discharge and is not usually associated with fever.

Careful analysis of the infections acquired by the immunodeficient adolescent may allow the physician to predict which branch of the immune system is defective. Cellular (T-cell) defects with or without antibody (B-cell) defects are usually more severe, becoming manifest as viral, fungal, and gram-negative bacterial infections in the first months of life; it is impossible that a child with such a defect would survive to puberty without intensive medical intervention. Defects in antibody production alone are not usually apparent until the transplacentally acquired maternal antibodies are depleted (at about 6 months of age), at which time infections with gram-positive encapsulated bacteria may start to occur. However, children with a partial or subclass antibody defect may have a more benign course, and may escape diagnosis until adolescence. Phagocytic cell defects may lead to bacterial infections of the respiratory tract, skin, and mucous membranes and patients are often symptomatic in infancy, although milder cases may not be recognized until adolescence. Disorders of complement are rare, but may make the adolescent patient susceptible to recurrent bacterial infections, particularly neisserial infections such as *Neisseria gonorrhoeae* or *Neisseria meningitidis,* if the later components (C6, C7, C8) are missing.

When an immunodeficiency is suspected in an adolescent, initial screening tests performed by most hospital laboratories may be used to gauge the patient's immune status (Table 92–3). A complete blood count and differential can determine whether there are adequate numbers of white blood cells, and also allow for examination of their morphology. Antibody function may be measured quantitatively by immunoglobulin levels (IgG, IgA, IgM) and qualitatively by titers of specific antibody to antigens to which the patient has been immunized. Delayed skin tests to agents such as mumps or tetanus test T-cell function. An elevated IgE level may suggest HIE syndrome, which is associated with neutrophil chemotactic defects, and which may also help distinguish an allergic from an infectious disease process. Total complement activity may be checked and specific components determined if this value is low.

PRIMARY IMMUNODEFICIENCIES

The primary immunodeficiencies categorized by the component of the immune system that is deficient are listed in Table 92–4; salient clinical and laboratory features are also included. The discussion that follows

Table 92–2. Clinical Features in Immunodeficiency

FREQUENCY OF OCCURRENCE	FEATURE
Usually present	Recurrent upper respiratory infections
	Severe bacterial infections
	Persistent infections with incomplete response to therapy
Often present	Failure to grow
	Infection with unusual organisms
	Skin lesions (rash, seborrhea, pyoderma, alopecia, eczema, telangiectasia)
	Recalcitrant thrush
	Diarrhea and malabsorption
	Persistent sinusitis, mastoiditis
	Recurrent bronchitis, pneumonia
	Evidence of autoimmunity
	Paucity of lymph nodes and tonsils
	Hematologic abnormalities (aplastic anemia, hemolytic anemia, neutropenia, thrombocytopenia)
	Weight loss, fever
Occasionally present	Chronic conjunctivitis
	Lymphadenopathy
	Hepatosplenomegaly
	Severe viral disease
	Arthralgia or arthritis
	Chronic encephalitis
	Recurrent meningitis
	Pyoderma gangrenosa
	Adverse reaction to vaccines
	Bronchiectasis, pneumatoceles

Table 92–3. Laboratory Tests for Suspected Immunodeficiency

SCREENING TESTS	ADVANCED TESTS
B-cell Deficiency	
IgG, IgM, IgA levels	B-cell enumeration by flow cytometry
Isoagglutinin titers	IgD and IgE levels
	Ab responses to vaccines (typhoid, pneumococcal)
Pre-existing antibody titers (tetanus diphtheria, *Haemophilus influenzae*)	Lateral pharyngeal x-ray films
	IgG subclass levels
T-cell Deficiency	
Lymphocyte count and morphology	T-cell enumeration and subsets (CD3 CD4, CD8)
Delayed skin tests: *Trichophyton*, mumps, *Candida*, tetanus toxoid	Lymphocyte proliferative responses to mitogens, antigens, allogeneic cells
	Enzyme assays (ADA, NP)
	Cytotoxic assays (NK, ADCC, CTL)
	Lymphokine assays (γ-interferon, interleukin-2)
Phagocytic Cell Deficiency	
Serial WBC with differentials	Random mobility and chemotactic assays
Granulocyte morphology	Bactericidal assay
NBT test of chemiluminescence	Surface receptors by flow cytometry (CD11b CD16)
IgE level	Granule constituents (lactoferrin, MPO)
Complement Deficiency	
CH_{50} activity	Normal (classic) and alternative complement activity assays
C3 level	Component assays—immunochemical or functional
C4 level	Inhibitor assays—immunochemical or functional

Ab, antibody; ADA, adenosine deaminase; ADCC, antibody-dependent cellular toxicity; C, complement; CD, cluster designation; CTL, cytotoxic T lymphocyte; Ig, immunoglobulin; MPO, myeloperoxidase; NBT, nitroblue tetrazolium; NK, natural killer; NP, nucleoside phosphorylase; WBC, white blood cells

describes some of these disorders, with particular emphasis on problems encountered by adolescent patients. More of these patients are surviving to adulthood because of such treatments as bone marrow transplants (see Chapter 54) and immunoglobulin replacement, and the number of survivors will increase further with the use of such therapies as recombinant cytokines, γ-interferon (now used for CGD), granulocyte colony–stimulating factor (GCSF) for congenital neutropenia, and interleukin-2 (IL-2) for T-cell deficiencies.

X-Linked (Bruton) Agammaglobulinemia

This form of panhypogammaglobulinemia (XLA) is characterized by low levels of immunoglobulins, low levels or no B cells, intact cellular immunity, and onset of infections some time after 6 months of age in male infants, when maternal antibody has disappeared. These infants have recurrent pyogenic infections of the lungs, sinuses, and bones with encapsulated bacteria. They are also susceptible to vaccine-induced poliovirus infection

and chronic echovirus encephalitis. The diagnosis can be confirmed by the profound deficiency of mature B cells, as assessed by flow cytometry.

These adolescents require lifelong replacement with immunoglobulin (IgG), either by intramuscular injection or intravenous infusion. IgG levels are monitored with the goal of keeping the trough level above 400 mg/dl. Prompt and adequate administration of antibiotics with each infection is crucial; continuous antibiotics are sometimes indicated. Despite these measures, many adolescents develop persistent sinusitis, bronchitis, and bronchiectasis, and many suffer hearing loss because of recurrent otitis media.

Other manifestations of XLA include aseptic arthritis, usually of the large joints, which resolves with IgG replacement therapy. Adolescents with XLA are also at greater risk for developing malignancy, usually leukemia, in adolescence or adulthood (see Chapter 53).

Selective IgA Deficiency

This disorder is defined as the absence or marked reduction (<15 mg/dl) of serum IgA with normal levels of other immunoglobulins and intact cellular immunity. Selective IgA deficiency is the most common (and mildest) immunodeficiency, occurring as often as 1 in 400 subjects. Selective IgA deficiency is usually sporadic but occasionally is familial. It is also reported in relatives of patients with CVID.

Most adolescents are asymptomatic and their IgA deficiency is evident only by laboratory testing, but others experience recurrent respiratory infections, chronic diarrhea, allergy, or autoimmune disease. Adolescents with complete IgA deficiency may develop anti-IgA antibodies as a result of exposure to IgA in plasma or serum, and these antibodies can cause anaphylactic reactions when a serum product or blood is subsequently given. Symptomatic adolescents with an IgA deficiency should also be tested for IgG subclasses (see later).

Treatment is usually not necessary, but continuous antibiotics may be needed for those with persistent respiratory infections. Administration of IgG or plasma may be contraindicated because of the possible anaphylaxis from sensitization to exogenous IgA, and a medical alert bracelet is recommended. A few patients with IgA deficiency have been reported to remit spontaneously.

IgG Subclass Deficiencies

Immunoglobulin subclass deficiencies are antibody deficiencies associated with increased susceptibility to infection and the absence or severe reduction of one or two IgG subclasses, but with normal levels of other subclasses. Normal or near-normal total IgG and other immunoglobulin levels are usually present, but there is decreased antibody responsiveness. Chronic respiratory infections, otitis media, chronic lung disease, and recurrent meningitis may occur, but milder cases may not be recognized until adolescence. IgG1 comprises 70% of the total IgG and therefore isolated IgG1 deficiency

Table 92–4. Clinical and Laboratory Features of Primary Immunodeficiencies

DISORDER*	CLINICAL FEATURES	AGE OF ONSET†	LABORATORY FINDINGS
B-cell (antibody) deficiency			
X-linked agammaglobulinemia (XL)	Recurrent pyogenic infections	Infancy	Absent Ig, absent B cells, normal T cells
Hyper-IgM immunodeficiency (XL)	Lymphadenopathy, recurrent bacterial infections	Infancy to early childhood	Low IgG, normal or elevated IgM, neutropenia
IgA deficiency	Most asymptomatic; respiratory infections	Infancy to adulthood	Low IgA, low IgG2 subclass in symptomatic adolescents
Common variable immunodeficiency	Recurrent sinopulmonary, gastrointestinal disease	Childhood to fourth decade	Low Ig, B cells present
X-linked lymphoproliferative syndrome (XL)	Severe mononucleosis with Epstein-Barr virus infection	Infancy to early childhood	Low Ig and B cells, decreased natural killer cells
Immunodeficiency with thymoma	Sinopulmonary infections, diarrhea	Fourth decade or older	Low Ig and few B cells, red cell aplasia
T-cell (cellular) deficiency			
DiGeorge syndrome	Congenital heart disease, tetany, characteristic facies, thrush	Infancy	Hypocalcemia, low T-cell numbers and decreased function
Nezelof syndrome (cellular immunodeficiency with immunoglobulins)	Bronchiectasis, viral and bacterial infections, diarrhea	Infancy	Low T-cell numbers and decreased function, low specific Ig
Combined immunodeficiency with adenosine deaminase or nucleoside phosphorylase deficiency (AR)	Bacterial and viral infections	Infancy	Lymphopenia, poor T-cell function, absent enzymes
Ataxia-telangiectasia (AR)	Ataxia, telangiectasia on conjunctivae and ears, sinusitis	Infancy to childhood	Decreased IgE, chromosome defects
Wiskott-Aldrich syndrome (XL)	Eczema, petechiae, melena	Infancy	Thrombocytopenia, increased IgA and IgE decreased IgM
Chronic mucocutaneous candidiasis	Thrush, nail infection caused by *Candida albicans*	Infancy to adulthood	Low T-cell numbers to *Candida* antigen, endocrine abnormalities
Short-limbed dwarfism	Dwarfism, sparse hair, infections	Infancy	Abnormal hair and skeleton, decreased T-cell function and numbers
Phagocytic disorders			
Hyper-IgE	Dermatitis, sinopulmonary infections	Infancy to adulthood	High IgE (>2000 IU/ml), eosinophilia
Leukocyte adhesion deficiency (AR)	Periodontitis, delayed umbilical cord separation	Infancy to adolescence (partial forms)	Leukocytosis, lack of complement receptors on leukocytes
Congenital (Kostman) or cyclic neutropenia	Sinopulmonary infections, bacterial sepsis	Infancy (Kostman) to adulthood (cyclic)	Neutropenia, eosinophilia, monocytosis
Chronic granulomatous disease (XL or AR)	Lymphadenopathy, pneumonia, abscesses	Infancy to adolescence	Failure to reduce nitroblue tetrazolium, defective bactericidal response
Chediak-Nigashi syndrome (AR)	Oculocutaneous albinism, peripheral neuropathy	Infancy to adolescence	Abnormal granules in all leukocytes
Myeloperoxidase (MPO) deficiency	Most asymptomatic; candidiasis	Childhood to adulthood	Lack of MPO in neutrophils, abnormal chemiluminescence
Complement deficiency			
C1q (AR)	Infections, autoimmune disease	Childhood to adulthood	Decreased total complement, absent C1q
C1r, C4, C2 (AR)	Autoimmune disease	Childhood to adolescence	Decreased total complement, absent components
C3, C5	Pyogenic infections, autoimmune disease	Infancy to adolescence	Decreased total complement, absent components
C6, C7, C8, C9 (AR)	*Neisseria* infections	Childhood to adulthood	Absent components, decreased total complement (except for C9)
Properdin deficiency (AR)	Meningococcal meningitis	Infancy to adolescence	Abnormal alternative pathway, normal (classic) pathway
Hereditary angioedema (AD)	Sudden swelling of face, laryngeal edema, abdominal pain	Childhood to adulthood	Lack C1 inhibitor, low C4, normal C3

*Mode of inheritance: XL, X-linked; AR, autosomal recessive; AD, autosomal dominant.
†Age at which significant symptoms occur that make diagnosis likely. Diagnosis may often be made earlier by laboratory evaluation.

results in panhypogammaglobulinemia. Selective or combined deficiency of IgG2 (<50 mg/dl) or IgG3 (<25 mg/dl) with or without IgG4 deficiency is the most common subclass deficiency. Adolescents with IgG2 deficiency (selective or combined with another subclass deficiency) often have impaired antibody responses to polysaccharide antigens and/or an associated IgA deficiency (<15 mg/dl). Adolescents with documented IgG subclass deficiencies may benefit from immunoglobulin injections or infusions, such as those used for adolescent patients with X-linked agammaglobulinemia. Subclass deficiencies in young children may be transient in nature and disappear with age.

Common Variable Immunodeficiency

This heterogeneous disorder occurs in both sexes and is characterized by the onset of recurrent bacterial infections in the second or third decade as a result of markedly decreased immunoglobulin and specific antibody levels. The presence of normal numbers of B cells distinguishes CVID from X-linked agammaglobulinemia. Cellular immunity is usually intact but may be impaired in some adolescent patients, and T-cell immunoregulatory abnormalities have been described. Autoimmune abnormalities, including Addison disease, thyroiditis, and rheumatoid arthritis, are not uncommon in these adolescents and their relatives. Diarrhea, malabsorption, and nodular lymphoid hyperplasia of the gastrointestinal tract are sometimes present, and bronchiectasis often develops. Immunologic abnormalities vary among adolescent patients—that is, excessive T-suppressor activity, deficient T-helper activity, intrinsic defects of B-cell function, and autoantibodies.

Treatment involves lifelong immunoglobulin replacement.

DiGeorge Syndrome (Thymic Hypoplasia)

This congenital immunodeficiency is characterized clinically by hypocalcemic tetany, aortic and cardiac anomalies, characteristic facies, and increased susceptibility to infection; pathologically, by the absence or hypoplasia of the thymus and parathyroid glands; and immunologically, by partial or complete T-cell immunodeficiency but normal or near-normal B-cell immunity. Recurrent infections begin soon after birth. The cause seems to be an interruption of the normal growth of pharyngeal pouch structures near the eighth week of gestation, and the development of this disorder is associated with maternal alcoholism, chromosome 22 abnormalities, and other factors. The degree of immunodeficiency varies considerably among adolescents, and T-cell function sometimes improves spontaneously.

Some success has been achieved with fetal thymic transplants and bone marrow transplantation, but the severity of the heart disease often determines the eventual prognosis. Partial T-cell deficiency is compatible with prolonged survival if the cardiac defects can be corrected.

Combined Immunodeficiency

This group of disorders is characterized by congenital and often hereditary deficiency of both B- and T-cell systems, lymphoid aplasia, and thymic dysplasia, and includes severe combined immunodeficiency (SCID), adenosine deaminase (ADA) deficiency, and Nezelof syndrome. Most patients have an early onset (within 3 months of age) of infection with thrush, pneumonia, and diarrhea and, if left untreated, a progressive downhill course, with death before the age of 2 years.

Treatment with immunoglobulin and antibiotics (including *Pneumocystis carinii* prophylaxis) is indicated, but is not curative. The treatment of choice is bone marrow transplantation, and a parent may be used as a bone marrow donor (haplotype match) for these adolescents if a HLA-matched sibling is not available (see Chapter 54).

More recently developed treatment involves replacement of the biologic factors that the adolescent may be lacking. Adolescents with ADA deficiency may now be treated with weekly subcutaneous injections of bovine ADA bound to polyethylene glycol (PEG), which greatly prolongs the half-life of this enzyme and makes it less antigenic. ADA deficiency has been treated in one patient to date by infusion of autologous lymphoid cells in which the defective gene has been replaced with a normal one. Interleukin-2, which may now be produced by recombinant methods, may also be bound to PEG and given as weekly intravenous injections to treat some adolescent patients with defective T-cell function.

Ataxia-Telangiectasia

This autosomal recessive, progressive, multisystem disorder is characterized by cerebellar ataxia, telangiectasia of the conjunctivae and skin, recurrent sinopulmonary infections, and variable immunologic disease.

Both neurologic symptoms and evidence of immunodeficiency vary in onset. Ataxia usually develops at about the time when children begin to walk, and leads to severe disability. Slurred speech, choreoathetoid movements, ophthalmoplegia, and muscle weakness generally progress as the disease advances. Telangiectasias develop between 1 and 6 years of age, most prominently on the bulbar conjunctivae and ears, and recurrent sinopulmonary infections may begin in early childhood, leading to recurrent pneumonia, bronchiectasis, and chronic lung disease. Endocrine abnormalities may occur, including gonadal dysgenesis, testicular atrophy, and diabetes mellitus.

There is a high degree of malignancy (especially leukemia, brain tumors, and gastric cancer) that may occur in children, adolescents, or adults, and an increased frequency of chromosome breaks, probably indicative of a defect in DNA repair. Heterozygotes for this disease are also at greater risk for malignancies, particularly breast cancer in females, but do not have the other associated manifestations. Adolescent patients often lack IgA and IgE and have cutaneous anergy and a progressive cellular immune defect. The serum α_2-fetoglobulin level is generally elevated.

Treatment of the immunodeficiency with antibiotics or gamma globulin is of some value, but there is no effective treatment for the central nervous system abnormalities. The course is therefore one of progressive neurologic deterioration with choreoathetosis, muscle weakness, and dementia, although some adolescent patients survive into the third or fourth decade.

Wiskott-Aldrich Syndrome

Wiskott-Aldrich Syndrome (WAS), an X-linked recessive disorder of male infants, is characterized by eczema, thrombocytopenia, and recurrent infection. The first manifestations are often hemorrhagic (usually bloody diarrhea), followed by the development of recurrent respiratory infections. Malignancy (especially lymphoma and acute lymphoblastic leukemia) is common in children who survive beyond the first decade; this risk increases with increasing age. Characteristic immunologic defects include poor antibody responses to polysaccharide antigens, cutaneous anergy, partial T-cell immunodeficiency, elevated levels of IgE and IgA, low levels of IgM, and normal IgG levels. Because of the combined deficiency in both B- and T-cell functions, infections occur from pyogenic bacteria, viruses, fungi, and *Pneumocystis carinii*. Hematologically, adolescent patients have small platelets and increased splenic destruction of platelets; accordingly, splenectomy may alleviate the thrombocytopenia (see Chapter 52). Vasculitis, glomerulonephritis, and inflammatory bowel disease have also been reported in adolescent WAS patients.

Treatment consists of splenectomy, continuous antibiotics, and intravenous immunoglobulin (not intramuscular, because of risk of hemorrhage). Bone marrow transplantation has been successful, and is the treatment of choice if an HLA-matched sibling donor is available.

Chronic Mucocutaneous Candidiasis

Chronic mucocutaneous candidiasis (CMC) is a cellular immunodeficiency characterized by persistent *Candida* infection of the mucous membranes, scalp, skin, and nails, and is often associated with an endocrinopathy, particularly hypothyroidism. Onset may be in infancy, with the occurrence of persistent thrush, or may be delayed until adolescence or even late adulthood. The disorder is somewhat more frequent in females than in males. The disease ranges in severity from involvement of a single nail to generalized mucous membrane, skin, and hair involvement, and disfiguring lesions of the face and scalp. Systemic candidiasis does not occur. Several clinical patterns exist, including an autosomal recessive form associated with hypoparathyroidism and Addison disease (*Candida*-endocrinopathy syndrome).

The characteristic immunologic findings are cutaneous anergy to *Candida* and absent proliferative responses to *Candida* antigen (but normal responses to mitogens), although antibody responses to *Candida* and other antigens are normal. Associated findings in some cases include bronchiectasis, hepatitis, and biotin deficiency with carboxylase enzyme deficiency.

Treatment consists of local (nystatin, clotrimazole) or systemic (ketoconazole, fluconazole, amphotericin B) antifungal drugs. Affected nails may have to be removed surgically. Immunotherapy with transfer factor, thymic epithelium, thymic hormones, or immune lymphocytes is not of permanent benefit. Bone marrow transplantation has been successful in a single case.

Hyper-IgE Syndrome

Hyper-IgE (HIE) syndrome is an immunodeficiency syndrome characterized by recurrent staphylococcal infections, particularly of the skin and lungs, and by markedly elevated levels of IgE. The staphylococcal infection may involve the skin, lung, upper airways, and other sites. Other common pathogens include *Candida albicans*, *Haemophilus influenzae*, streptococci, and pneumococci. Physical examination reveals eczematous skin disease, often starting in infancy, coarse facial features, and "cold abscesses," or those lacking the usual inflammatory features of an infection. Osteopenia and recurrent fractures may occur, possibly because of increased osteoclastic activity. All have exceptionally elevated IgE levels, usually in the range of 20,000 IU/ml. Other laboratory features include tissue and blood eosinophilia and an elevated erythrocyte sedimentation rate. Neutrophil chemotactic defects occur to a variable degree and may be caused by a serum factor. The basic defect in HIE may be an immunoregulatory T-cell abnormality, and abnormalities in both T- and B-lymphocyte functions have been reported.

Treatment consists of prompt administration of antibiotics to treat new infections; the goal is to prevent permanent lung injury, such as empyemas and pneumatoceles, that often develop as the adolescent patients get older. The use of prophylactic antibiotics, such as trimethoprim-sulfamethoxazole or dicloxacillin, is also recommended, as well as antifungal agents for some adolescents. Adolescent HIE patients have been treated with γ-interferon, which decreases IgE levels, but the clinical impact of this therapy is not yet known. Plasmapheresis, intravenous IgG, and γ-interferon have also been reported to have had some success.

Chronic Granulomatous Disease

This inherited disorder of leukocyte bactericidal function (see Chapter 52) is characterized by widespread granulomatous lesions of the skin, lungs, liver, and lymph nodes. The clinical pattern is one of recurrent infections by catalase-producing organisms, such as *Staphylococcus aureus*, *Serratia*, *Escherichia coli*, and *Pseudomonas* sp., as well as by fungi, such as *Aspergillus*. The organisms survive intracellularly and this continued antigenic stimulus may account for the granuloma formation.

The onset of disease is usually in infancy or early childhood, but it may not be diagnosed until the early teens. Clinical features include suppurative lymphadenitis, hepatosplenomegaly, pneumonia, and hematologic evidence of chronic infection. Persistent rhinitis, dermatitis, diarrhea, perianal abscesses, stomatitis, osteomyelitis, brain abscess, obstructive gastrointestinal and genitourinary tract lesions (from granuloma formation), and delayed growth also occur. The increased risk for fungal infections, especially by *Aspergillus,* can result in abscesses in the brain or liver.

The laboratory diagnosis of CGD, as well as its clinical management, are discussed in Chapter 52.

Leukocyte Adhesion Deficiency

Leukocyte adhesion deficiency (LAD) is an autosomal recessive disorder of leukocyte function characterized by recurrent or progressive necrotic soft tissue infection, severe periodontitis, poor wound healing, leukocytosis (even when not infected), and delayed (by more than 3 weeks) umbilical cord detachment. Severely affected infants have multiple infections with a rapidly progressive downhill course but moderately affected children have a less severe course, with many reaching adolescence. The severity is correlated with the degree of deficiency of specific glycoproteins on the surface of the leukocytes that anchor cells to surfaces, promote bacterial adherence, and serve as receptors for opsonic complement component C3bi. There are actually three different surface glycoprotein receptors lacking on these cells (CD11a, CD11b, and CD11c). Each is comprised of a β chain and one of three different α chains. The defect is in the β chain, with the result that none of the receptors are expressed on the surface.

The granulocytes and lymphocytes are defective in chemotaxis, natural killer activity, antibody-dependent cytotoxicity, and phagocytosis of bacteria. Diagnosis is established by demonstrating an absence or severe deficiency of these antigens on the surface of leukocytes, using monoclonal antibodies (anti-CD11) and flow cytometry.

Treatment consists of vigorous and often continuous antibiotic therapy. Bone marrow transplantation has been curative in a few cases. The gene responsible for the defect in LAD has been transfected in LAD cells *in vitro.* This allows these cells to express the CD11 proteins, thus making these adolescent patients candidates for genetic engineering.

REFERENCES

General References

Ellis EF, Middleton E, Reed CE: Allergy: Principles and Practice, 3rd ed. St. Louis, CV Mosby, 1988.

Groopman JE, Molina JM, Scadden DT: Hematopoietic growth factors: Biology and clinical applications. N Engl J Med 321:1449, 1989.

Samter M: Immunological Diseases, 4th ed, Vols I and II. Boston, Little, Brown & Co, 1988.

Stiehm ER: Immunologic Disorders in Infants and Children, 3rd ed. Philadelphia, WB Saunders, 1989.

Combined Disorders of Cellular and Humoral Immunity

Casper JT, Ash RA, Kirchner P, et al: Successful treatment with an unrelated-donor bone marrow transplant in an HLA-deficient patient with severe combined immune deficiency ("bare lymphocyte syndrome"). J Pediatr 116:262, 1990.

Pahwa R, Chatila T, Pahwa S, et al: Recombinant interleukin 2 therapy in severe combined immunodeficiency disease. Proc Natl Acad Sci USA 86:5069, 1989.

Rumelhart SL, Trigg ME, Horowitz SD, Hong R: Monoclonal antibody T-cell depleted HLA-haploidentical bone marrow transplantation for Wiskott-Aldrich syndrome. Blood 75:1031, 1990.

Disorders of Cellular Immunity

Herrod HG: Chronic mucocutaneous candidiasis in childhood and complications of non-candida infection: A report of the pediatric immunodeficiency collaborative study group. J Pediatr 116:377, 1990.

Mueller W, Peter HH, Wilken M, et al: The DiGeorge syndrome: I. Clinical evaluation and course of partial and complete forms of the syndrome. Eur J Pediatr 147:496, 1989.

Disorders of Immunoglobulin Production

Conley ME, Park CL, Douglas SD: Childhood common variable immunodeficiency with autoimmune disease. J Pediatr 108:915, 1986.

Lederman HM, Winkelstein JA: X-linked agammaglobulinemia: An analysis of 96 patients. Medicine 64:145, 1985.

Shackelford PG, Polmar SH, Mayus JL, et al: Spectrum of IgG2 subclass deficiency in children with recurrent infections: Prospective study. J Pediatr 108:647, 1986.

Stiehm ER: Human gamma globulins as therapeutic agents. Adv Pediatr 35:1, 1988.

Disorders of Phagocytic Cells

Anderson DC, Finegold MJ, Rothlein R, et al: The severe and moderate phenotypes of heritable Mac-1, LFA-1 deficiency: Their quantitative definition and relation to leukocyte dysfunction and clinical features. J Infect Dis 152:668, 1985.

Curnutte JT (ed): Phagocytic defects. I: Abnormalities outside of the respiratory burst. II: Abnormalities of the respiratory burst. Hematol/Oncol Clin North Am 2:1 (Pt I), 2:185 (Pt II), 1988.

Disorders of the Complement System

Frank MM: Complement in the pathophysiology of human disease. N Engl J Med 316:1525, 1987.

CHAPTER 93

Viral Infections

MEASLES, RUBELLA, AND OTHER VIRAL EXANTHEMS

MICHAEL RADETSKY

More than 75 viruses worldwide are known to produce exanthems. The majority of rash-producing viral infections that occur in North America are benign and require no therapy. However, the presence of an infectious rash is of great importance in clinical medicine because it gives the physician the ability to make a rapid, presumptive diagnosis based on physical findings alone. An early diagnosis would then facilitate (1) prognosis of the illness, (2) anticipation of complications, (3) assessment of communicability and prevention of spread, (4) selection of early treatment (when available) in the event of a serious manifestation or complication of infection, and (5) differentiation of other serious diseases with similar findings caused by pathogens that require specific therapy.

Viruses that produce rashes are excellent immunogens. With the exception of those viruses that persist in a latent form and have the capacity for reactivation (e.g., herpesviruses), a normal individual contracts any particular exanthematous viral infection only once. Furthermore, the early childhood immunizations for measles and rubella have created a pool of immune children who have not had infection with the wild virus. For these reasons, the incidence of acute exanthematous viral infections in adolescents is generally low. However, the exchange of secretions that occurs with close contact during adolescence affords the opportunity for transmission of viral agents of low communicability not previously encountered, such as Epstein-Barr virus (see Chapter 93). Also systemic viral disease, which is usually asymptomatic in infancy, may present with more vigorous manifestations in adolescents, including a visible rash. Finally, lack of immunologic responsiveness to childhood vaccines (primary vaccine failure) may become clinically apparent during adolescence, when epidemic spread occurs in schools, colleges, military camps, or other institutions in which young people are congregated together. Such a phenomenon has been seen recently with measles. Secondary vaccine failure (waning immunity) also may be a very important factor in adolescents' being susceptible to measles infection.

PATHOGENESIS

Viral infections affect the skin by three potential routes: local spread from an internal focus, systemic dissemination, or direct inoculation.

The classic viral exanthem results from a primary systemic viral infection with subsequent dissemination of the virus via blood (viremia) to the skin. The rash may be the result of viral replication in the epidermis, dermis, or dermal capillary endothelium or of host immune response to the viral infection, or both. Varicella and enteroviral infections are examples of viremic seeding of the skin. Erythema multiforme and the Stevens-Johnson syndrome may occur as postviral immunologic diseases with cutaneous findings. Measles and rubella are thought to produce both a direct viral effect and an immunologically mediated response.

The viruses causing warts, molluscum contagiosum, and primary herpes simplex infect the skin by direct inoculation and replicate in the epidermis. The cytopathic effects of viral replication account for the early lesions of the disease. Recurrent herpes simplex and varicella-zoster infections represent spread to the skin of viral elements residing in deeper sites, the sensory ganglia.

CLINICAL MANIFESTATIONS, DIAGNOSIS, AND TREATMENT

Not all acute exanthems are caused by viruses. Serious bacterial, rickettsial, and immunologic conditions can present with similar physical findings. For this reason, differentiation among causative organisms is vital. The history and clinical findings can be used to determine most of these causes or to indicate the strong probability of their presence. The data from history, including prodromal symptoms, characteristics of the rash, eye findings, oral mucous membrane involvement, hand and feet involvement, desquamation, and special suggestive or pathognomonic findings, usually lead to the correct diagnosis.

Exanthems due to Viral Pathogens

MEASLES

Although the incidence of measles has decreased by 99% since the introduction of measles vaccine in 1963, many recent outbreaks have been reported in school-aged children and adolescents. Two thirds of the new cases have occurred in previously vaccinated persons with low or absent antibody titers. A poor immune response to the primary immunization seems the most likely explanation for the persistence of the disease in this susceptible population.

Clinical measles in the unimmunized adolescent may be more severe than the condition is in younger children, with hepatitis and gastrointestinal symptoms as additional features of their illness. Measles in adolescents with primary vaccine failure may not have these more serious features.

1. *Prodrome.* 3 to 4 days of fever, conjunctivitis, coryza, and cough.

2. *Rash.* Reddish-brown, maculopapular, discrete, progressing to confluence; spreads downward from the face; generalized by day 3.

3. *Eyes.* Purulent conjunctivitis.

4. *Oral cavity.* Koplik spots (punctate white papules on a red base) on oral mucosa preceding and during the early stages of the rash; red macular enanthem on palate.

5. *Hands and feet.* Rash may be present.

6. *Desquamation.* Branny, fine scales; hands and feet do not desquamate.

7. *Pathognomonic features.* Koplik spots; the "five C's" of conjunctivitis, coryza, cough, "Koplik" spots, and crabbiness.

8. *Diagnosis.* Serology (greater than fourfold rise in hemagglutination-inhibition titers).

9. *Treatment.* None; secondary bacterial pneumonia may be a complication.

10. *Immunization.* The measles vaccine currently used in the United States is the Moraten vaccine, similar to the Schwarz strain first introduced in 1965. In children immunized after 15 months of age, protective efficacy is 95%.

Reimmunization policy (see Chapter 25). For susceptible individuals exposed to measles, two approaches are recommended: (1) live measles vaccine given within 72 hours of exposure; (2) immune serum globulin, 0.25 to 0.5 ml/kg (max = 15 ml) intramuscularly.

RUBELLA

1. *Prodrome.* Variable, 1 to 4 days of malaise and low-grade fever; temperature may be normal.

2. *Rash.* Pink, maculopapular, discrete; begins on face, generalized by 24 hours, disappears by 3rd day; may have appearance of acne on face; pruritic in older children.

3. *Eyes.* Mild to no conjunctivitis.

4. *Oral cavity.* Enanthem of red macules, pinpoint to blotches, on soft palate (Forschheimer spots) during first day of rash.

5. *Hands and feet.* May be involved.

6. *Desquamation.* Fine scales to no desquamation.

7. *Pathognomonic features.* Lymphadenopathy, especially posterior auricular and occipital.

8. *Diagnosis.* Positive viral throat culture; serology (multiple techniques).

9. *Treatment.* None.

10. *Immunization* (see Chapter 25). The rubella vaccine in current use is prepared in human diploid cell culture. In clinical trials, 95% or more of susceptible persons who received a single dose of rubella vaccine when they were 12 months of age or older developed antibody, and 90% of vaccines are expected to have protection against both clinical rubella and asymptomatic viremia for a period of at least 15 years. Vaccine virus is nontransmissible. It is available as a monovalent vaccine or in combination with measles vaccine alone or with measles and mumps vaccines.

Immunization is recommended not for the sake of the immunized host, but for the sake of preventing congenital rubella syndrome in the next generation. A history of natural rubella is unreliable. Therefore, all adolescents should be immunized unless there is a positive immunization history. Although there is no evidence to suggest that rubella vaccine induces congenital rubella syndrome when given to a pregnant female, women known or likely to be pregnant should not be immunized. Ten percent to 15% of susceptible adolescent women may have arthritis-like symptoms 3 to 25 days following rubella immunization. Immune serum globulin given after exposure to rubella does not prevent infection or viremia. (See Chapter 25 for further information.)

With the advent of routine immunization in infancy, clinical rubella has become a rare event. However, silent reinfection may be common, occurring in up to 80% of immunized individuals during rubella epidemics. In adolescent females, arthritis and arthralgia during clinical rubella are common. Arthralgias and frank arthritis are important adverse effects of the vaccine when administered to this group of older girls. Rubella encephalitis is generally uncommon, but older individuals are at a higher risk for this complication. There is no evidence that waning immunity following immunization is clinically important, and reimmunization during adolescence is not recommended.

ERYTHEMA INFECTIOSUM

Erythema infectiosum is caused by human parvovirus B19 (HPV). It is an epidemic disease of school children. Respiratory spread is presumed to be the route of infection. The period of viremia is usually silent or minimally symptomatic, and the clinical onset of erythema infectiosum begins 2 weeks later as a postinfectious phenomenon when the young person is no longer contagious. Adolescents tend to have a higher risk of joint involvement with this virus. Since HPV preferentially infects erythrocyte precursors in the bone marrow, reticulocytopenia and a falling hematocrit routinely occur, beginning 1 week before the appearance of the rash. This fall in red cell mass poses no risk to normal adolescents. However, in adolescents with any chronic hemolytic anemia (e.g., sickle cell disease), HPV induces an aplastic crisis, with severe anemia and shock (see Chapter 52). HPV during pregnancy carries a measurable risk of fetal demise or nonimmune hydrops fetalis. There is no immunization available.

1. *Prodrome*. None.

2. *Rash*. There are three phases. The first phase begins as bright red, erysipeloid exanthem of cheeks ("slapped cheeks"). During the second phase, 1 to 4 days later, a generalized erythematous maculopapular, discrete rash is prominent on extensor surfaces, with central clearing becoming lace-like. The third phase occurs subsequently as 1 to 3 weeks of fading and disappearance of the rash.

3. *Eyes*. Usually uninvolved.

4. *Oral cavity*. Usually uninvolved.

5. *Hands and feet*. Usually uninvolved; one case report of rash on palms and soles.

6. *Desquamation*. None.

7. *Pathognomonic features*. Slapped face appearance in a well adolescent; joint pain, joint swelling, or myalgias in adolescents.

8. *Diagnosis*. Elevated IgM or IgG titer rise to parvovirus B19.

9. *Treatment*. None.

VARICELLA

Five to ten percent of individuals do not have early childhood infection with varicella-zoster virus. When the infection does occur during adolescence, the risk of complications increases and includes pneumonia and encephalitis. Asymptomatic viral pneumonia may occur in up to 15% of adolescents.

Pregnant women have the highest rate of severe infection. Infants born to mothers whose rash appears 5 days before or 2 days after delivery may subsequently succumb to a fetal neonatal varicella infection and should be treated with varicella-zoster immune globulin (VZIG) and, possibly, acyclovir. Preliminary information indicates that oral acyclovir (10 mg/kg/dose qid) attenuates the symptomatic infection in adolescents. In the immunocompromised patient, intravenous acyclovir is required.

1. *Prodrome*. 1 to 2 days of fever, malaise, headache, anorexia; may have no prodrome.

2. *Rash*. Small vesicles on erythematous base ("dewdrops on a rose petal"), progressing rapidly to pustules and rupturing with crust formation; pruritic; only vesicular rash to appear on scalp; new crops appear daily; lesions at various stages of evolution seen simultaneously.

3. *Eyes*. Palpebral lesions and conjunctivitis may be present.

4. *Oral cavity*. Vesicles transiently appear with rapid rupture to shallow ulcers.

5. *Hands and feet*. May be involved, but lesions are usually few in number.

6. *Desquamation*. None.

7. *Pathognomonic features*. Only vesicular disease to appear in scalp or to be present in various stages of evolution simultaneously.

8. *Diagnosis*. Tzanck scraping of a lesion showing multinucleated giant cells or intranuclear inclusion bodies; viral culture of throat or lesion.

9. *Treatment*. Acyclovir. VZIG prevents or attenuates varicella in exposed susceptible individuals if given within 96 hours of exposure. It is supplied in vials of 125 units each in a volume of 1.25 ml. The dose is one vial per 10 kg of body weight intramuscularly, with a maximum of five vials in the adult.

10. *Immunization*. A live attenuated varicella vaccine is manufactured but is not yet licensed for general use. It is highly immunogenic and provides protective efficacy of 95% or greater. It may be given in conjunction with the measles-mumps-rubella vaccine, and the likely delivery vehicle will be a quadrivalent MMRV vaccine to be given at age 15 months. Knowledge of the duration of immunity is still incomplete, but data from Japan suggest that it provides a minimum of 10 years of protection.

EPSTEIN-BARR VIRUS (see following subchapter)

Epstein-Barr virus (EBV) is a ubiquitous virus that infects most individuals prior to adolescence with few or no symptoms. Clinically aparent infectious mononucleosis syndrome (IM) appears most frequently when the primary infection occurs during the second decade of life.

1. *Prodrome*. 1 to 3 days of malaise, headache, sore throat.

2. *Rash*. Erythematous papular, "sandpaper-like"; may be scarlatiniform, urticarial, or hemorrhagic; occurs in 5% to 10% of EBV infection and in 50% to 100% of patients with EBV infection who take ampicillin.

3. *Eyes*. May have mild conjunctivitis; commonly have periorbital edema.

4. *Oral cavity*. Pharyngitis and tonsillitis (may be membranous or exudative), palatal enanthem.

5. *Hands and feet*. Not usually involved.

6. *Desquamation*. None.

7. *Pathognomonic features*. Membranous tonsillopharyngitis, diffuse lymphadenopathy, splenomegaly.

8. *Diagnosis* (see following subchapter).

9. *Treatment*. Poor response to current antiviral agents (see following subchapter).

ENTEROVIRUSES

Enteroviral infections pose no special risks for adolescents. The manifestations of disease depend on the infecting viral serotype. Viral meningitis, poliomyelitis syndrome, myocarditis, and pericarditis are caused by virulent strains. Protection against the three strains of poliovirus is ensured by proper immunization.

1. *Prodrome*. Variable; ranges from no prodrome to 3 to 4 days of fever and malaise.

2. *Rash*. Generalized erythematous and maculopapular; may be morbilliform, petechial, vesicular, urticarial, scarlatiniform.

3. *Eyes.* Mild to no conjunctivitis.
4. *Oral cavity.* May be involved with red maculae, vesicles, or ulcers.
5. *Hands and feet.* Occasionally involved.
6. *Desquamation.* None.
7. *Pathognomonic features.* Hand-foot-and-mouth syndrome; rash associated with aseptic meningitis during the summer or fall months.
8. *Diagnosis.* Viral culture of throat or stool.
9. *Treatment.* None.

ADENOVIRUSES

The 42 serotypes of adenovirus can cause infections in susceptible adolescents. Fifty percent of infections are subclinical. Symptomatic disease is usually respiratory, with pharyngitis, bronchitis, and bronchopneumonia all possible. Epidemic keratoconjunctivitis may be severe and extremely contagious. Rarely, central nervous system (CNS) infection may occur. Enteric strains of adenovirus (types 40 and 41) are a cause of acute diarrhea.

1. *Prodrome.* 1 to 2 days of fever, often with respiratory syndromes.
2. *Rash.* Erythematous, rubelliform, maculopapular; may mimic measles; occasionally petechial; spreads from face downward to trunk and extremities; lasts 3 to 5 days.
3. *Eyes.* Mild to severe conjunctivitis; may cause painful keratitis.
4. *Oral cavity.* Enanthem often present; red maculae to petechiae; palate often involved; pharyngitis common; may be associated with conjunctivitis (pharyngeal-conjunctival fever).
5. *Hands and feet.* May be involved.
6. *Desquamation.* None.
7. *Pathognomonic features.* Rash and respiratory symptoms; pharyngeal-conjunctival fever.
8. *Diagnosis.* Viral throat culture.
9. *Treatment.* None; susceptible to ribavirin *in vitro*.

HEPATITIS (see Chapter 62)

Hepatitis B virus (HBV) is transmitted by blood. Adolescents who receive tainted blood or blood products, who share intravenous needles, or who have sexual relations with HBV carriers all are at risk for acquiring the infection. The marker for infection is the presence of the hepatitis B surface antigen (HBsAg) in blood. Full recovery from acute HBV hepatitis may be prolonged, and 5% to 10% of patients become HBV carriers, with a future risk of chronic hepatitis, cirrhosis, and hepatocellular carcinoma. Up to 70% of infants born to HBV carrier mothers acquire the virus during birth, and one half of these infants become chronic HBV carriers. The highest prevalence of HBV chronic carriage is in central Africa, East Asia, and the Pacific Islands and among Eskimo populations. Pregnant adolescents originating from these areas or who fall into another of the HBV risk groups should be tested for HBsAg. If test results are positive, HBV immune globulin (HBIG) and HBV immunization should be given to the newborn child to prevent transmission.

1. *Prodrome.* Arthralgia or arthritis may precede the rash.
2. *Rash.* Rash precedes jaundice; generalized, erythematous, maculopapular, and/or urticarial; lasts 4 to 7 days; in younger children, papular acrodermatitis may occur (Gianotti-Crosti syndrome).
3. *Eyes.* May have mild conjunctivitis.
4. *Oral cavity.* Usually normal.
5. *Hands and feet.* May be involved.
6. *Desquamation.* None.
7. *Pathognomonic features.* Subsequent hepatitis.
8. *Diagnosis.* Hepatitis B surface antigen serology.
9. *Treatment.* None.

Exanthems due to Nonviral Pathogens

Even though the major focus of this chapter is on viral exanthems, nonviral exanthems are included for differential diagnostic purposes.

STREPTOCOCCAL SCARLET FEVER (see Chapter 94)

1. *Prodrome.* 12 hours to 2 days of fever and sore throat.
2. *Rash.* Erythematous, punctiform, diffuse erythredema; sandpaper-like texture; most intense in neck, axillary, inguinal, and popliteal folds (Pastia sign); circumoral pallor.
3. *Eyes.* Mild, nonpurulent conjunctivitis.
4. *Oral cavity.* Acute tonsillopharyngitis, strawberry tongue, palatal enanthem, red lips.
5. *Hands and feet.* Involved.
6. *Desquamation.* Begins on face with fine flaking; second week the torso and then the extremities begin to peel with large flakes or sheets; may last 3 to 8 weeks.
7. *Pathognomonic features.* Strawberry tongue and exudative pharyngitis.
8. *Diagnosis.* Streptococcal throat culture; in surgical scarlet fever, wound culture should be done. A toxic shock–like illness due to virulent strains of group A streptococci has recently been described (see Chapter 94).
9. *Treatment.* Penicillin.

STAPHYLOCOCCAL SCALDED SKIN SYNDROME VARIANTS (see Chapter 94)

1. *Prodrome.* None.
2. *Rash.* Ranges from a diffuse, painful erythroderma with positive Nikolsky sign to scarlatiniform rash similar to that of group A streptococci (staphylococcal scarlet fever).
3. *Eyes.* Moderate to severe purulent conjunctivitis.
4. *Oral cavity.* Spared.
5. *Hands and feet.* Involved.
6. *Desquamation.* May be gross, with sheets of superficial epidermis, or may have diffuse flaking.
7. *Pathognomonic features.* Positive Nikolsky sign, combination of purulent conjunctivitis with normal oral mucous membranes.

8. *Diagnosis.* Skin biopsy showing intraepidermal cleavage plane; isolation of phage group 2 exfoliation-toxin–producing *Staphylococcus aureus.*

9. *Treatment.* Antistaphylococcal antimicrobials (see Chapter 96).

TOXIC SHOCK SYNDROME (see Chapter 94)

GONOCOCCAL DISEASE (see Chapter 97)

MENINGOCOCCEMIA

1. *Prodrome.* 0 to 1 day of fever, malaise, headache, vomiting.
2. *Rash.* Erythematous maculopapular, often becoming petechial; purpura may be present and is a grave prognostic sign.
3. *Eyes.* Mild to no conjunctivitis.
4. *Oral cavity.* Macular or petechial enanthem may be found.
5. *Hands and feet.* Involved.
6. *Desquamation.* None.
7. *Pathognomonic features.* Petechial or purpuric rash with signs of shock or meningitis.
8. *Diagnosis.* Blood culture, cerebrospinal fluid Gram stain or culture, Gram stain of aspirated skin lesions, urine antigen detection (sensitivity, 60%).
9. *Treatment.* Penicillin; supportive care for shock, meningitis, disseminated intravascular coagulation.

ROCKY MOUNTAIN SPOTTED FEVER (see Chapter 94)

ERYTHEMA MULTIFORME–STEVENS-JOHNSON SYNDROME

1. *Prodrome.* None.
2. *Rash.* Any morphologic feature possible; red maculae, papules, urticaria, petechiae, or bullae.
3. *Eyes.* Moderate to severely purulent conjunctivitis.
4. *Oral cavity.* Mild to severe involvement.
5. *Hands and feet.* Involved.
6. *Desquamation.* Mild to gross peeling.
7. *Pathognomonic features.* Rash following medications or a preceding illness compatible with *Mycoplasma pneumoniae infection,* herpes simplex, or other viral syndrome.
8. *Diagnosis.* The diagnosis is clinical and presumptive once other possible causes have been eliminated; skin biopsy may be helpful.

9. *Treatment.* None; corticosteroids do not alter the course of the illness.

LEPTOSPIROSIS

1. *Prodrome.* 4 to 7 days of fever and influenza-like symptoms; defervescence of 1 to 2 days; then onset of rash and headache.
2. *Rash.* Erythematous, maculopapular; jaundice seen in severe disease (Weil disease).
3. *Eyes.* Hyperemia.
4. *Oral cavity.* Mild to no involvement.
5. *Hands and feet.* Rarely involved.
6. *Desquamation.* None.
7. *Pathognomonic features.* Biphasic illness; aseptic meningitis; renal or hepatic involvement (Weil disease).
8. *Diagnosis.* Serology or isolation of organisms from urine (requires special growth media).
9. *Treatment.* Penicillin.

BIBLIOGRAPHY

Anderson LJ: Role of parvovirus B19 in human disease. Pediatr Infect Dis J 6:711, 1987.

Centers for Disease Control: Measles prevention: Recommendations of the Immunization Practices Advisory Committee (ACIP). MMWR 38(S-9):1, 1989.

Cherry JD: Viral exanthems. Curr Probl Pediatr 12(6):1, 1983.

Kirk JL, Fine DP, Sexton DJ, Muchmore HG: Rocky Mountain spotted fever. A clinical review based on 48 confirmed cases, 1943–1986. Medicine 69:35, 1990.

Krause PJ, Cherry JD, Deseda-Tous J, et al: Epidemic measles in young adults. Clinical, epidemiologic, and serologic studies. Ann Intern Med 90:873, 1979.

Krugman S, Katz SL, Gershon AA, Wilfert C: Diagnosis of acute exanthematous diseases. In Krugman S, Katz SL, Gershon AA, et al (eds): Infectious Diseases of Children, 8th ed. St. Louis, CV Mosby, 1985, pp 454–462.

Larkowitz LE, Preblud SR, Fine PEM, Orenstein WA: Duration of live measles vaccine–induced immunity. Pediatr Infect Dis J 9:101, 1990.

Mann JM, Preblud SR, Hoffman RE, et al: Assessing risks of rubella infection during pregnancy. A standardized approach. JAMA 245:1647, 1981.

Rapp CE, Jr, Hewetson JF: Infectious mononucleosis and the Epstein-Barr virus. Am J Dis Child 132:78, 1978.

Straus SE, Ostrove JM, Inchauspe G, et al: Varicella-zoster virus infections. Biology, natural history, and prevention. Ann Intern Med 108:221, 1988.

Todd JK: Staphylococcal toxin syndromes. Annu Rev Med 36:337, 1985.

EPSTEIN-BARR VIRUS INFECTIONS

JAMES F. JONES

HISTORICAL PERSPECTIVE AND BACKGROUND

Burkitt's identification of a high incidence of head and neck lymphoid tumors (Burkitt lymphoma, BL) in young males in Uganda suggested to Epstein a possible viral link in the development of those tumors. Epstein and colleagues failed to identify virus in tumor tissue *per se* but found herpes-like virus particles in cultures of tumor cells. The new virus was identified as a member of the herpes family by Werner and Gertrude Henle, who named the agent the Epstein-Barr virus (EBV) after two of its discoverers. The Henles subsequently developed immunofluorescent antibody techniques that identified anti-EBV antibodies in patients with BL and in adults, but not young children, in the general population in the United States. The presence of antibodies to the virus suggested acquisition after a common infectious disease. Anti-EBV antibodies in a previously seronegative laboratory worker following acute infectious mononucleosis (IM) led to the subsequently well-proven association among EBV and most cases of IM.

IM had been described as glandular fever in Europe in the late 1890s. The illness was also recognized in the United States; diagnosis was based on the classic clinical features (exudative tonsillitis, lymphadenopathy, and fever) and on relative or absolute lymphocytosis with greater than 20% atypical lymphocytes. After 1939, a positive heterophile test was used, and today a rapid slide test is available. Thus, the prototype illness associated with EBV became infectious mononucleosis.

EPIDEMIOLOGY

The epidemiology of IM, however, is not the epidemiology of EBV. Classic EBV-induced IM occurs primarily in adolescents and young adults, although several reports have suggested that typical IM may be more common in preadolescents than was suspected originally. The diagnostic hallmark in these cases is a positive heterophile test. Application of the specific serologic tests developed by the Henles to sera from young children, patients with heterophile-negative IM-like illnesses, and groups of all ages, has yielded the following information:

1. Over 90% of adults worldwide have anti-EBV antibodies; this level is attained by the age of 5 years in underdeveloped nations, but at the age of 30 in the United States and other developed countries.

2. Only 33% of persons with anti-EBV antibodies describe IM or an IM-like illness.

3. In the United States, infection occurs before 6 years of age in 15% of middle-class children and in 80% of underprivileged children (these figures may increase as more children attend child care facilities).

4. Subsequent antibody acquisition occurs infrequently in the 6- to 10-year age group, but occurs in 15% of adolescents annually between 11 and 15 years of age.

5. Intrafamilial virus transmission occurs in 20% to 26% of family members when someone in the family has IM; illness, however, may not occur at the same frequency.

6. Excretion of virus in the saliva occurs in 20% to 100% of asymptomatic, permanently infected children, adolescents, and adults.

There is, therefore, widespread exposure to the virus, but limited disease expression. The expression of disease depends on the individual clinical presentation with a particular infectious agent. Because infectious mononucleosis is the prototypic illness associated with EBV in the Western world, it is the disease that physicians expect to be associated with EBV, particularly in adolescents. Other illnesses associated with EBV seroconversion that occur in children and adolescents, and that may be as common or even more common than IM, include typical upper respiratory tract infections, pharyngitis, tonsillitis, lymphadenopathy, and unexplained exanthema (see previous subchapter). Observations about the expression of symptoms in families suggest that IM is the illness seen in multiple family members in certain families, but may be rare in others.

PATHOPHYSIOLOGY

Etiologic Agent

The structure of the virus on electron microscopy is that of a protein core surrounded by DNA, a nucleocapsid with 162 episomes, a protein matrix between the nucleocapsid, and an outer envelope with glycoprotein spikes. The viral genome is linear in the virion and consists of over 172,000 base pairs. The genome has been cloned and sequenced.

Mechanisms of Viral Action

There is considerable information about the events surrounding replication of the virus. After binding to the cell surface, entering the cytoplasm, and uncoating and entering the cell nucleus, the virus undergoes four basic stages of replication. The first stage is the production of proteins associated with the initiation and maintenance of latent infection (the EB nuclear antigens). The second and third stages are recognized by the production of early antigens and enzymes required for viral DNA synthesis, respectively. The last stage consists of the production of viral capsid antigens and membrane antigens. Assembly of these components is followed by the release of viral progeny and death of the cell (lytic infection).

A lytic infection does not always occur, however. There is also latent infection. A hallmark of EBV infection is the transformation of lymphocytes, with the viral genes encoding only the latent proteins. Multiple copies of the viral genome are maintained in the latent state, usually as free circular episomes. Only rarely does it appear that the viral genome is integrated into the host nuclear material. Latently infected lymphoid cells are found in the peripheral blood and the bone marrow, but rarely in peripheral lymph nodes. The virus may also persist in the latent state in salivary gland epithelial cells.

IMMUNE RESPONSE

The immune response to EBV is complex. This response results in the clinical and laboratory alterations of overt disease. The initial nonspecific response may be activation of the complement system with neutralization of virus. The initial cellular response appears to be mediated by natural killer cells. The role of monocytes and macrophages thought to be involved in response to viral infection in response to EBV is unknown. The soluble products of mononuclear cells (interferon, interleukins, and other cytokines) are also evident in early disease. The increase in peripheral blood lymphocytes is composed of CD8 lymphocytes primarily, which also constitute most of the atypical lymphocytes. There is also a marked proliferation of both infected and noninfected B lymphocytes, accompanied by the release of immunoglobulins. Some of these proteins are antinuclear or autoantibodies. As infection progresses and usually resolves, specific antibody and T-cell responses, particularly cytotoxic CD8+ cells that are antigen- and HLA-specific are detected. The resolution of illness is accompanied by the persistence of specific antibody responses (see Chapter 92) and specific CD8+ cells. These latter cells are important in the control of or response to reactivation of the latent infection.

It is commonly thought that IM is a disease of adolescence because of the uniqueness of the immune system at this time. Unfortunately, there are no data supporting this concept. The immunologic response is thought to have reached adult status by the age of 8 to 10 years, but IM is uncommon in this age range. Perhaps the uniqueness is of the immune response in younger children who do not have mature immune systems, rather than the uniqueness of the immune system in adolescence.

ILLNESS PRODUCTION

Infection with EBV begins with exposure to the virus through aerosol or saliva. The virus enters the oropharynx and binds either to immature epithelial cells or to B lymphocytes through the C3d receptor. The apparent natural ligand for the receptor is the d component of activated complement component C3. Pharyngeal epithelial cells are usually thought to be the primary site of binding and replication. In normal hosts, these cells include parotid cells and pharyngeal and buccal mucosal cells. In immunodeficient adolescent patients, epithelial cells of the tongue also become infected (hairy leukoplakia).

Infection of epithelial cells produces a lytic infection primarily, whereas infection of B lymphocytes leads to both lytic and latent infections. Injury to pharyngeal epithelial cells contributes in part to the pharyngitis. Mediator release, including interferons, allows enlargement of lymphoid tissue along with the proliferation of B and T lymphocytes. Mediator production and proliferative events account for the general symptoms, lymphadenopathy, and hepatosplenomegaly, as well as for the hematologic and immunologic changes that are hallmarks of EBV-related disease. For example, the muscle aches, fatigue, headache, and desire to sleep and be alone can be attributed to the presence of interferons. These cytokines also contribute to lymph node enlargement and activation of T lymphocytes, which make up most of the cells in the atypical lymphocytosis. These lymphocytes are mostly CD8-positive and function as cytotoxic-suppressor cells in controlling the B-cell proliferation and, presumably, infection of epithelial cells.

The CD8 population is also responsible for the production of other clinical and laboratory features seen in active disease, including hypogammaglobulinemia, leukopenia, thrombocytopenia, ineffective neutrophil oxidative burst responses, and aplastic anemia.

The mechanism responsible for elevated liver enzyme levels is unclear. The virus is not present in hepatic parenchymal cells, but there is a marked mononuclear cell infiltration of portal areas.

CLINICAL MANIFESTATIONS

As previously mentioned, IM is the "classic" disease associated with EBV in the United States and other developed countries. After exposure, the incubation period lasts 4 to 6 weeks. Illness begins with fatigue, malaise, and headache, followed by a sore throat and lymph node tenderness and swelling. In fact, lymphoid swelling throughout the ring of Waldeyer is common. Thirty per cent of patients have a "shaggy" exudate; its presence may strengthen the case for EBV in a given adolescent patient. Occasionally, marked edema of the pharynx and surrounding neck occurs. Fever up to 39.5°C or higher, lasting 7 to 10 days with a gradual decrease over 1 or 2 weeks is common.

Lymphadenopathy is not limited to the cervical chains and may occur in the axillary and inguinal regions, as well as in the mesentery and mediastinum. Splenomegaly occurs in 50% of adolescent patients and hepatomegaly in 10% to 25%. An interesting sign is eyelid edema, which may occur in 5% to 15% of adolescents with classic IM. The distribution of symptoms varies among adolescents and younger children. The classic skin eruptions of IM occur in 5% of adolescent patients, and more frequently in those taking ampicillin (see previous subchapter). The classic signs and symptoms are summarized in Table 93–1.

Classic EBV IM usually is readily recognizable. There

TABLE 93–1. Signs and Symptoms of Acute Infectious Mononucleosis

Lymphadenopathy	Malaise
Pharyngitis	Headache
Fever	Anorexia
Splenomegaly	Myalgias
Hepatomegaly	Chills
Palatal exanthem	Nausea
Jaundice	Abdominal discomfort
Rash	Cough
Sore throat	Vomiting
	Arthralgias

With permission from Jones JF: A perspective of Epstein-Barr virus disease. Adv Pediatr 36:307–346, 1989.

are numerous other possible clinical manifestations of EBV infection. Many of these problems precede, accompany, or follow classic IM. For example, an adolescent may present to the physician with bizarre behavior, including hallucinations, and be diagnosed as having schizophrenia, only to develop classic IM. Resolution of the IM accompanies complete resolution of the psychiatric symptoms of unknown pathophysiology.

Other possibilities include the development of known consequences of IM, such as aplastic anemia, without overt IM. In these cases, serologic evidence of acute

TABLE 93–2. Disease Processes Associated with EBV Infection

Neurologic effects
  Meningitis, encephalitis, meningoencephalitis
  Acute hemiplegia
  Acute cerebellar ataxia
  Psychoses: depression, schizophrenia
  Guillain-Barré syndrome
  Bell palsy
  Peripheral neuritis
  Acute transverse myelitis
  Sleep disturbances
  Cranial nerve involvement
Ophthalmologic consequences
  Follicular conjunctivitis
  Epithelial and strand keratitis
  Iridocyclitis
  Optic neuritis
  Retinitis without uveitis
  Choroiditis and panuveitis
Chest disease
  Pneumonia
  Lymphoid interstitial pneumonia
  Fibrosing alveolitis
  Pleural effusion
Hematologic consequences
  Thrombocytopenia
  Granulocytopenia
  Hemolytic uremic syndrome
  Aplastic anemia
  Chronic atypical lymphocytosis
  Hemophagocytic syndrome
Miscellaneous organ effects
  Myocarditis
  Pericarditis
  Adrenal infection
  Glomerulonephritis
  Pancreatitis
  Recurrent parotitis
  Papular acrodermatitis (Gianotti-Crosti syndrome)
  Urticaria (chronic and cold)

TABLE 93–3. Immunologic Consequences of EBV Infection

Autoantibody production
Autoimmune disease; Sjögren syndrome, rheumatoid arthritis (?)
Hypo- or hypergammaglobulinemia
Lymphoblastic lymphadenopathy

EBV infection and identification of viral DNA support causative role for the virus.

Table 93–2 lists EBV disease processes associated with EBV infection. It might be suggested that these manifestations are complications of IM. A complication, however, is a secondary process that occurs as a consequence of primary disease. Because these all occur in EBV-related disease that is not IM, and are a result either of direct virus involvement or of the host's response to the virus, they are not true complications. Airway obstruction caused by swollen pharyngeal lymphoid tissue is a complication. Anaerobic soft tissue infection of the pharyngeal wall is a complication, as are multiple abscesses secondary to the neutropenia that commonly accompanies EBV infection. Splenic rupture after trauma and subcapsular hematomas may also be considered complications.

Infections with other agents may occur concomitantly with EBV. For many years, a high incidence of β-hemolytic streptococcal infection was reported with IM. Most series suggested that up to 25% of cases were accompanied by streptococcal infections. Some authors raised the question of routine antibiotic therapy. More recent data suggest that fewer than 5% of adolescent IM patients have concurrent streptococcal infection, and therapy is advised only for culture-positive adolescent patients (see Chapter 94). *Mycoplasma pneumoniae* infections may also accompany primary IM, particularly if clinical pneumonia or pleural effusions are present (see Chapter 94). In addition, multiple herpesviruses may be present, with each contributing to the overall illness.

Because the virus infects a critical component of the immune system, and control of the infection depends on cytotoxic-suppressor T cells, natural killer cells, and other as yet unknown mechanisms, problems with the immune system may rarely occur (Table 93–3). The requirement for a normal immune response for resolution of EBV infection has been demonstrated by peculiar or prolonged courses in several congenital abnormalities (Table 93–4; see Chapter 92). Children with congenital abnormalities are particularly susceptible to tumor development.

Severe or chronic EBV diseases are being recognized with increasing frequency. The adolescent patient might have a classic case of IM. The hallmarks of these cases

TABLE 93–4. Congenital Abnormalities Associated With Severe or Fatal EBV Disease

X-linked and non–X-linked lymphoproliferation
Chediak-Higashi syndrome
Absent γ-interferon production
Ataxia-telangiectasia
Wiskott-Aldrich syndrome

are prolonged symptoms lasting months to years, versus a few weeks. The course of fever is prolonged or recurrent, with the oral temperature higher than 39°C. There are frequent hematologic and immunologic abnormalities—neutropenia, thrombocytopenia, hyper- or hypogammaglobulinemia. Pneumonia is common. The antibody titers are usually high, and have a distinctive pattern. Some of these adolescents have had prolonged illness with fulminant terminal courses associated with tumor development, particularly T-cell lymphomas. Occasionally, an adolescent with severe disease and evidence of virus replication may not produce specific anti-EBV antibodies.

PATHOLOGY

Histopathologic findings in typical IM are rarely reported. Lymphoid tissue is only obtained when the diagnosis is in question or surgery is performed to relieve respiratory tract obstruction, splenic abnormalities, or unrelated trauma. The common features of EBV-induced IM are reactive in nature and include follicular hyperplasia, expansion of T-cell zones (paracortical) with distortion of normal architecture, and focal preservation of sinuses. The sinuses, however, are filled with reactive cells and appear dilated. A number of peculiar cell types may be seen in the expanded paracortical region. These cells include Reed-Sternberg–like cells, transformed lymphocytes of varying sizes, and plasma cells. The changes are not uniform in adolescent patients, and may be highly suggestive of malignancy in some cases. Epithelioid changes are rare and can be differentiated from other disease processes.

MALIGNANCIES

Although the EBV was originally isolated from lymphoid tumors, virus-associated malignancies account for only a small percentage of disease in developed countries. The association of the virus with tumors in general remains a mystery. Does the virus induce changes in cells that lead to malignant transformation? Does the virus infect cells predetermined to be malignant, and contribute to the malignant transformation? Or, is the virus simply a passenger in malignant cells? BL cells don't always carry the EBV gene. Only 15% to 20% of Burkitt tumors in the United States carry the virus, whereas 90% or more of the African forms contain the virus. BL cells have chromosomal translocations involving immunoglobulin genes and the proto-oncogene c-myc. These translocations occur in tumors regardless of the presence of the virus.

The EBV genome is found in most, if not all, tumor cells in nasopharyngeal carcinoma (NPC). These tumors do not contain detectable chromosomal abnormalities. The relationship among other tumors listed in Table 93–5 and the presence of EBV in tumor cells is even less well appreciated.

Treatment of these malignancies is not addressed in this chapter. The reader is referred to relevant literature on the subject.

TABLE 93–5. Malignant Disease Associated With EBV

African and American (rare) Burkitt lymphoma
Nasopharyngeal carcinoma
Lymphoma (B and T cell); normal and immunodeficient hosts
Parotid gland tumor
Thymic epithelial lymphoma
Hodgkin disease (?)

TRANSPLANTATION

EBV-related disease in adolescent posttransplant patients (see Chapter 54) may take several forms. One is a severe primary infection in previously seronegative recipients. The infection may be airborne or may arise from latently infected donor cells. Adolescent patients receiving multiple transfusions are also at risk of receiving blood containing the virus. If the transplant is from a normal donor to a congenitally immunodeficient patient the outcome is often fatal, because the bone marrow may not function for a prolonged period and inherent immunity is absent or markedly diminished. Solid organ recipients have relatively or completely normal underlying immune function and respond to decreased suppressive therapy (see Chapter 54).

DIAGNOSIS

The diagnosis of EBV infection should be based on a high index of clinical suspicion. It should not be dependent on the heterophile or Monospot test. When positive, these nonspecific tests allow confirmation of 85% to 90% of typical EBV-associated infectious mononucleosis. These tests do not detect antibodies directed against EBV or any other specific infectious agent. Indeed, the epitope detected by heterophile antibodies is unknown. Although a positive slide test result may persist for several weeks to several months in rare cases of EBV-IM, false-positive test results may persist for years. False-positive in this context means that no specific evidence of EBV infection or of clinical IM has been found, and that blood specimens are negative for heterophile antibodies following ox cell absorption.

The lack of reliability of heterophile tests is particularly important in IM-like illnesses. These illnesses have some of the characteristics of IM but do not meet the usual diagnostic criteria, or they may have some of the hematologic or immune sequelae of IM but not the typical clinical disease pattern. These cases require specific diagnostic procedures to identify EBV or the other infectious agents that may produce these illnesses. Table 93–6 presents the heterophile antibody response and the types of serologic responses to EBV using the test system devised by the Henles.

Figure 93–1 illustrates the typical antibody response in acute infectious mononucleosis. It is not known whether similar responses occur in asymptomatic infected adolescents or in those with other EBV-related illnesses.

The interpretation of anti-EBV antibody titers (see Table 93–6) is based on the following premises:

TABLE 93–6. Serologic Diagnosis of EBV Infections

OLD WAY: HETEROPHILE ANTIBODY	AFTER ABSORPTION WITH	
	Guinea Pig Kidney	Beef RBCs
IM	+	−
Serum sickness	−	+
Normal serum	−	−

NEW WAY: SPECIFIC ANTIBODY	VCA IgG	VCA IgM	EA	EBNA
No past infection	−	−	−	−
Acute IM	+	+	+ (D)	−
Convalescent IM	+	+ or −	+ or −	−
Past infection	+	+ or −	Low + or −	+
Reactivated or chronic	+	+ or −	High +	Low + or −

IM, infectious mononucleosis; RBC, red blood cell; VCA, viral capsid antigen; EA, early antigen; EBNA, Epstein-Barr nuclear antigens.

With permission from Jones JF: A perspective of Epstein-Barr virus disease. Adv Pediatr 36:307, 1989.

1. Anti-VCA (viral capsid antigen) antibodies appear first.

2. Anti-EA (early antigen) antibodies appear next or are present with anti-VCA early in the course of illness.

3. With diminution (resolution) of symptoms, anti-VCA and anti-EA antibodies decrease and anti-EBNA (Epstein-Barr nuclear antigens) appears.

4. In the postinfection period, anti-VCA and anti-EBNA antibodies are always present; occasionally, anti-EA may similarly be present in low titers.

Other premises that may not always be correct are the following: antibodies to EBV persist for life; an antibody titer to EA greater than 80 is indicative of active disease (primary, chronic, or reactivated); and anti-EBNA antibodies are indicative of resolution and, therefore, of inactive disease. It must be emphasized that the titers described here may not be found in the

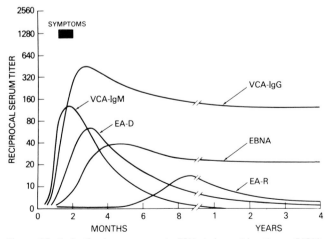

Figure 93–1. Antibody responses to EBV viral capsid antigens (VCA), early antigens (EA-D, EA-R), and nuclear antigens (EBNA) following exposure to the virus. (Jones JF, Straus SE: Chronic Epstein-Barr virus infection. Annu Rev Med 38:195, 1987. Reproduced, with permission, from the Annu Rev Med Vol. 38, © 1987 by Annual Reviews Inc.)

same range in every laboratory—higher or lower values may be normal for a given laboratory.

An anti-VCA titer of 640 or more, an anti-EA–diffuse or EA-restricted titer of 80 or more, or an anti-EBNA titer of 5 or less is unusual in asymptomatic adolescents; whereas they are seen in various conditions known or assumed to be immune dysfunctional viral states and reactivation of lytic infection. For instance, adolescents with severe EBV disease have anti-VCA levels greater than 10,000, anti-EA levels greater than 640, and low to absent anti-EBNA titers. Frequently, these patients have elevated IgA anti-EA levels and may have antibodies against specific virus-encoded enzymes, such as DNA polymerase and DNase. Except for the adolescents with severe disease, there is no correlation between anti-EBV titers and the severity of clinical IM.

Identification of the virus is performed by immunofluorescent antibody techniques or by examination of tissues, cells, secretions, and even plasma or serum for viral nucleic acid, using either *in situ* hybridization or the polymerase chain reaction, a gene amplification technique.

EBV may be isolated by culturing filtered saliva specimens with human cord blood lymphocytes and by inducing transformation of these target cells. Lymphoid cells from peripheral blood or bone marrow or tumor may themselves replicate, as detected by outgrowth in tissue culture. This latter phenomenon is rare in normal adolescents, but occurs commonly in immunosuppressed adolescent patients.

DIFFERENTIAL DIAGNOSIS

Infectious organisms other than EBV may produce typical IM and/or IM-like diseases. Although classic IM caused by these organisms is relatively uncommon, it may occur in 10% of cases, particularly in adolescents. The causative agents are cytomegalovirus, parvovirus, adenovirus, human immunodeficiency virus-1 (HIV-1), human herpesvirus-6 (HHV-6), *Toxoplasmosis gondii*, and *Mycoplasma pneumoniae*. Symptoms indicating IM infection by these organisms (and not by EBV) include lack of exudative pharyngitis, exposure history (e.g., incubation period, exposure to animals, sexual practices), peculiar physical findings (e.g., cough without rales), or peculiar laboratory findings (markedly elevated lymphocyte number without atypia (e.g., adenovirus infection).

It is important to note that an altered T-cell ratio (e.g., a CD4:CD8 ratio less than 1) is not diagnostic in these cases because a reversal of the normal ratio may be seen in EBV, CMV, and HIV infections. The alterations resolve in the case of isolated herpesvirus infections, however.

The importance of making the correct diagnosis is exemplified by adolescents who have severe EBV disease. Although the types and number of symptoms are similar to those of IM and other EBV syndromes, the severity of the disease is greater than usual. The major finding that severe disease is present is the magnitude and pattern of the anti-EBV antibody response. Presumably, instead of developing a latent infection, these adolescent patients continue to have a "permissive" or active lytic infection. If this assumption is correct, these severely ill adolescents may respond to chronic specific antiviral therapy.

THERAPY

Treatment for EBV-induced disease varies with the individual adolescent patient. There is no specific therapy for IM. Fluids, rest, taking adequate time for recovery, and realizing that recovery may be prolonged are the critical factors in treating EBV-IM.

EBV in its lytic, replicative phase is susceptible to acycloguanosine (acyclovir). The virus does not respond in the latent phase. In addition, the pathophysiology of the clinical syndrome may influence the efficacy of the drug. For instance, several trials in IM have shown little clinical benefit of the drug even though salivary excretion of virus was interrupted while the patient was on the drug. Once drug treatment stopped, excretion of the virus resumed. No influence on presence of virus in peripheral blood lymphocytes in short-term trials has been found. Spontaneous transformation of peripheral blood lymphocytes occurred in spite of therapy. These trials were of limited duration (1 to 4 weeks), however; the experience in severely ill patients with lytic infection is different. Symptoms markedly improved while patients were on the drug, but recurred with cessation of therapy.

IM, however, does respond to systemic corticosteroid therapy. These agents influence immune function, including CD8 cell function, and thus ameliorate many signs and symptoms of the disease. Most studies have reported no adverse effects, either clinically or in laboratory responses, after short-term corticosteroid therapy. The indications for systemic corticosteroid therapy are serious central nervous system involvement and airway obstruction. The hematologic and immunologic aspects of infection may respond in selected adolescent patients (e.g., improvement of neutropenia and thrombocytopenia).

Adolescents in whom immunodeficiency is suspected may have disease amelioration or possibly prevention by the administration of intravenous gamma globulin. Although adequate controlled trials have not been performed, except in organ or bone marrow transplantations, this mode of therapy is realistic in severe cases. Its use is based on the provision of neutralizing antibodies, which are either directly effective in inhibiting infection or are part of an antibody-dependent cell cytotoxicity system.

Active prevention of EBV at this time is impossible. The virus is highly ubiquitous, contacts may be unknown, and disease expression varies widely. Immunization is potentially practical. Current efforts are based on the development of vaccines directed against the outer glycoprotein envelope. Antibody development in immunized adolescents would then prevent infection by blocking binding to the C3d receptor.

Consideration should be given to the use of live vaccines with genetically altered strains (either naturally or by genetic engineering) that produce an active infection, but that do not allow the development of latency. If a successful vaccine is developed, the next challenge would be to define who should be immunized and when they should be immunized.

COURSE AND PROGNOSIS

Acute IM is usually described as a self-limited immunoproliferative disease with a duration of days to weeks and an uneventful outcome. The many complex illnesses accompanying EBV infection should dispel that concept. Even the typical case, in which acute illness is short-lived, may be followed by a prolonged convalescence, during which the performance of usual activity is prevented by systemic and central nervous system symptoms. In other adolescents, all symptoms and signs of illness disappear, but an overwhelming fatigue persists. Although this latter topic is discussed in detail elsewhere (see next subchapter), it is important to note that classic EBV-induced IM may persist for months or years before complete resolution of symptoms. If such a prolonged course occurs, adolescents are particularly likely to experience family, school, social, and self-perception problems. The family, school, and physician must be careful not to push a return to usual activities in these adolescents. They must be encouraged to rest and to resume activity gradually. Recurrences or exacerbations of symptoms during convalescence, including the reappearance of IgM anti-VCA antibodies, may also occur. Reports from early in this century, as well as more recent observations, suggest that premature resumption of normal activity may contribute to this phenomenon.

The problems of recurrent or persistent symptoms in the absence of overt illness and the resolution of laboratory alterations are particularly difficult. Persistent symptoms may be caused solely by the adolescent's biologic response to the disease or to the adolescent's and family's reaction to those symptoms. Occasionally, they may be a result of the adolescent's need to be ill or to the family's need for him or her to continue to be ill. More rarely, the illness is not caused by infection at all. It has been suggested that in these cases, there may be an accompanying psychosomatic illness. Frequently, comparisons of signs, symptoms, and the course of biopsychosocial illnesses are made.

Positive data for considerable psychosocial overlay are obtained from school performance (e.g., a decline in academic achievement), inability to participate in social or family activities, signs of persistent infection, and exacerbation of symptoms with activities considered to be normal. One cannot expect that the pattern of acute active disease is present in a prolonged convalescence. Thus, determining psychosocial symptoms during convalescence, rather than during the acute active phase, is appropriate.

The question of assumption of full activity is particularly important in relationship to athletics. It has been suggested that full training may be resumed from 2 weeks after resolution of symptoms to as long as 6 months. The adolescent who has persistently enlarged lymph nodes and spleen should not engage in full activity, particularly contact sports. Other indications of ongoing disease are persistently elevated liver enzyme levels (transaminases) or a persistent positive heterophile test. The best overall clinical guide is resumption of classroom and social activities without complaints. If parents observe that the adolescent is suffering excess fatigue, then resumption of full athletic activities is contraindicated. Poor athletic performance and a prolonged convalescence may occur in highly trained adolescent athletes. In addition, rhabdomyolysis has been reported as a consequence of heavy muscle activity during the course of EBV-induced IM.

The outcome of the complex neurologic, hematologic, or cardiac sequelae may be unfavorable. Death from these sequelae is a distinct possibility. Adolescents with severe organ failure (renal, cardiac, and pulmonary) may survive with intensive supportive therapy.

IATROGENIC PROBLEMS

The major physician error in caring for adolescents with EBV disease is to consider that it is always a benign, self-limiting illness. The second problem is failure to consider the virus as a possible cause of illness in a given adolescent. The third is to have considered EBV but to have relied on the results of a heterophile antibody or rapid slide test as the sole diagnostic procedure. A fatal outcome could be the result of these errors.

Additional problems may follow failure to recognize the emergent complications, which include acute sinusitis, pharyngeal wall or peritonsillar abscesses, systemic anaerobic infections, airway obstruction, and splenic hematomas or ruptures. Bacterial complications should be considered when the temperature course does not show an appropriate decline with decreasing systemic symptoms, or when typical signs of acute sinusitis are present (e.g., facial tenderness, purulent posterior pharyngeal mucus, midface edema). Because swelling of soft tissues in the neck may be part of the primary process, the otolaryngeal complications are best detected by close observation of respiratory effort, jaw muscle motion, and voice character. In such cases, early consultation by an otolaryngologist, experienced in the spectrum of EBV disease, is often mandatory.

Large splenic hematomas may mimic an acute abdomen. Appropriate imaging studies allow identification of this problem. Splenic rupture is an emergency and requires immediate surgical intervention.

BIBLIOGRAPHY

Davis S (ed): Critical Reviews in Oncology/Hematology, Vol 9. Boca Raton, FL, CRC Press, 1989.
Englund JA: The many faces of Epstein-Barr virus. Postgrad Med 83:167, 1988.
Grose C: The many faces of infectious mononucleosis: The spectrum of Epstein-Barr virus infection in children. Pediatr Rev 7:35, 1985.
Jones JF: A perspective of Epstein-Barr virus diseases. Adv Pediatr 36:307, 1989.
Kieff E, Liebowitz D: Epstein-Barr virus and its replication. In Fields BN, Knipe DM (eds): Virology, 2nd ed. New York, Raven Press, 1990, p 1889.
Miller G: Epstein-Barr virus. Biology, pathogenesis, and medical aspects. In Fields BN, Knipe DM (eds): Virology, 2nd ed. New York, Raven Press, 1990, p 1921.
Pearson GR: The humoral response. In Schlossberg D (ed): Infectious Mononucleosis, Vol 1. New York, Praeger, 1983, p 141.
Schooley RT, Dolin R: Epstein-Barr virus (infectious mononucleosis). In Mandell GL, Douglas RG Jr, Bennett JE, et al (eds): Principles and Practice of Infectious Diseases, 3rd ed. New York, Churchill Livingstone, 1990, p 1172.
Sumaya CV: Epstein-Barr virus infections in children. Curr Probl Pediatr 24:682, 1987.

CHRONIC FATIGUE

DEDRA BUCHWALD and MARK SCOTT SMITH

During the past decade, much attention has been focused on an illness called chronic fatigue syndrome (CFS). CFS is a disabling systemic illness characterized by severe persistent fatigue that is often associated with fevers, pharyngitis, myalgias, headache, neurocognitive difficulties, sleep disturbances, and depression. It is a provisional diagnosis, to be considered only after all other potential causes of illness have been reasonably excluded. CFS frequently has a sudden onset following a flu-like, presumably viral, illness. Most commonly, CFS affects young, previously healthy adults and is more common in females than in males. The cause of CFS remains obscure, although findings from a growing body of literature suggest that immunologic abnormalities, infectious agents, particularly viruses, and psychological factors may play an important role.

Historical review suggests that chronic fatigue may be an old clinical problem. Epidemic and sporadic cases of unexplained fatigue associated with various symptoms, including fever, sore throat, headaches, myalgias, and depression, have been reported for the last 100 years. In particular, epidemics of an illness remarkably similar to CFS, variously labeled myalgic encephalomyelitis, Icelandic disease, or Royal Free disease, have been described for half a century. A postinfectious syndrome of debilitating fatigue following exposure to various agents has also been reported. Finally, fibromyalgia, a chronic condition characterized by fatigue, myalgias, and tender points on examination, is similar if not identical to CFS.

Three epidemics affecting primarily adolescents have also been described. One epidemic occurred at the time of a poliomyelitis outbreak, and was characterized by an acute illness with multiple neurologic symptoms followed by symptoms such as memory loss, sleep disturbance, emotional lability, arthralgias, and prolonged disability. In another outbreak, among schoolgirls, symptoms including fatigue, myalgia, sore throat, and headache were frequently associated with prolonged convalescence. Another cluster of cases included children and adolescents, most of whom described a gradual onset over several months. All complained of marked fatigue and headache and most had neurologic complaints, including loss of short-term memory, dyslogia, paresthesias, and dizziness. Other prominent symptoms included disturbed sleep, arthralgias, myalgias, abdominal pain, recurrent sore throat, and lymphodynia. More recently, interest in chronic fatigue has increased following studies that described persistent fatigue in children, adolescents, and adults associated with markers of viral infection and reports describing an outbreak of unexplained fatigue in Nevada.

For all age groups, heterogeneous and loosely drawn case definitions have probably contributed to an apparent increase in the incidence of CFS. In 1988, a consensus panel convened by the Centers for Disease Control (CDC) in an attempt to identify a discrete and homogeneous syndrome, proposed formal diagnostic criteria for CFS. Although this more restrictive definition may facilitate research on CFS, the criteria probably exclude most patients who report symptoms of chronic fatigue.

The CDC case definition for CFS is intended for use by providers as a guide in evaluating adolescents with chronic fatigue of unknown cause. To meet these criteria, patients must have both of two major (Table 93–7) and eight of eleven minor symptoms *or* six of eleven minor symptoms *and* two of three physical findings (Table 93–8). These criteria are controversial, because they may not identify a discrete group of patients and because the presence of psychiatric dysfunction is both a minor symptom criterion and potential grounds for exclusion. Because these criteria were developed for adult populations they may not be appropriate for children and adolescents, in whom chronic fatigue syn-

TABLE 93–7. Major Criteria for CFS

New onset of debilitating fatigue that does not resolve with bed rest and impairs average daily activity below 50% of patient's premorbid level for at least 6 months
Exclusion of clinical condition that may mimic CFS, including the following:
Malignancy
Autoimmune disease
Infection:
    Localized (e.g., occult abscess)
    Chronic or subacute bacterial (e.g., endocarditis, Lyme disease, tuberculosis)
    Fungal (e.g., histoplasmosis, blastomycosis)
    Parasitic (e.g., toxoplasmosis, giardiasis)
    Human immunodeficiency virus infection
Psychiatric disease
Chronic use, abuse, or side effects of prescription or illicit drugs (e.g., antidepressant, alcohol)
Exposure to toxic agents (e.g., solvents, heavy metal)
Chronic inflammatory disease (e.g., sarcoidosis, hepatitis)
Neuromuscular disease (e.g., multiple sclerosis)
Endocrine disease (e.g., hypothyroidism, diabetes mellitus)
Other chronic pulmonary, cardiac, gastrointestinal, hepatic, renal, or hematologic disorders

TABLE 93–8. Minor Criteria for CFS

SYMPTOM CRITERIA
(To fulfill a symptom criterion, a symptom must have begun at or after the time of onset of increased fatigability, and must have persisted or recurred over a period of at least 6 months.)

Mild fever—oral temperature between 37.5° and 38.6°C—or chills
Sore throat
Painful axillary, anterior, or posterior cervical nodes
Unexplained generalized muscle weakness
Muscle discomfort or myalgia
Prolonged (24 hours or greater) generalized fatigue after levels of exercise that would have been easily tolerated in the patient's premorbid state
New or different generalized headaches
Migratory arthralgia without joint swelling or redness
Neuropsychological complaints (e.g., photophobia, transient visual scotomata, forgetfulness, excessive irritability, confusion, difficulty thinking, inability to concentrate, depression)
Sleep disturbance (hypersomnia or insomnia)
Description of the main symptom complex as initially developing over a few hours to a few days

PHYSICAL EXAMINATION CRITERIA
(Physical criteria must be documented by a physician on at least two occasions, at least 1 month apart.)

Low-grade fever—oral temperature between 37.6° and 38.6°C, or rectal temperature between 37.8° and 38.8°C
Nonexudative pharyngitis
Palpable or tender anterior or posterior cervical or axillary lymph nodes

drome is distinctly less common and in whom the average number of symptoms is lower. Additionally, if CFS is a variant of somatoform disorder, children and adolescents would also be expected to have fewer symptoms than adults.

PATHOPHYSIOLOGY

Many theories about the causes of CFS have been postulated, but strong evidence to support any of them is lacking. Most investigators believe that no single agent will prove to be the cause in most, or all, cases. A plausible hypothesis is that CFS occurs in a vulnerable individual in whom depression, atopy, viral infections, or other factors have resulted in some degree of immune compromise, which may not be measurable by standard testing (Fig. 93–2). Subsequently, latent viruses are reactivated and contribute to the morbidity directly by causing symptoms and indirectly by eliciting an ongoing immune response. In particular, it is possible that the production of cytokines is responsible for the symptoms of CFS. Cytokines are known to cause the flu-like symptoms associated with many acute infections and have also been shown to induce a CFS-like syndrome when administered for therapeutic purposes. As with any chronic illness, symptoms lead to disability that is both caused by and results in psychological dysfunction.

CLINICAL MANIFESTATIONS

In adults, a compelling piece of evidence that CFS is an "organic" illness is the sudden onset in 85% of

Figure 93–2. Possible pathogenetic model of CFS. EBV, Epstein-Barr virus; HHV 6, human herpesvirus-6.

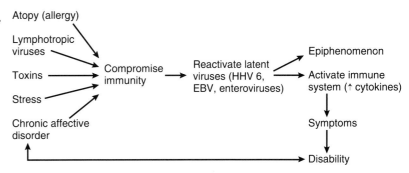

patients. Most adult patients stated that their illness began on a particular day, with a flu-like syndrome characterized by fever, pharyngitis, adenopathy, myalgias, and related symptoms; however, unlike the usual flu, they never fully recovered.

The most prominent symptom in adults is fatigue. Approximately 25% of adult CFS patients described themselves as regularly bedridden or shut in and unable to work, and one third could work only part-time. Patients were usually physically active, but since becoming ill even modest physical exertion resulted in an exacerbation of many of their symptoms. Although the exertion itself may be reasonably well tolerated at the time, 6 to 24 hours later most adults reported a marked worsening of their fatigue, cognitive function, adenopathy, pharyngitis, and fevers.

Other chronic symptoms frequently accompany the fatigue, such as fever, myalgias, sleep disorders, headaches, and pharyngitis (Table 93–9). Several points require emphasis. First, in adults, these symptoms are present much of the time. Second, many of these symptoms are sufficiently severe that they impair normal functioning. Third, in response to explicit questioning, most patients state that these symptoms were not a problem prior to their illness, but became common after the illness began.

Neuropsychiatric symptoms such as word groping, poor concentration, and impaired short-term memory are common, and one third of adults reported at least one episode of complete confusion or disorientation. One study found neurocognitive deficits in more than half of adults with CFS. Although neurocognitive symptoms are suggestive of organicity, they may also be frequent symptoms in major depression. Controlled studies of neurocognitive testing comparing CFS and depressed patients have not been performed.

A study of 15 adolescents with profound fatigue found that their daily activities decreased by at least 50%, and that the fatigue was associated with at least three other symptoms. These 9 girls and 6 boys had a mean age of

TABLE 93–9. Frequency of Occurrence of Symptoms in CFS

ADULTS		CHILDREN AND ADOLESCENTS	
Symptom	Frequency (%)	Symptom	Frequency (%)
Fatigue	100	Fatigue	100
Low-grade fever	60–95	Neurologic symptoms	27–100
Myalgias	20–95	Headache	73–97
Sleep disorders	15–90	Abdominal pain	47–97
Impaired cognition	50–85	Eye pain, photophobia	7–97
Depression	70–85	Recurrent sore throat	67–91
Headaches	35–85	Lymphatic pain	67–91
Pharyngitis	50–75	Myalgia	33–91
Anxiety	50–70	Arthralgia	27–88
Muscle weakness	40–70	Rash	7–88
Postexertional malaise	50–60	Fever, chills, night sweats	47–72
Premenstrual worsening	50–60	Fever	47
Stiffness, "gelling"	50–60	Depression	60
Visual blurring	50–60	Adenopathy	67
Nocturia	50–60	Nausea, vomiting	67
Nausea	50–60	Sleep disturbance	40
Dizziness	30–50	Anorexia	40
Arthralgias	40–50	Weight loss	40
Tachycardia	40–50	Rhinitis	27
Paresthesias	30–50	Diarrhea	20
Dry eyes	30–40	Weight gain	20
Dry mouth	30–40	Chest pain	20
Diarrhea	30–40	Palpitations	20
Anorexia	30–40	Anxiety	20
Cough	30–40	Dysuria	7
Finger swelling	30–40	Syncope	7
Night sweats	30–40		
Painful lymph nodes	30–40		
Rash	30–40		

14.5 years, and all were white. The mean duration of symptoms was over 18 months, ranging from 6 to 36 months. In 11 adolescents the onset of symptoms was associated with an acute febrile illness; 7 of these had positive Monospot test results.

In general, adolescents with CFS have fewer symptoms than do adults (see Table 93–9), reporting from 3 to 15 symptoms (mean, 6.5). As in adults, fatigue is the most prominent symptom. Most commonly, it is unremitting or intermittently prolonged, and marked hyperfatigability with exercise is characteristic. Although, on average, these adolescents reported more than 8 hours of sleep at night, one third reported insomnia and a few reported hypersomnia. Almost all noted a lack of refreshing sleep, with fatigue present when they arose in the morning.

After fatigue, headache is the most prominent symptom. Two thirds of the adolescents reported sore throat, adenopathy, and nausea or vomiting. Other symptoms, in decreasing order of frequency, included the following: dizziness, depression, abdominal pain, low-grade temperature, sleep disorder, anorexia, weight loss, myalgia, paresthesia, rhinitis, arthralgia, anxiety, diarrhea, weight gain, palpitations, chest pain, dysuria, rash, and syncope.

Daily activities are usually mildly to moderately reduced but may be severely restricted. In our study, fatigued adolescents missed an average of 34 school days during the prior 6 months that school was in session, and one third noted a marked decrease in school performance.

Physical Findings

Abnormalities in the physical examination of both adolescents and adults are unusual (Table 93–10). Fevers, low basal body temperatures, posterior and anterior cervical adenopathy, and tender points have all been described in adults (see Table 93–10). In adolescents, the physical examination is generally unremarkable, with the exception of nontender, shotty, anterior or posterior cervical adenopathy in 40%. Generalized myalgias and arthralgias are common, but, contrary to findings in adults, tender points are uncommon.

Psychological and Social Dysfunction

Investigative studies have consistently found a high prevalence of psychiatric disorder, primarily depression, in adult CFS patients. Those studies, which included control groups, demonstrated a markedly higher prevalence of psychiatric disorder in CFS patients than in control subjects. Studies that examined the temporal sequence of CFS and psychiatric disorder found that the psychiatric disorder often preceded the onset of fatigue. In a specialty fatigue clinic, it was found that 95% of patients did not meet CDC criteria for CFS, primarily because a psychiatric disorder was thought to be responsible for the fatigue syndrome. However, since depression may be a symptom of CFS, controversy remains regarding a primary or secondary role for psychiatric disorders in this illness.

In adolescents, multiple somatic complaints may be indicative of psychological or social dysfunction. Although our adolescent patients with CFS had an apparently normal premorbid medical and psychosocial history, many developed significant psychosocial morbidity, with social isolation and school absenteeism becoming major issues. Furthermore, psychosocial interviews revealed significant family problems in 4 of 15 adolescents and isolation from peers in 6 of 15. Psychiatric interviews using the Schedule for Affective Disorder and Schizophrenia, Children's Version, identified 5 of 15 adolescents, all girls, with major depression. Of interest, 4 of the 5 depressed girls experienced the onset of symptoms following documented acute infectious mononucleosis (see previous subchapter). Although the 10 fatigued adolescents who did not have major depression reported many of its secondary symptoms, key features were missing in most subjects. In addition, indicators of severity, such as guilt, suicidality, and functional incapacity, were relatively uncommon.

LABORATORY FINDINGS

Although diverse laboratory abnormalities have been reported in adults, mostly in uncontrolled studies, there have been no consistent findings associated with CFS. Leukocytosis and leukopenia are each seen in approximately 20% of cases, and lymphocytosis has been de-

TABLE 93–10. Physical Findings in CFS

ADULTS		CHILDREN AND ADOLESCENTS	
Findings	**Frequency (%)**	**Findings**	**Frequency (%)**
Tender points	33–75	Lymphatic tenderness	0–91
Inflamed pharynx	40–60	Abdominal tenderness	0–84
Posterior cervical adenopathy	20–40	Pharyngitis	7–81
Impaired tandem gait	15–25	Muscle tenderness	0–69
Macular rash	10–20	Anterior or posterior cervical adenopathy	40
Fever (>37.6°C) at a single office visit	10–20	Rash	0–22
Low body temperature (<36.1°C)	20–30		
Hepatomegaly	5–20		
Splenomegaly	5–20		
Axillary adenopathy	5–15		

scribed in up to 71%. Atypical lymphocytes were reported in 0% to 30% of patients and, in serial studies, in about 50%. Approximately 15% of CFS patients have positive findings in heterophile or Monospot tests, and 20% of patients have modestly elevated transaminase levels.

Immunologic Abnormalities

Unusual and often conflicting findings have been noted in many immunologic studies in adults (Table 93–11). Of the various circulating autoantibodies reported, the most common are antinuclear antibodies, found in up to one third of adult patients. Immunoglobulin levels yielded inconsistent findings, because both decreased and, less commonly, increased immunoglobulins of the IgA, IgD, IgG, or IgM class have been reported. An average of 53% of adult patients had low levels of circulating immune complexes, but only a minority of patients showed depressed complement and none had clinical manifestations of immune-complex mediated disease.

Several studies have noted abnormalities in the lymphokine and interleukin responses of adults with CFS. Leukocyte activity of the interferon-induced enzyme, $2'5'$-oligoadenylate synthetase, was elevated in a small number of CFS patients. Circulating interferon has been detected infrequently. Although one study found reduced synthesis of γ-interferon and interleukin-2 by mitogen-stimulated lymphocytes, others found elevated interleukin-2 levels in CFS patients.

Abnormalities of lymphocyte number and function have also been noted. Both elevated and diminished numbers of B, CD4, and CD8 cells and increased and decreased CD4:CD8 ratios have been found. Lymphocyte function may also be abnormal. In some studies, half of patients were anergic and significantly delayed hypersensitivity to multiple antigens was demonstrated. Decreased responsiveness *in vitro* to standard mitogen stimulation assays has also been reported. A controlled study found a significant reduction in the display of

CD3, a common membrane structure found on T cells. Because CD3 interacts with antigen and is considered important in the transduction of T-cell activation signals, this finding suggests a mechanism for the T-cell dysfunction observed in CFS. Finally, decreased numbers of natural killer (NK) cells and reductions in the normally dominant (NKH1-positive–T3-negative) subset have been reported. Natural killer cell function has been found to be increased, decreased, and normal, as measured by cytolytic activity against a number of different target cell lines. These abnormalities are interesting, given the central role played by these cells in viral infections.

Infections

CFS has been reported as a postinfectious syndrome in adult patients with several different infectious agents. Although early studies linked Epstein-Barr virus and CFS, further investigations, including two seroepidemiologic surveys, indicated that Epstein-Barr virus is unlikely to be a causative agent in most cases of CFS. Many studies found elevated IgG to viral capsid antigen and early antigen, generally in the absence of viral capsid antigen-IgM; however, there is extensive overlap between patients and healthy control subjects. A low or absent antibody to Epstein-Barr nuclear antigen, thought to be an unusual finding in healthy seropositive individuals, has been found in some CFS patients.

The enteroviruses have also been implicated as possible causative agents in CFS. Two intriguing studies reported finding circulating enteroviral antigen and IgM complexes in most adults and isolation of the virus in 22%. Moreover, enteroviral nucleic acid has been found in muscle cells more often in patients with CFS than in control subjects.

Several latent viruses—herpes simplex, cytomegalovirus, measles virus, and human herpesvirus-6—may be reactivated in patients with CFS. If true, it is unclear whether this reactivation contributes to the morbidity of CFS or whether it is an epiphenomenon. In addition, no evidence of infection with known retroviruses has been found.

Other Findings

Although allergies are a common feature of adults with CFS, this observation has not been noted in adolescents. Increased cutaneous reactivity to allergens, increased levels of circulating IgE and IgE-bearing T and B cells, and greater lymphocyte responsiveness to allergens have all been found in adults. The mechanisms linking allergy and CFS remain unknown.

Muscle studies of chronic fatigue patients have not demonstrated abnormal muscle enzymes or metabolic or enzymatic evidence of a defect in the intermediary energy pathway. Although muscle biopsies have shown structural abnormalities, and 75% of patients tested had abnormal single fiber electromyography, several techniques have documented normal muscle strength, endurance, and recovery. However, on graded exercise

TABLE 93–11. Frequency of Occurrence of Selected Laboratory Abnormalities in Adults With CFS

FINDINGS	FREQUENCY (%)
Hematologic	
Leukocytosis	0–21
Leukopenia	0–26
Lymphocytosis	0–71
Atypical lymphocytes	0–30
Positive heterophile	0–50
Immunologic	
Positive antinuclear antibodies	0–32
Decreased immunoglobulin classes	4–100
Increased immunoglobulin classes	11–40
Circulating immune complexes	0–73
Increased CD4:CD8 ratio	30–40
Decreased CD4:CD8 ratio	2–100
Anergy	0–54
Decreased number of natural killer cells	0–73
Decreased natural killer cell function	0–100

testing (which is effort-dependent), CFS patients had a markedly limited exercise capacity characterized by an inability to achieve their target heart rate, a lower exercise heart rate, and an abbreviated exercise duration.

In summary, the laboratory abnormalities observed in adults with CFS are diverse, sometimes conflicting, and frequently moderate in degree. Although there is evidence of diffuse immunologic dysfunction, reflecting both deficient function and hyperactivity, it has not been shown that these findings explain the symptoms and signs of CFS, or correlate with changes in symptoms over time. Most likely, when more systematic blinded studies using healthy control subjects are performed, some of the "abnormalities" currently thought to be characteristic of CFS may disappear.

In our experience, extensive laboratory testing in adolescents with CFS yields little helpful information. Urinalysis, complete blood count, erythrocyte sedimentation rate, and the alanine aminotransferase level were normal in all adolescents evaluated. Although one third of these adolescent patients had transient titers of Epstein-Barr–IgM, serologic testing for Coxsackie B viruses 1 to 6, cytomegalovirus, Epstein-Barr virus, human herpesvirus-6, and *Toxoplasma gondii* generally provided little evidence for an infectious cause of the chronic fatigue.

DIAGNOSIS

A detailed history, physical examination, and selected laboratory tests are indicated in adolescents with chronic fatigue that significantly affects daily activity. Equal emphasis must be placed on the psychosocial evaluation, searching, in particular, for anxiety and depression (see Chapters 100 and 102). Although no laboratory tests are diagnostic in CFS, a reasonable laboratory test battery to evaluate adolescent patients, based on studies in adults, consists of the following: (1) a complete blood cell count, with a manually performed differential white blood cell count; (2) erythrocyte sedimentation rate; (3) chemistry panel; (4) thyroid-stimulating hormone; (5) antinuclear antibodies; and (6) in some cases, circulating immune complexes and immunoglobulin levels. These tests may be helpful in supporting a diagnosis of CFS or in ruling out other diseases that can produce chronic fatigue. Extensive serologic testing for viruses is not usually helpful in identifying a causal link between fatigue and persistent or reactivated viruses.

In addition to screening for anxiety and depression, a psychosocial evaluation should review functioning of the adolescent in major life areas, including family and peer relationships and school and community activities. Observations of family interactions and illness behavior may also provide clues about facilitating and sustaining factors. Our experience suggests that a major complication in many adolescents is the assumption of the powerless "victim" role and avoidance behavior toward normal activities, similar to that seen in chronic pain syndromes. Identification of family dysfunction and adolescent avoidance behavior must be tactfully but firmly addressed in management efforts.

DIFFERENTIAL DIAGNOSIS

It is important to note whether the complaint of fatigue is registered by the adolescent or the parent. Sleeping late on weekend mornings, tiredness when family chores or activities are planned, and boredom with daily family interactions may all be attributes of the normal adolescent. On the other hand, a complaint of increased fatigability that interferes with activities that were previously enjoyed should be investigated carefully.

Although it is uncommon for systemic disorders to present solely with fatigue, conditions associated with fatigue during adolescence include pregnancy, anemia, inflammatory bowel disease, chronic renal failure, diabetes mellitus, hypothyroidism, connective tissue diseases, neoplasms, and infectious processes such as sinusitis or hepatitis. The existence of the frequently diagnosed "allergy-tension-fatigue" syndrome, in which allergy presumably causes chronic fatigue, is controversial.

Fibromyalgia, a syndrome characterized by diffuse musculoskeletal aching, well-defined tender points, and fatigue, has been described in adolescents (see Chapter 90). Prominent associated symptoms include sleep disturbance, irritable bowel syndrome, headache, and psychological dysfunction. In fatigued adolescents with prominent musculoskeletal symptoms, discrete tender points are unusual, and a clear distinction between CFS and fibromyalgia is often not possible.

Sleep disturbance, concentration and memory problems, and anhedonia in the fatigued adolescent should elicit further questions regarding depressed mood, weight loss, self-recrimination, and suicidality. Psychiatric conditions such as dysthymia, major depressive disorder, anxiety disorders, and substance abuse are commonly associated with chronic fatigue, and may not be readily apparent (see Chapters 100, 103, and 111). Because some adolescents underreport depressive symptoms, it is important to elicit a history from family members or other significant persons.

Psychophysiologic symptoms are also common in distressed adolescents without a psychiatric disorder. Disruptive experiences, such as the onset of puberty or starting a new school, may lead to negative self-appraisal, greater sensitivity to bodily changes, and somatization. Adolescents who are experiencing a loss, unresolved conflict, feelings of inadequacy, or other threats to well-being may focus concern on a symptom such as fatigue. Certain personality traits (e.g., overachievement), coping styles, and psychosocial or medical stressors may also operate in concert to produce chronic fatigue in the adolescent.

TREATMENT

There is no specific therapy for CFS. Treatment should be directed at relief of specific symptoms and reintegration into the individual's social network. Symptomatic therapy may include antipyretic and nonsteroidal anti-inflammatory agents. Anecdotal reports of successful treatment include antiviral and immunomodulating drugs, vitamins, holistic remedies, diet modifications, and rest. In adults, low doses of antidepressants such as fluoxetine in the morning and amitriptyline or doxepin taken at bedtime may be beneficial. Although the role of antidepressants in adolescents with chronic fatigue who do not meet criteria for major depression is undefined, we have used desipramine and fluoxetine with modest success. Two agents, acyclovir and a liver extract–vitamin B_{12}-folate preparation, have undergone vigorous evaluation, and neither was found to be more effective than placebo. In addition, two controlled studies of adults treated with intravenous immunoglobulin produced conflicting results.

A supportive approach aimed at enhancing self-efficacy and reconditioning is effective in many cases. Emphasis should be placed on regular sleep patterns, with avoidance of napping and significant changes in the sleep cycle. Diet should be well balanced, with meals appropriately spaced throughout the day. Physical activities previously enjoyed by the adolescent (e.g., bicycle riding, swimming) should be gradually increased in a structured manner, because complete inactivity appears to promote fatigue.

Because school fulfills an important social developmental role for normal adolescents, attendance should be encouraged and home tutoring, which promotes isolation and retards the development of psychosocial competence, discouraged. Evidence of school phobia may be present in adolescents with excessive school absence (see Chapter 103). A return to regular school activities is often most effectively accomplished by direct physician communication with school personnel and by specific planning for increasing the time spent at school. Frequently, arrangements for brief periods of rest and/or a modified curriculum can be negotiated.

Finally, continuity of care, coupled with education, instruction in coping skills, and counseling, are often neglected but important aspects of treatment for CFS. Reassurance and encouragement are powerful aspects of any treatment program. Periodic reassessment for organic and psychiatric disorders should be performed at regular intervals, but extensive laboratory testing without additional indications is not warranted.

COURSE OF ILLNESS AND PROGNOSIS

CFS is not a progressive disease. For most adults, symptoms are most severe during the first 6 months of illness, plateau relatively early, and recur with varying degrees of severity. Although longitudinal studies are lacking, it appears that most patients report a gradual recovery, usually punctuated with relapses precipitated by overexertion, stress, or infection. Death resulting directly from CFS has not been reported.

In adolescents, our data suggest a reasonably optimistic outcome for at least half of patients. On structured telephone interviews completed 13 to 32 months from study intake, four adolescents reported complete recovery, four were markedly improved, and seven were unimproved or worse. A median of 15 school days was missed over the previous 6 months. Initial tests for viral causation or for anxiety and depression did not predict functional status at follow-up.

BIBLIOGRAPHY

Buchwald D, Komaroff AL: Laboratory abnormalities in chronic fatigue syndrome. Rev Infect Dis 13:512, 1991.
David AS, Wessely S, Pelosi AJ: Postviral fatigue syndrome: Time for a new approach. Br Med J 296:696, 1988.
Holmes GP, Kaplan JE, Gantz NM, et al: Chronic fatigue syndrome: A working case definition. Ann Intern Med 108:387, 1988.
Holmes GP, Kaplan JE, Stewart JA, et al: A cluster of patients with a chronic mononucleosis-like syndrome. Is Epstein-Barr virus the cause? JAMA 257:2297, 1987.
Katz BZ, Andiman WA: Chronic fatigue syndrome. J Pediatr 113:944, 1988.
Komaroff AL: Chronic fatigue syndromes: Relationship to chronic viral infections. J Virol Methods 21:3, 1988.
Komaroff AL, Buchwald D: Symptoms and signs in chronic fatigue syndrome. Rev Infect Dis 13:58, 1991.
Manu P, Lane TJ, Matthews DA: The frequency of the chronic fatigue syndrome in patients with symptoms of persistent fatigue. Ann Intern Med 109:554, 1988.
Smith MS, Mitchell J, Corey L, et al: Chronic fatigue in adolescents. Pediatrics 88:195, 1991.
Straus SE: The chronic mononucleosis syndrome. J Infect Dis 157:405, 1988.

INFLUENZA INFECTIONS

CAROLINE BREESE HALL

HISTORICAL BACKGROUND

Influenza is known by various sobriquets, such as the "flu" or the "grippe." Influenza may have acquired its name from the Latin influere, which means to flow in, or possibly from the Italian influenza di freddo, meaning effect of cold or winter factor.

Influenza is a seasonal acute respiratory disease that occurs in epidemics, occasionally pandemics, or in local outbreaks. Despite the generic term flu, used to describe many respiratory and gastrointestinal illnesses, true influenza is caused by three immunologically distinct types of human influenza virus (A, B, and C). The disease produced by the influenza viruses may be mimicked by other respiratory viruses. However, the clinical, and especially the epidemiologic, characteristics of the illnesses caused by influenza A and B viruses can produce a distinctive picture.

Influenza, as the last of the ancient great plagues, has a colorful history. Epidemics of influenza were probably described from the time of Hippocrates. The epidemic in 1173 A.D. in Italy, Germany, and England is generally designated as the first recorded epidemic. The first pandemic involving Asia, Europe, and Africa occurred in 1580 A.D., and the first epidemic recorded in the Western Hemisphere was in 1647. However, the modern study of the disease and its epidemiology probably began with the pandemic of 1889, which was particularly severe throughout much of the world and resulted in one of the highest death rates ever recorded in the United States. The most infamous of influenza pandemics was that of 1918. Called the Spanish influenza, its toll was 20 million deaths worldwide, with 548,000 in the United States alone.

VIRUSES

The influenza viruses belong to the family of orthomyxoviruses and consist of three types, A, B, and C. Influenza C viruses appear to be less important in human infection, usually causing mild, asymptomatic infection. The influenza viruses are medium-sized, negative-stranded RNA viruses, with an envelope studded with spikes that contains eight virus-coded proteins. The nucleoprotein and matrix protein are antigenically type-specific and stable.

The hemagglutinin (H) and neuraminidase (N), integral in immunity to influenza, determine the subtype and undergo change. The envelope projections of hemagglutinin are glycoprotein rods consisting of a trimer of three polypeptides, which allow viral attachment. The surface "mushrooms" of neuraminidase, composed of a tetramer of polypeptides, appear to have several functions, including the release of new virions from host cells. Three separate hemagglutinins, H_1, H_2, H_3, and two neuraminidases, N_1 and N_2, have been identified. Changes in these proteins cause the observed annual antigenic variation. A major antigenic change, or shift, results in a new subtype, and probably occurs through genetic reassortment. A drift denotes minor changes in these surface proteins, probably through point mutations, which do not result in a change in the subtype. Both influenza A and B viruses drift, but a shift occurs only with influenza A viruses.

EPIDEMIOLOGY

Influenza has been called the last of the great plagues. Each year it appears throughout the world, causing appreciable morbidity and mortality. Predicting the type and path of influenza has become a scientific avocation. Influenza has been delineated epidemiologically and in the laboratory for over half a century. Surveillance is conducted by monitoring various epidemiologic parameters, such as absenteeism in schools and industries, and mortality reports from influenza and pneumonia. A network of World Health Organization laboratories also analyzes new strains in an effort to forecast the coming strains that should be included in the yearly inactivated vaccine.

The unpredictability of influenza, especially influenza

A, has made predictions and plans problematic. Outbreaks usually occur in January through March in the United States, but may appear from October to May. Furthermore, the epidemiologic nature of influenza has changed over the past decade. Previously, only one influenza type predominated each year, and in some years influenza activity was minimal. More recently, the United States has witnessed appreciable activity each year, and often more than one influenza type is prominent within a single season (Fig. 93–3). Influenza's overall impact can be correlated with the drift of the strains from year to year. A shift, characterized by an influenza A strain with a new H or N, generally results in a major epidemic or pandemic. No shift has occurred since the appearance of influenza A/H_3N_2 in 1968 and of A/H_1N_1 in 1977. Considerable drift, however, has subsequently occurred among these strains (A/H_3N_2 and A/H_1N_1) and also among the influenza B strains.

Because of this antigenic variation, and because of waning immunity, influenza may cause repeated infections. The highest attack rates are usually in young children, but the highest case-fatality rates occur at both ends of the age spectrum. Longitudinal family studies by Glezen and colleagues have depicted the appreciable morbidity produced by influenza annually (Table 93–12). The infection rate was higher in adolescents than in children under 2 years of age, and the proportion with symptomatic illness was similar. Lower respiratory tract disease occurred in about 10% of all illnesses. In adolescents, this rate appears to vary widely in different settings and with different strains, but may be estimated at 1% to 5%. The annual rates of influenza infection of 20% to 50%, observed in children in the Houston family studies, are frequently surpassed in adolescents attending boarding schools and in students in colleges and other institutions.

The attack rates in various age groups may vary according to the predominant strains of the season. This may be partly explained by the previous experience of older age groups with influenza strains of earlier years, which were antigenically similar. For example, the reappearance of influenza A/H_1N_1 in 1977 to 1978 occurred after an interim of 21 years. Older adults, particularly those over 52 years of age, tended to have some antibody to the H_1N_1 virus, resulting in little morbidity among the older population. Nevertheless, the higher attack rates of certain strains in particular age groups cannot

TABLE 93–12. Influenza Virus Infection and Illness Rates for Children Followed Longitudinally During a Houston Family Study, 1976–1984*

AGE (YEARS)	NUMBER OF CHILD-YEARS	NUMBER OF INFECTIONS (RATE, %)	NUMBER OF ILLNESSES (RATE, %)
<2	332	118 (35.5)	112 (33.7)
2–5	474	211 (44.5)	178 (37.6)
6–10	300	143 (47.7)	118 (39.3)
11–17	149	60 (40.3)	45 (30.2)
Total	1255	532 (42.4)	453 (36.1)

With permission from Glezen WP: Consequences to children from influenza virus infections. Pediatr Virol 4:1, 1989.

*Per 100 child-years.

Figure 93–3. Seasonal occurrence of influenza A/H₃N₂, A/H₁N₁, and B viruses over a 12-year period in the Rochester, New York area. (Data obtained from an ongoing Community Surveillance Program.)

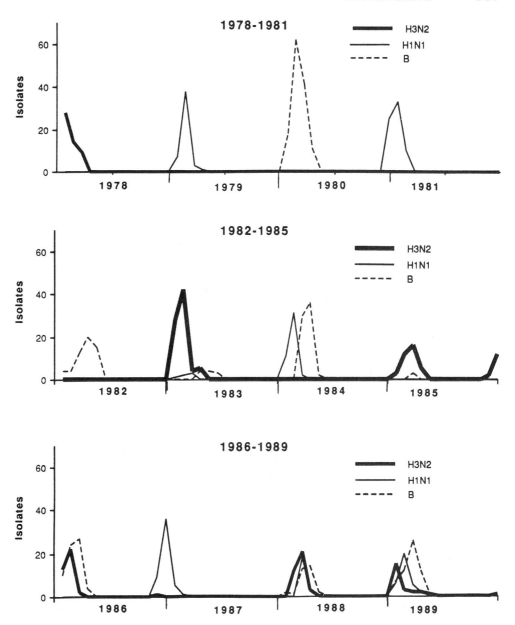

always be explained by previous experience and immunity. For instance, college-aged students were predominantly affected during the 1977 to 1978 winter, when influenza A/H₁N₁ first reappeared. A lower rate of infection was seen among young children, although they were equally susceptible.

PATHOPHYSIOLOGY

Spread of Infection

Influenza is spread by contact with infected respiratory secretions through large particle aerosols, by self-inoculation from contaminated hands, or even by small particle aerosols under certain conditions. Small particle aerosols may spread the virus over great distances, and can cause explosive outbreaks. One such outbreak was documented on a commercial airliner in 1977. After being held on board for 3 hours with an inoperative

ventilation system, 70% of the passengers developed an influenza-like illness within 72 hours that lasted an average of 6 days. Approximately 10% required hospitalization. Subsequent investigation revealed that the index case was a woman with fever and cough who was infected with influenza A/Alaska/77 (H₃N₂). The mean incubation period was 38 hours after exposure, and all illnesses occurred within 72 hours.

Pathogenesis

The incubation period appears to relate partly to the inoculating dose, but is short, from 18 to 72 hours. The ciliated columnar epithelial cells of the respiratory tract are the major site of infection. The replication cycle requires approximately 4 to 6 hours. Virus continues to be released until cell death. Spread of infection occurs by absorption of the new virions onto adjacent cells. Local edema, cellular infiltration, and necrosis of the epithelium result. Inflammation and necrosis of the nasal and tracheal ciliated cells occur early in the illness, and spread to the lower respiratory tract may subsequently occur. Repair and regeneration of the epithelium begin by the third to fifth day, with the maximum response approximately 2 weeks after onset of the infection. The reappearance of the cilia and mucus requires 15 days or more.

In most persons the major pathology occurs in the upper respiratory tract, frequently in the trachea and bronchi. The desquamation of the epithelium in the tracheobronchial tree and the prolonged regeneration time result in the pronounced cough, which commonly continues for weeks after the acute influenza illness. This is one of the frequent causes of tracheobronchitis or bronchitis in previously normal adolescents and young adults.

Influenza infection may be complicated by pneumonia from direct spread of the virus to the lower respiratory tract or as a result of secondary bacterial infection, or by a combination of both viral and bacterial infections. In most cases of influenza with viral pneumonia, especially in children, the virus spreads from the bronchi to involve the smaller airways and alveolae, producing an interstitial infiltration and some alveolar filling. This pneumonitis may be mild to moderate in severity and should be differentiated from the rare primary influenza viral pneumonia, which is usually fatal and occurs primarily in those with underlying cardiac or pulmonary diseases or in the elderly. This fatal influenza viral pneumonia is characterized by marked sloughing and necrosis of the epithelium in the tracheobronchial tree, as well as by hemorrhagic alveolar exudates, hyaline membrane formation, and lymphocytic infiltration.

Immune Response

Shedding of influenza virus generally continues for longer periods in children than in adults. Young and school-aged children may shed both influenza A and B viruses for a period of up to 2 weeks, although 1 week is more common. Interferon frequently appears in the respiratory secretions and sera of infected persons within 3 to 6 days, and is usually associated with diminished viral shedding. Secretory antibodies are frequently detectable within the first to second week after the onset of infection, are predominantly of the IgA class, and may persist for weeks to several months.

Serum antibodies are generally detectable by the second week after infection and peak by four weeks. Neutralizing (Nt), hemagglutination-inhibiting (HI), complement-fixing (CF), and enzyme-linked immunosorbent antibodies are produced after primary infection, and generally an anamnestic response is witnessed after reinfection. HI and Nt antibodies are long-lasting, persisting for months to years, but at diminishing titers. CF antibodies are primarily IgM and shorter lasting, disappearing within weeks to months.

The protection against infection correlates well with the level of serum antibody. Although variation exists, most individuals with a serum HI titer of 1:40 or an Nt titer of 1:8 or more are protected against infection. Nt antibody titers in nasal secretions also correlate with immunity. Lower levels of antibody and antibody that is cross-reactive against heterologous strains of influenza may offer some degree of protection, such as against systemic illness. The degree of protection offered by antibody produced by infection from one strain of influenza A to another strain of the same influenza A subtype depends on the degree of drift between the two strains, and thus on the degree of cross-reactivity of the antibody. Antibody formed toward the hemagglutinin appears to function primarily in preventing infection with the virus, whereas antibodies against the neuraminidase have a prominent role in diminishing the severity of illness. Antibodies against other components of the virus, such as the nucleocapsid and matrix proteins, have not been associated with protection against infection or illness.

Repetitive infection produces a gradual breadth and duration of immunity toward both influenza A and B strains. Because influenza B viruses demonstrate less antigenic drift and no shift, reinfection with influenza B viruses tends to be less frequent in older children and adults.

CLINICAL MANIFESTATIONS

Influenza

The classic picture of influenza is an acute, febrile illness associated with upper respiratory signs and systemic myalgias and malaise. The onset is typically so abrupt that the adolescent may note the hour when symptoms began. Fever develops, often with chills and peak temperatures of 39° to 41°C, and with severe myalgias, headache and, commonly, a mild, dry cough. Respiratory signs and symptoms are not initially very prominent, tending to be overshadowed by the systemic manifestations. Headache associated with retro-orbital pain and discomfort on eye movement, the feeling of "square eyes in round sockets," are often striking findings early. A mild erythema of the conjunctiva is frequent. Within 2 to 3 days, respiratory signs become more prominent with nasal congestion, a diffusely erythematous pharynx, and a worsening hacking cough. In uncomplicated influenza the fever commonly persists for 2 to 5 days but occasionally has a biphasic course, even without secondary bacterial infection or other complications. The signs and symptoms of influenza in adolescents have been distinctive enough to allow pediatricians in our community surveillance program to make the correct presumptive diagnosis in 55% of adolescents from whom influenza virus was subsequently cultured (Figs. 93–4 and 93–5). Upper respiratory tract signs predominated, and the complaint of sore throat was more common than overt pharyngitis. Fever was above 103°F (39.5°C) in 24% of those with fever with influenza A and in 16% of those with influenza B infections. Lower respiratory tract illness was present initially in about 10%. The diagnosis of tracheobronchitis was made more frequently later in the course, when persistent cough became the major reason for the visit, but

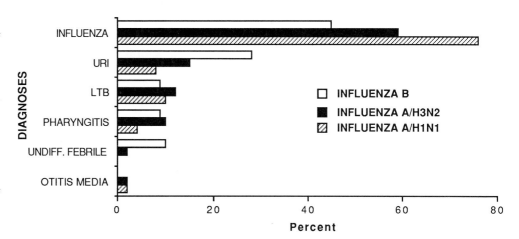

Figure 93–4. Primary diagnoses by private pediatrician at time of initial visit of teenagers from whom influenza virus was isolated. The proportion of patients with each diagnosis is shown according to the type of influenza infection, A/H$_3$N$_2$, A/H$_1$N$_1$, or B. URI, upper respiratory tract infection; LTB, laryngotracheobronchitis, undiff. febrile, undifferentiated febrile illness. (Data are from the Community Surveillance Program of the Rochester, New York area, patients 12 through 18 years of age, examined 1978–1989.)

when influenza virus was no longer likely to be cultured from the respiratory secretions.

In individuals with more immunity the illness may more closely resemble a cold, or infection may be asymptomatic. The frequency of the signs and symptoms varies according to age and sometimes according to the type of influenza (see Figs. 93–4 and 93–5). Young children tend to have a higher fever and more gastrointestinal signs, sometimes suggesting the diagnosis of gastroenteritis. Other manifestations of influenza predominantly found in younger children are febrile convulsions, croup, and otitis media. Croup can occur with both influenza A and B viral infections and in patients of a wide age range. Otitis frequently develops several days after the onset of the infection. Even adolescents may complain of ear congestion or pain, with or without a frank otitis media. Occasionally, tympanitis alone may cause ear pain.

Lower Respiratory Tract Disease

The overall rate of lower respiratory tract involvement in adolescents is difficult to assess, but may be about 5%. Most frequently this is tracheobronchitis. In previously normal adolescents, bronchitis or tracheobronchitis is usually the sequela of a viral or *Mycoplasma pneumoniae* infection and, during the influenza season, influenza A and B viruses are usually the primary cause. Adolescents presenting with a recent onset of acute bronchitis should be questioned about a preceding influenza-like illness in themselves and in their families.

Pneumonia associated with influenza infection in children is most frequently viral and, particularly in the young child, similar to that caused by the other respiratory viruses. In the adolescent, influenza is one of the few agents that may cause a viral interstitial pneumonia, although it is uncommon. The pneumonia tends to be relatively mild, sometimes not detectable by auscultation, but rarely may be moderately severe. This type of pneumonia should be differentiated from the frequently fatal primary influenza pneumonia, mentioned previously, which is rare in children. The latter is a bilateral pneumonia marked by rapid progression, severe hypoxia, respiratory failure, and a high mortality. Adults with chronic underlying diseases are primarily affected by this rare form of pneumonia, but occasionally a young, healthy adult succumbs to this unusual complication. A secondary bacterial pneumonia may occur in children and adolescents, caused most frequently by *Streptococcus pneumoniae,* followed by *Haemophilus influenzae* and *Staphylococcus aureus.* The bacterial

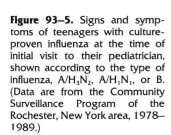

Figure 93–5. Signs and symptoms of teenagers with culture-proven influenza at the time of initial visit to their pediatrician, shown according to the type of influenza, A/H$_3$N$_2$, A/H$_1$N$_1$, or B. (Data are from the Community Surveillance Program of the Rochester, New York area, 1978–1989.)

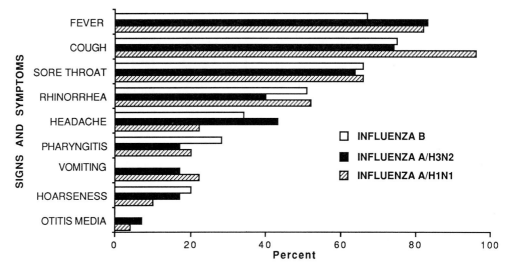

pneumonia may occur concurrently with a viral pneumonia or subsequent to an influenza illness, resulting in a double-humped febrile and clinical course. The initial influenza illness may be indistinctive enough to be missed, and the patient may appear to have a sporadic pneumococcal pneumonia.

In adolescents and young adults, lower respiratory tract involvement with acute influenza infection may occur more often than that which is clinically evident. Pulmonary function abnormalities following influenza have been frequently detected in adolescents with no evidence of pneumonia. Hyperreactivity and abnormalities of the peripheral airways may be detected during the acute infection, and usually persist for weeks.

Myositis

Acute myositis may occur with influenza A and B viral infections, and has been reported as a relatively common manifestation in previously healthy children during some outbreaks of influenza B viral infections. The myositis usually occurs 2 to 4 days after the onset of illness, with the development of pain and tenderness in the calves of the legs. Although other muscle groups may also be affected, the gastrocnemius and soleus muscles are most frequently, and almost always, involved. During an influenza B viral outbreak in the Rochester area, 21% of children with influenza B viral infection developed mild and transient myositis. Occasionally, the myositis may be more severe and associated with myoglobinuria and markedly elevated serum creatine phosphokinase (CPK) levels. Cases of acute rhabdomyolysis with renal failure have been reported, mostly in adults with influenza A viral infection.

Rare Manifestations of Influenza

Acute viral myocarditis and pericarditis have occasionally been associated with acute influenza viral infections in patients who were previously normal, as well as in those with underlying cardiac disease. Various neurologic manifestations have also occasionally been associated with influenza. Encephalitis and encephalopathy have uncommonly accompanied both influenza A and, more frequently, influenza B viral infections. Although encephalitis has been observed in all age groups, it is more frequent in adults and may be manifest at the time of the acute flu-like illness or subsequently. The clinical course may be severe, and may be marked by signs of cerebellar and brainstem dysfunction. Guillain-Barré syndrome and transverse myelitis are also rarely observed in association with influenza. Rash is rarely observed with influenza, but occasionally a child or adolescent presents with scattered petechiae. This, in association with a high fever, may evoke the suspicion of meningococcal disease.

DIAGNOSIS

The clinical diagnosis of influenza may be made with reasonable accuracy in the setting of a community epidemic, especially when accompanied by a rise in school absenteeism, and when the adolescent patient presents with the typical influenza syndrome. Few other common agents produce this acute syndrome in an otherwise healthy adolescent. Findings on physical examination are not specific for influenza, but the constellation of signs and symptoms amid the correct epidemiologic backdrop allows the specific diagnosis of influenza to be made surprisingly often. A history of abrupt onset of fever and the symptoms mentioned above in the adolescent patient, and in close contacts within the preceding week, are diagnostic clues.

Laboratory findings are not distinctive, especially initially. The white blood cell count (WBC) is usually normal at the onset of the illness but subsequently falls, often to below 5000/μl, with a lymphocytic predominance. The mean WBC in children with influenza A/H$_3$N$_2$ viral infection, when first seen by their private pediatrician an average of 2 days after onset of symptoms, was approximately 6000/μl. About one third had a WBC between 3000 and 5000/μl and only 7% had a WBC greater than 10,000/μl.

Specific diagnosis requires viral isolation, a rapid diagnostic test for influenza antigen, or a serologic test. A nasal wash specimen or a swab of the throat combined with a nose swab are generally the best and most easily obtained specimens, and should be immediately inoculated into viral transport media and sent to the laboratory as soon as possible. Viral isolation may be made within 3 days for one half to two thirds of specimens, and most all are identifiable within 5 to 7 days. Rapid identification of influenza antigen may be made on cells from the respiratory secretions using immunofluorescent or enzyme-linked immunosorbent assay (ELISA) techniques, but their sensitivity and specificity vary, and should be used in conjunction with viral isolation. Serologic diagnosis may be made by a number of assays, such as HI, Nt, and ELISA but, because a convalescent serum is required after 3 to 4 weeks, serology is rarely helpful in the clinical management of the adolescent patient.

DIFFERENTIAL DIAGNOSIS

Influenza may have various manifestations, sometimes resembling those of other viral agents. Usually the epidemiology of influenza is the most important differential factor, emphasizing the need for a local surveillance system that can inform community physicians about influenza's arrival, activities, and departure. The flu-like syndrome may be produced by other viruses, especially some enteroviruses and adenoviruses. Respiratory syncytial virus, the parainfluenza viruses, and rhinoviruses may cause respiratory illnesses or colds in adolescents, but are less likely to cause the abrupt onset of fever and profound systemic symptoms. The seasonal occurrence of these other viruses may also differ from that of influenza.

The acute onset of sore throat and fever, especially with adenitis, in adolescents is frequently caused by infectious mononucleosis (see subchapter on Epstein-Barr virus) or by group A β-hemolytic streptococci (see

Chapter 94). The initial presentation of these agents, however, generally includes a more prominent sore throat, often with exudate and petechiae, and with cervical adenitis. The primary agent that causes tracheobronchitis (and pneumonia) in adolescents similar to that caused by influenza is *Mycoplasma pneumoniae* (see Chapter 94). Other viral agents may also cause acute bronchitis, especially respiratory syncytial virus.

TREATMENT

Treatment of most cases of influenza in adolescents is symptomatic. Acetaminophen for the control of fever and myalgias is the mainstay of therapy. Aspirin should not be used for the treatment of influenza because of its association with an increased risk of Reye syndrome. Public awareness of this problem, and the labeling of aspirin, have resulted in a diminished use of aspirin for influenza and in a lower incidence of cases of Reye syndrome associated with its use in the treatment of influenza. However, the proportion of cases of Reye syndrome in adolescents has increased; this is believed to be a result of self-medication with aspirin by adolescents.

Specific treatment for influenza A virus, but not for influenza B virus, is possible with amantadine or rimantadine, the newer analogue of amantadine. Amantadine has been shown to be effective in diminishing the signs and symptoms of influenza in adults. Side effects of amantadine, such as insomnia, inability to concentrate, and dizziness, have limited its use for routine, uncomplicated influenza. Rimantadine is equally effective, but is associated with fewer side effects. Resistant strains, however, have developed during treatment of some children with uncomplicated influenza. The clinical significance of this is as yet unclear. Ribavirin has also been shown to be effective in the treatment of both influenza A and influenza B viral infections in college students, but this broad-spectrum antiviral agent is not currently approved for this use. Both ribavirin and amantadine or rimantadine have been used for the more severely ill, hospitalized patient, but the experience is thus far anecdotal. One *in vitro* study suggested that the two drugs may be additive in their antiviral effect against influenza A viral infection.

PREVENTION

For decades, the major emphasis in controlling the plague of influenza has been prevention through the use of inactivated influenza vaccines and, more recently, chemoprophylaxis with amantadine or rimantadine. Two types of inactivated influenza vaccines are now available, whole virus vaccines made from the intact, purified virus particles, and split virus vaccines, which are prepared by the additional step of disrupting the lipid-containing membrane of the virus. Large multicentered studies with these inactivated influenza vaccines in 1976 and 1978 showed that both types of vaccines were immunogenic and safe but, in younger children, the split product vaccines generally produced fewer side effects. Hence,

the subvirion vaccines are recommended for use in children under 13 years of age. Current vaccines, in contrast to the older vaccines, have few reactions. The efficacy of the vaccines is generally 70% to 80%, but depends on the antigenic similarity of the vaccine strain to the circulating strain.

Recommendations for the yearly use of the inactivated vaccines are primarily aimed at protecting individuals who are deemed to be at high risk for severe or complicated influenza. Targeted groups include those with functionally significant cardiac and chronic pulmonary disease, such as those with asthma, the immunosuppressed, and those with hemoglobinopathies (see Chapters 43, 52, 53, and 76). Others considered to be at high risk are those with diabetes mellitus or chronic renal or metabolic diseases and those receiving long-term aspirin therapy (see Chapters 30, 47, 50, 59, 60, 65, 88, and 90). In addition, normal adolescents are recommended for routine immunization if they are in close contact with high-risk patients. Other normal individuals may be immunized at the discretion of the physician and family. Because the influenza season frequently occurs at the time of important events in an adolescent's life, such as examination periods or championship sports events, immunization may be beneficial to some. Furthermore, many experts recommend influenza immunization for all students at boarding schools, colleges, and other such institutions.

Chemoprophylaxis against influenza A viral infection may also be accomplished using amantadine or rimantadine. Many studies have shown the efficacy of daily administration of these drugs to both children and adults in preventing influenza infection and illness. Chemoprophylaxis may be used when immunization has been missed, while waiting for protection to occur from immunization, and for the rare individual who cannot receive influenza vaccine. In those for whom maximum protection is desirable, chemoprophylaxis should be used with vaccination.

COURSE OF ILLNESS AND PROGNOSIS

The course of uncomplicated influenza in most adolescents is 3 to 5 days, occasionally longer. The most frequent sequela is tracheobronchitis, as mentioned above. Cough and abnormal pulmonary function studies, which are often clinically silent, may persist for several weeks. A less frequent complication in adolescents is a secondary bacterial pneumonia, which usually becomes manifest within a few days to 2 weeks after the onset of influenza. Staphylococcal complications, such as the toxic shock syndrome (see Chapter 94), may occur in previously healthy adolescents, especially after influenza B viral infection. A rare complication is the disseminated staphylococcal syndrome. This occurs primarily in previously normal adolescents, more frequently males, in whom *Staphylococcus aureus* may be isolated from the blood and other sites for prolonged periods.

Reye syndrome has been strongly linked with influenza. Approximately nine outbreaks of Reye syndrome have occurred during influenza B viral outbreaks, and a clustering of cases also occurred during the 1978 to 1979 outbreak of influenza A/Brazil/78/H_1N_1. The median age of cases occurring sporadically is approximately 6 years, whereas the median age of cases occurring in association with influenza is greater, about 11 years of age. The onset is usually 4 to 6 days (occasionally 2 weeks) from the onset of influenza. Typical features include nausea and vomiting, followed by a change in mental status, hepatomegaly, and elevated blood ammonia levels. The mortality may be 10% to 40%. The estimated risk of developing Reye syndrome after influenza is between 30.8 and 57.8 cases in 1 million infected students. As previously mentioned, children who receive aspirin for their prior influenza-like illness have higher incidence of Reye syndrome.

Individuals with underlying diseases may have a more prolonged or complicated illness, usually because of an increased chance of pulmonary or cardiac complications or because the febrile illness may aggravate the underlying condition. Whether pregnancy should be considered a high-risk condition for influenza has long been the subject of controversy (see Chapter 74). During the 1918 pandemic, an extraordinarily high mortality rate was reported for pregnant women who developed influenza, 25% in uncomplicated cases and 50% in those with pneumonia. More recent and better controlled studies, however, have suggested that pregnant women with influenza have the same complication rate as their nonpregnant counterparts. Influenza has not been shown to be teratogenic. Thus, in the recommendations for influenza vaccine, pregnancy is no longer considered as a high-risk condition.

BIBLIOGRAPHY

American Academy of Pediatrics: Report of the Committee on Infectious Diseases, 22nd ed. Elk Grove, IL, 1991, pp 274–281.

Brady MT, Sears SD, Clements ML, et al: Safety and efficacy of low-dose rimantadine for prophylaxis. J Respir Dis Dec. (Suppl):32, 1989.

Dietzman DE, Schaller JG, Ray CG, et al: Acute myositis associated with influenza B infection. Pediatrics 57:255, 1976.

Douglas RG, Jr: Prophylaxis and treatment of influenza. N Engl J Med 322:443, 1990.

Glezen WP: Consequences to children from influenza virus infections. Pediatr Virol 4:1, 1989.

Glezen WP, Decker M, Joseph SW, et al: Acute respiratory disease associated with influenza epidemics in Houston, 1981–83. J Infect Dis 155:1119, 1987.

Hall CB, Dolin R, Gala CL, et al: Treatment of children with influenza A infection with rimantadine. Pediatrics 80:275, 1987.

Hall CB, Douglas RG, Jr, Geiman JM, Meagher MP: Shedding patterns of children with influenza B infection. J Infect Dis 140:610, 1979.

Kilbourne ED: Influenza in man. In: The Influenza Viruses and Influenza. New York, Plenum, pp 157–218.

Kilbourne ED: Viral structure and composition. In: The Influenza Viruses and Influenza. New York, Plenum, 1987, pp 33–56.

Knight V, Gilbert BE: Ribavirin aerosol treatment of influenza. Antiviral chemotherapy. Infect Dis Clin North Am 1:441, 1987.

Little JW, Hall WJ, Douglas RG, Jr, et al: Airway hyperreactivity and peripheral airway dysfunction in influenza A infection. Am Rev Respir Dis 118:295, 1978.

Moser MR, Bender TR, Margolis HS, et al: An outbreak of influenza aboard a commercial airliner. Am J Epidemiol 110:1, 1979.

Wright PF, Cherry JD, Foy HM, et al: Antigenicity and reactogenicity of influenza A/USSR/77 virus vaccine in children—a multicentered evaluation of dosage and safety. Rev Infect Dis 5:758, 1983.

CHAPTER 94

Bacterial Infections

STAPHYLOCOCCAL INFECTION (TOXIC SHOCK SYNDROME)

JAMES K. TODD

Toxic shock syndrome is an acute, febrile, exanthematous illness associated with shock and multiorgan system involvement. It was formally described and associated with *Staphylococcus aureus* infection in 1978, although it is clear that sporadic cases had been reported previously. In 1980, toxic shock syndrome was associated with menstruation and tampon usage, especially in younger women. Although this association has been supported by subsequent studies, it is now clear that the removal of one tampon brand from the market and changes in tampon usage practices have not eliminated toxic shock syndrome as a problem in menstruating women, and that the disease also continues to occur in males as well as females of all ages, unassociated with menstruation. Toxic shock syndrome is a potentially life-threatening disease, which nonetheless can be managed successfully with the initiation of appropriate treatment if recognized early in its course.

EPIDEMIOLOGY

Toxic shock syndrome was originally described in seven children (three males and four females) in 1978. In 1980, epidemiologic data suggested an association in young women (many adolescents) with tampon use. Subsequently, an association was observed with a particular tampon brand, and it was removed from the marketplace. In spite of these actions, toxic shock syndrome has continued to occur, predominantly being seen in menstruating females using tampons, as well as in women using other inserted vaginal devices (e.g., diaphragms, contraceptive sponges) and in women in the postpartum period. Symptoms can occur at any age, but adolescents and young women seem to be at greatest risk. Table 94–1 presents the factors associated with an increased risk of toxic shock syndrome, including menstruation, and also emphasizes that males or females may get toxic shock syndrome associated with surgical wound infections or proven *Staphylococcus aureus* infections of any type (e.g., cellulitis, abscess, pneumonia, bacteremia). In addition, any adolescent patient with

shock or a fever and a rash, and with the other common symptoms of toxic shock syndrome (e.g., nausea, vomiting, diarrhea, myalgia, mucous membrane hyperemia), should have toxic shock syndrome included in the differential diagnosis. Although current passive surveillance techniques suggest that the incidence of toxic shock syndrome has decreased since 1980, it is still reported throughout the United States and the rest of the world and remains a very serious and potentially fatal infection.

PATHOPHYSIOLOGY

Toxic shock syndrome was initially associated with *S. aureus* infection, but its epidemiology suggests some unusual pathophysiologic aspects, because it was found to occur only in those patients who had proven focal sites of *S. aureus* infection. Figure 94–1 depicts the current understanding of the pathophysiology of toxic shock syndrome. Initially an adolescent patient must be colonized with certain *S. aureus* strains that are known to produce the causative toxins. It is clear that mere colonization is not enough to initiate disease, because many individuals can be shown to be colonized, and most normal individuals develop antibodies to these toxins without any known associated illness. The occurrence of toxic shock syndrome is associated primarily

TABLE 94–1. Clinical Risk Factors or Symptoms for Toxic Shock Syndrome

RISK FACTOR OR SYMPTOM(S)	SEX
Menstruation with tampon or other inserted vaginal foreign body	F
Use of barrier contraception (e.g., diaphragm, contraceptive sponge)	F
Postpartum period	F
Surgical or traumatic wound infection	M or F
Staphylococcus aureus infection	M or F
Fever, with hypotension or rash*	M or F

*Common presenting symptoms include fever, rash, hypotension, conjunctival hyperemia, pharyngitis, myalgias, vomiting, and diarrhea.

893

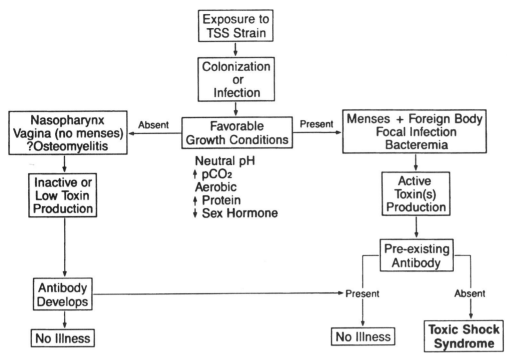

Figure 94–1. Pathogenesis of toxic shock syndrome. (With permission from Todd JK: Toxic shock syndrome. Clin Microbiol Rev 1:432–446, 1988.)

with menstruation and tampon use and with focal infections (e.g. cellulitis, abscess), suggesting that conditions at the site of these infections may differ from those of sites of colonization and may enhance the production of toxin. These conditions were actually measured in a number of patients with toxic shock syndrome. It was found that they consisted of a relatively normal pH within an aerobic environment, increased PCO_2, and the presence of protein. *In vitro* studies confirmed that these identical conditions are necessary for maximal production of toxin. Figure 94–1 also explains why, in certain infections in which these conditions are not present (e.g., osteomyelitis), or at sites of normal staphylococcal colonization (e.g., anterior nares), where the requisite conditions are not present, disease is unlikely to occur. In addition, only adolescents who do not have prior immunity to the toxins are at risk at the time of exposure.

The association of these specific growth conditions at sites of focal infections has been extended by the epidemiologic observation that TSS occurs most commonly in young women who are menstruating and using some type of inserted vaginal device. Normally, at times during the menstrual cycle not associated with menstruation, the vagina has an acidic pH and is anaerobic. During menstruation, menstrual blood tends to neutralize the pH of the vagina, but it remains anaerobic until a tampon (regardless of brand) is inserted, thus providing the oxygen necessary for toxin formation. This explains why toxic shock syndrome can occur in both males and females but is more likely to occur in menstruating females using an inserted vaginal device. The key role of tampons in pathogenesis seems to be that they carry oxygen to the vagina. Once an inserted vaginal device is in place, the longer it is left in place, the more time the organism has to express its toxic potential.

After the toxin(s) has been absorbed into the body, it appears to activate interleukin-1 (IL-1) and tumor necrosis factor (TNF), which may then mediate vascular leakage and hypotension and produce the rash. Subsequent multiorgan system involvement is associated with the severity of the hypotension. The pathophysiology of shock seems to be a high-output, low–peripheral resistance, decreased venous return phenomenon, typical of a disease caused by leaky capillaries.

MICROBIOLOGY

When it was first described, toxic shock syndrome was associated with a hypothetical exotoxin produced by *Staphylococcus aureus*. Since then, the primary toxin, called toxic shock syndrome toxin-1 (TSST-1), has been purified and shown to produce similar toxicity in animals. In addition, several staphylococcal toxins, including a number of the enterotoxins, have been epidemiologically associated with toxic shock syndrome. It is well documented that TSST-1–negative strains may cause classic symptoms of toxic shock syndrome. Other organisms, most commonly group A streptococci, have occasionally been associated with a clinical illness similar to TSS. Thus, it appears that both group A streptococci and *Staphylococcus aureus* can cause a syndrome that could be clinically defined as toxic shock syndrome.

CLINICAL MANIFESTATIONS

Table 94–2 summarizes the case definition of toxic shock syndrome. Major criteria include an acute fever associated with a generalized erythematous rash that, at convalescence, has characteristic desquamation of the fingertips, toe tips, palms, and soles. The other major

TABLE 94–2. Clinical Definition of Toxic Shock Syndrome

Major criteria (all must be present)
  Acute fever
  Exanthem (diffuse erythroderma)
  Desquamation (convalescent)
  Hypotension (orthostatic syncope, shock)
Minor criteria (three or more)
  Gastrointestinal (vomiting or diarrhea)
  Muscular (severe myalgia, elevated creatine phosphokinase [CPK] level)
  Mucous membrane hyperemia (vaginal, pharyngeal, conjunctival)
  Central nervous system (nonfocal altered consciousness unrelated to hypotension)
  Renal (elevated blood urea nitrogen or creatinine levels or >5 WBCs/high-power field)
  Hepatic (elevated liver function tests)
  Hematologic (platelets <100,000/mm^3)
Exclusionary data
  Negative nonpermissive cultures (other than *Staphylococcus aureus*)
  Serologic studies, excluding other causes

feature is hypotension, which may be characterized as a blood pressure lower than that for the 5th percentile for age, or orthostatic changes, including dizziness or syncope. At least three minor criteria reflecting multiorgan system involvement are required, as well as exclusionary data that exclude diseases within the differential diagnosis (e.g., bacteremia, other than *Staphylococcus aureus* or group A streptococci endotoxic shock, leptospirosis, measles, Rocky Mountain spotted fever, Kawasaki syndrome, and severe drug reaction).

The adolescent patient who has classic toxic shock syndrome presents early with fever, nausea and vomiting, diarrhea, and pharyngitis. The erythematous rash may be mild and may have gone unnoticed. Adolescent patients characteristically have early hyperemia of their mucous membranes (conjunctiva, pharynx, vagina). It is important to emphasize that not all rashes are typical of that of toxic shock syndrome. The classic rash is a scarlatiniform macular eruption that is often more pronounced on the face and trunk than on the extremities (especially if hypotension is present). The conjunctivitis is characterized by an absence of purulent exudate.

Because toxic shock syndrome can occur in males as well as females, it is important not to use menstruation or tampon usage as a marker for the disease. In all adolescent patients with the clinical symptoms listed above, it is important to look for a focus of infection, because the staphylococcal organism that most commonly causes this syndrome requires special growth conditions to express toxin and, therefore, disease. In adolescent females who have had menarche, this includes the potential of a vaginal focus. It is also important to emphasize that anyone, including young women, may develop toxic shock syndrome because of some other nonmenstrual focus (e.g., abscess, cellulitis), which should be sought assiduously. Occult sinusitis has been shown to be a potential focus of infection that can lead to toxic shock syndrome, so a thorough examination of all patients is in order to determine the site at which the organism is growing and producing toxin.

DIAGNOSIS AND TREATMENT

The basis of successful treatment of toxic shock syndrome is early diagnosis. Using the risk features shown in Table 94–1 and the diagnostic features in Table 94–2, early diagnosis should be possible. Such diagnosis may be missed if it is not well understood that TSS can occur in males or in females who are *not* menstruating. Therefore, menstruation is not a feature of the diagnostic definition, and should not be used exclusively as a marker for risk. Any adolescent patient who has a *Staphylococcus aureus* infection or who presents with shock or an erythematous rash should have toxic shock syndrome considered early in the differential diagnostic workup. If, on further evaluation, this diagnosis appears to be likely, initial treatment should consist of careful monitoring of the vital signs, including temperature, heart rate, respiratory rate, and blood pressure, and of the urine output. Initial laboratory screening tests should include a white blood cell and differential count, electrolyte, renal function and liver function tests, a platelet count, and disseminated intravascular coagulation (DIC) screen, as well as a CPK test, because muscle involvement is often a prominent clinical feature. In addition, it is important to identify any potential focus of *S. aureus* infection on physical examination and history and to provide appropriate drainage of the infectious site as soon as possible. This includes removal of any tampon in a menstruating adolescent with gentle vaginal irrigation to remove any residual toxin and surgical drainage of any abscess or sequestered focus of infection. Appropriate cultures should be taken as soon as possible, including blood cultures and any potential focus of infection, followed immediately by parenteral antistaphylococcal therapy (see Chapter 96). Intravenous fluids should be given in large volumes to compensate for any deficit and to reestablish blood pressure, perfusion, and urine output. This should initially include crystalloid (e.g., Ringer lactate or normal saline) and might include colloid in adolescent patients refractory to standard fluid therapy.

Because the capillaries appear to be leaky in those with toxic shock syndrome, large amounts of fluid continue to be lost in the interstitial space, and venous return continues to be poor in spite of the development of edema and the administration of larger than expected volumes of fluid. Under such circumstances, a central venous pressure catheter or Swan-Ganz catheter may help monitor fluid status. In general, continued administration of fluid results in an increased venous return and appropriate cardiac output, with abatement of signs of hypotension. In some cases, adult respiratory distress syndrome (ARDS) or myocardial failure may develop as a consequence of the initial shock. These are not usually caused by excessive fluid administration but are complications of the original disease. Continued administration of appropriate volumes of fluid, the provision of positive end-expiratory pressure (PEEP) for airways, or the administration of inotropic agents such as dopamine or dobutamine for cardiac failure may be necessary. In severely ill adolescent patients with refractory hypotension, parenteral steroids (methylprednisolone,

10 mg/kg/dose) and intravenous immune globulin (1 g/kg) may be used.

Once adolescents who have toxic shock syndrome begin to improve, they can maintain adequate hydration orally and their temperature returns to normal. At this time, they may be changed from intravenous to oral antimicrobial agents, with a rapid tapering of corticosteroids (if used). Relapses are rare during the acute period as long as the site of infection has been appropriately drained. Adolescents recovering from severe episodes of toxic shock syndrome may suffer from intensive care unit neurosis. They are concerned generally about the risk of recurrence and their ability to fight infection in the future. These concerns should be anticipated and can be allayed by expectant reassurance. During the second week of convalescence, adolescent patients usually develop peeling of the fingertips, toe tips, palms, and soles. Months later they may have transient hair loss, as well as creasing of the nails. Forewarning hospitalized adolescents that these benign and transient sequelae may occur can help allay future apprehension.

Recurrence of toxic shock syndrome has occurred commonly in menstruating women who were not adequately treated with antistaphylococcal antibiotics or who continue to use tampons during subsequent menstrual periods. The current recommendation is to avoid tampon use for the subsequent five menstrual periods and thereafter to remove any tampon or vaginal device immediately if any of the initial symptoms (e.g., fever, nausea, vomiting, diarrhea) of toxic shock syndrome appear. This advice is equally important to all adolescent females. In addition, it is probably advisable to counsel young women who are first beginning to use tampons about the risk of toxic shock syndrome and of early clinical signs. Frequent changing of tampons during the day and the use of pads at night provides an additional safety factor.

Toxic shock syndrome is not entirely preventable because it can occur in association with many types and sites of *S. aureus* infection. However, with early diagnosis and therapy, most adolescents can be treated successfully (Table 94–3).

TABLE 94–3. Principles of Prospective Management of Toxic Shock Syndrome

CLINICAL CONDITION	INITIAL EVALUATION*	ONGOING MONITORING	THERAPY
Presentation			
Infectious focus	Identify focus	Body temperature	Remove tampon, irrigate vagina, surgical drainage of abscess
	Cultures: blood, focus, urine, vagina		Antibiotic: IV antistaphylococcal antibiotic
Hypotension		Vital signs: blood pressure, urine output, central venous pressure, peripheral perfusion	Fluids: colloid and crystalloid to maintain normal pressures, urine output, expect two to five times normal maintenance fluids
			Severe cases: intravenous immune globulin (1 g/kg), methylprednisolone (10 mg/kg every 8 to 12 hours, IV)
Disseminated intravascular coagulation (DIC)		Clinical bleeding, signs of vaso-occlusion	Rarely necessary
Progression			
Edema		Weight	Fluids: maintain normal central venous pressure (CVP); likely to require colloid and fluids far in excess of expected†
Adult respiratory distress syndrome (ARDS) (24–48 hours)	Chest x-ray	Respiratory rate, color; chest x-ray, blood gases	Positive pressure: intubate, PEEP, increased F_{IO_2}†
Myocardial failure		CVP; echocardiogram; Swan-Ganz catheter; gallop rhythm	Inotropic agents: dopamine; maintain normal calcium level
Acute renal failure		Urine output, blood urea nitrogen (BUN), creatinine	Perfusion: maintain blood pressure; dialysis
Convalescence			
Infection			Antibiotic: 10 days total antistaphylococcal therapy
Expected sequelae			
Peeling fingers, toes, hands, feet; hair loss			Anticipatory guidance
Intensive care neurosis			Empathetic anticipation and reassurance
Recurrence		Clinical	Avoidance: no tampons for 4 to 6 months
			Anticipation: see physician for recurrent focus of infection, fever with menstruation

*Should include following laboratory tests: cultures (see above), complete blood cell and differential count, (DIC) screen, BUN, creatinine, urine analysis, liver function tests, CPK, electrolyte, calcium, phosphate, and serum protein levels, others (as indicated by condition).
†Avoid temptation to restrict fluids or administer diuretics at the expense of maintaining an adequate filling pressure.

BIBLIOGRAPHY

Davis JP, Osterholm MT, Helms CM, et al: Tri-state toxic shock syndrome study. II. Clinical and laboratory findings. J Infect Dis 145:441, 1982.

Fisher CJ Jr, Horowitz Z, Albertson TE: Cardiorespiratory failure in toxic shock syndrome: effect of dobutamine. Crit Care Med 13:160, 1985.

Shands KN, Schmid GP, Dan BB, et al: Toxic shock syndrome in menstruating women: Association with tampon uses and *Staphylococcus aureus* and clinical features in 52 cases. N Engl J Med 303:1436, 1980.

Todd J: Toxic shock syndrome. Clin Microbiol Rev 1:432, 1988.

Todd J, Fishaut M, Kapral F, Welch T: Toxic shock syndrome associated with phage-group I staphylococci. Lancet 2:1116, 1978.

Todd JK, Ressman M, Caston SA, et al: Corticosteroid therapy for patients with toxic shock syndrome. JAMA 252:3399, 1984.

Todd JK, Todd BH, Franco-Buff A, et al: Influence of focal growth conditions on the pathogenesis of toxic shock syndrome. J Infect Dis 155:673, 1987.

Todd JK, Wiesenthal AM, Ressman M, et al: Toxic shock syndrome. II. Estimated occurrence in Colorado as influenced by case ascertainment methods. Am J Epidemiol 122:857, 1985.

STREPTOCOCCAL INFECTIONS

MICHAEL E. PICHICHERO

MICROBIOLOGY

Streptococci are part of the normal flora of the upper respiratory and gastrointestinal tracts, skin, and mucous membranes of adolescents. Their ability to cause infection is determined by the species, strain, and host response. Streptococci cause various infections (Table 94–4). In addition, a carrier state can exist in which these bacteria can be cultured, but are not pathogenic.

Streptococci are gram-positive bacteria that grow in culture as pairs or chains of variable length. On sheep blood agar they appear as transparent to opaque, round, small colonies surrounded by a zone of hemolysis of red cells: complete hemolysis (β), partial (α), or absent (γ). The β-hemolytic streptococci include the pathogens of Lancefield groups A, C, and G. *Streptococcus viridans* produces variable hemolysis of the α or γ type; group D streptococci produce variable hemolysis. *Streptococcus pneumoniae (Pneumococcus)* produces α-hemolysis.

Biologic products elaborated by streptococci are important determinants of virulence. Antibody responses to these antigens are sometimes used to identify streptococci as the cause of an infection. In addition to hemolysins (including streptolysins O and S), streptococci may elaborate streptokinase, streptodornase, bacteriocins, deoxyribonuclease, exotoxins, hyaluronidase, nicotinamide adenine dinucleotidase, and proteinase.

EPIDEMIOLOGY

The spread of streptococci varies with the clinical infection. For groups A, C, and G streptococcal pharyngitis, close contact among adolescents is required. Spread within family units or in the classroom occurs by direct projection of large aerosolized droplets from the respiratory tract or by physical transfer of secretions containing the bacteria. The acute stage of pharyngitis is associated with the greatest period of contagion. Antibiotic therapy rapidly suppresses contagion so that, following 24 hours of treatment, adolescents are noninfectious and can return to normal activities. However, in some cases, even after a course of antibiotics, a subclinical infection persists or a carrier state may become established. Under these circumstances, contagion may recur and provide conditions for the continued endemic spread of these bacteria. Streptococcal pharyngitis is more frequent in the winter and spring than during the other seasons.

Among the streptococcal species, group A β-hemolytic streptococci are the most commonly associated with adolescent infections and are the only strain associated with acute rheumatic fever. Group A, probably group

TABLE 94–4. Infections Caused by Streptococci in Adolescents

SYSTEM OR AREA AFFECTED	INFECTION(S)
Upper respiratory tract	Tonsillopharyngitis Otitis media Sinusitis
Lower respiratory tract	Pneumonia Empyema
Skin and soft tissue	Impetigo Cellulitis Erysipelas
Cardiovascular	Endocarditis Myocarditis Pericarditis Phlebitis
Central nervous system	Meningitis Brain abscess
Musculoskeletal	Septic arthritis Osteomyelitis Pyomyositis
Abdominal	Peritonitis Appendicitis Liver abscess
Genitourinary	Pyelonephritis Urethrocystitis Vulvovaginitis
Ophthalmic	Conjunctivitis
Lymphatic	Lymphadenitis
Systemic	Septicemia

G, and group C streptococci are associated with post-streptococcal glomerulonephritis (see Chapter 65).

Impetigo or pyoderma produced by streptococci require trauma to the skin for infection to occur. The streptococci causing impetigo or pyoderma may be found in the nose or throat, but this usually occurs after the establishment of skin infection. Impetigo is generally a disease that occurs during the summer months. Streptococcal pharyngitis and impetigo are both more common in preadolescence than in adolescence.

Streptococcus viridans is part of the normal oral flora and is the bacterium most commonly associated with endocarditis. The spectrum of disease caused by this organism is not well defined, but includes uncomplicated transient bacteremia and dental caries. Manipulative procedures in the oropharynx are the source of *S. viridans* bacteremia. In nearly all cases the bacteremia is quickly cleared by natural host defenses. A previously damaged heart valve, a prosthetic heart valve, or injured endocardium may serve as the nidus of infection. Therefore, patients with valvular or congenital heart disease should receive antibiotic prophylaxis at the time of dental and selected other surgical procedures (see Chapters 47 and 96).

Group D streptococci *(Streptococcus faecalis, S. faecium,* and *S. durans)* are normal skin, gastrointestinal, and genitourinary flora. They are bacteria with low virulence and require special host conditions to produce disease. Bacteremia with subsequent deep-seated infection (e.g., endocarditis) usually originates from the genitourinary tract following manipulation, but seeding from the skin or biliary or intestinal tract can occur.

Streptococcus pneumoniae are normal upper respiratory flora, colonizing as many as 50% of adolescents. Pneumococci are the second most common cause of bacterial pneumonia in adolescents (after *Mycoplasma pneumoniae;* see next subchapter) and the most common cause of bacterial meningitis. Pneumococcal infections predominate in fall and winter and occur more frequently in adolescent males than in adolescent females.

PATHOPHYSIOLOGY

Group A β-hemolytic streptococci (GABHS) attach to the epithelial cells of the upper respiratory tract or the skin by a cell wall component composed of lipoteichoic acid. To initiate infections, GABHS must compete with indigenous flora for attachment sites. Invasion of tissues by GABHS may be enhanced through the production of toxins and enzymes by the bacteria. The changes in tissues infected with streptococci are those of an acute inflammatory response (e.g., migration of polymorphonuclear leukocytes, edema, erythema, and pain). Regional lymphadenopathy is common as the lymphoid tissue reacts to prevent the spread of the infection.

The rash and other toxic manifestations of GABHS scarlet fever have been attributed to the development of hypersensitivity to the erythrogenic toxins produced by these bacteria. In the skin, there is an acute dilatation of blood vessels and a superficial inflammatory infiltrate. The death of epidermal cells leads to desquamation.

Similar to GABHS, the pathogenesis of *Streptococcus viridans*, group D streptococcal, or *S. pneumoniae* infections involves bacterial attachment to susceptible tissues, followed by an inflammatory process.

CLINICAL MANIFESTATIONS

Streptococcal infections during adolescence most commonly involve the respiratory tract, skin, and soft tissues. Bacteremic dissemination with subsequent deep infections are rare in adolescence and therefore are not discussed in detail here. Rheumatic fever and glomerulonephritis are described elsewhere (see Chapters 50 and 65).

Respiratory Tract Infections

These conditions are also discussed in Chapters 40 and 43.

PHARYNGITIS

Fewer than 15% of adolescents who visit a physician with a sore throat are infected with streptococci. Approximately 50% of adolescents with tonsillopharyngitis are infected with a virus (Table 94–5). The remainder of sore throats in adolescents are generally referred to as idiopathic. A relationship between streptococcal infection and infectious mononucleosis has been noted (see Chapter 93). When urogenital gonorrhea is present in an adolescent, the possibility of *Neisseria gonorrhoeae* as the cause of pharyngitis should be considered. Similarly, when the history discloses a high risk for sexually transmitted disease (STD), or if another STD is present, pharyngitis secondary to *N. gonorrhoeae* should be considered.

Common signs and symptoms of acute GABHS pharyngitis are noted in Table 94–6. Classic GABHS pharyngitis presents with a severe sore throat of acute onset, accompanied by fever and cervical adenopathy. The adolescent may report fatigue, dysphagia, and anorexia. Symptoms of headache and occasionally abdominal discomfort can be elicited. Notably, GABHS pharyngitis is not accompanied by symptoms of the common cold; therefore, the presence of cough or rhinorrhea should be viewed as a negative factor for streptococcal pharyngitis and should lead to consideration of an alternate diagnosis. On physical examination, the pharynx is typically very inflamed with edema of the tonsils and profuse yellowish pharyngeal exudate. There may be palatal petechiae with or without an associated "strawberry" tongue. Cervical adenopathy involves the anterior chain, and the nodes are moderately tender to palpation. A scarlatiniform rash, if present, predominates in the axilla and inguinal areas, has a sandpaper feeling, and consists of multiple, very small, erythematous papules. Streptococcal pharyngitis may be associated with infection of the sinuses, otitis media, or pneumonia.

Symptoms of groups C and G streptococcal pharyn-

TABLE 94–5. Common Causes of Acute Pharyngitis

	FREQUENCY OF OCCURRENCE	EXAMPLES
Primary pathogens	15%	Group A β-hemolytic streptococci (GABHS) Group C streptococci Group G streptococci *Neisseria gonorrhoeae*
Possible primary pathogen	<5%	*Chlamydia pneumoniae* (TWAR) *Mycoplasma pneumoniae* *Archanobacterium haemolyticum*
Viruses	50%	Rhinovirus Adenovirus Influenza A and B Parainfluenza Coxsackievirus Coronavirus Echovirus Herpes simplex Epstein-Barr Cytomegalovirus
No pathogen isolated	30%	
Possible copathogens		*Staphylococcus aureus* *Haemophilus influenzae* *Moraxella catarrhalis* *Bacteroides melaninogenicus* *Bacteroides oralis* *Bacteroides fragilis* *Fusobacterium* spp. Peptostreptococci

gitis are similar to those of GABHS. Adolescents and young adults are particularly susceptible to groups C and G streptococcal pharyngitis. The symptoms may not be as severe as those of GABHS, but all the symptoms described above may be present.

OTITIS MEDIA

Most bacterial cases of otitis media and sinusitis are caused by *Streptococcus pneumoniae, Haemophilus influenzae* (see subchapter on *H. influenzae*), and *Moraxella (Branhamella) catarrhalis. S. pneumoniae* accounts for 25% to 35% and GABHS for 5% to 10% of cases of acute otitis media and sinusitis, and therefore both must be considered as possible causative factors in these conditions.

TABLE 94–6. Common Signs and Symptoms of Acute GABHS Pharyngitis

Rapid onset of symptoms ("scratchy throat" for several days is a negative factor for GABHS)
Fever (usually with rapid onset; 100.5° to 102°F [or 38° to 39°C])
Cervical adenopathy
Headache
Abdominal discomfort
Absence of cough (cough and nasal discharge are negative factors for GABHS)
Pharyngeal erythema
Pharyngeal exudate

The history of acute otitis media is generally one of acute ear pain, often associated with fever, diminished hearing, and cough. On physical examination pneumatic otoscopy should be employed. The findings of a red, bulging tympanic membrane with purulent material in the middle ear space should indicate a high likelihood of *Streptococcus pneumoniae* or GABHS otitis media. Otitis media caused by other major bacterial pathogens, such as *Haemophilus influenzae* and *Moraxella catarrhalis*, is more likely to produce a thickened appearing tympanic membrane with less erythema and a grayish exudate in the middle ear space (see Chapter 40). However, these distinctions on clinical examination are far from universal and cannot be relied upon to direct therapy.

PNEUMONIA

Streptococcus pneumoniae and GABHS may also cause pneumonia (see Chapter 43). The clinical presentation is generally that of a rapidly progressive illness with a lobar infiltrate. A greater degree of tissue necrosis is produced by GABHS, thereby causing a radiologic picture that is more severe than would be expected with *S. pneumoniae*. GABHS pneumonia results in the development of pleural effusions and/or empyema requiring chest drainage more frequently than pneumococcal pneumonia.

With *Streptococcus pneumoniae* and GABHS, fever in excess of 39°C, productive cough, and significant constitutional symptoms, such as dyspnea, malaise, and fatigue, are typical. On examination, the findings of a lobar consolidation in an ill-appearing adolescent should be anticipated.

Skin Infections

The most common form of skin and soft tissue infection caused by GABHS is impetigo. Typically, at the site of a previous injury, such as a scratch, abrasion, or insect bite, a small pustule develops that subsequently ruptures spontaneously with the development of a thin, honey-colored scab. Multiple sites of involvement are a result of scratching. The individual lesions are very superficial and involve the outermost layers of the epidermis.

Erysipelas is a superficial cellulitis characterized by a raised, irregular, advancing border. Systemic symptoms include fever, vomiting, and irritability. GABHS may be the only causative organism or may be present with *Staphylococcus aureus*, as in other forms of cellulitis. There are no unique clinical features to skin and soft tissue infections caused by GABHS compared with those of *S. aureus*; thus, both organisms should be considered.

Streptococcal scarlet fever must be differentiated from various viral exanthems, including the exanthem of infectious mononucleosis and enteroviral infection. Rubeola (measles), which is noted to be increasing in incidence in the adolescent population, should also be given consideration in the differential diagnosis. Other entities similar to streptococcal skin rashes at some phase in their evolution include erythema infectiosum (fifth disease), rubella, scalded skin syndrome (toxic epidermolysis), Stevens-Johnson syndrome, and Kawasaki disease, all of which are rare (see Chapter 93).

Bacteremia and Meningitis

Invasion of the blood stream or meninges rarely occurs following infection of the upper respiratory tract or skin with streptococci. An increased incidence of invasive streptococcal infection is observed in certain vulnerable hosts (e.g., adolescents who are postsplenectomy, those with sickle cell disease, or those who are immunodeficient). Signs and symptoms of streptococcal bacteremia and/or meningitis do not differ notably from those caused by other bacteria, which more commonly produce these conditions in adolescents.

ENDOCARDITIS

Fever, chills, malaise, anorexia, weight loss, myalgia, and arthralgia comprise the classic clinical presentation of endocarditis (see Chapter 50). A heart murmur is heard at some time in the course of the disease in nearly 100% of adolescents with bacterial endocarditis. Embolic phenomena result in petechiae, splinter hemorrhages, clubbing, Osler nodes, and Janeway spots, and are observed less frequently in adolescents than in adults with endocarditis.

LABORATORY DIAGNOSIS

Respiratory Tract Infections

PHARYNGITIS

The clinical diagnosis of streptococcal pharyngitis without culture confirmation misses at least 15% to 25% of cases. One advantage of obtaining a throat culture for determination of streptococcal infection is improved compliance of the adolescent with a therapeutic regimen. Many adolescents whose symptoms have improved after several days of penicillin do not continue the medication for the full 10-day treatment course prescribed. If the presence of streptococcal infection has been *proven* by culture, there is an increased chance of compliance (see Chapter 26).

The sensitivity, specificity, and overall accuracy of the new "rapid strep test" (latex agglutination and enzyme immunoassay test) have now been evaluated. Unfortunately, approximately 10% of assays using the rapid strep test yield false-negative results when, in fact, the adolescent does have GABHS infection. To avoid missing these adolescent patients, throat culture is necessary; if positive, treatment can be instituted for adolescents with hemolytic streptococcal infection. If a physician is intent on diagnosing GABHS and wishes to avoid missing adolescents who are infected, and thus vulnerable to developing rheumatic fever, a second swab should be processed as a routine throat culture when the rapid strep test result is negative.

OTITIS MEDIA

The only laboratory method currently available for the definitive diagnosis of otitis media is tympanocentesis. This procedure is infrequently used in the United States for those with uncomplicated acute otitis media. Tympanometry, pneumatic otoscopy, and audiometry are useful laboratory adjuncts to assist in the follow-up and objective characterization of morbidity associated with acute otitis media.

PNEUMONIA

Confirmation of the diagnosis of pneumonia (see Chapter 40) is made presumptively by chest radiography. The diagnosis of the causative pathogen through sputum analysis, transtracheal aspirate, or lung puncture is infrequently pursued because of variable reliability or perceived morbidity from the procedure.

Skin Infections

Laboratory confirmation of group A β-hemolytic streptococcal skin infection requires culture of the skin on sheep's blood agar. GABHS impetigo may occur concomitantly with *Staphylococcus aureus* skin infection.

Bacteremia and Meningitis

Group A β-hemolytic streptococcal bacteremia and *Streptococcus pneumoniae* bacteremia are rare in adolescents. Laboratory confirmation requires culture of blood or of the specific site that was secondarily seeded (e.g., cerebrospinal fluid for meningitis).

TREATMENT

Respiratory Infections

PHARYNGITIS

Treatment of GABHS pharyngitis prevents suppurative complications, reduces contagion, shortens its course, and usually prevents acute rheumatic fever and poststreptococcal glomerulonephritis. Treatment of groups C and G β-hemolytic streptococcal pharyngitis probably prevents suppurative complications, reduces contagion, and shortens the course of illness. The impact of treatment on preventing poststreptococcal glomerulonephritis caused by these serogroups is less well understood.

The incidence of bacteriologic and clinical failures with treatment regimens using penicillins has been rising over the past 20 years. There is variability among regions, but 20% to 30% of all adolescents with GABHS pharyngitis treated with penicillin, whether orally or by intramuscular injection, may develop a bacteriologic or clinical relapse. The incidence of relapse can be reduced by using alternate agents with broader antimicrobial coverage. Cephalosporins as an antibiotic class produce

GABHS pharyngitis failures in 2% to 10% of adolescent patients. Other drugs with superior bactericidal effects include dicloxicillin and amoxicillin-clavulanate. For eradication of the streptococcal carrier state, the combination of penicillin for 10 days and rifampin (300 mg twice daily for 4 days) for the last 4 days of the 10-day penicillin treatment course has proven effective. Sulfa drugs (e.g., trimethoprim-sulfamethoxazole; Septra, Bactrim) and tetracycline should not be used to treat GABHS disease, because they are ineffective.

The most common explanation for recurrent streptococcal pharyngitis is inadequate compliance (Table 94–7) with the therapeutic regimen (see Chapter 26). In the case of penicillin, which is generally prescribed three times daily, directions for optimal absorption (e.g., administration 1 hour before meals and 2 hours after meals) often compounds the compliance issue. Streptococcal recurrences may also involve repeated exposure within a family setting or among peers at school. Throat cultures of likely co-infected persons (e.g., siblings, parents, friends) may shed light on a particularly persistent case of streptococcal relapse. The presence of β-lactamase–producing "copathogens" in a specific adolescent may account for recurrence(s) of streptococcal infection after treatment with penicillin. Probable co-pathogens include *Staphylococcus aureus, Haemophilus influenzae, Moraxella catarrhalis*, and anaerobes. These normal pharyngeal flora elaborate β-lactamases that inactivate penicillin in the tonsillar milieu, thereby preventing penicillin's direct action on the streptococci. Retreatment of adolescent patients who do not respond to penicillin therapy should involve selection of an alternative antibiotic agent with a broader spectrum of activity, such as a cephalosporin. *Tolerance* to an antimicrobial refers to a phenomenon in which the concentration of antibiotic required to kill a specific bacterium is 16- to 32-fold greater than that required to inhibit growth. Tolerance of GABHS to penicillin has been described in several clinical studies; tolerance may be associated with penicillin treatment failure. Some streptococcal recurrences may occur because immediate antibiotic use (prior to the occurrence of 48 hours of symptoms) prevents the adolescent's host immunity from developing to the infecting GABHS strain. Eradication of streptococci before the development of a host

response thereby predisposes these adolescents to reinfection. Finally, a "carrier" state can occur with GABHS, in which the organism is no longer pathogenic; with their virulence potential lost, these bacteria become commensals.

Effective management of adolescent streptococcal pharyngitis should start with the importance of emphasizing compliance. When first-line therapy with penicillin fails, alternative antibiotics with appropriate activity (e.g., a cephalosporin) should be considered. In the case of frequent recurrences, cultures of family members and friends may be useful. To determine whether the adolescent is simply a carrier of streptococci, some experts recommend measuring antibody titers (antistreptolysin O and antiDNase B) and assessing changes over time. If all other options have been explored, low-dose, long-term antibiotic prophylaxis might be effective to reduce or eliminate streptococcal occurrences over the period of a winter season. Rheumatic fever prophylaxis doses are appropriate. In rare cases, tonsillectomy might be considered.

OTITIS MEDIA

Treatment of *Streptococcus pneumoniae* or GABHS as the cause of acute otitis media or sinusitis (see Chapter 40) in nearly all cases may be adequately accomplished with the use of oral penicillin. However, these streptococci are not the only significant bacterial pathogens in these conditions. Therefore, without definitive culture from middle ear or sinus fluid, therapy must employ broader spectrum agents that are effective against most (if not all) of the most likely pathogens. Alternate agents (Table 94–8) include amoxicillin, cefaclor, cefuroxime axetil, cefixime, and amoxicillin-cla-

TABLE 94–7. Explanations for Recurrent GABHS Pharyngitis

Inadequate compliance with therapeutic regimen
Reacquisition from close contact
β-Lactamase–producing oral microflora
Resistance or tolerance to antibiotic
Host immunity suppressed by "early" antibiotic use
Carrier state, no disease

TABLE 94–8. Efficacy of Selected Antimicrobial Agents for Common Bacterial Pathogens in Acute Otitis Media and Sinusitis

ANTIMICROBIAL AGENT	PATHOGEN				
	Streptococcus pneumoniae (30–40%)	*Haemophilus influenzae* (20%)	*Branhamella catarrhalis* (<20%)	*Streptococcus pyogenes* (<5%)	*Staphylococcus aureus* (<5%)
Ampicillin or amoxicillin	+	±	±	+	±
Cefaclor	+	±	±	+	+
Cefuroxime axetil	+	+	+	+	+
Cefixime	±	+	+	+	−
Amoxicillin plus avulanate	+	+	+	+	+
Erythromycin plus sulfisoxazole	+	+	+	+	+
Trimethoprim plus sulfamethoxazole	+	+	+	−	+

vulanate (see Chapter 96). In considering antimicrobial therapy for these clinical entities, consideration of the potential for serious adverse effects, gastrointestinal upset, dosing frequency, and cost must be weighed in the final clinical decision.

When initial empirical antimicrobial therapy is unsuccessful, resistant pathogens may be causative. Antibiotic tolerance, resistance, or host factors may be active. Persisting in retreatment with β-lactamase–susceptible antimicrobial agents, (e.g., amoxicillin) in the face of clinical failure, is an inappropriate strategy.

PNEUMONIA (see Chapters 43 and 96)

Treatment of early, mild GABHS pneumonia or of *Streptococcus pneumoniae* involves the use of penicillin orally or by injection. The length of such treatment is empirical. For *S. pneumoniae*, a 7- to 10-day course is usually instituted. A longer treatment course may be necessary for GABHS, because the pneumonic process tends to be necrotizing. However, duration of treatment should be based on the clinical response. Treatment failures may occur on all regimens. Advanced cases of GABHS and *S. pneumoniae* pneumonia require hospitalization and parenteral antibiotics.

Skin Infections

Skin infections with GABHS, if limited in extent and degree, can be treated adequately with topical hygiene, including removal of impetiginous crusts through warm soaks followed by the topical application of antibacterial ointments. Adolescents with a moderate number of streptococcal impetiginous lesions may be managed satisfactorily with the topical application of mucopurocin (Bactroban). When impetigo becomes extensive, oral antibiotic therapy combined with topical hygiene measures should be employed. Oral or injectable penicillin is successful if lesions are colonized only with GABHS. However, cocolonization with *Staphylococcus aureus* occurs more frequently than pure GABHS infection, so therapy with an agent effective against both bacteria (e.g., cefalexin, cefadroxil, amoxicillin-clavulanate, cefuroxime axetil) may be more appropriate.

Cellulitis and erysipelas caused by GABHS strains generally require the intravenous administration of antibiotics, at least until the infection subsides. Therapy can be completed using an oral regimen.

Bacteremia and Meningitis

Intravenous penicillin G is the treatment of choice for systemic and severe streptococcal infections. One to 2 million units every 4 to 6 hours, to a maximum of 10 million units daily, may be used. Repeat blood cultures and lumbar puncture for septicemia and meningitis, respectively, are necessary only if the clinical course is unsatisfactory. Tolerance has been observed in a small percentage of *Streptococcus pneumoniae* isolates from

the United States. It is best to have the microbiology laboratory evaluate strains causing systemic or severe infections for evidence of tolerance. That is, in cases of systemic or severe infection, one cannot rely on the almost universal susceptibility of streptococci to penicillin.

Endocarditis

Streptococcus viridans, group D streptococcal endocarditis, and the less frequently occurring GABHS or *S. pneumoniae* endocarditis, are generally treated with parenteral, aqueous penicillin G (10 to 20 million units per day, administered every 4 hours) for 4 to 6 weeks. Gentamicin is frequently used for antibiotic synergy at a dose of 5 mg/kg/day, divided every 8 hours. Concomitant aminoglycoside therapy is often undertaken for the initial 2 weeks of therapy.

COURSE OF ILLNESS
Respiratory Infections

PHARYNGITIS

Streptococcal pharyngitis symptoms subside without treatment, usually over a 3- to 5-day course. With treatment, symptoms abate within 24 to 36 hours. In the preantibiotic era, untreated streptococcal pharyngitis occasionally progressed to peritonsillar abscesses, cervical lymphadenitis, or bacteremia, with spread of infection to distant foci. The major concern with inadequately treated group A streptococcal pharyngitis involves the nonsuppurative sequelae of acute rheumatic fever and glomerulonephritis.

OTITIS MEDIA AND SINUSITIS

Untreated acute otitis media and sinusitis have a spontaneous resolution rate of 30% to 100%. Treatment shortens the clinical course and prevents the contiguous and distant spread of infection. Untreated otitis media can lead to mastoiditis or contiguous spread to the meninges, with subsequent meningitis. Similarly, untreated sinusitis can spread through the lymphatics to the meninges and result in meningitis.

PNEUMONIA

Untreated *Streptococcus pneumoniae* or GABHS pneumonia has a low spontaneous resolution rate with the consequences of significant morbidity, which includes parenchymal scarring, progression to empyema, or associated bacteremia with metastatic foci of infection. The symptoms and signs gradually resolve if lobar pneumonia caused by either of the major streptococcal species is treated adequately. If empyema occurs, a long clinical course can be anticipated in a significant number of adolescent patients, thereby requiring the prolonged parenteral administration of antibiotics. Chest tube drainage is frequently employed when empyema develops. Stripping of the pleura in cases of persisting effusion is now practiced infrequently.

Skin and Soft Tissue Infections

Streptococcal impetigo usually shows rapid resolution of clinical manifestations with appropriate topical and/or systemic therapy. Sequelae are infrequent. Untreated streptococcal skin infections caused by group A β-hemolytic strains may produce nonsuppurative sequelae.

Bacteremia and Meningitis

As a result of the polymorphonuclear response typically elicited by streptococcal infections, meningitis caused by *Streptococcus pneumoniae* or GABHS is more likely to have significant sequelae than other common bacterial causes of meningitis, such as *Neisseria meningitidis*. Neurologic sequelae, including deafness and gross motor, fine motor, and intellectual impairment, are unfortunately common.

Endocarditis

Even with proper treatment, endocarditis may lead to permanent valvular damage, thereby increasing the workload of the heart, with the subsequent risk of congestive heart failure. Damaged heart tissue is more susceptible to the reestablishment of relapsing endocarditis.

PROGNOSIS

Streptococcal infections may heal if left untreated, but pyogenic or nonsuppurative complications are common. Complete recovery from infection is the rule with early therapy, except in progressive and sometimes fulminant infections such as pneumonia, bacteremia, or meningitis, which may progress despite seemingly appropriate therapy.

BIBLIOGRAPHY

Bisno AL, Dismukes WE, Durack DT, et al: Antimicrobial treatment of infective endocarditis due to *viridans* streptococci, enterococci, and staphylococci. JAMA 261:1471, 1989.

Burman LA, Norrby R, Trollfors B: Invasive pneumococcal infections: Incidence, predisposing factors, and prognosis. Rev Infect Dis 7:133, 1985.

Denny FW: Current problems in managing streptococcal pharyngitis. J Pediatr 111:797, 1987.

Denny FW, Clyde WA: Acute lower respiratory tract infections in nonhospitalized children. J Pediatr 108:635, 1986.

Kays MA, Pichichero ME: Outpatient management of pediatric pneumonias. Semin Pediatr Infect Dis 1:340, 1990.

McMillan JA: Sore throats in teens: Strep and beyond. Contemp Pediatr 5:20, 1988.

Pichichero ME: Group A beta-hemolytic streptococcal pharyngitis: Immediate treatment with penicillin, rapid diagnosis and antibiotic selection. In Barkin RM (ed): The Emergently Ill Child: Dilemmas in Assessment and Management. Gaithersburg, MD, Aspen, pp 38–49, 1987.

Pichichero ME: Controversies in the treatment of streptococcal pharyngitis. Am Fam Physician 42:1567, 1990.

Sussman JI, Baron EJ, Tenenbaum MJ, et al. *Viridans* streptococcal endocarditis: Clinical, microbiological, and echocardiographic correlations. J Infect Dis 154:597, 1986.

Tuazon CU, Gill V, Gill F: Streptococcal endocarditis: Single vs. combination antibiotic therapy and role of various species. Rev Infect Dis 8:54, 1986.

Turner RB, Lande AE, Chase P, et al: Pneumonia in pediatric outpatients: Cause and clinical manifestations. J Pediatr 111:192, 1987.

MYCOPLASMA PNEUMONIAE INFECTIONS

JULIA A. McMILLAN and LEONARD B. WEINER

Mycoplasma pneumoniae has been recognized as a cause of respiratory disease in humans since Eaton and co-workers reported recovery of the organism from a patient with primary atypical pneumonia in 1944. It was not until the early 1960s that the Eaton agent was isolated on cell-free media and understood to be the same as the "pleuropneumonia-like organism."

Early epidemiologic studies demonstrated that *M. pneumoniae* is responsible for approximately 1 case of pneumonia in 1000 persons annually, and that pneumonia caused by *M. pneumoniae* tends to cluster during the second and third decades of life. Particularly susceptible populations include college students and military recruits.

Attempts to develop an effective vaccine against infection by *M. pneumoniae* were launched once the organism had been isolated and Koch's postulates had been fulfilled by infecting human volunteers with isolates grown in tissue culture. Although growth-inhibiting antibody provoked in some volunteers by inactivated vaccine appeared to be protective against subsequent illness caused by *M. pneumoniae,* a paradoxically severe infection occurred in subjects who did not develop protective levels of antibody. Immunization with organisms attenuated by multiple passages in the laboratory produced unacceptably high levels of symptomatic disease, and attempts to develop a vaccine against *M. pneumoniae* were abandoned until the last few years.

MICROBIOLOGY

M. pneumoniae is a member of the bacterial class Mollicutes. Mollicutes have in common the absence of cell walls, the ability to grow on cell-free media as long as sterols are provided for adequate growth, and susceptibility to protein synthesis-inhibiting antibiotics. Obviously, they are resistant to the effects of antibiotics that inhibit cell wall synthesis. *In vitro* growth of the Mollicutes can be inhibited by specific antibodies.

Although various other Mollicutes have been recognized as veterinary pathogens, only *M. pneumoniae*, *Mycoplasma hominis*, and *Ureaplasma urealyticum* are unequivocally believed to be pathogens in humans. *M. hominis* and *U. urealyticum* cause infection primarily in the genitourinary tract (although *U. urealyticum* is also thought to be a cause of respiratory infection in infants). Many now believe that a newly recognized mycoplasma, *M. genitalium*, causes both genitourinary and respiratory infections in humans, but *M. pneumoniae* is the only member of the class for which a significant clinical and epidemiologic role has been well defined.

EPIDEMIOLOGY

Serologic investigation has demonstrated that children of all ages are infected with *M. pneumoniae*. Infection in pre–school-aged children, however, is more likely to result in asymptomatic infection or mild upper respiratory tract symptoms. Although children over the age of 6 years have a lower incidence of pneumonia from all causes than infants and younger children, the proportion of cases of pneumonia among school-aged children that is caused by *M. pneumoniae* increases and continues to rise until approximately the age of 40 years. Among junior high and high-school students, as many as 20% of all cases of pneumonia are caused by *M. pneumoniae*, and among college students and military recruits the proportion rises to as high as 50% (see Chapter 43).

Seasonal outbreaks of *M. pneumoniae* infection are superimposed on low levels of endemic disease, and the rate of transmission of infection among family members during these outbreaks is high. School-aged children, adolescents, and young adults are most likely to be affected. Clinical evidence of pneumonitis may be subtle. Studies done in the 1950s and 1960s at the University of North Carolina, the University of Wisconsin, and Tulane University all demonstrated that most of the university students infected with *M. pneumoniae* whose symptoms led them to seek medical attention had pneumonia, whereas a much smaller proportion had upper respiratory infections, including simple coryza and pharyngitis.

M. pneumoniae infection in immunocompetent adolescent patients leads to the development of various specific antibodies, named for the methods by which they are detected in the laboratory. These include indirect hemagglutination, complement fixation, and growth-inhibiting antibodies. Cold agglutinin antibodies are anti-I–IgM autoantibodies that agglutinate human erythrocytes at 4°C. Although cold agglutinin antibodies

occur in patients with infections caused by other organisms, they can be detected in approximately 75% of adult patients with pneumonia caused by *M. pneumoniae*. None of the usual antibodies that are provoked in response to *M. pneumoniae* infection appears to be protective against future infection. Antibody undoubtedly plays a role in protection from significant disease, however, because symptomatic lower respiratory tract involvement occurs more frequently among young children than among adults infected with this organism. Marine recruits with detectable growth-inhibiting antibodies have been shown to be less susceptible to *M. pneumoniae* infection, and to have a more moderate course of their disease if infected, compared with those without preexisting antibody. In addition, severe infection by *M. pneumoniae* has been described primarily among those with hemoglobinopathies, drug-induced immunosuppression, and other immunocompromising conditions (see Chapters 53 and 76). However, both recurrent and repeat infections have been described in immunocompetent patients, despite the documentation of antibody response following a previous infection.

PATHOPHYSIOLOGY

M. pneumoniae infection is spread by respiratory droplets among close contacts. The organism penetrates the mucociliary blanket of the respiratory epithelium and attaches by way of a specific receptor on the host epithelial cell. The attachment protein of *M. pneumoniae* has been described, and its presence has been postulated to relate directly to the virulence of the organism. The infection that ensues does not involve penetration of the host cell, nor does the organism invade the blood stream. Damage to the respiratory epithelial cells is thought to occur because of the release of cytotoxic products from the organism. *M. pneumoniae* is known to release hydrogen peroxide, and the intracellular release of H_2O_2 and superoxide anions following attachment to host cells might be the primary mechanism of injury. In addition, *M. pneumoniae* infection is associated with a paralysis of the respiratory cilia, a condition that may persist longer than the acute symptoms and that might account for the paroxysmal cough that often continues after the patient is otherwise well.

The concomitant detection of autoantibodies during *M. pneumoniae* infection and the frequent description of extrapulmonary symptoms have led many to conclude that there is a cause-and-effect relationship between these observations. Autoantibodies and immune complexes have been detected in as many as 41% of adolescent patients with *M. pneumoniae* infection, and only rarely are extrapulmonary signs and symptoms found in association. Attempts to isolate *M. pneumoniae* from extrapulmonary sites, including cerebrospinal and joint fluids, have usually not been successful, and the search persists for documentation of immunologic mechanisms as the cause of non–respiratory tract disease.

Early studies of those with *M. pneumoniae* infection demonstrated that prolonged shedding of the organism following symptomatic improvement occurs in many adolescent patients. Although both tetracycline and erythromycin can be shown to inhibit *in vitro* growth of *M. pneumoniae*, and symptomatic improvement is seen in infected adolescents within 24 hours of the institution of therapy with either of these antibiotics, therapy is not always successful in eradicating the organism from the respiratory tract. It is thought that prolonged carriage, with or without antibiotic therapy, may contribute to the spread of infection.

CLINICAL MANIFESTATIONS

M. pneumoniae infection and the symptoms caused by infection may occur anywhere in the respiratory tract. Infection is typically heralded by general malaise and an aching sensation accompanied by sore throat, retrobulbar headache, and fever. There is nothing about these symptoms to distinguish respiratory infection by *M. pneumoniae* from that caused by other respiratory viruses (see Chapter 93).

In studies of university students, *M. pneumoniae* was isolated from 30% to 50% of patients with pneumonia, whereas approximately 10% of those with *M. pneumoniae* infection had bronchitis and fewer than 10% had upper respiratory infection (URI) symptoms or pharyngitis. In a more recent study, however, 34% of students complaining of sore throat during an outbreak had *M. pneumoniae* isolated from throat swabs. Students with *M. pneumoniae* pharyngitis could not be distinguished by virtue of any of their signs and symptoms from students with pharyngitis caused by group A streptococcus (see previous subchapter).

Adolescents who develop lower respiratory tract infection caused by *M. pneumoniae* may develop chills, chest pain, nausea, vomiting, and diarrhea. The cough is usually nonproductive, but a productive cough may occur later in the course of illness. Physical findings are usually less impressive than the subjective complaints of the adolescent patient, but may include rales and wheezing. Chest x-ray films often reveal unsuspected pulmonary infiltrates. Respiratory infection may also be localized in other portions of the respiratory tree and cause sinusitis, tracheitis, and tracheobronchitis. The total duration of illness in adolescents with *M. pneumoniae* infection is approximately 2 weeks. Although antibiotic therapy may cause a diminution of symptoms, it rarely abolishes all signs of illness. A persistent and irritating cough may continue for several weeks following the resolution of all other symptoms.

Ear pain and middle ear effusion have been persistently described as predominant findings in patients with *M. pneumoniae* infection, particularly among adolescents and young adults. Bullous myringitis has been seen during experimental infection and in some of the patients studied by Foy and colleagues, but this specific form of otitis is not a predominant finding among adolescents. Reports of rash associated with *M. pneumoniae* infection are difficult to interpret because of the frequently confounding treatment with antibiotics. There are, however, enough reports of an erythema multiforme–like rash in patients with pneumonia caused by this organism that it is difficult to deny the association.

The chest x-ray film in patients with *M. pneumoniae* pneumonia can be confused with that seen in viral or classic bacterial pneumonia. In general, however, a unilateral infiltrate is seen with only one lung field involved. An interstitial pattern may be seen, but an alveolar infiltrate is more common. Pleural fluid may be seen in as many as 20% of adolescents if lateral decubitus films are taken. The chest x-ray film combined with the history and physical findings may be helpful in that the onset of *M. pneumoniae* disease is generally more insidious than that of pneumonia caused by the usual bacterial pathogens, yet the x-ray film does not reveal the diffuse pattern more often associated with viral infection.

Systematic white blood cell studies in adolescents and young adults with *M. pneumoniae* infection are not available, but infected adult volunteers were found to have a mild to moderate increase in neutrophils that began approximately 4 days following infection and persisted for about 14 days.

NONRESPIRATORY DISEASE

A wide variety of nonrespiratory complications have been associated with *M. pneumoniae* infection. Often the association is made because of an elevation in complement-fixing antibody in adolescents who have no respiratory symptoms, and without recovering the organism from appropriate cultures. Hemolysis resulting from cold autoantibodies is rarely sufficient to cause clinical anemia. When it does occur, hemolysis is most evident approximately 2 to 3 weeks following the onset of respiratory symptoms, when the cold agglutinin titer is likely to be at its peak.

Infrequent but persistent reports of a wide variety of central nervous system manifestations in association with *M. pneumoniae* infection have been difficult to substantiate with diagnostic tests other than the complement-fixing antibody procedure. There are, however, at least two reports of direct isolation of *M. pneumoniae* from patients with meningoencephalitis. A similar loose association exists among *M. pneumoniae* infection and pericardial and myocardial disease, pancreatitis, hepatitis, and nephritis.

A clearer association exists between *M. pneumoniae* and arthritis. The isolation of *M. pneumoniae* from the joint fluid of a patient with hypogammaglobulinemia has provided convincing evidence that, in adolescents with respiratory complaints and inflammatory joint disease, *M. pneumoniae* should be considered as a cause. The arthritis described in immunologically normal patients is usually monarticular, but some have had multiple joint involvement suggestive of rheumatoid arthritis. *M. pneumoniae* arthritis may be slow to resolve, but most adolescents recover from their joint disease as their respiratory symptoms subside.

DIAGNOSIS

Awareness of the existence of *M. pneumoniae* disease activity in the community is perhaps the most useful diagnostic clue when seeing an adolescent who has clinical signs of pneumonia or pharyngitis. This information, when coupled with a history of insidious illness onset in an adolescent or young adult, suggests that the patient has respiratory symptoms caused by *M. pneumoniae*.

M. pneumoniae culture methods are complex and most clinical laboratories do not possess these capabilities, thus making confirmation of the organism difficult. Throat swabs and sputum specimens provide for equivalent recoverability, although many adolescents with *M. pneumoniae* pneumonia do not have a productive cough. Improved culture techniques often allow for a positive result within 4 to 7 days, but an even shorter turnaround time is necessary for clinically relevant results. When a specimen from an infected adolescent is placed in an appropriate *M. pneumoniae* cell-free broth medium, the organisms metabolize glucose in the medium as they grow, with a resulting decrease in pH and an indicator color change. Then these presumptive positive cultures are passed to a solid medium in which subsequent characteristic *M. pneumoniae* colonial growth can be observed. Further confirmation takes advantage of the hemadsorbing properties of *M. pneumoniae* colonies; guinea pig erythrocytes are overlayed on a solid medium, gently washed, and the colonies observed for hemadsorption. Alternatively, an agar plate immunofluorescence technique may be used to confirm the presence of *M. pneumoniae* colonies.

Rapid, nonculture identification for *M. pneumoniae* organisms and/or antigen detection have been successful using enzyme immunoassay, immunoblot, and DNA-RNA probe technologies. Because *M. pneumoniae* is known to persist in the oropharynx for weeks following clinical disease, with or without appropriate antibiotic therapy, positive culture or antigen detection must be correlated with other clinical and laboratory information. Surveillance testing of college-aged individuals has revealed that as many as 9% of asymptomatic students have positive pharyngeal cultures for *M. pneumoniae* during a time of the year when *M. pneumoniae* is prevalent.

Serologic diagnosis of *M. pneumoniae* infection can be accomplished by testing acute and convalescent specimens for a fourfold or greater increase. Complement fixation (CF), immunofluorescence, indirect hemagglutination, precipitin, growth inhibition, mycoplasmacidal antibody assay, and enzyme immunoassay (EIA) techniques have all been described. CF antibodies develop early in the course of disease and usually peak by 1 month. Subsequent decline is variable, but CF antibody is more short-lived than the other anti–*M. pneumoniae* antibodies. It is currently the most readily available antibody test for *M. pneumoniae* infection, but the glycolipid antigen that provokes a positive CF antibody has been found to cross-react with glycolipids on human cells, particularly in adolescents with pancreatitis and meningoencephalitis. In adolescents with these clinical conditions, therefore, CF antibody detection may be of limited usefulness.

The serum cold agglutinin titer can be useful in the diagnosis of *M. pneumoniae* disease. Titers greater than or equal to 1:32 are present in 50% to 90% of adolescents with *M. pneumoniae* pneumonia, but are less predictably elevated in adolescents with upper respiratory tract infection. Generally, the severity of pulmonary involvement correlates with the cold agglutinin response, and children are less likely than adolescents to develop a positive cold agglutinin response. The rapid cold agglutinin screening test can be accomplished at bedside by adding a small amount of blood to a tube containing anticoagulant and placing the specimen into ice water for 30 to 60 seconds. When examined immediately, coarse agglutination can be visualized at the sides of the tube as it is slowly tilted. This phenomenon disappears as the contents of the tube return to room temperature. Positive cold agglutinins can occur with pneumonia caused by viral and rickettsial agents; 18% of patients were positive in one study of military recruits with adenoviral pneumonia.

TREATMENT

Therapy for *M. pneumoniae* requires an antimicrobial agent whose action is not directed at bacterial cell wall constituents. Erythromycin and tetracycline are the drugs of choice, with erythromycin required for children younger than 9 years of age. Recommended oral dosage for adults and adolescents is 2 g/day in divided doses (for either drug). The earlier the antimicrobial treatment is initiated, the greater the clinical response. Furthermore, a greater therapeutic effect is noted in adolescents with more severe signs of lower respiratory tract involvement. Radiologic improvement lags significantly behind clinical response to therapy and, in contrast, the initial physical findings of pneumonia can be present before radiologic abnormalities develop.

There are no studies supporting the use of antimicrobial therapy for nonrespiratory manifestations of *Mycoplasma pneumoniae* disease. Because these are thought to be immunologic in nature, rather than a result of direct infection, and because they usually develop during the resolution phase of the respiratory symptoms, it is unlikely that treatment would be beneficial.

COURSE OF ILLNESS AND PROGNOSIS

Persistence of the organism is only minimally affected by antimicrobial therapy, so adolescents may remain contagious during and after treatment and the relapse rate is high. Furthermore, one study has indicated that prophylaxis of household contacts with tetracycline prevents pneumonia in those contacts but does not alter the rate of infection. Many minimally symptomatic adolescent patients also have prolonged shedding. Studies of the efficacy of treatment in patients with tracheobronchitis, pharyngitis, or upper respiratory manifestations of *M. pneumoniae* are lacking.

BIBLIOGRAPHY

Baseman JB, Dallo SF, Tully JG, Rose DL: Isolation and characterization of *Mycoplasma genitalium* strains from the human respiratory tract. J Clin Microbiol 26:2266, 1988.

Collier AM, Clyde WA, Jr: Relationships between *Mycoplasma pneumoniae* and human respiratory epithelium. Infect Immunol 3:694, 1976.

Denny FW, Clyde WA, Jr, Glezen WP: *Mycoplasma pneumoniae* disease: Clinical spectrum, pathophysiology, epidemiology, and control. J Infect Dis 123:74, 1971.

Evans AS, Allen V, Sueltmann S: *Mycoplasma pneumoniae* infections in University of Wisconsin students. Am Rev Respir Dis 96:237, 1967.

Foy HM, Grayston JT, Kenny GE, et al: Epidemiology of *Mycoplasma pneumoniae* infection in families. JAMA 197:137, 1966.

Hata D, Kuze F, Machizuki Y, et al: Evaluation of DNA probe test for rapid diagnosis of *Mycoplasma pneumonia* infections. J Pediatr 116:273, 1990.

Kahane I: *In vitro* studies on the mechanism of adherence and pathogenicity of mycoplasmas. Isr J Med Sci 20:874, 1984.

Lambert HP: Infections caused by *Mycoplasma pneumoniae*. Br J Dis Chest 63:71, 1969.

Lin J-SL: Human mycoplasmal infections: Serologic observations. Rev Infect Dis 7:216, 1985.

McCracken GH: Current status of antibiotic treatment for *Mycoplasma pneumoniae* infections. J Pediatr Infect Dis 5:167, 1986.

Mogabgab, WJ: *Mycoplasma pneumoniae* and adenovirus respiratory illnesses in military and university personnel, 1959–1966. Am Rev Respir Dis 97:345, 1968.

Murray HW, Masur H, Senterfit LB, Roberts RB: The protean manifestations of *Mycoplasma pneumoniae* infections in adults. Am J Med 58:229, 1975.

Smith CB, Chanock RM, Friedewald WT, Alford RH: *Mycoplasma* infection in volunteers. Ann NY Acad Sci 143:471, 1967.

Smith CB, Friedewald WT, Chanock RM: Shedding of *Mycoplasma pneumoniae* after tetracycline and erythromycin therapy. N Engl J Med 276:1172, 1967.

HAEMOPHILUS INFLUENZAE INFECTIONS

MARY T. CASERTA and MICHAEL E. PICHICHERO

Haemophilus influenzae has been a recognized human pathogen since 1892, when it was first isolated by Pfeiffer. Because of its presence in respiratory secretions studied during an outbreak of influenza, *H. influenzae* was originally thought to be responsible for epidemic influenza—hence, its initial designation as the "influenzae bacillus." Approximately 40 years later its role as a secondary invader following influenza virus infection became apparent, and its emerging role in many other infections came under closer study.

MICROBIOLOGY

H. influenzae is a small, nonmotile, nonspore-forming gram-negative bacillus found only in humans. Despite this clear description, clinical specimens may be difficult to identify correctly because of inconsistent Gram stain results and the pleomorphic, even filamentous, appearance of primary isolates. Also, the organism is somewhat fastidious, and transport time between obtaining clinical material and setting up appropriate cultures should be minimized to enhance isolation.

The aerobic growth of *H. influenzae* in the laboratory requires a medium supplemented with X factor (heat-stable iron-containing pigments) and Y factor (heat-labile nicotinamide adenine dinucleotide, NAD). Both these factors can be supplied by lysed erythrocytes present in chocolate agar (hence, the origin of the name *Haemophilus*—blood-loving). The absolute requirement for Y factor for aerobic growth distinguishes *H. influenzae* from *Haemophilus parainfluenzae*. The anaerobic growth of *H. influenzae* does not require Y factor, so this cannot be used as an identifying characteristic under anaerobic conditions.

H. influenzae bacteria also grow around colonies of *Staphylococcus aureus* as satellites because of the release of X factor into the culture medium by the hemolytic staphylococci. Aerobic culture growth appears to be optimum with 5% to 10% CO_2 supplementation.

There are two major biologic forms of *H. influenzae* that correlate with the two colony types seen on solid medium culture. There is a rough type (R), which corresponds to nonencapsulated organisms, and a smooth or mucoid type (S), which represents encapsulated strains. In addition to the presence or absence of a capsule, all strains of *H. influenzae* have a cell envelope composed of an outer membrane, a peptidoglycan layer, and an inner cytoplasmic membrane. The outer membrane consists of proteins, lipo-oligosaccharide, and phospholipid.

The encapsulated strains produce abundant amounts of an outer polysaccharide capsule. This feature allows for further subtyping of the encapsulated strains into six defined types. These are labeled a through f, based on the serologic identification of unique capsular components. Using this scheme, all nonencapsulated strains are referred to as nontypable.

The most recently developed subclassification system characterizes strains on the basis of the electrophoretic mobility of 16 major metabolic enzymes and designates various electrophoretic types. Despite the fact that encapsulated organisms may lose this characteristic on laboratory subculture, the use of this typing system has unequivocally demonstrated that the nonencapsulated strains exhibit a great deal of genetic diversity and are not merely "bare" encapsulated strains. Through these methods it has also been shown that type b strains are basically clonal and exhibit strong geographic patterns.

EPIDEMIOLOGY

Since the 1930s, *H. influenzae* has become accepted as an extremely important pathogen, with most disease caused by this organism occurring during infancy and childhood. *H. influenzae* type b is responsible for most cases of meningitis in children under 5 years of age, with an incidence of 19 to 63 cases in 100,000 children, or 12,000 cases annually in the United States. Other infections such as sepsis, epiglottitis, osteomyelitis, pneumonia, empyema, and pericarditis are also caused by *H. influenzae* type b, with an annual incidence for all invasive disease being 67 to 129 cases in 100,000 children. Invasive diseases caused by *H. influenzae* type b are also seen in adolescents. Based on a population study in Fresno County, California, the incidence of all invasive infections caused by *H. influenzae* in persons older than 14 years of age was 1.26 in 100,000 annually; the incidence of meningitis was 0.23 in 100,000 annually. Thus, although infants and children are at highest risk for acquiring infection from *H. influenzae* type b, it causes the same pattern of disease in those in older age groups.

Nontypable *H. influenzae* is also an important etiologic agent to consider in invasive infections in adolescents, with a higher frequency than previously believed. Nontypable strains have been found in 16% to 55% of cases of meningitis in patients older than 6 years of age, with three of eight isolates from adults in the Fresno County study being identified as nontypable. By comparison, there were no isolates of nontypable *H. influenzae* in the younger age groups. Nontypable *H. influenzae* is also responsible for a large proportion of cases of acute otitis media, sinusitis, and conjunctivitis, with reports of respiratory and genitourinary infections in both the pediatric and adult literature.

PATHOPHYSIOLOGY

H. influenzae is a normal inhabitant of the respiratory tract, with carriage rates of approximately 80%. The rate for colonization with type b organisms averages 5% in these carriers, but can be higher in closed communities. Approximately 1% of female genital tracts are colonized with nontypable *H. influenzae* strains.

Regardless of the age of the patient, *H. influenzae* type b gains entrance to the blood stream from the respiratory tract by unidentified mechanisms. Various parts of the organism play an important role in eluding host defenses and facilitating this spread, and have been studied extensively. The best characterized of these factors is the polysaccharide capsule, but, fimbriae and Ig A proteases may also be involved. Immunity to the type b strain is age-dependent and is responsible for the striking preponderance of infection caused by this organism in younger children. The appearance of anticapsular antibody in serum seems to correlate best with immunity to *H. influenzae* type b, but antibody to other cellular components such as the major outer membrane proteins and lipo-oligosaccharide also appears to be active in protection, especially against the nontypable

strains. Both colonization with multiple strains of *H. influenzae* and colonization with other gram-negative organisms that share similar antigenic structures appears to be immunizing.

In contrast to the pattern of invasive disease caused by type b organisms, most disease caused by nontypable strains of *H. influenzae* is in contiguous areas of the respiratory tract and develops via local extension of the organisms. This is especially true if there is any anatomic or functional breakdown in local host defenses. Sinusitis, otitis media, bronchitis, pneumonia, and genitourinary infections typify this mode of disease spread (see Chapters 40, 43, and 66). Meningitis and its recurrence in adults is often caused by nontypable organisms, and is usually preceded by disease in contiguous structures (e.g., sinusitis or otitis media).

CLINICAL MANIFESTATIONS

The typical clinical manifestations of invasive *H. influenzae* type b infection are fever and a toxic appearance associated with local symptoms corresponding to the site of invasive disease. Unfortunately, there are no clinical features that distinguish infection by *H. influenzae* from that caused by other organisms responsible for the same type of diseases, except perhaps the age of the patient and the epidemiology of the disease. Certain infections, however, merit special discussion, either because of their relevance to the adolescent population or because of their unusual nature.

Although the exact frequency of disease caused by *H. influenzae* in the adolescent age group is difficult to discern, nontypable organisms can be a common cause of community-acquired pneumonia in adults. Although this appears to be more of a problem in older patients with underlying pulmonary disease, a similar type of pathophysiology could operate in adolescents with chronic pulmonary pathology.

Urinary tract infections caused by *H. influenzae* have been reported in all age groups and appear to be related to underlying renal or urologic abnormalities (see Chapters 65 and 66). Routine urine culture techniques are not conducive to the growth of these organisms. Detecting "sterile" pyuria in a patient with an underlying urinary tract abnormality in association with other signs of infection should prompt the use of media that can support the growth of *H. influenzae* if this diagnosis is to be confirmed.

Genital infections caused by nontypable *H. influenzae*, including acute and chronic salpingitis and obstetric infections, have been well documented. Endometritis, chorioamnionitis, and maternal and neonatal bacteremia with neonatal pneumonia exemplify the possible range of disease. Although these infections have been associated with only mild symptoms in the pregnant female, with or without associated bacteremia, disease in the newborn can include respiratory distress, pneumonia, and shock, mimicking other more common causes of neonatal infections. *H. influenzae* as an etiologic agent of acute and chronic salpingitis has been recognized as a result of its isolation from fallopian tube aspirates obtained at laparoscopy. As is true with other organisms causing this infection, polymicrobial disease is the rule, with the frequency of isolating *H. influenzae* being low.

DIAGNOSIS

The diagnosis of *H. influenzae* infection can be firmly established by culturing the organism from a routinely sterile site. Because of the unique growth requirements noted previously, care should be taken in the handling of specimens to minimize transport time and selection of appropriate culture media for optimum isolation and identification of the organism. An alternative method of diagnosis of type b disease is by detection of capsular antigen in urine, serum, or other sterile fluid using a latex agglutination or counterimmunoelectrophoresis technique.

TREATMENT

Antibiotic therapy remains the mainstay of treatment for those with *H. influenzae* infections (see Chapter 96). Although resistance patterns vary across the country, it is now recognized that the resistance of type b organisms to ampicillin can be as high as 50% and range from 13% to 50%. This resistance is almost always caused by plasmid-mediated production of β-lactamase. Other mechanisms, such as altered penicillin-binding proteins, have been described. Chloramphenicol resistance is rare in the United States but has been detected in type b strains causing invasive disease.

Resistance to trimethoprim-sulfamethoxazole (TMP-SMX) is also seen in isolates of *H. influenzae*. Testing of this organism against TMP-SMX, however, involves certain technical problems that may overestimate resistance figures.

Third-generation cephalosporins are especially useful in the treatment of invasive *H. influenzae* type b disease, especially ceftriaxone and cefotaxime.

Second-generation cephalosporins such as cefuroxime are active *in vitro* against *H. influenzae* type b. Clinical failures have been documented, however, especially in meningitis. Despite these reports, cefuroxime remains a useful drug for milder disease caused by *H. influenzae*.

Nontypable strains of *H. influenzae* do not share the same frequency of antibiotic resistance as the type b strains noted above. In reports describing invasive isolates obtained from genital sources, the incidence of ampicillin resistance was found to range from only 3% to 7.5%. In a national collaborative study, the rate of β-lactamase production of non–type b strains was found to be 15%. Most of these isolates were obtained from the respiratory tract or eye. Because of these findings, ampicillin remains a useful single drug for infections caused by nonencapsulated strains, but resistance is an increasing problem.

PREVENTION

Routine vaccination of children using polysaccharide vaccines or oligosaccharide capsular components of *H. influenzae* type b linked to protein antigens is currently underway in the United States. The occurrence of *H. influenzae* type b disease in adolescents should therefore decline in the years ahead. Routine immunization beyond the age of 5 years is not recommended because of the dramatic decrease in natural infection by this organism after this age. Two groups of adolescents in whom immunization might be beneficial include those with sickle cell disease or cancer (see Chapters 52 and 53). Both groups have been shown to be at increased risk for invasive *H. influenzae* type b disease. At present, the American Academy of Pediatrics recommends vaccination with a conjugate vaccine in children older than 5 years of age with diseases associated with functional or anatomic asplenia.

BIBLIOGRAPHY

American Academy of Pediatrics: Report of the Committee on Infectious Diseases, 22nd ed. Haemophilus influenzae Type b conjugate vaccines: Recommendations for immunization of infants and children 2 months of age and older: Update (RE9203). Elk Grove, IL, AAP, 1991, pp 220–229.

Granoff DM, Basden M: *Haemophilus influenzae* infections in Fresno County, California: A prospective study of the effects of age, race, and contact with a case on incidence of disease. J Infect Dis 141(1):40, 1980.

Levin DC, Schwarz MI, Matthay RA, LaForce FM: Bacteremic *Haemophilus influenzae* pneumonia in adults. A report of 24 cases and a review of the literature. Am J Med 62:219, 1977.

Murphy TF, Apicella MA: Nontypable *Haemophilus influenzae*: A review of clincal aspects, surface antigens, and the human immune response to infection. Rev Infect Dis 9(1):1, 1987.

Schuit KE: Isolation of *Haemophilus* in urine cultures from children. J Pediatr 95(4):565, 1979.

Smith AL: Antibiotic resistance in *Haemophilus influenzae*. Pediatr Infect Dis 2(5):352, 1983.

Van Alphen L, van Damm A, Bol P, et al: Types and subtypes of 73 strains of *Haemophilus influenzae* isolated from patients more than 6 years of age with meningitis in the Netherlands. J Infect 15:95, 1987.

Wallace RJ, Baker CJ, Quinones FJ, et al: Nontypable *Haemophilus influenzae* (Biotype 4) as a neonatal, maternal, and genital pathogen. Rev Infect Dis 5(1):123, 1983.

Wilfert CM: Epidemiology of *Haemophilus influenzae* type b infections. Pediatrics 85(Suppl):631, 1990.

BORDETELLA PERTUSSIS INFECTION AND PERTUSSIS SYNDROMES

MAUREEN A. KAYS and MICHAEL E. PICHICHERO

The first reference to pertussis or whooping cough appeared in a discussion of a 1578 Parisian epidemic. Pertussis is an endemic and epidemic illness caused by *Bordetella pertussis*. *Bordetella parapertussis* and adenoviruses types 1, 2, 3, and 5 produce a similar clinical picture. Most sporadic cases and epidemics of whooping cough are caused by *B. pertussis*. Wrongly, many consider pertussis a diagnosis of the past, and only to be considered in infants.

EPIDEMIOLOGY

The use of pertussis vaccines has had a major effect on the epidemiology of pertussis. Prior to vaccination programs, there were 115,000 to 270,000 cases reported in the United States, with 5,000 to 10,000 deaths annually. Since the 1950s, with the advent of widespread pertussis vaccination, the endemic pattern of pertussis has ceased and a cyclic pattern of epidemics has dominated. Immunization beyond 7 years of age is not recommended (see Chapter 25). Thus, those with vaccine-induced immunity are aging, with accompanying waning immunity. As a consequence, adolescents and young adults are becoming both a reservoir for pertussis and a large susceptible population.

During the period from 1986 to 1988, state health departments reported 10,468 cases of pertussis to the Centers for Disease Control. Of these cases, 46% occurred in people between the ages of 10 and 14 and 12.7% occurred in those older than 15 years. The World Health Organization has estimated that 600,000 deaths annually result from pertussis. The actual incidence is uncertain, because the diagnosis is often not considered as a result of a low index of suspicion, the lack of a characteristic whoop, and the difficulties of laboratory diagnosis. The consequences are a delay in diagnosis and a delay in treatment and quarantine, allowing the further spread of disease. Most diagnosed illness still occurs in unimmunized infants. In susceptible populations, attack rates of 100% have been found.

The endemic nature of pertussis has little seasonal variation. Unlike other infectious diseases, females are more prone to infection than are males. The ratio of females to males with pertussis increases with increasing age. There is no variation among ethnic groups.

PATHOPHYSIOLOGY

Bordetella pertussis is a gram-negative coccobacillus. It was first cultured by Bordet and Gengou in 1906, and the Bordet-Gengou medium is still used for isolation of the organism. *In vivo* the organism is tropic for ciliated cells of the respiratory tract.

Transmission of infection is presumed to be airborne, through respiratory secretions from an infected individual to the respiratory tract of a susceptible host. *B. pertussis* bacteria have pili that allow for attachment to epithelial cells. They attach and replicate along the entire respiratory tree, causing cilial paralysis, cell death, and resultant shedding of the epithelium. The bacteria do not invade the submucosa or other sites.

Restricted to the respiratory tract mucosa, the bacteria secrete multiple toxins, which are presumed to cause the systemic symptoms of the disease. The primary toxin, formerly referred to as pertussis toxin, but now known as lymphocytosis-promoting factor (LPF), has many effects and is the subject of active research. These effects include histamine sensitization, lymphocytosis promotion, adjuvancy, a hypoglycemic effect, and mitogenicity. LPF may be responsible for the encephalopathy that rarely accompanies pertussis infection. Antibody to LPF is protective in animal models.

Filamentous hemagglutinin (FHA) is a surface protein on *B. pertussis* that may be important in the attachment of the bacterium to ciliated epithelium. In animal models, FHA antibodies inhibit adhesion of the organism, thereby preventing lethal respiratory infection. Agglutinogens and LPF are also important in the attachment of *B. pertussis* to host cells.

Tracheal cytotoxin is a toxin derived from the *B. pertussis* cellular envelope; it has specificity for ciliated epithelial cells. Host defenses are hampered by *B. pertussis* adenylate cyclase, adversely affecting phagocytic activity. Heat-labile toxin, a cytoplasmic protein, is dermonecrotic in animals and is probably involved in the epithelial necrosis seen in clinical disease in humans. Like other gram-negative bacteria, an endotoxin is present, with effects similar to those of other bacterial lipopolysaccharides. Through the action of these *B. pertussis* by-products, lymphocytes and polymorphonuclear leukocytes infiltrate the respiratory mucosa, with resultant inflammatory debris clogging the lumen of the bronchi. Peribronchial hyperplasia is followed by a necrosis of the mid-layer and basal layer of the epithelium. Pneumonia, atelectasis, and bronchiolar obstruction can therefore develop.

Cell-mediated immunity is altered by *B. pertussis*. The role of cell-mediated immunity in the pathophysiology of pertussis has not been determined. The antibody response to pertussis infection is marked. Antibody production is important in the human host's ability to resist and recuperate from infection.

CLINICAL MANIFESTATIONS

The incubation period of pertussis is from 6 to 20 days (mean, 7 days). The clinical illness is divided into three stages—catarrhal, paroxysmal, and convalescent. In the catarrhal stage the illness is subtle in onset, initially resembling a mild upper respiratory infection. Symptoms include rhinorrhea, mild conjunctival injection, tearing, occasional sneezing, and a mild cough. Transmission of the organism to susceptible hosts is greatest during the catarrhal stage, with decreasing infectiousness throughout the remainder of the illness.

At 1 week to 10 days, the illness enters the paroxysmal stage. The upper respiratory symptoms continue with a persistent, dry cough. The cough increases in severity, is more frequent at night, and occurs as episodic paroxysms. At the peak of the illness, many patients experience 10 to 20 coughing paroxysms each day. The cough is staccato-like, with little or no inspiratory effort between coughs. Completion of the paroxysm is sometimes marked by an inspiratory whoop. Vomiting is common after termination of a coughing paroxysm. Multiple stimuli invoke paroxysms. Between paroxysms, the patient appears minimally ill. Most of the morbidity and mortality of the disease occurs during this period. The paroxysmal stage continues from 1 to 4 weeks, becoming less severe over time. During the final convalescent stage persistent coughing can continue for 6 months, with recurrence during intercurrent respiratory infections. During convalescence the organism is not usually present, despite continued coughing.

In adolescents, pertussis may have an atypical presentation. The signs and symptoms may be considerably milder, with a persistent cough secondary to a tracheobronchitis. Although coughing may persist for weeks, complications are unusual. The atypical features make diagnosis difficult, unless epidemiology supports pertussis infection. Any adolescent with cough persisting for over 2 weeks, especially if coughing terminates with vomiting, should be suspected to have pertussis.

Table 94–9 outlines complications of hospitalized patients with pertussis by age group. Although infants have the highest mortality rate, adolescents suffer considerable morbidity. Secondary infection can develop and a rise in temperature may indicate superinfection, because pertussis does not typically cause significant febrile episodes. The violence of the coughing episodes can cause hemorrhagic effects to multiple systems, with resulting epistaxis, melena, petechiae, and subdural hematoma. The intensity of the cough appears to cause increased intravascular pressure and the rupture of small vessels. Hernias and rectal prolapse have also been described. Central nervous system manifestations are extremely uncommon in adolescents, occurring during the paroxysmal stage. Acute complications include seizures, paralysis, ataxia, aphasia, blindness, deafness, and decerebrate rigidity.

DIAGNOSIS

The diagnosis rests both on clinical and laboratory methods. In typical disease, with supporting epidemiologic evidence, the diagnosis can easily be made on clinical grounds alone during the paroxysmal stage. Atypical cases are often misdiagnosed.

Physical examination during the catarrhal phase is often unremarkable. In the paroxysmal stage, adolescents with pertussis are likely to be afebrile and to complain of a sore throat and a persistent cough.

Leukocytosis with an absolute lymphocytosis is present in classic pertussis. The increased white blood cell count is usually first noted at the end of the catarrhal stage, with elevations greater than 30,000 cells/dl commonly found. In atypical or modified illness, lymphocytosis may be milder or absent. Chest radiographic findings are nonspecific and reveal bronchopneumonia with segmental atelectasis, as is seen with many other lower respiratory pathogens (see Chapter 43).

The isolation of the organism from nasopharyngeal swabs remains the standard for diagnosis. The fastidiousness of the organism and contamination by other nasopharyngeal organisms make culture difficult. Specimens should be obtained from the nasopharynx using Dacron or calcium alginate swabs. Cotton swabs contain fatty acids that inhibit growth of the organism. Direct plating onto selective media by the addition of selected antimicrobial agents during the first month of illness is most effective for isolation of the organism. By 6 weeks after onset of the illness, only 15% to 20% of cases are culture-positive. Previous antibiotic treatment lowers isolation rates. Successful growth of the organism is more difficult if specimens are obtained from previously immunized persons. Despite best efforts, isolation in suspected cases is often unsuccessful. Under optimal

TABLE 94–9. Pertussis Patients Hospitalized or With Complications (United States, 1986–1988)*

| | | HOSPITALIZED | | COMPLICATION | | | | | |
| | | | | PNEUMONIA† | | SEIZURES | | ENCEPHALOPATHY | |
AGE GROUP	TOTAL NO.	No.	(%)	No.	(%)	No.	(%)	No.	(%)
<6 mo	3061	2129	(69.6)	522	(17.1)	79	(2.6)	32	(1.1)
6–11 mo	963	473	(49.1)	149	(15.5)	21	(2.2)	6	(0.6)
1–4 yr	1805	451	(25.0)	187	(10.4)	37	(2.1)	7	(0.4)
5–9 yr	1421	83	(5.8)	39	(2.8)	9	(0.6)	5	(0.4)
10–14 yr	395	24	(6.1)	12	(3.0)	1	(0.3)	3	(0.8)
≥15 yr	979	36	(3.7)	27	(2.8)	10	(1.0)	3	(0.3)
All ages‡	8682	3230	(37.2)	945	(10.9)	159	(1.8)	57	(0.7)

*Supplementary Pertussis Surveillance System.
†Radiographically confirmed.
‡Includes 58 patients of unknown ages.
From Centers for Disease Control: Pertussis surveillance—United States, 1986–1988. MMWR 39:57, 1990.

conditions, in a known outbreak, 80% of cases can be confirmed by culture.

Direct fluorescent antibody (DFA) tests attempt to identify the organism directly from nasopharyngeal specimens. There is controversy as to which is more sensitive, culture methods or DFA tests. The variability of results may occur because of the stage of the illness at which specimens are obtained. In early disease, when only a few organisms are present, culture is more sensitive. In late disease, or after antibiotic treatment, when viable organisms may not be present, DFA tests are more sensitive. DFA reader variation and false-positive rates can be significant.

Specific serologic responses to *B. pertussis* have been used to indicate vaccination response or illness. Enzyme-linked immunosorbent assays (ELISA) for IgM, IgA, and IgG antibodies against *B. pertussis* antigens have been measured. Confounding variables include age of the infected person, immunization status, and antibiotic pretreatment. As research on optimal methods continues, it is likely that a combination of serologic methods will be necessary for maximum sensitivity and specifity.

New diagnostic methods include DNA probes, which hybridize with a sequence present in the *B. pertussis* genome, detection of specific products elaborated by the organism, and counterimmunoelectrophoresis (CIE). Table 94–10 compares various laboratory procedures, but only culture and DFA are currently available for routine use.

DIFFERENTIAL DIAGNOSIS

Persistent and spasmodic cough is evident in asthma, bacterial pneumonia, cystic fibrosis, tuberculosis, and diseases causing extrinsic compression of the large airways (see Chapter 43). Foreign body aspiration may also present with coughing spasms. A thorough history, physical examination, and prudent use of the laboratory can distinguish among these entities.

Infections with *B. parapertussis*, *Bordetella bronchiseptica*, and adenoviruses types 1, 2, 3, and 5 have a similar clinical presentation, indistinguishable from that of clinical infection with *B. pertussis*. Isolation of the infecting organism or, in the case of adenoviral infection, a rise in complement-fixing antibody titer, differentiates these infections from those caused by *B. pertussis*.

TREATMENT

Erythromycin is the most effective antibiotic against pertussis. If started in the paroxysmal stage, the course of illness is probably not shortened; however, erythromycin aborts or attenuates the illness if given in the catarrhal stage. Erythromycin eradicates the organism from the nasopharyngeal tract, which shortens the duration of infectiousness. The recommended dosage for adolescents or young adults is 50 mg/kg/day, in three or four divided doses of erythromycin (the estolate ester)

TABLE 94–10. Sensitivity and Specificity of ELISA for Diagnosis of Pertussis

ANTIGEN PREPARATION	CRITERIA FOR POSITIVE RESULT	COMPARISON STANDARD	SENSITIVITY (%)	SPECIFICITY (%)
Whole cells	IgG or IgM 3.5× controls	Clinical*	55	NA
		CF	100	53
Sonicate of formalin-killed whole cells	IgM or IgA ≥ mean + 2 SD of pooled age-matched uninfected controls or difference in paired sera > 2 SD of repeated reference assays	Clinical	36	95
		Clinical	62	NA
		Agglutination	92	30
		Culture	48	66
		Culture	100	15
		Culture	89	52
Partially purified FHA	IgG and IgA 2× mean of healthy age-matched controls or twofold rise in paired sera	Clinical	82	97
		CF	100	25
	IgG or IgM > mean + 2 SD of healthy age-matched controls or twofold rise in paired sera	Clinical	64	NA
		Clinical	54	NA
		FA	77	63
		Culture	96	53
		Culture	88	62
Extract of treated cells	IgA ≥ highest vaccinated controls	Clinical	76	92
Purified LPF	IgG > upper c.i. of vaccinated controls without IgA	Culture or IgA	100	72†
Purified LPF and FHA	IgA or IgM anti-FHA or anti-LPF	Culture or FA	50	76
Purified LPF and FHA	Two tests (IgA +/or IgG) > 90th percentile of controls	Clinical	25	92
	Fourfold rise in paired sera or IgG antiLPF > mean + 3 SD or two tests (IgA +/or IgG) > mean + 2 SD of unexposed controls	Culture	100	100

CF, complement fixation; FA, fluorescent antibody; FHA, filamentous hemagglutinin; LPF, lymphocyte-promoting factor; NA, not available.
*Clinically suspected cases. Criteria for CF and agglutination differ in different studies.
†Standard includes IgA and/or IgG-positive.
With permission from Onorato IM, Wassilak SGF: Laboratory diagnosis of pertussis: The state of the art. Pediatr Infect Dis 6:147, 1987. Copyright by Williams & Wilkins, 1987.

for 14 days (maximum, 2 g/day). A relapse rate of as high as 10% can occur if treatment is stopped before the 2-week course of therapy has been completed.

Erythromycin is also the drug of choice in the prophylactic treatment of susceptible contacts and in those whose immune status is unknown. Information about the optimal duration of prophylaxis is insufficient, but treatment for 14 days after the last known contact with the index case should be adequate, even for those who are incubating the organism.

The pregnant patient with pertussis presents a special problem. If the mother is still infectious at the time of delivery, the neonate is at risk of acquiring the disease. Use of passive protection with pertussis immune globulin does not prevent or ameliorate the illness in the newborn. Historically, mothers were isolated from their newborns for as long as 5 weeks to prevent transmission of the organism. With the growing awareness of the importance of maternal-infant bonding, however, new recommendations became imperative. In Sweden, a group of 35 women with pertussis and their neonates were treated with erythromycin, starting at delivery. Breast feeding and other contacts were allowed. The risk of pertussis infection in the infant was eliminated. Of note, there were no alterations in neonatal gut bacterial flora while on erythromycin.

Supportive measures are extremely important. Care should be taken to avoid factors that provoke paroxysms. Hydration and maintenance of adequate humidity are imperative. The use of corticosteroids remains controversial. Bronchodilators (e.g., β-adrenergic inhalers) have been anecdotally reported as being somewhat helpful.

PREVENTION

Antibiotic management of pertussis is only a supplement to vaccination efforts. Goals of vaccination programs include the reduction of pertussis morbidity and the minimization of vaccine-associated morbidity. The whole cell vaccine used in the United States is not perfect and is under constant criticism. The most common vaccines in use today are whole cell preparations, differing slightly from the original vaccine introduced in the 1930s. With greater than 90% compliance, the vaccine has shown to have an efficacy varying from 60% to 90%. The success of the whole cell pertussis vaccine has led in substantial part to the 99% decrease in pertussis incidence in the United States. It was hoped that, with humans as the only reservoir for pertussis, the eradication of the disease would occur with complete immunization compliance, but the vaccine only confers transient protection. A Michigan study showed an efficacy of 80% 3 years after the last dose, 50% between 4 and 7 years, and 0% after 12 years. Thus, by middle adolescence, protection has significantly decreased and, by late adolescence, has disappeared completely.

The pertussis component is part of the DPT (diphtheria-pertussis-tetanus) vaccine. The whole cell vaccine is not recommended after 7 years of age, because reaction rates no longer justify its use. Research efforts are directed at the development of a more immunogenic but less reactogenic vaccine. Early trials with acellular pertussis vaccines in adolescents and adults have thus far demonstrated excellent immunogenicity, with acceptably low reaction rates. It is anticipated that one or several acellular pertussis vaccines will be licensed that are safe for booster doses in adolescents as their protection wanes (see Chapter 25).

BIBLIOGRAPHY

American Academy of Pediatrics: Report of the Committee on Infectious Diseases, 22nd ed. Elk Grove, IL, AAP, 1991, pp 358–369.
Bass JW: Erythromycin for treatment and prevention of pertussis. Pediatr Infect Dis 5:154, 1986.
Bass JW, Stephenson SR: The return of pertussis. Pediatr Infect Dis 6:141, 1987.
Bergquist S, Bernander S, Dahnsjo H, Sundelof B: Erythromycin in the treatment of pertussis: A study of bacteriologic and clinical effects. Pediatr Infect Dis 6:458, 1987.
Centers for Disease Control: Pertussis surveillance—United States, 1986–1988. MMWR 39:57, 1990.
Cherry JD, Brunnell PA, Golden GS, Karzon DT: Report of the Task Force on Pertussis and Pertussis Immunization—1988. Pediatrics 81(6):Part 2, 1988.
Fine PEM, Clarkson JA: Reflections on the efficacy of pertussis vaccines. Rev Infect Dis 9(5):866, 1987.
Granstrom G, Sterner G, Nord CE, Granstrom M: Use of erythromycin to prevent pertussis in newborns of mothers with pertussis. J Infect Dis 155(6):1210, 1987.
Nelson JD: The changing epidemiology of pertussis in young infants. Am J Dis Child 132:371, 1978.
Onorato IM, Wassilak SGF: Laboratory diagnosis of pertussis: The state of the art. Pediatr Infect Dis 6:145, 1987.

RICKETTSIA RICKETTSII
(ROCKY MOUNTAIN SPOTTED FEVER)

HILLEL K. JANAI, HARRIS R. STUTMAN, and MELVIN I. MARKS

HISTORICAL BACKGROUND

Although more than 600 cases are reported in the United States annually, Rocky Mountain spotted fever (RMSF) is rarely seen by physicians outside endemic areas. Nevertheless, because of its severity, RMSF has gained the attention of physicians all over the United States, and should be included in the differential diagnosis of any illness with fever and rash. Although the disease was first described among settlers in Montana in the late eighteenth century (and is named RMSF after this first-described foci of human infection), the latest literature report concerns a focus of the disease in Bronx, New York. The causative agent of this disease, *Rickettsia rickettsii*, is named after Howard Ricketts, the first physician to describe its microbiologic properties. Ricketts and collaborators reported that "spotted fever" was caused by microorganisms that are present in the patient's blood. The disease was found to be transmissible from humans to guinea pigs and monkeys, and could be prevented by filtration of the blood. Later studies showed that a tick bite could transmit the disease to guinea pigs and humans. Ricketts died of typhus in 1910, a rickettsial disease he described and studied.

EPIDEMIOLOGY

United States—RMSF

Figure 94–2 illustrates the geographic distribution of reported cases of RMSF in 1987 in the United States. States with more than 1 case in 100,000 population are Oklahoma, Kansas, Tennessee, and North and South Carolina. However, RMSF outbreaks may occur in endemic and nonendemic areas. Long Island, New York, has been endemic for years and, from 1971 to 1976, 124 new cases of RMSF were reported there, for an attack rate of 4.85 in 100,000 population. The seasonal patterns of RMSF correspond with tick activity, usually the summer months (April to September). Most cases occur in patients 20 years old or younger. Case fatality rates, currently 3% to 5%, have decreased significantly since the introduction of antibiotics effective against *Rickettsia rickettsii*. The mortality rate is reported as 23% among patients not receiving antibiotics, as compared to only 3% in patients receiving antibiotic therapy. The case fatality rate is 6.5% in persons older than 30 years and 2.0% in individuals under 30 years. This is a result of the more frequent "atypical" presen-

tation in older patients and of the lack of consideration of the diagnosis by physicians caring for older patients.

Rickettsial Diseases in Other Countries

Table 94–11 summarizes the different disease entities caused by rickettsial agents worldwide. Most of these diseases are characterized clinically by fever, rash, and severe headache, with the exception of Q fever, in which no rash is present. Q fever is also unique among rickettsioses because the disease is transmitted by the inhalation of infected particles from the environment surrounding infected animals, rather than by tick or flea bites.

In the Mediterranean area, rickettsial spotted fever is caused by *Rickettsia conorii*. Clinical manifestations, although of lesser severity, are similar to those of RMSF. Fever, rash, myalgias, and vomiting are prevalent, as well as the laboratory findings of thrombocytopenia and hyponatremia.

Ehrlichia canis, a known rickettsial pathogen in dogs that produces fatal canine thrombocytopenia, has been reported to infect humans and cause a disease characterized by fever, thrombocytopenia, leukopenia, and anemia. Rash is not a prominent feature. This is easily confused with RMSF when rash is present.

MICROBIOLOGY AND PATHOPHYSIOLOGY

RMSF is caused by *Rickettsia rickettsii*, a small (0.2 to 0.5 μm in diameter and 0.3 to 2.0 μm in length), obligate, intracellular bacterium. The bacteria can grow in the yolk sacs of embryonated eggs, and may remain viable in blood cultures stored at 4°C. When a tissue

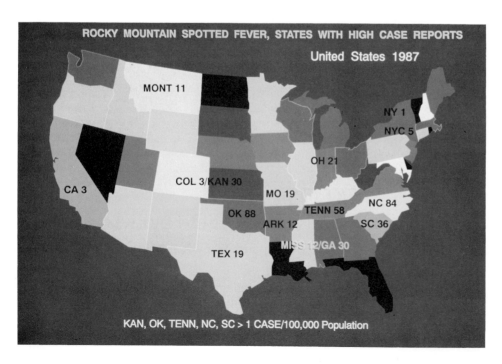

Figure 94–2. Geographic distribution of Rocky Mountain spotted fever in the United States (reported cases, 1987).

TABLE 94–11. Geographic Distribution of Rickettsial Diseases

AGENT	DISEASE	AFFECTED AREA(S)
Rickettsia typhi	Tick spotted fevers	Worldwide foci
R. rickettsii	Rocky Mountain spotted fever	Endemic regions (see Fig. 94–2)
Coxiella burnetii	Q fever	Worldwide
R. akari	Rickettsialpox	United States, Soviet Union, Korea
R. tsutsugamushi	Scrub fever (scrub typhus)	Southeast Asia, Australia
R. prowazekii	Louse-borne typhus	Worldwide
R. conorii	Tick spotted fevers	Mediterranean regions
Ehrlichia canis	Spotless tick fever (ehrlichiosis)	Southeast United States

sample is examined, the organism appears as a red coccobacillus with Giemsa stain.

The dog ticks *Dermacentor andersoni* and *Dermacentor variabilis* are the principal carriers of *R. rickettsii*. RMSF can also be transmitted by blood transfusion or by the aerosol route. A tick bite leads to inoculation of the pathogen. It takes from 4 to 12 hours for the rickettsiae to be shed from the tick salivary gland and to become reactivated by the skin's warm temperature. This interval is the best time to prevent RMSF by removing the tick and interrupting the inoculation. It has been determined that only 1 in 20 ticks harbors rickettsiae. Hence, early removal of a tick and gentle cleansing of the area is all that is recommended.

In the event of inoculation, the rickettsiae spread through the lymphatic system to the blood and then throughout the body. Rickettsiae tend to proliferate inside endothelial cells, invade adjacent endothelial cells, and spread into vessel wall smooth muscle. Thus, the major pathologic event is a generalized vasculitis. The vasculitic process is readily noted in the skin, but vasculitis affecting the heart, central nervous system, adrenals, and kidneys may be more difficult to diagnose and can result in significant morbidity and mortality.

CLINICAL MANIFESTATIONS

After an incubation period of 2 to 12 days, symptoms appear gradually; however, the onset is sometimes abrupt. Fever, headache, and myalgias are prominent. Mild to severe abdominal pain mimicking that of an acute surgical condition, chills, sore throat, and nausea and vomiting may occur. A macular or maculopapular rash, becoming gradually petechial, is first seen on the extremities, including the palms and soles, and then spreads centripetally to the rest of the body. Rarely, infection can present without rash, and diagnosis must be made by a high index of suspicion in any adolescent patient who has been to an RMSF endemic area and has fever, chills, and headache.

Other clinical manifestations, depending on the degree of tissue invasion and injury, can include meningitis, hepatitis, myocarditis, pneumonia, and nephritis. Thrombocytopenia and hyponatremia are commonly

reported. Thrombocytopenia is probably the result of disseminated intravascular coagulation that may develop, and the hyponatremia may be caused by capillary leaks secondary to vasculitis and/or inappropriate antidiuretic hormone secretion. The infection tends to progress gradually, reaching its peak of severity 7 to 14 days after onset.

Table 94–12 lists the most common symptoms and signs in patients with RMSF. It is noteworthy that those younger than 15 years of age usually present with clinical findings typical of the disease. Adolescents above the age of 15 years and adults may have an atypical clinical picture, often without rash, resulting in delay in the diagnosis and, as a result, more severe complications than those that occur in children.

DIAGNOSIS

The most suggestive clinical clues in the diagnosis of RMSF are tick exposure, headache, myalgia, and fever. Thrombocytopenia and hyponatremia are also highly suggestive of RMSF in adolescent patients with fever in tick season in endemic areas. Although cultivation of the organism is possible from blood and tissue, this procedure is complex and slow. The hazards of working with rickettsiae usually discourage laboratories from attempting its isolation.

The indirect immunofluorescent antibody (IFA) and indirect hemagglutination (IHA) assays are the most specific and sensitive tests currently available, but are used only by research laboratories. Latex agglutination (among commercially available reagents) seems to be the most specific and accurate method for documenting increases in antibody titers. Because there is cross-antigenicity between antigens of *Proteus* and *Rickettsia*, agglutination of *Proteus* OX19 can be used to estimate the presence and amount of *R. rickettsii* antibody, but the sensitivity and specificity are low.

A presumptive diagnosis is based on a *fourfold increase* of antibodies during convalescence, combined with the typical clinical illness and other laboratory

TABLE 94–12. Common Symptoms and Signs in RMSF

SYMPTOM OR SIGN	FREQUENCY OF OCCURRENCE (%)
Fever	99
Headache	91
Rash	88
Myalgia	83
Nausea, vomiting	60
Abdominal pain	52
Conjunctivitis	30
Diarrhea	19
Edema	18
Meningeal irritation	18
Pneumonitis	12
Jaundice	9
Myocarditis	5

Data from Helnick OG, Bernard KW, D'Angelo LJ: Rocky Mountain spotted fever: Clinical, laboratory and epidemiological features of 262 cases. J Infect Dis 150:480, 1984.

findings. New techniques for the detection of rickettsial DNA from blood, augmented by polymerase chain reaction methodologies, are being developed, and these procedures might be of future diagnostic value in the clinical laboratory.

DIFFERENTIAL DIAGNOSIS

In 1987, the Centers for Disease Control in Atlanta advised that a diagnosis of RMSF should be considered in endemic areas when an adolescent has an unexplained febrile illness, even if there is no history of a tick bite or travel to a tick-infested area. The differential diagnosis should obviously focus on the rash appearing on the palms and soles, but it must be remembered that the disease may present without rash. Table 94–13 summarizes the differential diagnosis for rash on the palms and soles in adolescents. The adolescent should be questioned about travel, sexual exposure, drug and medication ingestion, and tick bites, because these factors are especially relevant.

TREATMENT

Antibiotic Therapy

In severe cases, therapy for RMSF should be aimed initially at stabilizing the critically ill adolescent, including management of hyponatremia, severe thrombocytopenia, myocarditis, encephalitis, and adult respiratory distress syndrome. The two specific drugs of choice for RMSF are chloramphenicol and tetracyclines. In children 9 years or older and adolescents, tetracyclines are recommended because of the risk of the idiosyncratic and dose-related bone marrow toxicity of chloramphenicol. If tetracycline is used, postmenarchal adolescents should be screened for pregnancy. Because both drugs are rickettsiostatic, relapses may occur and therapy should be continued for 5 days after clinical signs have improved and the temperature has returned to normal, with a minimum course of 7 days.

COURSE OF ILLNESS AND PROGNOSIS

Although fever may persist for up to 5 days, most adolescents show clinical improvement within 48 hours after therapy is initiated. The mortality rate, once as high as 25%, has decreased to 5% or less in the United States. Death usually occurs in adolescent patients with delayed diagnosis, often because of atypical presentations, and usually is a result of cardiovascular or renal failure during the second week of illness.

Complications or sequelae are uncommon, especially with prompt diagnosis and therapy. The most severely affected adolescents may develop pneumonia or complications of carditis, including arrhythmias or congestive failure.

TABLE 94–13. Differential Diagnosis for RMSF in Adolescents

Meningococcemia	Enteroviral syndromes
Disseminated	(especially
gonococcemia	Coxsackie A virus)
Drug hypersensitivity	Ehrlichiosis
Erythema multiforme	Adenovirus
Measles	Scarlet fever
Secondary syphilis	

PREVENTION

Currently, there is no approved vaccine for RMSF. A formalin-inactivated vaccine has been evaluated in a placebo-controlled, double-blind study. The vaccine provided only partial immunity, but ameliorated the illness. Researchers have cloned the gene that codes for the protective antigen on the rickettsial surface. The gene product induces protection for mice and guinea pigs against an otherwise lethal injection of organisms. Human studies with the vaccine are in progress.

Until an effective vaccine is developed, eradication of the organisms that transmit the disease represents the first line of prevention. When camping in endemic areas, adolescents are advised to wear protective clothing and use an insect repellent. Ticks should be promptly removed. This is done by grasping the tick with tweezers or covered fingers (glove, tissue) and pulling. Engorged ticks can be removed by the same technique. Other methods, such as using lighted cigarettes, vaseline, or alcohol, are more likely to harm the adolescent by causing the tick to regurgitate possibly infected material before being dislodged. The hands should be washed carefully after handling ticks, because they may contain rickettsiae.

BIBLIOGRAPHY

Clements ML, Wisseman CL, Jr, Woodward TE, et al: Reactogenicity, immunogenicity, and efficacy of a chick embryo cell-derived vaccine for Rocky Mountain spotted fever. J Infect Dis 148:922, 1988.

Helnick CG, Bernard KW, D'Angelo LJ: Rocky Mountain spotted fever: Clinical, laboratory and epidemiological features of 262 cases. J Infect Dis 150:480, 1984.

Kelsey DS: Rocky Mountain spotted fever. Pediatr Clin North Am 26:367, 1979.

McCloskey RV: Ehrlichiosis—spotless spotted fever. Del Med J 61:335, 1989.

McDonald GA, Anacker RL, Mann RE, et al: Protection of guinea pigs from experimental Rocky Mountain spotted fever with a cloned antigen of Rickettsia rickettsii. J Infect Dis 158:228, 1988.

Salgo MP, Telzak GE, Currie B, et al: A focus of Rocky Mountain spotted fever within New York City. N Engl J Med 318:1345, 1988.

Trianabos T, Anderson BE, McDate JE: Detection of Rickettsia rickettsii DNA in clinical specimens by using polymerase chain reaction technology. J Clin Microbiol 27:2866, 1989.

Walker D: Rocky Mountain spotted fever: A disease in need of microbiological concern. Clin Microbiol Rev 2:227, 1989.

Westerman EL: Rocky Mountain spotted fever. A dilemma for the clinician. Arch Intern Med 142:1106, 1982.

Wolach B, Franco S, Bogger-Goren S, et al: Clinical and laboratory findings of spotted fever in Israeli children. Pediatr Infect Dis J 8:152, 1989.

CHAPTER 95

Giardia lamblia Infections

BURRIS DUNCAN

Giardiasis is an intestinal infection caused by *Giardia lamblia*, a flagellate intestinal protozoa. *G. lamblia* is recognized as one of the most ubiquitous parasites and is one of the ten most important causes of human enteric parastic disease, with over 200 million infections occurring each year. The prevalence of infection varies from 1% to 30%. In some areas where there is poor sanitation and hygiene, 50% to 70% of the community may harbor the infection. It is the most prevalent human parasite in the United States. Both domestic and wild animals can carry this parasite, and can contaminate lakes and streams. Such water is frequently ingested by campers and backpackers. Adolescents and young adults are frequent visitors to such areas, may be unaware of the potential problem, and often do not take the time to decontaminate water from clear mountain streams. *Giardia* has contaminated swimming pools and picnic foods, has even been found in the water supply of large urban centers, and has infected infants and toddlers in child care centers. Some hosts are merely asymptomatic carriers, whereas others have frequent recurrent bouts of crampy, abdominal pain associated with severe watery diarrhea; in some, the infection leads to malabsorption, with subsequent significant weight loss.

LIFE CYCLE, EPIDEMIOLOGY, AND PREVENTION

The *G. lamblia* protozoan has a trophozoite and a cyst stage, both of which are capable of multiplication by binary division; hence, the parasitic load can increase without repeated reinfection. The trophozoites are approximately 12 to 15 μ long (lymphocytes are about 9 μ long) and resemble a split pear with a broad, rounded anterior end and a narrowing, pointed posterior end. The two nuclei in the top half give the appearance of two eyes and are separated by a longitudinal bar that resembles a nose. Flagella emerging from the lower half resemble a tail (Figs. 95–1 and 95–2).

Trophozoites are easily destroyed once they leave the intestinal lumen, but cysts, protected by a thick hyalin wall, can survive for several months outside the host. Transmission is through cysts that have contaminated water or food, or from the hands of food handlers or other individuals through direct hand-to-mouth passage. The cysts are oblong, measure 8 to 12 × 7 to 10 μ, and have eye-like nuclei that are located at one end and are

separated by a longitudinal bar (Fig. 95–3). The cysts resist ordinary chlorination, and outbreaks can involve entire communities that rely only on chlorination to purify the water supply.

Ingestion of the cysts starts the life cycle in the host (Fig. 95–4). The thick hyalin wall of the cysts resist gastric acidity, and therefore they pass unharmed into the small bowel. In the more alkaline environment of the duodenum, in which the pH is between 6.38 and 7.02, the parasite increases its movement within the cyst and eventually breaks through the cyst wall, liberating two trophozoites. Trophozoites have a large sucking disk on their ventral surface and a centrally placed ostium. Two oscillating flagella just beneath this ostium assist the ventral sucking cup in finding and firmly attaching to the microvilli of the intestinal epithelium of the small bowel and in resisting expulsion by peristalsis. Repeated longitudinal binary division by the trophozoites can greatly increase the parasitic load, so the duodenum and upper jejunum can literally become carpeted with organisms (Fig. 95–5). It is no wonder that giardiasis can result in malabsorption, weight loss, and eventually malnutrition. Each trophozoite obtains its nutrition through the absorption of digested food particles in the intestinal lumen, and probably also from

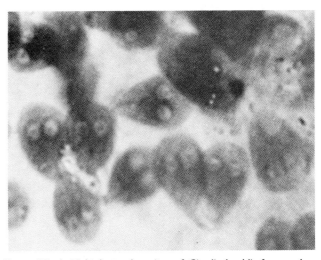

Figure 95–1. Multiple trophozoites of *Giardia lamblia* from a duodenal aspiration give the appearance of ghosts with large white eyes and a flowing tail. (With permission from Hoskins `LC, Winawer SJ, Broitman SA, et al: Clinical giardiasis and intestinal malabsorption. Gastroenterology 53:265, 1967.)

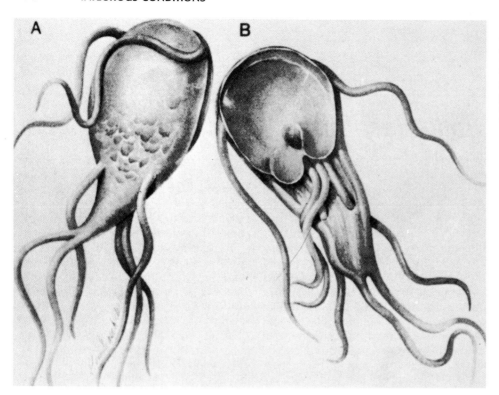

Figure 95–2. A drawing based on scanning electron microscopic observations of the dorsal (*A*) and ventral (*B*) surfaces of a *Giardia lamblia* trophozoite. The ventral sucker, mouth, and flagella are evident. (With permission from Burke JA: The clinical and laboratory diagnosis of giardiasis. CRC Crit Rev Clin Lab Sci 7(4):373, 1977.)

robbing intestinal brush border epithelial cells of already absorbed nutrients.

The flagella dislocate the trophozoite from one site and relocate it to a fresh site. When peristaltic activity increases, the trophozoites can no longer maintain their position in the upper bowel and are propelled into the lower tract, where they become dehydrated and then encysted. In this process, the flagella are shortened and retract, and a thick wall is formed around the shrinking cytoplasm. If peristaltic activity is greatly increased, the transit time may be shortened enough to allow the passage of trophozoites in the watery stool. On the other hand, if the trip is longer and the stool drier, encystation occurs and only the cyst stage may be found in the stool specimen. Trophozoites do not survive outside the host and, even if immediately ingested, would be destroyed by the acidic environment of the stomach. Thus, it is only through ingestion of the resistant cysts that the cycle is completed (see Fig. 95–4).

Giardiasis is found in all parts of the world, with an overall prevalence rate of 7.2%; in the United States, the rate is 7.4%. Sheep, cattle, dogs, domestic cats, mice, and beavers all can harbor species of *Giardia*, which are morphologically similar to *G. lamblia* and have caused symptoms in these animals that resemble those of human giardiasis. The contamination of streams and municipal water supplies by these animals has probably been responsible for outbreaks in campers and in those at ski resorts. Infected domestic and farm animals can transmit the parasite to humans. There is a reported 12% to 13% prevalence in homosexual males. It is presumed that transmission occurs through anal or oral sex (see Chapter 32).

Avoiding the ingestion of water contaminated by *Giardia* cysts or properly treating water suspected of harboring the cysts should prevent infection by this protozoan. Because the cysts can survive in cold or tepid water for many weeks, but are killed immediately at 50°C, travelers to endemic areas are advised to drink only boiled or properly treated bottled water. Cysts can survive ordinary chlorination, but are killed by a 2% iodine solution. Hence, the use of chlorine tablets should probably be replaced by the use of 2% tincture of iodine (five drops added to 1 quart of clear water, or ten drops added to cold or cloudy water and left to stand for at least 30 minutes). Drinking water should be protected from fecal contamination, and filtration and sedimentation processes should be implemented. Proper hygiene

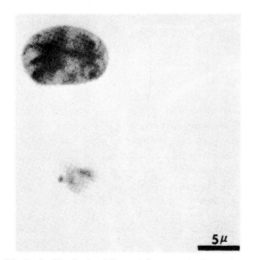

Figure 95–3. A *Giardia lamblia* cyst from a stool specimen. (With permission from Burke JA: The clinical and laboratory diagnosis of giardiasis. CRC Crit Rev Clin Lab Sci 7(4):373, 1977.)

Figure 95—4. The life cycle of *Giardia lamblia* in the human host. (With permission from Meyer EA, Jarroll EL: Giardiasis. Am J Epidemiol 111:1, 1980.)

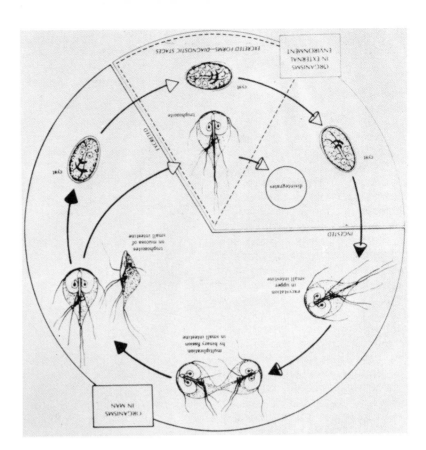

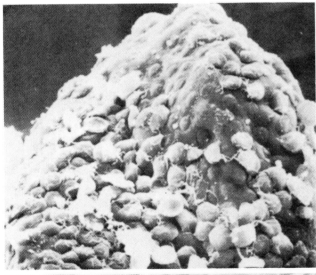

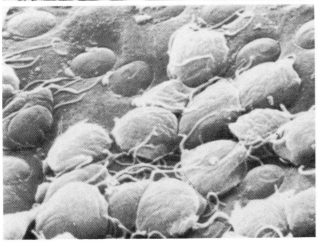

Figure 95—5. This apical portion of an intestinal villus is from a rat heavily infested with *Giardia muris*. The parasites virtually carpet the villus structure, and their disk prints can be seen in the lower picture taken through a scanning electron microscope magnified 2950 times. The nutritional effect of such an infestation is easy to imagine. (With permission from Erlandsen SL, Chase OG: Morphological alterations in the microvillous border of villous epithelial cells produced by intestinal microorganisms. Am J Clin Nutr 27:1277, 1974.)

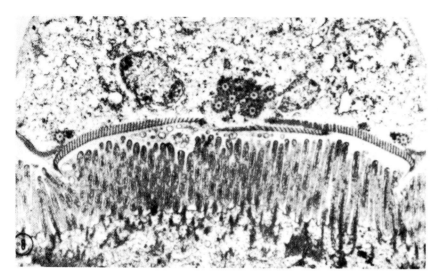

Figure 95–6. An electron microscopic view of a transversely sectioned *Giardia lamblia* attached to the microvillus. Disruption of the epithelium is evident at the margins of the suction disk. Cellular debris or food particles can be seen between the undersurface of the disk and the upper surface of the epithelium. (With permission from Erlandsen SL, Chase OG: Morphological alterations in the microvillous border of villous epithelial cells produced by intestinal microorganisms. Am J Clin Nutr 27:1277, 1974.)

measures in food handling and hand washing should decrease the potential spread of this parasite to the unsuspecting host.

PATHOPHYSIOLOGY

The exact pathogenesis of giardiasis is not well understood but is probably related to mechanical injury of the intestinal microvillus secondary to the vacuum attachment of the suction disks of multiple trophozoites. The rim of the disk interdigitates between the microvilli, with the floor of the disk resting on the brush border (Figs. 95–6 and 95–7). Villi are shortened at the site of attachment and epithelial cells, which are subject to the suction, show compression vacuolization and often se-

vere damage (Fig. 95–8). Cell injury causes a mild but reversible polynuclear inflammatory response in the lamina propria of the crypts of Lieberkühn. Although the reaction caused by a single organism is mild, a heavy infestation multiplies the injury thousands of times and is repeated recurrently as the trophozoites move from site to site. Mucosal invasion is rare, and therefore diarrheal stools do not contain blood or inflammatory cells.

The severity of symptoms, however, is not directly related to the intensity of the parasitic load, so other factors must be involved in the pathogenesis of giardiasis. Age seems to be a factor, since children and adolescents tend to have more severe symptoms than adults. The specific strain of *Giardia* may also be an important factor in determining the severity of symp-

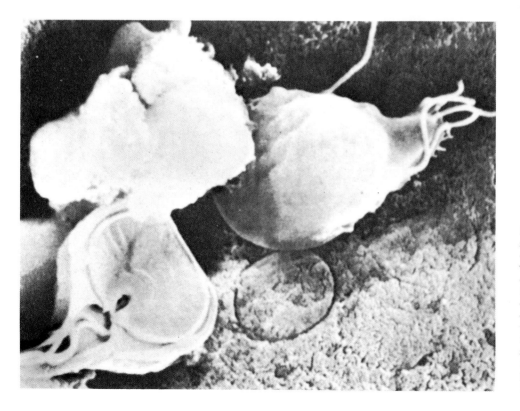

Figure 95–7. As seen through the scanning electron microscope, one of the *Giardia* is displaying its ventral surface and another its dorsal surface. The adhesive disk has recently detached, and the disk print is evident in the microvillous border of the intestinal tract. The parasite is ready to move on and attach to another site. (With permission from Warren KS: Geographic medicine in practice. Hosp Pract 1:110, 1980.)

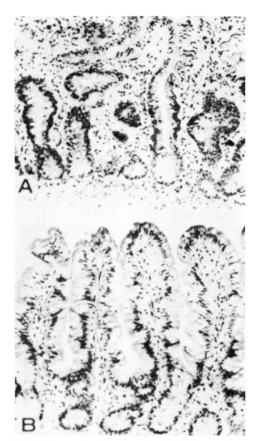

Figure 95–8. Pathologic alterations in giardiasis can be severe, as seen in this biopsy specimen taken from the duodenojejunal junction (A), but are reversible after successful treatment (B). (With permission from Ament ME, Rubin CE: Relationship of giardiasis to abnormal intestinal structure and function in gastrointestinal immunodeficiency syndromes. Gastroenterology 62:216, 1972.)

toms. Other host susceptibility factors include the following: achlorhydria, which promotes infection; non-immune gastrointestinal factors such as bile salts, which promote encystation of trophozoites, and intestinal mucus, which protects the organism; hypogammaglobulinemia, particularly a deficiency in IgM or in secretory IgA, which would allow attachment of the parasite; immunosuppression from chemical or radiation exposure or as seen in AIDS patients, which intensifies infection; and previous exposure to *G. lamblia*, which, if it results in the production of secretory IgA, should provide some protection against infectivity.

The spectrum of clinical manifestations of giardiasis is variable. Most infected individuals are asymptomatic. A survey in Arizona found *Giardia* cysts in stools of 9% of the population, but 80% of those infected had no suggestive symptoms. Clinical symptoms usually occur approximately 2 weeks after ingestion of the cysts, although they may not develop for several months after exposure. Some infected individuals have recurrent bouts of anorexia, abdominal bloating with excessive gas, crampy abdominal pain, and explosive watery, malodorous diarrhea. This picture may be mild or severe and may be of short duration or, if undiagnosed and untreated, may persist for months or even years. Some adolescents who present with a history of weight loss

appear malnourished secondary to anorexia or malabsorption and may have steatorrhea.

The enteritis initiated by the parasite causes alterations in intestinal secretion, absorption, and motility. The adolescent patient complains of nausea, anorexia, and watery, secretory diarrhea. Vomiting is present in less than one third of adolescent patients, and fever is not often present. These two negative features help distinguish this parasitic infestation from viral and bacterial causes of gastroenteritis. Food is poorly absorbed, particularly carbohydrates because of the injury to brush border cells, and consequently there is loss of disaccharidase enzymes. Undigested carbohydrates promote bacterial growth and metabolism, with the liberation of CO_2 resulting in abdominal bloating, belching, and flatulence. This causes adolescent patients to be irritable. In most adolescents and adults, the acute phase can last from 2 weeks to 4 months. Spontaneous resolution can occur within 4 to 6 weeks from onset of symptoms. Typically, the clinical picture is one of intermittent diarrhea, with watery to mushy and very foul-smelling stools. The abdominal symptoms of bloating, anorexia, nausea, and epigastric discomfort may be intermittent or continuous (Table 95–1). The adolescent may present with a picture very similar to that seen with celiac syndrome. Urticaria has been reported in association with giardiasis, as has an elevation of hepatic enzymes, but a causative relationship has not been firmly established.

DIAGNOSIS

The clinical presentation of giardiasis varies, so a high index of suspicion is necessary when an adolescent presents with gastrointestinal symptoms. Particularly suspect would be the adolescent hiker, backpacker, or child care worker. Because the incubation period may

TABLE 95–1. Frequency (%) of Complaints in Symptomatic and Asymptomatic Giardiasis by Age Group

COMPLAINT	AGE		
	<5 years (N = 144)	>5 years (N = 52)	Adult (N = 38)
None	39	69	76
Diarrhea	28	6	21
Intermittent diarrhea	45	19	24
Constipation	45	19	0
Abdominal cramps	10	21	18
Abdominal distention	26	10	13
Anorexia	36	13	11
Nausea	18	15	11
Vomiting	17	2	8
Malaise	12	6	18
Failure to thrive	47	0	0
Weight loss	41	0	5
Pale, greasy feces	11	2	5
Malodorous feces	10	2	5
Flatulence	0	0	5
Belching	0	0	8

With permission from Craft JC: Giardia and giardiasis in childhood. Pediatr Inf Dis 1(3):196, 1982. Copyright by Williams & Wilkins, 1982.

be weeks to months, the trip to the mountains may have been long forgotten by the time symptoms develop. Adolescents are often hesitant to talk about their stools and usually do not look at them, nor do they involve their parents in such personal matters. Hence, an accurate history and stool description are often difficult to obtain.

Similarly, laboratory diagnosis is often difficult. Confirmation of infestation still depends on identifying the parasite from a stool specimen, duodenal aspirate, cytologic imprint, or small bowel biopsy. Serologic testing on stool for the presence of parasitic antigen and on serum for antibodies against the organism is being developed and soon should be available.

Only G. lamblia cysts are found in formed stools, but both trophozoites and cysts may be found in watery or mushy stools. Although cysts withstand drying and temperature changes, their morphology may be altered if the stool specimen is not examined shortly after passage, unless it has been preserved in polyvinyl alcohol or 10% formalin. The trophozoites are more delicate and they cannot be seen unless the stool is very fresh and watery. The microscopic examination of a small amount of the liquid stool mixed with a drop of saline solution or methylene blue reveals the rapid, erratic motility of the pear-shaped trophozoites. A drop of iodine mixed with a small amount of stool stains the internal structure of cysts and trophozoites yellow-brown for easier identification. Cysts are ovoid and colorless, and have a highly refractile cell wall. Unfortunately, excretion patterns vary from many organisms in every milliliter of stool to no parasites excreted for several weeks. Furthermore, there is little correlation of the quantity of cyst excretion with stool consistency. Alternate-day examination can increase the positive yield.

Detection of Giardia antigen in stool specimens is a more reliable test than examination of stool and is not influenced by the presence of antidiarrheal compounds or other factors. Tests for antigen can be done on stool specimens that have been preserved in formalin for months. The enzyme-linked immunosorbent assay (ELISA) has a sensitivity of 94% and a specificity of 95%. Counter-immunoelectrophoresis (CIE) has a sensitivity of 88% and a specificity of 99%. These antigen tests have been used not only for diagnosis but also to assess the effectiveness of therapy.

Specific serum IgM and IgG antibodies to Giardia have been detected. Some preliminary evidence suggests that the predominant antibody in acute or nonpersistent infections is IgM, whereas persistent and asymptomatic carriers have anti-Giardia antibodies of the IgG class.

False-negative results can be caused by the presence of drugs that alter the morphology of the parasite. These include antibiotics, antispasmodics, kaolin, antacids, and oily laxatives. Barium also affects morphology. All these factors, plus variability in the skill of the technician, necessitate examining several stools. Examination of only one stool specimen misses 25% and examination of two specimens misses 10% of adolescents with giardiasis. Such high false-negative rates have led to the use of other diagnostic methods. One method involves examining duodenal secretions obtained by using the Entero-Test* capsule. Following a 4-hour fast, the adolescent swallows a gelatin capsule that contains a weighted silicone rubber bag and 140 cm of nylon yarn. One end of the yarn is held while the capsule is swallowed and then taped to the side of the adolescent's face. The gelatin capsule dissolves in the stomach and the weighted bag continues into the duodenum. Approximately 4 hours after ingestion, the yarn is pulled up out of the bag and the bile-stained mucus covering the distal end of the yarn is immediately examined for trophozoites. Cytologic smear of biopsies (touch cytology) and tissue biopsies have also been helpful in adolescents who are difficult to diagnose, but the invasiveness of the procedure limits its use.

The white blood cell and differential counts are usually normal. Eosinophilia is rarely seen. The sedimentation rate is normal. White blood cells and blood are not present in stool specimens. With the development of malabsorption, intestinal transit time is rapid, and the stools contain an excessive number of fat globules and an increased quantity of reducing substances. The fat-soluble vitamins A, D, and E, as well as folic acid and vitamin B_{12}, are poorly absorbed. Both lactose and D-xylose tolerance test results are abnormal. The lactose intolerance may persist for months, even after appropriate treatment has eliminated the parasite. If diarrhea persists after treatment, both persistent infestation and lactose intolerance should be considered. Roentgenograms of the small bowel have a variable and nonspecific pattern. Findings of an upper gastrointestinal series may be normal or may indicate a pattern consistent with a chronic malabsorption (i.e., thickening and flattening of mucosal folds, flocculation, and increased secretions).

MANAGEMENT AND TREATMENT

Because of the difficulty in confirming the diagnosis, and given a history that strongly suggests infection with G. lamblia, some physicians give a course of treatment on empirical grounds. Three drugs are currently available in the United States (Table 95–2) for the treatment of giardiasis: quinacrine (Atabrine), with a cure rate of 90% to 95%; metronidazole (Flagyl), with a cure rate of approximately 85% to 90%; and furazolidone (Furoxone), with a cure rate of 80% to 85%. Only furazolidone comes in a liquid form, although the other two can be specially formulated and put into suspension. Three other drugs are available in Europe and South America that can be given as a single dose. Tinidazole, ornidazole, and nitrimidazine are chemically related to metronidazole, and are reported to have a 90% to 95% cure rate.

All three drugs have a disulfiram (Antabuse) reaction with alcohol, and the adolescent should be aware of this. Because the teratogenic effect of these anti-Giardia medications is not known, their use in pregnancy is contraindicated. The Centers for Disease Control recommend that paromomycin, a nonabsorbable aminogly-

---

*Available from Health Development Corporation, 2411 Pulgas Avenue, Palo Alto, CA.

TABLE 95–2. Drug Treatment of Giardiasis

| DRUG | RECOMMENDED DOSAGE | |
	Adults	Children and Adolescents
Preferred		
Quinacrine HCl	100 mg, three times daily, for 5 days	6 mg/kg/day in 3 divided doses for 5 days (maximum, 300 mg/day)
Alternatives		
Metronidazole	250 mg, three times daily, for 5 days	15 mg/kg/day in 3 divided doses for 5 days
Furazolidone	100 mg, four times daily, for 7 to 10 days	6 mg/kg/day in 4 divided doses for 7 to 10 days

coside, be used for treating the severely symptomatic pregnant adolescent.

Each drug has its own side effects. Quinacrine is bitter, and treatment is frequently accompanied by dizziness, headache, vomiting, and diarrhea. Occasional reactions include jaundice, insomnia, nightmares, toxic psychosis, blood dyscrasias, urticaria, and other skin rashes. Metronidazole has not been approved by the Food and Drug Administration for the treatment of giardiasis. It frequently causes nausea, headache, dry mouth, and a metallic taste in the mouth. Occasionally, it is associated with vomiting, diarrhea, insomnia, weakness, stomatitis, vertigo, paresthesia, skin rashes, dark urine, and dysuria. Furazolidone frequently causes nausea and vomiting and occasionally causes hypotension, allergic reactions, pulmonary infiltrates, urticaria, fever, headache, hypoglycemia, and hemolytic anemia in glucose-G-phosphate dehydrogenase–deficient patients.

The need to treat asymptomatic carriers is controversial. Certainly from a public health viewpoint, it seems advisable to treat all those with jobs involving the possibility of spread to others. Many such jobs are held by adolescents, who often work in fast food establishments or restaurants, as lifeguards or swimming pool maintenance employees, and as helpers in child care centers or nursing homes.

BIBLIOGRAPHY

Abramowicz M (ed): Drugs for parasitic infections. Medical Lett Drugs Ther 32(814):23, 1990.

Ament ME, Rubin CE: Relationship of giardiasis to abnormal intestinal structure and function in gastrointestinal immunodeficiency syndromes. Gastroenterology 62:216, 1972.

Brown HW, Neva FA: Basic Clinical Parasitology, 5th ed. Norwalk, CT, Appleton-Century-Crofts, 1983.

Burke JA: The clinical and laboratory diagnosis of giardiasis. CRC Crit Rev Clin Lab Sci 7(4):373, 1977.

Craft JC: Giardia and giardiasis in children. Pediatr Inf Dis 1(3):196, 1982.

Duncan B: Diseases caused by intestinal protozoa. In Kelley VC (ed): Practice of Pediatrics, Vol 4. New York, Harper & Row, 1986, pp 15–25.

Erlandsen SL, Chase OG: Morphological alterations in the microvillous border of villous epithelial cells produced by intestinal microorganisms. Am J Clin Nutr 27:1277, 1974.

Hoskins LC, Winawer SJ, Broitman SA, et al: Clinical giardiasis and intestinal malabsorption. Gastroenterology 53:265, 1967.

Janoff EN, Craft JC, Pickering LK, et al: Diagnosis of *Giardia lamblia* infections by detection of parasite-specific antigens. J Clin Microbiol 27(3):431, 1989.

Kulda J, Nohynkova E: Flagellates of the human intestine and of intestines of other species. In Kreier JP (ed): Parasitic Protozoa, Vol II. New York, Academic Press, 1977, pp 69–104.

Kumkum, Khanna R, Nain CK, et al: Depressed humoral immune responses to surface antigens of *Giardia lamblia* in persistent giardiasis. Pediatr Infect Dis J 7(7):492, 1988.

Meyer EA, Jarroll EL: Giardiasis. Am J Epidemiol 111:1, 1980.

Payne FJ, Atchley FO, Wasley MA, et al: Association of *Giardia lamblia* with disease. J Parasitol 46:742, 1960.

Pickering LK, Engelkirk PG: *Giardia lamblia*. Pediatr Clin North Am 35(3):565, 1988.

Warren KS: Geographic medicine in practice. Hosp Pract 15(1):110, 1980.

CHAPTER 96

Selecting Antimicrobial Agents

KEITH R. POWELL

When antimicrobial agents first became available susceptibility testing had not been considered, and the pharmacokinetic properties of the antimicrobial agents were unknown. The early approach to antimicrobial therapy was to use an antimicrobial agent if the patient seemed to have a bacterial infection, and to use a large amount if the patient appeared very ill. As more antimicrobial agents became available, and their spectra of activity defined, the "bug-and-drug" approach became popular. That is, the antimicrobial agent was selected according to the known or suspected pathogen. If the pathogen could not be identified and the patient appeared quite ill, a "shotgun" approach was used.

Current therapy employs a new approach to the selection and use of antimicrobial agents in adolescents and patients of all ages. Selecting an antimicrobial agent should be based on considerations of the anatomic site of infection, the possible bacterial pathogens that cause infections at that site, and the ability of antimicrobial agents to achieve concentrations at the site effective against the causative bacteria. This new approach should also use available information about the antimicrobial activity and pharmacokinetics of antimicrobial agents. Using available information wisely maximizes the effectiveness of antimicrobial therapy, decreases their toxicity, and decreases the emergence of resistant bacteria.

The rudiments of antimicrobial therapy, such as drug selection for empirical therapy, serum concentrations, and antimicrobial activity, are summarized in Tables 96–1 and 96–2. The selection of an antimicrobial agent(s) can be optimized, however, if the relationship between the antimicrobial activity and pharmacokinetics of an antimicrobial agent is considered in conjunction with host factors. Because the adolescent's size is between that of a child and an adult, particular care must be taken not to overdose adolescents; doses should be administered based on mg/kg/dose and should not exceed adult doses stated in mg/dose or g/dose.

For most common infections in adolescents, antimicrobial agents can be given without the use of laboratory tests (Table 96–1). The site of infection can be found by examination, the likely pathogens causing such infections can be determined, and the outcome can be predicted if certain antimicrobial agents are used. A wide number of antimicrobial agents given orally can achieve effective concentrations at the site of infection and result in a clinical and microbiologic cure. No laboratory tests are necessary to manage such patients.

The rational use of antimicrobial agents requires an understanding of testing susceptibility and using susceptibility data and pharmacokinetics to optimize therapy. This chapter explains the general principles of antimicrobial therapy and provides pharmacokinetic data and information about antimicrobial activity that can be used in the application of these principles.

GENERAL PRINCIPLES

Antimicrobial Activity

The *in vitro* activity of an antimicrobial agent against a particular bacterium is determined by adding diminishing concentrations of the agent to a series of test tubes containing 10^5 bacteria/ml in a clear broth culture medium. When the concentration of the antimicrobial agent is too low to inhibit bacterial growth, the broth becomes turbid after overnight incubation. The lowest concentration of the antimicrobial agent that can prevent bacterial growth (i.e., the broth remains clear) is denoted as the minimum inhibitory concentration (MIC). Bactericidal activity is determined by quantitatively subculturing broth from test tubes that have remained clear onto agar plates. After additional incubation, the colonies of bacteria are counted. The lowest concentration of the antimicrobial agent that resulted in the death of 99.9% of the original inoculum is denoted as the minimum bactericidal concentration (MBC). MIC and MBC values are reported as μg of antimicrobial agent/ml of broth required to inhibit or kill the bacteria, respectively.

Most diagnostic laboratories do not routinely determine the MIC when antimicrobial susceptibility testing is requested. Instead, the clinical isolate is inoculated onto an agar plate and paper disks containing standard concentrations of selected antimicrobial agents are placed on the surface of the agar. The antimicrobial agents diffuse into the agar so that, as the distance from the disk increases, the concentration of the antimicrobial agent decreases. If the bacteria are susceptible to an antimicrobial agent, there is a zone around the disk in which the bacteria do not grow (zone of inhibition). The diameter of the zone of inhibition can be correlated to MIC values. Organisms are usually reported as susceptible, intermediate, or resistant. A report of intermediate susceptibility should be treated as resistant. Susceptible means that 95% of bacterial strains tested are inhibited by concentrations of the antimicrobial agent

TABLE 96–1. Initial Empirical Therapy for Selected Infections in Adolescents

CLINICAL DIAGNOSIS (SITE OF INFECTION)	MOST LIKELY PATHOGEN(S)	ANTIMICROBIAL AGENT(S)
Skin and soft tissue infections	*Streptococcus pyogenes* *Staphylococcus aureus*	Dicloxicillin, cephalexin, clindamycin, erythromycin (or intravenous equivalent)
Pyogenic arthritis	*Staphylococcus aureus* *Neisseria gonorrhoeae*	Nafcillin Ceftriaxone
Osteomyelitis	*Staphylococcus aureus*	Nafcillin
Otitis media, acute sinusitis	*Streptococcus pneumoniae, Haemophilus influenzae* (untypable), *Moraxella catarrhalis*	Amoxicillin augmentin, trimethoprim-sulfamethoxazole
Epiglottis	*H. influenzae*, type b	Ceftriaxone
Pneumonia	*Mycoplasma pneumoniae* *Streptococcus pneumoniae*	Erythromycin or tetracycline Penicillin
Infective endocarditis	*Streptococcus viridans* (subacute) *Staphylococcus aureus* (acute)	Nafcillin plus gentamicin
Acute diarrhea (white blood cells in fecal smear)	*Shigella, Salmonella*	Trimethoprim-sulfamethoxazole or ampicillin (if suspect *Shigella*, not for *Salmonella*)
Urinary tract infections, cystitis	*Escherichia coli*	Sulfisoxazole or amoxicillin; reculture in 36 to 48 hours and change if positive
Pyelonephritis	*Escherichia coli*	IV aminoglycoside
Sexually transmitted diseases, pelvic inflammatory disease	See Chapter 75	
Meningitis	*Streptococcus pneumoniae* *Neisseria meningitidis* *Haemophilus influenzae* (less common)	Ceftriaxone
Brain abscess	*Streptococcal* spp. (anaerobes) *Staphylococcus aureus*	Penicillin (use nafcillin if *S. aureus* suspected) plus metronidazole
Abdominal sepsis	Gram-negative anaerobes, Enterococcus (enteric)	Ampicillin plus an aminoglycoside plus metronidazole or clindamycin
Septic shock	*Neisseria meningitidis*	Ceftriaxone until cause known
Toxic shock syndrome	*Staphylococcus aureus*	Nafcillin (parenteral)
Lyme disease, acute	*Borrelia burgdorferi*	Tetracycline, ceftriaxone

that can be achieved in the serum if the usual dose is given by the usual route of administration to treat an infection by that organism. The cutoff for "susceptible by disk" is the MIC_{95}, or the concentration of antimicrobial agent required to inhibit 95% of all isolates of that species of bacteria. The MIC_{95} that correlates to susceptible by disk is included in Table 96–2 for the antimicrobial agents listed. The MIC_{95} values given in this table are used by most diagnostic microbiology laboratories. Thus, MIC_{95} values for antimicrobial agents not listed in Table 96–2 can usually be obtained from the laboratory. If a concentration of antimicrobial agent equal to or greater than 10 times the MIC can be achieved at the site of infection, a clinical and microbiologic cure is likely.

Bactericidal Versus Bacteriostatic

A bactericidal antimicrobial agent is not usually required to treat infections in normal adolescents. Exceptions include bacterial endocarditis, meningitis, and possibly osteomyelitis. Because the effectiveness of bacteriostatic agents depends on host bacterial clearance mechanisms, bactericidal agents are usually necessary in immunocompromised hosts.

Pharmacokinetics

The most widely used pharmacokinetic feature of an antimicrobial agent is usually its concentration in serum over time. It is also important to consider the distribu-

tion of individual antimicrobial agents into specific tissues or fluids, and whether the agents are active in these sites. The pharmacokinetic parameters that correlate best with a microbiologic cure are the peak serum concentration and length of time that the serum concentration remains above the MIC for the infecting bacterium. The peak serum concentration, the time after administration that the maximum concentration is reached, and the serum half-life of selected antimicrobial agents are included in Table 96–2.

Inhibitory Quotient

The relationship between the activity of an antimicrobial agent and its pharmacokinetics can be expressed as an inhibitory quotient (IQ):

$$IQ = \frac{\text{Concentration of antimicrobial agent}}{\text{MIC for the causative bacteria}}$$

When the concentration of the antimicrobial agent at the site of infection exceeds the MIC by 10-fold, the outcome is likely to be a clinical and microbiologic cure. For infections in well-perfused sites, the peak serum concentration can be considered as approximately equal to the concentration of the antimicrobial agent at the site. For infections in sites such as the central nervous system, it is necessary to know how well individual antimicrobial agents reach these sites. *The Use of Antibiotics* (see bibliography) is an excellent reference for information about the pharmacokinetics of antimicrobial agents.

TABLE 96–2. Dosage, Peak Serum Concentrations, and MIC$_{95}$ For Selected Antimicrobial Agents

| ANTIMICROBIAL AGENT | ROUTE OF ADMINISTRATION | DOSE | | Peak Serum Concentration (µg/ml) | Time From Administration to Peak | Susceptible MIC$_{95}$ (µg/ml) |
		Pediatric* (mg/kg/ dose, interval)†	Adult (mg/dose, interval)			
Penicillin G	IV	25,000–50,000 U, q4–6h	0.3–4 × 10⁶ U, q4–6h	240	5 minutes	≤0.1; *Listeria monocytogenes*, ≤2
Penicillin V	PO	6.25–12.5, q6h	250–500, q6h	3–5	½–1 hour	≤0.1
Ampicillin	IV	25–75, q4–6h	1000–2000, q6h	40	5 minutes	Gram-negative, ≤8; *Streptococcus*, ≤0.1; *Haemophilus influenzae*, ≤2
Amoxicillin	PO	10–15, q8h	250–500, q8h	4.7–7.5	2 hours	As for ampicillin
Nafcillin	IV	25–50, q6h	500–1500, q4–6h	11	5 minutes	≤1
Dicloxacillin	PO	3.125–6.25	250–500, q6h	15–18	½–1 hour	≤1
Mezlocillin	IV	50–75, q4–6h	3000, q4h	200–300	5 minutes	≤64
Cefazolin	IV	8.3–25, q6–8h	500–1500, q6–8h	188	5 minutes	≤8
Cephalexin	PO	6.25–12.5, q6h	250–1000, q6h	8–40	1 hour	≤8
Cefoxitin	IV	20–26.6, q4–6h	1000–2000, q4–6h; or 3000, q8h	110–125	5 minutes	≤8
Cefotaxime	IV	25–50, q6h	1000–2000, q4–6h	1 g, 40; 2 g, 80–90	5 minutes	≤8
Ceftriaxone	IV	50, q24h (CNS—50, q12h)	500–2000, q24h	1 g, 150	5 minutes	≤8
	IM			1 g, 50	2 hours	
Ceftazidime	IV	25–50, q8–12h	500–2000, q8–12h	1 g, 85	5 minutes	≤8
Amikacin‡	IV	5, q8h; or	5 mg/kg, q8h; or	20–40	½ hour	≤16
	IM	7.5, q12h	7.5 mg/kg, q12h	20	1 hour	
Gentamicin‡	IV	1–2.5, q8h	1–1.7 mg/kg, q8h	4–10	½ hour	≤4
	IM			7	1 hour	
Tobramycin‡	IV	1–2.5, q8h	1–1.7 mg/kg, q8h	4–14	½ hour	≤4
	IM			4	1 hour	
Trimethoprim (TMP)—sulfamethoxazole (SMX)	PO	3–6 TMP/15–30 SMX, q12h; 5 TMP/25 SMX, q6h for *Pneumocystis*	160 TMP/800 SMX, q12h for *Pneumocystis;* use "pediatric" dose	2–4/80–100	1–2 hours	≤2/38
	IV				5 minutes	
Sulfisoxazole	PO	37.5, q6h	500–1000, q6h	40–50	2–3 hours	≤100 (urinary tract infections only)
Erythromycin estolate	PO	10 q8h, or 15 q12h	250–500, q6h	4.2	2 hours	≤5
Erythromycin ethylsuccinate	PO	10, q6h	250–500, q6h	1.5	2 hours	≤5
Clindamycin	PO	2.5–7.5, q6h	150–450, q6h	2.5–3.6	1–2 hours	≤5
	IV				5 minutes	
Chloramphenicol‡	IV	12.5–18.75, q6h	12.5–25 mg/kg, q6h	19	2 hours	*H. influenzae*, ≤4
	PO			25	2 hours	Others, ≤12.5
Tetracycline	IV	Children older than 8 years, 6.25–12.5, q6h	250–500, q6h	8	5 minutes	≤4
	PO			4	3 hours	
Vancomycin‡	IV	10–15, q6h	15 mg/kg, q12h	30–40	2 hours	≤5
Metronidazole	PO		7.5 mg/kg, q6h	11.5	1 hour	≤4
	IV	7.5, q6h		20–25	½ hour	
Rifampin	PO	10–20, q24h	600, q24h	7	2 hours	≤1
Norfloxacin	PO	Not recommended	800, q12h	1.6	1–2 hours	≤4
Ciprofloxacin	PO	Not recommended	250–750, q12h	2.9	1–1½ hrs	≤1
	IV		200–400, q12h	3.8	5 minutes	

Note: Dosages are for patients with normal hepatic and renal function.
*If the dose calculated as mg/kg/dose for the adolescent exceeds the adult dose in mg/dose, the adult dose (smaller of the two) should be used.
†mg/kg/dose, unless noted otherwise.
‡Dosage should be adjusted according to serum concentration.

Serum Bactericidal Titer

The *in vivo* activity of an antimicrobial agent against the infecting bacteria can be approximated by determining the serum inhibitory titer. The test is performed much like the MIC. Rather than adding a known concentration of an antimicrobial agent to the test tubes containing bacteria in broth, serial twofold dilutions of serum are added. The serum bactericidal titer is determined by quantitatively subculturing broth in which there is no visible growth. The most dilute specimen of serum that results in the death of 99.9% of the original inoculum is the serum bactericidal titer. If a peak serum bactericidal titer of 1:8 can be achieved, a clinical and microbiologic cure can be anticipated. To interpret results, it is critical that blood be drawn when the peak serum concentration of the particular antimicrobial agent has been attained. The time that peak concentration is reached (see Table 96–2) varies not only with the antimicrobial agent, but also with the route of administration.

Role of the Laboratory in the Use of Antimicrobial Agents

When the site of infection can be identified and the likely pathogens anticipated, the practitioner can divide the peak serum concentrations of selected antimicrobial agents by the MIC$_{95}$ (both given in Table 96–2) to select an antimicrobial agent that is likely to work. For common infections such as cellulitis, lymphadenitis, local abscess, pneumonia, sinusitis, and otitis media, it is not usually necessary to perform laboratory tests. When usual therapy fails, when the adolescent is seriously ill or immunocompromised, or when the clinical situation is unusual, appropriate specimens should be obtained to culture for bacterial pathogens. When pathogens are isolated from specimens that are usually sterile, susceptibility testing is performed. If the isolate is an uncommon bacterium, or its susceptibility is unpredictable, the MIC should be determined for selected antimicrobial agents.

SPECIFIC ANTIBACTERIAL AGENTS

It is usually possible to use any one of many different agents and have an equally good outcome. Making a choice is based on considerations such as cost, toxicity, route and frequency of administration, and the potential for ambulatory therapy. Rather than trying to know *all* the possible alternative therapies, the practitioner is advised to learn how to use a selected number of antimicrobial agents well. Table 96–1 lists selected infections in adolescents, the pathogens usually associated with these infections, and antimicrobial agents that could be used for initial empirical therapy. General information about the classes of antimicrobial agents is presented in the next section. Peak serum concentrations that can be expected with the doses indicated and the antimicrobial activity against susceptible bacteria for selected agents from each general class are presented in Table 96–2. The practitioner should be familiar with potential toxicities, drug interactions, and the possible effects of the antimicrobials during pregnancy when prescribing any antimicrobial agent.

β-Lactams: Penicillins and Cephalosporins

β-Lactams inhibit cell wall synthesis. The precise mechanism of action is not known, although evidence indicates the inhibition of transpeptidation. Resistance to β-lactams can be based on the production of β-lactamases by bacteria, lack of binding sites on the bacteria for the antimicrobial agent, or inability of the antimicrobial agent to pass through the outer layers of the organism to reach appropriate binding sites. Some organisms bind β-lactams and are inhibited but do not undergo autolysis and death. Such organisms are said to be "tolerant" to β-lactams.

PENICILLINS

The natural penicillins, penicillins G and V, are most active against gram-positive aerobes and anaerobes. Most strains of *Staphylococcus* require the use of a penicillinase-resistant penicillin such as nafcillin (for intravenous use) or dicloxacillin (for oral administration). Ampicillin (parenteral) and amoxicillin (oral) have the activity of the natural penicillins but are also active against some gram-negative aerobes, such as *Escherichia coli*, *Salmonella* spp., and *Shigella* spp. (amoxicillin is not effective for shigellosis). Ampicillin (usually in combination with an aminoglycoside) is the drug of choice for infections by enterococci or *Listeria monocytogenes*. When combined with a β-lactamase inhibitor such as clavulonic acid (Augmentin) or sulbactam (Unasyn), activity against β-lactamase–producing organisms is regained. Extended-activity penicillins, such as ticarcillin, mezlocillin, and piperacillin, are generally active against *Pseudomonas* spp. and other Enterobacteriaceae but have less specific activity against gram-positive organisms. In general, extended-activity penicillins should be used in combination with an aminoglycoside when used to treat *Pseudomonas* infections.

CEPHALOSPORINS

Cephalosporins are classified based on antimicrobial activity into first-, second-, and third-generation cephalosporins. Generally, first-generation cephalosporins are effective against gram-positive cocci, except enterococci and penicillinase-producing *Staphylococcal* spp., and have limited activity against gram-negative organisms, except *Escherichia coli*, *Klebsiella pneumoniae*, and *Proteus mirabilus*. The second-generation cephalosporins are somewhat more active against gram-negative organisms including *Haemophilus influenzae*. Third-generation cephalosporins are even more active than second-generation cephalosporins against gram-negative organisms but are less active against gram-positive organisms than first-generation cephalosporins.

Imipenem (Primaxin) and aztreonam (Azactam) are relatively new β-lactams with limited clinical roles at present. Imipenem has an extremely broad spectrum of activity that includes most aerobic and anaerobic bacteria, but such a broad spectrum of activity is seldom required in clinical practice. Aztreonam is a monobactam with little activity against gram-positive bacteria or anaerobes but excellent activity against Enterobacteriaceae and *Pseudomonas aeruginosa*.

Other Agents

AMINOGLYCOSIDES

Aminoglycosides inhibit the synthesis of bacterial proteins through interaction with bacterial ribosomes. Resistance occurs through bacterial production of aminoglycoside-inactivating enzymes, or because of the inability of the aminoglycoside to enter through the bacterial cell wall. Aminoglycosides can have both ototoxic and nephrotoxic effects, and therefore serum concentrations should be monitored periodically. The main use of aminoglycosides is to treat serious gram-negative infections. Aminoglycosides should be used in combination with an extended-activity penicillin when treating *Pseudomonas* infections.

TRIMETHOPRIM-SULFAMETHOXAZOLE

This combination decreases bacterial folic acid synthesis (at different steps), which inhibits bacterial growth by decreasing bacterial nucleotide production. Bacterial resistance is based on the ability to overproduce substrate or a decreased ability to bind the antimicrobial agent. The most common side effects of sulfonamides are hypersensitivity reactions, which usually cause minor rashes but may result in Stevens-Johnson syndrome. Neutropenia is associated with large doses of sulfamethoxazole, and adolescents with G6PD deficiency are at risk for aplastic anemia (see Chapter 52). Trimethoprim-sulfamethoxazole is widely used to treat urinary tract and upper respiratory tract infections and is the drug of choice for the treatment of *Pneumocystis carinii* pneumonia.

ERYTHROMYCIN AND CLINDAMYCIN

Both these antimicrobial agents inhibit RNA-dependent protein synthesis at the step of chain elongation. The most common side effect seen with erythromycin is gastrointestinal upset. This may be reduced by avoiding the use of the erythromycin base and by administering one of the erythromycin salts or esters immediately before meals. Side effects with clindamycin are uncommon, but pseudomembranous colitis caused by the toxin of *Clostridia difficile* can occur. Neither drug enters the cerebrospinal fluid in therapeutic concentrations, and current data suggest that erythromycin does not enter synovial fluid well. Erythromycin has a wide spectrum of activity and is the drug of choice for infections caused by *Mycoplasma pneumoniae*, *Legionella* spp., *Corynebacterium diphtheriae*, *Bordetella pertussis*, *Chlamydia*

trachomatis, and *Campylobacter jejuni*. The administration of erythromycin to adolescent patients receiving theophylline can result in increased serum concentrations of theophylline. Clindamycin is active against most gram-positive aerobes and most anaerobes.

CHLORAMPHENICOL

This also inhibits protein synthesis by binding to the 50S ribosomal subunit. Resistance to chloramphenicol is based on bacterial production of an acetyltransferase that inactivates chloramphenicol, or the inability of chloramphenicol to enter bacteria. Although chloramphenicol is active against a wide range of bacterial pathogens, other antimicrobial agents are usually used because of the potential toxic effects of chloramphenicol. The most common side effect of chloramphenicol is dose-related bone marrow suppression. The most feared side effect is idiopathic aplastic anemia, which is usually fatal. Chloramphenicol should no longer be used empirically for children, adolescents, or adults.

TETRACYCLINE

This bacteriostatic agent binds to the 30S ribosomal subunit, resulting in the inhibition of protein synthesis. Tetracyclines are not altered by resistant bacteria, and resistance is usually a result of interference with the energy-dependent entry of tetracycline into the cell. The two major side effects of tetracycline are permanent discoloration and hypoplasia of the enamel of developing teeth. Tetracycline can also cause skeletal growth depression *in utero* and in premature infants. Therefore, tetracycline use is avoided in children younger than 9 years old (after which dental enamel of the permanent teeth has developed) and during pregnancy. Because some foods and dairy products can interfere with the absorption of tetracycline, oral forms should be given 1 hour before or 2 hours after meals. Antacids containing aluminum, calcium, or magnesium can also interfere with the absorption of tetracycline and should be avoided.

In adolescents and adults, tetracycline is a useful antimicrobial agent. Tetracycline is the drug of choice for brucellosis, chlamydial infections, lymphogranuloma venereum, epididymitis, granuloma inguinale, Lyme disease, relapsing fever, leptospirosis, pelvic inflammatory disease, plague, prostatitis, and rickettsial infections. Tetracycline is also effective against many other infectious organisms, including *Mycoplasma pneumoniae* (see Chapters 75 and 94).

VANCOMYCIN

This inhibits cell wall synthesis. Cross resistance with other antimicrobial agents has not been observed, and resistance has not been observed to develop during therapy. The side effects of vancomycin have been greatly reduced with the production of a more highly purified preparation. The "red neck syndrome" (fever, chills, pain at the injection site, and tingling and flushing of the face, neck, and thorax) occurs if the drug is administered too rapidly. Nephrotoxicity is a concern when vancomycin and an aminoglycoside are used concurrently. Vancomycin is used primarily to treat infections caused by *Staphylococcus* spp. that are resistant to semisynthetic penicillins. The most common setting for infections with these organisms in adolescent patients is in those with tunneled central venous catheters or prosthetic cardiac valves.

METRONIDAZOLE

This is reduced to intermediate products after being taken up by bacterial cells, and these products are toxic to the cell. The most common side effect of metronidazole is gastrointestinal upset. Metronidazole can potentiate the effects of warfarin and can also cause a disulfiram (Antabuse) reaction when alcohol is consumed. The urine may develop a brown discoloration. Central nervous system dysfunction has been associated with the use of metronidazole.

Metronidazole was originally introduced for the treatment of *Trichomonas vaginalis* infections (see Chapter 75) but has become an important agent for the treatment of anaerobic infections. Metronidazole remains the drug of choice for trichomoniasis and is also effective in amebiasis, amebic abscess (liver), and giardiasis (see Chapters 75 and 95). Metronidazole is the drug of choice for bacterial vaginosis *(Gardnerella vaginalis)* (see Chapter 75) and is often used in combination with another antimicrobial agent to treat brain, pulmonary, intraabdominal, and pelvic abscesses in which the presence of anaerobic bacteria is known or suspected. However, metronidazole cannot be recommended during the first trimester of pregnancy because of possible teratogenic effects.

RIFAMPIN

This inhibits a DNA-dependent RNA polymerase that prevents chain initiation. Mutation of the polymerase to one that is resistant to rifampin occurs rapidly, and therefore rifampin is seldom used alone. Rifampin should not be used during pregnancy. Adolescents should be told that their tears, urine, and feces may turn a red-orange color. Contact lenses should not be worn, because they can be permanently stained. Rifampin induces liver enzymes and may thereby reduce the effectiveness of a wide range of drugs. Patients using oral contraceptives should be instructed to use nonhormonal methods while receiving rifampin. The most widespread use of rifampin worldwide is for the treatment of mycobacterial infections, especially tuberculo-

sis. Rifampin is also routinely used prophylactically to prevent the spread of *Neisseria meningitis* and *Haemophilus influenzae* type b. Rifampin is active against gram-positive organisms and, when used in combination with an antistaphylococcal or antistreptococcal agent, is effective in eradicating persistent upper respiratory tract carriage.

QUINOLONE DRUGS

These agents inhibit bacterial DNA replication. Side effects are usually mild. The major limitation of the use of quinolone antimicrobials in children and adolescents has been the observation of lameness and permanent cartilage damage in weight-bearing joints of immature dogs. Although nalidixic acid (the first quinolone in general use) was widely used for the chronic suppression of urinary tract infections in children, there were no reports of associated joint disease. Nevertheless, these agents are not now approved for such use. Once the rapid phase of growth during puberty has been completed, however, it should be safe to use these antimicrobial agents. Currently, two broad-spectrum quinolones are licensed for use in the United States, norfloxacin (Noroxin) and ciprofloxacin (Cipro). These agents are given orally and are active against most gramnegative aerobic bacteria as well as *Staphylococcus* spp., *Streptococcus pneumoniae*, and *Streptococcus pyogenes*.

The newer quinolones are gaining widespread use in the treatment of upper and lower respiratory, urinary tract, and skin, soft tissue, bone, and joint infections caused by susceptible gram-negative bacteria. The use of quinolones can be justified in younger adolescents who have an underlying disease such as cystic fibrosis or spina bifida, or infection with *Pseudomonas aeruginosa* (most strains of *P. cepacia* and *P. maltophilia* are not susceptible to quinolones).

BIBLIOGRAPHY

Donowitz GR, Mandell GL: Beta-lactam antibiotics. N Engl J Med 318:419, 1988.

Kaye D (ed): Antibacterial agents: Pharmacodynamics, pharmacology, new agents. Infect Dis Clin North Am 3:375, 1989.

Kucers A, Bennett N: The Use of Antibiotics, 4th ed. Philadelphia, JB Lippincott, 1987.

Mandell GL, Douglas RG, Jr, Bennett JE (eds): Principles and Practice of Infectious Diseases, 2nd ed. New York, John Wiley & Sons, 1985.

National Committee for Clinical Laboratory Standards: Performance Standards for Antimicrobial Disk Susceptibility Tests, 3rd ed., 1984.

SECTION XXII

Emergency Conditions

CHAPTER 97

Adolescent Emergency Conditions

STEPHEN LUDWIG, STEVEN M. SELBST, and JANE LAVELLE

The transition from childhood to adulthood is a time of turmoil—physically, behaviorally, psychologically, and socially. It is no wonder that a large number of medical emergencies arise. Some occur because of the disparity between adolescents' physical prowess and their lack of mature judgment. Other emergencies are the product of interpersonal or intrapersonal conflict, and others involve the seemingly random misfortunes of illness and injury that occur across the entire age spectrum. This chapter presents some common adolescent emergencies and stresses the unique aspects of their presentation, diagnosis, and treatment. We focus on five areas: resuscitation, gynecologic, neurologic, toxicologic, and behavioral emergencies.

For adolescents with any type of emergency problem, one must first develop an appreciation for the patient population.

Developmental Issues

In the emergency department (ED) or office, the physician may see a wide range of ages and developmental levels. There is nonhomogeneity even within the group we label "adolescents." It is important to direct the approach to the developmental level of the individual adolescent. This may be difficult with a crisis situation in the ED, but it is precisely then, when time is short, that it becomes critical. The developmental issues of adolescence have been stated in various terms (see Chapters 9, 10, 11, and 68). These can be summarized and include becoming independent, developing peer group relationships and, later, individual intimate relationships, developing a sexual identity, and expanding the ability to think abstractly and into the future.

Tolmas has presented the following prerequisites for a pediatrician to work successfully with adolescents: (1) knowledge of the growth and developmental tasks young people must address; (2) a personal interest in teenagers and young adults; (3) respect for teenagers' confidentiality; (4) honesty and pragmatism in all aspects of behavior and conversation; (5) avoidance of value judgments; (6) a genuine attempt to keep from projecting one's own moral code (Tolmas, 1990, pp 146–147). These principles cannot be overlooked or violated because the adolescent is being treated in an emergency situation.

Anticipating Fears

In the ED, fear is a complicating factor in all medical and behavioral conditions. Whether a simple laceration or major multiple trauma, the adolescent is fearful. Sometimes the fear is expressed, but at other times it is unspoken or covered over by nonchalance or bravado. The ED physician must recognize the fear and respond to it. What are these fears? At the heart of all of the adolescent's fears are the developmental tasks listed above. The adolescent fears being unable to meet the developmental challenges. For example, there is fear about the pain of a broken leg, but there may be more fear that this will exclude the younger adolescent from the peer group or, for the older adolescent, keep him or her from achieving academic or career goals.

Evaluating Chief Complaints

Another important issue in the approach to the adolescent is the evaluation of the chief complaint—what you hear is not always what you get. For many different reasons the adolescent may not express the true chief complaint when arriving at the ED. Thus, the ED physician needs to be flexible and imaginative to elicit the true complaint. Sometimes the issue is lack of knowledge on the part of the teen or denial of the actual chief complaint.

Issues of Confidentiality

Chapter 20 has presented this issue in detail, but it also needs to be emphasized here. The ED may be the adolescent's preferred site of care, particularly for reasons of confidentiality. Moreover, the adolescent's illness may have advanced to an emergency stage because of fear of loss of confidentiality. The ED physician must speak with the adolescent patient alone at some time. The ED physician must abide by the adolescent's request to keep information confidential, as long as the adolescent will not do harm to himself or herself or to others. This is a central issue to the successful doctor-patient relationship.

Medicolegal Issues

There are many medicolegal issues that arise in the process of delivering medical care in the ED setting. These include not only issues of consent for treatment, but also reporting of criminal activity and infectious diseases, involuntary restraint, reporting of adolescent abuse, and refusal of consent. The ED has the potential for malpractice actions. It is also the interface between the community, governmental agencies, the media, and the hospital. It is important to know the laws of the state, county, and municipality in which the physician practices. Keeping track of these issues in an ED policy and procedure manual saves time and anxiety during a crisis situation.

RESUSCITATION EMERGENCIES

Causes of Death in Adolescence

Chapter 2 presents the causes of death in adolescence. Accidents and injuries are the predominant causes of death among adolescents. Statistical reports usually use the term "injury" to reflect nonintentional or noninflicted trauma. If intentional or inflicted forms of trauma, such as suicide and homicide, were included in the category of "traumatic death," the incidence would be several times greater than all other forms combined. Of the so-called "accidental" injury types, motor vehicle injuries rank first. There are also significant numbers of adolescents who die because of drowning, or firearm injuries. Of the nontrauma-related causes of sudden death: cardiovascular disorders, seizure-related trauma, intracranial hemorrhage, and asthma are the most frequent.

In any discussion of mortality statistics, it must be noted that causes of death might not be determined accurately. The adolescent who drives his or her car off the road may be listed as suffering a nonintentional injury, when in fact, the act was suicidal. In an inner city setting, motor vehicle deaths may be insignificant when compared with the incidence of homicide or fire deaths. Over the long term, it may be noted that the death rates from disease have fallen over the past 20 years. Death rates from injury have remained constant or, in some categories such as suicide and homicide, have increased (see Chapter 2).

Beyond mortality statistics, ED visits by adolescents and the reported diagnoses may be examined. One study indicated that nonfatal visits for inflicted traumatic injury parallel those resulting in homicide.

Pattern of Resuscitation

Resuscitation procedures for a traumatic or medical arrest follow a pattern; all emergency care differs from nonemergency care in this structured way. Figure 97–1 shows the pattern that requires assessment of the physiologic status, followed by immediate correction of physiologic abnormalities. After treatment, reassessment en-

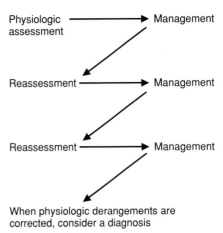

Figure 97–1. Pattern of emergency care.

sures that the therapeutic intervention has worked. This is followed by more treatment and further reassessment. Throughout this process there may be no directed attempt at establishing a specific diagnosis. Rather, efforts are aimed at the immediate correction of altered physiologic states.

Resuscitation Techniques for Trauma

Because trauma is the predominant cause of adolescent mortality, it requires primary consideration. Physicians trained in traditional medical specialties, such as pediatrics, internal medicine, or family medicine, might immediately search for their surgical colleague. Emergency medicine has taught us that there is a role for every physician in the care of the adolescent who has sustained trauma. Although the surgeon is ultimately in charge, and must make the decision of whether an adolescent requires surgery, other physicians can be involved. Indeed, if the morbidity and mortality of trauma are to be reduced, all physicians must be trained in basic resuscitative techniques. The most well-organized system for learning these procedures is the Advanced Trauma Life Support (ATLS) Course given by the American College of Surgeons. Figure 97–2 identifies the basic phases in the ATLS approach.

PRIMARY SURVEY

The primary survey is the first step in the assessment process. It includes checking the airway and maintenance of cervical spine control. The airway should be open and, if closed, should be opened with a chin lift or jaw thrust maneuver, or simply by removing debris from the airway. While doing this, the cervical spine must be held in a neutral position to avoid cervical cord injury. It should be assumed that any adolescent with injury above the clavicle may have cervical spine injury.

The second step in the primary survey is to expose the chest and assess ventilatory exchange. If ventilation does not seem to be occurring, artificial breathing support with supplemental oxygen must be given. The three

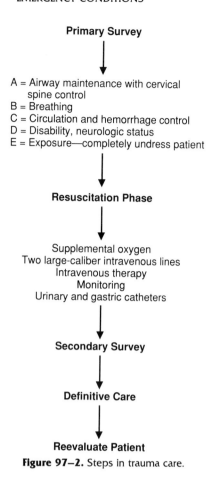

Primary Survey

A = Airway maintenance with cervical
      spine control
B = Breathing
C = Circulation and hemorrhage control
D = Disability, neurologic status
E = Exposure—completely undress patient

Resuscitation Phase

Supplemental oxygen
Two large-caliber intravenous lines
Intravenous therapy
Monitoring
Urinary and gastric catheters

Secondary Survey

Definitive Care

Reevaluate Patient

Figure 97–2. Steps in trauma care.

most common traumatic impedances to ventilation are tension pneumothorax, open pneumothorax, and flail chest with pulmonary contusion.

The third step is to assess circulation. This is done by evaluating the pulse, skin color, and capillary refill. There should also be a rapid survey for active points of blood loss that must be controlled.

The next step is a brief neurologic evaluation, using the pneumonic device AVPU. This reminds the examiner to check for A (alertness), V (responds to voice), P (responds to pain), and U (unresponsive).

The final step of the primary survey is to expose the adolescent adequately to ensure a thorough physical examination and assessment, looking for evidence of trauma or injury that may not have been thoroughly appreciated on initial evaluation.

LIFE SUPPORT

In the second phase of trauma resuscitation, the goal is life support or resuscitation. During this phase, further measures are instituted to support vital function. These include the institution of oxygen therapy, the establishment of two large-caliber intravenous lines, and the treatment of shock. Also important in this phase is the placement of cardiorespiratory monitors and urinary and gastric tubes. At this point, the adolescent's life support should be under control, and the physician is ready to continue to the next phase.

SECONDARY SURVEY

The secondary survey conducted by the physician is a head-to-toe survey, looking for additional injuries (Table 97–1).

STABILIZATION, TRANSPORT, AND DEFINITIVE CARE

The final phase includes providing definitive care on site or preparing the adolescent patient for transfer to another hospital unit or to a facility that can deliver a higher level of care. Table 97–2 lists the provisions that must be made for transfer or transport.

Resuscitation Techniques for Medical Arrests

When an adolescent arrests from a nontraumatic cause, the guidelines that should be used are those developed by the American Heart Association and presented in the Advanced Cardiac Life Support (ACLS) Course. Although this course was originally designed for the adult victim of myocardial infarction, its principles may be applied to adolescents in arrest. Figure 97–3 shows the basic steps of ACLS.

AIRWAY

The airway should be assessed and managed in an organized fashion. This starts with the basic life support skill of assessing the airway by proper positioning of the head and neck and looking, listening, and feeling air

TABLE 97–1. Injuries Identified by Careful Secondary Survey for Trauma

REGION OF THE BODY	POSSIBLE FINDINGS
Head	Pupillary reaction; signs of increased intracranial pressure
	Funduscopic examination for hemorrhage
	Examination for specific eye trauma
Maxillofacial	Cribriform plate fractures
	Cerebrospinal fluid leak
Cervical spine and neck	Recheck for cervical spine trauma
	Penetrating trauma
Chest	Sucking chest injury
	Flail chest
	Pneumothorax or hemothorax
	Pulmonary contusion
	Cardiac tamponade
Abdomen	Intraabdominal hemorrhage
	Fractures of lower rib cage
	Fractures of pelvic region
Rectum	Blood in bowel
	Displaced prostate
	Loss of sphincter tone
Extremities	Deformity, crepitance
	Neurovascular impairment
Nervous system	Glasgow coma scale
	Areas of paralysis or paresis

Adapted with permission from American College of Surgeons, Committee on Trauma: Advanced Trauma Life Support. Chicago, American College of Surgeons, 1989.

TABLE 97–2. Provisions for Transportation of Emergency Adolescent Patient

Determine need for patient transfer
Referring physician contacts receiving physician
    Identification of patient
    History of injury
    Initial findings
    Treatment and response
Receiving physician determines need for additional care and specifics
    of transfer
Transfer equipment must include
    Airway equipment
    Volume expansion fluids/blood
    Full set of resuscitation equipment/medications
Documentation must include
    Full records of referring hospital including fluid flow sheets and
      medication records
    Radiographs and laboratory studies
    Name and phone number of referring physician
    Name and phone number of receiving physician
Permission from patient and/or family documented in writing
Transfer flow sheet to monitor vital signs and treatments en route

Adapted with permission from American College of Surgeons, Committee on Trauma: Advanced Trauma Life Support. Chicago, American College of Surgeons, 1989.

movement through the airway. If the airway is not open, the rescuer must use the head tilt, chin lift, and jaw thrust maneuvers, or go through an obstructed airway sequence (Heimlich maneuver). Once the airway is open, ACLS recommends the use of mechanical devices to maintain open airway position. These include oropharyngeal and nasopharyngeal airways and translaryngeal artificial airways placed by orotracheal or nasotracheal intubation.

BREATHING

Once the airway is open, the next step in resuscitation is breathing. This again requires that a rapid assessment be made by looking at the chest wall rise and fall and noting respiratory rate, effort, and color. If the assessment shows that the adolescent needs assistance with oxygenation alone, then oxygen is given through supplementation to the self-breather. This is done with an oxygen mask or nasal prongs; when ventilation is also inadequate, oxygen must be given in conjunction with ventilatory support by means of a bag-mask device or anesthesia bag. Once any intervention is made, there is reassessment to ensure that the physiologic impairment has been corrected.

CIRCULATION

The next step is assessment of the adequacy of circulation. This is done by checking the pulses, pulse strength, color, and capillary refill. A decrease in measured blood pressure is a late sign of circulatory insufficiency. If circulation is inadequate, external cardiac compression should be immediately initiated. ACLS recommends the placement of an intravenous line, because more advanced procedures require the administration of fluids and drugs. Table 97–3 lists common drugs for resuscitation and their recommended dosages for adolescents. Once a cardiac rhythm has been initi-

ated, its pattern must be monitored on the ECG. Dysrhythmias are rare in children but may be seen in adolescents who have chronic heart disease or a toxicologic emergency affecting the heart. There is a discussion of dysrhythmias in Chapter 46.

STABILIZATION

In the stabilization phase, the focus is on the correction of acid-base balance, the placement of more invasive but important monitoring equipment, the definition and treatment of the underlying cause for the arrest (e.g., toxin, asthma, heart disease), and preparation of the adolescent for transfer to an intensive care unit or to a facility that can provide a higher level of care.

Helping the Family

Any resuscitative effort is accompanied by the responsibility of supporting the family. This is true for the successful resuscitation, as well as when death is the outcome. Often, adolescents are seen as having been in their "prime" prior to a sudden event. Even for those adolescents with a chronic fatal disease, the patient had lived long enough so that relationships had been established and the loss not fully anticipated. All parents experience guilt about their adolescent's illness or death. All parents want to know that their child did not suffer or feel pain, and that they and the medical staff did all that could be done. All parents need time and privacy to ventilate their feelings, and someone to listen to them and share their grief.

GYNECOLOGIC EMERGENCIES

Adolescents are maturing earlier and engaging in sexual activity at a younger age (see Chapter 5). Chapter 2 presents data on sexual activity and pregnancy, and Chapter 75 discusses gynecologic infections and sexually transmitted diseases (STDs). This section focuses on common gynecologic problems that bring adolescents to the emergency department, first considering more serious conditions and then those that cause the adolescent discomfort.

History and Physical Examination

The adolescent female with gynecologic disease often presents with symptoms that are nonspecific or not immediately referable to the reproductive tract. Conversely, she might present with gynecologic symptoms such as abdominal pain, which are eventually attributed to nongynecologic disease involving the gastrointestinal, genitourinary, or pulmonary systems. These adolescents are challenging to evaluate, and require a thorough history and physical examination.

HISTORY

Important data include the adolescent's age, sequence of presenting complaints, duration, characteris-

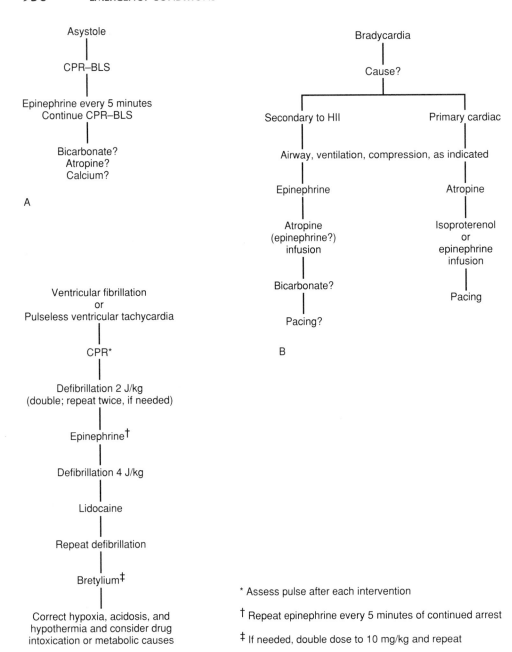

Figure 97–3. Algorithms for advanced life support. *A*, Asystole. *B*, Bradycardia. *C*, Ventricular fibrillation or pulseless ventricular tachycardia. CPR, cardiopulmonary resuscitation; BLS, basic life support; HII, hypoxic-ischemic insult. (With permission from American Heart Association: Textbook of Pediatric Advanced Life Support. Dallas, American Heart Association, 1990, Appendix D, pp 113–115. Copyright American Heart Association.)

tics and location of pain, and presence of associated symptoms, such as fever, nausea, vomiting, vaginal discharge, or bleeding. The age at menarche, cycle length and regularity, duration of menses, and associated pain or heavy bleeding always must be considered in the sexually mature female with abdominal pain. Whether the adolescent has ever been pregnant, has had abdominal surgery, or has had a recent abortion can be extremely important in determining the cause of pain. A complete sexual history, including contraceptive method, last sexual exposure, number of partners in the preceding 6 months, previous gonorrhea or pelvic inflammatory disease (PID), previous STD, and any symptoms in the partner, helps identify the patient at risk for STD, PID, or pregnancy and its complications.

PHYSICAL EXAMINATION

A pelvic examination is indicated for all sexually active adolescent females who present in the emergency department with abdominal pain, vaginal discharge or bleeding, dysuria, hepatitis, or STD exposure (see Chapter 69). Often, the adolescent may be having her first pelvic examination in the chaotic surroundings of a busy emergency department. One third have anxiety levels comparable to those of patients prior to surgery. Thus, a period of discussion should precede the examination, during which the procedure can be explained and individual preferences elicited. The younger the adolescent, the more likely she prefers having a family member present, but this is her option. The examination can be performed in the semisitting position with a mirror to

TABLE 97–3. Resuscitation Drugs

DRUG	CONCENTRATION	ROUTE	DOSE	FINAL DOSE*	NOTES
Epinephrine (1:10,000)	0.1 mg/ml	IV, ET, IO	0.01 mg/kg	0.1 ml/kg	Maximum standard dose = 1 mg (10 ml) May repeat every 5 minutes If no response, use 10× the dose (0.1 mg/kg) by using epinephrine 1:1000 at 0.1 ml/kg. If ET route, use 2–3× the dose (min = 1.0 ml)
Sodium bicarbonate (8.4%)	1.0 mEq/ml	IV, IO	0.5–1.0 mEq/kg	0.5–1.0 ml/kg	Use once in prolonged (> 10 min) arrest; then per arterial blood gas, or 0.5 mEq/kg every 10 minutes if blood gas measurements are not available
Atropine	0.1 mg/ml	IV, ET, IO, IM	0.02 mg/kg	0.2 ml/kg	Minimum dose (children) = 0.1 mg Minimum dose (adolescents) = 0.5 mg May repeat once in 5 minutes Maximum total dose (adolescents) = 2 mg
Lidocaine	10 mg/ml (1%) or 20 mg/ml (2%)	IV, IO, ET	1 mg/kg	Concentration dependent	Initial dose = 1 mg/kg Subsequent doses q 8–10 min = 0.5 mg/kg Maximum total dose = 3 mg/kg Toxicity can cause seizures, myocardial dysfunction
Naloxone hydrochloride	0.4 mg/ml, 1.0 mg/ml	IV, IO, ET, IM	0.01–0.1 mg/kg	Concentration dependent	Indications: suspected narcotic overdose Higher dose range preferred Usual initial adult dose = 2 mg May repeat q 3 minutes to maximum 10 mg
Dopamine drip	40 mg/ml or 80 mg/ml	IV, IO	2–20 μg/kg/min		For poor perfusion post cardiac arrest Dopaminergic, beta and alpha effects Do *not* mix with NaHCO₃
Dobutamine drip	250 mg/20 ml/vial	IV, IO	5–20 μg/kg/min		Minimal alpha effects; useful for poor perfusion post cardiac arrest
Epinephrine drip (1:1000)	1 mg/ml	IV, IO	0.1–1.0 μg/kg/min		For hypotension post cardiac arrest
Lidocaine drip	40 mg/ml (4%)	IV, IO	20–50 μg/kg/min		Use continuous infusion only after circulatory function established

ET, endotracheal; IM, intramuscular; IO, intraosseous; IV, intravenous.
*Final dose may vary since these drugs may come in several concentrations.
Adapted from the American Heart Association: Textbook of Advanced Cardiac Life Support. Dallas, American Heart Association, 1987; and Pediatric Emergency Information Poster: Department of Pediatrics, Rochester General Hospital and the Department of Pediatrics, University of Rochester, Strong Memorial Hospital Medical Center (EMSC/DHHS-MCH).

allow for a more active adolescent-physician relationship and to facilitate teaching the adolescent. The examination should include inspection of the external genitalia for skin lesions, clitoral size, and sexual maturity rating (SMR). This is followed by speculum examination using the Huffman (0.5 × 4.5-inch) or Pederson (1 × 4.5-inch) speculum. The adolescent will feel less discomfort during the speculum examination if the speculum is warmed first (e.g., by the physician warming it up in warm water). The cervical os normally appears red because of the ectropion or cervical columnar epithelium prominent in the adolescent female. Appropriate swabs should be taken for *Neisseria gonorrheae, Chlamydia trachomatis*, and vaginal bacterial culture in addition to a wet mount and potassium hydroxide preparation. Papanicolaou (Pap) smears are not routinely taken in the emergency department, although in the future this may be the place to screen this particular population. A rectal examination should be performed for masses, tenderness, or the presence of blood (see Chapters 69 and 75).

The information obtained by a thorough history and physical examination should allow the experienced physician to formulate a complete but directed differential diagnosis for the adolescent being evaluated. The remainder of this section discusses the diagnosis and treatment of gynecologic diseases in adolescent females. Both life-threatening and non–life-threatening diseases are discussed; fortunately, most are in the latter category. Those diseases that are immediately life-threatening should be considered and acted on appropriately.

The most common serious disease diagnosed in these adolescent patients is pelvic inflammatory disease. PID presents with a broad spectrum of clinical manifestations, some of which can mimic those of surgical emergencies. Table 97–4 summarizes the results of laparoscopy on patients with the clinical diagnosis of PID. Diseases masquerading as PID include ectopic pregnancy, ovarian torsion and cyst rupture, appendicitis, and endometriosis (see Chapter 70). Thus, many of those diagnosed with PID require surgical or gynecologic consultation.

Specific Gynecologic Emergencies

ECTOPIC PREGNANCY

The triad of pelvic pain, abnormal vaginal bleeding, and amenorrhea are considered pathognomonic for the

TABLE 97–4. Laparoscopic Observations in Patients with a Clinical Diagnosis of PID

DIAGNOSIS	STUDY 1	STUDY 2	STUDY 3	TOTAL NO. (%)
Salpingitis	532	103	25	661 (62)
Normal	184	51	0	235 (22)
Ovarian cyst	12	39	0	51 (5)
Ectopic pregnancy	11	27	1	39 (4)
Appendicitis	24	2	1	27 (3)
Endometriosis	16	1	1	37 (3)

With permission from Eschenbach D: Epidemiology and diagnosis of acute pelvic inflammatory disease. Obstet Gynecol 55 (Suppl):142S–152S, 1980.

diagnosis of ectopic pregnancy, but not all adolescent patients have a clear presentation. Ectopic pregnancy is the second most common cause of maternal death in the United States and is largely preventable with prompt diagnosis and treatment. There is usually a history of abnormal bleeding in the preceding 3 months and symptoms of the physiologic changes of pregnancy. Often, these adolescents have made previous visits to a physician for similar symptoms of unclear cause. In the adolescent patient with signs and symptoms of intravascular depletion, acute resuscitation should include continuous monitoring of the heart and blood pressure and the administration of oxygen and crystalloid intravenous fluids. Rarely, military antishock trousers (MAST) may be necessary to maintain blood pressure while the operating team is being mobilized.

In the stable adolescent in whom ectopic pregnancy is a possibility, blood should be drawn for a complete blood count, type, and cross, and for a qualitative and quantitative beta-human chorionic gonadatropin (β-HCG) measurement while arranging for a pelvic ultrasound examination. The abdominal and vaginal examinations indicate exquisite tenderness and may reveal uterine enlargement. Only 20% of adolescent patients have an appreciable mass. Anemia out of proportion to the history of bleeding helps substantiate the diagnosis, but may not reflect an acute hemorrhage. Because ectopic pregnancy may present with an HCG level as low as 10 mIU/ml, the laboratory should provide for a serum radioimmunoassay (RIA) β-specific HCG assay. Enzyme-linked immunosorbent assay (ELISA) methods have sensitivity ranges from 90% to 96% and are easily and quickly done (see Chapter 69). An emergency gynecology consultation should be sought to evaluate the need for culdocentesis or laparoscopy.

OVARIAN TORSION

Ovarian torsion may occur with a corpus luteal cyst, ovarian cyst, dermoid cyst, diseased adnexa, or tumor (see Chapter 71). The onset of pain is acute and severe, usually unilateral and discrete, and is often associated with simultaneous and persistent nausea and vomiting. There may be a previous history of ovarian cyst but usually no history of amenorrhea or abnormal vaginal bleeding, which helps distinguish this from ectopic pregnancy. The physical examination reveals cervical motion tenderness, adnexal tenderness, and a mass. The sever-

ity of pain may range from mild tenderness to a diffusely tender and rigid abdomen but is usually less severe than the pain associated with an ectopic pregnancy. If this diagnosis is suspected, an emergency gynecologic or surgical consultation must be obtained. Time is of the essence for the preservation of normal tube and ovarian function.

OVARIAN CYST

Ovarian cysts usually include follicular and corpus luteal cysts in addition to endometriomas and tumors (see Chapter 71). They are asymptomatic, unless complicated by rupture or torsion. The relationship of the occurrence of pain to the timing of the menstrual cycle is of utmost importance. The pain is often described as gradual and steady. Many adolescents report previous episodes of recurrent pain associated with ovulation, facilitating the diagnosis of a more severe attack. This is an unlikely diagnosis for the adolescent taking oral contraceptives on a regular basis. Mittelschmerz is the normal release of the follicular cyst at ovulation, resulting in brief, unilateral, sharp adnexal pain, and perhaps a small amount of bleeding due to estrogen withdrawal. Corpus luteal cyst rupture presents in the same way but occurs prior to menses. Physical examination reveals tenderness in the iliac fossa, but peritoneal signs are usually lacking. Pelvic examination reveals unilateral tenderness and perhaps fullness. Cyst rupture may be complicated by ovarian hemorrhage, which results in severe unilateral pain or peritoneal signs, depending on whether the hemorrhage is intraovarian or extraovarian. Rupture of endometriomas results in severe, bilateral, lower abdominal pain caused by hemoperitoneum. Adolescent patients who have symptoms that are inconsistent with simple cyst rupture or those who have suspected adnexal mass need immediate gynecologic evaluation.

ENDOMETRIOSIS

Ectopic endometrial tissue, or endometriosis, is probably the most common cause of chronic pelvic pain in older adolescents. These adolescents complain typically of dull, aching premenstrual pain, followed by severe cramping and associated dysuria, dyspareunia, rectal pressure, or tenesmus, depending on where the ectopic tissue is located. These adolescents should be referred to the adolescent medicine physician or gynecologist to be evaluated for the need for laparoscopy and/or hormonal suppressive therapy.

PELVIC INFLAMMATORY DISEASE

Pelvic inflammatory disease (PID) is an ascending, spontaneously occurring infection of the uterus and tubes in sexually mature females (see Chapter 75). Studies using laparoscopy and transvaginal culdocentesis have established the polymicrobial nature of the disease. Adolescents have a greater cervical ectopia of columnar epithelium, which may allow for increased infection by *Chlamydia trachomatis*. In addition, the local immune status remains unchallenged.

PID presents with a broad spectrum of clinical manifestations, making accurate diagnosis a challenge. Classic symptoms include the triad of lower abdominal pain of usually less than 1-week duration, abnormal vaginal discharge or bleeding, and fever. However, the adolescent's symptoms are often nonspecific, making it difficult to differentiate among gastrointestinal, urinary tract, and reproductive tract pathology (see Chapters 61–66, 70, and 71). Symptom frequency in acute PID has been studied. The presence of fever was the only significant finding, and the classic triad identified only 20% of those who had laparoscopy-proven PID.

A thorough pelvic examination is crucial in making the diagnosis, because this helps distinguish reproductive disease from gastrointestinal or urinary tract disease. Adolescents who have pelvic peritonitis often have anorexia, nausea, and vomiting, and usually fever. Physical examination generally reveals exquisite tenderness in both iliac fossae and suprapubic tenderness. Pelvic examination reveals vaginal discharge and perhaps an inflamed cervix, cervical motion tenderness, and adnexal tenderness or fullness. Cervical motion tenderness is a nonspecific finding as stretching of the broad and utero-sacral ligaments causes pain in any condition resulting in pelvic peritonitis. Criteria have been suggested in an attempt to identify that subset of adolescent patients with true salpingitis. Although it has not been proven that intravenous antibiotic therapy reduces the short-term and long-term sequelae of PID, or that hospitalization reduces future risk of recurrent disease, it seems prudent that the adolescent female be hospitalized for therapy and education if this diagnosis is strongly suspected (see Chapter 75).

Laboratory tests can help substantiate the physician's clinical diagnosis of PID. A white blood cell count greater than or equal to 10,500/mm³ is found in one third to one half of adolescents with PID, and two thirds of adolescents have a sedimentation rate greater than 15 mm/hour. Those adolescents with a sedimentation rate greater than 60 mm/hour are more likely to have an associated abscess. A cervical Gram stain positive for intracellular gram-negative diplococci and white blood cells helps confirm the diagnosis in one third of adolescents with PID. Chlamydial culture (not the rapid test) remains the standard for the diagnosis of chlamydial infection (see Chapter 69). Gonorrheal cultures should be obtained with cotton-tipped swabs, and Thayer-Martin and chocolate agar plates should be inoculated immediately. Obtaining urethral and rectal swabs for gonorrhea culture may increase the sensitivity of these tests. All adolescents should have pregnancy, wet mount, and rapid plasma reagin (RPR) tests done. Other laboratory tests include Tzanck preparations and herpes simplex virus rapid slide determination. Specific serology or HIV testing should be done on an individual basis.

Pelvic and perhaps vaginal probe ultrasonography may be a useful adjunctive tool in evaluating the adolescent female, especially for pelvic disease. The usefulness of ultrasound has been studied, and adnexal fullness was more commonly found in those fulfilling the clinical criteria for the diagnosis of PID. The presence of an abscess that was not suspected on physical examination was also frequently identified.

Therapy is directed at eradicating infection and preventing sequelae. Treating the most common pathogens requires a minimum of two drugs. Treatment suggestions are presented in Chapter 75. Additional instructions include fluids, bed rest, pelvic rest (i.e., no sexual activity), and follow-up at 48 to 72 hours to ensure improvement in clinical symptoms. It is recommended that all sexual partners within the preceding 2 months be evaluated and treated. The decision to admit the adolescent for intravenous therapy is made on the basis of uncertain diagnosis, fever, peritoneal signs, age, pregnancy, suspected noncompliance, suspected abscess, uncertain follow-up, and failed outpatient therapy.

COMPLICATIONS OF PELVIC INFLAMMATORY DISEASE (see Chapter 75)

Adolescent patients who have Fitz-Hugh–Curtis syndrome most often complain of right upper quadrant pain. However, pleuritic and shoulder pain resulting from diaphragmatic irritation secondary to perihepatitis might confuse the physician as to the true underlying cause. Usually these adolescents have silent or minimal pelvic disease. Any of the pathogens of typical PID can cause this disease and, therefore, the same therapy is instituted. Laboratory studies are notable for minimal elevation of liver enzyme levels, distinguishing this from infectious hepatitis (see Chapter 62).

Tubo-ovarian abscess occurs in 10% to 15% of adolescents with PID. Rupture of these abscesses occurs in approximately 5% to 15% of adolescent patients, and represents a true surgical emergency.

Disseminated gonorrhea typically presents as a polyarticular migratory arthritis of small and medium joints (see Chapter 90). Often, one joint is more obviously involved, and has swelling, warmth, and decreased range of motion. The pain of this arthritis seems less exquisite than that of other infectious arthritides. Joint fluid examination reveals an elevated white blood cell count, greater than 50,000/mm³, with a polymorphonuclear predominance, a low glucose level, and culture and Gram stain may or may not be positive. These adolescents may have the typical rash of gonorrhea characterized by small vesicles filled with purulent fluid on the distal surfaces of the extremities. The organism can usually be isolated from these vesicles. The adolescent presenting with symptoms of disseminated gonorrhea should be admitted for intravenous therapy.

Sequelae occur in 25% of adolescents with PID; these include involuntary infertility, increased risk for ectopic pregnancy, chronic pelvic pain, and abdominal adhesions predisposing to bowel obstruction. The risk of these sequelae in adolescents reinforces the need for accurate diagnosis and correct treatment, follow-up, and education.

TOXIC SHOCK SYNDROME

Toxic shock syndrome is a serious infection, occurring predominantly in young menstruating women using tampons, with one third of cases occurring in those 15 to 19 years of age (see Chapter 94). It also can occur in nonmenstruating females and in males. It is a toxin-mediated disease caused by *Staphylococcus aureus* that affects multiple organ systems. The adolescent presents typically with fever, pharyngitis, myalgia, vomiting, diarrhea, and abdominal pain on the third or fourth day of the menstrual cycle. There is a diffuse, macular, erythematous rash or erythroderma that develops over the first 2 days of illness. The conjunctival, oropharyngeal, and vaginal mucosa appear hyperemic. The adolescent patient may exhibit diffuse soreness of the skin and/or muscles on palpation.

The pelvic examination is normal, except perhaps for the presence of an abnormal vaginal discharge. Hypotension develops within 72 hours of the onset of illness. Laboratory studies reveal a leukocytosis and multisystem organ disease evidenced by renal and hepatic abnormalities. The criteria for diagnosing this illness are presented in Chapter 94. Cultures taken from the cervix and vaginal pool grow *S. aureus* in most affected adolescents. The diagnosis is based on the history and clinical findings, and is substantiated by laboratory abnormalities and vaginal culture yielding *S. aureus*. Treatment consists of a penicillinase-resistant penicillin or a β-lactamase resistant antimicrobial and local irrigation of the vagina if there is copious discharge or a foul-smelling tampon was removed. These adolescent patients may require large volumes of fluid in addition to vasopressor support to maintain adequate blood pressure. Admission to the intensive care unit for monitoring and support of vital functions may be necessary in the initial days of illness.

The differential diagnosis includes scarlet fever, meningococcemia, fulminant viral or bacterial sepsis, Rocky Mountain spotted fever, severe toxin-induced diarrhea, leptospirosis, and Kawasaki syndrome (see Chapter 93). Most adolescent patients recover within 2 weeks. The mortality rate varies widely and there is a small risk of recurrence.

Adolescents may also present to the emergency department with other illnesses, although not as serious as the preceding diseases, that may cause discomfort or concern. These include vaginal discharge, genital lesions, and menstrual disorders.

ACUTE VAGINITIS AND MUCOPURULENT CERVICITIS

The most common complaints in this group of adolescents include an increased malodorous vaginal discharge, perhaps associated with pruritus, burning, dysuria, and abnormal bleeding (see Chapter 75). Although these are not life-threatening conditions, they may herald an underlying STD and may cause the adolescent a considerable amount of discomfort.

The diagnosis of mucopurulent cervicitis is made when pelvic examination reveals mucopurulent discharge and an inflamed, friable cervix. The cause is the same as that of PID and therefore these adolescents should receive the same therapy. Cervical Gram stain usually reveals many white blood cells but appropriate cultures should be obtained, follow-up established, and treatment of the sexual partner accomplished.

The most common cause of vaginitis is probably *Candida albicans*. This infection manifests with severe pruritus and burning. Physical examination reveals vulvar inflammation and edema and a white, cottage cheese–like discharge, with patches seen along the vaginal walls. Predisposing factors include obesity, oral contraceptive use, antibiotic use, diabetes mellitus, pregnancy, immune deficiency, and poor hygiene. A saline mount with 10% to 20% potassium hydroxide (KOH) used to lyse cellular elements to make the hyphae more visible confirms the diagnosis. Any symptomatic adolescent patient with a positive KOH preparation should be treated with a miconazole vaginal suppository (200 mg once daily for 3 days, or 100 mg once daily for 7 days) or with clotrimazole (200 mg once daily for 3 days or 100 mg once daily for 7 days). In addition, sitz baths with baking soda and hydrocortisone may relieve severe symptoms.

Trichomonas vaginalis is often a multifocal infection involving the vagina, urethra, bladder, and Skene glands. It is one of the most frequently acquired STDs and is often found coexistent with other infections. Examination reveals a frothy, green-gray discharge, with a granular appearance to the vaginal walls and punctate cervical hemorrhages, accounting for the "strawberry cervix." A saline wet mount reveals pear-shaped, motile protozoa with three to five flagella. Metronidazole given as a single 2-g dose or as a 7-day regimen (250 mg three times daily) is the appropriate treatment. This drug has many side effects, including a disulfiram-like effect, so adolescents should be cautioned to avoid alcohol when taking this medication.

The coccobacillus *Gardnerella vaginalis*, along with other anaerobes, causes a vaginitis that results in a thin, gray discharge with a particularly offensive fishy odor. Physical examination is normal, except for the thin, malodorous discharge. The diagnosis is supported by a vaginal pH greater than or equal to 4.5, enhancement of the fishy odor after 10% KOH addition, and the presence of clue cells on Gram stain. The latter represent epithelial cells to which the coccobacilli have become adherent. Metronidazole (500 mg twice daily for 7 days, or a 2-g single dose) is the treatment of choice, and clindamycin may be used as an alternative. Treatment of the male sexual partner is not indicated.

GENITAL LESIONS

Genital herpes simplex is the most common cause of genital ulcerative lesions. Primary infections usually present with multiple, painful, and papular lesions, which become vesicular or ulcerative, or both, and are associated with mild lymphadenopathy. This primary disease is generally of longer duration than recurrent episodes and is often associated with systemic symptoms, including fever, malaise, and abdominal pain. Recurrent or secondary herpes is less severe and is not accompanied by systemic symptoms. These lesions typically clear in 10 to 21 days. Complications include urethral, vaginal, and perianal extension, urinary retention, and bacterial superinfection. The diagnosis is substantiated by Tzanck preparation in about 50% of cases but should be confirmed by viral culture, especially if therapy is undertaken.

Treatment of genital herpes with topical acyclovir has been shown to reduce the duration and severity of local symptoms and to decrease the duration of viral shedding. Five percent ointment should be applied to all lesions four to six times daily for 7 days. At present, topical therapy is not indicated for recurrent episodes. Oral acyclovir (200 mg, five times daily, for 10 days) may reduce symptoms and shedding even more effectively than topical acyclovir, but does not alter the subsequent risk for or severity of recurrence. Patients with severe disease may benefit from intravenous acyclovir. Other therapies include oral analgesics and cold, wet compresses with 1:40 Burow solution. Adolescents who have a history of severe, painful recurrences should be referred to a dermatologist or gynecologist for chronic suppressive therapy with acyclovir, 400 mg, twice daily, for 6 months to 1 year.

Syphilis presents with various genital lesions, including the painless ulcer or chancre, with adjacent lymphadenopathy of primary syphilis, or the silvery plaques or condylomata lata of secondary syphilis. Other manifestations include fever, generalized lymphadenopathy, maculopapular rash, and pharyngitis. Diagnosis is made by dark field microscopy of material from scraped lesions along with serologic testing, including nontreponemal and treponemal antibody testing. The only proven therapy for the eradication of syphilis is benzathine penicillin G, 50,000 U/kg, not to exceed 2.4 million U, given as an intramuscular injection, with repeat serologic testing at 3, 6, and 12 months. In adolescents with latent syphilis (syphilis of more than 1 year's duration), treatment is given weekly for 3 consecutive weeks with serologic follow-up for 2 years following treatment. In patients with suspected neurosyphilis, CSF evaluation with VDRL is mandatory and intravenous therapy with aqueous penicillin G (for 2 weeks) is recommended.

Chancroid, or *Haemophilus ducreyi* infection, results in painful, shallow ulcers, usually on the labia minora, but sometimes on the vulva, vaginal mucosa, or cervix. These lesions may coalesce to form an eroded area covered with a purulent exudate. There may be associated suppurative inguinal adenitis or bubo formation. Diagnosis is confirmed by laboratory culture and by smears that reveal gram-negative bacilli in a linear arrangement. The adolescent should be evaluated for syphilis, because the two infections may coexist. The currently recommended treatment is erythromycin (500 mg, four times daily, for 7 days) or single-dose ceftriaxone (250 mg). Sexual partners in the preceding 10 days of symptom onset should be evaluated and treated.

Granuloma inguinale is a rare STD caused by *Calymmatobacterium granulomatis*. The initial lesions appear as small, red, painless nodules that progress to ulcerations and eventually extend from the urethra to the rectum, interfering with urination, defecation, and sexual intercourse. Diagnosis is confirmed by tissue biopsy, which reveals characteristic Donovan bodies. Doxycycline (100 mg, twice daily, for 21 days) is the treatment of choice, with chloramphenicol or aminoglycoside as an alternative.

Lymphogranuloma venereum is an infection caused by *Chlamydia trachomatis*, usually presenting with unilateral, painful, inguinal adenopathy. The initial, small,

vulvar lesions often go undetected. Extensive tissue destruction and inguinal abscess formation occur if treatment is not initiated. Doxycycline (100 mg, twice daily, for 21 days) is the treatment of choice.

Molluscum contagiosum is an asymptomatic, probably viral disease that causes discrete, pink-gray unbilicated papules on the perineum and thighs. Adolescents should be referred to the dermatologist for cryotherapy.

Condyloma acuminatum presents with velvety, wart-like growths on the vulva associated with vaginal discharge and pruritus. Podophyllin (25%) may be applied to lesions smaller than 1 cm in diameter for a 4- to 6-hour period. Trichloroacetic acid, 25% to 85%, may be used in place of podophyllin, followed by cool normal saline or aloe vera gel. This solution may offer the advantage of causing less burning to the patient. All patients with warts should be referred for Pap smear and follow-up therapy.

Other disorders, including pediculosis, scabies, bartholinitis, skenitis, tumor, pemphigus, Lipschutz ulcer, Crohn disease, Stevens-Johnson syndrome, Behçet syndrome, amebiasis, staphylococcal infections, and tuberculosis, can produce vaginal ulcerations. These need to be considered in the unusual adolescent with ulcerative vaginal lesions.

COMMON MENSTRUAL DISORDERS

Menstrual disorders are common in young adolescents (see Chapter 70). Primary dysmenorrhea occurs in 70% of adolescents, and approximately 5% to 10% have dysfunctional uterine bleeding. The emergency physician needs to distinguish these two common problems from other conditions associated with abnormal or painful vaginal bleeding, such as spontaneous or septic abortion, ectopic pregnancy, abruptio placentae, placenta previa, ovarian cyst, PID, congenital uterine malformations, tumor, and bleeding disorders.

A complete menstrual history should be taken in these adolescents, including age of menarche, details of cycle interval, quantity of menstrual flow, duration, character, severity and onset of pain, and sexual history.

Dysmenorrhea or painful menstrual bleeding is most commonly primary without an underlying pathologic process, but can be secondarily associated with underlying disorders such as endometriosis, tumor, adenomyosis, fibroids, polyps, ovarian cysts, and congenital uterine abnormalities (see Chapter 70). Primary dysmenorrhea is the most common of these and is associated with dull, midline cramping lower abdominal pain that begins with the menses and lasts for a few hours to 2 days. There may be associated headache, nausea, flushing, and diarrhea. Onset occurs within 18 months of menarche and is associated with ovulatory cycles. Particularly severe pain with onset at menarche or experienced more than 3 years after menarche is suspicious, and an underlying cause is more likely to be uncovered. This subgroup of adolescents needs gynecologic referral for diagnostic evaluation and treatment.

The pathophysiology of primary dysmenorrhea and its evaluation and treatment are noted in Chapter 70.

Dysfunctional uterine bleeding is associated with anovulatory cycles and painless, excessive bleeding, and is the most common cause of heavy menstrual bleeding.

Only 5% to 10% of adolescents with excessive bleeding have an underlying pathologic condition. The differential diagnosis includes ectopic pregnancy, threatened abortion, pregnancy, placenta previa, abruptio placentae, and infection. These conditions are usually associated with lower abdominal pain. Hypothyroidism more commonly produces menorrhagia, but hyperthyroidism can also be a cause. Polycystic ovary disease should be suspected in the obese, hirsute adolescent who has a history of irregular periods with heavy bleeding. Tumors and fibroids are uncommon in adolescents, and vaginal adenosis, ovarian cyst polyps, and PID rarely present with heavy bleeding. The most commonly found coagulation disorders are von Willebrand disease and idiopathic thrombocytopenia purpura. Incorrect or surreptitious use of oral contraceptives, aspirin, or anticoagulants should be determined from the history.

All adolescents require attention to vital signs and evaluation for the degree of anemia and possible iron deficiency. Coagulation studies and pregnancy testing are done as indicated. Virginal adolescent girls with a history of bleeding less than 7 days and without anemia do not require pelvic examination, and should be referred to their primary care physician for follow-up. Sexually active adolescents or those with prolonged bleeding and anemia require pelvic examination. Treatment is discussed in Chapter 70.

Any adolescent patient with vaginal bleeding, with or without crampy abdominal pain and who is pregnant, should be referred for immediate gynecologic evaluation and treatment of suspected abortion.

PREGNANCY

Symptoms of pregnancy in the adolescent may be vague and nonspecific and include fatigue, nausea, headache, abdominal pain, and depression (see Chapter 74). The reason the adolescent seeks medical care is often unclear and the concern of possible pregnancy may become apparent only during the interview with the adolescent. Often, there is no history of amenorrhea, because adolescents may mistake vaginal spotting at the time of implantation with a menstrual period. They may experience irregular bleeding and may not keep careful track of their menstrual cycle. There should be a low index of suspicion for diagnosing possible pregnancy, and in adolescents early identification is of the utmost importance. Communication of a positive result should occur between the adolescent and physician. At this interview, the physician can identify from whom this adolescent may seek support and can share the burden of future decisions. It is ideal when the adolescent involves the baby's father and her and his parents or other surrogate in discussing the pregnancy and its resolution (see Chapters 69 and 74).

RAPE AND SEXUAL ABUSE (see Chapters 118 and 119)

The incidence of rape continues to increase in the United States, and it is estimated that 50% of all cases may involve adolescents. This is an emotional crisis for the adolescent, and the staff must respond in a sympathetic, gentle manner. In most emergency departments there are established protocols for evaluation of the rape victim, or each city may have a designated rape center for children and adolescents. The physician responsible for evaluating the victim needs to be familiar with the specifications and requirements of the local forensic laboratory. The physician should obtain consent for examination from the adolescent and should take the time to explain what to expect during the evaluation. An interview should follow the examination, discussing the presence or absence of injuries with the adolescent. The family and adolescent should be referred for counseling to avoid the long-term consequences of sexual abuse (see Chapter 119).

NEUROLOGIC EMERGENCIES
Status Epilepticus

More than 1 million people in the United States have recurrent seizures (see Chapter 83). About 3% to 8% of these patients experience status epilepticus some time during their lives. Status epilepticus can also occur in adolescents who have never had a previous seizure. Status epilepticus is defined as a generalized, tonic-clonic seizure that lasts more than 20 minutes, or a series of recurrent seizures that lasts more than 30 minutes, during which the adolescent does not regain consciousness.

Seizure disorders are common among adolescents (see Chapter 83). Status epilepticus is discussed here because it is a medical emergency that requires immediate intervention to prevent permanent brain injury. Morbidity and mortality are more likely with young children, but adolescents are also at risk. Although most cases of status epilepticus occur in young children, they can occur at any age, and those caring for adolescents must be prepared to manage the prolonged seizure. The incidence of status epilepticus is about equal among males and females.

PATHOPHYSIOLOGY

There are many causes for status epilepticus in adolescents (Table 97–5). In the large majority of cases no specific cause is found, and these episodes are labeled as "idiopathic." In about 20% of cases an underlying chronic disorder is known, and the status epilepticus is a result of noncompliance with antiepileptic medications

TABLE 97–5. Common Causes of Status Epilepticus in Adolescents

Idiopathic
Infection
  Meningitis/encephalitis
  Brain abscess
Anoxia
Trauma
Toxins
  Medications
  Nonprescription drugs
Vascular disorders
  Vasculitis
  Bleeding, embolism
Tumors

(see Chapter 26). In other cases acute infections, such as meningitis or encephalitis, or anoxic insults, such as smoke inhalation or near-drowning, precipitate status epilepticus. Intracranial abscesses secondary to undiagnosed or undertreated sinusitis infection have caused prolonged seizures in some adolescents. Certainly, head trauma is an important cause of status epilepticus in adolescents. Toxins are another important cause of prolonged seizures in adolescents. Some may result from prescribed drugs, such as theophylline, but some result from a suicide attempt or recreational use of street drugs. These are discussed later in more detail. More unusual causes are vasculitis, bleeding diatheses, and cardiac disease with embolic phenomena.

Finally, brain tumors and vascular problems of the central nervous system are rare but possible causes of status epilepticus in adolescents.

Death from status epilepticus may result from the underlying cause of the seizure, such as a tumor or infection. However, the prolonged seizure itself can cause permanent brain injury because of associated hypoxia. This hypoxia may be secondary to respiratory insufficiency from muscle spasm during the seizure or from increased systemic cellular energy needs. Other complications can occur during the seizure, such as hypertension or hypotension, acidosis, or cerebral edema, and these may contribute to the morbidity and mortality of the event. Certainly, there can be complications such as respiratory depression or arrhythmia that result from drug therapy used for control of the seizure. The neurologic sequelae from status epilepticus are related to the duration of the seizure, and one that continues for several hours is more likely to be devastating than one that is quickly controlled.

MANAGEMENT AND DIAGNOSIS

The management of status epilepticus must proceed quickly, even before the assessment of the adolescent is complete. Although it is important to consider the differential diagnosis and search for the cause of the seizure, this cannot take precedence over immediate attempts to stabilize the adolescent with a sustained tonic-clonic generalized seizure. The first priority is to preserve vital functions. The airway must be open to allow adequate exchange of oxygen. The adolescent should be positioned so that the head is flexed and the neck extended. A towel roll under the shoulders may help maintain this open airway. Also, it may be necessary to use the chin lift or head tilt maneuver to open the airway. In some cases, a plastic oral airway may help maintain the unobstructed airway, but other objects, such as a stick or fingers, should not be placed in the adolescent's mouth, because this does not improve the patency of the airway and could cause further obstruction or injury to the patient or caretaker. Next, the oropharynx should be suctioned, because secretions or vomitus may obstruct the airway. Oxygen should be delivered by face mask, even in the absence of cyanosis. A clear, soft, plastic face mask is recommended so that vomitus can easily be noted and suction applied promptly. Assisted ventilation with a bag-valve-mask device may be useful but difficult to use effectively in the adolescent who is seizing actively. Frequent assessment of air exchange is needed, and endotracheal intubation might be necessary (rarely) if poor air exchange persists.

Next, the circulation should be assessed and a cardiac monitor attached to the adolescent. Blood pressure should be measured, and temperature should be controlled (by giving an antipyretic if needed, or using a heat lamp if body temperature is too cool). A peripheral intravenous (IV) line should be placed, but fluid resuscitation is usually not needed. Maintenance fluids can be started or the IV line can be used to obtain blood for analysis and to keep the vein open for medications. Immediate venous blood studies should include tests for serum electrolyte and glucose levels, toxicology screen, and probably tests for blood urea, nitrogen, and calcium levels if no known seizure disorder exists. Determination of the anticonvulsant level is needed if the adolescent has been on anticonvulsant medications. Liver enzyme and ammonia level determinations are optional blood tests, and are not sent initially unless Reye syndrome is suspected. Although hypoglycemia is unusual in an adolescent, a Dextrostix test is still a helpful and fast screening test. If infection is likely, a complete blood count and culture are needed. An arterial blood gas is not done initially and is desirable only if the seizure is prolonged. (A urine toxicology screen should also be done when urine is obtained.)

While such treatments are ongoing, it is important to protect adolescents from undue harm caused by the convulsive movements. The patient should be placed on a soft, flat surface with no sharp objects nearby and should be protected from rolling off the stretcher. Although turning the adolescent on the side may prevent aspiration of vomitus, it may also hamper ventilation. Thus, a nasogastric tube may be placed to empty the stomach quickly and to prevent subsequent vomiting.

A brief history should be obtained from those accompanying the adolescent while the resuscitation proceeds. It is crucial to learn whether the adolescent has a known convulsive disorder or other medical problems that could precipitate a seizure. For instance, a history of diabetes mellitus makes hypoglycemia likely, and an asthmatic taking theophylline is at risk for seizures from this medication. Similarly, those accompanying the adolescent may be aware of a possible suicide attempt or of the use of recreational drugs or alcohol. A history of recent trauma and signs of possible infection (e.g., fever, chills) should be sought. Next, an abbreviated physical examination is needed. The physician should assess the adolescent's general medical condition and specifically seek signs of infection or trauma. The neurologic assessment should determine any focal deficit, such as asymmetric pupils or unilateral hypertonia. If the "seizure" only seems to occur in the presence of a family member or professional, pseudoseizure should be suspected. Also, those with pseudoseizures rarely fall to the floor or injure themselves in other ways.

It is only after this initial stabilization and assessment that attempts are made to stop the seizure. Anticonvulsant medications should be given intravenously and then allowed sufficient time to work; the actual dose given is known. Intramuscular injections of anticonvulsant agents are less useful because the onset of action is

TABLE 97–6. Medications for Status Epilepticus

DRUG	DOSE	CAUTIONS	COMMENTS
Lorazepam (Ativan)	0.05–0.1 mg/kg intravenously; may repeat in 10 minutes × 2	Respiratory depression, hypotension, excessive sedation	Maximum, 4 mg/dose Maximum total dose is 8 mg
Diazepam (Valium)	0.2–0.5 mg/kg intravenously slowly; repeat every 10–15 minutes × 3	Respiratory depression likely with phenobarbital Short half-life (20 minutes); must give longer acting drug once seizures are controlled	Maximum, 10 mg/dose Maximum total dose is 20–30 mg
Phenytoin (Dilantin)	18–20 mg/kg intravenously slowly	Hypotension and cardiac depression if infused rapidly; monitor EKG/blood pressure	Maximum, 1000 mg/dose Infuse slowly (50 mg/minute)
Phenobarbital	20 mg/kg intravenously	CNS and respiratory depression (especially with diazepam)	Maximum, 800 mg/dose

delayed. Perhaps the most useful agent for status epilepticus is lorazepam (Ativan). Studies have shown that this drug stops seizures within 2 to 3 minutes in 80% to 100% of adolescent patients when given intravenously. It has a long half-life, 10 to 12 hours, and causes respiratory depression, hypotension, or excessive sedation in approximately 12% of patients. The drug is repeated at 10 minutes if seizure persists. Diazepam (Valium) is another effective drug that has a rapid onset of action, but it is rapidly redistributed in the body and seizures are likely to recur in 20 or 30 minutes unless another long-acting anticonvulsant is subsequently given. Side effects include sedation, hypotension, and respiratory arrest. Although such respiratory depression is not desirable, it may actually be easier to ventilate an adolescent who is neither breathing nor seizing than one with persistent seizure activity.

Phenytoin (Dilantin) is a less useful drug for managing status epilepticus because its effects may take 20 minutes to occur when given intravenously. It may be useful after the seizure is ended with lorazepam or diazepam. It is not a strong sedative, so it may facilitate monitoring of the adolescent's level of consciousness. Thus, some recommend its use if the seizure is caused by trauma. When given, the drug should be infused slowly (at a rate not to exceed 50 mg/minute) to prevent the side effects of cardiac arrhythmias and arrest. Phenobarbital is another anticonvulsant, most useful after the seizure is ended. It also requires 10 to 20 minutes for its antiepileptic effect when given intravenously. This drug can cause hypotension and respiratory depression, especially when combined with diazepam. Both phenytoin and phenobarbital may be valuable if the adolescent is already using these medications and a subtherapeutic drug level is thought to be the cause of the status epilepticus. First, the rapid-acting benzodiazepines can be administered. Other agents such as paraldehyde, lidocaine, or general anesthesia are rarely used for status epilepticus. Table 97–6 summarizes the commonly used anticonvulsants and their doses.

In addition to anticonvulsants, other treatment may be needed. If hypoglycemia is noted, 50 ml of 50% dextrose should be given quickly. If hypertension is thought to be the cause of seizure, intravenous diazoxide, 2 mg/kg given rapidly, is indicated.

If the seizure cannot be controlled after appropriate medications, the physician must look for a cause for the failure. Reassessment of ventilation, as well as a search for metabolic derangements, are indicated. Once the seizure ends, frequent reassessment of the adolescent is critically important. Further tests should be considered, such as an arterial blood gas to assess oxygenation and possible metabolic acidosis. If infection is suspected, lumbar puncture is indicated when the adolescent is stable. Antibiotic administration may be necessary prior to the lumbar puncture if this test cannot be performed quickly. Other therapies depend on the suspected cause of the seizure. Although skull radiographs have little value in the management of the adolescent with seizures, a CT scan may be helpful if there is a suspicion of head trauma or intracranial mass, or if focal deficits are found on the neurologic examination. An EEG is not useful in the acute management of someone with a seizure disorder unless pseudoseizure is considered. Admission to the hospital is indicated for all adolescents with status epilepticus. Safe transport of the adolescent from the ED to the inpatient unit is crucial.

Coma

Coma is a clinical state in which the adolescent shows decreased responsiveness to environmental stimuli. Levels of coma can be objectively measured using the Glasgow Coma Scale (Table 97–7), which evaluates the

TABLE 97–7. Glasgow Coma Scale

PARAMETER	SCORE
Eyes open	
Spontaneously	4
To speech	3
To pain	2
None	1
Best verbal response	
Oriented	5
Confused	4
Inappropriate	3
Incomprehensible	2
None	1
Best motor response	
Obey commands	6
Localize pain	5
Withdrawal	4
Flexion to pain	3
Extension to pain	2
None	1

patient's ability to open the eyes, respond verbally, and respond with an appropriate motor action. This scale can be used to predict outcome and to transmit information about the level of consciousness to others caring for the adolescent.

PATHOPHYSIOLOGY

Coma can be caused by lesions in the central nervous system that depress or damage the cerebral cortex, white matter, or upper thalamus, or that cause localized damage to the ascending reticular activating system (a polysynaptic neuronal network that lies in the central core of the brainstem, thalamus, and hypothalamus). These structures can be damaged by direct trauma, displacement, or compression by mass lesions, increased intracranial pressure, or blood flow compromised because of damaged blood vessels that perfuse the brain.

CLINICAL MANIFESTATIONS

The adolescent with coma may have other findings in addition to an altered state of consciousness. Associated findings such as hypotension, hypertension, respiratory distress, and focal neurologic findings depend on the cause of the coma.

DIFFERENTIAL DIAGNOSIS

There are many causes of coma in the adolescent, and these should be considered while stabilization and management are ongoing.

Head Trauma. This is probably the most common cause of coma in the adolescent. Homicides are a leading cause of death in older adolescents, and this intentional trauma is increasing because of increased adolescent involvement in the drug trade. Nonintentional head injury is also common from a fall or motor vehicle accident. When trauma is the cause of coma, head injury is usually obvious. Occasionally, more subtle injuries cannot initially be detected. An epidural hematoma may occur after a blow to the head that did not seem significant at first. Some adolescents have a period of brief unconsciousness followed by a "lucid interval" and then prolonged coma. A subdural hematoma is more common than an epidural bleed and this usually results from significant head injury with immediate loss of consciousness. When there is diffuse, severe, head trauma, brain swelling results, with increased intracranial pressure and loss of consciousness. In addition, a more minor injury such as a concussion can cause brief coma, which lasts less than a few hours, or a contusion (local hemorrhage in the brain), which causes more persistent coma.

Intoxications. These are also common causes of coma in adolescents, and may be intentional or inadvertent. They are discussed in detail elsewhere in this chapter.

Infectious Causes. These must also be considered. Meningitis and encephalitis are possible causes, and history of fever in association with coma make these more likely. Adolescents with these illnesses may present with seizures that can themselves produce prolonged unconsciousness. However, with these, there is

often a history of tonic-clonic activity, and the postictal state should eventually terminate or further seizure activity recurs, which makes the diagnosis obvious.

Intracranial Mass Lesions. These are a less common cause of coma. However, brain tumors should be considered, as some destroy the reticular activating system or compress the brainstem (see Chapter 53). Sometimes there is hemorrhage into the tumor, with resulting coma. More likely, tumors cause coma gradually, secondary to increased intracranial pressure. Similarly, undetected or untreated sinusitis can result in a subdural empyema, which can precipitate coma in some adolescents.

Metabolic Problems. Various types can lead to coma. For example, the adolescent with diabetes mellitus is at risk for coma (see Chapter 59). Those with diabetic ketoacidosis have hyperosmolarity and lactic acidosis. Certainly, a past history of this disease is helpful, and some adolescents comply poorly with treatment regimens. Some may deliberately withhold insulin treatments as a suicidal gesture. The history of vomiting and polyuria with dehydration makes this diagnosis likely, before laboratory tests confirm the acidosis and the hyperglycemia. Hypoglycemia and resulting coma are also possible from an insulin reaction. Hepatic encephalopathies are more unusual causes of coma in adolescence. Although Reye syndrome is now seen infrequently, it should be considered, because adolescents accounted for 50% of cases in the mid 1980s. Only 56 cases were reported in the United States in 1987 and 1988 (perhaps because of warnings against aspirin use for viral illness), but about 50% to 60% of these became comatose. Most presented with an antecedent illness (varicella, respiratory illness) within 3 weeks of the onset of vomiting and neurologic symptoms. The encephalopathy develops coincident with or soon after persistent vomiting occurs. This progresses from irritability, combativeness, and confusion to delirium, stupor, and coma. The adolescents are usually afebrile and do not have jaundice or scleral icterus.

Environmental Factors. Finally, some adolescents may become comatose because of environmental hazards. Anoxia for any reason can result in coma, and adolescents may be victims of near-drowning or smoke inhalation. There is usually a history suggestive of these causes. However, carbon monoxide poisoning can be subtle when the cause is exposure to automobile exhaust fumes in a closed space or a faulty home heater. In addition, some adolescent athletes may develop heat stroke when exercising on a very hot day. In these cases, varying levels of coma are associated with seizures, hemiparesis, pupillary changes and hyperpyrexia ($\geq 41°C$). The coma may be abrupt or there may be progression from headache, dizziness, weakness, confusion, and combativeness.

DIAGNOSIS AND MANAGEMENT

As with many other emergencies, treatment of coma must begin before a definitive diagnosis can be established. The first priority when caring for a comatose adolescent is to evaluate the airway. If the airway is clear, but cyanosis is present, supplemental oxygen should be administered. If head trauma is suspected, the neck should be immobilized. The adolescent's breathing is then assessed. Assisted ventilation may be necessary if cyanosis doesn't improve quickly or if chest expansion seems inadequate. Insertion of an oral or nasal airway may prevent or relieve obstruction. Endotracheal intubation should be considered when the adolescent has a depressed gag reflex, has obvious difficulty with oral secretions, has a Glasgow Coma Scale score of 8 or less, or has significant respiratory depression. While assessing the adolescent's respiratory effort, consider the breathing pattern. If deep Kussmaul respirations are present, diabetic coma is possible. Similarly, hyperventilation may be a sign of increased intracranial pressure (ICP) and impending herniation.

If circulation is inadequate, fluid resuscitation with normal saline must begin immediately. Otherwise, intravenous access should still be established but fluids should be given cautiously, especially if head trauma is likely. While vascular access is established, blood should be obtained and sent for analysis of electrolytes, blood urea nitrogen, creatinine, and glucose levels, and a toxicology screen. A Dextrostix test is done immediately. Ammonia and liver studies may be indicated if the cause is unclear or if Reye syndrome is suspected, and an arterial blood gas determination may be desirable to assess acid-base status. Measurement of serum osmolality to evaluate the osmolar gap is also recommended. An increased osmolar gap may imply ethanol or methanol intoxication. Other laboratory tests are guided by the history and physical examination. Urine for routine analysis and a toxicology screen should be sent later.

The vital signs are then assessed. The temperature and blood pressure should be taken. A Foley catheter should be placed and an electrocardiogram obtained.

A brief history should be obtained from the family member while the adolescent is being stabilized. The physician needs to know whether the adolescent has any known medical illnesses, such as cardiac disease, diabetes mellitus, or a chronic neurologic disorder. Also, history of recent infection or exposure to infection is important. Certainly, any history of trauma should be sought, as well as the possibility of intentional or accidental ingestion of alcohol, drugs, or prescribed medications. Moreover, history of a recent headache or change in personality may suggest a brain tumor, other mass lesion, or central nervous system bleed.

Next, a rapid but careful physical examination may further elucidate the cause of coma. The signs of cerebral herniation should be sought, because this must be treated immediately. If there is unilateral pupillary dilatation and contralateral hemiplegia, uncal herniation is likely, and immediate treatment with hyperventilation (to a PCO_2 20 to 25 mmHg) and dehydrating agents (mannitol) are mandatory. Also, if there is evidence of increased intracranial pressure, such as bradycardia, hypertension, and respiratory irregularities (Cushing triad), this, too, should be treated immediately with hyperventilation and elevation of the head to about 30 degrees, followed by the infusion of mannitol.

If these life-threatening emergencies are not present, the physical examination can be carried out. The head may show obvious trauma, such as battle signs or "raccoon eyes." The skin may reveal bruises, suggesting

less obvious head trauma. Also, petechiae may indicate the presence of an infection or bleeding disorder, with resulting intracranial hemorrhage. Skin examination may also reveal needle marks or a characteristic rash of the glue abuser (perioral pustular dermatosis). Paint may be noted on the face, indicating the abuse of spray paint cans for inhalation. The eyes should be inspected for papilledema or hemorrhage. The tympanic membranes may show hemotympanum, suggesting a basilar skull fracture. Clear rhinorrhea from the nose may also indicate a basilar skull fracture. The adolescent's breath should be evaluated, and the smell of alcohol or the fruity smell of diabetic ketoacidosis may be found. The neck should be evaluated for evidence of nuchal rigidity, unless head trauma is suspected. Central nervous system infection in the comatose adolescent cannot be ruled out, however, even in the absence of meningismus. The chest should be examined with the focus on possible infection, trauma, or heart disease, with possible embolism to the brain. The abdomen may reveal tenderness (if occult trauma is present) or hepatomegaly, which is initially found in about 50% of adolescents with Reye syndrome.

A careful neurologic examination may elucidate the cause of coma. In general, metabolic disorders cause partial dysfunction at many levels of the central nervous system rather than focal deficits. Tremor, asterixis, and myoclonic activity are more likely with a metabolic problem. Focal neurologic signs suggest tumors, abscess, or hematoma. The pupillary examination is important, and preserved pupillary reaction to light usually implies a metabolic cause rather than a structural problem. However, some toxins (e.g., amphetamine, cocaine, atropine) can cause nonreactive, large pupils. Small pupils are rarely caused by head trauma, but may be seen with narcotic or barbiturate ingestion. As noted earlier, a unilateral, dilated, unresponsive pupil indicates third nerve compression and uncal herniation of the temporal lobe. The oculomotor responses should be tested. If the brainstem is still intact, the doll's eye reflex is present. The absence of this reflex and of corneal reflexes implies a brainstem lesion. Posturing may be present, which signifies structural dysfunction in the hemispheres (decorticate) or midbrain and upper pons (decerebrate).

If no explanation for the coma is obvious, treatment should begin with an intravenous dose of naloxone (2 mg) and glucose (50 ml of 50% dextrose). This universal treatment has few complications, even if intoxication or hypoglycemia are not responsible for the coma. If the adolescent responds to glucose, an infusion of 10% dextrose in water should be continued. If the adolescent responds to naloxone, it should be repeated every 2 to 3 minutes unless an infusion is started.

Specific causes of coma require specific treatment. If head trauma is suspected, the cervical spine must be evaluated radiographically while the neck remains stabilized. A portable, lateral, cervical spine film should be obtained. Neurosurgical consultation should also be obtained. If increased intracranial pressure is suspected, hyperventilation is continued. Intravenous mannitol (0.5 g/kg) may reduce brain swelling, but the use of steroids remains controversial. They are not indicated in the acute management of head trauma.

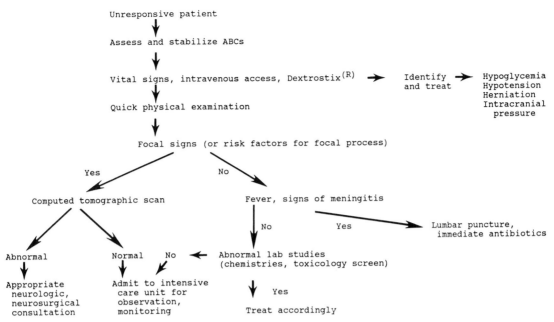

Figure 97–4. Approach to the adolescent in coma. (Adapted from Riviello JJ: Coma. In Selbst SM, Torrey SB [eds]: Pediatric Emergency Medicine for the House Officer. Baltimore, Williams & Wilkins, 1988, pp 57–67.)

If central nervous system infection is suspected, a lumbar puncture should be done unless focal neurologic signs or an increased intracranial pressure are present. In such cases a CT scan is indicated, but antibiotic therapy should not be delayed while the lumbar puncture is deferred.

Diabetic hypoglycemic coma can be managed with intravenous glucose and fluids. Insulin, saline, and perhaps sodium bicarbonate are used for diabetic ketoacidosis. The management of Reye syndrome is supportive and depends on the stage. If the adolescent is comatose, intubation and hyperventilation are required until he or she is transferred to another unit capable of managing this complicated syndrome.

Carbon monoxide poisoning is treated with 100% oxygen after the adolescent is removed from the source. Transfer to a facility in which hyperbaric oxygen can be delivered should be considered.

Heat stroke is treated with active cooling of the adolescent to 38.5°C. This can be achieved by giving an ice bath or massaging with ice while fans are directed onto the adolescent. The cardiovascular system should be supported and fluids given at maintenance rates unless insufficient cardiac output is noted.

If ingestion is suspected or the cause of the coma is unclear, lavage should be performed through a 30 to 40 French orogastric hose. This should be done after the airway is protected with a cuffed endotracheal tube. A small nasogastric tube is certainly not sufficient to remove pill fragments, if present. The adolescent patient should be positioned in the left lateral decubitus position and lavaged with 200- to 300-ml aliquots of saline. This is continued until the fluid is clear of particulate matter, which may require several liters. Then 50 to 100 g of activated charcoal in 8 ounces of water is given down the tube, followed by cathartics such as magnesium sulfate (30 g). Ipecac should not be used to empty the stomach in comatose adolescents, who might be unable

to protect their airway. Specific antidotes for some poisonings may be available. Treatments for some common intoxications are presented in the next section.

Adolescents with coma, even if brief, require admission to the hospital for further observation. If coma persists, admission to an intensive care unit is warranted. Further tests such as an electroencephalogram or CT scan can be arranged if the cause of the coma is unclear. Safe transport of the adolescent for all laboratory studies should be ensured. Consultation with a neurologist is recommended. Figure 97–4 summarizes the approach to the adolescent in coma.

THE INTOXICATED ADOLESCENT

Adolescents are unlikely to ingest substances accidentally, like toddlers. Still, they are frequently the victims of poisoning by intentional overdose of medications as a suicide attempt or by the use and abuse of mind-altering agents (see Chapter 111). A 1985 national survey has revealed the frequency of substance abuse among adolescents (see Chapter 2). Substance abuse reaches across all socioeconomic and educational backgrounds. The chances are great that those caring for adolescents will see some who suffer the side effects of these substances and who require acute care.

Substance abuse can precipitate several medical problems for adolescents beyond the direct effect of the drug used, including infections such as hepatitis, endocarditis, aspiration pneumonia, and AIDS. Substance abuse can be responsible for serious trauma from automobile accidents, violent behavior, or falls, and can result in psychiatric problems such as depression, withdrawal, and drug-induced psychosis. Substance abuse among adolescents is discussed elsewhere in this text (see Chapter 111). Here we focus on the immediate life-threatening emergencies that can result from the intentional overdose or abuse of common drugs.

Diagnosis and Management

The intoxicated adolescent may be comatose or very hostile, and might have obvious trauma. If the adolescent is comatose or has serious trauma, he or she must be stabilized, as described previously. If the adolescent is awake, alert, and perhaps hostile, some additional guidelines are recommended. Agitated behavior can be the result of hypoxia, head trauma, or the intoxication itself. An attempt should be made to calm the adolescent without using physical threats. If the adolescent is truly violent or cannot be calmed, restraint is necessary. This should be performed with adequate personnel to prevent injury to the staff and to the adolescent. One person should handle each extremity while another manages the head and neck for placement of the adolescent into four-point leather restraints. Occasionally, sedation is needed. If the adolescent is armed with a weapon, he or she should not be examined or confronted by medical personnel until disarmed by police or security guards.

A history should be obtained to discover which drugs were taken, as well as the intent of their use. It is important to learn whether the overuse was intentional or accidental, recreational or experimental, and episodic or habitual. An accurate drug history may not be obtainable, but it is helpful to question the adolescent alone, apart from the family and friends. After obtaining consent, the adolescent patient's clothing and belongings should be checked for possible clues about the substance ingested. The adolescent may not know what has been taken, however, because street drugs are often misrepresented. Also, many suicide attempts may involve the ingestion of multiple drugs in various doses.

The adolescent should then be examined completely, as described for the patient in coma. Further treatment is guided by the history and findings on physical examination. Consultation with a social worker is often valuable so that long-term plans for counseling can be made.

Specific Intoxications

RECREATIONAL DRUGS

Alcohol

Alcohol (ethanol) is a sedative-hypnotic that can produce aggressive behavior, ataxia, impaired mentation, slurred speech, lethargy, and vomiting. The level of intoxication depends on the blood alcohol level. Levels above 100 mg/dl may impair function, whereas levels of 400 mg/dl are toxic. However, deaths have been reported with levels as low as 200 mg/dl. Death may be a result of the drug itself, trauma, or vomiting and aspiration that are associated with alcohol use. The blood ethanol level may be estimated by calculating the osmolal gap. This is given by the following formula:

$$\text{osmolal gap} = \text{measured serum osmolality} - \left(2\,[\text{serum Na}] + \frac{[\text{BUN}]}{2.8} + \frac{[\text{serum glucose}]}{18} \right)$$

An osmolal gap of 22 to 25 mOsm/kg exists for every 100 mg/dl of ethanol in the serum.

Treatment of alcohol intoxication consists mainly of supportive measures. Although alcohol is absorbed quickly from the gastrointestinal tract, a peak blood concentration is reached 30 to 120 minutes after ingestion. This may be delayed further if food is in the stomach. Thus, emesis with 30 ml ipecac is recommended unless the patient is comatose, convulsing, or has no gag reflex. In these cases, activated charcoal lavage (as described previously) is recommended. A cathartic such as magnesium sulfate should follow. ED observation is recommended until the effects of the drug wear off. The rate of reduction in blood alcohol level varies from 10 to 25 mg/dl/hour.

Hemodialysis is used for only those who are very severely intoxicated.

Amphetamines (Sympathomimetics)

Sympathomimetics are administered by many routes, including "snorting," smoking, placement in body orifices, and the oral, intravenous, or subcutaneous route ("skin popping"). Amphetamine (speed) abuse is now on the rise since the introduction of "ice," a smokable methamphetamine. The effects are seen within minutes after intravenous administration or smoking. These drugs are abused for their ability to maintain wakefulness and elevate mood (in small doses). Mild intoxication causes palpitations, chest pain, headache, agitation, and a tremulous state. On examination, hypertension, tachycardia, hyperthermia, tachypnea, and dilated pupils are found. These can become extreme problems with severe intoxication and arrhythmias and seizures can result.

Management is directed toward the above problems, with the use of verapamil for supraventricular tachyarrhythmias and of oral nifedipine for mild hypertension, or intravenous nitroprusside when severe. Seizures should be managed as described earlier. If hyperthermia is present, the adolescent should be actively cooled with sprays or cooling blankets, rather than antipyretics.

Gastric decontamination should be accomplished with lavage and activated charcoal if the agent was administered orally. Ipecac is not indicated because of the risk of seizures from the drugs. The adolescent should be admitted to the hospital if the overdose is significant.

Barbiturates

Barbiturates are central nervous system depressants that can produce mild sedation, euphoria, or coma. The adolescent who has barbiturate overdose exhibits sluggishness, slurred speech, emotional lability, poor judgment, and irritability. With a significant overdose, hypothermia, hypotension, shock, and respiratory depression are possible. Barbiturates are often used in combination with amphetamines.

Withdrawal symptoms include restlessness, tremor, abdominal cramps, nausea, and vomiting. Seizures may occur after 48 to 72 hours of abstinence from short-acting barbiturates and after 7 to 8 days of abstinence from long-acting barbiturates. Death occurs from overdose in about 12% of cases.

Management includes emesis, charcoal, and catharsis for minor ingestions. For significant overdoses, the airway is secured with intubation and vascular access established. Gastric lavage with saline followed by charcoal administration is indicated. Repeat charcoal doses with cathartics and urinary alkalinization are recommended. Hypotension must be corrected with fluid administration. Continuous monitoring in an intensive care unit should be arranged. Charcoal hemoperfusion is reserved for severe cases.

Cocaine

Cocaine can be inhaled or smoked, or taken orally, intranasally, or intravenously. In the mid 1980s the use of "crack cocaine," or free cocaine base in powder or pellet form, became widespread. This inexpensive drug has allowed many adolescents to become cocaine users. When crack is smoked, blood levels similar to those from intravenous dosing are achieved. The effects are rapid in onset and brief in duration, and crack is highly addictive. Significant cardiovascular effects include hypertension and tachycardia; the former may result in intracranial and subarachnoid bleeding. Arrhythmias are common, including sinus, atrial, or ventricular tachycardia. Ventricular fibrillation is believed to be the cause of sudden death in some cocaine users. Myocardial ischemia and myocarditis tend to be manifested later, after the cocaine has been eliminated from the body. Hypotension and shock occur in those with severe intoxication. Central nervous system manifestations include headaches, seizures (usually soon after taking cocaine), agitation, dizziness, ataxia, vertigo, and blurred vision. Pulmonary problems such as pneumothorax and pneumomediastinum also occur, usually from a ruptured alveolar bleb during coughing or forced Valsalva maneuver while snorting or smoking cocaine. The adolescent with these problems complains of chest pain.

Treatment is aimed at correcting seizures, as described earlier. Tachyarrhythmias are managed with propranolol. Severe hypertension is treated with vasodilators such as intravenous nitroprusside, 0.5 to 5 μg/kg/minute, and moderate hypotension can be treated with oral nifedipine, 10 to 20 mg. Hypotension is treated with fluid resuscitation. Agitation may be treated with intravenous diazepam, 5 to 10 mg. If hyperthermia is present, exposed skin should be sprayed with tepid water while a fan is directed at the adolescent.

Gastrointestinal decontamination is usually not indicated but, if cocaine has been ingested, activated charcoal should be used. Ipecac is to be avoided because of the likelihood of seizures. Repeat charcoal and whole bowel irrigation with solutions such as GoLYTELY are recommended if packets of cocaine with large doses have been ingested. Surgical intervention may be needed if these packets rupture and signs of toxicity are manifested. Emesis is not recommended if packages of cocaine have been ingested.

Inhalants

Glue, cleaning fluid, paint, and typewriter correction fluid are often inhaled for their mind-altering effects. These substances are inexpensive and easily available to adolescents. Adolescents who abuse these substances often present with altered mental status, such as euphoria, hallucinations, confusion, restlessness, and slurred speech. Adolescent users may have gastrointestinal complaints, such as nausea, vomiting, and abdominal pain. Also, respiratory problems from pneumonitis can be seen. Syncope, cardiac arrhythmias, carbon monoxide poisoning, methemoglobinemia, and cardiac arrest are also possible.

These symptoms are abrupt in onset but brief in duration. Thus, management is primarily supportive. After separation from the causative agent, airway management, oxygen, vascular access, arrhythmia treatment, and blood pressure stabilization are priorities. Careful monitoring is needed until the effects wear off, usually within a few hours.

LSD (Lysergic Acid Diethylamide)

LSD was popular in the 1960s, but still remains a street drug of abuse in the 1990s. Adolescents usually take this drug orally and may present with a "bad trip," which produces anxiety, paranoia, and possibly acute psychotic reactions. Some users have flashbacks, with similar but less intense feelings than those caused by the original intoxication, without new exposure to LSD. Life-threatening problems include associated trauma, hypertension, tachycardia, hyperthermia, coagulopathy, coma, and respiratory arrest.

Management includes initial stabilization, as described earlier, and cardiac monitoring. Some believe that the psychological dangers of induced emesis or forced lavage outweigh the benefits of these attempts to empty the stomach. Activated charcoal in a slurry can be offered to the adolescent for voluntary consumption, but gastric lavage is mandatory only with severe overdose. Marked agitation can be treated with diazepam (5 to 10 mg), and a quiet environment is suggested. Hospital admission, although rarely needed, is recommended if intoxication is severe, ED observation is not possible, or a risk of suicide is present.

Marijuana

Marijuana is the most commonly used recreational drug in the United States after alcohol. Marijuana is usually smoked and this produces euphoria, relaxation, and altered space and time perception. Only in high doses are panic, paranoia, delusions, hallucinations, or psychoses reported. Its use may cause sinus tachycardia, but, again, orthostatic hypotension occurs only with high doses. Marijuana cigarettes are occasionally laced with cocaine or phencyclidine, so toxicity from these agents may be seen.

Although in common use, few marijuana users present

to the ED for treatment of acute intoxication. The mild anxiety or panic reactions that may be seen respond to supportive care in a quiet room. Sedative drugs are used occasionally. Admission to the hospital is rarely necessary.

Opioids

Opioids (e.g., morphine, codeine, heroin, meperidine, paregoric, diphenoxylate [Lomotil], propoxyphene) are infrequently abused by adolescents. The classic signs of poisoning include central nervous system depression, respiratory depression, and miosis. Adolescents may be hypothermic, hypotensive, and bradycardic. Some are at risk for aspiration pneumonia because of coma, centrally mediated vomiting, and impaired gag reflex. Neurogenic pulmonary edema has been reported with heroin use, as has bronchospasm.

Management focuses on control of the airway, cardiovascular support, and use of intravenous naloxone (2 mg) to reverse the opioid effects. When intravenous access is not available, the naloxone can be placed down an endotracheal tube, with comparably rapid effects. If no effect is initially seen, the naloxone should be repeated every 3 minutes until 10 mg has been given or the adolescent's condition improves. If no response occurs after 10 mg, opioid toxicity is unlikely. If naloxone reverses the central nervous system and respiratory depression, a continuous infusion of naloxone may be considered. The dose is calculated as two thirds of the dose used to reverse respiratory depression, given every hour in a continuous infusion.

In addition, gastric lavage with activated charcoal, should be performed immediately when oral ingestion is suspected. Hospitalization is required if there has been central nervous system or respiratory depression.

Phencyclidine (PCP; Angel Dust)

Phencyclidine is popular among adolescents because it is inexpensive and accessible and produces mind-altering, hallucinogenic effects. It is frequently added to other drugs. PCP is usually smoked, and one cigarette can contain 1 to 100 mg, depending on the source. Coma can result from the ingestion of 5 to 10 mg, respiratory depression and seizures from 10 mg, and death from 1 mg/kg. The presentation of adolescents intoxicated with PCP is variable. There may be staggered gait, slurred speech, blank stare, muscle rigidity, and nystagmus. Hypertension and tachycardia are possible. Bizarre and violent behavior may precede or follow coma. This may include confusion, delusions, hallucinations, or mutism. Adolescents are prone to sustaining injuries. The behavior may wax and wane, but symptoms usually resolve in a few hours. Severe complications such as hyperthermia, rhabdomyolysis, intracranial hemorrhage, apnea, and death may also occur.

Initial treatment involves emptying the stomach with gastric lavage in a quiet room. Activated charcoal should follow. Pharmacologic agents such as diazepam or haloperidol may be used for sedation rather than restraints, which could worsen the rhabdomyolysis. Urinary acidi-

fication has been recommended. Complications such as seizures and hypertension must be treated and, if rhabdomyolysis is noted, vigorous intravenous hydration is indicated. Adolescents who have seizures, rhabdomyolysis, hyperthermia, and significant injuries should be admitted to the hospital. Observation of mental status is required for several hours, and adolescents with severe poisoning and derangements in mental status also need admission.

SUICIDAL OVERDOSES

Acetaminophen

Some adolescents consume large amounts of acetaminophen with the goal of committing suicide or calling attention to psychoemotional problems (see Chapter 101). Adolescents are twice as likely as young children to develop potentially toxic blood levels following ingestion.

The clinical course has been divided into four stages. During stage 1, the first 24 hours after ingestion, adolescents have nausea, vomiting, diaphoresis, and malaise. During the next 24 hours (stage 2), the adolescent feels better and symptoms resolve. However, liver enzyme levels may rise if treatment was not administered earlier. In stage 3, 48 to 96 hours postingestion, marked hepatotoxicity can be seen in those with a major overdose (less than 1% of adolescent patients). Then, in stage 4 (day 7 or 8 postingestion), hepatic abnormalities usually resolve. Only 2% to 4% progress to hepatic failure and death; the severity of intoxication can be predicted by the amount ingested. Severe toxicity in adolescents occurs when 10 to 15 g of acetaminophen are ingested. Determining the acetaminophen level 4 hours postingestion is usually the most reliable indicator for toxicity, because the amount ingested is not always known.

Management involves gastric lavage. If multiple drug use is suspected, activated charcoal should be used. If the ingestion is known to be purely acetaminophen, however, charcoal should not be used, because it could bind the antidote, N-acetyl-L-cysteine. Cathartics such as magnesium sulfate are useful.

N-Acetyl-L-cysteine as a 5% solution (140 mg/kg) given orally reduces the toxicity of acetaminophen if administered within 24 hours of ingestion. Thus, if the ingestion was significant, it is acceptable to begin treatment and terminate the acetylcysteine if the level is eventually found to be below the toxic range. (Treatment is begun if ingestion has occurred within the previous 24 hours.) If the acetaminophen level is found to be in the toxic range, using the nomogram (Fig. 97–5), the adolescent is admitted and the antidote is continued in doses of 70 mg/kg every 4 hours for 17 doses. Diuresis, dialysis, and hemoperfusion are not helpful. Consultation with a local poison center is advised.

Aspirin Poisoning

Aspirin is another agent commonly ingested by adolescents who wish to commit suicide or call attention to their problems. Usually, ingestions of less than 150

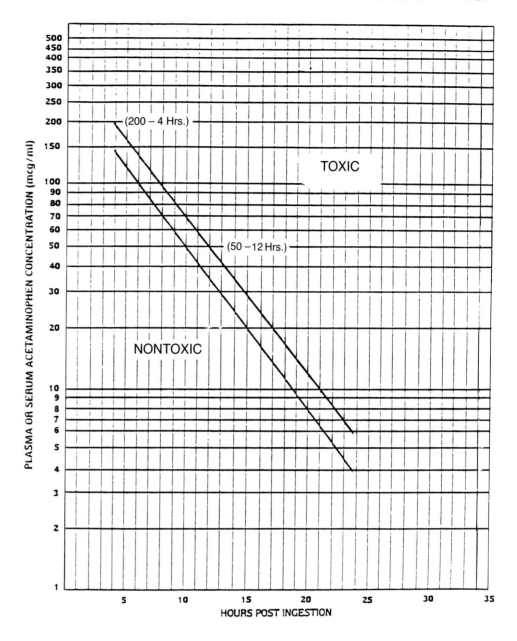

Figure 97–5. Nomogram for estimating the severity of acute acetaminophen poisoning. (Modified with permission from Fleisher GR, Ludwig S (eds): Textbook of Pediatric Emergency Medicine, 2nd ed. Baltimore, Wiliams & Wilkins, 1988, p 575; as adapted from Rumack BH, Matthew H: Acetaminophen poisoning and toxicity. Pediatrics 55:871–876, 1975. Copyright, American Academy of Pediatrics, 1975.)

mg/kg are benign, whereas those in the 150- to 300-mg/kg range produce moderate toxicity. More than 300 mg/kg causes severe toxicity, and 500 mg/kg can be fatal. Signs and symptoms of intoxication include nausea, vomiting, tinnitus, hyperpnea, lethargy, and irritability. Seizures or coma can occur with severe intoxication. Fluid and electrolyte disturbances occur, and hyperglycemia and dehydration are possible. Respiratory alkalosis may be seen in those with mild poisoning, but metabolic acidosis usually predominates in a mixed acid-base picture.

Management involves gastric lavage followed by charcoal administration. Fluid therapy is needed to restore electrolyte balance and sodium bicarbonate is used to treat acidosis. Alkalinization of the urine is helpful, but hemodialysis and hemoperfusion are reserved for those with serious overdoses. The Done nomogram (Fig. 97–6) can help predict toxicity based on an aspirin level drawn at least 6 hours after ingestion.

BEHAVIORAL EMERGENCIES

The adolescent patient may be brought to the ED for a behavioral emergency. The cause of these range from the long-standing effects of dysfunctional family life to the sudden effects of exploratory behaviors in otherwise psychologically healthy adolescents. Behavioral manifestations vary from acting out to serious suicide attempts. The common denominators are an adolescent who feels anxious and out of control and a family unable to provide support and control. This section discusses three problems, suicide, child abuse, and acute psychosis. It is estimated that the number of visits for these problems has doubled in the past 10 years.

Suicide

Suicide is a leading cause of death during adolescence, and some accidents are actually unrecognized suicides. The demography of suicide is discussed in Chapter 2.

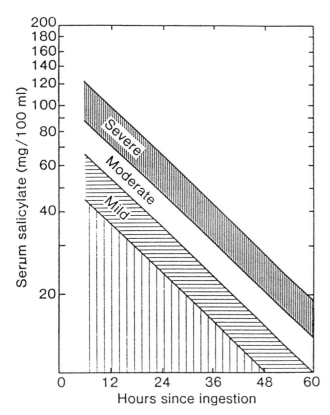

Figure 97–6. Done nomogram for estimating the severity of acute salicylate poisoning. (With permission from Done AK: Salicylate intoxication. Significance of measurements of salicylate in blood in cases of acute ingestion. Pediatrics 26:800, 1960. Copyright, American Academy of Pediatrics, 1960.)

The ED recognition of and response to a suicide attempt are important. This is particularly true when considering that many adolescents have seen a physician for a "medical" complaint in the weeks prior to their suicide attempt. Thus, in working with adolescents in the ED setting, one must be vigilant for signs and symptoms that might reflect a risk for suicide (Table 97–8).

Once a suicide attempt has been made, the ED phase includes medical treatment of the insult, assessment of the adolescent's intention, and assessment of the means used. It is never appropriate for the ED physician to assume that this attempt was "only a gesture," and to discharge the patient from the ED. We require that every attempt be reviewed by a psychiatrist and cleared for discharge. Whether an adolescent goes home depends on many factors beyond the realm of the usual ED physician's assessment. One needs to assess the family and supporting social structure for their strengths and ability to protect the adolescent from further self-inflicted harm. All adolescents discharged from the ED following suicidal behavior must have a specific follow-up plan, and preferably a scheduled appointment with a health care provider.

Child Abuse (see Chapters 118 and 119)

Abuse of children is usually thought of as involving young children and infants. However, most state child

TABLE 97–8. ED Findings Indicating High Risk for Suicide

Recent suicide attempt in past
Multiple ED visits for trauma
Suicidal threat made
"Accidental" ingestion in child older than 5 years
Signs of depression
Medical concerns accompanied by depression
Recent withdrawal behavior
Underlying psychiatric condition
    Psychosis
    Conduct disorder
    Attention deficit disorder
    Substance abuse
    Mental retardation
Family history of suicide
Recent cluster suicides in community

abuse laws seek to protect children through the adolescent age of 18 years. Adolescents may not be as prone to the broken bones and central nervous system injury as the younger child, but are just as vulnerable to soft tissue and sensory organ injuries, and perhaps more vulnerable to sexual abuse (Chapter 119), emotional abuse, and neglect (Chapter 118). In 1989, in Pennsylvania, 52% of substantiated injuries related to abuse occurred in those in the 10- to 12-year-old age group. Of these, 40% were for physical abuse, 58% for sexual abuse, and less than 1% for emotional abuse and 1% for neglect. In Pennsylvania, there were five deaths in this age group in 1989 and five deaths in 1988.

Figure 97–7 illustrates the steps of ED case management for suspected child abuse. The physician must be alert to the problem of abuse. The incidence of abuse is such that every traumatic injury in an adolescent should be screened for the possibility of it being abuse-related. Also, every sexually transmitted disease, pregnancy, or complaint of genital pain or finding of similar trauma should be screened for its abuse potential. All states require physicians to report any suspicion of

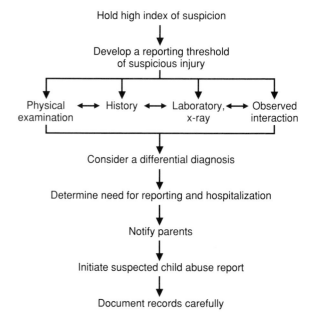

Figure 97–7. Management steps in suspected child abuse cases.

abuse. An actual case need not be documented—there need only be a suspicion. All states protect physicians who report in good faith. On the other hand, physicians who refuse to "get involved" run the risk of further injury or death of the adolescent, as well as specific and general liability for themselves. Often, it is assumed that adolescents can protect themselves, and that a child abuse report would be superfluous. Such an assumption is incorrect and dangerous.

Acute Psychosis

Acute psychosis is a relatively infrequent occurrence in the ED but, when it occurs, it often produces a great deal of turmoil. Acutely psychotic patients are usually brought by their families or by the police for medical clearance. Often, there is violent behavior or threatened violence that motivates the family or others into action. The role of the ED physician is to ensure that there is no organic basis for this type of behavior. Table 97–9 presents suggestions about differentiating organic from functional psychosis. One confounding factor is the use of drugs or alcohol. Adolescents with functional psychosis may begin to use drugs and/or alcohol to gain some control of the symptoms. Finally, when this form of self-medication does not work, they lapse into frank psychosis. On the other hand, some adolescents use drugs recreationally, only to sustain a dramatic organic psychosis. These two conditions may be difficult to differentiate and can be distinguished only by careful history taking. The history is usually the key to distinguishing between organic and functional psychosis. As with functional psychosis, there is a long preceding history of maladjustment or other form of ailing mental health.

Violent behavior is often present in the acutely psychotic patient, and it stimulates immediate attention and a large degree of staff anxiety. One helpful step is to place the violent adolescent in a stimulus-neutral environment. A quiet room, isolated from other patients, is ideal. Having a well-trained security staff is also helpful if physical protection of the staff becomes necessary.

TABLE 97–9. Organic versus Nonorganic Psychosis

The following suggest organic brain syndrome:
  Disorientation
  Clouding of consciousness
  Abnormal vital signs
  No previous psychiatric history
  Visual hallucinations
  Illusions

The following suggest nonorganic psychosis:
  Fully alert
  Normal vital signs
  Previous psychiatric disorder
  Family history of psychiatric disorder
  Auditory hallucinations

Adapted with permission from Dubin WR, Hanke N, Nickens HW (eds): Psychiatric Emergencies. (Clinics in Emergency Medicine, Vol 4.) New York, Churchill Livingstone, 1984, pp 21–33.

Often, approaching violent adolescents with quiet confidence allows them to relax enough to permit a screening physical examination to be done. Explanation of the procedures allows adolescents to bolster their self-control. Sometimes a psychotic adolescent may be so out of control that physical or pharmacologic restraint becomes necessary. We prefer the latter, because physical restraint may be difficult to enforce and is more likely to result in injury to the adolescent or staff. Consultation with psychiatric staff regarding pharmacologic agents and their dosage is suggested.

BIBLIOGRAPHY

Agnello V: Toxic shock syndrome: The emerging picture. Ann Intern Med 94(2):264, 1981.

American College of Surgeons; Committee on Trauma: Advanced Trauma Life Support. Chicago, American College of Surgeons, 1989.

American Heart Association: Textbook of Advanced Cardiac Life Support. Dallas, American Heart Association, 1987.

American Heart Association: Textbook of Pediatric Advanced Life Support. Dallas, American Heart Association, 1990.

Augenstein WL (editor): Emergency aspects of drug abuse. Emerg Med Clin North Am 8:467, 1990.

Blum R: Contemporary threats to adolescent health in the United States. JAMA 257:3390, 1987.

Bruce DA, Schut L, Sutton LN: Neurosurgical emergencies. In Fleisher GR, Ludwig S (eds): Textbook of Pediatric Emergency Medicine, 2nd ed. Baltimore, Williams & Wilkins, 1988, pp 1112–1126.

Centers for Disease Control: Sexually transmitted diseases treatment guidelines. MMWR 38:1, 1989.

Coran AG, Harris BH (eds): Pediatric Trauma. Philadelphia, JB Lippincott, 1990.

Dubin WR, Hanke N, Nickens HW (eds): Psychiatric Emergencies. (Clinics in Emergency Medicine, Vol 4.) New York, Churchill Livingstone, 1984.

Eschenbach D: Epidemiology and diagnosis of acute pelvic inflammatory disease. Obstet Gynecol, 55(Suppl):142S, 1980.

Felter R, Izsak E, Lawrence HS: Emergency department management of the intoxicated adolescent. Pediatr Clin North Am 34:399, 1987.

Golden N: The use of pelvic ultrasonography in the evaluation of adolescents with pelvic inflammatory disease. Am J Dis Child 141:1235, 1987.

Goldstein D: Acute and chronic pelvic pain. Pediatr Clin North Am 36:3, 1989.

Hausman AJ, Spivak H, Roeber JF, et al: Adolescent interpersonal assault admission in an urban municipal hospital. Pediatr Emerg Care 5:275, 1989.

Henretig FM, Cupit GC, Temple AR, Collins M: Toxicologic emergencies. In Fleisher GR, Ludwig S (eds): Textbook of Pediatric Emergency Medicine, 2nd ed. Baltimore, Williams & Wilkins, 1988, pp 548–598.

Katzman D: Chlamydia trachomatis Fitz-Hugh-Curtis syndrome without salpingitis in female adolescents. Am J Dis Child 142:996, 1988.

Lacey DJ, Singer WD, Horwitz SJ, et al: Lorazepam therapy of status epilepticus in children and adolescents. J Pediatr 108:771, 1986.

National Academy of Science: Injury in America. Washington, DC, National Academy Press, 1985.

Neuspiel DR, Kuller LH: Sudden and unexpected national death in childhood and adolescence. JAMA 254:1321, 1985.

Results from the National Adolescent Study Health Survey. JAMA 261:2025, 1989.

Riviello JJ: Coma. In Selbst SM, Torrey SB (eds): Pediatric Emergency Medicine for the House Officer. Baltimore, Williams & Wilkins, 1988, pp 57–67.

Shafer M-A., Sweet R: Pelvic inflammatory disease in adolescent females. Pediatr Clin North Am 36:3, 1989.

Shaw KR, Sheehan KH, Fernandez RC: Suicide in children and adolescents. Adv Pediatr 33:313, 1987.

Shields WD: Status epilepticus. Pediatr Clin North Am 36:383, 1989.

Strasburger VC, Greydanus DE (eds): The at-risk adolescent. In Adolescent Medicine: State of the Art Reviews. Philadelphia, Hanley & Belfus, 1990, pp 1–198.

Talbot C: The gynecologic examination of the pediatric patient. Pediatr Ann 15:501, 1986.

Tolmas HC: The role of the private practitioner. In Strasburger VC, Greydanus DE (eds): Adolescent Medicine: State of the Art Reviews. Philadelphia, Hanley & Belfus, 1990, pp 146–151.

Washington AE, Sweet R, Shafer M: Pelvic inflammatory disease and sequelae in adolescents. J Adolesc Health Care 6:298, 1985.

PSYCHOLOGICAL ISSUES

Introduction

In this section, those conditions and problems that may affect or are a result of disturbances in psychological function are presented. These chapters discuss problems that account for large numbers of health visits and thus have the potential to consume a significant amount of the physician's time. Among adult general medical practices, at least 50% and perhaps as many as 75% of health visits are related to or precipitated by psychosocial factors. Physical symptoms are often the first and only presenting manifestations for a variety of problems whose underlying causes are social or emotional, or both. Many of these problems can and should be evaluated and treated by the primary physician. It is estimated that approximately 10% of adolescents could benefit from psychiatric intervention. Many of these adolescents will require referral to mental health colleagues. Negotiating successful psychiatric referrals is an art that requires knowledge about the psychological condition and the patient's functioning. The successful physician will understand the adolescent's symptoms within the context of the tentative psychiatric diagnosis and the adolescent's life circumstances. The physician must be able to develop a differential diagnosis based on an understanding of biologic and psychological conditions.

These chapters present current information about the common psychiatric problems and emotional symptoms of adolescents. As with other sections of this volume, when possible a uniform format is followed, detailing epidemiology, natural history, diagnostic criteria, differential diagnosis, the presumptive etiology, and treatments. The reader will note that the majority of these chapters are written by psychiatrists or psychologists. This is consistent with other sections of the text and the philosophy of the editors. The authors are the recognized experts in their respective areas. Some of the concepts may be new to physicians and those less familiar with adolescent psychiatric disturbance and will require careful reading. We believe the investment will be worthwhile.

We have chosen to use standard psychiatric nomenclature and have framed the chapters as much as possible within contemporary biologic psychiatry for the following reasons:

1. It facilitates communication among professionals and disciplines and allows the interested reader to more easily investigate suggested readings and the literature.

2. It underscores our belief that mental health is integral to adolescent, and indeed all, health care.

3. It allows the practitioner to develop meaningful differential and preliminary diagnoses more carefully—a process that we believe is vital to providing quality health care. The more the physician appreciates the deviation from normal development (extent of psychopathology), the greater the likelihood of his or her appropriately treating or referring the adolescent patient with emotional or behavioral symptoms. Increasing evidence suggests the biologic and genetic underpinnings of many major psychiatric conditions.

We have also included certain problems such as adoption, divorce, grief and bereavement, interpersonal violence, physical and sexual abuse, and organ transplantation that do not represent psychiatric disturbance; rather, these common psychosocial issues carry great risk of affecting children and adolescents adversely. In standard psychiatric nomenclature, they are usually considered conditions that do not represent disturbance, but may require treatment. Clearly they represent situations that frequently confront the physician caring for teenagers.

A word about the organization of this section is in order. Its focus on pathologic conditions should not leave the reader with the unwarranted assumption that adolescence is a pathologic state or that all adolescents have serious emotional problems. Rather it is an attempt to focus the physician's thinking on identifying youth who require psychological help. Normal adolescent development is carefully detailed in Chapters 8, 9, and 11.

The reader will also note that the chapters on eating disorders will be found in the section under medical conditions. This choice does not minimize our belief that these conditions are serious psychiatric disturbances. Rather it reflects the fact that adolescents with these conditions usually present to nonpsychiatric physicians with physical symptoms—usually weight loss or vomiting. We have not included a chapter on nonintentional trauma in this section despite the fact that accidents are the leading cause of death in youth. The statistics are presented in Chapters 2 and 3. We believe that at present there is insufficient information about the emotional or behavioral etiologic causes of these most distressing problems to go beyond a description. When sufficient information becomes available about the biopsychosocial basis for nonintentional trauma, it will be included in future editions of this volume.

Psychological Evaluation

CHAPTER 98

Approaching the Adolescent with Psychological Symptoms

CHRISTOPHER H. HODGMAN

It is the thesis of this text that adolescent medical care also means adolescent psychological care. In many respects, adolescence is the healthiest period in the entire lifespan. Its morbidity is heavily influenced by psychological determinants: impulsiveness, unreadiness to assume responsibility with resultant poor compliance (see Chapter 26), and above all an inability to accept one's own vulnerability. All these tendencies are found in younger and older patients as well, but they seem especially marked during the adolescent period, when mortality largely stems from trauma—accidents, suicide, homicide—(see Chapter 2) under major psychological influence. With few exceptions, adequate medical care for the adolescent involves psychological support. Approaching the adolescent with psychological problems is, therefore, essentially like approaching any other adolescent patient and can be studied in the same context.

HISTORICAL PERSPECTIVE

It was not medicine, but law, in which the necessity to recognize psychological aspects of adolescent behavior first became apparent. Eighteenth-century laws governing "infants of tender age" (who were therefore not fully responsible for their behaviors) versus adults (presumably fully responsible) were seen as inappropriate for older children and adolescents by the nineteenth century. Previously, for example, English laws had permitted execution of an 8-year-old child for stealing a loaf of bread. Recognition of the inappropriateness of such an approach led to the juvenile justice system, which, in turn, encouraged adolescent psychology (see Chapter 1).

BIOPSYCHOSOCIAL CARE

The biopsychosocial model implies that all symptoms have psychological components; it is increasingly evident that the contrary is generally true as well (see Chapter 24). Early, ambitious claims for psychological causes of many common medical conditions provoked disrepute because they were overly inclusive and untestable. The observed complexity of human illness dictates conservative assumptions; the value of the biopsychosocial

approach is that all influences on health are seen as relevant and all health problems are recognized as having psychological elements. If this assumption is incorporated into routine adolescent care from the outset, the caregiver and the adolescent alike assume that psychological elements are part of everyday medical treatment. Adolescents and their families are, therefore, more likely to raise such issues with the physician.

EPIDEMIOLOGY

The biopsychosocial model implies an epidemiologic approach to the adolescent patient. Although it is most practical to begin with a presenting problem, it is essential to acknowledge and consider the role of the setting in which the problem has occurred. In large teaching hospitals, it is easy to forget the many things that are important: the adolescent's community and neighborhood; the family and its history (parents and their relationship, siblings, and the adolescent patient's place in the sibship); the peer group, which is relatively difficult to bring into the hospital; the school (often seen as irrelevant); academic competence as a measure of overall function; and financial and social status.

DIAGNOSTIC SYSTEMS

For the generalist unfamiliar with modern concepts of psychopathology, a constantly changing psychiatric nomenclature is challenging and disconcerting. Earlier diagnostic systems incorporated assumed psychodynamic elements in psychopathology—issues often clinically insightful but difficult to measure or test. As biologic treatments have become increasingly important, diagnostic terms that can be replicated have become even more essential. Hence, newer diagnostic systems incorporate objective, descriptive elements with greater demonstrable reliability among observers. As such descriptions are generally accepted, the nomenclature changes; accordingly, the Diagnostic and Statistical Manual (DSM) of the American Psychiatric Association has passed through successive changes—DSM-III, DSM-III-R, and the soon-to-be-published DSM-IV. The need to correlate the diagnoses made from this manual with the International Classification of Diseases (ICD-

10) so that replication can take place internationally is also recognized in the text.

CLINICAL MANIFESTATIONS

Although texts must follow a nomenclature, adolescent patients do not. As with physical illnesses, similar psychological symptomatology may have a variety of causes. First, it is necessary to elicit that symptomatology. The presenting illness may make this relatively simple. However, what if the adolescent patient cannot, or chooses not to, discuss psychological complaints? If the caregiver assumes the biopsychosocial model, eliciting epidemiologic data can be a helpful route to psychological complaints. A few examples readily show how typical problems can be elicited during routine data collection: questions about the adolescent's relationship to the community or neighborhood can be used to learn about conduct disorders in a previously well-behaved youngster; questions about the adolescent patient's family, parents, and siblings can be used to uncover distressing changes that the adolescent is unable to discuss comfortably and accurately; questions about the peer group, friends, and social life can reveal substance abuse, socialized delinquency, or social isolation. Inquiries about school may be used to approach significant changes in school performance that need investigating.

Studies of office practices have revealed that such complaints (conduct disorders, family problems, substance abuse, delinquency) may actually constitute the greatest concerns for adolescents. Not asking about the community, the family, and social contacts may suggest to the adolescent or his or her family that these matters are not considered relevant, and the office visit may end without determination of the primary problem.

After routine inquiry into ordinary life circumstances, it is essential not to omit direct investigation into psychopathology *per se* in the broad areas subsumed in the various chapters of this section. Evidence suggests that such inquiry does not generally occur in the context of most medical care. To ask about psychopathology, whether or not a direct answer results, indicates a readiness on the part of the practitioner to discuss such issues if they should arise at a subsequent time.

DIAGNOSIS

The Diagnostic Sequence

INITIAL CONTACT

The first contact with the adolescent may determine the effectiveness of subsequent care. It may be desirable to inform adolescent patients and their parents through a note, a notice enclosed with other mailings, or appointments that the practitioner welcomes direct contacts from individual adolescents. The desirability of involving both parents in the care should also be indicated. These contacts might occur through the use of a specific telephone hour for direct adolescent calls, keeping in mind local school schedules. The availability of the caregiver for direct telephone contact is sometimes more effective than a secretarial appointment system. The physician's professional card with his or her name and telephone number is often helpful for both adolescents and their parents when they wish to contact the physician. Finally, a policy may be established that does not require parental involvement or permission for initial contacts; in that case, however, parental consent at the onset of care or annually may be desirable to permit such sessions to be billed. Continuing interviews without parental knowledge may be unacceptable ethically and legally unless the caregiver is prepared to prove its necessity in a court of law (see Chapter 20).

BEGINNING THE INTERVIEW

Interviewing in general is discussed in Chapter 22, in which the desirability of having individual interviews with adolescents at as young an age as possible is stressed. The effects of developmental stage on the interview are discussed in Chapters 8, 9, and 22.

The interviewing process really begins with the first call to the office but certainly when the adolescent and his or her family are greeted in the waiting room. It is usually worthwhile to see all the individuals who come in with the adolescent, since their presence suggests their importance. It is also worthwhile to observe social amenities in the interview, striving to support self-respect in the adolescent and the family (e.g., offering appreciative comments that they have come despite poor weather, difficult traffic, known scheduling problems, and so on).

Interviewing Parents

It is valuable to recall that the parents of a troubled youngster are also troubled and often need parenting themselves. Assuming that everyone has problems and needs help is usually the most productive stance. It is also important to recall that the caregiver needs the support of the parents; the adolescent can usually do better without the caregiver than without the parents, so contests between adults must be avoided or the therapy will fail. In warring households, particularly, youngsters become adept at setting parents against each other to escape attacks upon themselves, so they will almost automatically seek to set the interviewer against the parents. This must be avoided. When particularly outrageous parental behavior or language is reported by the patient, it is often useful to observe that "there is probably another side to it." To accept the whole story burdens the youngster with guilt, for there is indeed almost always "another side to it." Adolescents will often relax if they can trust that the caregiver will not side with them blindly.

It is most essential, then, to create a positive alliance with the parents as well as with the adolescent. To do so usually involves finding out about the parents' own needs. A way to do this without implying fault is to ask for limited data about each parent directly, identifying the information and supporting the responses. In pediatric ambulatory care, it has been shown that attending to mothers as individuals in their own rights, rather than attending only to their parental roles, actually leads to improved compliance with the pediatrician's directions for the care of the child. Indicating an awareness of how difficult parenting some adolescents can be, and truly believing it, can be very helpful.

One parent may attempt to turn the caregiver against the other parent, for example, by implying that the other parent is uninterested or unavailable. Avoid accepting this as fact. Also avoid having the parent summon the spouse in a hostile manner: "The doctor wants to find out what you did wrong!" It is usually best for the physician to make appointments directly with the spouse, either in person or by telephone contact.

Information From Others

It is important for the busy caregiver to seek all the assistance possible to make an accurate diagnosis. It may seem that a call to an agency, a school, or another caregiver will be burdensome, but such steps can save much effort. It is essential for information collection to be efficient; it is easier when the caregiver knows personnel in the systems approached, because a single contact can help organize data collection on behalf of the adolescent. When the adolescent has school problems, for example, one should assume that testing has been done, or at least that the accounts of the adolescent's current and past classroom behavior can be obtained. When a history of delinquency is found, one should assume that there may be a court or police record with much information (see Chapter 108). If the youngster is receiving welfare assistance, the Department of Social Service probably has important reports. If at all possible, one should learn how to identify multiproblem families early to get multiagency input, saving endless inquiries. In most instances, the physician should seek the authority of greatest competence, for example, the school principal, the head of family court investigations, or the welfare supervisor. The names of competent personnel in the community and the region in which one practices should be gathered. Even if they are uninvolved with a specific case, they may know the place in which to seek information. They may be able to intercede and can serve as available "character references" for the caregiver when information is sought. Prior to collecting information from an agency, a school, or a community organization, the physician should explain to both the adolescent and his or her parents the fact that these data are critical so that one can best understand the adolescent's concerns. The specific agencies and the specific persons to be contacted, and the reasons for these contacts, should be clarified. Written permission should be obtained from both the adolescent and his or her parents for each group contacted. If the practitioner plans to personally visit an agency, both the adolescent and his or her parents should be informed about the details of the visit—that is, when it will occur, who will be seen, and the reason for the contact. Some adolescents will choose to introduce their practitioners to the key school authorities. Since control is such a vital issue for adolescents, it is important for them to be given as much control as is appropriate.

Evaluation Instruments Unique To Adolescents

Paper-and-pencil or computerized structured instruments are valuable for the primary caregiver because they cover major relevant areas methodically. Sometimes they lead to so much data that they overwhelm the user. Relatively few structured instruments have been designed for adolescents only; most are also used for older children and young adults. Currently, such rating scales are most frequently employed by pediatricians in the assessment of depression, as well as attention deficit disorder and other school-related difficulties.

In depression, the Beck Depression Inventory is employed from midadolescence into adulthood, and the analogous Children's Depression Inventory is used in young adolescence. Among other useful tests are the Children's Depression Scale (ages 9 to 18 years) and the Reynolds Adolescent Depression Scale (ages 8 to 13 years). Most such scales are relatively brief but inclusive. Suicide and "hopelessness" scales have been developed as well. Although depression and suicide scales should never be considered as definitive by the practitioner, they encourage more complete investigation of adolescents deemed at risk.

Similarly, teachers and parents are usually willing to complete brief scales to evaluate hyperactivity, such as those of Conners. Their use permits methodical measurement of behavior outside the clinic or office. A distinct change in ratings after the adolescent takes medication does not definitely establish its suitability (since even normal children may respond similarly), but it offers useful information nonetheless.

Other scales include measures of anxiety, obsessive-compulsive behavior, and eating disorders. Most are not used in the general caregiver's office because of the relative infrequency of such conditions, but their availability should be recalled when appropriate. The use of routine parent or teacher screening devices is most productive if their brevity encourages compliance. Longer diagnostic and guided interview schedules are also valuable in special instances. There is evidence that self-completion by adolescents of paper-and-pencil or computerized scales encourages more honest reporting, which can then be followed up by direct interviews. Indeed, it is essential that positive answers or damaging admissions, or both, evoke a careful response from the caregiver. Again, however, access to excessive data may discourage careful and appropriate evaluation and review.

Differential Diagnosis

Although differential diagnosis of individual conditions is discussed in each specific area, certain general principles apply throughout the behavioral area. Diagnoses are still made by the history because there are as yet few biologic *sine qua nons*. Many conditions present similarly at a given moment and can be clarified only as time passes. Observation of the longitudinal course, for example, is often required to distinguish among psychoses or the somatoform disorders. For the non–mental health provider, functional-behavioral appellations may be more useful for the first assessment. School failure (see Chapter 107), delinquency (see Chapter 108), runaway behavior (see Chapter 108), sexually inappropriate acts (see Chapter 108), substance abuse (see Chapter 111), and impulse-prone (see Chapter 108), suicidal (see Chapter 101), or violent (see Chapter 117) behaviors all dictate an energetic response, whatever their formal causes may prove to be. These are *not* diagnostic labels, they are merely descriptions of problems that require responses. Each behavior can conceal a variety of conditions requiring different treatments. In fact, the use of any behavioral appellation should be a challenge to the practitioner to uncover its underlying causes. At the same time, diagnostic labels risk overlooking multiple causes—the "single-cause explanation" often oversimplifies. A common example is the treatment of substance abuse alone, without attention to an underlying causative depression, or the treatment of depression alone, without controlling substance abuse and its consequences. It is important, then, to recall that more than one form of psychopathology can be present.

Despite the complexities, apparent imprecision, and unfamiliarity of the psychiatric diagnostic nomenclature, it is well to remember the value of a correct diagnosis. Precisely because a diagnosis involves a *prediction*—that a certain condition will progress in a certain way—the clinician needs to be prepared for that eventuality in order to manage it when it occurs (e.g., it is important to distinguish between unipolar and bipolar depression: in the latter, antidepressants can precipitate mania, which must therefore be anticipated, see Chapter 100).

THEORIES OF ETIOLOGY

This text assumes that most psychopathologic conditions involve multiple levels of causation. Indeed, many such conditions can be seen as "final common pathways" (see Chapter 12). An apt example is depression, (see Chapter 100), which may follow important psychological losses or other psychodynamic stresses; physical illness of many sorts, including infection, metabolic insult, neoplasms (see Chapter 53), or trauma (see Chapter 97); exposure to toxic substances; medications with unintended side effects; nutritional deficiencies (see Chapter 7); seasonal and other environmental changes; and still other factors, including very significant hereditary influences. Effective assessment of a condition such as depression may thus involve a wide variety of investigations. The availability of apparently "specific" medication may shortchange such explorations; medication alone is sometimes successful, but too often only for a short time. Accordingly, etiologic factors in each condition will be presented in subsequent chapters in as broad a context as appropriate.

TREATMENT

Similarly, varied therapeutic approaches offer varying advantages. Just as depression may originate from many factors, studies have demonstrated that a variety of treatments of depression are of proven worth. Thus supportive psychodynamically derived psychotherapy, in which the emotional origins of depression are explored, is of demonstrable value, as is informed supportive therapy, particularly in reactive depressions. Cognitive therapy, in which repeatedly self-destructive thought patterns are identified and altered, has also been proved effective in reversing the "learned helplessness" behind much depression. Behavioral and physical treatments can be useful in depression, as can a variety of psychopharmacologic approaches. (see Chapters 123–125). Similar varieties of treatment for the other most common forms of adolescent psychopathology will be discussed in this section.

Prevention

Prevention of psychiatric problems is often mentioned only in passing, but evidence suggests that it may in fact be more efficacious than often believed. It is possible to claim too much for prevention, but one must also acknowledge that, by its nature, successful preventive treatment is often forgotten. Examples of primary prevention (see Chapter 36) in adolescents include education about cigarette smoking and drug use and abuse (see Chapters 37 and 38). Diminution of adolescent male smoking patterns in the United States suggests that primary prevention can succeed, whereas an increase in adolescent female smoking habits suggests how far it has to go. Secondary prevention involves the identification of an individual pathologic condition. Examples in adolescence include the delinquent population, who are at greater risk for everything from dental caries, defective vision, and poor hearing to sexually transmitted diseases (including acquired immunodeficiency disease [AIDS]). Tertiary prevention—forestalling complications by effective treatment—is also greatly needed in vulnerable adolescent populations. Evidence suggests that preventive approaches are indicated at the primary care office, at school, and at home, and that more imaginative approaches to this task must be developed.

Early Intervention

With respect to psychological complaints, the accessibility of care and its responsiveness are significant. It has been demonstrated that many psychological complaints are never mentioned in the pediatric office because the parent or adolescent considers the caregiver uninterested or unequipped to handle such complaints (see Chapter 24). The practitioner signals his or her availability by asking routine questions in behavioral areas, by the use of questionnaires or behavioral computer-assisted investigation of emotional issues, and by active follow-up of positive answers. Unless useful responses are available, however, identification of psychological problems will be discouraged.

When to suspect that there is a psychological basis for symptomatology depends on (1) a readiness to consider such symptoms as a possibility, (2) a knowledge of typical symptom patterns that include a psychogenic cause, (3) knowledge of how to treat and the readiness to do so, and (4) a readiness to refer and a suitable pathway that will make referral likely to succeed (see Chapter 24). When the caregiver indicates that a psychological cause may explain the adolescent's difficulties, it is particularly important to include psychological factors among the initial differential possibilities presented to the adolescent and his or her family, rather than later as a matter of elimination. It is always easier if tests or consultations for psychopathologic conditions are included in the initial work-up, if such a possibility is as reasonable as any other. Similarly, including commonplace psychological formulations such as *stress* or *depression* in the differential diagnosis emphasizes the multifactorial nature of the cause. Modern views do indeed consider biologic and psychological factors as closely related (see Chapters 12–16); success in achieving the patient's acceptance of such formulations also lies in the caregiver's assertions, and justified belief, that psychological conditions are amenable to successful treatment and can often be considered preferable alternatives to more "respectable" purely organic conditions.

Acceptance of a psychological formulation will be much greater if the logic behind it and the data to support it are marshalled in as much detail as provided in a somatic diagnosis. The adolescent and his or her family should learn that a psychological diagnosis is made on positive grounds and not by exclusion. An eventual psychiatric assessment is made much harder if a series of dramatic investigatory procedures for physical illness is instituted first, since they tend to confirm a nonpsychological hypothesis in the patient's and the family's minds. Negative test results often do not convince; instead, they tend to confirm the probability of an organic cause in impressionable families (see Chapter 24).

Above all, psychological explanations must not be inadvertently presented as implied rejections of the patient and family. It is particularly important that psychological symptoms be mentioned in the context of expected treatment. They will not seem like rejections if they are presented with plans for the adolescent's further evaluation and care. Too often psychological symptoms are made trivial, as "just imaginary, all in your head," and so on, as if such a formulation will make the complaints vanish. It cannot be repeated too often that "psychological" complaints are (1) as real as any other symptoms (e.g., there is no such thing as "imaginary pain"); (2) as common as or more common than so-called somatic symptomatologies in the typical caregiver's office; and (3) at least as treatable as other pathologic conditions and often more so. If the caregiver is convinced of all these truths, the presentation to the patient and family will be much more likely to be accepted.

Treatment

A clear majority of "psychological" complaints, broadly construed, are treated in the primary caregiver's office (see Chapter 24). A host of complaints of psychological origin can be treated there, often with success. An important rule, then, is that referral need not be an automatic response to a psychiatric diagnosis. Rather, acknowledging that a problem is psychological should dictate a mutual decision as to the next step. Including the adolescent and family in that decision minimizes any potential sense of rejection. Emergency room studies have revealed that mutual decision-making should be stressed. Otherwise, it may appear, on the one hand, that referral is in fact rejection ("I do not want to go on caring for you"), or, on the other hand, that a failure to refer is dismissal ("Your problem does not warrant expert care—referral is not worth the trouble") (see Chapter 24).

Specific therapeutic approaches will be detailed for individual conditions. It is important to emphasize that the basic feature of most successful treatments is the human link between the adolescent and the caregiver—technique is less central than intent, which is to help the adolescent. Specifics of therapeutic technique too often eclipse the physician-patient relationship. In the end, for the treatment to be used and to be successful, the adolescent patient must want to comply.

Some specific problems in the therapeutic interview are mentioned in Chapter 22. Several generic problems occur in many relationships with adolescents. They include *splitting*—as already mentioned, this is a tendency for the adolescent to set adults concerned with his or her care against one another. As already noted, this occurs particularly in youngsters brought up with ongoing parental discord; it is also common in the borderline state (see Chapters 11 and 109). The fact that splitting has occurred may be signaled by a feeling in the caregiver of significant anger at another adult involved in the adolescent's care—parent or parents, other professional personnel, or other authority figures. The best solution for splitting is to confront it by direct contact among the individuals set at odds by the adolescent patient's care or basic situation. A second common problem is the *crush*—an intense attachment of the adolescent for another individual, often the therapist, which appears to have intense hetero- or homosexual content. Beneath the sexuality, however, one can usually discern the dependent nature of the relationship; it is this dependence that needs consideration and treatment. It is helpful to remember that extreme dependence in an adolescent is usually transient and at some level is abhorred by the adolescent as regressive behavior. Finally, *hostility* is a very common hazard in treatment of the adolescent. Curiously, it often reflects the very same process as the crush—that is, dependent feelings, which in this instance evoke anxiety and anger in the adolescent. Above all, the therapist who recognizes such hostility should avoid the understandable counterhostility it evokes. This does not mean that the caregiver must accept or tolerate abusive behavior; rather, it indicates a need for continued interpretation and reconfiguration of the treatment relationship.

Referral

It is important to stress that successful referral usually does *not* mean termination of the original treatment effort or relationship (see Chapter 24). This is true in referrals of all types, but is especially so in psychiatric matters because of the implied "value judgment" perceived by many or most adolescent patients and families. A psychopathologic condition is still generally perceived as failure in our society, so referral can be seen as rejection or abandonment.

When should referral occur? The time to refer is when the primary caregiver feels too uncomfortable (e.g., with a suicidal adolescent patient), uncertain (e.g., in an unclear diagnostic situation), inexperienced (e.g., in many psychopharmacologic applications), or overburdened (e.g., when more time will be required than the caregiver can invest). Referral may also be wise, at least for consultation, when one senses that one is "in over one's head"—that is, overinvolved, too caring, or too worried to make the necessary objective decisions. This may be especially common with long-term adolescent patients in pediatric practice.

Before referral, it is important to know the potential financial aspects of mental health care for the specific patient and his or her insurance coverage. It is embarrassing to make a referral only to discover that it is not financially feasible. One should recall that many insurance policies do not support mental health care, whether for ongoing treatment or simply for adequate diagnosis. Successful referrals require preparation by the caregiver to ascertain the availability of a suitable mental health professional for the needed care. The choice of a specific specialist often comes down to the question of availability. A consultation may be indicated simply to choose appropriate and available alternatives (see Chapter 24). In most geographic areas, there is a dearth of skilled psychiatrists, psychologists, or other professionals able to work effectively with an adolescent and his or her family. In such instances, consultation or coordinate care may be the only realistic solution. Competence is generally more important than specific professional identity; all things being equal, a competent professional will find ways to undertake the proper therapy. It is important to recognize, however, that a referral to certain resources carries an expectation of certain kinds of care. Too often a psychopharmacologically oriented psychiatrist is uninterested in the family support necessary to achieve compliance, whereas a family therapist may be indifferent to the worth of medication. Indeed, some "experts" often carry their positions to extremes, as when an inpatient facility "never" uses medications lest they "destroy the relationship," or a substance abuse facility "never" stresses the underlying pathologic condition for which the abused substances were self-medication. All these considerations heighten the need for the primary caregiver to stay actively involved until referral is successfully accomplished and necessary goals have been achieved.

Given the nature of psychological complaints, some referrals are bound to fail (see Chapter 24). In these cases, a continuing relationship with the primary caregiver is essential, permitting reevaluation of the problem and assessment of a more constructive alternative solution. This is why scheduling a follow-up visit by the primary caregiver should be routine. At times, the best referral fails because it becomes a power struggle among the patient, parents, and the caregiver. In such an instance, consultation with the mental health specialist can help determine whether or not alternative approaches (e.g., parent counseling) might be more successful.

At other times, it may be apparent that a particular therapist is the "wrong fit" for the adolescent patient. If an alternative is available, the primary caregiver who has stayed in touch with the situation is in the best position to limit the damage and make the change.

Finally, if no more appropriate alternative can be found, the only solution may be for the primary caregiver to render the ongoing care. In this instance, indirect consultation with a skilled mental health practitioner may bring success (see Chapter 24). Groups of pediatricians have counseled one another in the treatment of mental health problems, often quite ably; it is frequently easier to perceive what is required in treatment if one is not immersed in it. At other times, issues of psychosis or safety may supervene. Here, again, consultation with a skilled mental health professional may guide the primary caregiver to a successful resolution of a difficult problem.

In all instances, the investment of the primary caretaker must be in the adolescent patient and his or her family *as individuals* rather than "cases." Such an investment is not only essential for success but also is ultimately among the greatest gratifications in adolescent care.

BIBLIOGRAPHY

Beck A: Beck Depression Inventory: Center for Cognitive Therapy, 133 S. 36th Street, Philadelphia, PA 19104.

Conners CK: Conners Parent-Teacher Questionnaire. New York, Plenum Publishing, 1978.

Goldstein SE, Yager J, Heinicke CM, Pynoos RS (eds): Preventing Mental Health Dysfunctions in Childhood, Sect III. Washington, DC, American Psychiatric Association, 1990.

Green M, Haggerty RJ (eds): Ambulatory Pediatrics 4. Philadelphia, WB Saunders, 1990.

Jellinek MS, Herzog DB (eds): Psychiatric Aspects of General Hospital Pediatrics. Chicago, Yearbook Publishers, 1990.

Prugh DG: The Psychosocial Aspects of Pediatrics. Philadelphia, Lea & Febiger, 1983.

CHAPTER 99

Psychological Assessment of Adolescents

RICHARD J. LAWLOR

GENERAL CONSIDERATIONS

Erikson describes adolescence as a normative crisis of development and suggests that the purpose of this period (consisting of 1 decade or longer) is the ultimate development of a stable sense of identity (see Chapter 9). Many fluctuations in functioning will be seen along the way to achieving this sense of identity. These minor fluctuations are normal and do not indicate the presence of a psychopathologic condition. Adolescence, however, is not a period of universal turmoil, and the presence of chronic distress is an indication of psychological difficulty and the need for evaluation of the underlying problem (see Chapter 8). Parents of such adolescents often seek advice from physicians; one component of assessment is often a referral for psychological testing. Testing, in conjunction with a full psychological or psychiatric evaluation, can often assist in the development of a proper diagnosis of the problem (see Chapter 8) and can lead to effective recommendations for treatment or intervention.

TYPICAL REASONS FOR REFERRAL

Typical referral questions are generally related to issues of cognitive functioning that often become manifested in academic performance, behavioral problems, disturbances of mood and affect, problems with thinking or thought processing, or psychosomatic or eating disorders. Alternatively, the referral may be needed to determine the depth and extent of personality disorganization. Cognitive functioning difficulties usually relate to issues of intellectual competence or learning disabilities (see Chapter 107). Behavioral problems are typically associated with one of the disruptive disorders of adolescence (see Chapter 108), personality disorders (see Chapter 109), or substance abuse problems (see Chapter 111). Depressive and anxiety disorders of adolescence are a significant problem in this age group (see Chapters 100, 102, and 103) and can severely interfere with academic functioning, achievement of normal developmental milestones, and development of a stable sense of identity. Although far less common, psychotic disorders (see Chapter 110) may pervasively disrupt cognitive skills, emotional functioning, and thought processes and content. Finally, adolescents may present with symptoms suggestive of somatization disorder (see Chapter 112), conversion disorder (see Chapter 112), eating disorder (see Chapter 60), psychogenic pain disorder (see Chapter 113), factitious disorder (see Chapter 112), or malingering. Because adolescents with these psychiatric problems almost always present to the physician because of unconscious or denied psychological conflict, psychological testing may be most useful. Psychological testing and a complete psychological or psychiatric examination is often a crucial part of the evaluation. Testing is uniquely helpful in several situations. Interviewing may fail to elicit information because of the adolescent's resistance, inability to verbalize effectively, or lack of insight into the problem (see Chapter 98). Testing can often help clarify the underlying problem. Testing is also particularly helpful in adolescents who may be in the prodromal stage of an emotional disorder when the overt manifestations are not yet clear. Testing can suggest or identify the underlying conflict or disturbance. At times one must know the specific level of ability or achievement so that an adolescent patient's capacity to understand medical regimens or to participate effectively in treatment can be assessed. Finally, testing is often extremely useful in clarifying the underlying dynamics of the problem when interviewing has not been successful. Physicians who have an understanding of the process of psychological testing will be better able to maximize the effectiveness and usefulness of the examination.

INITIATING THE PSYCHOLOGICAL REFERRAL

Defining the Role of the Psychologist

Since most physicians have had limited experience working with mental health professionals (psychologists, psychiatrists, psychiatric social workers, psychometricians, or special education consultants), and since most mental health professionals have even less experience working with adolescents within a medical context, it is critical that the referral process and the expectations of both professionals are clear. It is important that the mental health consultant know the specific reasons for the consultation. For example, is the consultee seeking strictly an evaluation and opinion regarding diagnosis or is the request also that the psychologist undertake therapy with the adolescent? Should the psychologist or the referring physician present the results of the evaluation to the adolescent and his or her parents? Sometimes the referring physician may wish to present the findings jointly with the psychologist. These issues should be clarified early in the consultation process to help assure a smooth and effective evaluation.

Specifically, the psychologist needs to know the physician's, the adolescent's, and the family's perceptions of the presenting problems. These perspectives may differ. Previous psychological evaluations (especially if recent) are important. Knowledge of previous testing may avoid a duplication of certain tests. In other circumstances it may be appropriate to compare the current results with those of a previous evaluation, making repetition necessary. At times the referring physician already has extensive family and other background information; this information may be very useful to the consulting psychologist. At other times there may be little background information, and an extensive family and developmental history will be needed as part of the psychological assessment.

Prior to the evaluation, the physician must discuss with the adolescent and his or her parents the proposed psychological evaluation, the reasons for the request and, in a general way, the proposed uses of the expected information. Sometimes the adolescent and his or her parents may be resistant. The physician can almost always deal with it in an unhurried discussion with them (see Chapters 24 and 98). One must obtain parental permission. This is especially important in inpatient settings in which the parents may not always be present and consultations may proceed rapidly.

Once these preliminary issues are completed, the most important task is to clarify, delineate, and at times reformulate the referral questions into ones that are sufficiently specific to be amenable to psychological evaluation. For example, a general request for a "personality evaluation" of an adolescent whose school performance has declined suddenly cannot be addressed in a useful way by any particular test or combination of tests. Information that is useful to the referring physician can be obtained if the question is rephrased into more specific questions addressing issues such as possible depression, an underlying thought disorder, or preoccupation with marital conflict within the family.

The psychologist may need to help the physician refine the referral questions in order to perform a meaningful evaluation. Telephone contact can easily bring clarification and can allow the physician to elaborate the initial referral questions. It will also help the psychologist to understand and clearly address the concerns of the physician (see Chapter 24).

Table 99–1 presents a suggested format for requesting a psychological evaluation.

SPECIFIC ASSESSMENT INSTRUMENTS

An exhaustive review of the psychological literature on tests available for specific types of assessments is

TABLE 99–1. Request for Psychological Evaluation

Presenting problem or problems
  Prior psychological evaluation and treatment
  Brief summary of adolescent's background
Perception of problem
  As viewed by physician, adolescent, parent
  Might inpatient treatment be necessary?
Specific questions to be answered
  Direct contact with psychologist may be useful
Expectations for service
  Evaluation only
    Psychologist presents results, physician presents results, both present results
  Evaluation and recommendations for treatment; indicate if you need assistance with identifying services
  Evaluation and treatment

beyond the scope of this chapter, but the most common general areas of assessment and some of the leading tests in these areas can be reviewed briefly.

Intellectual Functioning

Wechsler Scales

The most commonly used tests of intelligence employed in clinical settings are the various Wechsler Scales. They consist of three different scales that are used with individuals from 2 years of age through late adulthood. The scales used with younger and older adolescents are the Wechsler Intelligence Scale for Children—Revised (WISC-R; 1974) and the Wechsler Adult Intelligence Scale—Revised (WAIS-R; 1981). These tests are administered individually and yield three separate scores: a verbal intelligence quotient (IQ) score, a performance IQ score, and a full-scale IQ score. The tests do not cover every aspect of cognitive functioning, but they do provide a valid predictor of ability and potential for success in an academic environment. Various patterns of scores on individual subtests of these scales often provide useful information about personality functioning and can generate hypotheses for further evaluation of neuropsychological (cortical) functioning. Discrepancies between the verbal and the performance scales and the degree of variation of subscales within the verbal and performance scales provide useful information about specific areas of cognitive strengths or weaknesses. This information may be useful in order to help the physician better understand the adolescent's specific areas of difficulty.

Academic Achievement

Many tests assess levels of school or academic performance. In conjunction with measures of intellectual or cognitive ability, they can provide important information about a potential learning disability, reasons for academic underachievement, an inability to learn and follow a medical treatment regimen, or an ability to benefit from specific types of academic or therapeutic programs. Some of the more common tests include the Wide Range Achievement Test—Revised (WRAT-R), the Peabody Individual Achievement Test—Revised, and the Woodcock-Johnson Psycho-Educational Battery. Each of these tests measures somewhat different aspects of academic functioning, such as word recognition, reading, comprehension, spelling, mathematics, written language skills, knowledge of the world, and so on. The pattern of scores is often helpful in determining whether poor academic performance is due to cognitive deficits, emotional problems, drug or alcohol involvement, learning disabilities, behavior problems, or motivational difficulties.

Neuropsychological Assessment

In the past 25 years, significant advances have occurred through psychological techniques, in the assessment of brain-behavior relationships (see Chapter 10). These neuropsychological assessment techniques can shed light on more specific organic (cortical) deficits that underlie learning disabilities following head injuries or toxic brain conditions and help elucidate possible organic factors that might be involved in certain psychopathologic conditions. Neuropsychological results can also provide baseline data from which to measure and plan cognitive rehabilitation programs. It may be important and necessary to differentiate between functional illness and an acute or chronic neurologic impairment in order to decide whether psychological, medical, or surgical intervention is required.

The three most common batteries of tests currently used in assessment of adolescents are the Halstead-Reitan Battery for Children (used for younger adolescents through age 14 years), the Halstead-Reitan Neuropsychological Battery (used for adolescents 15 years and older and adults), and the Luria Nebraska Battery. Each of these batteries consists of many individual tests or scales designed to assess specific sensory, perceptual, motor, and cognitive functions. Patterns and levels of functioning on each of the tests are assessed; the psychologist makes comparisons across tests and hypotheses about strengths and weaknesses in underlying cortical functioning. These findings then lead to specific suggestions regarding either remediation or development of alternative methods for helping the adolescent perform in the areas in which deficits appear.

There are also many other individual tests of various aspects of neuropsychological functioning that are sometimes used by neuropsychologists to assess specific areas of brain-behavior functioning or to complete the testing battery, or both. Personality functioning is often assessed in neuropsychology laboratories; the most common test used is the Minnesota Multiphasic Personality Inventory (MMPI), though some laboratories also use various projective tests (see further on).

Personality Functioning

STRUCTURED TESTS AND BEHAVIORAL CHECKLISTS

Hundreds of specific tests are available to evaluate various aspects of personality functioning and traits of adolescents. They range from self-report scales, checklists, and structured tests with various age group norms, to projective tests of various types. These tests may be used singly or in combination with batteries designed to comprehensively assess many dimensions of the adolescent's personality functioning.

The most widely used and researched of the structured objective personality tests given to adolescents is the MMPI, which consists of 566 statements to be endorsed by the adolescent as true or false. This instrument was developed with adults in the late 1930s; adolescent norms began to be used widely in the 1960s and 1970s. If an adolescent as young as 12 or 13 years of age has at least a sixth-grade reading level, it is possible to use this instrument to assess a wide variety of personality states and traits. It is also expected that an adolescent version of the new MMPI-2 will be available soon.

Other objective measures that are sometimes used with adolescents include the Personality Inventory for Children, the Millon Adolescent Personality Inventory, and the Child Behavior Checklist. The Personality Inventory for Children can be used with adolescents up to age 16 years and is a 600-item true or false inventory that is completed by the child's parent or caretaker. The test itself measures a variety of intellectual and emotional areas and is especially useful in the early stages of assessment for helping to isolate particular problem areas for further study.

The Millon Adolescent Personality Inventory is designed to overcome what some psychologists see as the primarily adult focus of the questions on the MMPI. The questions on the Millon Inventory reflect more the concerns and language of teenagers. It is also shorter (150 true or false items) than the MMPI and thus can hold the attention of some adolescents more easily, especially those with psychoses or attention disorders. It yields measures of various personality styles, expressed concerns of the adolescent, and various behavioral problem areas.

The Child Behavior Checklist assesses both social competencies and behavioral problem areas. The parent rates 113 descriptive statements on a three-point scale ranging from not true to frequent. This test is useful primarily in defining areas for further assessment.

PROJECTIVE TESTS

Although not as widely used as in the past, projective techniques, such as the Rorschach, various thematic tests, and measures using incomplete sentence blanks, can provide useful information, especially if one suspects the presence of an underlying thought disorder. The underlying assumption of all devices in this category is that the adolescent will respond to relatively ambiguous stimulus situations (such as inkblots, less than fully clear pictures, or the stems of sentences) by projecting his or her own personality traits, concerns, and states onto the stimulus.

The Rorschach consists of ten cards, each containing a symmetrical inkblot. The adolescent responds by conveying what the blot looks like to him or her. Various complicated scoring systems are used with this test. The interpretive approaches range from assessing underlying personality dynamics to the more narrow focus of using the test as a strictly perceptual-cognitive task designed to assess the adolescent's perceptual-cognitive style. The clinician then attempts to generalize from these styles ways in which the adolescent is likely to respond to various situations outside the test setting.

Thematic tests consist of a variety of different sets of pictures to which the adolescent is asked to respond by telling a story about what is going on, the people's behaviors and feelings, and the likely outcome of the story. Again, the projective hypothesis is that the adolescent will project his or her personality functioning.

The most widely used of the many thematic tests is the original Thematic-Apperception Test. This test is believed to identify important needs, conflicts, and pressures within the personality. The test has no accepted scoring system and is generally used by clinicians to develop hypotheses about underlying personality dynamics, which are later investigated through other psychometric tests and interviews.

Sentence completion tests require adolescents to complete the sentence based upon a stem presented to them. The way the sentence is completed is thought to reflect underlying concerns, preoccupations, attitudes, and feelings—the most frequently used version for adolescents is the Rotter Incomplete Sentence Blank—High School Form. Again the responses are generally useful to develop hypotheses that require further evaluation.

MENTAL STATUS EXAMINATION

The mental status examination is a formal interview technique that allows the clinician to thoroughly assess various aspects of the adolescent's mental functioning and includes the following categories: appearance and behavior, affect and mood, speech and thought perceptions, orientation, memory and concentration, intelligence, and insight and judgment. This chapter will not cover the details of the mental status examination; however, this examination provides a useful technique for obtaining a picture of the adolescent's functioning in several areas at a given time. As such, it can be used for comparison with previous or subsequent levels of functioning.

PSYCHOLOGICAL REPORT

Psychological reports range from brief (less than one page) summaries of the results of the psychological evaluation to lengthy multipage documents. The basics of any report will include specific reasons for the referral and the specific questions to be assessed, the instruments used, behavioral observations of the adolescent during the testing, the test results and interpretation, and a summary, along with conclusions and recommendations. It is important that the report clearly address the questions that were raised, even if all questions cannot be adequately answered. The report should proceed from the original problems and questions to conclusions about these problems, with recommendations for how the problem can best be addressed.

The report should be addressed to the referring clinician but should be written with as little "jargon" as possible so that its information can be shared meaningfully with the adolescent and the family. Under ordinary circumstances, both the adolescent and his or her parents should participate in a feedback session in which the results and recommendations are clearly and thoroughly discussed and some agreement is reached on how to proceed. There are circumstances, particularly when an adolescent may be psychotic, when the physician may wish to present the detailed, comprehensive feedback to the parents and only involve the adolescent in a brief summary presentation of the findings and results. It is important to allow sufficient time for the family to raise questions and to deal with both the informational and emotional impact of the results. Each family member should be involved in these discussions, and any differences in understanding, reactions to, and expectations should be thoroughly explored. If these issues are adequately dealt with, there is a greater likelihood of acceptance and follow-through with the recommendations. A careful, comprehensive disposition conference will ensure that the family is satisfied and that the results of the psychological evaluation are useful in identifying a treatment for the adolescent.

BIBLIOGRAPHY

Achenbach TM: The classification of children's psychiatric symptoms: A factor-analytic study. Psychol Monogr, 80:1, 1966.

Erikson E: Identity: Youth and Crisis. New York, WW Norton, 1968.

Exner JE: The Rorschach: A Comprehensive System, Vol 1. Basic Foundations. New York, John Wiley & Sons, 1986.

Marks PA, Seeman W, Haller D: The Actuarial Use of the MMPI with Adolescents and Adults. Baltimore, Williams & Wilkins, 1974.

Millon T, Green CJ, Meagher RB, Jr. Millon Adolescent Personality Inventory. Minneapolis, MN, National Computer Systems, 1977.

Rotter JB, Rafferty JE, Lotsof AB: The validity of the Rotter Incomplete Sentences Blank, High School Form. J Consult Psychol 18:105, 1954.

Siassi I: Psychiatric interviews and mental status examinations. In Goldstein G, Hersen M (eds): Handbook of Psychological Assessment. New York, Pergamon, 1984, (pp 259–275).

Wechsler D: WAIS-R Manual: Wechsler Adult Intelligence Scale—revised. New York, Psychological Corporation, 1981.

Wirt RD, Lachar D, Klinedinst JK, Seat PD: Multidimensional Description of Child Personality: A Manual for the Personality Inventory for Children. Los Angeles, Western Psychological Services, 1977.

Disorders of Mood and Affect

CHAPTER 100

Depression: Unipolar and Bipolar

NEAL D. RYAN

It is only over the past 2 decades that systematic research has considered whether children and adolescents experience depressive disorders, and if so, whether they are related to adult depressive disorders. This is in sharp contrast to the great strides that have been made in the study of adult depression throughout this century. In part, the delay in studying juvenile-onset depression resulted from excessive reliance on psychological theories that remained totally untested long after adult psychiatry had benefited from a strong nosologic and descriptive approach. These theories postulated that children lacked the necessary psychological structures or cognitive abilities to become truly depressed. Since depression was theoretically not possible, systematic exploration for it was delayed.

Depression, like all other psychiatric disorders, is a syndrome for which we do not yet know the pathophysiologic cause. Nevertheless, starting in the mid-1970s, investigators examined several clinic-referred populations to study whether there were children and adolescents who fit adult criteria for major depression (which at that time were the Research Diagnostic Criteria (RDC) and Diagnostic and Statistical Manual of Mental Disorders: Third Edition [DSM-III] criteria, which for affective disorders were similar to the present Diagnostic and Statistical Manual of Mental Disorders: Third Edition–Revised [DSM-III-R] criteria). Once depressed children were identified, studies to define the similarities or differences between the adult and juvenile forms of this disorder were initiated.

Obviously, syndromic similarity does not guarantee that adult and child and adolescent forms of a disorder are related. For example, an entirely reasonable hypothesis is that children and adolescents might fit adult criteria for major depression or other mood disorders and yet on longitudinal follow-up have a brief, time-limited disorder or a disorder that does not recur in the adult pattern. As discussed further on, this is not the case, and there are multiple lines of evidence suggesting strong continuity from childhood through adolescence and on to adult forms of depression and bipolar disorder.

Even if child and adolescent forms of mood disorders are related to adult forms, there is no *a priori* reason why there should not be systematic differences in the symptomatic picture with physical and psychological maturation. Without specific testable hypotheses about the variation of symptomatology with maturation during adolescence, largely unmodified adult criteria have been employed in most studies of juvenile depression. The possibility remains, however, that as we understand the pathophysiology of adolescent depression, we will indeed determine that the symptomatic picture varies with age.

"Masked depression" was hypothesized when it was believed unlikely that children and adolescents showed adult forms of depression. It was believed that the same disorder across the age span had a dramatically different presentation in childhood, a "masked" presentation. As already discussed, this was a reasonable hypothesis. Unfortunately, however, there were no systematic criteria for deciding which child or adolescent had a masked depression. Basically, masked depression was all-inclusive. Conduct problems (see Chapter 108), hyperactivity (see Chapter 106), enuresis, encopresis, and other childhood psychiatric disorders all were proposed as masked depressions. Thus, the concept was too broad and all-inclusive to be testable. Recent data do not support the concept that most disturbances of behavior are indeed related to depressive disorders, though it is certainly a possibility in some cases.

EPIDEMIOLOGY

There has been no ideal study to assess the prevalence of the incidence of affective disorders in children and adolescents. Previous studies have included a number of methodologic limitations, including (1) relatively small sample sizes, (2) use of instruments that were not designed to identify depression and are not particularly informative about the core symptoms of depression, (3) obtaining information only from the adolescent and not from the parents, (4) low response rate, and (5) wide variation in the definition of what constitutes a case. The National Institute of Mental Health (NIMH) has begun the pilot phase of a project to study the epidemiology of child and adolescent psychiatric disorders in multiple sites.

Within the methodologic limitations of past studies, there is some convergence of the data. The prevalence of major depressive disorder in prepubertal children is between 1% and 3% and the male-to-female ratio is approximately 1:1, with a predominance of males in some studies. In adolescents the rate in most studies is higher, ranging from less than 1% to 6%. Most investigators report a 4% to 6% point prevalence or 6-month prevalence of major depressive disorder in adolescents. If dysthymic disorder and other depressive syndromes that are not sufficiently severe to meet the criteria for major depression are included, the rate approximately doubles. There seems to be a slight preponderance of girls over boys in the rates of major depressive disorder in adolescence.

Bipolar affective disorder is rare throughout life with an estimated lifetime prevalence of approximately 1%. It is extremely rare for this disorder to occur before puberty. The period of greatest onset is between 15 and 25 years of age. Because depression is relatively less frequent in children and adolescents than in adults, the percentage of children and adolescents who present with a major depression and who will eventually have bipolar disease is much greater than the percentage of adults who present with a major depression for the first time and who will subsequently have bipolar disease. One study estimated that 20% or more of first-episode depression that presents during elementary school will, upon follow-up, turn out to be bipolar disease.

DIAGNOSTIC CRITERIA

Overview

As already discussed, adult criteria are used to diagnose affective syndromes in children and adolescents with very minor variations made in the threshold values for a few criteria symptoms. The current criteria are from the DSM-III-R, and in the next few years they will be taken from the DSM-IV. Nevertheless, the majority of adolescents diagnosed with major depression or bipolar disorder fit the same category by any of these classification schemes. Learning current criteria is likely to serve the clinician well for a decade or more.

DSM-III-R, the current official manual of mental disorders of the American Psychiatric Association, defines a *mood syndrome* as a group of mood and associated symptoms that occur together for a minimal time. A mood episode is a mood syndrome that is not caused by known organic factors and is not part of a nonaffective psychotic disorder (e.g., schizophrenia). A mood disorder is the pattern of mood episodes. The diagnosis of mania (described in detail further on) requires a manic mood episode and, in general, one or more depressive mood episodes. The mood disorder diagnosis of recurrent major depression requires one or more episodes of major depression and no episode of mania. Following the pattern of the DSM-III-R, a description is made of different types of mood episodes, and then mood disorders are defined from them.

Depression

A *major depressive episode* is defined by the DSM-III-R as the presence of at least five of nine symptoms at the same time for at least a 2-week period that represents a change in previous level of functioning. One of the five symptoms required must be either depressed mood or loss of interest or pleasure (Table 100-1).

The nine symptoms that meet the criteria for a major depressive episode are (1) *depressed or irritable mood*

TABLE 100–1. Criteria for Major Depression and Bipolar Disorder

MAJOR DEPRESSION

Diagnosis requires five symptoms for at least a 2-week period with the presence of symptom No. 1 or No. 2 required.
1. Depressed or irritable mood
2. Diminished interest or pleasure
3. Weight loss or weight gain
4. Insomnia or hypersomnia
5. Psychomotor agitation or retardation
6. Fatigue or loss of energy
7. Feelings of worthlessness or excessive guilt
8. Decreased concentration or indecisiveness
9. Thoughts of death, suicidal ideation, or suicide attempt

BIPOLAR DISORDER

Diagnosis requires one or more manic episodes, which are periods of abnormally and persistently elevated, expansive, or irritable mood with at least three of the following symptoms:
1. Inflated self-esteem or grandiosity
2. Decreased need for sleep
3. More talkative or pressured speech
4. Flight of ideas or racing thoughts
5. Distractibility
6. Increased goal-directed activity
7. Excessive involvement in pleasurable activities with a high potential for painful consequences

Adapted with permission from American Psychiatric Association: Diagnostic and Statistical Manual of Mental Disorders, 3rd ed., revised. Washington, DC, American Psychiatric Association, 1987, pp 217, 222.

in adolescents most of the day nearly every day as indicated by the adolescent patient's self-report or the observation of others, (2) diminished interest or pleasure in all or almost all activities most of the day nearly every day (this symptom is also called *anhedonia*), (3) significant weight loss or weight gain when not dieting or a decrease or increase in appetite nearly every day (in adolescents consider failure to make expected weight gains), (4) insomnia or hypersomnia nearly every day, (5) psychomotor agitation or retardation nearly every day, (6) fatigue or loss of energy nearly every day, (7) feelings of worthlessness or excessive or inappropriate guilt, (8) diminished ability to think or concentrate or indecisiveness, and (9) recurrent thoughts of death, recurrent suicidal ideation, or a suicide attempt or specific plan for committing suicide. The only two changes made to the adult criteria when applying these guidelines to adolescents are (1) to allow irritable mood to stand for the equivalent of a depressed mood as the first symptom and as one of the two necessary criteria (along with inability to experience pleasure), and (2) to allow failure to make expected weight gains as equivalent to the adult weight loss criterion.

Each episode within major depressive episodes is further subcategorized as either melancholic or nonmelancholic. The criteria for the melancholic subtype includes the presence of at least five of the following nine symptoms: (1) loss of interest or pleasure in all or almost all activities, (2) lack of reaction to usually pleasurable stimuli, (3) depression regularly worse in the morning, (4) early morning awakening (at least 2 hours before usual time of awakening), (5) psychomotor retardation or agitation, (6) significant anorexia or weight loss, (7) no significant personality disturbance before first major depressive episode, (8) one or more previous major depressive episodes followed by complete or nearly complete recovery, and (9) previous good response to adequate specific psychopharmacologic therapy.

The significance of the presence or lack of a melancholic subtype in adolescent depression is not well established. Clinically, adolescents with the melancholic subtype experience the most severe depressions, and at least one study has indicated they may paradoxically have a poorer response to somatic therapies. In addition, it is clear that the criteria for the melancholic subtype are designed for adult patients and are not as directly applicable to youthful depressive disorder. Adolescents with depression are likely to present during their first episode, even though in most the disease recurs multiple times, so they are less likely to have had full recovery after prior episodes or to have been previously treated with antidepressants. By DSM-III-R criteria, personality disorders cannot be diagnosed until early adulthood, and so the criteria of no personality disorder is not meaningful for adolescents.

The diagnosis of a major depressive disorder requires one or more major depressive episodes and no lifetime episode of mania (see further on). It is subcategorized into single-episode and recurrent types.

Dysthymia

The diagnosis of dysthymia requires a persistent, depressed mood most of the day more days than not for a period of at least 1 year, with associated depressive symptoms, but these symptoms must be of insufficient severity to meet the criteria for major depression. The adolescent must not have been free of symptoms of depression for more than 2 months during the interval. The diagnosis is not made if there is evidence of the adolescent's meeting the full syndromal criteria for major depression during the first year of the disorder. There also must be at least two of the following symptoms in addition to the depressed mood: (1) poor appetite or overeating, (2) insomnia or hypersomnia, (3) low energy or fatigue, (4) low self-esteem, (5) poor concentration or difficulty making decisions, and (6) feelings of hopelessness or helplessness.

According to the DSM-III-R, "The boundaries of dysthymia with major depression are unclear, particularly in children and adolescents." It appears that adolescents who first meet criteria for dysthymia subsequently experience a major depression (by definition after more than a year of the persistent low-grade dysthymia). They probably have a particularly morbid course, with more episodes of major depression and little time fully recovered from the depression and dysthymia.

Bipolar Disorder

A manic episode is defined by the presence of a period of abnormally and persistently elevated, expansive, or irritable mood in the presence of at least three of the following seven symptoms (four are required if the mood is irritable but not elevated or expansive):

(1) inflated self-esteem or grandiosity, (2) decreased need for sleep, (3) more talkative than usual or pressured to keep talking, (4) flight of ideas or subjective experience that thoughts are racing, (5) distractibility, (6) increase in goal-directed activity (either socially, at work or school, or sexually) or psychomotor agitation, and (7) excessive involvement in pleasurable activities that have a high potential for painful consequences.

If the mood disturbance is sufficiently severe to cause marked functional impairment in school, social activities, or relationships with others or is severe enough to require hospitalization, the episode is a manic one; otherwise, the episode is a hypomanic one. Just as for a diagnosis of major depression, the criteria for a manic or hypomanic episode require that at no time should there have been 2 weeks or more of delusions or hallucinations without the presence of prominent mood symptoms (a symptom that would indicate a disorder in the schizophrenic spectrum). In addition, the disorder must not be superimposed on schizophrenia or a schizophreniform disorder or other psychotic disorder, and the disturbance must not be initiated and maintained by an organic factor. The DSM-III-R notes specifically that somatic antidepressant treatment, including tricyclic antidepressants, other antidepressants, and electroconvulsive therapy (ECT) that precipitate mania are not considered causative organic factors and so do not rule out the diagnosis of mania.

The diagnosis of bipolar disorder (also called manic-depressive disorder) requires one or more manic episodes over a lifetime and virtually always is accompanied by one or more depressive episodes over the lifetime. However, the first affective episode certainly can be that of mania, so the diagnosis can be made at the first episode of mania even if a depressive episode has not yet occurred. Bipolar disorder is subclassified into (1) mixed, in which symptoms of mania and depression are intermixed or alternating every few days or less in the current episode; (2) manic, in which the current episode is a manic episode; and (3) depressive, in which the current episode is a depressive episode.

Cyclothymia

The DSM-III-R defines cyclothymia as a chronic mood disturbance of at least 1 year's duration involving numerous hypomanic episodes and numerous periods of depressed mood or anhedonia of insufficient severity or duration to meet the criteria for a major depressive disorder. Although this disorder does occur in adolescents, it is probably rare and almost entirely unstudied in this age group.

DIAGNOSIS

The criteria symptoms that compose the various affective disorders according to the current classificatory schema DSM-III-R are described in detail in the following paragraphs. The criteria for major depression and bipolar disorder are summarized in Table 100–1. Other affective disorders (e.g., dysthymia without superimposed major depression and cyclothymia) are poorly studied in adolescents and therefore will not be discussed at length.

Differential Diagnosis

The differential diagnosis of major depression includes alcohol abuse, substance abuse, cocaine or stimulant withdrawal (see Chapter 111), endocrinopathies (see Chapter 55), medication side effects (e.g., reserpine, steroids), and, very rarely, occult malignancies. Primary sleep disorders with irritability may be confused with depression (see Chapter 86). The prodromal phase of schizophrenia (Chapter 110), obsessive-compulsive disorder (see Chapter 105), and other psychiatric disorders may also provide a psychiatric picture that is difficult to classify and may be diagnosed as major depression, only becoming clarified with the progression of time.

Adjustment disorder with depressed mood is a diagnosis made only after a psychosocial stressor that could reasonably be expected to cause disturbance of affect and if the symptomatic picture does not meet the threshold for major depression. If the symptom complex becomes severe enough to meet the criteria for major depression, that diagnosis is made regardless of the presence or lack of a precipitating event.

The differential diagnosis of bipolar disorder includes other psychotic disorders (especially schizophrenia), and hallucinations of organic cause (hallucinogens, phencyclidine piperdine [PCP], and so on). In younger children, the differential diagnosis of bipolar disorder and attention deficit hyperactive disorder may be particularly difficult and, again, may only be clarified with time.

Assessment of Symptoms of Depression and Mania

Although, as already presented, virtually the same diagnostic criteria are applied to depression in adolescents as are applied in adults, different assessment techniques are required.

The clinician should interview both the parents and the adolescent (see Chapter 98). In general, the best information is obtained if the two are interviewed separately at some point during the evaluation. When interviewed together exclusively, data vital to making the diagnoses may be frequently censored by one or the other party. Multiple studies have uniformly found that the parent and the adolescent provide different, largely nonoverlapping data. Not infrequently, the adolescent will be a better informant about the internal affective state (i.e., depressed mood or inability to experience pleasure) and the parents are better informants about the adolescent's behavior (angry outbursts, decreased socialization, and so on). However, no general rule can be given as to how to combine the data from parent and adolescent; the clinician must use his or her best clinical judgment, which varies from symptom to symptom and from adolescent to adolescent.

Although contact with the teacher and school system is frequently helpful in the diagnosis of a disorder, the teacher's report, except to note falling grades, is not in general a critical issue in making the diagnosis of depression. This is in sharp contrast to the diagnosis of attention deficit disorder with hyperactivity, in which information from the adolescent's teacher is almost essential for the diagnosis. Teachers may not observe disturbances of mood as well as they observe disturbances of behavior.

Interview with the Adolescent

Although the same symptomatic criteria are used, the interview techniques appropriate to an adult require some modification for the adolescent patient.

Assessment of the cognitive ability of the adolescent is important. Certainly, the younger adolescent may be confused by abstract psychological concepts. Obviously, the clinician has to determine the symptoms by asking questions in terms familiar to the individual adolescent. The less cognitively mature adolescent may have an idiosyncratic description of his or her own dysphoric affective state and may not generalize it into the term *depression*. An example will make this clear. One adolescent, when asked if he felt sad or depressed replied "no." When asked if he was blue, he replied "yes." These questions were repeated, with the same answers. Finally when asked to clarify, he explained that he felt depressed after his grandfather died. The major depression that he was now experiencing was a bad feeling, but a different feeling; therefore, it was not a depressed feeling, it was a blue feeling. He was unable to generalize that two different dysphoric feelings could both be described as "depressed."

A frequent issue arises in the assessment of insomnia in which the adolescent reports difficulty falling asleep, yet the parent says he or she has looked in and the adolescent has been sleeping well and does not seem to have difficulty falling asleep. The report of the adolescent qualifies for the disturbance of sleep symptom despite the parent's failure to confirm it. In other words, it is likely the adolescent is reporting lighter sleep, more awakenings, nonrestorative sleep (failure to feel refreshed after sleep), or some other sleep-related problem, even though when periodically observed by the parent, the adolescent is not uniformly awake.

The symptom of decreased concentration is frequently manifested in impaired grades. However, the possibility that the adolescent experiences this symptom should not be dismissed simply because good grades are maintained. For example, one adolescent, the child of immigrant Korean greengrocers, maintained straight As only by studying 6 hours a night rather than the usual 2 hours.

A frequent error occurs in assessing how much of the day the adolescent is depressed when the adolescent says that he or she feels depressed, for example, 2 hours a day. If this line of questioning stops here, the interviewer will miss the fact that this is frequently the report of an adolescent who feels severely depressed 2 hours a day but has persistent depression the entire rest of the day. If, in contrast, the adolescent is asked whether the rest of the time he or she feels normal or whether he or she feels better but still quite depressed, this fluctuating mood that never reaches euthymia will be readily elicited. It cannot be overemphasized how frequently this error is seen and how readily the adolescent can clearly respond when questioned in this manner.

Although the experienced clinician may make few errors in the assessment of suicidal inclination, the young clinician trainee frequently makes the following error: An adolescent reports suicidal thoughts or plans (see Chapter 101). The interviewer becomes markedly anxious and looks for any alternative hypothesis other than that the adolescent is indeed suicidal. The interviewer then asks questions like, "You are not really thinking about hurting yourself are you? You are just saying that to get attention are you not?" This makes it clear to the adolescent that the interviewer does not want to hear the truth. The adolescent will then agree that this was merely an attempt to get attention, and the symptom will not be correctly evaluated. Certainly some adolescents report suicidal thoughts or plans merely to get attention, but assuming that this is the explanation forecloses obtaining the truth. The appropriate response is that it is important for the adolescent and the clinician to discuss these feelings because the clinician wants to help the young person receive the appropriate care. Without unbiased, open-ended questioning, one could easily convey to the adolescent that the interviewer does not want to hear about these thoughts or plans that are frightening to both the adolescent and the interviewer.

Once the clinician thinks about the possibility of an adolescent having mania, the diagnosis is usually relatively clear. The presentation for evaluation is frequently a result of dangerous impulsive behavior. In distinction to the adolescent with impulsive behavior secondary to hyperactivity, this is not usually a lifelong trait but more typically a disorder with a relatively distinct onset.

Symptoms of mania this author has seen include (1) a 14-year-old who had never driven before and who when he became manic took his parent's car and started driving on the freeway; (2) a 14-year-old boy of slight build who suddenly started taunting and getting into fist fights with much larger adolescents; and (3) an older adolescent girl who previously was sexually monogamous who over one weekend had sex with four different boys. None of these symptoms alone make the diagnosis of mania a certainty, but each should raise suspicion of this disorder.

ETIOLOGY

As repeatedly emphasized, the pathophysiology of affective disorders is not yet understood; therefore, causative factors are understood only in a statistical sense. When the clinician is caring for an adolescent with depression who has a strong family history of affective disorders, a difficult family and social environment, and recent psychosocial stressors, the cause of depression in that adolescent will forever remain unknown. Nevertheless, epidemiologic studies provide a statistical understanding of correlates and possible causes for depression.

Risk Factors for Depression

Both positive and negative life events have been shown to be risk factors for adult depression. Several studies of child and adolescent depression have shown that this is also the case for younger individuals. This is a difficult area to demonstrate rigorously because in almost all studies the proportion of the depression related to life events is relatively modest, accounting for perhaps 10% of the variance. In addition, the meaning of the particular life event to the individual must be considered.

The one particular life event that shows up recurrently among many adult studies is the early death of the mother, which causes a severalfold increase in the likelihood of depression in adulthood and, though it has not yet been demonstrated, would presumably cause a similar increase in the likelihood of depression in childhood and adolescence. Obviously the large majority of adolescents who experience depression have not lost their mothers at early ages.

Other factors associated with child and adolescent depression in some studies include family dysfunction and low self-esteem in the individual. These are correlative findings, and the direction of causation is unclear. These studies cannot distinguish whether the individual had poor self-esteem before the onset of depression and then experienced depression or had depression first and then experienced poor self-esteem. Interestingly, in studies of adolescent depression, low intelligence quotient (IQ) scores and poor physical health are not risk factors for depression per se.

Familial Transmission

Family studies, adoption studies, and twin studies all show robust familial transmission of adult major depression (though studies of adults who have their first depressive episode after 45 years of age show no increase in familial "loading"). There is clearly a strong genetic transmission component to bipolar disorder (documented through adoption and twin studies). The mechanism of familial transmission is less certain in adult nonbipolar depression. Some studies demonstrate environmental transmission, but genetic transmission is also likely to be important.

There are no adoption or twin studies examining adolescent major depression. Several family transmission studies have been performed. Both the "top-down" studies (adults with depression and normal probands are ascertained and then the rates of disorder in their children are examined) and "bottom-up" studies (normal and depressed child and adolescent probands are ascertained and then rates of disorder in adult relatives are examined) show a strong familial transmission of major depression from adults to adolescents. From both sets of studies, a consistent picture emerges—the younger the age (from childhood through mid-20s) at onset of the first episode of major depression in a proband, the greater the average "loading" for affective disorders in the proband's family (the more likely that there is affective disorder in the proband's family). When this is combined with the epidemiologic data that imply the prevalence of depression is least in children, somewhat greater in adolescents, and even greater in adults, a relative protective effect of childhood and adolescence is suggested, so only those youth with the greatest "loading" manifest depression.

Psychobiologic Markers

For the past 20 years, investigators have used psychobiologic markers (see Chapter 12) as a way of validating and delineating adult depressive disorders. Several of the broad strategies that have been applied to adults have now been investigated in children and adolescents.

One strategy looks at the hypothalamic control of pituitary and adrenal hormones. The first such system looked at was the hypothalamic-pituitary-adrenal axis. In adults with major depression, multiple studies have shown a subset that hypersecretes cortisone. Other studies have shown that subjects with depression show more rapid cortisol escape from the suppression induced when oral dexamethasone is given. Dexamethasone, a synthetic steroid, suppresses the hypothalamic release of corticotropin-releasing factor (CRF) and the pituitary release of adrenocorticotropic hormone (ACTH) and so suppresses circulating cortisone. Adults with a major depressive disorder escape from this suppression much more rapidly than do adults who are not depressed. This appears to be a "state" marker, an abnormality that is present during the episode but not before or after. Unfortunately, these abnormalities in the hypothalamic-pituitary-adrenal axis appear to be quite nonspecific. They are also found in other psychiatric disorders, in Alzheimer disease, and in very modest weight loss that is independent of a psychiatric disorder.

The results of applying these tests to children and adolescents with major depressive disorder have been equivocal. There is as yet little indication of basal cortisol hypersecretion. Some studies have suggested an increased rate of early escape from dexamethasone suppression, whereas other large studies have failed to find a higher rate of escape from dexamethasone suppression than is seen in normal children. Because of the variability of these findings in children and adolescents and their nonspecificity in adults in relation to major depression, it is hard to know what final role studies of the hypothalamic-pituitary-adrenal axis will have in the understanding of juvenile affective disorders.

These tests, like the other psychobiologic tests discussed further on, are of considerable theoretical interest in understanding the pathophysiology of depression. However, they are not of value to the clinician. A diagnosis can neither be ruled in nor ruled out by using any of them at present.

Another area of study using the same neuroendocrine strategy is the growth hormone (GH) axis. Numerous adult pharmacologic challenge tests of GH secretion (including clonidine, insulin, and desipramine stimula-

tion, all of which probably have as a final common pathway the stimulation of postsynaptic α_2-receptors) show that adults with major depression demonstrate lesser stimulation with these compounds than do normal controls. Similar findings have been found after desipramine stimulation in adolescents with a suicidal major depression and after clonidine stimulation in prepubertal children with a major depression. Although these studies tend to implicate α_2-receptors, one study in prepubertal children and one study in adults showed a correlation between the response to clonidine and the response to growth hormone releasing hormone (GH-RH) in the same individuals, suggesting that changes in somatostatin might be implicated instead. The finding of decreased GH secretion after these stimuli appears to be a "trait" marker for depression—it is present during the depression and after the recovery from the depression, and in one, as yet unpublished, study it appears to be present in high-risk children before their first episode of depression. This finding in adults has also been reported with some forms of anxiety disorder. This test is not yet of clinical utility.

Changes in sleep architecture have been one of the most robust markers of depression in adults. Studies have consistently found that a subset of depressed adults have shortened rapid eye movement (REM) latency and decreased δ wave sleep. Similar findings have been observed in several groups of older adolescents and in hospitalized inpatient prepubertal children. It is likely that there is an age interaction, with the normal sleep architecture being relatively preserved at younger ages. At present, this test is not useful in the diagnosis of depression in any age group.

TREATMENT

Pharmacologic Treatment of Nonbipolar Depression

Pharmacologic treatment strategies are covered in detail elsewhere in this book. Only a brief summary is included here.

Controlled studies in adolescents have examined various tricyclic antidepressants, including nortriptyline, imipramine, amitriptyline, and fluoxetine. Unfortunately, the results of these studies are inconclusive as yet, primarily because the total number of subjects entered in all studies to date is small. Plasma level–response studies (in which fixed or weighed, adjusted dose of medication is given, after which the correlation between plasma level and clinical response, which is assessed without regard to plasma level, is examined) have given equivocal findings, some suggesting that there is a relationship between plasma level and clinical response and others suggesting that there is not. Medication and placebo studies have been largely negative to date. Open clinical studies have certainly suggested that in some individuals the tricyclic antidepressants seem to be efficacious.

Several possibilities emerge:

1. These medications may on average be as efficacious

in adolescent major depression as they are in adult major depression, but inadequate sample size may have caused the failure to demonstrate this.

2. The choice of dosages, titration strategies, and so on may turn out to be suboptimal in the different trials completed to date.

3. The medications may well work in a subset of adolescent major depression that is yet to be defined, and this effect may be masked by the inclusion of adolescents who also meet criteria for major depression but have a different, medication-nonresponsive disorder.

4. The disorder of major depression may be constant from childhood through adolescence to adulthood, but because of maturational changes in the brain or changes in the sex steroid milieu of the brain, the antidepressants that work through re-uptake blocking mechanisms may be less efficacious in adolescents than in adults. Neural pathways, thought to be important in the pathophysiology of major depression, are still developing and changing throughout adolescence. Noradrenergic pathways are not fully developed until early in the third decade of life. The ratio of serotonergic to noradrenergic balance in the brain is changing throughout adolescence.

5. Estrogens have widespread effects on multiple neurotransmitter systems and are at their peak during this age period. Maturational changes are a very strong candidate for age-related changes in pharmacologic responsivity, and though they are hard to test, particularly in a disorder like depression without truly adequate animal models, they can always be evoked as an explanation for differential response.

Controlled studies of other pharmacologic treatments have not yet been undertaken. One open clinical study has suggested a possible place for lithium augmentation of tricyclic antidepressants in adolescents with unipolar depression that is unresponsive to tricyclic antidepressants alone and for monoamine oxidase inhibitors when used judiciously. Because of the problematic nature of the interaction of monoamine oxidase inhibitors and some medications and tyramine-containing foods, with potential for serious morbidity or mortality secondary to strokes or heart attacks with the hypertensive crisis, it is unlikely that a physician not experienced with their use would wish to undertake this treatment. Nevertheless, this group of medications has considerable potential for serious depressions that are refractory to other treatments.

Psychotherapeutic Treatment of Nonbipolar Depression

Unfortunately, the clinician is in a similar situation with psychological treatment as with pharmacologic treatment—no controlled studies have as yet been performed. In adult depression, a synthesis of multiple studies of psychotherapy alone or combined with medication suggest that both have a place in the treatment of adult depression and that the combination may be more efficacious than either alone. The forms of psychotherapy that have demonstrated efficacy in adult depression are the interpersonal therapy developed by Klerman and Weissman and cognitive therapy developed by Beck and colleagues. Interpersonal therapy concentrates on the decreased pleasant social interactions found in adults with major depression because of their inability to experience pleasure, their lack of motivation for social interactions, and so on. Cognitive therapy focuses on the negative cognitive distortions consistently experienced by depressed individuals—that is, viewing everything bad as a confirmation of the fact that life is impossible and will never get better and ignoring good events in their life. Both of these specific approaches seem to be better in controlled studies of adults than in nonspecific talking therapy. It is likely that these techniques can be extended to adolescents with appropriate modifications for their lesser compliance through take-home exercises (see Chapter 26), their different levels of cognitive ability, their different social milieu, and so on. Several studies are being undertaken to examine these psychological treatments in a controlled manner.

Given the findings of impaired social functioning even after the adolescent recovers from major depression, specific therapies addressing these impairments have considerable validity. Specifically, the adolescent who functions badly with friends or at home during or after depression may well be considered for either individual or family psychotherapy.

Treatment of Bipolar Disorder

There are no controlled studies of the treatment of bipolar depression in adolescents, so the following is an extrapolation from adult studies and from adult and adolescent clinical experience.

Although psychotherapy can be a very useful adjunct to pharmacologic treatment, psychotherapy alone is not an effective treatment for either the manic or depressed phases of a bipolar disorder. Occasionally, the clinician will be forced to intervene to obtain pharmacologic treatment for the adolescent with bipolar disease who is already in psychotherapy, potentially against the advice of the therapist. This is always difficult, but imperative, given the highly morbid potential course of this disorder.

The pharmacologic treatment of first choice is lithium carbonate. Additionally, carbamazepine or valproic acid, or both, may be useful in addition if lithium alone is inadequate. In general, treatment of a bipolar disorder is best undertaken by a physician who is experienced caring for adolescents with this disorder. Both the clinical course and the pharmacologic treatment tend to be complicated and difficult.

OUTCOME

Longitudinal studies suggest that adolescents with major depression will have significant morbidity with frequent recurrence of affective syndromes.

Natural History of Depression in Adolescence

The classic study following school-aged children (aged 8 to 12 years) with major depression and similar children with adjustment disorder with depressed mood referred to a child guidance clinic in the Pittsburgh area clearly demonstrates that major depression beginning during school age is a highly recurrent disorder. In that study, 70% of the children showed a recurrence within 5 years of the initial diagnosis. The children who had adjustment disorder with depressed mood (which by definition meant that they did not have sufficient symptoms to meet the criteria of major depressive disorder but had some stressful life event at the time of the onset of symptoms, in distinction to those children who met the criteria for major depression) had a benign course with relatively rapid remission of the present episode and little or no depressive symptomatology when followed longitudinally. Those children with "double depression," which consisted of a major depression superimposed upon a chronic dysthymic course, showed the most morbid longitudinal outcome. They had more episodes of depression and a much shorter average period of remission from the dysthymia and major depression.

Studies of psychosocial functioning during depression demonstrate marked impairment in all spheres of social functioning in adolescents, including at school, with friends, and with family during episodes of major depression. Although the adolescents, on average, improved after resolution of the depression they did not, on average, return fully to their baseline states. These findings suggest that one of the important areas for "talking therapy" in adolescent depression is likely to be around regaining exactly these social skills.

Predictors of Bipolarity in Adolescents Presenting With Major Depression

As already discussed, the rate of eventual bipolar disease will be relatively high when the first episode of major depression occurs in adolescence. Therefore, a most important concern consists of the symptoms and other variables that predict an eventual bipolar outcome. In a study that has now been replicated, it has been shown that an eventual bipolar outcome in an adolescent presenting with a first episode of major depression is predicted by a high family "loading" of bipolar affective disorder (paralleling adult findings), the development of manic or hypomanic symptoms when treated with tricyclic antidepressants (paralleling adult findings), very rapid onset of symptoms of depression, and psychotic symptoms (hallucination or delusions). In these two studies, two thirds of adolescents with a psychotic depression had bipolar disease on follow-up. The prediction of bipolarity is of paramount importance because the pharmacologic treatment strategies are different for bipolar and unipolar depression, and the predicted long-term outcome is different. The individual with bipolar disease will have increasingly virulent episodes of depression, as well as episodes of mania, and may be at an elevated risk for suicide even over the already-elevated risk from unipolar depression.

Comorbidity

In clinic-referred samples of children and adolescents with major depression, there is a greater than expected frequency of comorbid psychiatric diagnoses, even given the incomplete knowledge of the epidemiology of childhood psychiatric disorders. There are three possible explanations, and each probably helps to elucidate this phenomenon.

First, the increased frequency of comorbidity may be an artifact resulting from referral biases. Psychiatric or psychological referral is likely to be initiated based on some function of the total impairment, the number of symptoms, or the effect of the adolescent's behavior on the parents and other adults. If any one disorder is severe enough, there is a high likelihood of referral. However, if an adolescent has two disorders, each of which is not very severe, he or she may still have enough symptoms to be referred to the mental health system. This mechanism undoubtedly operates across the spectrum of mental disorders, so it is a factor even when comorbidity also results from other mechanisms having to do with the cause of the disorder. This mechanism alone may account for inconsistent reports of an increased comorbidity of eating disorders in depression—for example, in clinic-referred samples that have been hard to demonstrate through family studies.

Another mechanism that may be responsible for some of the observed comorbidity is that of a shared familial transmission liability that is causative in both disorders (whether the liability is transmitted through genetic or environmental mechanisms). In familial transmission studies of adult depression and anxiety disorders, it appears that exactly this mechanism—a shared, familial transmission liability—accounts for the overrepresentation of each disorder seen within the same families and within the same individuals. In clinic-referred samples of adolescents there is also a high rate of comorbidity of anxiety and depressive disorders.

Finally, through a unidirectional pathway, one disorder can increase the risk for a second disorder. One proposed theoretical example of this, which has not yet been demonstrated, is the possibility that children with attention deficit disorder and hyperactivity eventually become demoralized as they become older, and subsequently a depressive syndrome develops. In other words, primary hyperactivity may lead to increased risk of depression, whereas primary depression would not necessarily lead to an increased risk of hyperactivity. However, the other two mechanisms described probably also contribute to the reported high comorbidity between attention deficit disorder and depression.

SUMMARY AND CONCLUSIONS

The pathophysiology of depression, bipolar disorder, and all other psychiatric disorders is as yet unknown.

Nonbipolar depression probably has both genetic and environmental contributions. Bipolar disorder appears to have a strong genetic component. These clinical syndromes are diagnosed by inclusion and exclusion criteria. Therefore, current diagnostic criteria will not exactly correspond to the underlying pathophysiology or pathophysiologies that will ultimately be discovered. Nonbipolar depression probably has different causes in different individuals—as of yet we cannot distinguish among possibly several different underlying disorders that present with similar syndromic pictures.

Multiple lines of evidence strongly suggest that adolescent depression is continuous with adult forms of the disorder. Nevertheless, treatment strategies of demonstrated efficacy in adult forms may require modification for application in adolescents. An aggressive approach to these disorders is indicated because of significant social and functional impairment and an elevated risk of suicide.

BIBLIOGRAPHY

Fleming J, Offord D: Epidemiology of childhood depressive disorders: A critical review. J Acad Child Adolesc Psychol 29:571, 1990.

Kovacs M, Feinberg TL, Crouse-Novak MA, et al: Depressive disorders in childhood. I. A longitudinal prospective study of characteristics and recovery. Arch Gen Psychiatry 41:229, 1984.

Kovacs M, Feinberg TL, Crouse-Novak M, et al: Depressive disorders in childhood. II. A longitudinal study of the risk for a subsequent major depression. Arch Gen Psychiatry 41:643, 1984.

Puig-Antich J: Affective disorders in children and adolescents: Diagnostic validity and psychobiology. In Meltzer HY (ed): Psychopharmacology: The Third Generation of Progress. New York, Raven Press, 1987.

Ryan N, Puig-Antich J, Rabinovich H, et al: The clinical picture of major depression in children and adolescents. Arch Gen Psychiatry 44:854, 1987.

Ryan ND: Heterocyclic antidepressants in children and adolescents. J Child Adolesc Psychopharmacol 1:21, 1990.

Ryan ND, Puig-Antich J: Affective Illness in Adolescence. Frances AJ, Hales RE (eds): American Psychiatric Association Annual Review, Vol 5. Washington, DC, American Psychiatric Press, 1986.

Strober M, Carlson G: Bipolar illness in adolescents with major depression: Clinical, genetic, and psychopharmacologic predictors in a three- to four-year prospective follow-up investigation. Arch Gen Psychiatry 39:549, 1982.

Strober M, Morrell W, Burroughs J, et al: A family study of bipolar I disorder in adolescence. Early onset of symptoms linked to increased familial loading and lithium resistance. J Affect Disord 15:255, 1988.

Weissman MM, Gammon GD, John K, et al: Children of depressed parents. Increased psychopathology and early onset of major depression. Arch Gen Psychiatry 44:847, 1987.

CHAPTER 101

Suicide and Suicidal Behaviors

DAVID SHAFFER and ROGER HICKS

Many of the common childhood psychiatric conditions—for example, the developmental disorders and attention deficit (see Chapter 106) and conduct disorders (see Chapter 108)—are chronic and continue to cause problems as the child reaches and passes through adolescence. There are also a number of other conditions with a typical onset during adulthood, for example, major depression (see Chapter 100), schizophrenia (see Chapter 110), and alcohol dependence (see Chapter 111), that may have an earlier onset in the adolescent years. However, suicidal behavior is a problem that is characteristic of adolescence. Suicide attempts, or "gestures" as they are sometimes called, are relatively uncommon before puberty; they increase in incidence at 12 to 13 years of age and reach a peak between 16 and 17 years of age before declining to lower levels in adulthood. Adolescents who attempt suicide account for a majority of new emergency or crisis referrals to adolescent medical and psychiatric or behavioral ambulatory programs and for a high proportion of admissions to both adolescent general medical and psychiatric units.

Completed suicide attempts begin to occur with some frequency in midadolescence, reaching a peak incidence in the early twenties that is maintained for most of the remainder of adult life (Fig. 101–1). Although this better fits a model of an illness with a characteristically adult onset that less commonly has an early onset in adolescence, suicide is one of the three most important causes of adolescent mortality (Table 101–1; and see Chapter 2). The problems of attempted and completed suicide are closely related. Approximately one third of those who successfully commit suicide have made a prior attempt; thus, those who attempt suicide are at greatest risk for later suicide completion. This chapter will address both conditions. The first section reviews risk factors for and epidemiology of completed suicide, and the second section reviews the characteristics of and summarizes the knowledge about the treatment of adolescents who attempt suicide.

COMPLETED SUICIDE
Incidence

Adolescent suicide is uncommon; the rate in 1988 for 15- to 19-year-olds was 11.3 deaths/100,000 population.

Prepared with assistance from Grant R49 CCR202598–01 from the Centers for Disease Control and from Grants ROI MH 38198–04 and ROI MH416898–02, and Research Training Grant MH 16434 and Research Center Grant MH 43878–02 from the National Institute of Mental Health.

Suicide is among the three leading causes of death for both black and white teenagers (see Chapter 2 and Table 101–1).

Age

As already noted, suicide is very unusual before puberty and becomes increasingly common in adolescence (Fig. 101–1), with the sharpest rate of increase occurring after age 16 years. More than one half of all adolescents who commit suicide are aged 18 or 19 years. A likely reason for the rapid increase in suicide rates after age 16 years is the increasing importance of alcohol and drugs as risk factors; the abuse of both is more common among older adolescents than among younger ones (see Chapter 111).

Gender

In the United States, as well as in most but not all other countries, successful suicide is more common in males than in females at all ages except among the very young. Approximately five times more male teenagers commit suicide than do female adolescents. One likely reason is the close relationship between completed suicide and aggressive behavior and alcohol and substance use and abuse. Both of these risk factors are more prevalent among males than among females. The differences in method between males and females are another factor that may contribute to sex differences as well as to the variation in sex ratios that is found in different countries. Self-poisoning is a preferred female method of manifesting suicidal behavior. In the West, with its advanced emergency treatment resources and strict regulations governing the availability of potentially lethal agents such as barbiturates, the suicide attempt is rarely "successful." Most countries in which rates of male and female suicides are similar are in the Third World, where treatment is less widely available or where the preferred ingestational agents include herbicides, such as paraquat, for which there are no effective treatments.

Ethnic and Cultural Factors

In the United States, whites have higher suicide rates than do blacks at all ages, including adolescents. The difference between black and white rates is greatest in

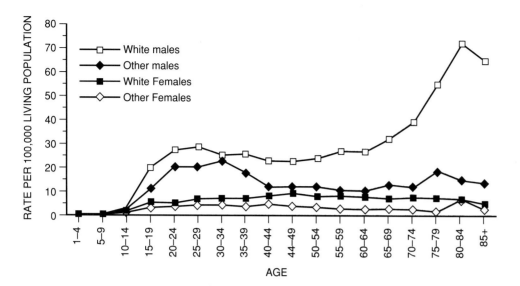

Figure 101–1. Suicide rate per 100,000 living population for all ages, 1988.

the southern states and least in the north central and western states. The incidence of suicide also varies considerably among different Native American groups. Some of these groups have rates that are more than 20-fold higher than the national average; for others the rate is no different from that of the nation as a whole.

The mechanisms that mediate cultural differences are by no means clear; they do not appear to be a function of selective underreporting or of the strong association between social class and ethnicity. Cultures in countries such as Japan, which historically sanctioned suicide under certain circumstances, do not have the highest suicide rates. Roman Catholicism carries strong prohibitions against suicide, but predominantly Catholic countries include those with the lowest and those with the highest suicide rates. It is possible that the rate is influenced by other, less explicit beliefs—for example, that suicide is cowardly or a sign of insanity, which could inhibit the behavior in individuals who might otherwise be predisposed toward committing suicide.

Secular Trends

Over the past 2 decades, suicide has become increasingly common in young persons. As shown in Figure 101–2, the increase has been greatest (threefold) among males between the ages of 15 and 19 years, with the rate increasing nearly every year during this period. There has been no significant increase in the rate among children younger than 15 years of age, nor among female adolescents. Possible causes for the selective increase in suicide among older males include the increase in alco-

hol and drug use and abuse among that group during the past 3 decades.

Methods of Suicide

The methods commonly used to commit suicide vary in different countries. In the United States, adolescents of both sexes are most likely to commit suicide with a firearm. The next most common method for boys is hanging, whereas for girls it is jumping from a height. Deliberate ingestion of poisons, which is by far the most common method used by adolescents who attempt suicide, accounts for relatively few completed suicide attempts in adolescents.

Precipitants

Most teenagers commit suicide shortly after experiencing an acute stress, such as getting into trouble in one way or another—for example, after an arrest or after being discovered cheating or truant from school. Other common precipitants include peer humiliation, such as being expelled from a party, losing a fight with a peer, a threatened or actual breakup with a boyfriend or girlfriend, or the approach of an event that has been anticipated with fear. Many suicide victims have been drinking heavily just prior to death. Deliberate, well-planned completed suicides without obvious recent antecedents do occur but are uncommon.

Risk Factors

FAMILY HISTORY

There are significantly higher rates of both suicide completions and suicide attempts in first-degree family members of adolescents who attempt or complete suicide. A positive family history is most common among adolescents who were depressed at the time of their death. Twin studies in adults who commit suicide show

TABLE 101–1. Three Leading Causes of Death (United States) in 15- to 19-Year-Olds in 1988 (Deaths/100,000 Population)

WHITES	RATE	BLACKS	RATE
Accidents	50.3	Homicide	44.7
Suicide	12.3	Accidents	29.4
Homicide	5.6	Suicide	6.0

Figure 101-2. Changes in adolescent suicide rate, 1964 to 1988.

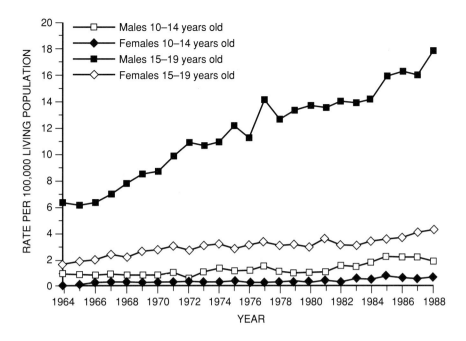

IMITATION AND MEDIA EFFECTS

The conclusion that suicide, especially among adolescents, can be imitated or induced in vulnerable individuals is drawn from several different sources, including (1) documented examples of "copy-cat" suicides that have occurred within a few hours after a teenager viewed a film, read a book, or saw a news story pertaining to a suicide; (2) the occurrence of suicide clusters in a high school or other self-contained community thought to have an imitative basis; (3) the broadly consistent body of research that has shown a relationship between short-lived increases in the suicide rate and repeated, prominent coverage of a suicide in newspapers or television; and (4) a similar effect after fictional television programs featuring adolescent suicide. There is no suggestion that any of these influences affect normal children. Research among adolescents involved in a suicide cluster indicated that adolescents who were in the category of "copy-cat" suicides commonly had a past history of a psychopathologic condition or previous suicidal behavior. The vulnerability of teenagers to imitation has implications for suicide prevention programs that show filmed examples of suicidal behavior or interviews with adolescents who have attempted suicide and have survived. Such films may be misinterpreted by vulnerable teenagers and can have inadvertently negative effects.

PERINATAL MORBIDITY

One group of investigators examined the birth records of consecutive suicides in adolescents and noted an excess of obstetric complications and the prevalence of maternal smoking and alcohol ingestion. This relationship could be due to some consequence of central nervous system damage before, during, or after delivery, including exposure to a teratogen during pregnancy; to the heritability of a psychopathologic condition; or to the effects of inappropriate parenting.

higher rates of concordance for suicide among monozygotic twins, suggesting that the high family incidence is not solely a function of imitation or suggestion but may be a marker of inheritance of a mood disorder or other predisposing characteristic (see Chapter 100).

SUICIDE AND MENTAL ILLNESS

A number of research approaches have shown a strong relationship between suicide and psychiatric illness in adults who commit suicide. Epidemiologically based studies show a high suicide rate among identified psychiatric patients, a very low suicide rate in study samples of individuals who are free of psychiatric disorders, and high rates of psychiatric disorders among adults who complete suicide. The range of research has been more limited among adolescents. However, all of the epidemiologically based psychological autopsy studies among adolescents have found that a majority of adolescents who commit suicides had evidence of a psychiatric disorder during the period prior to death.

The predominant psychiatric diagnosis differs between the sexes and also between older and younger adolescents who commit suicide. Male teenagers 17 years and older are most commonly diagnosed as exhibiting alcohol and substance abuse, which is a factor in as many as three quarters of all cases, prior to the adolescent committing suicide. Approximately one third of these individuals have an associated and often long-standing conduct disorder, and about one quarter of them have been diagnosed as having a major depression. Quite often conduct disorder and depression coexist. In these cases, the features of conduct disorder usually predate the features of depression. Substance and alcohol use and abuse are uncommon in younger boys and female adolescents regardless of age; the most common diagnoses among these suicide victims are depression, anxiety, and conduct disorders.

NEUROTRANSMITTER ABNORMALITIES

In the past decade, a number of biologic correlates of suicide have been identified in adults who commit suicide and those who attempt suicide. The most frequently replicated finding is the presence of significantly lower concentrations of the serotonin metabolite 5-hydroxindoleacetic acid (5-HIAA) in the cerebrospinal fluid of those who attempt suicide and those who complete suicide than in age- and sex-matched nonsuicidal control subjects. This finding does not seem to be a function of the psychiatric diagnosis because it has been found in suicide victims who have a variety of psychiatric diagnoses. Nor is it an artifact of analyzing spinal fluid; although 5-HIAA in cerebrospinal fluid comes from both brain and spinal cord, autopsy studies show high correlations between the two. There is some evidence that low serotonin levels are associated with impulsive labile and aggressive behavior, and these character traits may be more important correlates than is psychiatric diagnosis (see Chapter 109).

Despite the large number of studies that have reported on these findings, a number of unanswered questions remain. The specific behavioral correlates of low serotonin states have yet to be documented in large samples; there are conflicting reports about whether 5-HIAA levels are stable or fluctuate with mental state, and it is not known in what proportion of teenaged or adult suicide victims such abnormalities occur.

In one promising development, one group of investigators noted a 1-year suicide completion rate of 21% among adults who attempted suicide in whom the level of 5-HIAA in the cerebrospinal fluid was less than 90 µg/ml, compared with only a 2% death rate among adults with higher levels who attempted suicide. If, as has been postulated, declining or stable low levels of 5-HIAA predict a poor prognosis, secondary or tertiary prevention could be served by routine cerebrospinal fluid monitoring of patients who have made a suicide attempt, with special care being given to those with abnormally low levels of 5-HIAA.

Conclusions

A consideration of the risk factors described previously suggests that suicide does not occur randomly and that there is no universal potential for it. Instead, suicide victims are drawn from certain predisposed groups, including drug and alcohol abusers, individuals with depressive illness, and those with aggressive personality disorders. These conditions are not in themselves sufficient to determine suicide risk. Most deaths from suicide occur in such individuals shortly after a stressful event or intoxication has induced some extreme emotion. Further, whether or not a predisposed individual who experiences stress will engage in suicidal behavior is influenced by (1) access to the means of committing suicide and (2) possibly by factors such as whether the individual's family and peers view suicide as a legitimate, understandable, or sanctioned behavior or as a less understandable or romantic act.

ATTEMPTED SUICIDE

Incidence

Most of the information available on the incidence of suicide attempts in nonreferred populations has been derived from self-completion forms, the accuracy of which is always suspect. However, several such studies have been consistent in reporting a lifetime prevalence of between 6% and 10% in 17-year-olds. By contrast, interview studies with adults report a cumulative prevalence of between 2% and 3%. The reasons for these discrepancies are not clear. It may be that adolescents overrepresent what they view to be a suicide attempt or that adults forget or do not report some attempts committed during adolescence.

Clinical Features

Studies among both psychiatric and adolescent medical clinic patients suggest that adolescents who attempt suicide fall into one of two groups. The first, consisting of predominantly older adolescents who are more likely to have a clear-cut psychiatric illness (most often depression), indicate feelings of hopelessness and despair and have made a potentially lethal attempt. Many also suffer from drug and alcohol abuse. The second group is more common and consists of younger persons, predominantly females. These individuals make less serious attempts that are often precipitated by an acute interpersonal crisis. They are likely to have a diagnosis of adjustment disorder (see Chapter 109). It must be emphasized that these descriptions are drawn from adolescents who attend an ambulatory program and may not be representative of the many adolescents who make a suicide attempt and do not seek or who are not referred for psychiatric evaluation, but may be cared for by their primary care physicians.

It is clear that not all adolescents who attempt suicide are depressed, and similarly that not all depressed adolescents are suicidal. Comparisons between suicidal and nonsuicidal depressed adolescents suggest that those who are suicidal are generally more aggressive and less likely to be withdrawn. They are also more likely to have a positive family history for alcoholism and to have parents who have themselves experienced suicidal ideation.

Family Background

Reports on the family characteristics of adolescents who attempt suicide have similarly been drawn from psychiatric ambulatory or emergency medical room populations and may not be representative of all those who attempt suicide. Common findings include high rates of parental psychiatric illness and marital conflict; however, these are common findings among the parents of disturbed adolescents and may not be specific for those who attempt suicide. Uncontrolled studies have reported parental characteristics such as secretiveness, coldness, uncommunicativeness, rigidity in communicating with offspring, and rigidity and reluctance to accept change or tolerate crisis. Adolescents who attempt suicide often describe their parents as hostile or indifferent or as having extreme and unrealistic expectations of the amount of control that they should exert, alternating between indifference and laxity.

Prognosis and Natural History

REPEAT ATTEMPTS

Between 20% and 50% of adolescents who attempt suicide for the first time will make a repeat attempt. The best predictors of repeat attempts are male gender and the use of a method other than ingestion. It is generally believed, but not clearly supported by the limited available research, that those who repeatedly attempt suicide carry a higher risk of eventually completing suicide.

LATER SUICIDE

Although only a minority of adolescents who attempt suicide progress to commit suicide, follow-up studies show that their suicide rate is considerably higher than that of the general population. Observed rates for adolescent males range from approximately 9% for a group who had been depressed or who had made a suicide attempt and were admitted to a psychiatric inpatient unit, to less than 1% of adolescent males who presented to an emergency room but who, presumably because they were deemed to be less disturbed, were not admitted to a psychiatric hospital. Similar rates for females range from 1% for former psychiatric inpatients to 0.1% for those who received no inpatient psychiatric care. Symptoms that were significantly more common among those who eventually completed suicide include the features of severe depression, such as psychomotor retardation, social withdrawal, hopelessness, hypersomnia, and a belief that they had mental illness. However, these symptoms have limited specificity, for they are also commonly found in adolescents who attempt suicide but do not go on to commit suicide.

Initial Assessment and Management

The initial evaluation should determine (1) whether the adolescent can be safely discharged home or whether he or she needs inpatient care and (2) whether the adolescent needs to be referred to a mental health professional or can be adequately cared for by a general physician.

The decision to hospitalize is often made on purely medical grounds (see Chapter 19). However, if the adolescent's medical condition is stable, it is necessary to determine the likelihood of whether the adolescent will make a further, perhaps successful, attempt and whether his or her mental state requires specialized inpatient care.

Although some programs suggest that all adolescents who attempt suicide should be admitted to a general adolescent inpatient unit for at least 24 hours, others follow criteria or guidelines for admission. The following criteria suggest admission to a hospital for evaluation and supervision (Table 101–2).

1. Gender: Males should generally be admitted for detailed evaluation before discharge. Females who have made several previous attempts at suicide and for whom there has been no resolution of the conditions that are causing them to be suicidal should be admitted.

2. Mental state: Teenagers of either sex should be admitted to a hospital if there is evidence of significant depression, feelings of hopelessness, evidence of psychosis, or a recent history of social withdrawal and uncommunicativeness. Adolescents who declare that they still wish to die should be admitted. An intoxicated adolescent should be retained in the emergency room until he or she can be reevaluated when sober.

3. Nature of the attempt: Hospitalization is indicated if the attempt employed a method other than an ingestion or superficial cuts to the skin, for example, an attempted hanging, jumping from a high place, or the use of a firearm. If the ingestion was potentially lethal or thought to be lethal by the adolescent, admission is advised.

4. Past history: A history of a previous suicide attempt made within the last year or an established history of volatile, unpredictable behavior, or both, are indications for close supervision.

5. Home background: The lack of a caring or responsible setting to which to discharge the patient is another indication for hospitalization.

It may be reasonable to discharge the adolescent home if his or her physical condition permits and if none of the preceding criteria are met. However, discharge should take place only after the following precautions have been taken:

1. Salient features in the history (details of the method used, the history of other recent attempts, evidence of disturbed behavior prior to the attempt) must be corroborated by the teenager's usual caretaker.

2. The caretaker must help the adolescent's family to

TABLE 101–2. Criteria for Hospitalization

SEX
All males and females who have made recurrent attempts, are serious about killing themselves, and lack ongoing family support

MENTAL STATE
Moderate to severe depression
Psychosis
Pervasive wish to die

NATURE OF ATTEMPT
Violent means
Serious ingestion attempt

PAST HISTORY
Previous suicide attempt
Volatile behavior

HOME BACKGROUND
Lack of stable living arrangement
Lack of responsible adult in the home

immediately remove or secure any firearms or potentially dangerous medications present in the home.

3. Concrete and precise arrangements must be made for a follow-up appointment. It is not sufficient to instruct the teenager or his or her family to call the office tomorrow to make an appointment. If the adolescent or the family does not make or keep the appointments, the responsible health care professional should contact them.

4. The teenager must be given a written telephone number to call in the event that he or she again feels like committing suicide.

5. The adolescent should sign a simple written statement or "contract" promising not to attempt to take his or her life before attending the next appointment.

Treatment

If the adolescent is in a high-risk category (see preceding discussion), hospital admission is indicated. As previously discussed, no adolescent who attempts suicide should be discharged from an emergency room or a physician's office without a history being taken from a parent or caretaker as well as the adolescent. In all cases, a definite appointment should be made for the next visit and given in writing, rather than leaving the adolescent or his or her parent with a telephone number of the program.

Many adolescents who attempt suicide and are treated medically in a hospital emergency room and are offered an appointment do not keep the appointment. Noncompliance with treatment recommendations is determined by a number of factors, including having a parent with an untreated psychiatric disorder and very likely the style and procedures used in the emergency room. Patients who are given a specific appointment are significantly more likely to keep it than are those who are simply provided with the telephone number of the ambulatory program. If the adolescent fails to keep his or her appointment, outreach efforts are justified.

Many different therapies have been advocated for the adolescent who attempts suicide; however, there have been no controlled studies in either adolescents or adults to demonstrate that one approach is any better than another. It is customary to use a problem-oriented approach based on the evaluation of the adolescent's mental state, the circumstances that led to the attempt, the family situation, the psychiatric status of the parents, and the nature of family interactions. Some of these problems—not uncommonly found in suicidal adolescents—may suggest specific interventions. Both behavioral and family therapy (see Chapters 124 and 125) have been recommended to reduce parent-adolescent conflict. Cognitive behavioral therapy has been recommended to investigate the options that are open to the adolescent patient. For example, if suicide is seen as the only solution to an otherwise hopeless problem, one would help the adolescent weigh more rationally the reasons for living and dying, to teach alternative problem-solving solutions and, through the use of role playing or other techniques, rehearse strategies that can be used when a crisis situation next arises. An adolescent who resorts to a suicide attempt in order to effect change within the family may benefit from assertiveness training. Group therapy may be used when there is a need to reduce a sense of isolation or to provide peer support and opportunities to share problems. However, given the evidence that suicide may sometimes be a modeled behavior, groups with adolescents who have attempted suicide should be constituted and run with caution by skilled and experienced professionals.

There is no evidence to date that tricyclic or monoamine oxidase antagonist antidepressants are effective in adolescents, and because of their low therapeutic index, they are generally contraindicated among adolescent ambulatory patients who have made a prior suicide attempt.

PREVENTION

Curriculum-based "Suicide Education" Programs

Concerns about an increase in the incidence of suicide among male adolescents has led to the widespread introduction of suicide education curricula in high schools in the United States. The programs, which are most commonly directed toward teenagers and school staff but in many cases also toward parents, aim to (1) raise awareness of the problem of teenaged suicide, (2) increase the knowledge about the clinical features of presuicidal youngsters, (3) provide both behavioral and informational advice about how to refer adolescents identified as being at risk of possible suicidal behaviors to appropriate resources, and (4) encourage any suicidal youngsters to obtain appropriate help.

Most suicide education programs operate on the assumption that potentially suicidal students are more likely to discuss their feelings and intentions with other students than with adults. It follows that a further goal is to teach students that if they are told about a friend's intent to commit suicide, even if in confidence, it is important that they inform a responsible adult.

Many program developers believe that suicide is a consequence of stress, and relatively few take the view that suicidal behavior may be related to a mental illness. The relationship between suicidal thoughts and disturbed behavior or distorted thinking is minimized, and suicide is often presented as a misguided, but understandable, response to common adolescent stresses. Although this view is not supported by systematic research, it allows programs to present a nonstigmatizing model of suicidal behavior that, it is hoped, will encourage disclosure by potentially suicidal adolescents.

Several concerns have been voiced about these programs. The first is that there is evidence that these programs are in fact ineffective at changing attitudes about suicide among those young persons who are contemplating suicidal behavior. Second, they are directed toward unselected adolescents, the overwhelming proportion of whom are not at risk, rather than toward groups at high risk for suicidal behavior. Third, there is evidence that a proportion of high-risk adolescents who are exposed to the programs respond to them in a negative fashion. This latter factor, coupled with the evidence (see preceding discussion) that adolescents may imitate suicidal behaviors, raises concern that programs that increase awareness of the problem of suicide or that present suicide as an understandable response to common adolescent problems may inadvertently facilitate the expression of suicidal ideas.

Crisis Services (Hotlines)

Although substantial evidence exists that suicide crisis services used by adolescents who have a high suicide potential, their impact on the number of suicides within a community is generally negligible. The low impact of such services appears to be a function of inadequate use by adolescents who are either contemplating suicide or who have attempted suicide, for only a minority of those who attempt suicide and those who complete suicide use hotlines. Some of the reasons for this include

1. *The mental state of individuals who are close to suicide*: These adolescents experience extremes of fear, jealousy, rage, and intoxication with alcohol or drugs. The potential distortions of thinking from an underlying mental illness may be incompatible with the logical behavior of calling a hotline. This is regrettable because it is precisely in such individuals at high risk that one might expect a crisis call to be most effective, to engage the caller, and interrupt the affect.

2. *Lack of knowledge about the availability or usefulness of crisis centers*: This has been shown to be the case in most adolescents who attempt suicide. This lack of knowledge could be remedied by appropriate advertising in high-incidence areas.

3. *Limited appeal, or perhaps selective resistance by important groups*: The impact of suicide crisis centers must be confined to those who call, namely, young adult females, which is a group with a low overall risk for suicide. Teenaged and young adult males, the group at greatest risk, do not use hotlines.

4. *Ineffective techniques*: Many callers who are considering suicide do not have the psychological resources to make and keep appointments. Hotlines that offer only information services may fail these callers if the call is not linked to a specific strategy. Aggressive techniques, including making appointments with an appropriate agency and following up to ensure appointments are kept, might improve the impact of the hotlines.

5. *Responder techniques vary significantly*: There are differences in empathy, knowledge of resources for suicidal youth, and the ability to make diagnostic decisions among those who answer the hotlines.

Intervention After an Adolescent Suicide

An intervention with family survivors, the school, or the community after an adolescent commits suicide could serve several preventive functions: (1) providing

TABLE 101–3. Adolescents at Risk for Suicide

Boys who have made a previous suicide attempt regardless of their mental state or the method used
Depressed adolescents of either sex
Girls who attempt suicide using a method other than ingestion

a structure for trying to understand the death of the young person, thus alleviating some grief, guilt, and isolation experienced by family survivors; (2) minimizing the scapegoating (i.e., whose fault was it?) that can affect parents, teachers, the school, or peers close to the deceased; and (3) reducing the likelihood of imitation, either within the family or within the community, or both.

There has been very limited research in this area, although uncontrolled studies suggest that the introduction of brief (2 months' duration), volunteer-led survivor support groups are perceived as helpful and are associated with a decline in symptomatology among survivors. Research with bereaved parent support groups, such as the Compassionate Friends does not indicate that attendance helps reduce the duration or intensity of bereavement responses. Adaptation styles that have been shown to speed recovery from grief, such as immersion in another activity or bearing a "replacement" child, are less common among individuals who attend self-help groups for long periods.

There are many questions outstanding with respect to intervention after adolescent suicide in schools, for example, is it good or bad to hold large assemblies, to arrange small groups among close friends, to ignore or downplay the death? There has been no systematic research in this area to date.

Screening for High-risk Cases

Calculations based on both follow-up and case control studies of teenagers suggest that the groups at highest risk for suicide are as listed in Table 101–3. These groups are potentially easy to identify, either by systematic screening in high school or in pediatric offices or when they present for care in emergency rooms or in psychiatric or adolescent medicine clinics. Screening teenagers who already are suicidal, evaluating them carefully with well-proven clinical methods, and providing them with problem-oriented treatment may not be a quick fix and may not catch all vulnerable adolescents, but it is probably the only safe, sure way to prevent suicide.

BIBLIOGRAPHY

Asberg M, Nordstrom P, Traskman-Bendz L: Cerebrospinal fluid studies in suicide. In Mann JJ, Stanley M (eds): Psychobiology of Suicidal Behavior. New York, The New York Academy of Sciences, 1986, pp 243–255.
Brent DA, Perper JA, Kolko DJ, Zelenak JP: The psychological autopsy: Methodological considerations for the study of adolescent suicide. Am Acad Child Adoles Psychiatry 27(3):362, 1988.
Gould MS, Shaffer D: The impact of suicide in television movies: Evidence of imitation. N Engl J Med 315(11):690, 1986.
Motto JA: Suicide in male adolescents. In Sudak HS, Ford AB,

Rushforth NB (eds): Suicide in the Young. Littleton, MA, John Wright, 1984, pp 227–244.

Phillips DP, Carstensen LL: Clustering of teenage suicides after television news stories about suicide. N Engl J Med 315(11):685, 1986.

Salk L, Sturner W, Reilly B, et al: Relationship of maternal and paternal conditions to eventual adolescent suicide. Lancet 8429(1):624, 1985.

Shaffer D. (1974) Suicide in Childhood and Early Adolescence. Journal of Child Psychology and Psychiatry, 15, pp 275–291.

Shaffer D, Garland A, Gould M, et al: Preventing teenage suicide: A critical review. J Am Acad Child Adolesc Psychiatry 27:675, 1988.

Shaffer D, Vieland V, Garland A, et al: Adolescent suicide attempters: Response to suicide prevention programs. JAMA 264:3151, 1990.

Stanley M, Mann JJ: Biological factors associated with suicide. In Frances AJ, Hales RE (eds): American Psychiatric Association Annual Review. Washington, DC, American Psychiatric Press, 1988, pp 334–352.

Trautman PD, Shaffer D: Treatment of child and adolescent suicide attempters. In Sudak HS, Ford AB, Rushforth NB (eds): Suicide in the Young. Littleton, MA, John Wright, 1984, pp 307–323.

CHAPTER 102

Fears and Phobias

BARBARA G. MELAMED

Fear and anxiety are normal emotions. To a large extent, they serve a useful purpose by helping the adolescent set limits (e.g., refusing to participate in a dangerous activity because of fear of the negative consequences of the contemplated action) or serving to motivate (e.g., studying or practicing a musical instrument because of awareness that anxiety will result from poor performance). Perhaps because of the heightened sense of introspection during adolescence, worries about performance, social interactions, physical appearance, and health are increasingly common. There are times, however, that these emotions may become excessive and interfere with daily activities, social relationships, or learning. Anxiety, often with the appearance of intense physical symptoms, may overwhelm the adolescent. Unrealistic fear may preoccupy the individual and prevent participation in once enjoyable activities. The idea that certain types of stimulation may be intrinsically likely to produce intense vigilance and even fearful reactions has been demonstrated in both animal and human research. Qualities such as novel, sudden, and intense stimuli may be predominant in serving as prepared cues for avoidance. This preparedness theory of fear, which has recently received renewed attention, is based on the evolutionary darwinian notion of survival of the species.

As social learning influences began to be explored, the influence of family and peers on both the acquisition and maintenance of fearful behavior was stressed. This is particularly relevant to the adolescent, in whom puberty, self-consciousness, and perhaps entering a new school and becoming more focused on peer group acceptance take prominence. A more current trend has been to view the genetic predisposition for anxiety and related dispositions, such as shyness, as necessary but not sufficient for creating disturbances. It is the transactions among the individual, the family, and real-life stressors that determine the extent of maladaptiveness. The normal influence of hormonal changes that occur in adolescents must also be considered. The most appropriate form of intervention, therefore, is a combination of psychotherapy for the individual; involvement of family, school, and community agencies; and in certain conditions, the use of psychopharmacologic agents.

EPIDEMIOLOGY

Anxiety symptoms are quite common at all ages and in both sexes. The frequency and specificity of adoles-
cent anxiety disorders is not well studied. Early epidemiologic studies on the Isle of Wight indicated that 3.2% of adolescents (aged 14 to 15 years) had "emotional disorders," with another 1.9% showing mixed emotional and conduct disorders. The lack of consistent reporting on incidence is in part due to the lack of an appropriate Diagnostic and Statistical Manual of Mental Disorders, Third Edition (DSM-III) diagnosis for adolescent anxiety, with practitioners preferring to use adjustment disorder as a diagnosis.

Age

The age-related tendency of transient fears in children and adolescents indicates that the stages of fear follow a natural progression that seems to parallel changes in developmental capacities. The fears and worries of pre-adolescents may include bodily injury and concerns about physical appearance and acceptance by peers. At this stage, girls seem to have more fears than do boys. School phobia (the fear of going to school) is always a cause for concern; in younger children, it may be a signal that something is preventing the child from separating from the parent (see Chapter 103). The illness of a family member or maternal overprotection may lead to school phobia and frequent absences from school. Children may also try to avoid going to school because they are afraid of examinations, of making mistakes, or of being criticized. Often children will complain of ailments, such as headache or stomachache, the existence of which cannot be disproved, so that their parents will allow them to stay home. There has been a demonstrated relationship in adolescents between somatic complaints and social phobias, though the directional causality has not been studied. There is longitudinal evidence that despite the fact that there is a tendency to view prepubertal disturbance as transitory and benign, there is a phenotypic continuity between adolescent and adult psychopathology (see Chapter 8).

The nature of an individual's reactions to repeated medical procedures or chronic illness also has much to do with their cognitive abilities and adolescent concerns. Some younger children seem to believe that painful medical procedures, illness, and hospitalization are punishments for wrongdoing or the result of a deliberate desire on the part of the health practitioner to hurt them. Older children who are very upset or frightened about pain may regress to this more primitive level of reasoning. Adolescents' fears are more likely to be the result of unpleasant memories of previous visits to the doctor or dentist. Anticipating pain, the patient may build up anxiety when a visit is impending. As they approach puberty, children become more concerned about social situations and bodily harm.

Sex

Sex differences have also been studied but without a careful systematic theoretical perspective. In studies of adolescents with anxiety disorders, diagnosed according to DSM-III, it has been determined that there are no differences in male:female ratios regarding separation anxiety disorders, social phobias, or obsessive-compulsive disorders (see Chapters 103 and 105). Neuroses are thought to be more common in adolescent females than in adolescent males. Females more commonly exhibit simple phobia, agoraphobia, and panic disorder, whereas more males are diagnosed with overanxious disorder.

Gender differences in reporting style may confound the issue. Female adolescents are more likely to report a greater number of fears, including fear of lightning, test-taking, going outdoors alone, and blushing, whereas boys are more likely to report a fear of talking. Females generally reach the peak age of reporting each fear earlier than do males, which may be related to the slightly earlier age of puberty in females. However, no sex differences are evident about worries concerning personal adequacy, animals, economic factors, or health. The most common worries of adolescents, in descending order of rank, are family, school, and social relationships.

Prevalence

The prevalence of adolescents diagnosed with anxiety disorder is also not well studied and is confounded by the fact that adolescents may also be diagnosed as having adult anxiety disorders (except generalized anxiety disorder). Simple phobias are common in both children and adolescents. Social phobias, in which the adolescent fears and avoids social encounters that involve scrutiny and evaluation, occur during adolescence, with a peak period of onset occurring after puberty. In a study of normal fourth and fifth graders, the school emerged as the most frequently stressful event. Cross-cultural validation for the onset of social phobias in adolescence is further supported by a Japanese study comparing 6034 normal subjects and finding by questionnaire that fear of blushing and being looked at was at a maximal level in the midteenaged years, with a subsequent gradual decrease in both males and females across age.

In addition, agoraphobia (the fear of being in places or situations from which escape might be difficult, or embarrassing, or in which help might not be available in the event the adolescent suddenly experiences symptoms), previously thought to be rare before early adulthood, has been found by retrospective study to have an age of onset before age 20 years in 26% of a large sample of adults with agoraphobia, with 22% having a reported onset between 10 and 19 years of age. In fact, though panic attacks accompanied by agoraphobia are unusual before puberty, their onset is often traced to adolescence. Concurrent diagnoses of panic in consecutive admissions to an outpatient child and adolescent anxiety disorder clinic found a 9.6% rate of occurrence. There was a 2:1 male to female ratio. The most commonly occurring comorbid disorder was depressive disorder, though approximately one half of the patients showed no history of prior psychiatric disturbance.

Socioeconomic Status

The Isle of Wight study of the prevalence of emotional disorders of adolescence did not show a consistent difference with social class. Adolescents of higher socioeconomic status worried more about school achievement and money, whereas children of lower socioeconomic status were prone to worry about imaginary and health concerns.

CLINICAL MANIFESTATIONS AND DIFFERENTIAL DIAGNOSIS

When is a fear serious enough to merit "disorder" status? The general consensus is that when an adolescent's fear is found (1) to be excessive, (2) to last over a relatively long period, (3) to be age-inappropriate, and (4) to create problems in living for the parents or child, or both, therapeutic intervention should be considered.

There have been two broad classification approaches to diagnosis. First, there are clinically derived categories such as those of the American Psychiatric Association (Diagnostic and Statistical Manual of Mental Disorders: Third Edition—Revised; DSM-III-R) or multiaxial diagnosis of the group for the World Health Organization. A second approach is developed from an empirically oriented effort in which classification occurs through multivariate statistical procedures.

Because anxiety disorders are common among adolescents and because many other areas of life are affected (such as academic performance and peer relationships), it is unfortunate that there have been so few empirical studies that focus on the nature or phenomenology of these disorders. To date, reliability studies have yielded different levels of agreement for the DSM-III-R diagnostic category of "Anxiety Disorders of Childhood or Adolescence." Problems in reliability clearly present serious constraints on establishing diagnostic validity. Most reliability studies have been based on small samples (Table 102–1).

Three anxiety conditions are unique to children and adolescents. Avoidant disorder exists when anxiety is focused on contact with strangers, resulting in persistent avoidance of or shrinking from both adults and peers. Overanxious disorder focuses on excessive worry and fearful behavior that is not limited to a specific situation or object (see Chapter 103). Separation anxiety disorder

TABLE 102–1. Diagnostic Criteria of Avoidant Disorder, Simple Phobia, and Pain Disorder

AVOIDANT DISORDER

Excessive shrinking from contact with unfamiliar people that interferes with social functioning in peer relationships

Desire for social involvement with familiar people and generally warm, satisfying relationships with them

Not due to avoidant personality disorder

SIMPLE PHOBIA

Persistent fear of specific stimulus (object or situation)

Exposure to stimulus provokes immediate anxiety

Stimulus is avoided or endured with intense anxiety

Fear or avoidant behavior interferes with normal routine or relationships or causes morbid distress

Recognition that fear is excessive or unreasonable

Stimulus unrelated to obsessive-compulsive disorder or posttraumatic stress disorder

PANIC DISORDER

Discrete periods of unexpected intense fear or discomfort not triggered by being focus of attention

Four attacks within 4-week period or one attack and 4 weeks of fear of future attack

At least four symptoms during an attack:

  Shortness of breath or smothering sensation
  Dizziness, unsteady feelings, or fainting
  Palpitation or tachycardia
  Trembling or shaking
  Sweating
  Choking
  Nausea or abdominal distress
  Depersonalization or derealization
  Paresthesias
  Flushes or chills
  Chest pain or discomfort
  Fear of dying
  Fear of going crazy or doing something uncontrolled

No organic etiology

Adapted from American Psychiatric Association: Diagnostic and Statistical Manual of Mental Disorders, 3rd ed, revised. Washington, DC, American Psychiatric Association, 1987, pp 62–63, 237–238, 244–245.

indicates excessive anxiety about separation from family members (see Chapter 103).

In addition, adult anxiety diagnostic categories may be applied to adolescents. These include phobic disorder, in which fear and avoidance are associated with a specific situation or object, and panic disorder, in which the panic attacks do not only occur when the adolescent is exposed to particular phobic stimuli or a life-threatening situation or during physical exertion (see Chapter 103). Finally, obsessive-compulsive disorder, which is diagnosed by recurrent obsessions or compulsions (see Chapter 105), is less common.

DIAGNOSTIC ASSESSMENT

Differential Diagnosis

Because fear and anxiety are common to many psychiatric disorders, the conditions that make up differential diagnosis of the adolescent with undue anxiety are many. The duration, magnitude, and impact of the symptoms on lifestyle will help the clinician differentiate normal from abnormal behavior. Short-lived anxiety that follows an identifiable life stress may represent an adjustment disorder. A variety of psychoactive sub-

stances can cause anxiety, and a detailed inquiry about their use is vital (see Chapter 111). Adolescents with learning disabilities (see Chapter 107), with or without concurrent attention deficit hyperactivity disorder, may become anxious when they recognize their limitation or are placed in situations that require learning. At times, adolescents in the midst of an acute psychotic break may experience intense anxiety by the appearance of confused thought, hallucination, or ideas of reference (see Chapter 110). One of the major questions of difficulty is the distinction between anxiety and major depression or in many instances the comorbidity of these disorders (see Chapters 100 and 103). Another area in which adolescent diagnosis is difficult is in distinguishing between social anxiety and avoidant personality disorder. These diagnoses in DSM-III-R are not mutually exclusive. The clinical literature would suggest that in the avoidant personality disorder the adolescent reports less desire to interact with people if his or her irrational need for unconditional acceptance is not met. In contrast, the socially phobic individual reports the same type of anxiety regarding social interactions but desires continued contact.

Fear can be manifested in a variety of ways, including behavioral avoidance responses, verbal self-reporting, and physiologic reactions. No one response necessarily connotes fear, and often there is inconsistency between response domains. This is further complicated by the time at which the fear response is assessed. Any rigorous definition of fear seems to require a broad multidimensional analysis, with care taken to specify when measures are of anticipation anxiety, actual reaction to stress, or recovery from a frightening experience.

DIAGNOSIS

Direct Interviews With Adolescents

Until recently, there were relatively few standardized formats available for adolescents. Clinicians used parent interviews and a variety of questionnaires to diagnose anxiety. These measures include questions about the nature of the problem, the length of suffering, situational cues, intensity of avoidance, and change in symptom patterns over time. The adolescent is asked about his or her relationship with parents, the relationship between his or her parents, as well as relationships with other adults, teachers, and so on. School performance (achievement and social relationships), close friends, part-time jobs and recreational activities, dating and patterns of heterosexual activities, living arrangements, and religiosity are important areas to be covered.

An increased number of structured interviews have become available; however, few are specifically for use with adolescents (Table 102–2).

The Anxiety Disorders Interview Schedule for Children (ADIS-C) is more specific for diagnosing childhood and adult anxiety disorders in adolescents than either the Diagnostic Interview for Children and Adolescents (DICA) or the KIDDIE-SADS. Its κ-coefficients are

TABLE 102–2. Structured Interviews for Children's Anxiety Disorders

NAME	REFERENCE
The Anxiety Disorders Interview Schedule for Children (ADIS-C)	Silverman and Nellis, 1988
Diagnostic Structured Interview Schedule for Children (DISC)	Costello et al, 1984
Diagnostic Interview for Children and Adolescents (DICA)	Herjanic and Reich, 1982
KIDDIE-SADS	Puig-Antich et al, 1978
Interview Schedule for Children (ISC)	Kovacs, 1983

0.83 for the child and 0.78 for the adult form, which indicates a high level of agreement among raters for specific diagnostic categories.

Self-Report Questionnaires

The advantage of self-administered and objectively scored questionnaires is the ease of acquisition and potential for the collection of normative data on large populations of adolescents. These norms provide a means of standardizing scores for interpretations that are relevant to youth of varying ages and sociocultural diversity. Many of these tests require adequate comprehension to ensure that the questions are understood; therefore, oral administration may be preferred to group administration, particularly for younger or mentally impaired youngsters (Table 102–3).

Behavioral Observation

There are four categories of behavioral observation: behavioral avoidance tests (BAT), observational codes, behavioral checklists, and global behavioral ratings.

The BAT typically is used with very specific fears, such as fear of snakes or dogs or water phobias. The adolescent is asked to perform the same graded series of approach behaviors toward the phobic object both before and after treatment. The BAT is administered in a standard, carefully controlled fashion, making the scoring of the approach behavior relatively straightforward. Although the BAT does not always correlate well with the individual's self-report measures of fear, it successfully differentiates those treated for their fears from controls who have received no treatment.

Several observational codes have been developed to

TABLE 102–3. Self-administered Questionnaires

NAME	REFERENCE
Fear Survey Schedule for Children	Scherer and Nakamura, 1968
Revised Children's Fear Survey Schedule	Ollendick and Hersen, 1983
Louisville Fear Survey Schedule	Miller et al, 1972
State-Trait Anxiety Inventory for Children	Spielberger, 1973

measure behaviors presumably associated with anxiety. The Observer Rating Scale of Anxiety (ORSA) is a 29-category code that includes behaviors such as crying, trembling hands, stuttering, and talking about being afraid. Using a time-sampling procedure, an observer records the presence or lack of each behavior during each observational interval. The Behavior Profile Rating Scale (BPRS) is a similar code designed particularly for dental settings. Recording intervals are 3 minutes in length, and each behavior on the scale is weighted according to the degree it would disrupt the dentist's examination and treatment of the child. High interrater reliability exists, and dentists' ratings of an individual's fear of dentistry have correlated positively with the child's subsequent BPRS scores. Both the ORSA and the BPRS have differentiated treated children and untreated children. They tend to correlate with parental ratings on the Behavior Problem Checklist and may predict neurotic tendencies.

Behavioral checklists involve a standard set of specific behaviors that are rated by someone who knows the adolescent well. Usually each behavior is checked as occurring or not occurring, or it is rated on a scale ranging from low to high frequency.

Several investigators have used global behavioral ratings as measures of behavior that are assumed to be related to anxieties or fears, as well as measures of cooperativeness and anxiety. Global behavioral ratings have correlated positively with measures of maternal anxiety at the young child's first dental visit and scores on the BPRS. Although they are sensitive to various treatment manipulations, global ratings should be used cautiously because they have been found to be especially susceptible to observer bias. Table 102–4 lists observational tests.

Psychophysiologic Measures

Although the psychophysiologic measurement of anxiety is a well-researched area in adults, it has received considerably less attention in adolescents. Existing information seems to parallel that provided by adults; physiologic correlates of anxiety are typically low to moderate in nature and are inconsistently reported from study to study.

Although the literature clearly suggests that various measures of anxiety often do not intercorrelate, palmar sweat prints (PSP) have proved useful and reliable in several studies as one measure of interventional effects. Several investigators have reported PSP to be sensitive to situational stresses (e.g., surgery) and to various treatment manipulations (e.g., a modeling film of an individual's experience prior to and during surgery).

TABLE 102–4. Behavioral Observation Ratings

NAME	REFERENCE
Conners Teacher Rating Scale	Conners, 1969
Child Behavior Checklist	Achenbach and Edelbrock, 1983
Revised Behavior Problem Checklist	Quay and Peterson, 1983

ETIOLOGY

Instinctual or Preparedness Theories

It was assumed that innate fears should be immutable, common to all members of a species, and present at all times and at all ages. Some fears, particularly those among animal species, may meet the requirements, but since fears fluctuate in humans and are age-related, it is difficult to sort out whether fears are innate or learned. Even in humans, certain fears seem to be prepared (i.e., triggered by specific stimuli, such as fear of snakes, fear of strangers, and so on), which were avoided for the preservation of the species. This has come to be known as the preparedness hypothesis. There is some evidence that certain phobias seem to be resistant to extinction based on their survival value. The persistence of some fears throughout and beyond childhood is of interest, particularly with regard to studies of neurotic adults. The persistence of a circumscribed fear or the presence of multiple or diffuse fears leads to a degree of incapacitation that is often the hallmark of a neurotic disturbance. Adult psychiatric population studies have shown that early fear of social situations was a major concern in these individuals. This fear was accompanied by fears related to loss of approval, feelings of rejection by others, loss of status, and humiliation. It is possible that we are born with individual differences relating to the ease of becoming conditioned to a situation (e.g., timidness) or a general failure to become habituated to a nonmeaningful set of events.

Genetic Predisposition

There are well-founded reasons for believing that individuals are born with substantial differences in the ease with which they acquire new fears and the persistence with which fears endure. The individual differences in the acquisition of fears have received more attention than the differences in the habituation rate. One study found considerable evidence that neurotic disorders can be incorporated within the personality dimensions of extraversion-introversion and a second dimension of neuroticism, which is thought to relate to emotional stability or instability. Neurotic tendencies are correlated with high sensitivity to environmental events, and increasing degrees of introversion represent increasing sensitivity to punishment rather than to reward. Studies of the psychophysiology of behavioral inhibition across time and situations suggest that there may be a lowered threshold for sympathetic arousal in these children and adolescents for unfamiliar situations or individuals.

The lack of high concordance rates in familial studies does not substantiate direct inherited transmission of anxiety disorders. Even though epidemiologic data show that mothers diagnosed with both depression and panic disorder have a high proportion of children with major depression (26%) and separation anxiety (37%), it may be inadequate parenting as well as biologic predisposition that influences concordance. In fact, there is evidence that many children who have parents with psychiatric conditions and depression are at risk for anxiety. In addition, sexually abused children are at risk for greater fear and anxiety symptoms.

In a recent study, it was found that family transmission may be a key variable, since the children of parents who were agoraphobic, with high avoidance scores as opposed to low avoidance scores, had higher rates of identifiable behavioral problems that persisted at the end of a year, which may be early markers of anxiety-related problems. The mothers may model overprotective and anxious stances and instill anxious attachment.

Nonspecific factors, including temperament, are probably key in the genetic transmission of anxiety. Introverted children are more apt to experience problems with anxiety. Others have also suggested that shyness is an inherited characteristic and that the importance of child-rearing practices may influence the risk of the actual manifested disorder. It has been seen in twin and adoption studies that mothers with low sociability and the report of low family cohesion predict social anxiety, thus supporting the importance of environmental contributions. The mothers with low sociability may not have exposed their children to varied social situations, thereby perpetrating a cycle of social fear.

Learned Transmission

Social learning theorists, such as Bandura, have experimentally demonstrated that fears may be learned vicariously by the direct or simulated (videotaped) observation of others. Mothers and children's fears are highly correlated. Mothers in particular have been influential in that they may demonstrate phobic behavior nonverbally or verbally with their own children or allow the child to avoid potentially frightening situations such as dental visits or haircuts. Recently, evidence has accumulated for the importance of peer modeling in both the transmission and the reduction of phobias. If a child observes a group of peers acting in a phobic manner, in the presence of a puppy for instance, the child may also become afraid.

Conditioning Phenomenon

Early evidence for the learning of fears came from the classic conditioning paradigm of Watson and Raynor. A child was originally shown to have no fear of a white rat, then after the rat was presented (unconditioned stimulus) in the presence of a contiguous loud, aversive noise, the child demonstrated fearful behaviors, such as crying and withdrawal (unconditioned response) anytime a white rat appeared. In addition, this response became further generalized, and the child exhibited these fearful behaviors in the presence of any similar stimulus, including white cotton and white fur (conditioned response). There are many clinical examples in which children have become traumatized following a car accident or have exhibited avoidance behavior in relation to doctors or dentists following unpleasant procedures, such as injections or operations.

TREATMENT

Prevention

The need to recognize the normality of transitional fears before turning to professional help is stressed because overreaction may reinforce phobias. Children and adolescents who are allowed to experience fear as a normal response learn self-mastery in fearful situations. Exposing the adolescent to potentially fearful experiences rather than being overprotective will facilitate the competence to cope with anxiety.

Pharmacologic Methods

There is widespread use of imipramine, an antidepressant used in the treatment of children with obsessive-compulsive disorders. The usual tranquilizers, such as alprazolam and diazepam, have anxiolytic effects but are likely to lead to dependency and are prescribed less often (see Chapter 125). Panic disorder is often treated with fluoxetine hydrochloride. Side effects and dependency reactions from this drug are not fully evaluated. Phenelzine sulfate or monoamine oxidase inhibitors have negative side effects when taken with certain foods. Pharmacotherapy may help adolescents begin to interact with the environment if there has been marked withdrawal and avoidance. Research would suggest that drugs plus behavioral therapy, which teaches the adolescent to cope with the anxiety, is more effective than drugs alone. For example, in a study of young cancer patients, the use of diazepam actually enhanced the fear of lumbar puncture unless it was combined with the presence of a coach, parent, or psychologist to help the adolescent use new or available coping strategies during the procedure.

Behavioral Methods

Systematic Desensitization. In this technique, fears are graduated in a hierarchy from least to most frightening. The adolescent is then asked to imagine them while using progressive relaxation or assertiveness techniques to compete with the sympathetic nervous system response of fear. This mechanism has been called reciprocal inhibition. Emotive imagery or identification with a hero figure have been employed for younger adolescents. The procedure has been successful in helping children overcome fears of the dark, animals, and dentists (see Chapter 124).

Imaging Procedures. Adolescents with good imaging abilities may profit from this technique. They are encouraged to imagine themselves successfully in the feared situation. Those with poor imaging abilities may need "*in vivo* exposure," in other words, reintroducing them to the actual avoided situation. This modeling is often accomplished by videotaped models of peers showing successful coping. The therapist can use guided participant modeling techniques with extremely phobic patients. In this case, the therapist accompanies the adolescent during the approach, models effective coping, and guides the individual in making the correct response.

Relaxation Training. Adolescents can be taught to relax by practicing muscular tension and relaxation during imagined situations. Occasionally, controlled breathing is substituted; patients are taught to breathe in a slow and regular fashion. In this way, they are less likely to hyperventilate and enhance a fear response. Controlled breathing can be taught by having them watch an adolescent model or by tracking a respiration simulator.

Modeling. The opportunity to observe examples of others dealing with similar stressful situations is called modeling. Bandura postulates that these experiences serve to elicit former coping responses, inhibit the tendency to make avoidance responses, or actually teach new behaviors that were not in the adolescent's repertoire. He feels that in addition to the instruction, motor coding through behavioral practice is important in learning modeling techniques.

Cognitive Self-strategies. A number of procedures (which have come to be known as stress inoculation) that rely heavily on cognitive self-control are called cognitive self-strategies. The adolescent first learns what it is about the situation that is worrisome—that is, he or she identifies the potential stressors. The responses that can be used to overcome the anxiety are then identified, such as distracting imagery and cognitive coping statements such as "I will make a plan to reduce my anxiety." An important third step is the behavioral rehearsal of these strategies in situations that are as similar as possible to the actual target problem. If the patient has an opportunity to practice coping strategies in advance of the confrontation, he or she is likely to have better self-efficacy for overcoming the real-life situation. The adolescent will rate the likelihood of being able to perform the feared act as higher if he or she has more self-efficacy. Adolescents who are encouraged to actively participate during a filmed exposure to a model overcoming a dental injection phobia are more likely to deal with their anxiety than are those who just passively observe the models of coping behaviors.

Operant Methods

Extinction. Some fears actually disappear over time. This may result from the presentation of the eliciting stimuli (either the unconditioned fear stimulus [loud noises]) or the conditioned stimuli (those that are present in time or place and have also become capable of eliciting fear responses) without the occurrence of painful or aversive events (unconditioned or conditioned responses).

Flooding. In flooding, the adolescent remains in the phobic situation long enough to experience the fear and see that it does not have a reality base. It is not often used with adolescents because of concerns that extinction will not occur and sensitization may cause a worsening of the problem. In reality, much of the work on school phobias, which is based on getting the adolescent back into the classroom as soon as possible, would support the usefulness of flooding. Many of these programs involve a graduated exposure, in which the patient stays only for a short while and progressively increases the length of time, or in which the parent, who is at first present, is gradually encouraged to leave the adolescent alone.

Nontraditional Treatment

Self-help groups have been formed spontaneously among adult patients with various phobias, particularly agoraphobia. In principle, since adolescents are very vulnerable to peer pressure, the opportunity to learn that others are phobic and hear about how they overcame the problem may serve to reduce anxiety and encourage cooperation with treatment strategies. In addition, the use of group therapy to improve peer acceptance and assertiveness skills will be most helpful to the phobic adolescent who has become isolated as a result of avoiding usual activities.

Inpatient Hospitalization

In rare cases in which suicide or severe concurrent depression is present, hospitalization may be indicated. When anorexia nervosa has become a threat to life, hospital supervision and family therapy may be needed, in addition to dealing with the irrational fears of overweight or the body image delusions of these patients (see Chapter 60). Adolescents with extreme phobias or manifestations of obsessive-compulsive disorders are also best treated in the hospital, so that when an exposure or flooding treatment program is in progress, safety can be ensured.

COURSE OF ILLNESS AND PROGNOSIS

Age of onset and severity as an indication of "treatability" vary with the diagnosis. Many adolescent fears are developmental and disappear without treatment as the individual matures. If phobic behavior interferes with the adolescent's functioning or becomes generalized to many other situations or individuals, treatment is indicated. Particularly problematic are adolescent social fears or separation anxiety, which may signal the risk for adult neurotic disturbances. Few long-term data are available to allow one to predict the long-term outcome in adulthood (see Chapter 103).

BIBLIOGRAPHY

Achenbach TM, Edelbrock CS: The classification of child psychopathology: A review and analysis of empirical efforts. Psychol Bull 46:759, 1978.
Bandura A: Principles of Behavior Modification. New York, Holt, Rinehart & Winston, 1969.
Eysenck HJ: The Biological Basis of Personality. Springfield, IL, Charles C Thomas, 1967.
Freud S: The analysis of a phobia in a five year old boy. Collected Papers, Vol 3. London, Hogarth Press, 1905.
Last CG: Anxiety disorders in childhood and adolescence. In Last CG, Hersen M (eds): Handbook of Anxiety Disorders. New York, Pergamon Press, 1988, pp 531–540.
Last CG, Strauss C: Panic disorder in children and adolescents. Anxiety Disord 3(2):87, 1989.
McNally RJ: Preparedness and phobias: A review. Psychol Bull 101:283, 1987.
Morris RJ, Kratochwill TR: Treating Children's Phobias. New York, Pergamon Press, 1983.
Rutter M, Lebocici S, Eisenberg L, et al: A tri-axial classification of mental disorders in childhood: An international study. J Child Psychol Psychiatry 10:41, 1969.
Silverman W, Cerney JA, Nelles WB, Burke AE: J Am Acad Child Adolesc Psychiatry 27:772, 1988.
Watson J, Raynor R: Conditioned emotional reactions. J Exp Psychol 3:1, 1920.

Measures

Achenbach TM, Edelbrock CS: Manual for the Child Behavior Checklist and Revised Child Behavior Profile. Burlington, VT, University of Vermont, Department of Psychiatry, 1983.
Conners CK: A teacher rating scale for use in drug studies with children. Am J Psychiatry 126:884, 1969.
Edelbrock C, Costello A: Structured psychiatric interviews for children and adolescents. In Goldstein G, Hersen M (eds): Handbook of Psychological Assessment. New York, Pergamon Press, 1990.
Herjanic D, Reich W: Development of a structured psychiatric interview for children: Agreement between child and parent on individual symptoms. J Abnormal Child Psychol 10:307, 1982.
Kovacs M: The interview schedule for children (ISC): Interrater and parent-child agreement. Unpublished manuscript, University of Pittsburgh, 1983.
Miller LC, Barrett CL, Hampe E, Noble H: Factor structure of childhood fears. J Consult Clin Psychol 39:264, 1972.
Ollendick TH, Hersen M: A historical overview of child psychopathology. In Ollendick TH, Hersen M (eds): Handbook of Child Psychopathology. New York, Pergamon Press, 1983, pp 3–12.
Puig-Antich J, Orvaschel H, Tabrizi RN, Chambers WJ: Schedule for Affective Disorders and Schizophrenia for School-age Children. New York, New York State Psychiatric Institute, 1978.
Quay HC, Peterson DR: Interim Manual for the Revised Behavior Problem Checklist. Coral Gables, FL, University of Miami, 1983.
Scherer MW, Nakamura CY: A fear survey schedule for children (FSS-FC): A factor analytic comparison with manifest anxiety (CMAS). Behav Res Ther 6:173, 1968.
Silverman WK, Nellis WB: The influence of gender on children's ratings of fear in self and same-aged peers. J Genet Psychol 149:17, 1988.
Spielberger C: Manual for the State-Trait Anxiety Inventory for Children. Palo Alto, CA, Consulting Psychologists Press, 1973.

CHAPTER 103

School-related Anxiety and Related Conditions

HAROLD S. KOPLEWICZ and RICHARD GALLAGHER

Of all the settings in which an adolescent spends time, the school occupies the vast majority of waking hours. Nearly all the developmental tasks are partially completed in the school setting (see Chapter 9). Obviously, education and academic performance are carried out there, but social contact, negotiation of sexual relationships, and self-supervision of behavior are also conducted in this setting. Thus the school setting is an important component of the adolescent's life.

Psychological disorders that interfere with school attendance or performance of educational and social tasks in school have a dramatic impact on later adult success and adaptation. Such disorders hinder adequate social contact, impede concentration, and prevent appropriate independence. Separation anxiety, overanxious disorder, and school refusal have such a broad impact. We refer to them as school-related anxiety disorders because they are manifested in the school setting. They are disorders that are likely to be encountered by primary care physicians because they are frequently accompanied by somatic complaints such as recurrent pain, headaches, and abdominal pain. Often they go unrecognized as psychological disorders because adolescent patients and their families may acknowledge only the physical distress and deny the psychological characteristics. Familiarity with these disorders, their impact on adolescent life, and their appropriate treatment is an important component of adolescent health care.

First we will discuss two specific anxiety conditions, separation anxiety and overanxiousness, and the symptom of school refusal, an approach to assessment and treatment, and finally outcome for this group of problems.

SEPARATION ANXIETY DISORDER

Separation anxiety disorder (SAD) was recognized early. It was studied extensively by Bowlby and colleagues as early as the 1940s. It is a variant of normal reactions to loss of contact with a parental or attachment figure.

Clinical Manifestations

The cardinal features of SAD in youth are distressing anxiety when away from a parental figure and extensive worries that some event threatens the integrity of the family. In childhood, behavioral manifestations can include difficulties sleeping alone, intense distress at the prospect of being left with caretakers during the preschool years, and frequent absences from school and refusal to spend time with peers outside of the home during the school-aged years and adolescence. Since separation is required for school attendance, physical symptoms are often expressed. Gastrointestinal complaints are common in childhood, whereas cardiovascular symptoms (see Chapters 45–50) and headaches (see Chapter 84) are more likely to occur during adolescence. Such physical complaints are notably cyclical and patterned. They often emerge on Sunday evening or Monday morning just before school and dissipate over the weekend when school is not in session.

An adolescent who has SAD often demonstrates unremarkable behavior as long as the primary attachment figure is present. Adolescents are generally able to remain in a different part of the house, travel to many settings, talk and behave freely, and, at times, even attend school when the location of the primary attachment figure is known. Distress and alterations of behavior often emerge rapidly when the prospect of separation occurs. In milder forms of the condition, brief periods of separation can be tolerated, but the adolescent almost always needs frequent physical or verbal contact to be assured that the parent is fine. Therefore, during the episodes of separation, the adolescent may return from other activities or frequently telephone to be assured of the parent's (or other attachment figure's) safety.

Distress is experienced at the prospect of separation and intense behavioral problems are often demonstrated as the adolescent may try very hard to prevent separation. Behavioral problems in the adolescent may include severe outbursts of temper, major arguments, and violence against a parent or authority figure who demands separation. In many cases, the adolescent who has SAD may become possessive and prevent the parent from maintaining a normal work and social life. As a result, the disorder can have serious effects by contributing to the disruption of marital and family relations.

The frequency of SAD varies with age. Generally, SAD is found more frequently in children than in adolescents. In one study of adolescents who were evaluated at an anxiety disorder clinic, the average age of children in whom the primary diagnosis was SAD was 9 years, whereas other anxiety disorders appeared on the average in older children. Symptom expression also varies with age. Significantly, adolescents with SAD report physical complaints on school days as the primary symptom. Younger children reported worries of harm, refusal to attend school, and distress on separation as the primary symptoms. Another characteristic of the adolescent who has SAD, which seems to vary from the child who has SAD, is their ability to attend school. Not all children who have SAD refuse to attend school, though the majority do; however, older adolescents who have SAD are more likely to refuse to attend school. Thus some adolescents are capable of separating long enough to attend classes, especially if they find the school highly supportive, and phone contact with the parent can be maintained at intervals during the day. Other separations that involve a less predictable schedule and allow less freedom of contact are more problematic.

The criteria for diagnosis as specified in the Diagnostic and Statistical Manual-III-R (DSM-III-R) are presented in Table 103–1 in abridged form.

OVERANXIOUS DISORDER

Overanxious disorder (OAD) has received significantly less scrutiny in the research literature than have phobic disorders and SAD. OAD is characterized by more pervasive anxiety, as tension and worries are not limited to one set of situations. The child or adolescent with this problem is excessively concerned about the outcome of past and future events, has excessive worries about evaluation by others, and is markedly self-conscious. Little is known about its epidemiology or course, since research has begun only in the past 5 years.

OAD has a pervasive impact. Anxiety may be high because of concern about grades, appearance, how others will react, and the potential negative consequences of any action. The adolescent who has OAD is not generally reassured by the presence or statements of parents, so he or she has persistent fears that something terrible will occur. Despite the lack of comfort provided by statements from others, the youth with

---

TABLE 103–1. Separation Anxiety Disorder

I. Excessive anxiety concerning separation shown by at least three of the following:
  a. Unrealistic worry of harm befalling major attachment figure
  b. Unrealistic worry that event will cause separation
  c. Reluctance or refusal to go to school
  d. Reluctance or refusal to go to sleep
  e. Avoidance of being alone
  f. Nightmares about separation
  g. Physical symptoms
  h. Distress at anticipating separation
  i. Distress when separated
II. Lasts more than 2 weeks
III. Onset before 18 years of age
IV. Occurs independently of psychotic disturbance

Adapted with permission from American Psychiatric Association: Diagnostic and Statistical Manual of Mental Disorders, 3rd ed., revised. Washington, DC, American Psychiatric Association, 1987, p 61.

OAD is still likely to seek out reassurance and requests may become burdensome.

Certain situations are particularly problematic for many persons with OAD. The completion of homework and performance of tests are difficult. Frequently, the adolescent may feel unduly pressed to complete homework according to unrealistically high standards. At times, reworking of homework causes excessive time demands and stress. For days before a test, on the day of a test, and following the test, the adolescent experiences intense worries and high levels of anxiety. Sometimes anxiety becomes debilitating so that performance is hindered and the person "freezes." Social situations are also fraught with worries and concern. Paradoxically, because the adolescent experiences such high levels of tension with school work and social situations, he or she often avoids these situations or procrastinates to the extent that homework or preparation for examinations cannot be completed in a timely fashion. Avoidance and conflicts can lead to complaints of physical discomfort, which are genuinely experienced but also serve to facilitate avoidance of social or school situations.

Adolescents who experience OAD are generally older than those who experience SAD. In one anxiety disorder clinic, the average age of youth who presented with OAD was 13 years. As a group, adolescents who had OAD also had many more secondary anxiety disorders, including simple phobias, social phobias, and panic disorders. Thus as a group, teenagers who have OAD have greater potential for disruption of their day-to-day lives. Less stress may be placed on family members because attachment and contact are not necessary in this disorder. As a result, many adolescents who have OAD may suffer in silence. However, many share their distress through constant requests for reassurance, avoidance of assignments, and repeated focus on their performance.

As already indicated, OAD as a primary diagnosis seems to be more prevalent in adolescence than in childhood. The adolescent profile and the childhood profile are not the same. Although children with the disorder share most of the symptoms with adolescents, the adolescent patient is more likely to have worries about the effects of past behavior and its appropriateness than does the child with the condition. In both age groups, worries about the future and competence, needs for reassurance, frequent tension, and somatic complaints that have no physical basis are highly prevalent. However, the adolescent with more experience and a sense of history seems to add worries about previous actions to the excessive concerns.

The profile of accompanying disorders also differs in childhood and adolescence. Children are much more likely to exhibit conjoint SAD. Adolescents are more likely to report specific phobias and meet the criteria for affective disorders, including major depression. The prevalence of major depression has been reported to be as high as one half of the adolescent population who have OAD. The clinical picture for adolescents includes acknowledgment of more of the symptoms associated with OAD, more phobic fears of specific situations or objects, and more depressive symptoms with vegetative signs (i.e., disturbances of sleep, appetite, concentration, and libido). This suggests that OAD is a more severe disorder when encountered in adolescence. The

DSM-III-R criteria used for diagnosis are listed in Table 103–2.

SCHOOL REFUSAL

"School refusal" is a descriptive phrase that refers to behavior that has many causes. "School refusal" is often a symptom of SAD and OAD. However, it should not be assumed that "school refusal" and SAD or OAD are synonymous. Therefore, a full discussion of "school refusal," its definition, and its many psychiatric sources is required.

An adolescent who refuses to attend school presents a significant challenge to the youth's parents, school personnel, mental health professionals, and primary care physicians. It is a problem that can have a profound impact on an adolescent's capacity to complete important developmental tasks, including separation from the family and the establishment of independence in the face of decreased supervision by adults. Additionally, persistent refusal to attend school is predictive of limited life success, for it has a negative effect on adult employment status and social adjustment. Adolescents with a long history of school absence earn significantly less money as adults, demonstrate twice the rate of behavioral problems, and experience more psychiatric problems of anxiety and depression than do adolescents who attend school regularly. For the primary care physician, it is one of the most important mental health disturbances in adolescence. Complaints of illness and discomfort are its main manifestation, and research indicates that primary care physicians are contacted much more frequently and much earlier in the course of this condition than are mental health professionals or school personnel.

Epidemiology

Since persistent school absence has a negative outcome, much attention has been directed toward its understanding and treatment. Rates vary, but it is conservatively estimated that 10% to 15% of a school population will be absent on any given day. Of those absences, most are the result of physical illness. How-

TABLE 103–2. Overanxious Disorder

I. Unrealistic worry for a period of more than 6 months shown by at least four of the following:
   a. Unrealistic anxiety about future
   b. Excessive concern about past behavior
   c. Unrealistic worry about competence
   d. Somatic complaints
   e. Marked self-consciousness
   f. Excessive need for reassurance
   g. High tension
II. Symptoms are in addition to any other disorder
III. If patient is older than 18 years, symptoms not due to generalized anxiety disorder
IV. Not due to psychotic disorder

Adapted with permission from American Psychiatric Association: Diagnostic and Statistical Manual of Mental Disorders, 3rd ed., revised. Washington, DC, American Psychiatric Association, 1987, pp 64–65.

ever, up to 25% of children and adolescents who are absent are not ill and do not have a legitimate excuse; 15% are believed to be truant, and 10% represent "school refusers." The history of the study of school absence reflects increasing attention to subgroups differentiated on the basis of psychological and behavioral characteristics.

Initially, unexcused absences were thought to reflect poor moral upbringing and an antisocial attitude toward school and authority, especially when present in adolescence. However, psychological investigations initiated in the 1930s indicated that not all persons with persistent absences held antisocial beliefs and demonstrated amoral behavior. Although school absence was a shared symptom, a significant percentage of the absences were found in children and adolescents who valued school, adhered to social convention, and were generally accomplished intellectually. This group of youth were also likely to be found at home or with family members, as opposed to others who were involved in social groupings or work settings away from home and family. When psychological status was reviewed, the group at home not only possessed effective academic abilities but also valued education. As a group, however, members reported that they found the school setting highly distressing and anxiety-arousing. These students were found to be highly self-conscious, easily aroused to anxiety, and often obsessively fearful that harm would befall themselves or others in their family. As a result of their experiences, they remained home to avoid anxiety while they watched over their status and that of valued family members.

Subsequent to the initial studies, two major divisions were devised for children with unexcused absences: (1) truants, defined as those who stay away from school to participate in social or work activities and demonstrate disruptive behaviors and attitudes that devalue education and (2) "school refusers," defined as those who value school but cannot attend because of anxiety or other emotional disturbances, even though they value education as an essential means to success. The issue of truancy will not be addressed in this discussion, except to indicate that it generally results from conduct problems and not anxiety or affective disorders.

One percent to 5% of the school population consists of "school refusers." There are three age-related peaks of incidence, which are associated with specific school or life changes: (1) 5- to 7-year-old children who demonstrate problems with the initial separation from home for full-day schooling, (2) 11-year-old children who seem to have trouble with changes in school building (from elementary to junior high) and increased demands for independence that result when multiple teachers and classrooms must be negotiated in middle and junior high school settings, and (3) 14-year-old adolescents whose refusal is associated with the emergence of affective illnesses as a prevalent psychiatric disorder.

Clinical Manifestations

Although adolescents who refuse to attend school represent a small percentage of the school population, they can represent a significant proportion of the adolescent population in contact with primary care physicians. The reasons that they present to the physician rarely include discussions of their emotional experience but involve somatic distress. Vaguely described stomachaches, headaches, and pain often are noted. Their caretakers often consult physicians for evaluation and advice. In this way, the primary physician can be the first contact person and can influence the course of the disorder. Review of case studies indicates that adolescents who refuse to attend school generally have a history of several months to 2 years of poor attendance before school guidance personnel or mental health professionals are consulted. Thus persistent somatic complaints and contact with a physician can be used as an early sign of "school refusal."

Differential Diagnosis

It is clear that there are many psychiatric contributions to "school refusal" as a problem. The task in evaluating an individual who demonstrates "school refusal" is determining which psychiatric problem or problems are responsible. The differential diagnoses of the psychiatric causes of "school refusal" are listed in Table 103–3.

A large percentage of adolescents who refuse to attend school have anxiety disorders. Separation anxiety disorder is a major cause of "school refusal" in adolescence, as school is just one of many settings in which separation concerns are raised. However, as discussed later, not all adolescents who have SAD refuse to attend school. Persistent "school refusal" was found in only 73% of one sample of patients with SAD. The prevalence of "school refusal" among patients with OAD is unclear. Specific components of this disorder contribute to discomfort with aspects of school, including performance and social interactions, but it seems rare that worries reach the level that result in avoidance of school. A person who has both SAD and OAD, a fairly common occurrence, is likely to refuse to attend school.

The anxiety disorder associated most consistently with refusal to attend school, especially in adolescence, is school phobia. This is a misnomer because the adolescent is not afraid of the school itself but some aspect of situations encountered in school. School phobia has

TABLE 103–3. Differential Diagnoses of "School Refusal"

ANXIETY DISORDERS
Separation anxiety disorder
Overanxious disorder
School phobia
   Simple phobia of public speaking and tests
   Social phobia of school
Panic disorder
Obsessive-compulsive disorder

AFFECTIVE DISORDERS
Major depressive disorders
Dysthymia

OTHER PSYCHIATRIC DISORDERS
Schizophrenia
Autistic disorder and pervasive developmental disorder
Developmental learning disorders
Adjustment reactions
Personality disorders

TABLE 103–4. Panic Disorder

  I. Discrete periods of unexpected intense fear or discomfort not triggered by being focus of attention
  II. Four attacks within 4-week period or one attack and 4 weeks of fear of future attack
 III. At least four symptoms during an attack:
    a. Shortness of breath or smothering sensation
    b. Dizziness, unsteady feelings, or fainting
    c. Palpitation or tachycardia
    d. Trembling or shaking
    e. Sweating
    f. Choking
    g. Nausea or abdominal distress
    h. Depersonalization or derealization
    i. Paresthesias
    j. Flushes or chills
    k. Chest pain or discomfort
    l. Fear of dying
    m. Fear of going crazy or doing something uncontrolled
 IV. No organic etiology

Adapted with permission from American Psychiatric Association: Diagnostic and Statistical Manual of Mental Disorders, 3rd ed., revised. Washington, DC, American Psychiatric Association, 1987, pp 237–238.

been described in two forms. The first form of school phobia results because the adolescent fears evaluation. School arouses anxiety because of the emphasis on grades and level of performance. These students experience intense worries that they will do poorly on assignments and tests. Often they have had experiences in which intense concern has prevented clear thinking so that they have failed despite long periods of preparation. Other aspects of junior or senior high school may result in newly experienced anxiety, for example, class presentations, teachers asking questions in class, and graded homework assignments. This type of anxiety has been called test or performance anxiety, which is a variant of OAD. In severe cases, refusal to attend school has been documented. The second form has been called social phobia of school. Social phobia is a clearly delineated diagnostic disorder. Its criteria primarily include fear of social situations because of concern that others will critically review behavior. Adolescents with social phobia worry about making mistakes that will humiliate them. Although this seems similar to performance anxiety, it has a broader scope, for the person may fear simple conversation as well as completion of formal assignments. In adolescence, the disorder results in shy withdrawal from others. In severe cases, refusal to attend school is common as a means to avoid social contact.

Two other anxiety disorders contribute to "school refusal." Panic disorders and obsessive-compulsive disorder (see Chapters 102 and 109) contribute a small percentage to the school refusal population. Panic disorder is usually encountered in adulthood, but it seems to emerge in late adolescence in most cases and is found in children on rare occasions. In childhood and adolescence, the youth experiences intense anxiety episodes that cause such dramatic changes in physiologic arousal that the youth believes that a serious illness or death is imminent (Table 103–4). These experiences are so frightening that the adolescent develops strategies to remain in a secure setting at all times. The adolescent, as well as the adult, often requires close contact with a parent or other trusted person to make certain that appropriate treatment would occur if physical illness were to develop. As a result, the person usually does not travel alone or leave circumscribed areas. In cases reported in adolescence, refusal to attend school is frequent. This disorder differs from other forms of anxiety. Although many settings are avoided, the youth fears the physiologic arousal rather than the setting.

Obsessive compulsive disorder (OCD) (see Chapter 109) contributes to "school refusal" both directly and indirectly. An adolescent with OCD experiences repetitive thoughts that are unreasonable but cannot be ignored—that is, obsessions. The content of the thoughts often includes ideas that the adolescent cannot touch certain objects for fear of serious contamination, that the adolescent will do or has done something repugnant (such as kill other persons), or that the adolescent is dirty and unacceptable to other persons. The adolescent may also engage in ritualistic, repetitive behaviors to make certain that negative consequences do not occur—that is, compulsions. The authors have encountered patients in whom the presence of obsessive thoughts contributed to "school refusal" because the school building or some aspect of the school environment was believed to be a source of contamination. More commonly, indirect refusal to attend school has resulted when youth are unable to halt compulsions and meet the school schedule. Others experience severe difficulties in completing school assignments because they have obsessive ideas that they have not read, written, or understood the material well enough. In these latter cases, "school refusal" occurs when the adolescent totally avoids school work in an effort to avoid obsessions and compulsions.

Affective illnesses are often encountered as contributing factors in the adolescent refusing to attend school (see Chapter 100). In the adolescent population, depressive disorders are frequently encountered in conjunction with the anxiety associated with school attendance. Studies report depression to be present in 45% to 70% of adolescents who refuse to attend school, a much higher rate than that encountered during childhood.

The refusal to attend school demonstrated by the depressed adolescent follows a different course from that encountered in the primarily anxious youth. Refusal is one arena in which the decreased energy, interest, and activity associated with depression is expressed. The adolescent may have difficulty with the mental activities of school and may find social interaction problematic. This may lead to anxiety about school assignments and social contact with teachers and peers. The depressed adolescent may find the school setting anxiety-arousing because formerly easy tasks are difficult and are completed with many more errors.

Depression can interfere with school in several ways (see Chapter 100). First, cognitive performance on tasks that require concentration, speed of processing, and memory is decreased. Second, when depressed, a person is more sensitive to the reactions of others, with a heightened sensitivity to rejection. Third, experiences are evaluated more negatively when a person is depressed so that neutral events may take on an aversive quality. Thus the depressed adolescent can no longer

achieve at the same level, is more sensitive to teasing and mild interactional slights, and evaluates events and personal performance negatively. Depression can increase the negative feelings experienced by the adolescent. As a result, negative events such as lowered performance on tests or perceived rejection by others often make the depressed adolescent experience greater sadness. In turn, all the situations associated with increased depression become associated with heightened sadness and further insults to the adolescent's self-esteem. These situations may then arouse anticipatory anxiety and therefore become settings to avoid. Thus when depressed, the adolescent can refuse to attend school in order to avoid negative experiences.

The initial presentation of depression associated with "school refusal" is similar to that of the primarily anxious person. The person does not attend for many days and justifies absence with vague complaints about feeling poorly. The physical complaints occur daily for depressed adolescents, compared with on school days only for the anxious adolescent. Exaggerated responses to illness are common so that contact with a primary care physician is often based on physical complaints. When evaluated through interview or objective self-report measures, the adolescent will indicate high levels of anxiety that are at least as high as those indicated by students who are experiencing only anxiety. However, in addition, the student will acknowledge and possibly report symptoms of depression (see Chapter 100). The presence of depressive symptoms in addition to anxiety indicate the need for treatment that is different from that offered to the person who presents with anxiety only.

Less frequently, "school refusal" may be encountered with other psychiatric conditions. The social withdrawal and deterioration of cognition associated with schizophrenia often results in the individual refusing to attend school when the disease becomes active (see Chapter 110). Relatively high-functioning adolescents with autistic disorders often experience separation anxiety or social phobia when their school setting is changed. These adolescents may find the added demands of multiple teachers and the increased demands of peer relationships in junior and senior high school settings highly anxiety-arousing, even though they may have functioned adequately in small elementary school settings. Students with learning disabilities or other developmental disorders are also at risk for refusing to attend school because they find their limited success in meeting academic demands highly frustrating and discouraging (see Chapter 107). As a result, they can experience anxiety disorders about performance, which leads to school avoidance.

A group of particular concern for pediatricians are adolescents who have physical disabilities or serious medical disorders (see Chapter 30). The authors have encountered several adolescent patients in whom aspects of their medical disorder or physical disability contributed to their refusal to attend school and their anxiety in that setting. Those who have physical disabilities have often expressed extreme self-consciousness about their physical differences, which led to intense distress in school and other "public" settings. With chronic illnesses, some students experience fears that their disease will become active in school, so they avoid school because it is unsafe. For example, petit mal seizures in school may lead to social discomfort because the adolescent believes that others are staring. Additionally, fear of having a grand mal seizure in school may cause an adolescent to avoid this setting to make certain that only trusted people (family) are present when it occurs. Adolescents with diabetes mellitus may fear hypoglycemic attacks and refuse to attend school. Thus "school refusal" can develop as an adjustment reaction to a physical disorder.

DIAGNOSTIC ASSESSMENT

The assessment of adolescents with symptoms of anxiety or refusal to attend school requires different strategies, depending on the presenting complaint. The adolescent who presents to a primary physician because of persistent physical distress (a common route) requires a two-stage assessment process. If the adolescent or parent acknowledges psychological distress and requests guidance in its treatment, the adolescent may not require a complete physical evaluation, and the first step may be unnecessary.

When a persistent physical complaint is present, physical evaluation is essential. The extent of the evaluation is determined by the symptoms, their history, and results of a complete physical examination. This first step is designed to exclude common sources of headache, stomachache, fatigue, and pain and to obtain support for a psychological origin of the complaints.

The physician looks for the presence of anxiety or other psychiatric complications and for any temporal relationships of symptoms with common stress or events (see Chapters 98 and 112).

A first step that can prove useful and is often acceptable to the adolescent patient and the family is a behavioral analysis of the physical symptoms and their occurrence. Simply put, this approach requests information regarding the time, place, and situation in which the physical symptom is experienced during a typical week. Interviews to determine the adolescent's weekday and a weekend schedule provide the broad outlines of the demands of the adolescent's life and the individuals with whom he or she comes into contact. Descriptions of the likelihood of experiencing the physical symptoms in each of these situations can provide cues as to what may be arousing anxiety or distress. If certain situations have been reduced or dropped from the schedule because of physical symptoms, it is often these settings that arouse distress. Interviews are probably the most time-efficient way to gather such data, but a weekly diary of activities and symptoms has been used effectively.

Once it has been established that symptoms have situational fluctuations, and a physical cause is unlikely, a consultation with a mental health professional may be indicated. The clinician must determine the nature of the disorder and the breadth and depth of the anxiety experienced. Large categorical clusters of situations most often encountered by adolescents include separation experiences, school, social contact with peers, social contact with adults, and performance of typical activities such as homework, tests, and leisure pursuits. If distress is acknowledged, an arbitrary delineation of the amount of distress can be used. Wolpe developed the use of Subjective Units of Distress. The person is to rank situations on a scale from 0 to 100 as to the amount of distress experienced, with "0" equal to "no anxiety" and "100" equaling "intolerable" levels. Finally, once the categories are evaluated, exact situations are reviewed. For example, if separation and school are indicated as problem areas, it is determined if separation from both parents is problematic and if the adolescent is able to attend some classes but not others. Such specific delineation helps make the differential diagnosis.

When refusal to attend school is an accompanying characteristic of the presenting problem, it must be remembered that this is a behavior, not a disorder. One must review for anxiety and also consider other disorders, especially depression. In chronic "school refusal," case studies suggest the need to explore family relationships to determine whether "school refusal" is inadvertently being supported by a pathologic parent-child relationship. A highly anxious, socially isolated parent often encourages an adolescent to stay home to provide support, company, and, sometimes, protection. The latter circumstance is most often present when one spouse, usually a husband, is substance-dependent and is abusive to the other spouse. It is also possible that anxiety disorders have a hereditary component and therefore "run in families."

The clinical interview described can be replaced or supplemented with standardized measures of anxiety to assist with diagnosis, but care must be used. For the purpose of determining the level of anxiety relative to peers, self-report questionnaires are useful. Two such measures with appropriate levels of reliability and validity are the Revised Children's Manifest Anxiety Scale and the State-Trait Anxiety Scale—Youth Version. Both provide indications of the amount of anxiety experienced by the adolescent by sampling a number of situations that may arouse anxiety. The Revised Fear Survey Schedule asks the adolescent to indicate the level of fear experienced when considering many situations in the school and home and social and physical situations, among others. On all of these measures, anxious adolescents obtain scores that are higher than other adolescents, so they provide an initial point for evaluation. To determine specific characteristics of anxiety for the purposes of diagnosis and to determine if other disorders are present, structured interview schedules that follow the criteria of DSM-III and DSM-III-R are recommended. Specialized training is required to administer the measures, but they have proved valuable in differential diagnosis. The most widely used are the Schedule for Affective Disorders and Schizophrenia for School-Aged Children (KIDDIE-SADS), the Diagnostic Interview for Children and Adolescents (DICA), the Interview Schedule for Children, and the Diagnostic Interview Schedule for Children (DISC).

ETIOLOGY

The development of anxiety disorders in children and adolescents is not clearly understood. Many theories exist, but none has unequivocal support. It is helpful to group these disorders into four clusters: (1) physiologic, (2) developmental-cognitive, (3) psychodynamic, and (4) learning and modeling. Of course, it is possible that all of the theories have utility and explain some aspect of anxiety disorders. A full elaboration of these ideas is beyond the scope of this chapter, but a brief review is given.

The physiologic theories focus on the functional nature of anxiety and how it is a natural process that serves protective purposes. In this model, anxiety serves to signal danger and, in the case of young organisms, motivates them to return to the protection of parents and safe settings. At certain stages of development, the avoidance of situations motivated by anxiety is appropriate. However, in the case of those who have anxiety disorders, the natural process has gone awry, or those with anxiety disorders have a disordered sensitivity. It is suspected that a low threshold for anxiety may be a temperamental characteristic of some youth, which can be traced to infancy. Such a low threshold may also have a genetic base. Family studies indicate that the children of adults with anxiety disorders exhibit more anxiety disorders when compared with the children of healthy adults and, conversely, the parents of children with anxiety disorders are more likely to have SAD than are the parents of other psychiatrically disturbed children and unaffected children.

The developmental-cognitive model is a recently proposed theory based on therapeutic work with adults who have anxiety disorders. Foa and Kozak propose that individuals work to develop an emotion-processing set of cognitions that help them plan responses to emotional arousal. A memory of feared situations is stored for future reference and includes data on the nature of the stimulus, the physiologic and behavioral response to that stimulus, and the consequential meaning of that stimulus and those responses for subsequent outcome. Disorders develop when cognitive distortions are present in the emotion-processing system such that the feared stimulus is predicted to result in greater harm than is true, that the person will have inadequate responses available to avoid negative consequences, and that the physiologic arousal has broader meaning (e.g., an impending heart attack) than is the case. Whether or not such distortions are responsible for anxiety disorders in youth has only been raised but not studied.

A more traditional and long-standing theory of anxiety has been that developed with the earliest development of psychoanalytic theory. Within this model, certain situations are feared and avoided because they arouse intense unconscious connections that are feared.

The learning approach suggests that anxiety develops because the adolescent learns to avoid situations by experiencing intense discomfort on one occasion, which generalizes to other situations that share similar qualities. Traumatic experiences contribute to the development of anxiety disorders, though they may not be essential. Observational learning can also contribute to inappropriate arousal and avoidance through the process of modeling. If important members of the adolescent's family or social group demonstrate anxiety in certain situations or encourage the adolescent to avoid these settings, he or she may demonstrate similar anxieties and avoidance. This may be an alternative process through which anxiety disorders are transmitted across generations, rather than through genetic transmission. Other factors seem to maintain avoidance and anxiety. Members of the adolescent's environment may covertly or overtly reward avoidance, as in cases in which a dependent, lonely parent treats the adolescent to special presents or activities if he or she does not attend school. Such reinforcement prevents the youth from entering the feared situations and learning to cope with the distress experienced. The avoidance response itself is also thought to be rewarded when an immediate decrease in anxiety is experienced as soon as the adolescent turns from an approach to a feared situation.

TREATMENT

The approaches used in the treatment of anxiety disorders and "school refusal" have varied. Intensive psychodynamic approaches explore the unconscious sources of anxiety through the use of free association, dream analysis, and interpretation. The revelation of unconscious sources of anxiety is reported to decrease their control over behavior. Behavioral therapy techniques use relaxation procedures, exposure to the feared situations, skills training to enhance social responses, and operant procedures to facilitate motivation for approaches to the anxiety-arousing situations (see Chapter 124). Family therapy has also been used. It attempts to alter relations in the family to make certain that (1) parents are the established authority, (2) parents are working at shared goals in child-rearing, and (3) all relationships are conducted in a way that facilitates normal contact with the adolescent's environment. Thus these efforts seek to make certain that avoidance of situations is not supported by the family in any way (see Chapter 123). Finally, psychopharmacologic efforts reduce or eliminate the experience of anxiety so that the adolescent is not likely to avoid distressing settings.

There has been very little research about the effectiveness of psychotherapeutic interventions and family therapy. In contrast, behavioral therapy approaches have used scientific designs but have still involved only single cases. One large sample study reported that although brief psychodynamic psychotherapy and brief behavioral therapy resulted in improvements of parental reports of the child's anxiety symptoms, there were no differences between the two approaches. Importantly, adolescents who were older showed much less response to treatment than did children less than 11 years of age. Follow-up study compared the outcomes of children and adolescents who received one of three treatments: (1) outpatient behavioral therapy, (2) inpatient hospitalization, and (3) home tutoring with outpatient psychotherapy. At the start of treatment, groups were found to match regarding the level of symptoms, intelligence, and socioeconomic background. Most of the patients were older than 11 years of age, with the average age being 13 years. At follow-up 1 year later, the behavioral therapy group had a significantly higher school attendance rate. Behavioral therapy was significantly more effective than hospitalization or home tutoring with outpatient psychotherapy. Ninety-three percent of the behavioral therapy group returned to school, compared with 38% for the hospitalized group and 10% for the home tutored group. Further analysis indicated that home tutoring had a dramatically poor outcome, with no student ever reaching the criteria of 80% or better attendance. In fact, only 33% of this group were free of separation problems at follow-up, compared with 100% of the behavioral therapy group and 93% of the hospitalized group.

The usefulness of many pharmacotherapeutic agents has been studied, although only a few have proved successful (see Chapter 125). Neuroleptics, anxiolytics, and antihistamines are neither appropriate nor effective. A benzodiazepine, alprazolam (Xanax), has been reported as useful in decreasing separation anxiety and panic disorder. The tricyclic antidepressant imipramine has been studied most rigorously and has proved useful in decreasing separation anxiety and its associated refusal to attend school in double-blind, placebo control studies. Use of medications requires careful monitoring.

The principles behind our approach to treatment of "school refusal" and anxiety endorse (1) exposure to the anxiety-arousing situation; (2) gradual increases in exposure; (3) the use of techniques to counter anxiety, including medication, relaxation, and developing coping strategies; and (4) the development of cooperative relationships among adults in the adolescent's life so that participation in anxiety-arousing situations is supported and mandated. The same principles can be applied to other disorders when avoidance of particular settings is hindering functional adjustment. Early intervention to make certain that avoidance of situations does not become habitual is essential. In the case of "school refusal," this means that school attendance in some form is essential. Variations can include relatively brief attendance at the guidance office, individual tutoring in the library, and participation in one or two classes. Evidence suggests that total avoidance of school and any separation experience through home tutoring should be avoided. This is especially important information for the physician because parents and adolescents often request medical justification for home tutoring.

Implementing plans requires several steps. First, the adolescent must attend school. This often requires negotiation with parents and the adolescent to establish a new or newly endorsed family rule. Second, the parents may need help establishing enough authority to ensure school attendance. Parents must be prepared to face arguments and temper outbursts. To decrease the power of these outbursts, consequences for violation need to be established. Third, if physical complaints play a role in the disorder, how they influence attendance needs to be determined. Generally, the adolescent must attend unless certain physical signs are present. Often this means that an adolescent must attend unless the parents

have documented a specific elevation in temperature (101°F is safe). Attendance should still be required during the evaluation of the physical complaints. Fourth, negotiation with school personnel is required. This is necessary to facilitate the development of a modified schedule and to establish a comfortable contact person for the adolescent. School personnel are usually experienced with adolescents who refuse to attend school. It is inappropriate to develop a treatment plan without this contact. Contact is often initiated with the principal but is usually maintained through a guidance counselor or school psychologist. Finally, once the previous steps are taken, a consistent team composed of the physician, family, and school must remain in contact so that firm, but supportive, efforts are maintained to help the adolescent continue attendance. If this approach meets with failure in a relatively short time, a mental health consultation for psychopharmacologic treatment in conjunction with behavioral therapy should be obtained.

OUTCOME AND PROGNOSIS

The outcome for SAD, OAD, and social phobia is not clearly known. Studies suggest that they may not be benign conditions. In severe cases, adult versions of SAD are present, which prevent a full work and school life. Retrospective reports by adult patients with agoraphobia, generalized anxiety disorder, and panic disorder indicate that a large percentage of them (10% to 50%) experienced SAD or other childhood anxiety disorders. Many parents of children and adolescents with anxiety disorders share similar problems. These data suggest that persistent problems with anxiety may be an outcome for many persons who experience such disorders in childhood. One report demonstrated a higher than expected lifetime occurrence of panic disorder and social phobia for children with SAD evaluated 18 years later.

Adult outcome of OAD is not clearly understood; however, it is strongly suspected that many adults with generalized anxiety disorder experienced OAD in childhood and adolescence. Generalized anxiety disorder shares many characteristics with OAD. Some researchers believe that OAD may portend a lifelong difficulty with anxiety. Peer relations are influenced so that social interactions are restricted and interpersonal relations are problematic.

The information on "school refusal" is clearer, though the few longitudinal studies have methodologic problems. However, data indicate that those who regularly miss large periods of time in school or who never graduate are at high risk for poor work attendance, poor adjustment, and lower social status than would be predicted by intelligence and status of families of origin. In the short term, these adolescents persist with problems in school attendance, and up to 70% experience other psychiatric disorders, including difficulties leaving home alone (22% in one sample), no return to school (20% in another study), and depression.

BIBLIOGRAPHY

Ballenger JC, Corek DJ, Steele JJ, Cornish-Motigne D: Three cases of panic disorder with agoraphobia in children. Am J Psychiatry 146:922, 1989.

Berg I, Jackson A: Teenage school refusers grow up: A follow-up study of 168 subjects, ten years on average after in-patient treatment. Am J Psychiatry 133:532, 1985.

Bernstein GA, Garfinkel BD: School phobia: The overlap of affective and anxiety disorders. J Am Acad Child Psychiatry 25:235, 1986.

Blagg, NR, Yule W: The behavioural treatment of school refusal—a comparative study. Behav Res Ther 22:119, 1989.

Foa EB, Kozak MJ: Emotional processing of fear: Exposure to corrective information. Psycholo Bull 99:20, 1986.

Gittleman R, Koplewicz HS: Pharmacotherapy of childhood anxiety disorders. In Gittleman R (ed): Anxiety Disorders of Childhood. New York, Guilford Press, 1986, pp 180–206.

Hersov L, Berg, I: Out of School: Modern Perspectives in School Refusal and Truancy. Chichester, England: John Wiley & Sons, 1980.

Last CG: Anxiety disorders of childhood and adolescence. In Last CG, & Hersen M (eds): Handbook of Anxiety Disorders. New York, Pergamon Press, 1988.

Miller LC, Barnett CL, Hampe E, Noble H: Comparison of reciprocal inhibition, psychotherapy, and waiting list control for phobic children. J Adolesc Psychol 79:269, 1972.

Trueman P: The behavioral treatment of school phobia: A critical review. Psychol Schools 21:215, 1984.

Measures

Costello EJ, Edelbrock CS, Dulcan MK, Kalac R: Testing of the NIMH Diagnostic Interview Schedule for Children (DISC) in a Clinical Population (Contract No. DB81-0027). Final report for the Center for Epidemiological Studies, National Institute for Mental Health. Pittsburgh, PA, University of Pittsburgh Press, 1989.

Herjanic B, Reich W: Development of a structured psychiatric interview for children: Agreement between child and parent on individual symptoms. J Abnorm Child Psychol 10:307, 1982.

Kovacs M: The Interview Schedule for Children (ISC): Form C and the Follow-up Form. Unpublished manuscript. Pittsburgh, PA, University of Pittsburgh, 1978.

Ollendick TH: Reliability and Validity of the Revised Fear Survey Schedule for Children (FSSC-R). Behav Ther Research 21:685, 1983.

Puig-Antich J, Chambers W: The Schedule for Affective Disorders and Schizophrenia for School-aged Children. Pittsburgh, PA, Western Psychiatric Institute and Clinic, 1978.

Reynolds CR, Richmond BO: What I think and feel: A revised measure of children's manifest anxiety. J Abnormal Child Psychol 6:271, 1978.

Spielberger C: Manual for the State-Trait Anxiety Inventory for Children. Palo Alto CA, Consulting Psychologists Press, 1973.

Wolpe J: The Practice of Behavior Therapy. New York, Pergamon Press, 1973.

CHAPTER 104

Post-traumatic Stress Disorder

ROBERT S. PYNOOS and KATHI NADER

Post-traumatic stress disorder (PTSD) may have a critical and long-lasting impact on the lives of adolescents. Perhaps more so than in any other age group, during adolescence this condition may constitute a psychiatric emergency. Adolescents are at risk of engaging in dangerous, self-destructive or violent traumatic reenactments, or of making impulsive decisions that alter their future. Recognition of the salient features of the disorder by physicians who provide care for adolescents, as well as prompt treatment or referral, can avert some of the most deleterious consequences of PTSD in this age group.

PTSD occurs in response to traumatic experiences in which an individual is faced with a catastrophic event. There is typically life threat to self or to a significant other, grotesque mutilation or death, serious injury, or physical coercion. PTSD may result from exposure to such events as rape, sexual or physical abuse, criminal assault, sniper attack, military combat, severe accidents, natural and technological disasters, the witnessing of sibling, peer, or family member suicide or homicide, or acts of community violence. PTSD can occur concomitantly with physical injury that requires trauma surgery, reconstructive surgery and rehabilitation, and becomes an important issue in hospital care and outpatient recovery in such cases.

EPIDEMIOLOGY

As yet, there have not been epidemiologic studies to determine the incidence or prevalence of PTSD specifically among adolescents in the general population. Homicide, suicide, and death by accident are leading causes of death in the adolescent age group, suggesting a significant level of exposure to types of events associated with PTSD. In addition, the extent of familial and community violence would also indicate a significant risk of exposure. There are also many adolescents who are immigrants from either war-torn countries where they have witnessed atrocities or from disaster-stricken areas where the level of morbidity and mortality had been high.

A recently completed epidemiologic study of young adults in a major metropolitan area found that nearly 40% of this population had reported lifetime exposure to at least one event that could be considered "traumatic" by Diagnostic and Statistical Manual of Mental Disorders: Third Edition–Revised (DSM III-R) criteria.

These included experiences of life threat, serious accidents or disaster, witnessing death or injury to another, victimization by criminal assault or rape, and combat. Although the study did not clearly measure the degree of life threat or exposure to these events, the rate of post-traumatic stress disorder subsequent to these stressors was approximately 20%. In the case of rape, 80% of the victims developed PTSD. There are factors that are associated with risk of exposure to traumatic events as well as factors that influence the development or chronicity of PTSD after exposure. For example, personality characteristics or substance abuse may lead adolescents to be involved in situations where violence or recklessness may lead to traumatic injury or death. Family history of anxiety or panic disorders may be associated with a greater likelihood of developing the disorder after exposure.

CLINICAL MANIFESTATIONS

Recent studies have confirmed that the clinical syndrome in adolescents is similar to the adult presentation of the disorder, although in adolescents the presentation may be uniquely influenced by age-specific developmental considerations. Like adults, adolescents respond to traumas with symptoms of (1) re-experiencing, (2) numbing or avoidance, and (3) increased states of physiologic arousal (Table 104–1). These symptoms may radically alter the life trajectory of the adolescent, with interpersonal, educational, and legal ramifications.

"Re-experiencing phenomena" refers to symptoms where elements of the traumatic experience recur in a distressful and intrusive manner in the adolescent's mental life. This is manifested in intrusive images and thoughts, traumatic dreams, flashbacks or behavioral reenactments, and psychological and physiologic reactivity to traumatic reminders. An intrusive image is an intense perceptual recollection that is hard to dispel and often incorporates horrifying or helpless moments of the traumatic experience. For example, a family returning home from a picnic was confronted with an intruder robbing their house. The father was shot, and died while his 13-year-old daughter tried to stop his bleeding. The girl was flooded with recurrent, intrusive images of her father's head wound and with unrelenting thoughts of her unsuccessful efforts to revive him. Intrusive images can be intensified by unnecessary, secondary exposure to graphic details. The brother, in the above case, had

TABLE 104–1. Diagnostic Criteria for Post-Traumatic Stress Disorder

A. The person has experienced an event that is outside the range of usual human experience and that would be markedly distressing to almost anyone, e.g., serious threat to one's life or physical integrity; serious threat or harm to one's children, spouse, or other close relatives and friends; sudden destruction of one's home or community; or seeing another person who has recently been, or is being, seriously injured or killed as the result of an accident or physical violence.

B. The traumatic event is persistently re-experienced in at least one of the following ways:
   (1) Recurrent and intrusive distressing recollections of the event (in young children, repetitive play in which themes or aspects of the trauma are expressed)
   (2) Recurrent distressing dreams of the event
   (3) Sudden acting or feeling as if the traumatic event were recurring (includes a sense of reliving the experience, illusions, hallucinations, and dissociative [flashback] episodes, even those that occur upon awakening or when intoxicated)
   (4) Intense psychological distress at exposure to events that symbolize or resemble an aspect of the traumatic event, including anniversaries of the trauma.

C. Persistent avoidance of stimuli associated with the trauma or numbing of general responsiveness (not present before the trauma), as indicated by at least three of the following:
   (1) Efforts to avoid thoughts or feelings associated with the trauma
   (2) Efforts to avoid activities or situations that arouse recollections of the trauma
   (3) Inability to recall an important aspect of the trauma (psychogenic amnesia)
   (4) Markedly diminished interest in significant activities (in young children, loss of recently acquired developmental skills such as toilet training or language skills)
   (5) Feeling of detachment or estrangement from others
   (6) Restricted range of affect, e.g., unable to have loving feelings
   (7) Sense of a foreshortened future, e.g., does not expect to have a career, marriage, or children, or a long life.

D. Persistent symptoms of increased arousal (not present before the trauma), as indicated by at least two of the following:
   (1) Difficulty falling or staying asleep
   (2) Irritability or outburst of anger
   (3) Difficulty concentrating
   (4) Hypervigilance
   (5) Exaggerated startle response
   (6) Physiologic reactivity upon exposure to events that symbolize or resemble an aspect of the traumatic event (e.g., a woman who was raped in an elevator breaks out in a sweat when entering any elevator).

E. Duration of the disturbance (symptoms in B, C, and D) of at least 1 month.

Specify delayed onset if the onset of symptoms was at least 6 months after the trauma.

With permission from American Psychiatric Association: Diagnostic and Statistical Manual of Mental Disorders, 3rd ed, revised. Washington, DC, American Psychiatric Association, 1987, pp 250–251.

chased the robber, and did not see his father's mutilated body. However, at the preliminary hearing, the district attorney, unannounced to the boy, asked him to identify his father from the photographs taken at the crime scene. The boy, who had been free of traumatic images, now could not dispel this grotesque memory of his father.

Traumatic re-enactment behavior refers to the repetition of actions, taken or imagined, during moments of the traumatic event. These re-enactments often occur in response to self-induced or external traumatic reminders. A 17-year-old boy had been in an automobile accident that killed his best friend after their car was hit from the blind side and rolled over. Compulsively, he began to ride a "corkscrew" roller coaster at a nearby amusement park. Examination of this behavior revealed that he was repeating the experience of rolling in the car, only this time with a guaranteed safe outcome. As he rode the roller coaster, he practiced keeping his eyes open. This is an example of "thrill-seeking" re-enactment behavior that represents an effort to anticipate the accident and prevent the fatal outcome.

Avoidant behavior and psychological numbing indicate continued restriction or regulation of emotions or behavior in an effort to control the recurrent impressions and the associated affect. Adolescents may become avoidant of specific thoughts, locations, concrete items, or themes in their cognitive or physical activities that remind them of the traumatic events. They may exhibit reduced interest in what had been pleasurable activities, experience a sense of aloneness, even estrangement from others, and develop a fear of any overwhelming affects. Memory disturbances, including omissions, distortions, and even dissociation may act to control the sense of life threat or harm to another. Adolescents may also exhibit loss of newly acquired skills and learning.

Traumatic avoidance may selectively restrict daily activity. Avoidance may remain bound to highly specific traumatic cues or evolve into more general phobic behavior. Furthermore, adolescents may experience a profound change in their attitude toward the future. They may become more pessimistic, expect future harm, envision a foreshortened future, and alter plans for school, career, marriage, and family.

Increased states of arousal refer to tonic and phasic alterations in physiologic status, including disturbances in sleep, increased irritability and anger, difficulty concentrating, hypervigilance, exaggerated startle response, and heightened physiologic reactivity to reminders. The sleep disturbance may reflect relative changes in sleep stages, mark the onset of parasomnia and, untreated, may last for months, even years. Environmental noises may easily arouse the adolescent. Sleep may be fitful and not restful, and fatigue may interfere with daytime concentration. Expressions of irritability and anger merit particular attention, because they may reflect a disregulation of aggression. These disturbances may strongly influence ongoing personality development during these crucial years.

There are also associated features of the disorder, including guilt, grief, worry about a significant other, and renewed symptoms from a previous life experience. Expressions of guilt may intensify the level of distress over the traumatic occurrence. Worry about the safety of a significant other may be an additional source of extreme stress for adolescents and their families. Adolescents worried about a younger sibling have reported greater post-disaster distress and more somatic complaints than their peers. There is an interplay between post-traumatic stress reactions and bereavement. These trauma reactions often keep the adolescents' mind focused on the circumstances of the death, interfering with grief resolution and adaptation to subsequent life changes. The current traumatic event may serve as a powerful reminder of a past experience, and thereby provoke a recurrence of symptoms of an earlier trauma or loss.

NEUROBIOLOGIC AND NEUROCHEMICAL CORRELATES

The understanding of PTSD in adolescents must be rooted in sound developmental neurobiology. The tonic and phasic physiologic changes in arousal and anxiety appear to be associated with alterations in a number of biologic systems. Most of these have thus far only been investigated in adults with PTSD, and there is a need to extend these studies to adolescents.

The neurophysiologic findings include (1) disruption of sleep architecture, (2) enhanced or modified acoustic startle eye-blink response, (3) altered event-related evoked potentials, (4) lowered threshold for peripheral autonomic arousal, and (5) increased physiologic reactivity to self-induced or external traumatic reminders. The physiologic alterations tend to reinforce other symptoms of the disorder. These changes may also have medical consequences; for example, there are reports of persistent increased heart rate and blood pressure following combat exposure and other adult traumas.

The neurochemical correlates of PTSD include (1) excessive peripheral sympathetic reactivity associated with increased adrenergic function, (2) a central adrenergic regulatory dysfunction, (3) possible alterations in serum testosterone levels and other sexual hormones, (4) opioid system dysfunction, especially from chronic or repeated trauma, with suggested tonic depletion and phasic reversible stress-induced analgesia, and (5) alterations in the serotonin system, important in the apprehension and response to threat.

DIFFERENTIAL DIAGNOSIS

Post-traumatic stress disorder shares symptoms with other common psychiatric disorders and may coexist with other conditions. When the clinician is unaware that a traumatic experience has occurred, especially one that has taken place in the distant past, the differential diagnosis may be long. Knowledge of potentially traumatic experiences when considering the overall symptom picture may help to alleviate misdiagnosis. By the time adolescents reach adulthood, there may be a multiplicity of clinical presentations. Even after a single traumatic experience, with time, it becomes more difficult to ascertain the specific influence of the trauma.

Anxiety and depression are common adjuncts to PTSD, and the associated disorders may appear in conjunction with post-traumatic stress reactions. As secondary adversities accumulate or when an associated bereavement is accompanied by self-punitive thoughts and a pervasive anhedonia, major depression, a common cause of secondary comorbidity in PTSD, should be independently assessed and treated (see Chapter 100). Pre-existing depression may predispose adolescents to react with unjustified guilt, even when their exposure was minimal.

A wide range of anxiety symptoms commonly occur following traumatic experiences (see Chapters 102 and 103). During a traumatic event, adolescents may experience increased attachment behaviors, such as worries about the safety of family members or friends. Specific symptoms of separation anxiety may be present (e.g., morbid fears of catastrophe befalling family members, nightly checking on the safety of a family member, continued apprehension about a sibling or parent being out of sight). Prior threats to important attachment bonds (e.g., parental illness, separation, or divorce) or constitutional proneness may contribute to post-trauma anxiety reactions. Simple phobias, which result from frightening or injurious encounters, may differ from PTSD by the absence of re-experiencing phenomena or tonic changes in arousal behavior. On rare occasions, a conversion disorder may occur involving an area of the body injured during a violent trauma (see Chapter 112).

After violence, rituals such as checking door locks occur in response to obsessional concerns about safety (see Chapter 105). Obsessional thoughts of contamination or washing rituals may occur after sexual assault. Rarely, obsessive-compulsive disorder develops in the context of PTSD by secondary generalization. Schizophrenia, the delusional disorders, and brief reactive psychoses are readily distinguished from PTSD on the basis of minimal criteria overlap, dissimilarities between psychotic intrusive thoughts and PTSD re-experiencing, and the presence of otherwise intact reality testing in PTSD (see Chapter 110).

PTSD can exacerbate or even mimic those disorders characterized by behavioral manifestations. Before diagnosing oppositional-defiant disorder, conduct disorder (see Chapter 108), or attention-deficit hyperactivity disorder (see Chapter 106), it is important to rule out PTSD as the cause of the adolescent's deteriorating school performance, alteration in attentional ability, or new-onset irritability or aggression. Traumatic events can also exaggerate pre-existing conduct or learning disorders, which in turn can hamper the ability of the adolescent to process traumatic experiences (see Chapter 107). Such reciprocal exacerbation may be especially characteristic of substance-abusing adolescents, who may come to rely on drugs as a maladaptive coping strategy.

A history of recurrent or repeated trauma may serve as one of several complex antecedents to borderline personality disorder (BPD) (see Chapter 109). Therefore, symptoms of self-mutilation, sexual or aggressive play, and suicidal behaviors in adolescents with incipient BPD or narcissistic or antisocial disorders should always raise the question of re-enactment behavior and prompt a search for traumatic antecedents. Repeated victimization may result in demonstrable contradictory behaviors across different contexts or, in their extreme, multiple personality or other dissociative disorders (see Chapters 118 and 119).

Severe parental psychopathology may add to the risk of exposure to traumatic stressors due to psychotic, violent, or suicidal parental behavior or assertive mating with a violent or abusive partner. In addition, the adolescent's own personality may also influence exposure. For example, an adolescent with pre-existing conduct disturbances or substance abuse may frequent situations where there is added risk of violence (see Chapter 111). Adolescents who have been severely traumatized, for example, by a violent massacre, may demonstrate subsequent dangerous, volatile, and substance-abusing behavior that prompts a host of diagnoses without consideration of PTSD as a primary diagnosis. Severe trauma-avoidant behavior may lead the clinician away from exploring traumatic antecedents.

Finally, it is important to recognize the normative nature of many reactions, especially during the initial weeks following a traumatic event. The diagnosis of an adjustment disorder is appropriate when the stressor is less extreme than in PTSD, the full criteria for PTSD are not met, and there is less interference with personality functioning.

DIAGNOSIS

Diagnosis of PTSD is made according to the criteria listed in Table 104–1. As discussed in Chapter 22, obtaining historical information from parents and others may be very useful. There is often parent-adolescent discordance in the report of behavioral changes and subjective distress, or in memory regarding portions of the traumatic event.

ETIOLOGY

By definition, PTSD results from exposure to severely distressing event(s). It is unknown why some individuals are more vulnerable or less resistant to them than are others. Adolescents may be at risk because of certain unique aspects of their development. Because of the complex developmental challenges of adolescence, the intrusion of a trauma may provoke a "true case" of adolescent turmoil. Traumatized adolescents may embark upon a period of post-traumatic acting-out behavior, in the form of school truancy, precocious sexual activity, substance abuse, delinquency, or self-endangering re-enactment behavior.

The disregulation of aggression in this age group can have serious deleterious consequences, including suspension from school, serious injury to another or oneself, and arrest. With the increasingly easy access to guns, automobiles, and drugs, the adolescent's post-trauma behavior can become dangerous, even life-threatening. A 17-year-old boy fought off the assailant who was sexually assaulting his mother. He attacked him with a kitchen knife and was disarmed before the rapist fled the house. When the police arrived, they drew their guns on the adolescent who again held the knife and ordered him to spread eagle on the ground. The boy was able to signal to the police that the assailant was escaping, and he was captured. One month later, this boy, who had no prior delinquent behavior, drove after another boy who had upset him, and ended up in a high-speed chase with the police, who finally pulled him over and drew their guns on him. Fortunately, one of the officers recognized him from the previous incident, and a more calamitous outcome was avoided. Furthermore, as Van der Kolk has written, the adolescent is vulnerable to trauma-induced narcissistic rage, and is at risk for taking revenge into his or her own hands; for example, committing an atrocity in response to witnessing the killing of a friend.

The core symptoms of PTSD as well as the secondary ramifications of the trauma may both disturb the adolescent's peer relationships. Post-traumatic irritability, inhibition, or aggression can strain sibling and peer relationships. Temporary dislocation and permanent relocation of residence can interrupt peer friendships, which are an important source of social support, especially for adolescents.

Post-trauma changes in personality also affect interpersonal relations. After a hostage-taking in which all of her family members were killed, teenage friends complained that a formerly popular and social 16-year-old girl had become serious and no longer carefree. The girl was openly judgmental of her peers when they seemed unappreciative of their family members. Simple irritability or confusing behaviors may result in ostracism and thus affect self-esteem, and may limit the adolescent to aberrant rather than mainstream relationships.

Many of the developmental disturbances may reflect subjective changes in self-concept, cognition, and conscience. For example, a trauma-induced sense of discontinuity in the sense of self (feeling one is not the same person as before) can have a disrupting influence on the adolescent task of integrating past, present, and future expectations into a lasting sense of identity. There may be increased confusion about one's self-definition, sexual definition, and occupational definition. For example, a 17-year-old boy who had failed in his attempt to subdue the man who had sexually assaulted his mother subsequently misconstrued his ineffectualness for cowardliness and weakness, especially in allowing the assailant to disarm him. In his first year of college, he found his dating and sexual behavior radically altered by intrusive images of the rapist on top of his mother. He altered his ambition to become a lawyer and became preoccupied with plans to become a gun merchant, with the fantasy that he would always be better equipped than the assailant if they were to meet again.

There may also be serious disturbances in adolescent consolidation of feelings of masculinity and femininity. A boy who was in a fast-food restaurant massacre experienced intense and prolonged psychosexual distress. There were pretrauma influences that arose out of his early childhood and parental divorce; however, the current violent trend had origins within his terrible sense of being emasculated by his experience. He had witnessed his best friend's mother die from a single bullet wound, while her husband survived multiple gunshots. He had also viewed shotgun mutilation to another woman's breast. The experience of lying helpless on the floor during the rampage took on vulnerable, repulsive, passive feminine attribution. Preteen and adolescent girls may be especially troubled by their own physical ineffectualness and vulnerability or be disturbed, even in their sense of femininity, by their intense aggressive impulses and fantasies of revenge.

Trauma during adolescence may pose a serious challenge to critical steps in cognitive development. It has been reported that one effect of chronic childhood trauma is a persistent reduced use of symbolic expression. Adolescents may find that age-appropriate increases in symbolic thinking may elicit a wider spectrum of traumatic reminders, thus evoking intense traumatic emotions and ongoing fears of renewed anxiety. In addition, disturbances in attention and concentration may lead to diminished academic achievement. There may be long-term educational consequences, for example, when, after a trauma, there is a deterioration in school achievement in the junior year of high school that subsequently jeopardizes opportunities for college.

There may also be a disturbance in the adolescent's evolving sense of morality and conscience, as well as in his or her relationship to society's regulations and authority. These disturbances may be manifested in confusion about the ultimate sources of moral knowledge. Because of their compelling need to judge the courage of their own actions and to scrutinize the motivation and behavior of others, adolescents are prone to assume inordinate guilt and shame, or to be preoccupied with their anger and rage at others or with the failure of society in general. In particular, revenge fantasies disturb their evolving sense of moral self.

The adolescent is alert to issues of human accountability, including the role of society in administering just punishment. If, for example, no assailant is arrested or prosecuted, the adolescent's respect for the principles of social justice may be undermined. This occurs at a critical time, when the adolescent is having to accept becoming increasingly under its purview.

One of the overall influences on the adolescent's life trajectory is the skewed valence placed on either dependence on family and society or self-reliance. Adolescents may exhibit a premature movement toward independence and extreme self-sufficiency or an intensified dependence on family and a reluctance to establish an independent life. The adolescent may drop out of school, marry early, or radically change his or her career choice or abandon plans to work or attend school away from home. Adolescents may anticipate how the traumatic experience will affect their adult behavior, including their parental behavior.

TREATMENT

Treatment of PTSD may be viewed along a continuum from prevention to long-term intervention. The type and extent depend on the nature of the trauma, the premorbid psychological health of the adolescent including vulnerabilities and resilience, availability of ongoing social support, and the extent of other life stressors. The four phases of possible treatment include (1) prevention and psychologic first aid, (2) specialized initial consultation, (3) brief therapy, and (4) long-term therapy. Intervention may involve four different sites, including the individual adolescent, the family, peer group, and school.

In working with families and children at risk for psychiatric morbidity, prevention goals include (1) ameliorating traumatic stress reactions and facilitating grief work, (2) preventing interferences with development and the resulting maladjustments, and (3) promoting competence in effectively adapting to the crisis situation. Successful preventive intervention requires access to children who are identifiably at risk, treatment of populations undergoing normative reactions to extreme stress, and prevention of the onset of disorders, or reduction of their duration and progression when they do exist.

The goal of psychological first aid is to provide important initial emotional relief through immediate psychological services. Table 104–2 includes a listing of proposed specific interventions to address common adverse traumatic reactions in adolescence. We believe that after a major disaster or act of community violence, the school setting is an optimum site for any organized intervention program, and have described an implementation plan.

The initial consultation is a key meeting with the adolescent, and it may significantly increase the adolescent's compliance with future treatment. The emotional meaning, as well as the personal impact, is imbedded in the details of the experience, and the clinician must be prepared to hear everything, however horrifying or sad. Special interviewing techniques may be necessary to assist adolescents to thoroughly explore their subjective experiences, and to help them understand the meaning of their responses. These special interviewing techniques include encouraging the adolescent to recount his or her subjective experience moment by moment, with special attention to the cognitive, affective, and physiologic reactions that had occurred. The goal is to help adolescents understand the meaning of their responses. They are assisted in identifying traumatic reminders that elicit intrusive imagery, avoidant behavior, or psychophysiologic reactions. The aim is to help adolescents to anticipate, understand, and manage everyday reminders, so that the intensity of these reminders and their ability to disrupt daily functioning recedes over time. Lastly, the interviewer invites exploration of the secondary changes in their lives as a result of the trauma, in order to promote their actively addressing these issues.

The clinician needs to communicate an availability to help the adolescent approach the most threatening moments and, to suggest by his or her interventions, that working through the adolescent's subjective experience offers more emotional relief than does continued traumatic avoidance. One key is to assist adolescents in recognizing the age appropriateness of their reactions when they tend to want to dismiss them as "childish."

TABLE 104–2. Specific First Aid Interventions for PTSD Prevention—Adolescents (Grades 5, 6, and up)

SYMPTOMATIC RESPONSE/ISSUE	FIRST AID
Detachment, shame, guilt	Discussion: event, feelings, limitations
Self-consciousness	Adult nature of responses
Post-traumatic acting-out	Link behavior and event
Life-threatening reenactment	Address impulse to recklessness
Abrupt shifts in relationships	Understanding expectable strain
Desire for revenge	Address plans and consequences
Radical changes in attitude	Link changes and event
Premature entrance to adulthood	Postponing radical decisions

Adapted with permission from Pynoos RS, Nader K: Psychological first aid and treatment approach to children exposed to community violence: Research implications. J Traum Stress 1(4):445–473, 1988.

Brief therapy allows the exploration of changes in emphasis or meaning of the multiple moments of the experience. It permits a contextual understanding of the trauma within the life situation and culture of the adolescent, the family and peer group. If increased arousal behavior leads to direct functional impairment, e.g., reduced attention and learning secondary to a chronic sleep disturbance or altered personality due persistent hypervigilance or exaggerated startle, then the use of medication to modify arousal behavior can be an important part of an overall treatment plan. Although antidepressants have been used in the treatment of PTSD, agents such as clonidine and propranolol, which directly suppress brain-stem systems involved in fear-enhanced arousal, may be the more specific agents to treat these symptoms.

The family provides the key site for reinstating a sense of safety and security. Family members may require their own therapeutic intervention before they can adequately attend to their adolescent's reactions. A primary goal of family therapy is to help family members validate and legitimize each other's psychologic course, thereby facilitating continued mutual support (see Chapter 123). Otherwise, there can be estrangement or impatience among family members. Parenting skills can be enhanced through education regarding post-traumatic stress reactions, realistic expectations about the course of recovery, differing psychological agendas, the management of temporary regressions, and the importance of encouraging open communication with their adolescents. Adolescents can learn to inform parents about the specific nature of their traumatic reminders, and parents can learn to provide extra support at these critical moments.

The small group offers opportunities to reinforce the normative nature of reactions and recovery (including grief), share mutual concerns and traumatic reminders, address common fears and avoidant behavior, increase tolerance for disturbing affects, provide early attention to depressive reactions, and aid recovery through age-appropriate and situation-specific problem solving. Especially for adolescents, groups can be a valuable tool to address temporary disturbances in peer relationships.

Pulsed intervention is an especially effective means of providing ongoing care to the traumatized adolescent. The major goal of this intervention is to maintain normal developmental progress. The clinician would see the adolescent at certain critical junctures, decided on through ongoing communication with the family and adolescent, by anticipated reminders of the event, and normal developmental challenges. Long-term therapy is sometimes indicated, especially when there has been prior trauma, the trauma was massive and violent, intense psychosexual disturbances are generated, major divergences in impulse control and impaired development of conscience result, or severe identificatory conflicts and persistent sadness follow; for example, a murder-suicide of the parents.

CLINICAL COURSE

The following clinical vignette illustrates a typical course of PTSD in a young adolescent.

A 12-year-old boy was vacationing with the family of his best friend when they stopped for lunch at a fast-food restaurant. An assailant took the customers and staff hostage for more than an hour, killing 21 people and injuring 20 with a semi-automatic weapon, a shotgun, and a hand gun. Eventually, a S.W.A.T. team shot and killed the assailant and stormed the restaurant. During the massacre, the boy, who remained under a table, witnessed the deaths of his best friend, the best friend's mother, and others who were shot in the restaurant. He was shot in both arms and feared that he would be killed, too. Even when the S.W.A.T. team entered, because they wore boots and army fatigues similar to the assailant, the boy thought they were there to continue the killing.

Afterwards, he was disturbed by thinking he heard the sounds of the repeated gunfire. He feared that harm would come to his family, and dreamed of them dying in earthquakes or other disasters. He saw and heard his dead friend on the television set in his room. Later the boy began to exhibit new, violent behaviors (kicking and hitting). He took a knife into areas known to be frequented by armed youths. He also provoked his schoolmates into fights or became aggressive toward them for no obvious reason. He refused to discuss the massacre and became estranged from family members and friends. He continued to be defiant and to display antisocial behaviors, and he began to use drugs. He was hospitalized because of increasing depression and aggressive behaviors at home and at school. He remained delayed in his physical and emotional development.

When first seen by the authors, the boy was emblazoned in traumatic reminders, including a "Dead Kennedy" sweatshirt, army boots, and a paper facsimile of an initial bracelet similar to the one cut off his best friend's wrist by the paramedics. Attention to these clothing details and their possible traumatic references assisted the consultant in engaging the boy in a discussion of his traumatic experience. In subsequent sessions, some of his most notable behavior became understandable in terms of their traumatic references. For example, one S.W.A.T. team member had reached down to grab the boy by the arm, jerked him up and forcibly prevented the boy from swinging at him. Thereafter, whenever someone put a hand on his arm, the teenager felt impelled to slug the person. Furthermore, before leaving the restaurant he repeatedly tapped his friend on the thigh in a vain attempt to revive him. Similarly, whenever he was touched on the thigh, he became violent. He was preoccupied with fantasies of jumping up and slugging the assailant to senselessness.

The clinical course of PTSD in adolescents is variable, depending on the severity, duration, and personal impact of the original traumatic experience; the coping and resiliency of the individual adolescent; the influence of previous trauma; the additive demands of grief and secondary stresses; the presence of adverse influences on recovery; and the impact on critical stages of development.

DSM III-R criteria require that core symptoms persist for at least 1 month before the diagnosis can be made. This time interval was chosen to permit early detection of the disorder and, at the same time, exclusion of persons with only a transient stress reaction. For those with mild exposure or minimum personal impact, the symptoms usually diminish rapidly within days or weeks of the event. However, adolescents who have faced severe life threat or witnessed horrifying violence or injury to a family member are likely to suffer a more prolonged course. Initial exposure and severity of reaction is strongly predictive of later course, although a delayed onset of symptoms can occur.

The effect of multiple adversities after major disasters or from massive trauma can greatly modify the complex of symptoms, their duration and resolution, specifically by increasing the rate of comorbidity, especially concurrent PTSD and major depressive disorder or generalized anxiety disorder. One catastrophic event can be associated with multiple adversities such as of severe life threat, loss of a family member or friend, loss of residence and relocation, involuntary unemployment of a parent, and change in the family's financial status. The chronic traumas inflicted by war involve a complex interplay of traumatic experiences superimposed on deprivation, malnutrition, family disruption, loss, immigration, and resettlement.

Adolescent intrinsic factors also influence the clinical course. Influenced by their phase of development and prior experience, adolescents vary widely in their attempts to interpret the event and their symptoms, to regulate their emotions, and to search for meaning, information, and assistance. Some appear to overgeneralize the traumatic reminders, while others display accurate cognitive discrimination. Although effective coping reduces distress, maladaptive coping, such as drug abuse, may exacerbate it or become a problem itself. Culture may influence coping behaviors; for example, Kinzie and colleagues found no increase in substance abuse or delinquency among adolescent Cambodians, even though they had a high prevalence of PTSD years after enduring massive trauma and family loss.

Some adolescents may interpret their post-traumatic stress reactions as an indication that something is wrong with them and may feel that their peers are not similarly affected. They may unrealistically expect their recovery time to be shorter. These expectations can intensify adolescents' distress and prevent them from seeking needed support. In addition, the way in which adolescents process traumatic reminders and manage the accompanying renewal of anxiety may also significantly affect their recovery. The presence of significant psychopathology in a parent or a guardian can jeopardize adolescents' own efforts to achieve an adaptive resolution.

Finally, because judicial proceedings adjudicate blame, there is a link between judicial outcome and trauma resolution that affects the course of recovery. For example, by the time of sentencing, adolescents who are preoccupied with fantasies of revenge may feel unburdened of the responsibility for obtaining justice.

BIBLIOGRAPHY

Breslau N, Davis GC, Andreski, P, et al: Traumatic events and posttraumatic stress disorder in an urban population of young adults. Arch Gen Psychiatry 48:216, 1991.

Dohrenwend BP, Dohrenwend BS, Warheit GJ, et al: Stress in the community: A report to the President's Commission on the Accident at Three Mile Island. Ann NY Acad Sci 365:159, 1981.

Famularo R, Kinscherff F: Propranolol treatment for children with acute post-traumatic stress disorder. Am J Dis Child 142:1244, 1988.

Giovacchini PL: Psychic discontinuity during adolescence: Discussion of panel presentations, American Society of Adolescent Psychiatry, May 1986. In Feinstein SC, Escman AH, Looney JG, et al (eds): Adolescent Psychiatry Volume 14: Developmental and Clinical Studies. Chicago, University of Chicago Press, 1987, pp 417–422.

Herman JL, Perry JC, van der Kolk BA: Childhood trauma in borderline personality disorder. Am J Psychiatry 146:490, 1989.

Kinzie JD, Sack WH, Angell RH, et al: The psychiatric effects of massive trauma on Cambodian children. J Am Acad Child Adolesc Psychiatry 25:370, 1986.

Krystal JH, Kosten TR, Perry BD, et al: Neurobiological aspects of PTSD: Review of clinical and preclinical studies. Behavioral Therapy 20:177, 1989.

Putnam FW: Dissociation as a response to extreme trauma. In Kluft RP (ed): The Childhood Antecedents of Multiple Personality. Washington, DC, American Psychiatric Press, 1985, pp 65–97.

Pynoos RS: Post-traumatic stress disorder in children and adolescents. In Garfinkel BD, Carlson GA, Weller EB (eds): Psychiatric Disorders in Children and Adolescents. Philadelphia, W. B. Saunders, 1990, pp 48–63.

Pynoos RS, Nader K: Children's exposure to violence and traumatic death. Psychiatric Annals 20:334, 1990.

Pynoos RS, Nader K: Issues in the treatment of post-traumatic stress in children and adolescents. In Wilson JP, Raphael B (eds): The International Handbook of Traumatic Stress Syndromes. New York, Plenum Press (in press).

Stilwell BM, Galvin M, Kopta SM: Conceptualization of conscience in normal children and adolescents, ages 5–17. J Am Acad Child Adolesc Psychiatry 30:16, 1991.

van der Kolk BA: Psychological Trauma. Washington, DC, American Psychiatric Press, 1987.

CHAPTER 105

Obsessive-Compulsive Disorder

BRUCE BLACK

Obsessive-compulsive disorder (OCD) is a common psychiatric condition affecting individuals of all ages, including adolescents. Although it has been known and described for hundreds of years, the advent of effective behavioral and pharmacologic treatments has led to increased interest and recognition that it is many times more prevalent than was previously thought.

EPIDEMIOLOGY

Until the 1980s, OCD was thought to be extremely rare. In the early 1980s, the National Institute of Mental Health Epidemiological Catchment Area (NIMH-ECA) survey—a large, community-based survey of more than 18,000 adult subjects—estimated the 6-month prevalence of OCD to be 1.6% and the lifetime prevalence to be 2.5%. Similar figures were generated by a study in Great Britain using similar survey methodology. There has been some controversy regarding these figures. The NIMH-ECA survey used trained lay interviewers who administered structured diagnostic interviews (the Diagnostic Interview Schedule). Diagnostic thresholds of severity of distress or impairment are arbitrary and are open to significant subjective variability. When individuals determined to have OCD in the ECA study were reinterviewed by psychiatrists, the prevalence rates dropped by 65% to 75%. Thus the lay interviewers may have overestimated the prevalence of the disorder.

An epidemiologic survey of 5600 high school students used more rigorous methodology, with self-administered screening questionnaires and then detailed interviews by experienced psychiatrists of those students scoring above a predetermined cutoff on the questionnaire, 0.3% of the students were diagnosed as meeting Diagnostic and Statistical Manual of Mental Disorders, Third Edition—Revised (DSM-III-R) criteria for OCD.

The average age at onset in most studies is in the late teenaged years to the early 20s. Males tend to have an earlier age of onset than do females and may have a more malignant course of illness. Among adults, female patients outnumber males by a ratio of 1.5:1, whereas in prepubertal children boys outnumber girls by 2:1. In adolescence, the sex ratio is approximately equal.

CLINICAL MANIFESTATIONS

OCD is characterized by recurrent obsessions or compulsions that occupy significant amounts of time; inter-fere with the individual's social, occupational, or academic functioning; or cause significant distress. *Obsessions* are recurrent intrusive, distressing, and senseless thoughts. *Compulsions* are repetitive, senseless, stereotyped behaviors that are performed according to certain rules or in a stereotyped fashion and are generally linked to an obsessive thought in some way. Individuals may feel that they need to perform the compulsive behaviors in order to prevent some dreaded event from occurring or to neutralize the anxiety associated with an obsessional thought. Not all patients with OCD have both obsessions and compulsions, although most do.

There are a number of characteristic presentations of the disorder, although each individual is unique, and many will not fit into any of these categories. The most common presentation is an obsessional fear of contamination with germs or infection (or sometimes chemicals, body fluids, toxins, radiation, or some unnameable noxious contamination), resulting in compulsive, repetitive washing or showering, usually in a ritualized manner, in order to become free of this contamination. These individuals may spend hours each day washing and commonly suffer adverse dermatologic conditions. They may also spend large amounts of time laundering clothes or washing dishes, floors and walls, doorknobs, and so on. Avoidance of possible contamination (by avoiding touching other persons, doorknobs, potentially contaminated dishes, utensils, foods, and so on) is a common symptom in these adolescent patients and may also be a cause of significant functional impairment. There may also be obsessive fears of harming others by inadvertently contaminating them.

Obsessional doubt and compulsive checking is another common manifestation. Adolescents with OCD may fear that they will do or have inadvertently done something that will harm themselves or others and compulsively check to try to reassure themselves that this has not happened. For example, these individuals may fear that they will cause a fire by leaving a clothes iron, stove, or light fixture turned on and will go back to check many times to try to be sure that they have turned it off, or they may fear that they absentmindedly ran over someone while driving and go back to look for the body, then fear they missed it and have to go back to look again, and again, and so on, driving around and around. At the heart of this pattern is an inability to ever be certain. Even after going back and looking at the switch or feeling the stove burner or examining the road dozens of times, the individuals may fear that they did not check it right, that they just thought they did, and that they need to check it again. Other individuals with OCD may have a less well formed fear ("something terrible will happen") or an apparently nonsensical fear ("my mother will get cancer and die") and perform obsessive touching, counting, arranging, sorting, or collecting, or nonsensical obsessive checking of order, symmetry, or matching of colors or numbers in order to avert the dreaded event or reduce the associated anxiety. These compulsive acts may be repeated dozens or even hundreds of times and may occupy many hours or even most of the adolescent's waking hours.

Some individuals suffer primarily from pure obsessive thoughts, especially of a sexual, violent, or blasphemous nature, and may perform so-called cognitive rituals, (i.e., stereotyped, repetitive, forced counterthoughts intended to ward off or neutralize the unwanted thoughts).

The characteristic symptoms of OCD are exaggerated forms of what are, to some extent, normal everyday thoughts, feelings, and behaviors that have somehow become fixed in the mind like a broken record repeating itself over and over and never coming to a conclusion. Obsessive thoughts and compulsive behaviors have also been referred to as "mental tics" and as "hiccups in the brain." In hearing about obsessive-compulsive symptoms, most individuals, though recognizing the bizarreness of the symptoms, also recognize the symptoms as somehow familiar. Almost everyone has occasionally been confronted with nagging doubts such as, "Did I really turn off the oven this morning or do I just think I did because I did so yesterday?" Many individuals have little ritualized ways of getting dressed in the morning, fixing breakfast, or making the bed, and are uncomfortable altering these rituals. Superstitions are common in many apparently healthy individuals (and rampant in some groups, e.g., athletes), and bizarre fears and compulsions are common in normal, healthy children ("step on a crack, break your mother's back"). Even most adults recognize occasional intrusive, bizarre, or senseless thoughts. What distinguishes OCD from these normal thoughts and behaviors is the degree of associated anxiety; the senselessness, intrusiveness, and repetitiveness of the obsessive thoughts and associated compulsions; the severe, nagging uncertainty or doubt; the amount of time occupied by obsessive thoughts or compulsive behaviors; and the associated functional impairment.

Although obsessive thoughts and compulsive behaviors are the primary diagnostic features of the disorder, the anxiety and distress that adolescent patients suffer and the impairment in their day-to-day functioning are the more clinically relevant features. Severe subjective distress is commonly associated with the persistence of intrusive, apparently senseless, thoughts, with the fear that one is crazy, and particularly with efforts to resist compulsions—that is, to not wash or check or touch. Characteristically, tension and distress increase steadily as the individual tries to resist the impulses that he or she recognizes as senseless, and then is relieved by giving in. Giving in to the impulses, however, leads to increased feelings of powerlessness and demoralization.

For many adolescent patients, the effort expended in resisting the compulsions waxes and wanes. Some individuals, particularly children, adolescents, and more severely affected patients, make little or no effort to resist performing compulsive behaviors.

The severity of obsessive-compulsive symptoms, distress, and impairment covers the whole spectrum from minimal to completely debilitating. The DSM-III-R criteria require that "the obsessions or compulsions cause marked distress, are time-consuming (take more than an hour a day), or significantly interfere with the person's normal routine, occupational functioning, or usual social activities or relationships with others." However, these threshold criteria for diagnosis are arbitrary. There is no empirical evidence that someone who spends 65 minutes a day washing the hands has a disorder, whereas someone who only spends 55 minutes does not.

The individual's recognition that the obsessive thoughts or compulsive behaviors are senseless or excessive is generally regarded as one of the characteristic diagnostic features of OCD and as a feature distinguishing OCD from psychotic disorders such as schizophrenia. Indeed, most individuals who have OCD will volunteer that their symptoms seem senseless, and most affected individuals seem in all other respects to be free of psychotic symptoms and to have an intact ability to distinguish reality from nonreality (intact "reality-testing"). However, this is not always so clear, particularly in younger patients or in the more severely affected. Many patients will volunteer that a dreaded event is completely unlikely to occur whether they perform their compulsive behaviors or not, but, if pressed, will acknowledge that they are not really sure about this. Many children or young adolescents will overtly insist that their ritualistic behaviors are in fact necessary and reasonable.

In addition to OCD as already described, a number of other disorders of habit have been considered "OCD-spectrum disorders." Chief among these are trichitillomania (compulsive hair-pulling), onychophagia (compulsive nail-biting), and compulsive skin-picking. Bulimia nervosa (see Chapter 60), anorexia nervosa (see Chapter 60), somatization disorders (see Chapter 112), compulsive masturbation, self-mutilation, kleptomania, and compulsive gambling have also all been considered as possible variants of OCD.

DIFFERENTIAL DIAGNOSIS

Overvalued ideas, superstitions, and rigid, fixed behavior patterns are not uncommon in healthy adolescents. Preoccupations with various specific fears or concerns are common in other anxiety disorders (e.g., with the death of a parent in separation anxiety disorder (see Chapter 103), or with how one is perceived by others in social phobia disorder). Preoccupations with thoughts of hopelessness, worthlessness, or guilt are common in major depressive disorder (see Chapter 100). In both of these cases, however, the thoughts are not experienced as senseless, and they seem congruent to the context of the other symptoms of the disorder. Stereotyped behaviors are common in autism, pervasive developmental disorder, and schizophrenia (see Chapter 110), but reality testing is grossly impaired in these conditions, and the other characteristic features of OCD are generally not present. However, compulsive behaviors in some autistic individuals may respond to medications shown to be effective in the treatment of OCD.

Comorbidity with other anxiety disorders is common, occurring in 40% to 60% of adolescent patients. Major depression also occurs with an increased prevalence in OCD patients. Motor tics may occur in up to one third of children and adolescents with OCD, and more than 50% of individuals with Tourette syndrome also suffer from obsessions and compulsions. Furthermore, a familial relationship between OCD and Tourette syndrome has been demonstrated (see further on).

Many individuals with other anxiety disorders (see Chapter 103), including panic disorder, social phobia, and overanxious disorder of childhood and adolescence, will report some obsessions and compulsions but may not suffer sufficient distress or impairment from those symptoms in order to meet the diagnostic criteria for OCD.

Generally, OCD has been very much underdiagnosed, though this is related to clinicians' lack of awareness of the features of the disorder and lack of appreciation of its prevalence. The primary cause of underdiagnosis is no doubt the secretiveness that many patients maintain in regard to their symptoms. Because of a fear that they will be considered crazy or ridiculous, many patients are quite expert at keeping their symptoms secret, even from family members or from psychiatrists who have been treating them for associated anxiety for many years. Although the disorder certainly continues to be underdiagnosed and undertreated relative to its prevalence in the population, there has also been some overdiagnosis (by inexperienced clinicians and especially by poorly informed family members) in recent years as a result of the tremendous publicity the disorder has received.

DIAGNOSIS

The diagnosis of OCD is based entirely on a history of the characteristic symptoms as reported by the individual or other observers of the adolescent's behavior, or both. History obtained from the adolescent patient's family or teacher is essential in the evaluation. Currently, there are no laboratory tests that contribute to confirming or eliminating the diagnosis of OCD. The diagnostic criteria most commonly used and accepted in the United States are those of the DSM-III-R (Table 105–1). There are a variety of diagnostic instruments that can be of value in gathering the history in this disorder. Structured and semistructured diagnostic interviews, such as the Schedule for Affective Disorder and Schizophrenia, Lifetime Anxiety Version (SADS-LA), the Diagnostic Interview Schedule for Children (DISC), and the Diagnostic Interview for Children and Adolescents (DICA), are useful adjuncts to ensure a complete history of relevant symptoms. A variety of specialized rating scales are available for use by both adolescents and clinicians to rate the presence or lack

TABLE 105–1. Diagnostic Criteria for Obsessive Compulsive Disorder

A. Either obsessions or compulsions
Obsessions: (1), (2), (3), and (4)
(1) Recurrent and persistent ideas, thoughts, impulses, or images that are experienced, at least initially, as intrusive and senseless, e.g., a parent's having repeated impulses to kill a loved child, a religious person's having recurrent blasphemous thoughts
(2) The person attempts to ignore or suppress such thoughts or impulses or to neutralize them with some other thought or action
(3) The person recognizes that the obsessions are the product of his or her own mind, not imposed from without (as in thought insertion)
(4) If another Axis I disorder is present, the content of the obsession is unrelated to it, e.g., the ideas, thoughts, impulses, or images are not about food in the presence of an eating disorder, about drugs in the presence of a psychoactive substance use disorder, or guilty thought in the presence of a major depression
Compulsions: (1), (2), and (3)
(1) Repetitive, purposeful, and intentional behaviors that are performed in response to an obsession or according to certain rules or in a stereotyped fashion
(2) The behavior is designed to neutralize or to prevent discomfort or some dreaded event or situation; however, either the activity is not connected in a realistic way with what it is designed to neutralize or prevent or it is clearly excessive
(3) The person recognizes that his or her behavior is excessive or unreasonable (this may not be true for young children; it may no longer be true for persons whose obsessions have evolved into overvalued ideas)
B. The obsessions or compulsions cause marked distress, are time-consuming (take more than an hour a day), or significantly interfere with the person's normal routine, occupational functioning, or usual social activities or relationships with others

From American Psychiatric Association: Diagnostic and Statistical Manual of Mental Disorders, 3rd ed, revised. Washington DC, American Psychiatric Association, 1987.

of, as well as the relative severity of, various obsessive thoughts and compulsive behaviors and also to rate the overall levels of distress and impairment. The most common rating scales are the Leyton Obsessional Inventory, the Maudsley Obsessive Compulsive Inventory, and the Yale-Brown Obsessive Compulsive Scale.

Whether or not standardized scales are used, every initial assessment of an individual affected with OCD must include some evaluation of the current severity of distress, anxiety, avoidance of feared objects or situations (e.g., avoiding touching doorknobs or leaving home for fear of contamination), resistance of compulsive impulses, and functional interference and impairment, since these are the real targets of treatment rather than the simple presence or lack of obsessions or compulsions.

Three patient presentations illustrating the features of OCD follow:

Stephanie was a 14-year-old girl referred by a non-physician psychotherapist because of suicidal ideation. She denied signs and symptoms of depression other than occasional suicidal thoughts but stated that she had thought of killing herself because of a fear that she was crazy. With some encouragement from the interviewing physician and with protestations that "you will think I am crazy," she reported that she spent most of her waking hours counting. She counted the white dividing lines in the road whenever riding in a car. She counted the footsteps of anyone walking by her at home or in school. She counted words on the page when she was reading or writing school work. Certain features of her environment, for example, corners of walls, had to be touched in a certain way and counted as she passed them. When there was nothing else to count, she counted her breaths. All counting had to end on an even number. Her preoccupation with counting had caused significant difficulty concentrating in school, and she was spending less and less time with friends. Her parents, who were previously unaware of her obsessive-compulsive symptoms, refused to accept their seriousness or the diagnosis of OCD. They felt Stephanie was just being "silly," and instructed her to stop doing these things. They refused further treatment.

John was an 11-year-old boy brought for evaluation because of touching objects repetitively. He initially denied the behaviors attributed to him by his family, but gradually revealed that he was preoccupied by fears that his mother or his dog would die, or that he would contract cancer, die, and go to Hell. He engaged in a variety of compulsive behaviors and feared that if he failed to perform these behaviors correctly, his fears would come true. He repeatedly touched certain objects, such as the television set or toilet seat, an odd number of times before using them. In school, he would cross and recross "t's" and dot and re-dot "i's" dozens of times until they were done "just right," and trace certain words over and over. His written school work, when he was able to complete it, was illegible and full of holes. When he wrote a word containing any letter from his mother's name, he would stop and touch this letter 5, 7, or 9 times. He read and reread single sentences in his schoolbooks dozens of times, feeling that he had not grasped the meaning of the sentence properly. He presented many other complex ritualistic obsessive thoughts and compulsive behaviors involving magic numbers, counting, colors, symmetry, and religious thoughts. John was failing in school because of an inability to complete assignments, and had no friends. He spent many hours per day carrying out his compulsive behaviors.

John's symptoms had continued to worsen for several years despite intensive individual and family psychotherapy. After 8 weeks on fluoxetine, John announced that "the touching stopped—I don't want to do it any more." All symptoms resolved entirely, and he remained asymptomatic after 8 months of treatment.

Melissa was a 13-year-old girl who collected used lottery tickets off the street and from neighbors in her urban neighborhood. She had stored 10,000 of these in shoeboxes in her room. She spent 3 to 4 hours per day counting and recounting these tickets and sorting them by ticket number or color.

ETIOLOGY

The cause of OCD is unknown. However, some neurobiologic abnormalities have recently been demonstrated. Positive-emission tomography (PET) brain imaging studies in adults with OCD have shown increased cerebral glucose metabolism in the frontal cortex and basal ganglia, and in some studies these abnormalities have correlated with symptom severity. A recent study has shown increased levels of arginine vasopressin, somatostatin, and corticotropin releasing hormone (CRH) in the cerebrospinal fluid of individuals with OCD. Similar findings have been reported in patients with anorexia nervosa. In animals, central nervous sys-

tem administration of these neuropeptides promotes grooming and perseverative behaviors that resemble behaviors of OCD patients, and increases arousal, which may play a role in the prominent anxiety of OCD patients.

The possible role of abnormal regulation of the serotonin neurotransmitter system has been suggested as a key pathophysiologic mechanism in the etiology of OCD. This hypothesis is supported most strongly by the observation that though most antianxiety and antidepressant medications are ineffective in treating the symptoms of OCD, medications that are potent inhibitors of the reuptake of serotonin into central presynaptic nerve terminals are effective (see further on). Furthermore, clinical response to these medications may correlate with pretreatment biochemical markers of serotinergic function and posttreatment alterations in both peripheral and central serotonergic markers.

Genetic factors in the pathogenesis of OCD have been suggested by several findings. First, family genetic studies have shown that approximately 25% of immediate family members of OCD probands also have OCD and that there is also an increased prevalence of other anxiety disorders. Second, the concordance rate for OCD in monozygotic twins is 63%. Finally, there is a significantly increased incidence of obsessions and compulsions in the relatives of Tourette syndrome patients, even when the proband Tourette syndrome patients do not have obsessive-compulsive symptoms. Within the families of patients with Tourette syndrome, OCD and Tourette syndrome appear to be etiologically related. Some studies report that the two disorders may be phenotypic variants of the same genotype. Segregation and linkage analysis studies suggest that the mode of transmission is consistent with autosomal dominant inheritance with variable penetrance.

TREATMENT
Pharmacotherapy

Most psychotropic medications are ineffective in the treatment of OCD; however, three pharmacologic agents—clomipramine, fluoxetine, and fluvoxamine—have been shown in placebo-controlled studies to be effective in reducing the frequency and severity of obsessions and compulsions and the associated impairment in adult patients. Clomipramine is a tricyclic antidepressant medication; fluoxetine and fluvoxamine are nontricyclic antidepressants that are structurally similar to each other. Although clomipramine shares the antidepressant activity and side effect profile of other tricyclic antidepressants, it is distinct from them in its very potent blockade of reuptake of the neurotransmitter serotonin into central presynaptic nerve terminals. Fluoxetine and fluvoxamine are also potent and selective blockers of serotonin reuptake. Antidepressant and antianxiety medications that do not produce this potent blockade of serotonin reuptake are not effective in the treatment of OCD. The therapeutic efficacy of these medications in the treatment of OCD is unrelated to coexisting depression, that is, they are equally effective in treating OCD symptoms whether or not the individual is also depressed. Only clomipramine and fluoxetine are currently available in the United States, and only clomipramine is approved by the Food and Drug Administration (FDA) for treatment of OCD. Clomipramine has also been more extensively studied in children and adolescents. It has been shown to be superior to placebo and to desipramine, another tricyclic antidepressant, in children and adolescents with OCD.

Neither clomipramine nor fluoxetine can be recommended as preferable to the other for treatment of OCD in adolescents at this time. Although only clomipramine has been proved effective in adolescents, preliminary clinical experience and open trials suggest that fluoxetine is equally effective and that it is tolerated better than is clomipramine. Both medications can produce troublesome side effects, which can be particularly difficult to manage in anxious patients. Because side effects generally have a rapid onset and therapeutic benefits a delayed onset, patients frequently feel worse before they feel better. Physicians prescribing either medication should be familiar with their use in this population, including dosage titration, drug interactions, and management of side effects. Both medications should be started at low doses and increased gradually.

In patients with less than adequate medication responses, trials with other medications or medication combinations may sometimes be fruitful. Although further follow-up studies are needed, it appears that many if not most patients successfully treated with medication will relapse if medication is discontinued. Long-term maintenance treatment may therefore be necessary.

Clomipramine has also been shown to be effective and superior to treatment with desipramine in the treatment of trichitillomania. It seems likely that both clomipramine and fluoxetine may have some efficacy in the treatment of any of the so-called OCD spectrum disorders.

Psychotherapy

Behavioral psychotherapy consisting of *in vivo* exposure, and response prevention have been shown to be effective in the treatment of approximately 70% of selected adults with OCD. This form of treatment may be most effective for patients with washing, touching, or checking rituals and less effective for patients with obsessions only. Patients must be highly motivated to participate in treatment. Most adolescent patients treated with behavioral therapy seem to maintain the therapeutic gains after treatment is discontinued, at least when reassessed 1 to 3 years after treatment. Unfortunately, behavioral treatments are very specialized, time-consuming, and expensive. Furthermore, there have been no systematic or controlled studies of behavioral treatment of OCD in children or adolescents.

Psychotherapies other than behavioral therapies, particularly individual psychodynamic psychotherapy or psychoanalysis, were widely recommended as the treatment of choice for OCD prior to the 1980s and are still occasionally recommended. There is no empirical evidence that such treatments are of any value.

Response rates with behavioral and pharmacologic treatments are generally similar, with about 30% to 50% of patients much improved at the end of treatment, 20% to 40% showing some improvement, and 10% to 20% showing little or no improvement. Although both behavioral and pharmacologic treatments have been advocated as the treatment of choice, there is no clear scientific rationale at this time for recommending one as superior to the other. There have been no studies directly comparing efficacy or patient acceptance of behavioral and pharmacologic treatments at any age, or comparing either treatment alone to combined treatment. Individual patient characteristics and preferences and the availability of skilled clinicians to provide one treatment or the other should be considered, as well as the expense and length of treatment. Many patients will not have a completely adequate treatment response to pharmacotherapy or behavioral therapy alone, particularly more severely impaired individuals. Combined behavioral and pharmacologic treatment is indicated for these patients. For severely disabled patients who fail to respond to aggressive behavioral and pharmacologic treatment, surgical cingulotomy may be an effective treatment.

Clinicians can also be very helpful to adolescents and their families by providing information regarding OCD and advising families on how to cope with the adolescent's symptoms. A variety of excellent pamphlets and booklets are available. Lay organizations for individuals with OCD and their families have been developed in recent years, and local chapters are in existence in most major urban areas in the United States. Participation in these organizations can be a very valuable source of support and information for patients and their families.

COURSE OF ILLNESS AND PROGNOSIS

Little information is available on the long-term course of OCD. Most patients seen in clinical settings appear to have a chronic course, but there may be many individuals in the community with a more episodic course who never come to treatment. There do seem to be some individuals who experience an episode of OCD, recover without treatment, and never relapse. Epidemiologic studies to date have demonstrated that the great majority of OCD sufferers at all ages never come to treatment. Although treatment is effective in relieving symptoms for many patients, and behavioral treatments seem to lead to prolonged remission, little is known about the very long-term course of the disorder after behavioral treatment or with long-term maintenance pharmacotherapy.

BIBLIOGRAPHY

American Psychiatric Association: Diagnostic and Statistical Manual of Mental Disorders, 3rd ed., revised. Washington, DC, American Psychiatric Association, 1987.

Flament M, Whitaker A, Rapoport JL, et al: Obsessive compulsive disorder in adolescence: An epidemiological study. J Am Acad Child Adolesc Psychiatry 27(6):764, 1988.

Leonard HL, Swedo SE, Rapoport JL, et al: Treatment of obsessive-compulsive disorder with clomipramine and desipramine in children and adolescents: A double-blind crossover comparison. Arch Gen Psychiatry 46(12):1088, 1989.

Pauls DL, Pakstis AJ, Kurlan R, et al: Segregation and linkage analysis of Tourette's syndrome and related disorders. J Am Acad Child Adolesc Psychiatry 29(2):195, 1990.

Rapoport JL (ed): Obsessive-Compulsive Disorder in Children and Adolescents. Washington, DC, American Psychiatric Press, 1989.

Rapoport JL: The Boy Who Couldn't Stop Washing: The Experience and Treatment of Obsessive Compulsive Disorder. New York, Dutton, 1989.

Rasmussen SA, Eisen JL: Epidemiology of obsessive compulsive disorder. J Clin Psychiatry 51(Suppl)2:10, 1990.

Swedo SE, Schapiro MB, Grady CL, et al: Cerebral glucose metabolism in childhood-onset obsessive-compulsive disorder. Arch Gen Psychiatry 46(6):518, 1989.

Swedo SE, Rapoport JL, Leonard H, et al: Obsessive-compulsive disorder in children and adolescents. Arch Gen Psychiatry 46(4):335, 1989.

Turner SM, Beidel DC: Treating Obsessive Compulsive Disorder. New York, Pergamon Press, 1988.

Disturbances of Behavior, Learning, and Thought

CHAPTER 106

Attention Deficit Hyperactivity Disorder

BRUNO J. ANTHONY and SHERIDAN PHILLIPS

Attention deficit hyperactivity disorder (ADHD) is one of the most common psychiatric disorders of childhood and often persists into adolescence and adulthood. The diagnostic challenge with adolescents is to detect the more subtle manifestations of ADHD at that developmental level.

Impairments in (1) attention, (2) regulation of activity, and (3)impulse control are the key characteristics of ADHD. This constellation of problems has been noted by clinicians for at least 90 years but was not identified and generally recognized as a diagnostic category until the term *minimal brain dysfunction* emerged in the early 1960's. It was subsequently catalogued as hyperkinetic reaction of childhood in the second edition of the Diagnostic and Statistical Manual of Mental Disorders (DSM-II). Since that time, the disorder has been variously entitled attention deficit disorder (ADD), then ADD with two subtypes (with and without hyperactivity), and now ADHD. Each revision of the DSM changed the diagnostic criteria. Although important, these refinements in diagnostic criteria make analysis of the literature quite difficult and limit our understanding of ADHD during adolescence.

It has been suggested that ADHD may best be conceptualized as a chronic disease that generally persists into adulthood. These individuals are likely to experience continuing problems with antisocial behavior, academic attainment, employment success, interpersonal skills, and self-esteem. As with any other chronic disease, the clinician's task includes not only management of ADHD during adolescence but also anticipation of continuing difficulties during adulthood. The goal of intervention during adolescence is to prevent or minimize subsequent problems. Because ADHD typically is present from childhood and because limited data are available for adolescents, we will discuss ADHD in both childhood and adolescence. Historical information about earlier behavior may be crucial in making the diagnosis during adolescence.

EPIDEMIOLOGY

Stringent application of the current Diagnostic Manual for Mental Disorders: Third Edition–Revised (DSM-III-R) criteria for ADHD indicates that approximately 5% of North American children have this disorder. The negative impact of ADHD continues to be evident in adolescence for approximately 75% of these children. A recent study of all children and adolescents in the Canadian province of Ontario reported a prevalence of 3.3% for females and 9% for males using the DSM-III criteria for ADHD. The rates for females did not vary substantially by age. For males, however, the prevalence of ADHD for 12- to 16-year-olds was 7.3%, in contrast to the 10% rate found for boys aged 4 to 11 years.

CLINICAL MANIFESTATIONS

The clinician treating adolescents will encounter four presentations of ADHD. First, ADHD may develop initially during adolescence. This occurs infrequently and generally only subsequent to neurologic trauma. Usually it is unclear whether such symptoms truly reflect ADHD or organic brain syndrome. Second, the disorder may have been present during childhood but masked by factors such as superior intelligence. During adolescence, academic tasks increase in quantity and complexity, and social expectations demand greater responsibility and self-control. The disabling effects of ADHD may thus become increasingly evident. Third, the disorder may have been identified during childhood but not successfully treated. Our increasing understanding of interventions mandates reevaluation of the adolescent. Fourth, ADHD may have been diagnosed and managed appropriately during childhood. Even then, management often requires readjustment during adolescence.

Core Symptoms

Children and adolescents with ADHD demonstrate symptoms of inattention, impulsiveness, and overactivity. *Attention problems* are usually described by parents and teachers as difficulty in listening, concentrating, and resisting distraction. Observation of children with ADHD shows them to spend more time "off-task" than do normal children. These problems with sustained attention show up most clearly under conditions in which required activities are boring and dull.

Impulsiveness refers to difficulties in witholding behavior in response to situational demands. Children with ADHD often fail to wait for instruction or for their turn in some activity. They make careless errors, take risks by failing to consider consequences, and have difficulty delaying immediate gratification to obtain larger rewards at a later time. This lack of behavioral regulation makes these children appear demanding to adults and selfish and indiscreet to peers.

Hyperactivity refers to developmentally inappropriate levels of motor/or vocal behavior, or both. Phrases used to describe this overactivity include "always on the go," "cannot sit still," and "talks incessantly." This excess activity is seen as "task-irrelevant" and purposeless and even occurs during sleep. Teachers report that these children are always restless and out of their seats playing with objects. Impulsiveness and hyperactivity covary closely and it has been suggested that these two symptom areas are united by a global constuct of behavioral disinhibition or disturbed regulation or inhibition of behavior.

Associated Problems During Childhood

Children with ADHD have a higher likelihood of physical, cognitive, academic, and behavioral problems than do normal children. They are also more likely to meet criteria for other neuropsychiatric disorders (see section on comorbidity).

Physical Problems. Children with ADHD have more minor physical anomalies than do normal children and display more neurologic "soft" signs, particularly those reflecting poor motor inhibition (e.g., overflow movements), and often display poor handwriting. They are more likely to experience general health problems and suffer more accidents. Sleep difficulties are common (see also Chapter 86). Evidence for an increased frequency of enuresis and encopresis in ADHD is equivocal.

Cognitive Problems. On standardized intelligence tests, children with ADHD tend to score 7 to 15 points below normal, which may reflect the effects of inattention, impulsiveness, and lack of sustained effort on test performance. There is little evidence for particular problems in perceptual or memory processes. Rather, children with ADHD do poorly on tasks requiring "executive" processes, such as planning, organization, and strategic problem-solving. Speech problems are common, especially when elaboration is required.

Academic Problems. Poor school performance is an almost universal occurrence in children referred for ADHD. As many as 50% of these children score significantly less than expected levels of academic achievement. Follow-up studies have shown that they are more likely to experience school failure, with up to 35% having been retained in a grade at least once before reaching high school. Specific learning disabilities are far more common in children with ADHD, with a prevalence in clinic-referred groups ranging from 20% (using the most conservative definition of learning disabilities) to almost 60%. In epidemiologic populations, the prevalence estimates are around 10%.

Conduct Problems. There is a high incidence of de-fiant, aggressive, and antisocial behaviors in children with ADHD (see also Chapter 108). Among adolescents referred to clinics, the percentage with aggressive, oppositional, or conduct problems can reach 70%. However, in nonreferred samples, the percentage drops to approximately 20%.

Social Relations. Parents frequently report difficulties in relating to their children with ADHD. These children tend to be less compliant, more negative, and more talkative than are normal children. Parents tend to use negative, controlling, and directive behaviors more frequently; however, these behaviors decline when the ADHD symptoms are reduced through medication. Thus negative family interactions appear to develop in part from the parents' increasing frustration with the ADHD behaviors and their consequent use of less adaptive behavioral management procedures.

It is estimated that more than 50% of children with ADHD have significant problems in social relationships with peers. Their interactions with other children tend to be intrusive, negative, and unpredictable, and they lack adequate knowledge of social skills and appropriate behavior. Peers also tend to respond to the immature and provocative behaviors with controlling and directive behavior and frequently avoid or reject ADHD children.

Attention Deficit Hyperactivity Disorder During Adolescence

More than one half of the children diagnosed with ADHD during childhood continue to meet the criteria for this disorder during adolescence or exhibit significantly impaired adjustment in academic, peer, and family domains, or both. However, the clinical picture alters somewhat with development. First, many adolescents with ADHD do not display the increased levels of purposeless motor behavior seen in children with this disorder. Instead, adolescents more often exhibit fidgety behavior that is more responsive to situational demands. Second, impulsiveness also tends to present in a different fashion. Rather than difficulties in withholding responses, adolescents display poor frustration tolerance and wide mood swings, often resulting in explosive anger and arguments. Third, difficulties with sustained attention and following instructions surpass overactivity as the most prevalent symptom cluster. Organization and planning deficits become more evident with the increased self-management required of middle-school and high-school students.

Problems associated with ADHD also change with developmental stage. Low self-esteem emerges as a major problem during adolescence, with an estimated prevalence as high as 40%. The frequency of severe conduct problems increases; lying, stealing, physical cruelty, truancy, and destruction of property occur significantly more often than in normal adolescents. Substance use (increased cigarette, alcohol, and drug use) becomes a problem for those adolescents with ADHD who also engage in significant antisocial behavior (see also Chapter 111). Academic progress continues to be disrupted, with these adolescents being far more likely to be retained in a grade than are normal children. The presence of a co-occurring conduct disorder is associated with a higher prevalence of school suspensions and expulsions.

The normal problems of adolescence are magnified by the ADHD behaviors, leading to intensified conflict with parents. However, Barkley has reported surprising stability of mother-child interactional problems across the developmental stage. Mothers who are more intrusive and commanding tend to display the same patterns across time and elicit more negative behaviors in their adolescent offspring. Noncompliant children with ADHD continue to show poor interactions with their parents in adolescence. Areas of family conflict center around independence, a significant issue for adolescents in general (see Chapter 9). The difficulty that the adolescent with ADHD has in planning and organizing and with impulsiveness delays both the ability to deal with increased responsibility and the adolescent's parent's willingness to grant it. Peer problems are common. Compared with individuals who do not have ADHD, peer rejection occurs more frequently. Adolescents with ADHD report spending more free time alone or with younger children than do normal adolescents.

Differential Diagnosis

The differential diagnosis of ADHD is complicated by the common occurrence of the core symptoms of inattention and impulsiveness, as well as overactivity to some degree, in normal children and adolescents. Thus it is important to consider developmental changes in the expression of the syndrome because symptoms of ADHD occur most often in preschool children, decreasing through young adulthood. Barkley suggests that decreasing the cutoff score for a DSM-III-R diagnosis of ADHD from 8 of 14 symptoms to 6 of 14 provides better sensitivity and specificity of classification for adolescents. Care should be taken in assessing adolescents from inadequate, disorganized, or chaotic home environments, since such environmental factors may exacerbate ADHD symptoms.

Differential diagnosis should also consider that symptoms of ADHD can result from neurologic conditions (e.g., head trauma, seizures, acquired immunodeficiency syndrome [AIDS]-related dementia), physical disease (e.g., hyperthyroidism), and substance abuse. Adolescents with mood disorders (see Chapter 100) may also display psychomotor agitation and difficulty concentrating.

DIAGNOSIS

The DSM-III-R diagnostic criteria for AHDH are presented in Table 106–1. The items are arranged in order of descending discriminating power. This single-category system is broader than previous systems and has led to a greater number of children being diagnosed with the disorder. The category "without hyperactivity" has been deleted. This acknowledged the lack of evi-

TABLE 106–1. Diagnostic Criteria for Attention Deficit Hyperactivity Disorder

Note: Consider a criterion met only if the behavior is considerably more frequent than that of most people of the same mental age
A. A disturbance of at least 6 months during which at least eight of the following are present:
  (1) Often fidgets with hands or feet or squirms in seat (in adolescents, may be limited to subjective feelings of restlessness)
  (2) Has difficulty remaining seated when required to do so
  (3) Is easily distracted by extraneous stimuli
  (4) Has difficulty awaiting turn in games or group situations
  (5) Often blurts out answers to questions before they have been completed
  (6) Has difficulty following through on instructions from others (not due to oppositional behavior or failure of comprehension), e.g., fails to finish chores
  (7) Has difficulty sustaining attention in tasks or play activities
  (8) Often shifts from one uncompleted activity to another
  (9) Has difficulty playing quietly
  (10) Often talks excessively
  (11) Often interrupts or intrudes on others, e.g., butts into other children's games
  (12) Often does not seem to listen to what is being said to him or her
  (13) Often loses things necessary for tasks or activities at school or at home (e.g., toys, pencils, books, assignments)
  (14) Often engages in physically dangerous activities without considering possible consequences (not for the purpose of thrill-seeking), e.g., runs into street without looking
Note: The preceding items are listed in descending order of discriminating power based on data from a national field trial of the DSM-III-R criteria for disruptive behavior disorders.
B. Onset before the age of 7 years
C. Does not meet the criteria for a pervasive developmental disorder

CRITERIA FOR SEVERITY OF ATTENTION DEFICIT HYPERACTIVITY DISORDER

Mild: Few, if any, symptoms in excess of those required to make the diagnosis *and* only minimal or no impairment in school and social functioning

Moderate: Symptoms or functional impairment intermediate between "mild" and "severe"

Severe: Many symptoms in excess of those required to make the diagnosis *and* significant and pervasive impairment in functioning at home and school and with peers

From American Psychiatric Association: Diagnostic and Statistical Manual for Mental Disorders, 3rd ed, revised. Washington, DC, American Psychiatric Association, 1987.

dence that such children truly constitute a distinct diagnostic entity. Pending further research, the vaguely defined category of "undifferentiated attention deficit disorder" was created to encompass disturbances consisting only of developmentally inappropriate inattention. Guidelines for specifying the severity of the disorder are provided and are based on a combination of the pervasiveness of the symptoms across situations (i.e., home, school), and the number of symptoms.

Plans for DSM-IV include reinstatement of independent dimensions of the disorder (attention and impulsiveness-hyperactivity) and the three subtypes. The ADD-H subtype will not be defined solely by the lack of hyperactivity but will rather consist of core symptoms of inattention plus additional symptoms that are unique to the subtype (e.g., daydreaming, forgetfulness, low energy, reduced motivation).

Comorbidity

As mentioned earlier, core symptoms of ADHD frequently occur with other psychiatric disorders. However, only the presence of pervasive developmental disorder or mental retardation specifically precludes a diagnosis of ADHD (see Chapters 31, 107, and 110). ADHD can be a comorbid condition with other psychiatric disorders. Only about 36% of children diagnosed with ADHD do not have an additional psychiatric diagnosis. Because treatments need to be individualized, it is important to identify all psychiatric conditions.

Disruptive Disorders. Adolescents with a coexisting disruptive disorder (oppositional defiant [ODD] or conduct disorder [CD]) are more likely to have a family history of conduct disorder (see Chapter 108), antisocial personality disorder, major depression (see Chapter 100), or substance abuse (see Chapter 111). Data from clinical populations suggest an overlap as high as 65% for ADHD and ODD. For CD, comorbidity with ADHD increases from 20% to 30% in childhood to as high as 60% in adolescence.

Anxiety Disorders. ADHD does not appear to be linked with anxiety disorders. Although anxiety disorders become the most prevalent psychiatric disorder in adolescence (see Chapters 102 and 103), less than 20% of adolescents with ADHD meet the diagnostic criteria for any type of anxiety disorder.

Mood Disorders. There is mixed evidence linking depressive disorders (see Chapter 100) and ADHD, but they are more prevalent in children with ADHD than in normal children. However, follow-up studies of children with ADHD have consistently reported no evidence of increased depressive illness among adolescents.

Specific Developmental Disorders. Estimates of the percentage of children with ADHD who are likely to have learning, language, and motor problems range widely, depending in part on the definitions employed (see Chapter 107). Using conservative criteria, 19% to 26% of clinic-referred children with ADHD have at least one type of specific reading, spelling, or mathematics disorder.

Subtyping

The issue of subtyping is closely related to comorbidity. The diagnosis of ADHD encompasses a heterogeneous group of individuals. Although they are all characterized by a combination of developmentally inappropriate levels of inattention, overactivity, and impulsiveness, they also possess a variety of other behavioral and emotional difficulties. This diversity has prompted attempts to subdivide this disorder in order to create more homogeneous, clinically meaningful groups.

Hyperactivity. Several lines of evidence suggest that ADD exists without hyperactivity.

1. These groups have different behavioral sequelae. Individuals who have ADD without hyperactivity (ADD–H) appear socially withdrawn, cognitively sluggish, apathetic, and prone to daydreaming. In contrast, those with hyperactivity (ADD+H) are more disinhibited, noisy, disruptive, and impulsive, with more aggressive, oppositional, antisocial activity and less self-control. Children and adolescents with ADD+H also have greater peer relationship problems. These individuals are more often placed in classes for emotional disturbance, while ADD–H individuals are placed in learning-disabled programs. Compared with adolescents with ADD–H, adolescents with ADD+H are more likely to require behavioral intervention and a higher dose of stimulant medication to manage their symptoms.

2. The prevalence of ADD–H does not appear to decline with age, as is the case for ADD+H.

3. Family history studies, though not entirely consistent, suggest that relatives of adolescents with ADD+H have a greater history of ADD and substance abuse, whereas relatives of adolescents with ADD–H may have a significantly greater prevalence of anxiety disorders.

4. Those with ADD–H show difficulties with the efficiency of information processing—the ability to selectively process information accurately and rapidly; adolescents with ADD+H encounter problems with sustaining attention and effort to a task as well as with impulse control.

Aggression. Although aggressive and ADHD behaviors are independent but closely related dimensions of child behavior, hostile and defiant children with ADHD tend to be rated as more severely maladjusted than children with "pure" ADHD and have poorer peer and family relationships. Some evidence suggests that children with ADHD *without* concurrent aggressive behavior tend to display significant deficits in attention, whereas those with concurrent aggression do not.

Follow-up examinations of children with ADHD in adolescence reveal significant differences on the basis of co-occurring aggressive symptoms. Sixty percent of children with ADHD also are diagnosed with CD or ODD in adolescence. However, the adolescents with ADHD who also display aggressiveness show significantly higher rates of substance abuse (predominantly cigarettes, marijuana, and alcohol; see Chapter 111) and school suspensions, expulsions, and drop-out. Both aggressive and nonaggressive adolescents with ADHD show an increased number of grade retentions, suggesting that academic difficulties are associated more with the presence of ADHD symptoms than with conduct problems.

Outcome in adolescents and young adults is significantly worse for children with ADHD and aggressiveness. These children are more likely to be diagnosed with CD, to continue to be rejected by peers, to show evidence of poorer educational adjustment and attainment, and to engage in more substance abuse. In clinic samples, as many as 46% of first-degree relatives of children with ADHD and another disruptive disorder also had ODD, CD, or antisocial personality disorder, compared with only 13% of relatives of children with "pure" ADHD. In adolescents with ADHD and aggressiveness, there is an increased incidence of substance abuse in fathers and affective disorder in mothers. Despite these differences in family psychopathology and outcome severity, children with ADHD with and without aggression are not differentially affected by stimulant medication. In general, the data suggest that aggressive behavior is an important feature to be identified in children with ADHD because it is strongly associated with greater maladjustment and a significantly worse prognosis.

Other Subtypes. Less information is available about the utility of other subtypes. The symptoms of ADHD in children with co-occurring anxiety or depression may respond better to an antidepressant medication than to stimulant medication. At present, the data do not suggest that categorizing children with ADHD on the basis of learning disabilities adds any useful information regarding their treatment, prognosis, or cause beyond the information available regarding their specific cognitive problems.

Assessment

Adequate evaluation requires careful measurement of the core symptoms and co-occurring behavioral and emotional difficulties, as well as cognitive and social-familial factors. Developmental issues need to be considered, as well as the variation in behavior across different situations. Gathering information from multiple informants is particularly important for adolescents because the number of significant contacts increases during this developmental stage. Therefore, information obtained from the adolescent patient via direct interviews and self-reporting should be supplemented with parent interviews and checklists, as well as reports from the school and, if necessary, objective tests of intellectual, academic, and neuropsychological functioning. Although reports from different informants may not show strong agreement, these disagreements appear to reflect differences in the situations in which the adolescent is observed and the observer's familiarity with the adolescent.

Adolescent Interview

The direct interview with the adolescent should solicit information about ADHD symptoms, other behavioral problems, emotional status, and family issues. Information gathered from adolescents through interview or self-report measures is more reliable than that gained from children in these circumstances; however, adolescents with ADHD still tend to underreport the prevalence and severity of their symptoms and conflicts with both family and peers (see Chapters 22 and 108). Observation of behavior in an office or clinic may be misleading, since adolescents with ADHD often fail to show behavioral problems in one-to-one office situations.

Parent Interview

Interviews with parents should gather descriptive information on their view of the adolescent's problems and their influence on the family and its functioning. In addition, a careful developmental and medical history is critical in order to rule out the possibility that ADHD symptoms arose secondary to central nervous system (CNS) trauma or infection or endocrine imbalance (e.g., hyperthyroidism see Chapter 55); and to evaluate co-existing medical conditions, especially those that might be contraindications for pharmacotherapy. Barkley provides a useful form to record this information, which prompts the interviewer to cover the most relevant information needed to assess an adolescent presenting with ADHD. The form includes a checklist of DSM-III-R symptoms for ADHD as well as for other psychiatric disorders that may coexist with ADHD.

The interview with the parent should gather information on psychiatric, learning, and developmental problems in the family, as well as the presence of marital problems. Besides aiding in the diagnosis, such information is often important in understanding the clinical presentation of the child with ADHD. Parental discord and psychopathologic conditions, especially depression, often lead to increased negative and oppositional behavior in the child or adolescent with ADHD.

Rating Scales

Rating scales are useful in clinical practice because they (1) provide a simple and efficient method of gathering information from individuals who have known the adolescent over time and in a variety of circumstances, (2) allow comparison of the behavior to normative data, and (3) provide a convenient method to evaluate the response to clinical intervention.

Because of the high comorbidity of ADHD and other psychiatric signs, symptoms, and disorders, instruments that cover a wide range of behavioral problems are particularly useful in initial diagnostic work. The Child Behavior Checklist (CBCL) is the best-standardized and normed of these general instruments and has parallel forms for use by parents, teachers, trained observers, and adolescents themselves. More circumscribed scales are available that assess core ADHD symptoms. These scales are useful in monitoring the program of treatment, particularly pharmacotherapy. The best known of these are the Conners Scales. Two adolescent self-report scales, developed by Robins and colleagues, may be particularly useful in the assessment of family conflict and communication, because families having adolescents with ADHD are at high risk for interpersonal conflict. Table 106–2 presents a summary of several rating scales.

Objective Tests

Standardized tests of intelligence and academic achievement should be obtained when educational problems are suspected (see Chapter 99). Under Public Law 94-142, public schools are required to provide such evaluation services when warranted, though there may be a lengthy waiting period (see also Chapter 30).

Since ratings of inattention can be highly influenced by other co-occurring behavior, such as aggression, withdrawal, and oppositional behavior, it is often useful

TABLE 106–2. Rating Scales Useful in Evaluation of Attention Deficit Hyperactivity Disorder

MEASURE	TARGET BEHAVIOR	RATER	AGE RANGE (YEARS)
Child Behavior Checklist (CBCL)	General behavioral problems	Teacher, parent, adolescent	6–11, 12–16
CBCL Youth Self-report	General behavioral problems	Adolescent	11–18
Conners Scales (full measure)	ADHD core symptoms	Teacher, parent	3–17
Conners Abbreviated Symptom Questionnaire	ADHD core symptoms and conduct problems	Teacher, parent	3–17
Conners Child Attention Problem Scales	Specific ADHD core symptoms and conduct problems	Teacher, parent	3–17
IOWA Conners Teacher Rating Scales	Specific ADHD core symptoms and conduct problems	Teacher	3–17
Conflict Behavior Questionnaire	Family conflicts and communication	Parent, adolescent	Adolescent
Issues Checklist	Issues leading to family conflict	Parent, adolescent	Adolescent

to use objective measures of attention. Although a variety of neuropsychological tests have been used in research studies to examine the attentive and impulse-control problems in children with ADHD, their clinical reliability remains unclear.

Some investigators have proposed a model for the adequate assessment of attention that involves a battery of tests measuring four significant aspects of this complex construct. This battery produces a profile of attention deficits. The components and the tests include the following:

1. The ability to *focus* on targets in the face of simultaneous, irrelevant information. Tests: Talland Letter Cancellation, Stroop Test, Coding subtest of Wechsler Intelligence Scale for Children-Revised (WISC-R) (Digit-Symbol Substitution subtest of the Wechsler Adult Intelligence Scale-Revised [WAIS-R] for patients older than 16 years of age).

2. The ability to *sustain* attentive focus and alertness over time. Test: Continuous Performance Test.

3. The ability to *shift* attentive focus in response to environmental contingencies. Test: Wisconsin Card Sorting Test.

4. A component labeled *encode* that refers to the ability to direct attention to further processing of stimuli once stored in short-term memory. Tests: Digit Span and Arithmetic subtests of the WISC-R.

ETIOLOGY

The causes of ADHD are unknown; however, converging evidence points to the importance of the frontal lobes in the pathophysiology of ADHD.

Brain Damage

Although ADHD was originally conceptualized to result from brain damage, only a small percentage of ADHD cases can be linked to neurologic findings that are consistent with brain injury (trauma, infection, identifiable CNS disease). The association of ADHD with low birth weight or perinatal complications, or both, is reduced when maternal smoking, alcohol use, and economic disadvantage are considered.

Poor Parenting

Although poor parenting practices are more common in families of children and adolescents with ADHD and serve to maintain hyperactive and oppositional behavior in the affected adolescent, they do not appear to be a cause of ADHD symptoms. After the adolescent begins taking stimulant medication, the use of critical, commanding, and negative behavior by parents is reduced in conjunction with a reduction in noncompliant behavior by the child or adolescent. Thus the negative behavior of the parent seems to be more a response to the difficult and disruptive actions of the child than a causative agent of ADHD.

Environmental Toxins

There is no evidence that ADHD results from the ingestion of food additives or refined sugar. However, modest but consistent correlations have been reported between ADHD and the level of maternal cigarette and alcohol use during pregnancy. However, because parents with ADHD smoke and drink more than do parents without ADHD, the relationship between cigarette smoking and alcohol may reflect the strong genetic link in ADHD (see further on) rather than the toxicity of these substances. The low level of correlation between increased levels of lead and hyperactivity and inattention preclude it as a major cause of ADHD.

Genetic Factors

Evidence from family aggregation and twin pair studies indicates that genetic factors play a significant role in ADHD. It has been found that relatives of patients with ADD (DSM-III) are seven times more likely to have ADD than are the relatives of normal controls, and these individuals are more than four times as likely to have ADD than are relatives of children with other psychiatric disorders. The risk for ADD was similarly increased in the families of both children and adolescents with ADD, supporting the continuity of the disorder across different developmental stages. Relatives of those with ADD were also at higher risk for antisocial disorders and mood disorders. Twin studies uniformly show a higher concordance of ADHD between monozygotic twins than between dizygotic twins, with heritability estimated between 30% and 50%.

Catecholamine Disturbance

Because many of the drugs that are useful in treating ADHD alter catecholamine levels in the brain (primarily involving increased release and inhibition of reuptake of dopamine and norepinephrine), investigators have looked for disturbances in catecholamines. Little evidence for consistent differences between ADHD and normal children in peripheral levels of monoamines or their metabolites has been found. Also, altering different catecholamine systems (dopamine, norepinephrine, serotonin) through specific agonists and antagonists has produced generally insignificant effects on ADHD behavior. These results, plus the unlikelihood that the functioning of one neurotransmitter can be changed without altering the functioning of others, and the fact that effective medications for treatment of ADHD affect more than one system, argue against a single transmitter hypothesis. However, alteration in noradrenergic function as a result of medication seems most related to clinical change and may be basic to ADHD. Several investigators point to the extensive noradrenergic innervation of the cortex, the effect of norepinephrine on dopamine synthesis, and the role of the frontal lobes in ADHD (see further on) to suggest a model of the disorder involving reduced inhibitory, noradrenergic frontal activity acting to modulate dopamine-sensitive lower structures.

Neuroanatomic Disturbance

Neuroanatomic and neurobiologic data generally support a model for ADHD involving disordered pathways between prefrontal and limbic structures mediated by both dopamine and noradrenergic systems. This neural system may represent the final common pathway for ADHD symptoms. Early work demonstrated reduced perfusion and less brain matter in orbitofrontal areas of the cortex, as well as diminished blood flow to the striatum in children with ADHD. One group of investigators used positron-emission tomography (PET) to examine cerebral blood glucose metabolism in adults with a history of ADHD (DSM-III) in childhood. They observed a significant overall reduction in glucose metabolism in their patients compared with that in matched controls; areas of greatest depression included, but were not limited to, the premotor and superior frontal regions of the cortex. Prefrontal areas appear important for attention, and premotor cortex is involved in voluntary movement and the suppression of more automatic behavior. Damage to these areas can result in a variety of behaviors similar to ADHD symptoms — distractibility, restlessness, and, most strikingly, deficits in the inhibition of inappropriate responses. Support for a frontal lobe pathophysiology in ADHD also arises from neuropsychological test data. Several studies have found

that children with ADHD score more poorly on tests that are sensitive to frontal lobe functions; however, there is debate as to whether these findings reflect problems specific to ADHD or to co-occurring learning disabilities. The most consistent differences between children with ADHD and normal children occurs on the Continuous Performance Test, which involves processes most likely mediated by the orbitofrontal and subcortical striatum.

TREATMENT

Overview

Until a cure for ADHD is identified, intervention will necessarily focus on treating its symptoms. Recommendations specific for adolescents are somewhat limited because adolescents have been relatively neglected in research studies on treatment. One must extrapolate from reports on children and the few studies that have examined adults. It is clear, however, that treatment should occur in the context of a comprehensive management plan that includes thorough and ongoing communication with adolescents and parents. Stimulant medication is frequently an important component. Teenagers and parents should fully participate in the decision to use stimulant medication. We recommend a blinded, placebo-controlled trial incorporating behavioral measures and assessment of inappropriate attributions of medication effects.

Behavioral intervention is indicated if the clinician detects problems in the family's interactions or abilities to solve problems or if the teenager demonstrates deficient social or study skills. More intelligent teenagers may have the least developed study skills because academic work in elementary school may not have demanded much effort of them; the very bright teenager may thus benefit the most from specific study skill training. Maladaptive perceptions of the teenager, whether they are self-perceptions or those of parents and teachers, are also appropriate targets for intervention. Although behavioral intervention has not yet been documented to be efficacious for teenagers with ADHD its utility has been demonstrated with other populations, and thus it currently appears warranted when adolescents are experiencing problems in these areas.

Including a behavioral specialist in the clinical practice setting provides an optimal context for treatment because it facilitates coordination of behavioral and pharmacologic therapy and promotes the adolescent's and parents' acceptance of behavioral intervention. A behavioral specialist can also help with the assessment and implementation of controlled medication trials.

Advocacy is often an important component of successful treatment. Parents, school systems, and patients often have strong opinions about the use of stimulant medications. Health care providers can promote better care for patients with ADHD by providing more information about the disorder and its treatment to educators and the general public.

When Public Law 94-142 mandated special education services for a wide variety of learning, developmental, and behavioral-emotional disturbances, ADHD problems *per se* were overlooked. Most children with ADHD are currently provided with services only if they meet the criteria for other mandated disturbances.

Pharmacologic Intervention

Medication Effects. Seventy percent to 80% of children and 60% of adults with ADHD benefit from stimulant medication, with significant improvement in both academic and social behavior at school and a reduction in disruptive and negative behavior at home. In addition to increasing "on-task" behavior and decreasing noncompliant and aggressive behavior, medication also reduces the *variability* of behavior. Medication also typically improves mother-child interaction and reduces the amount of peer rejection. Note that these results are derived from studies of relatively short-term effects; long-term efficacy of medication is discussed further on.

Selecting and Titrating Medication. Methylphenidate (Ritalin) is the most common stimulant prescribed for individuals with ADHD. Fixed dosages are typically recommended. An algorithm has been developed for determining the appropriate dose of methylphenidate and other medications. (The interested reader is referred to the article by Davy and Rodgers.)

d-Amphetamine (Dexedrine) is an alternative CNS stimulant. Pemoline (Cylert) has also been used successfully. Little long-term data are available. Note that a teenager who does not respond well to one stimulant may respond well to another; as many as 20% of patients who respond poorly to the first stimulant prescribed subsequently respond well to a different one.

The peak behavioral effects of both methylphenidate and *d*-amphetamine occur within 1 to 2 hours and dissipate within 3.5 to 5 hours. Given a common dosage schedule of 7 A.M. (with breakfast) and 12 P.M. (with lunch), neither medication provides optimal coverage for the key academic periods of the school day. Coordination of school and medication schedules is important, but matching peak medication effects and academic demands may be difficult. Longer-acting stimulants such as sustained-release Ritalin (SR-20), longer-acting *d*-amphetamine (Dexedrine Spansule), and pemoline may provide useful therapeutic alternatives.

A double-blind trial has demonstrated the need to individualize therapy. Idiosyncratic responses to medication were common, and the *pattern* of responses varied. It appears difficult to predict the specific effects of a given drug on attention span, "on-task" academic behavior, and aggression in a given adolescent. The effects of different medications on each area must be individually assessed. The "best" drug represents a compromise between the desirable effects of the medication on the specific presenting symptoms and undesirable side effects. Therefore, a blinded, placebo-controlled trial is strongly recommended. It is possible to approximate a blinded trial by designating the stimulant "medication A" and a placebo, such as a multivitamin, "medication B." This is best done by the clinician dispensing the medication, with appropriate labels. However, a blinded, placebo-controlled trial can still be

successfully approximated, even when prescribed medications are filled at a local pharmacy.

Objective data should be collected from several sources (e.g., parent, teacher, and patient) across several settings (minimally, school and home); measures should include both behavior targeted for change and potential side effects. Several commonly used rating scales have been reviewed. Clinicians may need to reword some items to make them more appropriate or acceptable to teenagers or abridge forms to foster compliance. Adolescents should be included in data collection. A teenager's objective record of his or her ability to meet academic demands or to cope with social interactions (e.g., frequency of arguments with peers and parents), and his or her experience with side effects is valuable in assessing the costs and benefits of medication. Although it requires time to individualize appropriate instruments and teach the teenager how to use them, the importance of obtaining such data makes the effort worthwhile.

The key characteristics of good behavioral measures are specificity and simplicity. The method should use clear and concrete items that refer to specific behaviors (e.g.," completes class assignment"). Specific ratings of discrete behaviors are most accurate. Cooperation and compliance will be greatly enhanced by using shorter checklists or rating scales (e.g., a nine-point scale ranging from *never* to *always*), including the student's name on the form, providing an ample supply of forms, and using an unusual color of paper for the form.

Accurate baseline data are crucial, since "before" and "after" data are collected. Since practice effects are very likely to occur as raters become more familiar with these instruments, baseline data should be recorded for at least 2 weeks, and only the second week's data should be used to compare baseline versus intervention periods. Data collection sometimes must continue for many weeks if an initial low dose proves ineffective, and the dosage is systematically increased until an optimal effect is achieved. Medication trials are best conducted during a fairly stable time in the school year (i.e., October to May), avoiding major holidays. The clinician should inquire throughout the trial whether each week was relatively normal or whether there were unusual circumstances that might invalidate data from that week, such as parent-teacher conferences or other activities that reduce academic requirements. Visiting relatives may alter social interaction and demands at home.

Extended Monitoring and Terminating Medication. Medication should be closely monitored for 3 to 6 months to detect changes in efficacy or side effects. For example, some investigators have noted that there may be an increase in side effects over time with the longer-acting stimulants. The clinician should also be aware that generic forms of a drug may not always be bioequivalent.

Adolescents should be reevaluated annually to determine whether continued medication is warranted. Such reassessment should be scheduled in the middle of the school year. Substituting a placebo for the medication is an ideal way to assess the need for ongoing pharmacotherapy. Data from 2 weeks of medication (discarding the first week) and 1 week of placebo should be sufficient to reassess efficacy. Objective measures should be used.

Because relatively few studies have been conducted specifically with adolescents, little is known about the potential effect of puberty on response to medication. Obviously, any change in efficacy or side effects reported by parents or teenagers requires reevaluation. It may be necessary to change dosage or medication. The decision to terminate medication should be based on a controlled trial using objective data that confirm that medication is no longer necessary. Currently available evidence indicates that medication is beneficial for most teenagers with ADHD.

Short-term Side Effects and Contraindications. Decreased appetite is the most common side effect of CNS stimulants and is experienced by more than 50% of children. Sleep disturbance is reported by 5% to 60% of these patients. It must be emphasized that these same side effects are frequently reported during placebo periods, underscoring the importance of using a controlled medication trial. Rating the severity of any side effect is useful because most are mild. A variety of less common, mild, transient side effects have been reported. They include mood changes (increased anxiety, irritability, and tearfulness), state changes (social withdrawal, dizziness, reduced alertness, and drowsiness) and physical symptoms (abdominal discomfort, headaches, myalgia, rash, dry mouth, nausea and vomiting, eye/and muscle twitches, and bed wetting). Reports of such co-occurrences are not consistent across studies and are not linked to specific drugs. Side effects appear to be idiosyncratic to each patient's drug combination. Most of these are transient and cease after 1 to 2 weeks. If the symptoms persist, a slight reduction in dosage may be helpful. Other alternatives include switching to another drug or even reintroducing the same drug following a brief hiatus, because symptoms will often not recur following readministration. It is estimated that only 2% of children with ADHD cannot tolerate any form of stimulant medication.

Sometimes medication (especially methylphenidate) occasionally improves behavior early in the day but results in deterioration in the late afternoon and evening despite a noontime dose. This "rebound" effect may respond to an additional low dose in the late afternoon or to a reduction in the noontime dose if the afternoon dose affects sleep.

The initiation or exacerbation of nervous tics is a potentially serious side effect of stimulant medication. Less than 1% of children with ADHD have developed a tic disorder secondary to stimulant medication, but 13% of children with ADHD have experienced an exacerbation of preexisting tics. While this side effect typically resolves following withdrawal of medication, there has been one report of Tourette syndrome developing as a consequence of stimulant medication. One must obtain a personal and family history of tics and Tourette syndrome before beginning stimulant medication. When there is a positive history, the teenager and his or her parents should be fully informed of the potential risk of at least exacerbating these symptoms so that they can assess the advisability of stimulant medication. Stimulant medication should only be considered in such cases when ADHD is a major disability for the teenager, and behavioral and educational intervention have been unsuccessful in moderating its effects.

The choice of specific medication should also take into consideration the possibility of concurrent problems. Thought disorders and psychosis (see Chapter 110) and anxiety disorders (see Chapter 103) can be exacerbated by stimulant medication. Antidepressants may be more effective than stimulants for children with ADHD and anxiety disorders and depression. The use of monoamine oxidase (MAO) inhibitors and clonidine has been found to improve the behavior of some children with ADHD. Finally, stimulant medications heighten the activity of antidepressants and MAO inhibitors. Given the complexity of making these differential diagnoses, selecting appropriate medications, and considering the interactive effects of medications, psychiatric consultation is generally warranted when such comorbidity is present.

Interactions of stimulants with other medications have not been studied extensively, but few serious interactions have been reported. Stimulants may lower seizure thresholds, necessitating an increase in the level of anticonvulsants. Stimulants may antagonize the effects of hypnotic drugs and may also increase their toxicity. Alternatively, some antihistamines can inhibit the effect of CNS stimulants and thus reduce their efficacy. Specific dietary intake, including food additives and sugar, does not influence the effect of stimulant medication.

Long-term Effects. There appear to be few, if any, long-term effects of stimulant medication; however, data are limited. There appears to be no appreciable impact on eventual height and weight in adulthood. It is unclear whether the initial suppression of growth is secondary to reduced appetite or a direct influence on growth hormone. Nevertheless, careful assessment of height and weight gain are important.

There also is little evidence to support a relationship of stimulant medication to subsequent abuse or addiction to these or other drugs.

At present, there are no data regarding the potential impact of medication on cardiovascular outcome in adulthood or on health in general.

Special Concerns for Adolescents. Since stimulant medication does not cure ADHD, some investigators have questioned that the predominant focus of treatment should be the school. Expanding the arena of treatment beyond time spent in school seems particularly applicable to teenagers, whose academic programs deliberately demand that increasing amounts of learning occur outside the structured school day. In addition, evening and weekend activities involving peers become even more salient for teenagers than they are for children. This suggests that adolescents' medication regimens should parallel those of adults, using longer-acting drugs and fewer unmedicated periods than with children.

Compliance with Pharmacotherapy

Compliance with stimulant medication is also an important issue (see Chapter 25). Most parents, teachers, and adolescents have a bias about its use in ADHD. Some refuse to accept it. For those who do accept it, up to 50% may not comply fully, sometimes taking only one half the prescribed amount.

Even when the teenager and his or her parents have had a positive experience with stimulant medication during childhood, the onset of adolescence can substantially alter attitudes and compliance. Adolescents often resist being different from their peers; it has been shown that even adolescents with a well documented history of ADHD consistently underreport the nature and severity of their symptoms, including their conflicts with others. Teenagers are particularly likely to reject a regimen that they perceive to be imposed by adults, whether they be parents or physicians. Even if teenagers do not view medication as a source of "external control," some may dislike the modulating effects of medication because some adolescents may enjoy feeling spontaneous, impulsive, and wild. Finally, the teenager with ADHD must deal with the issues surrounding "taking drugs" that confront all adolescents who require chronic medication.

One must present the use of stimulant medication within the appropriate developmental context. The teenager must be included in the decision-making process and must be increasingly acknowledged as the key player in management as he or she progresses through adolescence. The use of a blinded, placebo-controlled medication trial that provides clear evidence of a beneficial effect may be a key factor in obtaining parental compliance.

Disadvantages and Limitations of Medication. There are two important limitations of medication. Academic *behavior* may improve, whereas scores on achievement tests do not. Possible explanations include problems inherent to achievement tests, imperfect medication compliance, and methodologic flaws in study design. Lastly, perhaps stimulant medication simply affects actual learning less than academic behaviors, thereby altering teacher perceptions of academic success (a desirable goal in and of itself).

Medication does not, in and of itself, improve peer interaction. Although aggression, impulsiveness, and disruptiveness are reduced, stimulants do not aid the adolescent in initiating more positive peer interactions or having more friends.

Behavioral Intervention

A wide variety of psychosocial interventions are currently available to treat adolescents and their families (see Chapters 98, 123, 124, and 125). Of these, behavioral therapy is the only form of psychosocial treatment that has been evaluated for use with children and adolescents with ADHD.

Behavioral therapy includes traditional behavioral approaches to management, such as contingency contracting, as well as more recent cognitive-behavioral variants that employ a problem-solving model and may incorporate concepts from family-systems theory (see Chapters 123 and 124). Behavioral therapy has been shown to be effective for adolescents with conduct problems, social skill deficits, study skill deficits, and family conflicts. Since these are some of the most common problems experienced by teenagers with ADHD, behavioral therapy is a logical treatment choice. However, few systematic investigations have focused specifically on behavioral treatment of adolescents with ADHD.

Controlled studies of behavioral intervention with patients with ADHD have been conducted primarily with children. Although results are mixed, contingency management and parent-teacher training have typically yielded more consistent improvement in noncompliance and oppositional behavior than in academic achievement, prompting increased investigation of cognitive-behavioral interventions (e.g., self-instruction and self-control techniques). To date, neither approach has yielded results that rival those found with medication.

Although behavioral therapy is a promising intervention that warrants considerably more study, it requires time, effort, expense, and considerable professional expertise. Given the documented utility of pharmacologic treatment of ADHD, and serious limitations in research data, it appears that behavioral interventions are best used in conjunction with medication as part of an individualized treatment plan. Behavioral therapy is most appropriate if there are problems in the family's interactions or ability to solve problems, if the teenager has deficient study or social skills, or if the clinician detects maladaptive perceptions of the adolescent—either self-perceptions or those of parents or teachers.

COURSE AND PROGNOSIS

Approximately 75% of children with ADHD experience problems in the general areas of academic and occupational success, interpersonal relationships, self-esteem, and impulsiveness and restlessness. Approximately 60% of these individuals will continue to have difficulties as adults. Typical problems include lower levels of academic and vocational attainment, employment instability, maladaptive relationships with family and peers, subjective feelings of restlessness, and an increased frequency of auto accidents and trouble with the law.

Although current studies suggest a relatively poor prognosis for teenagers with ADHD, data are far from conclusive. Most reports are severely limited by methodologic flaws common to retrospective studies. Investigators also frequently fail to present sufficient information about the details of intervention, making it difficult to draw firm conclusions. One hopes that current treatments addressing adequate stimulant medication, learning deficits, and coexisting social, behavioral, and family problems will improve the long-term prognosis.

BIBLIOGRAPHY

American Psychiatric Association: Diagnostic and Statistcal Manual of Mental Disorders, 3rd ed, revised. Washington, DC, American Psychiatric Association, 1987.
Barkley RA: Attention-Deficit Hyperactivity Disorder: A Handbook for Diagnosis and Treatment, 2nd ed. New York, Guilford, 1990.
Biederman J, Faraone SV, Keenan KED, Tsuang MT: Family-genetic and psychosocial risk factors in DSM-III attention deficit disorder. Child Adolesc Psychiatry 29:526, 1990.

Brown RT, Borden KA, Wynne ME, et al: Compliance with pharmacological and cognitive treatments for attention deficit disorder. J Am Acad Child Adolesc Psychiatry 26:521, 1987.

Campbell SB, Werry JS: Attention deficit disorder (hyperactivity). In Quay HC, Werry JS (eds): Psychopathological Disorders of Childhood, 3rd ed. New York, John Wiley & Sons, 1986.

Davy T, Rodgers CL: Stimulant medication and short attention span: A clinical approach. J Dev Behav Pediatr 10:313, 1989.

Pelham WE, Greenslade KE, Vodde-Hamilton M, et al: Relative efficacy of long-acting stimulants on ADHD children: A comparison of standard methylphenidate, Ritalin SR-20, Dexedrine Spansule, and Pemoline. Pediatrics 86:226, 1990.

Phillips S: Psychosocial intervention with adolescents. In Friedman SB, Fisher M, Schonberg SK (eds): Comprehensive Adolescent Health Care. St. Louis, Quality Medical Publishing, in press.

Phillips S: The use of stimulant medication with children. J Dev Behav Pediatr 10:319, 1989.

Zametkin AJ, Nordahl TE, Gross M, et al: Cerebral glucose metabolism in adults with hyperactivity of childhood onset. N Eng J Med, 323:1361, 1990.

Zametkin AJ, Rapoport JL: Neurobiology of attention deficit disorder with hyperactivity: Where have we come in 50 years? J Am Acad Child Adolesc Psychiatry 26:676, 1987.

CHAPTER 107

Underachievement and Learning Disabilities

LARRY B. SILVER

This chapter will review the multiple factors that can result in academic underachievement and will then focus in greater detail on the learning disabilities as the primary cause for this underachievement.

Success in school is one of the primary goals of adolescence. School success has a major impact on the future economic well-being and emotional life of the individual as an adult. Learning disabilities can have a major impact on the adolescent's ability to learn, perform, and succeed in school.

ACADEMIC UNDERACHIEVEMENT

It is estimated that at least 20% of most students have difficulty performing academically at an age-appropriate level. For some of these individuals, the underlying problem is mental retardation (see Chapter 31). For others, the below normal performance is a result of primary emotional or behavioral problems. For still others, there are family, social, or cultural factors that contribute to the underachievement. Some children and adolescents have specific deficits in their learning performance. They are usually sensorially intact and of average or above average intellectual ability. These young persons have learning disabilities, which will be discussed later in this chapter.

Level of Intelligence

Adolescents who have mental retardation should have been identified as children and should be in the appropriate special education program (see Chapter 31).

There are two other problems relating to the level of intelligence that can have an impact on academic achievement—the adolescent with "borderline" intelligence and the adolescent with a "mismatched" intelligence.

Under Public Law 94-142 (Education for all Handicapped Children), an adolescent with an intelligence quotient (IQ) of 70 or less can be classified as having mental retardation, and an adolescent with an IQ of 85 or more who has academic difficulties might meet the criteria of a learning disability. Most schools have no system for formally identifying what used to be called the "slow learner"—those adolescents with an IQ be-tween 71 and 84. These individuals often fall between regular education and special education programs. They might struggle through the lower levels of regular classes or be placed in what are often called basic classes.

There are two ways that an adolescent can be "mismatched." The individual might have a solid, average intellectual ability. However, the family might live in a neighborhood in which the IQ of the student population averages 120. This adolescent may struggle to keep up because the level of expectation is designed for the "average" student, who in other school systems would be above average. The other problem is for the adolescent of superior intelligence who is not recognized as gifted and is kept in regular classes. This individual might be unchallenged or become bored, resulting in behavioral problems and possible underachievement.

It is essential that the school system identify those adolescents who do not have mental retardation but who have academic problems because of their level of intelligence. Proper programs are needed. Individual and family counseling can minimize the academic difficulties and prevent emotional problems.

Emotional and Behavioral Problems

The public school system considers an adolescent to have behavioral problems if the student's difficulties prevent the student from learning in the classroom or prevent other students from learning in the classroom. The adolescent is considered to have an emotional problem if he or she has a psychiatric disorder that interferes with attendance or performance in school. Each of these problem areas is discussed elsewhere in this book.

Family, Social, and Cultural Problems

The family system, the community, and the school environment have an impact on the adolescent's values, motivation, and performance in school. Each must be considered when an individual is underachieving.

Economic, environmental, or emotional stress within

the family can result in an adolescent becoming dysfunctional in school. The parents' interest in and level of value placed on the adolescent's educational success can also have a great influence on the individual's drive and motivation in school.

The value of education held by individuals in the community has an equally important impact on the adolescent. Perhaps this impact is greatest from peers. If peer values minimize the importance of attending or succeeding in school, the adolescent may adopt these values as his or her own in order to gain peer acceptance or to avoid peer rejection.

The environment of the school also affects the adolescent. If the teachers are overwhelmed, if they have lost interest in teaching, or if the primary attitude of the student body is that of indifference to learning, it will be difficult for an individual adolescent to do other than conform to the expected level of performance. Success not only is not expected but also can lead to peer hostility or rejection.

LEARNING DISABILITIES

Definition

The Diagnostic and Statistical Manual of Mental Disorders: Third Edition—Revised (DSM-III-R) identifies individuals with learning disabilities as having a "developmental learning disorder." The public school system uses the guidelines of Public Law 94-142, and refers to these individuals as having a learning disability. The clinician may use the DSM-III-R codes for third-party forms, but may use the term *learning disability* when interacting with the family or school system.

Developmental learning disorders are listed in the DSM-III-R under the Axis II diagnosis of "specific developmental disorders." These disorders are characterized by inadequate development of specific academic, language, speech, and motor skills not resulting from demonstrable physical or neurologic disorders, a pervasive developmental disorder, mental retardation, or deficient educational opportunities. These disorders are subgrouped as follows:

Academic Skills Disorders:
 Developmental arithmetic disorder
 Developmental expressive writing disorder
 Developmental reading disorder
Language and Speech Disorders:
 Developmental articulation disorder
 Developmental expressive language disorder
 Developmental receptive language disorder

Motor Skills Disorder:
 Developmental coordination disorder

The definition of a learning disability as stated in the Federal law is:

> *. . . a disorder in one or more of the basic psychological processes involved in understanding or using language, spoken or written, which may manifest itself in an imperfect ability to listen, think, speak, read, write, spell,*

> *or to do mathematical calculations. The term includes such conditions as perceptual handicaps, brain injury, minimal brain dysfunction, dyslexia, and developmental aphasia. The term does not include children who have learning problems which are primarily the result of visual, hearing, or motor handicaps, or mental retardation, of emotional disturbance, or of environmental, cultural, or economic disadvantage.*

Historical Background

Prior to the 1940s in the United States, children and adolescents who had academic difficulties were considered to have mental retardation or emotional disturbance or to be socially and culturally disadvantaged. During the 1940s, a fourth possibility for these difficulties was introduced—individuals might have problems with academic performance for neurologic reasons, that is, the cause of the difficulty was presumed to be related to brain function. Two different research approaches explored these presumed neurologically based learning disorders.

One group of researchers noted that these children had the same types of learning difficulties as identified brain-damaged individuals. They concluded that these children also had brain damage; however, it was so subtle or minimal it could not be confirmed clinically. The term *minimal brain damage* was introduced. Other researchers explored the possibility that the learning difficulties resulted from a brain that functioned differently, possibly because of being "wired" differently rather than being damaged. The term *minimal brain dysfunction* was used to reflect this concept. Recent research supports this concept of brain dysfunction rather than brain damage.

Initially, the types of academic difficulties were described based on the primary skill disorder. Reading disorders were called dyslexia; writing disorders were called dysgraphia; and arithmetic disorders were called dyscalculia. Later efforts focused on the underlying learning difficulties or learning disabilities that caused the problems with reading, writing, and arithmetic. The term *learning disability* was introduced. Currently, this is the preferred term.

Prevalence

The true prevalence of learning disabilities is not known because of the many case definitions used in different studies. There remains controversy over which definition to use. The Centers for Disease Control attempted to establish the prevalence of this disorder. These researchers concluded that because the definition of and the criteria for learning disabilities have not been standardized, consistency in the design of prevalence studies has not been maintained. Thus accurate analysis of data over time is not possible. Without good prevalence data, they concluded that between 5% and 10% was a reasonable estimate of the percentage of persons affected by learning disabilities. Until a uniform definition and diagnostic criteria are used, more accurate data will not be available.

Studies consistently note a male predominance in this disorder. The male to female ratio ranges from 3:1 to 5:1 and higher. Recent studies suggest that this predominance of males over females may, in part, be explained by referral bias. Because males are more likely to "act out," they are more likely to be referred for study. Females appear to tolerate deficits in reading and spelling skills more easily than do males, showing less antipathy to reading and less emotional impact. One recent study that attempted to correct for referral bias found no specific cognitive differences or patterns of problems between the sexes.

Associated Disorders

Adolescents with neurologic disorders such as Tourette syndrome, neurofibromatosis, or seizure disorders show a higher incidence of learning disabilities than would be expected. (see Chapter 83). Children with learning disabilities might show other evidence of neurologic dysfunction. The most frequently found disorder is attention deficit hyperactivity disorder (see Chapter 106). It is estimated that between 20% and 25% of children with learning disabilities have this disorder.

Most adolescents with learning disabilities have secondary emotional, social, and family problems. It is important to be aware of these associated difficulties when developing a differential diagnosis for an individual with academic problems and before designing a treatment plan.

Clinical Manifestations

Most eductional test instruments and special educational literature use a cybernetics model for understanding learning and learning disabilities. It is understood that any learning task involves more than one process and that any learning disability can involve more than one area of dysfunction. However, separating learning into steps, rather than describing the overall problems with reading, writing, or mathematics, clarifies the process.

The first step in this model is input, in which information is entered into the brain. Once the information is recorded, that which is received is processed and interpreted, a process called integration. Next, the information must be used or stored and later retrieved, the memory process. Finally, this information must be sent out through language or motor activities, the *output* process.

Input Disabilities. Input is a central brain process and does not pertain to peripheral visual or auditory problems. This process of perceiving one's environment is referred to as "perception." An adolescent might have a visual or auditory perception disability.

Visual Perception Disabilities. An adolescent may have difficulty in organizing the position and shape of what he or she sees. Input may be perceived with reversed or rotated letters. The letters d, b, p, and q

might be confused with each other, as might the letters n and u. This confusion with position of input shows up almost immediately when the child begins to read, write, or copy letters or designs.

Another adolescent might have a "figure-ground" problem, that is, difficulty in focusing on the significant figure instead of the other visual inputs in the background. Reading requires this skill of focusing on specific letters or groups of letters, then tracking from left to right, line after line. Adolescents with this disability may have reading problems. They may skip words, read the same line twice, or skip lines.

Judging distance or depth perception is another visual perception task that can be dysfunctional. An adolescent may misjudge depth, bumping into things, falling off chairs, or knocking over a drink because the hand reached too far for it.

Auditory Perception Disabilities. As with visual perception, an adolescent may have difficulty with one or several aspects of auditory perception. An adolescent who has difficulty distinguishing subtle differences in sounds will misunderstand what is said and may respond incorrectly. Words that sound alike are often confused—*blue* and *blow* or *ball* and *bell*. For example, a boy is asked, "How are you?" and answers, "I am 15 years old." He thought he heard "old" instead of "are" or in addition to "are."

Some individuals have difficulty with auditory "figure-ground." The adolescent might be watching television in a room in which others are playing or talking. A parent or teacher may call out or speak to this person. It might not be until the third paragraph the teacher or parent verbalizes that the adolescent begins to pick this voice (figure) out of the other sound inputs (background). It appears that he or she never listens or pays attention.

Some persons cannot process sound inputs as fast as normal individuals can. this is called an *auditory lag*. At a normal rate of speech, the individual may miss part of what is said. If a parent or teacher is talking, he or she must concentrate for a fraction of a second longer on what has been heard while trying to remember what comes next. As a result, he or she falls behind at times and has to jump ahead. Thus parts of what is said are missed. For example, a teacher explains a mathematics concept. The student with this disability receives and understands steps one, two, and three then misses step four, picking up on step five. The result is that he or she is lost and cannot grasp the concept.

Integration Disabilities. Once information enters the brain, it has to be understood. At least three steps are required to do this: sequencing, abstraction, and organization. The process of integrating input thus requires these three steps. An adolescent might have a disability in one area or in all areas. If the difficulty is with processing information brought in visually, the disability is referred to as a visual sequencing, a visual abstraction, or a visual organization disability. If the difficulty is with auditory input, it is called an auditory sequencing disability, and so on. In general, such disabilities usually involve all input areas.

Sequencing Disabilities. An adolescent with a sequencing disability might hear or read a story, but in recounting it, may start in the middle, go to the beginning, then shift to the end. Eventually the whole story comes out, but the sequence of events is wrong. Alternatively, he or she might see the word "dog" and read it as "god." Spelling words with all of the right letters in the wrong order can also reflect this disability.

An individual might memorize a sequence—the days of the week or months of the year, for example—and then be unable to use single units out of the sequence correctly. For example, asked what comes after August, the adolescent cannot answer spontaneously but must go back over the whole list, "January, February ..." before knowing the answer. The same may be true when using the alphabet, always having to start with "a" and working up to the letter being used.

Abstraction Disabilities. Abstraction is the ability to derive the correct general meaning from a particular word or symbol and is a very basic intellectual task. Once information is recorded in the brain and is placed in the right sequence, one must be able to infer meaning. Most individuals with learning disabilities have only minor difficulties in this area.

Some of these individuals, however, do have problems with abstraction. They may not infer the full meaning of material. Often, they do not understand jokes and do not laugh. They confuse idioms or puns. Sometimes they appear to be paranoid because they take what is said literally and think people are critical or angry with them. If the adolescent has a significant disability in abstraction, he or she is apt to be functioning at a significant retarded level.

Organization Disability. Once information is recorded, sequenced, and understood, it must be integrated with a constant flow of new information and also related to previously learned information. Some individuals have difficulty pulling multiple pieces of information into a full or complete concept. An adolescent may learn a series of facts but not be able to answer general questions that require using these facts. Such an individual's life may reflect this "dys-organization." His or her notebook, reports, locker, or room may be disorganized. Work needed at home may be left in school; work for school may be forgotten at home. Organizing time may also be a problem.

Memory Disabilities. Once information is received, recorded in the brain, and integrated, it has to be stored so that it can be retrieved later. This storage and retrieval process, or memory, can be two types: short-term memory and long-term memory.

Short-term memory is the process of retaining information for a brief time while attending to or concentrating on it, for example, calling the information operator for a long-distance telephone number. Most individuals can retain the 10 digits long enough to dial the number if it is done right away. However, if someone starts talking when the person is in the process of dialing, the number may be forgotten. Long-term memory refers to the process by which one stores information that has been repeated often enough that it can be retrieved by thinking of it.

Most individuals with a memory disability have a short-term one. Like abstraction, a long-term memory disability would interfere so much with learning that such individuals would more likely be functioning at a retarded level. An adolescent with a short-term memory problem may require many more repetitions to retain what the average child could retain after a few repetitions. Yet, the same individual may have no problem with long-term memory, surprising parents with details from years ago.

A short-term memory disability can occur with information received visually, a visual short-term memory disability, or with information received from auditory input, an auditory short-term memory disability. Often the two are combined. For example, the adolescent might review a spelling list one evening and know it well because he or she is concentrating on it. The next morning in school it is forgotten. Alternatively, a teacher might go over a mathematical concept in class until it is understood. Yet, when the student does homework that night, he or she has forgotten it.

Output Disabilities. Information is expressed by means of words, language output, or muscle activity (writing, drawing, gesturing, motor output). An adolescent may have a *language disability* or a *motor disability*.

Language Disabilities. Two forms of language are used in communication—spontaneous language and demand language. Spontaneous language occurs in situations in which one intitiates whatever is said. In this instance, one has the opportunity of selecting the subject, organizing one's thoughts, and finding the correct words before speaking. In a demand language situation, someone else sets up a circumstance in which one must communicate. For example, a question is asked, and it is necessary to simultaneously organize, find the right words, and answer more or less appropriately.

Adolescents with a specific language disability usually have no difficulty with spontaneous language. They may, however, have problems with demand language. The inconsistency can be striking. The adolescent may initiate all sorts of conversation, may never keep quiet, and may sound quite normal. However, when put into a situation that demands a response, the same individual might answer "Huh?" or "What?" or "I do not know," or he or she may ask for the question to be repeated in order to gain time or not answer at all. If forced to answer, the response may be so confusing or circumstantial that it is difficult to follow. The individual may sound totally unlike the person who spoke so fluently before.

Motor Disabilities. Difficulty coordinating groups of large muscles is called a gross motor disability. Difficulty in performing tasks that require coordination of groups of small muscles in an integrated way is called a fine motor disability.

Gross motor disabilities may cause the individual to be clumsy, stumble, fall, bump into things, or have trouble with generalized physical activities like running, climbing, or swimming. The most common form of a fine motor disability relates to writing. There is an inability to get the many muscles in the dominant hand to work together. Adolescents with this "written language" disability have slow, difficult to produce, poor handwriting. They often have problems with spelling. These motor disabilities might cause problems with life tasks such as buttoning, zipping, or tying.

When an adolescent has a visual perception problem, the brain, which has incorrectly recorded or processed information, may misinform the muscles during activities that require this eye-body coordination. This is referred to as a visual motor disability.

Learning Disability Profile

Obviously the learning process is much more complex, but this simple model for describing specific learning disabilities can be helpful. Each individual with a learning disability will have his or her own profile of learning abilities and disabilities. Thus each person must be evaluated and understood differently; it is important to know each person's profile so that interventions can be planned, whether they be educational or clinical.

Establishing the Diagnosis

When an adolescent is evaluated because of academic difficulties, especially when the difficulties are associated with behavioral problems in school or with the family, or both, the clinician must consider the possibility of a learning disability. This possibility is even greater if the adolescent patient also has clinical evidence of attention deficit hyperactivity disorder (see Chapter 106).

The history as obtained from the family, plus a review of the school records and any evelation reports are all essential. One looks for inconsistencies in performance or between one or more areas of performance.

The adolescent can be the best diagnostician. Questions can focus on basic academic skills or tasks. An adolescent with reading difficulties may say that he or she skips words, reads the same line twice, or skips lines (suggestive of a visual perception problem) or that he or she reads a chapter in a book but does not remember what was read (suggestion of a reading comprehension problem, the cause of which must be found). A student who has difficulty with mathematics may say that he or she does not understand mathematical concepts, cannot learn the times tables, or makes silly mistakes like transposing the sequence of numbers, misreading the signs, or confusing the lines or columns. He or she may forget the sequence of steps required or the necessary formulae. Adolescents with a written language problem will describe or demonstrate that they hold their pencil differently or that their hand gets tired easily. They write slowly and often complain, "My hand doesn't work as fast as my head is thinking."

These adolescents will report that they have difficulty with spelling or grammar or both, as well as capitalization and punctuation. If asked, the adolescent may describe difficulty understanding what the teacher says, misunderstanding what friends say, remembering what he or she has learned by listening, or problems expressing himself or herself when speaking.

During the office contact, the clinician might actually observe difficulty with listening and understanding what is said or with the adolescent expressing himself or herself clearly. The adolescent might have difficulty doing basic eye-hand tasks or may be unable to read well or do other academic tasks.

Once the diagnosis of a learning disability is suspected, it can be confirmed through a battery of psycho-educational tests. These should be performed by the patient's school system but may have to be done privately and taken to the school. The physician may need to be supportive of the parents and be an advocate to push for these studies and for the necessary programs if the diagnosis is established.

The psychological assessment may consist of a neuropsychological or a clinical psychological evaluation. One is interested in the individual's IQ, especially to determine whether there are any discrepancies or "scatter" within the subtests. Other tests assess perceptual, cognitive, and language abilities. The educational diagnostician measures the individual's current level of academic skills using an achievement test and evaluates for the presence of a learning disability by using a specific diagnostic test. The most frequently used tests follow (see Chapter 99):

Psychological Tests
Wechsler Intelligence Scale for Children (WISC) (ages 6 to 16 years)
Wechsler Adult Intelligence Scale (WAIS) (ages 16 years and older)
Stanford-Binet Intelligence Scale (ages 2 years to adulthood)

Achievement Tests
Wide-range Achievement Tests
Peabody Individual Achievement Test
Woodcock-Johnson Psychoeducational Battery
Metropolitan Achievement Tests
Stanford Diagnostic Achievement Tests

Educational Diagnostic Tests
Woodcock-Johnson Psychoeducational Battery

The results of the psychological and educational evaluations should establish the presence or lack of a learning disability. If present, the results will also clarify the specific areas of learning abilities and learning disabilities.

The public school system addresses an issue other than whether an adolescent has a learning disability. The issue is whether this individual is eligible for services. This decision is based on the concept of a discrepancy—that is, does the student have a significant discrepancy between his or her academic and intellectual potential and his or her current academic performance to warrant special services? Each school system has its own criteria for eligibility based on the degree of discrepancy. If the adolescent has a learning disability but is not far enough behind to qualify for services, the family may have to provide these services privately.

The clinician must rule out any medical disorder that might explain the academic difficulties. Conditions such as vision and hearing impairment (see Chapter 40), endocrine dysfunction (e.g., hypothyroidism; see Chapter 55), or chronic illness (see Chapters 30 and 121) should also be considered in the differential diagnosis.

If the history and clinical observations suggest a learning disability, the clinican plays a key role in alerting and educating the parents so that they can go to their school system for formal diagnostic studies and essential services. The clinican must be an advocate for his or her patient and family, encouraging the school to do the necessary assessments and to provide the necessary interventions.

Treatment

The treatment of choice for learning disabilities is special education. These interventions should be provided by the school system. The student could be in a regular classroom and receive individual help with his or her learning disabilities for a part of each day. Alternatively, he or she could be assigned to a special education classroom and be "mainstreamed" for part of the day to attend regular classes. Some individuals may attend full-time self-contained special education programs.

The special education professional will provide specific interventions for disabilities in the areas of reading, writing, and mathematics. In addition, efforts are made to develop successful study skills and strategies based on the individual's areas of learning strengths and weaknesses. The overall goal is to build on the learning abilities while working to correct or compensate for the learning disabilities.

The regular classroom teachers are expected to understand the individual's disabilities and to make the necessary accommodations in the classroom to allow him or her to succeed. Other professionals might participate in the treatment plan. A speech pathologist might work on the auditory perception or language disabilities. An occupational therapist might work on the visual perception or motor disabilities.

At home, the parents should try to understand their son's or daughter's learning abilities and disabilities so that they can build on the adolescent's strengths while trying to understand and compensate for the disabilities. With this information they can work to pick chores, sports, activities, and so on that build on the adolescent's strengths, thereby maximizing the possibility of success, rather than magnifying the adolescent's weaknesses and increasing the possibility of failure. Several books are listed in the bibliography that describe how parents can use this approach.

If there are emotional, social, or family problems, they must be addressed in a multimodal treatment plan. When performing individual, group, family (see Chapter 123), or behavioral therapy (see Chapter 124), it is important for the clinician to be aware of the impact of the learning disabilities on the individual's life as well as the impact of the disabilities on the treatment itself. For example, auditory perception or demand language disabilities will have an impact on any form of listening-talking therapy.

Course of the Disability and Outcome

Learning disabilities are lifetime disabilities. For most persons, if not all, the disability will persist throughout life. The child with learning disabilities becomes the adolescent with learning disabilities who becomes the adult with learning disabilities. Thus treatment planning will change with each developmental stage, including adulthood.

With early recognition and appropriate special education intervention, most individuals can overcome or learn to compensate for their learning disabilities. These interventions may be needed throughout the individual's education. Today there are such services available in postsecondary programs, vocational programs, colleges, and graduate and professional schools.

Without recognition or treatment, the outcome can be poor. Studies of children and adolescents diagnosed as having a conduct disorder show that approximately one third have unrecognized or recognized and poorly treated learning disabilities (see Chapter 108). Similar findings have been observed with adolescent boys in detention centers and in juvenile courts. The current view is that the learning disabilities do not cause behavioral problems, delinquency, or substance abuse. It is the lack of appropriate recognition and treatment, with the resulting experiences of failure and emotional stress, that contribute to the problems. Adolescents with learning disabilities who receive the appropriate help have no greater incidence of behavioral or delinquency problems or substance abuse than do normal adolescents. Adolescents with learning disabilities who are not diagnosed, or who are diagnosed but who receive minimal or inadequate services, might have a higher incidence of these problems.

Adolescents with learning disabilities have a chronic medical illness and must be viewed as such (see Chapters 30 and 121). Like diabetes mellitus, arthritis, or other chronic medical illnesses, if picked up early and treated properly the adolescent has the maximal possibility of growing up to have fewer complications and a greater level of health and quality of life. Early recognition and diagnosis, followed by the appropriate treatments, can result in a happy, productive, successful adult. Missing the diagnosis of learning disability or providing inadequate help or no help can result in an emotionally dysfunctional, underachieving adult who may work at less than his or her potential throughout life. It is critical that the clinician suspect this diagnosis with every patient who is doing poorly in school and that he or she follow through with establishing the diagnosis and implementing the necessary therapy.

BIBLIOGRAPHY

Fleischner JE, Garrett U, Silver LB: Developmental arithmetic disorders. In Kaplan H, Sadock B (eds): Comprehensive Textbook of Psychiatry, 5th ed. Baltimore, Williams & Wilkins, 1989, pp 1801–1804.

Galaburda AM, Sherman GF, Rosen GD, et al: Developmental dyslexia: Four consecutive patients with cortical abnormalities. Ann Neurol, 18:222, 1985.

Lerner JW: Educational interventions in learning disabilities. J Am Acad Child Adolesc Psychiatry 28:326, 1989.

Osman BB: No One to Play With. The Social Side of Learning Disabilities. New York, Random House, 1982.

Osman BB: Learning Disabilities. A Family Affair. New York, Random House, 1979.

Shawitz SE, Shawitz BE: Hyperactivity/attention deficits. In Kavanagh JF, Truss TJ, Jr, Learning Disabilities: Proceedings of the National Conference (eds): Parkton, MD, York Press, 1988.

Shepherd MJ, Charnow DA, Silver LB: Developmental reading disorder. In Kaplan H, Sadock B (eds): Comprehensive Textbook of Psychiatry, 5th ed. Baltimore, Williams & Wilkins, 1989, pp 1790–1796.

Shepherd MJ, Charnow DA, Silver LB: Developmental expressive writing disorder. In Kaplan H, Sadock B (eds): Comprehensive Textbook of Psychiatry, 5th ed. Baltimore, Williams & Wilkins, 1989, pp 1796–1800.

Silver LB: Psychological and family problems associated with learning disabilities: Assessment and intervention. J Am Acad Child Adolesc Psychiatry 28:319, 1989.

Silver LB: The Misunderstood Child. A Guide for Parents of Learning Disabled Children. New York, McGraw-Hill, 1984.

CHAPTER 108

Disorders of Conduct and Delinquency

DOROTHY OTNOW LEWIS

Almost every other neuropsychiatric condition of childhood and adolescence can, at some time, be manifested as a disorder of conduct. Mental retardation, hyperactivity, and the disorders we now categorize as schizophrenia, mania, depression, and organic brain damage may all periodically, or even throughout their course, appear to be simply behavioral problems. Since most other diagnoses have specific treatment implications and better prognoses, it is imperative that the clinician rule out all other possibilities before the diagnosis of conduct disorder is made. The more knowledgeable the clinician, the less frequently the diagnosis of conduct disorder will be made.

Many adolescents with disorders of conduct are known to the juvenile justice system and are designated delinquent. The term delinquent, however, is a legal rather than a medical term; it designates youngsters whose behaviors have been adjudicated illegal by a juvenile court. There are two types of offenses: status and nonstatus. Those offenses that are illegal only if performed by children (e.g., running away) are status offenses; those offenses that are considered crimes when committed by adults (e.g., burglary, robbery, murder) are nonstatus offenses. Although for the most part adolescents are considered minors until 18 years of age (see Chapter 20), whether or not a given youngster is tried as an adult for a particular offense depends on the nature of the act and on the jurisdiction in which the act is committed. However, conduct disorder and delinquency are similar in that both terms cover a multitude of problems, as well as a multitude of different neuropsychiatric conditions.

The current concept of conduct disorder has evolved from a rather pejorative label to a description of types of behaviors. Prior to the current classification system (Diagnostic and Statistical Manual of Mental Disorders: Third Edition—Revised; DSM-III-R), adolescents with disturbances of behavior could be considered to have antisocial personality (a permanent condition) or unsocialized aggressive reaction (amenable to change). The term *conduct disorder* was introduced in 1980 and was used to designate behaviors ranging from relatively minor infractions of rules to violent acts. Conduct disorder was divided into four different categories: (1) aggressive, (2) nonaggressive, (3) socialized, and (4) undersocialized. Individuals classified as aggressive and undersocialized were described as failing to bond with others or to establish a normal degree of empathy and affection. The determination of a "normal degree of empathy and affection" was left to each clinician.

DSM-III-R attempts to use behavioral data exclusively to make the diagnosis of conduct disorder. In DSM-III-R, conduct disorder is defined as a disturbance of behavior lasting at least 6 months in which the basic rights of others or the major age-appropriate norms and rules of society are violated, or both. For the diagnosis to be made, an adolescent should manifest 3 of 13 problematic behaviors, ranging in severity from truancy and running away to rape and assault (Table 108–1). There is no lower age limit for the diagnosis, and the upper age limit is vague (e.g., a person 18 years old or older who does not meet the criteria for antisocial personality may be diagnosed with conduct disorder). In the interest of greater objectivity, the categories of aggressive-nonaggressive and socialized-undersocialized have been superceded by the categories (1) solitary aggressive, (2) group type, and (3) undifferentiated. The severity of the disorder is rated on a three-point scale: mild, moderate, and severe.

The DSM-III-R criteria for conduct disorder are signs not symptoms. No distinctions are made among adolescents who, because of episodic paranoid misperceptions, lash out in response to imagined insults; those who fight because of impulsiveness and emotional lability secondary to organic impairment; and those who fight because they are teased. Similarly, no distinction is made among the adolescent who stays away from school because of anxiety, the adolescent who stays away because of cognitive difficulties, or the adolescent who stays away because of the need to babysit for younger siblings while his or her mother is hospitalized. Clearly, all the 13 behavioral criteria for diagnosing conduct disorder occur as part of numerous situations and other diagnoses, the common manifestations of which may be some form of antisocial behavior. Underlying disorders include mental retardation, mood disorders, organic syndromes, multiple personality, and the disorders subsumed under the term *schizophrenia*. The clinician must therefore remember that adolescents have a relatively small repertoire of behaviors with which to express their thoughts and feelings. The more astute the clinician, the more likely that he or she can discern underlying neuropsy-

TABLE 108–1. Diagnostic Criteria for Conduct Disorder

Has stolen without confrontation of a victim on more than one
    occasion (including forgery)
Has run away from home overnight at least twice while living in
    parental or parental surrogate home (or once without returning)
Often lies (other than to avoid physical or sexual abuse)
Has deliberately engaged in firesetting
Is often truant from school (for older person, absent from work)
Has broken into someone else's house, building, or car
Has deliberately destroyed others' property (other than by
    firesetting)
Has been physically cruel to animals
Has forced someone into sexual activity with him or her
Has used a weapon in more than one fight
Often initiates physical fights
Has stolen with confrontation of a victim (e.g., mugging, purse-
    snatching, extortion, armed robbery)
Has been physically cruel to people

With permission from American Psychiatric Association: Diagnostic and
Statistical Manual of Mental Disorders, 3rd ed, revised. Washington, DC,
American Psychiatric Association, 1987, p 55.

chiatric vulnerabilities that present on the surface as
simply conduct disorder.

EPIDEMIOLOGY

The incidence and prevalence of conduct disorder are
uncertain. Clearly, behaviors that are perfectly normal
at age 5 years may be considered characteristic of
conduct disorder in adolescence. Thus frequent temper
tantrums during the preschool years are of far less
concern than are similar behaviors during adolescence.
Some studies have indicated, however, that unmanageable behaviors are the most common reasons for psychiatric referrals during the very early years of life.

The question arises how predictive behavioral problems in early childhood are of subsequent conduct
disturbance. On the whole, destructiveness, bullying,
and even stealing tend to diminish between the ages of
5 years and 9 years. In contrast, serious behavioral
problems at 4 years of age, characterized by high levels
of activity and parental problems controlling the child,
are associated with conduct disturbance in later years.
The persistence of unmanageable behaviors from preschool to elementary school is more common in boys
than in girls.

Aggressive behaviors at 8 to 10 years of age are quite
good predictors of aggression during adolescence.
Aggression during the elementary school years is among
the most ominous early signs of severe psychopathology
and almost invariably an indicator of serious family
disturbance. In spite of these findings, it is essential to
recognize that the majority of behaviorally disturbed
young children do *not* grow up to be sociopathic adults.
However, they appear at risk for developing a variety
of other (nonsociopathic) psychiatric conditions.

There is a demonstrable relationship between a delinquent's degree of early neuropsychiatric impairment and
family violence and the severity of the delinquent's adult
violent behaviors. Data from a variety of different
studies indicate strong linkages among serious behavioral problems, a variety of neuropsychiatric signs and
symptoms, family psychopathology, and ongoing major
problems in social adaptation.

CLINICAL MANIFESTATIONS AND DIFFERENTIAL DIAGNOSIS

Unfortunately, the behaviors with which adolescents
with conduct disorder present are often so objectiona-
ble, even dangerous, that they rarely elicit sympathetic
responses from clinicians. Disobedience, truancy, repeated physical aggression, firesetting, stealing, running
away, cruelty to animals, lying, inappropriate sexual
behaviors, and substance abuse may all be characteristic
of adolescents diagnosed with conduct disorder. These
troublesome behaviors usually obscure the kinds of
underlying vulnerabilities that contribute to the picture
of conduct disorder. However, if the clinician can overcome an understandable initial dismay at the adolescent's presenting symptoms and make the effort to look
beneath these behaviors, he or she will almost invariably
discover combinations of psychiatric, neurologic, cognitive, and intrafamilial vulnerabilities that contribute
to the child's maladaptation.

PSYCHIATRIC VULNERABILITIES

The psychopathology underlying the antisocial behaviors of adolescents with conduct disorder is rarely obvious. Rather, their psychiatric signs and symptoms most
often place them on the borderline of numerous different kinds of diagnoses. Unfortunately, when these signs
and symptoms fail to meet the full set of criteria for
other established diagnoses, they tend to be overlooked.
Thus episodic psychotic, affective, or organic symptoms
are often ignored, and such adolescents are usually
diagnosed simply on the basis of their antisocial behaviors. They present with a sullenness or bravado and
would rather be considered "bad" than "crazy." Some
of the most pathologic behaviors of adolescents with
conduct disorder (their recurrent aggressive acts) are so
frightening that the underlying psychopathologic condition is overlooked. Probably the most common cause of
recurrent violent acts by adolescents is their misperception that they have been insulted behind their backs or
that they have been looked at in a threatening or
demeaning way. Ironically, the most recurrently violent,
paranoid, grandiose youngsters are also the best at
concealing their underlying psychiatric disturbance with
a boastful, ostensibly callous facade. The more paranoid
the youngster, the more likely that he or she will respond
with "I don't care" or "he deserved it" when asked how
he or she feels about the victim. Thus the youngsters
who are most out of touch with reality are also those
most likely to alienate the clinician and be dismissed as
severely sociopathic. Their sullenness and paranoia are
often dismissed by the inexperienced examiner simply
as manifestations of a lack of empathy.

Although few adolescents with conduct disorder appear to be schizophrenic, many of the most repetitively

antisocial individuals are found to have first- and second-degree relatives who have a history of psychosis. The identification of psychotic symptomatology in such youngsters is especially difficult during adolescence. Bender observed that many children who were identified as psychotic in childhood appeared to be simply antisocial in adolescence. It would seem that the adolescent's reluctance to reveal symptoms, coupled with the clinician's greater tolerance for aberrant behaviors in adolescent patients, together impede the recognition of psychotic symptomatology in this age group. It is common for the very same kinds of violent bizarre behaviors that during childhood were recognized as psychotic and requiring treatment to be reinterpreted in adolescence as signs of a character pathology. In childhood, such individuals are often placed in residential treatment settings, and it is common for them to respond to low doses of antipsychotic medication. During adolescence, when these individuals are physically larger, the very same behaviors they demonstrated earlier are more threatening and, whatever the cause, they frighten caretakers. Many aggressive youngsters who were previously diagnosed as borderline psychotic are therefore expelled from treatment centers, and their symptomatology is reinterpreted as being merely a sign of character pathology or a reflection of social disadvantage. The experienced clinician has an appreciation of the fact that by and large adolescence is *not* normally characterized by turmoil (see Chapter 8). When severe behavioral problems occur (especially adaptational problems starting in the early years), the likelihood of underlying psychopathology, ranging from organic dysfunction to an incipient psychotic disorder, must be considered. Most behaviorally disturbed children come from extremely chaotic households. Nevertheless, the more intact or resilient the adolescent, the more likely that he or she will be able to function adequately in society in spite of such stressors.

The irritability and rage that often accompany episodic depression, especially when aggravated by alcohol or drug ingestion, can also present as a conduct disorder. Bipolar mood disorders may present as episodic destructive behaviors or sporadic episodes of robbery and burglary (see Chapter 100). In female delinquents, manic episodes are frequently manifested by sexual promiscuity and a heedlessness for the possible consequences of such behaviors. Thus, conduct disorder may be an overt manifestation of a biologically and psychodynamically treatable mood disorder. In fact, the alcoholism diagnosed in the parents of many adolescents with conduct disorder is often the adult manifestation of a depressive illness and not merely an indicator of a dissolute way of life.

Suicidal behaviors, both deliberate and unconscious, are frequent in the adolescent population with conduct disorders (see Chapter 101). Although these behaviors are not necessarily manifestations of depression, they still must be taken seriously. They are often expressions of extreme frustration, pain, anger and, of course, impulsiveness. They should not be dismissed as manipulative behaviors. The experienced clinician is aware of the fact that successful suicides often occur subsequent to initial suicide attempts. The attempt must therefore be taken seriously. The death rate among delinquent adolescents is extraordinarily high and is almost invariably violent in nature (i.e., suicide, homicide, accidents).

Drug and alcohol abuse are common among adolescents with conduct disorder (see Chapter 111). It is not unusual to obtain a history of drug and alcohol abuse beginning at age 11 or 12 years. Children raised in some of the most emotionally and physically abusive households have sometimes started drinking as early as 8 years of age. There is a current tendency to send young substance abusers to substance abuse programs and to look no further for the causes of the abuse. Substance abuse is used by different children and adolescents for different reasons, including attempts to self-medicate anxiety, depression, psychosis, and hyperactivity. A diagnosis of substance abuse alone in a youngster with conduct disorder sometimes reflects a failure to explore underlying symptomatology. This tendency to overlook the psychopathology underlying substance abuse is lamentable, because the kinds of underlying disorders in question (e.g., depression, psychosis) are often responsive to specific pharmacologic interventions. Since drug programs may be concerned about the use of medication, the depressed or borderline psychotic adolescent in such a program is unlikely to receive the kind of medication that might diminish his or her subjective need for alcohol or drugs (see Chapter 111).

One of the psychiatric conditions that is most frequently overlooked in the population of adolescents with conduct disorder, especially the violent population, is multiple personality. Although it is a disorder that begins very early in life, most individuals with this disorder are in treatment many years before the condition is recognized. This disorder is probably far more common among episodically violent youngsters than we realize, since many violent youngsters have histories of having been physically and sexually abused (Chapters 118 and 119), and the most extreme forms of abuse are associated with the development of multiple personality. Furthermore, adolescents with multiple personality are usually accused of chronic lying. This is because many of the antisocial behaviors occur while the adolescent is in an alternate state, and he or she really does not remember them.

Many of the other symptoms and signs of conduct disorder—such as episodic destructiveness, extreme moodiness, impaired memory for behaviors, wandering off and not returning home for hours or days, finding something in one's possession and denying knowledge of how it got there—are also characteristic of adolescents with multiple personality disorder. The fact that we do not make the diagnosis more often has been more a reflection of our failure to consider it (or, worse, our belief that it does not exist) than a reflection of its rarity. In the author's experience, the extreme mood changes of youngsters with multiple personality, if not attributed to a conduct disorder, are likely to be misdiagnosed as bipolar illness. Similarly, the memory lapses, if not dismissed as fabrications, are often attributed to seizure disorders (see Chapter 83).

A study comparing incarcerated adolescents with adolescents in psychiatric hospitals found that the two groups had very similar signs, symptoms, and behaviors. It is of note that they were even comparably violent. The major variable that distinguished which adolescents went to correctional schools and which adolescents were hospitalized was race. The clinician must appreciate the fact that incarcerated adolescents are very similar to adolescent psychiatric patients and that the very same treatment modalities that are effective for one group can be expected to be helpful in the treatment of the other group if made available.

MEDICAL AND NEUROLOGIC VULNERABILITIES

It has been shown that delinquent adolescents tend to have far more adverse medical histories than do nondelinquent children; in addition, the more behaviorally disturbed the adolescent, the more likely it is that he or she has suffered central nervous system (CNS) injury and has been abused. Although most youngsters with conduct disorder do not have obvious or localized neurologic damage, a careful medical and neuropsychological assessment will reveal subtle indicators of CNS dysfunction.

Such youngsters often demonstrate attention problems, hyperactivity, and a variety of minor neurologic problems, such as an inability to skip, poor fine motor coordination, and impaired short-term memory. These kinds of nonlocalized indicators of CNS dysfunction are often dismissed by neurologic consultants as noncontributory to behavioral problems. Their importance rests on the fact that children with such vulnerabilities also often have trouble modulating feelings, making appropriate judgments, and controlling behavior.

Few adolescents with conduct disorder suffer from epilepsy, though there is some evidence that psychomotor seizures (complex partial seizures) are more common in violent delinquents than in the general population, and abnormal electroencephalograms are more common in the prison population than in the general population (see Chapter 83). Psychomotor symptoms, such as impaired memory for nonviolent as well as violent behaviors, olfactory hallucinations, and vivid recurrent episodes of déja vu are fairly common findings in the aggressive delinquent population. Many seriously delinquent children (as well as many incarcerated adults) will be found to have equivocal or diffusely abnormal electroencephalograms. These kinds of signs and symptoms suggest that in some youngsters with conduct disorder, abnormal electrical activity in the brain, possibly in the limbic system, probably contributes to difficulties in modulating behavior. As in the case of psychoses, the signs and symptoms of adolescents with conduct disorder usually are not distinct enough to meet criteria for specific neurologic diagnoses. Rather these signs and symptoms, all of which may have treatment implications, place them on the borderline of a variety of different neurologic diagnoses.

COGNITIVE VULNERABILITIES

The low-normal intelligence quotient (IQ) scores on standard intelligence tests of many youngsters with conduct disorder place them on the borderline of a potentially treatable diagnosis—mental retardation. The clinician should not dismiss low scores on standardized testing as evidence of merely cultural deprivation, rather than as a need for remediation, simply because a youngster comes from a disadvantaged background. Whatever the explanation for cognitive limitations may be, they do impede social functioning. Poor judgment, impaired abstract reasoning, and difficulty planning ahead and anticipating consequences all contribute to behavioral problems.

Learning disabilities are especially common in the delinquent population with conduct disorder (see Chapter 107). Adolescents with language and reading problems have special difficulty putting their angry thoughts and feelings of frustration into words rather than actions. School thus becomes a place of failure and disappointment rather than of gratification and learning. Without proper assistance, such adolescents often drop out of school early and "hang around" the streets, and their relatively minor behavioral problems often escalate and become seriously delinquent behaviors.

Since adolescents with conduct disorders are often on the borderline of cognitive impairment or intellectual deficiency, they tend to receive neither the attention reserved for the severely impaired nor that afforded the intellectually gifted.

In summary, adolescents with severe conduct disorder usually have a multiplicity of different neuropsychiatric and cognitive vulnerabilities that place them on the borderline of numerous other diagnoses simultaneously. Because these vulnerabilities are not obvious, there is a serious risk that the behaviors these adolescents exhibit will overshadow their vulnerabilities. In addition, these young people may not receive the careful diagnostic evaluation that would identify conditions that are treatable.

DIFFERENTIAL DIAGNOSIS

Any condition or combination of conditions that lowers impulse control, diminishes "reality-testing," increases suspiciousness, and impairs judgment is likely to result in a disorder of conduct. At some stage in the evolution of many neuropsychiatric conditions—ranging from schizophrenia to encephalitis—antisocial, even aggressive, behaviors may occur. Therefore the differential diagnosis of conduct disorder is broad.

Most often, in the author's experience, conduct disorder is a transitional designation used by clinicians when underlying causes for aberrant behaviors have not yet been identified. Hence the diagnosis of conduct disorder in psychiatry, at this point in our understanding, is analogous in many ways to the diagnosis of fever of unknown origin in pediatrics and internal medicine.

DIAGNOSTIC EVALUATION

The clinician evaluating the delinquent adolescent or the adolescent with conduct disorder has a special responsibility. The clinician's findings often determine whether or not a youngster will obtain treatment or be relegated to the juvenile correctional system. Because the signs and symptoms of a neuropsychopathologic condition underlying behavioral disorders are often subtle, and because it is usually the combination of vulnerabilities and environmental stressors that leads to chronic disorders of behavior, patience, time, and good will are essential in the clinician. Both adolescents and their parents tend to be defensive and need much reassurance that the examiner, whatever his or her discipline, is not critical either of the behaviors leading to consultation or of the underlying causes of these behaviors (see Table 108–1 for diagnostic criteria).

Interview with the Adolescent

The clinician who sits back and asks nondirective questions of the already defensive adolescent is likely to elicit little information (see Chapter 22). The more open-ended and general the questions, especially if they involve feelings or relationships, the more anxious the adolescent is likely to become. Asking straightforward factual questions, such as where the adolescent was born and where and with whom the youngster lived from birth onward, is a fairly nonthreatening way of starting and also of getting a sense of the stability or lack thereof in the adolescent's life. Reasons for moves and reactions to these moves then can then be explored. A discussion of feelings is best approached by gathering seemingly factual data, for example, "So you lived with your grandmother while your mother was in the hospital. How long was that? To whom would you say you are closest?" or "That must have been hard, moving back with your mother when you were 8 years old after living with your grandparents all your life. What was that like for you?"

One of the best ways of acquiring relevant psychological as well as medical information is in the context of a careful medical history. Many adolescents, especially those who have had prenatal problems, can furnish information regarding their birth. The mothers of seriously delinquent youngsters often have notoriously poor prenatal care, and adolescents may know whether or not they were premature or had other perinatal problems.

The clinician evaluating the behaviorally disordered adolescent is especially interested in any injuries or illnesses affecting the CNS. It is not enough to ask whether or not an adolescent has had any serious accidents. Usually the response to such a question is negative or it elicits a single injury. The clinician must take the time to inquire specifically about car accidents, bicycle accidents, falls from high places, and blows to the head. After ascertaining that a youngster has received such an injury, the clinician must allow further time to inquire about other car accidents or other bicycle injuries the youngster has sustained. In each instance the examiner must be prepared to ask about whether the adolescent was "knocked dizzy" or knocked unconscious. Questions about alterations of consciousness must also be asked in several different ways. "Have you ever fainted? Have you ever blacked out? Have you

ever been told you stared off into space and were out of it?" All questions must be asked.

Similarly, questions regarding seizures must be asked several different ways (see Chapter 83). It is not unusual for an adolescent to deny ever having had a seizure, only to tell the examiner later that he or she did have epilepsy or a convulsion. If an adolescent has been violent episodically, it is also important to know whether he or she can tell in advance when the aggression will occur, how he or she feels afterward, and whether all aspects of the event are recalled.

The medical history is a good vehicle for covering aspects of the mental status examination. Even the most disturbed adolescent when asked if he or she hears or sees things other people do not hear or see is likely to deny the experience, often with the comment, "What do you think I am? Crazy?" However, if first asked about visual problems, such as the need for eyeglasses, the adolescent is more likely to respond to a follow-up question such as, "Have your eyes ever played tricks on you? Have you ever seen a person or an animal and you know your eyes have played tricks on you?" Similarly, auditory hallucinations are often best elicited in the context of questions regarding earaches or ear infections. One of the most useful questions that can be posed in this context is, "Have you ever had the experience of thinking people said something bad about you or your mother, and they say they did not?" One of the most common causes of recurrent violent acts by adolescents is the paranoid misperception that they are being talked about, belittled, or threatened.

Severe physical abuse (see Chapter 118) is a common finding in the history of aggressive, behaviorally disturbed adolescents. Nonetheless, adolescents are usually very protective of their parents. Moreover, they usually believe that they deserved any battering they received. When asked about the worst punishment ever received, most will say "I was grounded" or "I could not watch television." However, a subsequent series of matter-of-fact questions specifically inquiring if an adolescent was ever hit with a belt, belt buckle, cord, hanger, and so on will often be answered in the affirmative.

The behaviorally disturbed adolescent often shows evidence of accidents and battering all over his or her face, head, arms, legs, and body. The examiner should ask about the cause of every visible scar and then should ask, "Are there any scars I cannot see?" With appropriate attention to issues of privacy, the clinician should examine the youngster's back, chest, and buttocks for signs of abuse. The author has examined youngsters with scars on the bottoms of their feet and even on their penises, where caretakers had threatened castration.

The clinician must avoid questions that invite yes or no answers. It is more useful to ask, "How does beer or wine or alcohol affect you? Does it ever make you angry or aggressive?" than to ask, "Do you drink alcohol?" Similarly, questions about drugs can be posed in terms of how "pot" or "weed" or "reefer" affects the adolescent. Then questions such as "What else have you tried? How much do you use? How does it affect you?" are acceptable. Adolescents who report visual or auditory hallucinations while drinking or taking drugs should also be asked, "When has something like this happened without alcohol or without drugs?" Again, yes or no questions should be avoided. Adolescents who do not drink or use drugs or who have not ever hallucinated will respond to these questions without taking offense.

One of the hardest areas to ask about is sexual abuse (see Chapter 119). However, sexual abuse is common in the histories of behaviorally disturbed youngsters, especially in those who have themselves committed sexual offenses. The clinician may soften the threat of these kinds of questions by observing that research has indicated that many children as they were growing up were bothered sexually by someone older than themselves. Then the clinician can ask, "What sorts of experiences did you have when you were a child?" Questions about who taught the youngster about sex and whether or not the adolescent ever had a sexual relationship with someone much older than he or she will often elicit information regarding sexual abuse that the adolescent did not regard as abusive (e.g., "My mother had a girlfriend. She used to visit a lot and she showed me what to do.") As in the case of inquiring about accidents and injuries, inquiries about sexual abuse that elicit positive responses should be followed by, "Who else bothered you sexually?"

Space precludes a description of the entire interview. Certain principles of interviewing should be observed whatever the topic to be covered (see Chapter 22). These principles include the need to interact actively and not permit long awkward silences; the need to begin with fairly factual, concrete questions before moving into areas of feelings and attitudes; the need to ask specific, detailed questions rather than general questions; the need to avoid questions inviting yes or no responses; the need always to assume that there is more to learn and therefore to ask, "What other? Who else? When else?" after receiving positive responses.

Interview with the Parents

Parents whose adolescents have behavioral problems often feel very guilty. Since stresses within the family are frequent concomitants of behavioral problems, family members often believe that they have a lot to hide. Again, the clinician will alleviate anxiety by focusing initially on factual material (e.g., the adolescent's perinatal or medical history) and gradually moving toward more sensitive subjects (see Chapter 22).

Parents can provide information regarding the family history of diseases that often underlie and contribute to behavioral problems. Although it is important to ask specifically whether any family members—aunts, uncles, cousins, grandparents—had trouble with their nerves or were ever hospitalized, a negative response is often inaccurate. The examiner must inquire whether anyone was depressed, committed suicide, had problems with alcohol or drugs, or was very flamboyant, successful, or artistic. Finally, asking briefly about specific family members (e.g., "Tell me about your brothers and sisters What do they do for a living?") will often prove far

more informative than general questions focused on the entire family.

Both the behaviorally disturbed adolescent and his or her parents are more comfortable blaming the adolescent for family excesses. Thus, when asking a parent about abuse, it helps to acknowledge the fact that the adolescent has been hard to manage. Questions such as, "I know that Johnny has been a handful to raise. Has he ever made you go further than you meant while disciplining him? How about his father? Has Johnny ever made his father lose his temper? What happened?"

The more time spent with the parents, and the more empathic the clinician, the more likely that the parent will share relevant information. The clinician should also remember that siblings and other relatives can also be invaluable sources of information. Finally, the clinician should not assume that an incarcerated father is simply a sociopath or that a mother with a problem with substance abuse is simply an alcoholic or a drug addict. Just as antisocial behavior or substance abuse in the adolescent can obfuscate underlying psychopathology, these behaviors can also mask similar disorders in the parents.

Information from Other Sources

Given the fact that social maladaptation usually begins early, most behaviorally disturbed adolescents have long histories of conduct disorder and attempts to address it. For this reason, the clinician must make every effort to obtain all previous medical, educational, social, and psychiatric or psychological records. A review of these records at the very beginning of the evaluation often provides a focus for the rest of the evaluation and prevents unnecessary repetition of tests and procedures (see Chapters 22 and 106–111).

In addition to a comprehensive medical and psychiatric history and examination, it is sometimes helpful to have a neurologic examination and electroencephalographic studies performed. If a neurologic consultation is to be useful, however, the primary clinician, whatever his or her specialty, must gather enough data to make a knowledgeable referral that contains specific questions for the neurologist based on a thorough initial assessment.

The kinds of neuropsychological problems characteristic of behaviorally disturbed adolescents are often better documented with psychological, neuropsychological, and educational evaluations. Tests such as the Halstead-Reitan and Luria Nebraska batteries often elicit subtle neurologic and cognitive impairments missed by standard psychiatric or neurologic examinations. Similarly, detailed educational assessments of specific learning skills can often identify previously overlooked vulnerabilities that contribute to maladaptive behaviors. Whatever specialized procedures are employed, the primary clinician has the responsibility of assimilating diverse findings and determining the ways in which they contribute to the adolescent's maladaptation.

As mentioned, the differential diagnosis of adolescents with conduct disorder is almost as broad as the field of child psychiatry and includes organic impairment, mood disorders, psychoses, and cognitive impairment. Usually the adolescent with conduct disorder has a multiplicity of vulnerabilities, each of which must be identified and addressed if behavior is to improve.

THEORIES OF ETIOLOGY

Biochemical, Physiologic, and Medical Perspectives

Although the understanding of the relationship of specific neurotransmitters to behaviors is in its infancy, some of the most promising and intriguing studies suggest the existence of an association between diminished CNS levels of serotonin and impulsive, aggressive behaviors (see Chapters 10 and 12).

Other investigators have hypothesized that delinquent youngsters are born with or acquire abnormal autonomic reactivity. They hypothesize that such individuals are slower than others to recover from aversive stimuli and thus are harder to influence with positive or negative reinforcement.

Numerous animal and human studies suggest that testosterone plays a role in aggression (see Chapter 13). The males of most species are far more aggressive than the females. In addition, in animals, castration of the male at certain developmental stages diminishes aggression. In humans, however, findings regarding the relationship of testosterone levels to aggression are equivocal. Nevertheless, if one examines the play of small children or the criminal behavior of adults, males are demonstrably more aggressive than females. Of note, numerous other hormones, including the corticosteroids and the female sex hormones, have been implicated in changes in aggressive behavior. There is also preliminary evidence that gonadal hormones and neurotransmitters are interrelated and together affect behavior (see Chapter 13).

Psychosis, Conduct Disorder, and Aggression

Most individuals with psychiatric disturbances are not violent, but many have a variety of adaptational difficulties. As alluded to previously, violence, it seems, is associated not so much with a specific psychiatric disorder as it is with the symptom of paranoid misperceptions and misinterpretations. Whatever the cause of the paranoia, paranoid individuals are more likely than others to lash out in response to real or imagined threats. At this time, the syndrome we call schizophrenia probably encompasses many different kinds of psychoses, manifested by a continuum of maladaptive symptoms (see Chapter 110). The signs, symptoms, and behaviors of these antisocial youngsters suggest that their own pathologic condition falls somewhere along this spectrum. As stated, manic-depressive psychoses also may

be manifested initially by antisocial aggressive behaviors.

Genetic Perspectives

Reports during the 1960s and 1970s suggested that chromosomal abnormalities, specifically the XYY syndrome and XXY (Klinefelter) syndrome were associated with criminality. More recent studies suggest that most individuals with XYY and XXY chromosomal constellations do not exhibit criminal behavior. Since there is a higher proportion of individuals with these kinds of anomalies in institutional settings, it is likely that they are especially vulnerable to problems of adaption that, depending on their environments, may or may not be manifested as antisocial behaviors. Similarly, studies reporting a high prevalence of criminality in adopted offspring of criminal fathers should be examined critically. Men with psychiatric disturbances who act aggressively are more likely to be incarcerated than are women who have similar psychiatric impairments.

Parental Factors

There is a consensus that parental maladaptation is closely related to adolescents' behavioral problems. Although early studies focused primarily on parental alcoholism and sociopathy, more intensive examination of parental signs, symptoms, and behaviors suggests that many parents of delinquents and children with behavior disorders suffer from serious psychiatric disorders (including psychoses) that impair their ability to provide the kinds of nurturing and protection necessary for a child's normal development. Their difficulties in setting limits and providing consistent nonviolent discipline are only part of the problem. They have such difficulty organizing their own lives that little energy is left to invest in the physical, much less emotional and educational, well-being of their children. In and out of prisons and mental hospitals, they cannot provide the stability and predictability necessary for their children to learn to order their own behaviors.

Without question, the most devastating consequence of parental dysfunction is the tendency to take out anger and frustration in physical abuse of their children. In this way they provide a model of abuse, inflict the kinds of diffuse CNS injury associated with behavior problems, and instill a rage that is often displaced onto others in the child's environment.

Interaction of Biopsychosocial Factors

Conduct disorder is obviously not a discrete diagnostic entity. It is usually the final common pathway, the behavioral result of the interaction of psychological, neurologic, and cognitive vulnerabilities and an abusive violent family environment. When such vulnerable youngsters are raised in especially violent societies such as our own in which access to weapons is easy and in which the media depicts violence constantly, their ability to adapt in socially acceptable ways is further diminished. Although violence in the media in and of itself probably does not cause ordinary healthy adolescents to behave in aggressive ways, it may be especially stimulating to adolescents whose impulse control and "reality-testing" are already compromised. There is also evidence that more disturbed, aggressive youngsters gravitate toward violent entertainment.

TREATMENT

In spite of the fact that numerous different treatment approaches have been tried, no single modality has proved more effective than any other. This is not because adolescents with conduct disorders cannot be treated. It is, rather, because each adolescent with conduct disorder has a distinct constellation of neuropsychiatric and cognitive vulnerabilities and environmental stressors. Each of these must be elucidated and addressed for behavior to improve.

In spite of the myriad signs, symptoms, and stressors contributing to maladaptive behaviors, single-treatment modalities continue to be developed. They have included attempts to train parents in effective ways of communicating and interacting with their offspring, using moderate discipline and positive reinforcement rather than physical punishment. Other treatment modalities have focused on providing behaviorally disturbed youngsters with the problem-solving skills they lack. This method stresses improving the adolescent's ability to identify problems, recognize causality, appreciate potential consequences of behaviors, and find new ways of coping with stress. Other treatment programs have taken into account the severe problems within most families of delinquents and have attempted to create community support in the form of concerned individuals acting as mentors, advocates, and friends.

Some attempts have been made to treat youngsters with conduct disorder with specific medications, ranging from amphetamines to lithium carbonate. These biologic interventions, like the previously mentioned family, individual, and community programs, are helpful for some behaviorally disturbed adolescents but not for others. This is because of the different types of neuropsychiatric pathology underlying behavior disorders. Clearly, stimulant medication is more likely to be of help in the behaviorally disturbed youngster with an attention deficit disorder than in the youngster with an incipient psychosis. In short, medications such as stimulants, antipsychotics, antiepileptics, lithium carbonate, antidepressants, and even the β-blockers must be selected according to the needs of the individual adolescent and should be regarded as potentially useful adjuncts to a comprehensive therapeutic regimen.

If a treatment program is to be successful it must be based on sophisticated individual clinical evaluations. It must be multimodal, addressing the medical, psycho-dynamic, emotional, cognitive, educational, family, and social needs of each behaviorally disturbed adolescent. Moreover, the vulnerabilities and needs of adolescents with serious conduct disorder are usually chronic. Therefore interventions cannot be limited to months or even 2 or 3 years. These youngsters require ongoing, constant support throughout adolescence and even into early adulthood if they are to function adequately in society.

Clearly the treatment of disorders of conduct, based as it must be on the identification and ongoing treatment of vulnerabilities, is time-consuming and costly. As in so many other pathologic conditions, prevention is potentially far simpler and more effective. The prevention of perinatal difficulties and insults to the CNS during childhood would go far in improving the child's ability to cope, even with extreme environmental stressors. Programs are needed to inform and educate adolescents, males as well as females, regarding the extraordinary physical and emotional demands of infants and children. Teenagers must be helped to make responsible choices regarding their preparedness to become parents. Programs are needed to assist those young parents already overburdened by the unanticipated needs of their children. Most important, society as a whole, and parents in particular, must be helped to appreciate the extraordinary neurologic and psychological damage caused by physical abuse and intrafamily violence and the association of abuse with the development of violence. Each clinician can educate and support the adolescents in his or her practice—both those who are already parents and those who will become parents—in the interest of diminishing behavior disorders and violence in the next generation.

COURSE OF ILLNESS AND PROGNOSIS

To date, there have been no studies of treatment programs based on comprehensive clinical evaluations and ongoing treatment for the specific biopsychosocial vulnerabilities of individual delinquents. Therefore it is impossible to report with confidence the results of appropriate treatment. The results of individual modalities (e.g., parent training) are more or less successful, depending on the severity of the antisocial behaviors and the adolescent's and family's ability to make use of a particular service. The more chaotic the environment, the less the family will be able to make use of a single modality approach.

In the author's experience, when antisocial behavior is regarded as a signal of underlying vulnerabilities, and when the clinician refuses to settle for a diagnosis of conduct disorder, the likelihood is greatly increased of discovering other kinds of conditions amenable to specific treatment. The greater the sophistication and experience of the clinician, the less often the diagnosis of conduct disorder alone will be made.

BIBLIOGRAPHY

Bender L: The concept of pseudopsychopathic schizophrenia in adolescents. Am J Orthopsychiatry 29:491, 1959.

Coccaro EF, Siever LJ, Klar HM, et al: Serotonergic studies in patients with affective and personality disorders. Arch Gen Psychiatry 46:587, 1989.

Kazdin AE: Conduct Disorders in Childhood and Adolescence, Vol 9. Newbury Park, CA, Sage Publications, 1987.

Lewis DO (ed): Vulnerabilities to Delinquency. New York; Spectrum Publications, 1981.

Lewis DO, Lovely R, Yeager C, Della Femina D: Toward a theory of the genesis of violence: A follow-up study of delinquents. J Am Acad Child Adolesc Psychiatry, 28(3):431, 1989.

Mednick SA: The learning of morality: Biosocial bases. In Lewis DO (ed): Vulnerabilities to Delinquency. New York, Spectrum Publications, 1981, pp 187–204.

Patterson GR: Coercive Family Processes. Eugene, OR, Castalia Publishing, 1982.

Robins LN: Deviant Children Grown-Up. Baltimore, Williams & Wilkins, 1966.

Rutter M, Giller H: Juvenile Delinquency: Trends and Perspectives. New York, Guilford Press, 1984.

West DJ: Delinquency: Its Roots, Careers and Prospects. Cambridge, MA, Harvard University Press, 1982.

CHAPTER 109

Personality Disorders

DRAGAN M. SVRAKIC and C. ROBERT CLONINGER

Personality disorders (PDs) are often recognizable in adolescence or earlier, and they continue throughout most of adult life. As a result, most PDs defined by official classification systems—notably, the Diagnostic and Statistical Manual of Mental Disorders: Third Edition—Revised (DSM-III-R)—can be observed and should be diagnosed in adolescents. Some clinicians are hesitant to diagnose PDs in adolescents because of unfounded concerns about stigmatization, but this practice usually serves only to delay effective treatment of the adolescent and education of the family.

The inherently imprecise definition appears to be the major problem in the overall diagnosis of PDs. For example, to arrive at a correct diagnosis, one must carefully evaluate "significant socioprofessional or subjective distress" (DSM-III-R)—an extremely arbitrary diagnostic criterion. Similarly, many of the features of various PDs may be seen during an episode of another mental disorder (e.g., chronic depression), and yet it is essential to distinguish between state (e.g., depression-related) and trait (e.g., personality) manifestations. The PD diagnosis is justified only when the features are typical of a person's long-term functioning and are not limited to the discrete episode of other mental disorders or situational factors. Understandably, the clinician is cautious.

Several other points are important. First, though some authors have suggested that adolescent "identity crises" are normal aspects of development, many studies have shown that adolescent turmoils and crises are not normal phenomena that resolve spontaneously (see Chapter 8). The treatment of such adolescent maladjustment is discussed later. Second, mental development, cognitive maturation, and identity formation do not follow discrete stage-like processes; each of these aspects of maturation can change continuously and at different rates (see Chapter 9). Third, early adolescence, which is traditionally regarded as the most painful period in the entire course of adolescence, is characterized by fewer, rather than more, personality difficulties. Finally, and contrary to common belief, research has shown that adolescent-parent relationships are not necessarily characterized by a generalized "generation gap"—parents and their children share similar value systems, whereas

adolescent-peer similarities characterize areas of "adolescent culture," such as fashions in preferred music or grooming. Accordingly, we have included a brief discussion about adjustment and identity disorders in this chapter.

The DSM-III-R classifies three clusters of PDs (Table 109–1). The following discussion of etiologic, pathogenetic-developmental, diagnostic, and treatment aspects of PDs, as well as the previous presentation of the dimensional approach to personality and PDs, is relevant to the majority of individual PDs. We discuss the diagnostic criteria and clinical picture of borderline PD (BPD) in more detail for the following reasons:

1. There is great clinical, behavioral, and phenomenologic similarity between BPD and identity problems in adolescence, and the differential diagnosis between these disorders is of critical importance. In fact, many authors agree that the major task of adolescent psychiatry and the "major dilemma of adolescence" is to distinguish BPD from identity and adjustment disorders.

2. The borderline level of personality organization is likely to be the "baseline" for individual PDs.

3. Space limitations preclude further discussion. The bibliography provides sources for detailed clinical and diagnostic descriptions of other PDs.

NORMAL AND DEVIANT PERSONALITIES

The term *deviant personality* refers strictly to uncommon styles of interacting with other individuals and situations. Normal and deviant personalities are inherently relative concepts, as both represent arbitrary subdivisions within the full spectrum of human behaviors (see Chapter 11). PDs are context-dependent disorders. Depending on the context, the same personality trait could be diagnosed as normal or deviant. For example, the same traits that are ideal for a fighter pilot might lead to severe maladaptation if the pilot were assigned to a desk job as an accountant. Finally, maladaptation might be a temporary, first response to a new stimuli, which can later, through the process of adaptive learning, develop into a well-adapted behavior.

The traditional clinical criterion for the differentiation of normal and deviant personalities is the presence of long-term and pervasive maladaptation that is recognizable through its subjective, social, and occupational

Supported in part by Grant MH31302 from the National Institute of Mental Health, Grants AA07982 and AA08028 from the National Institute of Alcoholism, and a grant from the MacArthur Foundation Mental Health Research Network I (Psychobiology of Depression).

TABLE 109–1. Characteristics of Personality Disorders

CLUSTER A
(often appear odd or eccentric)

1. *Paranoid Personality Disorder*—pervasive pattern of unwarranted tendency to interpret the actions of people as deliberately demeaning or threatening
2. *Schizoid Personality Disorder*—pervasive pattern of indifference to social relationships and a restricted range of emotional experience and expression
3. *Schizotypal Personality Disorder*—pervasive pattern of peculiarities of ideation, appearance, and behavior and deficits in interpersonal relatedness

CLUSTER B
(often appear dramatic, emotional, or erratic)

1. *Antisocial Personality Disorder*—pervasive pattern of irresponsible and antisocial behavior beginning in childhood or early adolescence and continuing into adulthood
2. *Borderline Personality Disorder*—pervasive pattern of instability of self-image, interpersonal relationships, and mood
3. *Histrionic Personality Disorder*—pervasive pattern of excessive emotionality and attention-seeking
4. *Narcissistic Personality Disorder*—pervasive pattern of grandiosity (in fantasy or behavior), hypersensitivity to the evaluation of others, and lack of empathy

CLUSTER C
(often appear anxious or fearful)

1. *Avoidant Personality Disorder*—pervasive pattern of social discomfort, fear of negative evaluation, and timidness
2. *Dependent Personality Disorder*—pervasive pattern of dependent and submissive behavior
3. *Obsessive-Compulsive Personality Disorder*—pervasive pattern of perfectionism and inflexibility
4. *Passive-Aggressive Personality*—pervasive pattern of passive resistance to demands for adequate social and occupational performance

Data from American Psychiatric Association: Diagnostic and Statistical Manual of Mental Disorders, 3rd ed, revised. Washington, DC, American Psychiatric Association, 1987.

consequences. In accordance with this, the contemporary DSM-III-R or International Classification of Diseases (ICD-10) definition of PDs is the following:

Personality traits are enduring patterns of perceiving, thinking, and relating to the environment and oneself, and are exhibited in a wide range of important social and personal contexts. It is only when personality traits are inflexible and maladaptive, and cause either significant functional impairment or subjective distress that they constitute personality disorders.

We note here that both the DSM-III-R and the ICD-10 classification systems are categorical—that is, they adopt the classic medical model that a disorder is either present or not. Categorical models are optimal when attributes are distributed discontinuously, for example, in gastric ulcer. However, when characteristics of the disorder are personality traits that vary quantitatively and have different adaptive significance in different situations, any "yes" or "no" decision regarding the existence of a psychopathologic condition is arbitrary. Dimensional models, which conceptualize deviant personality types as extremes on a continuum, appear to be more informative and practical because they avoid the need for multiple, overlapping diagnoses and are as easily applied to the common atypical and mild cases as they are to the rare prototypical and severe cases.

CLASSIFICATION OF PERSONALITY DISORDERS

DSM-III-R Classification System

The DSM-III-R classifies 12 "official" PDs (see Table 109–1) and two disorders, self-defeating and sadistic PD, as "entities for further research." Eleven are listed in the table; the other is multiple personality disorder. With respect to the group of PDs, the advantages of the DSM-III-R classification are:

1. The DSM-III-R is an atheoretical system that does not rely on etiopathogenetic assumptions but classifies PDs according to the clinical picture; this, in turn, motivates etiopathogenetic investigations.
2. The multiaxial diagnostic approach of the DSM-III-R ensures that the PDs are not overlooked, even when they occur with clinically more impressive Axis I disorders, and allows the establishment of both diagnoses when the two disorders coexist.
3. The DSM-III-R is a consistently polythetic classification (i.e., use criteria are comprised of many alternative items). An approach that requires a single pathognomonic profile of a PD is incompatible with the heterogeneity of PD symptomatology.

The disadvantages of the DSM-III-R classification are:

1. As already mentioned, the DSM-III-R is a categorical system and is not an optimal diagnostic instrument for PDs. When it becomes available, the DSM-IV is unlikely to introduce a dimensional approach to PDs.
2. The DSM-III-R has improved the diagnostic reliability of PDs, but these disorders still attain the lowest reliability of any major category of mental disorders.
3. The DSM-III-R classifies some disputable PDs, such as schizotypal PD (insufficiently well differentiated from schizophrenic disorders), avoidant PD (insufficiently well differentiated from social phobia), and dependent PD (insufficient knowledge to make it a separate nosologic entity).
4. We note here that the DSM-III-R accurately points to the childhood origins of antisocial PD but inaccurately assumes that conduct disorder in children antedates adult antisocial PD (see Chapter 108). Antisocial behavior has different antecedents at different ages; thus conduct disorder does not necessarily represent an early phase of adult antisocial PD. Conversely, adoption and follow-up clinical studies suggest that attention deficit disorder in childhood may increase the risk of postpubertal delinquency and antisocial PD (see Chapter 106).

ADJUSTMENT AND IDENTITY DISORDERS

Adjustment disorder and identity disorder of adolescence are not usually considered to be PDs. However, both disorders may reflect an underlying PD or may lead to severe maladaptation. In addition, the diagnosis of adjustment disorder is widely used to avoid more precision—that is, to avoid making the PD diagnosis that is really warranted. Hence, we will discuss these disorders in some detail.

Adjustment Disorder

CLINICAL MANIFESTATIONS

Adjustment disorders usually begin acutely and are characterized by regressive behavior, such as clinging to peers or parents and impulsive "acting-out." Anxiety, depression, eating and sleep disorders, somatic complaints, and impairment in occupational functioning are common. The disorder is a *reaction* to an identifiable psychosocial stressor that occurs within 3 months of onset of the stressor and *persists for no more than 6 months*. Several studies have shown that 8% to 15% of the adolescent population at some point manifests adolescent adjustment disorder.

According to psychodynamic theory, the main cause of adjustment disorder is "regression in the service of egomastery." In other words, when adolescents are faced with external problems or demands with which they have difficulty coping, they may revert to means of coping that were effective at an earlier age. The clear reactive and regressive nature of the change in behavior represents the hallmark of the DSM-III-R concept of adolescent adjustment disorder. Practical problems of differential diagnosis arise, however, because of the low reliability of evaluating the significance of past life events retrospectively. Regardless of age, individuals have a natural tendency to try to explain psychiatric complaints as consequences of coincidental life events, even when longitudinal studies show that such events are neither necessary nor sufficient to explain the symptoms.

DIAGNOSIS

The diagnostic features and types of adjustment disorders (DSM-III-R) are listed in Table 109–2.

TABLE 109–2. Diagnostic Criteria for Adjustment Disorder

Adjustment disorders are classified by their predominant symptoms: anxious mood, depressed mood, disturbance of conduct, mixed disturbance of emotions and conduct, mixed emotional features, physical complaints, withdrawal, and work (or academic) inhibition.
1. A reaction to an identifiable psychosocial stressor (or multiple stressors) that occurs within 3 months of onset of the stressor or stressors
2. The maladaptive nature of the reaction is indicated by either:
   a. impairment in occupational (including school) or in usual social activities or relationships with others
   b. symptoms that are in excess of a normal and expected reaction to the stressor or stressors
3. The disturbance is not merely one instance of a pattern of over-reaction to stress or an exacerbation of another mental disorder
4. The maladaptive reaction has persisted no longer than 6 months
5. The disturbance does not meet the criteria for any specific mental disorder and does not represent uncomplicated bereavement

With permission from American Psychiatric Association: Diagnostic and Statistical Manual of Mental Disorders, 3rd ed, revised. Washington, DC, American Psychiatric Association, 1987, p 330.

TREATMENT AND OUTCOME

Treatment is not always necessary but can facilitate correct resolution of conflicts and thus enable further personality development. Mild adjustment disorders usually respond to reassurance or short-term psychotherapy. With more severely maladapted adolescents, the choice of technique is likely to be influenced by the nature of the stressor and on the symptoms manifested. However, there are no systematic empirical studies that show whether one treatment is better than another treatment or even no treatment. Regardless of their theoretical orientation, clinicians-therapists generally agree that collaboration with the family is nearly always critical.

Identity Disorder

Identity disorder of adolescence has been called identity disturbance, identity crisis, identity confusion, and identity diffusion. Erikson and Kernberg seem to be responsible for this confusion in terminology. Both authors write about "pathologic identity diffusion," but Erikson understands it as a transient developmental crisis, whereas Kernberg regards it as the hallmark of borderline personality organization. As described in the DSM-III-R, identity disorder of adolescence resembles the traditional concept of an identity crisis and is thus closer to Erikson's concept.

CLINICAL MANIFESTATIONS

The distinguishing clinical feature of identity disorder is severe distress arising from uncertainty about a variety of identity-related issues (e.g., career choice, long-term goals, value system). Impairment in personal and socio-professional functioning distinguishes it from adjustment problems. Identification with different ideologies and roles is intense and transient, changing frequently as adolescents struggle to find their optimal role in life. Clinically, two forms of identity disorder are regularly observed—acute-brief and chronic-severe. The latter form tends to persist into adult life and suggests a borderline psychopathologic condition. The implication is that each particular instance of adolescent problems should be regarded as an alarm signal that indicates the need to evaluate the adolescent in depth.

DIAGNOSIS

The DSM-III-R diagnostic criteria for identity disorder are listed in Table 109–3. They include a duration of at least 3 months, and the lack of other mental disorders, such as mood disorders, schizophrenia, and especially BPD (which *may* be diagnosed after 16 years of age). Anxiety, depression, impulsiveness, low self-esteem, and oppositional behavior ("negative identity") complete the clinical picture.

TREATMENT

The course of adolescent identity disorder is relatively brief in most cases, and in its classic acute form is usually

TABLE 109–3. Diagnostic Criteria for Identity Disorder

1. Severe subjective distress regarding uncertainty about a variety of issues relating to identity, including three or more of the following:
   a. long-term goals
   b. career choice
   c. friendship patterns
   d. sexual orientation and behavior
   e. moral value systems
   f. group loyalties
2. Impairment in social or occupational (including academic) function as a result of the symptoms
3. Duration of at least 3 months
4. Occurrence not exclusively during the course of a mood disorder or of a psychotic disorder, such as schizophrenia
5. The disturbance is not sufficiently pervasive and persistent to warrant the diagnosis of borderline personality disorder

With permission from American Psychiatric Association: Diagnostic and Statistical Manual of Mental Disorders, 3rd ed, revised. Washington, DC, American Psychiatric Association, 1987, pp 90–91.

responsive to simple forms of psychotherapy, such as acceptance, support, or simply a provision of a chance to reconsider major decisions (so-called psychosocial moratorium). If a PD underlies identity disorder and the confusion lasts more than 1 year, symptomatic pharmacotherapy and intensive individual psychotherapy are indicated.

OUTCOME

Identity disorder is usually, but not always, characterized by an acute onset. If the disorder begins in late adolescence, it is usually resolved by the mid-20s. However, identity disorder becomes chronic and interferes with personal and socioprofessional relationships in a substantial minority of cases. In such chronic cases, identity disorder in adolescence heralds the adult diagnosis of BPD or some other severe psychopathologic condition.

Assessment Methods

Adjustment and identity disorders indicate the need to evaluate the adolescent in depth (see Chapter 98). A differential diagnosis to rule out affective disorders or PDs is critical. Furthermore, it is important to measure in detail behavioral autonomy and developmental competence in adolescence in order to evaluate prognosis and to assess subsequent change over time. A reliable and valid instrument, the autonomous functioning checklist, has been developed for this purpose. The DSM-III-R establishes two axes that are supposed to evaluate the severity of stressors (Axis V) and the level of adaptive functioning (Axis IV); these axes may be used for the evaluation of an adolescent's personality or behavioral problems, or both. However, one should be cautious with the two axes because some recent data indicate that they have low reliability.

BORDERLINE PERSONALITY DISORDER

The hallmarks of BPD are extremely unstable mood, unstable interpersonal relationships, and marked iden-

tity disturbance. Thus BPD is a more pervasive disorder than is identity disorder of adolescence.

EPIDEMIOLOGY

Borderline personality disorder has been ranked the most common of the PDs, despite or perhaps because of its low discriminant validity from other PDs. The prevalence is said to be about 2% to 4% in the general population and about 15% to 20% in the outpatient and inpatient psychiatric population. Some studies suggest that 10% to 30% of hospitalized adolescents meet the criteria for BPD. Many studies have shown that BPD tends to run in families. For example, relatives of inpatients with BPD are 10 times more likely to manifest BPD than are relatives of other psychiatric patients. "Borderline families" also show an increase in other forms of pathologic character conditions, as well as alcoholism and nonmelancholic unipolar depression. No support exists for a genetic relationship to either schizophrenic or affective psychoses. BPD occurs more frequently in females than in males (ratio from 2:1 to 9:1).

CLINICAL MANIFESTATIONS

An identity disturbance that is observable in BPD is *chronic* uncertainty about self-image, sexual orientation, or long-term goals and values. Instability of mood is evidenced by marked, frequent, and brief mood swings from the baseline level to depression, irritability, or anxiety. Intense anger, lack of impulse control and anxiety tolerance, and chronic feelings of emptiness and boredom are common. Dependent and stormy interpersonal relationships are characterized by the alternation of overidealization and total devaluation. Intolerance to being alone and recurrent self-destructive behavior, including suicide and suicide attempts, reflect the painful nature of these patients' lives.

The clinical picture of BPD in adolescence also includes running away from home, promiscuity, substance abuse, educational difficulties, a pervasive sense of futility, hypochondriasis and, in some cases, "clinging" behavior.

DIFFERENTIAL DIAGNOSIS

The differential diagnosis of PDs as a group aims at establishing the distinction between these disorders and neuroses, psychoses, psychoactive substance use, and organic psychosyndromes.

There is considerable overlap between BPD and other PDs, particularly histrionic, narcissistic, antisocial, and dependent PDs. Moreover, many authors conceptualize BPD as a level of personality organization, rather than a "true" PD, or as a dimension measuring the severity and instability of other PDs. Indeed, the majority of PDs manifest the borderline level of personality organization—that is, primitive defenses, partial object relations, poor impulse control, poor anxiety tolerance, occasional impairments in "reality-testing," and an inability to reach a stable identity. Hence, the differential diagnosis among PDs is based on identifying the individually specific type of adaptation that is clinically observable (e.g., a histrionic, antisocial, dependent, or avoidant type of adaptation to the external world). These behavioral features (i.e., symptoms) are widely used as diagnostic and nosologic criteria. However, it seems that both the vertical continuum of different levels of personality organization (e.g., normal, neurotic, borderline) and the horizontal continuum of specific adaptive strategies (symptomatology) define a comprehensive matrix for systematic assortment of normal, neurotic, and deviant personality types (see Chapter 10).

With respect to the distinction between PDs and neuroses, the following general observations should be helpful: (1) in contrast to neurotic patients, who seek psychiatric help complaining of suffering and symptoms (egodystonic symptomatology), PD patients often accept their own deviant behavior as desirable and natural for them (egosyntonic symptomatology); (2) the psychodynamics of PDs do not reveal the classic neurotic pattern of "conflict-anxiety-defense-symptom" but rather the primitive personality structure, which is in itself the cause of permanent maladaptation; (3) PDs are primarily manifested in the interpersonal domain. Thus, in technical terms, neurotic symptoms are "autoplastic" (i.e., leading to distress or change in one's self), whereas PD symptoms are "alloplastic" (i.e., leading to distress or change in others).

More specifically, BPD should be differentiated from symptomatic neuroses in adolescence, which may affect adolescent functioning to such an extent that it resembles a more serious personality pathologic condition. Narcissistic PD should be differentiated from frequent infantile narcissistic reactions in adolescence, which usually include unrealistic grandiose expectations. Further, avoidant PD should be differentiated from social phobia; the latter involves concerns about humiliation in specific public situations rather than general problems in social and personal relationships. Finally, dependent PD should be distinguished from adjustment disorder in adolescence (the latter is characterized by a transient increase in dependent behavior) and from agoraphobia (the latter is often associated with active demands for situational support, rather than pervasive, long-lasting, and passive dependency).

The differentiation of PDs from adolescent psychoses, especially schizophrenic spectrum disorders, usually is not difficult. One should keep in mind, however, that a PD may precede psychoses and impede the treatment of psychoses and may develop in response to chronic disability. Except for schizotypal and paranoid disorders, there is no evidence that PDs predispose to psychosis (see Chapter 110).

Many studies have shown a considerable overlap between symptoms of BPD and affective disorders—nonmelancholic unipolar depression in particular. The distinction between the two disorders can be, and frequently is, difficult, leading to further doubt about the discriminant validity of BPD as a discrete entity.

Finally, it is worth reminding ourselves that the establishment of the diagnosis of any PD is questionable without somatic and neurologic examination of the adolescent to exclude various organic mental disorders or the organic personality syndrome.

Diagnosis. The diagnostic criteria for BPD are listed in Table 109–4. The reported reliabilities of the DSM-III-R criteria for BPD vary between 0.29 and 0.81. In general, the reliability of the diagnosis based on these criteria is usually very low. In many instances, the diagnosis of BPD relies on the exclusion criteria for other PDs.

Several semistructured interviews (e.g., Diagnostic Interview for Borderline Patients [DIB], The Schedule for Interviewing Borderlines [SIB], The Structured Interview for DSM-III-R personality disorders [SIDP-R], Personality Disorders Examination [PDE]) and self-reports (Personality Disorders Questionnaire–Revised [PDQ-R]) have improved the diagnostic reliability of BPD somewhat. Some of the instruments cited (e.g., SIDP-R) require additional diagnostic information from the family members or significant others, which is helpful in individuals who do not have accurate or objective images of themselves.

ETIOLOGY

We will briefly review genetic, biologic, and developmental factors implicated as contributing to PD (see Chapter 11).

Genetic Factors

Many pathologic personality traits are strongly genetically determined. Substantial heritability has been detected for neuroticism; extraversion; antisocial, histrionic, and obsessive traits; and for impulsiveness, sociability, and proneness to aggression and fear.

The majority of PDs—particularly histrionic, schizotypal, borderline, antisocial, and obsessive-compulsive PDs—tend to run in families. In addition, in 15,000 pairs of American twins, the concordance for PDs

---

TABLE 109–4. Diagnostic Criteria for Borderline Personality Disorder

Pervasive pattern of instability of mood, interpersonal relationships, and self-image, beginning by early adulthood and present in a variety of contexts, as indicated by at least *five* of the following:
1. Pattern of unstable and intense interpersonal relationships characterized by alternating between extremes of overidealization and devaluation
2. Impulsiveness in at least two areas that are potentially self-damaging (e.g., spending, sex, substance use, shoplifting, reckless driving, binge eating)
3. Affective instability: marked shifts from baseline mood to depression, irritability, or anxiety, usually lasting a few hours and rarely more than a few days
4. Inappropriate, intense anger or lack of control of anger
5. Recurrent suicidal threats, gestures, or behavior, or self-mutilating behavior
6. Marked and persistent identity disturbance manifested by uncertainty about at least two of the following: self-image, sexual orientation, long-term goals or career choice, type of friends desired, preferred values
7. Chronic feelings of emptiness or boredom
8. Frantic efforts to avoid real or imagined abandonment

With permission from American Psychiatric Association: Diagnostic and Statistical Manual of Mental Disorders, 3rd ed, revised. Washington, DC, American Psychiatric Association, 1987, p 347.

among monozygotic twins was at least twice as high as among dizygotic twins (about 0.20 and 0.40, respectively).

The most probable mode of inheritance is polygenic.

Biologic Factors

NEUROTRANSMITTERS

Many neurotransmitters and neuromodulators interact in the regulation of motivated behavior. However, it appears that only one of the monoamines plays a major role in the modulation of each of the three personality dimensions described by Cloninger. This may account for the tridimensional nature of personality structure. Specifically, dopamine appears to be the major neuromodulator of the brain behavioral activation system. Low basal dopaminergic activity is believed to be associated with high impulsiveness and frequent exploratory activity—traits that are particularly pronounced in histrionic and antisocial PDs.

Low basal serotonergic activity is believed to underlie risk-taking behaviors and suicidal tendencies. High basal serotonergic activity is believed to underlie fearfulness, shyness, and fatigability—traits that are particularly pronounced in borderline, avoidant, and dependent PDs.

Norepinephrine appears to be the major neuromodulator of the brain behavioral maintenance system. Low basal noradrenergic activity is believed to be associated with high reward dependence and hypersensitivity—traits that are particularly pronounced in histrionic, narcissistic, and dependent PDs.

HORMONES, ENZYMES, AND NEUROPEPTIDES

Several authors have reported high rates of dexamethasone nonsuppression (dexamethasone suppression test [DST]) and deficient thyroid-stimulating hormone (TSH) response to TRH infusion (TRH test) in BPD and obsessive-compulsive PD. However, it is likely that both a positive DST and a TRH test characterize obsessive and borderline adolescent patients with coexisting depression.

Several studies have found that low platelet monoamine oxidase (MAO) activity is associated with impulsive-aggressive personality traits in adolescents and young adults. Unfortunately, little is known about hormonal and biochemical aspects of normal and deviant development in adolescence.

OTHER RELEVANT BIOLOGIC FINDINGS

Electroencephalographic abnormalities (i.e., slow wave activity and spike phenomena) have been shown in antisocial and borderline patients and in juvenile delinquents, whereas decreased rapid eye movement (REM) latency characterizes sleep patterns of BPD. Similarly, "soft" neurologic signs are more common in borderline and antisocial personalities. These findings are difficult to interpret, however, because of concurrent histories of head trauma in antisocial subjects and of depression in borderline subjects. It is not possible to distinguish cause from consequence in available data.

Developmental Factors

Developmental theories emphasize the importance of familial and nonfamilial environmental influences in the genesis of PDs. Specifically, it has been suggested that various types of early psychic trauma (e.g., loss of a parent, separation, child abuse) interferes with normal personality development. Such experiences facilitate the persistence of immature coping mechanisms and contradictory self- and object-images in the inner world. Available data are difficult to interpret with confidence, however, because genetic and environmental backgrounds are often confounded in children reared in more or less intact homes.

If adolescents tend to see things as either all good or all bad ("splitting"), they also tend to be inappropriately aggressive or fearful. In other words, immature adolescents have difficulty objectively evaluating the threats and risks that they experience. As a result, deviant personality traits and behavioral tendencies develop that are objectively maladaptive.

According to psychodynamic theories, such developmental failure can be described in terms of ego and superego deficiencies. The former are manifested as nonspecific ego weakness (lack of impulse control and anxiety tolerance), specific ego defect (such as indistinct self-object boundaries and transient misjudgment of reality), primitive object-relations (alternation between "all good" and "all bad" experiences), and identity disturbance (such as borderline-like identity diffusion). An inadequately developed superego is either generally sadistic (e.g., in obsessive PD) or rigid in some areas but completely lacking in other areas, permitting the conflict-free expression of immature impulses and behaviors (e.g., in BPD and histrionic, antisocial, and narcissistic PDs).

In contradiction to many social theories of personality development, studies of twins and adoptees show that the nonfamilial experiences that are unique to every individual are much more important than the family environment shared by siblings in influencing the personality style of different individuals. Conversely, social learning in the family may influence how successful an individual is in adapting his or her personality style to the life situation.

In summary, we emphasize that the key factors in the genesis of personality are the polygenic contributions and nonshared environmental effects. Family environment may, however, be important in determining whether an extreme personality variant leads to personality disorder or successful adaptation.

TREATMENT

We discuss briefly some specific topics regarding the treatment of adolescents with PDs. Because long-term treatment is often required, referral to mental health colleagues is generally indicated.

Psychotherapy

According to the literature, it appears that practically all types of psychotherapy are used in the treatment of PDs. However, our experience indicates it is not adequate to "do anything, but just do it." As in the case of neurotic and psychotic disorders, specific PDs require specific techniques that selectively address the problems of the disorder in question.

Classic psychoanalysis is usually contraindicated, especially for borderline, schizoid, and severely narcissistic adolescents, for two main reasons. First, it tends to flood the adolescent's mind with fantasies and urges that interfere with integrative processes. Second, such patients easily regress in response to the lack of structure in psychoanalysis.

Kernberg and Masterson have demonstrated that long-term, individual, intensive, psychodynamically oriented psychotherapy is a useful technique in the treatment of borderline and narcissistic persons. If some other method is used, the therapist should keep in mind that a structured therapeutic situation, reliability, consistency, and a relationship that addresses both emotional and cognitive aspects of motivated behavior appear to be crucial in the treatment of adolescents with PDs.

In addition to the personal relationship between the patient and the clinician, the therapy also focuses on everyday problems and should offer practical help in the resolution of such problems; such help includes instruction and discussion of alternative adaptive strategies in specific situations, along with encouragement of practice ("homework") in order to provide the behavioral conditioning that is necessary to modify emotional responses and feelings.

The therapeutic goal is specifically designed for each particular individual. Initially, the therapy focuses on identifying the adolescent's psychological needs and problematic behaviors. Next, the adolescent is helped to learn alternative adaptive strategies that will allow change in the problematic behavior in a way that satisfies the patient's particular profile of psychological needs. The third phase aims at more general emotional development or personality synthesis, or both. This phase, like the second, is a step-by-step strategy that frequently meets numerous obstacles as different situations and problems arise. Such obstacles can be viewed as opportunities to learn additional adaptive strategies. At each step, it is necessary for the adolescent to identify the emotional needs that motivate maladaptive behaviors, to learn alternative adaptive behaviors, and to practice them until the new behaviors feel natural and satisfying emotionally and interpersonally. In other words, learning must take place at both conceptual and unconscious behavioral-emotional levels. If everything goes well, one may hope that over time, usually 2 to 4 years, the adolescent will achieve sufficient and more or less stable maturity.

Pharmacotherapy

In general, two strategies for a pharmacologic approach to PDs exist. The first one is causal pharmacotherapy, which attempts to correct a biochemical disturbance thought to underlie certain deviant personality traits. For example, high serotonergic activity may underlie avoidant personality traits; down-regulation of serotonergic activity is thus expected to correct them. The theoretical basis for causal pharmacotherapy of PDs thus arises from modern biology of behavior. However, causal pharmacotherapy of PDs still relies on biochemically untested personality models and, at the moment, represents a useful theoretical framework for pharmacologic challenge or follow-up studies, or both. In addition, little is known about long-term pharmacotherapy of personality traits.

The second approach is *symptomatic pharmacotherapy*—that is, the treatment of specific target symptoms shared by various PDs, such as mood dysregulation, psychotic symptoms, and disturbance of impulse control. Symptomatic pharmacotherapy cannot be usefully organized around diagnoses of PDs, for its efficacy is better evaluated on the behavioral (symptom) level.

Most medications have a shorter mean half-life in children than they do in adults. Thus adolescents may fail to respond because of undertreatment.

Several studies suggest the advantages of lithium carbonate over neuroleptics in the treatment of chronic impulsive-aggressive behavior and hostility in childhood and adolescence; lithium is also efficient in the treatment of sporadic, unprovoked physical aggression behaviors in children, who seem to tolerate this drug much better than adults do.

Between 25% and 30% of children with attention deficit disorder experience antisocial aggressive behavior; most of them exhibit low arousal (as measured by electrodermal activity and auditory evoked potentials) and respond well to catecholamine agonists, such as methylphenidate. A subgroup of hyperactive children are hyperaroused and respond poorly to catecholamine agonists; rather, they seem to benefit from cholinergic drugs.

Benzodiazepines and tricyclic antidepressants (TCAs) may aggravate hostile, impulsive, and self-destructive behavior in borderline patients, including borderline adolescents.

Several studies show that adolescent patients whose aggressiveness and impulsiveness is poorly controlled but somewhat understandable in context should be treated with low-dose neuroleptics. In contrast, patients whose impulses are of "seizure-like" quality and make no sense should be treated with lithium carbonate. Some adolescents manifest episodes of unprovoked angry outbursts in the context of cerebral instability and abnormal electroencephalograms. This "ictal impulsiveness" responds well to anticonvulsants and benzodiazepines. The former are recommended because tolerance to the anticonvulsive effects of benzodiazepines may develop. In fact, the use of benzodiazepines in aggressive behavior is controversial.

In patients with BPD, mood disturbance is manifested mainly as rapid and intense mood swings. Both the intensity and the frequency of these mood disturbances are well controlled by lithium carbonate because of its more favorable spectrum of side effects. If, for any reason, lithium is not used, neuroleptics may be helpful.

Most adolescents with PD manifest atypical depression—that is, they meet the DSM-III-R criteria for depression or dysthymia but also have some atypical symptoms (hyperphagia, hypersomnolence). Atypical depression is often not responsive to TCAs but rather to neuroleptics or monamine oxidase (MAO) inhibitors, or both.

Adolescents with high cognitive anxiety may have a high tolerance for antianxiety drugs and alcohol, whereas those with high somatic anxiety may have a low threshold for sedation with these same drugs. Yet cognitive anxiety seems more responsive to benzodiazepines, whereas somatic anxiety seems more responsive to MAO inhibitors. Somatic anxiety, especially vegetative signs of depression and anxiety, can be treated with β-blockers as well. Severe, psychotic-like anxiety (which is relatively rare in PDs) seems to respond best to low doses of neuroleptics.

Many presenting symptoms of the adolescent with PD are transient and stress-related, brief state manifestations of underlying trait vulnerabilities. Temporarily psychotic adolescents with PDs are likely to respond to and comply with low doses of neuroleptics.

Table 109–5 summarizes drug choices for various target symptoms of PDs.

Hospital Versus Outpatient Treatment

According to our clinical experience, adolescents with PDs should be treated primarily as outpatients. Indications for hospital treatment occasionally appear in some cases of borderline, antisocial, or schizotypal PD, usually when the disorganization of behavior is so dramatic that intensive psycho- and pharmacotherapies are required. Additional indications for hospitalization include the emergence of psychotic symptoms, psychoactive substance use with no possibility of abstinence, high risk of suicide or assault and, finally, when the adolescent must be removed from an environment that has turned extremely hostile or intolerant, and vice versa.

In recent years, 10% to 25% of psychiatric hospital admissions have been diagnosed as BPD. Indications for long-term hospitalization are controversial. This treatment strategy seems indicated for patients with chronic regression who have not responded to treatment and are unable to function any place but a well-structured hospital. Therapeutic community models seem efficient in the long-term treatment of such cases. Adolescents with borderline personality structure may easily acquire "hospitalism" because the hospital setting may be far more preferable for them than a vegetative existence at the periphery of the local community.

Outcome

Borderline personality disorder is rarely diagnosed after the age of 30 years. Because many "borderline-like" features may accompany adolescent crisis, a reliable diagnosis cannot be made before the age of 16 years, when more stable personality patterns develop. Longitudinal studies suggest that the most disruptive behaviors tend to diminish during the 30s and later.

TABLE 109–5. Choice of Drugs According to Target Symptoms of Personality Disorders

TARGET SYMPTOM	DRUG OF CHOICE	CONTRAINDICATIONS
Mood Dysregulation		
Aggression-impulsiveness		
Affective aggression (hyperirritability)	Lithium carbonate, serotonergic drugs Neuroleptics	?Benzodiazepines
Predatory aggression (hostility)	Neuroleptics Lithium carbonate	Benzodiazepines
Organic-like aggression	Imipramine Catecholamine agonists	
Ictal aggression (abnormal electroencephalogram)	Carbamazepine Phenytoin Benzodiazepines	Neuroleptics
Emotional lability	Lithium carbonate Neuroleptics	?TCAs
Depression		
Atypical depression-dysphoria	MAO inhibitors Neuroleptics	?TCAs
Classic depression	TCAs (full doses)	
Anxiety		
Chronic cognitive	Serotonergic drugs MAO inhibitors Benzodiazepines	
Chronic somatic	MAO inhibitors β-blockers	?Benzodiazepines
Emotional detachment	Sulpiride ?TCAs MAO inhibitors	?TCAs
Psychotic Symptoms		
Acute and brief psychotic episodes	Drug choice depends on the clinical picture; doses usual or lower than usual	
Chronic and low-level psychotic-like symptoms	Low-dose neuroleptics	

TCAs, tricyclic antidepressants.

However, the symptomatology of BPD remains fairly stable over time. Masterson demonstrated that the course of treated adolescents with BPD is different from that already described and is characterized by a better outcome.

Complications

Brief reactive psychotic episodes are common. Adolescents with BPD are unlikely to experience schizophrenic or severe affective psychoses in the course of time.

Dysthymia frequently accompanies BPD. Clinical studies suggest that 20% to 60% of adolescents with BPD have concomitant depressive symptoms, mostly dysthymic disorder (see Chapter 100).

Several studies have shown that 48% to 67% of adolescents with BPD also meet the criteria for psychoactive substance use disorder. Conversely, 13% to 16% of patients who abuse drugs, including heroin, manifest BPD (see Chapter 111).

Finally, the risk of suicide is higher in individuals with BPD than in the general population but not as high as in those who have affective illness (see Chapter 101).

BIBLIOGRAPHY

American Psychiatric Association: Diagnostic and Statistical Manual of Mental Disorders, 3rd ed, revised. Washington, DC, American Psychiatric Association, 1987.

Cloninger CR: A systematic method for clinical description and classification of personality variables: A proposal. Arch Gen Psychol, 44:573, 1987.

Erikson EH: Childhood and Society. New York, Norton, 1950.

Feinstein S: Identity and adjustment disorder of adolescence. In Kaplan H, Sadock B (eds): Comprehensive Textbook of Psychiatry, 4th ed. Baltimore, Williams & Wilkins, 1985.

Gunderson J: Personality disorders. In Nicholi A (ed): The New Harvard Guide to Psychiatry, Cambridge MA, Belknap Press, 1988, pp 337–357.

Kernberg O: Borderline Conditions and Pathological Narcissism. Jason Aronson, New York, 1975.

Klar H, Siever L: The psychopharmacologic treatment of personality disorders. Psychiatr Clin North Am, 7 (4):791, 1984.

Masterson J: From Borderline Adolescent to Functioning Adult: The Test of Time. Brunner/Mazel, New York, 1980.

Sigafoos A, Feinstein C, Diamond M, Reiss D: The measurement of behavioral autonomy in adolescence: The Autonomous Functioning Checklist. In Feinstein S (ed): Adolescent Psychiatry, Vol 15. Chicago, University of Chicago Press, 1988, pp 432–462.

Sigvardsson S, Bohman M, Cloninger CR: Structure and stability of childhood personality: Prediction of later social adjustment. J Child Psychol Psychiatry 28 (6):929, 1987.

Wolf S, Chick J: Schizoid personality in childhood: A controlled follow up study. Psychol Med 10:85, 1980.

CHAPTER 110

Schizophrenia

PETER SZATMARI, MARK SANFORD, and HEATHER MUNROE BLUM

The onset of schizophrenia in adolescence is an extremely disturbing event. Not only are the symptoms frightening, but the illness disrupts development and threatens future adjustment. The important tasks of adolescence, such as the successful completion of school, the development of heterosexual relationships, and the maturing of family relationships are all profoundly affected by the disorder. In spite of this, relatively little has been written specifically about schizophrenia that has its onset in adolescence. This is surprising in view of the fact that both Bleuler and Kraepelen recognized that schizophrenia often begins during this period. Although the true mean age of onset is somewhat later, it is clear that many schizophrenic symptoms begin in adolescence or, alternatively, that there are premorbid personality deviations associated with the adult development of the disorder.

The presentation, course, and treatment of schizophrenia in adolescence is in many ways different from that in adulthood. The developmental issues of adolescence, both biologic and psychosocial, complicate a psychiatric illness that is already confusing by its very nature. The objective of this chapter is to briefly review the clinical features of adolescent-onset schizophrenia. Reference is made to the adult literature on schizophrenia only when no information is available on the condition in adolescence and when clinical experience suggests that such extrapolation is appropriate. An important theme of this chapter is that in many ways, schizophrenia is itself a "developmental" disorder and has many features in common with other such disabilities.

EPIDEMIOLOGY

Recent reviews of the epidemiologic studies of schizophrenia report that prevalence rates range from 0.6 to 8.3/1000, depending on the study. Results from the recent Epidemiologic Catchment Area Study have reported higher rates (0.6% to 1.2%) based on results from lay interviewers who used a structured interview.

There are very few data describing the prevalence of adolescent-onset schizophrenia. There are no community studies, and most information comes from clinics that provide biased estimates of prevalence. For example, one study reported that 5% of 500 adolescents referred had psychotic illness, the vast majority of which were schizophrenics. It is unlikely, however, that this estimate can be generalized to other settings. A hospital-based survey identified adolescents treated for "psychotic" disorders in Gotheburg, Sweden. Among teenagers aged 13 to 19 years, schizophrenia was found in 2 to 3/1000. Most of these psychotic disorders had an onset after 16 years of age, and there were twice as many boys as girls. Approximately 16% of the adolescents had demonstrated major psychiatric problems prior to adolescence—a nonspecific mixture of difficulties in attention, emotional, and behavioral disorders.

Although the prevalence of schizophrenia appears to be equal in men and women during the adult years, there are important sex differences. For example, males appear to have an earlier age of onset and first hospitalization than do females. In males, the clinical presentation of schizophrenia starts to increase around 15 years of age and reaches a peak between 21 and 29 years of age. In females, it begins to increase in the early twenties and reaches a peak between 30 and 35 years of age. An early age of onset is also associated with a worse outcome, greater cognitive impairment, and structural brain changes (see further on). Thus adolescent-onset schizophrenia may represent an important and perhaps etiologically distinct subtype of schizophrenia.

CLINICAL MANIFESTATIONS

The diagnostic boundaries of schizophrenia have recently undergone considerable change. In the past, schizophrenia was probably overdiagnosed in North America when compared with Europe and other countries. Indeed, a number of elegant studies concluded that individuals diagnosed as schizophrenic in North America are often identified as "depressed" in the United Kingdom. This has led to a refinement of the diagnostic criteria for schizophrenia, with an increased emphasis on the presence of "mood-incongruent" hallucination, delusions, and thought disorder. The criteria for schizophrenia according to the Diagnostic and Statistical Manual of Mental Disorders: Third Edition—Revised (DSM-III-R) now closely parallel definitions used by the World Health Organization.

Schizophrenia in adolescence presents with either an acute or an insidious onset. In the former, the apparent onset of the illness is sudden (over hours or days), with severe disorganization of the adolescent's behavior and thinking; it may be preceded by a major life event, such as leaving home. The adolescent may be agitated and incoherent, or the disorder can be less florid, consisting of paranoid disturbances with auditory hallucinations. An acute onset frequently takes family members by surprise, though in retrospect, they may identify changes in thinking and behavior over previous weeks. Alternatively, the onset may be insidious, with gradual deterioration in social functioning, withdrawal from friendships, diminished self-care, and unusual preoccupations or concerns. Depressed mood and social anxiety are common, and the core symptoms of schizophrenia may be poorly formed or transitory. Thus the psychopathologic condition may be underestimated. Similarly, individuals with significant premorbid disturbances (especially schizotypal disorder, in which odd preoccupations, unusual behavior, and excessive fantasy predominate) can present diagnostic problems for the clinician because in these cases there is less deviation in usual functioning and behavior.

Specific disturbances in the personal experience of the adolescent are central to the diagnosis and involve several aspects of mental functioning, such as abnormalities of perception, experiences of unity of self, thought, and experiences of time and bodily integration. However, among the most common and specific disturbances are particular forms of delusions, auditory hallucinations, and disruptions in the form of thinking. These are the basis of modern diagnosis, such as the DSM-III-R classification system and the International Classification of Disease, 9th revision (ICD-9) system (Table 110–1).

Delusions are abnormalities in the content of thought—a false belief that is firmly held, even in the face of clearly contradictory evidence given the individual's age, knowledge, and cultural background. It is the illogical nature of the thought supporting the belief, rather than its bizarre quality, that is the essential feature. Delusions in schizophrenia often follow a period of delusional mood—the experience that something "odd" or "sinister" is occurring. Delusions seen in adolescent schizophrenia commonly begin as over-valued ideas. These ideas are preoccupations without the fixity of belief that is characteristic of true delusions. Alternatively, they may arise de novo as fully formed ideas (sudden delusional ideas) or in connection with a commonplace perception (delusional precept). The content matter of delusions in schizophrenia is broad. Common types of delusions are persecutory and grandiose delusions or delusions that some external agency is controlling the adolescent's thoughts or body. The adolescent may believe that particular individuals or groups are placing thoughts in his or her mind (thought insertion) or withdrawing thoughts (thought withdrawal), or alternatively that the adolescent patient's thoughts themselves are being communicated directly to others without speech (thought broadcast).

An hallucination can be defined as "a false perception that is not a sensory distortion or misinterpretation but that occurs at the same time as real perceptions." Hallucinations occur in all sensory modalities (i.e., visual, auditory, tactile, gustatory, and olfactory) and are generally experienced by the adolescent as a "true" perception. For instance, the auditory hallucinations of

TABLE 110–1. Diagnostic Criteria for Schizophrenia

DSM-III-R	ICD-9
One week's duration of	Characteristic disturbances
(1) Two of the following:	Of thought
Delusions	Of perception
Hallucinations	Of mood
(persistent)	Of conduct
Incoherence or marked	Of personality
loosening of	(preferably two during the
associations	same illness)
Catatonic behavior	
Flat or grossly	Symptoms are
inappropriate	Fundamental disturbance of
affect	personality disorder
OR	Thought disorder (e.g.,
(2) Bizarre delusions:	perplexity)
Thought broadcast or	Delusions
being controlled by a	Feelings of control by alien
dead person	forces
OR	Perceptual abnormalities
(3) Auditory hallucinations:	(e.g., hallucinations)
Persistent and mood-	Feelings of passiveness
incongruent running	Autism
commenting voice or	Affective abnormalities (e.g.,
two or more voices	inappropriate or
conversing together	incongruous affect)
	Ambience
Functional impairment	Catatonia
At work	Clear consciousness and
In social relationships	intellectual capacity usually
In self-care	retained
No schizoaffective disorder or	
mood disorder with psychotic	
features	
Six months' duration of	
disturbance	

schizophrenia are experienced as voices or sounds, almost always arising outside the body and heard through the ears. All types of hallucinations may occur, though visual, tactile, gustatory, and olfactory hallucinations should raise the suspicion of an organic illness. Auditory hallucinations are the most common and take many forms—muffled sounds, garbled voices, a voice repeating the adolescent's thoughts (écho de penseés), and several voices discussing the adolescent patient or speaking directly to him or her.

Disordered thought and speech, though common, frequently present a problem, because they can occur in other disorders (i.e., mania, language disorders) and thus are not central to schizophrenia. Mild thought blocking or marked loosening of associations can be present. In thought blocking, the adolescent is observed to stop speaking in midsentence and resume after an interval. Loosening of associations consists of a breakdown of the usual connections between thoughts. The adolescent's speech moves from one subject to another without an apparent link (as opposed to manic flight of ideas in which some link, either by "clang" or theme, is maintained). Loosening of associations may be so severe that it renders the patient incoherent.

These symptoms are essential to the diagnosis of schizophrenia. However, delusions, hallucinations, and thought disorder may occur in other psychotic disorders, and none is pathognomonic for schizophrenia. Furthermore, an array of other abnormal experiences and oddities of behavior are also present. These experiences may predominate early in the presentation. Examples would include affective disturbances such as intense anxiety, flat or incongruous affect, ecstasy experiences, illusions, apraxia, distortions in the experience of time, depersonalization and derealization, and more subtle forms of thought disturbance (i.e., excessive fantasy, unusual symbolization, or concrete thinking).

DIFFERENTIAL DIAGNOSIS

There are a number of other disorders and conditions in which psychotic phenomena can occur. It is extremely important to be aware of these conditions in formulating the differential diagnosis (Table 110–2).

Hallucinations in Psychiatrically Disturbed Adolescents

Hallucinations do occur, albeit rarely, in adolescents with conduct and emotional disorders. They are mostly auditory and vary in duration from a week to several years. Precipitants are clearly identified and include change of school, admission to hospital, or threatened separation from parents, or a combination of factors. Hallucinations in response to bereavement are also common.

The differentiation of these nonspecifically disturbed adolescents with hallucinations and those with schizophrenia usually poses little problem. Hallucinations in schizophrenia are most often accompanied by delusions, thought disorder, and an overall deterioration in social and cognitive functioning. Hallucinations among nonspecifically disturbed adolescents are often isolated, stable phenomena and occur in response to some clearly identifiable precipitant.

Affective Disorders

Major affective disorders are not uncommon during adolescence (see Chapter 100). Adolescents with unipolar and bipolar disorders may present with psychotic phenomena, including hallucinations and delusions. In many cases it is difficult to distinguish these phenomena from schizophrenia. In affective psychosis, the hallucinations and delusions usually have a depressive or grandiose nature, occur early in the presentation of the disorder, and are consistent with the overall clinical picture. The psychotic phenomena and the mood associated with schizophrenia are "incongruent" with the prevailing mood—that is, the adolescent is either affectively flat or inappropriately silly. Another helpful distinguishing characteristic is the family history. The presence of a first- or second-degree relative with a clear-cut affective disorder can be quite helpful in the differential diagnosis. The clinical course is, however, the most important feature. Although the adolescent with an affective disorder may appear psychotic initially, a subsequent episode will be clearly depressive or manic. In view of the difficulties in differential diagnosis, the physician must always keep an open mind and seriously entertain the possibility of an affective disorder, even when the presentation strongly suggests schizophrenia.

Schizotypal Disorders

The diagnosis of "schizotypal personality disorder" appeared for the first time in the adult section of DSM-III. It was first described in first-degree relatives of schizophrenics, suggesting that these disorders have a genetic relationship to schizophrenia. The term *personality disorder* may be inappropriate in adolescence, since the diagnosis requires that the symptoms or behaviors be characteristic of the individual's overall functioning and not limited to discrete episodes or developmental periods. The symptoms include magical thinking (i.e., superstitiousness, clairvoyance, telepathy, and so on), ideas of reference, social isolation, recurrent illusions, odd patterns of speech, poor rapport, paranoid ideation, and undue social anxiety or hypersensitivity to real or imagined criticism. Many of these symptoms represent subclinical, or subthreshold, psychotic phenomena. Unfortunately, there are no natural history studies of schizotypal disorders in adolescence, and it remains to be seen how many schizotypal adolescents progress to schizophrenia.

Asperger Syndrome

Asperger syndrome is a type of pervasive developmental disorder characterized by impairments in reciprocal two-way social interaction and verbal and nonverbal communication, as well as a restricted range of imaginative activities. It is generally considered to be a mild variant of autism. Children with Asperger syndrome often have serious social impairments, are extremely isolated, and relate to others in unusual or eccentric ways. They also exhibit impairments in the pragmatics of communication (i.e., the ability to hold a conversation) so that their speech will appear tangential and lacking in cohesion. On this basis, adolescents with Asperger syndrome are often misdiagnosed as having a thought disorder.

TABLE 110–2. Differential Diagnosis

Hallucinations in adolescents with nonspecific
  psychiatric disorder
Bereavement (see Chapter 116)
Affective disorders (see Chapter 100)
Schizotypal disorders
Asperger syndrome
Drug abuse (see Chapter 111)
Organic Conditions
  Wilson disease
  Thyroid disease
  Addison disease
  Systemic lupus erythematosus
  Porphyria
  Herpes encephalitis
  Temporal lobe disease
  Degenerative disorders

Adolescents with Asperger syndrome frequently present with intense preoccupations or hobbies that often have a bizarre quality. For example, they may be overly interested in the weather, bus timetables, horror movies, or science fiction. These adolescents often demonstrate flat affect, overvalued ideas, and ideas of reference. These symptoms may lead to an appearance of psychosis, particularly under conditions of extreme stress.

Age of onset is the chief distinguishing characteristic between Asperger syndrome and schizophrenia. Children with Asperger syndrome invariably present in the preschool years (most often prior to 3 years of age) with impairments in social responsiveness toward adults, delayed language, insistence on sameness, rituals, and so on. These symptoms attenuate with development; thus the natural history of children with Asperger syndrome is improvement. Adolescents with schizophrenia have a better early developmental history but experience a deterioration in adaptive functioning.

Drug Abuse

Drug use disorders must be included in the differential diagnosis of schizophrenia (see Chapter 111). Many psychoactive drugs obtained "on the street" can induce psychotic phenomena. Drugs of particular importance are stimulants, lysergic acid diethylamide (LSD), cocaine, and phencyclidine. These drugs produce an intense, florid psychosis, with acute deterioration and extravagant hallucinations and delusions of a persecutionary nature. The adolescent may underestimate drug use or may not admit to it. Drug screening and a history of conduct disorder can all be used to distinguish these disorders. It is also important to remember that the onset of schizophrenia can *lead* to drug use, often in response to troubling symptoms. The possibility that drug abuse exists should always be entertained in any psychotic illness beginning abruptly in adolescence.

Organic Psychoses

Several organic conditions are associated with psychotic illness in adolescence. Wilson disease should be considered, particularly when the psychosis is associated with a movement disorder or liver disease (see Chapters 62 and 83–89). The Kayser-Fleisher ring and blood levels of serum copper and ceruloplasmin are very helpful as diagnostic tests (see Chapter 62). Other organic conditions associated with schizophrenia are thyroid disease (see Chapter 55), Addison disease (see Chapter 55), systemic lupus erythematosus (see Chapter 90), acute intermittent porphyria (see Chapter 83), herpes simplex encephalitis, and temporal lobe tumor or disease. Sometimes degenerative disorders can begin in adolescence (i.e., adrenoleukodystrophy) and psychotic phenomena may occur as part of the degenerative process (see Chapters 83–89). Organic conditions are very rare but should always be considered a possibility nevertheless. Routine medical screening is only occasionally helpful in identifying these particular conditions. Rather, one should approach psychosis in adolescence with a high index of suspicion that an organic disorder is present and use the history and physical examination to substantiate the need for further medical investigation.

DIAGNOSIS

Interview with the Adolescent

At any age, a schizophrenic psychosis is a terrifying and perplexing experience. This is especially true for the adolescent who may have little understanding of what is occurring, and therefore frequently presents as confused, secretive, and resistant to assessment. The clinician should be warm, firm, and direct, explaining to the adolescent the nature of the investigations and treatments that will be undertaken, as well as interpreting the adolescent's most disturbing experiences. The clinician should be frank and label psychotic experiences as abnormal, rather than attempt false reassurance. Adolescents who have psychosis are very sensitive to information overload, and it is therefore important to communicate with them in a direct and simple manner. When the psychosis is under control, it is then appropriate to discuss in greater detail possible causes and treatments. The clinician taking the history must focus both on life experiences and symptoms. It is important to place the illness in a developmental context so that the adolescent and his or her family are reassured that the clinician is as interested in the adolescent's aspirations and current functional impairments as in the symptoms. This broad approach will also enable the clinician to recruit the adolescent into the ongoing treatment process.

The assessment is conducted in the course of several interviews (see Chapter 22). It should include a detailed gathering of information about family life, peer relationships, academic and work experiences, and recent stressors (Table 110–3). An important area to assess is the adolescent's attributions regarding the illness—that is, is it seen as a "disease," a character flaw, or some punishment for previous wrongdoing? The mental state examination should document abnormal experiences and carefully assess mood, orientation, and cognitive functioning. The extent of suicidal or homicidal ideation should also be elicited (see Chapters 101 and 117). A physical examination, with particular emphasis on the neurologic system, is indicated in all adolescent patients presenting with psychotic illness. There is considerable

TABLE 110–3. Assessment of Schizophrenia

FROM THE ADOLESCENT	FROM THE PARENTS
Model of illness	Developmental history
Family life	Family history
Peer relationships	Premorbid functioning
School history	Details regarding onset
Recent stressors	Model of illness
Mental status	Family level of expressed emotion
Suicidal or homicidal risk	and style of communication
Drug and alcohol use	
Past medical history	
Review of symptoms	
Physical examination	

evidence that adolescents with schizophrenia suffer from a higher prevalence of other medical conditions and that they often go untreated in the chronic phase of the illness.

Interview with Parent(s)

It is essential to include parents in the assessment process. Not only does the illness have a great impact on the family, but family members can give a detailed developmental history (including premorbid personality) and a family history (often unknown to the adolescent). They can also provide an objective account of odd behaviors that may not be described by the adolescent. It is important to recognize, however, that in the acute phase of the illness, parents often may be unable to give reliable information. These data should be gathered over time, with opportunities to review previously collected information. Premorbid abnormalities of thought and behavior are identified by the parents, or by a review of school records, in 30% to 50% of adolescent patients. These abnormalities include emotional disorders, social withdrawal, solitary aggressive or antisocial acts, hyperactivity, and eccentricity of behavior. These features do not constitute a recognizable syndrome, except when a diagnosis of schizotypal disorder can be made. It is often the parent's account that enables the clinician to date the onset of the illness. The clinician can also judge the family's knowledge about schizophrenia and critical or unaccepting attitudes toward the patient. These factors are very important in management, as will be discussed later.

Psychological Testing

Psychological testing may be helpful in situations in which the diagnosis is not clear, particularly if one is considering an organic cause (see Chapter 99).

ETIOLOGY

There is no known cause for schizophrenia, whether the onset is during adolescence or adulthood. It is probably more accurate to think of a heterogenous group of causes that have a final common pathway. Although various attempts have been made to identify specific causes for separate subgroups, this approach has not yet been successful. Several lines of investigation are being actively pursued at present and they will be briefly reviewed.

Genetics

There has long been a recognition that schizophrenia is a "familial" disorder—that is, it tends to cluster in certain families more than one would expect from chance alone. Whether this clustering is due to genetic

or environmental factors has been difficult to determine. We now know that the risk of schizophrenia in the children of a schizophrenic parent is about 10% increasing to 50% if both parents are schizophrenic. Monozygotic twins have a higher concordance for schizophrenia than do dizygotic twins, and the risk of schizophrenia does not vary if one lives with one's natural schizophrenic parents or is adopted (see Chapter 114).

Although genetic factors seem important, the mode of transmission has not been determined (i.e., dominant, recessive, or multifactorial), nor is it clear whether genetic factors play a role in the *majority* of adolescents who have schizophrenia. Recently, linkage analysis has demonstrated cosegregation of schizophrenia and a genetic marker on chromosome 5. Unfortunately, this finding has not been replicated independently.

Structural Brain Changes

A number of radiologic investigations have demonstrated structural brain abnormalities in the brains of schizophrenic adults. Most commonly, these changes include large ventricles and widened sulci but also more subtle, localized changes to the frontal or temporal lobes. These abnormalities are apparently unrelated to age or prolonged use of medication. Another consistent finding is that schizophrenics appear to be at high risk for a variety of complications during pregnancy and birth. It is conceivable that these events lead to ventricular changes and other structural abnormalities.

Dopamine

The antipsychotic effect of neuroleptic medication is related to its ability to block dopamine receptors in the brain. This has led to speculation that dopamine systems might be responsible for the syndrome. Dopamine is a neurochemical transmitter that is highly concentrated in certain brain areas, particularly in the subcortical regions. Thus the notion that schizophrenia might be "caused" by an excess of dopamine is based on this finding. Independent confirmation of this hypothesis has been difficult to obtain, however. Measurement of dopamine metabolites and receptors has provided conflicting evidence. Recent advances in brain imaging with radioactive dopamine ligands may provide more definite information.

Neurodevelopmental Models

Recently, it has been suggested that schizophrenia be seen as a "neurodevelopmental disorder." Sex differences in age of onset, the high frequency of obstetric complications, and abnormalities on computed tomography might all reflect developmental markers of damage to subcortical (particularly dopamine-rich) areas. A lesion (either genetic or obstetrically induced) in the first few months of life might lie dormant until maturation of the related part of the brain is complete. Stress and maturational vulnerability would then combine to "trigger" the onset of schizophrenia in adolescence or young adulthood.

TREATMENT

The beneficial effect of drugs in the treatment of schizophrenia was first recognized with the introduction of reserpine and chlorpromazine in the 1950s. There are now a large number of antipsychotic drugs available. The important classes are the phenothiazines (e.g., chlorpromazine, thioridazine, fluphenazine), the thioxanthenes (e.g., thiothixene hydrochloride, flupenthixol), the butyrophenones (e.g., haloperidol), the diphenylbutylpiperidines (e.g., pimozide), and the dibenzoxazepines (e.g., loxapine). These drugs constitute the first line of treatment for schizophrenic psychosis.

A new class of drugs, the dibenzodiazepines (e.g., clozapine) have the apparent advantage of a lack of neurologic side effects; some adolescent patients are said to respond preferentially to them. However, the potential of fatal agranulocytosis has restricted their use to individuals who are resistant to other medications. The antipsychotic drugs have tranquilizing effects, neuroleptic effects (i.e., a tendency to produce specific symptoms of neurologic dysfunction, specifically extra pyramidal symptoms), and specific antipsychotic effects. They reduce or eliminate the "positive" symptoms of schizophrenia (hallucination, delusions, and thought disorder), usually over 1 to 3 weeks or longer. The drugs have demonstrated efficacy in the treatment of acute schizophrenia, and it is now firmly established that continuation of these drugs prevents relapse into psychosis in up to 85% of cases. A small but significant number of adolescent patients relapse even when taking medication and are drug-resistant. However, drug therapy in association with supportive psychotherapy, social skills training, and family education is the cornerstone of treatment in the prevention of relapse (see further on).

No individual drug or class of drug is superior in its antipsychotic effect, as long as an equivalent dosage is given. The choice of drug is guided by side effects and clinical benefit. For instance, the thioxanthenes are reputed to have specific antidepressant effects and are a good choice in anergic and depressed patients. High-potency drugs produce antipsychotic effects with less sedation and are indicated in acute states, although very agitated adolescents might benefit from more phenothiazines with more sedative effect (such as chlorpromazine). Adolescent patients with a history of prior extrapyramidal symptoms, or poor compliance with anticholinergic agents, may do better with low-potency drugs. It is always wise to use a drug that has shown a good previous response with few side effects. Age is also a factor in the choice of drug, as young males are prone to the development of extrapyramidal symptoms. Therefore, many clinicians prefer drugs with a lower tendency to produce these symptoms (e.g., thioridazine, chlorpromazine, or perphenazine).

High doses have no advantage over low to moderate doses in the majority of cases and may lead to unwanted side effects. Lower doses are effective in the maintenance phase, and ongoing monitoring of the dose allows for time-limited increases to control fluctuating symptom levels in response to stressful life events. The prescribing clinician should be aware of the standard doses of one or two drugs from each of the different classes. Formulae for calculating dosage equivalents for different drugs are unreliable. Thus the dose must be titrated to the correct level for each individual. The clinician should resist the impulse to adjust the dose upward after a short period when there has been no reduction of psychotic symptoms. Improved sleep and reduction in general agitation are expected early, but true antipsychotic effects are usually not seen for 1 to 3 weeks, regardless of dosage. In the maintenance phase, approximately one half or less of the initial dose will suffice. In the younger adolescent, it is wise to start with a lower dosage and increase very gradually in accordance with the clinical response.

Medications can be given by the oral route or through intramuscular injection. The intramuscular route has the advantage of increased compliance and lower total dose requirement. Compliance with antipsychotic medication is a major problem in all age groups, but particularly in the adolescent (see Chapter 26). The clinician should always choose a single antipsychotic agent rather than resorting to multiple agents, which is without merit. It is essential that the clinician provide the adolescent and his or her family with a full account of the rationale for treatment and the consequences of noncompliance or discontinuation of drugs. However, many adolescents will refuse injections or the orally administered drugs, especially early in the course of the disorder when denial of illness often occurs. If the adolescent discontinues the medication prematurely, the clinician should encourage attendance for regular surveillance, and both the adolescent and the family should be advised of the early symptoms of recurrence. The current state of knowledge suggests that it would be best for the adolescent to continue maintenance medication for 2 to 3 years following the initial psychosis. Monitoring should continue for a period of 1 year beyond the cessation of medication administration.

Side Effects of Medications

The most important side effects of antipsychotic agents are extrapyramidal—that is, dystonia, drug-induced parkinsonism, akathisia, "rabbit syndrome" (repetitive perioral movements), "paradoxic" dyskinesia, and tardive dyskinesia. "Rabbit syndrome" and "paradoxic" dyskinesia are uncommon. The other extra pyramidal syndromes occur with greater frequency, and it is essential that the prescribing physician know the characteristic signs and symptoms of these disorders.

The acute extra pyramidal syndromes can be effectively controlled with anticholinergic agents, such as benztropine or amantadine. Akathisia is more likely to respond to propranolol. All syndromes are dose-related and may respond to a reduction in the total daily dose. The antipsychotic effect is related to the drug's relative potency as a dopamine blocker, and thus extra pyramidal symptoms are more common with the more potent drugs (such as the butyrophenones, thioxanthenes, and piperidine phenothiazines). Less potent drugs generally have more anticholinergic effects, the most serious being postural hypotension and confusional states secondary to central anticholinergic effects.

The neuroleptic malignant syndrome is a life-threatening disorder manifested by confusion, hypertension, hyperpyrexia, hyperreflexia, leukocytosis, elevated creatine phosphokinase levels, and coma. The adolescent patient requires intensive care and may respond to emergency treatment with a dopamine agonist (such as bromocriptine). Other serious side effects include interference with new learning (especially with more sedative drugs), lowering of the seizure threshold (producing epileptic seizures), agranulocytosis, jaundice, and some rash and skin photosensitivity. Tardive dyskinesia is the most important long-term side effect and is hypothesized to result from supersensitivity of dopamine receptors. The risk for this movement disorder varies according to individual vulnerability, duration of treatment, and level of dose. The early signs involve dyskinetic movements of the face and mouth and vermicular movements of the tongue. Reduction of medication may lead to a worsening of the dyskinesia, but in many instances, there will be improvement over time.

It is generally held that anticholinergic medication should not be initiated routinely with antipsychotic agents but rather should be instituted at the first sign of extrapyramidal symptoms. Several trials have demonstrated that undetected extrapyramidal symptoms are common in clinical populations. Given the high risk of developing these symptoms in the adolescent age group, anticholinergic drugs may be instituted at initiation of treatments (especially when using high-potency antipsychotic agents). These drugs should be continued for 2 to 3 months and withdrawn gradually, preferably along with some reduction of the antipsychotic dosage. Only infrequently will extrapyramidal symptoms reemerge following discontinuation of the anticholinergic agent.

Psychosocial Treatments

Although few treatment studies have concentrated on adolescents with schizophrenia, several well-conducted experiments on the effects of psychosocial treatments for young adult males with schizophrenia have been completed. The interest in psychosocial treatment stems from an acknowledgment that pharmacotherapy plays a necessary, but insufficient, role in reducing relapse. Twenty-five percent to 40% of schizophrenic patients continue to relapse in the first year following hospital discharge, even when the administration of antipsychotic drugs has been assured. These rates compare with relapse rates averaging 68% or greater without pharmacotherapy. Notions of the interconnectedness between biologic and psychosocial factors have led to the implementation of a wide range of psychosocial interventions in conjunction with maintenance pharmacotherapy. In addition, social factors are often implicated in the rehospitalization of schizophrenics, and social characteristics have been described as the best predictors of 5-year clinical and social outcome in the International Pilot Study of Schizophrenia. Although only minimal effects have been attributed to either psychotherapy or supportive therapy for schizophrenia, these therapies (in conjunction with pharmacotherapy) have been the standard form of treatment for schizophrenia. Recently, the important role of social factors in predicting the course and outcome of schizophrenia has led to increased enthusiasm regarding psychosocial interventions. Psychosocial treatments with the most promise include (1) patient-centered psychosocial skills training and (2) family psychoeducational programs.

Patient-centered social skills training programs come in a range of formats but generally focus on teaching the patient problem-solving techniques and include a basic set of procedures derived from learning principles. Such programs focus extensively on teaching patients life skills and effective communication styles, in addition to activities aimed at improving skills in daily living, stress management, vocational skill development, and ways of effectively engaging in leisure and recreational activities. Studies that have compared the effects of social skills training with other patient-centered treatments have demonstrated that social skills training interventions can be effective, especially with young adult males.

Family psychoeducational programs compose the second class of psychosocial intervention and are also offered in a variety of formats. Many are based on groups of family members, with or without the ill person present. These groups may be conducted in a time-limited fashion or may be extended and open-ended. The common denominator, however, is the emphasis on providing knowledge and education concerning the diagnosis, symptoms, etiology, course, and treatment of schizophrenia. In addition, there is an emphasis on family communication style and behavioral training in the development of positive communication styles for family members. This emphasis stems from research originating in Britain, which identified that the emotional climate, or communication style, of the family is related to the course of schizophrenia. Thus programs have been developed to alter the communication style of family members. A number of controlled studies have demonstrated that when family psychoeducational programs are used as outpatient treatment, as well as for select inpatient groups, the communication style of these families can be altered, and an associated decrease in the relapse rate can be obtained.

An important issue in planning the psychosocial treatment of schizophrenia centers on whether or not enriched forms of treatment lead to further improvement in outcome. One study explored whether social skills training plus family psychoeducation, used in conjunction with pharmacotherapy, led to improved outcomes over the use of pharmacotherapy plus social skills, or pharmacotherapy plus family psychoeducation. The 1-year follow-up of this study demonstrated that first-year relapse rates among adolescents exposed to treatment demonstrated a main effect for family treatment (19% relapse), a main effect for social skills training (20% relapse), and an additive effect for the combined treatment (0% relapse), relative to controls (41% relapse). Only the combined treatments sustained remission in households that were high in expressed emotion (a measure of communication style that includes dimensions of criticism, hostility, and emotional overinvolvement). Although the second-year follow-up of these patients demonstrated that the effects of psychosocial interventions may become attenuated over time, a positive effect clearly exists for combined social skills training and family psychoeducation in conjunction with pharmacotherapy. This study represents a major advancement in understanding the potential effects of psychosocial interventions.

COURSE, OUTCOME, AND PROGNOSIS

Although schizophrenia has traditionally been viewed as an illness with poor outcome, the heterogeneity of the disorder is undeniable. Studies of course and outcome span several countries and numerous decades. In comparing the results of outcome studies conducted at different points in time, it must be remembered that not only has the definition of schizophrenia become more stringent over time, but treatment of these conditions has improved with advances in psychopharmacology and psychosocial treatment.

The 5-year follow-up of the British section of the International Pilot Study of Schizophrenia indicated that approximately one fifth of patients did not experience any further episodes of major mental disorder after the episode of inclusion. At the other extreme, one tenth of patients never recovered from the episode. More than one third of patients spent more than half of the follow-up period in episodes of major mental disorder. Overall, about one half of the patient sample was considered to have good symptomatic and social outcomes at 5-year follow-up. Conversely, it should be noted that even among patients considered to have a good outcome, many continued to experience some degree of symptomatic or social disability.

As has been mentioned, the variability in course and outcome of the disorder is substantiated across cultures and over time. Attempts have been made to identify those factors that predict good versus poor outcome. Early age of onset, low familial socioeconomic status, length of time to treatment, and male sex are all equated with poor outcome. The social environment also has a role in predicting poor versus good outcome. Adolescent patients residing in family environments with high expression of emotion are more likely to experience relapse. An intriguing finding from the International Pilot Study of Schizophrenia is that patients in developing countries have a more favorable prognosis than do patients in highly developed countries. Explanations of this finding have taken a number of directions. Some speculate that the illness itself is different in developed versus developing countries. An alternate, and perhaps more plausible hypothesis, suggests that the lower expressed emotion and clearer, more simplified role expectations of family life in developing countries bode well for the outcome of the disorder.

There is also considerable evidence to suggest that social and life history variables have a well-demonstrated effect upon course and outcome. Factors such as community acceptance, living arrangements, social relationships, employment, and economic status all influence how well a person with schizophrenia will do over time.

In examining social and life history factors affecting outcome, consideration should be given to the effect of important life events. Relapsing schizophrenic patients may experience more important life events than those who continue in remission. Life events appear to contribute an incremental component to the stress of discharged patients, which is in many cases associated with subsequent rehospitalization. Individuals with schizophrenia may experience a subtle event as more stressful than would the general population. For example, a seemingly minor change in routine and environment may be enough to create a significant stress for a person with a schizophrenic condition.

The effect of treatment interventions on the course and outcome of schizophrenia has, of course, received much attention. Hospitalization occurs in various forms and with various effects. In general, it is effective in treating the acute stage of the illness and for relatively short periods, whereas long-term hospitalizations generally produce negative effects and contribute to chronicity and institutionalization. Partial hospitalization programs, such as day care programs, have been effective ways of reintegrating the adolescent patient into the community following the remission of the acute episode of the illness.

Much remains to be learned about the prognosis of schizophrenia and factors associated with optimal course and outcome. Although a number of factors are predictive of outcome, only about 30% of the variance in short-term course and outcome has been explained by the available data.

BIBLIOGRAPHY

American Psychiatric Association: Diagnostic and Statistical Manual of Mental Disorders, 3rd ed, revised. Washington, DC, American Psychiatric Association, 1987.

Baldessarini R: Drugs and the treatment of psychiatric disorders. In Gilman AG, Rall TW, Murad F (eds): Goodman & Gilman's The Pharmacological Basis of Therapeutics, 6th ed. New York, Macmillan, 1980.

Eaton WW, Day R, Kramer M: The use of epidemiology for risk factor research in schizophrenia: An overview and methodologic critique. In Nasrallah HA (ed): Handbook of Schizophrenia, Vol 3. Amsterdam, Elsevier, 1988.

Gillberg C, Wahlstrom J, Forsman A, et al: Teenage psychoses:

Epidemiology, classification and reduced optimality in the pre-, peri-, and neonatal periods. J Child Psychol Psychiatry 27:87, 1986.

Hogarty GE, Anderson CM, Reiss DJ, et al: Family psychoeducation, social skills training, and maintenance chemotherapy in the aftercare treatment of schizophrenia. Arch Gen Psychiatry 43:633, 1986.

Prudo R, Munroe Blum H: Five year outcome and prognosis in schizophrenia: A report from the London Field Research Centre of the International Pilot Study of Schizophrenia. Br J Psychiatry 150:345, 1987.

Szatmari P, Bartolucci G, Bremner R: Asperger's syndrome and autism: Comparisons on early history and outcome. Dev Med Child Neurol 31:709, 1989.

Vaughn CE, Leff JP: The influence of family and social factors on the course of psychiatric illness. Br J Psychiatry 129:125, 1976.

World Health Organization: Mental Disorders: Glossary and Guide to Their Classification in Accordance with the Ninth Revision of the International Classification of Disease. Geneva, World Health Organization, 1978.

CHAPTER 111

Substance Use and Abuse

S. KENNETH SCHONBERG

DRUG ABUSE

Initial experiences with drugs that alter mood and behavior are a normative, but often unhealthy aspect of the process of adolescence. In the passage from childhood to adulthood, virtually all teenagers will at a minimum experiment with drugs of abuse, ranging from alcohol and marijuana to more overtly dangerous substances. Most will have little in the way of adverse effects, although all will experience some risk, and a not insignificant minority will suffer ill health, injury, serious behavioral disruption, and even death as a consequence of this behavior.

Epidemiology

Exact data on the incidence of drug abuse among adolescents are unavailable. All available data are gathered by survey and are hence in large part dependent on the veracity of the teenage respondents. The best available information is gathered from annual surveys of high school seniors. A deficit inherent to this information is that those young people who have dropped out of school cannot be included within the surveys. This deficit is of lesser importance in assessing the more common intoxicants, alcohol and marijuana, but assumes significance in attempts to quantify the extent of abuse of drugs such as cocaine and heroin, which are more likely to be associated with greater behavioral disruption and school failure. Nevertheless, this information is helpful in clarifying the extent of the drug abuse problem and demonstrating changing patterns of drug use over time. In some ways, information gathered from adolescents attending school has some advantages in that it assesses those teenagers most likely to be encountered in the routine practice of medicine.

Before graduation from high school, over 90% of adolescents will have consumed alcohol (see Chapter 2). Of greater significance, approximately two thirds of high school seniors will report drinking at least once per month, with about half of these young people drinking to the point of intoxication and nearly 5% drinking on a daily basis (Table 111–1). Alcohol is the most frequently abused substance among adolescents. Such use often begins early in the teen years, with almost 10% of young people reporting a first use prior to seventh grade and over half having had a first experience prior to their sophomore year in high school (Table 111–2).

The early onset of drinking, its frequency, and consequences suggest early vigorous efforts are needed to delay and mediate this behavior.

Approximately half of high school seniors have used marijuana, with about 40% reporting use in the past year and nearly 20% in the past month (see Table 111–1). Although there has been a gradual decline in the number of teenagers using marijuana, first experiences with marijuana most often occur during middle school and early high school years, implying that marijuana and alcohol prevention need to be timed simultaneously.

Reported cocaine use among adolescents has also declined during the past decade; however, it is here that in-school surveys most underestimate the prevalence. Although less than 15% of high school seniors have tried cocaine, with far less than 1% using it daily (see Table 111–1), that small minority of adolescents who become cocaine addicted represent a significant clinical problem. Adolescent use of heroin and other opiates is far less common than it was in the late 1960s and early 1970s. Less than 1% of high school seniors now report ever having used opiates. The multitude of physical problems routinely encountered 2 decades ago now rarely present to the physician.

Similarly, sequelae of inhalant abuse (i.e., the sniffing of cleaning fluid, glue, gasoline, or other volatile hydrocarbons), although not uncommon (about 17%), rarely cause disability requiring medical attention. Most inhalant abuse is confined to preteens and early adolescents, who find it easier to obtain these readily available products rather than more potent intoxicants.

Lifetime prevalence of amphetamine use (about 20%), sedatives (about 8%), and tranquilizers remains high, but often represents semitherapeutic use as self-medication, not dissimilar to that encountered in adults, rather than serious abuse with major direct health consequences. Hallucinogen abuse (about 9%) has remained rather constant over the past 2 decades, although the drug most frequently abused is now phencyclidine (angel dust) rather than lysergic acid diethylamide (LSD). The lifetime prevalence of tobacco use remains quite high (>65%), with nearly 20% of teenagers smoking daily, despite intense efforts to create a "smoke-free" generation.

In sum, the vast majority of adolescents at some time use a mood-altering drug, and some experience a major adverse consequence. The physician must understand these consequences and intervene in order to minimize the risks to the adolescent patient.

TABLE 111–1. Prevalence of Drug Use—Class of 1988

	EVER USED (%)	PAST MONTH (%)	DAILY (%)
Alcohol	92	64	4
Marijuana	47	18	3
Cocaine	12	3	0.2
Hallucinogens	9	2	0.0
Inhalants	17	3	0.2
Heroin	1	0.2	0.0
Stimulants	20	5	0.3
Sedatives	8	1	0.1
Tranquilizers	9	2	0.0
Cigarettes	66	29	18

Data from Johnston LD, O'Malley PM, Bachman JG: Illicit Drug Use, Smoking, and Drinking by America's High School Students and Young Adults, 1975–1987. Rockville, MD, National Institute on Drug Abuse, 1988.

Risk Factors

Although the data would indicate that virtually all adolescents are at some risk from drug abuse, certain young people, by virtue of genetics, family circumstances, peer relationships, and individual personality traits, are at increased danger of serious abuse and addiction. These familial and personal issues should cause the physician to be more vigilant for the signs and symptoms of drug-related difficulties.

Children and adolescents whose parents are substance abusers are far more likely to abuse drugs themselves. This relationship is almost certainly the result of both genetic factors and role-modeling behaviors. Studies of adoptees have demonstrated that one alcoholic biologic parent increased the likelihood of alcoholism in the young person three to four times. The parent–child correlation for alcoholism was stronger for the biologic relationship than for the adoptive family. Monozygotic twins show a higher concordance for alcohol abuse than dizygotic twins. These studies are strongly suggestive of a genetic predisposition for alcoholism, which may or may not be applicable to other drug abuse behavior and addictions. However, whether secondary to genetics or role modeling, any parental drug use increases the likelihood that the adolescent will engage in similar behavior.

In addition to the effect of parental drug use behavior, parental attitudes toward drug use and the quality of the parent–child interaction also influence the behavior of the adolescent. Parents who condone or express a liberal attitude toward drug use are more likely to have children who are drug involved. Parenting that is inconsistent or excessively permissive or, conversely, severely disciplinarian, offering little praise or worth to children, has been associated with adolescent substance abuse. Adolescents from families with a history of antisocial behavior or criminality are at higher risk for substance abuse.

Other important issues inherent to the adolescent include peer relationships, antisocial behaviors, and psychopathology. The vast majority of young people are initiated into drug-taking behavior by friends rather than strangers. The drug abuse behaviors of the peer group and, in particular, close friends are quite predictive of the practices of the adolescent. Although it is unclear whether the drug use of friends evoked similar behavior in the adolescent or the friends were specifically chosen because of their drug use characteristics, an assessment of the activities of the peer group is often a less threatening and most revealing entry into the discussion of the adolescent's personal practices. There is also the expected relationship between drug abuse and other antisocial behavior. Young people who have a history of delinquency, truancy (see Chapter 108), school failure (see Chapter 107), or promiscuity (see Chapter 68) are far more likely to be abusing drugs than their more conventional friends.

Those young people who begin their drug use prior to the age of 15 years (even with the so-called "gateway" drugs—tobacco, alcohol, and marijuana) tend to develop more dysfunctional drug use patterns. In addition, those individuals who initiate their drug use early or late (after the age of 24 years) are more likely to have underlying psychiatric disorders. A history of a major depressive episode or an anxiety disorder doubles the risk for drug abuse and dependence (see Chapters 100 and 103). At times adolescents who are depressed or anxious turn to drugs in an effort to medicate themselves. Most often these attempts at self-medication cause further social, academic, and vocational difficulties for the adolescent and exacerbate the underlying psychopathology. Comorbidity, the presence of both substance abuse and a psychiatric illness, is particularly ominous because serious drug-related dysfunction is more likely and pharmacotherapy for the underlying disorder is extremely problematic.

DIFFERENTIAL DIAGNOSIS

An adolescent with a psychiatric disorder may also abuse substances; at times this may represent an attempt to self-medicate. As discussed above, many of the symptoms of psychoactive substance use are common in other disorders. The treatment approach is likely to differ depending on whether the psychiatric condition is primary or secondary to the substance use. Thus, it is important to evaluate adolescents' symptoms carefully. Other conditions included in the differential diagnoses of an adolescent thought to be using any substance include disorders of affect (see Chapter 100), conduct (see Chapter 108), personality (see Chapter 109), atten-

TABLE 111–2. Grade at First Use—Class of 1988

	ALCOHOL (%)	MARIJUANA (%)	COCAINE (%)
6th	8	3	0.1
7–8th	23	10	0.4
9th	25	11	2
10th	18	10	2
11th	12	8	4
12th	6	5	4
	92	47	12.5

Data from Johnston LD, O'Malley PM, Bachman JG: Illicit Drug Use, Smoking, and Drinking by America's High School Students and Young Adults, 1975–1987. Rockville, MD, National Institute on Drug Abuse, 1988.

TABLE 111–3. Diagnostic Criteria for Psychoactive Substance Dependence

A. At least three of the following:
  (1) Substance often taken in larger amounts or over a longer period than the person intended
  (2) Persistent desire or one or more unsuccessful efforts to cut down or control substance use
  (3) A great deal of time spent in activities necessary to get the substance, taking the substance, or recovering from its effects
  (4) Frequent intoxication or withdrawal symptoms when expected to fulfill major role obligations at work, school, home, or when substance use is physically hazardous
  (5) Important social, occupational, or recreational activities given up or reduced because of substance use
  (6) Continued substance use despite knowledge of having a persistent or recurrent social, psychologic, or physical problem that is caused or exacerbated by the use of the substance
NOTE: The following items may not apply to cannabis, hallucinogens, or phencyclidine (PCP):
  (7) Characteristic withdrawal symptoms
  (8) Substance often taken to relieve or avoid withdrawal symptoms

B. Some symptoms of the disturbance have persisted for at least 1 month, or have occurred repeatedly over a longer period of time.

With permission from American Psychiatric Association: Diagnostic and Statistical Manual of Mental Disorders, 3rd ed, revised. Washington, DC, American Psychiatric Association, 1987, pp 167–168.

tion (see Chapter 106), anxiety (see Chapters 102 and 103), academic performance (see Chapter 107) and thought (see Chapter 110).

DIAGNOSIS

According to Diagnostic and Statistical Manual of Mental Disorders: Third Edition–Revised (DSM III-R) criteria, psychiatric disturbances due to the use of psychoactive substances are classified as disorders of dependence or abuse, with further specification of the particular substance. Both symptoms and maladaptive behavioral changes are considered. The criteria for dependence and abuse are listed in Tables 111–3 and 111–4. During adolescence it may more difficult to distinguish abuse or dependence from less serious use. Adolescents have a relatively short history of use compared to adults and may not experience all of the negative consequences required to meet the diagnostic criteria for dependence. Because local substance use patterns vary widely among youth, an individual may not consider his or her use abnormal. Many of the social, family, and psychological problems associated with use may have existed prior to or be a result of use, making disentanglement difficult. Finally, adolescents' cognitive skills are less developed (see Chapter 9), which may limit their understanding of the extent and scope of their problems.

Comorbidity or Dual Diagnoses

Certain psychiatric conditions are found more frequently among populations of drug abusers than would be expected by chance. There is a strong association of drug abuse with affective disorders (see Chapter 100),

with the strongest link to alcohol. One study of adolescents treated on an inpatient chemical dependency unit found that conduct disorder accounted for 50% of the dual diagnoses. There appears to be a greater likelihood of substance abuse in those adolescents who have both attention deficit hyperactivity disorder (see Chapter 106) and conduct disorder (see Chapter 108). Alcoholism has been found to be common in the families of those with borderline personality disorder (see Chapter 109).

Diagnostic Evaluation

Every adolescent seeking health care should receive evaluation and counseling regarding potential sequelae of substance abuse (see Chapter 25). An appreciation of the risk factors for serious consequences of drug abuse will help the physician identify those adolescents who are most likely to experience major drug-related dysfunction. Psychoactive drugs will touch on the lives of every teenager, either through personal use or as a result of the behaviors of peers.

This evaluation is a natural adjunct to questioning regarding other aspects of adolescent behavior, such as developing sexuality, socialization, and educational plans and accomplishments. As with the assessment of other behavioral issues, the clinician is most dependent on the interview, rather than the physical examination or the laboratory findings. Rarely will previously unsuspected drug abuse be uncovered because of a physical finding or an unanticipated laboratory result.

Interview

In order to obtain reliable information about an adolescent's personal drug abuse behavior, it is critical that the interview take place in an appropriate setting with a clear understanding regarding confidentiality and its limits (see Chapter 22). An appropriate setting must ensure privacy, with parents excluded from this portion of the interview process. It is important also to obtain information about parental drug-related concerns and to question the teenager privately. This portion of the history must proceed with some understanding among

TABLE 111–4. Diagnostic Criteria for Psychoactive Substance Abuse

A. A maladaptive pattern of psychoactive substance use indicated by at least one of the following:
  (1) Continued use despite knowledge of having a persistent or recurrent social, occupational, psychologic or physical problem that is caused or exacerbated by use of the psychoactive substance
  (2) Recurrent use in situations in which use is physically hazardous (e.g., driving while intoxicated)
B. Some symptoms of the disturbance have persisted for at least 1 month, or have occurred repeatedly over a longer period of time
C. Never met the criteria for Psychoactive Substance Dependence for this substance

With permission from American Psychiatric Association: Diagnostic and Statistical Manual of Mental Disorders, 3rd ed, revised. Washington, DC, American Psychiatric Association, 1987, p 169.

physician, adolescent, and parents regarding what information will remain confidential.

Although the privacy of certain aspects of adolescent health care is protected by the law, such as those dealing with sexuality, no such protection exists regarding information about drug abuse (see Chapter 20). Each physician must establish his or her own criteria for the limits of confidentiality. If all information will be shared with the family, it is unlikely that the teenager will answer sensitive questions honestly, and the clinician thus will lose important information. If no information will be shared, then an opportunity will be lost to involve the family in the care of the adolescent whose behavior is out of control and overtly self-destructive. There must be a balance, with that balance adjusted to the age of the patient, the circumstances of the family, and the comfort of the physician. Whatever that balance, it is best discussed with teenager and family prior to the interview.

No single style of questioning suits all physicians and all adolescents (see Chapter 22). The best format is the one that provides comfort to the adolescents and the physician and fosters honest answers. Often, it is best to begin questioning with inquiries regarding behaviors of peers and schoolmates. This provides insight into the teenager's daily milieu and an easier entry into discussions of the personal practices of the adolescent. Most often, when questioned about the use of drugs by others at social events, parties, and school settings, the adolescent will feel less threatened than if the interview began with direct questions about personal behavior. If the physician is able to respond to this information without alarm or dismay, the stage will be set to question the adolescent directly about his or her own drug use in these settings.

Information should be sought on not only the specific drugs the adolescent has used but also the extent of use, the settings in which drugs were used, the risks involved, and the degree of social, educational, and vocational disruption attributable to drug use behavior. This additional assessment of drug-related dysfunction is necessary to determine the extent of the need for intervention and counseling and to assist in convincing the teenager or the family that intervention is necessary. Evidence of school failure, delinquency, truancy, belligerence, automotive accidents, concurrent psychopathology, or other disruption of adolescent development may provide the impetus for remediation.

Physical Examination

Certainly, there are sequelae of substance abuse that produce physical findings. Intravenous drug abuse, of a variety of psychoactive drugs, in particular, produces both cutaneous stigmata, track and needle marks, and wide-ranging organ system disease with accompanying physical findings. The patient presenting for care with impaired sensorium often represents a diagnostic dilemma that requires the clinician to search for signs which would indicate causation, among them drug abuse. However, it is most rare that the diagnosis of substance abuse is made on the basis of an unanticipated

physical finding. In the main, the physician must be aware of the somatic sequelae of the abuse of a variety of psychoactive drugs and the consequences of differing methods of drug administration. The physical examination of the drug abuser is directed by information gathered from the interview.

Laboratory Assessment

The use of the laboratory in the detection of drug abuse in adolescents remains controversial. Although new methodologies allow one to detect drugs in body fluids with a high degree of accuracy, there are serious ethical and practical concerns to the routine screening of all adolescents in an effort to discover those who are less than candid about their drug use behaviors. There is little controversy regarding periodic testing in the adolescent in treatment for substance abuse. Similarly, the young person who is clearly out of control may require involuntary testing for drug abuse. However, the routine screening of all adolescents who present for care, as one might do for tuberculosis, has not been widely accepted.

A variety of methodologies are available to detect the metabolites of drugs of abuse in body fluids. In general, the simpler and less costly methods are less accurate; tests that are more complex and costly usually have increased reliability. Tests range from simple color or spot tests that can be performed in a physician's office to gas chromatography–mass spectrometry (GC-MS), which requires sophisticated and very expensive technical equipment only available within laboratory settings.

The color or spot test is performed by adding a small amount of urine to a reagent, which then turns a specific color if a particular drug is present. Such tests are inexpensive, do not require sophisticated equipment, and give immediate results. A variety of metabolites yield similar color reactions, making false-positive tests common, and a large quantity of drug metabolite is necessary, resulting in false-negative tests if abuse has not been recent or extensive.

Enzyme-multiplied immunoassay technique (EMIT), available at most commercial medical laboratories, is the method most commonly employed in clinical practice. Radioimmunoassay techniques are based on the principle that a drug labeled with a radioactive substance will compete for binding sites with a similar drug that is unlabeled. The more unlabeled drug present, the less radioactivity will be detected. Because the amount of radioactivity present can be measured, these tests are semiquantitative. A wide variety of drugs of abuse can be detected by this method, including marijuana (cannabinoids), opiates, barbituates, amphetamines, phencyclidine, and LSD. Cross-reactions with other drugs do occur, yielding false positives and false negatives; adulteration of a urine sample may yield uniformly negative results.

Gas chromatography–mass spectrometry is extremely accurate, time consuming, requires technical sophistication, and is expensive. This technique is most often reserved for those medical-legal circumstances where the validity of results is critical. It is seldom employed in routine clinical practice.

Despite issues of false positives and false negatives, the controversies surrounding the routine use of the laboratory to screen for adolescent drug abuse do not relate primarily to concerns regarding accuracy, but rather practical and ethical considerations. Those adolescents who are more deeply involved with drugs and unwilling to respond honestly to questions regarding their behavior are the patients most likely to have the intent and expertise to sabotage the testing process. To avoid adulteration of a urine sample or the substitution of a "clean" or old specimen for a freshly collected sample, urine collection should proceed under direct observation of the physician or a member of the office staff. Often such supervised collection of specimens, although acceptable in a legal setting, run counter to the inclination of the doctor–adolescent relationship and are embarrassing to adult and young person alike.

An additional practical concern is that even for those drugs that are assessed in routine testing (alcohol is frequently not assessed), tests most often remain positive for only a few days. The adolescent who is able to remain abstinent for a few days in anticipation of a visit to the physician may very well escape detection.

Beyond concerns regarding privacy, modesty, and deceptive results are ethical considerations. Although parental consent is sufficient for the performance of procedures on children who lack the capacity to make informed judgments, parental permission alone is not usually regarded as sufficient as the basis for treatment or evaluation of the older competent adolescent. There would be little concern regarding testing the adolescent with informed voluntary consent; however, the adolescent who would deny drug use but then voluntarily submit to testing that would detect drug abuse would not be commonly encountered. It seems wisest to limit screening to those situations where evidence of behavioral dysfunction is of a sufficient magnitude to overcome the practical and ethical drawbacks of routine screening.

Counseling, Treatment, and Referral

It should be assumed that all adolescents are in need of some counsel regarding the potential dangers of drug abuse. The vast majority of teenagers will at some point use alcohol or marijuana, and a not insignificant minority will try potentially more dangerous substances. Even that minority of young people who will remain totally abstinent may be at risk because of the drug use of their peers. The physician must question and counsel all adolescents, and determine which young people are experiencing drug-related difficulties that require more intense interventions and possible referral for therapy.

For that majority of adolescents who are not experiencing major disruption from drug abuse, counseling should focus on the very real risks of morbidity and mortality associated with intoxication. The leading causes of death and injury during the teen years (accidents, violence and, to a lesser degree, suicide attempts) are all associated with the use of alcohol and marijuana (see Chapters 2 and 3). Approximately 40% of 25,000 accidental deaths among adolescents in the United States can be linked to alcohol. The majority of these accidental deaths are secondary to automotive collisions; an intoxicated teenage driver is frequently at fault. The preventive counsel of teenagers would not be complete without some exploration of the attitudes and behaviors of the adolescent at social events, parties, while driving, or while a passenger in a motor vehicle. Does the teenager drink and drive? How might the adolescent or the family respond to a circumstance where a safe ride home cannot be assured? Is the discussion of a parent–adolescent "contract" about drinking and driving a possibility within a particular family? Such questioning and discussion has multiple potential benefits. It may lead to safer behavior by the adolescent. It certainly forces the adolescent to think about drug-related behaviors. It reinforces the fact that drug use is a health concern and of sufficient importance to the physician so as to be addressed in the process of health care. It also allows for an even broader discussion about the use of drugs in other circumstances and the modification of drug use behaviors. The conversation permits further insight into the attitudes and practices of the young person. This questioning and exchange of perspectives should be a routine part of adolescent health care.

For some young people, who either present for routine care or specifically for a drug abuse problem or other behavioral disruption, drug use behavior goes beyond the normative and requires specific intervention. In this respect, the appraisal of adolescent drug use is no different than the evaluation of other behavioral difficulties; that is, specific information is required to aid the physician in determining the extent of the problem and in reaching a dispositional decision. Dispositional alternatives include intervention by the primary care physician, referral to an individual who specializes in the treatment of substance abuse, hospitalization for detoxication or the care of somatic consequences of drug use, and referral to a residential drug treatment program or inpatient psychiatric facility.

The determination of the severity of an adolescent's drug abuse problem is at times complicated by the fact that denial is often a symptom of serious drug abuse. This denial is a genuine psychological symptom of substance abuse and does not truly represent willful deceit by the patient. This denial deprives the physician of one of the most important sources of information, the adolescent patient. The family, too, may deny the degree of disruption secondary to drug abuse; when both teenager and parents minimize difficulties, it is easy to overlook the appropriate diagnosis. A degree of skepticism is indicated when aspects of the adolescent's behavior and performance are not in accord with the information presented at interview.

Although there is no formula for determining which young people require intervention, certain factors are helpful in detecting adolescents with drug-related difficulties, and among them which are most likely to require referral for care. The specific drugs being used, the frequency of use, and the setting are important. The young person who drinks a beer once a month is clearly different from the adolescent who is using hallucinogens, is addicted to opiates, or smokes crack cocaine multiple times each day. For some young people, the extent of their drug use alone, without the need for any corroborating information, is sufficient to mandate intense and immediate intervention.

Early onset of drug use, certainly prior to leaving the elementary grades, is one reason for increased concern. Early drug use is not only often a sign of difficulties within the family constellation, but also allows for a more prolonged disruption of adolescent psychosocial development. Information about the behaviors of the adolescent's peer group is most helpful in assessing the difficulties of a particular teenager. The young person who moves toward greater involvement with a cohort of drug-using friends is often self-selecting for peers with similar interests and will have greater difficulty in interrupting a behavior that has become so closely linked with all aspects of his or her social life. An assessment of the adolescent's function within the family is of great value in determining disruption. Drug abuse by the teenager often leads to tensions and hostilities with parents. The extent of such tensions is not only a measure of the problem, but also a measure of the family's ability to be supportive and participate in a therapeutic program.

Important in determining disposition is the adolescent's own attitudes toward drug abuse. Denial and minimization of the problem and acceptance of drug abuse as a way of life are not good signs and often indicate that intervention may need to be involuntary and intense. In contrast, the adolescent who is able to express an understanding of the relationship between his or her drug use and other life difficulties is a better candidate for voluntary treatment.

The presence of other psychiatric disturbances makes prognosis less favorable. The adolescent with a disorder of thought or mood or who is character disordered is most difficult to treat, even by those most skilled in drug abuse intervention (see Chapters 100, 108, and 110). The young person with a "dual diagnosis," that is, drug dependency and another psychiatric disturbance, almost always requires referral for treatment and is likely to require a period of inpatient care. The presence of a dual diagnosis also has implications in the selection of an appropriate drug treatment program. Many drug treatment programs do not include psychiatrists or psychologists within the therapeutic team and, in fact, some programs have a specific antiprofessional philosophy, relying exclusively on ex-addicts and peers for therapy. Such programs would be inappropriate to the needs of an adolescent with coincident psychiatric illness.

Finally, an assessment of other aspects of adolescent function will not only provide insights into the degree of drug-related difficulties but also may provide the evidence necessary to convince a teenager or a family about the need for intervention. Factors that need be considered include academic performance, vocational accomplishments, and difficulties with the police or other indications of delinquent behavior.

Synthesis of information on these factors allows the physician to determine which young people are having drug-related difficulties, who may be adequately treated within the office setting, who requires referral, and who may need hospitalization.

Some adolescents whose drug use goes beyond the acceptable may still be managed within the office setting. Although the degree of drug-related disruption that can be managed by the primary care provider will vary with the skills and orientation of that provider, certain guidelines are applicable. In general, those teenagers who are experiencing minimal disruption of their progress through adolescence, despite their drug use, who express a willingness to address their problem, and who have reasonable family supports are the best candidates for office management. Components of such management include frequent follow-up visits with urine testing to document abstinence and, often, adjunctive support to the young person through such programs as Alcoholics Anonymous or Narcotics Anonymous. Although controversy exists as to the role of urine testing in screening for drug abuse, testing is a part of the management of the teenager with a known drug abuse problem. Many teenagers will use such testing as reinforcement for that part of their personality that would wish to remain drug-free. Routine urinalysis emerges as an aid to the adolescent rather than a methodology for detecting deceit.

As with other behavioral problems and, for that matter, all medical problems, when doubt exists as to the seriousness of drug abuse or the advisability of office management, consultation with a specialist should be sought. The primary care provider has an obligation to identify a drug abuse specialist within the community in the same manner as one identifies other referral resources for health problems that require special expertise. A particular caution applicable to choosing a drug abuse specialist is that at times those individuals are affiliated with a single treatment program or modality. When available, it is best to refer to an individual who does not have a particular bias toward or affiliation with only one specific treatment.

Whether on the basis of direct referral by the primary care physician or only after consultation with a drug abuse specialist, some adolescents will require care from a program that specifically treats drug abusers. Many programs are available and no concrete rules can be offered for selecting among them. Within some communities, there are few options and either geography or financial considerations will dictate a particular choice. However, when options do exist, guidelines to select the better programs include (1) the program insists on total abstinence, (2) that drug abuse is addressed directly with an appreciation that addiction is an entity unto itself, (3) the family is included in the treatment, and (4) drug abuse is recognized as a chronic illness with provisions for long-term follow-up after the young person has been returned to the community. Knowledge of the components and practices of available treatment programs not only provides the practitioner with the ability to select among options but also is of value in facilitating acceptance of a referral by the adolescent and the family.

Finally, some adolescents require hospitalization for the somatic consequences of drug abuse. At times it is those somatic consequences that have brought the teenager to medical attention. Alternatively, illness is discovered during the process of evaluation. In either case, such hospitalizations are an excellent opportunity for therapeutic intervention beyond addressing the somatic illness. Often illness or the fear of disability or death will provide the motivation for addressing the causative drug abuse behavior. A period of forced abstinence within an inpatient setting and the successful treatment of withdrawal symptoms may represent overcoming a hurdle to treating the underlying behavior. The physician's knowledge of the somatic consequences of substance abuse and the ability to treat them are a valuable asset in addressing what is primarily a behavioral problem.

Consequences of Specific Drugs of Abuse

The majority of consequences of substance abuse are behavioral and generic (i.e., not specific to a particular drug). The impact of addiction on the lifestyle of the adolescent and the fabric of the family is generally similar regardless of the addicting drug. Understanding the epidemiology and sequelae of different drugs will help the physician establish credibility with adolescents, their parents, and other health professionals, and assist in the search for the conditions associated with particular drugs.

The acute management of intoxication of recreational drugs is explored in Chapter 97.

MARIJUANA

Pharmacology

Marijuana is obtained from the hemp plant, cannabis sativa. The active ingredients, which include delta-9-tetrahydrocannabinol (THC) and other cannabanoids, are found within the leaves and flowering shoots of the plant. A resinous exudate called hashish is derived from female plants and contains greater concentrations of THC.

Although THC and its derivatives can be taken orally, it is usually smoked. Intoxication occurs rapidly, with peak plasma concentration reached within 10 minutes. Although plasma levels fall rapidly after 60 minutes, the effects on behavior and performace may last 4 to 6 hours. Metabolites of the drug may be detected within the urine within 1 hour after inhalation, and toxicologic test results for marijuana remain positive for periods of up to 3 or 4 days in even occasional users. Storage of the drug within adipose tissues may lead to positive toxicologic tests for up to a month after cessation of heavy use.

Epidemiology

Marijuana use has decreased slightly over the last decade. Approximately half of all high school seniors will report some use of marijuana during their lifetime, with nearly one in five reporting use in the past month (Table 111–1). About 25% of these teenagers report a first experience prior to entrance into the tenth grade (Table 111–2). Although not among the most addicting or physiologically dangerous drugs of abuse, regular marijuana use is associated with behavioral dysfunction and trauma while intoxicated.

Health Consequences

Marijuana has behavioral and somatic consequences. It causes mild acceleration of the heart rate and minimal elevations of blood pressure. Acute inhalation causes bronchodilation; chronic use causes irritation and bronchoconstriction, and has been associated with neoplastic changes in the lungs.

Heavy marijuana use has been associated with reduced sperm counts and decreased levels of circulating testosterone. In laboratory animals, interference with ovulation and decreases in pituitary gonadotropins have been demonstrated. Infertility in adolescent users has not been demonstrated.

Metabolites of marijuana cross the placenta and have been demonstrated to cause fetal growth retardation and congenital anomalies in animal studies. The teratogenetic effects of marijuana have not been clearly demonstrated in humans, but would certainly be a concern for the pregnant teenager (see Chapter 74).

The most important effects of marijuana use are on behavior and performace. Smoking acutely affects the ability to judge time, speed, and distance. Motor coordination, reaction time, and the ability to track a moving object are impaired. These effects last for hours. The impairment of sensory motor skills combined with disinhibition and euphoria is thought to contribute to accidents, homicide, and suicide.

Marijuana intoxication also interferes with attention, the ability to acquire and store information, problem-solving skills, and short-term memory. Use during the school day is of concern. The "amotivational syndrome" described in heavy users is characterized by an inability to sustain any goal-directed activity and may lead to marked deterioration in all aspects of the adolescent's academic, vocational, and social spheres.

ALCOHOL

Pharmacology

Ethyl alcohol is produced from the fermentation of various grains and fruits by yeast. The varying concentrations in the more commonly consumed alcoholic preparations are beer, 3% to 6%; wine, 8% to 12%; and liquors (vodka, rum, whiskey, scotch, and so on), 40% to 50%. A bottle of beer, a glass of wine, and a shot of liquor are roughly equivalent in their total alcohol content.

Alcohol is rapidly absorbed from the gastrointestinal tract, with drug effect noted in about 10 minutes. The consumption of alcohol with foods, particularly protein and fat, tends to delay absorption, while carbonated mixers accelerate this process. Drug effect usually lasts for about an hour, but varies with the total amount consumed. Because alcohol is usually consumed over time with repetitive doses, intoxication is quite often prolonged.

Alcohol is metabolized in the liver through oxidation to acetaldehyde. It is excreted both in the urine and in expired air. For either therapeutic or medical–legal reasons, alcohol levels can be determined from blood, urine, or expired air. A blood alcohol level of approximately 0.05% is sufficient to cause intoxication; legal definitions of intoxication vary by state. Levels of 0.10% or greater are often used as a legal determinant of intoxication, whereas levels of 0.30% and greater are capable of producing stupor and death.

Alcohol also produces central nervous system depression, and suppression of antidiuretic hormone leading to diuresis. Tolerance to alcohol develops over time, and addiction to alcohol with an abstinence syndrome, although uncommon in adolescents, is frequent among adult alcoholics.

Epidemiology

Alcohol is the psychoactive drug most commonly used by both adolescents and adults (alcohol use among adolescents has not diminished in the past decade). Over 90% of high school seniors have had some lifetime experience with drinking, and two thirds report use over the preceding month. Of those who report use during the past month, about half admit to drinking to the point of intoxication, with nearly 5% drinking on a daily basis. Alcohol use begins early, with some 10% of young people having a first experience in elementary school and over half before entrance into high school.

Health Consequences

The acute physiologic sequelae from alcohol usually relate to the ingestion of an excessive amount of alcohol over a brief period of time. Considering the extent of alcohol use by adolescents, acute overdose requiring medical intervention is not common (see Chapter 97). Both acute gastritis and acute pancreatitis may result from a large, single ingestion. Acute erosive gastritis is marked by abdominal pain, vomiting, and gastrointestinal bleeding, usually with hematemesis. Often symptoms subside without specific intervention, but particularly if bleeding persists, the adolescent will require vigorous antacid therapy and further diagnostic evaluation to localize bleeding. Acute alcohol-induced pancreatitis similarly presents with severe abdominal pain and vomiting, which is accompanied by elevations of serum amylase and lipase (see Chapter 62). Management includes analgesia and the correction of any fluid and electrolyte imbalance that may evolve secondary to profuse vomiting.

Accidents, primarily automotive accidents, are the leading cause of death among adolescents, followed by homicide and suicide. A significant portion of these accidental deaths as well as homicidal and suicidal behavior relates to intoxication (see Chapter 2). From this perspective, alcohol is the leading cause of death for adolescents. Alcohol use also contributes to a large number of nonfatal injuries. Delinquency, belligerence, and sexuality are all influenced by intoxication.

Although the vast majority of older adolescents drink, and all should be considered at risk from intoxication, only a small number become young alcoholics. Physiologic addiction to alcohol, as determined by the occurrence of a withdrawal syndrome upon abstinence, is rare. Adolescent alcoholism should be defined by behavioral rather than physiologic criteria. For treatment purposes, daily drinkers should be considered alcoholics. Usual concommitants of daily drinking often include blackout spells, school failure, deterioration of social relationships, and frequent accidents.

A larger group of teenagers may be classified as problem drinkers. Problem drinkers become drunk six or more times per year or suffer negative consequences from drinking such as trouble with the police, friends, family, and school work. Adolescents involved in accidents secondary to intoxication would also be included within this category. Although rarely in need of inpatient treatment, these problem drinkers should be considered for behavioral interventions specifically designed to interrupt their drinking behavior.

Although physiologic addiction to alcohol is rare during adolescence, consistent daily drinking may lead to tolerance and addiction. Abstinence then results in minor (early) and major (late) withdrawal syndromes. The minor withdrawal syndrome may begin as soon as 8 hours after the cessation of drinking and lasts no longer than 1 to 2 days. Symptoms are generally benign and include tremors, mild diaphoresis, and restlessness; brief, self-limited seizures are rare. The major withdrawal syndrome, or delirium tremens, is extremely uncommon in adolescents and is characterized by hallucinations, profuse sweating, and fluid and electrolyte disturbances.

Fetal alcohol syndrome may occur. It is characterized by mild to moderate mental retardation, microcephaly, poor coordination, hypotonia, attention deficit disorders with hyperactivity, and distinguishing facial features. Although more often associated with heavy drinking early in pregnancy, no level of fetal exposure to alcohol has been determined to be safe. Any pregnant teenager should be advised to be abstinent and most certainly to avoid alcoholic excess. At times a young woman will alter her behavior for the sake of her fetus in circumstances where she would not have changed for her own benefit alone (see Chapter 74).

COCAINE

Pharmacology

Cocaine hydrochloride is a crystalline white powder derived from the leaves of Erythoxolon coca, a plant indigenous to South America. It is well absorbed from mucous membranes and is most frequently abused by nasal inhalation or "snorting." Subcutaneous or intravenous administration is less common. Because cocaine powder decomposes when heated, it is smokeable only after conversion into its freebase or "crack" form. Crack cocaine is rapidly absorbed through the lungs, resulting in an instantaneous and intense high.

Cocaine produces an intense euphoria, accompanied by tachycardia, vasoconstriction, hypertension, decreased fatigability, and increased motor activity. Effects are usually short lived, lasting only minutes, and may be followed by periods of depression. Tolerance to the psychic effects develops over time, necessitating increased dosages. No clear abstinence syndrome has been described.

Cocaine is detoxified in the liver and excreted in the urine. It can be detected in the urine by enzyme-multiplied immunoassay (EMIT) for up to 2 to 3 days after use.

Epidemiology

Cocaine emerged as one of the more popular drugs of abuse of the 1980s. At its peak, nearly 20% of high school seniors had had some lifetime experience with cocaine, although daily use was reported at far less than 1%. For cocaine, as well as other hard drugs, data on daily use may be deceptively low, because frequent use is not compatible with continued attendance in school, where most drug abuse surveys are conducted. Reported cocaine use among adolescents has declined with current surveys, indicating an approximate 12% lifetime experience.

Health Consequences

Cocaine and crack cocaine abuse has been associated with deterioration of academic performance, social relationships, and all other goal-directed behavior. Prostitution to obtain money for drugs or sex for direct payment with drugs is not infrequent. Sexually transmitted disease including infection with the human immunodeficiency virus (HIV) may result (see Chapters 75 and 76). The cocaine-abusing adolescent may become increasingly involved in criminal behaviors to support this habit.

Tolerance and dependence emerge rapidly with continued use. Although no specific abstinence syndrome has been described, cocaine withdrawal is marked by intense cravings for the drug that coincide with demonstrable changes in neurotransmitters within the brain. Despite the absence of physical signs of withdrawal, the intensity of drug-seeking behavior and agitation upon abstinence would suggest that differentiating between psychological dependence and physiologic addiction is only of semantic, rather than practical, importance.

Physiologic sequelae of cocaine use rarely come to medical attention. Because inhaled cocaine is a powerful local vasoconstrictor, ulceration and infections of the nasal mucosa and secondary sinusitis do occur. Smoked products (i.e., crack cocaine), may cause bronchitis, wheezing, and pharyngeal irritation. Although users will admit to such symptoms on questionnaires, the symp-

toms rarely result in the need for medical care. The intravenous abuse of cocaine carries the same risks of infectious complications, including hepatitis and the acquired immunodeficiency syndrome (AIDS), that are associated with the intravenous abuse of other drugs.

Despite publicity that would suggest the contrary, the fatality rate directly attributable to the pharmacologic effects of cocaine remains quite low. When fatal reactions do occur, they are often of such an acute nature as to result in death prior to any possible medical intervention. Such deaths are most often secondary to cardiac arrhythmias, seizures, strokes, and respiratory arrest.

Cocaine use during pregnancy has been associated with prematurity, abruptio placentae and spontaneous abortions. An increased incidence of congenital malformations, in particular bony defects of the skull, has been suggested but remains unproven. Babies born to mothers who are actively using cocaine are found to have depressed interactive behavior and irritability when aroused. At this time there is no clear evidence that given proper nurturance the infant exposed to cocaine *in utero* will have been permanently damaged.

OPIATES
Pharmacology

A wide variety of naturally occurring, semisynthetic, and synthetic compounds are included in the opiate family. All produce analgesia and euphoria. Opium is obtained from the opium poppy, *Papaver somniferum*, grown principally in Asia. Morphine is a derivative of opium. Heroin, the most frequently abused opiate, is produced by the acetylation of morphine. Methadone, a synthetic opiate, has been used medically as both an analgesic and an antitussive, and more recently as a treatment for heroin addiction. It is also widely abused. Other semisynthetic and synthetic opiates include oxycodeine (Percodan and Percoset), hydromorphine (Dilaudid), and meperidine (Demerol). All are capable of producing euphoria and addiction in addition to analgesia, and all have been abused. However, the majority of adolescent opiate abuse involves either heroin or methadone.

Heroin in pure form is a crystalline white powder. When sold as a drug of abuse, it is almost always adulterated. Lactose, other sugars, and quinine are the most often used fillers or diluents. It is most frequently sold in small glassine envelopes or "bags," each of which will usually contain from 1 to 20 mg of heroin. Methadone, a pharmacologic preparation, is available in both liquid and tablet form. The most frequently used therapeutic preparation is a tablet in which cellulose is admixed with the drug as a method to prevent dissolution and intravenous injection.

Heroin may be abused via nasal inhalation ("snorting"), subcutaneously ("skin popping"), or intravenously ("mainlining"). Methadone differs from both morphine and heroin in that it is effective when taken orally. Although the oral route is most frequently employed by abusers, intravenous administration is also possible. The onset of action varies with both the drug abused and the route of administration. Intravenous abuse of heroin results in an almost instantaneous euphoria, with effects lasting for some hours. Methadone taken orally has an onset of action of approximately 30 minutes, and a plasma half-life and some mood-altering effects lasting nearly a full day. Tolerance to all opiates emerges rapidly with repetitive use, with increasing amounts required to produce euphoria and to prevent withdrawal symptoms.

Opiates are detoxified by conjugation with glucuronic acid within the liver and are excreted in the urine. By-products of heroin can be detected in the urine for approximately 48 hours after last use, and methadone for about 1 day longer.

Epidemiology

Heroin abuse among adolescents has become far less common than it was at its peak in the late 1960s and early 1970s; however, it is probably more frequently abused than is detected by in-school surveys. Such surveys would suggest that less than 1% of high school seniors have ever tried opiates and that addiction among this population is almost nonexistent. The consequences of heroin abuse among adolescents are now rarely encountered in medical practice.

Health Consequences: Heroin and Methadone

Although all of the opiates are potentially addicting, the use of heroin accounts for the vast majority of somatic consequences associated with this family of drugs. The health consequences of methadone abuse are less serious than those associated with heroin and differ slightly.

Somatic consequences of heroin abuse result from both the pharmacologic actions of the drug and the method of administration. Heroin and other opiates are not in themselves particularly harmful. Decreased gastrointestinal motility is noted with all opiates; chronic constipation and hemorrhoids are quite frequent among heroin abusers. There is an increased frequency of duodenal ulcers among adult heroin addicts; often the ulcer is not discovered until perforation has taken place. The addict may falsely attribute abdominal discomfort to withdrawal symptoms and increase the dose or frequency of the abused drug, masking the symptoms.

Anovulation and amenorrhea are common in female adolescent heroin addicts. Contraception must be included in rehabilitation programs when the young woman abstains from heroin (see Chapter 73).

The most serious pharmacologic consequences of heroin abuse are overdose (see chapter 97) and addiction.

Several weeks of daily opiate use are required to produce addiction characterized by an abstinence syndrome. Components of withdrawal include dilated pupils, goose flesh, yawning, lacrimation, bowel hyperactivity, diarrhea, mild hypertension, tachycardia,

abdominal pain, insomnia, anxiety and, at times, intense cravings for opiates. Seizures are exceedingly rare. Adolescent patients with chronic pain are often treated with opiates for extended periods of time without experiencing withdrawal symptoms. In these circumstances, withdrawal symptoms are most frequently mild, and it is often the anxiety symptoms rather than the degree of discomfort that represents the major obstacle to detoxification.

Withdrawal may be treated in a variety of ways. Some therapeutic communities use no pharmacologic agents, treating withdrawal with reassurance and activities to divert attention from symptoms. Both methadone and diazepam have been widely used to treat abstinence-related symptoms. Methadone (30 to 40 mg as a single daily dose) is sufficient to prevent withdrawal symptoms in all but the most heavily addicted young people. An initial dose of no greater than 20 mg will prevent any possibility of overdose in the teenager who was inventing or greatly exaggerating addiction. If lethargy does not develop within 2 to 4 hours of the initial dose and symptoms persist, an additional 10 to 20 mg may be offered. The daily dose should be reduced at a rate of 5 mg per day until abstinence is achieved. As the dose is reduced, some symptoms of withdrawal may emerge, especially craving for the drug and difficulty sleeping. Alternatively, one may use diazepam 10 mg every 4 to 6 hours for 3 to 4 days. This regimen will control most symptoms of withdrawal, with the exception of diarrhea and occasionally insomnia. The successful treatment of the abstinence syndrome is only the first step in assuring a continued drug-free state. Without continuing support, most adolescents will not be able to sustain an opiate-free lifestyle.

Although it is not known how many adolescents try heroin once or twice but not again, or alternatively succeed in remaining abstinent after a medically supervised detoxification or a self-imposed withdrawal, it is clear that most adolescents once addicted have great difficulty sustaining an opiate-free existence. Although ambulatory support programs such as Narcotics Anonymous may be successful, the majority of opiate-involved adolescents will require more intense interventions. Therapeutic communities and methadone maintenance appear to be most likely to provide long-term abstinence.

Most therapeutic communities use a highly structured rehabilitative process, often under the direction of ex-addicts. Clients must remain in treatment for periods of 6 to 18 months, with most programs requiring at least 1 year before graduation and release. Many adolescents have difficulty in tolerating the incarceration and abrasive therapy inherent to the therapeutic community approach and will resist such placement or remain for only a brief period of time. In addition, such placements may be inappropriate for the adolescent with co-existent psychopathology, because most therapeutic communities provide little or no traditional psychiatric support.

Methadone maintenance, used less frequently for adolescents, substitutes methadone for the abused narcotic. Within a therapeutic program, methadone is given in a single daily dose and does not produce euphoria in the tolerant individual. Although many patients do quite well while remaining in a maintenance program, receiving their methadone under supervision with counseling and support, only a minority will successfully be detoxified and remain drug-free. For many, the maintenance program becomes permanent therapy; hence the reluctance to commit young people to this treatment modality. In addition, it should be noted that, unlike therapeutic communities where the treatment approach is not drug-specific, methadone maintenance is exclusive to narcotic addiction.

The majority of health consequences associated with the opiate abuse are secondary to the method of administration. Nasal inhalation may result in ulcers of the nasal mucosa, which rarely lead to serious local infections and perforation of the nasal septum. Continued abuse through such "snorting" is uncommon, because it is difficult to sustain a large habit without causing severe nasal irritation and the onset of drug action is delayed and erratic. Subcutaneous "skin-popping" and intravenous "mainlining" abuse may lead to skin abscesses, cellulitis, and subcutaneous fat necrosis. Adulterants admixed with the heroin can cause severe local reactions, including skin ulcers and necrosis. The subcutaneous deposition of carbon particles from a needle tip that has been flamed in an attempt at sterilization leads to permanent hyperpigmentation above blood vessels, which resemble "railroad tracks."

Pulmonary granulomas and hypertension are rare complications of the injection of adulterants. To discourage intravenous abuse, methadone may be combined with nalloxone. The nalloxone has no pharmacologic effect taken orally. If injected intravenously, the nalloxone will precipitate withdrawal symptoms. Methadone may also be combined with insoluble compounds (such as cellulose) which, if injected, may produce vascular occlusions.

Infectious complications are more common and important. Acute hepatitis is the most common infectious complication of heroin abuse in adolescents (see Chapter 62). Approximately one third of adolescents with a history of opiate addiction will have evidence of persistent hepatic dysfunction. Elevations of levels of serum transaminase may persist for months to years. Liver biopsies in these teenagers reveal findings consistent with a diagnosis of chronic persistent hepatitis.

The intravenous drug abuser presenting with a fever of unknown origin must be evaluated for bacterial endocarditis. Infective endocarditis may be encountered in the addict with or without a pre-existing cardiac lesion, and may affect either the right or left side of the heart. A variety of infectious agents have been isolated; however, *Staphylococcus aureus* is most common. Fungal infections carry a poorer prognosis.

Septic embolization from an infected tricuspid valve has been associated with metastatic infection in the brain, spleen, kidneys, and lungs. Intracranial microabscesses may occur even in the absence of carditis as a result of the direct seeding of infectious material. Focal neurologic signs may be absent, and the only evidence of the infection will be fever and personality change. Reaching the appropriate diagnosis requires both a high index of suspicion and sophisticated imaging techniques, because it is easy to overlook such personality change in the addict with a history of aberrant behavior.

Intravenous abuse may result in infection with HIV (see Chapter 76). Currently over 10% of adolescents diagnosed with AIDS have a history of intravenous drug abuse. Any adolescent with a history of intravenous abuse should be counseled regarding HIV infection and offered diagnostic testing.

Opiate use during pregnancy has been associated with an increased incidence of spontaneous abortion, stillbirths, and small for gestational age newborns. Opiate withdrawal during the last trimester of pregnancy has been linked to fetal distress, suggesting that attempts at abstinence should occur early in pregnancy or, alternatively, methadone maintenance be offered to those adolescents approaching term. A fetal abstinence syndrome with feeding difficulties, irritability, diarrhea, and occasional seizures is not uncommon and may occur within hours to weeks after delivery. The later onset of this abstinence syndrome is associated with either the abuse or therapeutic use of methadone.

INHALANTS

A variety of volatile hydrocarbons produce intoxication when inhaled or "sniffed." Although this behavior remains relatively common among adolescents (lifetime prevalence for any use is reported by approximately one in five high school seniors), inhalant use is primarily confined to preteens and young adolescents. Persistence into late adolescence or adult life is often a marker of underlying psychopathology.

These drugs are easily accessible and include gasoline, cleaning fluid (trichloroethylene), airplane glue, and aerosol propellants from spray cans. Less readily available compounds but still widely abused agents include the volatile nitrites such as amyl, butyl, and isobutyl nitrite.

These substances may be inhaled directly from a can or a spray bottle or plastic bag. A saturated cloth may be placed over the mouth and nose. All of the inhalants are absorbed readily through the lungs and produce a rapid intoxication, often within seconds, lasting for up to 10 to 15 minutes.

Health Consequences

Somatic consequences from inhalant abuse are uncommon, but both a "sudden sniffing death" syndrome and acute organ toxicities have been reported. Sudden sniffing death (thought to be from cardiac arrhythmias) has been associated with a variety of inhalants including halogenated hydrocarbons (freons), cleaning fluids, typewriter correction fluid, and certain glues. Suffocation may occur if a plastic bag placed over the head is used as the vehicle for inhalation, and loss of consciousness is precipitated by the high concentration of inhaled substance.

Cleaning fluid has been associated with acute hepatic and renal toxicity. Although uncommon, cleaning fluid sniffing should be considered as a possible cause in the adolescent presenting with the sudden onset of vomiting, abdominal pain, jaundice, and laboratory evidence of hepatic dysfunction, or as a cause of acute renal dysfunction, including oliguria or anuria.

AMPHETAMINES

Although about 20% of high school seniors will report some lifetime experience with amphetamines, most use is limited to semitherapeutic attempts at weight reduction or staying awake to study for an examination. Extensive or daily use of these drugs is now quite uncommon (see Table 111–1). Amphetamines may be taken orally or intravenously. Among this class of drugs is a series of compounds derived from the parent compound alphamethyl-phenylethylamine, including DL-amphetamine (Benzedrine), dextroamphetamine (Dexedrine), and methamphetamine. There are also a series of amphetamine "look-alikes," with similar actions, such as phenylpropanolamine (PPA).

When amphetamines are taken orally, the onset of action is approximately 30 minutes. Effects include exhilaration, euphoria, increased wakefulness, improved ability to concentrate, and decreased appetite. With intravenous abuse, effects are instantaneous and more intense. Amphetamines are detoxified in the liver through deamination and hydroxylation and excreted through the kidneys. Metabolites may be detected in the urine for periods of up to 2 to 3 days.

Health Consequences

Beyond the rare occurrence of an acute overdose syndrome, usually secondary to intravenous abuse (see Chapter 97) most medical consequences represent an exaggeration of therapeutic effects. With chronic use, adolescents may experience insomnia, agitation, weight loss, tachycardia, and hypertension. The symptoms encountered often mimic those found in hyperthyroidism. The findings abate rapidly with discontinuation of the drug.

An organic mental syndrome has been associated with both the prolonged use of amphetamines and the abrupt discontinuation of the drug. Confusion, severe agitation, and paranoia may occur. With withdrawal of amphetamines, similar symptoms may be encountered and complicated by extreme changes in mood, including depression, somnolence, voracious appetite, belligerence, and suicidal or homicidal behaviors.

Intravenous abuse is subject to the same risks as with the abuse of other drugs, including not only infectious complications but also embolic phenomena from injecting particulate matter. In addition, severe hypertension, cerebrovascular accidents, and angiitis have been associated with intravenous abuse.

Although uncommon, fetal anomalies (limb deformities and biliary atresia) have been reported secondary to amphetamine abuse during the first trimester. Babies born to mothers abusing amphetamines in the days immediately prior to delivery may withdraw, resulting in tremulousness, irritability, hypoglycemia and, rarely, seizures.

BARBITURATES AND OTHER DEPRESSANTS

The abuse of barbiturates and other depressants is no longer common among adolescents. Although somewhat less than 10% of high school seniors report some lifetime use of depressants, more frequent use or daily use with addiction is rare.

A wide variety of barbiturates are commercially available for therapeutic use as sedative/hypnotics and as anticonvulsants. The parent compound for these formulations is barbituric acid. The duration of action of long-acting barbiturates (phenobarbital) is approximately 12 to 24 hours; intermediate acting (amobarbital), 8 to 10 hours; and short-acting (pentobarbital), 4 to 8 hours. Other nonbarbiturate drugs within this category include both methaqualone (Quaalude) and glutethimide (Doriden). Street names for these drugs change rapidly and new terms emerge for old compounds. Among the names in common usage are "reds" (secobarbital); "yellow jackets" (pentobarbital); "blues" (amobarbital); "cibas" or "goofballs" (glutethimide); and "ludes" or "soapers" (methaqualone). It is difficult to predict the actual drug abused from the street name offered by the abuser, because he or she is often unaware of the exact nature of the compound abused.

These drugs are most often taken orally; intravenous or subcutaneous use is less common. They are primarily metabolized in the liver and excreted in the urine. Glutethimide is an exception; after metabolism in the liver, it is excreted into the intestine via the biliary system with a far lesser amount of metabolite appearing in the urine.

The length of time following use during which one may detect the drug or its metabolites varies widely with the duration of action of the abused compound. Short-acting barbiturates may be undetectable in the urine after 48 to 72 hours, whereas long-acting compounds may be present for periods of 1 week or longer.

Health Consequences

The barbiturates produce an intoxication characterized by slurred speech, short attention span, nystagmus, and ataxia. The intoxicated state is easily confused with alcoholic inebriation and, as with alcohol, trauma while intoxicated is possible. Serious medical consequences include those related to intravenous abuse, overdose, and addiction.

Risks associated with intravenous abuse are similar to those described for opiate abuse.

Serious overdose is not uncommon, because all produce respiratory depression. It is not uncommon that the depressant drugs are combined with alcohol. The management of the acute overdose syndrome is detailed elsewhere (see Chapter 97).

Although now rarely encountered, the abstinence

syndrome from barbiturates is potentially life-threatening. Any adolescent using 500 mg or more per day of a barbiturate or any other sedative is at risk of an abstinence syndrome if the drug is abruptly discontinued. The abstinence syndrome is characterized by anxiety, restlessness, tremors, and abdominal cramps, with symptoms emerging approximately 12 hours after the last dose. Within 24 hours the adolescent may become weak, with hyperactive reflexes and orthostatic hypotension. Over the next 24 hours, symptoms may progress to major motor seizures and shock. Abuse of long-acting barbiturates is characterized by a delayed onset of symptoms, sometimes as long as 1 week after the last dose.

The abstinence syndrome is prevented by the administration of barbiturate in a dose approximating that which was abused and then slowly decreasing that dose over days. Although it is very difficult to estimate the correct dose to administer, one should attempt to estimate the daily consumption and divide it into four equal doses. Phenobarbital is substituted for the abused barbiturate on a milligram-for-milligram basis. The initial dose may be given orally. Intramuscular administration is preferred if there has been either a delay in seeking care or abstinence symptoms are present. The desired end-point of initial treatment is the emergence of signs of mild barbiturate toxicity manifested by slurred speech, ataxia, and nystagmus. This will assure that sufficient medication is being administered to prevent the abstinence syndrome. If signs of toxicity do not emerge within 2 hours of the initial dose, the total daily dose should be recalculated, adding 120 mg (30 mg per 6-hour dose). The dose should be increased each 6 hours until toxicity emerges. The dose at which toxicity appears is the daily maintenance dose. After the maintenance dose is established and continued for a full day, the daily dose is then decreased at a rate of 120 mg per day (30 mg per dose) until abstinence is achieved. Caution must be observed during the initial stages of treatment, to be certain that the patient is not overmedicated. If respiratory depression or extreme lethargy emerge, medication should be withheld.

Treatment for the abstinence syndrome must proceed within a narrow therapeutic range. If withdrawal proceeds too rapidly, convulsions and shock may be encountered. If treatment is overzealous, there is a risk of iatrogenic respiratory depression and coma. The management of this abstinence syndrome is often best left, when possible, to the clinician experienced in treating barbiturate withdrawal.

Barbiturates cross the placenta, and a neonatal abstinence syndrome has been described in babies born to mothers using barbiturates during the last trimester. Features of the neonatal abstinence syndrome include hyperactivity, excessive crying, tremors, hyperreflexia, sneezing, and hiccups. The onset of symptoms is usually delayed for some days to a week after delivery, presumably as the result of hepatic immaturity in the newborn, allowing for a delayed excretion of barbiturate. Treatment for the neonatal abstinence syndrome may include sedation and diminished input of environmental stimuli. In addition to the abstinence syndrome, occasional anatomic abnormalities and minor malformations have been noted in babies born to mothers using or abusing barbiturates during pregnancy.

TRANQUILIZERS

Tranquilizers, including the benzodiazepines and meprobamate, are the most widely prescribed group of drugs in the United States. Not surprisingly, approximately 10% of high school seniors have had some lifetime experience with these drugs. The majority of such use is semitherapeutic. Excluding such self-treatment for anxiety or insomnia, extensive abuse and addiction among adolescents is quite uncommon.

This family of drugs include the benzodiazepines—flurazepam, oxazepam, lorazepam, alprazolam and, in particular, diazepam (Valium)—and meprobamate. They are almost always abused orally and are readily absorbed from the stomach, detoxified in the liver, and excreted in the urine. They may be detected in blood or urine for periods of up to 3 days after use.

Health Consequences

Acutely, these drugs cause ataxia, dizziness, weakness, and drowsiness. Memory and psychomotor function are impaired with decreased ability to drive or operate machinery. Major medical complications are restricted to acute overdose and an abstinence syndrome.

Addiction to tranquilizers is rarely encountered in adolescents. Features of the abstinence syndrome would include insomnia and irritability, progressing to tremulousness, diaphoresis, tachycardia, hypertension, confusion, and rarely a convulsion. Treatment of the benzodiazepine withdrawal syndrome consists of reinstituting tranquilizer therapy and slowly tapering medications over a period of a few weeks. Meprobamate abstinence may be treated by the substitution of phenobarbital and use of the protocol outlined for barbiturate addiction.

The benzodiazepines and meprobamate cross the placenta; however, uncertainty persists regarding their teratogenicity. The benzodiazepines have been associated with an increased rate of oral clefts. Reports of cardiac, brain, and limb abnormalities associated with meprobamate use during pregnancy remain unsubstantiated.

HALLUCINOGENS

A variety of compounds bearing little or no resemblance to one another are capable of producing an hallucinatory state. Included are lysergic acid diethylamide (LSD, "acid"); phencyclidine (PCP, "angel dust"); peyote cactus (which contains mescaline); jimson weed ("loco weed"), which contains atropine/scopolamine; mushrooms containing psilocybin; and a synthetic catecholamine 2,5-dimethoxy-4-methylamphetamine (DOM or "STP"). Although 10% of adolescents will at one time or another try one of these compounds, frequent use is uncommon and is most often a marker of either underlying psychopathology or serious polydrug abuse. Metabolites of these drugs are not always routinely sought in urine toxicology screens, but may be detected for days to (in the case of phencyclidine) a week after ingestion.

Health Consequences

Because the hallucinogens do not represent a homogenous group of drugs, physiologic complications of abuse vary with the drug ingested. The consequences of the hallucinatory state are, however, in the main generic. Acute hallucinatory states may be marked by bizarre behavior, extreme belligerence, death-defying acts, and panic reactions; these may place the young person and others at risk of injury or death. Although some hallucinogens may produce physiologic alterations that are life-threatening and hence require immediate attention (see specific hallucinogens below), a primary concern is preventing acute injury.

The adolescent should be placed in a quiet, nonthreatening environment to minimize sensory stimuli and decrease the potential for misinterpretation and reaction to ongoing activities. This may be difficult in the busy emergency room. One should try to reassure the adolescent that the hallucinatory experience is drug-related, self-limited, and that he or she will not be harmed. These efforts to "talk down" the adolescent who is experiencing a "bad trip" are a worthwhile initial effort, but are often unsuccessful. Although hallucinations are not in themselves dangerous, those patients who continue to manifest dangerous behaviors are candidates for physical or pharmacologic restraint. Both have the potential for added difficulties. Attempting physical restraint will almost certainly add to the paranoia and belligerence of the adolescent and therefore risk injury to both patient and staff. Ideally, physical restraint should not be attempted until overwhelming force is available to minimize the potential for injury. Pharmacologic restraint carries the risk of further disorientation and producing iatrogenic physiologic compromise. Although the choice of a specific tranquilizing agent is best left to the comfort and experience of the clinician, in general benzodiazepines and haloperidol are least likely to accentuate physiologic deficits. Phenothiazenes should be avoided because their anticholinergic effects may be additive to the physiologic difficulties produced by some of the hallucinogens.

"Flashbacks" (the reccurrence of the hallucinatory experience at a later date, when no drug has been taken) has been most frequently associated with the use of LSD, but are possible with all hallucinogens. Because flashbacks may occur at any time without warning, they represent a potential danger, particularly in the adolescent who has a history of repetitive abuse. Although there is no specific therapy for flashbacks, mild tranquilization and reassurance by the physician that these episodes do not represent emerging psychosis is often most helpful to the patient. At times such reassurance is difficult to offer, because there is an association between psychosis and hallucinogen abuse (see Chapter 110).

Lysergic Acid Diethylamide (LSD, "Acid"). This is the most notorious of the hallucinogens and is effective orally in minute doses. It may be ingested in solution with other liquids, on a sugar cube, or absorbed on to a piece of blotter paper ("blotter acid") and swallowed, paper and all. Beyond the hallucinatory experience and the trauma associated with disorientation, major physiologic complications do not occur. Rarely, seizures have been reported with high doses and a prolonged psychotic state after use. Suicides while under the influence of LSD have also been reported. Reports of chromosomal damage and teratogenicity have not been substantiated.

Phencyclidine (PCP, "Angel Dust"). Although no longer available commercially, this compound is easily manufactured in illegal laboratories. It is available as a white crystalline powder that may be ingested, snorted intranasally, dissolved and injected, or sprinkled on tobacco or marijuana and smoked. The onset of action is almost instantaneous with injection, but delayed for minutes to a half hour with smoking, inhalation, or ingestion. The duration of action may be prolonged, lasting hours to days with large doses. In addition, prolonged drug-related psychosis lasting up to a month has been reported.

In contrast to LSD, phencyclidine has the potential to cause serious physiologic disturbance. Effects of PCP include tachycardia, hypertension, ataxia, nystagmus, and dysarthria (see Chapter 97). Overdose is associated with seizures, coma, and respiratory arrest.

Mescaline (Peyote Cactus). This is a naturally occurring alkaloid found in the peyote cactus; it may also be synthesized. With great frequency, street drugs sold as mescaline are in fact other drugs, in particular, LSD or PCP.

Visual hallucinations most commonly follow mescaline use; auditory hallucinations are less common. The effects of orally ingested mescaline appear slowly and may persist for 12 to 18 hours. Use may result in pupillary dilatation; hypothermia and hypotonia are common. High doses frequently cause severe headaches; respiratory and cardiac depression and hypotension are rare. Teratogenic effects have been reported in laboratory animals but not confirmed in humans.

Psilocybin (Mushrooms). Certain mushrooms contain psilocybin and psilocin. These compounds have chemical structures and hallucinatory effects similar to LSD. The toxicity of these substances is extremely low. Dryness of the mouth and nausea are the only common side effects.

Jimson Weed. The plant *Datura stramonium* is known by a variety of names, including loco weed, devil's weed, stinkweed, and green dragon. Portions of the weed may be ingested, chewed, or smoked. The active ingredients include the belladonna alkaloid, atropine, and scopolamine. Beyond hallucinations and disorientation, the side effects of this drug are identical to atropine intoxication and include dry mouth, mydriases, hyperpyrexia, tachycardia, hypertension, and urinary retention. Although an occasional adolescent may require catheterization because of urinary retention, other aggressive therapy, including the administration of physostigmine, is rarely indicated. If sedation is necessary, phenothiazines are contraindicated because their additive anticholinergic effect may result in cardiovascular collapse.

BIBLIOGRAPHY

American Medical Association; Report of the Council on Scientific Affairs. JAMA 257:3110, 1987.

American Medical Association Committee on Alcoholism and Addiction; Dependence on amphetamines and other stimulant drugs. JAMA 197:1023, 1966.

Anon: Mescaline. PharmChem Newsletter 1:1, 1972.

Arnow R, Dane AK: Phencyclidine overdose: An emerging concept of management. JACEP 7:56, 1978.

Beck JE, Gordon DV: Psilocybin mushrooms. PharmChem Newsletter 11:1, 1982.

Bergman RL: Navajo peyote: Its apparent safety. Am J Psychiatry 128:51, 1971.

Bright GM, Hawley DL, Siegel PP: Ambulatory management of adolescent alcohol and drug abuse. Semin Adolesc Med 1:279, 1985.

Chasnoff IJ: Drug use in pregnancy: Parameters of risk. Pediatr Clin North Am 35:1403, 1988.

Cherubin CE: A review of the medical complications of narcotics addiction. Int J Addict 3:163, 1968.

Comerci GK, MacDonald DI: Prevention of substance abuse in children and adolescents. Adolescent Medicine—State of the Art Reviews 1:127, 1990.

Coupey SM, Schonberg SK: Evaluation and management of drug problems in adolescents. Pediatr Ann 11:653, 1982.

Johnston LD, O'Malley PM, Bachman JG: Illicit Drug Use, Smoking, and Drinking by America's High School Students and Young Adults, 1975–1987. Rockville, MD, National Institute on Drug Abuse, 1988.

Kandel D, Logan J: Patterns of drug use from adolescence to young adulthood: I. Periods of risk for initiation, continued use, and discontinuation. Am J Public Health 74:660, 1984.

Mace S: LSD. PharmChem Newsletter 7:1, 1978.

McGlothlin WH, Arnold DO: LSD revisited. Arch Gen Psychiatry 24:35, 1971.

National Research Council, Institute of Medicine, Division of Health Science Policy and Relman A (ed): Marijuana and Health. Washington, DC, National Academy Press, 1982.

Newcomb M, Maddahian E, Bentler P: Risk factors for drug use among adolescents: Concurrent and longitudinal analyses. Am J Public Health 76:525, 1986.

Shervette RE, Schydlower M, Tampe RM, Fearnow RG: Jimson "loco" weed abuse in adolescents. Pediatrics 63:520, 1979.

Smith DE, Wesson DR: Phenobarbital technique for treatment of barbiturate dependence. Arch Gen Psychiatry 131:1337, 1977.

Stephenson JN, Moberg MA, Daniels BJ, et al: Treating the intoxicated adolescent. JAMA 252:1884, 1984.

Substance Abuse: A Guide for Health Professionals. Elk Grove Village, IL, American Academy of Pediatrics, 1988.

Washton AM, Gold MS (eds): Cocaine: A Clinician's Handbook. New York, Guilford Press, 1987.

Weiner M: Inhalant abuse. PharmChem Newsletter 8:36, 1979.

Weiner MJ: Adolescent Substance Abuse—Risk Factors and Prevention Strategies. Maternal and Child Health Technical Information Bulletin, National Center for Education in Maternal and Child Health, February, 1991.

Yamaguchi K, Kandel D: Patterns of drug use from adolescence to young adulthood: II. Sequences of progression. Am J Public Health 74:668, 1984.

Yamaguchi K, Kandel D: Patterns of drug use from adolescence to young adulthood: III. Predictors of progression. Am J Public Health 74:673, 1984.

Psychosomatic Conditions

CHAPTER 112

Somatization, Conversion, and Related Disorders

RICHARD LIVINGSTON

Somatization means experiencing feelings as physical symptoms. A teenager says, "This class is a real headache" and the class may in fact give him or her a headache. Emotions, particularly when extreme, are experienced viscerally, for example, sadness fatigues, anger tenses, elation lifts, and fear contracts organs or whole organisms.

This chapter concerns adolescents who have symptoms for which no adequate of simple medical explanation is apparent; therefore a psychological etiology is presumed. Current psychiatric nomenclature includes three groups of conditions in this category: (1) somatoform disorders, for those adolescents who are genuinely experiencing symptoms, and (2) factitious disorders and (3) malingering for those adolescents whose symptoms are fabricated.

The conditions defined by the Diagnostic and Statistical Manual of Mental Disorders: Third Edition—Revised (DSM-III-R) and discussed in this chapter include somatization disorder, hypochondriasis, conversion disorder, body dysmorphic disorder, undifferentiated somatoform disorder, factitious disorder with physical symptoms, and malingering. Somatization disorder is a syndrome characterized by multiple medically unexplained physical symptoms. Hypochondriasis is an obsessional fear that one has a particular disease. Conversion disorder describes inexplicable physical symptoms. Body dysmorphic disorder is marked by preoccupation with some imagined defect in one's personal appearance. Undifferentiated somatoform disorder includes other presentations of one or only a few unexplained symptoms. Factitious disorder and malingering are characterized by the conscious fabrication of symptoms.

Among adults, relatively little epidemiologic information is available about these disorders, with the exception of somatization disorder, which is known to occur in 1% to 2% of women and much more rarely in men. Hypochondriasis is primarily identified in males. Factitious disorders and malingering also are somewhat more common in males. The sex ratios for the other disorders in this group are not known.

Even less is known about the epidemiology of these disorders in adolescents, and developmental issues complicate case identification. The monosymptomatic somatoform disorders—conversion disorder, hypochondriasis, and undifferentiated somatoform disorder—may

be relatively easier to identify because they tend to have acute or subacute onsets. The polysymptomatic somatization disorder has a more gradual onset, and the diagnosis may not be evident until later in its course.

Somatization disorder typically begins in adolescence, but as many as 20% of cases may begin earlier in life. Conversion disorder is uncommon in very young children, but it occurs at about 10 years of age and beyond and is about equally prevalent in both sexes before adulthood. Body dysmorphic disorder typically begins during adolescence but more commonly has its onset in early to midadulthood.

Factitious (feigned or fabricated) disorders among the very young are usually caused by someone else, as in the so-called Munchausen syndrome by proxy, in which another person (usually a parent) causes the adolescent's symptoms. Rarely is this true of adolescents, but there are recent reports of anorexia nervosa by proxy among adolescents. Usually, however, factitious symptoms during adolescence are fabricated by the adolescent.

Although there is much to learn about risk factors for the somatoform disorders, some information is available to identify individuals at risk for purposes of early identification and early prevention. A family history of criminality, alcoholism, or somatization disorder is one known risk factor. Abnormal illness behavior and unusual patterns of health care use in families are other factors that should raise the possibility. In some studies, conversion disorder is increased among young persons from impoverished rural families and in those whose parents are depressed or have anxiety disorders. The presence of comorbid conditions (discussed later) that are known to be associated with increased prevalence of somatoform disorders also constitutes a risk factor

CLINICAL MANIFESTATIONS

Somatization Disorder (Briquet Syndrome)

Somatization disorder consists of multiple physical complaints for which no medical basis is evident. These complaints are often presented dramatically and in exaggerated fashion but may also be presented with a striking degree of indifference. Associated features may include a vague and imprecise cognitive style, labile but shallow mood and affect, and seductive or other attention-seeking behavior. Interpersonal difficulties and discipline problems are common, and an additional diagnosis of conduct or oppositional defiant disorder may be warranted.

Attention deficit hyperactivity disorder is also very common in this group (see Chapter 106). Anxiety and depressive symptoms are often present, usually episodically and associated with obvious psychosocial stressors. These conditions should be diagnosed when present, because treatment varies with the specific comorbid symptom.

Two sets of criteria are used for the diagnosis of somatization disorder. The DSM-III-R criteria require a history of many complaints or a belief that one is sickly beginning early in life and persisting over time *and* at least 13 symptoms from a specific list. (Table 112–1). These symptoms are counted as significant only if (1) no medical cause has been found for the symptoms or the impairment, (2) the occurrence of the symptom has not been during a panic attack only *and* (3) the symptom has caused the individual to take medication other than over-the-counter pain medicines *or* see a doctor *or* alter his or her life in some way, such as missing a significant amount of school. The list of symptoms is divided into groups that include gastrointestinal symptoms, pain, cardiopulmonary symptoms, conversion or pseudoneurologic symptoms, sexual difficulties, and female reproductive symptoms. Seven particularly common symptoms have been identified as useful for screening, with the suggestion that the presence of two or more of these screening items indicate a high likelihood of the disorder. The screening items include (1) vomiting other than during pregnancy, (2) pain in the extremities, (3) shortness of breath when not exerting energy, (4) amnesia, (5) difficulty swallowing, (6) a burning sensation in the sexual organs or rectum other than during intercourse, and (7) painful menstruation.

Another set of criteria that is currently in use for somatization disorder is the Washington University research criteria for Briquet syndrome, which is more specific and more stringent than the DSM-III-R criteria, requiring 25 symptoms in at least 9 of 10 groups for a definite diagnosis and 20 symptoms for a probable diagnosis. The following lists the symptoms for the various groups: Group 1, frequent headaches or regarding oneself as sickly; group 2, pseudoneurologic symptoms; group 3, fatigue, a lump in the throat, weakness, and other miscellaneous symptoms; group 4, panic-type symptoms; group 5, gastrointestinal symptoms; group 6, abdominal pain and vomiting; group 7, menstrual problems; group 8, sexual difficulties; group 9, various pains; and group 10, symptoms of depression. Most of the available research on somatization disorder is from studies that use these criteria or the similar Research Diagnostic Criteria.

The associated histrionic personality features, relationship difficulties, and antisocial behaviors apparently are observed in adolescents with somatization disorder, regardless of the criteria by which they are identified. It

TABLE 112–1. Diagnostic Criteria for Somatization Disorder

A. History of many physical complaints or belief that one is sickly, beginning before age 30 and persisting for several years
B. At least 13 symptoms:
Gastrointestinal
　1. Vomiting (not pregnant)
　2. Abdominal pain (not dysmenorrhea)
　3. Nausea
　4. Bloating
　5. Diarrhea
　6. Food intolerance
Pain
　7. Pain in extremities
　8. Back pain
　9. Joint pain
　10. Pain during urination
　11. Other pain (excluding headaches)
Cardiopulmonary
　12. Shortness of breath at rest
　13. Palpitations
　14. Chest pain
　15. Dizziness
Conversion or pseudoneurologic
　16. Amnesia
　17. Difficulty swallowing
　18. Loss of voice
　19. Deafness
　20. Double vision
　21. Blurred vision
　22. Blindness
　23. Fainting or loss of consciousness
　24. Seizure
　25. Trouble walking
　26. Paralysis or weakness
　27. Urinary retention or difficulty urinating
Sexual
　28. Burning sensation in sexual organs or rectum (except during intercourse)
　29. Sexual indifference
　30. Pain during intercourse
　31. Impotence
Female reproductive (judged excessive)
　32. Painful menstruation
　33. Irregular menstrual periods
　34. Excessive menstrual bleeding
　35. Vomiting other than during pregnancy

With permission from American Psychiatric Association: Diagnostic and Statistical Manual of Mental Disorders, 3rd ed, revised. Washington, DC, American Psychiatric Association, 1987, pp 263–264.

is important to note, however, that the sets of criteria identify overlapping but not identical populations. In a research population at the author's center, for example, patients identified by DSM-III-R criteria seemed to have more symptoms in the pseudoneurologic and pain categories, whereas the patients who met criteria for Briquet syndrome appeared to have, in addition to a greater variety of complaints, more gastrointestinal symptoms, sexual difficulties, and mood problems.

Regardless of precise diagnostic criteria, the essentials for clinical diagnosis are the same: a complex medical history with a wide variety of medically unexplained physical symptoms.

Somatization disorder may begin before puberty in up to 20% of cases, but it more typically has its onset during middle to late adolescence. In younger children and adolescents, recurrent unexplained abdominal pain for which no medical cause is evident appears to be a

TABLE 112–2. Comparison of Somatization Disorder, Factitious Disorder, and Malingering

	SOMATIZATION DISORDER	FACTITIOUS DISORDER	MALINGERING
Presumed motive	No presumption necessary	Assume and maintain sick role	Overt personal gain
Source of signs and symptoms	Subjectively experienced	Fabricated or deliberately caused	Fabricated or deliberately caused
Predominant associated personality traits	Histrionic	"Unstable," borderline, mixed histrionic and antisocial	Antisocial
Comorbid psychiatric diagnoses	Attention deficit hyperactivity disorder, depression, anxiety, dissociative disorders	Personality disorder, substance abuse disorders	Conduct disorder, substance abuse disorders
Recommended treatment	Primary medical care with psychiatric consultations as needed	Psychiatric care desirable; patients often resistant	Diagnosis and disposition

common initial presentation, though this well-known childhood form of somatization also may present as an isolated complaint or in association with other psychiatric disorders, such as depression and separation anxiety. Since we know relatively little about the sequence of symptom development, any medically unexplained symptom should at least raise suspicion. It would also be prudent for the physician to have a high index of suspicion for somatization disorder developing in female patients with histrionic personality traits (see Chapter 109) and with the associated conditions of attention deficit disorder (see Chapter 106) and behavioral problems. A careful review of systems should be performed on a *regular basis*. As this list grows to include more and more unexplained symptoms for which the individual adolescent has sought care, missed school, or otherwise experienced impairment, the presence of the disorder is thus gradually confirmed (Table 112–2).

Hypochondriasis

Hypochondriasis is an anxiety-based disorder in which the adolescent presents with a preoccupation, specifically the fear or belief that he or she has a certain serious disease. These adolescents have had sensations or symptoms that they have interpreted as evidence of illness, but the physician's history and examination will not support the diagnosis of any disease that accounts for the reported symptoms.

The adolescent's fear or conviction of illness will persist after the physician has reassured him or her to the contrary. The DSM-III-R requires that the symptoms in question cannot merely be symptoms of panic disorder (see Chapters 102 and 103) (palpitations, chest pain, hyperventilation, tingling in the fingers or perioral region, and so on), that they must last at least 6 months, and that they cannot be of delusional intensity (beliefs

TABLE 112–3. Diagnostic Criteria for Hypochondriasis

Preoccupation with fear of having, or the belief one has, a serious disease
Lack of medical evidence to support diagnosis of physical disorder and symptoms are not just symptoms of panic attack
Fear or belief present despite medical reassurance
Duration of at least 6 months
Belief is not of delusional intensity

With permission from American Psychiatric Association: Diagnostic and Statistical Manual for Mental Disorders, 3rd ed, revised. Washington, DC, American Psychiatric Association, 1987, p 261.

are considered delusional when the individual is absolutely convinced they are true and will not acknowledge the possibility that they are not) (Table 112–3).

Associated features include a history of seeking care from several physicians, anxious or depressed mood, or both, and overattentiveness to the body and its functions (which is also common in the other somatoform disorders). Clinical experience suggests that currently common hypochondriacal fears among adolescents include acquired immunodeficiency syndrome (AIDS), other sexually transmitted diseases, pregnancy, skin cancer, and eating disorders. Any of these concerns may of course present in the much more common form of a milder concern, lacking the intensity and potential for impairment associated with diagnosable hypochondriasis.

Conversion Disorder

Conversion disorder describes the monosymptomatic somatoform disorder characterized by alteration or loss of physical function that is experienced and presents as a physical illness, classically neurologic, but instead is presumed to be psychological. The source of the symptom is presumed to be symbolic expression of a psychological need or resolution of a conflict.

Conversion symptoms may also appear as part of the clinical picture of somatization disorder, mood disorder, or schizophrenia; the diagnosis of conversion disorder is reserved for those cases in which these other disorders are not evident.

In addition to the loss or alteration of physical functioning, the DSM-III-R requires a temporal relationship between the symptom and an identifiable stressor (Table 112–4). The criteria also require that the individual must not be aware of intentionally producing the symptoms

TABLE 112–4. Diagnostic Criteria for Conversion Disorder

Loss of, or alteration in, physical functioning suggesting a physical disorder
Psychological factors judged causal because of temporal relationship between a psychosocial stressor that appears related to psychosocial conflict or need and the symptom
Person is not consciously or intentionally producing the symptom
Symptom is not culturally sanctioned and cannot be explained by a physical disorder
Not limited to pain or sexual functioning

Adapted with permission from American Psychiatric Association: Diagnostic and Statistical Manual of Mental Disorders, 3rd ed, revised. Washington DC, American Psychiatric Association, 1987, p 259.

TABLE 112–5. Diagnostic Criteria for Body Dysmorphic Disorder

Preoccupation with imagined defect in appearance in a normal-appearing individual
Belief not of delusional intensity
Not exclusively during anorexia nervosa or transsexualism

Adapted with permission from American Psychiatric Association: Diagnostic and Statistical Manual of Mental Disorders, 3rd ed, revised. Washington, DC, American Psychiatric Association, 1987, p 256.

and that the symptom cannot be explained as a culturally sanctioned response pattern (such as seizure-like behavior as a usual part of certain religious ceremonies.)

It is important to note that conversion symptoms are commonly noted in individuals who have a related physical disorder; the most common example of this in adolescence is probably pseudoseizures in individuals who have a seizure disorder (see Chapter 83). Pseudoseizures and paralysis appear to be conversion symptoms more often identified in males, whereas females are more likely to present with syncope.

In a classic presentation, the conversion symptom has an acute or subacute onset within hours, days, or weeks of the identified stressor, along with fairly obvious relationship to the stressor. For example, a conscientious teenaged boy might experience paralysis of the arm after experiencing the unacceptable desire to hit his mother, or an individual who has witnessed an overwhelmingly traumatic event might become blind.

Associated features may include striking indifference toward the symptom. A history of extreme stressors is often present but is not volunteered spontaneously. Unresolved grief after a death or other serious loss, is probably the most common stressor associated with conversion in adolescence.

Academic underachievement, depressed mood, dependent personality traits, and maternal overprotectiveness have all been associated with conversion disorder.

Body Dysmorphic Disorder

Body dysmorphic disorder, also known as dysmorphophobia, is an obsessional but not delusional preoccupation with some imagined defect in physical appearance. It most commonly involves the face or overall body build. The DSM-III-R requires that the symptoms are not present exclusively during the course of anorexia nervosa (see Chapter 60) or transsexualism (see Chapter 120) (Table 112–5).

Commonly, affected adolescents present to plastic surgeons, dermatologists, or otolaryngologists and request corrective surgery, or they present to physicians in primary care and request such a referral. Associated features include depressive symptoms and social anxiety.

The pattern of symptom development has not been well studied. Clinical experience suggests that individuals with histrionic personality traits who have an excessive concern for appearance or those with obsessive-compulsive traits that include perfectionism may be more susceptible.

Undifferentiated Somatoform Disorder

The category of undifferentiated somatoform disorder includes somatoform symptoms that do not fit into the preceding patterns. For this diagnosis, the DSM-III-R requires that physical complaints be present that either cannot be explained on the basis of a physical disorder or are grossly in excess of what would be predicted from physical findings. The overall disturbance must last for at least 6 months to meet these diagnostic criteria, though it is not required that any single symptom last that long. The DSM-III-R specifically excludes symptoms that occur exclusively during the course of another somatoform disorder, a specific sexual disorder, a mood or anxiety disorder, sleep disorder, or a psychotic state (Table 112–6).

This diagnosis includes a heterogeneous group of physical complaints, but it is important to note that it may initially be the most correct diagnosis in young persons who are early in the course of developing somatization disorder.

Factitious Disorder And Malingering

Factitious disorder is the diagnosis assigned when an adolescent feigns symptoms or intentionally produces signs or symptoms of illness because of a presumed psychological need to assume or maintain a sick role. The same is true of malingering, except that in malingering there is a recognizable overt personal gain, such as avoiding taking a test for which a student is unprepared or avoiding criminal charges. Malingering is not a psychiatric diagnosis but a conclusion about behavior. Factitious disorder, in contrast, is considered a psychiatric disorder.

The chronic and extreme form of factitious disorder is known as Munchausen syndrome. The condition in which a parent feigns or intentionally produces an adolescent's symptoms has been called Munchausen syndrome by proxy; this condition is usually identified in younger children, but it is important to note that it is occasionally seen in adolescence, with the parent ma-

TABLE 112–6. Diagnostic Criteria for Undifferentiated Somatoform Disorder

One or more physical complaints, e.g., fatigue, loss of appetite, gastrointestinal, urinary

Either:
 No organic pathologic condition identified to account for symptoms
 If related organic pathologic condition is present, symptoms or resultant impairment are in excess

Duration of at least 6 months

Not due to disorder of sexual dysfunction, mood, anxiety, sleep, psychosis, or another somatoform disorder

Adapted with permission from American Psychiatric Association: Diagnostic and Statistical Manual of Mental Disorders, 3rd ed, revised. Washington, DC, American Psychiatric Association, 1987, p 267.

neuvering to produce signs of illness without detection or even with the adolescent's awareness in the context of an extremely enmeshed and symbiotic parent-child relationship.

Common presentations of factitious disorder in the office or emergency room include abdominal pain, syncope, subjective fever, and complaints of blood in sputum, urine, or feces. The history may suggest some knowledge of medical terminology, but details will often be inconsistent and occasionally presented in the context of bizarre and apparently uncontrollable story telling, which has been called pseudologia fantastica.

The physician's suspicions are often aroused by excessive requests for pain medication or by the addition of new complaints when the initial presentation has been found to be without medical basis.

A wide variety of means are used to fabricate signs of disease and commonly include the introduction of blood or other foreign substances into specimens of urine or other body fluids, ingestion of drugs, self-injection with saliva or even feces, application of irritants to the skin, and use of a heating pad or hot liquids to elevate body temperature artificially. Even when observed directly in such behaviors, these individuals characteristically deny the allegation and leave the facility to seek care elsewhere.

Factitious disorder and malingering usually are not discovered immediately but become apparent more gradually as physical disorders are ruled out, suspicions are aroused, and confirming evidence is sought. Factitious symptoms are sometimes discovered in an individual who in fact has somatization disorder, supporting the concept that these disorders are in the same spectrum of conditions. More often, comorbid psychiatric disorders include conduct disorder, antisocial personality disorder or traits, histrionic traits, borderline personality, and so forth.

DIFFERENTIAL DIAGNOSIS

As long as the physician believes that there is significant uncertainty, the diagnosis can be considered (and labeled) provisional. Multiple diagnoses should be made when appropriate.

There are several uncommon medical disorders that may present, especially early in the course, with vague, fleeting or strange symptoms. Among them are systemic lupus erythematosus (see Chapter 90), multiple sclerosis (see Chapter 88), juvenile rheumatoid arthritis (see Chapter 90), acute intermittent porphyria, inflammatory bowel disease (see Chapter 63), Wilson disease (see Chapter 62), partial complex seizure disorder (see Chapter 83), or almost any degenerative central nervous system condition or autoimmune-inflammatory disorder. All of these disorders, like somatization disorder, tend to have a gradual onset, waxing and waning symptoms, and variable findings on objective physical and laboratory examination. Over time, the clinical picture will usually stabilize enough to make the diagnosis feasible, underscoring the need for ongoing care by one physician.

In as many as 30% of adults who appear to have a conversion symptom, a medical diagnosis will eventually be found to explain the previously unexplained phenomenon. Available evidence suggests that the number is much smaller among children and adolescents—that is, what looks like a conversion symptom probably is.

Somatization is common in several psychiatric disorders. Young persons with severe *separation anxiety disorder* or *depression* are prone to have several physical complaints, particularly stomachache, headache, and palpitations. This is also true, to a lesser extent, for the other anxiety disorders (overanxious disorders, avoidant disorder, social phobia);(see Chapter 103).

Very odd or unusual symptoms and conversion-like symptoms are sometimes reported by individuals with schizophrenia or other psychotic disorders. Dysmorphic body image of an extremely unusual nature or delusional in degree also raises the possibility of a psychotic disorder (see Chapter 110).

Panic disorder can begin in childhood or adolescence and may present during a panic attack with hyperventilation, palpitations, chest pain, tingling in the hands, perioral numbness, or other symptoms, or it can occur between attacks with a hypochondriacal concern about heart disease.

EVALUATION AND DIAGNOSIS

History

History-taking should always include the psychiatric and familial factors associated with these disorders, with focal questions as indicated for a particular diagnosis. Relationships, mood disorder, and substance use must be explored.

A thorough review of symptoms must be obtained regularly. Because the polysymptomatic somatization disorder often begins with a monosymptomatic version, the possible development of the more complex disorder must be pursued regularly even after a diagnosis of another somatoform disorder has been made. Any item answered positively must be pursued. "Did you miss school or work? Did you go to the doctor? Was there a diagnosis? Did you take medicine? If so, what was it?"

Interviewing individuals of any age who have somatization symptoms can be a frustrating experience and requires patience and a willingness to tolerate imprecision, vagueness, and some dramatics as well. The gen-

TABLE 112–7. "Red Flags": Indicators of Possible Somatoform Disorders

No signs of illness on examination when history strongly suggests there should be

Incapacity or distress not in proportion to findings (either too much or too little)

Signs or symptoms appear responsive to suggestion

Obvious temporal relation to stressor, life event, or threat

Prior history of unexplained symptoms

Associated psychiatric symptoms-disorders: depression, anxiety, conduct disorder, attention deficit hyperactivity disorder

Unusual medical knowledge on the part of adolescent or parent

Family history of alcoholism, criminality, somatization

eral approach is as described in this text, with a few extra points of emphasis.

1. The physician should assume, unless there is evidence of fabrication, that the adolescent experiences the symptoms as described and should refrain from questioning the reality of the adolescent's subjective experiences.

2. The cognitive style of many of these adolescent patients is such that it is useful to provide second chances periodically; for example, "Think back on what we have covered so far — is there anything else you remember that I should know?"

3. Since many adolescents with somatization symptoms are highly suggestible, leading questions should be avoided.

4. Hostile or flattering remarks about one's self or other physicians do not require a response but should be heard as expressions of frustration or hope.

5. The adolescent will usually provide the best information about his or her emotional symptoms (depression and anxiety); teenagers with somatization symptoms are often at one extreme or another in this area. Some are alexithymic—that is, unaware of emotions or unable to express them. Others are highly emotional and are much more accustomed to feeling than to thinking.

In addition to the current complaints and a review of systems and emotional symptoms, the adolescent should provide information about adaptive functioning (school attendance, academic performance, employment, sports, and other activities and friendships), and the impact of their symptoms on these areas and also on the family. Information about trouble with authority, other problem behavior, and substance use should also be included.

Often parents are better informants about behavioral difficulties than is the adolescent, and they will report instances that the youth will minimize, rationalize, or "forget." Parent interviews should also provide confirmation or expansion of information about the physical symptoms, past medical and developmental history, and the overall pattern of symptom development. It is particularly important to obtain the history of the quest for care and to get a sense of the adolescent's expectations and frustrations. Finally, relevant family medical history is pursued, followed by a basic inquiry about psychiatric disorders, alcoholism, and criminality in the immediate family and also in the previous two generations.

Whenever possible, it is wise to obtain medical records from other physicians and facilities. It is often helpful to see records of attendance and performance at school; having the adolescent take each report card to the office for copying can become expected routine.

Examinations

MEDICAL

A standard thorough physical examination must be performed on the initial visit to establish the relationship with the adolescent, to seek physical findings, and to provide a basis for comparison: physicians who are familiar with the usual "pseudoguarded" abdomen of a particular hysterical adolescent patient will quickly detect the difference if real peritonitis should occur.

With histrionic adolescents, it is worthwhile to have a professional present in the examining room during the examination. Histrionic adolescents frequently show social behavior that is perceived as seductive, which makes physicians uncomfortable. They are interested in approval not seduction, and the behavior is easily ignored when the physician and adolescent are not alone.

On subsequent visits when a full examination is not required, focal examination should be pursued to the extent required to determine whether there are signs associated with the reported symptoms.

Occasionally it is necessary to perform maneuvers to establish unequivocally the psychogenic origin of some particular symptom (Table 112–8). When required, it should be performed in a matter-of-fact way, not as confrontation or "proof" to convince the adolescent or family.

The mental status examination should be performed and recorded in detail, with examples and particular attention to appearance and manner (dramatic, eccentric, flighty), lability and depth of affect and its appropriateness to content, suggestibility, reality perception, preoccupations, emotional reactiveness and impulsiveness, suicidal ideation, cognitive style (vague or precise), egocentricity, judgment as reflected in behavior, and capability for good judgment as reflected in response to problems such as "What would you do if you smelled smoke in a crowded theater?"

A few specific mental status findings should be mentioned as associated with certain conditions, although none should be considered entirely specific or pathognomonic. Vorbeireden, the consistent giving of "near-miss" or approximate answers, is associated with factitious disorder. La belle indifférence, the display of incongruously little affect in describing pain or other symptoms, is common in somatoform disorders. Asthenia, a general state of fatigue, weakness, and lack of vigor, is often present in somatoform disorders but should also give rise to consideration of mood, anxiety, and endocrine disorders.

PSYCHOLOGICAL TESTING

Cognitive testing for intelligence and educational achievement should be requested if it has not recently been performed, because attention deficit disorder, learning disabilities, and academic underachievement in general are common in adolescents with somatization symptoms and may not have been identified previously, particularly in girls.

Personality testing may be useful in identifying or confirming patterns in relationships and behavioral style. The Minnesota Multiphasic Personality Inventory (MMPI) has hysteria (HY) and hypochondriasis (HS) scales, on which elevated scores may identify individuals with somatization disorder, whereas the often-associated behavioral disorders may generate an additional elevation on the Pd (psychopathic deviance) scale. Other patterns may be less suggestive of somatization disorder. One would expect a depressive, phobic, or obsessive

TABLE 112–8. Organic versus Nonorganic Neurologic Examination Findings

	ORGANIC	NONORGANIC
Anesthesia	More loss distally; gradual transition to normal; different level of loss for each sensation (e.g., touch proximal to pain); finger-nose or heel-shin coordination may be impaired by damaged proprioception; vibration sense follows whole bone	Uniform "stocking" or "glove" loss, may begin or end at anatomic landmark; withdrawal from painful stimuli when asleep; finger-nose–heel-shin coordination intact; loss of vibration sense follows claimed area of loss
Bilateral loss of vision	No tracking of tachistoscope	Involuntarily tracks tachistoscope
Unilateral loss of vision	With red glass over "good" eye, reads black letters but not red	Reads both red and black letters with red glass over "good" eye
"Tunnel vision"	Visual fields follow typical disease patterns	Visual fields same size regardless of distance from target
Deafness	No response in sleep to sudden loud noise	Response to sudden loud noise in sleep
"Whisper" speech	"Bovine" cough (abrupt and qualitatively different)	Loud normal cough
Paralysis-weakness		
General	"Classic" symptom picture specific to cause; does not move paralyzed part in sleep	Subjective impression of withholding strength; fluctuating weakness at different times; responds to suggestion; does not fit neuroanatomically; moves paralyzed part in sleep
	Sudden flexion or extension toward resistance followed by involuntary opposite movement	Sudden flexion toward resistance followed by extension or vice versa
Arms	When hand is held over face and dropped, it hits face	When hand is held over face and dropped, it falls to side of face
Legs	With examiner's hands on inner thighs of supine patient, the patient is instructed to resist with "good" leg; no response in other leg	With examiner's hands on inner thighs of supine patient, the patient is instructed to resist with "good" leg; other leg adductors contract
Gait	Patient circumducts affected leg	Patient drags affected leg, holds it

individual with a monosymptomatic somatoform picture to generate a profile more suggestive of depression or anxiety (see Chapter 99).

On the Tridimensional Personality Questionnaire, the two groups that one would predict to have somatization disorder are (1) high novelty-seeking, high reward-dependence, and low harm-avoidance (histrionic) and (2) low novelty-seeking, low reward-dependence, and high harm-avoidance (obsessional).

ETIOLOGY AND PATHOGENESIS

Somatization disorders are a heterogeneous group of disorders for which the available evidence suggests a multifactorial etiology.

A familial cluster pattern has been identified for somatization disorder: somatization, alcoholism, antisocial personality, and attention deficit hyperactivity disorder. Twin studies show greater concordance for somatization among monozygotic twins than among dizygotic twins, with co-twins also showing an increased prevalence of anxiety disorders. Further evidence for a genetic contribution comes from studies in which the daughters of alcoholic or criminal fathers who were adopted are clearly more likely to have somatization disorder.

There is also evidence that the origins of somatization disorder are not entirely genetic. Similarity of experience also influences the concordance rate in twins. There is evidence that parenting is significantly impaired in some adults who have somatization disorder, and parenting skills are certainly impaired by alcoholism and antisocial personality disorder. Attention deficit hyperactivity often persists throughout adult life, with symptoms including poor sustained attention and poor impulse control, neither of which is likely to improve the performance of parental duties. Both genetic and environmental components of the familial risk may be increased by the tendency toward assortative mating: individuals with somatization disorder, alcoholics, and individuals with criminal tendencies tend to marry one another; these marriages tend to be stormy and unstable, with frequent separation or divorce. The inability of some of these individuals to hold a job for long, frequent moves, and constant exposure to unpredictable adult behavior (sometimes including violence, physical abuse, or sexual victimization) create an environment that is unlikely to foster any strong sense of safety and security.

Adolescents with somatization disorder are much more likely to have experienced more negative life events than those who do not have this disorder.

Yet another environmental factor is the presence of models—that is, adults with medical symptoms from whom children and adolescents may model symptom formation (consciously or not) and from whom they learn how to behave when ill.

A separate issue associated with illness on the part of a parent or grandparent, particularly if the condition is perceived by the young person as life-threatening or debilitating, is the potentially extreme anxiety it can induce. Early adolescence usually corresponds with a blossoming ability for abstraction, which brings an altered awareness of time, a futuristic orientation, and the capacity to perceive death as permanent. With this new cognitive set, the possibility of mortality has greater impact on some individuals (see Chapter 9).

Conditioning and learning theory suggests other causes. One can hypothesize a primary gain (reduction of emotional distress) for many psychogenic symptoms, particularly conversion symptoms, and perhaps for all symptoms. Secondary gains (overt benefit) may also occur, with or without primary gain. Either or both will reinforce the illness behavior and continued assumption of the "sick role." The benefit of the sick role is that the adolescent is released from usual obligations, is absolved of responsibility for the condition, and is entitled to care. In a dysfunctional family, focusing on a sick member may restore equilibrium temporarily, another perhaps less obvious benefit. Physicians reinforce maintenance of the sick role (or somatization generally), in several ways, all of which are ordinarily thought of as "good doctoring," for example, by pursuing a medical explanation for a symptom through a progressively more expensive or invasive battery of procedures, by offering medical names for complaints resulting from somatization (e.g., "spastic colon") and by providing greater affect and social warmth to these individuals when they show distress.

Biologic factors that may contribute directly include those associated with the physical experience of the stress response or of anxiety in general (autonomic overactivity) and adrenalin symptoms. Abdominal pain, diarrhea, sweating, palpitations, chest pain, and a host of other symptoms may result.

Adolescents who have somatization symptoms report more adverse life events in general, but there may be a more specific association between somatization and sexual abuse. Some believe that sexually abused youth exhibit somatization symptoms and experience emotional distress, (compared with physically abused youth, who misbehave), so the possibility of sexual victimization must at least be considered in all cases.

In addition to these explanations of conversion, somatization is also considered psychodynamically to be a defense mechanism. One classic psychoanalytic theory holds that somatization symptoms function to maintain repression of an intolerable traumatic memory or unacceptable wish.

In the vast majority of cases, consideration of more than one of the etiologic factors will be helpful. The author hypothesizes that the key elements in the pathogenesis of somatization disorder include a genetic predisposition, attention deficit disorder, sexual abuse or other life events that provoke overwhelming anxiety, and positive reinforcement of illness behavior.

TREATMENT

General Considerations

Treatment goals are defined according to the natural history of the disorder. For acute or episodic disorders, it is reasonable to aim for a complete remission of symptoms and prevention of recurrence. Of the disorders discussed in this chapter, this applies to most cases of conversion disorder, mild cases of hypochondriasis, and nonchronic cases of undifferentiated somatoform disorder. For chronic conditions, more realistic treatment goals include reducing symptoms, preventing complications, and minimizing disability. This applies to somatization disorder, body dysmorphic disorder, factitious disorder, and the more severe cases of hypochondriasis and undifferentiated somatoform disorder.

Physicians should also think of maintaining a satisfactory physician-patient and physician-family relationship as a goal for all patients with somatization symptoms, which is often a truly challenging task. Great diplomacy is required to accurately communicate suspicions or conclusions about the nature of these illnesses without alienating the adolescent patient or the family. A few principles are included here: accept the adolescent's subjective experiences as stated (not applicable to malingering or factitious disorder), explain the somatoform disorder as a real disorder, and offer a concrete plan or treatment with the explanation of the diagnosis. Initial denials may not last, so keep the possibility of communication open to those who deny. Identification and treatment of underlying or comorbid psychiatric disorders is always indicated.

Most cases of somatoform disorders in adolescents will be best managed by primary care physicians, with consultation with a child and adolescent psychiatrist when indicated (see Chapters 24 and 98). In many cases, the primary physician will be tempted to refer the adolescent for psychiatric evaluation immediately, and for some individuals, this is wise (Table 112–9). In most instances, however, these patients and their families then discontinue treatment entirely or change primary physicians. "Doctor-shopping" is very common; physicians are advised to communicate with one another frequently about these individuals.

Many of these adolescent patients are suggestible and most are in need of positive reinforcement for healthy behavior. Praise is often *very* helpful, for example, admiring the "courage it takes to keep going to school every day despite your terrible cramps and back pain."

Although there are certainly indications for medication among adolescents with somatization symptoms (Table 112–10), certain characteristics of this group make caution imperative when using medicines. Drug abuse is a common complication, so careful record-keeping and a high index of suspicion are needed. The imprecise cognitive style and learning disabilities may interfere with understanding and remembering instruc-

---

TABLE 112–9. Indications for Psychiatric Consultation or Referral of Adolescents with Somatization Symptoms

1. Depression or Anxiety—Severe
   (a) Unresponsive to primary measures
   (b) Causing functional impairment
2. Suicidal Behavior
   (a) Attempt or plan, with low probability of rescue and high lethalness of method
   (b) Frequent attempts
   (c) Lack of psychosocial support system
   (d) Alcoholism or other addiction present or suspected
3. Hallucinations, delusions, or formal thought disorder
4. Factitious disorders
5. Self-mutilation (especially if more than one occasion)
6. Prominent dissociative symptoms
   (a) Trance-like states
   (b) Psychogenic amnesia
   (c) Responds at different times as if two or more different persons, apparently outside adolescent's awareness
7. Adolescent experiences overwhelming stressors or adverse events
8. Adolescent's behavior causing conflict among staff or other patients, or both

TABLE 112–10. Psychotropic Medications in Adolescent Somatoform Disorders

MEDICATIONS	INDICATIONS	CAUTIONS
Heterocyclic antidepressants	Severe depression, frequent panic attacks	Limit supply if suicidal or impulsive; simplify dosage schedule if possible (e.g., single dose at bedtime)
Fluoxetine, clomipramine	Obsessional preoccupations	Relatively new drugs; risks and benefits in this population not established
Stimulants (methyl-phenidate, d-amphetamine, pemoline)	Attention deficit hyperactivity disorder if causing significant academic-behavioral impairment	Methylphenidate and pemoline have less abuse potential than does amphetamine; parent dispensing doses and sustained-release forms may improve compliance when indicated
Benzodiazepines	Extreme, debilitating anxiety; alcohol detoxification (rarely in adolescents)	High abuse-dependence potential in this population; patients often resist attempts to discontinue
Propranolol	Social fears or other severe anticipatory anxiety	Usual side effects and asthma-allergy cautions
All classes	Best used when indications are firm, e.g., distress or impairment are significant	Patients tend to use multiple medications, so interactions can be an issue; cognitive vagueness requires careful education and reeducation; insist old psychotropics be disposed of

tions for medication use; written instructions, repeated verbal directions, and careful labeling may help. Noncompliance is common and should be checked periodically (see Chapter 26). Finally, because complaints fluctuate so in this population, medication should be reserved for clearly indicated target symptoms or signs of illness and should not prescribed "empirically" or to placate the patient with somatization symptoms.

Somatization Disorder

The principal treatment for somatization disorder includes brief and regular visits with the primary physician—frequent enough to minimize "doctor-shopping." Once every week or two will often suffice. In times of stress, more frequent visits will be needed. During these visits, the physician should attend to complaints, perform indicated examinations, inquire about life circumstances, and reinforce healthy behavior. *Medications and costly or invasive surgical or diagnostic procedures should be reserved for adolescents who have not only subjective complaints but also objective signs of disease.*

Like everyone else, the person with somatization can experience "real" medical problems, and the physician who knows the adolescent well usually will quickly detect the difference between the usual "functional" symptoms and the presentation with medical disorder.

The all-too-common suicidal behavior of some of these individuals is rarely medically or psychiatrically serious but requires thorough evaluation. Most often it is an overdose of medication or wrist-cutting, performed with a low probability of lethalness and a high probability of rescue, during a crisis in a relationship. Psychiatric hospitalization is not usually required and if it is deemed necessary, should be as brief as possible. Occasionally a comorbid major depression will be present, however; if it is, it should be treated aggressively as with any other major depression.

Occasionally the symptoms in a young person with somatization symptoms will cause such disruption of school routines that admission to day treatment or a hospital for intensive behavioral modification is indicated.

Hypochondriasis

Treatment of hypochondriacal young individuals is not well studied but should be undertaken on an individualized basis using basic principles. Hypochondriacal fears may seem to have either more of a phobic quality or more of an obsessive quality. The phobic quality will be evidenced by anxiety symptoms, which may include panic attacks or partial panic attacks, with fear of disease the dominant theme. These adolescents may respond to imipramine or other tricyclic antidepressants, or to phenelzine, alprazolam, and other agents typically used for panic attacks, alone or in conjunction with other treatments (behavioral treatments, such as systematic desensitization, or traditional psychotherapy). In the obsessive type of hypochondriasis, preoccupations, inability to banish the thought, compulsive reading about the disease, and ritualized "prevention" behaviors like excessive hand washing will be prominent. This form is more likely to respond to treatment with fluoxetine or clomipramine, as in obsessive-compulsive disorder (see Chapter 105).

In psychotherapy or counseling for hypochondriasis, the therapist should use an empathic, non patronizing method and a realistic and cognitive approach for most adolescents, leading them toward more realistic thinking without arguing with them unproductively.

Brief, regularly scheduled physician visits may minimize anxiety. Practical advice, such as for the adolescent to refrain from discussing his or her concerns over illness with friends, may help prevent social disability. Strong positive reinforcement for school attendance may help prevent academic failure in more chronic cases.

Conversion Disorder

Pseudoneurologic symptoms can be managed successfully by primary care physicians with assistance from a psychiatric consultant. Any underlying acute psychiatric disorder—for example, depressive illness—must be identified and treated aggressively. If a psychodynamic basis is hypothesized, the presumed underlying fear or conflict should be addressed in both individual and family therapy as indicated; this may require some continued psychiatric treatment.

"Lost" adaptive function can often be restored, without the adolescent feeling discounted or humiliated, through a short course of "therapy" coupled with strong positive suggestions that improvement is forthcoming and enthusiastic positive reinforcement for effort and success. Physical therapists and occupational therapists who are asked to provide restorative therapy must be fully informed of the plan. Prolonged loss of function can result in atrophy or contractures, which will improve with physical therapy.

Recurrence, lack of improvement, and emergence of new symptoms are not usual. They generally occur only when a chronic underlying psychiatric disorder is present (such as somatization disorder or schizophrenia) or when improvement will result in return to an intolerable situation (such as a home in which the adolescent is subject to ongoing physical or sexual abuse). These possibilities must be investigated when there is no improvement.

Body Dysmorphic Disorder

Because the preoccupations of body dymorphic disorder resemble obsessions, antiobsessional medications (clomipramine or fluoxetine) may be helpful in severe cases. Any other associated psychiatric disorder should be identified and treated first, since it is possible that such treatment will reduce the symptoms or their impact.

Regular brief office visits may be helpful, especially when social anxiety is high. During these visits, individualized interventions should be provided as needed. Individuals who fear their "defect" is growing may be helped by periodic photography and measurements. Some will need realistic information about mail-order "remedies," nutritional fads, and so on.

Psychiatric referral is not usually successful because the adolescent often will not accept it; such a referral should be considered only if the impairment is severe. The referral will most likely be followed through if the primary physician has a solid relationship with the patient before the suggestion is made.

Undifferentiated Somatoform Disorder

Adolescent patients with undifferentiated somatoform disorder are a heterogeneous group and should be treated using the principles given for the somatoform category most closely resembling their pathologic condition.

Factitious Disorders

In those rare instances in which an adolescent's factitious symptoms are produced by another individual (Munchausen syndrome by proxy), the top priority in treatment must be to keep the adolescent safe from further harm. In the hospital, the suspected offender should never be with the adolescent unless under direct professional observation. Legal measures through social agencies must be sought to provide continued protection.

When the adolescent is causing his or her own symptoms, consideration of other diagnoses may facilitate treatment. If the individual otherwise appears to have somatization disorder, treatment should follow the guidelines for somatization disorder but with a high index of suspicion for factitious origin of future symptoms. If, in contrast, the primary psychopathologic condition is a conduct disorder, which is fairly common among both young persons with factitious symptoms and malingerers, the general approach for conduct disorder will be more suitable (see Chapter 108).

The more deep-seated cases of factitious disorder, in which there is a frantic or desperate effort to stay under medical care at any cost, are fortunately rare among adolescents. Psychiatric referral should be attempted but will seldom be embraced unless the adolescent feels significantly anxious or depressed.

Communication among physicians can sometimes assist in the early identification of these adolescents and may decrease the probability of unnecessary exploratory surgery and other iatrogenic complications, but the use of aliases by these adolescent patients' and physicians' natural concerns about confidentiality can impede this informal communication process.

Malingering

Once malingering is discovered, disposition is the issue. If an underlying psychiatric or medical disorder is present, appropriate treatment should be offered. Disclosure of malingering to the parents is a clinical judgment to be made on an individual basis. Disclosure in most instances is recommended. This is particularly important in those cases in which the malingering is part of a pattern of dishonest behaviors and conduct problems and when the condition causes adverse impact upon the parents or others. Occasionally one sees less serious malingering by an otherwise "good kid in a bind"; after careful thought, the physician may elect to inform the adolescent patient privately of the findings and provide an opportunity for a "rapid and face-saving recovery."

BIBLIOGRAPHY

Ford CV: The somatizing disorders. Psychosomatics 27:327, 1986.
Goodyer I, Taylor DC: Hysteria. Arch Dis Child 60:680, 1985.
Guze SB, Cloninger CR, Martin RL, Clayton PJ: A follow-up and family study of Briquet's syndrome. Br J Psychiatry 149:17, 1986.
Livingston R, Taylor JL, Crawford SL: A study of somatic complaints and psychiatric diagnosis in children. J Am Acad Child Adolesc Psychiatry 27:185, 1988.
Monson RA, Smith GR: Somatization disorder in primary care. N Engl J Med 308:1464, 1983.
Volkmar FR, Poll J, Lewis M: Conversion reactions in childhood and adolescence. J Am Acad Child Psychiatry 23:424, 1984.
Weller RA, Weller EB, Herjanic B: Adult psychiatric disorders in psychiatrically ill young adolescents. Am J Psychiatry 140:1585, 1983.

CHAPTER 113

Psychogenic Pain Conditions

PATRICK J. McGRATH and JOANNE GOODWIN

Historically, *psychogenic pain* has referred to pain accompanied by major disruptions in lifestyle for which no organic cause could be found. The condition, as thus understood, is inherently ill-defined because one of the essential features, the lack of a physical cause, involves negative evidence and makes no allowances for the fact that pain can be of unknown origin. Many pains reported by adolescents are of unknown origin and may be due to normal variation in physiologic functioning rather than organic or psychological disease (see Chapter 16).

The American Psychiatric Association altered the criteria for a diagnosis of psychogenic pain in the Diagnostic and Statistical Manual of Mental Disorders: Third Edition—Revised (DSM-III-R). The disorder labeled *psychogenic pain disorder* in the DSM-III, which was published in 1980, was renamed *somatoform pain disorder* in the DSM-III-R. The authors state that this change was made to acknowledge that "the disorder frequently appears in the absence of clear evidence of the etiologic role of psychological factors."

The criteria for a diagnosis of psychogenic pain disorder in the DSM-III included the presence of clear evidence that psychological factors were involved in the etiology, through either an obvious temporal relationship between pain and an environmental stimulus (with the pain allowing avoidance of an unpleasant activity) or a condition in which the presence of pain enabled the person to receive support.

In contrast, the DSM-III-R criteria require only that (1) an individual (in this instance, an adolescent) be preoccupied with pain for at least 6 months and (2) that there be no evidence of an organic pathologic condition or a pathophysiologic mechanism that accounts for the pain, or if an organic pathologic condition is present, the individual's response must appear highly exaggerated in light of the apparent physical cause (Table 113-1).

In the International Classification of Diseases (ICD), psychogenic pain is defined as pain with mental origin. The assumption that pain is psychologically induced is made when more specific psychiatric or medical diagnoses are not possible.

The definition of pain of psychological origin according to the International Association for the Study of Pain implies that positive evidence for psychological causation is required but does not provide any guidelines for determining psychogenicity. In summary, current diagnostic criteria for psychogenic pain require only a diagnosis of exclusion—that is, simply the lack of or-

ganic cause in the presence of unexplained social or psychological problems. As such, these criteria define a "catchall" category, a diagnostic label that can be applied when investigations fail to yield positive evidence for another disorder. Unfortunately, the diagnosis of somatoform pain disorder is not much clearer. Although it does have the advantage of not insisting that the pain is psychogenic, somatoform pain disorder does imply that there is a psychological substrate.

We propose that clearer criteria for psychogenic pain be established and that the impact of the disorder be separated from the cause. The diagnosis of psychogenic pain should be made on the basis of positive evidence—that is, the role played by psychological factors in the genesis of the pain must be clear. Generally, this involves observation of a temporal relationship between a specific event or noxious stimulus and the onset of pain. Such a temporal relationship in the occurrence of pain is the only reasonable way to diagnose psychogenicity. Diagnoses lacking such positive evidence may well be incorrect.

The diagnosis of psychogenic pain does not rule out organic disease. Because psychogenic and organic disorders can coexist, the diagnosis of one does not rule out the possibility of the other. Moreover, disease that has a clearly organic cause may be responsive to stress without being caused by psychological factors.

When it does occur, psychogenic pain is not intentionally produced; it may be of equal intensity and causes as much suffering as pain of organic origin.

The second aspect of what is usually termed *psychogenic pain* is the impact of the pain on the social role. The World Health Organization (WHO) has developed a classification system for the consequences of disease (International Classification of Impairment, Disabilities, and Handicaps). The classification itself is not particularly useful for adolescent pain, but the model upon which it is based is very useful. According to this model, disease and its effects can be conceptualized as occurring in four planes of experience. The first plane is that of the occurrence of an abnormality (disease). The second plane of experience occurs when someone (usually the affected individual) becomes aware of the abnormality or a symptom develops. Pain would be one such symptom. This is termed an *impairment*. The third plane of experience, *disability*, occurs when there is "any restriction or lack (resulting from an impairment) of ability to perform an activity in the manner or within the range considered normal." The fourth plane of experience,

TABLE 113–1. Diagnostic Criteria for Somatoform Pain Disorder

Preoccupation with pain for at least 6 months
Either:
No organic pathology or pathophysiologic mechanism to account for the pain
If related organic pathology is present, the complaint or resulting impairment is grossly in excess of expected

With permission from American Psychiatric Association: Diagnostic and Statistical Manual of Mental Disorders, 3rd ed, revised. Washington, DC, American Psychiatric Association, 1987, p 266.

handicap, occurs when the experience is socialized. Handicaps are concerned with the social disadvantages experienced by the individual as a result of impairments and disabilities.

In summary, impairments are at the organ level, disabilities are at the level of the person, and handicaps are at the level of the social role. Adolescents who are described as having psychogenic pain frequently have extensive handicap, primarily in school, peer, and family relationships. Table 113–2 provides two examples of pain (headache and back pain) and the causes and consequences in the light of the WHO model.

Confusion arises when there is discordance within planes of experience or across planes of experience. For example, if a physician receives a report from an adolescent of pain from headache, but the adolescent is smiling while giving the report, the behavior and the self-report are discordant. Similarly, if an adolescent has a disease or a disorder that is not expected to cause pain, and yet there is a high level of pain reported, the clinician is likely to be in a quandary. As we have insisted, this confusion is not a reasonable reason to label the pain *psychogenic*. For example, smiling while reporting headache may be caused by anxiety. Discordance should be an occasion for further assessment.

Conceptualizing the cause of the pain and the handicap resulting from the pain as independent phenomena frees the clinician to formulate a specific plan to address both the psychological cause of the pain and to reduce or eliminate the handicap. The two are independent and both must be targeted.

The epidemiology of psychogenic pain is not known. However, there is good evidence that most of the more prevalent pain problems occurring in adolescents—for example, recurrent abdominal pain and migraine—arise in psychologically normal adolescents. Moreover, the prevalence of handicap, as evidenced by school absence

TABLE 113–2. Headache and Back Pain and Their Causes and Consequences (International Classification of Disabilities, Impairments, and Handicaps)

DISEASE OR DISORDER	IMPAIRMENT	DISABILITY	HANDICAP
Organic cause	Pain	Activity or ability	Social function
Migraine	Headache	Inability to study	Educational failure
Unknown	Back pain	Difficulty participating in sports	Peer isolation

due to at least one common pain, headache, is very low. We believe that psychologically caused pain with serious handicap is quite rare in adolescents. However, adolescents who do have psychogenic pain with handicap are likely to seek medical care repeatedly and thus will be overrepresented in medical settings.

CLINICAL MANIFESTATIONS

Psychologically caused pain with handicap may be manifested as abdominal pain, headache, dysmenorrhea, or limb, chest, or back pain that results in school, peer or family handicap, or all of these.

The most easily determined handicap is school or work handicap, which is evidenced by excessive absenteeism. The occurrence of pain that results in school absence is often termed *school phobia* (see Chapter 103). With young children, the pain is usually easily overcome by insistence on return to school. In adolescence, the pain is usually much more firmly established; the dynamics are likely to be more complex, and the pain will not disappear so easily. A handicap in peer relationships is difficult to assess in adolescents because many adolescents will claim to have numerous friends even if they are isolated from or neglected by their peers. Withdrawal from family relationships and duties can also constitute a handicap. Assessment of handicap in family functioning is usually made on the basis of reports from family members. The degree of handicap is not related to the amount of pain, or is handicap always related to disability (the specific activities interfered with by pain).

Although migraine headaches are excluded by both the ICD and DSM-III-R manuals because causality can be traced to physiologic factors, there is no evidence that psychologically caused migraine headache with handicap is really different from other forms of pain with handicap.

Associated features may include "doctor shopping" as a consequence of failure to find adequate pain relief. Some adolescent patients experience iatrogenic complications, with particularly excessive use of analgesics or minor tranquilizers. Excessive use of analgesics is often associated with continuous headache. For this reason, a careful survey of all medication being taken is important. Adolescents who are taking analgesics regularly without relief should be weaned by gradual reduction. An initial increase in headaches should be anticipated. Chronic use of minor tranquilizers has no place in pain relief and should be eliminated gradually.

DIFFERENTIAL DIAGNOSIS

Adolescents who have pain from serious organic causes can also be suffering from frank psychological problems; the identification of one problem does not rule out the existence of the other.

Pain may be experienced by individuals suffering from psychotic disorders, but it is not usually the predominant feature. Pain and depression (see Chapter 100) frequently coexist, and the predominance of one or the other is not always clear. However, it is probably best to treat each rather than assume that one is the result of the other.

Adolescents may experience physical symptoms involving pain, such as headaches or stomachaches as part of a posttraumatic stress disorder (see Chapter 104). In such cases, the cause of symptoms may be linked to the experience of a highly stressful event (e.g., sexual abuse) in the past (see Chapter 118).

In conversion disorder, the primary feature involves a loss of or alteration in physical functioning (e.g., conversion blindness) (see Chapter 112). Alteration in functioning or a usual pattern of symptoms is not sufficient to diagnose conversion disorder.

Malingering and factitious disorder involve the intentional production of symptoms in order to achieve a desired goal. Psychogenic pain is not intentionally produced. These conditions are rare (see Chapter 112).

DIAGNOSIS

The diagnosis of psychologically caused pain with handicap requires a relatively detailed understanding of the events and responsibilities in the adolescent's life to clarify psychological factors that led to the development of pain. The best evidence for psychogenic pain is derived when the pain is related temporally to other events. For example, pain that begins following a family argument or prior to attending school, may be psychogenic. Pain diaries (Table 113–3), in which antecedent and consequent events in relation to pain are recorded over time, can be helpful (see Chapter 16). They can provide clear evidence of psychogenicity if pain is related to events. A diary will provide the adolescent with a better understanding of the relationship between pain and life situations. Diaries can also provide a useful starting point for physician-adolescent discussions.

In many cases, neither a psychological nor an organic cause will be found for the pain. It is often difficult for both the physician and the adolescent to tolerate acknowledgement that a specific cause has not been found, but we believe that honest communication promotes a cooperative approach to the problem.

Establishing rapport with an adolescent is particularly important in order to facilitate gathering sufficient information to make a positive diagnosis. A very thorough history and careful physical examination serve both to gather information and to build rapport. Comments that may create defensiveness, such as the implication that the pain is not real or the suggestion that "It is all in your head," must be avoided; rather the physician should attempt to gather information and provide advice in a nonjudgmental, supportive fashion. The strategy should be to develop a collaborative relationship with the adolescent and the family. Finally, the adolescent's experience of pain should not be underrated in any way simply because an organic cause is not apparent.

With the difficulties in documenting details regarding the adolescent patient's life prior to the onset of pain, and the advantages of obtaining a broad picture of the family's style and functioning, interviewing parents is most helpful. It is important to avoid blaming the family for the adolescent's pain. Efforts should be made to focus on familial strengths rather than weaknesses and to emphasize methods in which the family unit can help the adolescent understand and cope with the pain. The extent and limit to which information is confidential must be discussed with both the adolescent and the parents (see Chapter 20).

In adolescents for whom school activities are involved, corroborating information should be obtained from teachers regarding the patient's academic progress, including recent changes in the ability of the adolescent to respond to academic demands. Information regarding interpersonal qualities and possible peer difficulties should also be sought. Usually, a series of telephone calls is the most effective and efficient way to obtain these data.

School absence should be determined accurately by specific questions. General questions such as, "Are you missing much school?" are likely to be responded to by equally general answers such as "No, not much."

ETIOLOGY

Since psychogenic pain is the outcome of psychological factors, the cause varies from adolescent to adolescent and is generally not attributable to one particular causal agent but rather to the interaction of current stresses, personality and family factors, and the adolescent patient's psychosocial history. Three general factors that contribute to the cause of psychogenic pain will be considered here: (1) anxiety, (2) family variables, and (3) social learning processes.

Anxiety

It has long been recognized that stress may precipitate or exacerbate pain. The mechanism by which one or more stressful events engender psychogenic pain is unclear; however, it has been suggested that autonomic changes may mediate an alteration in muscle tension or vascular changes. Physiologic changes occurring with the

TABLE 113–3. Antecedent-Consequence Pain Diary

DATE-TIME	WHAT HAPPENED BEFORE THE PAIN?	LEVEL OF PAIN 0–10 (10 = WORST)	WHAT HAPPENED THEN?
Feb 22—7 A.M.	Woke up for school	6	Argued with mother
Feb 22—7:15 A.M.	Went to bed	7	Slept until 10 A.M., then went to mall
Feb 22—9:30 P.M.	Went home	5 then 7	Went to bed

experience of one traumatic event may then be triggered when similar events are experienced (see Chapter 102). Circumstances that trigger the anxiety-pain response in adolescents include academic demands, social stressors, and family distress.

Psychogenic pain may serve as an avoidance or escape mechanism when a student experiences anxiety related to school attendance. Performance anxiety relating to academic expectations may be an outcome of undetected learning disabilities (Chapter 107). The experience of pain provides the adolescent relief from the frustration and anxiety of trying to keep up academically because it justifies absenteeism. School phobia is usually accompanied by pain, but the pain may or may not play a prominent role in the disorder. School phobia in adolescents is most likely to be accompanied by a history of absenteeism and a troubled or unstable family background (see Chapter 103).

Sexual abuse has been implicated as an etiologic factor in some cases of psychogenic pain, but the extent of this relationship is not known (see Chapter 118).

Overall, however, the evidence that stress plays a major role in the etiology of pain is mixed. One group of investigators studied a population of children and adolescents suffering from recurrent abdominal pain and found little evidence that stress contributed to pain. Another group examined adolescents with headaches and found that anxiety and stress levels were no different from those of the control group. In contrast, however, one investigator found a significant relationship between stress levels and pain. This study examined 2000 adolescents over a 17-month period and found an interaction among stress, gender, and pain symptoms. Girls manifested more symptoms, and life events and interpersonal problems were significantly correlated with symptoms. Additionally, it was found that adolescents in families experiencing discord were more likely to report somatic symptoms.

The Family

Using a systems model, family therapists have delineated common aspects in families who exhibit psychosomatic tendencies. The most outstanding feature is the enmeshed system in which they function. Family relationships are characterized by constant intrusion into each others' lives, weak boundaries between members, and extreme proximity. Personal autonomy is subjugated to demands for family loyalty. Typically such families are child-oriented and overprotective, with an abnormal amount of attention being focused on the adolescent's psychological and physiologic functioning. If the adolescent experiences pain, possibly as a function of intense somatic concerns within the family, members tend to mobilize in an attempt to protect the adolescent, thus rewarding the behavior. Both pain and handicap may become absorbed into the family system, and the illness becomes the adolescent's "identity card"; thus the family system maintains pain and handicap.

We have studied adolescents with chronic nonmalignant pain who were missing school. The adolescents in this study were required to perform an exercise task while their mothers supervised. Mothers of adolescents with handicap were more intrusive (both discouraging and encouraging their children more often) than were mothers of adolescents without handicap. The direction of the effect is not clear, however. The overinvolvement displayed by the mothers of adolescents who were missing school may be either the cause or the result of the handicap.

Social Learning Processes

Social learning processes, which include modeling, reinforcement, and punishment, are assumed to influence both the display of pain behaviors and the use of coping skills. These processes have been studied in adult populations, but as yet little research has been directed toward the adolescent population. Psychogenic pain is sometimes maintained when pain behavior is directly rewarded, for example, when an adolescent is allowed to remain home from school because of pain and spends the day watching television. Parental modeling probably plays a role in the likelihood of an individual adolescent experiencing psychogenic pain with handicap. Adolescents who have problems with pain often report that their parents experienced problems with pain as well, but the data for familial aggregation of most pains or handicap from pain are not very strong. The relative contributions of biologic and social learning factors are not clear.

TREATMENT

Treatment of psychogenic pain with handicap presents many challenges. Treatment can be directed toward the presumed causes of the problem or toward the symptoms. The primary care physician has both medical and psychological strategies available for intervention. Low-dose amitryptyline is the most widely accepted and validated medical treatment (see Chapter 125). A flexible dosage schedule may maximize the effectiveness and help reduce the side effects. The use of analgesics is not widely recommended. As already mentioned, adolescents who are using analgesics, such as acetaminophen or other nonsteroidal anti-inflammatory drugs, on a daily basis may experience headache. These adolescents are likely to benefit from elimination of all analgesic use. The occasional use of analgesics may be helpful, however, and is unlikely to be harmful. The use of opioids is controversial. The conventional wisdom is that opioids should never be used. However, some investigators have reported on the successful long-term use of opioids in adult patients with a variety of noncancerous pain syndromes. No comparable work with adolescents has been reported. We suggest caution (see Chapters 16 and 111).

Some primary care physicians do not consider themselves competent in the psychological treatment of adolescents who have pain. However, there is an important role for the primary care physician in caring for adolescents who do have psychogenic pain and handicap. Firm expectations that pain does not necessarily lead to handicap and therapeutic optimism that the pain will get better are key elements of the psychological treatment. If pain and handicap continue, especially if no definitive cause can be found, referral for further mental health and physical investigation is warranted. Frequently there are major difficulties in convincing the family that a mental health referral is appropriate. Families usually interpret such a referral as an indication that they are not believed or are thought to have mental illness.

We have found that a mental health referral framed in terms of routine procedure for all who are handicapped by pain is usually accepted (see Chapter 24). In addition, referral for evaluation of both organic and psychological aspects of the problem should proceed simultaneously. If one refers adolescents who have pain for psychological investigation only after all medical investigations have produced negative results, handicap may be more firmly established because of social isolation and school failure. The referral may be seen by both the adolescent and the parents as one of desperation, "We cannot find anything wrong with you so we are sending you to the 'shrink'." Finally, the primary care physician should continue to follow adolescents who are referred to a mental health specialist. Follow-up is useful for coordination and explanation of consultations, as well as for reducing the sense of abandonment that the adolescent may feel (see Chapter 24).

Specific behavioral interventions are often most appropriate when the disorder is clearly related to a specific anxiety-inducing agent or situation, as may be the case in pain related to school or performance anxiety (see Chapter 124).

Psychogenic pain that is related to interpersonal difficulties or family stresses may benefit most from family therapy (see Chapter 123). There are no data to favor one specific form of brief therapy over another. The quality of the therapist and his or her skill in dealing with adolescents who have pain and their families may be the most important factor. Often the objective of family therapy in such cases is to enhance the adolescent's sense of autonomy and independence and to challenge the enmeshed family system. Treating such families is often difficult; change does not occur quickly and the families may be disinclined to remain in therapy.

Individual therapy is beneficial in helping the adolescent who has pain to cope with the condition by changing attitudes and behaviors. Even though there may be issues of confidentiality that must be addressed, we have found that involving the parents in regular updates on the progress of therapy is often extremely helpful.

COURSE OF ILLNESS AND PROGNOSIS

The course of psychogenic pain with handicap is not known. It may appear suddenly, following a minor illness or injury, and then gradually increase in severity. There is often a tendency for the individual to assume an invalid's role. Adolescents may therefore become increasingly restricted in their social roles if successful intervention is not provided. Little is known, however, about long-term outcome.

BIBLIOGRAPHY

American Psychiatric Association: Diagnostic and Statistical Manual of Mental Disorders, 3rd ed; revised. Washington, DC, American Psychiatric Association, 1987.

Aro H: Life stress and psychosomatic symptoms among 14 to 16 year old Finnish adolescents. Psychol Med 17:191, 1987.

Collin C, Hockaday JM, Waters WE: Headache and school absence. Arch Dis Child 60:245, 1985.

Cooper PJ, Bawden H, Camfield PR, Camfield R: Anxiety and life events in childhood migraine. Pediatrics 79:999, 1987.

McGrath PJ, Unruh AM: Pain in Children and Adolescents, Vol 1. Pain Research and Clinical Management. New York, Elsevier, 1987.

McGrath PJ, Goodman JT, Firestone PR, et al: Recurrent abdominal pain: A psychogenic disorder? Arch Dis Child 58:888, 1983.

Merskey H (ed): Classification of chronic pain: Descriptions of chronic pain syndromes and definitions of pain terms. Pain 3(Suppl):S1–S226, 1986.

Pilowsky I, Barrow CG: A controlled study of psychotherapy and amitryptyline used individually and in combination in the treatment of chronic intractable "psychogenic" pain. Pain 40:3, 1990.

Portenoy R, Foley KM: Chronic use of opioid analgesics in nonmalignant pain: Report of 38 cases. Pain 25:171, 1986.

World Health Organization: International Classification of Impairments, Disabilities and Handicaps. Geneva World Health Organization, 1980.

Nonpsychiatric Conditions with Psychological Implications

CHAPTER 114

Adoption

ADELE D. HOFMANN

Estimates of the total United States adoptee population—children, teenagers, and adults—range between 2.5 and 5 million individuals. The June 1980 Current Population Survey and the 1981 National Health Interview Survey reported 2.1% to 2.9% of all children in the United States to be adopted and 3.8% of married couples to have an adopted child in the home.

The fact of adoption is a very real issue in the lives of a substantial number of adolescents, and one that significantly complicates progress through normal developmental tasks. The reality of a dual parentage, the experience of early life abandonment, and limited knowledge about one's genetic, biologic, and cultural past all make the inevitable questions of "Who am I?" and "Where did I come from?" much more difficult to answer than they are usually during adolescence. Adoptive parents also face issues of their own, particularly when challenged by their sexually maturing adopted adolescents. These include reactivation of the parents' sense of loss over their own infertility, fear of loss of their adopted adolescent's love, and parents' concern over emergence of unknown genetic history eventuating in problem behavior. Adopted adolescents who want to know about their origins in detail or who wish to contact their birth mothers are particularly apt to provoke parental anxiety.

For many years, the typical model for adoption was that of a single young woman who bore an out-of-wedlock child and placed the child for adoption in infancy because she was unable to support the baby; the infant was then adopted by an infertile couple. At the time of adoption, the biologic parent surrendered all custodial rights voluntarily, and the adoptive parents assumed full legal guardianship. The adoptee probably was told about his or her entry into the family at approximately 5 years of age, when he or she first asked, "Where did I come from?" But since that time parents and child had never discussed the adoption again.

Traditional social policy once considered early and permanent severance of all ties between the biologic parents and the adoptee as a necessary step in providing the best possible outcomes. It was believed that only in this way would the child bond with the new family effectively, the adoptive parents unreservedly commit themselves to the child, and the biologic parent put her "mistake" behind her and move on with her life. Adoptees who wanted more information about their birth parents or even sought reunion were generally perceived as being emotionally disturbed. More contemporary perspectives, however, provide a different view.

There are, of course, many variations on this model, such as cross-cultural adoptions, transracial adoptions, adoptions of older children, adoptions of those who are disabled, and adoptions of "hard-to-place" children and adolescents. Open adoption is another, relatively new option, in which the identities of all participants are known to each other and varying degrees of contact are maintained. Although each of these alternatives raises specific issues, space limits this discussion to the basic paradigm.

DEVELOPMENTAL ISSUES IN ADOPTION

Cognitive Conceptualization of Adoption

The adoptee's conceptualization of what being adopted means is highly dependent on cognitive maturation and shifts dramatically from early childhood to adolescence. Preschoolers do not distinguish between birth and adoption as paths to parenthood. It is not until around age 6 years that children are capable of perceiving the difference, but even then they cannot appreciate the reason for it. Between the ages of 8 and 11 years, the child's concept expands to include a beginning awareness of the motivation of the parents to have the child, but this is limited to the perception that the adoptive parents want a baby to care for and love. The actual origins of the baby are only vaguely appreciated and tend to be limited to either the biologic parents' untimely death or their dire poverty.

Only with the cognitive maturity of middle adolescence is there a relatively sophisticated and abstract appreciation of adoption as a sociolegal form of substitute child care based on protecting the rights and welfare of the child, of infertility as a reason to adopt, and of nonmarital birth and parental immaturity as reasons for surrender. Consequently, explanations and information given in preschool years will be inadequate answers if presented to the young person and can be a precipitating factor in an adolescent's wish to search for his or her birth parents.

Adoption and the Stage of Family Romance

As children advance into the stage of latency, they normally go through a period in which they become disappointed in their parents (see Chapter 9). Formerly idealized parents are now perceived as being less than perfect and as being capable of making mistakes. The child's realization that the adults he idealizes and depends on for nurture, protection, and love are just plain ordinary human beings is a major disillusionment. In countering this realization, adolescents ordinarily go through a stage in which they devalue their parents, demoting them in status, and elaborate the thought that they themselves may have been adopted, stolen, or separated from parents of aristocratic or even royal birth. All the good attributes once assigned to the real family are now transferred to this fantasied paragon family. The ultimate dream is that one day reunion will occur and the adolescent will be restored to his rightful status and regal life.

This fantasy performs several functions. First, it reduces any anxiety due to incestuous and aggressive impulses that the adolescent may have toward his or her parents by lessening feelings of parent-child intimacy and placing distance between them. For the same reasons, it can serve to help the adolescent achieve independence from the absolute authority of parents. It also can represent an attempt at compensating for the loss of idealized parental love as age brings more realistic assessment.

For the average youngster, this illusion can be very consoling and assists him or her in smoothly and safely progressing to a more mature stage. The fantasy is safe because he or she knows at heart that these thoughts are just make-believe and that they ultimately will be surrendered.

This is not the case with an adopted child, where an initial abandonment did indeed take place. It also is possible that he or she, in fact, could be returned to the biologic home. At the same time, the youngster is now at the stage in which he or she is beginning to be aware that his or her origins were not romantically ideal and that life would not necessarily be any better if he or she returned to his or her beginnings. There may even be an early appreciation of the fact that his or hers was not a wanted birth. It may be very difficult for some adoptees to negotiate this developmental stage, because the reality of fantasied possibilities is too threatening and may be one of the factors contributing to later adolescent acting-out behaviors.

Gender Differences

Adopted girls are much more keenly interested in their origins and in much more conflict about it than are boys. Indeed, boys often seem to be quite indifferent. This difference probably is not so much caused by being adopted but rather comes from the identification conflict experienced by a girl whose adoptive mother—and role model—is unable to bear children, as do other women. In establishing her identity, the adopted adolescent female must first identify with her mother and imitate her behaviors. She must then go one step further and achieve a sense of bodily integrity and generativity by developing the confidence that she is more whole than her mother and *is* capable of bearing a child. This is not

a concern for the boy, because paternal infertility is not very obvious and he can model himself after his father without any sense of incompleteness. As a consequence, young women are much more likely to initiate a search for their birth parents than are young men.

Adolescent Developmental Tasks

Adopted adolescents commonly, even normatively, experience feelings of uncertainty and incompleteness about their identities due to a lack of knowledge about their biologic and genetic pasts, with the result of compromised self-esteem. This issue has been referred to as identity "lacunae" or genealogic bewilderment. Anxiety and confusion are heightened further when the natural parents are perceived as inferior because they could not take care of the adoptee and gave him or her up; when there is the fear of possible genetic handicap; and when the youth is unable to incorporate his or her ancestors into his or her self-image. Although relatively few adopted adolescents actually want to initiate a birth parent search, the vast majority definitely wants considerably more information about their biologic backgrounds than they actually receive, and find that such information is critical to resolving genealogic bewilderment and gaining an uncompromised identity.

Emancipation also poses special issues for the teenage adoptee. In the course of normal development, some degree of distancing from parents is an essential step to becoming independent and autonomous. Commonly, this involves rejecting parental values, supervision, and control, sometimes in a provocative manner. A deep sense of belonging irrevocably to the family makes this process safe. But when the adolescent is adopted, the sense of irrevocable belongingness is not quite so secure. The knowledge that one did not come into this world a wanted person and was once abandoned gives a certain credibility to this possibly happening again.

The majority of adoptees in competent and well-functioning families negotiate these added developmental burdens very well. Others, particularly when adopted after age 2 years, in less intact homes, or more difficult by temperament, may not have such an easy time. Some may manifest their heightened anxiety in being super good to insure that abandonment does not occur again. Others go to the opposite extreme, testing earlier adoptive parental proclamations of being specially chosen and cherished. A third pattern is evidenced by those adolescents who take on negative roles and behaviors in acting out their fantasies about who their biologic parents were and why they were surrendered, reflecting the conclusion that negative identities are better than no identities at all. These adolescents may threaten to search for their birth parents to manipulate or punish their adoptive ones. This is no different than the youth who threatens to run away. But here the adolescent all too well senses that the adoptive parents have an even greater vulnerability. The adoptive parents will see the wish for birth parent reunion as an indication of their personal failure as parents or as a sign of the adolescent's ingratitude.

But even very emotionally healthy adoptees in very

stable families seek information about their births. When these adolescents believe that they do not have sufficient knowledge about their genealogic pasts to complete their identities satisfactorily, they may communicate these concerns in various ways. Some roam around restlessly, almost aimlessly, in a symbolic search of what their true character might be without being aware of the reason. Others are preoccupied with existential concerns and feelings of isolation and alienation due to the break in the continuity of life through the generations. Many also have a strong sense of entitlement to full knowledge of their origins and autonomous self-definition without regard to the wishes of either the birth or adoptive parents. In turn, this may lead to life adjustment as a rebel or an unconventional life path. Quests, pilgrimages, causes, and crusades all have a special attraction for adopted adolescents and young adults, appealing to their search for their origins, their roots in answering the question "Who am I?"

The threat of searching for the birth parent rarely is taken so far that it might come to completion, at least during adolescence. All that adolescent adoptees want is more information, not reunion. Moreover, even if wanted, reunion is perceived as too risky. First, the adoptee might find out "really bad things" about himself or herself; and second, he or she might hurt the adoptive parents to an unacceptable degree.

ADOPTIVE PARENTS' ADJUSTMENT TO THE ADOPTEE

To be successful, the adolescent's quest for independence requires parental approval. Parents have to refrain from projecting their ego ideal onto the teenager; they also have to resist trying to make up for their own past failures through the life of the adolescent; and have to come to terms with no longer being idealized by the adolescent. Adoptive parents' reactions to their emancipating adolescents vary. Those who have worked through their feelings about their infertility are less likely to overidentify with the youth and be injured during the adolescent's separation than those who have not. Parents with unresolved conflicts and still emotionally vulnerable may be less able to cope. They may have so much investment in the longed for and long-awaited child that they cannot let go. This may be complicated further by the thought that any acknowledgment of the emerging separateness of their adolescent may only reemphasize "this is not our child; we could not have one."

Because of the great scrutiny to which adoptive parents are subject by adoption agencies, they may feel they are "good" parents and have a reputation to live up to. When they have not worked through their own loss and maintain a facade of "good" parenting, their own sense of self-esteem is compromised. Then, when parents look to the adoptee to bolster their uncertain self-image, realistic limit setting may be made more difficult, especially an adolescent's challenge over who is in control.

Adoptive parents may be particularly challenged by their adopted adolescent's emerging sexuality. In normal adolescence, parents invest in and identify with the vigor and rise of their offspring. The adopted adolescent, however, can never confirm the parents' own sexual identity; rather, he or she is a constant reminder of what they lost. In turn, this may be projected as unconscious anger at the adolescent and be manifested in various ways, from being overrestrictive or excessively punitive to distancing themselves from the youth as he or she distances from them.

Adoptive parents also may question who their adopted child is and fear some unknown genetic influences. Indeed, they may blame any behavior they do not approve of on inherited traits over which they have no control. Any disappointment they may feel will be attributed to "bad" genes: "What else could we expect? He's not our child." This is a particular area of concern in relation to a daughter's possible "promiscuity" with fantasies that she may mirror the biologic mother's "promiscuity" as evidenced by an unwanted birth. In fearing unpredictable adverse behaviors, adoptive parents can be excessively restrictive over any type and degree of acting out, even if trivial. But in relationship to sexuality, this can equally well prompt the opposite in subtle encouragement of their daughter's becoming pregnant, thereby allowing the parents to live out their own lost fertility vicariously.

OUTCOME OF ADOPTION

An important issue relates to the impact of adoption on the adolescent. This is probably an unanswerable question in the true experimental sense. However, there is a large body of research that has used populations of adoptees, including twins. Although not designed to investigate the effect of adoption *per se* (rather to search for effects of environmental versus genetic influences), these studies can be useful in that they generally demonstrate that adoptees have no more psychiatric disturbances than does the population at large. Adopted adolescents show greater individuality in personality and temperament when compared with other family members than do adolescents who are raised by their biologic parents. Concordance among biologic children and their parents is only marginally better. Personality and temperament in general are highly individualistic and relatively independent traits; a shared environment contributes very little to their development.

Studies of intelligence show a moderate but temporary degree of concordance between adoptees and their adoptive parents during childhood, provided the child was placed as an infant. But this is transient, and by adolescence any similarity is gone. Even this early concordance is not observed when adopted children are placed after the age of 4 years. Moreover, if these latter youngsters initially were institutionalized or placed in multiple foster homes, they start out their adoptive lives with significantly lower intelligence quotients than do younger adoptees; this deficit persists at least through age 16 years. Comparative studies have not been done beyond this age.

Studies of psychological health indicate that children

and adolescents adopted as infants are just as likely to become healthy adults and are even less likely to seek out mental health services than are nonadopted adults, despite a general belief to the contrary. It is true that juvenile adoptees are overrepresented in mental health clinics; it also is true that these youngsters may evidence transient elementary school maladjustment and may exhibit somewhat more acting-out as adolescents. However, with the exception of attention deficit hyperactivity disorder (see Chapter 106)—which is more prevalent among adoptees as a group—there is no greater incidence of permanent emotional disturbance of any other type; moreover, the incidence of psychosis is even less than it is for nonadoptees. The best conclusion that can be drawn from these data is that the greater number of adopted youngsters seen in mental health clinics is a reflection of heightened parental concern and perhaps adjustment problems in the children. Adoptive parents are likely to be more concerned than are natural parents about the possibility of hidden negative genetic traits or are more likely to overreact to normal adolescent emancipating and experimenting behaviors.

The optimistic outcome for children adopted as infants is not true for youngsters who began life in institutions or multiple foster home placements and were not adopted until after age 2 years. Although able to develop good family attachments, these children are apt to have behavioral problems in school, where they demonstrate more attention-seeking behavior, are more restlessness and disobedient, and have poorer peer relationships than do other children. These difficulties persist through adolescence and, presumably, on into adulthood as well. Late adoption, then, does not auger well for good adjustment in the world outside the family.

It also is true that the recognized genetic risks of schizophrenia (see Chapter 110), the affective disorders (see Chapters 100–105), and alcoholism (see Chapter 111) exist as much for adopted individuals as anyone else. These may be significant considerations when the mental health of the biologic parents is unknown. At the same time, the incidence of risk is no greater among adoptees than among the general population.

MANAGEMENT ISSUES

Contemporary understanding increasingly recognizes that, as far as the adopted adolescent is concerned, adoption is a dynamic process with continuing needs for dialogue over time, in concert with the adoptee's cognitive and psychosocial maturation. The young person's increasing awareness that he or she was abandoned and that perhaps no one wanted him or her as a child is profoundly diminishing to self-esteem. The two central questions of the adopted adolescent are "Who were my parents?" and "Why did they give me up?" When such questions remain unanswered, the gaps are filled with fantasies, commonly of being the "bad" product of "bad" parents. The more information that is given over time, the earlier it is given, the more it is given in a positive frame, and the more opportunity there is for discussion about it at different stages in the adoptee's life, the greater the likelihood that the adopted adolescent can identify with a good parental image.

Understanding these matters, the health provider can incorporate the special issues of adopted adolescents into anticipatory guidance with parents and youth. They also should be looked for as contributory factors in instances of adjustment difficulties and behavioral problems. The most important management issues are encouraging adoptive parents to maintain an open dialogue with their youngster, not to be threatened by this, and educating them about normal adolescence and the tasks of emancipation and identity formation. Adoptive parents also need to understand their own vulnerabilities and how these may be tested during these years. The parents need to be reassured that these are normal adolescent behaviors and that adopted youths will grow up to be emotionally healthy adults, much like every one else. They need to know that adopted adolescents and young adults really need to know more about their biologic, genealogic, and cultural pasts as they mature, and that this is an important part of their identities. Most of all they need to know that even birth parent reunion will not weaken the love and commitment adopted children feel for their adopted parents; indeed, the relationship is often strengthened.

THE BIRTH PARENT SEARCH

It is estimated that more than two thirds of all young adult adoptees want more information about their background. One in five would like birth parent reunion. Studies of searching adoptees find them generally to be well adjusted and functional adults, with the search connected to completing identities rather than to any deep-rooted disturbance.

Currently, there is strong support for providing adoptive parents with ongoing reports concerning the birth parents, in order to answer the children's questions and for providing all but identifying information to mature adolescents and all adults directly. A 1981 statement of the American Academy of Pediatrics reflects contemporary thought in stating that, while most adoptees have warm, loving, and bonded relationships with adoptive parents, they also may have a compelling desire to learn more about their birth parents; many adult adoptees and contemporary adoption specialists see this search as essential to the establishment of a healthy identity. The Academy further notes that there is a growing body of law speaking to constitutional privacy rights and individual access to any record containing personal information and suggests that this right may well have applicability in relation to sealed birth records. In conclusion, the Academy recommends that adoptive parents should be provided full, nonidentifying information, with periodic updates if possible, in order to helpfully answer their adopted child's questions as he or she grows. The more open the communication, the less likely are serious identity problems. Withholding data only gives adolescent adoptees the feeling that full information would reveal the "awful truth." The Academy also supports the right of legally mature adoptees to have full and open access to their birth records.

Laws governing birth record information, however, largely reflect the traditional view that once they are sealed, they are sealed forever except for compelling reason. Although there are a few notable exceptions, most states continue to prohibit opening an adoptee's birth record without a court order. If an adult adoptee (or adoptive parents on a minor adoptee's behalf) wishes information from this record, he or she first must submit a petition. The court then will decide on the merits of the claim. Approval tends to be limited to situations where there is a clear need for medical or, in some instances, mental health data. Released information is restricted to relevant facts only, and any possible birth parent identifiers carefully excluded.

The law, however, is beginning to change. Great Britain, Finland, and Israel have completely open birth records. In the United States, adult adoptees may obtain copies of their original birth certificates in Alabama, South Dakota, and Virginia. In Minnesota, adoptees over the age of 21 years may open their sealed records if the birth parent agrees.

California enacted a particularly responsive law in 1983. Any adoptee over age 18 years may receive a report on his or her medical background simply on request, but without birth parent identifiers; this report may be obtained at a younger age on the adoptive parents' request. Birth parents are encouraged to keep the agency informed of their current address and any new health problems that could affect the child. At age 21 years, adoptees may also request and receive their birth parents' name and address if the birth parent has given permission. Reciprocally, birth parents may obtain the identity of the adoptee at age 21 years, if the adoptee agrees. The statute further provides a mechanism whereby birth parents may deposit letters, photographs, or other items of personal property with the State Department of Social Service. These may be released to adoptees at age 18 years on request or to adoptive parents for those of younger years. Similar materials may be reposited by the adoptee or adoptive parents for the birth parent. In either case, all identifiers must be removed before releasing.

Adoption agencies are a ready source of information, more so than are the courts. They also have a significant amount of data that was collected at the time the child was placed. Increasingly, these agencies are willing to share this information (short of birth parent identification) with mature adolescent and adult adoptees or adoptive parents of younger children. This may be sufficient for the majority of individuals who seek background information only. Once majority age is reached, the adoptee has the additional option of seeking assistance from adoptees' search organizations for both obtaining further information and attempting reunion. Most prominent among these organizations is the Adoptees Liberty Movement Association (ALMA), with branches in many cities. ALMA provides specific information on searching and helpful information about adoptees' rights. Their main address is P.O. Box 154, Washington Bridge Station, New York, NY 10033, and their telephone number is (212) 581–1568.

BIBLIOGRAPHY

Brinich PM, Brinich EB: Adoption and adaptation. J Nerv Ment Dis 170:489, 1982.

Brodzinsky DM, Singer LM, Braff AM: Children's understanding of adoption. Child Dev 55:869, 1984.

Dukette R: Value issues in present-day adoption. Child Welfare 58:233, 1984.

Hofmann AD, Gardiner A: Adopted adolescents and the birth parent quest. Pediatr Ann 18:238, 1989.

Lindholm BW, Touliatos J: Psychological adjustment of adopted and nonadopted children. Psychol Rep 46:307, 1980.

Loehlin JC, Horn JM, Willerman L: Modeling IQ change: Evidence from the Texas Adoption Project. Child Dev 60:993, 1989.

Nichtern S: The pursuit of the fantasy family: Generational aspects. Adolesc Psychiatry 11:27, 1983.

Nickman SL: Losses in adoption: The need for dialogue. Psychoanal Study Child 40:365, 1985.

Scarr S, Weinberg RA: The Minnesota adoption studies: Genetic differences and malleability. Child Dev 54:260, 1983.

Sorotsky AD, Baran A, Pannor R: The Adoption Triangle. Garden City, NY, Anchor Press/Doubleday, 1979.

CHAPTER 115

Divorce

NEIL KALTER

The clinical and research literature focused on the potential effects of parental divorce on the trajectory of child development is barely two decades old. Prior to the early 1970s, children's responses to divorce, death of the father, and even the extended absence of the father from the family home due to military service or occupational demands were contained in the "father absence" literature. This conceptual combination obscured crucial differences in children's reactions to these very difficult life events. However, beginning with the pioneering efforts of Wallerstein and Kelly, parental divorce was differentiated from other forms of family stress and the "children of divorce" literature was firmly launched.

It is likely that this advance was spurred by the dramatic increase between 1960 and the early 1970s in the percentage of adolescents affected by divorce. During that period the total percentage of youngsters younger than the age of 18 years who had experienced at least one parental divorce rose from approximately 10% in 1960 to over 20% by 1973. Previous estimates based on projected divorce rates, which have in fact materialized, indicate that now nearly one third of children in the United States experience parental divorce. There are no indications that this will change substantially in the foreseeable future, despite a slight decline in the divorce rate in the 1980s.

EFFECT OF DIVORCE ON ADOLESCENTS

Until recently, the crisis and trauma theory was the prevailing view of how divorce affected youngsters. In this theory, divorce was a crisis in the life of an adolescent and was compared to natural disasters such as floods and earthquakes. This crisis created emotional trauma for nearly all adolescents. Powerful feelings and conflicts were stimulated; transient maladaptive behaviors might then result. It was believed, however, that nearly all girls and the great majority of boys would regain their full developmental stride within the 2-year period following the initial parental separation. Any long-term difficulties were considered to be caused by inadequate coping styles and defenses established soon after parental separation. Beginning in the middle 1970s, other theories of how divorce may affect youngsters were developed. Parental discord, economic pressures

on the family, and the nature of postdivorce parent–child relationships were seen as potential continuing stresses on children and adolescents.

The cumulative effects of multiple life stresses associated with parental divorce may be understood in terms of the long-term developmental vulnerabilities that they create for youngsters. Although the immediate crisis of parental separation is painful and distressing to nearly all adolescents, parental divorce results in a host of life events, each stressful in its own right, that unfold for many years after the parents part. It is the number and intensity of these psychosocial stressors that account for the formation of psychological symptoms and the long-term, divorce-related psychosocial sequelae for an estimated 30% to 45% of adolescents of divorced parents. Thus, adolescent psychopathologic conditions following divorce may be viewed as a diverse array of stress-stimulated disorders.

A distillation of the divorce literature suggests the following key psychosocial stressors that may, but do not always, attend parental divorce. These are listed in decreasing order of their psychological importance: (1) ongoing parental discord; (2) the presence of an emotionally distressed (especially custodial) parent; (3) loss of the relationship with one (typically the noncustodial) parent; (4) parental dating (especially by the custodial parent); (5) remarriage (especially of the custodial parent); and (6) downward economic mobility, often resulting in residential shifts and less availability of parental supervision.

Although there are other factors that enter into an adolescent's postdivorce adjustment (e.g., the youngster's predivorce temperament, relationship with each parent, general adjustment, and the availability of extended family or professional help after parental separation), the number and intensity of these divorce-related stressors will determine to a great degree the adolescent's success in adapting to divorce.

Adolescents' Reactions to Divorce

It is crucial to differentiate the feelings adolescents have about their parents' divorce from the *psychological symptoms* that may develop. The stresses associated with divorce evoke many widely shared feelings and conflicts among adolescents. However, emotional pain and conflict do not necessarily result in symptom formation. It is only when emotional distress overwhelms the adolescent's capacity to cope with and defend against inner turmoil that symptoms emerge. These may take the form of action-oriented, externalizing behaviors (e.g., aggressive behavior, sexual promiscuity, substance abuse [see Chapter 111]), or quieter, yet subjectively more upsetting, internalizing problems (e.g., depression [see Chapter 100], psychosomatic complaints, anxiety). A distressed adolescent is vulnerable to developing psychological symptoms, but distress in itself is a normal reaction to the vicissitudes of difficult life circumstances such as divorce.

What then are the feelings and conflicts divorce stimulates in adolescents? Regardless of how troubled or overtly conflicted the marriage has been, adolescents usually are surprised when they learn of their parents' intention to separate and seek a divorce. Initially, adolescents often deny the permanence of the parental separation, harbor powerful wishes for their parents to reconcile, and may try to convince their parents to get back together. Many adolescents are furious at one or both parents for separating and thus disrupting their lives with parental conflicts, changed family circumstances, and the possibility of having to move from the family home (and even change schools, a painful prospect for most adolescents). This anger can be expressed by the adolescent through becoming sullen, uncooperative, or directly argumentative with one or both parents. Other adolescents are visibly saddened by the end of their family as they have known it. They may cry, miss the parent who has moved away, or implore parents plaintively to settle their differences and continue the marriage.

These initial reactions to their parents' divorce, although painful, do not necessarily cause significant developmental problems for adolescents. However, transient symptoms may result because these emotional reactions provoke internal conflicts. Anger toward parents is unsettling and opposed to the teenager's love for them. Many youngsters (especially boys) are uncomfortable with permitting themselves to be aware of, let alone express, intense sadness.

When an adolescent enjoys an open and emotionally close relationship with his or her parents, direct expression of the pain and conflict is tolerated better by both the teenager and the parents alike. More commonly, adolescents defend against becoming consciously aware of their distress, and emotional suffering and conflicts therefore may be expressed indirectly. This may take externalizing forms such as becoming uncooperative or argumentative with teachers (rather than directly with parents) or using illicit substances (as a way of acting against parental wishes and values). Other teenagers rely on internalizing rather than action-oriented defenses. They may turn their anger inward and become depressed or develop psychosomatic complaints such as "tension" headaches or stomach aches (see Chapters 112 and 113).

At the very least, it is likely that conscious painful feelings or conflicts aroused by these emotional reactions will result in some temporary difficulties. Grades may drop, involvement in extracurricular activities may suffer, and relationships with family members and peers may be strained. The majority of adolescents appear to

regain their developmental equilibrium within a year or so, and continue to progress well developmentally. This successful outcome is especially likely if parents can (1) tolerate their teenager's distress and support them emotionally, and (2) minimize the six key stresses associated with divorce.

As the divorce process moves beyond the initial crisis phase, the likelihood of the adolescent becoming exposed to acutely stressful divorce events and processes actually increases. Parental tension frequently intensifies as parents try to reach a settlement regarding the division of property, child support payments, and custody and visitation arrangements. Parents are likely to begin to date, develop serious relationships, and remarry. Finances often become strained. As the parents confront these realities, one or both parents may become emotionally distraught and thus less psychologically available to their children. Under these pressures, a parent may turn to his or her teenager for support. New and difficult roles are then imposed on teenagers: man of the house, co-parent, confidant about adult issues (finances, jobs, dating), and ally or pawn in the parental differences are among the most common. Thus, at precisely the time in their development that youngsters require their parents' assistance in becoming emotionally independent, they are pulled more strongly into the parents' emotional conflicts The noncustodial parent, typically the father, also may see the children less as the divorce process unfolds beyond the initial crisis phase.

These divorce stresses provoke in adolescents many painful feelings and inner conflicts. Adolescents often are angry about being drawn into parental battles and may feel guilty about either participating in them or refusing to do so. They are tempted and at times encouraged to take sides in parental conflicts, which stirs intense loyalty conflicts within them. Teenagers are often curious about their parents dating, but at the same time they may resent it. They are confronted by their parents' becoming overtly sexual beings at the same time as they are beginning to address their own sexuality. Parental dating evokes competitive feelings toward the parent's partner for both the parent's time and affection. A distraught parent is also problematic for the adolescent. Adolescents feel less supported emotionally by a markedly depressed or anxious parent. The roles they may be expected to assume make them resentful and may interfere with their own developmental task of putting emotional distance between them and their parents. The loss of a close relationship with the noncustodial parent is also difficult for the adolescent.

Some adolescents develop psychological symptoms, and not just short-term responses to parental divorce. Commonly observed externalizing symptoms are acrimonious differences with their parents or teachers, school truancy (see Chapter 103), substance abuse (see Chapter 111), sexually precocious or promiscuous behavior (see Chapter 68), and conflicts with the law (see Chapter 108). Internalizing symptoms such as somatic complaints with no physical basis (see Chapter 112), depression (see Chapter 100), and anxiety are also frequently observed. As a result, there may be a drop in school grades, suspension from school, withdrawal from extracurricular activities, social isolation from peers, addictions or overdoses, pregnancy or venereal disease, and suicide attempts. Although there are no firm statistics regarding the incidence of these difficulties, the above sequence reflects a rough order of the frequency with which they occur.

Once these psychological symptoms and their accompanying developmental sequelae occur, the impact on adolescent and adult development is markedly deleterious without professional help. Psychiatric disturbances that tend to emerge include conduct disorders (see Chapter 108), substance abuse disorders (see Chapter 111), dysthymia, anxiety disorders (see Chapter 103), somatization disorder (see Chapter 112), and personality disorders.

The focus here has been on parental divorce occurring during a youngster's adolescent years. It is important to recognize, however, that many children have already experienced divorce prior to becoming a teenager. These children may enter adolescence having been exposed to multiple divorce stresses and are thus overburdened by the painful feelings, conflicts, and psychological symptoms that arise in the context of these stresses. For these youngsters, the considerable developmental challenges of adolescence can be experienced as overwhelming. Problems may be intensified or the youngster may retreat emotionally and act as well as appear younger than his or her years. Development may become stalled. Children who seem to have adjusted well to divorce prior to adolescence may still develop psychological problems of the types described earlier as the normal vicissitudes of this period rekindle old issues, or as new divorce stresses arise.

ASSESSMENT

Clinicians need to be wary about relying too heavily on interview-based impressions of an adolescent in assessing the level of distress, the nature of conflicts, and the presence of psychological symptoms. Despite the necessary assurances of confidentiality, teenagers frequently are well defended emotionally against being aware of their own difficulties or are reluctant to discuss problems with an adult.

Instead, a thorough interview with at least one parent, preferably both, is required. These interviews can begin with an assessment of the number and intensity of divorce-related stresses (e.g., parental discord, the presence of a distraught parent, etc.) facing the adolescent. This can provide clues regarding the extent to which the teenager may be distressed and overburdened by divorce issues. Such an interview also should cover the teenager's family relationships, school performance, social involvement with peers, and mood states. Parental suspicion of substance abuse or sexual behavior should be explored. School reports and the perceptions of teachers and school guidance counselors are also often helpful.

On the basis of information obtained from parents and school personnel, the clinician can decide whether or not an intervention is warranted. The nature of the intervention will depend on the clinician's conclusion regarding the adolescent's current adjustment.

INTERVENTIONS

Although many have argued for preventive interventions timed as close to the parental separation as possible, an emerging view is that such efforts are only minimally effective. The notion that brief interventions early in the divorce process can inoculate youngsters against developing psychological symptoms and their sequelae does not fit with the view of divorce as a process that extends over many years. As the divorce process unfolds, new stresses for youngsters arise that had not been dealt with in an earlier intervention.

The range of possible interventions, regardless of when in the evolving divorce process one intervenes, includes parent guidance, brief support groups for adolescents, individual psychotherapy (see Chapter 124) and family therapy (see Chapter 123). Generally, the first two options are most effective for teenagers before acute symptoms develop.

In parent guidance, often done intermittently (at times over a period of years), the clinician can sensitize parents to the nature of divorce stresses on adolescents and the feelings and conflicts they tend to evoke. Parents can be helped to minimize the stresses while helping their teenagers cope effectively with those that are present.

Support groups conducted in school settings and mental health clinics can be enormously helpful to youngsters. This peer-mediated intervention helps (1) normalize the feelings and conflicts adolescents have about their parents' divorce, (2) clarify divorce-related confusions, (3) examine and rework painful feelings and conflicts, and (4) develop coping strategies for distress subsequent to divorce. Support groups may be more helpful than individual or family therapy when symptoms are mild or have not yet arisen, because participating in such groups is experienced as less stigmatizing than being in therapy.

However, when an adolescent becomes moderately to acutely symptomatic, either individual or family therapy is warranted. If the difficulties are primarily the result of ongoing divorce stresses (e.g., parental discord) and family relationships have changed as a result of the divorce (e.g., a parent using the teenager as a confidant, an ally in battles with the former spouse, etc.), family therapy can be extraordinarily helpful. Parent guidance sessions in conjunction with family therapy can educate parents about the nature of the divorce experience for adolescents and the needs teenagers have to be able to successfully adapt to divorce. At times, adolescents will accept participating in family therapy more readily than individual therapy because they experience the former as putting them less directly in full focus.

For other teenagers, individual therapy is the best choice. When conflicts have become firmly integrated into the youngster's psychic development, and when external sources of stress currently are minimal, individual treatment is indicated. At times, the adolescent's need to separate and gain emotional distance from parents may indicate individual psychotherapy, often with separate parent guidance sessions, because a family approach may be unacceptable to the youngster. It is also sometimes useful to combine family and individual therapeutic approaches, either concurrently or sequentially.

There are no long-term outcome studies comparing adjustment subsequent to parental divorce in adolescents when an intervention has occurred versus the absence of any intervention. Many clinicians agree, however, that each of the interventions described here are notably helpful in avoiding long-term problems related to divorce.

BIBLIOGRAPHY

Biller HB: Father absence, divorce and personality development. In Lamb ME (ed): The Role of the Father in Child Development, 2nd ed. New York, John Wiley & Sons, 1981, pp 489–552.

Glick PC: Children of divorced parents in demographic perspective. J Social Issues 35:170, 1979.

Hetherington EM: Divorce: A child's perspective. Am Psychol 34:851, 1979.

Kalter N: Long-term effects of divorce on children: A developmental vulnerability model. Am J Orthopsychiatry 57:587, 1987.

Kalter N: Growing Up With Divorce. New York, The Free Press, 1990.

Kalter N, Schaefer M, Lesowitz M, et al: School-based support groups for children of divorce: A model of brief intervention. In Gottlieb BH (ed): Marshalling Social Support. Newbury Park, CA, Sage, 1988, pp 165–185.

National Center for Health Statistics: Births, marriages, divorces and deaths for 1989. Monthly Vital Statistics Report 38:1, 1990.

Wallerstein JS, Kelly JB: The effects of parental divorce: The adolescent experience. In Anthony EJ, Koupernik C (eds): The Child in His Family: Children at Psychiatric Risk, Vol 3. New York, John Wiley & Sons, 1974.

Wallerstein JS, Kelly JB: Surviving the Breakup. New York, Basic Books, 1980.

CHAPTER 116

Grief and Bereavement

OLLE JANE Z. SAHLER

Intellectually, death is an inevitable, universal experience that comes to all living things; emotionally, death is the end of a relationship that can never be restored. Much as adults may try to shield them from the pain of loss, adolescents seldom escape experiences with death, whether among family members or friends. In past times, the presence of multiple generations within the same household made death a more commonplace event in the lives of young people than it is today. It has been suggested that such experiences made death easier to bear. Whether it is or is not true that the intensity of the loss was less in the past—most likely the bereaved would argue that the pain is and always has been almost unbearable—it is true that the trappings of death (presence of the casket in the house, laying out of the body by a family member, photographs of the dead body) are less familiar than they were years ago.

Because grandparents and other older relatives now usually die in a nursing home, often in another state, an adolescent's first encounter with death may be the premature death of a parent, friend, or sibling—and frequently the death is sudden, accidental, or traumatic, allowing no time to prepare for the loss. Having had so few experiences with death, the adolescent may have special difficulty coping with acute bereavement because there is little understanding that the pain of grief eventually will diminish with time. Health care and other professionals who understand the phases of normal bereavement can be helpful to the adolescent both by providing support as the process unfolds and by identifying those in need of more active treatment. Indications for treatment or referral are the same as for any behavioral or emotional symptoms (i.e., appropriate if they persist and interfere with day-to-day functioning).

As responsible adults we must examine critically the strengths and weaknesses of our own education about death and guide young people, not because we hope to take away all their hurt, but because we hope to make the path to resolution slightly less arduous. The task is neither trivial nor easy; indeed, it demands considerable emotional energy.

CONCEPTS OF DEATH

The development of a mature concept of death is the result of a relatively predictable, stepwise process that is modified by personal experience. Thus, because those who have lived through the death of a friend or close relative understand death differently from those who have not, children or adolescents of the same age but with different life experiences can have differing ideas about death.

To understand both adolescents' views of death as well as their usual reactions to the death of friends or family members, it is useful to review how most children in our society typically progress through the various developmental stages of comprehending death. Such a perspective can assist the clinician in interpreting responses that might be considered immature or unusual; in actuality, such responses often represent regressions to earlier stages of understanding, a common occurrence among individuals of any age who are attempting to cope with overwhelming stress.

Our ability to study the understanding of death among infants and very young, preverbal children is limited by their inability to participate in the usual kinds of activities (sentence completion, doll play) used for such research. However, from our observations of children in the hospital, it has been found that discomfort when separated from significant familiar others (e.g., parents) and fear of pain are common emotions. They appear as early as 8 to 10 months of age, when the child begins to distinguish among individuals, associating some with painful procedures and differentiating them from those who provide comfort and care. Just how much these issues are in the minds of young children is illustrated by a comment made by a 2½-year-old "veteran" patient trying to comfort an 18-month-old child who had just been hospitalized: "It's OK, your mommy and daddy will be back. And they don't hurt you too much here."

From about the age of 2 to 6 years, children are in the Piagetian stage of preoperational thinking. Although able to use language to indicate wants and explain events, children of this age are prelogical in their thinking. They believe inanimate objects and natural events are alive and act through conscious desire. They also are influenced by "magical thinking," the belief that events in the external world are the direct result of their own thoughts and wishes; such thinking endows them with tremendous perceived personal powers for both good and evil.

It is of interest that children learn the word *dead* at about age 3 years, long before they learn the word *alive*. But their use of *dead* is not to designate an irreversible biologic state, but rather a state other than alive. That is, to young children, all things are alive in the same way that they themselves are alive. It is only when they find a dead bird, for example, and take it to their parents, who shake their head and say, "Poor bird is dead," that children begin to recognize that this word somehow means not flying, not chirping—not alive. But part of the reason for taking dead birds or animals to parents is for them to make what is dead alive again. For, at this age, children do not understand that death is irreversible; for them, being dead now does not preclude being alive at some time in the future. Thus, burying cans of food along with a dead pet seems fully consistent: otherwise, what will the animal eat tomorrow? During this stage, children also see death as contingent on old age, where being old is some age beyond the child's own current age. Therefore, they do not consider themselves vulnerable to death because they are young.

Because children believe death is reversible, there is likely to be little or no emotion associated with their first experience with death. Helping them gain some conception of the permanence of death and some understanding of grief is facilitated, for example, by encouraging parents not to replace a dead pet immediately, but rather to allow the child time both to understand that that particular animal is gone and to grieve the loss. Otherwise, the child may develop the confused notion that everything (and everyone) that dies can be replaced.

The heavy burdens imposed by the child's sense of pervasive control over the environment is illustrated by the inner turmoil of the 3-year-old who, when visiting his grandfather in the intensive care unit, was asked by his parents to "Cheer Grandpa up. Make him feel better." After the grandfather died later that day, the child asked, tearfully: "Why did Grandpa die? I tried to make him feel better." It was not until the parents were able to reassure him that he had, indeed, done his job (cheered his grandfather and made him feel better in that way), but that the doctors, whose job it was to make his grandfather physically well, had been unable to do so, that he felt comforted and at ease. This vignette is a classic example of the egocentrism of young children: the sense that they are the force behind events in the environment that, in reality, are entirely beyond their control.

During the late stage of preoperational thought, children view death as a personified being, often a witch or monster who comes in the night to steal people away. The literalism of their language makes it imperative that metaphors such as "Grandma went to sleep" or "Aunt Mary went on a long trip" not be used to explain death, because children can come to fear going to bed at night or going on family outings.

During the early school years, in what Piaget had termed the stage of concrete operations, children learn by experimenting with the external world: that is, what they truly are able to understand is what they can see or manipulate. It is not uncommon for children of this age to develop what has been termed a "morbid curiosity" about death: the bird buried in the back yard is dug up daily for viewing; how else to understand the process of decomposition, something that might otherwise be beyond comprehension? These experiences also help to solidify the notion of irreversibility: it seems increasingly less probable to the child that what has decomposed can come back to life.

By about the age of 8 years, children begin to understand that they, themselves, may die. Experience plays a major role in this step: it is unlikely that the average child would proceed beyond the primary grades in a reasonably sized school without experiencing the death of a schoolmate or a schoolmate's sibling. The idea that one must be old to die gives way to an understanding that even the young, like themselves, are vulnerable.

Perhaps as a result of the combination of experiences provided by nature and the facts learned in health class, at about the age of 9 or 10 years, children develop a logical, biologic understanding of death. Being dead means that the heart stops beating and there is no pulse; breathing stops, the body becomes cold, and movement or activity are no longer possible; the child knows that he or she, like anyone and everyone, can die, and being dead is forever. There is a matter-of-factness to discussions about death among preadolescents, and concerns about personal death center primarily on never-to-be-had experiences and lost relationships with family and friends.

The capacity for formal operational or abstract thought, which allows the individual to contemplate issues and phenomena that are beyond experience and to develop hypotheses that take into account all combinations of possibilities, develops during adolescence (see Chapter 9). Thus, the teenager, as part of a process that occurs over time, eventually comes to understand theoretical moral, political, and philosophical ideas, and to comprehend such concepts as liberty, justice, the ideal world, and death.

During adolescence, the concept of death becomes inextricably intertwined with the concept of life's purpose. Who put me here? Why am I here? What is it that I am destined to accomplish? These are questions adolescents ask themselves. Particularly during middle adolescence, when intense mastery acquisition increases their sense of self-importance, they come to view themselves as of great importance to many others as well. Further, they come to regard themselves, particularly their feelings, as special and unique. This belief in personal uniqueness and universal importance viewed in the context of "Why am I here anyway unless it is to do wonderful things?" becomes a conviction that they will not die—"How could I die when I have not yet done the things I am fated to do?" This sense of immortality is an illustration of the "personal fable," a highly private story of invulnerability or invincibility that adolescents tell themselves. It is not until the adolescent develops intimate relationships with others and, through mutual sharing, learns that others have the same personal fantasies (for example, of immortality) that the intensity of the personal fable diminishes. Despite its decreased intensity, however, the personal fable (of immunity from bad things) probably is never fully overcome even during adulthood, or perhaps overcome only in the very last stages of life, when the inevitability of personal death finally may be understood.

Adolescents both approach death by flirtatious participation in death-defying activities and avoid it as a serious topic of conversation or consideration for themselves. When adolescents do think or write about death, they often imbue it with a mystical, magical, or romantic dimension by describing it as an act that overpowers evil or leads to reunion with a lost love. The irreversibility of death frequently is denied or mitigated by espousing reincarnation, resurrection, or transmigration of souls; such beliefs serve to reconcile personal feelings of invincibility with de facto irrevocability. The fascination adolescents have with courting danger, with supremacy of the underdog, and with surviving disaster to accomplish superhuman feats has been attributed to late-night television and bionic man story lines. In truth, however, stories like that of David and Goliath are evidence that these ideas are timeless: by definition, youth are those individuals caught in the transition between the fairy tales of childhood and the struggle to exert power and authority in the adult world.

EDUCATION ABOUT DEATH

What, when, and how to teach about death is a major curriculum issue in many school districts. Parental scrutiny of death education is probably second only to parental scrutiny of sex education. Whereas for sex education the arguments raised both by opponents ("If teenagers know about it, they will do it") and by proponents ("If teenagers know about it, they will make more responsible choices") have been fairly consistent over the years, the issues are less clear for death education. Indeed, the reasons why death education is not a good idea have ranged from "It will make more students feel that death is not bad and lead to more suicide" to "It's just too uncomfortable to talk about" (although *who* finds it too uncomfortable for discussion may refer more to the parent than to the adolescent).

That death is inevitable is rarely debated. Nor can anyone deny that a student is highly likely to experience the death of a friend or loved one. Indeed, in a recent random sampling of students in a small city high school done in 1989, 89% of the students who completed the questionnaire had experienced the death of at least one family member or friend. Furthermore, among those students, the average number of experiences with death was 3.5. Sixty-nine per cent of students reported the death of one or more grandparents; 13% reported the death of friends or distant family members; 12% reported the death of a parent or sibling; and 6% reported the death of a pet as a major loss. When asked how old they were when they first realized that they, themselves, could die, answers ranged from 3 years to 11 years of age, with an average of 7.2 years. When asked what was good about death, the majority listed an end to suffering; several listed going to heaven/God; one wrote "nothing" (this was a student who had lost a parent). Bad things about death focused on the survivors' feelings of loss; a few students took the perspective of the deceased, with comments such as "unfinished business" or "uncertainty about what will happen." When asked to list three words brought to mind by the word "grieving," most listed forms of worrying, sadness, pain, regret, loneliness, and emptiness; a few listed variations of weak, unhealthy, and selfish.

Schools often provide formal death education, which,

per se, can be useful in two ways: (1) familiarizing students with rituals and the purposes they serve; and (2) providing an emotional outlet for that subgroup experiencing unresolved grief. The content of such courses varies widely and may include historical perspectives; cultural and ethnic differences in the meaning of death, belief in afterlife, and mourning practices; visits to graveyards and funeral homes; and the writing of obituaries either for other people or for one's self. This last exercise is sometimes seen as too personally intrusive by parents, perhaps because the issue is closer to home for the middle-aged than for the adolescent. Yet, if put in the context of "when you die sometime in the future," it permits teenagers to fantasize about what they will accomplish in life and what legacy of achievements they would like to leave behind as a way of reconciling the issue of "Why am I alive?" with the inevitability of death.

Death education will be most successful if the teacher is at ease with the instructional modules used; that is, the specific content is probably less important than the feelings of respect for the dead, comfort with the grieving process, and understanding and acceptance of different points of view about dying, death, and mourning that the teacher is able to convey. This task is not simple; the audience often will resort to grim humor to hide its anxiety.

There should be no expectation that such education, even when done well, will necessarily have any significantly mitigating effect on personal feelings of loss, despair, or loneliness during the acute phase of actually grieving the death of someone close. Cognitive understanding and emotional response serve very different and equally valid purposes; while both aid in ultimate grief resolution, neither can be substituted for the other.

The very fact that death education does not take away the pain of grieving is sometimes cited as a major reason for excluding it from the curriculum; that is, "What good does it do?" Yet so many students are faced with coping with death and from middle elementary school age know that they themselves will die someday, that to not teach about it as an integral part of life does them a major disservice by giving the message that it is too terrible to talk about. That message then becomes operationalized as "When you or someone close to you is dying, silence is the only socially acceptable response." To educators, the dilemma should not be do we teach about death or not, but rather, how do we help our students understand that our teaching about death is actually an expression of our caring for them?

Indeed, in answer to the question of what the school could do to help a student cope with the death of someone close, the most popular response in our survey was "nothing"; other responses were an even mix of suggestions for greater school involvement by understanding mood swings and incomplete homework assignments when a student had lost a friend or family member and of suggestions to leave the student alone. Parents were seen as having a more active role than the school both by talking, comforting, and explaining and by leaving alone.

The range and variety of answers as to what constitutes helpful intervention by the two main institutions (family and school) in adolescents' lives reflect the common dilemma that potential information-giving and support systems face when confronted with helping someone cope with a significant stress: there is no prescription that accommodates everyone, especially as they move beyond the stage of childhood when hugs cured most ills. Indeed, the growing need for independence and resistance to comforting provided by adults make it especially crucial that adolescents be allowed to maintain their fragile identity during crisis by asking "How can I help?" rather than providing a set intervention. A response such as "leave me alone" should be accepted graciously but coupled with the assurance that help will continue to be available if, at some time in the future, the adolescent chooses to use it. It also can be beneficial to touch base occasionally, to let them know they are being thought of and to reiterate the offer of help. Doing so by a written note gives adolescents greater control over accepting or rejecting such offers without feeling directly confronted. The wording of such a note is crucial and needs to convey that the adolescent's own abilities to cope are respected and may well be sufficient. Furthermore, such statements allow adolescents to titrate the amount, kind, and timing of intervention provided. Clearly, as with coping with any stress, the most productive therapeutic relationship will be established when the contract is between the caregiver and the adolescent, not the caregiver and the parent or some other "helpful" adult or friend; and it may take a long time for the adolescent to perceive a true need for such intervention.

REACTIONS TO THE DEATHS OF OTHERS

Death of a Grandparent

The expectation that members of earlier generations will die before those of later generations and the frequent presence of incurable chronic or debilitating conditions make the death of a grandparent an inevitable and less unacceptable event in the natural history of life. Despite such expectation, however, it can bring great sadness, especially if the grandparent played a major role as a parent surrogate or best friend; it also may be the adolescent's first experience with the death of someone emotionally close.

Intervention. Among adolescents, just as with adults, resolution of grief is facilitated by the opportunity to make peace where there may have been conflict, to provide tokens of esteem or gratitude by gestures of caring, and to say goodbye. For example, during the time when the death is anticipated, participation by the adolescent in providing comfort care or diversional activities serves as a way of paying back the grandparent for past gifts or emotional support and can leave a lasting positive feeling about their mutual relationship. The busy, peer-oriented lives of adolescents who fear and thus detest physical disfigurement and cognitive impairment can leave little room for quiet sitting by the bedside of an incontinent, aphasic stroke victim. How-

ever, despite their reluctance, they should be encouraged to make at least brief visits and give a rehearsed, if necessary, recitation about their latest athletic, academic, or social activities. Although the amount of parental patience required to support a teenager in performing such tasks will be substantial, the lifelong benefits of good memories—for everyone—is well worth the effort.

These kinds of experiences also provide adolescents with the opportunity to learn how to talk and interact with someone who is dying within the familiar and supportive environment of home. In addition, adolescents watching their parents cope with the illness and death of a father or mother provides a powerful model for what their own behavior will be like in later years, when they are faced with similar situations. Indeed, parents should be encouraged to share their mixed feelings of frustration, love, gratitude, guilt, and obligation that form the basis for the parent–child role reversal that is so common in contemporary American society. What better time is there to critically evaluate the values that are important to that particular family, pass on those that are growth promoting, and place aside those that are inhibiting and unhealthy?

In some instances, grandparents have lived at a distance from the adolescent and the death may have only limited emotional impact. Parents may resent or misunderstand the lack of grief displayed by their adolescent or they may confuse acting-out, belligerent or withdrawn behavior in the adolescent as a reaction to the death rather than the effects of their own grieving, which may be deep and render them emotionally unavailable to their adolescent. Such projection among parents is not uncommon and can lead to a sense of guilt in the adolescent for not feeling more deeply. Although the dynamic is complex, it may be helpful for the parent to have private confidential discussions with the adolescent in which honesty is encouraged; this also may help the parent to differentiate his or her own feelings of loss and unresolved conflict from the less emotionally charged feelings of the adolescent.

Death of a Parent

The death of a parent is probably the most disruptive death for an adolescent to experience, because adjustment to such loss requires major reorganization of family structure and function. The loss of the mother results in the need to replace the nurturing homemaker, a position often assumed by or thrust on the oldest daughter; such increased responsibility at home frequently is given precedence over age-appropriate after-school and peer-related activities. Death of the father, especially if he was the major breadwinner, often results in a dual loss for the children: not only is he lost, but the mother may have to assume either greater or new responsibilities in the workplace, making her less available for home-oriented activities. Thus, older sons, especially, may have to obtain employment to supplement the family income and older daughters may have to take on increased burdens at home to help compensate for the mother's unavailability. Reduced financial security may lead to postponement or cancellation of plans for education after high school; indeed, in some instances, leaving high school may be necessary.

Adolescents in these circumstances must cope not only with their own feelings of loss both of the parent and of participation in typical teenage life, but also with the depression of the surviving parent. Added to this is the burden that widowed parents, often unwittingly, place on their children by confiding financial and even romantic problems. That is, the bereaved parent may seek an inappropriately close emotional relationship with the adolescent to replace the lost marital relationship.

Intervention. Sadness (sometimes to the point of depression), decreased productivity at school, and feelings of isolation from peers are common acute symptoms of adolescent bereavement. How sustained these reactions are in the otherwise healthy teenager is often a reflection of how well or poorly the surviving parent is coping with the loss. Frequently, it is only when a symptomatic child is brought for evaluation that poor parental coping is uncovered through careful history-taking; seeing the parent alone and exploring the depths of his or her own feelings may be the clinician's most productive diagnostic strategy.

There are, however, issues specific to the teenager that deserve attention. These include rage against demands to be mature prematurely; grief over lost friendships with peers; and overcoming obstacles in forming a new relationship with the surviving parent, especially if the deceased parent formerly served as an intercessor. Uncovering such feelings, particularly if the adolescent perceives that they are circumstantially unacceptable ("I must be a bad person to feel this way") may require a great deal of skill. It can, however, be very freeing to the adolescent to learn that these are natural and common feelings. Helping them problem-solve about their dilemmas within the bounds of reality—especially financial reality—can provide adolescents with a sense of mastery over a situation that seemed hopeless before.

A frequently neglected but medically important aspect of counseling is assessment of the teenager for risk factors for similar premature death, especially if it was the result of cardiovascular disease (see Chapter 49), alcoholism (see Chapter 111), or another genetic or familial disorder. If the risk factor index is low, the finding can be reassuring. If the index is high, preventive measures can be undertaken to reduce the risk and give the adolescent a feeling of potential control over suffering a similar fate.

Monitoring over time is essential to assess the progress of bereavement. Although deep sadness, feelings of unreality or preoccupation with the dead parent, and disruption of everyday life are common for a period of weeks, the intensity of these feelings should diminish progressively over several months and be coupled with an increasing interest in the future. Teenagers should, however, be warned about the reemergence of feelings of deep sadness and loneliness that often accompany special events (such as a graduation), holidays, and anniversaries even years after the death.

Lastly, but most importantly, because parent-child relationships are typically love–hate relationships, especially during adolescence, the teenager may need to confront and resolve negative feelings toward the dead parent. Under the best of circumstances, the death is expected and the adolescent can be helped to make peace with the dying parent while there is still time for this to happen in person. In instances of sudden death or other situations where this is not possible, anger and guilt may be pervasive; resolution may require referral for formal mental health intervention.

Death of a Sibling

The death of a brother or sister might be termed the "rivalrous death"—not the death of a rival, because, in fact, the idealized image of the child may serve as a yardstick against which the parents measure the behavior, attitudes, and accomplishments of the living child. Comments such as "If John were alive, he wouldn't have done X" can be extremely frustrating to the surviving sibling, who knows not only that John would have done X, but indeed that he did do X—and more than once. Comparisons between siblings can be difficult enough when they are alive together and both vulnerable—and likely—to do things that are displeasing to the parents. The situation can become intolerable to the survivor when the principle of "nisi nil bonum" (nothing but good about the dead) is exercised by parents who selectively remember only the dead adolescent's good behaviors, leaving no room for imperfection among the living children. Formal counseling may be necessary to help parents understand the detrimental effects of, and cease making, such comparisons.

The death of a chronically ill brother or sister can be a relief to the sibling who felt jealous and deprived of parental love and attention while the child was alive. Understanding that these feelings are natural and reconciling them with the deep sadness expressed by the parents may be difficult; it also may be impossible to share these feelings with the parents because they seem so unacceptable.

Intervention. Helping the surviving sibling put "unacceptable" feelings into words so that they can be explored and resolved is a major goal of any intervention strategy. Even when the teenager does not admit to or actively denies feelings of rivalry or relief at the death of a sibling, the clinician should mention these reactions as normal and not necessarily an indication of not loving or not missing the brother or sister who died. If the teenager persists in denial, the clinician should merely state that feelings can change and should these or others that somehow seem "bad" arise in the future, they can be discussed if desired.

Many bereaved teenagers benefit from the suggestion that they put their feelings into a story or poem or into making some kind of remembrance that would be a memento of their special relationship (acknowledging both its burdens and pleasures) with their dead brother or sister. Indeed, creating such a memento may be a useful outlet for working through the death of anyone with whom the adolescent felt a close bond.

Death of a Peer

The death of someone close in age and relationship to the teenager can be very personally assaultive. Such a death intrudes into their sense of personal invincibility and invulnerability and is a potent reminder of their own susceptibility to death. Interestingly, teenagers die most often when they are breaking society's rules (e.g., driving too fast or under the influence of drugs or alcohol). A fatal accident may be seen as confirmation of intrinsic "badness" that deserved punishment. However, when there was no fault for which death seems just reward, the question "Why him?" or "Why her?" may be unanswerable. Bitterness, anger, and resentment may be masks for the real—and frightening—thought: "It could have been me."

Concerns about their own health, safety, and welfare tend to be high among adolescents immediately after the death of a peer and for some time afterward. Among some students, especially after an accidental death or suicide, this concern about personal vulnerability is expressed as a need to participate in reckless or death-defying activities, primarily as a way of assuring themselves that death cannot happen to them.

Intervention. The death of a peer may mark the first time the adolescent must deal with the social conventions of expressing sorrow, attending a funeral, and deciding about memoralization outside the confines of the family. Frequently, the school, as a social institution, serves to facilitate both group and individual grieving processes.

Schools, like people, are highly variable in their initial response to the report of the death of a student, especially when it is sudden or unexpected. Some districts have established policies regarding announcement of the death that include advance notification of faculty and prompt provision of support services for those identified as having particular problems coping with the death. How individual teachers, however, respond in their classrooms ranges from immediate resumption of academic work after the announcement has been made to cancellation of class to permit discussion about the student, manner of death, probable feelings of the family and, most importantly, feelings among the students themselves. Often, unfortunately, a teacher's reaction is more a reflection of how he or she is coping—or not coping—with the death than a reflection of the needs of the students. It is not unusual, years later, for a now-adult to report: "It was awful and I will never forget it. We were never allowed to discuss the death in class. It was as if my classmate had never lived. I wondered for a long time if I would be forgotten so quickly, too."

An illustration of the power of the classroom teacher is provided by the experience of a small rural town after the suicide of an eighth-grade, "All-American" girl. Following the death, the school district sponsored a mandatory conference about how to deal with the growing number of suicide notes being written by students. Only one teacher reported that he had neither found nor been given any notes; he had had, however, innumerable conversations with many very sad and shocked teenagers. When the faculty was polled, it became apparent that he was the only one who talked about the suicide in his classes the morning after it was discovered. His final comment to his students was "If you ever feel alone, remember that you're not. I'm always here for you." In response, his students flocked to his open door.

Immediately following a death, students tend to visit the family or attend the funeral in mutually supportive groups rather than individually. This is not surprising, because this may be the first time an adolescent has had such experiences without parental presence. This also may be the first time the adolescent has written a letter of condolence; for some, construction of a group letter as part of a class exercise may be less intrusive and may facilitate participation by those who are uncomfortable responding as individuals. Regardless of whether the letter is written individually or not, learning that placing themselves in the position of the family and deciding what they would want to read if the letter were addressed to them can help them determine what they will include and is an invaluable experience for the future.

Because commitment to friends and to the group is a hallmark of adolescence, memorialization takes on special meaning and serves to help perpetuate a sense of continued presence of the student. Memorials which will last "forever," living memorials, and memorials related to special interests usually are chosen, much as they are by adults. It is not unusual, at high school graduation, for the student to be remembered in the year book, even if the death was several years before. "I have not forgotten you" might well be translated as "Please don't forget me."

THE DYING TEENAGER

Children and adolescents with chronic or terminal illness go through the usual stages of learning about and understanding death, but frequently at an accelerated pace; thus, they often have an appreciation of death that exceeds that of age-matched peers (see Chapters 30 and 121). Clearly, meeting other adolescents in the hospital or clinic who have similar diseases, often becoming good friends, and then experiencing loss through death of these friends confers a real life understanding of dying. By their own desire, it is not unusual for children as young as 7 or 8 years of age to participate in decisions regarding further, especially experimental, treatment for terminal illness. Such participation includes receiving not only information about the benefits of therapy but also counseling from their parents or physicians that nontreatment is expected to lead to disease progression and death. Although they understand death and its irreversibility, with the assurance that they will be as comfortable as possible, many children and adolescents choose to receive only comfort care—preferably in the familiar surroundings of home, with their family and friends—during the last days of their life. Conversely, especially among some adolescents, further treatment is desired or even demanded. As in the situation with the adolescent who is coping with the death of a family member or friend, determining where the patient is in dealing with his or her illness, both cognitively and emotionally, is essential to providing personally appropriate support and treatment.

Adolescent patients live until they die. Interest in the future and hopes for a cure remain high even during the stage of progressive inexorable deterioration. Sometimes their seeming lack of concern about their bleak future is interpreted as denial. An alternative interpretation, however, is that for individuals who live for tomorrow and for whom next month is light years away, a prognosis of survival for a year is almost the length of another lifetime. Inherent in their reaction is also their implicit trust in the adult world of parents and professionals to find the key to successful treatment. Perhaps, too, they have a magical fear that saying it out loud will make it come true.

These alternative interpretations are exemplified by a 13-year-old boy with cystic fibrosis. During the first four of his five hospitalizations during the last 7 months of his life, he refused to discuss his illness, and instead focused first on such issues as what he would do when he finished high school, then his classroom placement for the following year, then going on fishing trips with his father during the summer and, finally, plans that he had made for the week after he was discharged from the hospital. Although the time frame became progressively constricted, he always oriented his thoughts toward the future. It was only when he was admitted for what was to be the last time that he gave any indication of what had, probably, been on his mind for a long time. Among his first words were, "I don't want to die." When asked what had been going through his mind when he thought about dying, he replied: "They've got to find a cure real quick, like this weekend. Do you think they'll find it this weekend?" When asked whether his doctor had been honest with him about his condition he replied, "No. But you tell him I want him to be the same now as always. No different this weekend from any other time." He died late that Sunday evening.

Intervention. Probably the most feared question an adolescent can ask is "Am I going to die?" Clinicians struggle with how to respond, not wanting to give a trivial response such as "everyone dies," nor to play God by saying yes or no. Although some might argue that it avoids the issue, "Tell me what you're thinking" opens the door for all the concerns about pain, fear of the unknown, separation, and loss that we know underlie the question and allows us to ultimately satisfy the adolescent's need for particular reassurances.

More often, however, our patients do not ask the question. Yet our fear of it comes between us and we begin to withdraw. Self-preservation and feelings of personal and professional inadequacy are the most common explanations for abandonment of the dying. Because they are facing death, perhaps we think they could not possibly be interested in the mundane issues of everyday life; perhaps we fear some display of overwhelming sadness that we will be helpless to relieve; or perhaps we are egocentric and self-important enough to think that any anger they have is directed at us and our inability to cure. Regardless of the reason, however, there is no question that unless we make an overtly conscious effort not to, we avoid the dying.

Yet the dying themselves have told us how much they want to be a continuing part of everyday life, because, after all, is that not what living is all about? Thus, the fundamental principle of caring for the dying adolescent is to remain actively involved by listening, reflecting, sharing, engaging, answering questions and posing others, relieving pain, providing encouragement, and, above all, being present.

The second principle is that people cope with death the way they have coped with other crises throughout their lives. Although we must allow time for quiet talk or angry outbursts if the adolescent wishes, we also must respect the need for privacy. Health care professionals tend to be verbal. To demand of people who are not naturally verbal that they share their innermost feelings with us may satisfy our needs but merely imposes additional stress on them at a time when they are already overburdened.

The third principle is to maintain hope. It may be that the adolescent's hope is that tomorrow or even the next minute will be easier to bear than today or this minute; it may be that the afterlife will be a blessed relief. Somehow, the word hope has become synonymous in the minds of many health providers with the wish for cure. We must not confuse what we may hope for with what the patient hopes for.

The fourth principle is to help the adolescent die as he or she wishes: at home or in the hospital, receiving comfort care or active treatment, but always with dignity and the sense that the life lived will not be forgotten.

Adolescents have a great sense that they are destined to leave an indelible mark on the world and an exquisitely fragile ego identity that makes them feel constantly on the edge of oblivion. Death is an intruder that can rob them of fulfillment. They cope with their anxiety about death by flirting with it much as they flirt with a desired companion at a party; confronted face-to-face, however, they are tongue-tied and run away. Death is the freely chosen subject of abstract love poems and art class projects but not a comfortable topic of real conversation. Death education can tell them what they will feel and do but cannot really prepare them for the overwhelming sense of loss, fright, and betrayal they will actually experience.

The desire to help adolescents avoid pain and suffering often leads to attempts to shield or distract them from the deep emotions associated with death. Yet, it is their sensitivity to death—in others and themselves—that is a hallmark of their emerging sense of self in relationship to others and within the context of human experience. And, as they grow and develop their own personalities and styles of coping, what they need most is not pity or well-meaning but empty pats on the back, but rather the tools of self-reflection, honest exploration of their feelings, and guided problem-solving to help them overcome the grief presented by each death experience they have: to learn how to reorient themselves; move on without the grandparent, parent, sibling, or friend they once had; and view themselves as still the same person but one challenged by new circumstances. Maintaining the integrity of the individual is also essential for the adolescent who is dying. In the words of my young friend: "The same now as always."

BIBLIOGRAPHY

Adams DW, Deveau EJ: When a brother or sister is dying of cancer: The vulnerability of the adolescent sibling. Death Studies 11:279, 1987.

Bluebond-Langner M: Private Worlds of Dying Children. Princeton, NJ, Princeton University Press, 1978.

Corr CA, McNeil JN: Adolescence and Death. New York, Springer Publishing, 1986.

Easson WM: The Dying Child, 2nd ed. Springfield, IL, Charles C Thomas, 1981.

Sahler OJZ: The Child and Death. St. Louis, C. V. Mosby Co., 1978.

Schowalter JE, Patterson PR, Tallmer M, et al: The Child and Death. New York, Columbia University Press, 1983.

Wass H, Corr CA: Childhood and Death. New York, Hemisphere Publishing, 1984.

Wass H, Corr CA: Helping Children Cope with Death: Guidelines and Resources, 2nd ed. New York, Hemisphere Publishing, 1984.

Wass H, Corr CA, Pacholski R, Forfar JO: Death Education: An Annotated Resource Guide, Vol 2. New York, Hemisphere Publishing, 1985.

CHAPTER 117

Violence

DEBORAH PROTHROW-STITH and HOWARD R. SPIVAK

At the age of 17 years, KM, a senior in an inner-city high school, had attended more funerals than dances—sixteen in all. Friends, primarily young men ranging from 12 to 21 years of age, had been murdered. One of her friends (RD), a 19-year-old former boyfriend of her sister, was stabbed to death in a barbershop during an argument over who was next in line for a haircut. Like many of her other dead friends, this young man had a long history of injuries from fighting. In spite of repeated contacts with health care settings for the treatment of these injuries, no attempts had been made to reduce his risky behaviors.

During a routine physical examination, KM provided this information on the number of funerals she had attended. Further questioning revealed that she was depressed but had initiated treatment by joining a peer education and support group.

When we consider violence and homicide, we generally think of drug deals or robberies (carefully premeditated behavior) or psychotic maniacs with automatic weapons standing on street corners. But this, in fact, is not the case. The more common event involves two young men of the same race, who have been drinking, who know each other and get into an argument involving a weapon, during which someone is injured or dies. This situation is unlikely to be influenced by the punitive consequences offered as a deterrent by the criminal justice system. However, it does involve behaviors that are greatly influenced by risk factors of poverty, racism, gender roles, developmental stresses, weapon carrying, and, maybe most importantly, the learned use of violence as a primary way of coping with conflict and anger. Understanding these risk factors can provide important insights for clinicians in developing preventive, early identification and intervention strategies for this serious, growing problem, which has its greatest impact on young people. Those young people like RD, who are directly involved in violent behavior, and those like KM, who are indirectly affected by this violence, require the concern and attention of clinicians.

Homicide has become the third leading cause of death for teenagers and young adults in the United States; it is the leading cause of death for young black men (see Chapter 2). Young black men are at greatest risk for death and injury from violence. Their death rate from homicide is from 7 (for 15 to 24 years of age) to 12 (25 to 44 years of age) times higher than national rates. The United States, with the fifth highest homicide rate in the world, has a particular problem with violence. In 1980, homicide and aggravated assault accounted for almost 25,000 deaths, 350,000 hospitalizations, 1½ million hospital days, and almost $0.75 billion in health care costs in the United States. Furthermore, homicide is now the fourth leading cause of potential years of life lost, yet another reflection of the fact that it is a problem particularly devastating to young people.

For every homicide, there are as many as 100 nonfatal intentional injuries observed in emergency rooms and numerous similar injuries that never come to the attention of the health care system. The magnitude of this problem compels us to focus greater attention on prevention and intervention services. Although traditionally delegated to the criminal justice system, violence and its consequences present to health care providers more frequently than to the police—an observation that requires health and public health professionals to be better prepared.

CLINICAL MANIFESTATIONS

Although the media generally present violence as coldly premeditated or randomly directed to innocent bystanders or as the consequence of criminal activity such as drug dealing, the epidemiologic characteristics of violence and homicide reflect a very different clinical picture. Altering the misconceptions of violence being predominantly interracial, stranger related, or involving criminal intent is an important first step toward addressing the problem in a constructive manner.

Although blacks are dramatically overrepresented in homicide statistics, with 44% of homicide victims being black, this does not reflect an interracial phenomenon. In over 80% of cases, homicides occur between people of the same race. In general, blacks kill blacks, whites kill whites, Hispanics kill Hispanics.

Numerous studies confirm that a large majority of homicides and violent events occur between people who know each other. Between 50% and 60% of homicides occur either between family members or acquaintances. This observation is probably an underestimate, because a significant number of assailants remain unknown to the legal system. Nonetheless, approximately 20% to 25% of homicide assailants are family members, and 30% to 35% are friends or acquaintances.

One half or more of homicides occur in the context of an argument. Often, these arguments are spontaneous and can be over an issue as minor as name-calling. This can be compared with only 15% of homicides that are

1113

precipitated by the commission of another crime, such as robbery or drug commerce, or are premeditated homicide.

Alcohol use and possibly other drug use, such as cocaine or "crack" cocaine, play an important clinical role as well (see Chapter 111). Over one half of homicide victims have elevated blood alcohol levels, and similar observations have been made for homicide assailants when the assailant is identified soon enough after the event, to allow for accurate determination of their blood alcohol levels. Studies have also shown that alcohol, as well as other drugs, affects the level or threshold for violent behavior among users.

Obviously, the carrying of weapons is a key factor in violence and homicide. Guns, particularly handguns, followed by knives, are the primary weapon involved in most homicides. There is evidence that weapon carrying among teenagers is a growing phenomenon. One recent study in Boston observed that over one quarter of high school students (37% of boys, 17% of girls) reported occasionally carrying weapons to school. The increased presence of weapons is clearly important in influencing the risk of violent behavior leading to serious or fatal outcomes.

Lastly, the consequences and clinical manifestations of violence present more commonly in the health and human service system than to the police and criminal justice systems. Although the most severe violence-related outcome, homicide, generally and consistently presents in the criminal justice context, nonfatal intentional injuries are significantly more likely to present to health care and emergency room providers and do not necessarily concurrently present to the police. For example, one study in Ohio observed that four times as many intentional injuries presented in emergency rooms than to police and were often "treated" without police involvement.

THEORIES OF CAUSE

There has also been a growing recognition of the risk factors that contribute to or influence the use of violence. Understanding these risk factors is important to clinicians who have the opportunity to identify at-risk or high-risk individuals who could benefit from interventions and who can create opportunities for primary prevention. When one examines the known violence-related risk factors, it becomes clear that some of these factors reflect societal and cultural level phenomena that put groups or communities at high risk, whereas others reflect personal phenomena that put specific individuals at higher risk for violence.

At the larger societal level, the most prominent risk factors include race and racism, socioeconomic issues such as poverty, gender and sex roles, adolescent development, and the media (because they portray violence in an unrealistic, often glamorous manner).

As noted earlier, a common misconception about violence is that it is interracial. Relatively few homicides, however, occur between people of different races, and this appears to hold true for more serious nonfatal intentional injuries as well.

Without question, racism contributes to the levels of anger, stress, and frustration experienced by communities and may in fact contribute to the level of violence experienced in communities of color. It is important to point out that several studies that have corrected homicide rates for socioeconomic status have observed that the disparity in homicide rates between blacks and whites virtually disappears. This strongly suggests that the use of violence may be more substantially influenced by the effects of poverty than racial factors.

Poverty is clearly a major risk factor for exposure to or experience with violence. In addition to the observations that reflect the likelihood that homicide disparities are more rooted in poverty than race, others have consistently observed low socioeconomic status to be significantly associated with death by homicide as well as risk of nonfatal intentional injury. The Centers for Disease Control (CDC) consistently report that homicides most often occur in urban areas characterized by low socioeconomic status, high population density, poor housing, and high unemployment rates. Homicide rates have been observed to rise in communities about 1 year after a rise in unemployment rates.

Gender is also an important risk factor. Most homicide victims (77%) and a large majority of assailants are male. This pattern may not be as strong in nonfatal events; however, less data are available. Women represent the majority of victims of sexual violence, although in most other forms of interpersonal violence, men are in the majority, as both victims and assailants. This may relate to weapon-carrying behavior because males are more likely to carry weapons. There is concern that women may be influenced by the increasing number of violent female heroes in the media and increased marketing of weapons directed toward women, which may narrow the disparity in risk between men and women.

Age is another major risk factor. Homicide rates begin to rise in mid-adolescence, peak in the late 20s and early 30s, and fall off dramatically by the mid-40s. Adolescents are at particularly high risk for violence because of the rapid psychological and developmental changes that occur in the transition to adulthood. Adolescents face a number of major developmental tasks: (1) individuation from family through a period of narcissistic preoccupation; (2) development of a sexual identity that includes a period of overidentification with gender role extremes; (3) development of a moral and personal value system, often through experimentation; and (4) preparation for future employment and responsibility (see Chapter 9).

Many of the behaviors involved or associated with these tasks clearly predispose adolescents to violence. Their self-preoccupation, an important stage in separation from family, has a strong component of self-consciousness, making a teenager particularly vulnerable to embarrassment. Adolescents' preoccupation with themselves, their appearance, and their image all make them extremely susceptible to overreacting to even a mild insult. Although adolescent boys and girls can and do choose fighting to defend their honor, linking this with identification with the extreme gender role stereotype often sets the stage for teenage boys to use violence.

Peer pressure, an important factor in facilitating success in many developmental tasks, can further enhance the likelihood of violent behavior. If fighting is expected by peers, then an adolescent will have considerable difficulty disregarding the pressure to fight. When the lack of visible future options of poverty and racism are superimposed on this process, it is not surprising to see high levels of risk-taking behaviors related to violence (e.g., weapon carrying) among inner city and minority adolescents.

When fighting and violence become integral parts of a peer group culture, as is the case with gangs, then members literally have no choice. Gangs are a seductive vehicle for meeting adolescents' needs and for protection, belonging, nonfamily social structure, accomplishment, and survival. Gang norms define manhood and maturity in concrete and readily available ways, particularly with the use of violence. The lack of available pro-social peer group settings in many poor communities furthers the attractiveness of gang membership. The absence of healthy alternative visions of manhood and maturity is, in and of itself, a risk factor that exacerbates the perceived legitimacy of violence.

Last, but far from least, is the influence of media. The average television-viewing teenager is exposed to over 9000 violent events each year. Media heroes most frequently choose violence as a primary mechanism for dealing with conflict, anger, or stress; few heroes model pro-social problem-solving strategies. Violence is commonly represented in the media as successful and entertaining, and heroes rarely, if ever, die or feel pain. Although not all people respond to or learn from the media equally, those individuals with other societal and personal risk factors may be more influenced by this media exposure, because it supports or legitimizes their choice of violence.

These broader societal risk factors create the context for understanding why certain communities or groups are a greater risk for violence than are others. There are also personal factors that place certain individuals at particularly high risk for violent behavior.

Several personal risk factors have already been discussed. Alcohol and other drug use (such as cocaine and "crack" cocaine) lowers an individual's threshold for use of violence. Chronic users are at greater risk, but even occasional use can be, in some circumstances, a risk. Weapon carrying is an even more serious risk factor. The availability of firearms (there are over 20 million unregistered handguns in the United States) is a factor, but the decision to actually carry a weapon is still, in general, an individual choice. The carrying of guns and knives is becoming an increasingly common behavior, particularly among urban teenagers. Frequently, the reason given for weapon carrying is self-protection. The rise in violence-related fatalities and serious injuries may very well be a direct consequence of increased weapon carrying, rather than an actual increase in the amount of fighting among teenagers.

Increasing evidence suggests that violence is a learned behavior—a primary choice in response to stress and conflict. Exposure to family violence early in life, even if the violence is not directly experienced and only observed, has been associated with adolescent violent behavior (see Chapter 118). While the human service system is designed to protect and often remove young children from family violence, little has been developed to address the long-term consequences resulting from this exposure. These children may, in fact, be the most vulnerable to the media violence exposure as a substantiation of their personal experience. There is growing evidence that children and young people demonstrate the behavior that they observe on television. More recently, several studies show that children are equally likely to mimic and learn nonviolent problem-solving strategies from television exposure as well, but the opportunities for viewing pro-social behaviors are extremely limited.

Psychological and descriptive characteristics of victims of violent injuries provide further understanding of other contributing individual risk factors. Early exposure to family violence, incomplete schooling, illiteracy, depression, chronic alcohol and drug use, and low self-esteem are all significant risk factors for being a victim of homicide. Strong similarities in behavior and psychological profiles between homicide assailants and victims of serious assaults have also been observed. One study that longitudinally followed victims and assailants reported that a number of subjects changed roles from victim to assailant or vice versa during the study period. This suggests that individuals with high-risk characteristics can present initially as either a victim or assailant, but may be at risk for either role in the future. It also illustrates that differentiation or identification of an individual as a possible victim or assailant may be hazy at best. Among adolescents, it is often difficult in a specific episode to identify the instigator of a fight. The relationship between instigating and getting hurt is not consistent because the one who starts the fight may very well be the one who gets hurt.

Finally, despite the overwhelming evidence of the psychological context of violence, organic factors also may contribute to an individual's risk for violence. There is a body of literature suggesting a link between central nervous system impairment and the occurrence of violent behavior. For example, several studies have identified associations between a history of severe head trauma and the display of violent behavior (see Chapter 108). It is important to note that this group represents a relatively small portion of the population of individuals with violence-related problems, but this factor should be considered as a potential risk factor.

CLINICAL EVALUATION

Clinicians must obtain adequate information about adolescents in order to identify risk level and establish an intervention plan. Because much of the information needed is sensitive and may reflect illegal behaviors, obtaining it must be handled sensitively and often requires several sources of information and repeated efforts. This information may appear only after trust has been established. Parent interviews, record reviews, and other objective and subjective testing options may be helpful.

Basic information should include

1. Family history of violence
2. Family history of weapon possession and use
3. Substance abuse history for adolescent and other family members
4. Weapon availability and weapon-carrying behavior
5. Mental status—depression, aggression, school performance and attitude, self-esteem, and severe psychopathologic condition such as thought disorder
6. Family and individual stress issues
7. History of fights
8. Injury history—both unintentional and intentional. (This area should address whether the adolescent identifies himself or herself as victim or assailant, whether injuries were self-inflicted, and whether revenge was considered or attempted. Record review and, in particular, emergency room records may be most helpful.)
9. Biologic factors

An assessment is particularly important when adolescents are seen for treatment of an intentional injury. Intent to seek revenge is a crucial factor in determining risk for recurrence; it is not uncommon among homicide victims to find a long history of intentional injuries prior to the fatal event. It is currently standard practice to assess future risk for adolescents who present with self-inflicted injuries. A similar approach should be developed for individuals with non–self-inflicted intentional injuries. Assessment at the time of treatment for the acute intentional injury should include

1. Circumstances of the event
2. Victim-assailant relationship
3. Use of drugs or alcohol
4. Underlying emotional factors
5. Injury history
6. Predisposing biologic factors
7. Intent to seek revenge
8. Weapon-carrying behaviors and weapon access

Psychological testing may be helpful in the complete evaluation of an adolescent. Tests can confirm or identify underlying pathology such as depression, learning disabilities, psychotic disorders, or indications of organic components in individuals displaying violent behavior (see Chapter 99). A strong note of caution is necessary because these tests cannot be used to predict the likelihood of future violent behavior or the circumstances under which violence might be displayed. They should be used to identify treatable psychological disorders and to engage the at-risk adolescent patient in the mental health system. These tests may also provide insight into the environment and circumstances that have placed patients at risk. Subjective observations from the persons administering the tests sometimes provide the most useful information about possible points of intervention.

The clinical evaluation of violent adolescents has been inadequate. As a result, diagnostic categories are limited and do not reflect the complexities presented by patients. Often, the adolescent patient's problem list lacks appropriate acknowledgment of victimization, aggression, or violence-related risk. Even diagnostic labels for acute intentional injuries inadequately define the circumstances of the injury.

Clinical assessment and documentation of the findings are extremely important. Clinicians should gather clinical data, as they do with adolescents who have other medical problems. This is essential to developing adequate treatment strategies.

TREATMENT

Broad-based collaboration of professionals and community agencies is ideal for addressing the problem of interpersonal violence. At present, there are only a few such professionals or agencies. This should not discourage attempts to address the problem because a few can make a significant contribution. A multidisciplinary group of professionals can implement primary violence prevention programs in schools, clinics, and community agencies. Providers can screen and identify high-risk individuals. Appropriate referrals will mandate increased services and improved rehabilitative services. In this context, the medical and public health communities can provide impetus for change in collaboration with other appropriate human service, mental health, education, community, and criminal justice institutions.

There are many ways individual providers can incorporate violence prevention within their medical practices. Violence prevention can be incorporated with anticipatory guidance of children. Violence is learned behavior, and parents can be enlisted to help prevent violent behavior in their children. Parents have many opportunities to teach their children acceptable ways of handling anger. With guidance, parents can teach their children positive, nonviolent strategies for directing and resolving anger. Physicians can remind parents that they teach by example. Methods for discipline, regulating television viewing, and negotiating conflicts between siblings, and ways for parents to display and respond to their anger can be addressed during these encounters. One helpful strategy is to teach parents to role play with children, asking them to act out a situation that caused a conflict and use nonviolent ways to prevent or resolve the conflict. Children learn from and enjoy these activities.

The practitioner should discuss violence and anger directly with older children and adolescents. Raising awareness of the risks of fighting and the factors that lead to violent situations can lead the way to more detailed discussion. Studies indicate that many youth have fears and concerns about risks of violence. Adolescents may carry weapons for self-protection. Discussing these fears and helping adolescents identify and develop alternative strategies for avoiding violent situations may assist them in better understanding their options. Anger is a normal emotion, and adolescents require concrete options for creative and productive responses to it.

Beyond primary prevention, clinicians have the opportunity to play an important role in screening and early identification of youth at high risk for violent behavior. An understanding of the risk factors will help them recognize youth at risk for violence. Screening for a history of family or peer violence, substance abuse, depression and low self-esteem, carrying weapons, and history of central nervous system injury or pathology can identify youth who may be helped by referral to mental health and other related services.

This effort of primary care health providers must be linked to the increased development and availability of intervention services directed toward violent behavior. Merely identifying high-risk youth without appropriate referral resources would be frustrating. Educational, mental health, and support services for adolescents need to be enhanced, and intervention strategies addressing the underlying emotional and behavioral components of violent behavior must be developed. These services can be modeled after the current approaches to depression and suicide.

The current "stitch them up and send them out" approach to youth with intentional injuries must be modified. Health care institutions, particularly emergency departments, are the major site of contact with persons with violence-related problems. Diagnostic and intervention services for victims of rape, physical and sexual abuse, and suicide attempts are standard care in these settings (see Chapters 118 and 119). The extent of support services for children and families displaying these symptoms is considerable. Yet, many intentional injuries do not clearly fit these categories. Adolescent peer violence and spouse abuse generally are managed from the perspective of treating the injury without investigating the circumstances or underlying issues and behaviors that may have led to it. Suturing a superficial stab wound and sending an adolescent home does nothing to alter the cycle of violence; moreover, it communicates a sense that violence is inevitable. Such adolescent patients present a double risk in that they are victims today, and may be assailants in the future. Intentional injury victims often explicitly express their intent to seek revenge, much as depressed adolescents will discuss their suicidal intent.

Individual clinicians cannot address violence in isolation. The public health community must become involved.

PUBLIC HEALTH EFFORT

Individual level interventions alone are unlikely to be successful. A larger collaborative effort can increase the level of awareness and understanding of the community. One approach is based on the cognitive learning theory model, in which knowledge and understanding are thought to lead to changes in attitudes and behavior. At the core of the intervention is The Violence Prevention Curriculum for Adolescents. This ten-session unit provides descriptive information on the risks of violence and homicide, and alternative conflict-resolution techniques. Its goal is to create a classroom ethos that is nonviolent and values violence prevention behavior.

In the curriculum, anger is presented as a normal, essential, and potentially constructive emotion. Rather than eliminating the anger itself, the curriculum focuses on changing the response to anger into a healthy one. It seeks to raise the individual's threshold for violence by creating peer pressure for nonviolent behavior and by extending the individual's repertoire of responses to anger. It also acknowledges the existence of institutional sources of anger, such as racism. Students are taught not to become passive agents, but rather to be creative in their responses to anger.

Creative alternatives to fighting are stressed. Classroom discussion during one session, for example, focuses on the good and bad outcomes of fighting. Invariably, the list of bad outcomes is longer than the good, concretely illustrating the need to identify alternatives. This exercise emphasizes that fighting is a choice and that it is important to consider the real risks inherent in the decision.

Another public health approach used in addressing health problems involves attempts to manipulate the environment to reduce risk. For example, the use of safety locks on firearms (analogous to safety caps on medication bottles) might be indicated. Although this would not necessarily be expected to significantly reduce premeditated intentional injuries, it might reduce the extent of unintentional firearm injuries, as well as providing a moment for second thought in unplanned violent events. It is important to keep in mind that this sort of environmental intervention is limited in its potential effect when the intent to hurt someone is a primary factor in a violent episode.

The public health system also can advocate more extensive mental health services for violent behavior. Increased collaboration with institutions that deal with violent individuals, such as the police and courts, is needed. Improving access to supportive services for these individuals is important for the human service system.

Improved control of weapons is a targeted intervention. The availability of lethal weapons is associated with the most serious consequences of violence. Reduced access to guns or more stringent regulation of firearm licensing may contribute to a reduction of the more serious injuries. The medical and public health sectors can help increase public awareness of the serious complications of easy access to weapons.

Increased efforts to reduce the level of substance abuse also can potentially decrease the extent of violence. The role of physicians and the broader medical and public health community is more obvious with substance abuse prevention efforts than with violence. The medical community can help to educate the public about the link between alcohol and violence.

The public health community and its agents can help change or modify media messages about violence. The pervasive image of the "violent hero" is a dangerous, unrealistic, and glamorous model for children and adolescents. Media heroes who display nonviolent strategies to resolve conflict are difficult to find. The news media's portrayal of stereotypic violence makes awareness and understanding of the problem difficult.

BIBLIOGRAPHY

Akbar N: Homicide among black males: Causal factors. Public Health Rep 95:549, 1980.
Barancik JI: Northeastern Ohio trauma study: I. Magnitude of the problem. Am J Public Health 73:746, 1983.
Centers for Disease Control: Homicide among young black males—U.S. 1978–1987. MMWR 39:869, 1990.

Centers for Disease Control: Violent deaths among persons 15–24 years of age—United States, 1970–78. MMWR 32:453, 1983.

Dennis RE: Homicide among black males: Social costs to families and communities. Public Health Rep 95:556, 1980.

Poussaint AF: Why Blacks Kill Blacks. New York, Emerson Hall, 1972.

Prothrow-Stith D: Interdisciplinary interventions applicable to prevention of interpersonal violence and homicide in black youth. In Surgeon General's Workshop on Violence and Public Health. Washington, DC, US Department of Health and Human Services, Publication No. HRS-D-MC86-1, 1986, pp 35–43.

Prothrow-Stith D, Spivak H, Hausman AJ: The violence prevention project: A public health approach. Science, Technology and Human Values 12:67, 1987.

CHAPTER 118

Physical and Emotional Abuse

AMY C. RICHARDSON

Physical and emotional abuse and neglect of adolescents are common but underrecognized events. Abuse of adolescents has been overshadowed by the more widely appreciated phenomenon of abuse of younger children. Early statistics incorrectly suggested that the abuse of adolescents was a rare event. For example, the first edition of *The Battered Child* by Kempe and Helfer in 1968 cites a study in which only 33 of 504 cases of abuse involved children older than 12 years of age. To some extent, the failure of health professionals to appreciate the extent of adolescent abuse and neglect may relate to the lack of a watershed article to bring the subject to public attention, as "The Battered Child Syndrome" did for child abuse in 1962. It may also relate to a tendency of society to perceive that adolescents are in some way responsible for their being abused.

DEFINING ABUSE

Many definitions of abuse are available. In general, physical abuse implies injury of a nonaccidental nature with a significant risk of death, disfigurement, or prolonged disability. To meet the legal definition of abuse (as opposed to assault), the injury must have been inflicted by the parent, caretaker, or legal guardian. Sometimes the boundary between excessive punishment and intentional injury is a vague one, creating conflict between the helping professional and legal system. Neglect implies the failure of the caretaker to minimally provide adequate food, shelter, clothing, education, and health care. The minimal standards for neglect may seem unreasonably low for health care providers and child advocates. Emotional abuse is the most difficult form of abuse to define and diagnose. It may include acts of omission, such as rejection or lack of discipline, or commission, such as degrading comments or public humiliation. The identification of this type of abuse is further complicated by the problem of establishing a direct link between the abusive acts by the parent and the negative effects on the child. For example, the legal definition of emotional abuse in New York State requires demonstration of substantially diminished psychological or intellectual functioning, provided that such impairment may be clearly attributable to the unwillingness or inability of the parent to exercise a minimum degree of care.

It is important to recognize that the legal, social, medical, and research definitions of various types of abuse may vary. Legal definitions focus on minimum standards of care, while social definitions focus on optimal care. Legal definitions may require standards of proof that a medical diagnosis may not be able to meet because there are few physical findings pathognomonic of abuse. Medical diagnosis frequently relies on establishing patterns of injury (including physical *and* behavioral indicators) over time. Research definitions must rely on relatively rigid, reproducible criteria that may actually underestimate abuse. There is also significant state-to-state variation with regard to the upper age limit for child abuse (from 12 years of age to 18 years of age). Legally defined abuse also measures only harm at the hands of parents, guardians, or caretakers, and does not address the broader spectrum of violence directed toward adolescents.

EPIDEMIOLOGY

The exact incidence of physical and emotional abuse and neglect in the adolescent population is unknown. Most studies are believed to underestimate true frequency of the problem. Over 1.5 million children each year are believed to have been abused or neglected (see Chapter 119). Adolescents (age 12 years and older) account for approximately 39% of all reports of physical abuse, 52% of emotional abuse reported, and 47% of reports of neglect.

The *National Study of Incidence and Prevalence of Child Abuse and Neglect: 1988* replicated a similar study conducted in 1980. Information on suspected incidents of abuse and neglect was compiled from a variety of sources, including protective and law enforcement agencies, schools, and hospitals. Using the slightly more inclusive 1986 definitions of abuse in which the endangerment standard was revised to allow inclusion of cases where the child's health or safety was endangered through abuse or neglectual treatment, the findings were strikingly similar to those reported in 1980. There was no difference in the incidence of *neglect* by age; however, there was a marked increase in the incidence of physical and sexual abuse among older children and teenagers. The rate of physical abuse among those younger than 2 years of age was approximately 2.8 in 1000 children and 7.5 in 1000 among 12- to 17-year-olds. Although overall neglect was not higher among the teenagers, educational and emotional neglect did increase. Adolescents were at lower risk for fatal injuries resulting from abuse, but were at a greater risk of moderate injury. Other risk factors included living in a low income family, being female, and being from a large family. There were no differences in the incidence of abuse and neglect by racial and ethnic groups or the area of residence.

Abused adolescents are at risk for multiple types of abuse. The National Clinical Evaluation Study evaluated 19 intervention programs for subpopulations of abused children. Their sample contained 701 adolescents and demonstrated a significant overlap of types of abuse (see Chapter 119). Of their adolescent sample, 54.8% had experienced more than one form of abuse or neglect; 74.2% experienced physical abuse, neglect, or emotional abuse alone or in combination with another form of abuse.

There are differences in reporting practices between children and adolescents. Adolescents are more likely to have been reported by professionals (52% of the reports), compared with younger children (44%). Among the professionals, medical personnel report only 5.9% of the abused teenagers, compared with 12.2% of the younger children. Schools (18.2%) and law enforcement personnel (16.4%) account for the increased reporting for adolescents among professionals. Among younger children, schools (10.7%) and law enforcement agencies (11.1%) report fewer cases of abuse. Overall, it appears only 43% of all the abuse cases are known to child protective services.

CLINICAL MANIFESTATIONS

The clinical manifestations of abuse are not specific to adolescents. Bruises (including black eyes), lacerations, facial injuries, and welts are the most common physical findings. Adolescents have fewer fractures, burns, and internal injuries than young children. The overlap of physical abuse and neglect with sexual abuse suggests that physical manifestations of sexual abuse may also be present (see Chapter 119).

The list of behavioral and emotional manifestations attributed to abuse and neglect is long. It includes aggression, acting out, running away, withdrawal, substance abuse and harmful health behaviors, including smoking and suicide attempts, and symptoms suggestive of depression. None of these is pathognomonic of abuse, although abuse should be considered in the differential diagnosis when evaluating a teenager for behavioral symptoms.

DIAGNOSIS

Because there are no pathognomonic physical findings, the diagnosis of physical or emotional abuse relies heavily on the inclusion of abuse/neglect in the differential diagnosis and the interview of the adolescents (Table 118–1). Although adolescents are generally more verbal than are younger children, the interview process must not be hurried, and requires time to establish a trusting relationship in order to obtain a good disclosure. It is important to remember the purpose of the inter-

TABLE 118–1. Interviewing the Abused Adolescent

GENERAL
Allow sufficient time for an unhurried interview
Acknowledge the adolescent's feelings and the risks involved in disclosure
Avoid making unrealistic promises
Explain the steps in an abuse investigation
Do not interpret a recantation as evidence of a false allegation
PSYCHOSOCIAL HISTORY
Explore family structure and dynamics
Search for family stressors
Assess adolescent's mood, social functioning, suicide and runaway risks
Consider other forms of domestic violence
Obtain information from other pertinent agencies, including schools, police, and medical facilities
HISTORY OF THE ABUSE
Obtain detailed information about the incident(s) of abuse, including
    Time(s)
    Place(s)
    Person or people involved
    Type(s) of abuse
Delineate precipitants of abuse
Define patterns of abuse, including duration and frequency
Assess imminent risk to the adolescent's safety
Consider possibility of sexual abuse

view. Pursuing the initial suspicions of abuse or neglect may require only sufficient information to justify reporting to the local agency mandated to evaluate the suspicion. In other circumstances (e.g., in areas with lack of sufficient legal and protective services), the health provider may need to obtain more detailed information about the adolescent and family. Coordination of efforts is important in all circumstances in order to minimize the duplication of the interview and examination.

In those situations in which the health provider suspects that abuse or neglect are involved, he or she needs to be direct and as matter of fact as possible in acknowledging his or her suspicion to the adolescent. As with many other sensitive issues, beginning with a gentle statement is useful. For example, "I have noticed a lot of bruises on your back that could have happened in a lot of ways. Tell me what happened."

It is helpful to acknowledge that the disclosure of the abuse is courageous and involves potential physical and emotional risk for the adolescent. Although health care providers may wish to rescue children and teens who have been or are being abused, it is important to avoid promises (such as "I'll make sure you'll be safe") that may be impossible to keep. The process of investigating and managing cases of alleged abuse is complex and one that sometimes overwhelms even experienced professionals. It is therefore crucial to keep the adolescent informed as to the steps in the process (e.g., filing the report, court hearings, and so on) and the reasons for various interventions, so that he or she does not feel doubly victimized by the system. Under the stress of disclosure and investigation, some children and teenagers will recant their initial story. This should not immediately be interpreted as a false allegation.

The disclosure interview should initially focus on the details of the abuse, including precipitant and patterns of abuse. Specific questions about the possibility of sexual abuse must be included (see Chapter 119). The effects of the abuse on the adolescent's life should also be explored; specifically, mood, school functioning, peer relations, health habits, and any thoughts about or plans to commit suicide or run away.

As part of the complete assessment, the family structure, dynamics, strengths, and supports should be delineated. Stressors, such as financial problems and parental substance use, and other forms of family violence, such as spouse or sibling abuse, should be evaluated.

Information from a variety of other sources may be helpful in the evaluation of alleged abuse. Schools may provide information regarding attendance, performance, and peer relations. A history of suspicious injuries, problems with growth or development, and behavioral concerns may be obtained from hospitals or other health care facilities, particularly the adolescent's primary care physician. In some cases, police agencies, shelters for runaways, and other social service agencies may also be useful resources.

A detailed physical examination with careful documentation of all physical findings is critical. Physical injuries should be documented in detail, including size, color, and location of bruises and other skin findings. Good color photographs that include appropriate identifying information provide documentation of injuries. The examination is essential for three primary reasons: (1) to identify and treat any serious injuries, (2) to document any injuries for medicolegal purposes, and (3) to identify any other chronic or acute medical conditions requiring further evaluation, treatment, or follow-up. If sexual abuse is also suspected, gynecologic evaluation is necessary (see Chapters 69 and 119). Laboratory evaluation of the allegedly abused or neglected adolescent must be determined by the history and physical findings. As with younger children, the evaluation of bruising requires exclusion of coagulation and platelet disorders. Radiologic examination should be appropriate to the physical findings and history. Looking for old or unsuspected fractures is generally unwarranted.

THEORIES OF CAUSE

Two general patterns of abuse in adolescents have been observed. First, abuse identified in adolescents may represent a continuation of abuse that began during childhood or the deterioration of dysfunctional parenting into frank abuse (e.g., physical punishment now severe enough to produce serious injury). However, a substantial proportion of abuse identified in teenagers begins in adolescence, perhaps in response to the developmental challenges of this period.

This is supported to some extent by data indicating that, relative to younger children, families in which adolescent abuse are reported are less often headed by females, more often have a male caretaker, require less public assistance, and are larger. This has been interpreted by some as suggesting that adolescent abuse is, to a greater extent than among younger children, dis-

sociated from the poverty stressors and more associated with other factors, such as developmental stresses.

The very characteristics of adolescence itself may make abuse in this age group different from child maltreatment. Adolescents are physically larger and stronger and thus may be able to directly resist the abusive adult. Indeed, some teenagers may become involved in reciprocal physical violence with their parent(s). Teenagers have broader social networks outside the family. They begin to develop an independent identity and separate from the family. However, most adolescents remain economically dependent on their parents, and may increase the family's financial stresses through needs or desires for clothing, automobiles, entertainment, etc. The need for adjustment to the adolescent's changing role in the family, struggles over control and separation, changes in the teen's physical and cognitive capabilities, and continued financial dependence may overwhelm some parents and culminate in abuse.

OUTCOME

Accumulating evidence from diverse sources indicates that there are serious behavioral and psychiatric sequelae resulting from adolescent maltreatment. Converging evidence from clinical populations of abused children and adolescents, psychiatric patients, and from nonclinical populations strongly suggests that individuals are adversely affected by abuse and neglect. At this time, research does not permit one to separate the potentially confounding affects of abuse *per se* from the influences of environment, family, brain damage and genetic factors. It also appears that the impact of physical and sexual abuse differ.

Among psychiatric patients, reports of prior physical abuse are more common than one would expect to find in a general population. Studies have demonstrated that physical abuse is significantly more common among females with borderline personality disorder (see Chapter 109) and may resemble post-traumatic stress disorder (see Chapter 104). An association with adolescent delinquency and physical and sexual abuse is supported by a variety of studies. More adolescent delinquents report significant physical abuse than their nondelinquent peers. Follow-up studies of abused children have demonstrated that they are more likely to come to the attention of the courts because of delinquency (see Chapter 108). There is also evidence to suggest that violent delinquents are more likely to have experienced abuse than nonviolent delinquents. Some investigators have attempted to link violent behavior and early trauma by suggesting that central nervous system and intellectual deficiencies noted among more violent abused adolescents are a result of early maltreatment. Data in this area are unclear.

Among populations of physically and sexually abused children and adolescents (a select sample), there is a greater prevalence of emotional problems severe enough to warrant treatment. Identified problems include difficulty handling aggressive impulses; negative self-image; and difficulty relating to peers and adults, forming attachments, and trusting (see Chapter 119).

TABLE 118–2. Therapeutic Considerations

Severity of abuse and imminent risk to adolescent's safety
Concomitant psychiatric dysfunction
Duration and chronicity of abuse
Adolescent's age and behavioral symptoms
Other therapeutic issues, including substance abuse
Adolescent's living situation
Family's willingness to join in therapy
Adolescent's need for immediate response

These observations of an adverse effect of abuse among diverse clinical populations are supported by a small number of studies conducted with nonclinical adolescent populations. Adolescents reporting prior physical and sexual abuse also report engaging in significantly more potentially self-destructive behaviors. Their risks for suicide attempts, suicidal ideation, the use of a wide variety of legal and illegal substances, and having run away are significantly greater than their nonabused peers. Data on emotional symptoms are, however, less clear. One study has demonstrated that physically abused adolescents report significantly more trouble sleeping, difficulty with anger, and trouble making friends than nonabused peers. Together, these data strongly suggest that abuse and neglect may seriously interfere with making a healthy transition into adulthood. It is unclear whether adolescent abuse will be transmitted across generations.

TREATMENT

The research literature provides little comparative data on specific treatment modalities for abused adolescents, although it is clear that treatment is necessary. In general, treatment should be tailored for each teen and his or her family. Recommendations regarding the type and length of therapy must take into account the severity and chronicity of the abuse, the age of the adolescent, the extent of the adolescent's symptoms and psychopathology, and the willingness of the family to participate in the therapy. The teen's specific living arrangement (e.g., living at home, in foster care, in a runaway shelter) must also be considered. There should be some immediacy to the therapeutic intervention, with the initial goal of providing the adolescent with specific, concrete strategies for avoiding potentially abuse situations, without making the teen feel responsible for his or her own abuse. Some adolescents may require only supportive follow-up by a primary health provider experienced in caring for adolescents (Table 118–2). Others will require psychotherapeutic intervention, ranging from brief outpatient treatment to intensive inpatient care.

BIBLIOGRAPHY

American Association for Protecting Children: Trends in Child Abuse and Neglect: A National Perspective. Denver, CO, The American Humane Association, 1984.
Blum RW, Runyan C: Adolescent abuse: The dimensions of the problem. J Adol Health Care 1:121, 1980.
Daro D: Confronting Child Abuse—Research for Effective Program Design. New York, The Free Press, 1988.
Farber ED, Joseph JA: The maltreated adolescent: Patterns of physical abuse. Child Abuse Negl 9:201, 1985.
Garbarino J: Troubled youth, troubled families: The dynamics of adolescent maltreatment. In Cicchetti D, Carlson V (eds): Child Maltreatment: Theory and Research on the Causes and Consequences of Child Abuse and Neglect. New York, Cambridge University Press, 1989, pp 685–706.
Garbarino J, Sebes J, Schellenbach C: Families at risk for destructive parent-child relations in adolescence. Child Dev 55:174, 1984.
Hibbard RA, Ingersoll GM, Orr DP: Behavioral risk, emotional risk and child abuse among adolescents in a non-clinical setting. Pediatrics 86:896, 1990.
Lourie IS: The phenomenon of the abused adolescent: A clinical study. Victimology 2:268, 1977.
U.S. Department of Health and Human Services, Office of Human Development Services: Study Findings: Study of National Incidence and Prevalence of Child Abuse and Neglect: 1988. Washington, DC, US Government Printing Office, 1988.
U.S. Department of Justice, Office of Juvenile Justice and Delinquency Prevention: Child Abuse: Prelude to Delinquency? Washington, DC, US Government Printing Office, September, 1986.

CHAPTER 119

Sexual Abuse

ROBERTA A. HIBBARD

Sexual abuse of children and adolescents has taken on a variety of meanings and implications in both health care and legal arenas. Molestations, incest, date rape, and statutory rape are among the forms of sexual abuse of adolescents. Health care providers must be aware of the clinical manifestations, treatment, and interventions to identify and manage suspected victims. This chapter discusses adolescent sexual abuse in the context of all child sexual abuse. Few studies distinguish children from adolescents, but when possible, features specific to adolescents are presented. *Child* in this context refers to anyone 18 years old or younger. Revictimization of children during adolescence and presentation for care of an adolescent who was victimized as a child necessitate knowledge regarding sexual abuse from childhood through adolescence.

DEFINING SEXUAL ABUSE

Sexual abuse usually refers to unwanted sexual activity. Types of sexual abuse are defined by the specific activities, and the relationship or age of the victims and perpetrators. Child sexual abuse is often defined as the involvement of dependent, developmentally immature children and adolescents in sexual activities that they do not understand, to which they are unable to give informed consent, or that are inappropriate for family roles. The developmental level of the adolescent (normal or delayed) may limit the adolescent's understanding and the implications of sexual activity. The adolescent lacks the authority to say "no" in many situations.

Sexual abuse is a complex concept that is difficult to define adequately or simply. Many definitions refer to the exploitation of minors for the sexual gratification of adults. Molestation refers to noncoital sexual activity with an adult, and may include viewing, genital or breast fondling, or oral–genital stimulation. Sexual assault is any contact of an offender with the genitalia of a nonconsenting victim. A sexual assault is considered rape when the penis of an assailant is introduced to the victim's genitalia, either without consent or by threat of force or compulsion. This does not necessarily imply ejaculation or hymenal injury; vulvar intercourse is a common form of rape among children and adolescents. Incest is the sexual relationship between individuals who are related and not legally able to marry. This is often expanded to include step-relatives and parental figures who are in the home. Legal definitions of minor–adult sexual contact, such as statutory rape, may vary somewhat from state to state. Consensual intercourse, the illegality of which is based only on one's status as a minor, may or may not be abusive, depending on the circumstances.

The emergence of adolescents' sexuality can present special problems in defining and understanding the sexual abuse of adolescents. Normal development of adolescents involves sexual experimentation. An adolescent may agree to participate in sexual activity, without understanding fully what may happen or what the consequences are. The "sex stress syndrome" describes the adolescent claiming sexual abuse in order to avoid telling parents about consensual sexual activity. Careful assessment generally distinguishes the true victim from the adolescent hiding consensual activity. Although sexual abuse can still be defined within appropriate family roles, the adolescent's ability to consent to and understand sexual activity is changing. When is the adolescent truly consenting with an understanding of the actions? Such issues are of paramount concern in date rape.

EPIDEMIOLOGY

The Study of National Incidence and Prevalence of Child Abuse and Neglect report in 1988 revealed that over 1.5 million children were victims of all child abuse in 1986 (see Chapter 118); 25% were between 12 and 17 years of age. It was estimated that almost 156,000 cases of sexual abuse occurred in 1986 among adolescents, involving 15 youth per 1000 aged 12 to 14 years and 13.5 youth per 1000 aged 15 to 17 years. Although this reflected a significant increase in the rate of sexual abuse among children and adolescents since the earlier report in 1980, this increase occurred predominantly in older children and teenagers. Surveys of adults about their childhood experiences repeatedly suggest that 20% to 30% of adult women experience sexual victimization as children or as adolescents; approximately 10% to 15% of men report sexual victimization before the age of 19 years. In several studies of junior and high school students in nonclinical settings, almost 20% of students reported some type of abuse and 8% reported sexual victimization. Studies of date rape reveal almost 80% of college women and 60% of college men report unwanted sexual activity on a date. Fifteen percent of women and 7% of men report unwanted sexual intercourse on those dates.

Some attention has been paid to apparent underreporting of sexual abuse in males. Retrospective studies suggest one third of victims are male, yet males account for only one fifth of the reported cases. Differences in reporting may be indicative of the stigma of homosexual abuse. A highly critical societal attitude may heighten the anguish and embarrassment of having been involved in sexually deviant behavior. Despite societal concerns, there is little information to suggest a relationship of homosexual abuse to the ultimate development of homosexuality (see Chapters 32 and 120).

Sexual abuse occurs in individuals of all ages, sexes, races, and socioeconomic levels. Children and adolescents account for one third of all alleged sexual abuse victims. Of reported alleged sexual abuse, females account for approximately 85% of the victims. The median age of sexual abuse in females is approximately 10 years, with bimodal peaks at 5 to 6 years and a second peak at 14 to 15 years. Adolescents are prime targets for both physical and sexual abuse.

Adolescents are most often abused by relatives and young males whom they know. Approximately 75% of reported sexual abuse involves an older person known to the victim. Males are identified as perpetrators in more than 90% of the cases, but there is increasing recognition of adolescents and females as perpetrators of sexual abuse. In many reports, the mean age of perpetrators is 25 years or younger.

Adolescents tend to be subjected to more violence and trauma when they are sexually abused than are young children. Although physical trauma and evidence of sexual abuse is not always apparent, it is more likely to be found in the adolescent rape victim than in a younger sexually abused victim.

RISK FACTORS

Risks for victimization have been identified primarily from survey studies and retrospective reviews of patients reporting sexual abuse as children. Risk factors involving issues of family dynamics are difficult to define sharply, but many patterns emerge. Poor family communication, minimum supervision, and unmet emotional needs in the adolescent may increase the susceptibility to sexual abuse. Strict attitudes in the home about sex (such as punishment for masturbation or viewing sexually explicit material) is associated with a higher risk than more relaxed sexual attitudes. Confusion between sex and affection plays a role in abuse that occurs in homes where the father demonstrates little affection. The mother's role as a protector is an important one. A threefold increase in risk is noted when the victim has never lived with the natural mother. Those who have stepfathers are also identified as being at increased risk for sexual abuse. This risk is explained by abuse both by stepfathers as well as other men; some increase in risk occurs even before the child has a stepfather and suggests that the child may be in a sexually opportunistic environment. Any one of these environmental conditions may be an important risk factor for a given adolescent.

Adolescence per se has been considered a risk factor for sexual victimization. The developmental pressures and emerging sexuality in the task of separating from parental ties may place the early and middle adolescent in physical and social situations where rape and assault are more likely to occur. Risk-taking behaviors were commonly observed in adolescent sexual assault victims in one study—such activities as social interactions with strangers in unprotected surroundings, hitchhiking, and late evening interactions. Although unrealistic, adolescents who are physically mature may be expected to be able to protect themselves cognitively and physically from all such circumstances.

ACQUAINTANCE RAPE

There has been considerable investigation into the phenomenon of date rape and examination of risk factors. Because of the prior relationship of the individuals involved, date rape is considered a grossly underreported offense. Several potential risk factors have been suggested. There are conflicting data about the occurrence of date rape on a first date versus in a long-term relationship; 24% to 47% of reported date rape cases occur on first dates, but the percentage of all dates that are first dates is unknown. It is important to recognize that at any point in time in a relationship, date rape is a possibility. Some studies identify no relationship with the length of time the partners have known each other or with the age differential. Some increased risk for date rape has been identified when the man has initiated the date, pays for the date, and drives. Heavy use of alcohol or drugs by either person also places the adolescent at risk. "Parking" places the adolescent at the highest risk for date rape; this is linked to an apparent misinterpretation and miscommunication about expectations of sexual activity. Men frequently overestimate the date's interest in sex and feel "led on." Men seem to justify rape more often than do women.

Adolescents are often lenient in condoning nonconsensual sexual intercourse, particularly when partners are dating. Identification of nonconsensual sex as rape depends on who was encouraging sexual activity, the amount and type of force used, and the relationship between partners. Several studies demonstrate that adolescents of both genders expect that forced sexual relations may be legitimate and acceptable in a variety of circumstances. Because many adolescents misperceive social cues as an invitation for sexual intercourse, early education for both males and females on how to interpret behaviors more accurately as cues for sexual intimacy should be considered.

CLINICAL MANIFESTATIONS

Adolescents experience a heightened sexual awareness that may be filled with confusion, conflict, and contradictions. As the sexual roles develop, the adolescent seeks gender identification and the capacity for intimacy (see Chapters 9 and 120). Attaining independence is a major task. Mid-adolescence may be filled with the inability to control the course of events in one's life. Sexual abuse during this crucial phase may have serious implications. Coercion, misrepresentation, secrecy surrounding sexual activity, and an awareness of the taboo making adolescents different from peers may all contribute to the deleterious effects. Abusive relationships may teach adolescents to use sexual pleasure as a means of attaining social status or receiving approval and affection. Adolescents are often perceived differently from younger children when abuse is disclosed. The adolescent's behavior is often considered provocative, erratic, and limit testing. If runaway behavior or family violence (see Chapter 117) precipitates disclosure of sexual abuse, the adolescent is often considered the perpetrator, whose behavior encouraged the abuse. Thus, the young adult has not only the developmental issues of sexual identification and emancipation to address, but also may experience guilt and humiliation, much of which may be the result of societal biases against the adolescent.

The clinical manifestations of sexual abuse vary considerably from one adolescent to another, but all may encompass medical or psychological sequelae. Indicators of abuse are those behavioral or physical characteristics that suggest the possibility of sexual abuse but do not necessarily prove it. These are signs of problems or stress in the young person, one cause of which may be sexual abuse.

The behavioral manifestations commonly cited include such problems as depression (see Chapter 100), withdrawal, acting-out sexually, promiscuity, prostitution, drug and alcohol use (see Chapter 111), poor school performance, or any significant change in the adolescent's behavior. Abusive experiences may predispose adolescents to behavioral and emotional problems, sleep disturbances (see Chapter 86), drug and alcohol abuse (see Chapter 111), eating disorders (see Chapter 60), school failure and suicidal ideation (see Chapter 101). Low self-esteem, social isolation, delinquency, and runaway behavior are known among some sexual abuse victims. The physical indicators of abuse include genital complaints, sexually transmitted disease (see Chapter 75), genital pain, pregnancy in the very young adolescent (see Chapter 74), or other forms of trauma. If one does not ask the pregnant adolescent who the father of the child is, one will not ever discover that it is a relative or the result of unwanted sexual activity. These are obviously nonspecific findings, but some are more indicative of sexual abuse than others. All, without any other explanation, should raise suspicions of the possibility of sexual abuse of the young person.

Studies examining the strength of associations between behavioral and emotional problems and self-reported abuse have identified and confirmed that some indicators are strongly associated with sexual abuse. In a nonclinical school setting, students reporting sexual abuse did not report the emotional problems any more frequently than did those indicating no abuse. However, those students (boys and girls) reporting sexual abuse were almost five more times likely to report using laxatives and vomiting to control weight, and were three times more likely to report having attempted suicide. Students reporting both physical and sexual abuse reported a fivefold increase in laxative use (see Chapter

60), a fourfold increase in attempting suicide (see Chapter 101), and an almost tenfold increase in considering suicide. These findings in a nonclinical setting support those findings from clinical settings, suggesting the behavioral and physical sequelae of sexual abuse. Of particular concern are the associations with possible eating disorders, runaway behavior, and suicidal risk. There have been reports of lower self-esteem among those who have been sexually abused; there are conflicting data, however, to support those findings. Studies in nonclinical settings have not consistently supported the finding of lower self-esteem among adolescents reporting sexual abuse, particularly when age and gender are considered.

Although many of these symptoms should suggest the possibility of sexual victimization, it is important to recognize that there may be other causes. Several specific presentations, however, warrant questioning about possible sexual abuse in every situation, because of the much higher prevalence of a history of abuse among those presenting with such symptoms. These include hysterical seizures (see Chapter 83), eating disorders (see Chapter 60), runaway behavior, attempted suicide (see Chapter 101), multiple personality disorder (see Chapter 109), and post-traumatic stress disorder (see Chapter 104).

Sexually abused adolescents reporting the stresses of rape were fearful for their lives and of bodily harm. Guilt, shame, and self-blame were of greater concern than was anger directed at the perpetrator. The most important issue was to be accepted and treated like their peers. The "rape trauma syndrome" describes the constellation of behavioral, psychological, and somatic reactions of adult females to sexual abuse. Common symptoms include humiliation, anxiety, anger, embarrassment, and self-blame. Somatic symptoms are commonly experienced. Long-term effects include changing home location frequently, enhanced use of psychosocial supports, and development of trauma phobias. Adolescents' responses to rape may be considered developmentally based manifestations of the same process. Fears of leaving the home, interacting with strangers, and developing relationships with boys are followed by denial, permitting increasing socialization. Psychosomatic complaints of headaches, dizziness, or abdominal pain are often manifested.

It is estimated that 20% to 50% of sexual abuse victims suffer some major long-term sequelae from sexual victimization. In order to identify those experiences, one must ask whether they have occurred and thus address early victimization experiences in treatment. A disproportionate percentage of psychiatric clinic visits or psychiatric hospitalizations for adolescents represent those who have a history of having been sexually abused. It is postulated that the effects may not appear immediately after a sexually victimizing experience, but may develop over time. Subsequent situations may act as developmental triggers in expression of stress or distress from previous victimization. Sexual abuse has a serious mental health impact in an important portion of victims. The assessment of traumatic experiences demands tact, thoroughness, and good listening skills.

DIAGNOSIS AND ASSESSMENT

In order to identify the alleged sexual abuse victim, one must be receptive to the diagnosis and willing to accept the fact that sexual abuse does occur both during and before adolescence. If one does not have a high level of suspicion, one cannot identify the possibility that sexual abuse has occurred. The components of the evaluation for suspected sexual victimization are no different than those for any other evaluation. Each adolescent deserves a complete history, physical examination, assessment, and management plan. Health care providers should be involved in the medical diagnosis and treatment of suspected sexual abuse. They are making medical evaluations and recommendations, not legal determinations as to whether or not criminal activity was involved. However, health care providers in all states are mandated by law to report all suspected sexual abuse to the appropriate social or legal authorities (usually child protective services) in the community. Cooperation and communication with those social and legal professionals offer the best chance for appropriate protection and treatment of suspected abuse victims.

The interview should include a complete medical history. When sexual abuse is suspected, if the adolescent is able and willing to disclose inappropriate sexual activity, that information should be obtained. The health care provider performing the physical and initial psychosocial assessment does not need to obtain details about the abuse directly from the adolescent, but it is helpful to know the nature of the sexual activity in order to direct the physical examination. The interviewer should avoid asking leading questions and should allow the adolescent to disclose as much information in his or her own words as possible. Straightforward, matter-of-fact questions generally elicit most information. It is not the role of the health care provider to perform an investigative interview concerning alleged sexual abuse. In most situations when the abuse has been disclosed to other professionals, and when sexual abuse will have to be reported to social and legal authorities, the health care professional should avoid reinterviewing the adolescent about details that may make the adolescent feel uncomfortable. Interviewing in a mental health and therapeutic setting, however, is somewhat different, necessitating careful but extensive collection of detailed information. The complete history should include past medical history, including past sexual activity, use of tampons or feminine pads, and a menstrual history. Any surgeries or significant injury or trauma resulting in physical findings to the genital area are important to note. Signs or symptoms suggestive of stress, genital pain, or sexually transmitted diseases (STDs) need to be ascertained.

The physical examination should be complete, including a detailed genital, anal, and for some females, a gynecologic examination. It is important to allow the adolescent to have a support person in the room during the examination if he or she desires. The general examination should identify trauma anywhere on the body—bites, bruises, petechiae, strangulation marks, or signs of being physically tied about the wrists or ankles.

The detailed genital examination should be performed within the context of a routine complete physical examination for both males and females. In the young female adolescent who has not been previously sexually active and is premenarcheal, a pelvic examination may not be necessary, because specimens for cultures and for evidence of seminal fluid may be obtained without inserting a speculum. Collection of forensic evidence is indicated if an assault occurred within 72 to 96 hours of presentation to medical care, and should be done according to protocol set by individual communities or hospitals. Components of such protocols are described in detail elsewhere. Details of the genital and gynecologic examination are described in this text (see Chapter 69). All adolescent victims of suspected sexual abuse should be cultured for sexually transmitted diseases, including *Neisseria gonorrhoeae* and *Chlamydia trachomatis*. Testing for human immunodeficiency virus (HIV) and syphilis depends on the epidemiology and prevalence of such problems in the community as well as risk based on the clinical history. If one sexually transmitted disease is identified, the diagnosis of others must be sought. Pregnancy testing is an important consideration in menarcheal females (see Chapter 69). Pregnancy prophylaxis and sexually transmitted disease prophylaxis in the acute rape victim are usually included in forensic evidence protocols (see Chapter 75).

The physician's examination, short of detecting a sexually transmitted disease or evidence of sperm on wet mount, can rarely "prove" or "disprove" sexual contact. Even when sexual contact is evident, the examining physician cannot state the identity of the perpetrator. Most victims of nonviolent sexual abuse have normal physical examinations. It is often difficult to ascertain whether an adolescent has actually had vaginal or rectal penetration. Penetration means penetration of the genitalia and does not imply ejaculation or hymenal injury; in vulvar intercourse, the labia are penetrated. Fondling, oral/genital contact, and vulvar intercourse rarely leave physical findings. One study recently reported that the child and adolescent victims in 77% of legally proven cases of sexual assault with penetration had no physical evidence of abuse. The physician's emphasis should be on identifying and treating medical complications, reporting suspected abuse to the appropriate authorities, and seeing that the adolescent victim receives the appropriate mental health service and intervention. Protection and appropriate treatment are the major issues.

TREATMENT

Treatment issues include primary and secondary prevention, as well as early intervention for suspected victims, medical treatment, and mental health services. Coordination of the evaluation and treatment of an adolescent victim of sexual abuse is critical in assuring appropriate and optimal delivery of services and intervention. The best interest of the adolescent must be addressed when coordinating services and optimizing the outcome. Successful sexual abuse evaluation and treatment programs are multidisciplinary. Physicians, nurses, social workers, and mental health providers should have close working relationships with child protective service agencies, welfare departments, and police and judiciary systems. Medical treatment is directed at specific and medical sequelae of abuse, sexually transmitted disease, pregnancy, and physical trauma. The availability of short-term and long-term psychological services is necessary, and the physician may wish to refer adolescents, depending on his or her counseling skills.

A majority of treatment is directed at the psychological impact of sexual abuse. There are four trauma-causing factors that need to be addressed: traumatic sexualization, betrayal of the adolescent, the sense of powerlessness, and stigmatization of having been a sexual assault victim. There are many impact and treatment issues that need to be addressed. The "damaged goods syndrome" is common—the adolescent feels that his or her body has been permanently harmed and subsequent normal sexual relations are impossible. There are also issues of guilt, fear, depression, low self-esteem, repressed anger and hostility, and the impaired ability to trust. Pseudo-maturity is often a difficulty, and the adolescent must learn self mastery and control. Treatment must eventually examine what the sexually abusive experiences were and what the expectations of the adolescent are now, and why the sexual abuse has been revealed at this time, particularly if it occurred long ago. Generally, both the adolescent and parents need to be involved in treatment. There must be some assessment of the adolescent's present and past functioning and of the parent's feelings about what happened. It is very important to help the parents learn to treat the adolescent as they had before the abuse. The adolescent is not a different person simply because he or she has been the victim of sexual assault.

There are a variety of treatment programs and approaches available. Many will recommend both individual and family therapy and support group therapy for the same family (see Chapters 98 and 123). There are professional and self-help groups. It is also important in many situations, particularly family situations, for the perpetrator to receive treatment. When the perpetrator is a family member, effective treatment must occur before the family is reunited. It is important not to place any blame on the adolescent victim in such a setting. The goal of a treatment program is to address the sexually abusive experience and put it into a perspective in the child and family's life. The ultimate goal and hopeful outcome is that the adolescent and family go on to lead a normal life.

LONG-TERM OUTCOME

The impact of sexual abuse on eventual adult outcome is influenced by numerous variables. There are many unknowns preceding and following abusive experiences, so direct cause and effect cannot be determined. Many associations are noted, suggesting that sexual victimization relates to adjustment disorders in later life (see Chapter 104). Some studies suggest that the greatest impact results from a longer duration of abuse, abuse perpetrated by a close relative, the type of genital contact involved, the use of force or aggression in the assault, and the degree of the adolescent's participation in the sexual activity. Environment and support play an important role, particularly at the time of disclosure. The receptivity of the parents and the system to the adolescent's disclosure may have a considerable impact. Evidence also suggests that sexual victimization as an adolescent has a more significant impact than abuse at a younger age. There are so many variables involved that, for any given individual, it is impossible to predict the long-term outcome. Strong emotional and psychosocial supports are imperative for a good outcome. Later, more normal sexual experiences and the attitudes of the family and community may temper the adverse effect.

There is a clear association between sexual victimization in the family and ongoing sexual abuse in future generations. Cycles of violence have been identified—it is important to break the cycle of abuse as soon as possible. It is true that, in many situations, the victims of sexual abuse appear to have adapted and adjusted very appropriately. There are many women in their middle age and senior years who have never previously disclosed the sexual victimization they experienced as young people who disclose it as older individuals. These women apparently have led very normal, well-adjusted lives. The significant potential for short- and long-term negative impact, however, warrants appropriate and timely intervention and provision of service needed.

Sexual abuse affects far more adolescents than one would like to believe. Recognition of the problem and its potential effect on an adolescent can facilitate identification and management, to offer the best opportunity for optimal outcome.

BIBLIOGRAPHY

Browne A, Finklehor D: Impact of child sexual abuse: A review of the research. Psychol Bull 99:66, 1986.

Burgess AW, Groth AN, Holmstrom LL, et al: Sexual Assault of Children and Adolescents. Lexington, MA, D.C. Heath and Co, 1978.

Burgess AW, Holmstrom LL: Rape trauma syndrome. Am J Psychiatry 131:981, 1974.

Cavallin BJ: Treatment of sexually abused adolescents, views of a psychologist. Seminars in Adolescent Medicine 3:39, 1987.

Emans SJ, Goldstein DP: Sexual abuse. In Pediatric and Adolescent Gynecology, 3rd ed. Boston, Little, Brown and Co, 1990, p 539–568.

Hibbard RA, Brack CJ, Rauch S, et al: Abuse, feelings, and health behaviors in a student population. Am J Dis Child 142:326, 1988.

Hibbard RA, Orr DP: Incest and sexual abuse. Seminars in Adolescent Medicine 1:153, 1985.

Hibbard RA, Ingersoll G, Orr D: Behavioral risk, emotional risk, and child abuse among adolescents in a non-clinical setting. Pediatrics 86:896, 1990.

Kanda M, Thomas JN, Lloyd DW: The role of forensic evidence in child abuse and neglect. Am J Forensic Med Pathol 6:7, 1985.

Kluft RP (ed): Treatment of victims of sexual abuse. Psychiatr Clin North Am 12:237, 1989.

Muehlenhard CL, Linton MA: Rape and sexual aggression in dating situations: Incidence and risk factors. J Counseling Psychol 34:186, 1987.

Wisdom CS: The cycle of violence. Science 244:160, 1989.

CHAPTER 120

Sexual Orientation

ANKE A. EHRHARDT and ROBERT H. REMIEN

Sexual orientation norms vary in different societies and at different times. The United States has undergone radical changes during the twentieth century in the patterns of sexual behavior that are acceptable and are actually practiced.

Adolescent sexual behavior is usually assessed by age of first sexual intercourse and by patterns of sexual practices and number of partners (see Chapters 2 and 68). Findings of recent national surveys provide estimates of the average age of initiation of sexual intercourse in the United States. Most adolescents report having engaged in sexual intercourse by age 19 years, with a higher percentage of males than females at any age and with earlier intercourse among black than among white teenagers.

The stereotype of adolescents who are indiscriminate is not supported by existing data. Many adolescents have only one sexual partner. Adolescent men tend to have more partners than do adolescent women, but even for them, the most common pattern can be described as serial monogamy, rather than a pattern of simultaneous affairs with more than one partner. Furthermore, sexual intercourse for adolescents often occurs sporadically rather than on a regular basis. Conversely, once sexual intercourse has been initiated, sexual activity usually continues. Thus it is uncommon for teens to become completely abstinent once they have engaged in sexual intercourse.

Adolescence is also a time when there is psychological separation of the young person from the parents. Adolescents who are greatly influenced by peer behavior and perceived peer norms may view the parent(s) as obstacles in their "belonging." Power struggles over freedoms and privileges ensue, and communication may be characterized by conflict. Adolescents, while desiring accurate information about their sexuality, may find it difficult to discuss the topic with their families. Often the physician is the only "informed" adult in whom the adolescent can confide his or her feelings and thoughts about sexuality. It is important, therefore, that health care workers be knowledgeable and feel comfortable discussing sexual behavior with adolescents.

SEXUAL ORIENTATION

Sexual orientation refers to a person's sexual responsiveness to partners of the same or opposite gender and one's sense of self in society (see Chapter 32). The concept of sexual orientation includes at least three distinctive aspects: sexual imagery (fantasies and attractions); actual sexual behavior; and a person's sexual identity as heterosexual, bisexual, or homosexual.

The adolescent years are a crucial time for the establishment of adult sexual identity. This process is often accompanied by worry, confusion, and uncertainty. It is normal for adolescents to experiment and rehearse sexual behaviors. Many adolescents may have both heterosexual and homosexual attractions and experiences, which do not necessarily predict a specific adult sexual identity. Some homosexual behaviors, such as mutual touching or masturbation, are considered by some scientists and clinicians to be a normal aspect of the transition from childhood to heterosexual adulthood. In fact, homosexual experimentation is common during adolescence, and many more adolescents engage in homosexual behavior than become homosexually oriented.

DIFFERENTIAL DEFINITIONS

Homosexuality needs to be differentiated from gender identity disorders and especially from transsexualism and transvestism (see Chapter 32).

Gender identity disorders reflect a person's profound sense of discomfort and confusion about his or her anatomical body and a persistent sense of belonging to the opposite sex. In cases of transsexualism, gender-identity confusion is so profound that the person persistently desires to change his or her gender and to seek surgical and hormonal sex reassignment. The ultimate goal is to become the gender opposite to that which was originally assigned and in which one was raised. When transsexualism is expressed in adolescence, specialized counseling and treatment are always indicated, although some believe considerations of hormonal and surgical procedures need to be postponed until the person is an adult, whereas others believe hormone therapy during late adolescence may be indicated. However, transsexual adolescents need acceptance and nonjudgmental counseling and support for their dilemma, rather than punitive moralizing that may alienate and isolate them even further.

Transvestism is recurrent and persistent cross-dressing by a man who is typically heterosexual. Cross-dressing in women's clothes is often linked to sexual excitement.

This research was supported in part by NIMH/NIDA Grant #1P50 MH-43520, HIV Center for Clinical and Behavioral Studies, New York, New York.

For the transvestite, cross-dressing may begin in childhood or adolescence and progress into adulthood. Treatment may be initiated by the transvestitic man himself or by his female partner.

Homosexuality usually does not include a problem with one's gender identity as a man or a woman, although confusion and worry, especially during the initial phase of establishing one's homosexual identity, may include concern over adequacy and appropriateness of gender. Cross-dressing does occur in some homosexual men and, to a lesser extent, among lesbian women.

THEORIES OF CAUSE

At the present time, there is still a lack of a conclusive and generally accepted theory about the development of sexual orientation. Researchers and clinicians have more often focused on assessing the factors that may lead to homosexuality rather than to heterosexuality, on the assumption that homosexual behavior is "deviant" and "abnormal." Although many arguments proclaiming the "pathology" of homosexual behavior are based on personal, cultural, political, or moral grounds, scientific arguments promoted in support of homosexuality as deviance have stood up poorly to close empirical and theoretical scrutiny. According to Marmor, the concept of homosexuality as pathology is based on three major premises: (1) that homosexual behavior is a disorder of sexual development resulting from disturbed family relationships, (2) that it represents an obvious deviation from the biological norm, and (3) that homosexuals are found to be emotionally disturbed, unhappy people when studied psychodynamically. Past and current theories reflect these premises.

Family Constellation

Several theories suggesting the importance of early experiences in the life of a child have been proposed to explain adult homosexuality. The focus of these theories has been on the long-term importance of either traumatic or rewarding childhood sexual experiences that set the stage for adult homosexual orientation. These experiences may be between the child and his or her peers or with an adult. Most often, the focus has been on the family constellation.

Psychoanalysis has been the most influential theory for clinicians in shaping their concepts and clinical approaches to homosexuals and homosexual experiences. Psychoanalysis basically proposes that homosexuality stems from an arrested development based on a complex family constellation of a mother who keeps her son too close and a father who is too threatening and distant. Freud's theory on female homosexuality is less well developed, as is the case in most sexual orientation theories.

The basic flaw of family constellation theories is that they derive their evidence from retrospective accounts of adult patients without proper controls. When put to the test of empirical evidence, these theories typically do not hold up and lack conclusive evidence. For instance, in a large survey about the lives of homosexual and heterosexual men and women, most assumptions about specific family constellations and early experiences as being different for homosexuals than for heterosexuals were not supported.

Biologic Deviance

Another set of theories is based on the assumption that homosexuals are biologically different from heterosexuals. Recently, the main focus of these theories has been differences in sex hormones, either prenatally or in adulthood. The premise is that male homosexuals have lower levels of androgens than do heterosexual men, and that lesbians have either lower estrogens or increased androgens. As summarized in comprehensive reviews, one can safely conclude from the exisiting literature that male and female homosexuals do not differ from heterosexuals in their serum levels of sex hormones.

Although the debate on differences in peripheral serum levels of sex hormones has been largely settled, theories of biologic differences have continued. Currently, most of the discussion in this area is focused on prenatal sex hormonal differences that may affect the developing brain. The empirical evidence is usually based on animal experimental models, studies involving men and women with atypical prenatal histories, or on experimental hormonal studies of adult homosexual and heterosexual men and women that may indicate a presumptive prenatal anomaly. The findings of these studies are controversial and often contradictory, and do not warrant any conclusion that homosexuals as a group can be described as biologically different from heterosexuals.

Interactional Theories

It appears that one can assume at this point that adult men and women with homosexual orientations vary in their histories, just as do heterosexual men and women, and that etiologic roots are complex, with different pathways for various "homosexualities" and "heterosexualities." It may well be that specific constitutional predispositions set the stage for a greater likelihood of developing a homosexual or heterosexual orientation dependent on postnatal life events and choices. Rather than searching for one underlying important variable that will explain complex behavioral clusters as sexual orientation, we should adopt the approach of an interactional or transactional model that integrates constitutional and environmental events and may explain different types of homosexual and heterosexual orientation.

One theory combines both biologic events and social development. It proposes that early maturing adolescents are more likely to form homosexual attachments than are other adolescents. Early adolescence is a time of strong same-sex friendships. It is argued that early pubertal development increases sexual fantasies and attractions. Because early maturers have not begun to interact socially with opposite-sex peers, the sexual attractions become focused on same-sex friends. This theory needs empirical testing. Studies on clinical populations with precocious puberty do not support the proposed association of early maturation and homosexuality.

Gender Role Development

Gender role behavior includes play, interests, attitudes, and choices that may be either masculine or feminine. More frequently than straight men, gay men consistently retrospectively report a childhood history of "feminine" behavior. Lesbians recall having been tomboys more often than do straight women. "Feminine" behavior in boys leads to peer isolation and teasing, while tomboys are usually integrated and appreciated by their female peers. In adulthood, most homosexual men and women exhibit gender role behavior that is either completely unremarkable or more or less typically feminine or masculine within the spectrum of acceptable gender expression in our society. Gay men and lesbian women usually do not have problems about their gender identification.

A small subgroup of male homosexuals undergo a traumatic childhood because they exhibit extremely "feminine" behavior. Those boys typically come to the clinical attention of counselors and therapists because they are desperately unhappy and want to be girls. Based on a relatively small group of prospective studies, it appears that a substantial number of those extremely "feminine" boys often become homosexuals in adulthood.

Extremely masculine behavior in girls is much rarer and typically does not alienate girls from their peers in the way that "feminine" boys are alienated from their peers. While there are fewer data on the developmental course of such girls, it appears that female gender role development plays a different role in the establishment of sexual orientation in women than in men. One such follow-up study of very masculine girls and their controls revealed no differences at puberty.

It is unclear how different patterns of gender role development interact with adult sexual orientation. There is no conclusive evidence on why some boys exhibit extreme "feminine" behavior in childhood or why some girls exhibit extreme "tomboyish" behavior. Etiologic considerations include critical events and possibly prenatal dispositions leading to specific temperamental patterns.

Homosexuality as a Mental Illness

Before 1973, homosexuality was included in the list of "mental disorders" in the *Diagnostic and Statistical Manual for Mental Disorders (DSM)* published by the American Psychiatric Association. It was not until December 1973 that the Board of Trustees of the American Psychiatric Association voted to delete homosexuality from subsequent editions of the *DSM*.

This decision was made following considerable debate. The final consensus, albeit controversial in the psychiatric profession, is that homosexuality in and of itself does not constitute a mental disorder and that sexual orientation should be considered irrelevant to the issue of mental illness. As with heterosexual individuals, psychiatric assessment of homosexuals should be made on the basis of specific psychiatric criteria.

Several studies have shown that homosexual persons do not experience more mental illness than do heterosexual persons, although they may report more unhappiness and problems of self-acceptance, which is not surprising in a society that consistently exhibits homophobia and discrimination. Therefore, the establishment of an adolescent's or a young adult's sexual identity and the support and acceptance received from a clinician are of paramount importance.

ESTABLISHMENT OF SEXUAL IDENTITY

Although the process of sexual identity development begins in childhood and often continues into adulthood, adolescence is a critical time for its establishment. Many of a teenager's thoughts, feelings, and desires are focused on his or her sexuality. It is during middle to late adolescence that gay and lesbian teenagers begin to question the notion that their thoughts and feelings might mean that they are indeed homosexual. This stage of "identity confusion" is characterized by conflict and self-doubt, and may lead to significant depression, interpersonal difficulties, school failure, substance abuse, and even suicide in some instances (see Chapter 32). Because of the stigma so strongly associated with homosexuality, this can be an extremely difficult time for a teenager facing these issues. As a result, the adolescent may actively conceal his or her thoughts and feelings and avoid discussing them with anyone. This can contribute to a lack of knowledge and inaccurate information about homosexuality, leading to unfavorable outcomes and increased isolation. It is in this stage that adolescents are at highest risk for extreme "acting out," such as dropping out of school and running away from home. It is also a time when intervention by a nonjudgmental, accepting professional can have its greatest beneficial impact. When and how to intervene in such cases will be discussed in greater detail below.

The individual (adolescent or adult) struggling with a possible homosexual identity may cope in one or several typical ways. He or she may simply deny it to himself or herself, as well as to others. He or she may try to "fix" it by becoming immersed in heterosexual activities to varying degrees or, alternatively, by seeking professional help to change his or her orientation. Avoidance of coming to terms with one's homosexual identity can take various forms, such as shying away from interactions with opposite-sex peers or from exposure to other "identified" homosexual individuals, groups, or to any available information on homosexuality. In its more extreme form, avoidance may involve adapting an "antihomosexual" stance, which can lead to such behaviors as ridiculing or even physically attacking known homosexuals. Extreme escapism, such as substance abuse, is another maladaptive strategy. Some individuals may cope by redefining their behavior or rationalizing it. They may, for instance, attribute their behavior to a situation such as being "too high" on alcohol or other drugs, or they may excuse their behavior by telling themselves that it is only temporary or a phase that they are going through.

Assuming a homosexual identity and presenting oneself as homosexual is seen as an emerging stage in a larger process of "coming out." The process of coming out can be a long one, typically extending well into adulthood. Self-disclosure of one's homosexual identity occurs in restricted circumstances initially, typically by first coming out to close confidantes. Early supportive contacts can facilitate the ongoing process of coming out, ultimately culminating in self-acceptance and confidence in one's identity as valid, and the desire and ability to enter into same-sex love relationships.

Women usually establish their sexual identity later than men, often in their twenties and thirties. Cass describes the achievement of "identity synthesis" in the following way: "You are prepared to tell almost anyone that you are homosexual. You are happy about the way you are, but feel that being a homosexual is not the most important part of you. You mix socially with homosexuals and heterosexuals, with whom you are open about your homosexuality." This of course is not meant to indicate that one must tell everyone of his or her sexual identity, just as a person need not disclose his or her heterosexuality, political party affiliation, or preferences in food in every and all situations. Self-disclosure of sexuality will depend on many factors, including the prevailing community atmosphere and the cultural and geographic circumstances in which an individual finds himself or herself (see Chapter 32).

CLINICAL MANAGEMENT

Approaching and Discussing the Topic of Sexual Orientation

Developing adolescents have many questions about their bodies and the changes that occur in them, but will almost never ask. Often an adolescent is too self-conscious or embarrassed to raise the topic and is relieved when the physician introduces it. The physician who is prepared to listen and to accept information in a nonjudgmental way can be extremely helpful in clarifying mixed or conflicting feelings in adolescent patients. When approaching adolescents about issues of sexual identity, it is important to initiate a discussion about how the adolescent sees himself or herself; specifically, whether a young girl sees herself as heterosexual or lesbian and whether a young man sees himself as heterosexual or gay. The physician fulfills a unique role in determining whether this is a young person who has questions about his or her sexual identity. What is more important, however, is what their feelings, behaviors, and uncertainties are (see Chapter 32).

Within the context of obtaining a medical and behavioral history, the matter of sexual identity can be broached by the clinician. One may, for example, say to a young man, "Some of the boys I talk to tell me about wanting to have a sexual experience. Do you feel that way? With girls? With another boy? Has that ever happened to you?" This approach lets the adolescent know that this is not new or shocking to the physician, and establishes an atmosphere in which the adolescent can discuss a subject that might otherwise by considered totally taboo.

If the adolescent confides homosexual experiences, one can expand the conversation by asking the adolescent how he or she feels about this situation and how it might affect relationships with friends. Seeing oneself as different from one's peers is an experience more common for gay youth than for heterosexual youth. However, it is important to remember that the adolescent years are formative for the development of sexual identity in all adolescents, and every effort should be made to avoid early self-labeling by the patient that ultimately may not be accurate.

Sexual Identity Crisis

When feelings of ambivalence and doubt result in a true sexual identity crisis, it is important that this condition is recognized and that the adolescent be helped in addressing those feelings. A sexual identity crisis occurs when the adolescent experiences distress over his or her own sexual identity. As described earlier, deep concern about sexual identity can lead to worry, depression, isolation, and "acting out behaviors" (e.g., substance abuse, sex with multiple partners, poor school performance). The physician can be a key person for open dialogue with the adolescent and can initiate a plan that ensures that proper assistance will be given for resolving such conflicts and anxieties.

Counseling and Treatment

Homosexual behavior should not be seen as a disorder and, therefore, does not require treatment. However, adolescents may need help and support, which may be provided by the physician or knowledgeable mental health counselor. The physician should include in his or her counseling a discussion about the risks of sexually transmitted diseases (STDs) and human immunodeficiency virus (HIV) from unsafe sexual behavior and how the adolescent can exert protection (see Chapters 32, 75, and 76).

CASE PRESENTATION

Tom, a 15-year-old boy, saw the physician for a physical examination at his mother's request. The physician had only seen Tom once before, 2 years earlier, but had also treated Tom's younger brother (age 11 years) and sister (age 9 years) and, therefore, knew the family. Tom's mother had noticed that Tom had recently become quiet, lethargic, and withdrawn. Previously a good student, he had done very poorly in several of his examinations recently. His appetite was poor and he had lost several pounds during the past several weeks. When questioned, he denied there was anything wrong. Tom's mother was concerned that he might have a physical problem and wanted him to be evaluated.

When Tom came in for his examination, he appeared to be underweight and sullen. Upon initial questioning, Tom denied experiencing any physical or psychologic difficulties. In the course of the examination, the clinician raised the issue of sexuality. He said that he knew Tom was at the age when boys usually experience many different sexual feelings that at times can become confusing, and he wondered if he had any questions in this area. Tom said he didn't and that he had a "girlfriend" but had never had sex. He admitted that he did feel some pressure to have sex because all the boys at school talked about it, but that he didn't really feel that he wanted to. He confessed that he was wondering if this was normal.

The physician assured Tom that it is okay to not be sexually active and that it is normal not to feel ready for it. He also explained that very often boys his age boast about having sex even when they have not really had it. Sensing that there was more that was bothering Tom, he went on to say that very often boys his age also experience an attraction to other boys, and wondered if this had ever happened to Tom. Tom seemed to become embarrassed. After considerable discussion, Tom admitted to an incident a month earlier in which he and a neighborhood boy were involved in a discussion about sex that culminated in mutual masturbation; he assured the physician that he was definitely not "queer." Nevertheless, Tom had been feeling quite confused and upset by the experience. Although he likes this boy a lot, he is afraid that others will think that he is gay if they see him with the boy or if they find out about what happened. At school, the other boys had been teasing this boy because he is slightly effeminate. In fact, Tom himself has joined them, ridiculing the boy in order to protect his own image. He feels quite guilty about this. Tom does not want to become homosexual, and is also concerned about setting the right example for his younger brother and sister. He wanted reassurances from the doctor that he wasn't really "queer," and made him promise not to tell anyone about this discussion, including his parents.

The physician correctly saw Tom's need for continued discussion and the opportunity for counseling, if he so desired. The medical examination revealed no abnormalities, and it was therefore safe to assume that his withdrawal, lethargy, weight loss, and dysphoria might be related to his concerns about his sexuality. Medical follow-up, of course, would continue. The physician assured Tom that the behavior in which he engaged was normal for boys his age, and that it didn't necessarily mean that he was gay. He went on to say, however, that Tom should consider it an open question as to whether or not he would become gay or perhaps bisexual in the future; that it was normal to be questioning his own sexuality at this time; and that if he did develop stronger homosexual attractions, it would not be wrong. He recommended that Tom speak with a counselor.

It was important for the physician to alleviate some of Tom's guilt and anxiety by "normalizing" his feelings and experience, and also by letting Tom know that homosexual feelings and behavior are okay. By providing the opportunity for counseling, he was letting Tom know that it is good to talk about these issues with someone who has experience, because Tom probably had other feelings and thoughts that he had not been able to express. It was not clear whether Tom would develop a gay, heterosexual, or bisexual identity. It was important, however, for the physician to tell him that whatever his identity would be, there was no need for him to experience guilt or shame.

The physician suggested that it would probably be helpful to Tom if he eventually spoke with his parents about some of these issues, but that he would respect his confidence and would not tell his parents about the details of their discussion. It was important that Tom knew he could trust the doctor. The physician's nonjudgmental stance and willingness to maintain confidentiality allowed for continued discussions.

BIBLIOGRAPHY

Bell AP, Weinberg MS, Hammersmith SK: Sexual Preference: Its Development in Men and Women. Bloomington, IN, Indiana University Press, 1981.

Cass CV: Homosexual identity formation: Testing a theoretical model. J Sex Res 20:143, 1984.

Ehrhardt AA: Abnormal puberty: Psychological implications and treatment issues. In Shaffer D, Ehrhardt AA, Greenhill LL (eds): The Clinical Guide to Child Psychiatry. New York, The Free Press, 1985, pp 145–168.

Green R: "The Sissy Boy Syndrome" and the Development of Homosexuality: A 15-Year Prospective Study. New Haven, CT, Yale University Press, 1986.

Herdt G (ed): Gay and Lesbian Youth. New York, Harrington Park Press, 1989.

Luria Z, Friedman S, Rose MD: Human Sexuality. New York, John Wiley & Sons, 1987.

McCauley E, Ehrhardt AA: Psychotherapy in the clinical management of females with gender identity disorders. J Nerv Ment Dis 172:353, 1984.

Marmor J: Homosexuality and the issue of mental illness. In Marmor J: Homosexual Behavior: A Modern Reappraisal. New York, Basic Books, 1980, pp 391–401.

Meyer-Bahlburg HFL: Sex hormones and male homosexuality in comparative perspective. Arch Sex Behav 6:297, 1977.

Meyer-Bahlburg HFL: Sex hormones and female homosexuality: A critical examination. Arch Sex Behav 8:101, 1979.

Miller HG, Turner CF, Moses LE (eds): AIDS: The Second Decade. Washington, DC, National Academy Press, 1990.

Storms M: A theory of erotic orientation development. Psychol Rev 88:340, 1981.

Williams K, Goodman M, Green R: Parent-child factors in gender role socialization in girls. J Am Acad Child Adolesc Psychiatry 24:720, 1985.

CHAPTER 121

Chronic Illness and Psychological Health

GREGORY K. FRITZ

Robert Louis Stevenson has been quoted as saying, "Life is not a matter of holding good cards but of playing a poor hand well." Adolescents with a chronic illness are engaged in this process on a daily basis, and their physicians have the potential to improve their chances for a successful outcome. The psychological impact of chronic illness on adolescent development is best conceptualized and evaluated in terms of its effect on the developmental tasks of adolescence. Psychosocial interventions are available to prevent, minimize, or treat the psychosocial problems of chronically ill adolescents. This chapter reviews both the areas of impact and the interventions, concluding with a discussion of the process of effective interdisciplinary collaboration to help these patients (see Chapter 30).

PSYCHOLOGICAL IMPACT OF CHRONIC ILLNESS

Four specific developmental tasks of adolescence are widely recognized, and chronic illness potentially affects all of them. Attainment of physical maturity is a central process in adolescence that has been described in detail earlier in this volume. In healthy adolescents, the variation in timing of pubertal events has an impact on subsequent psychosocial adjustment, especially for boys. Early maturing boys are rated as more popular, confident, and socially mature than boys who mature later, although the pattern is less consistent for girls.

Many chronic illnesses have an impact on adolescent physical development and intensify normal concerns. Congenital heart disease, endocrine disorders and inflammatory bowel disease can lead to delayed growth and maturation; cystic fibrosis, rheumatoid arthritis and many neurologic disorders have associated physical stigmata; visible side effects are common with prednisone and many chemotherapeutic agents (see Chapter 30). The adolescent's exquisite sensitivity to bodily changes and a fragile body image may hinder compliance with treatments that disfigure or otherwise make the adolescent look different from peers (see Chapter 26). Anxiety about physical sequelae of chronic illness also has an external source, because the negative reactions to phys-

ical disabilities that pervade society are especially intense in junior and senior high schools. Adolescents with a chronic illness may experience insensitivity or even cruelty at one time or another. Unfortunately, the affected adolescent may have to initiate meaningful social interactions. Humor, directness, and confidence are important skills for chronically ill adolescents. Some studies have suggested that adolescents who are marginally affected by an illness or disability have more serious psychosocial adjustment problems than do adolescents whose physical disabilities are more obvious and severe, presumably because of the associated ambiguity and the fact that their own and others' expectations do not take the chronic condition into account.

Development of autonomy and separation from parents is a gradual process that results in living independently. The degree to which rebellion, upheaval, turmoil, and disagreements with parents are essential components of this individuation process is widely debated. Most empirical studies do not support the inevitability of "storm and stress" during adolescence (see Chapter 8). Major alienation or conflict should be viewed as signs of potential problems (occurring in 4% to 5% of all adolescents) and not inevitable aspects of growing up.

A chronic illness can have a significant effect on an adolescent's autonomy. The illness dictates a degree of dependence on adults, both parents and physicians, that is not required of healthy adolescents. Because adolescents (and parents) both desire and fear independence, the enforced dependency experienced by a chronically ill adolescent may be frustrating, but also may be gratifying. The adolescent with a physical disorder can use it to express rebellious independence (by flaunting noncompliance, missing appointments, and so on) or, alternatively, to influence adults to make allowances and to care for them. Parents may be overprotective and excessively involved in the teenager's life as a result of guilt about their belief that they are somehow responsible for the adolescent's disorder. In extreme cases, the opposite occurs: the parents reject an ill adolescent and justify their actions as hastening the adolescent's separation from them. Adolescent compliance problems, risk-taking, retaliation, and manipulation may result when the illness and the treatment of the illness are a struggle for independence. In contrast, compliance (with contraceptive therapy in a general adolescent population and salicylate therapy among adolescents with rheumatoid arthritis) has been shown to increase with increasing adolescent autonomy. Autonomy is based on internalized standards and a sense of self that are fostered by the adolescent's ongoing love and respect for his or her parents. Autonomy, seemingly the antithesis of compliance, actually promotes the adolescent's active participation in and acceptance of therapeutic goals—hence, some physicians' preference for the term "adherence" to "compliance" (see Chapter 26).

Adolescence is a period of establishment of sexual identity and mature relationships with both sexes. The investment of adolescents in peer group relationships is a gradual process, with stages leading to increasing personal intimacy. In early adolescence, fashions, language, activities, and manners of the peer group are rigid, and the young teenager who is forced to deviate from them can be ostracized. Contacts with the opposite sex begin as group activities, progress to awkward dating, and may lead to intense "first love" in middle or late adolescence (see Chapter 68). A rich fantasy life, masturbation, crushes on idealized older teenagers or adults, and sexual exploration are common, normal components of the adolescent's development toward a stable sexual identity. Narcissism (self-love and preoccupation) is prominent in adolescence and may lead to transient homosexual experimentation.

An extensive literature documents the pervasive tendency of healthy, able-bodied people of all ages to not recognize the sexuality of those with physical disability. When chronically ill adolescents are hospitalized in rooms shared with the opposite sex, examined without draping or privacy, or thought not to need sex education or contraception, the covert message is that they are asexual (see Chapter 30). When urogenital involvement, sterility, or physical maturation delay complicates the picture, the adolescent may be uncomfortable and self-conscious to the point of withdrawal from sexual exploration. Any change in an adolescent's body integrity evokes concern about loss of masculine or feminine self-image, which can then be manifested in an immature, "cute-but-asexual" bearing or compensatory seductive or "macho" posturing. Unavoidable school absence or a hastily authorized home tutor may isolate the ill adolescent even further from the peer culture. The isolation can be aggravated by the healthy teenagers' ignorance about medical facts and their own fears of disability. Healthy peers may avoid or actively exclude the chronically ill adolescent and foreclose opportunities for that adolescent to experiment sexually and to develop social skills with the peer group.

Adolescents are preparing for a productive place in society. Much of adolescence is devoted to developing the factual knowledge, cognitive abilities, technical expertise, and personal maturity needed to join the work force and to raise a family. The presence of a chronic illness may interfere with the preparatory tasks of adolescence through reduced or irregular school attendance. The illness can result in decreased energy to invest in broadening experiences, where a special interest or talent can be discovered, such as in music, 4-H activity, religious youth groups, or other extracurricular activities. Chronically ill teenagers, even those who are able, often do not participate in volunteer work programs or experiment with part-time jobs to the same degree as do their healthy peers, thereby delaying their initiation into the world of productive work.

The task of preparing for the future may be especially difficult for the adolescent with a progressive or potentially fatal illness. Well-meaning adults may feel that preparation for an uncertain future is pointless and adopt a "have fun every day you can" attitude. For the adolescent with cancer or cystic fibrosis, central concerns are the need to contribute to society and to leave a mark of his or her existence on the world. Thus, seriously ill adolescents are often enthusiastic to create something, to participate in a meaningful teaching program, or to help other less fortunate individuals.

The degree to which psychological problems are caused by the stresses of chronic illness is under intense study. Nolan and Pless, in a review of over 50 studies of the psychosocial consequences of a variety of disorders present at birth, concluded that although the epidemiologic evidence is imperfect, a causal relationship does exist between the presence of a chronic disorder and increased risk of later emotional problems. Chronic illness during childhood and adolescence is associated with significantly greater use of social, mental health, and special education services by the families of the chronically ill. Adolescents with a chronic disorder may be at twice the risk of experiencing psychosocial problems compared to their healthy peers, data that warrant clinicians' heightened alertness.

There is ample evidence documenting that most chronically ill adolescents make a satisfactory adjustment to their illnesses and are relatively free of major psychopathology.

Mattsson has provided a practical definition of what constitutes reasonable adjustment to a chronic disorder in adolescence: (1) age-appropriate dependence on the family, (2) minimal need for secondary gain from the illness, (3) acceptance of the limits and responsibilities imposed by the disease, and (4) the development of compensatory sources of satisfaction.

There is always the potential that the experience of coping with a chronic illness can have a positive influence on the adolescent's planning for the future. Greater maturity, enhanced empathy, and familiarity with the medical environment, developed in the course of living with a chronic illness may be advantageous for the adolescent. Physicians and other medical personnel may be important, positive role models for chronically ill adolescents.

A wide range of psychological defense mechanisms which have been thought to be pathologic when they appear in other circumstances are associated with chronically ill adolescents' successful coping; these include isolation, denial, and projection. The importance of recognizing creative, "abnormal" solutions to the problem of growing up with a chronic illness cannot be overemphasized. Developmental theories, standards, and assessment instruments that were developed for healthy, able-bodied adolescents may not accurately evaluate the psychosocial status of chronically ill adolescents. Ultimately, one must rely on clinical judgment to determine if a particular adolescent's status represents an adaptive solution or a troubled outcome that necessitates intervention.

INTERVENTIONS TO PROMOTE ADJUSTMENT

Adolescents' developmental vulnerability to the effects of chronic illness and the documented increased risk of psychosocial morbidity have prompted early intervention efforts. Beyond a growing recognition that psychosocial adjustment issues span disease categories, intervention programs are still being actively studied. A comprehensive home-care service program provided by pediatricians and nurse practitioners in the Bronx has improved adjustment in chronically ill children and adolescents. However, a rigorous evaluation of the effects of routine social service intervention in a children's hospital found no differences in psychosocial outcome between those who received the intervention and control subjects. The need to individualize psychosocial intervention was underlined in another study that demonstrated significant benefits from a group workshop approach for working class diabetic teenagers, but no benefits from the same program for poor diabetic adolescents.

Educational Approaches

Education as a means to increase the intellectual understanding and management skills of both the adolescent and the family is the first step in promoting successful adjustment to a chronic disorder. Fantasies about the physiology, treatment, or medical implications of an illness are often more disabling to an adolescent with an active imagination than the reality of the disorder. Knowledge empowers the teenager by replacing fantasy with fact. Education is especially important in addressing compliance problems (see Chapter 26). Knowledge in one area (i.e., nutrition) does not predict the level of knowledge about another aspect of a chronic illness (i.e., insulin use) such as in diabetes mellitus. Sufficient knowledge does not ensure adequate skill in the management tasks required.

Adolescents who have diabetes mellitus are as knowledgeable about diabetes as their mothers and know more than their fathers. However, they make more errors in insulin administration and blood glucose self-testing. Inadvertent noncompliance occurs when adolescents are unaware of making errors and believe they are following the physicians' recommendations.

Education should attempt to anticipate obstacles to compliance (unrealistic goals, peer pressure, and so on), present information at the individual adolescent's cognitive level, and use written handouts wherever possible. It is important not to view health education as a static process that, once accomplished, can be "checked off" and ignored. Reevaluation and repetition, with modifi-cations as appropriate to the teenager's cognitive and social maturation, are essential components of the educational process.

Adequate knowledge is very important for effective management of a chronic illness, but for adolescents it is not the only factor that determines compliance. Adequate social skills to handle the awkward times among peers, a supportive family environment, and a trusting, supportive relationship with the physician all have been shown to contribute to improved compliance. Care must also be taken with adolescents not to make a simple equation of "problems in the course of the illness mean patient noncompliance." The physiologic changes during adolescent development can alter previously stable diabetes mellitus, cardiac disease, seizure disorders and, perhaps, other conditions even with excellent adherence to the treatment regimen.

Supportive Approaches

A number of approaches support the chronically ill adolescents' ability to cope with the disorder. The physician can offer an outlet for the ventilation of feelings associated with the chronic disorder. The need to express strong feelings and have them understood is powerful; for chronically ill adolescents, the limiting factor often is how much emotional expression they believe others can tolerate. Such expression is easiest in safe situations—and these may not include interactions with either the physician or the family. The adolescent may fear displeasing the physician or may be uncomfortable in the presence of authority figures, and therefore be reluctant to discuss his or her feelings. Adolescent discussion groups provide a unique alternative, combining the power of the peer group with the security of numbers and the presence of others who are experiencing similar stressors. Such groups ideally involve adolescents at various stages of the illness, allowing the more experienced adolescent patients the satisfaction of helping newly diagnosed patients. Tapes, journals, and drawings can be used for emotional expression as well and should be encouraged.

At no other age is the supportive physician–patient relationship a more critical component of medical care. Yet teenagers may be among the most difficult patients for whom the physician believes a solid alliance exists. A strong relationship with an adolescent is based on complete honesty, respect of confidentiality (see Chapter 20), a friendly, interested manner, and appropriate use of humor. Once established, a strong relationship allows discussion of identified problems with the adolescent.

Psychotherapy

Formal psychotherapy, be it individual or family therapy, is frequently recommended after psychiatric evaluation. The mental health professional proposing psychotherapy should articulate particular problems to be addressed or goals to be pursued in the process of therapy. A clear treatment plan that makes sense to the adolescent, the family, and other professionals caring for the adolescent is essential at the outset of therapy. Without such an explicit plan the therapy is likely to fail and to result in misunderstanding, ambivalence, or unrealistic expectations on the part of one or all parties. Psychotherapy always entails difficult periods in which there is little progress, significant resistance, and discouragement. When other professionals hear from the adolescent or the family of this discouragement, they can help the adolescent or family to continue treatment by supporting the rightness of the decision, the appropriateness of the initial plan, and the competence of the therapist. Individual psychotherapy with an adolescent requires that there is a delicate balance between the adolescent's desire for and right to confidentiality and the parents' or professional's need to know about progress and problems. This is best accomplished by the therapist periodically summarizing relevant general issues to adults in the presence of the adolescent, while avoiding specific details of the therapy. Maximal change occurs in therapy when there is an optimal level of tension or anxiety. Too much anxiety or stress means that little "psychic reserve" exists and defenses must be maintained at a high level. Too little perceived anxiety is associated with reduced motivation for change and minimal progress. When change does occur, it should be noted and reinforced.

Behavioral approaches in psychotherapy are especially useful with chronically ill adolescents (see Chapter 124). Behavior modification, relaxation techniques, hypnosis, and biofeedback are discussed in Chapter 124.

Psychoactive Medications

Chronically ill adolescents may manifest significant symptoms of anxiety or depression in association with fluctuations in the course of their illness. Although it may be difficult to differentiate whether somatic symptoms, pain, anorexia, insomnia, fatigue, etc, are due to disease activity or part of a psychopathologic process, it is clear that some chronically ill adolescents experience diagnosable levels of anxiety and depression that merit vigorous treatment. In addition to psychotherapeutic efforts, psychoactive medications have a role in these cases. Unfortunately, few empirical studies or clinical reports can guide the clinician's use of anxiolytic agents or antidepressants in chronically ill adolescents. Those that exist are generally encouraging regarding the safety and efficacy of such drugs when used conservatively in this population.

Benzodiazepines have been useful in the short-term treatment of a variety of behavioral disturbances in healthy children and adolescents, with side effects usually found to be minimal. Alprazolam was useful among a group of pediatric cancer patients when used to treat anticipatory anxiety and acute anxiety associated with stressful procedures (see Chapter 16). Even at very low doses, the benefit of alprazolam was significant. Mild drowsiness is the most common side effect, and when used in a relatively brief regimen, behavioral disinhibition, rebound anxiety, or withdrawal effects are not a problem.

Tricyclic antidepressants such as impramine or amitriptyline are increasingly used in treating chronically ill adolescents who are significantly depressed (see Chapter 100). A daily dose is recommended, and blood levels should be used to determine when a therapeutic level is reached. Electrocardiographic changes should be monitored, and trials of high-dose tricyclic antidepressants should occur when the adolescent is hospitalized. Tricyclic antidepressants have also been reported to potentiate the effects of analgesics and to reduce anxiety, so their potential beneficial range is broad. The risks from side effects, which are usually dose-related and include anticholinergic effects, sedation, gastrointestinal symptoms, and potential cardiovascular side effects, need to be evaluated individually for each adolescent patient. The same applies for drug interactions, especially when the adolescent is already on a complex medication regimen. Tricyclic antidepressants should be prescribed cautiously at low doses for patients on dialysis or with compromised renal function (see Chapter 65), and blood level monitoring is mandatory if these agents are to be used with this group of adolescents. Coordination with other physicians is essential.

MENTAL HEALTH REFERRAL

Major emotional distress, poor functioning, and psychopathology should not be considered acceptable or inevitable for chronically ill adolescents any more than they are for healthy teenagers. Patients' psychological symptoms and distress should be explored and followed up, with involvement of a mental health professional when appropriate. Indications for mental health referral include (1) suicidal threats or ideation; (2) significant noncompliance, despite efforts to improve it; (3) regression to immature behavior lasting more than several weeks; (4) behavior that isolates the adolescent, or signs of significant withdrawal; (5) persistent signs of depression (see Chapter 100); and (6) unexplained feelings (such as anger, rejection, or protectiveness) regularly evoked in the physician by the adolescent. The last point is that the physician's own reactions provide important data about the adolescent (see Chapters 24 and 98).

Adolescents with chronic illness deserve a multidisciplinary group of professionals who are aware of and respect each other's strengths and differences (see Chapter 27). Successful interdisciplinary collaboration between primary care professionals and mental health professionals requires personal familiarity and an established professional relationship in which realistic expectations are used as standards of practice.

BIBLIOGRAPHY

Gliedman J, Roth W: The Unexpected Minority: Handicapped Children in America. New York, Harcourt Brace Jovanovich, 1980.

Johnson SB: Knowledge, attitudes and behavior: Correlates of health in childhood diabetes. Clin Psychol Rev 4:503, 1984.

Litt IF, Cuskey WR, Rosenberg A: Role of self-esteem and autonomy in determining medication compliance among adolescents with juvenile rheumatoid arthritis. Pediatrics 69:15, 1982.

Mattsson A: Long-term physical illness in childhood: A challenge to psychosocial adaptation. Pediatrics 52:801, 1972.

McAnarney ER, Pless IB, Satterwhite B, Friedman SB: Psychological problems of children with chronic juvenile arthritis. Pediatrics 53:523, 1974.

Nolan T, Pless IB: Emotional correlates and consequences of birth defects. J Pediatr 109:201, 1986.

Pfefferbaum B, Overall JE, Boren HA, et al: Alprazolam in the treatment of anticipatory and acute situational anxiety in children with cancer. J Am Acad Child Adolesc Psychiatry 26:532, 1987.

Schowalter JE: Psychosocial reactions to physical illness and hospitalization in adolescence. J Am Acad Child Adolesc Psychiatry 16:500, 1977.

Simmons CH, Parsons RH: Developing internality and perceived competence: The empowerment of adolescent girls. Adolescence 18:917, 1983.

Stein REK, Jessop DJ: Does pediatric home care make a difference for children with chronic illness? Findings from the Pediatric Ambulatory Care Treatment Study. Pediatrics 73:845, 1984.

CHAPTER 122

Psychological Care of Adolescents Undergoing Transplantation

MARGARET L. STUBER

Although kidney transplantation has been the treatment of choice for end-stage renal disease for more than a decade, transplantation of other solid organs was uncommon until the mid-1980s (see Chapter 54). Then, largely owing to the availability of improved immunosuppression with cyclosporine, liver and heart transplantation programs began to proliferate. Bone marrow transplantation (BMT) programs similarly increased in number as advances in both chemotherapy and immunology improved patient survival. In addition, BMT was applicable to leukemia, solid tumors, and immunologic and metabolic disorders in addition to aplastic anemia.

With 2-year survival figures in the 70% to 80% range for heart and liver transplants, major centers are now developing programs for lung, pancreas, and combined organ transplantation. The continued introduction of new medications and surgical techniques promises further breakthroughs and advances. Bone marrow transplants use computer-matched unrelated donors to extend the availability of bone marrow from individuals other than family members.

However, these scientific opportunities create challenges in the treatment of adolescents. An immediate issue is the decision to have transplantation. Many of the protocols are experimental. Should the adolescent make the principal decision? What if the family and the adolescent disagree? Should a transplantation ever be done despite the objections of the adolescent patient (because in most other medical conditions there is often no other life-saving alternative, such as dialysis in end-stage renal patients)? Are there some adolescents who should not receive a transplant?

After the decision has been made for an adolescent to receive a transplant, there may be new problems. The scarcity of available donor organs creates a new category of patients: adolescents waiting for a curative procedure that may not be able to be performed in time to save the adolescent's life. A small adolescent may have to wait for several months to receive an organ of the right size. There may be no one available who has perfectly matched bone marrow. Being "on the list"

represents a hope rather than a promise for a number of adolescents.

Transplantation itself introduces psychological issues. Although the transplantation may preserve the life of the adolescent, the young person is dependent on daily medication and frequent medical supervision. Can these adolescents, who have often been chronically ill before transplantation, ever be "normal"? How do they cope with the side effects (hirsutism secondary to the use of cyclosporine or the truncal obesity secondary to the use of steroids)? This chapter will consider these common, but often perplexing, problems facing adolescents undergoing transplantation.

PSYCHIATRIC ISSUES IN THE DECISION TO TRANSPLANT

Most transplantation programs include a psychiatric evaluation of the candidate and the family prior to listing a candidate for a donor organ in order to anticipate the psychosocial needs of the candidate and family. The information is also used in the team's decision to accept the adolescent as a candidate for transplantation. Domains that should be evaluated include (1) previous functioning in school, home, and peer group; (2) understanding of the illness, transplantation, and aftercare; (3) commitment to the transplantation and long-term care; (4) availability of support from family, peers, and social network; (5) affective and coping style; (6) history of alcohol, tobacco, and drug use; (7) history of psychiatric problems; and (8) history of medical compliance.

Although it is generally accepted that prior noncompliance, significant psychopathologic disorder, or a chaotic family situation predicts psychosocial complications, missed follow-up visits, and increased need for nursing, social work, and psychiatric assistance, there are relatively few good prospective studies to establish psychiatric predictors of medical and psychosocial outcome. Most available data are studies performed with adult populations. Research of the predictors of outcome for children and adolescents undergoing transplantation is being done, but there is insufficient evidence currently. The present studies are examining the significance of

This work was supported in part by Clinical Oncology Career Development Award #89-92 from the American Cancer Society.

(1) health beliefs or attributional style; (2) perceived social support from family or peers; (3) pretransplantation behavioral or emotional problems; (4) self-concept and self-esteem; and (5) family adaptability and cohesion. Evaluation batteries that can predict psychosocial and compliance problems of transplantation candidates with sufficient accuracy to plan suitable interventions should be available soon. However, it is difficult to establish absolute or even relative psychiatric contraindications to transplantation. When the alternative is death, very few transplantation teams are willing to reject an otherwise suitable adolescent for psychosocial reasons alone. However, utilization of scarce resources (especially organs, and also operating rooms, intensive care beds, and state and federal funding) demands that the criteria for transplantation be considered carefully. Three possibilities for contraindications would be (1) informed refusal of the transplantation by the adolescent patient, (2) unavailability of family or other social support system, and (3) history of serious noncompliance with medical treatment.

Informed Refusal. Many adults may not believe that an adolescent can make an informed choice to die rather than to undergo transplantation. However, the data indicate that some adolescents can and do make that choice. A number of legal and ethical dilemmas are raised. If it is established with sufficient data that the prognosis is significantly diminished when a fully informed adolescent refuses transplantation, transplantation teams may have to give that opinion precedence over the wishes of the parents, in the interests of the adolescent's wishes and appropriate allocation of scarce resources. The developmental stage and competence of the adolescent must be considered. Very young adolescents may not fully understand the complexity and seriousness of the decision not to undergo transplantation.

Lack of Support. Even with an adolescent candidate who is fully dedicated to complying with the transplantation regimen, the absence of adequate support at home is a significant risk to long-term outcome after transplantation. Reluctant as health providers may be to refuse an adolescent the possibility of transplantation on the basis of parental absence or illness, transplantation teams must evaluate the adequacy as well as the expense of creating an alternative supportive network for the adolescent through foster care and social work and psychiatric support.

Noncompliance History. A history of noncompliance in a young adolescent, although worrisome, is rarely sufficient grounds for denial of transplantation, especially if the adolescent has a supportive family. However, older adolescents who have established histories of behavioral problems are likely to have problems, regardless of the level of parental commitment. Even when additional supports are provided, such as groups or ongoing counseling, these adolescents are at extremely high risk for continued noncompliance and medical complications. Unless these adolescents become deeply committed to transplantation, they are very poor candidates.

DEVELOPMENTAL CONSIDERATIONS

The fundamental developmental tasks of adolescents pose the principal conflicts for transplantation patients. It is difficult for adolescents to pursue separation and individuation when their illness requires (1) prolonged hospitalization in a highly dependent state; (2) parental involvement in highly personal body functions and decisions; (3) extended isolation precautions, hampering normal peer interactions; (4) lengthy school absences, during a phase of school perceived as pivotal to future school and career; and (5) lifelong medications that lead to self-definitions as "sick" and create a dependency on physicians and insurance companies.

Although all these issues also pertain to children and adults undergoing transplantation, the impact is greater for adolescents, who are actively forming their identity structure and sense of self (see Chapter 9). This critical time is particularly vulnerable to the massive physical and psychological assault involved in removing and replacing a body part.

One aspect of the threat to identity may be a sense of invasion or foreignness introduced when one has a part of someone else's body within one's own body. From the limited research in this area, it appears that the type of organ involved is quite salient to the emotional response to replacement. For example, people seem much more disturbed by the idea of receiving a new heart than by receiving a new liver. This can be seen in cartoons and films, which play on our cultural belief that the heart contains the positive emotions, essential beliefs, or even the soul, of an individual. These beliefs appear prevalent throughout American culture, and affect adolescents as well as adults and children.

Adolescents may also respond emotionally to the idea that someone else had to die to give them this chance to live. Many recipients of donor organs want to communicate their gratitude (and guilt) to the donor family directly. This is forbidden by the national organ procurement organization in the interests of both families. Letters may be sent through an intermediary group, such as the regional organ procurement agency, with identifying information removed to prevent emotional responses from overwhelming appropriate boundaries between the two families. Some adolescents respond to this selfless act of someone else's giving an organ to them by becoming more empathic, more giving to others in need than they were prior to transplantation. Others are overwhelmed temporarily by a sense of responsibility to live for both people. Sensitive discussion usually can help the adolescent accept the gift, and go forward with his or her life.

Another common response to having a foreign organ is to develop a belief that the body eventually incorporates the new part, making that organ (and all it symbolically represents) part of the recipient. Unfortunately, this level of psychological acceptance can result in assumptions leading to concrete actions, such as the adolescent's ceasing to take immunosuppressive medications, which are perceived as no longer necessary. Such responses are being increasingly noted as both adolescent and adult recipients survive 2 or more years from the initial transplantation date.

CLINICAL ISSUES

A number of the psychological issues confronting adolescents undergoing transplantation represent variations or intensifications of issues that have been described in other populations of medically ill adolescents (see Chapters 30 and 121). Although not unique to transplantation, these issues can have serious implications for survival, as well as for the quality of life. They include anxiety, low self-esteem, noncompliance, and depression.

Anxiety. Transplantation involves a period of extreme dependency, with isolation from peers, and parental involvement in intimate body functions. The uncertainty of the waiting period and the experimental nature of many of the procedures can be extremely anxiety-provoking. Adolescents frequently respond with either an exaggerated dependency on family or intensified need for control. Previously independent, secure adolescents may now need parental input on seemingly small matters. Formerly reasonable adolescents may now refuse all advice or assistance. These defensive attempts to bind anxiety are rarely successful and result in frustration for all concerned.

Low Self-esteem. The illnesses that lead to transplantation and the subsequent surgery, isolation, and immunosuppressive medications may all contribute to adolescents' doubts about themselves. A cushingoid or hirsute adolescent is less likely to try out for cheerleading or for varsity tennis. Absence from much of a semester at school decreases a student's self-assurance about schoolwork, and may result in repeating a grade. Merely taking medication daily can be a painful reminder that this adolescent is different from his or her peers. All of this may be compounded by the effects of chronic illness, such as short stature, delayed puberty, or diminished muscle strength (see Chapter 30).

Noncompliance. Issues of anxiety, control, self-esteem, and body image also contribute to problems with medical compliance (see Chapter 26). Adolescents are often resistant to being told what to do by adults, and may test the limits set by the adults. They may experiment with their medications to reduce unwanted side effects. Noncompliance can also be used in an attempt to manipulate parents, friends, or schools. Adolescents may resort to exaggerated complaints to get or maintain the special attention they believe they are unable to receive through usual channels. Unfortunately, failure to take immunosuppressive drugs often has no overtly symptomatic impact until the rejection is far enough advanced as to cause irreversible scarring. Adolescents may, therefore, cause graft destruction when they were simply attempting to eliminate cosmetically unappealing side effects or to regain some control over their bodies and schedules. Such incidents can be fatal.

Depression. Although adolescents undergoing transplantation are frequently discouraged, or even demoralized, it is unusual for them to be overtly suicidal, or to suffer from the full symptom picture of major depression (see Chapter 100). Organic causes must always be considered, especially if an adolescent without a prior history of impulsivity, depression, dysthymic disorder, or personality disorder becomes seriously depressed. Common causes include encephalopathy (hepatic, ischemic, or toxic) and affective responses to steroids (which are neither dose-related nor predicted by history). Significant depression or organic encephalopathy can be differentiated from the energy-conserving withdrawal of a seriously ill, exhausted patient by (1) careful evaluation of the adolescent, assessing for hopelessness, guilt, and negative self-image; and (2) formal mental status examination to assess possible delirium. The most common reason for significant depression in adolescents without a psychiatric history or organic brain impairment is the belief that they are really dying, but no one is telling them the truth. This may be difficult to uncover, because adolescents may lack trust in adults. Intervention is possible once the specific cause is recognized.

PSYCHIATRIC INTERVENTIONS

The best approach to most of the psychological problems related to transplantation is prevention. Early contact with mental health professionals allows assessment and prediction of anticipated issues, as well as establishment of a working relationship to anticipate common problems. Psychiatric consultation during the decision-making process can enhance the adolescent's sense of participation in, and therefore commitment to, the decision for transplantation. The time spent waiting for availability of an organ can be used to discuss and to process information about the procedure and the hospitalization, the postoperative care, and the long-term prognosis. Questions about isolation procedures, diet, scars, and pain can thus be addressed in advance in a neutral setting, rather than urgently in the intensive care unit (ICU). Informational books or pamphlets, at an appropriate reading level, and preferably including humor, are very helpful.

A useful early intervention is for the adolescent to meet with an adolescent of similar age and diagnosis who is approximately a year post transplantation. These "survivors" can provide information to adolescent candidates. Groups, camps, parties, or one-to-one contact by telephone or in the ambulatory setting can be developed to facilitate this communication. Both adolescents benefit, because the adolescent who has already undergone transplantation gains self-esteem in being the "expert."

Specific training in relaxation, self-hypnosis, or guided imagery is extremely helpful if introduced early. When provided the opportunity to practice these techniques prior to hospitalization, adolescents can use them to handle the anxiety, pain, and insomnia that generally accompany postoperative recovery. A trained, experienced therapist can introduce and teach these techniques and manage the adolescent's emotional response, which appears in a relaxed or trance state. Hypnosis and imagery are powerful tools and should not be used any more casually than one would use other (medical) hypnotic or anxiolytic agents.

Psychiatric follow-up after transplantation is frequently overlooked, sometimes with dire consequences. Adolescents who are at risk for noncompliance or significant depression due to family stressors, psychopathologic problem, or other medical complications must be followed closely. It is generally simpler (and thus more likely to work) if the adolescent and the family can combine the psychiatric follow-up with a medical visit. After a number of months post transplantation, medical management may require only infrequent ambulatory care visits. However, the relationship with a mental health worker may require consistent reinforcement. Scheduling of ambulatory care visits should be arranged for both medical and psychiatric care. Family therapy, if indicated, may require additional, separate visits (see Chapter 123). These visits may be conveniently arranged with a therapist near the family's home. If a therapist not within the same institution as the transplantation team is seeing the adolescent, communication between the therapist and treatment team must be established, with the agreement of the family. Such communication is essential to appropriate management, because it demonstrates to the adolescent and his or her family the medical team's belief that psychotherapy is an important part of the overall medical care of this adolescent.

The role of the mental health worker with team members is the least clear and often perceived as the most frustrating aspect of mental health consulting to transplantation teams (see Chapters 24 and 27). Although transplantation nurses and physicians are generally eager to have psychiatric intervention for difficult adolescent patients, they are often reluctant to ask for assistance for themselves, despite an obviously extremely stressful work environment. Discomfort with the enormous responsibility of transplantation candidate selection may increase the resistance to interpretations of group or unconscious processes influencing decision-making. Nonetheless, this is a key function for mental health workers working with transplantation teams. The selection of transplantation recipients is a complex decision. Medical personnel, trained to provide help to specific patients, have difficulty when asked to decide between adolescent patients for their assistance. Psychiatric consultants must resist the push to make social worth determinations, in the guise of assessment of mental health. However, they must also assist the team in managing the burden of deciding whether a beloved, but deteriorating, adolescent patient gets a third or fourth transplantation, when other adolescents are waiting for their first organ. Interpretations of process must be offered tactfully and skillfully by a member of the team. Support can only be accepted if team members know it is offered with respect among colleagues. When psychiatric input is totally integrated into the team's functioning, both team and patients benefit (see Chapter 24).

LONG-TERM CONSIDERATIONS

Initial psychiatric research with transplantation recipients has focused on adjustment and morbidity during and shortly after the transplantation, with the goal of providing better intervention and identifying predictors of noncompliance. As transplantation has become established and survival has improved, research is focusing on the adjustment of the long-term survivors. Questions are being asked about the long-term psychiatric, as well as medical, sequelae of these intense, life-saving interventions.

Long-term follow-up studies of adolescents after renal transplantation suggest that psychological adjustment is relatively good overall, with the principal predictors of psychologic outcome being medical status and social support. This is consistent with some early findings with adult bone marrow transplant survivors and pediatric heart transplant survivors. However, there have been anecdotal reports of suicide attempts in adolescents following liver transplantation, and others of passive suicide by discontinuation of medication. A number of studies are now in progress, examining long-term outcome and predictors in bone marrow and liver transplantation recipients. Early findings suggest alterations in the adolescent's future expectations, approach to intimacy, and career selection.

Little is yet known about the impact of transplantation on adolescent identity formation and later vocational and interpersonal function. Many transplant survivors believe that the transplant was to have made them entirely well, and they are resentful that there are residua. It is not clear whether this misunderstanding stems entirely from denial on the part of the adolescent, or whether the transplantation team minimizes the sequelae, which are seen as minor in comparison to what is gained. The continued medication, side effects, hospital visits, biopsies, and scars that are common to transplant survivors serve as repeated reminders that they are not "normal" adolescents, but "different." Some adolescents are able to view this difference in a positive light, stating that they now appreciate life more and are more empathic with other people. Others find it difficult to establish a positive sense of themselves and their bodies. This can interfere with establishment of good peer relationships.

In addition to the psychological impact of medical residua, there may be psychiatric sequelae of the transplant itself. Organ transplantation is experienced by some adolescents as a traumatic event, resulting in symptoms of post-traumatic stress (see Chapter 104). These symptoms (e.g., anxiety, irritability, isolation, and withdrawal) could affect peer interactions and appropriate role and identity formation negatively. If the adolescent responds to medications and continued medical follow-up as people do to traumatic reminders, with denial and avoidance, further noncompliance problems can be anticipated. Research in this area is proceeding at several centers, with the goal of designing appropriate interventions.

BIBLIOGRAPHY

Cromer BA, Tarnoski KJ: Noncompliance in adolescents: A review. Developmental and Behavioral Pediatrics 10:207, 1989.
Didlake RH, Dreyfus K, Kerman RH, et al: Patient noncompliance:

A major cause of late graft failure in cyclosporine-treated renal transplants. Transplant Proc 3:63, 1988.

Ettinger RB, Marik JL, Malekzadeh M, et al: Improved cadaveric renal transplant outcome in children. Pediatric Nephrology 5:137, 1991.

Krener PG: Psychiatric liaison to liver transplant recipients. Clin Pediatr 26:93, 1987.

Lawrence KS, Fricker FJ: Pediatric heart transplantation: Quality of life. J Heart Transplant 6:329, 1987.

Olbrisch MS, Levenson JL, Hamer R: The PACT: A rating scale for the study of clinical decision-making on psychosocial screening of organ transplant candidates. Clinical Transplantation 3:164, 1989.

Siegal BR, Hanson P, Viswanathan R, et al: Renal transplant patients' health beliefs. Transplant Proc 21:3977, 1989.

Wolcott DL, Wellisch DK, Fawzy FI, Landsverk J: Adaptation of adult bone marrow transplant recipient long-term survivors. Transplantation 41:478, 1986.

Zitelli BJ, Miller JW, Gartner JC, et al: Changes in life-style after liver transplantation. Pediatrics 82:173, 1988.

Treatment Approaches

CHAPTER 123

Family Therapy

SUSAN McDANIEL and JUDITH LANDAU-STANTON

The more serious, intransigent psychosocial problems of adolescents can be treated successfully with family therapy. Physicians with special interest in family treatment may wish to attend postgraduate family therapy training programs and acquire the skills needed to conduct this therapy. Others do family assessments and family counseling, but refer the more difficult cases to family therapy–trained colleagues. The threshold for referral is different for each practitioner, but in general family therapy may be appropriate for severe or multiproblem families, families that stimulate unresolved personal issues for the physician, or families that have been refractory to treatment by the adolescent physician. Often, a one-time consultation with a family therapist may provide the information or intervention that then allows the physician to continue his or her treatment of the patient. Some physicians have a family therapist that works part-time in the office, so that both consultation and treatment for patients are easily accessible.

We believe that all adolescent mental health problems should be assessed and treated with consideration for the issues and resources inherent in the adolescent's family and natural support system. Just as family-oriented medical care is an approach to all medical interactions, whether with one patient or with multiple interested parties, so family therapy is an approach to treating mental health problems regardless of the number of people involved in treatment. It is more an orientation or philosophy than a modality of treatment. Both family therapy and family-oriented medical care (see Chapter 23) are grounded in systems theory, a theory that emphasizes understanding symptoms in the context of significant biologic, psychological, and social relationships. Well-trained family therapists may use family members when a patient is symptomatic, but they also consider whether psychotropic medication or some other treatment might be useful as part of the overall systemic treatment plan. Family therapists also view the referring physician as an important resource in understanding and treating the patient's problem. Virtually any psychological, interpersonal, or behavioral problem may be referred to a family-oriented mental health professional. In addition, nonphysician family therapists are likely to consult a psychiatrist on psychotic or high-risk patients, patients with significant affective disorders, or other problems with significant biologic factors such as psychosomatic disorders.

Family therapy has been shown to be effective for a wide range of adolescent disorders including anorexia (see Chapter 60), drug and alcohol abuse (see Chapter 111), school problems (see Chapter 103), runaways (see Chapter 108), suicide attempts (see Chapter 101), psychotic disorders, grief reactions (see Chapter 116), somaticizing (see Chapter 112), and other psychosomatic problems (see Chapter 113). Family therapy has a variety of forms, from psychoanalytic and behavioral, to the problem-focused approaches of structural and strategic, to transgenerational and integrative approaches. Research has yet to document the superiority of any one particular form, although all have shown some success with various adolescent problems.

The family therapies based on systems theory—structural, strategic, systemic, and transgenerational—all attempt to transform dysfunctional interactional patterns, to encourage resolution of the adolescent's symptoms and to facilitate individual and interpersonal growth for all family members. Family therapy is an optimistic approach that draws on individual and family strengths to solve problems and that encourages people to function at their best. Because all relevant people are involved in treatment, family therapy tends to be brief (e.g., six to ten sessions) and to sustain the change that is needed to support the adolescent's growth. Adolescents change quickly as part of normal development. The therapist's task is to optimize this change for the sake of the adolescent and the family.

Structural family therapy, as described by Minuchin, is a problem-focused approach that emphasizes establishing appropriate boundaries between subsystems in families, i.e., between parents and their children. Adolescents who function as a parent's confidante, or as a parent's parent, are likely to become symptomatic in some way. Structural family therapists work to correct problems in the family hierarchy through techniques such as reenactment (in which family members demonstrate or directly discuss their concerns), enactment (in which family members attempt in session to change the problem behavior), unbalancing (a technique used by the therapist to alter the power alliances in the family), elevating (in which the balance of power is realigned), and the use of intensity (selectively increasing the degree of affect in the room to facilitate emergence of new behavior in family members). Minuchin has described the effectiveness of his approach with both disadvantaged juvenile delinquents and with psychosomatic adolescents. Minuchin demonstrated that the blood sugar level of juvenile diabetics rose when their parents had a fight into which they were drawn. Others have described similar family dynamics with children who have asthma. The structural family therapy approach to such families involves containing the conflict between the parents or caregivers and not allowing the fight to be "detoured" through the adolescent.

Strategic family therapy is also problem-focused and characterized by the search for an effective strategy to help the adolescent and family reach their goals in treatment. Strategic family therapy as espoused by Haley and Madanes, like Minuchin's therapy, focuses on the importance of an appropriate family hierarchy. They also use metaphor, play, and indirect techniques such as paradox to achieve symptom relief. Haley has described his approach in treating severe behavior problems, psychosis, and other serious adolescent problems that can be related to issues around "leaving home." Other strategic therapists focus on patients' use of language and make frequent use of the technique of reframing, which involves introducing a different way of looking at a problem, an alternative reality that may lead to new behaviors and new solutions. Systemic therapy, first described by Palazzoli and associates, evolved from strategic therapy and uses paradox and positive connotation, which is a form of reframing that emphasizes the positive intentions of each family member in what they are doing to help the adolescent. This approach, like strategic therapy, is effective with adolescents who exhibit severe or psychotic symptomatology.

Transgenerational approaches to family therapy tend to be longer-term therapies, because they focus on multigenerational patterns of problems and family loyalties as the key to the resolution of symptoms. However, many systems-oriented therapists draw from several of these approaches to family therapy in treating adolescents. Some integrative therapists, such as Stanton and Landau-Stanton, use an intergenerational perspective in the brief treatment of a range of adolescent problems, from substance abuse to suicidality and problems resulting from immigration and cultural transition.

An adolescent who had suicidal behavior treated with a suicide watch may illustrate many of the techniques that are common in systems-oriented family therapy with an adolescent. (See Figure 123–1 for a genogram of this case.)

E, age 18 years, had been hospitalized for attempted suicide on six occasions since the age of 12 years. She was the youngest of four sisters—ages 25, 23, 20, and 18 years. The family expressed extreme concern about the danger to E's life with this latest, serious attempt. Her mother, a bright, attractive woman in her late 40s, felt inadequate to deal with her daughter's problems and wanted E placed out of the home. E's father, a quiet, overweight, and almost voiceless figure, had no idea how to handle the situation and refused to take sides with either his wife or his daughter.

During the initial family session with the therapeutic team (including E and her extended family, her primary nurse, the social worker, the referring pediatrician, and E's teacher), it was discovered that each of the daughters, in turn, had given their parents trouble. The oldest had had a disruptive and troublesome adolescence. As soon as she had successfully left home, the second daughter, who had been on drugs, made a hasty marriage at age 18 years to an older man of whom the parents did not approve. The third daughter had

a baby out of wedlock at age 18 years after an adolescence fraught with rebellion and suicidal threats. At that point, the third daughter moved out of the house. Soon after, E, age 16 years at the time, made a serious suicide attempt, which was followed by a 2-month hospitalization. It was evident to the therapeutic team that E was continuing a long-standing pattern by escalating her symptomatology around the transition of leaving home. Her first suicidal gesture was at age 12 years, shortly after the death of her paternal grandmother, with whom her father had been very close. E's dramatic history was even more problematic than that presented by her sisters; because she was the last child to face leaving home, the transitional conflict was severe. Consequently, any attempt to continue treating E independently of her family had to fail—much as such attempts had in the past. Involvement of the whole family system in therapy was the only logical recourse.

In the first family session, the parents appeared helpless and discouraged and E seemed testy and provocative, as if she were in charge of the family. To correct this inappropriate hierarchy, the team enumerated the parents' strengths and resources, and had the father describe in great detail situations at work when, as a manager, he had had to take charge of a difficult situation. Citing analogous strengths in the mother, the team elevated the parents and then moved to establish a 24-hour/day, 7-day/week suicide watch to keep E safe by never leaving her alone. At first, E's parents expressed concern about their ability to sustain such an intensive effort. The various members of the team agreed to provide appropriate back-up to the parents, as well as assistance in organizing their extended family and friends to participate in the safety watch. In particular, the three living grandparents were invited in to provide additional relief to the parents. The parents were very pleased about the support that family and friends provided, once the team helped them to organize their efforts.

In the course of the early sessions, E made frequent attempts to disrupt the tentative efforts of her parents to cooperate in addressing her problem. The therapist worked to improve the parents' teamwork and prevent E from splitting their efforts. In this way, the parents were able to resume their appropriate roles in providing limits for E when she was unable to do so for herself. E slowly calmed down in response to these interventions. Once her parents were feeling more confident about their skills in working together and keeping E safe, E was described as sacrificing herself and drawing the fire for her sisters who needed to leave home. Her parents, feeling safer and in control of the situation, were able to reassure her that they would handle any of her sisters' ongoing problems.

Within several weeks E had markedly improved; she was no longer suicidal and, for the first time, she and her parents were talking and listening to each other. For this to be achieved, however, it was essential for the whole treatment team to be cautious and reinforce the interventions with absolute consistency. Eventually, the family was ready to believe that E was no longer disobedient or suicidal, and informed the team that they were feeling far better about themselves as well. At that point, the team validated the parents' wisdom and their newfound perception of their daughter.

This therapy used a systems approach to enable the parents to work together and feel competent with E as well as assisting them in using the family and community resources available to them. This approach ensures that the adolescent feels safe, heard by the parents, and encourages the family to learn new skills for coping with

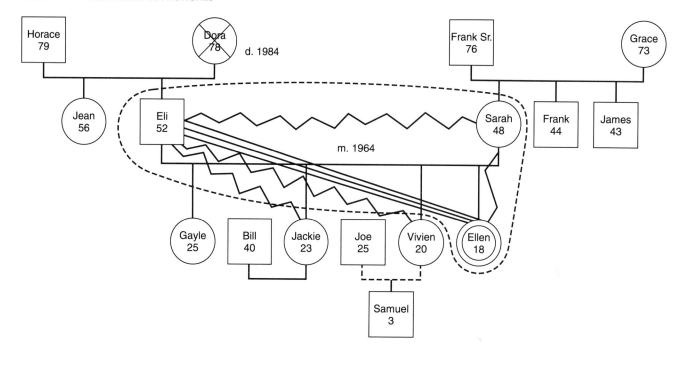

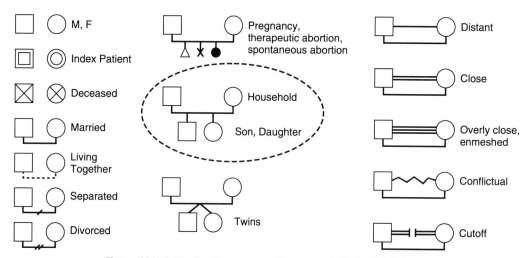

Figure 123–1. The family genogram. (See case study for details.)

subsequent problems. In addition, exploring the theme of major loss and unresolved grief was important to a successful outcome for this adolescent, as is often true with families of suicidal adolescents and families of adolescents who have trouble emancipating.

Systems theory offers a comprehensive approach to the medical problems of adolescents, from their day-to-day medical care to the serious and severe psychosocial problems that require family therapy intervention. Adolescence, with its characteristically rapid growth, presents the physician with a special opportunity to involve family members in brief, creative, and effective treatment of both psychosocial and many medical problems encountered during this stage of development.

BIBLIOGRAPHY

Fishman HC: Treating Troubled Adolescents: A Family Therapy Approach. New York, Bain Books, 1988.

Haley J: Leaving Home. New York, McGraw-Hill, 1980.

Landau-Stanton J, Stanton MD: Treating suicidal adolescents and their families. In Mirkin MP, Koman SL (eds): Handbook of Adolescents and Family Therapy. New York, Gardner Press, 1985, pp 309–328.

Madanes C: Strategic Family Therapy. San Francisco, Jossey-Bass, 1981.

Minuchin S, Fishman C: Family Therapy Techniques. Cambridge, Harvard University Press, 1981.

Minuchin S, Rosman BL, Baker L: Psychosomatic Families. Cambridge, Harvard University Press, 1978.

Palazzoli MS, Boscolo L, Cecchin G, Prata G: Paradox and Counterparadox. New York, Jason Aronson, 1978

CHAPTER 124

Behavior Therapy

ANNE M. BOWEN and ANTHONY SPIRITO

Behavioral interventions were first applied systematically in the 1950s and early 1960s and were equated with the principles of operant and classical conditioning. The development of a number of behavioral techniques applicable to specific problems (e.g., systematic desensitization for phobias) led many nonbehavior therapists to mistakenly view behavior therapy as a set of techniques. At this time, behavior therapists place no limit on clinical procedures that may be employed, except that such procedures must be amenable to experimental evaluation.

The primary assumption of the behavioral approach is that behavior (normal and abnormal) is logical and can be modified according to the principles of learning. The goal of the behavior therapist is the explanation, control, and prediction of behavior. Emphasis is placed on modification of observable behaviors, continuous assessment, and evaluation of treatment outcome. Observable behaviors include motor (e.g., swearing, number of tics per minute), cognitive (e.g., verbal reports of thoughts), and physiologic variables (e.g., heart rate, respiratory rate, sweating).

Behavioral interventions have been useful in treating a variety of medical and behavioral conditions in adolescence. Behavioral techniques have been shown to improve compliance with medical treatments such as chest physiotherapy in adolescents who have cystic fibrosis and dietary compliance in adolescents who have diabetes mellitus (see Chapter 26). Psychological factors may be modified to improve the course of diseases. For example, behavioral approaches to stress reduction are helpful with mild hypertension, recurrent abdominal pain, and pain management (see Chapter 16). Adolescents can learn methods to distract themselves and control pain during bone marrow aspirations and spinal taps (see Chapter 16). A variety of psychological problems are also amenable to behavioral treatment, including affective disorders, eating disorders (see Chapter 60), substance abuse (see Chapter 111), and disorders of conduct (see Chapter 108).

To provide the reader with an understanding of the process of behavior analysis and intervention, the following section briefly discusses social learning theory and then provides an overview of methods used in teaching behavioral skills. The last section provides the reader with a general overview of behavioral techniques with references to books or papers that discuss the theory and application of the technique more extensively. The reader should keep in mind that the combi-nation of environmental-social variables and person variables are unique for each adolescent, so the use of behavioral techniques requires assessment of all areas of functioning.

BEHAVIORAL ASSESSMENT AND BEHAVIOR CHANGE

Human behavior has been conceptualized comprehensively within the behavioral framework by Albert Bandura's social learning theory. Social learning theory suggests that behavior is controlled by the interaction of environmental variables (antecedent and consequent) and organismic variables. In order to appropriately apply behavior change techniques and plan for maintenance and generalization of behavior change, comprehensive assessment of these variables is necessary. The following section includes a brief overview of important aspects of the social learning perspective to aid the reader in understanding variables that should be assessed. For a comprehensive overview of behavioral assessment in general, see Hersen and Bellack; for children specifically, see Mash and Terdal.

Antecedent Stimuli. Antecedents of behavior (controlling stimuli) include specific aspects of both the physical and the social environment. Antecedent stimuli influence behavior since they indicate potential consequences of different behaviors or elicit emotional responses. For example, parents may be more likely to punish a young person's disruptive behavior if only family members are present than if nonmembers are present. As a result, adolescents are more likely to "act out" if company is present. An adolescent may also exhibit maladaptive behaviors in a chaotic home, but act appropriately in a structured psychiatric setting where behavioral consequences are strictly outlined. In order to adequately understand the controlling stimuli for various situations, the therapist must know situational factors such as the differences across and within situations. Variables that may be important include time, place, presence or absence of specific people, and the emotional and cognitive state of the adolescent.

Organismic Variables. The organismic (individual) variables are those that the adolescent brings with him or her to a specific situation, such as past learning history, cognitive factors, genetic influences, and physiologic state. Cognitive factors may include a person's attitudes, beliefs, and expectations about situations, attention to specific aspects of the environment, and so forth. For example, if an adolescent believes that using drugs and alcohol to excess is necessary for acceptance by a desired peer group, then he or she may engage in these behaviors regardless of side effects. In addition, if an adolescent believes that most things that happen to him or her are due to random events, then he or she is not likely to try and change maladaptive behaviors. Physiologic factors such as fatigue, the effects of psychoactive drugs, and anxiety or depression will also contribute to the maladaptive interpretation of situations. Genetic factors such as a family history of bipolar disease might influence a therapist's understanding of extreme agitation in an adolescent. Behavioral assessment of individual variables may include monitoring of blood pressure, heart rate, drug screening, and the use of paper and pencil tests for evaluation of cognitions. For example, feelings of hopelessness might be assessed by a questionnaire that asks questions about how the adolescent views the future.

Response Variables. Accurate assessment of frequency, duration, and intensity of specific behaviors in different settings and at different times will allow the therapist to assess the presence of maladaptive behaviors, behavioral deficits, or inappropriate stimulus control. For example, an adolescent may be socially isolated because he or she is aggressive (maladaptive behavior) or because he or she does not know the appropriate way to join a group or approach a peer (behavioral deficit). An example of inappropriate stimulus control is the adolescent who possesses the appropriate social skills to join a group, but acts aggressively instead.

It is also important to assess both emotional responses (e.g., anger, depression, fear) and instrumental (i.e., voluntary) behaviors, because these are controlled by different events. The antecedent stimuli can more strongly control the emission of emotional responses, while the anticipated consequences are more important with voluntary behaviors. For example, an adolescent who has school phobia will become fearful (emotional response) at the thought or sight (antecedent stimulus) of his or her school, regardless of his or her achievement or social status (individual factor). Conversely, adolescents may feign sickness (instrumental behavior) in order to skip school if they are social outcasts or are receiving poor grades. The treatment of these distinct problems would differ in that treatment of the phobia would involve changing the adolescent's responses to the thought or sight of school (antecedent), while treatment for the school avoidance would target social problems or poor grades (consequences).

Consequence Variables. Behavioral difficulties may arise because rewards and punishers (consequences) are inappropriate or used improperly. For example, the use of physical punishment in adolescence is frequently inappropriate, because it results in reciprocal aggression (negative consequence) rather than compliance (positive consequence). Other problematic reinforcements for adolescents include the social rewards from peers for drinking and drug abuse. Consequences that may not appear to be reinforcing include the attention many adolescents receive from parents for inappropriate be-

haviors such as skipping school, while no attention is given for maintaining a job or curfew. Finally, the therapist should keep in mind self-reinforcing systems. For example, if an adolescent expects perfection and berates himself or herself for anything less, then external rewards may be useless.

In summary, the appropriate use of behavioral techniques as well as the development of comprehensive treatment strategies requires evaluation of the extent of the problem behaviors, including frequency, intensity, and duration. Next, the assessment of environmental and social antecedents and consequences of the target behaviors is necessary, remembering that the strength of these variables will be influenced by learning history, genetics, and the physiological state of the adolescent. A comprehensive behavioral analysis will generally elucidate a variety of target behaviors, as well as interactions between these behaviors and the controlling stimuli. The choice of target behaviors for treatment and in what order they are treated depends on factors such as whether the behavior is dangerous (e.g., suicidal behavior) or irritating, whether changing a specific behavior might produce beneficial results in other areas, and the ease with which a behavior may be changed. In order to apply behavioral change techniques appropriately, it is important to remember that behavioral change is a process that occurs in stages.

Comprehensive Model of Change

Prochaska and DiClemente propose that behavior change is a process that occurs in four stages: precontemplation, contemplation, action, and maintenance. An adolescent in the precontemplation stage does not "see" a reason for changing his or her behavior and, generally, he or she has more "cons" than "pros" for changing. During contemplation, the pros and cons for change may be more equal and the adolescent may be thinking about changing. Developmental and environmental factors are generally important in starting an adolescent moving from precontemplation to contemplation. For example, an adolescent may begin thinking about giving up drugs because he or she was arrested (environmental factor). The action and maintenance stages are characterized by the adolescent activity of trying to change his or her behavior and maintaining those changes.

Appropriate use of different therapeutic techniques depends on the adolescent's stage of change. A solid therapeutic relationship, often between physician and adolescent patient, may be most important for helping an adolescent move from precontemplation into contemplating change. Providing information may also be helpful in moving a patient into action. Behavioral techniques have been found to be most useful during the action and maintenance phases of change. A therapist must balance the use of intervention techniques to match the adolescent's stage of change. In other words, a therapist who implements behavioral strategies with an adolescent in precontemplation will find these patients may resist self-monitoring and refuse to implement techniques. Conversely, a young person may become impatient if he or she is ready for action, but the therapies concentrate on developing insight.

A problematic pattern seen frequently in adolescent psychotherapy is when parents are ready to have their youngster change his or her behavior, but they believe the adolescent must do all the changing. In other words, the parents are in the action stage for their adolescent, but in the precontemplation stage for their own behavior. The adolescent in the precontemplation stage does not see any need for change. In this situation, environmental changes must occur in order to help the adolescent move into the contemplation and action stages. This may be accomplished if the parents can be convinced to change their behavior (e.g., set consistent limits) or by the therapist's interventions (e.g., clinic-based rewards, or developing a relationship with the adolescent). These factors suggest that treatment outcome may be enhanced if as much attention is paid to developing rapport with the adolescent as to learning about controlling variables during the assessment phase.

TEACHING BEHAVIOR CHANGE TECHNIQUES

In general, several steps are necessary in order to be most effective in promoting and maintaining behavior change. Adolescents should not only learn new ways to respond or to structure their environments, but also they must change their hierarchy of responding. In other words, the problematic pattern of responding may have been reinforced for many years and may have been adaptive during an earlier stage of development. The result becomes a predisposition to respond, automatically, with the maladaptive response in a specific situation. In order to change this hierarchy, a systematic approach to teaching the new behavior should be implemented that includes reading, hearing, seeing, and practicing.

The therapist first provides a rationale for the procedures being taught, and then provides readings that outline the technique and its rationale. The desired behavior is demonstrated by the therapist for the adolescent to observe and to ask questions. For example, in social skills training, the therapist has an assistant or the adolescent play the role of a friend who is asking the adolescent to buy him or her something very expensive. The therapist demonstrates an assertive refusal to the request. The next step is for the young person to practice the new behavior, while the therapist plays the role of the friend.

Generalization of the assertive response is taught by having the adolescent refuse a variety of requests that become more and more subtle. The therapist provides specific feedback that labels appropriate and inappropriate responses. Finally, the adolescent's skill is assessed while he or she performs the role play without feedback. Homework assignments are given and the adolescent is asked to keep track of his or her behavior. For example, the adolescent is asked to record both the number of times he or she refused unreasonable requests and the number of times he or she failed to refuse. The

therapist may also ask for a brief description of the request in order to help the adolescent improve his or her skill.

TECHNIQUES OF INTERVENTION

In this section, specific behavioral techniques are discussed according to whether they target (1) overt behaviors that may need to be increased or decreased; (2) organismic variables, especially cognitions; and (3) social interactions. Although these techniques are presented in isolation, a comprehensive treatment plan must include evaluation and possibly modification of controlling stimuli in other areas as well as medical interventions. For example, relaxation is discussed as a treatment for chronic pain, but pain behaviors may be increased by rewards such as staying home from school and having people attend to the adolescent. In such cases, consultation with educational personnel as well as assessment of social skills may be helpful. The reader is referred to a recent volume edited by Feindler and Kalfus, which presents case studies on the use of behavior therapy for a variety of presenting problems, such as depression, anger control, and so on.

Symptom and Situational Intervention

RELAXATION AND BIOFEEDBACK

Relaxation and biofeedback are discussed together, because relaxation is frequently taught with biofeedback training. These procedures have been found to be useful in the treatment of a variety of somatic complaints, such as (1) chronic pain, headaches, temporomandibular syndrome (see Chapter 16); (2) cardiovascular problems; (3) gastrointestinal symptomatology (e.g., recurrent abdominal pain); and (4) insomnia, and as a first step in the treatment of phobias. For a comprehensive guide to biofeedback, see Schwartz and associates.

Although there is no commonly accepted procedure for relaxation training, it generally includes deep muscle relaxation or mental imagery. In order to individualize the training, the therapist can conduct an assessment of the adolescent's preference for imagery versus deep muscle relaxation. Assessment might include having the adolescent tighten and loosen his or her fist while describing the feeling or having them imagine their favorite color spreading up their arm. This allows the therapist to identify the adolescent's preferences, as well as the words he or she uses to describe the feelings. In this way, the therapist can individualize the relaxation procedure. Mental imagery may include having the adolescent imagine a favorite location or activity.

Relaxation training generally begins by having the patient sit quietly in a comfortable chair in a quiet room. During deep muscle relaxation, the adolescent is told to tighten and loosen specific muscle groups while concentrating on the feeling in that muscle. One technique that we have found useful is to begin with deep muscle relaxation and then use imagery to maintain the teenager's relaxed state. It is usually helpful for the therapist to emphasize repetitive aspects of the preferred scenery, such as waves rolling onto a beach. Attention to the teenager's rate of breathing also aids the therapist in modifying the rate and duration of the session.

Finally, the session is generally audio taped and the audio tape is given to the adolescent to take home and use during the week. He or she is asked to practice once daily and to record how relaxed he or she is on a ten-point scale, prior to and after practicing. In this way, the adolescent keeps a record of practice sessions and their progress can be monitored. During subsequent therapy sessions, the procedure and the audio tape can be modified as needed.

Biofeedback may be used as an adjunct to relaxation training for muscle tension, Raynaud disease (see Chapter 90), or hypertension (see Chapter 67). It may also be used alone for problems such as urinary or fecal incontinence, or neuromuscular re-education. Biofeedback provides the patient with auditory or visual feedback about the target behavior (e.g., heart rate, temperature, or electromyography). For example, in Raynaud disease patients, a temperature probe might be attached to the young person's toe and the adolescent might be signalled by the off-set of a sound when the toe temperature reaches a certain level.

DESENSITIZATION (SYSTEMATIC, CONTACT, FLOODING)

Anxiety-based disorders such as (1) phobias, including agoraphobia, simple and social phobias (see Chapters 102 and 103); (2) panic attacks; (3) obsessive-compulsive disorder (see Chapter 105); and (4) post-traumatic stress disorder (PTSD) (see Chapter 104) are generally considered appropriate for desensitization. In these conditions, anxiety is controlled primarily by the antecedent stimuli such as examination taking, public speaking, social situations, or the perpetrator of the traumatic event. In addition, the anxious response may be precipitated by cognitions, such as obsessive thoughts about dirt in the case of the obsessive compulsive or by thinking about a traumatic event in the PTSD patient. For a more extensive overview, see Goldfried and Davison.

The basic premise of desensitization is that the individual's anxiety response can be attenuated by exposure to the feared stimulus. Systematic and contact desensitization are similar in that they include gradual exposure to increasingly feared stimuli. The general principle is that as fear decreases at one level, there will be generalization of the nonanxious response to the next level, making it easier to master. In both techniques, the adolescent develops a hierarchy of feared situations either by measuring his or her physiologic response to the discussion of potentially fearful situations or by having him or her rate subjective fear to specific situations.

Systematic desensitization begins by teaching the adolescent patient relaxation (see earlier) and then having him or her imagine the feared situations, from the least fear-inducing to the most fear-inducing. The patient is asked to rate how fearful he or she feels during each presentation; relaxation is reinduced when necessary. A specific scene is represented until the patient is able to maintain his or her relaxed state, then the next scene is presented. Contact desensitization differs from systematic desensitization in that the patient is placed in physical contact with the feared stimulus. This, too, begins with exposure to the least fear-inducing situation, and the patient remains in this situation or returns to it until he or she no longer feels anxious. He or she then moves to the next level on the hierarchy. It may be useful with extremely fearful patients to begin with desensitization in imagery and then progress to contact desensitization.

Flooding involves placing the adolescent in the most feared situation. It is extremely important that the patient remain in the situation until both verbal and physiologic signs of anxiety have been eliminated. The rationale is that if he or she leaves the aversive situation prior to complete calm, the escape will reinforce the fear and an even higher level of anxiety will result. Flooding is a very unpleasant procedure and it can be risky, especially with adolescents who have cardiovascular problems. As a result, it should be used infrequently and only in those adolescent patients who have had a thorough medical examination. The reasons to use a flooding procedure include an adolescent who has a single phobia (e.g., airplane phobia) who must fly immediately or an obsessive-compulsive youngster whose feared stimuli are cognitions.

HABIT REVERSAL AND MASS PRACTICE

Habit reversal or massed practice procedures may be useful in reducing the frequency or intensity of tics caused by chronic tic disorder and Gilles de la Tourette syndrome. These techniques may be useful alone or in conjunction with medication and changing reinforcement contingencies around the tics. For a more in-depth discussion, see the Hobbs, Dorsett, and Dahlquist chapter in Hersen and VanHasselt.

Massed practice is a technique in which the adolescent is asked to spend approximately 5 minutes practicing the tic during multiple sessions per day. The theory that led to the development of this paradoxical approach is that tics are reinforced by the reduction of a hypothetical drive. An alternative explanation might be that tics are caused by an increase in the level of neurotransmitters, and massed practice depletes the neurotransmitters.

Habit reversal assumes that tics are the result of an increase in frequency of a normal behavior until this behavior is automatic. As a result, it involves two basic steps in treatment. First, the patient's awareness of the tic is increased by having him or her describe it in detail while looking in a mirror and also monitoring its occurrence across situations. Second, the patient is taught a subtle competing response that is practiced daily in front of a mirror and then used throughout the day. For example, an adolescent who has an eye-blink tic might be taught to oppose the tic by holding his eyelids open for 3 seconds. This procedure is coupled with social reinforcement for performance of the competing response. Results of studies using this technique have reduced the incidence of the tic by as much as 90% to 100%.

CONTINGENCY CONTRACTING

Contingency contracting is an important treatment modality for improving parent–adolescent relationships, increasing compliance with medical treatments (see Chapter 26), improving conduct (see Chapter 108), and eating disorders (see Chapter 60). A contingency contract includes a specific definition of a behavior and the consequences of performing that behavior. For example, if the adolescent who has anorexia nervosa fails to eat and retain a certain number of calories during a meal, then he or she must remain in bed until the next meal. Additionally, if a certain number of calories per day are eaten, then he or she may be granted a special privilege.

An important component of successful contingency contracting is the development of appropriate consequences. If the consequence for coming home late is grounding, but the adolescent's parents fail to follow through, then the adolescent learns that coming in late is not a problem. Problems also arise if consequences are too severe. In our clinic, adolescents are brought in because their parents have grounded them for months, and it "just isn't working." Evaluation of the situation generally shows that the adolescent has learned to nag until their parents let him or her go out, or parents are "too busy" to make sure the adolescent stays home. In addition, from the adolescent's perspective, he or she is grounded forever, so he or she may as well sneak out to a party. Thus, it is important that there be a clear limitation on the length of grounding, which is negotiated and understood by the adolescent and his or her parents.

Maladaptive Cognitions

Cognitive behavioral therapy (CBT) targets organismic variables such as negative attributions, irrational thoughts, and deficits in problem-solving skills. One premise of CBT is that the way a person feels and acts is related to the way he or she thinks about a situation. If the adolescent is taught to identify irrational thoughts and problem situations and then given specific statements that include overt behavioral goals, he or she will be more able to change the behavior. CBT may be a component of therapy for problems such as depression (see Chapter 100), obesity (see Chapter 60), eating disorders (see Chapter 60), anxiety, and so forth. Three techniques most commonly taught in CBT are problem-solving training, self-statements, and anger management.

PROBLEM SOLVING

Many adolescents come into therapy because of difficulty in resolving problems on a day-to-day basis. The therapist may find that each session involves resolving a new problem with the adolescent, such as parental nagging about homework, disputes about going on dates, or disputes over television shows. Each session may resolve the new problem, but the specific solution is not useful in other situations. This may indicate a deficit in problem-solving skills in general.

Problem-solving skills training involves a step-by-step approach that includes introducing simulated and real problems of increasing complexity during therapy sessions. The adolescent is taught specific steps, which include (1) recognizing the problem; (2) defining the specifics of the problem, including his or her own reactions and the situations that set the stage for the problem; (3) generating a variety of alternative solutions while avoiding evaluating the solutions; (4) a thorough evaluation of long- and short-term consequences of the solutions; and (5) choosing one or a combination of solutions. Finally, the patient is asked to develop a procedure for implementing and evaluating the solution.

SELF-STATEMENTS

Self-statements may include specific verbalizations about a situation or specific instructions as to how to perform. For example, an adolescent who has been verbally abusive in the past may be taught self-statements such as "If I swear at my mother, I will get into trouble; but if I ask calmly, I might get my way." Self-statements for an adolescent who has school phobia might include talking about engaging in a distracting behavior. For example, the adolescent might say "I'm starting to get nervous about school; I need to take things one step at a time, so I'll go take my shower."

Self-instructional training is another aspect of self-statements that involves having the adolescent repeat instructions for a task aloud. Typically, the therapist models the appropriate steps for completing a task, while saying the instructions aloud. The adolescent is then taught to perform the same steps, while repeating the instructions aloud. The adolescent is taught to say the steps progressively more quietly until he or she mouths the words and finally is told to think them.

ANGER MANAGEMENT

Anger management is one aspect of changing cognitions and self-statements, but it is included separately because this is an important target area during adolescence and specific methods of teaching anger management are well developed. Anger management training has been found to be successful for treating adolescents diagnosed as conduct disorder–aggressive type (see Chapter 108), oppositional disorder, and attention deficit disorder (see Chapter 106). Feindler and Ecton's cognitive–behavioral program includes formats for teaching anger control to individuals and groups. It involves teaching the adolescents that thoughts and feelings about specific situations are what cause their anger. They are then taught to identify the relevant situations and triggers. The next steps in the program include relaxation training and assertiveness training. Assertion skills include standing up for their rights in a calm manner and using self-statements to maintain a calm approach to a problem situation. Finally, the adolescents are taught to plan ahead regarding how they intend to handle problem situations, and then evaluate themselves with regard to the approach they used (see Chapter 117).

Interpersonal Conflicts

Adolescents may have interpersonal conflicts with parents, adults in other settings, or peers. Three areas are considered in this section: teaching age-appropriate management skills to parents, communication training, and social skills training.

PARENTING SKILLS

Although parenting skills do not necessarily include the adolescent, appropriate parenting may motivate an adolescent who has a conduct disorder to think about changing his or her own behavior (i.e., move from precontemplation to contemplation and action in the behavior change model). In addition, problems may develop if parents maintain preadolescent parenting strategies (e.g., physical punishments and inflexible rules) as their adolescent develops and desires more freedom in decision making.

Parents and adolescents need to be taught skills such as contingency contracting and problem solving and negotiation. In this way, the adolescent can begin to participate in decision-making processes and develop skills necessary for independent living. An important aspect of parenting an adolescent includes establishing appropriate punishments that parents can enforce. Appropriate punishments include fines, work consequences (e.g., cleaning the garage), privilege loss (e.g., no car for a week), and natural consequences (e.g., summer school).

COMMUNICATION TRAINING

Teaching specific communication skills has been found to be helpful in improving parent-adolescent relationships. In general, Robin and Foster include teaching adolescents and parents to use "I" statements and not accuse or blame others or be defensive. For example, "I feel angry when you make rules without an explanation," rather than "That rule isn't fair, you're a jerk and I hate you!" Other skills include talking directly to one another, not through others, avoiding lecturing, and staying on the topic. Finally, another important issue is the tone of voice. Frequently parents complain that their adolescent "smarts off" or "has a bad attitude." Adolescents can be taught to make requests in a calm, objective manner, as can parents.

SOCIAL SKILLS TRAINING

Social skills deficits may lead to a variety of problems for adolescents, including social isolation, diminished happiness, and social aggression. For comprehensive programs for social skills intervention, the reader is referred to Michelson and colleagues and Schneider, Rubin, and Ledingham. Areas common to many social skills training programs include teaching assertiveness skills, conversation skills, and interpersonal problem solving. Assertiveness training teaches adolescents to make and to refuse requests and to express their thoughts, feelings, and ideas, with an emphasis on avoiding aggressive verbal behavior. Conversation skills may include teaching the adolescent to talk more, use minimal encouragers such as "okay" and "I see." Nonverbal skills include smiling, nodding, and making eye contact with the person to whom they are talking. Finally, interpersonal problem solving is taught, including teaching the adolescent to be aware of the effect of his or her behavior on others and to choose appropriate behaviors.

BIBLIOGRAPHY

Azrin NH, Nunn RG, Frantz SE: Habit reversal vs. negative practice: Treatment of nervous tics. Behavior Therapy 11: 169, 1980.

Bandura A: Social Learning Theory. Englewood Cliffs, NJ, Prentice Hall, 1977.

Craighead WE, Kazdin AE, Mahoney MJ: Behavior Modification: Principles, Issues and Applications. Boston, Houghton Mifflin, 1981.

D'Zurilla TJ: Problem Solving Therapy: A Social Competence Approach to Clinical Intervention. New York, Springer, 1986.

Feindler EL, Ecton RB: Adolescent Anger Control: Cognitive–Behavioral Techniques. New York, Pergammon Press, 1986.

Feindler EL, Kalfus G (eds): Adolescent Behavior Therapy Handbook. New York, Springer, 1990.

Goldfried MR, Davison GC: Clinical Behavior Therapy. New York, Holt, Rinehart & Winston, 1976.

Hersen M, VanHasselt VB: Behavior Therapy with Children and Adolescents. New York, John Wiley & Sons, 1988.

Hersen M, Bellack AS: Behavioral Assessment: A Practical Handbook, 2nd ed. New York, Pergamon Press, 1981.

Mash RJ, Terdal LH: Behavioral Assessment of Childhood Disorders, 2nd ed. New York, Guilford Press, 1988.

Meichenbaum D: Cognitive–Behavior Modification: An Integrative Approach. New York, Plenum Press, 1977.

Michelson L, Sugai D, Wood RP, Kazdin AE: Social Skills Assessment and Training with Children. New York, Plenum Press, 1984.

Prochaska JO, DiClemente CC: Toward a comprehensive model of change. In Miller WR, Heather N (eds): Treating Addictive Behaviors. New York, Plenum Press, 1986, pp 3–27.

Robin AL, Foster SL: Negotiating Parent Adolescent Conflict: A Behavioral–Family Systems Approach. New York, Guilford Press, 1981.

Routh DK: Handbook of Pediatric Psychology. New York, Guilford Press, 1988.

Schneider BG, Rubin KH, Ledingham JE: Children's Peer Relations: Issues in Assessment and Intervention. New York, Springer Verlag, 1985.

Schwartz MS and associates: Biofeedback: A Practitioner's Guide. New York, Guilford Press, 1987.

CHAPTER 125

Psychotropic Drug Treatment

DENNIS P. CANTWELL

The use of psychopharmacologic agents in young children and adolescents began in the late 1930s with Bradley's classic studies of the effects of stimulants on children who today would most likely be diagnosed as having attention deficit disorder with hyperactivity. Thus such therapy actually predates many of the developments of psychopharmacologic treatment of adults. However, advances in pediatric psychopharmacology have not been as rapid, particularly among the adolescent population.

There are many important reasons for this lag. Historically, psychotropic agents were not considered as first line interventions, rather their use was considered an admission of failure, since psychodynamic psychotherapy was considered to be the treatment of choice.

There are also public and professional concerns and prejudices against using psychotropic drugs in children and adolescents. Medical specialists who see adolescents on a regular basis may not be trained in up-to-date adolescent psychopharmacology and may have subtle conscious and unconscious biases against the use of psychotropic agents. There is a vocal antimedication faction in the United States, consisting of numerous nonscientific fringe groups that emphasize "horror stories" about the side effects of psychotropic medication. They view these drugs as "chemical strait jackets" for bright, exuberant, active adolescents who really have no mental illness.

In addition, prior to the use of the Diagnostic and Statistical Manual of Mental Disorders, Third Edition Revised (DSM-III-R), there was no adequate, reliable, valid classification system of child and adolescent psychopathology, making comparison of data very difficult. There also was a prevailing view that much of adolescent psychopathology was "normal adolescent turmoil" (see Chapters 8 and 9). That is, symptoms that would lead to the diagnosis of depression or schizophrenia in an adult were considered to be part of the normal developmental process for adolescents.

There is less knowledge about the efficacy and safety of many psychotropic agents in the adolescent population. Most FDA studies of new medications that are submitted for approval are conducted first with those older than 18 years of age. Only later do individual studies extend the use of approved psychotropic agents to adolescents and children. In many cases younger children are treated before adolescents. Adolescents' inability to provide informed consent limits their use as research subjects. Together these factors have resulted in less knowledge about the psychopharmacology of adolescents than that of adults and in some cases that of children. Nonetheless there have been major advances in child and adolescent psychopharmacology in the past 10 to 15 years.

GENERAL PRINCIPLES OF ADOLESCENT PSYCHOPHARMACOLOGY

There are general principles that apply when one is considering the use of medication with any adolescent patient, irrespective of the disorder or the type of medication (Table 125–1). First, a comprehensive diagnostic evaluation of the adolescent and the family is necessary in order to make a specific diagnosis (see Chapters 22 and 98). At a minimum this should include a detailed interview with the parents about the adolescent; detailed psychiatric interviews with the adolescent; physical and neurologic examinations, if appropriate; collection of information from the school; appropriate laboratory testing, including psychological testing as appropriate (see Chapter 99); and interviews with the parents about development of the adolescent (see Chapter 9), family structure (see Chapter 23), family dynamics, family interaction, and the greater psychosocial environment of the adolescent (see Chapter 98).

Second, if medication is going to be used as part of the therapeutic intervention, collect proper baseline information of all domains that are likely to be affected by the medication. Every psychotropic agent affects a number of mental and physical functions. Generally, the target behaviors in the management of adolescent psychopathologic conditions include activity level, cognitive function, academic achievement, disruptive behavior, and mood (such as anxiety and depression). Psychotropic drugs also affect physiologic systems; heart rate, blood pressure, height, weight, and at times specific information such as electrocardiogram results have to be measured at baseline so that they can be monitored over time.

There are a number of parent, teacher, clinician, and patient rating scales that have been developed for use in monitoring adolescent psychopathologic behavior. These include broad-based measures as well as specific measures of certain symptoms, such as depression, anxiety, or side effects. A more complete discussion of

TABLE 125–1. Guidelines for Use of Psychotropic Medication

Perform comprehensive diagnostic evaluation
If condition suggests medications may be useful:
Perform baseline evaluations
    Behavior
    Psychological
    Biologic
Involve adolescent patient, family, and school
Select class of medication
Select specific drug
Titrate dose
Monitor effects
    Behavior
    Psychological
    Biologic
Consider withdrawal if indicated
Consider drug holiday if indicated

these instruments can be found in a special issue of the *Psychopharmacology Bulletin*. All psychotropic drugs affect cognitive function, whether intended as a target behavior or resulting as a side effect. It is important to have some assessment of general intelligence and academic achievement. There are a variety of tests of cognitive functions that have found some utility in psychopharmacologic studies, including the reaction time task, the continuous performance task, the paired associate learning task, the short-term memory task, studies of discrimination learning, the matching familiar figure test, and the Porteus mazes. Certain psychotropic medications may have a dulling effect on cognitive function. It is important that improvement in the behavior of disturbed adolescents not be obtained at the expense of cognitive function. This is especially true with those adolescents who may be mildly retarded or who have borderline intellectual functioning.

Involve the significant others in the adolescent's life in the treatment process, including family members and caretakers as well as school personnel. The physician should explain in great detail the anticipated positive and negative effects of the psychotropic medication. Because parental reports are usually part of the monitoring process, the physician must know parental expectations of the drug. If the parents have ideas about obscure organic causes of their adolescent's disorder and have expectations that the medication will eradicate the basic cause of the disorder, then they may report that the medication is ineffective even when the medication may be doing physiologically exactly what it was intended to do. It is not unlikely that with an individual adolescent patient the physician may have to change the type of medication or the dosage in order to get the optimal effect of the most efficacious drug. The parents should be made aware of this and encouraged to observe the adolescent for both positive and possible negative responses to the drug.

It is important that the physician not let the issue of the use of medication become part of an "organic versus dynamic" etiologic debate. Most likely, if the medication is effective, it will improve some aspect of the adolescent's problem and may increase the efficacy of the overall treatment package, giving parents hope that the problem can be helped. Improvement through medica-

tion can decrease guilt on the part of the parents. Parents may feel totally responsible for the adolescent's behavior, and seeing medication make a difference may alleviate some unrealistic guilt. The approach of the physician prescribing the medication should be one in which the parents and the adolescent are involved as partners in the therapy. The physician may tell the family, "Medication might help. It has to be given a fair trial, but everybody will have to keep trying. The medication will not be able to do everything."

It is true that adolescents may rebel and be noncompliant because taking the medication may be seen as taking something from an authority figure (see Chapter 26). However, adolescents who receive an adequate explanation, who have support from parents and teachers, and who believe that the medication may help their problem accept medication more readily. The adolescent patient needs to understand that even if the medication is effective, it does not substitute for his or her own efforts to overcome the basic problem.

Involvement of the school is an important part of monitoring any adolescent receiving psychotropic medication. The importance of the teacher as an observer cannot be overestimated. Teachers are in a position in which they see a number of adolescents in the same setting doing the same tasks. They have observed the adolescent patient before and after medication was started. Relying on reports solely from parents, particularly with short-acting drugs that may have their maximum effectiveness during school time, may give a distorted picture.

The type of medication is selected after the comprehensive diagnostic evaluation has been completed; the diagnostic formulation has been made; proper baseline assessments have been taken; and the family, the school, and the adolescent patient have become involved in the therapeutic process. This is easiest when solid scientific evidence demonstrates that the drug is safe and effective for the particular disorder in the adolescent population. There are three levels of indication, depending on the type of studies that have been done: a definite indication, a possible indication, and a nonindication. A definite indication exists if there are substantial numbers of double-blind, placebo-controlled studies performed with a particular drug for a particular disorder in the adolescent age range. Most psychotropic drugs do not have this level of indication for use in the adolescent age range, either because no double-blind, placebo-controlled studies have been done or because results are conflicting. A nonindication simply means that there is no evidence one way or another from placebo-controlled, double-blind studies that the drug is effective for a particular condition in the adolescent age range. Thus, most of the indications that we have for psychotropic drug use in the adolescent age range are possible indications.

A drug can be considered to be a possible indication in a number of ways. First, open trials may suggest that the drug is effective for a particular disorder in the adolescent age range. Open studies are more useful for chronic conditions that are nonremitting than they are for relapsing and remitting conditions. For example, if 100 depressed adolescents are treated openly with antidepressants for a year, there is reasonable expectation that some will improve as part of the natural history of the mood disorder, and the medication may have had little to do with the improvement. In some cases, medication may indeed have played a very active role. The absence of placebo control does not allow one to make that decision. If a condition is known not to have spontaneous remissions, very large effects in open trial suggest that the use of the medication is potentially helpful.

Second, if the pathophysiologic etiology of a certain disorder is suspected and a drug is known to affect that pathophysiologic process, then there is at least a theoretical reason why the medication might be considered to be used for a particular disorder. As an example, stimulants are known to be effective for a substantial number of patients who have attention deficit hyperactivity disorder (ADHD). Moreover, the stimulant medication seems to affect primarily the attentional process in this disorder. The DSM-III diagnosis of attention deficit disorder without hyperactivity was conceptualized as a similar attentional problem in the absence of motoric overactivity and possibly impulsivity. One could hypothesize then that stimulants might also be effective in this condition, and this might be a possible indication for the use of stimulant medication (see Chapter 106).

Finally, if an adolescent disorder seems to be the same as a disorder that occurs more commonly in adults, one might consider the use of a medication that is effective for adults, even in the absence of placebo-controlled, double-blind studies with adolescent populations. For example, lithium is effective for adults in the treatment of bipolar mood disturbance (see Chapter 100). The onset of mania is common in adolescence, and it seems to be the same disorder occurring at an earlier age. Although there are not substantial numbers of double-blind, placebo-controlled studies with adolescents, one would seriously consider the use of lithium for a manic adolescent. Likewise, because stimulants are known to be effective in prepubertal children with ADHD, one would consider their use in adolescents, since the disorder seems to be the same disorder manifesting itself in slightly different ways (see Chapter 106).

Next, the specific drug is selected. Generally, it is best to use a drug that has been on the market for a longer period of time and with which one is familiar. Drugs that have been on the market for only a short period of time may acquire certain "fad" status. When compared with standard drugs, they usually are no more efficacious in terms of percentage of adolescents who might respond, but they may have a different side effect profile or have some particular unique psychopharmacologic action, such as selectively affecting one particular neurotransmitter. Nevertheless, except in rare instances, it is best to rely on old and trusted drugs as a first choice rather than on new medications for which there is limited information on long-term usage.

Titration of the dosage is the next step. In a nonurgent situation, begin with a small dose and increase the dose regularly until a good clinical response has been obtained, a known effective blood level has been obtained, or side effects necessitate either decrease in the medication or its withdrawal. Knowledge of the duration of

action is necessary. Short-acting drugs (short half-life), such as the short-acting stimulants, must be prescribed on a two times or a three times a day basis, depending on how long the physician wishes the medication to be active. Medications with longer serum or tissue half-lives (such as the tricyclic antidepressants) need not be prescribed as often; one has the expectation that there will be a predictable long-term effect with a specific dose. For most disorders of adolescents and for most psychotropic medications there are very few laboratory or other measures with which to titrate the medication. In general, the physician uses clinical judgment based on comprehensive information obtained from the parents, from the adolescent patient, from the school, and from direct observation of the adolescent to decide whether or not the medication is effective. In certain instances, such as the use of lithium for mania, the optimal therapeutic blood range is known.

The physician should monitor the therapeutic effects and any side effects of the medication and decide whether continuation treatment or maintenance treatment is necessary. This decision depends on the condition being treated and the specific drug. For example, a chronic condition such as ADHD that is being treated with a stimulant requires continuing treatment. In contrast, once an adolescent has responded to pharmacologic treatment for depression, the physician generally decides to discontinue the agent (see Chapter 100).

If improvement does occur, frequent monitoring needs to be done at regular intervals. Ratings of symptoms as reported by parents, teachers, the adolescent patient, and the clinician should be done at regular intervals as well as ratings of any potential side effects. These would include appropriate measures of learning, depressive affect, anxious affect, height, weight, pulse, blood pressure, and so forth. Psychoeducational and cognitive testing may be done as often as once a year to see whether there is a markedly noticeable effect on cognitive function and actual academic achievement.

In some cases, adolescents treated with chronic psychoactive medication should be given a drug-free trial to allow reevaluation. Placebo substitution is preferable, but simple discontinuation of the medication is also acceptable (see Chapter 106). The need to do this varies with the drug and the disorder. With a condition likely to persist over time (such as ADHD), it is often useful to have the adolescent start a new school year in a new class with a new teacher without medication to get baseline ratings over the course of the year. Any medication should be discontinued only when the clinical picture indicates that the adolescent no longer requires it. This is a matter of clinical judgment. Age does not enter into the decision to discontinue medication any more than it enters into the decision to start a medication. The decision to start a medication should be based on the fact that the adolescent has a disorder that is known to, or may likely, respond to a particular psychotropic drug and on the knowledge that the medication is safe. A drug should be stopped when those conditions no longer apply.

One of the major goals of any psychopharmacologic intervention with an adolescent should be the promotion of more normal patterns of maturation and development. In most cases, adolescents with psychiatric disorders are in treatment using other forms of therapy in addition to, not instead of, psychopharmacologic intervention. The use of psychopharmacologic agents with adolescents should not be viewed as an either-or situation. Unfortunately, very little research has studied the combined effect of psychopharmacologic intervention and other forms of intervention as compared with the effect of nonpsychopharmacologic interventions when given alone.

SPECIFIC USES OF PSYCHOPHARMACOLOGIC AGENTS IN ADOLESCENCE

In this section, the indications for use of psychotropic medications in the adolescent population are reviewed (Table 125–2). To the extent possible, the indication levels listed previously are used: definite indication, possible indication, and nonindication, as defined by Cantwell. The reader is referred to recent references for more details about each of the medications discussed.

Psychostimulants

Attention deficit disorder (ADD) with hyperactivity (see Chapter 106) is generally considered to be the only definite indication for the use of psychostimulants during adolescence. Cantwell has considered the following as possible indications: ADD residual state, ADD without hyperactivity, conduct disorders, and mental retardation and pervasive developmental disorder with concomitant symptoms suggestive of ADD. Popper lists ADD residual state as a possible indication and lists, under conjectural indications, ADD without hyperactivity, conduct disorders, specific developmental learning disorders, and "emotional lability." Dulcan adds ADD without hyperactivity and ADD in mental retardation, in fragile X syndrome with tics or Tourette disorder, and in pervasive developmental disorder. Dulcan also considers definite neurologic injury causing trauma to the brain with attendant ADHD symptoms as a possible indication. Thus, there is only minor disagreement with regard to indications for the use of psychostimulants in adolescents with different types of psychiatric disorders.

The undesirable effects of all common psychostimulants are similar. These include insomnia; loss of appetite, leading either to weight loss or to weight gain that is less than expected; social withdrawal; blood pressure and pulse elevation; headaches; abdominal pain; a rebound effect with an increase in ADD-like symptoms above baseline level; and an impairment of cognitive level effortful tasks at high dosages.

These adverse effects are relatively common but generally tend to be either short-lived or easily managed. Undesirable effects such as motor tics or a full-blown Tourette syndrome, psychosis, significant elevations of heart rate or blood pressure, and significant impairment of height are clinically more significant but much less common. Magnesium pemoline (Cylert) is associated with elevation of liver enzyme levels in about 3% of subjects; adventitious movements, night terrors, and other potential neuropsychiatric effects are less common. There is no good evidence that the appropriate use of psychostimulants in adolescents predisposes to recreational use of drugs or to psychological or physical dependence. Likewise, increased frequency of seizures is not a significant problem.

The stimulants that are commonly used in adolescents include methylphenidate, amphetamines, and magnesium pemoline. The first two are available in both short- and long-acting forms; pemoline is available in only one form, which is relatively long-acting. Clinical effects on behavior and cognitive function are relatively similar among the three major preparations, but they are not identically similar in individual patients (see Chapter 106). Thus, one patient may respond better to an amphetamine than to methylphenidate or pemoline, and the opposite may occur in other patients. Currenly there are no clinical or laboratory predictors of differential response.

Dosage is titrated clinically to produce maximum clinical benefit with the least side effects. The short-acting forms of the stimulants generally have a duration of about 4 hours, the long-acting forms, generally between 6 and 8 hours. Monitoring should include aspects of behavioral and cognitive function from as many settings as possible (home, school, and the clinic) and should also include height, weight, pulse, and blood pressure. General physical and neurologic monitoring is necessary to detect any changes in physical symptoms over time or the appearance of any tics or involuntary movements. With pemoline, liver function tests should be obtained twice a year. The value of routine laboratory tests such as blood counts, electrolytes, and so on is questionable in the usual case treated with stimulants.

There is a range of dosages that have been used in the treatment of adolescents, and the optimal dose for each patient needs to be titrated on an individual basis. There are no good guidelines in the literature for the ultimate dose that is useful for different adolescents with different clinical problems, or even for different adolescents with the same clinical problems, such as ADHD.

Fenfluramine is structurally similar to amphetamine but exerts its effect primarily on serotonin. Its major use has been in individuals with autism or autism spectrum disorders of a variety of different etiologies, including those with fragile X syndrome. The symptoms that are positively affected by fenfluramine in a minority of these children include the ADD symptoms of hyperactivity and attention span problems, and some of the more autistic-like behaviors such as affective relatedness and stereotypies. Side effects tend to be similar to those of other stimulants. Generally, there is no reason to use fenfluramine instead of the commonly available and used preparations described above.

Antidepressants

The antidepressants are medications that were introduced primarily for the treatment of mood disorders in

TABLE 125–2. Commonly Used Psychotropic Medications

CLASS AND GENERIC AGENTS	DEFINITE INDICATIONS	POSSIBLE INDICATIONS
Psychostimulants		
Methylphenidate	ADHD	ADD, residual type
Amphetamines		ADD, without hyperactivity
Pemoline		Conduct disorders
		Pervasive developmental disorder with attentional hyperactivity
		Specific learning disorder with attentional/hyperactivity symptoms
		Fragile X syndrome with tics
		Tourette syndrome
Fenfluramine		Autism (spectrum) disorders
Antidepressants		
Heterocyclics		Major depressive disorder
Clomipramine	Obsessive-compulsive disorder	ADD, without hyperactivity
Amitriptyline		AHD, residual type
Nortriptyline	Primary enuresis	Conduct disorder
Protriptyline	ADHD	Specific learning disorder with attentional/hyperactivity symptoms
Imipramine		Separation anxiety disorder
Desipramine		Panic disorder
		Eating disorders
Monoamine oxidase inhibitors		Major depressive disorder
		ADHD
		Bulimia
Newer agents		
Fluoxetine		Obsessive-compulsive disorder [ADULTS]
Bupropion		Major depressive disorder
		ADHD in children/adolescents
Antimanic Agents		
Lithium carbonate	Mania	Bipolar affective disorder
		Chronic aggressive acting out with conduct disorder
		Atypical cyclic disorders
Antianxiety Agents		
Benzodiazepines	Night terrors	Overanxious disorder
	Somnambulism	Separation anxiety disorder
	[ADULTS]	Tic disorders
	Anxiety disorders	
	Panic disorder	
Antihistamines	Agitation	Anxiety states
β-Blockers	[ADULTS]	[ADULTS]
	Anxiety disorders	Performance anxiety
Buspirone		Overanxious disorder
		Separation anxiety disorder
Barbiturates		
Others (chloral hydrate, paraldehyde)		
Neuroleptics		
Chlorpromazine	Schizophrenia	ADHD
Trifluoperazine	Mania	Pervasive developmental disorder
Fluphenazine	Severe aggression, self-mutilation, agitation	Retardation with impulsivity
Thioridazine		
Prochlorperazine		
Haloperidol	Tourette syndrome	
Pimozide	Tourette syndrome	
Other Agents		
Clonidine		Tourette syndrome
		Mania
		ADHD
Anticonvulsants	Seizure disorders	
		[ADULTS]
Valproic acid		Mania
Carbamazepine		Mania

adults. These include the heterocyclic antidepressants, the monoamine oxidase inhibitors, and other newer drugs such as fluoxetine and bupropion. Almost all the literature concerning adolescents has concentrated on the heterocyclic antidepressants. There are few data in adolescents on monoamine oxidase inhibitors and even fewer on the newer drugs.

Cantwell suggests that the definite indications for the heterocyclic antidepressants in adolescents are enuresis and ADHD and that possible indications include ADD residual state, ADD without hyperactivity, conduct disorder, separation anxiety disorder (see Chapters 102 and 103), depression (see Chapter 100), specific developmental disorders of learning (see Chapter 107), and the eating disorders (see Chapter 60).

Popper lists the same definite indications, adds panic disorder to possible indications (see Chapters 102 and 103), and lists conduct (see Chapter 108) and specific developmental learning disorders under conjectural indications. Ryan adds obsessive-compulsive disorder (see Chapter 105) and phobic disorders (see Chapter 102) under probable indications and includes under conjectural indications dysthymia, "affective conduct disorder" (see Chapters 100 and 108), borderline personality disorder (see Chapter 109) and in particular "affective borderlines," trichotillomania, and other disorders of impulse control with compulsive manifestations, as well as sleep terror and sleep walking disorders. For one heterocyclic antidepressant, chlorimipramine, obsessive compulsive disorder must also be considered a definite established indication (see Chapter 105).

Ryan suggests that the monoamine oxidase inhibitors are difficult to use in the adolescent population. Adolescents who might be treated with monoamine oxidase inhibitors also tend to have erratic diets, making them susceptible to significant side effects. In adults, monoamine oxidase inhibitors are effective for treating the major depressive disorders, ADHD, and bulimia. Until more data are available on their use in adolescents, these agents should probably be limited to individuals who have failed to respond to more traditional treatments.

Newer antidepressants, such as fluoxetine and bupropion, differ considerably from the heterocyclic antidepressants and from the monoamine oxidase inhibitors. Fluoxetine is primarily serotonergic, whereas bupropion is primarily dopaminergic. Bupropion has a unique chemical structure that is unrelated to the heterocyclic antidepressants. Fluoxetine has two rings in its structure, but it is unrelated to the other heterocyclic antidepressants. There is very little reported experience with these agents among adolescent populations.

The undesirable effects of the heterocyclic antidepressants include the anticholinergic effects (dry mouth), mild slowing of cardiac conduction, mild increase in heart rate, sedation, and orthostatic hypotension. Retention of urine, gastrointestinal symptomatology, and sleep disturbance with occasional nightmares are also reported by some individuals. These undesirable effects are generally not clinically significant.

Adverse effects that are considerably less frequent but potentially more dangerous include the production of heart block, lowered seizure threshold, hypertension

of clinical significance (generally occurring only if there is preexisting hypertension), central nervous system confusional states, anger, and possible precipitation of a psychotic episode, particularly manic episodes in those who are predisposed to develop mania. Minimization and management of these unwanted effects have been described by Ryan and by Klein and associates.

The practical aspects of management consist of the usual medical and neurologic evaluations (including recording of baseline height, weight, pulse, and blood pressure) and the observation and recording of involuntary movements (including possible tics and dyskinetic movements). Baseline electrocardiograms (ECGs) are mandatory for patients younger than the age of 18 years. Some clinicians suggest baseline electroencephalogram (EEG) for patients younger than 18 years of age.

Along with monitoring of clinical symptomatology, physical signs such as involuntary movements, height, weight, pulse, and blood pressure need to be monitored. ECGs or rhythm strips should be recorded with each dose increase. Routine laboratory tests including assessment of thyroid and liver function are recommended on a yearly basis, and patients should be warned about drug interactions, particularly with alcohol. Patients should also be warned that the heterocyclic antidepressants may cause drowsiness or decreased alertness and affect the use of automobiles, bicycles, motorcycles, machine shop tools, and so forth. Dosages of specific heterocyclic antidepressants vary with the diagnosis and are described in detail in other texts. Measurement of blood levels of the medications and their primary metabolites may be useful with some disorders but is not useful for others.

Antimanic Drugs

In a substantial number of cases mania begins for the first time in adolescence (see Chapter 100). Lithium carbonate was introduced as a medication that was effective in adults for the active manic phase of manic-depressive disease. Since that time, subsequent studies have suggested other established and possible indications, although there are slight differences between what clinicians and researchers consider the indications for the adolescent age range.

Although it is true that there are no double-blind, placebo-controlled studies of the use of lithium carbonate for mania in adolescents, Cantwell still considers this to be a definite indication for lithium use. He suggests that there are two possible indications.

1. Adolescents who present clinically with cyclical disorders that are not necessarily classically manic in their clinical picture
2. Certain types of aggressive behavior, including that found in the mentally retarded (data suggest that these may be responsive to lithium)

Shekim (in a personal communication) presents a considerably broader list: possible indications include bipolar disorder, both mania and hypomania, treatment for the acute phase and maintenance treatment; bipolar depression; chronic aggressive acting out behavior with conduct disorder; and cyclic symptomatology of aggressiveness mixed with a strong affective component. He also describes cyclic variations in vegetative symptoms as a possible indication. These include violent imagery and nightmares, restless sleep, difficulties in falling asleep, excessive appetite and thirst on the "high" side and on the "low" side, decreased dream recall, and an unusually sound and lengthy sleep with dysphoric affect on awakening. Augmentation of antidepressant treatment of unipolar depression and episodic and chronic cluster headaches, and episodic disorders, usually of a behavioral nature with a positive family history of bipolar disorder that has been responsive to lithium, are also considered possible indications by Shekim.

In their discussion of the use of lithium in adolescents, Campbell and colleagues also mention bipolar disorder, major depression, behavior disorders in adolescents whose parents are lithium responders, and some cases of autism and mental retardation with aggressive behavior that is either self-directed or directed against other people. (The anticonvulsant carbamazepine and valproic acid have also been suggested as effective antimanic drugs. These are discussed in the section on anticonvulsants.)

Somewhat more controversial as antimanic agents in adolescents are the recommendations of Weinberg. He suggests thioridazine as the primary drug of choice for what he considers "minor manic states" and also as the drug of choice as an additional drug in adolescents for those manic states that are induced by tricyclic antidepressant medication. He also suggests methylphenidate and pemoline as antimanic medications, with methylphenidate being considered the primary drug for chronic hypomania and for excessive daytime sleepiness, which he describes as hypovigilance. Pemoline is considered the secondary drug for chronic hypomania and for excessive daytime sleepiness. Weinberg suggests that methylphenidate may be added to antidepressant treatment in those adolescents who have rapidly cycling bipolar illness or cyclothymic disorder.

UNDESIRABLE EFFECTS

The undesirable effects of lithium are rather predictable and are generally dose related and related to blood level of the medication. Mild irritation of the gastrointestinal tract is relatively common. Less frequent are acneform skin rashes, a fine hand tremor, polydipsia and polyuria, and dehydration, which may be induced by lithium especially in hot weather or with strenuous exercise. The dehydration may be complicated by excessively high lithium levels. There are other side effects that are relatively rare. Some of them are potentially serious, others are not. A leukocytosis may occur, which may or may not be clinically significant. Blood sugar level likewise may rise, although its clinical significance other than for those who have diabetes is not clear. Endocrine changes, such as the formation of a goiter and an increase in calcium, may occur. Although central nervous system symptoms, such as slurred speech, drowsiness, dizziness, muscle weakness, and ataxia, may occur even with blood levels in the therapeutic range, they are usual symptoms of toxicity or overdose.

There is a question about whether long-term lithium use leads to possible kidney damage. All data relate to adults who have been managed on chronic lithium for bipolar illness. The weight of the evidence suggests that significant kidney problems most likely do not occur. Nevertheless, with an adolescent population and with the potential for being on lithium over the lifetime, the physician should consider the possibility of symptoms developing over a longer period of time that may not develop in adults.

PRACTICAL ASPECTS OF MANAGEMENT

Most clinicians recommend an initial and a follow-up workup beyond the ordinary examinations and laboratory tests that would routinely be done for an adolescent patient. Included would be baseline ECG and EEG as well as measurements of electrolyte levels and thyroid and kidney functioning (serum creatinine and creatinine clearance and urine specific gravity on first morning specimen). Blood levels of lithium need to be monitored monthly after the dose is stabilized unless physical or neurologic symptoms suggest otherwise. Routine physical and neurologic examinations and laboratory studies, including measurement of thyroid-stimulating hormone (TSH), are probably all that is necessary, but blood pressure, pulse, dyskinetic movements, blood creatinine levels, and specific gravity of the urine need to be followed more often.

Patients should be warned about a sudden intake of salt, which might lower blood lithium levels. This can be managed by maintaining consistent salt intake. In contrast, dehydration can cause increased lithium levels and possible toxicity. Adequate fluid intake must be maintained at all times, particularly in very hot weather and before and during significant exercise. Concurrent use of alcohol or marijuana should be prohibited, and the adolescent must be reminded that lithium can affect driving and the ability to operate difficult machines, as might be found in shop classes in high school.

Blood levels of 0.8 to 1.5 mEq/L are often needed for acute treatment, and some authors suggest that an even higher dosage leading to blood levels closer to 2.0 mEq/L may be necessary in some cases. The maintenance levels probably can be less, in the range of 0.6 to 1.2 mEq/L. Adolescents appear to have higher renal clearance, leading to the need for higher doses.

The mechanism for discontinuation of treatment needs to be individualized. Some authors suggest treatment for 6 months and then tapering to establish the need for continual treatment. There are data, however, with bipolar illness to suggest that recurrence of manic symptoms is more frequent when lithium is discontinued than when lithium is maintained.

Antianxiety Agents

Those drugs that have antianxiety properties in adolescents have other psychopharmacologic properties as well. Thus, as with antidepressants, there are indications for usage of medications that are traditionally labeled antianxiety agents other than for anxiety problems. The antianxiety agents are a very heterogeneous group of medications. Coffey details at least four separate groups: the benzodiazepines, the antihistamines, the β-blockers, and buspirone. Biederman includes the benzodiazepines; barbiturates; compounds such as chloral hydrate, paraldehyde, and meprobamate, which are structurally related to alcohol; sedative antihistamines; buspirone, and β-blockers. These are drugs that have been studied primarily in adults, with very few controlled studies of their use in the adolescent population. Coffey suggests that the established psychiatric indications for the use of benzodiazepines include night terrors and somnambulism. In adults, generalized anxiety disorder, panic disorder, anticipatory anxiety, situational anxiety, and alcohol withdrawal are also established indications for the use of benzodiazepines. In adolescents, overanxious disorder (see Chapters 102 and 103), the other anxiety disorders, anxiety states, and tic disorders all are possible indications. Various behavior disorders might be considered under the heading of conjectural usages. For the antihistamines, agitation is an established indication. Anxiety states are possible indications, and behavior disorders are conjectural indications. For the β-blockers, generalized anxiety disorder and situational and anticipatory anxiety are established indications in adults. Probable indications for the β-blockers would include lithium-induced tremor and performance anxiety in adults. Conjectural uses would include impulsivity and aggressive behavior associated with central nervous system damage, anxiety states, and symptoms of withdrawal from alcohol in the adult population (as an adjunct to benzodiazepines). Buspirone could be considered a probable indication for overanxious disorder and other anxiety disorders.

UNDESIRABLE EFFECTS

The undesirable effects have to be considered separately for the four major classes of antianxiety agents. For the benzodiazepines, the common effects include fatigue, drowsiness, and other symptoms of sedation. These are usually not serious. On a theoretical basis, memory impairments and impairment of psychomotor function could possibly lead to difficulty with school performance. However, this has not actually been demonstrated.

Clinically, there has been a suggestion that certain adolescents, particularly those who have evidence of central nervous system damage, who are emotionally labile, and who have problems with impulse control (see Chapter 108), may have symptoms of increased anxiety, excitement, hyperactivity, aggressive behavior, and rage outbursts. This is thought to be due to behavioral disinhibition. This has not been systematically studied, and apparently there are no predictors of this type of response. Benzodiazepines have potential for abuse, therefore adolescents who may already be having problems with substance abuse may be more at risk (see Chapter 111).

Blood abnormalities such as leukopenia, thrombocytopenia, and agranulocytosis rarely have been reported. Hallucinations and seizures have been described with withdrawal from various drugs; and since the benzodi-

azepines are drugs of potential abuse, physical and psychological dependence can occur. These effects are relatively rare and have not been systematically studied in adolescence. Withdrawal symptoms are more likely with rapid withdrawal. Therefore, the benzodiazepines, especially those that are short acting, should be tapered relatively slowly.

The undesirable effects of antihistamines seem to be relatively benign. Sedation is common. Anticholinergic side effects occur but are rarely of clinical significance. Coffey has suggested that seizures, delirium, psychosis, gastrointestinal upset, movement disorders, a "spaced out" feeling, and behavioral inhibition can occur, but that they are relatively rare. Among psychotropic drugs for adolescence, the undesirable effects of the antihistamines are probably less than those of other drugs.

Coffey suggests that the main adverse effects of the β-blockers can be grouped into five categories: central nervous system, respiratory, cardiovascular, metabolic, and sexual side effects. Those that are considered common are slowing of the heart rate, impotence and decreased libido, feelings of tiredness and weakness, and a Raynaud disease–like picture with tingling, numbness, and pain in the fingers. Bronchospasm may lead to asthma-like symptoms. (Use of these agents in individuals with asthma should be in conjunction with a physician experienced in treating asthma [see Chapter 43].) Mild to moderate dysphoria and depression may be a problem. Symptoms such as congestive heart failure occur primarily, if not exclusively, in individuals who already have heart disease. Hallucinations are extremely uncommon. Apparently the majority of these side effects may be more common with propranolol and less common with atenolol. Other effects such as hypoglycemia, diarrhea, nausea, dizzy spells, low blood pressure, and disruption of sleep are relatively uncommon.

The adverse effects of buspirone are less well known than the adverse effects of the drugs just mentioned, because it is relatively new. It apparently has only about one third of the sedation action of benzodiazepines, and Coffey suggests that adverse effects may include such symptoms as restlessness, lightheadedness, headaches, nausea, dizziness, central nervous system symptoms such as excitement and confusion, and mood changes such as anger and depression.

PRACTICAL ASPECTS OF MANAGEMENT

The reader is referred to Coffey's detailed review for dosage regimens for different drugs for different conditions. A large number of benzodiazepines vary in half-life, commercially available preparations, and cost. Special properties of β-blockers include their selectivity to β_1 receptor blockade, their route of elimination in either the kidney or the liver, half-lives ranging from 3 to 24 hours, and number of times they need to be given during the day.

In general, the antianxiety agents do not require much in the way of a special medical or laboratory workup. For those in whom β-blockers may be used, cardiovascular and respiratory symptoms and disorders, as well as a personal and a family history of mood disorders and diabetes, must be carefully inquired about. Vital signs need to be recorded initially and monitored carefully during the course of treatment. The need for a baseline ECG is unclear.

Most clinicians believe that all the antianxiety agents should be considered only for short-term use. Most are used in conjunction with other forms of therapeutic intervention. Thus, it should be relatively rare to have to repeat medical, neurologic, and laboratory monitoring over a long period of time in adolescents who are being treated with these antianxiety agents. The interested reader is referred to a review by Cantwell and Baker for more details.

Neuroleptics

The neuroleptics have been on the market since the introduction of chlorpromazine (Thorazine) in 1952. There are few primary care practitioners seeing adolescents who use neuroleptics on a regular basis. Most of the conditions for which neuroleptics are indicated in the adolescent age range are conditions that require management by a specialist.

Cantwell has suggested that the definite indications in this age range are schizophrenia (see Chapter 110), mania, and Tourette syndrome. As possible indications, Cantwell includes the pervasive developmental disorders, certain symptoms in the mentally retarded population, and ADHD.

Popper and Famularo include psychotic disorders, Tourette disorder, and symptoms of aggression, agitation, self-mutilation, and destructiveness, which are not manageable by nonpharmacologic means, as definite indications for the use of neuroleptics. As possible indications, they suggest ADHD, pervasive developmental disorder, and impulsive behavior that can occur with other disorders, such as mental retardation.

A recent comprehensive review by Teicher and Glod lists a large number of established indications in adults. They contend that these conditions can also be validly considered to be established indications in the adolescent age range, even though most if not all of them have not been systematically studied in adolescence. The primary indications are acute psychotic illnesses. These include the manic phase of bipolar illness (see Chapter 100), schizophrenia (see Chapter 110), schizophreniform disorder, and schizoaffective or drug-induced psychosis.

Although lithium is the treatment of choice for manic psychosis, the clinical effect of lithium may be delayed, and the use of neuroleptics may depress the excitement of the manic state until lithium begins to exert its effect. For children with pervasive developmental disorders, such as infantile autism and the autistic spectrum disorders, and in the retarded population, secondary symptoms are treated with neuroleptics. These secondary symptoms are varied and may include hyperactivity, aggressive behavior, and others. Clearly in the autistic population, as demonstrated primarily by Campbell and Spencer, neuroleptics are quite effective with many of the secondary symptoms and also may affect some of the social withdrawal, stereotypic behavior, and abnormal object relationships. However, their action in the autistic spectrum disorders and in mental retardation

generally is not "antipsychotic" in the true sense of the word.

Tourette syndrome is another major indication for neuroleptics such as haloperidol (Haldol) or pimozide. Psychotic depression generally requires the use of neuroleptics in addition to more standard antidepressant treatment. Other indications for use can be considered only probable or conjectural. In adults, borderline personality disorder is best treated psychopharmacologically with low dosages of high potency neuroleptics. Fewer data are available on the other personality disorders (see Chapter 109). Episodes of aggressive behavior and behavioral dyscontrol may be treated with neuroleptics in some cases. Some data suggest that children with ADHD who are treated with stimulants plus neuroleptics probably do just as well, if not slightly better, than those treated with stimulants alone. Moreover, data suggest very strongly that the supposed cognitive dulling effects of the neuroleptics in the ADHD individual may be overstated. Finally, in severe anxiety, if other treatments have failed or are contraindicated, neuroleptics may also be indicated.

UNDESIRABLE EFFECTS

Many different therapeutic preparations of the neuroleptic drugs are available commercially. They vary in the class of drug that they represent, in their potency, and in their likelihood of producing the side effects of sedation, low blood pressure, anticholinergic effects, extrapyramidal symptoms, and seizures. These have been detailed systematically by Teicher and Glod.

Because numerous neuroleptics are available, it is difficult to generalize about undesirable effects. Common unwanted effects of the neuroleptics include weight gain; sedation; orthostatic hypotension; constipation; blurred vision; dry mouth; motor symptoms (which may be parkinsonian in nature, acute dystonic reactions, or akathisia); skin reactions, such as easy burning in the sun and rashes; agitation; and sexual side effects (difficulties in maintaining erection and ejaculation problems).

More serious side effects include involuntary movements of the tardive dyskinetic nature or the withdrawal dyskinetic nature. Retinopathy resembling retinitis pigmentosa can occur at high doses. (This reaction is limited mainly to the use of thioridazine.) Hepatic dysfunction, such as hepatitis and obstructive jaundice, has been reported. Leukopenia and possible lowering of the seizure threshold can occur, although these may not be as frequent as once thought. Some of the indications in adolescents, however, for the use of neuroleptics may be associated with unsuspected EEG abnormalities and undiagnosed seizure behaviors. A lupus-like disorder, worsening of disorders such as glaucoma and cystic fibrosis, and the appearance of gynecomastia, galactorrhea, and amenorrhea may also occur.

A serious effect is the neuroleptic malignant syndrome, manifested by severe parkinsonian-like rigidity or catatonia and altered mental status, hyperpyrexia, and autonomic dysfunction (irregular pulse and blood pressure, rapid heart rate, and cardiac arrhythmias). This may occur early in treatment or after a relatively long period of the patient's receiving a stable dose. Neuroleptic malignant syndrome is of rapid onset and continues for approximately a week after discontinuation of neuroleptic treatment. The number of reports in the adolescent population is relatively small compared with the number of reports in adults. Either this particular negative effect is rarer in the adolescent age range or it is milder in nature and escapes diagnosis.

Pimozide produces ECG changes in a substantial number of individuals treated for Tourette syndrome. Cardiac function should be monitored carefully in those taking pimozide; although other preparations may lead to cardiovascular abnormalities, they are relatively rarer. Both Haldol and pimozide have been reported to cause anxiety symptoms and dysphoria in patients treated for Tourette disorder. The symptoms usually disappear when the drugs are discontinued.

PRACTICAL ASPECTS OF MANAGEMENT

Since the indications for the use of various neuroleptics are broad, no general statements can be made about dosage and management that would apply to all drugs for all conditions. More detailed references are available for the interested reader. In addition to the routine evaluation done for all adolescents who are taking a psychotropic agent, it is important for the clinician to systematically monitor dyskinetic effects prior to the institution of neuroleptics and to follow them over time. Standardized rating scales are available for this purpose, such as the abnormal involuntary movement scale (AIMS) and the Simpson scale. For those who are taking medication on a continual basis, monitoring of weight, blood pressure, pulse, and extrapyramidal and dyskinetic movements and doing routine blood examinations including liver enzyme testing once a year are indicated. Certain medications, such as clozapine, require a very specific type of monitoring. It is unlikely that many primary care practitioners of adolescent medicine treat individuals with chronic neuroleptic drugs; however, knowledge of its side effects is important.

Clonidine

Clonidine is a drug that has only recently been used for psychotropic purposes in the adolescent population. Although Hunt and colleagues suggest that the only established indication for the use of clonidine is hypertension, possible uses include Tourette syndrome, the manic phase of bipolar disorder in adults, ADD (particularly in those with hyperactivity, overarousal, and associated symptoms of oppositional and conduct disorder), and withdrawal from nicotine and opiates. They list the following conditions as conjectural usages: ADHD in adults, bipolar disorder in children and adolescents, psychosis in adults, significant aggressive behavior in adults who are agitated or psychotic, borderline personality disorder, panic disorder, social phobia, and anxiety and hyperarousal in post-traumatic stress disorder.

In their placebo-controlled study of clonidine in children and adolescents with Tourette syndrome, Leckman and colleagues demonstrated a statistically significant improvement at the end of 12 weeks in those patients assigned to clonidine versus placebo. (They administered 3 to 5 μg/kg/day of clonidine.) The patients receiving clonidine improved an average of slightly more than 25%, as compared with the placebo response of 11%. Motor tics improved in the clonidine group at an average rate of about 35%. Clonidine was effective in improving both Tourette syndrome and behavior problems. Impulsivity, hyperactivity, conduct problems, and learning problems improved. Clonidine is at this time probably a second choice drug for the treatment of Tourette syndrome. (Haldol remains the treatment of choice.) Further research is necessary to determine whether there are particular subgroups of patients with Tourette syndrome for whom clonidine would be most effective.

Clonidine is useful for the treatment of ADHD in both children and adolescents. Most likely, its major use will be in children with ADHD who also have tics or Tourette syndrome or who could be characterized as being extremely overactive or hyperaroused. It is possible that those children with ADHD who have comorbid diagnoses of oppositional and conduct disorder may also be those in whom clonidine may be most effective. On the other hand, clonidine may have less of an effect on the attentional process and other cognitive mechanisms in children, adolescents, and adults with ADHD than the psychostimulants do.

Although clonidine may be useful in adults with psychotic disorder, bipolar disorder, panic, posttraumatic stress, social phobic disorders, and aggressive behavior, more research is needed. Unfortunately, there are essentially no data in the adolescent population of any of these conditions.

UNDESIRABLE EFFECTS

Clonidine is relatively short-acting, with notable effects lasting 3 to 6 hours. Administration four times a day may be required. Clonidine is available in a transdermal patch, and this may prove useful. Sedation is the most common side effect. Other symptoms include gastrointestinal disturbance, headaches, dizzy spells, and hypotension. Depression may occur in as many as 5% of pediatric and adolescent patients. Other potentially more serious symptoms include rebound hypertension, skin irritation with the transdermal preparation, and cardiac arrhythmia.

PRACTICAL ASPECTS OF MANAGEMENT

As with all psychotropic agents, a baseline physical and neurologic examination; a medical, neurologic, and developmental history; and blood pressure and pulse measurements are routinely obtained. Some authors suggest including a complete blood count with differential and measurement of electrolytes, thyroid function, fasting blood sugar, and liver enzyme, as well as an ECG. Besides monitoring the psychotropic effects of the drug over time, blood pressure, pulse, and body weight should be monitored carefully.

Hunt and colleagues detail a dosage regimen for oral

clonidine over a 12-day period, followed by use of a transdermal patch. Although there appear to be selected clinical symptoms in certain populations that may be amenable to treatment with clonidine, more research is needed before any definitive statements can be made about clonidine's long-term efficacy and safety.

Anticonvulsants

Some anticonvulsants may be useful as psychotropic medications. Carbamazepine and valproic acid are the most notable.

Adolescent patients with epilepsy and other forms of seizure disorders have elevated rates of psychopathology. Interictal periods in children and adolescents with epilepsy and seizure disorders often are characterized by alterations in behavior, mood, and cognitive functioning, and some believe that control of the seizure disorder may lead to control of these associated problems.

Carbamazepine and valproic acid have demonstrated antimanic properties in adults. Whether this is also true in adolescents and children has not been established, but anecdotal literature suggests so. Evidence for its use in major depressive disorder, ADD, conduct disorder, and anxiety disorders is largely anecdotal.

UNDESIRABLE EFFECTS

The side effects of anticonvulsants are generally well known by practicing physicians and vary with the specific agent (see the review by Trimble). Ethosuximide and phenobarbital, which are not used primarily for purely psychiatric indications, can cause psychiatric symptoms (psychosis in the case of ethosuximide, and mood disorders with suicidal behavior in the case of phenobarbital).

A practical aspect of the use of anticonvulsants is a relatively straightforward medical workup that is similar for all anticonvulsants and includes CBC with differential and liver and renal function tests. Monitoring serum anticonvulsant levels is often useful and is usually indicated.

In general, the physician sees two rather different types of patients: those who have active seizure disorders and associated psychiatric symptomatology and those who do not have active seizure disorders but who have psychiatric symptomatology for which the anticonvulsants are being prescribed. In the former case, a primary physician or a neurologist is the primary manager of the neurologic condition, and a psychiatrist may be the primary manager of the nonneurologic aspects. Optimal seizure control is of greatest importance in the first group of patients, with attention also paid to the asso-

ciated psychiatric symptomatology. In the latter cases, in which there is no active seizure disorder, there is little information to guide the practitioner in the use of anticonvulsants for purely psychiatric reasons. This is best left to experienced psychiatrists. Recent literature may be helpful.

BIBLIOGRAPHY

Aman MG, Kern R: Review of fenfluramine in the treatment of the developmental disabilities. J Am Acad Child Adolesc Psychiatry 28(4):549, 1989.
Biederman J: Psychopharmacology in children and adolescents. In Wiener J (ed): Textbook of Child and Adolescent Psychiatry. Washington, DC, American Psychiatric Press, 1991.
Campbell M, Spencer EK: Psychopharmacology in child and adolescent psychiatry: A review of the past five years. J Am Acad Child Adolesc Psychiatry 27(3):269, 1988.
Campbell M, Perry R, Green WH: Use of lithium in children and adolescents. Psychosomatics 25(2):95, 1984.
Cantwell DP: The Hyperactive Child: Diagnosis, Management, and Current Research. New York, Spectrum Publications, 1975.
Cantwell DP: Pediatric psychopharmacology: Parts I & II. In Flach FF (ed): Directions in Psychiatry, Vol 3, Lessons 31, 32. New York, Hatherleigh, 1983, pp 1–6.
Cantwell DP, Baker L: Anxiety disorders in adolescents. In Hsu LKG, Hersen M (eds): Recent Developments in Adolescent Psychiatry. New York, John Wiley & Sons, 1988, pp 161–199.
Coffey BJ: Child psychiatry problems. In Tupin JP, Shader RI, Harnett DS (eds): Handbook of Clinical Psychopharmacology. Northvale, NJ, Aronson Press, 1984, pp 211–244.
Coffey BJ: Anxiolytics for children and adolescents: Traditional and new drugs. J Child Adolesc Psychopharmacol 1(1):57, 1990.
Dulcan MK: Using psychostimulants to treat behavioral disorder of children and adolescents. J Child Adolesc Psychopharmacol 1(1):7, 1990.
Hunt RD, Capper L, O'Connell P: Clonidine in child and adolescent psychiatry. J Child Adolesc Psychopharmacol 1(1):87, 1990.
Klein DF, Gittelman R, Quitkin F, Rifkin A: Diagnosis and Drug Treatment of Psychiatric Disorders: Adults and Children, 2nd ed. Baltimore, Williams & Wilkins, 1980.
Leckman J, Hardin M, Riddle M, et al: Clonidine treatment of Gilles de Tourette's disorder. Arch Gen Psychiatry 48:324, 1991.
Popper CW: Child and adolescent psychopharmacology. In Michels R, Cavenar JO, Brodie HK, et al (eds): Psychiatry, Vol 2. Philadelphia, JB Lippincott, 1985, pp 1–23.
Popper CW, Famularo R: Child and adolescent psychopharmacology. In Levine MD, Carey WB, Crocker AC, Gross RT (eds): Developmental-Behavioral Pediatrics. Philadelphia, WB Saunders, 1983, pp 1138–1159.
Popper CW, Frazier SH (eds): J Child Adolesc Psychopharmacol 1(1–3), 1990.
Rapoport J, Conners CK, Reatig N (eds): Psychopharmacol Bull 21(4), 1985.
Ryan ND: Heterocyclic antidepressants in children and adolescents. J Child Adol Psychopharmacol 1(1):21, 1990.
Teicher MH, Glod CA: Neuroleptic drugs: Indications and guidelines for their rational use in children and adolescents. J Child Adolesc Psychopharmacol 1(1):33, 1990.
Trimble MR: Anticonvulsants in children and adolescents. J Child Adolesc Psychopharmacol 1(1):107, 1990.
Weinberg WA: Learning disabilities, affective illness, and disorders of vigilance in relationship to management of epilepsy in children and adolescents. Int Pediatr 2:194, 1987.

CHAPTER 126

Pearls from Clinical Practice

CHRISTOPHER H. HODGMAN

What is a "pearl"? At its most definitive, a counterintuitive, difficult-to-prove, generally nonquantitative finding, often originating in an error made but not forgotten, a "pearl" not infrequently emerges from a series of unrewarding confrontations with a given medical phenomenon.

In retrospect, "pearls" often appear self-evident. But they are rare precisely because they have been consistently overlooked. Today's "pearl" may be commonplace tomorrow if it embodies a sufficiently broad concept.

As in nature, medical pearls can be cultivated; this makes continued practice rewarding, because new findings are available the longer a problem is studied.

PSYCHOSOCIAL CARE

There is much resistance to psychosocial care: it may be seen as "soft," a compromise, or an adverse value judgment. Caregivers often hesitate to include psychiatric possibilities in the initial evaluation because these might seem dismissive. The likelihood of psychiatric hypotheses rises with unsuccessful management, with an unpleasant personality in the adolescent or family, and with frustration or irritation on the part of the caregiver. But guilt over such responses may lead to a steadfast refusal even to consider psychosocial causes or problems.

Given such values in modern "scientific" medicine, even the "expert" feels a need to find esoteric biologic explanations for unusual findings. Indeed, the seasoned specialist is often expected to do so; most experienced clinicians recall instances when their own "expertise" resulted in misleading diagnostic or therapeutic excess. At the same time, such clinicians often realize that psychosocial care is more "scientific" than exclusionary biologic management; as a result, a significant proportion of "pearls" involve psychosocial care.

Demonstrating that symptoms have a psychological rather than a biologic basis fails to impress most adolescents for whom illness has resulted in psychological gain. The results of laboratory tests may convince everyone except the adolescent that symptoms are psychological in origin. Indeed, the more dramatic and impressive the test—even if negative—the more likely that a symptom will be confirmed for the patient, precisely because such a procedure was "required." Ordering tests does not "satisfy" the patient but, paradoxically, increases anxiety, concern, and secondary gain.

In rarer instances, a preoccupation with biologic measures can be dangerous: adolescents prone to factitial or self-damaging behaviors because of the gratifications of resulting medical care learn to use positive laboratory findings to that end. Too often, an esoteric mechanism is educed to explain laboratory findings of behavioral origin (e.g., borderline endocrine abnormalities in anorexia nervosa) or factitial manufacture (e.g., "hematuria" from self-injury, "hypoglycemia" from exogenous insulin, "fever of unknown origin" from a misused thermometer). In many instances, it is precisely the apparent interest of a finding that misleads.

A major feature of psychosocial care is a developmental approach. Thus, awareness of Piagetian concepts of formal operational thinking can protect a clinician from assuming that a bright 12-year-old who has diabetes mellitus can understand the principles of dietary exchanges—or, conversely, that pregnancy in a 14-year-old is necessarily the result of accident or ignorance.

Finally, a psychosocial approach encourages the clinician to ask questions about behavioral matters. It has been found that a majority of emotional complaints are not brought to the attention of office primary care physicians because mothers perceive the physicians to lack interest, expertise, or commitment to emotional care. (Too often, parents are told that their adolescent will "grow out of" behavioral problems, although studies have demonstrated the contrary.) In particular, clinicians generally do not ask about disconcerting matters such as depression or suicide, even though asking routinely about these problems informs the adolescent of the physician's readiness to address them if they ever arise (see also Chapter 24).

EPIDEMIOLOGY

Single-cause thinking is the enemy of mature care. Too often, a diagnostician stops thinking after a specific entity has been uncovered. In particular, the co-occurrence of "physical" and "mental" conditions is too rarely considered.

A prime example of this is depression in physical illnesses (see Chapters 30 and 121). The two diagnoses are seldom diagnosed concurrently: preoccupation with one tends to dismiss the other. Studies show that more physical problems than normal are common in depressed patients, and the converse; but actual practice tends not to reflect these findings.

A similar phenomenon occurs in substance abuse (see Chapter 111). Alcohol and many drugs are self-medication for depression on the one hand and cause depression on the other. Unfortunately, this truth is commonly overlooked in treatment programs; if the underlying depression or the complicating substance abuse are missed, successful care is jeopardized.

Another bane of single-cause diagnosis is found among conversion disorders (see Chapter 112), which can occur in concert with physical illness (pseudoseizures in the adolescent who has epilepsy) or with other psychiatric diagnoses (conversion paralyses in adolescents who have psychoses). In some instances, one of the adolescent patient's illnesses may serve as a model for the other, so disentangling the two is necessary for successful management.

CLINICAL MANIFESTATIONS

Each anatomic system provides important clinical lessons. Space permits only selective examples, but the principles involved apply to many other systems:

Skin. Skin conditions often mirror other pathology (see Chapter 39). Although an adolescent's medical or psychiatric pathology may be far more serious, treating acne or a rash successfully may be the essential prerequisite for compliance with other care. Clinicians in every specialty who treat adolescents should know about common adolescent skin problems and their treatment.

Atopic dermatitis may be dramatically improved by eliminating hot showers and excessive dedication to cleanliness.

Psoriasis is often artfully concealed by the adolescent patient. Its successful treatment has wide emotional implications.

Sensory Organs. Deafness and visual problems (see Chapter 40) often accompany academic (see Chapter 107) and behavioral problems. They are frequently denied because of embarrassment or because of gradual, imperceptible onset. Subtle perceptual handicaps are also often overlooked, particularly in youths whose intelligence permits at least average performance (when superior work could otherwise be anticipated).

Respiratory System. Hyperventilation, although not strictly a respiratory condition, may be so perceived by the adolescent and the family. An explanation of the symptoms of hypocapnia can make the condition more respectable, encouraging treatment.

Asthma must be distinguished from inspiratory stridor, in itself a condition that can induce anxiety (see Chapters 43, 102, and 103). In serious, repeated asthmatic episodes, poor compliance with medications should be pursued (see Chapter 26). It is remarkable how often this possibility is not actively considered, perhaps because the gravity of the event can distract the clinician from its cause. In potentially lethal asthmatic episodes, there may be a possibility of parasympathetic overresponse due, for example, to depression.

Circulatory System. In repeated episodes of cardiac failure, the possibility of excessive salt intake should be considered. Youthful cardiac patients and those who have a variety of other serious conditions may engage in a kind of "medical Russian roulette" to prove that they do not need to follow doctors' orders, to express anger or depression, or to manipulate their environment. The resulting consequences necessitate vigorous medical response, inadvertently rewarding their destructive origins.

Hematologic System. Hemophilia and other bleeding disorders often evoke poor compliance or physically self-harmful behaviors from mechanisms of denial similar to those mentioned above.

In blood dyscrasias and other oncologic conditions, the possibility of depression should be reviewed as a factor complicating response and compliance. At the same time, because most such conditions do not evoke depression, it is important to consider active treatment when depression does occur, rather than assuming that it is an inevitable consequence of serious, life-threatening illness (see Chapters 30 and 121).

Endocrine System. Failure to grow normally after infancy can be due to psychogenically induced inhibition of growth hormone secretion. A significant change in environment can be salutary.

Thyroid dysfunction and psychological function are closely related. Emotional trauma has triggered episodes of hyperthyroidism and even thyroid storm; similarly, hyper- and hypothyroidism or their treatments can trigger mental, particularly affective, illness (e.g., mania in response to thyroid replacement therapy for hypothyroidism).

Adrenal cortical and psychological functions are similarly related. Not only are hyper- and hypoadrenalism associated with adverse mental states, but corticosteroid therapy can inadvertently lead to mood disorder and even psychotic (usually manic) states.

Diabetes mellitus management is particularly related to age and psychological maturity (see Chapter 59). As noted previously, a younger patient may be unable to manage the abstract thinking necessary for good diabetic care; an inability to follow directions that appear obvious to the clinician may be maturational rather than deliberately obstructive. An adolescent patient may be able to repeat and seem to understand diabetic instructions without actually doing so; it is best to observe actual, uncoached performance.

Diabetic complications that are of emotional origin include surreptitious administration of insulin in hypoglycemic episodes, deliberate hypoinsulinism to induce weight loss, and use of denatured insulin or a substitute for insulin in repeated episodes of ketoacidosis. It is likely that such factitial complications will be repeated in stereotyped fashion to produce the desired outcome again; too often, the gravity of each episode distracts the clinician from the common, self-induced denominator.

Gastrointestinal System. Anorexia nervosa (see Chapter 60) and regional ileitis (see Chapter 63) are significantly coincident. Treatment of one may improve the other.

In bulimia, shame over the symptomatology is so intense as to constitute a diagnostic feature in itself. If evidence of dental enamel scouring or "chipmunk cheeks" (parotid gland irritation and swelling) are noted, frequent emesis should be considered. With regular, heavy use of phenolphthalein-containing laxatives, attempts to stop may result in distressing, objectively evident edema, thus reinforcing continued use.

Constipation is sometimes the first symptom of depression.

Genitourinary System. Genitourinary disorders are particularly prone to instrumentation and development of polysurgical addiction. Self-induced findings and stereotyped symptoms lead to multiple diagnostic instrumentations, which in turn become an end in themselves for the patient.

Enuresis is frequently a family matter. If the parent had similar problems at the same age, parental investment in the enuresis should be considered; a guarded prognosis is held until the adolescent reaches the age at which the parent's enuresis ceased.

Reproductive System. Many adolescents have an unclear picture of their reproductive anatomy or physiology (see Chapter 68). Girls are likely to think of the midcycle as "safe." Boys have an even less clear concept of internal anatomy than girls.

Contraception involves a reasonable knowledge of physiology; it often fails because the possibility of pregnancy is not believed to be possible, because of impulsivity, or because of a wish to become pregnant (more common than many clinicians believe).

DIAGNOSIS

Diagnostic features in various organ systems are mentioned above. A few additional comments about the diagnostic process itself may be appropriate.

In many instances, the chief barrier to successful diagnosis is the unwillingness of the diagnostician to consider unattractive possibilities. For example, anger at the adolescent patient for violating an implicit contract may delay the diagnosis of failure of compliance (see Chapter 26). Whenever possible, routine use of laboratory determinations should be incorporated in management to reveal failure to comply. Examples in conditions already cited include theophylline levels in asthmatic maintenance, glycosylated protein determinations in diabetic maintenance, or urine specific gravity to detect weight gain from excessive intake of water. Other examples are seizure medication levels, antidepressant levels (to forestall accumulation of potentially lethal dosages), and lithium levels in questionably compliant bipolar patients.

Poor compliance can sometimes be determined by direct question. In many instances, assertive denial will be followed by the tacit confirmation of improved compliance.

Laboratory tests can be diagnostically misleading. A penchant for testing may reveal relatively trivial abnormalities in thyroid determinations in severe anorexia nervosa (see Chapter 60) for example, which may lead to fruitless searches for endocrine disease when direct questioning would have revealed the proper diagnosis.

Insistence on the "whole syndrome," as in anorexia nervosa or depression, for example, deprives many adolescents of timely interventions (before the "whole syndrome" has become established).

An adolescent patient's or parent's "hunches" are too often discarded as "unscientific," when they contain important kernels of diagnostic truth.

The clinician must avoid the "nominative fallacy": that an unpleasant diagnosis will cause the outcome presumed by the diagnosis. For example, psychotic youths are diagnosed as having "adjustment reactions," as if to label them schizophrenic would assure that destiny. Poor treatment decisions are likely to ensue (see Chapter 110).

TREATMENT

Some examples exemplify worthwhile therapeutic approaches to common problems.

In patients with conversion symptoms, it is often better to "accept" the ostensible pathologic complaint rather than to attempt to show the adolescent that it is nonphysiologic. The patient can be told that "stress" or "tension" are involved, while face-saving physiotherapy is applied to the "paralyzed" limb. Attention to underlying dependent, regressive needs can be given simultaneously. It is unusual for symptom substitution (replacement of original complaint by a new problem) to occur if such needs are addressed.

In adolescents who have anorexia nervosa, tests of the clinician's resolve are frequent. Because many anorectics have features of the borderline personality (see Chapter 109), splitting (the setting of one member of the team against another) is to be expected. Even in obsessively honest patients, delusional or wish-fulfilling misperceptions render accounts of calorie intake unreliable. Control is generally the issue for such adolescent patients; whatever the therapist's philosophy of treatment, it is likely to be more successful if offered with both self-assurance and flexibility, assuring the adolescent that success will be the outcome.

Psychotropic medications often incorporate a significant placebo effect. Antidepressants, for example, are often only modestly better than placebo—both being reasonably successful not only for depression, but for anxiety attacks, phobias, and school refusal, as well as for some pain syndromes. Dosages generally must reach antidepressant levels. Side effects are generally necessary if dosage is sufficient; they can add to the nonspecific "placebo" effect if properly introduced to the patient.

Minor tranquilizers should seldom be used with adolescents, because of their tendency to disinhibit young patients (often worsening the behaviors they are intended to treat), their cross-reactions with alcohol, and their street value (see Chapter 125).

Major tranquilizers such as the phenothiazines or butyrophenones have the advantage of nonaddictiveness as well as some sedation. They can be particularly useful in the immobilized, post-surgical or orthopedic patient.

Psychotropic medication must be used in sufficient amount, by clinicians acquainted with the side effect profiles, with support, and with sufficient teaching so that the patient knows what to anticipate.

Practical psychotherapy is very much part of most pediatric treatment. Thus it has been established that support alone can be quite effective in depression; that hypochondriasis can be treated successfully by patience, a willingness to see the patient frequently, and readiness to discuss matters other than symptomatology; and that factitial illness often responds to supportive confrontation. In each of these instances, the readiness of the clinician to be available and supportive is essential.

Referrals for psychiatric consultation and treatment are most likely to succeed if the referring clinician arranges for a follow-up appointment after the first visit with the consultant, as well as telephone contacts thereafter. Such arrangements prevent the patient from feeling rejected or that the referral constitutes a value judgment (see Chapter 24).

APPENDICES

Reference Data for Physical Assessment of Adolescents

RICHARD R. BROOKMAN

There is a vast amount of reference data pertinent to the physical assessment of adolescents. Unfortunately, there has been no uniform approach to collecting or reporting these data. Some data are listed according to age or age groupings, such as data collected in the National Center for Health Statistics' Health Examination Surveys. Some age listings make it impossible to isolate data related to the adolescent developmental period. For example, some data are reported for the age groups 5 to 14 years and 15 to 24 years. Occasionally in the 1960s and increasingly since the 1970s, data related to growth or physiologic function have been reported by stage of pubertal maturation or sexual maturity rating (SMR).

These appendices include selected mean values and ranges or percentiles for many parameters of growth, physical fitness, and nutrition. Wherever possible, data are correlated with chronologic and/or skeletal age, sexual maturity rating, sex, and race.

Readers are also referred to Vaughan VC, Litt IF: Child and Adolescent Development: Clinical Implications. Philadelphia, WB Saunders, 1990.

Physical Growth

TABLE A–1. Height Standards by Age and Sex, American Youth

	MALE						FEMALE					
	Centimeters (Percentile)			Inches (Percentile)			Centimeters (Percentile)			Inches (Percentile)		
AGE	5th	50th	95th	5th	50th	95th	5th	50th	95th	5th	50th	95th
8	118	127	136	46	50	54	117	126	136	46	50	54
8½	121	130	139	48	51	55	120	129	140	47	51	55
9	123	132	142	49	52	56	122	132	143	48	52	56
9½	125	135	145	49	53	57	125	135	146	49	53	58
10	128	138	148	50	54	58	128	138	150	50	55	59
10½	130	140	152	51	55	60	130	142	153	51	56	60
11	133	143	155	52	57	61	134	145	156	53	57	62
11½	135	146	159	53	58	63	137	148	160	54	58	63
12	138	150	162	54	59	64	140	152	163	55	60	64
12½	140	153	166	55	60	66	143	155	166	56	61	65
13	143	157	170	56	62	67	145	157	168	57	62	66
13½	146	160	173	57	63	68	147	159	170	58	63	67
14	149	163	177	59	64	70	149	160	171	59	63	68
14½	152	166	180	60	66	71	150	161	172	59	64	68
15	155	169	182	61	67	72	151	162	173	59	64	68
15½	158	172	184	62	68	73	151	162	173	60	64	68
16	161	174	185	64	68	73	152	162	173	60	64	68
16½	163	175	187	64	69	74	152	163	174	60	64	68
17	165	176	187	65	69	74	153	163	174	60	64	68
17½	166	177	188	65	70	74	153	163	174	60	64	68
18	166	177	188	65	70	74	154	164	174	61	65	68

Data from National Center for Health Statistics: Growth curves for children birth–18 years, United States. Vital Health Stat [11] 165:20–63, 1977.

TABLE A–2. Weight Standards by Age and Sex, American Youth

	MALE						FEMALE					
	Kilograms (Percentile)			Pounds (Percentile)			Kilograms (Percentile)			Pounds (Percentile)		
AGE	5th	50th	95th	5th	50th	95th	5th	50th	95th	5th	50th	95th
8	20	25	35	45	56	76	20	25	35	43	55	77
8½	21	27	37	47	59	82	21	27	38	46	59	83
9	22	28	40	49	62	87	22	29	41	48	63	90
9½	23	30	42	51	66	93	23	31	44	51	67	97
10	24	31	45	54	69	100	24	33	47	54	72	104
10½	26	33	48	56	74	107	26	35	51	57	77	112
11	27	35	52	59	78	114	27	37	54	60	82	119
11½	28	38	55	62	83	121	29	39	57	64	87	127
12	30	40	58	66	88	128	31	42	61	67	92	134
12½	32	42	62	70	93	136	32	44	64	71	97	141
13	34	45	65	74	99	143	34	46	67	75	102	148
13½	36	48	69	79	106	151	36	48	70	79	107	155
14	38	51	72	84	112	159	38	50	73	83	111	161
14½	41	54	76	90	119	167	40	52	76	87	115	167
15	43	57	79	95	125	175	41	54	78	90	118	172
15½	46	60	83	100	131	182	42	55	80	93	121	176
16	48	62	86	105	137	189	43	56	81	96	123	179
16½	50	64	87	110	142	195	44	56	82	98	125	181
17	52	66	91	114	146	201	45	57	83	99	125	182
17½	53	68	94	116	150	207	45	57	83	100	125	182
18	54	69	96	119	152	211	45	57	83	100	125	182

Data from National Center for Health Statistics: Growth curves for children birth–18 years, United States. Vital Health Stat [11] 165:20–63, 1977.

TABLE A–3. Median Ages (years) of Fusion of Selected Epiphyses

	MALE	FEMALE
Humerus		
Trochlea	15.2	12.3
Capitellum	15.2	12.4
Lateral epicondyle	15.3	12.6
Medial epicondyle	16.3	14.1
Proximal end	18.2	15.6
Proximal radius	16.2	13.5
Distal radius	18.0	15.8
Proximal ulna	15.3	12.6
Distal ulna	17.8	15.9
Metacarpals	16.4	14.6
Phalanges	15.9–16.4	13.6–14.4
Femur		
Greater trochanter	15.9	13.9
Proximal	16.2	14.2
Distal	16.6	14.7
Distal tibia	16.8	14.8
Proximal tibia	16.9	14.8
Distal fibula	16.8	14.8
Proximal fibula	17.2	15.2

Adapted from Roche AF: Some aspects of adolescent growth and maturation. In McKigney JI, Munro HN (eds): Nutrient Requirements in Adolescence. Cambridge, MA, MIT Press, 1976, p 38.

TABLE A–4. Linear Growth Velocity (cm/year) During Puberty

MALE						FEMALE		
Percentile			Approximate Age	Year Relative to PHV	Approximate Age	Percentile		
3rd	50th	97th				3rd	50th	97th
3.6	5.0	6.2	11	−3	9	4.0	5.4	6.9
3.4	4.9	6.4	12	−2	10	3.8	5.4	7.0
4.4	6.4	8.0	13	−1	11	4.6	6.6	8.4
7.2	9.4	11.8	14	PHV	12	6.2	8.3	10.4
3.6	5.8	8.0	15	+1	13	3.4	5.2	7.4
1.0	2.6	4.4	16	+2	14	0.6	2.2	4.0
0.0	1.0	2.0	17	+3	15	0.0	0.7	1.7

PHV, peak height velocity.
Adapted from Barnes HV: Physical growth and development during puberty. Med Clin North Am 59:1305, 1975.

TABLE A–5. Velocity of Weight Gain (kg/year) During Puberty

MALE						FEMALE		
Percentile			Approximate Age	Year Relative to PWV	Approximate Age	Percentile		
3rd	50th	97th				3rd	50th	97th
1.4	3.1	6.2	11	−3	9.5	1.3	3.0	5.8
1.6	4.0	6.8	12	−2	10.5	1.8	3.5	6.4
2.8	5.4	8.6	13	−1	11.5	3.0	5.6	8.6
6.1	9.0	12.8	14	PWV	12.5	5.5	8.3	10.6
3.3	5.7	9.0	15	+1	13.5	0.8	5.3	7.6
0.4	2.6	4.8	16	+2	14.5	0.1	2.2	5.0
0.0	1.0	2.3	17	+3	15.5	0.0	1.0	3.4

PWV, peak weight velocity.
Adapted from Barnes HV: Physical growth and development during puberty. Med Clin North Am 59:1305, 1975.

TABLE A–6. Percentage of Body Fat by Age and Sex

AGE	MALE (Percentile)			FEMALE (Percentile)		
	10th	50th	90th	10th	50th	90th
9	12	17	23	10	15	24
10	12	18	23	10	16	24
11	10	17	22	12	19	26
12	9	15	21	13	20	26
13	7	13	20	16	22	28
14	6	11	18	18	23	29
15	7	11	18	18	23	29
16	6	12	18	20	24	29

From Widdowson EM: Changes in body composition during growth. In Davis JA, Dobbing J (eds): Scientific Foundations of Paediatrics, 2nd ed. London, William Heinemann, 1981.

TABLE A–7. Triceps Skinfold Measurements (mm) by Age, Sex, and Race*

AGE	WHITE MALES (Percentile)			BLACK MALES (Percentile)			WHITE FEMALES (Percentile)			BLACK FEMALES (Percentile)		
	5th	50th	95th	5th	50th	95th	5th	50th	95th	5th	50th	95th
12	5.2	9.7	23.2	3.8	7.4	23.2	6.1	12.0	25.1	6.0	10.6	25.6
13	4.8	9.4	22.6	3.6	7.2	25.2	6.6	12.7	25.4	6.0	9.8	27.2
14	4.3	8.2	21.2	3.6	6.4	19.2	7.3	14.2	26.8	5.5	12.5	24.6
15	4.3	7.8	21.3	3.9	6.4	14.7	7.5	15.1	29.9	7.2	12.8	25.8
16	4.2	7.6	20.5	4.0	6.7	12.8	8.1	16.0	29.1	7.0	13.1	31.5
17	4.1	7.7	20.7	4.2	6.1	15.8	8.5	16.3	29.5	7.1	13.4	25.8

*See also Chapter 6.
Data from National Center for Health Statistics: Skinfold thickness of youths 12–17 years, United States. Vital Health Stat [11] 132:23, 1974.

TABLE A–8. Percentile Values of Body Mass Index, NHANES I*

AGE (Year)	MALE (Percentile)			FEMALE (Percentile)		
	5th	50th	95th	5th	50th	95th
10	14.2	16.6	22.2	14.3	17.1	24.2
11	14.6	17.2	23.5	14.6	17.8	25.7
12	15.1	17.8	24.8	15.0	18.3	26.8
13	15.6	18.4	25.8	15.4	18.9	27.9
14	16.1	19.1	26.8	15.7	19.4	28.6
15	16.6	19.7	27.7	16.1	19.9	29.4
16	17.2	20.5	28.4	16.4	20.2	30.0
17	17.7	21.2	29.0	16.9	20.7	30.5
18	18.3	21.9	29.7	17.2	21.1	31.0
19	19.0	22.5	30.1	17.5	21.4	31.3

$$\text{Body mass index (BMI)} = \frac{\text{Wt (kg)}}{\text{Ht}^2 \text{ (m)}}$$

*NHANES I indicates National Health and Nutrition Examination Survey, 1971 to 1974.
Adapted from Hammer LD, Kraemer HC, Wilson DC, et al: Standardized percentile curves of body-mass index for children and adolescents. Am J Dis Child 145:260, 1991.

For additional data regarding adolescents, refer to the following:

Frisancho AR: Anthropometric Standards for the Assessment of Growth and Nutritional Status. Ann Arbor, MI, University of Michigan Press, 1990. (Includes growth data by race for white and black subjects ages 1–75 years.)
Ryan AS, Martinez GA, Baumgartner RN, et al: Median skinfold thickness distributions and fat-wave patterns in Mexican-American children from the Hispanic Health and Nutrition Examination Survey (HHANES 1982–1984). Am J Clin Nutr 51:925S, 1990. (Includes data by age for white, black, and Mexican-American youth ages 1–19 years.)
Roche AF, Guo S, Baumgartner RH, et al: Reference data for weight, stature, and weight/stature in Mexican-Americans from the Hispanic Health and Nutrition Examination Survey (HHANES 1982–1984). Am J Clin Nutr 51:917S, 1990. (Includes data for youth ages 1–19 years.)

TABLE A–9. Biochemical Correlates of Growth by Sexual Maturity Rating and Age in Males
(range of serum concentrations)

	URATES* (μmol/L)	PHOSPHORUS* (mmol/L)	CREATININE* (mg/dl)	ALKALINE PHOSPHATASE* (IU/L)	ALKALINE PHOSPHATASE† (IU/L)	
					White	Black
SMR						
I	121–384	1.10–1.46	0.44–0.71	85–171	54–110	43–130
II	123–390	1.02–1.54	0.52–0.82	114–171	42–106	53–204
III	165–428	1.19–1.53	0.50–0.90	107–220	53–141	46–240
IV	224–429	1.03–1.49	0.43–1.01	71–220	41–158	32–228
V	218–454	0.95–1.27	0.50–1.01	35–185	21–120	23–228
Age (years)						
8	75–323	1.10–1.62		71–178		
9	189–322	1.05–1.70	0.42–0.78	78–213		
10	136–353	1.08–1.50		78–178	58–110	
11	134–408	1.12–1.45	0.41–0.76	85–206	55–105	
12	120–390	1.06–1.55	0.42–0.87	78–220	55–207	
13	142–427	1.04–1.62	0.45–0.91	85–227	49–240	
14	172–441	0.99–1.57	0.36–1.04	71–234	36–192	
15	199–458	0.96–1.47	0.47–1.01	50–171	41–195	
16	234–462	0.93–1.33	0.49–1.13	35–171	32–142	

*Data from Clayton BE, Jenkins P, Round JM: Paediatric Chemical Pathology. Clinical Tests and Reference Ranges. London, Blackwell, 1980.
†Data from Bennett DL, Ward MS, Daniel WA: The relationship of serum alkaline phosphatase concentrations to sex maturity ratings in adolescents. J Pediatr 88:633, 1976.

TABLE A–10. Biochemical Correlates of Growth by Sexual Maturity Rating and Age in Females
(range of serum concentrations)

	URATES* (μmol/L)	PHOSPHORUS* (mmol/L)	CREATININE* (mg/dl)	ALKALINE PHOSPHATASE* (IU/L)	ALKALINE PHOSPHATASE† (IU/L)	
					White	Black
SMR						
I	182–361	1.05–1.53	0.47–0.66	57–163	51–90	69–108
II	161–389	1.03–1.55	0.41–0.79	50–192	49–134	65–138
III	167–380	1.03–1.41	0.44–0.88	64–163	36–108	26–148
IV	166–397	0.92–1.36	0.50–0.86	43–107	16–60	18–144
V	163–376	0.90–1.30	0.54–0.86	28–92	23–76	13–70
Age (years)						
8	129–371	1.06–1.54		78–163	59–102	
9	187–357	1.06–1.43	0.41–0.67	78–185	49–136	
10	227–367	1.09–1.43		71–199	51–118	
11	188–402	1.01–1.52	0.38–0.81	71–192	72–147	
12	158–407	0.98–1.50	0.42–0.81	78–213	65–148	
13	150–384	0.91–1.49	0.45–0.85	50–206	25–144	
14	152–391	0.85–1.39	0.50–0.86	36–114	22–91	
15	178–387	0.88–1.35	0.51–0.87	21–128	17–91	
16	192–359	0.87–1.34	0.57–0.89	28–71	13–56	

*Data from Clayton BE, Jenkins P, Round JM: Paediatric Chemical Pathology. Clinical Tests and Reference Ranges. London, Blackwell, 1980.
†Data from Bennett DL, Ward MS, Daniel WA. The relationship of serum alkaline phosphatase concentrations to sex maturity ratings in adolescents. J Pediatr 88:633, 1976.

TABLE A–11. Calcification and Eruption of Deciduous and Permanent Teeth

	AGE (YEARS) AT SHEDDING OF DECIDUOUS TEETH		AGE (YEARS) AT COMPLETION OF CALCIFICATION	AGE (YEARS) AT ERUPTION OF PERMANENT TEETH	
	Maxillary	Mandibular		Maxillary	Mandibular
Central incisors	7–8	6–7	9–10	7–8	6–7
Lateral incisors	8–9	7–8	10–11	8–9	7–8
Cuspids (canines)	11–12	9–11	12–15	11–12	9–11
First premolars (bicuspids)			12–13	10–11	10–12
Second premolars (bicuspids)			12–14	10–12	11–13
First molars	10–11	10–12	9–10	6–7	6–7
Second molars	10–11	11–13	14–16	12–13	12–13
Third molars			18–25	17–22	17–22

AVERAGE NUMBER OF ERUPTED PERMANENT TEETH

Age (years)	White Males	Black Males	White Females	Black Females
9	13.8	14.3	14.8	17.0
10	16.5	19.0	17.2	20.1
11	20.4	23.7	22.8	24.9
12	24.6	24.9	25.8	25.6
13	26.7	27.3	27.1	27.9
14	27.8	27.8	27.9	28.3
15	28.0	28.0	27.8	28.2
16	28.0	28.7	28.3	29.1
17	28.7	29.6	28.6	29.3

Adapted from Behrman RE, Vaughan VC III (eds): Nelson Textbook of Pediatrics, 13th ed. Philadelphia, WB Saunders, 1987, p 30; and National Center for Health Statistics: Decayed, missing, and filled teeth among persons 1–74 years, United States. Vital Health [11] 223:6–7, 1981.

APPENDIX B

Pubertal Maturation (see also Chapter 5)

TABLE B–1. Mean Age at Pubertal Events,* Females

SMR	ENGLAND†	ENGLAND‡	UNITED STATES§	OHIO ‖ White	OHIO ‖ Black
B-II	11.2	10.8	11.2	10.8	10.6
B-III	12.0	12.0	12.4	12.1	13.7
B-IV	12.9	13.0	13.1	14.9	14.3
B-V	15.0	14.0	14.5	15.7	15.2
PH-II	11.6		11.9	11.1	11.0
PH-III	12.3		12.7	12.3	11.6
AH		12.5	13.1		
PH-IV	12.8		13.4	14.7	14.3
PH-V	14.6		14.6	15.7	15.2
PHV		12.2	12.5		

AH, axillary hair; B, breast development; PH, pubic hair distribution; PHV, peak height velocity; SMR, sexual maturity rating.
*For menarche, see Table B–2.
†Data from Tanner JM, Whitehouse RH, Marubini E, et al: The adolescent growth spurt of boys and girls of the Harpenden Growth Study. Ann Hum Biol 3:109, 1976.
‡Data from Billewicz WZ, Fellowes HM, Thomson AM: Pubertal changes in boys and girls from Newcastle upon Tyne. Ann Hum Biol 8:211, 1981.
§Data from Lee PA: Normal ages of pubertal events among American males and females. J Adolesc Health Care 1:26, 1980.
‖ Data from Brookman RR, Rauh JL, Morrison JA, et al: The Princeton Maturation Study. Unpublished data, 1976.

TABLE B–2. Attainment of Menarche (Percentage of Females) by Age and Race

AGE (years)	ALL	WHITE	BLACK
6–9	0.2	0.2	0.2
10	1.2	0.8	4.0
11	12.8	11.6	21.3
12	43.3	41.7	51.2
13	73.2	72.9	74.1
14	91.7	91.4	93.5
15	98.3	98.2	98.7
16–17	99.7	99.6	100.0
Median age	12.77	12.80	12.52

Data from National Center for Health Statistics: Age at menarche, United States. Vital Health Stat [11]133:2–3, 1973.

TABLE B–3. Mean Age at Pubertal Events, Males

SMR	UNITED STATES*	OHIO† White	OHIO† Black
G-II	11.9	12.1	11.3
G-III	13.2	13.4	—
G-IV	14.3	14.4	14.9
G-V	15.1	15.6	15.6
PH-II	12.3	12.5	12.1
PH-III	13.9	13.4	—
AH	14.0		
PH-IV	14.7	14.9	14.9
PH-V	15.3	15.9	16.0
PHV	13.8		

AH, axillary hair; G, genital development; PH, pubic hair distribution; PHV, peak height velocity; SMR, sexual maturity rating.
*Data from Lee PA: Normal ages of pubertal events among American males and females. J Adolesc Health Care 1:26, 1980.
†Data from Brookman RR, Rauh JL, Morrison JA, et al: The Princeton Maturation Study. Unpublished data, 1976.

TABLE B–4. Age of Attainment of Pubertal Events, American Males

SMR	PERCENTILE		
	5th	50th	95th
G-II	10.0	12.0	13.5
PH-II	10.0	12.5	14.0
G-III	12.0	13.2	14.5
PWV	12.0	13.5	15.5
PH-III	12.0	13.5	15.0
PHV	12.0	14.0	15.5
VC	12.5	14.0	15.5
G-IV	13.0	14.5	15.5
PH-IV	13.5	14.5	16.0
PH-V	13.5	15.2	16.5
G-V	13.5	15.5	16.5

G, genital development; PH, pubic hair distribution; PHV, peak height velocity; PWV, peak weight velocity; SMR, sexual maturity rating; VC, voice change.

Adapted from Lee PA: Normal ages of pubertal events among American males and females. J Adolesc Health Care 1:26, 1980.

TABLE B–5. Mean Testicular Volume (cc) During Puberty

SMR	LEFT	RIGHT
II	6.4	7.0
III	14.6	14.8
IV	19.8	20.5
V	28.3	30.2

SMR, sexual maturity rating.

Data from Daniel WA, Feinstein RA, Howard-Peebles P, et al: Testicular volumes of adolescents. J Pediatr 101:1010, 1982.

TABLE B–6. Skeletal (Bone) Age and Sexual Maturity Rating, Males

SKELETAL AGE (Years)	GENITAL STAGE (Percent)				
	I	II	III	IV	V
10	54	43	3	0	0
11	35	48	16	1	0
12	23	51	24	2	0
13	10	44	36	9	1
14	4	19	32	36	9
15	1	3	12	42	42
16	½	½	1	28	70
17	0	0	1	12	87
18	0	0	1	7	92

Adapted from Harlan WR, Grillo GP, Cornoni-Huntley J, et al: Secondary sex characteristics of boys 12 to 17 years of age: The U.S. Health Examination Survey. J Pediatr 95:293, 1979.

TABLE B–7. Skeletal (Bone) Age and Sexual Maturity Rating, Females

Skeletal Age (Years)	PREMENARCHAL Breast Stage (Percent)				
	I	II	III	IV	V
10–11	100	0	0	0	0
12	69	31	0	0	0
13	23	64	13	0	0
14	9	47	33	11	0
15	0	21	49	27	3
16	0	10	37	45	8
17	0	0	54	46	0

Skeletal Age (Years)	POSTMENARCHAL Breast Stage (Percent)				
	I	II	III	IV	V
14	0	0	29	14	57
15	0	4	32	45	19
16	0	0	20	47	33
17	0	0	10	41	49
18	0	0	5	33	62
>18	0	0	3	26	71

Adapted from Harlan WR, Harlan EA, Grillo GP: Secondary sex characteristics of girls 12 to 17 years of age: The U.S. Health Examination Survey. J Pediatr 96:1074, 1980.

TABLE B–8. Mean Sexual Maturity Rating by Age, Sex, and Race

AGE (Years)	PITTSBURGH*		CINCINNATI†	
	White	Black	White	Black
Males				
10	—	1.5	0.3	1.5
11	1.7	1.9	1.4	2.0
12	2.2	2.4	2.1	1.7
13	2.8	3.1	3.2	3.3
14	3.1	3.4	3.9	4.8
15	—	3.9	4.5	4.3
16	—	4.6	4.7	4.6
Females				
10	—	2.4	1.9	2.0
11	2.0	2.5	2.3	2.9
12	2.7	3.0	2.9	3.0
13	3.4	3.3	3.2	4.4
14	3.9	4.2	4.0	4.7
15	—	4.1	4.4	4.6
16	—	—	4.7	4.8

*Data from Nankin HR, Sperling M, Kenny FM, et al: Correlation between sexual maturation and serum gonadotropins: Comparison of black and white youngsters. Am J Med Sci 268:139, 1974.

†Data from Brookman RR, Rauh JL, Morrison JA, et al: The Princeton Maturation Study. Unpublished data, 1976.

Physical Fitness and Nutrition

TABLE C–1. Electrocardiogram Measurements

Age (Years)	HEART RATE/MINUTE			P WAVE (sec)			PR INTERVAL (sec)			QRS COMPLEX (sec)		
	5th Percentile	Mean	95th Percentile	5th Percentile	Mean	95th Percentile	5th Percentile	Mean	95th Percentile	5th Percentile	Mean	95th Percentile
8–11	55	79	107	.061	.075	.092	.10	.14	.17	.05	.073	.084
12–15	55	75	102	.064	.081	.095	.11	.14	.16	.04	.068	.080

MEAN SUM (tenths of millivolts) OF R WAVE IN V_5 AND S WAVE IN V_2 BY SEX MATURITY RATING

SMR	Male		Female	
	Mean	95th Percentile	Mean	95th Percentile
I	41.0	63.6	40.1	53.7
II	42.3	64.3	39.9	51.0
III	41.2	58.3	32.9	44.7
IV	43.3	60.1	28.3	40.5
V	42.0	60.2	28.0	43.9

Adapted from Rigby ML, Shinebourne EA: Growth and development of the cardiovascular system: Functional development. In Davis JA, Dobbing J (eds): Scientific Foundations of Paediatrics, 2nd ed. London, William Heinemann, 1981; and Stafford EM, Weir MR, Pearl W, et al: Sexual maturity rating: A marker for effects of pubertal maturation on the adolescent electrocardiogram. Pediatrics 83:565, 1989.

TABLE C–2. Mean Hematologic Values by Age, Sex, and Race

AGE (years)	HEMATOCRIT (%)		HEMOGLOBIN (g/dl)		RBC ($\times 10^{12}$/L)		WBC ($\times 10^9$/L)		MCV (fl)		MCH (pg)		MCHC (g/dl)	
	White	Black	White	Black	White	Black	White	Black	White	Black	White	Black	White	Black
Male														
9–11	38.3	36.7	13.2	12.3	4.6	4.5	7.1	6.3	82.8	81.7	28.5	27.5	34.5	33.7
12–14	40.3	39.1	13.9	13.1	4.8	4.7	7.0	6.0	84.5	83.8	29.1	28.2	34.4	33.6
15–17	43.0	41.8	14.8	13.8	5.0	4.8	7.4	6.2	86.8	86.6	29.9	28.6	34.5	33.0
18–24	44.7	43.7	15.4	14.6	5.1	5.0	7.4	6.7	88.2	88.4	30.5	29.6	34.5	33.4
Female														
9–11	38.5	37.1	13.3	12.4	4.6	4.4	7.2	6.6	84.1	85.0	28.9	28.4	34.3	33.4
12–14	39.0	37.5	13.3	12.5	4.5	4.4	7.3	6.1	86.5	85.9	29.4	28.5	34.1	33.2
15–17	39.5	37.8	13.4	12.5	4.5	4.4	7.9	6.5	87.7	86.8	29.8	28.6	34.0	33.0
18–24	39.6	38.0	13.4	12.6	4.4	4.3	7.6	6.9	89.6	87.8	30.4	29.0	33.9	33.1

MCH, mean corpuscular hemoglobin; MCHC, mean corpuscular hemoglobin concentration; MCV, mean corpuscular volume; RBC, red blood cell mass; WBC, white blood cell mass.

Data from National Center for Health Statistics: Hematological and nutritional biochemistry reference data for persons 6 months–74 years of age: United States, 1976–80. Vital Health Stat [11]232:15–77, 1982.

TABLE C–3. Hematocrit by Age, Sex, Race, American Youth

AGE (years)	WHITE MALE (Percentile)			BLACK MALE (Percentile)			WHITE FEMALE (Percentile)			BLACK FEMALE (Percentile)		
	5th	50th	95th	5th	50th	95th	5th	50th	95th	5th	50th	95th
12	36	41	45	35	40	45	37	41	44	36	40	44
13	37	42	46	36	42	47	37	41	46	34	40	47
14	38	43	48	37	42	48	37	40	45	35	40	45
15	39	44	50	38	44	50	37	41	46	33	39	45
16	41	45	50	40	45	50	37	41	45	33	38	44
17	41	46	50	40	46	50	37	41	45	33	39	45

Data from National Center for Health Statistics: Hematocrit values of youths 12–17 years, United States. Vital Health Stat [11]146:21–23, 1974.

TABLE C–4. Hematocrit (Mean %) by Sexual Maturity Rating

SMR	WHITE MALE	BLACK MALE	WHITE FEMALE	BLACK FEMALE
I	39.5	37.7	39.1	37.3
	(37.1–41.8)	(35.2–40.2)	(36.1–42.1)	(34.6–39.9)
II	39.8	38.4	39.2	38.9
	(36.7–42.8)	(36.0–40.9)	(37.1–41.3)	(35.7–42.1)
III	40.9	39.7	39.6	39.0
	(38.2–43.5)	(37.3–42.0)	(37.0–42.2)	(35.2–42.6)
IV	42.3	41.1	39.2	38.4
	(39.7–44.8)	(38.3–43.8)	(36.9–41.6)	(34.9–42.8)
V	43.8	42.7	39.2	38.7
	(41.1–46.4)	(39.6–45.9)	(36.2–42.2)	(35.9–41.5)

Adapted from Daniel WA: Hematocrit: Maturity relationship in adolescence. Pediatrics 52:388, 1973; and Copeland KC, Brookman RR, Rauh JL: Assessment of Pubertal Development. Columbus, OH, Ross Laboratories, 1986.

TABLE C–5. Measurements of Iron by Age, Sex, Race, and Sexual Maturity Rating

	WHITE MALE (Percentile)			BLACK MALE (Percentile)			WHITE FEMALE (Percentile)			BLACK FEMALE (Percentile)		
	10th	50th	90th	10th	50th	90th	10th	50th	90th	10th	50th	90th
Serum iron (μg/dl)												
*Age (Years)**												
9–11	51	87	130	42	79	113	59	91	132	61	83	123
12–14	62	95	139	60	91	134	58	96	144	47	95	142
15–17	69	105	159	68	103	151	49	97	157	46	96	140
18–24	69	109	167	69	113	155	58	101	160	49	91	138
Iron binding capacity (μg/dl)												
*Age (Years)**												
9–11	329	378	439	344	390	451	323	379	436	321	375	421
12–14	343	398	464	337	386	458	332	392	463	341	395	463
15–17	332	388	456	323	374	443	328	387	456	353	404	483
18–24	315	369	434	316	378	445	318	387	477	317	386	503
Transferrin saturation (%)												
*Age (Years)**												
9–11	13	23	35	12	20	30	15	25	38	16	22	35
12–14	15	24	35	16	22	34	15	25	37	10	25	36
15–17	18	28	40	17	26	44	13	25	41	10	24	36
18–24	18	29	44	20	31	43	14	26	41	13	22	34
SMR (Mean)†												
II		30			31			26			29	
III		37			32			26			27	
IV		31			33			31			24	
V		37			32			30			28	
Mean iron intake (mg/day)												
SMR†												
II		9.6			11.1			8.1			10.9	
III		14.5			11.6			10.3			10.3	
IV		13.2			12.0			10.3			9.8	
V		15.3			12.7			10.5			10.4	

SMR, Sexual maturity rating.
*Data from National Center for Health Statistics. Hematological and nutritional biochemistry reference data for persons 6 months–74 years of age: United States, 1976–80. Vital Health Stat [11]232:87–113, 1982.
†Data from Daniel WA, Gaines EG, Bennett DL: Iron intake and transferrin saturation in adolescents. J Pediatr 86:288, 1975.

TABLE C–6. Serum Metals by Age, Sex, and Race (µg/dl)

	WHITE MALE (Percentile)			BLACK MALE (Percentile)			WHITE FEMALE (Percentile)			BLACK FEMALE (Percentile)		
	10th	*50th*	*90th*	*10th*	*50th*	*90th*	*10th*	*50th*	*90th*	*10th*	*50th*	*90th*
Zinc												
9–11 years	69	84	102	70	82	99	68	83	98	66	81	100
12–14 years	69	85	102	73	85	103	70	84	101	66	84	100
15–17 years	71	87	110	65	87	103	67	84	105	64	79	95
18–24 years	75	92	116	72	89	107	67	83	101	63	78	95
Copper												
9–11 years	99	120	148	114	130	160	95	118	142	95	126	150
12–14 years	83	105	132	93	116	145	88	108	131	90	120	153
15–17 years	82	97	120	84	107	133	89	107	144	90	126	188
18–24 years	82	102	118	87	111	156	91	123	218	102	144	241

Data from National Center for Health Statistics: Hematological and nutritional biochemistry reference data for persons 6 months–74 years of age: United States, 1976–80. Vital Health Stat [11]232:114–117, 1982.

TABLE C–7. Serum Albumin by Age, Sex, and Race (g/dl)

AGE (Years)	WHITE MALE (Percentile)			BLACK MALE (Percentile)			WHITE FEMALE (Percentile)			BLACK FEMALE (Percentile)		
	10th	*50th*	*90th*	*10th*	*50th*	*90th*	*10th*	*50th*	*90th*	*10th*	*50th*	*90th*
9–11	4.5	4.9	5.1	4.4	4.8	5.0	4.4	4.8	5.2	4.3	4.6	5.0
12–14	4.6	4.9	5.2	4.4	4.7	5.0	4.5	4.8	5.2	4.3	4.6	5.0
15–17	4.6	5.0	5.4	4.4	4.8	5.1	4.5	4.9	5.2	4.2	4.5	5.1
18–24	4.7	5.0	5.4	4.5	4.8	5.3	4.3	4.7	5.1	4.0	4.5	4.9

Data from National Center for Health Statistics: Hematological and nutritional biochemistry reference data for persons 6 months–74 years of age: United States, 1976–80. Vital Health Stat [11]232:120–121, 1982.

TABLE C–8. Average Number of Decayed, Missing, and Filled Teeth by Age, Sex, and Race*

AGE (years)	DECAYED		MISSING		FILLED	
	White	Black	White	Black	White	Black
Male						
12	0.9	2.1	0.2	0.7	2.9	0.4
13	1.7	3.1	0.3	1.3	2.6	1.2
14	1.4	3.4	0.4	0.8	3.3	1.0
15	1.4	3.0	0.5	0.5	3.6	0.8
16	1.9	3.4	0.5	1.0	4.9	1.4
17	1.9	3.4	0.5	1.2	5.8	2.7
Female						
12	1.4	1.8	0.2	1.1	2.1	0.9
13	1.6	2.4	0.3	0.8	3.4	0.7
14	1.9	2.4	0.5	3.3	4.1	1.6
15	1.4	4.1	0.5	2.1	5.0	1.6
16	1.8	3.4	1.2	1.7	5.5	1.6
17	2.1	4.4	1.5	2.2	6.0	1.6

*See also Chapter 41.
Data from National Center for Health Statistics. Decayed, missing, and filled teeth among persons 1–74 years, United States. Vital Health Stat [11]223:25, 1981.

Endocrinology of Puberty

TABLE D–1. Thyroid Function Tests by Sexual Maturity Rating

	SEXUAL MATURITY RATING				
	I	II	III	IV	V
Male					
T$_4$ (μg/dl)	10.7	9.4	8.9	8.5	8.4
T$_3$ (ng/dl)	139	121	134	146	131
TSH (μU/ml)	8.5	8.7	10.8	12.5	15.7
Female					
T$_4$ (μg/dl)	10.1	10.3	10.2	8.9	10.8
T$_3$ (ng/dl)	140	143	139	137	128
TSH (μU/ml)	10.5	9.8	7.4	8.3	8.9

T$_3$, triiodothyronine (RIA); T$_4$, thyroxine (radioimmunoassay [RIA]); TSH, thyroid-stimulating hormone (RIA).
Adapted from Abbassi V, Aceto T, Hung W: Thyroid function in relation to age. In Johnston TR, Moore WM, Jeffries JE (eds): Children Are Different: Developmental Physiology, 2nd ed. Columbus, OH, Ross Laboratories, 1978, pp. 80–89.

TABLE D–2. Plasma Growth Hormone (ng/ml) by Sexual Maturity Rating*

	SEXUAL MATURITY RATING			
	I	II	III–IV	V
Male	2.2	2.1	6.5	2.7
Female	3.3	1.9	3.5	2.3

*Mean 6-hour concentration.
Adapted from Miller JD, Tannenbaum GS, Colle E, et al: Daytime pulsatile growth hormone secretion during childhood and adolescence. J Clin Endocrinol Metab 55:989, 1982. © The Endocrine Society.

TABLE D–3. Plasma Somatomedin C (U/ml) by Sexual Maturity Rating

	SEXUAL MATURITY RATING				
	I	II	III	IV	V
Male	0.7–1.1	0.8–2.2	1.4–2.4	1.4–2.4	2.0–3.2
Female	0.8–1.8	0.6–2.6	2.0–4.2	2.0–4.2	2.0–4.2

Adapted from Rosenfield RI, Furlanetto R, Bock D: Relationship of somatomedin-C concentrations to pubertal changes. J Pediatr 103:723, 1983.

TABLE D–4. Serum Concentrations of Gonadotropins (mIU/ml) by Sexual Maturity Rating

	SEXUAL MATURITY RATING				
	I	II	III	IV	V
Male					
FSH					
Mean	4.5	5.9	8.1	8.5	8.0
Range	0.5–10.2	0.5–10.0	1.0–18.0	1.0–20.0	1.0–20.0
LH					
Mean	3.9	6.8	8.5	9.5	11.5
Range	0.2–10.3	0.5–12.0	0.5–15.0	0.6–20.0	0.5–25.0
Prolactin					
Range	3.6–10.3	2.4–18.9	3.0–15.2	4.3–18.1	3.1–15.7
Female					
FSH					
Mean	4.2	5.5	8.0	8.0	12.3
Range	0.5–8.1	0.7–10.0	0.8–15.0	1.2–20.0	1.3–20.0
LH					
Mean	2.9	3.9	8.4	11.3	18.9
Range	0.2–7.5	0.4–11.5	0.5–15.0	0.6–34.0	0.5–80.0
Prolactin					
Range	3.8–13.5	3.1–11.7	3.8–19.2	4.2–16.8	5.0–18.0

FSH, follicle-stimulating hormone; LH, luteinizing hormone.
Adapted from Copeland KC, Brookman RR, Rauh JL: Assessment of Pubertal Development. Columbus, OH, Ross Laboratories, 1986. (Ranges derived from several studies.)

**TABLE D–5. Serum Concentrations (ng/dl)
of Sex Steroids by Sexual Maturity Rating**

	SEXUAL MATURITY RATING				
	I	**II**	**III**	**IV**	**V**
Male					
Estrone					
Mean	2	3	3	4	3
Range	1–6	1–7	1–7	2–7	1–7
Estradiol					
Mean	2	1	2	4	3
Range	<1–3.5	<1–4	<1–3	1–6	1–5
Progesterone					
Mean	30	36	40	40	35
17-Hydroxyprogesterone					
Range	30–36	34–40	52–62	78–93	—
Testosterone					
Mean	10	18	52	170	350
Range	3–110	2–300	27–910	92–840	200–1000
Dihydrotestosterone					
Mean	3	4	13	26	13
Range	2–20	2–28	6–36	5–51	1–76
Androstenedione					
Mean	54	49	85	69	90
Range	13–79	17–81	48–122	40–111	50–200
Dehydroepiandrosterone					
Mean	192	300	396	396	450
Range	2–326	50–558	119–592	178–645	180–700
Female					
Estrone					
Mean	4	5	7	12	3
Range	1–8	1–9	1–11	1–19	2–8
Estradiol					
Mean	2	3	13	16	8
Range	<1–3	<1–6	<1–27	1–30	1–40
Progesterone					
Range	10–13	16	16–23	30–161	29–75*
17-Hydroxyprogesterone					
Range	32–38	38–52	55–69	101–127	11–80*
Testosterone					
Mean	11	19	28	48	38
Range	2–18	14–65	19–80	20–85	20–85
Dihydrotestosterone					
Range	2–16	3–24	9–25	9–32	—
Androstenedione					
Mean	35	72	103	176	141
Range	10–100	38–106	40–150	40–210	58–224
Dehydroepiandrosterone					
Mean	133	326	427	498	741
Range	19–300	45–1600	125–1700	153–1620	389–1093

*Follicular phase.
Adapted from Copeland KC, Brookman RR, Rauh JL: Assessment of Pubertal Development. Columbus, OH, Ross Laboratories 1986. (Ranges derived from several studies.)

**TABLE D–6. Serum Concentrations (ng/dl)
of Sex Steroids by Age**

	AGE (Years)				
	8–10	**10–12**	**12–14**	**14–16**	**16–18**
Male					
Estrone					
Mean	3.3	3.2	2.7	3.9	4.0
Range	2.0–5.4	2.1–4.9	1.7–4.4	2.1–7.0	2.5–7.0
Estradiol					
Mean	<0.5	<0.5	1.0	1.5	1.8
Range	0–1.1	0–1.5	0–2.5	0.2.4	0.9–3.0
Progesterone					
Mean			39	34	56
Range			20–60	20–50	30–75
17-Hydroxyprogesterone					
Mean	36	39	42	80	97
Range	18–60	12–75	15–219	12–200	42–200
Testosterone					
Mean	9	13	78	340	532
Range	3–26	3–48	10–437	150–772	264–900
Dihydrotestosterone					
Mean	3	4	13	32	50
Range	0–7	3–7	9–20	20–52	20–75
Androstenedione					
Mean	18	45	62	80	108
Range	13–31	31–65	45–99	48–140	70–140
Dehydroepiandrosterone					
Mean	85	135	229	333	380
Range	21–283	46–505	84–583	175–634	180–600
Female					
Estrone					
Mean	4.6	4.4	5.9	8.9	6.7
Range	3.1–7.0	2.8–6.8	3.7–14.0	2.1–14.0	1.4–14.0
Estradiol					
Mean	<0.5	1.6	4.2	8.6	8.4
Range	0–3.1	0–6.3	0.5–12.2	1.0–25.2	1.0–28.4
Progesterone					
Mean	6	8	37	189	161
Range	3–32	3–55	10–450	5–1400	23–1500
17-Hydroxyprogesterone					
Mean	35	42	84	94	108
Range	15–90	18–111	24–234	27–234	34–240
Testosterone					
Mean	8	18	26	34	41
Range	4–20	5–47	11–60	16–72	20–65
Dihydrotestosterone					
Mean	6	8	12	14	15
Range	4–10	5–12	7–19	10–30	10–32
Androstenedione					
Mean	32	65	123	133	151
Range	22–47	42–100	80–190	77–224	80–300
Dehydroepiandrosterone					
Mean	82	261	473	555	550
Range	24–289	50–916	93–2000	250–2000	250–2000

Adapted from Winter JSD: Prepubertal and pubertal endocrinology. Falkner F, Tanner JM (eds): In Human Growth. 2. Postnatal Growth. New York, Plenum, 1978, p 196. (Ranges derived from several studies.)

TABLE D–7. Plasma Gonadotropins and Sex Steroids by Sexual Maturity Rating and Age from Longitudinal Studies

	SEXUAL MATURITY RATING*				
	I	II	III	IV	V
Male					
FSH (mIU/ml)	1.0–4.1	1.3–4.5	1.7–6.3	1.8–7.8	1.1–3.3
LH (mIU/ml)	0.5–2.3	0.5–2.5	0.6–2.5	1.2–2.7	1.1–3.3
Androgens (nmol/L)†	0.3–3.3	0.5–9.0	0.7–13.6	4.5–19.1	—
Female					
FSH (mIU/ml)	1.9–8.1	1.4–8.2	2.2–11.4	1.3–10.7	1.3–15.2
LH (mIU/ml)	0.5–1.8	0.5–4.3	0.5–7.7	0.6–33.6	0.5–80.0
E_2 (pmol/L)	37–156	61–494	40–639	96–669	113–1299
	AGE (Years)				
	11.5–12.0	12.0–12.5	12.5–13.0	13.0–13.5	13.5–14.0
Male					
FSH (mIU/ml)	1.0–3.7	1.0–6.1	1.4–5.0	1.5–6.2	1.5–7.8
LH (mIU/ml)	0.5–1.0	0.5–2.3	0.6–2.5	0.6–2.5	0.6–3.3
Androgens (nmol/L)†	0.4–4.7	0.4–17.5	0.5–17.5	0.5–19.1	1.2–9.1
Female‡					
FSH (mIU/ml)	1.4–11.4	1.8–9.3	1.8–10.4	3.4–8.1	2.1–10.2
LH (mIU/ml)	0.5–5.7	0.5–7.0	0.6–9.6	0.6–33.6	1.0–7.8
E_2 (pmol/L)‡	50–494	37–708	76–1193	81–1299	115–924

E_2, estradiol; FSH, follicle-stimulating hormone; LH, luteinizing hormone.
*Genital stage for male; breast stage for female.
†Using antiserum with 100% cross-reaction with testosterone, 76% cross-reaction with 5 α-dihydrotestosterone, negligible reaction with others.
‡Excludes postmenarcheal females.
Adapted from Clayton BE, Jenkins P, Round JM: Paediatric Clinical Pathology. Clinical Tests and Reference Ranges. London, Blackwell, 1980.

TABLE D–8. Response of Plasma Gonadotropin Levels (mIU/ml) Following Stimulation with Synthetic LH-RH by Sexual Maturity Rating

	SEXUAL MATURITY RATING*				
	I	II	III	IV	V
Male					
FSH					
Basal	0.5–0.8	0.5–1.8	1.0–2.6	1.0–3.4	1.0–3.9
Peak	1.0–3.0	1.3–4.7	1.2–5.1	2.3–4.3	1.6–8.6
LH					
Basal	0.2–0.97	0.6–1.2	0.5–1.2	0.6–2.4	0.5–4.0
Peak	0.6–1.8	4.5–7.5	5.4–7.8	7.2–24.0	7.6–23.0
Female					
FSH					
Basal	0.5–0.9	0.7–3.6	0.8–2.4	1.2–2.8	1.5–4.3
Peak	1.0–3.2	1.5–13.0	2.2–7.1	2.6–8.0	2.7–10.0
LH					
Basal	0.2–1.0	0.4–1.35	0.5–1.3	0.6–2.6	1.4–3.2
Peak	2.1–3.8	3.1–13.5	4.5–12.5	7.1–25.0	8.6–23.0

FSH, follicle-stimulating hormone; LH, luteinizing hormone; LH-RH, luteinizing hormone releasing hormone.
Adapted from Dickerman Z, Prager-Lewin R, Laron Z: Response of plasma LH and FSH to synthetic LH-RH in children at various pubertal stages. Am J Dis Child 130:634, 1976.

Index

Note: Page numbers in *italics* refer to illustrations; page numbers followed by t refer to tables.

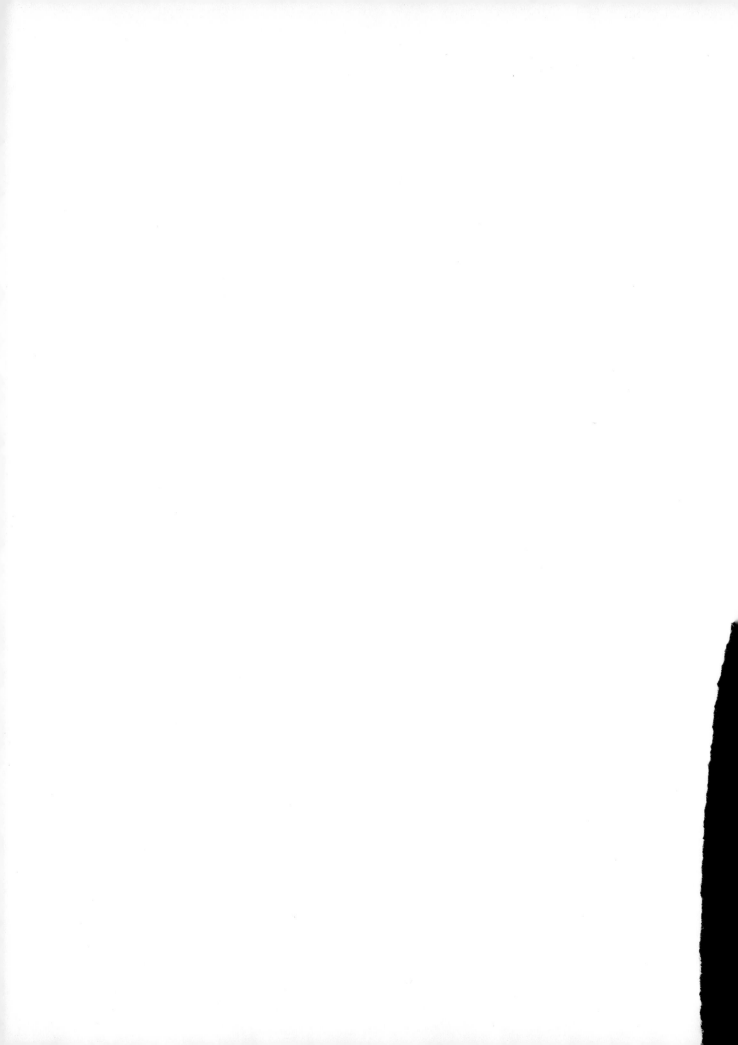

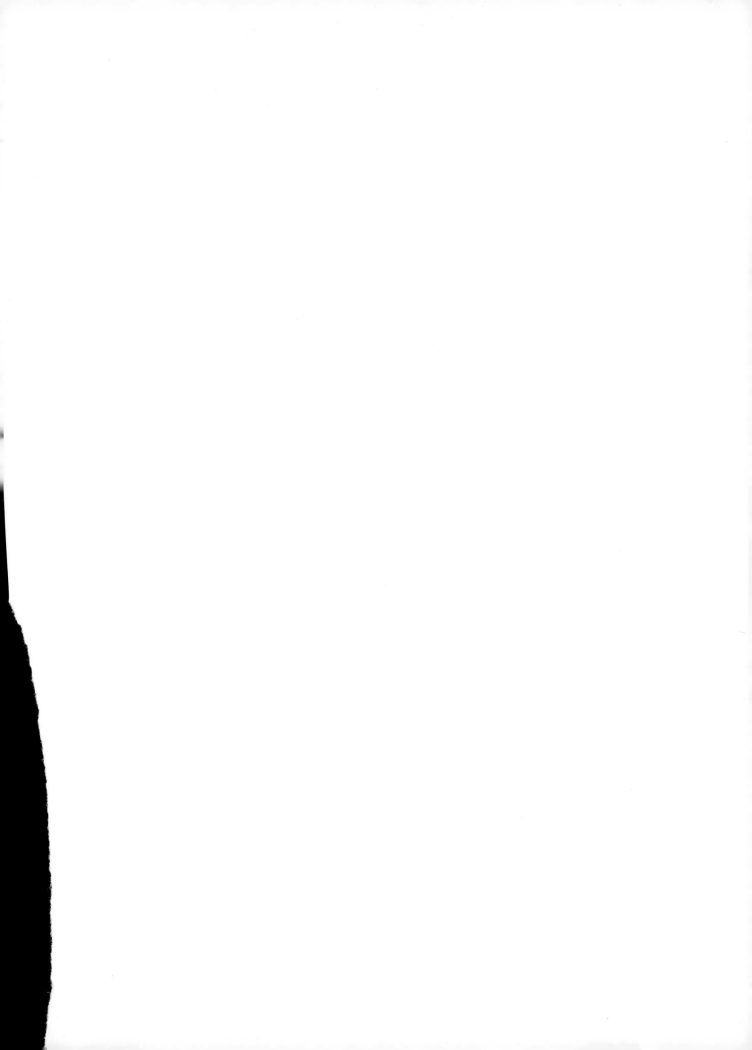